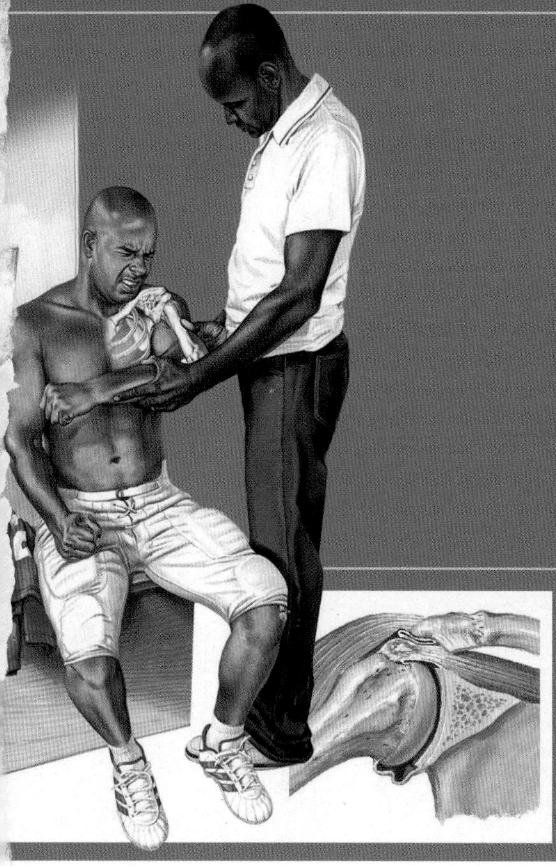

NETTER'S SPORTS MEDICINE

3rd EDITION

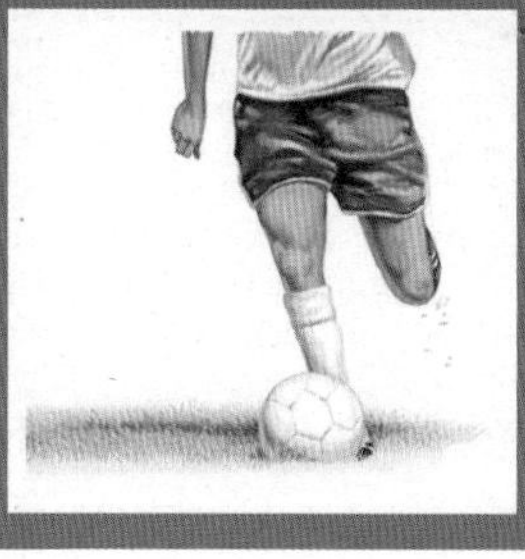
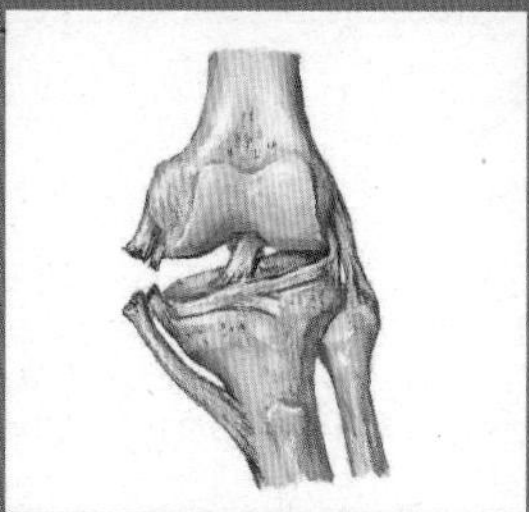
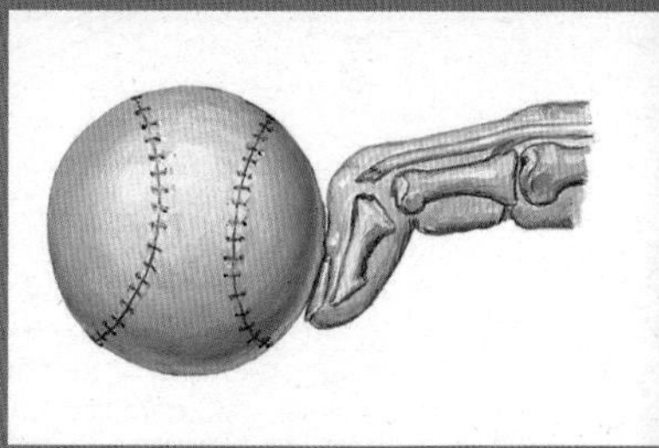

EDITORS

Christopher C. Madden, MD, FAMSSM, FACSM

Margot Putukian, MD, FACSM, FAMSSM

Eric C. McCarty, MD

Craig C. Young, MD, FAMSSM, FACSM

ILLUSTRATIONS BY

Frank H. Netter, MD

CONTRIBUTING ILLUSTRATORS

Carlos A.G. Machado, MD

John A. Craig, MD

Kristen Wienandt Marzejon, MS, MFA

Tiffany S. DaVanzo, MA, CMI

James A. Perkins, MS, MFA

ELSEVIER

ELSEVIER
1600 John F. Kennedy Blvd.
Ste 1800
Philadelphia, PA 19103-2899

NETTER'S SPORTS MEDICINE, THIRD EDITION ISBN: 978-0-323-79669-9

Content Strategist: Marybeth Thiel
Publishing Services Manager: Catherine Jackson
Senior Project Manager: Daniel Fitzgerald
Designer: Patrick Ferguson

Printed in India.

Last digit is the print number: 9 8 7 6 5 4 3

DEDICATION

Netter's Sports Medicine is dedicated to the evolving field of sports medicine, to the broad readership of previous editions of *Netter's Sports Medicine*, and to the *Team Physician's Handbook* and to the many thousands of sports medicine physicians and health professionals who have loyally followed and evolved with its content over three spectacular editions. *Netter's Sports Medicine* evolved from the original efforts embodying the *Team Physician's Handbook* and all that it represented in the early field of sports medicine, and it continues to expand its content and reach to modern-day sports professionals worldwide.

The Netter editions bring with them a broader and deeper approach to the comprehensive field of sports medicine. Many new topics, chapters, and authors are combined with high-quality Netter and other graphics, displayed in a colorful, user-friendly, easy-to-access format. *Netter's Sports Medicine* serves as both a user-friendly ready reference and a detailed resource for all sports medicine professionals.

This book is also dedicated with respect and honor to the original creators of the *Team Physician's Handbook:* W. Michael Walsh, MD; Morris B. Mellion, MD; and Guy L. Shelton, PT, whose vision and wisdom made this work possible. May their love of sports medicine, conduct in the field, and integrity as human beings set an example for us all to follow.

And to the most wonderful, loving family I can imagine: Jessica, my wise and beautiful wife, and Sage, my dedicated and inquisitive daughter. They are both my best teachers, and they bring me infinite happiness. Also, to my mother, Susan Madden, and my late father, Spencer Madden, whose love, patience, belief, and guidance presented me with limitless opportunity.

—Christopher C. Madden, MD, FAMSSM, FACSM

This book is dedicated to my parents, John and Elissa, who taught me to work hard, enjoy life, and respect other people; to my brother, Peter, and sister, Lisa, as well as their families; and to my husband and best friend, Joe Hindelang, as well as my stepson, Joel, and his new family. I treasure the time with family and friends and the memories we have and build. This book is also dedicated to all the sports medicine mentors I've had throughout my career, including my fellowship directors, Dave Hough and Doug McKeag, the founders of AMSSM, and my colleagues (many of whom are contributors to and editors of this book). I am so grateful for your friendship and support and the opportunity to participate in this project with all of you.

—Margot Putukian, MD, FACSM, FAMSSM

My dedication of this book goes to my best friend and loving wife, Miriam, who is ever supportive, patient, and enduring in her love, especially in an effort such as this book, with the hours it takes and late nights to make it happen. To my dear children, Madeleine, Cleveland, Shannon, and Torrance, who are the light and diversion to the busy life as an academician, surgeon, and team physician. To my parents, Cleve and Jackie, who gave me great inspiration in pursuing excellence. To my many teachers, mentors, coaches, and orthopedic partners who along the way have taught me so much and continue to live within me. Finally, to my ultimate mentor and the one who gave so much, my savior, Jesus Christ.

—Eric C. McCarty, MD

This is dedicated to my parents, Margaret and Jimmie, who instilled in me the thirst for knowledge, and to my teachers, who had the patience to give me that knowledge, especially to Drs. Jim Puffer, Bob Dimeff, and John Bergfeld. And finally, and most importantly, to my beautiful and wonderful wife, Sharon Busey, who has given me the love, support, and time to complete this project—I couldn't have done this without you.

—Craig C. Young, MD, FAMSSM, FACSM

EDITORS

CHRISTOPHER C. MADDEN, MD, FAMSSM, FACSM

Clinical Professor
Family Medicine
University of Colorado Health Sciences
Denver, Colorado
Private Practice
Longs Peak Sports Medicine and Family Practice
Longmont, Colorado

MARGOT PUTUKIAN, MD, FACSM, FAMSSM

Internist/Sports Medicine Specialist
Chief Medical Officer
Major League Soccer
New York, New York
Senior Advisor
National Football League, Head, Neck & Spine Committee
Team Physician, US Soccer

ERIC C. MCCARTY, MD

Professor
Chief of Sports Medicine and Shoulder Surgery
Department of Orthopedics
University of Colorado School of Medicine
Associate Professor Adjunct
Department of Integrative Physiology
University of Colorado, Boulder
Director of Sports Medicine
University of Colorado Department of Athletics
Head Team Physician
Colorado Avalanche Hockey Club
Fellowship Director
University of Colorado Sports Medicine and Shoulder Fellowship

CRAIG C. YOUNG, MD, FAMSSM, FACSM

Professor and Medical Director of Sports Medicine
Departments of Orthopaedic Surgery & Community and Family Medicine
Medical College of Wisconsin
Milwaukee, Wisconsin
Honorary Senior Researcher
WITS Institute for Sports & Health (WISH)
University of Witwatersrand
Johannesburg, South Africa
Team Physician
Milwaukee Brewers, Milwaukee Bucks
Company Physician
Milwaukee Ballet, Skylight Opera
Milwaukee, Wisconsin
Pool Physician
US National Freeski, Ski & Snowboard Teams, US Olympic Committee
President (2007–2008) American Medical Society for Sports Medicine

ABOUT THE EDITORS

Christopher C. Madden, MD, FAMSSM, FACSM, is in private practice on the Front Range of the Rocky Mountains in Colorado. His sports medicine practice is broad, and he has special interests in head injuries, biomechanics, environmental and altitude medicine, backcountry sports, endurance and ultraendurance medicine, snowboarding injuries, and cycling and mountain biking injuries. He also maintains a solid commitment to and presence within the full spectrum of primary care and family medicine, where his overarching approach exemplifies a complementary, mutual inclusivity of the two fields and enables him to serve his patients broadly. Chris has edited and written on a variety of topics in sports publications, ranging from previsit patient education to professional textbooks. He is on clinical faculty and teaches sports medicine and primary care to family medicine residents from the University of Colorado Family Medicine Residency Programs. He is active in the American Medical Society for Sports Medicine, where he is a past president, fellow, and past member of the board of directors. In 2011, Chris received the American Medical Society for Sports Medicine's (AMSSM) highest award, the Founders Award, which is given to "the individual, group or organization who exemplifies the best we can be or do in Sports Medicine." Chris is also a fellow with the American College of Sports Medicine, where he has served on the Education Committee, and has served on and chaired panels at various annual meetings. An avid backcountry enthusiast, Chris loves to mountain bike, trail run, snowboard, ski, hike, mountaineer, rock climb, practice yoga, travel, read, and spend time with his family.

Margot Putukian, MD, FACSM, FAMSSM, received her BS degree in biology from Yale University, where she participated in soccer and lacrosse. She received her MD from Boston University and then did both her internship and residency at the Primary Care Internal Medicine Program at Strong Memorial Hospital in Rochester, New York. She completed her fellowship in sports medicine at Michigan State University. Margot worked as the director of Primary Care Sports Medicine at Penn State University before starting her current position in January 2004 as the director of athletic medicine and head team physician for Princeton University. Margot also serves as a team physician for US Soccer and the Men's US National Lacrosse Team. Margot is a charter member of the American Medical Society for Sports Medicine (AMSSM), where she served as president from 2004 to 2005, and is currently the president of the AMSSM Foundation. Margot is a medical consultant for Major League Soccer. She currently serves as the chair for the Clinical Sports Medicine Leadership committee for the American College of Sports Medicine (ACSM) and served previously on the board of trustees for ACSM. She served previously on the NCAA Competitive Safeguards and Medical Aspects of Sport Committee and is currently serving as the chair of the Sports Science and Safety Committee for US Lacrosse. She currently serves on the NFL Head, Neck & Spine Committee. Margot has participated in several Team Physician Consensus Statements, NATA Statements, and the Third and Fourth International Consensus Conferences on Concussion in Sport in Zurich, Switzerland, in addition to the Fifth International Consensus Conference on Concussion in Sport in Berlin, Germany. She has served on the editorial board for *Medicine and Science in Sports and Exercise*, the *Journal of Athletic Training*, *The Physician and Sportsmedicine*, and *Athletic Training and Sports Health Care*. She is the proud recipient of the 2007 Dr. David Moyer Team Physician's award presented by the Eastern Athletic Trainers' Association, the 2015 AMSSM Founders Award, and the 2016 ACSM Citation Award.

Eric C. McCarty, MD, is a nationally and internationally recognized sports medicine trained orthopedic surgeon and shoulder specialist. He serves as the Chief of Sports Medicine and Shoulder Surgery and is a Professor in the Department of Orthopedics at the University of Colorado School of Medicine. His passion for treating the active individual stems from his experience at the University of Colorado where he excelled and received numerous honors for his exploits in the classroom as well as on the football field, where he was a first-team all-conference linebacker in the prominent Big Eight Conference, and he was also an Academic All-American. Dr. McCarty attended medical school at the University of Colorado. After graduation he completed his training in orthopaedic surgery at Vanderbilt University in Nashville, Tennessee. From there he completed an intensive year of fellowship training in sports medicine and shoulder surgery at the internationally renowned Hospital for Special Surgery in New York City. He subsequently returned to Vanderbilt as a faculty member in the Department of Orthopaedics. In 2003, Dr. McCarty was recruited back to Colorado from Vanderbilt University to take over the sports medicine and shoulder program in the Department of Orthopedics at the University of Colorado School of Medicine and to serve as the head team physician for the University of Colorado and University of Denver athletic programs. In recent years he has also been the medical director and head team physician for the Colorado Avalanche Hockey Club. His specialized practice involves the care of these collegiate and professional athletes as well as recreational and highly competitive athletes from the community and the Rocky Mountain area. In addition to his busy clinical practice, Dr. McCarty is very active in research, teaching, and writing in the field of sports medicine and knee and shoulder surgery. He has over 200 publications in the field of sports medicine. He has received competitive grants for his research and frequently gives talks at both the national and international level. He has been the recipient of numerous national research awards including the AOSSM Cabaud Award, AOSSM Herodicus Award, AOSSM O'Donoghue Sports Injury Research Award, AOSSM Douglas Brown Award, and AOSSM Aircast Award as well as the ASES Neer Award on two occasions. Additionally, he received the prestigious Kappa Delta Award from the AAOS in 2012 and 2019. He is also very active in national and international sports medicine and arthroscopic societies, including AOSSM, ISAKOS, AANA, and ASES with various positions of leadership in those societies. Since his playing days, Dr. McCarty continues to maintain a very active lifestyle with his family. He enjoys the activities he grew up with in Colorado including hiking, cycling, climbing, and skiing. This carries over into his unbridled dedication of returning his patients to their desired activity/sport. His passion for his work as a team physician, surgeon, educator, and researcher is quite evident in his enthusiasm for what he does.

Craig C. Young, MD, FAMSSM, FACSM, is a professor and the medical director of sports medicine at the Medical College of Wisconsin. He received a BS degree (cum laude) in biological sciences from the University of California, Irvine. He is a graduate of the University of California, San Diego School of Medicine. He completed a residency in family medicine at UCLA and a sports medicine fellowship at the Cleveland Clinic Foundation. Dr. Young has served as a team physician for the Milwaukee Brewers since 1994 and for the Milwaukee Bucks since 2016. He has served as a company physician for the Milwaukee Ballet since 1992. He has also served as a physician at the US Olympic Training Center (Chula Vista) and has been a pool physician for the US National Ski and Snowboard Teams since 1996. In 2007, he was appointed by the US Olympic Committee as a team physician for the 23rd World Winter University Games in Torino, Italy. Dr. Young is board certified in both family practice and sports medicine. He was the president of the American Medical Society for Sports Medicine (AMSSM) from 2007 to 2008. He was the 2012 recipient of AMSSM's highest award, the Founders Award, which is given to "the individual, group or organization who exemplifies the best we can be or do in Sports Medicine," and the 2013 David O. Hough Memorial Lecture Award for excellence and dedication to education in sports medicine. He was president of the Major League Baseball Team Physicians Association from 2013 to 2014 and selected to be team physician for the Major League Baseball All-Stars for the 2018 Japan tour. He has been on the editorial board of the *Clinical Journal of Sport Medicine* (since 2004) and a section editor for *Current Sports Medicine Reports* (2009–2017). His clinical interests include dance medicine, wilderness medicine, female athletes, adolescent athletes, and endurance athletes. His research interests include dance medicine and injury prevention.

ABOUT THE ARTISTS

FRANK H. NETTER, MD

Frank H. Netter was born in 1906 in New York City. He studied art at the Art Students' League and the National Academy of Design before entering medical school at New York University, where he received his MD degree in 1931. During his student years, Dr. Netter's notebook sketches attracted the attention of the medical faculty and other physicians, allowing him to augment his income by illustrating articles and textbooks. He continued illustrating as a sideline after establishing a surgical practice in 1933, but he ultimately opted to give up his practice in favor of a full-time commitment to art. After service in the United States Army during World War II, Dr. Netter began his long collaboration with the CIBA Pharmaceutical Company (now Novartis Pharmaceuticals). This 45-year partnership resulted in the production of the extraordinary collection of medical art so familiar to physicians and other medical professionals worldwide.

In 2005, Elsevier, Inc., purchased the Netter Collection and all publications from Icon Learning Systems. There are now over 50 publications featuring the art of Dr. Netter available through Elsevier, Inc.

Dr. Netter's works are among the finest examples of the use of illustration in the teaching of medical concepts. The 13-book Netter Collection of Medical Illustrations, which includes the greater part of the more than 20,000 paintings created by Dr. Netter, became and remains one of the most famous medical works ever published. *Netter's Atlas of Human Anatomy*, first published in 1989, presents the anatomical paintings from the Netter Collection. Now translated into 16 languages, it is the anatomy atlas of choice among medical and health professions students the world over.

The Netter illustrations are appreciated not only for their aesthetic qualities, but, more important, for their intellectual content. As Dr. Netter wrote in 1949, "...clarification of a subject is the aim and goal of illustration. No matter how beautifully painted, how delicately and subtly rendered a subject may be, it is of little value as a medical illustration if it does not serve to make clear some medical point." Dr. Netter's planning, conception, point of view, and approach are what inform his paintings and what makes them so intellectually valuable.

Frank H. Netter, MD, physician and artist, died in 1991.

Learn more about the physician-artist whose work has inspired the Netter Reference collection: https://netterimages.com/artist-frank-h-netter.html.

CARLOS A.G. MACHADO, MD

Carlos A.G. Machado was chosen by Novartis to be Dr. Netter's successor. He continues to be the main artist who contributes to the Netter Collection of medical illustrations.

Self-taught in medical illustration, cardiologist Carlos Machado has contributed meticulous updates to some of Dr. Netter's original plates and has created many paintings of his own in the style of Netter as an extension of the Netter collection. Dr. Machado's photorealistic expertise and his keen insight into the physician/patient relationship inform his vivid and unforgettable visual style. His dedication to researching each topic and subject he paints places him among the premier medical illustrators at work today.

Learn more about his background and see more of his art at: https://netterimages.com/artist-carlos-a-g-machado.html.

PREFACE

We are grateful for the opportunity to carry on the widespread popularity of the first two editions of *Netter's Sports Medicine*, the history of *Team Physician's Handbook*, and the widely respected anatomic graphic works of Frank Netter, MD. The third edition continues to strike a purposeful balance between serving as an accessible ready reference and a more detailed study and clinical guide, embracing a carefully organized, bulleted outline format complemented by colorful Netter graphics, tables, figures, pictures, diagnostic imaging, and other medical artwork. The text hosts a national and international author base that represents the best in sports medicine today.

Serving as a sports medicine physician or other professional is a unique privilege and an awesome challenge. *Netter's Sports Medicine* is written for the multitude of physicians and other healthcare professionals who provide care to a variety of athletes and active individuals in almost any setting imaginable, from general population to committed athlete, pediatric to senior athletics, Little League to professional sports, weekend warrior to Olympic champion, and backcountry mountainside to Super Bowl field.

The book is designed to serve as a comprehensive sports medicine resource and a ready reference in the busy outpatient office, in the training room, on the sideline, and behind the scenes as a quality learning and review resource for self-improvement and for sports medicine board certification. Insightful, expert, anecdotal experience fills the void where the most current evolving evidence in sports medicine falls short, and careful considerations of controversies are mindfully weighed and presented. The sports medicine literature continues to expand in breadth and depth since the first and second editions of *Netter's Sports Medicine* and its predecessor three editions of the *Team Physician's Handbook*, and many new chapters and chapter sections were added and revised to reflect the evolution of our exciting field. The text is divided into user-friendly sections for quick reference, and each chapter includes a Recommended Readings section limited to quality, author-recommended sources. We welcome many new, respected authors who joined us to produce this book, and we are fortunate to continue our lasting relationship with numerous previous, well-respected authors, who are leaders in their respective areas of emphasis. We thank all the authors who contributed chapters to past texts and whose previous work continues to provide a strong foundation to build upon.

Whether you are a primary care physician attempting to manage a common or unique musculoskeletal injury in a time-challenged ambulatory setting, an orthopedic surgeon trying to gain insight about a medical or psychological problem foreign to the cast or operating room, an athletic trainer trying to figure out a diagnosis in the training room, or a physical therapist pursuing further in-depth sports medicine knowledge, we sincerely hope you find this reference all it is meant to be and more, and we thank you for opening the cover and sharing with us what we feel is one of the highest-quality sports medicine works produced to date. Please enjoy.

CONTRIBUTORS

Jeffrey T. Abildgaard, MD
Orthopaedic Surgery and Sports Medicine
OrthoArizona
Phoenix, Arizona

Giselle A. Aerni, MD
Founder
Madam Athlete LLC
www.madamathlete.com
Red Lion, Pennsylvania
Team Physician
Sports Medicine
Gettysburg College
Gettysburg, Pennsylvania

Kathryn Alfonso, DO
Resident Physician
Physical Medicine & Rehabilitation
Mayo Clinic
Rochester, Minnesota

Brian F. Allen, MD
Fellow
Primary Care Sports Medicine Fellowship
University of Minnesota
Minneapolis, Minneapolis

Joanne B. "Anne" Allen, MD
Sports Medicine
University of North Carolina–Wilmington
Wilmington, North Carolina

Annunziato Amendola, MD
Professor
Orthopaedic Surgery
Duke University
Durham, North Carolina

Irfan Asif, MD
Professor and Chair
Family and Community Medicine
University of Alabama Birmingham (UAB) School of Medicine
Birmingham, Alabama

Chad Asplund, MD
Professor
Family Medicine and Orthopedics
Mayo Clinic
Minneapolis, Minnesota

Joshua Baker, MD
Emergency Medicine Attending
Ralph H. Johnson VA Medical Center
Charleston, South Carolina

Casey G. Batten, MD, FAMSSM
Director
Primary Care Sports Medicine
Kerlan Jobe Institute
Los Angeles, California

Taurean G. Baynard, MD
PGY-III Orthopaedic Surgery Resident
Medical College of Wisconsin
Milwaukee, Wisconsin

John Wilson Belk, BA
Research Assistant
Orthopaedics
University of Colorado
Denver, Colorado

Christopher C. Bell, MD
Sports Medicine Physician
Sports Medicine
Intermountain Healthcare
Salt Lake City, Utah

Holly J. Benjamin, MD, FAAP, FACSM, FAMSSM
Professor of Pediatrics, Orthopedic
Surgery and Rehabilitation Medicine
Director of Primary Care Sports Medicine
University of Chicago
Chicago, Illinois

Bret E. Betz, MD
Assistant Professor
Department of Emergency Medicine and Orthopaedics and Sports Medicine
University of Cincinnati College of Medicine
Cincinnati, Ohio

Anthony Beutler, MD
Professor
Family Medicine
Uniformed Services University
Bethesda, Maryland
Associate Medical Director and Fellowship Director
Musculoskeletal Clinical Program
Intermountain Healthcare
Provo, Utah

O. Josh Bloom, MD, MPH
Carolina Family Practice & Sports Medicine
Medical Director
Carolina Sports Concussion Clinic
Cary, North Carolina
Adjunct Instructor
Family Medicine
University of North Carolina
Chapel Hill, North Carolina
Clinical Associate
Family and Community Medicine
Duke University
Durham, North Carolina

Zach D. Bowers, DO
Resident
Orthopaedic Surgery
San Antonio Military Medical Center
San Antonio, Texas

Eric N. Bowman, MD, MPH
Assistant Professor
Department of Orthopaedic Surgery
Vanderbilt University Medical Center
Nashville, Tennessee

Jonathan T. Bravman, MD
Associate Professor
Director of Sports Medicine Research
CU Sports Medicine
Division of Sports Medicine and Shoulder Surgery
Department of Orthopaedics
University of Colorado
Denver, Colorado

Aaron D. Campbell, MD, MHS, MBA
Family & Sports Medicine
Associate Medical Director Far West Region
St. Luke's Clinic
Boise, Idaho

Michael K. Case, MD
Surgeon
Otolaryngology
Gundersen Health System
La Crosse, Wisconsin

Anthony S. Ceraulo, DO, CAQSM
Assistant Professor
Orthopedics
Division of Sports Medicine
Duke University
Durham, North Carolina

Jorge Chahla, MD, PhD
Assistant Professor
Rush University Medical Center
Chicago, Illinois

Cindy J. Chang, MD, FAMSSM, FACSM
Orthopaedics and Family & Community Medicine
University of California–San Francisco
San Francisco, California

Robert F. Chapman, PhD
Professor
Department of Kinesiology
Indiana University
Bloomington, Indiana

Sarah M. Cheney, BS
MD Candidate
Georgetown University School of Medicine
Washington, DC

Leon Y. Cheng, MD
Physician
Family Medicine
Palo Alto Medical Foundation
Sunnyvale, California

Stephanie Chu, DO
Associate Professor
Family Medicine
University of Colorado
Aurora, Colorado

Thomas O. Clanton, MD
Director
Foot and Ankle Sports Medicine
Orthopaedic Surgery
The Steadman Clinic
Vail, Colorado

Daniel C. Cole, PA-C
Physician Assistant
Vermont Orthopaedic Clinic
Rutland Regional Medical Center
Rutland, Vermont

Justin J. Conway, MD
Head Team Physician
Mount Saint Mary College
Crystal Run Healthcare
Newburgh, New York

David B. Coppel, PhD, FACSM
Professor
Department of Neurological Surgery
University of Washington
Seattle, Washington

David D. Cosca, MD
Assistant Clinical Professor, Retired
Sports Medicine
UC Davis Medical Center
Sacramento, California

Jason Cruickshank, ATC, CSCS
Athletic Trainer
Esports Neurocognitive/Strength and Conditioning Specialist
Cleveland Clinic
Cleveland, Ohio

Ginger L. Cupit, DO
Primary Care Sports Medicine Fellow
Family and Community Medicine
University of California–San Francisco
San Francisco, California

Stephen Dailey, Jr., MD
Assistant Professor
Department of Orthopaedics and Sports Medicine
University of Cincinnati
Cincinnati, Ohio

Michael Dakkak, DO
Fellow
Primary Care Sports Medicine
Orthopedics
Cleveland Clinic
Cleveland, Ohio

Katherine L. Dec, MD, FAAPMR, FAMSSM
Professor
Physical Medicine and Rehabilitation
Professor
Orthopaedic Surgery
Assistant Sports Medicine Fellowship Director
Virginia Commonwealth University Health Systems
Head Team Physician
Longwood University
Richmond, Virginia

William Dexter, MD, FACSM
Director
Sports Medicine Program
Department of Family Medicine
Maine Medical Center
Portland, Maine
Professor
Department of Family Medicine
Tufts University School of Medicine
Boston, Massachusetts

Robert J. Dimeff, MD
Staff Physician
Texas Orthopaedic Associates
OrthoLoneStar
Dallas, Texas

Jon Divine, MD, MS
Professor
Department of Orthopaedics and Sports Medicine
University of Cincinnati
Cincinnati, Ohio

Sameer Dixit, MD, FACP, FAMSSM
Assistant Attending Physician
Primary Sports Medicine
Hospital for Special Surgery
New York, New York

Timothy R. Draper, MD
Associate Program Director
Sports Medicine Fellowship
Cone Health
Team Physician
Guilford College
Greensboro, North Carolina
Clinical Assistant Professor
Family Medicine
University of North Carolina
Chapel Hill, North Carolina

Jonathan A. Drezner, MD
Professor
Department of Family Medicine and Center for Sports Cardiology
University of Washington
Seattle, Washington

Siatta B. Dunbar, DO, CAQSM
Physician
Sports and Orthopedics
MHealth Fairview
Burnsville, Minnesota

Cynthia D. Dusel, MSN, FNP-C, ONP-C
Nurse Practitioner
Orthopaedic Surgery
The Medical College of Wisconsin
Milwaukee, Wisconsin

Katie M. Edenfield, MD
Clinical Associate Professor
Community Health and Family Medicine
University of Florida
Gainesville, Florida

Kevin Eerkes, MD
Clinical Associate Professor of Medicine
Department of Internal Medicine
NYU School of Medicine
New York, New York

Amy Eichner, PhD
Advisor on Drugs and Supplements
US Anti-Doping Agency
Assistant Professor of Human Performance Optimization
Uniformed Services University
College of Allied Health Sciences
Colorado Springs, Colorado

Daniel Eichner, PhD
President
Sports Medicine Research and Testing Laboratory
President
SDTL
South Jordan, Utah

Ashraf M. Elbanna, MD
Orthopaedic Surgeon
Memorial Healthcare
Owosso, Michigan

Ahmed Emara, MD
Fellow
Clinical Research
Orthopaedic Surgery
Cleveland Clinic Foundation
Cleveland, Ohio

Mark J. Erickson, DDS
Staff Surgeon
Oral and Maxillofacial Surgery
Gundersen Health System
La Crosse, Wisconsin

Nicolai Esala, DO, CAQSM
Primary Care Sports Medicine Physician
Orthopedic Urgent Care
TRIA Orthopedics
Maple Grove, Minnesota

Paul Escher, MD
Resident Physician
Otolaryngology-Head and Neck Surgery
University of Iowa Hospitals and Clinics
Iowa City, Iowa

Scott A. Escher, MD
Department of Family Medicine
Section of Sports Medicine
Gundersen Health System
La Crosse, Wisconsin

Shayne D. Fehr, MD
Associate Professor
Orthopaedic Surgery
Medical College of Wisconsin
Milwaukee, Wisconsin

Kai Fehske, MD
Trauma Surgery
University of Wuerzburg
Wuerzburg, Germany

John E. Femino, MD
Clinical Professor
Department of Orthopedics and Rehabilitation
University of Iowa Hospitals and Clinics
Iowa City, Iowa

Karl B. Fields, MD, CAQ SM, FAMSSM
Emeritus Sports Medicine Fellowship Director
Sports Medicine Clinic
Cone Health System
Director of Undergraduate Medical Education
Greensboro AHEC
North Carolina AHEC Systems
Greensboro, North Carolina
Professor
Family Medicine and Sports Medicine
University of North Carolina
Chapel Hill, North Carolina
Editor in Chief Sports Medicine
UpToDate
Boston, Massachusetts

Adam N. Finck, PT, DPT, SCS, OCS, CSCS
Clinic Director
Champion Sports Medicine
Birmingham, Alabama

Andrew Fithian, MD
Resident
Orthopaedic Surgery
Stanford University
Stanford, California

R. Robert Franks, Jr., DO, FAOASM
Director
Rothman Concussion Institute
Sports Medicine
Rothman Institute
Associate Professor
Family Medicine
Thomas Jefferson University
Philadelphia, Pennsylvania
Volunteer Clinical Associate Professor
Family Medicine
Rowan-SOM
Stratford, New Jersey

Jessie R. Fudge, MD, FACSM
Physician
Activity, Sports and Exercise Medicine
Kaiser Permanente Washington
Everett, Washington

Paul S. Fuller, BS, LAT, ATC
Certified Athletic Trainer
Champion Sports Medicine
Birmingham, Alabama

Mikaela C. Gabler, MS, CSCS
Associate Instructor
Indiana University
Bloomington, Indiana

Matthew R. Gammons, MD
Director of Sports Medicine
Vermont Orthopaedic Clinic
Rutland Regional Medical Center
Rutland, Vermont

Kyle Goerl, MD, CAQSM
Medical Director
Lafene Health Center
Kansas State University
Team Physician
Kansas State Athletics
Manhattan, Kansas
Clinical Assistant Professor
Department of Family and Community Medicine
KU SOM-Wichita
Wichita, Kansas

Sophia Gonzalez, PT, DPT, SCS, ATC
Instructor of Clinical Physical Therapy
Division of Biokinesiology and Physical Therapy
University of Southern California
Los Angeles, California

Marci A. Goolsby, MD
Sports Medicine Physician
Hospital for Special Surgery
New York, New York

Andrew William Gottschalk, MD, CAQ
Director
Primary Care Sports Medicine
Sports Medicine Institute
Ochsner Health System
Head Medical Team Physician
New Orleans Pelicans
National Basketball Association
Team Physician
New Orleans Saints
National Football League
New Orleans, Louisiana

Laura Gottschlich, DO
Associate Professor
Departments of Orthopedic Surgery & Community and Family Medicine
Medical College of Wisconsin
Team Physician
Milwaukee Bucks
Milwaukee Ballet
Milwaukee Lutheran High School
Milwaukee, Wisconsin

David Graygo, MPT
Manual Physical Therapist
Esports Ergonomic Specialist
Cleveland Clinic
Cleveland, Ohio

Gary A. Green, MD
Medical Director
Major League Baseball
Head Team Physician
Pepperdine University
Medical Doctors of St. John's
Pacific Palisades, California

Leslie Greenberg, MD
Family Physician
Family and Community Medicine
University of Nevada School of Medicine
Associate Professor
Family and Community Medicine
University of Nevada Reno School of Medicine
Reno, Nevada

Mederic M. Hall, MD
Professor
Orthopaedics and Rehabilitation
University of Iowa
Iowa City, Iowa

Kimberly G. Harmon, MD
Professor
Family Medicine and Orthopaedics and Sports Medicine
University of Washington
Seattle, Washington

George D. Harris, MD, MS
Physician
Family Medicine and Sports Medicine
Fellow
American Medical Society for Sports Medicine
American Academy of Family Physicians
Gastonia, North Carolina

Jennifer S. Harvey, MD, CAQSM
Primary Care Sports Medicine Physician
Orthopedics and Sports Medicine
Novant Health
Kernersville, North Carolina
Medical Director of Sports Medicine
High Point University
High Point, North Carolina

Disa L. Hatfield, PhD
Associate Professor
Department Chair
Exercise Science
Department of Kinesiology
College of Health Sciences
University of Rhode Island
Kingston, Rhode Island

Bruce Helming, MD
Clinical Assistant Professor
Family & Community Medicine
Assistant Head Team Physician
Intercollegiate Athletics
Physician
Campus Health Service
University of Arizona
Tucson, Arizona

John C. Hill, DO, FACSM, FAMSSM, FAOASM, FAAFP
Professor
Director Emeritus of Primary Care Sports Medicine Fellowship
University of Colorado School of Medicine
Denver, Colorado

Corey K. Ho, MD
Assistant Professor
Department of Radiology
University of Colorado—Anschutz Medical Campus
Aurora, Colorado

Eugene S. Hong, MD, CAQSM, FAAFP, FAMSSM
Professor of Orthopedics and Family Medicine
Chief Physician Executive MUSC Health
Medical University of South Carolina
Charleston, South Carolina

Thomas M. Howard, MD
Physician
North Carolina
Flexogenix
Cary, North Carolina
Adjunct Associate Professor
Family Medicine
Campbell University Jerry M. Wallace School of Osteopathic Medicine
Lillington, North Carolina

Kenneth J. Hunt, MD
Associate Professor and Chief
Foot and Ankle Surgery
Department of Orthopaedic Surgery
University of Colorado, School of Medicine
Aurora, Colorado

Mustafa Husaini, MD
Assistant Professor
Department of Medicine
Cardiovascular Division
Washington University in St. Louis School of Medicine
St. Louis, Missouri

Brian A. Jacobs, MD
Family Medicine of South Bend
Team Physician
South Bend Cubs
South Bend, Indiana
Team Physician–Rugby, Boxing
University of Notre Dame
Notre Dame, Indiana

David J. Jewison, MD, MAT, CAQSM
Assistant Professor
Department of Orthopedics
Team Physician
University of Minnesota
Minneapolis, Minnesota

Bevila John-Daniel, MD
Adult Psychiatrist
Psychiatry
Compass Health Network
Eldon, Missouri

Robert Johnson, MD
Professor
Department of Family Medicine and Community Health
University of Minnesota
Minneapolis, Minneapolis

Nathaniel S. Jones, MD, CAQ-SM
Associate Professor
Orthopaedic Surgery and Rehabilitation
Loyola Stritch School of Medicine, Loyola University Chicago
Maywood, Illinois

Susan M. Joy, MD
Co-Director
Sports Medicine Center
Kaiser Permanente
Sacramento, California

Christopher C. Kaeding, MD
Professor
Orthopaedic Surgery
Executive Director
OSU Sports Medicine Center
The Ohio State University
Columbus, Ohio

John W. Karl, MD, MPH
Orthopaedic Surgeon
Vermont Orthopaedic Clinic
Rutland Regional Medical Center
Rutland, Vermont

Donald Kasitinon, MD
Assistant Professor
Departments of Physical Medicine and Rehabilitation and Orthopaedic Surgery
University of Texas Southwestern Medical Center
Dallas, Texas

Morteza Khodaee, MD, MPH
Professor
Family Medicine and Orthopedics
University of Colorado School of Medicine
Denver, Colorado

Christopher Kim, MD
The Iowa Clinic
West Des Moines, Iowa

Dominic King, DO
Orthopaedic Surgery
Cleveland Clinic
Cleveland, Ohio

Robert Kiningham, MD, MA
Professor
Family Medicine
University of Michigan
Ann Arbor, Michigan

Yuka Kobayashi, DO
Assistant Professor
Department of Orthopaedic Surgery
Department of Family Medicine
Medical College of Wisconsin
Milwaukee, Wisconsin

Chitra Kodery, DO
Clinical Assistant Professor
Department of Family and Sports Medicine
Rutgers, New Jersey Medical School
Newark, New Jersey

William J. Kraemer, PhD
Professor
Human Sciences
The Ohio State University
Columbus, Ohio

Matthew J. Kraeutler, MD
Resident
Orthopaedic Surgery
St. Joseph's University Medical Center
Paterson, New Jersey

Benjamin Krainin, MD
Primary Care Sports Medicine Fellow
Family Medicine
University of Colorado
Aurora, Colorado

Erica L. Kroncke, MD
Physician
Sports Medicine
Orthopedic & Sports Medicine Specialists
Green Bay, Wisconsin

Joseph D. Lamplot, MD
Assistant Professor
Department of Orthopaedics
Emory University
Atlanta, Georgia

Mark E. Lavallee, MD, CSCS, FACSM, FAMSSM
Chairman
Sports Medicine
USA Weightlifting
Colorado Springs, Colorado
Member
Executive Medical Committee
International Weightlifting Federation
Lausanne, Switzerland
Clinical Assistant Professor
Department of Family Medicine
Drexel University College of Medicine
Philadelphia, Pennsylvania
Faculty
UPMC Pinnacle Sports Medicine Fellowship
UPMC Pinnacle
Harrisburg, Pennsylvania

Lior Laver, MD
Orthopaedics and Sports Medicine Service
Hillel Yaffe Medical Center
Technion University Hospital
Hadera, Israel
ArthroSport Sports Medicine
Tel-Aviv, Israel

Aaron Lear, MD, MSc, CAQ
Faculty Physician
Family/Sports Medicine
Cleveland Clinic Akron General
Akron, Ohio
Associate Professor
Family Medicine
NEOMED
Rootstown, Ohio

Constance M. Lebrun, MDCM, MPE, CCFP(SEM), FCFP, Dip. Sport Med, FACSM, FAMSSM
Professor and Enhanced Skills Programs Director
Department of Family Medicine
Faculty of Medicine & Dentistry
University of Alberta
Consultant Sport Medicine Physician
Glen Sather Sports Medicine Clinic
Edmonton, Alberta, Canada

Benjamin D. Levine, MD
Professor
Internal Medicine & Cardiology
UT Southwestern Medical Center
Director
Institute for Exercise and Environmental Medicine
Texas Health Presbyterian Hospital Dallas
Dallas, Texas

Lewis G. Lupowitz, PT, DPT, CSCS
Physical Therapist
Orlin & Cohen Orthopedic Group
Woodbury, New York

Christopher C. Madden, MD, FAMSSM, FACSM
Clinical Professor
Family Medicine
University of Colorado Health Sciences
Denver, Colorado
Private Practice
Longs Peak Sports Medicine and Family Practice
Longmont, Colorado

Andrew S. Maertens, MD
Chief Orthopedic Surgery Resident
University of Colorado—Anschutz Medical Campus
Denver, Colorado

Steven A. Makovitch, DO
Clinical Instructor
Department of Physical Medicine and Rehabilitation
Harvard Medical School
Spaulding Rehabilitation Hospital
Boston, Massachusetts

Steven L. Martin, MD
Orthopedic Surgeon
Blue Ridge Surgery Center
Seneca, South Carolina

Robert Virgil Masocol, MD, FAAFP
Associate Physician
Sports Medicine
Kaiser Permanente
Elk Grove, California

Dawn Mattern, MD, FAAFP, FAMSSM
Medical Director
Sports Medicine/Physical Therapy/Occupational Therapy
Trinity Health
Minot, North Dakota

Eric C. McCarty, MD
Professor
Chief of Sports Medicine and Shoulder Surgery
Department of Orthopedics
University of Colorado School of Medicine
Associate Professor Adjunct
Department of Integrative Physiology
University of Colorado, Boulder
Director of Sports Medicine
University of Colorado Department of Athletics
Head Team Physician
Colorado Avalanche Hockey Club
Fellowship Director
University of Colorado Sports Medicine and Shoulder Fellowship

Eric C. McCarty, Jr.
Research Assistant
CU Sports Medicine
University of Colorado School of Medicine
Boulder, Colorado

Torrance A. McCarty
Research Assistant
CU Sports Medicine
Boulder, Colorado

Adrian McGoldrick, BCh, MRCGP, FFSEM
Former Senior Medical Officer
Irish Horseracing Regulatory Board
The Curragh
County Kildare, Ireland

Todd M. McGrath, MD
Sports Medicine
Assistant Attending Physician
Hospital for Special Surgery
New York, New York

Ian D. McKeag, MD, MS, CAQSM
Assistant Professor
Family & Community Medicine
University of Alabama Birmingham (UAB) School of Medicine
Birmingham, Alabama

Omer Mei-Dan, MD
Associate Professor
Department of Orthopedics
Division of Sports Medicine
University of Colorado SOM
Boulder, Colorado

Catherine Miller, PT, DPT, MA, ATC
Coordinator of Physical Therapy/Athletic Trainer
University Health Services
Princeton University
Princeton, New Jersey

Mark D. Miller, MD
Department of Orthopaedic Surgery
University of Virginia
University of Virginia Health System
Charlottesville, Virginia

Travis Miller, DO
Sports Medicine Physician
Orthopedics
Penn State Health
Wyomissing, Pennsylvania

Marc A. Molis, MD, FAAFP
Physician
Sports Medicine
UnityPoint Clinic
Urbandale, Iowa

Whitney E. Molis, MD
Pediatric and Adult Allergy, P.C.
Allergy
Des Moines, Iowa

Alexa Moriarty, MS, RD, CSSD, RYT
Clinical & Sports Dietitian
University Health Services
Princeton University
Princeton, New Jersey
Owner
Expert Nutrition and Wellness LLC
Cranford, New Jersey

Torb Morkeberg, DO
Post Graduate Year 1
Family Medicine and Community Health
University of Minnesota–St. John's Family Medicine Residency
Maplewood, Minnesota

George A. Morris, MD
Vice President
Performance Excellence
CentraCare
St. Cloud, Minnesota
Pool Physician
US National Ski & Snowboard Teams

Kinshasa C. Morton, MD, CAQSM
Assistant Professor
Department of Family Medicine and Community Health
Rutgers University
New Brunswick, New Jersey
Assistant Team Physician
Rutgers University
Piscataway, New Jersey

Rebecca Ann Myers, MD
Physician
Private Practice
Family and Sports Medicine
Longs Peak Family Practice
Longmont, Colorado
Assistant Clinical Professor
Department of Family Medicine
University of Colorado
Denver, Colorado

Michael K. Neilson, DO
Sports Medicine Physician
Direct Orthopedic Care
Meridian, Idaho

Mark W. Niedfeldt, MD
Associate Clinical Professor
Family and Community Medicine
Medical College of Wisconsin
Milwaukee, Wisconsin
Private Practice
Mark W. Niedfeldt, MD, LLC
Mequon, Wisconsin

Francis G. O'Connor, MD, MPH
Professor
Military and Emergency Medicine
Uniformed Services University Consortium for Health and Military Performance
Bethesda, Maryland

David E. Olson, MD, CAQ Sports Medicine
Assistant Professor
Department of Family Medicine and Community Health
University of Minnesota
Associate Medical Director
University of Minnesota Athletics
Minneapolis, Minneapolis

Amy Jo F. Overlin, MD
Sports Medicine Physician
Orthopedics and Sports Medicine
Banner University Medical Center
Phoenix, Arizona

Cecilia Pascual-Garrido, MD, PhD
Associate Professor
Washington University School of Medicine
St. Louis, Missouri

Jon S. Patricios, MBBCh, MMedSci, FACSM, FFSEM (UK), FFIMS
Professor and Director
Wits Sport and Health (WiSH)
Faculty of Health Sciences
University of the Witwatersrand
Director
Waterfall Sports Orthopaedic Surgery
Netcare Waterfall City Hospital
Johannesburg, South Africa

Tatiana Patsimas, MD
Fellow
Department of Family Medicine
University of Colorado
Aurora, Colorado

Stephen R. Paul, MD, MA, FAMSSM
Professor
Family and Community Medicine
Director Athletic Medicine
Campus Health-Intercollegiate Athletics
Assistant Head Team Physician
Intercollegiate Athletics
University of Arizona
Tucson, Arizona

Bradley J. Petek, MD
Fellow
Division of Cardiology
Massachusetts General Hospital
Boston, Massachusetts

Charles S. Peterson, MD
Sports Medicine Physician
Department of Orthopedics and Sports Medicine
Arizona Sports Medicine Center, Abrazo Health
Mesa, Arizona
Team Physician
Arizona Diamondbacks, Arizona Cardinals
Spring Training Physician
Chicago Cubs
Pool Physician
US Ski Team

David J. Petron, MD
Professor
Department of Orthopaedics
University of Utah
Salt Lake City, Utah

Sourav K. Poddar, MD
Associate Professor
Director
Primary Care Sports Medicine
Family Medicine and Orthopedics
University of Colorado School of Medicine
Denver, Colorado

Emily B. Porter, MD, ATC
Physician
Family and Sports Medicine
SSM Health–Dean Medical Group
Madison, Wisconsin

Andrew G. Potyk, BS
Research Fellow
CU Sports Medicine
Boulder, Colorado

Amy P. Powell, MD
Professor
Orthopaedics
University of Utah
Salt Lake City, Utah

Margot Putukian, MD, FACSM, FAMSSM
Internist/Sports Medicine Specialist
Chief Medical Officer
Major League Soccer
New York, New York
Senior Advisor
National Football League, Head, Neck & Spine Committee
Team Physician, US Soccer

Andrew V. Pytiak, MD
Fellow
CU Sports Medicine
University of Colorado School of Medicine
Denver, Colorado

Tauqeer Qazi, MD, CAQSM
Sports Medicine Physician

Courtney A. Quinn, MD
Inova Sports Medicine
Department of Orthopaedic Surgery
Inova Health System
Fairfax, Virginia

William G. Raasch, MD
Professor
Department of Orthopedic Surgery
Medical College of Wisconsin
Milwaukee, Wisconsin

Jeremiah W. Ray, MD, FACEP, CAQSM
Head Team Physician
Health Sciences Clinical Associate Professor
Physical Medicine and Rehabilitation
Health Sciences Clinical Associate Professor
Emergency Medicine
University of California, Davis
Davis, California

Tracy R. Ray, MD, CAQSM, FAMSSM
Physician
Sports Medicine
Piedmont Athens Medical Center
Athens, Georgia

Claudia L. Reardon, MD
Professor
Department of Psychiatry
University of Wisconsin School of Medicine and Public Health
University Health Services
Madison, Wisconsin

Andrew Reisman, MD
Head Team Physician
Student Health Services
Chief Medical Officer for Athletics
University of Delaware
Newark, Delaware

Dustin L. Richter, MD
Assistant Professor
Sports Medicine
Department of Orthopaedic Surgery
University of New Mexico
Albuquerque, New Mexico

Erin Riley, MS, RD, CSSD
Sports Dietitian
Athletic Medicine
Princeton University
Princeton, New Jersey

William O. Roberts, MD, MS
Professor
Department of Family Medicine and Community Health
University of Minnesota
Minneapolis, Minnesota

Kelly Ryan, DO, CAQSM, FAAFP
Faculty
Family Medicine/Sports Medicine
Medstar Franklin Square Medical Center
Baltimore, Maryland
Associate Professor
Georgetown School of Medicine
Washington, DC

Thomas R. Sachtleben, MD
Primary Care Sports Medicine Physician
Sports Medicine
Orthopaedic Center of the Rockies
Fort Collins, Colorado
Primary Care Sports Medicine Physician/Team Physician
Colorado State University
Fort Collins, Colorado

Marc R. Safran, MD
Professor
Orthopaedic Surgery
Chief
Division of Sports Medicine, Orthopaedic Surgery
Stanford University
Stanford, California

Inigo San-Millan, PhD
Assistant Professor
Medicine–Division of Endocrinology, Metabolism and Diabetes
University of Colorado
Aurora, Colorado
Associate Research Professor
Human Physiology and Nutrition
University of Colorado
Colorado Springs, Colorado

Jonathan Schaffer, MD, MBA
Managing Director of eCleveland Clinic
Information Technology Division
Joint and Reconstructive Orthopaedic Surgeon
Orthopaedic Surgery
Cleveland Clinic
Cleveland, Ohio

Mark Schickendantz, MD
Center for Sports Health
Department of Orthopaedic Surgery
Cleveland Clinic
Cleveland, Ohio

Brock E. Schnebel, MD
Clinical Professor
Department of Orthopedics
University of Oklahoma School of Medicine
Head Team Physician
University of Oklahoma Athletic Department
McBride Orthopedic Hospital and Clinic
Oklahoma City, Oklahoma

Jodi Schneider, MS, ATC
Assistant Athletic Trainer
University of North Carolina–Chapel Hill
Chapel Hill, North Carolina

Joshua C. Scott, MD
Primary Care Sports Medicine
Kerlan Jobe Institute
Los Angeles, California

Selina Shah, MD, FACP, FAMSSM
Sports, Dance, and Performing Arts Medicine Physician
Walnut Creek, California
Team Physician
USA Artistic Swimming, US Figure Skating
Company Physician
Diablo Ballet, New Ballet–San Jose, AXIS Dance Company, Blue Devils Drum Corps

Ian Shrier, MD, PhD
Associate Professor
Family Medicine
McGill University
Senior Investigator
Lady Davis Institute
Jewish General Hospital
Montreal, Quebec, Canada

Kartik Sidhar, MD
Fellow Physician
Primary Care Sports Medicine
University of Colorado
Denver, Colorado

Marc R. Silberman, MD
Director
Sports Medicine
New Jersey Sports Medicine and Performance Center
Gillette, New Jersey

Charles "Chip" Simpson II, DPT, CSCS, SCS
Sports Medicine Physical Therapist
Nashville, Tennessee

Edward J. Smith, DO
Assistant Professor, Sports Medicine
Department of Family Medicine and Community Health
University of Minnesota
Minneapolis, Minnesota

Matthew V. Smith, MD
Associate Professor
Department of Orthopaedics
Washington University
St. Louis, Missouri

R. Lance Snyder, MD
Sports Medicine Surgeon
Jacksonville Orthopedic Institute
Orthopedics
Baptist South
Jacksonville, Florida

Kurt P. Spindler, MD
Director
Research and Outcomes
Cleveland Clinic Florida
Director
Outcomes Management Evaluation
Professor
Surgery
CCLCM Case Western
Co-Director
Musculoskeletal Research Center

Jack Spittler, MD
Assistant Professor
Family Medicine
University of Colorado
Aurora, Colorado

James P. Stannard, MD
Hansjörg Wyss Distinguished Professor and Chairman
Department of Orthopaedic Surgery
University of Missouri-Columbia
Associate Dean and Chief Medical Officer
Procedural Services
Chairman
Department of Orthopaedic Surgery
Medical Director
Missouri Orthopaedic Institute
University of Missouri
Columbia, Missouri

Sasha Steinlight, MD
Physician
Medical Services
Princeton University
Princeton, New Jersey

Chaney G. Stewman, MD
Fellowship Director
Primary Care Sports Medicine
Family and Community Medicine
ChristianaCare
Team Physician
University of Delaware
Newark, Delaware
Clinical Assistant Professor
Sidney Kimmel Medical College
Philadelphia, Pennsylvania

Ryan S. Stolakis, MD
Faculty Physician
Family Medicine
Wellspan York Hospital
York, Pennsylvania

Mark Stovak, MD, FAMSSM, FACSM, FAAFP, CAQSM
Professor
Family and Community Medicine
University of Nevada, Reno School of Medicine
Reno, Nevada

Colin D. Strickland, MD
Associate Professor
Department of Radiology
University of Colorado—Anschutz Medical Campus
Aurora, Colorado

Jennifer D. Stromberg, MD
Clinical Associate
Community and Family Medicine
Duke University
Durham, North Carolina

Venkat Subramanyam, MD
Assistant Professor of Emergency Medicine
Assistant Professor of Orthopedics
University of Connecticut Health Center
Farmington, Connecticut

Karen M. Sutton, MD
Associate Professor
Orthopaedic Surgery
Weill Cornell Medical School
Attending
Orthopaedic Surgery
Hospital for Special Surgery
New York, New York

Tunde K. Szivak, PhD
Assistant Professor
Exercise & Rehabilitation Sciences
Merrimack College
North Andover, Massachusetts

Gwendolyn A. Thomas, PhD
Assistant Research Professor
Kinesiology
Penn State University
University Park, Pennsylvania

Jane S. Thornton, MD, PhD, CCFP(SEM), Dip Sp Phy (IOC)
Clinician Scientist
Family Medicine
Western University
Sport and Exercise Medicine Physician
Fowler Kennedy Sport Medicine Clinic
London, Ontario, Canada

John M. Tokish, MD
Orthopaedic Surgery and Sports Medicine
Mayo Clinic Arizona
Phoenix, Arizona

Eric Traister, MD
Physician
Longs Peak Sports Medicine
Longmont, Colorado

James A. Underwood, MD
Physician
Physical Medicine and Rehabilitation
Virginia Commonwealth University
Richmond, Virginia

Carole S. Vetter, MD
Professor
Orthopaedic Surgery
Medical College of Wisconsin
Milwaukee, Wisconsin

Armando F. Vidal, MD
Associate Professor
Sports Medicine and Shoulder Service
Department of Orthopedics
University of Colorado School of Medicine
Aurora, Colorado

Ryan J. Wagner, DO
Physician
Department of Orthopedics and Sports Medicine
ThedaCare Orthopedic, Spine and Pain Center
Appleton, Wisconsin
Team Physician: Wisconsin Herd and Wisconsin Timber Rattlers

Bryant Walrod, MD
Associate Professor
Family Medicine
The Ohio State University
Columbus, Ohio

Kevin D. Walter, MD
Associate Professor
Departments of Orthopaedic Surgery & Pediatrics
Associate Primary Care Sports Medicine Fellowship Director
Department of Physical Medicine and Rehabilitation
Medical College of Wisconsin
Program Director
Pediatric & Adolescent Sports Medicine
Children's Hospital of Wisconsin
Milwaukee, Wisconsin

Jeffry T. Watson, MD
Physician
Hand Center
Colorado Springs Orthopaedic Group
Colorado Springs, Colorado

Jaimi Weber, DO
Sports Medicine Fellow
Department of Family Medicine–Sports Medicine
University of Minnesota
Minneapolis, Minneapolis

Kevin E. Wilk, PT, DPT, FAPTA
Associate Clinical Director
Physical Therapy and Rehabilitation
Champion Sports Medicine
Director of Rehabilitative Research
American Sports Medicine Institute
Birmingham, Alabama

Robert A. Williams, Jr., PT, DPT, CSCS
Physical Therapist
Orthopaedic Rehab Specialists
Jackson, Michigan

Michelle Wolcott, MD
Associate Professor
Orthopedics
University of Colorado School of Medicine
Aurora, Colorado

Rick W. Wright, MD
Dan Spengler, MD Professor and Chair
Department of Orthopaedic Surgery
Vanderbilt University Medical Center
Nashville, Tennessee

Craig C. Young, MD, FAMSSM, FACSM
Professor and Medical Director of Sports Medicine
Departments of Orthopaedic Surgery & Community and Family Medicine
Medical College of Wisconsin
Milwaukee, Wisconsin
Honorary Senior Researcher
WITS Institute for Sports & Health (WISH)
University of Witwatersrand
Johannesburg, South Africa
Team Physician
Milwaukee Brewers, Milwaukee Bucks
Company Physician
Milwaukee Ballet, Skylight Opera
Milwaukee, Wisconsin
Pool Physician
US National Freeski, Ski & Snowboard Teams, US Olympic Committee
President (2007–2008) American Medical Society for Sports Medicine

CONTENTS

ONLINE CONTENTS

Visit your ebook (see inside front cover for details) for the following printable patient education brochures from *Ferri's Netter Patient Advisor,* 3rd edition.

SECTION I

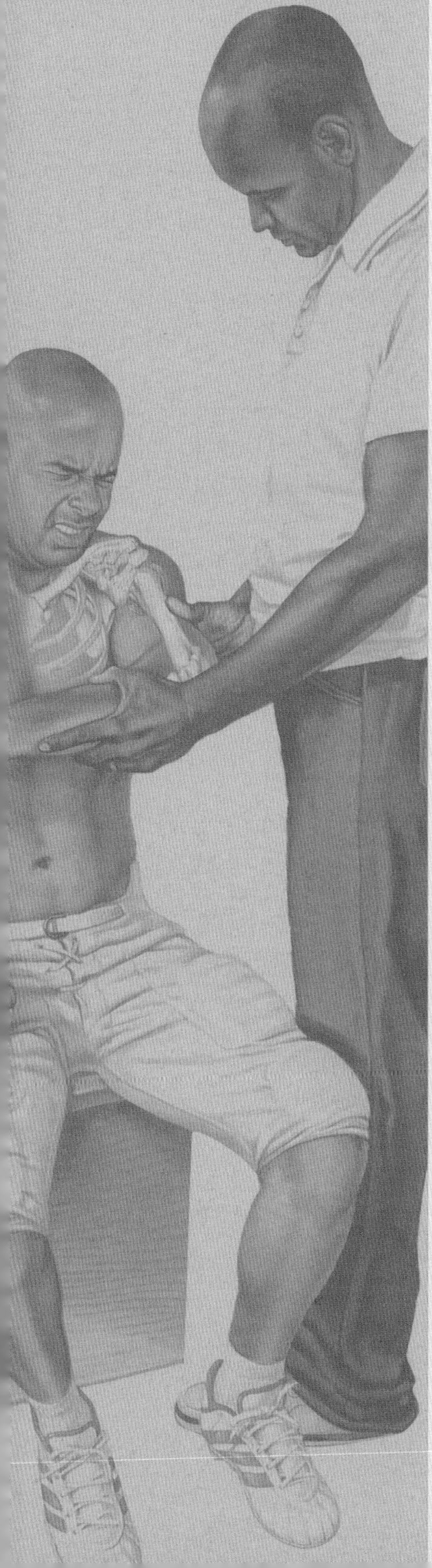

Medical Care and Supervision of the Athlete

THE TEAM PHYSICIAN 1

Margot Putukian • Christopher C. Madden • Craig C. Young • Eric C. McCarty

BEING A TEAM PHYSICIAN: A SPECIAL PRIVILEGE, AN AWESOME CHALLENGE

Special Role

- Team physicians have a unique responsibility of leadership while taking care of athletes.
- Core skills include leadership; team building; shared decision-making and collaboration; good communication; and a mission guided by selfless service, trust, and integrity.
- Athletes, their parents, and their team administrators expect team physicians to help guide decisions in terms of clearance to participate in the sport, as well as to assess and manage healthcare issues to ensure safe participation of athletes.
- Such decisions may be required in a setting of intense time pressure, such as when required on the sidelines.
- Team physicians may play a leadership role within an organization and may provide care for individuals and teams at mass-participation sporting events. In addition, team physicians have responsibilities and duties that are both medical and administrative, and these frequently include ethical and medicolegal issues.
- This chapter discusses the requirements of a team physician in terms of medical qualifications, education, and roles and responsibilities.

THE SPORTS MEDICINE TEAM

- Care of an athlete is a team effort, wherein members of a sports medicine team support each other for the benefit of the athlete and the athletic team.
- An athletic trainer occupies a unique position at the center of the athletic healthcare triangle.
- A team physician cares for the athletic team and also serves as a key player on the sports medicine team comprising the athlete, the team physician, the coach, the athletic trainer, and other supporting health professionals. Similar to the athletic team, sports medicine services are best provided following a team approach (Fig. 1.1).

Availability

- Availability is a cornerstone for the success of a team physician.
  - On the sidelines, at events, and during travel.
  - In the training room.
  - In the office: Team physicians may have to include special accommodations in their office schedules for athletes who require urgent medical attention.
  - After office hours and weekends: Most athletic activity happens outside a normal work day; thus, team physicians must accommodate this in their coverage considerations.
  - Video and digital communications, such as telehealth and email, may sometimes be appropriate settings to provide care and communicate with athletes.

DEFINITION OF THE TEAM PHYSICIAN

- Six major professional associations focusing on clinical sports medicine issues collaborated to develop guidance documents for team physicians.
- These "Team Physician Consensus Conference" Statements (TPCCs) cover various topics for team physicians, including the definition of team physicians: **TPCCs** (https://www.acsm.org/acsm-positions-policy/official-positions) and **Sideline Preparedness for the Team Physician: Consensus Statement** (https://pubmed.ncbi.nlm.nih.gov/11323559/).
  - The TPCCs defines the qualifications, roles, and responsibilities of team physicians along with providing guidelines for individuals and organizations seeking to select a team physician.
  - Other TPCCs are listed in "Recommended Readings" and provide resources that cover specific topics and populations.
- The team physician must be a medical doctor (MD) or doctor of osteopathy (DO) with an unrestricted license in good standing and knowledge of on-field emergency care and basic cardiopulmonary resuscitation (CPR) techniques, as well as musculoskeletal injuries and medical and psychological issues that affect athletes.

RESPONSIBILITIES OF THE TEAM PHYSICIAN

Medical Care

- The most important role of the team physician is to address the physical and psychological needs of an athlete.
- In addition to the essential requirements described in the TPCCs, it is desirable that the team physician has additional training and education in sports medicine, with medical specialty and fellowship training and additional American Council of Graduate Medical Education (ACGME)/American Osteopathic Association (AOA) certification in sports medicine, and additional experience, including:
  - Ongoing continued medical education in sports medicine
  - Experience in sports medicine
  - Membership and participation in a sports medicine professional association or society
  - Training in advanced cardiac and trauma life support
  - Ongoing involvement in education and research in sports medicine
- Understanding the complexities of medicolegal, disability, and compensation issues that can occur in sports medicine is helpful.
- To perform effectively, the team physician must maintain a broad and up-to-date knowledge base that addresses athletics and medicine.
  - All team physicians should feel comfortable in providing emergency care at sporting events.
  - Training in CPR and automated external defibrillator (AED) use is essential, and additional knowledge of advanced cardiac life support (ACLS) and advanced trauma life support (ATLS) is useful.
  - In addition, the team physician should have knowledge in the following areas:
    - **Medicine:** full-spectrum primary care, including musculoskeletal system, growth and development, cardiovascular and pulmonary medicine, infectious disease, gastroenterology, nephrology, neurology, and other medical areas pertaining to exercise and sports
    - **Psychology and behavior:** mental health issues such as depression, anxiety, eating disorders, alcohol and other drug use/abuse, and psychological response to injury
    - **Pharmacology:** therapeutics, supplements, performance enhancers, recreational drugs, interactions among these agents, and effects on performance

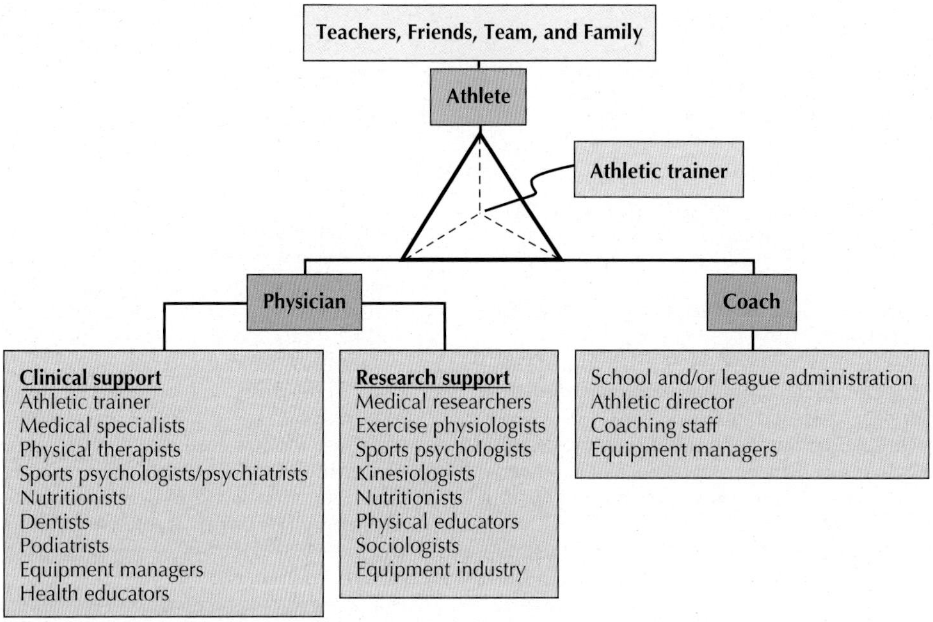
Teachers, Friends, Team, and Family
Athlete
Athletic trainer
Physician
Coach
Clinical support
Athletic trainer
Medical specialists
Physical therapists
Sports psychologists/psychiatrists
Nutritionists
Dentists
Podiatrists
Equipment managers
Health educators
Research support
Medical researchers
Exercise physiologists
Sports psychologists
Kinesiologists
Nutritionists
Physical educators
Sociologists
Equipment industry
School and/or league administration
Athletic director
Coaching staff
Equipment managers

Figure 1.1 The sports medicine team. The athletic trainer works under the supervision and license of the physician, often with a plan of care and/or standing orders. (Modified from Mellion MB. *Office Sports Medicine*. Philadelphia: Hanley & Belfus; 1996.)

- **Nutrition and exercise science:** nutrition, exercise physiology, biomechanics, sport-specific issues (e.g., altitude and other environmental issues)
- **Sexual violence issues:** advocate for safe environment and support any athletes exposed to abuse; collaborate with teams, sports organizations, and institutions on policies and procedures to reduce sexual violence within the institution
- **Sport- and population-specific issues:** including gender, age, disability, or other unique population factors

Additional Medical Responsibilities

- Coordinating assessment and management of injuries and illness on game day, including making decisions about clearance and same-day return to play
- Understanding the importance of the preparticipation physical evaluation (PPPE), emergency planning, pandemic planning, and issues of sudden death and heat illness, as well as recovery and rest

Administrative Responsibilities

The team physician has a range of important administrative responsibilities:

- Establish a chain of command for injury and illness management, including:
  - Involvement in planning and implementation of emergency action plans
  - Involvement in and awareness of protocols and equipment required for sideline preparedness
  - Coordinating assessment and management of game-day injuries and illnesses, including return-to-play decision-making
- Clearance for non–game-day participation and return-to-play decision-making
- Understand the importance of injury and illness prevention
- Understand the importance of collaboration with other healthcare providers, including athletic trainers, physical therapists, nutritionists, strength and conditioning specialists, psychologists, and other specialists, in the care of an athlete
- Understand the role of nutrition, supplements, and performance-enhancing agents
- Create protocols for use of medications, both prescription and over-the-counter, that comply with state and federal licensing, laws and practice acts, and policies established by sports organizations and schools
- Important decisions regarding PPPE and what it may include (e.g., screening for mental health issues, concussion baseline testing, and cardiac screening)
  - Such decisions are often complex and may involve several other stakeholders.
- Additional considerations include preventive measures:
  - Immunizations
  - Educational efforts (e.g., concussion, heat-related illnesses, nutrition, and cardiac illnesses)
  - Injury and illness prevention (e.g., anterior cruciate ligament [ACL] injury prevention or prophylaxis for communicable skin diseases)
- An important administrative responsibility of the team physician is to work with the organizing body (e.g., school, university, or club) to develop an agreement that clearly defines the roles and responsibilities of the team physician, as well as the reporting structure for other healthcare providers (e.g., the team physician makes clearance decisions, and the athletic trainer reports to the team physician and not the coach)

Ethical and Medicolegal Responsibilities

The team physician has a range of responsibilities that reflect the many relationships involved in the care of an athlete:

- Responsibilities toward the athlete, the team, and the institution and its representatives must be considered.
- All physicians have ethical responsibilities, but those of team physicians may be somewhat unique given the complex and often public nature of sports participation.
- As stated in the TPCCs, "the overriding principle for all physicians, including team physicians, in managing ethical issues, is to provide care focused on what is best for the patient and only for the patient." Several examples of ethical challenges are provided next.

Informed Consent

- Information provided by team physicians to an athlete and/or his or her parent or guardian must be complete and inclusive of all options so that the athlete can make an informed decision.
- Information should include a discussion of short- and long-term risks and benefits and balance the athlete's autonomy, desires, and optimal medical treatment.
  - For example, an athlete with a meniscus tear amenable to repair should be provided with all information so that he or

she can make an informed decision (e.g., short-term benefits of meniscectomy and return-to-play versus potential long-term benefits of repair).
  - Team physicians should provide information with a goal of protecting athletes from injury, re-injury, permanent disability, and themselves.
- Athletes must be counseled and thoroughly informed when there is a valid medical contraindication to participation or resumption of participation.

Confidentiality

- Team physicians must respect the rights of patients and safeguard their confidentiality within the constraints of the law, respecting both the Health Insurance Portability and Accountability Act of 1996 (HIPAA) and the Family Educational Rights and Privacy Act (FERPA).
- Relationship with athletes may have to be clarified in advance. Challenging examples may include:
  - Medical conditions that limit or affect participation
  - Psychological issues that may limit or affect participation
  - Medical issues that may affect other participants
  - Drug testing results

Conflict of Interest

- There are some situations where team physicians may experience a conflict of interest or a perceived conflict of interest.
- These include situations where a team physician is hired by a professional organization to care for team members, wherein there is a financial relationship with particular organizations, which may lead to a conflict with the care provided to the athlete.

Influence of Others

- Influence of others, such as teammates, parents, coaches, and administrators, may conflict with the medical care provided to the athlete.
- Team physicians should remain aware of potential implicit and explicit influences, including those provided by the community and media.

Marketing, Publicity, and Advertising

- A potential ethical issue for team physicians may occur when a company or individual offers compensation for services and medical care provided by them.
- Team physicians may be sponsored by a company or industry with the biased expectation that they will use one product over another.
- Ethical issues can arise when team physicians are expected to endorse or use new technology (e.g., equipment, treatment modality, or medications) without substantial evidence of efficacy or safety.

Drug Use

- Team physicians may be asked to prescribe or administer pain medications in order to allow an athlete to participate.
- Athletes using illegal, illicit, or performance-enhancing drugs may pressure team physicians to supply, administer, or help cover up the use of such drugs.

Medicolegal Issues

- Certain medicolegal issues may be unique for team physicians. Specific concerns may include the following:
  - Team physicians should clearly define professional autonomy over medical decisions
  - Issues regarding HIPAA and FERPA compliance
  - Guidelines, standards, policies, and regulations set by school and governing bodies
  - Rules, regulations, and/or laws of local, state, or federal government
  - Issues regarding the management of on-field (e.g., cardiac, concussion, cervical spine, or heat) injuries or illnesses
  - Issues regarding clearance to play and/or restriction from play, waivers, and return-to-play decision-making
  - Issues regarding medical documentation

RECOMMENDED READINGS

Available online.

2 THE CERTIFIED ATHLETIC TRAINER AND THE ATHLETIC TRAINING ROOM

Jodi Schneider

DEFINITION OF AN ATHLETIC TRAINER

- Athletic training encompasses the prevention, examination, diagnosis, treatment, and rehabilitation of emergent, acute, or chronic injuries and medical conditions. Athletic training is recognized by the American Medical Association (AMA), Health Resources Services Administration (HRSA), and Department of Health and Human Services (HHS) as an allied healthcare profession (see National Athletic Trainers' Association [NATA] https://www.nata.org/about/athletic-training)
- Athletic trainers (ATs) are highly qualified, multiskilled healthcare professionals who render service or treatment under the direction of a physician (see Chapter 1: "The Team Physician") in accordance with their education, their training, and their state's statutes, rules, and regulations (see NATA https://www.nata.org/about/athletic-training)
- They are uniquely qualified, allied healthcare providers who are optimally suited as front-line gate keepers and first responders for all athletic-related healthcare issues.
- ATs provide services including injury and illness prevention, emergency care, on-field and clinical diagnosis, patient education, and rehabilitation and therapeutic intervention of acute and chronic injuries and illnesses.
- ATs also act as a liaison between the physician, patient, coaching staff, and support staff to coordinate effective patient-centered care, establishing effective communication as one of the most important responsibilities of an AT.

Settings

- Traditional
  - High school, college, and professional sports
- Nontraditional
  - Hospital/orthopedic practice
  - Military/special forces
  - Occupational medicine
  - Performing arts
  - For additional information on nontraditional settings for ATs, please visit https://www.nata.org/professional-interests/emerging-settings (accessed March 2021).

EDUCATION

- To sit for the board of certification examination, candidates must graduate from a professional program that has been accredited by the Commission on Accreditation of Athletic Training Education (CAATE). At this time students may choose a bachelor's-level or a master's-level professional program, but effective in 2022, all CAATE-accredited programs will be fully transitioned to being offered at the master's level. Athletic Training Curriculum Competencies (5th edition CAATE), 2011 (https://caate.net/wp-content/uploads/2014/06/5th-Edition-Competencies.pdf; accessed March 2021) as follows:
  - Evidence-based practice
  - Prevention and health promotion
  - Clinical examination and diagnosis
  - Acute care of injury and illness
  - Therapeutic interventions
  - Psychosocial strategies and referral
  - Healthcare administration
  - Professional development and responsibility
- Seventy percent of ATs possess a master's or doctorate degree
- Post-professional education
  - Residency/fellowship: An emerging aspect of an AT's education is optional post-professional residencies or fellowships. These programs are designed to provide an advanced level of clinical and didactic education in specialized areas.

Licensure

As of March 2020, 49 states plus the District of Columbia require licensure or registration to practice as an AT. Efforts continue to enact licensure in California.

ROLES AND RESPONSIBILITIES OF AN ATHLETIC TRAINER

Domains of Practice, Board of Certification (BOC), 2015

Injury/Illness Prevention and Wellness Protection

- "ATs identify and understand intrinsic (patient history, demographics, education) and extrinsic factors (environmental, social, sport specific) that are relevant to the client, patient or population" (Henderson, 2015)
  - Education of patients, coaches, and administrators
  - Implement and assist in the administration of preparticipation physical examination with physicians
  - Preseason musculoskeletal screening
  - Playing surface, environmental, and weather safety monitoring
  - Screening and referral for mental health and psychological concerns
  - Effective recognition and referral to appropriate care providers
  - Supplement monitoring, education and oversight of weight management protocols, and safety in weight-class sports
  - Coordination with administration, coaches (including strength and conditioning), sports dietitians, and physicians in developing and implementing monitoring and education

Examination, Assessment and Diagnosis

- "Implementing systematic, evidence-based examinations and assessments to formulate valid clinical diagnoses and determine patients' plan of care" (Henderson, 2015)
- Acute and chronic injury evaluation on and off the field and effective referral to a physician when necessary
- Concussion evaluation, protocol management, and referral to physician

Immediate and Emergency Care

- "The profession of athletic training is unique in that the Athletic Trainer is often present at the time of an injury or emergency. ATs have a vast knowledge of medical conditions that can quickly become emergencies, and because ATs are often on-site, they are the primary healthcare professionals qualified to intervene" (Henderson, 2015).

- Development and implementation of emergency action plans based on the most up-to-date consensus/position statements and best practices. For a detailed list of up-to-date NATA position statements, please visit http://www.nata.org/position-statements.
- Coordination and pre-event communication with local emergency services departments.
- Prompt and proficient emergency care based on current standards of care.

Therapeutic Intervention

- "Rehabilitating and reconditioning injuries, illnesses and general medical conditions with the goal of achieving optimal activity level using the applications of therapeutic exercise, modality devices and manual techniques" (Henderson, 2015)
- Identification, management, and treatment of injuries and illnesses using evidence-based practices and appropriate referrals
- Returning patients to full preinjury function as soon as safely possible
- Determining the ability to safely return with functional testing
- Communication and coordination of rehabilitation and transition to full function with strength and conditioning and coaching staff
- Communication and coordination with external rehabilitation providers when appropriate

Healthcare Administration and Professional Responsibility

- "Integrating best practices in policy construction and implementation, documentation and basic business practices to promote optimal patient care and employee well-being" (Henderson, 2015)
- Development and implementation of policies and procedures of the sports medicine facility, emergency action plans, and medical coverage of events
- Maintain professional relationships to coordinate patient care with:
  - Coaching staff, including strength and conditioning staff
  - Administrators
  - Dietitians
  - Psychologists/counselors
  - External providers
- Timely and accurate medical record keeping
- Maintenance of supplies and budget of the athletic training facility

HOW AN ATHLETIC TRAINER AND A PHYSICIAN FUNCTION AS A TEAM

- ATs work under the direction of the team physician based on state practice acts
  - AT license requires a written plan of care (which varies from state to state depending on the legislation) to guide the day-to-day practice of an AT and can include:
    - Time frame for referral to physician
    - Emergency care procedures
    - Nonprescription medication administration
    - Treatment protocols and modality usage
  - Communicate effectively to provide collaborative patient-centered care
    - AT coordinates effective referrals to physician
    - Physician and AT work together to make return-to-play decisions
    - AT communicates frequently on day-to-day progress and status to physician to facilitate modifications to care plan as necessary
- The team physician and AT work together and develop policies and procedures specific to the institution/facility
  - Developing, communicating, and enforcing physician-led chains of command and establishing subsequent AT supervisory positions within the sports medicine department
  - Development of facility-specific emergency action plans and clearly communicating them to all members of the athletic department
  - Development and implementation of appropriate medical coverage policies
  - Standard operating procedures for sports medicine facilities and the staff
- Members of interdisciplinary treatment and performance teams
  - No greater demonstration of commitment to patient-centered care than development and participation in interdisciplinary treatment and performance teams. Aligning medical, coaching/performance, and academics to provide complete personal care and support to athletes. ATs and physicians are crucial and invaluable members of these teams not only because they provide medical care but because of the level of relationship that develops from day-to-day interaction with the athletes. This also provides ATs and physicians varied perspectives to help direct patient care and support.
    - Examples include:
      - Mental health
      - Eating concerns
      - Sport performance
      - Academic performance
      - Life skills/transition to post-athletic life

COLLEGIATE ATHLETIC MEDICINE/SPORTS MEDICINE DEPARTMENT MODEL

- Responsibility to provide an effective sports medicine structure/model free of conflict of interest. Determination of the best model varies from setting to setting.
- Several different models have been utilized across the United States, the most common being sports medicine housed within the athletic department. Recently, there has been a shift to housing sports medicine departments within university health services in an effort to decrease conflict of interest and provide better athlete-centered care. For a comprehensive description of other models, along with their advantages and disadvantages, please see "Inter-Association Consensus Statement on Best Practices for Sports Medicine Management for Secondary Schools and Colleges" in the Recommended Readings section.

RECOMMENDED READINGS

Available online.

3 THE PREPARTICIPATION PHYSICAL EVALUATION

Morteza Khodaee • Tatiana Patsimas • Margot Putukian • Christopher C. Madden

PREPARTICIPATION PHYSICAL EVALUATION (PPPE)

- History and physical examination, with additional testing as indicated, that is performed before participation in sport, that meets several objectives, and that is one of the most important functions provided by the sports medicine physician.
- Often, this is the first interaction between the physician and the athlete; for many young adults, it may be the first exposure to the healthcare system.
- It does not replace regular physical examinations, although many athletes think that it covers all healthcare needs.
- It encompasses clearance for participation in the sport and provides education and information to athletes regarding issues such as nutrition, supplementation, training and conditioning, injury prevention, and rehabilitation.
  - Addition of a 12-lead electrocardiogram (ECG) examination as part of the standardized screening process is controversial.
- Special considerations of PPPE include age specificity, sex specificity (special concerns for female vs. male athletes), sport specificity (specific demands of each sport should be considered), athletes with special needs, and athletes with physical or intellectual disabilities.

OBJECTIVES OF THE PPPE

- Emphasize cardiovascular, neurologic, and musculoskeletal issues
- Identify any life-threatening or disabling conditions (e.g., underlying cardiovascular or neurologic abnormalities)
- Identify any conditions that may put an athlete at risk of injury or illness (e.g., underlying ligamentous instability, musculoskeletal abnormalities, organomegaly, exercise-induced bronchospasm, or acute medical illness)
- Assess an injury that has not been appropriately rehabilitated
- Assess medical conditions and strength and flexibility deficits that put an athlete at risk of injury
- Assess general health status (e.g., immunizations), fitness, and maturity
- Meet insurance or legal requirements
- Screen for menstrual dysfunction, stress fractures, or disordered eating (female athlete triad, disordered eating in male athletes)
- Introduce athletes to the healthcare system and concepts of preventive medicine
- Offer an opportunity to address issues such as recreational and performance-enhancing substance use and abuse, sexuality issues, mental health issues, and health promotional activities (alcohol and drug abuse, seat belts, helmets, and self-breast or self-testicular examination)

TIMING

- The PPPE should be performed at least 6 weeks before the beginning of the sport season to allow adequate time for further evaluation of identified problems and treatment or rehabilitation of any conditions or injuries.
- If athletes are unavailable 4–6 weeks before the beginning of an early fall season, examinations performed at the end of the previous school year may be considered. Athletes should report any interval injuries, illnesses, and new medications between their examinations and the beginning of the fall season.
- A detailed medical history may be completed by athletes and/or parents in advance, which may improve the accuracy of the information (e.g., immunization records) and examination efficiency. Internet resources can facilitate the history and interval injury reporting process. An electronic format (ideally a national database) has several benefits, including communication and administration of the PPPE.

FREQUENCY

- Variable recommendations depend on individual athletes (i.e., age, gender, sport [single or multiple]; their health [underlying medical conditions or injury history], and cost); availability of records from past PPPEs (continuity of care); and requirements of state, city, or athletic governing body.
- **General guidelines** (no consensus about optimal frequency)
  - Comprehensive baseline PPPE before initiating a new sport or attaining a new level (e.g., entry into high school, college, or professional level), and every 2–3 years thereafter.
  - Subsequent annual PPPEs may be limited to injuries or illnesses disclosed by an interim health questionnaire, which focuses on issues associated with heat, head, heart, and mental health; yearly evaluation of the cardiopulmonary system may be appropriate.
  - If an athlete is participating in multiple sports during the year, consider more frequent evaluations.
  - Several **states** require an annual full screening examination (no standard requirements).
  - The **National Collegiate Athletics Association** (NCAA) requires an initial comprehensive PPPE on entrance, followed by interim history in the intervening years; limited additional examinations focusing only on new problems.
  - The **American Heart Association** (AHA) recommends initial comprehensive PPPE on entrance for high school and college athletes. The AHA recommends another comprehensive PPPE after 2 years for high school athletes and follow-up interim history and blood pressure measurements annually, along with focused additional examinations for new problems for college student athletes.
  - The American Medical Society for Sports Medicine (AMSSM) emphasizes a shared decision-making process involving the athletes or their legal representatives and clinicians for any potential limitation for initial sports participation or return to play.

METHODOLOGY

Office-Based

Potential advantages: patient-centered, physician–patient familiarity, privacy, and continuity of care

Potential disadvantages: greater cost, limited appointment time, limited physician interest/experience, and lack of communication of pertinent information to school athletic staff

Coordinated Medical Team-Based (Table 3.1)

Potential advantages: specialized personnel, time and cost efficiency, and good communication with school athletic staff

Potential disadvantages: rushed examinations, lack of privacy, and inadequate follow-up of identified problems

Table 3.1 REQUIRED AND OPTIONAL STATIONS AND PERSONNEL FOR COORDINATED PREPARTICIPATION PHYSICAL EVALUATION

Required Stations	Personnel
Sign-in, height and weight (BMI[a]), blood pressure, and vision	Ancillary personnel (coach, nurse, and community volunteer)
History review, physical examination[b], and clearance	Physician
Optional Stations	**Personnel**
Nutrition	Dietitian
Dental	Dentist
Injury evaluation[c]	Physician
Flexibility	Trainer or therapist
Body composition	Physiologist
Strength	Trainer, coach, therapist, and physiologist
Speed, agility, power, balance, and endurance	Trainer, coach, and physiologist

[a]Body mass index (BMI) can be calculated from height and weight (for specific age- and gender-adjusted categories, see www.cdc.gov/growthcharts).
[b]Physical examination can be subdivided if more than one physician is present.
[c]A musculoskeletal injury evaluation station may be used to provide a more complete evaluation when a musculoskeletal injury is detected during the required musculoskeletal screening examination.

Two types of group PPPEs: multistation (multiple physicians, each at a specialized station) and "locker room" (single or multiple physicians performing complete examinations individually, each in their own area [e.g., locker room]).

Recommendations

- At the final station of a station-based examination, an experienced team physician should be available to review all data and to determine clearance or provide appropriate recommendations.
- Communication between other primary or consulting physicians, athletic trainers, coaches, and parents may be enhanced by carefully documenting the problems and specific recommendations in the clearance section of the PPPE form.
- Cases of special concern may warrant a telephone conversation between the team physician and other involved healthcare providers.
- The 2019 *Preparticipation Physical Evaluation* monograph (see "Recommended Readings") considers "gymnasium examination" to be inadequate to achieve the goals and objectives of the PPPE process.

Personnel

Physicians

- PPPEs should be performed by an MD/DO physician, nurse practitioner, or physician assistant, with final clearance by an MD or DO physician.
- Regulations by certain states at the high school level allow other practitioners (e.g., chiropractors or naturopathic clinicians) to perform PPPEs.
- Primary care physicians perform a majority of PPPEs because of their ability to evaluate all organ (i.e., cardiopulmonary, musculoskeletal, neurologic, ophthalmologic, gastrointestinal, genitourinary, and dermatologic) systems.
- Specialists such as orthopedic surgeons, cardiologists, and ophthalmologists or optometrists are key consultants and may be present on site during the screening-station format examination.

Ancillary

- Medical staff, including athletic trainers, physical therapists, nurses, exercise scientists, dietitians, and sports psychologists, may be involved, particularly during the screening-station format PPPE.
- Nonmedical staff, including coaches, school administrators, and community volunteers, are particularly helpful during the screening-station format PPPE.

MEDICAL HISTORY

- There is an emphasis on screening for cardiovascular and musculoskeletal problems, prior head injuries and other neurologic problems, and significant recent illnesses. In addition, prior heat illness, pulmonary problems, medication problems, inadequate immunizations, allergic reactions, skin problems, and menstruation abnormalities and eating disorders in female athletes should be addressed (PPPE: History Form in English and in Spanish available at https://services.aap.org/en/community/aap-councils/council-on-sports-medicine-and-fitness/preparticipation-physical-evaluation; accessed January 2021). The medical history is an essential component of the PPPE that detects abnormalities in a majority of athletes.
- Joint completion of history forms by athletes and parents/guardians is recommended when possible, particularly if the athlete is unclear about family or personal history. In addition, the parent/guardian should be present or available during the PPPE for additional questions that may arise. However, athletes should be alone with the provider when questions regarding high-risk behaviors and mental health are addressed.
- **Cardiovascular history** (Box 3.1):
  - Screen for causes of sudden cardiac death (SCD; Fig. 3.1). The most common cause in people aged <35 years is hypertrophic cardiomyopathy (HCM; Fig. 3.2); in people aged ≥35 years, the most common cause is coronary artery disease (CAD). The PPPE is scrutinized by certain physicians for its ability to detect underlying causes of SCD, particularly in younger patients. However, the AHA states that a certain form of preparticipation screening for high school and college athletes is justifiable and compelling based on ethical, legal, and medical grounds.
- Personal history is important.
  - History of exertional chest pain, tightness, or chest pressure; any unexplained syncope or near-syncope; and excessive and unexplained dyspnea/fatigue or palpitations associated with exercise are all significant.
  - Prior recognition of a heart murmur.
  - Determine past history of invasive or noninvasive cardiac tests ordered by a physician.
  - Prior history of hypertension or prehypertension noted during examinations.
- **Family history is important.**
  - Twenty-five percent of first-degree relatives of patients with HCM exhibit morphologic evidence of HCM in ECG.
  - Other known genetic cardiac conditions associated with SCD (e.g., long QT syndrome, other ion channelopathies, Marfan syndrome, clinically or significant arrhythmias).
  - Premature death (sudden and unexpected or otherwise) before 50 years of age attributable to heart disease in ≥1 relative.
  - Disability from heart disease in close relatives aged <50 years.
  - Hypertension.

Neurologic Concerns

- It is important to ask questions about previous head or neck injury, concussion, neurologic symptoms, exercise-related syncope, stingers/burners, and seizure disorder.

BOX 3.1 THE 14-ELEMENT AMERICAN HEART ASSOCIATION RECOMMENDATIONS FOR PREPARTICIPATION CARDIOVASCULAR SCREENING OF COMPETITIVE ATHLETES

Personal Medical History

- Chest pain/discomfort/tightness/pressure related to exertion
- Unexplained syncope/near-syncope[a]
- Excessive and unexplained dyspnea/fatigue or palpitations associated with exercise
- Prior recognition of a heart murmur
- Elevated systemic blood pressure
- Prior restriction from participation in sports
- Prior heart testing ordered by a physician

Family History

- Premature death (sudden and unexpected or otherwise) in ≥1 relative aged <50 years attributable to heart disease
- Disability from heart disease in a close relative aged <50 years
- Hypertrophic or dilated cardiomyopathy, long QT syndrome, or other ion channelopathies or Marfan syndrome or clinically significant arrhythmias; specific knowledge of genetic cardiac conditions in family members

Physical Examination

- Heart murmur[b]
- Femoral pulses to exclude aortic coarctation
- Physical stigmata of Marfan syndrome
- Brachial artery blood pressure (sitting position)[c]

[a]Judged not to be neurocardiogenic (vasovagal) in origin; is of particular concern when occurs during or after physical exertion.
[b]Refers to heart murmurs judged likely to be organic and unlikely to be innocent; auscultation should be performed in both supine and standing positions (or with Valsalva maneuver), specifically to identify murmurs of dynamic left ventricular outflow tract obstruction.
[c]Preferably taken in both arms.
From Maron BJ, Thompson PD, Ackerman MJ, et al. 2007 Update. *Circulation* 2007;115:1643-1655. From Assessment of the 12-Lead ECG as a Screening Test for Detection of Cardiovascular Disease in Healthy General Populations of Young People (12-25 Years of Age): A Scientific Statement from the American Heart Association and the American College of Cardiology.

- The NCAA has a recommended symptom score, cognitive examination, and balance assessment as "best practices" for every athlete as part of his or her baseline physical examination.
- Concussion history, including the number, symptoms, and time out of activity, as well as a history for "modifiers" for concussion (e.g., migraine history, learning disability history, or history of depression/anxiety) should be considered as part of the baseline PPPE.
- Any positive response mandates a more thorough history, physical examination, and evaluation.

Musculoskeletal Concerns

- Complete history is essential.
- History of previous ligamentous injuries, documentation of surgery, rehabilitation, and time out of play
- History of prior advanced imaging (e.g., radiographs, magnetic resonance imaging [MRI], computed tomography [CT], or bone scan) for a musculoskeletal problem
- Any positive response mandates careful attention during physical examination, including assessment of ligamentous instability, strength and flexibility deficits/mismatches, and completeness of rehabilitation, as well as consideration for obtaining medical records related to the evaluation.
- If an athlete has had prior surgery, obtain medical records related to the evaluation and a documentation that the operating surgeon has cleared the athlete to return to competition and/or determine the athlete's rehabilitation status.

Previous Medical Illnesses (Examples)

- Heat exhaustion/illness
- Infectious mononucleosis
- Hepatitis
- HIV disease
- Diabetes
- Sickle cell disease/hemoglobinopathy
- Asthma
- Allergic reactions
- Kawasaki disease

Female Athlete Triad—Relative Energy Deficiency in Sport (RED-S)

Screening Questions

- Menstrual history:
  - Age of menarche
  - Date of last menstrual period
  - Number of periods in the past 12 months
- Bone health history:
  - History of stress fractures
  - History of bone injuries
  - Risk factors for osteoporosis
- Nutrition history and risk factors for disordered eating:
  - Discrepancies between ideal versus current body weight
  - Body image concerns
  - Pathologic eating behaviors

Additional Concerns

- Additional concerns not always included on the PPPE form may be addressed on an individual basis. If you do not ask, you might never find out.
- Nutritional issues: fluids, game-day nutrition, and general nutrition
- Supplements and performance-enhancing agents
- Sexuality concerns: pregnancy, sexually transmitted diseases, and sexual orientation (best addressed in a private setting)
- Recreational drugs and alcohol use
- Preventive medicine (e.g., seat belts, helmets, self-breast or self-testicular examination, cholesterol screening, and gynecologic examinations/Pap smear)
- Mental health and psychosocial issues: stress management, anxiety, depression, suicide (consider including screening questionnaires such as the Patient Health Questionnaire-9 [PHQ-9] or Generalized Anxiety Disorder-7 [GAD-7] for depression and anxiety, respectively)

PHYSICAL EXAMINATION (BOX 3.2)

- The physical examination should be comprehensive. It should focus on areas of greatest importance in sports participation and address any problems uncovered while recording an athlete's history.
- Adequate exposure during the examination is important.
- The **physical examination form** (PPPE: Physical Examination Form available at https://downloads.aap.org/AAP/PDF/PPE-Physical-Examination-Form.pdf, copyright 2019, accessed January 2021) is generally comprehensive and covers the scope of such examination, but it should not limit the clinician if additional examination is deemed pertinent.

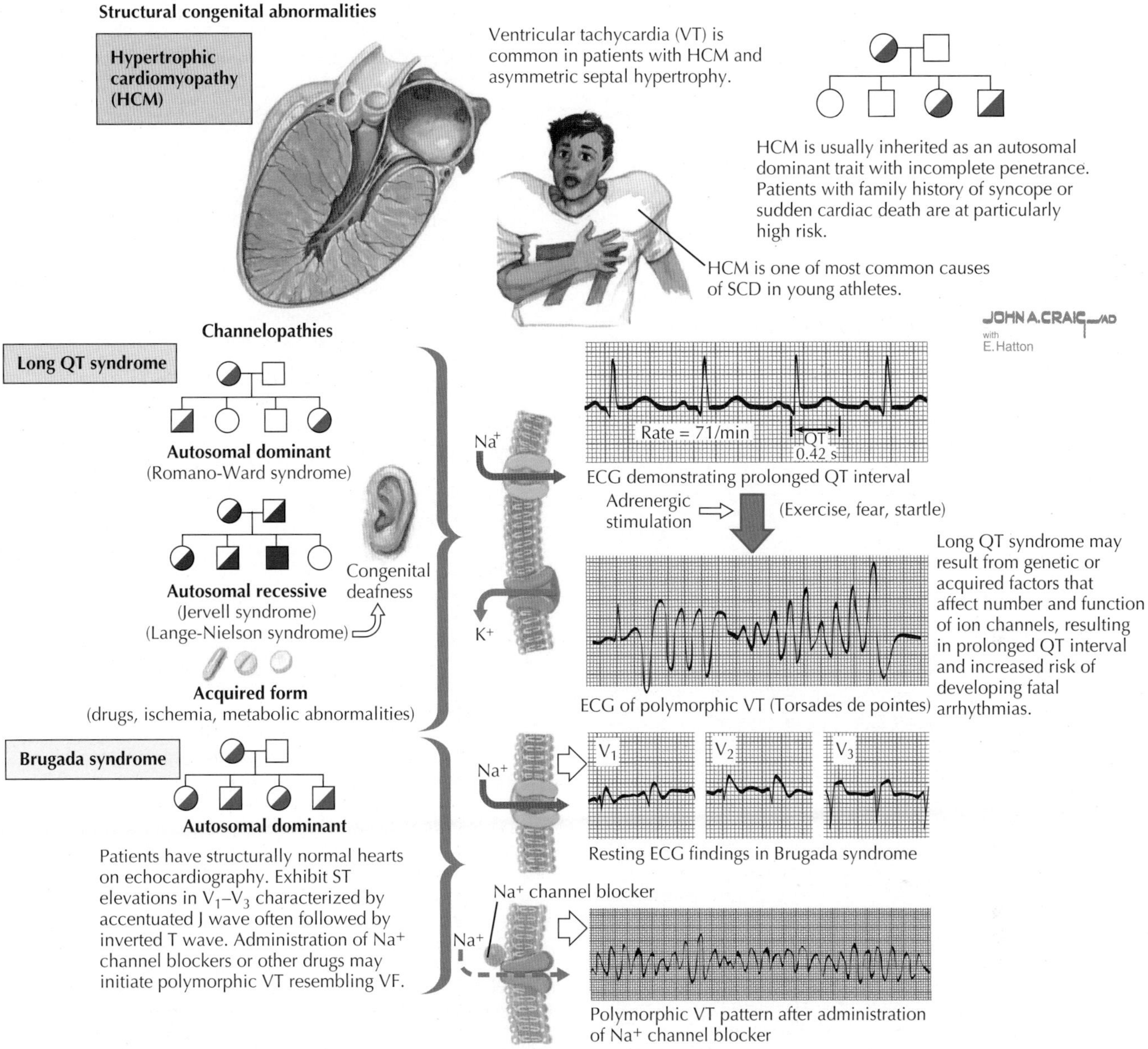
Structural congenital abnormalities
Hypertrophic cardiomyopathy (HCM)
Ventricular tachycardia (VT) is common in patients with HCM and asymmetric septal hypertrophy.
HCM is usually inherited as an autosomal dominant trait with incomplete penetrance. Patients with family history of syncope or sudden cardiac death are at particularly high risk.
HCM is one of most common causes of SCD in young athletes.
JOHN A.CRAIG AD with E.Hatton
Channelopathies
Long QT syndrome
Autosomal dominant
(Romano-Ward syndrome)
Autosomal recessive
(Jervell syndrome)
(Lange-Nielson syndrome)
Congenital deafness
Acquired form
(drugs, ischemia, metabolic abnormalities)
Na+
K+
Rate = 71/min
QT
0.42 s
ECG demonstrating prolonged QT interval
Adrenergic stimulation
(Exercise, fear, startle)
Long QT syndrome may result from genetic or acquired factors that affect number and function of ion channels, resulting in prolonged QT interval and increased risk of developing fatal arrhythmias.
ECG of polymorphic VT (Torsades de pointes)
Brugada syndrome
Autosomal dominant
Patients have structurally normal hearts on echocardiography. Exhibit ST elevations in V1–V3 characterized by accentuated J wave often followed by inverted T wave. Administration of Na+ channel blockers or other drugs may initiate polymorphic VT resembling VF.
V1
V2
V3
Resting ECG findings in Brugada syndrome
Na+ channel blocker
Polymorphic VT pattern after administration of Na+ channel blocker

Figure 3.1 Sudden cardiac death.

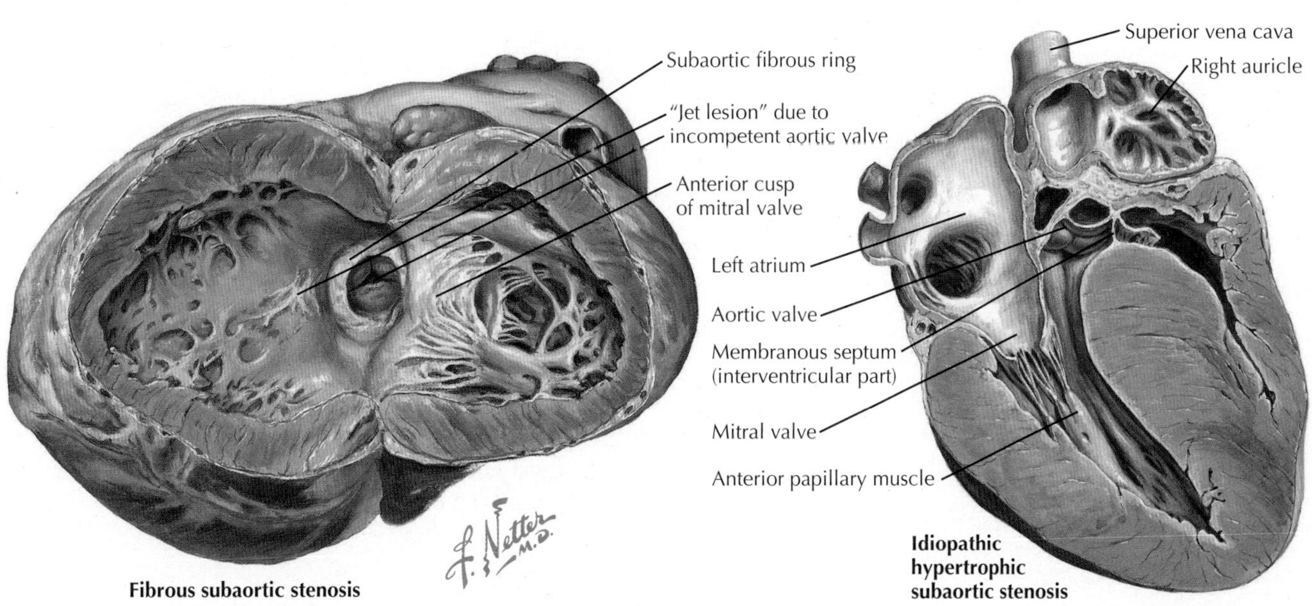
Subaortic fibrous ring
"Jet lesion" due to incompetent aortic valve
Anterior cusp of mitral valve
Superior vena cava
Right auricle
Left atrium
Aortic valve
Membranous septum (interventricular part)
Mitral valve
Anterior papillary muscle
F. Netter M.D.
Fibrous subaortic stenosis
Idiopathic hypertrophic subaortic stenosis

Figure 3.2 Hypertrophic cardiomyopathy.

Height and Weight

- In athletes with excessive weight change, explore the possibility of eating disorders or steroid abuse.
- Body mass index (BMI) should be calculated (gender and age specific; see www.cdc.gov/growthcharts). Understand the indications and limitations of using BMI.
  - Underweight (<5th percentile)
  - Overweight (85th–94th percentile)
  - Obese (≥95th percentile)

Head, Eyes, Ears, Nose, and Throat (HEENT)

- Optical examination is important: check visual acuity in all athletes, pupils for anisocoria, conjunctiva for anemia.
- Certain athletes may have a predilection for ear issues (e.g., swimmers [otitis externa], scuba divers [otic barotrauma], and wrestlers [auricular hematoma]).

BOX 3.2 STANDARD COMPONENTS OF THE PREPARTICIPATION PHYSICAL EVALUATION

- Height
- Weight
- Eyes: visual acuity and pupil size
- Oral cavity
- Ears
- Nose
- Lungs
- Cardiovascular system: blood pressure; femoral and radial pulses; and heart rate, rhythm, and murmurs
- Abdomen: masses, tenderness, and organomegaly
- Skin: rashes and lesions (infectious)
- Musculoskeletal system: contour; range of motion; and symmetry of neck, back, shoulder/arm, elbow/forearm, wrist/hand, hip/thigh, knee, leg/ankle, and foot

Modified from *Preparticipation Physical Evaluation,* 5th ed. Elk Grove Village, IL: American Academy of Pediatrics; 2019.

- Allergy sufferers and athletes with history of nose trauma need nasopharyngeal examinations.
- Smokeless tobacco users need oropharyngeal examinations.

Cardiovascular Assessment

A cardiovascular assessment is essential for both the initial PPPE and annual reevaluations (see Box 3.2).

Brachial artery blood pressure measurement (with appropriate cuff size and ideally in both arms): if elevated, recheck after the athlete rests quietly for 15 minutes and later, if needed (Table 3.2). The following are blood pressure categorizations for children and adolescents according to the 2017 American Academy of Pediatrics (AAP) guidelines.

- Classification categories of hypertension in children aged 1–13 years old:
  - Normal (<90th percentile for age, sex, and height)
  - Elevated blood pressure (≥90th but <95th percentile for age, sex, and height or 120/80 mmHg to <95th percentile, whichever is lower)
  - Stage 1 hypertension (≥95th percentile for age, sex, and height to <95th percentile + 12 mmHg or 130/80 to 139/89 mmHg, whichever is lower)
  - Stage 2 hypertension (≥95th percentile for age, sex, and height + 12 mmHg or ≥140/90 mmHg, whichever is lower)
- Classification categories of hypertension in children aged ≥13 years old:
  - Normal (<120/80 mmHg)
  - Elevated blood pressure (systolic blood pressure [SBP] between 120 and 129 with diastolic blood pressure [DBP] <80 mmHg)
  - Stage 1 hypertension (130/80 to 139/89 mmHg)
  - Stage 2 hypertension (blood pressure ≥140/90 mmHg)

Palpate radial and femoral pulses:

- Decreased or nonpalpable femoral pulses should raise suspicion for coarctation of the aorta.
- Irregular pulse should raise suspicion for arrhythmia and requires ECG evaluation.

Table 3.2 CLASSIFICATION OF HYPERTENSION

Age and Phase	90th–94th Percentile[b] High Normal[a] Prehypertensive[c]	95th–99th Percentile[b] Significant HTN[a] Stage 1 HTN[c]	>99th Percentile[b] Severe HTN[a] Stage 2 HTN[c]
6–9 yr			
Systolic[b]	104–121	108–129	>115–129
Diastolic[b]	68–81	72–89	>83–89
10–12 yr			
Systolic[b]	112–127	116–135	>123–135
Diastolic[b]	73–83	77–91	>84–91
13–15 yr			
Systolic[b]	117–135	121–142	>128–142
Diastolic[b]	76–85	80–93	>87–93
16–17 yr			
Systolic[b]	121–140	125–147	>132–147
Diastolic[b]	78–89	82–97	>90–97
≥18 yr			
Systolic[c]	120–139	140–159	≥160
Diastolic[c]	80–89	90–99	≥100

HTN, Hypertension.

[a]American Academy of Pediatrics, Task Force on Blood Pressure in Children. Report of the Second Task Force Control on Blood Pressure in Children—1987. *Pediatrics.* 1987;79:1-25. Updated in 1996;98(4 Pt 1):649-658.

[b]The blood pressure range is obtained from the Fourth Report on the Diagnosis, Evaluation, and Treatment of High Blood Pressure in Children and Adolescents. For specific blood pressure levels by age, gender, and height, see http://www.nhlbi.nih.gov/files/docs/guidelines/child_tbl.pdf.

[c]From the Seventh Report of the Joint National Committee on Detection, Evaluation, and Treatment of High Blood Pressure, 2003.

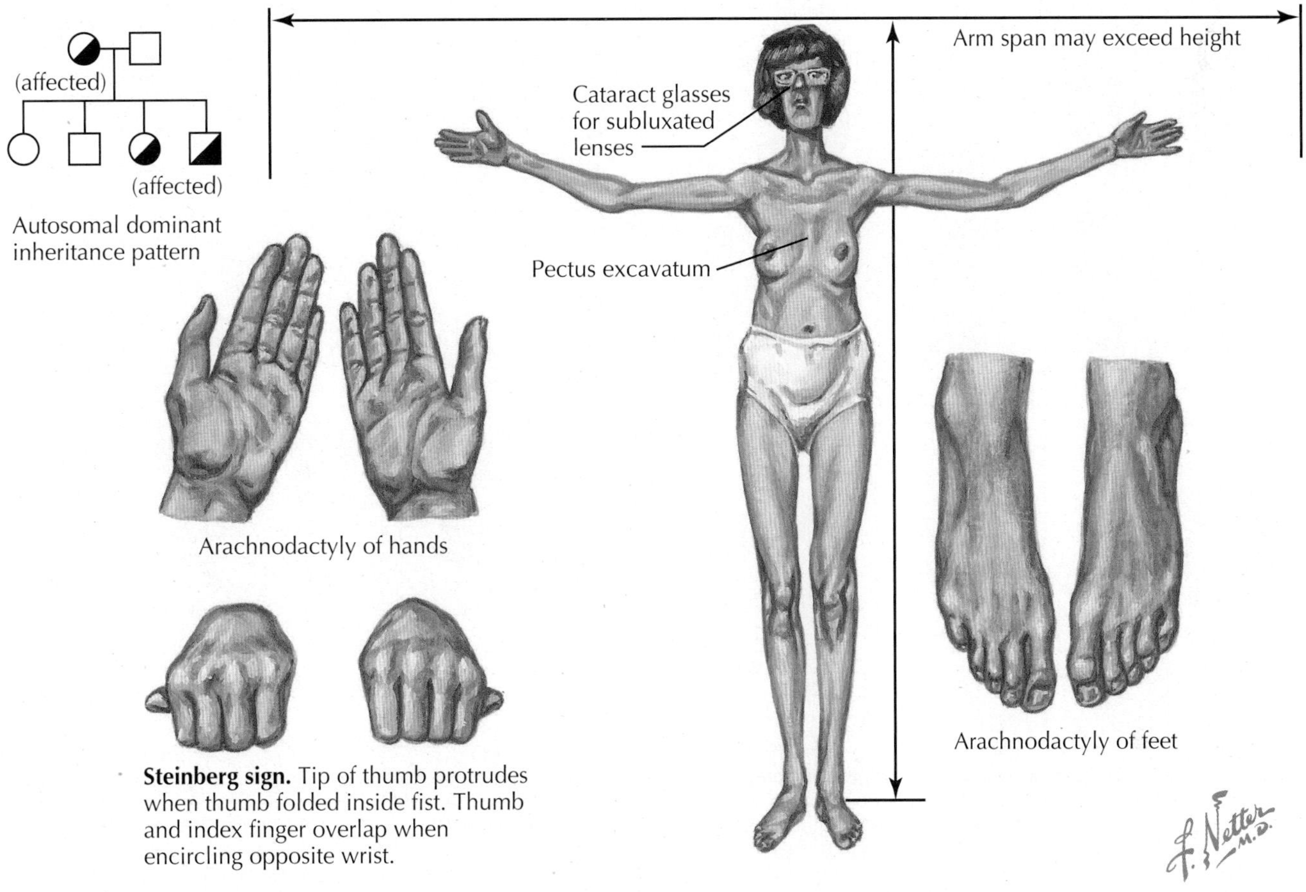
(affected)
(affected)
Autosomal dominant inheritance pattern
Cataract glasses for subluxated lenses
Arm span may exceed height
Pectus excavatum
Arachnodactyly of hands
Arachnodactyly of feet
Steinberg sign. Tip of thumb protrudes when thumb folded inside fist. Thumb and index finger overlap when encircling opposite wrist.
F. Netter M.D.

Figure 3.3 Marfan syndrome.

Heart auscultation in supine and standing positions: note the presence and character of any murmurs

- **HCM murmur:** systolic murmur heard best at lower left sternal border in the standing position; increases with maneuvers that decrease venous return to the heart
- Provocative maneuvers help differentiate functional murmurs from pathologic murmurs.
  - To decrease venous return: Valsalva maneuver and squat-to-stand
  - To increase venous return: deep inspiration, stand-to-squat, and isometric hand grip
- General recommendations for murmurs requiring further evaluation before the athlete can participate:
  - Any systolic murmur grade ≥III/VI in severity
  - Any diastolic murmur
  - Any murmur that gets louder with Valsalva maneuver

Marfan syndrome stigmata (Fig. 3.3): Tall stature, arachnodactyly, kyphoscoliosis, anterior chest deformity, arm span greater than height, decreased upper body length to lower body length ratio, heart murmur or midsystolic click, ectopic lens, thumb sign (the thumbs protrude from the clenched fists), wrist sign (the distal phalanges of the first and fifth digits of one hand overlap when wrapped around the opposite wrist), and family history of Marfan syndrome

Pulmonary Assessment

- Focus on detecting abnormal breath sounds: wheezes, crackles, rubs, and abnormal inspiratory to expiratory ratio
- Asthma screening (e.g., exercise challenge test) has been suggested but is impractical in most preparticipation settings.

Abdominal/Gastrointestinal Assessment

Should be performed with athlete in the supine position. Examples of problems requiring further evaluation before participation include organomegaly (liver and spleen), masses, bruits, tenderness, and/or rigidity and possible pregnancy in females.

Genitourinary Assessment

- Male: Per the fifth PPPE Monograph. Indications for performing the male genital examination include history of groin pain, inguinal bulge, possible testicular lump, or possible undescended testicle. If warranted by history or other findings, examine in a private setting. Chaperones may be present during this part of the examination per patient and/or provider preference.
- Female: routine examination is not recommended; if warranted by history or other findings, examine in a private setting.
- Tanner staging is no longer recommended in PPPE monograph as a standard element; however, it may be useful for counseling on growth and development and anabolic steroid use.

Musculoskeletal Examination

- Musculoskeletal examination is important to identify musculotendinous, bone, or joint problems that may limit athletic participation or predispose to acute injury or long-term complications (e.g., shoulder instability, anterior cruciate–deficient knee, unrehabilitated ankle sprain, or juvenile rheumatoid arthritis).
- General screening examination is most efficient for asymptomatic athletes with no prior musculoskeletal injuries (Fig. 3.4).

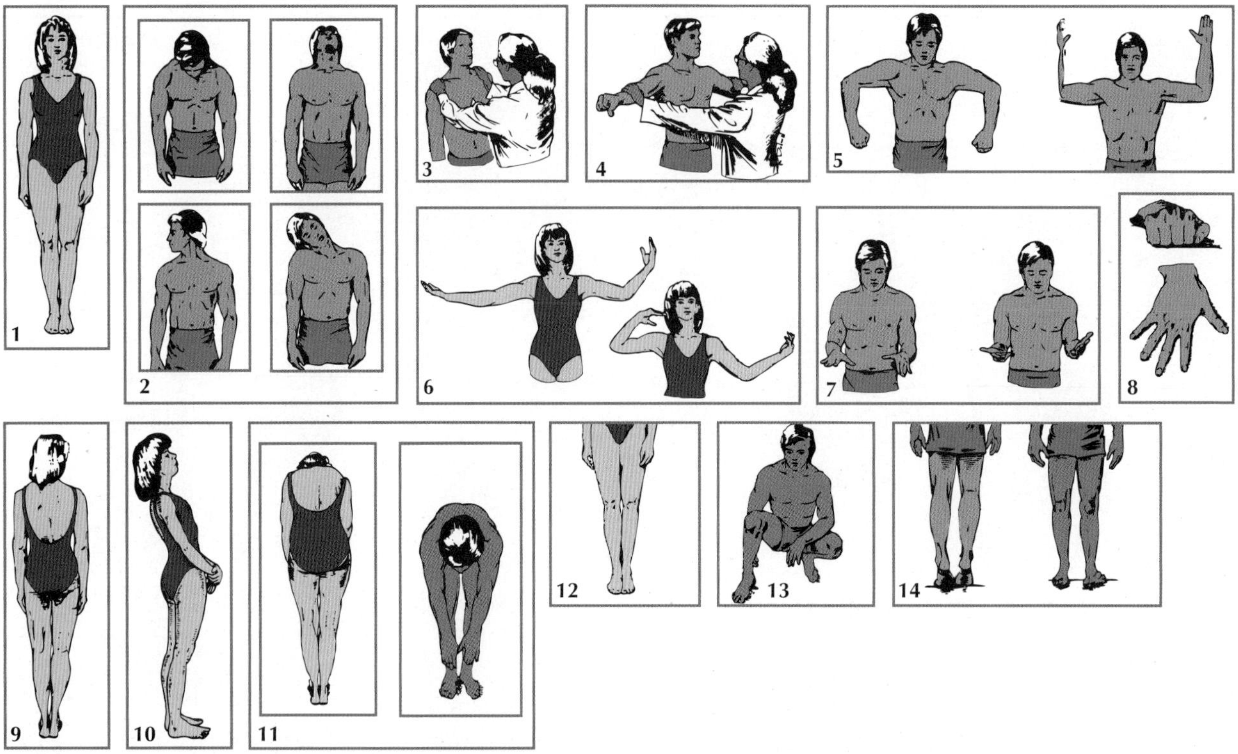
1
2
3
4
5
6
7
8
9
10
11
12
13
14

Figure 3.4 General musculoskeletal screening examination comprising the following: (1) inspection, athlete standing and facing the examiner (symmetry of trunk, upper extremities); (2) forward flexion, extension, rotation, and lateral flexion of neck (range of motion, cervical spine); (3) resisted shoulder shrug (strength, trapezius); (4) resisted shoulder abduction (strength, deltoid); (5) internal and external rotation of shoulder (range of motion, glenohumeral joint); (6) extension and flexion of elbow (range of motion, elbow); (7) pronation and supination of elbow (range of motion, elbow and wrist); (8) clench fist and then spread fingers (range of motion, hand and fingers); (9) inspection, athlete facing away from the examiner (symmetry of trunk, upper extremities); (10) back extension with knees straight (spondylolysis/spondylolisthesis); (11) back flexion with knees straight, facing toward and away from the examiner (range of motion, thoracic and lumbosacral spine; spine curvature; hamstring flexibility); (12) inspection of lower extremities, contraction of quadriceps muscles (alignment, symmetry); (13) "duck walk" four steps (motion of hip, knee, and ankle; strength, balance); (14) standing on toes and then on heels (symmetry, calf; strength; balance). (© Rebekah Dodson.)

- Joint-specific examination: recommended for problematic areas; most accurate and most time consuming.
- Back flexion is recommended in screening for thoracolumbar deformities such as scoliosis (Fig. 3.5).
- Sport-specific examination: some advocate need for focusing on commonly injured or stressed areas in particular sports (e.g., shoulder examination for throwers, tennis players, and swimmers and knee examination for basketball, football, and soccer players); also includes measures of endurance, strength, and flexibility in orthopedic screening but is time consuming and requires in-depth knowledge of particular sports.
- Consider screening for flexibility (e.g., back, hamstrings, and Achilles tendon) because clinical anecdotal evidence suggests that increasing flexibility reduces risk of overuse problems (e.g., mechanical back pain, patellofemoral pain, and medial tibial stress syndrome); however, no study has supported a decreased risk of acute injury (e.g., sprains, strains, and dislocations).
- Functional movement screening (FMS) may be added to PPPE to assess movement quality based on the sport, accessibility, and available resources.

Neurologic Assessment

Neurologic assessment (gross motor) is generally performed through musculoskeletal evaluation. Perform a more comprehensive neurologic examination in athletes with unexplained strength deficits, paresthesia, history of burners/stingers, history of head injury/concussion, or any focal or generalized neurologic deficit.

- The NCAA and others have recommended a baseline symptom score, cognitive examination, and balance assessment for all athletes; an example of this is the Sideline Concussion Assessment Tool-3 (SCAT-3).
- Consider baseline assessment of vestibular ocular motor movement screening (VOMS) for athletes participating in contact and collision sports.

Other Assessments

Assessment for other problems such as lymphadenopathy, thyromegaly, physical findings of eating disorders, and skin conditions should be considered on an individual basis.

Fitness and Performance Evaluation

- Secondary (ideal) objective of PPPE
- Performed more often in the group screening-station format
- Measures any or all of the following parameters:
  - Body composition (e.g., skinfold, underwater weighing, and circumferences)
  - Flexibility (e.g., sit-and-reach and goniometry)
  - Strength (e.g., manual muscle testing, hand or leg dynamometer, bench press or leg press, push-ups, pull-ups, or sit-ups)
  - Endurance (e.g., 12-minute and 1.5-mile run)
  - Power (e.g., vertical and standing broad jump)
  - Speed (e.g., 40-yard dash) and agility (e.g., agility run)
  - Balance (e.g., stork stand, balance beam walking, and Balance Error Scoring System [BESS] included in SCAT-3)

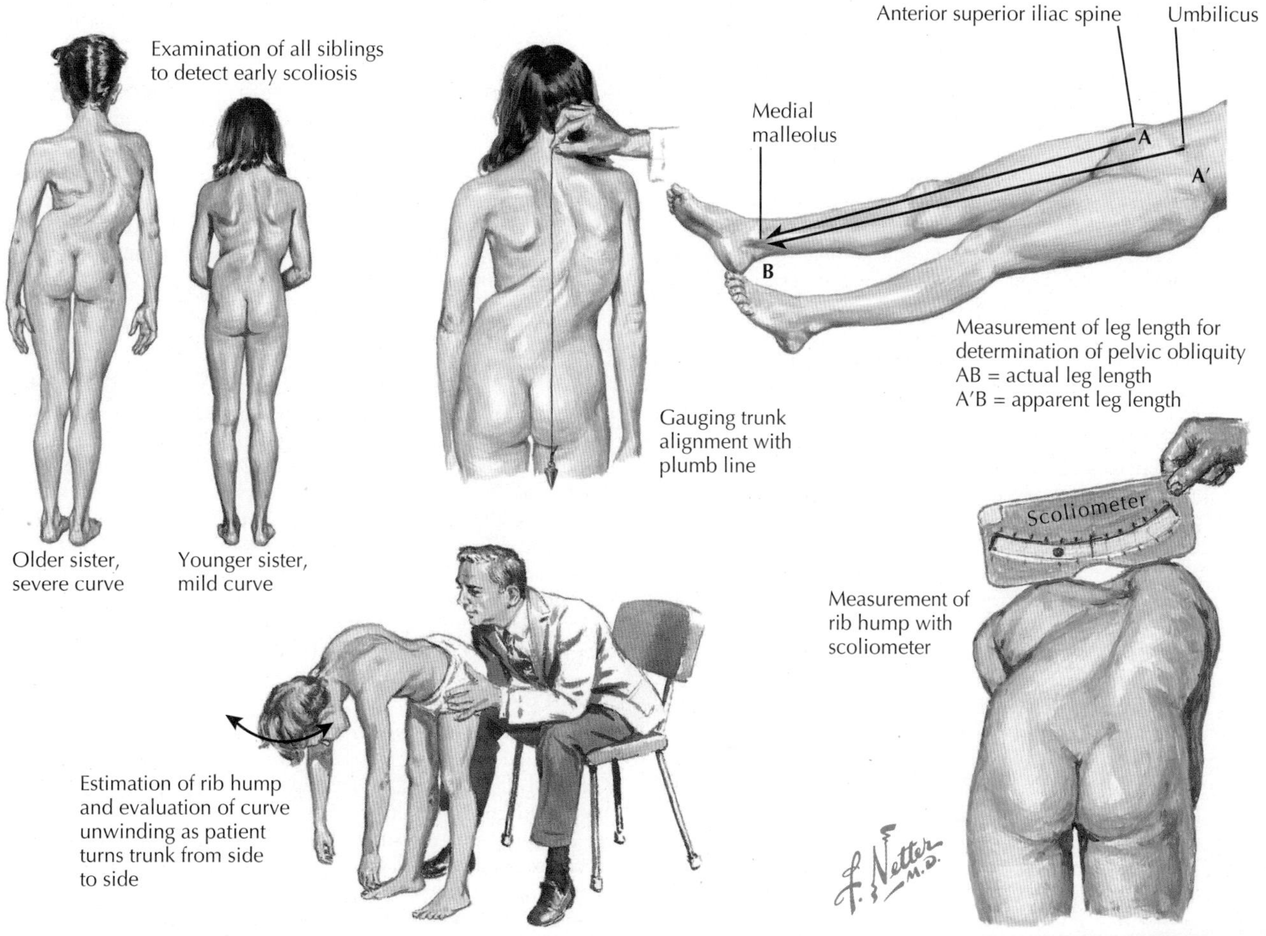
Examination of all siblings to detect early scoliosis
Older sister, severe curve
Younger sister, mild curve
Gauging trunk alignment with plumb line
Anterior superior iliac spine
Umbilicus
Medial malleolus
A
A′
B
Measurement of leg length for determination of pelvic obliquity
AB = actual leg length
A′B = apparent leg length
Scoliometer
Measurement of rib hump with scoliometer
Estimation of rib hump and evaluation of curve unwinding as patient turns trunk from side to side

Figure 3.5 Clinical evaluation of scoliosis.

- Vision performance testing and/or VOMS has been added in certain settings:
  - Dynamic visual acuity
  - Depth perception
  - Visual tracking or pursuit
  - Eye–hand and eye–body coordination

SCREENING TESTS

Difference Between Routine Screening and Diagnostic Testing

A complete blood count in an asymptomatic female athlete is a screening test, whereas a complete blood count in a female athlete with poor eating habits, heavy menstrual periods, fatigue, and pale conjunctiva becomes a diagnostic test.

- Does the burden of suffering resulting from the condition warrant screening?
- If the answer is "yes," ask the following:
  - What is the sensitivity of the proposed screening test?
  - Are the potential risks and cost of the test acceptable?
  - If the screening test identifies the condition, are proven and acceptable treatments available? Is there a clear advantage of initiating such treatment during the asymptomatic phase of the condition?

Routine Screening Tests

Routine screening is not recommended, but specific screening tests (e.g., sickle cell screening required by the NCAA and hemoglobin and ferritin for distance runners) are recommended as indicated.

Laboratory tests: urinalysis, complete blood count, chemistry profile, lipid profile, ferritin, sickle cell trait, sexually transmitted disease, infectious hepatitis, and urine drug screening

Radiographs: chest, cervical spine, and joint radiographs

Cardiopulmonary tests: ECG, echocardiogram, exercise stress test, spirometry, exercise spirometry, and other exercise challenge tests. Although certain studies suggest that using new ECG screening protocols (e.g., Seattle criteria) may decrease false-positive screens, recommendation of ECG screening for athletes still remains controversial, even in select populations. In 2014, the AHA published *Assessment of the 12-Lead ECG as a Screening Test for Detection of Cardiovascular Disease in Healthy General Populations of Young People (12–25 Years of Age)*. It states:

- Screening with 12-lead ECG in association with comprehensive history taking and physical examination to identify or raise suspicion of genetic/congenital and other cardiovascular abnormalities may be considered in relatively small cohorts of young healthy people aged 12–25 years but not necessarily limited to athletes (e.g., in high schools, colleges/universities, or local communities), provided that close physician involvement and sufficient quality control can be achieved; if undertaken, such initiatives should recognize known and anticipated limitations of 12-lead ECG as a population screening test, including the expected frequency of false-positive and false-negative test results, as well as the cost required to support these initiatives over time (Class IIb; Level of Evidence C).
- Mandatory and universal mass screening with 12-lead ECG in large general populations of young healthy people aged 12–25 years (including on a national basis in the United

States) to identify genetic/congenital and other cardiovascular abnormalities is controversial and an area where further research is necessary (Class III, no evidence of benefit; Level of Evidence C).

The "Italian Experience"

In Italy, a systematic, state-subsidized national program for mandatory annual PPPE of all athletes aged 12–35 years has been in place for approximately 35 years. Minimum annual tests include a general examination and 12-lead ECG. Elite competitive athletes undergo a more comprehensive medical and physiologic evaluation that includes routine ECG, the findings of which are as follows:

- Detection of few definitive examples of potentially lethal cardiovascular abnormalities remains the norm.
- A reported 2.2%–2.5% of athletes are disqualified (approximately 51% because of cardiovascular abnormalities).
- A study by Basso and colleagues suggests that the Italian national screening program can decrease the incidence of SCD among young athletes. During the study period, SCD occurred in 55 screened athletes versus 265 nonscreened nonathletes.
- Right ventricular dysplasia causes more athletic deaths than HCM. Reasons for the discrepancy in North American data (where HCM causes more deaths in athletes aged <30 years) are unresolved. In addition, possible disqualification of athletes through screening may contribute to this discrepancy.

With the rarity of potentially lethal cardiovascular abnormalities in young athletes and the overwhelming number of sports and athletic participants in the United States, screening of the Italian magnitude would be challenging in most settings.

ESC and IOC

The European Society of Cardiology (ESC) and International Olympic Committee (IOC) recommend combining noninvasive testing (e.g., 12-lead ECG) with the standard history-taking and physical examination for cardiovascular screening in large populations of young trained athletes.

ECG and/or Echocardiogram

ECG should be considered in athletes with any significant cardiac symptoms or abnormal findings on examination or with a family history of sudden death (unknown cause), SCD, or other cardiac conditions that are known predisposing factors for SCD (e.g., right ventricular dysplasia, HCM, long QT syndrome, and Marfan syndrome) in a family member aged <50 years, particularly a first-degree relative. Approximately 90% of people with HCM exhibit abnormal ECG findings.

Baseline Neuropsychological (NP) Testing

Baseline NP testing may be considered and recommended, if available, for athletes in sports considered to have a risk of head injury. The utility of neuropsychological testing as a stand-alone test, as well as the need for baseline testing, remains controversial. Nevertheless, baseline NP testing is valuable as part of a comprehensive concussion protocol injury (see Chapter 45: "Head Injuries").

Special Considerations for Transgender Athletes

Although the medical eligibility screening of transgender athletes is largely the same as the preparticipation physical evaluation described earlier, providers should be aware of additional health concerns that disproportionately affect this group of patients. Compared with cisgender counterparts, transgender individuals are at higher risk for depression, anxiety, disordered eating, and other mental health illnesses, and they should be appropriately screened for these conditions at the PPPE. Additionally, providers should screen for discrimination, bullying, and abuse in this population.

Providers should also be aware of local sports eligibility policies regarding transgender athlete participation and should advocate for their patients' competition status when necessary. One important way in which providers can help transgender athletes achieve appropriate competition status is by helping them apply for a therapeutic use exemption (TUE) from antidoping organizations (ADOs) if the athlete is taking testosterone, spironolactone, or other banned substances as part of their hormone therapy.

Patients With Disabilities

The PPPE and clearance to participate for athletes with disabilities is important and should be performed with an understanding of the medical and musculoskeletal issues that are present for the condition, as well as understanding the sport-specific demands for the athlete (Preparticipation Physical Evaluation: The athlete with special needs form available at https://www.aap.org/en-us/Documents/PPE-Athletes-with-Disabilities-Form.pdf; copyright 2019, accessed January 2021; for additional information related to athletes with disability, see Chapter 14: "The Athlete With Physical Disability"). A common example is athletes with Down syndrome, with possible atlantoaxial instability.

Down Syndrome

Patients with Down syndrome and their parents should be closely questioned regarding signs or symptoms of atlantoaxial instability. Cervical radiographs, including flexion and extension views, may be considered (Fig. 3.6).

- In asymptomatic patients, neurologic signs or symptoms may be more predictive of risk of injury progression than radiographic abnormalities.
- The AAP acknowledges the potential but unproven value of lateral plain radiographs of the cervical spine but does not recommend routine screening radiographs.
- Special Olympics requires cervical spine radiographs before athletic participation in all patients with Down syndrome in judo, equestrian sports, gymnastics, diving, pentathlon, butterfly stroke, diving starts in swimming, high jump, Alpine skiing, snowboarding, squat lift, and soccer.
- However, there is a lack of general agreement on the criteria for exclusion from sport.

CLEARANCE FOR PARTICIPATION

- Clearance falls into **four categories:**
  1. Full participation without restrictions
  2. Participation pending further testing/evaluation
  3. Participation just in certain sports
  4. Disqualification
- Differentiation of categories is important.
- Familiarity with the demands of a specific sport is essential; use of a classification system for sports by contact and strenuousness is helpful in this regard (Table 3.3 and Fig. 3.7).
- **Published guidelines for medical conditions and sports participation** are helpful, but clinical judgment should be used in applying general guidelines to individual athletes (Box 3.3).
- Additional considerations:
  - How does the condition/illness affect the athlete's risk of morbidity or mortality?
  - How will the condition/illness affect other participants?
  - Are there any limitations or modifications within the sport that allow the athlete to continue participation despite the injury or illness? If so, is it reasonable to allow participation with limitations until the condition resolves?

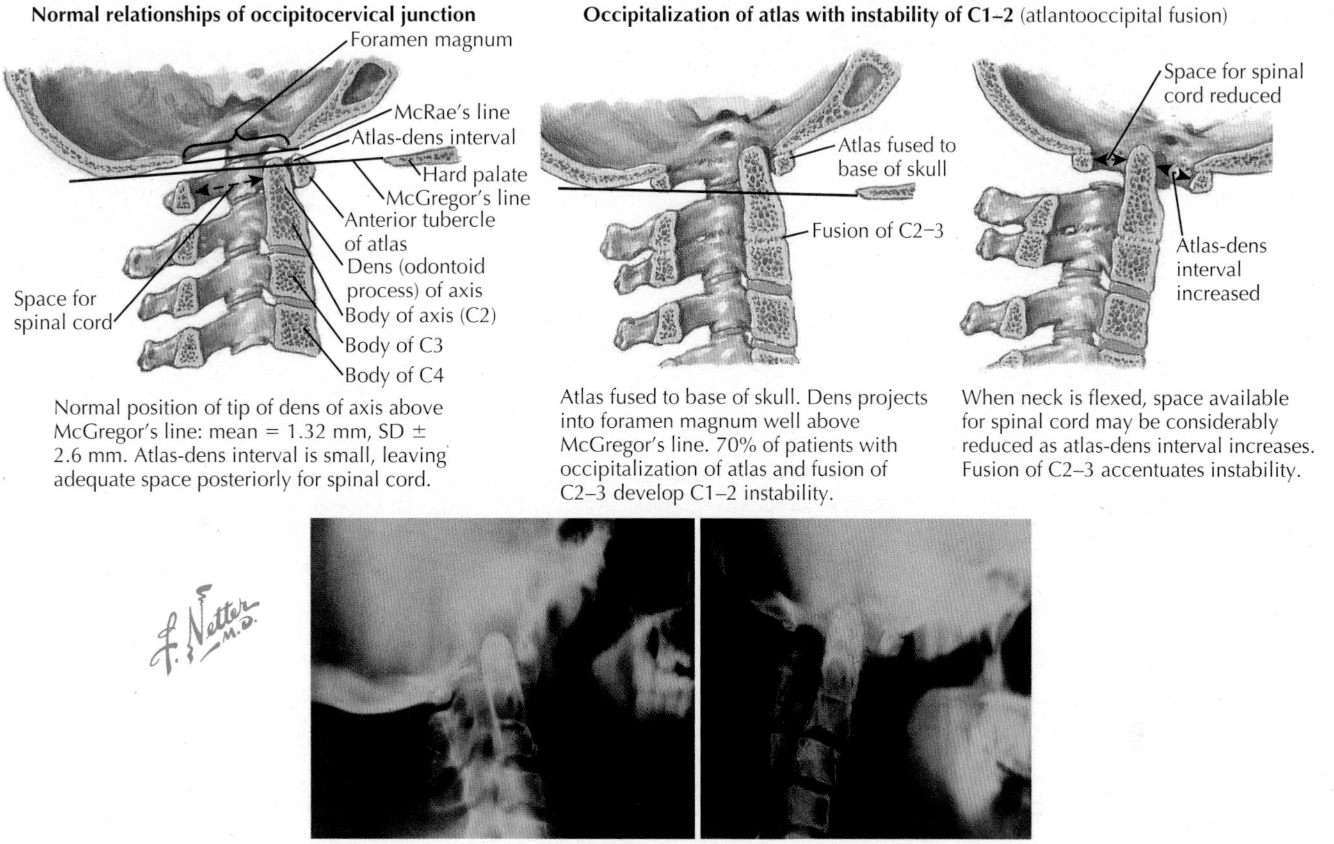
Normal relationships of occipitocervical junction
Foramen magnum
McRae's line
Atlas-dens interval
Hard palate
McGregor's line
Anterior tubercle of atlas
Dens (odontoid process) of axis
Body of axis (C2)
Body of C3
Body of C4
Space for spinal cord
Normal position of tip of dens of axis above McGregor's line: mean = 1.32 mm, SD ± 2.6 mm. Atlas-dens interval is small, leaving adequate space posteriorly for spinal cord.
Occipitalization of atlas with instability of C1–2 (atlantooccipital fusion)
Atlas fused to base of skull
Fusion of C2–3
Atlas fused to base of skull. Dens projects into foramen magnum well above McGregor's line. 70% of patients with occipitalization of atlas and fusion of C2–3 develop C1–2 instability.
Space for spinal cord reduced
Atlas-dens interval increased
When neck is flexed, space available for spinal cord may be considerably reduced as atlas-dens interval increases. Fusion of C2–3 accentuates instability.
F. Netter M.D.

Lateral radiographs in extension *(left)* and flexion *(right)* of patient with occipitalization of atlas and hypermobile dens extending well into foramen magnum (basilar impression).

Figure 3.6 Congenital anomalies of the occipitocervical junction.

- Most athletes are cleared for full participation without restriction or with minimal additional evaluation (e.g., reassessment of visual acuity, blood pressure, or ligamentous instability; correction of improper rehabilitation; and additional musculoskeletal consultation).
- Explain reasons for further evaluation to the athlete and parent/guardian (if athlete is <18 years old).
- Extensive updated information about a medical condition and the risk of participation often requires attention to specifics of the medical problem and the individual athlete, as well as a breakdown of sport-specific requirements.
- Decisions to disqualify may require additional specialist consultations, as well as one or two "second expert opinions." A total of three opinions is suggested.

AREAS OF CONCERN

Ethical Issues Associated With PPPE

Ethical issues to consider as a team physician include:

- Confidentiality (e.g., compliance with Health Insurance Portability and Accountability Act [HIPAA], Family Educational Rights and Privacy Act [FERPA], disclosing medical information, and drug testing results)
- Informed consent (e.g., discussion of all treatment options and balancing athletes' desire to participate versus providing optimal medical treatment)
- Influence of third parties (e.g., pressure from teammates, coaches, administrators, parents/guardians, or other people from the community)
- Drug use (e.g., using pain medications to allow participation; pressure to supply, administer, or provide counsel regarding illegal drugs; and illicit or performance-enhancing drugs)

Medicolegal Issues Associated With PPPE

Right to participate:

- Under enactments such as the Americans with Disabilities Act and the Federal Rehabilitation Act, an athlete may have a legal right to participate against medical advice.
- If athletes choose to participate against medical advice, **an exculpatory waiver** or **prospective release** is highly recommended. Despite questions of validity, these forms of written contracts are intended to demonstrate that the athlete was fully informed of his or her condition, as well as the potential risks of participation. "Guidelines" for various medical conditions (e.g., Concussion Guidelines and AHA/American College guidelines [formerly Bethesda Guidelines]) "are not intended to establish absolute mandates" and are better considered as recommendations for the team physician to consider when providing clearance decisions. Occasionally, these guidelines can provide support for the decision to restrict participation, and in others, the team physician may deviate from the recommendations based on individualized factors that might allow an athlete to participate. It is important that the physician fully informs the athlete of the potential risks and has it acknowledged in a written format so that there is no doubt that a discussion took place.

Table 3.3 SPORTS ACCORDING TO RISK OF IMPACT AND EDUCATIONAL BACKGROUND

	Junior High School	High School/College
Impact Expected	American football Ice hockey Lacrosse Wrestling Karate/judo Fencing Boxing	American football Soccer Ice hockey Lacrosse Basketball Wrestling Karate/judo Downhill skiing Squash Fencing Boxing
Impact May Occur	Soccer Basketball Field hockey Downhill skiing Equestrian Squash Cycling	Field hockey Equestrian Cycling Baseball/softball Gymnastics Figure skating
Impact Not Expected	Baseball/softball Cricket Golf Riflery Gymnastics Volleyball Swimming Track and field Tennis Figure skating Cross-country skiing Rowing Sailing Archery Weightlifting Badminton	Cricket Golf Riflery Volleyball Swimming Track and field Tennis Cross-country skiing Rowing Sailing Archery Weightlifting Badminton

- Compliance with school and governing body guidelines, standards, rules, regulations, and policies
- Compliance with privacy laws (HIPAA and FERPA) and local state and/or federal rules, regulations, and laws
- Documentation

"Good Samaritan" statutes: certain states have made an effort to protect volunteer examiners (PPPE) under "Good Samaritan" statutes.

Mandated reporting: Those providers performing a PPPE are mandated reporters of suspected abuse or neglect, as they would be in any other patient encounter.

Sexual harassment:

- Athlete expectations, lack of privacy during examinations, and inappropriate examinations (e.g., breast or gynecologic examination in nonprivate settings) may contribute to such allegations.
- Clear communication with athletes, respect for their privacy, and presence of a chaperone (in certain situations) during examinations minimize potential problems.

Confidentiality

- Good communication with other healthcare providers, parents, athletic trainers, and coaches is important, but it must take place with respect for the athlete's confidentiality.
- The newest PPPE form includes multiple pages—clearance considerations and recommendations are available as pages separate from the detailed history and examination.

Team Physician Versus Personal Physician

- Team physicians may perform the PPPE but have minimal control over evaluation of specific problems uncovered in the PPPE, particularly in high schools, smaller colleges, and managed care settings.
- Space is provided near end of the recommended PPPE form to write specific recommendations for further evaluation before clearance (see Preparticipation Physical Evaluation: Clearance Form available at https://downloads.aap.org/AAP/PDF/PPE-Medical-Eligibility-Form.pdf, copyright 2019). Communication and documentation are essential for the physician and the athlete (and parent/guardian, if applicable), as well as with other physicians.

Communication

- The team physician's **primary responsibility is toward the athlete, and parent/guardian if the athlete is younger than 18 years, in terms of discussion and decision-making.** Secondary responsibility is toward the university, school, or organization. This distinction is often critical at the professional level. It is important, at times, to explain primary and secondary responsibility to the coaching staff and administration in terms of sharing information. Emphasis must be placed on concerns regarding long-term safety and health.
- The team physician must respect the athlete's confidentiality with some understanding that if he or she is unable to participate in practice or play, this information should be shared with the coach and other medical care providers. Communication with athletic trainers, administrators, parents, and others, including the press, may be important. First, discuss with the athlete what information must be disclosed.
- The team physician can arrange for follow-up communication. Have a plan for follow-up care and establish it in writing, if appropriate. Arrange for additional evaluation and final clearance once additional testing requirements are met. Arrange for further rehabilitation, functional testing, return to play with modifications, and progression, as necessary. Inform the athlete regarding the risks and concerns of continued participation, and do not assume that the athlete will choose to participate. Follow-up care is essential.

RECOMMENDED READINGS

Available online.

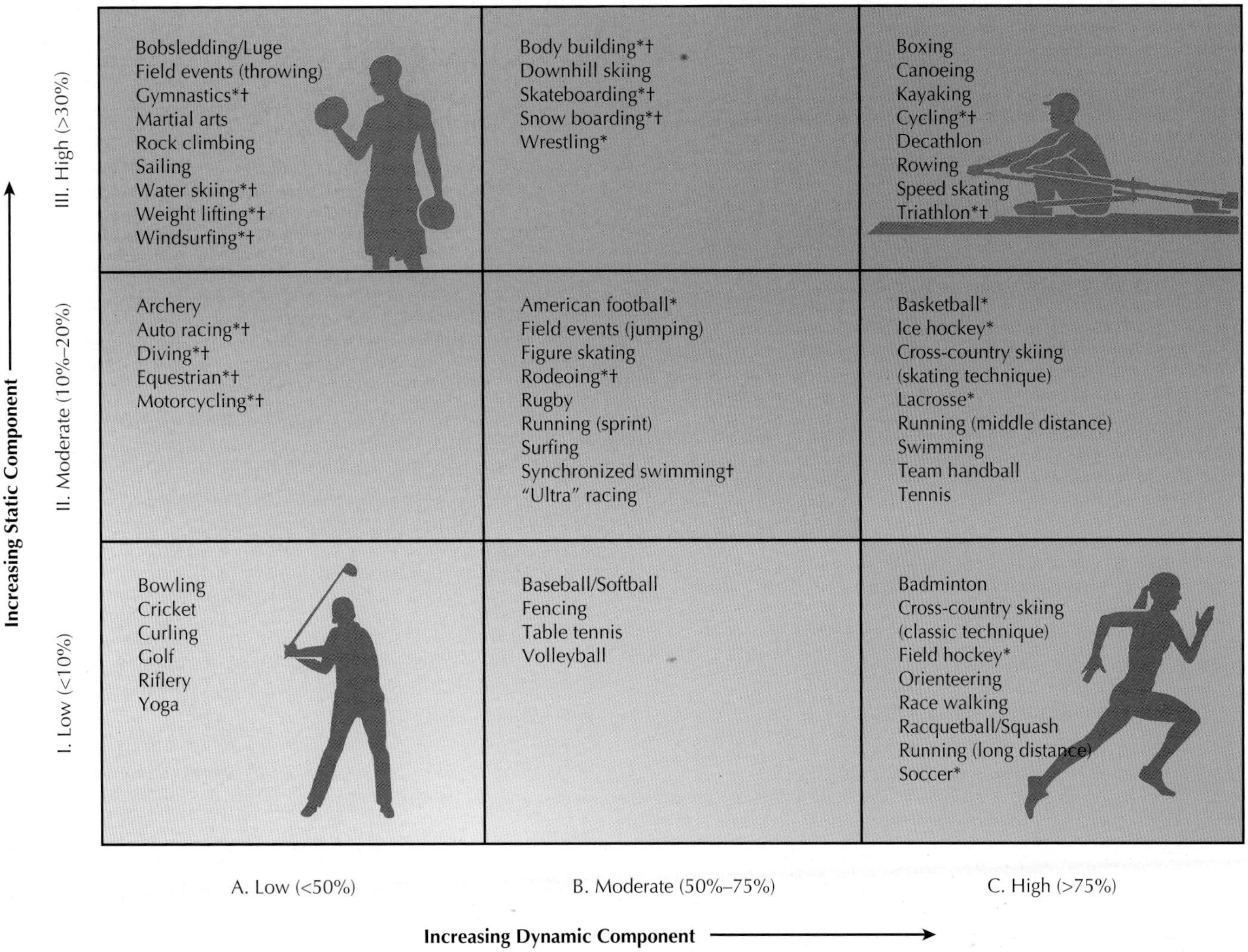
Increasing Static Component
III. High (>30%)
II. Moderate (10%–20%)
I. Low (<10%)
Bobsledding/Luge
Field events (throwing)
Gymnastics*†
Martial arts
Rock climbing
Sailing
Water skiing*†
Weight lifting*†
Windsurfing*†
Body building*†
Downhill skiing
Skateboarding*†
Snow boarding*†
Wrestling*
Boxing
Canoeing
Kayaking
Cycling*†
Decathlon
Rowing
Speed skating
Triathlon*†
Archery
Auto racing*†
Diving*†
Equestrian*†
Motorcycling*†
American football*
Field events (jumping)
Figure skating
Rodeoing*†
Rugby
Running (sprint)
Surfing
Synchronized swimming†
"Ultra" racing
Basketball*
Ice hockey*
Cross-country skiing (skating technique)
Lacrosse*
Running (middle distance)
Swimming
Team handball
Tennis
Bowling
Cricket
Curling
Golf
Riflery
Yoga
Baseball/Softball
Fencing
Table tennis
Volleyball
Badminton
Cross-country skiing (classic technique)
Field hockey*
Orienteering
Race walking
Racquetball/Squash
Running (long distance)
Soccer*
A. Low (<50%)
B. Moderate (50%–75%)
C. High (>75%)
Increasing Dynamic Component

Figure 3.7 Classification of sports based on peak static and dynamic components achieved during competition; however, higher values may be reached during training. The increasing dynamic component is defined in terms of the estimated percentage of maximal oxygen uptake ($\dot{V}O_2$ max) achieved and results in an increasing cardiac output. The increasing static component is related to the estimated percentage of maximal voluntary contraction reached and results in an increasing blood pressure load. The lowest total cardiovascular demands (cardiac output and blood pressure) are shown in the palest color, with increasing dynamic load depicted by increasing blue intensity, and increasing static load by increasing red intensity. Note the graded transition between categories, which should be individualized on the basis of player position and style of play. *Danger of bodily collision (see Table 3.3 for more detail on collision risk). †Increased risk if syncope occurs. (Modified from Mitchell et al. with permission. Copyright © 2005, *Journal of the American College of Cardiology*. From Recommendations for Competitive Athletes with Cardiovascular Abnormalities: Task Force 1: Classification of Sports: Dynamic, Static, and Impact: A Scientific Statement from the American Heart Association and American College of Cardiology. *Circulation.* 2015;132[22]:e262-266.)

BOX 3.3 MEDICAL CONDITIONS AND SPORTS PARTICIPATION

Athletes With the Following Diagnoses May Participate in Sports:

Asthma

Athletes with asthma or exercise-induced bronchospasm (EIB) may participate in sports, as long as their asthma or EIB symptoms are well controlled.

- All athletes with asthma or EIB should have an asthma action plan and a rescue inhaler on-site.
- Athletes taking systemic steroids for asthma management may need a therapeutic use exemption (TUE) from the World Anti-Doping Agency (WADA).
- Counsel on increased risk of respiratory distress while scuba diving.
- Athletes with severe-persistent asthma may require activity modifications.

Diabetes Mellitus (DM)

Athletes may participate in any sport while paying attention to necessary adjustments to diet, blood glucose concentration, and insulin regimen (if applicable). Regardless of exercise type, these athletes should be vigilant of their blood glucose before, during, and after exercise, and they should continue to monitor blood glucose concentrations throughout the evening, given increased risk of late-onset hypoglycemia.

- A combination of aerobic exercise and resistance training may improve glycemic control in patients with type 2 DM. However, each patient's exercise goals and parameters should be individualized to his or her level of training and comorbidities.
- Counsel athletes with type 1 DM that aerobic exercise generally leads to lower blood glucose concentrations, which can be addressed by decreasing basal insulin or increasing

Continued

BOX 3.3 MEDICAL CONDITIONS AND SPORTS PARTICIPATION—cont'd

carbohydrate consumption before exercise. Conversely, anaerobic exercise may lead to a transient increase in blood glucose concentrations, which may require modest insulin corrections.
- Each athlete should have an emergency hypoglycemia action plan.

HIV Infection

Athletes may participate in any sport, as appropriate for the athlete's overall health status.
- The risk of transmission through contact sports, particularly among those on antiretroviral agents, is very low.
- Universal precautions should be maintained to avoid contact with blood and bodily fluids. These include the use of gloves by healthcare workers and the use of cleaning supplies with antiviral properties to remove blood off of floors, mats, uniforms, etc.
- Any bleeding wounds should be completely covered.

Migraines

Generally, athletes with migraine headaches may participate in sports as tolerated.
- Counsel the athlete that exertion may be a trigger for their migraines.
- Advise them that patients with migraines may experience prolonged symptoms following a sport-related concussion.
- Review the patient's migraine medication list for any substances that may require a TUE.

Obesity

Overweight or obese athletes may participate in sports.
- Counsel the athlete on increased risk of cardiovascular strain and heat illness, as well as the importance of hydration and acclimatization.
- Provide nutrition recommendations as needed.

Seizure Disorder, Well-Controlled

There are no restrictions on sports participation in patients with a well-controlled seizure disorder. However, all patients with a seizure disorder should avoid very high-risk activities such as skydiving and scuba diving.
- In patients with a poorly controlled seizure disorder, patients who have recently started or stopped antiepileptic drugs, or patients who are within 2 months of their first seizure, restrictions may be required (see later).

Sickle Cell Trait

Athletes with sickle cell trait may participate in all sports.
- Counsel on the risk of exertional heat illness, rhabdomyolysis, and sudden death.
- Counsel on the importance of hydration and acclimatization.
- Encourage the athlete to report cramping or muscle aches immediately to coaching and medical staff.

Undescended or Solitary Testicle

Athletes with a single or undescended testicle may participate in sports.
- Recommend the use of a protective cup during high-risk activities.

Viral Hepatitis

Athletes with viral hepatitis may participate in any sport as appropriate for the athlete's overall health status.
- Universal precautions should be maintained to avoid contact with blood and bodily fluids, including the use of gloves by healthcare workers at games and the use of agents with antiviral properties to clean any blood off of floors, mats, uniforms, etc.
- Any bleeding wounds should be completely covered.

Athletes With the Following Diagnoses May Conditionally Participate in Sports as Outlined:

Bleeding Disorder

Athletes with bleeding disorders should be individually assessed to determine their eligibility for sports. Generally, patients with mild to moderate bleeding disorders may participate in vigorous exercise with appropriate supervision and planning.
- Assess the degree of the athlete's bleeding disorder, and ask about personal history of bleeds.
- Counsel the patient that a blow to the head can be life threatening.
- To minimize risk of injury, patients should undergo appropriate conditioning and strengthening before beginning a sport.
- Provide factor prophylaxis if appropriate.
- Have an emergency plan in case of acute bleed during sports.
- Encourage the use of appropriate protective equipment.

Transient Brachial Plexopathy (Burner or Stinger)

Athletes with a history of brachial plexopathy who are free of neck pain and radicular symptoms and who have full strength and range of motion may participate in sports.

Celiac Disease

Athletes with celiac disease should undergo a nutritional workup, as well as assessment of associated conditions such as anemia. These deficits should be adequately treated to allow full participation in sports.

Cerebral Palsy

Individual assessment of functional abilities related to sports-specific activities is recommended.

Cervical Cord Neuropraxia (CCN)

Individual assessment is recommended before returning to contact sports.
- Do not clear for sport if the athlete is demonstrating deficits in strength.
- Evaluate for cervical spine stenosis. If the athlete has documented spinal cord stenosis, recommend neurosurgical evaluation before returning to sport.

Congenital Heart Disease

Individual assessment by a cardiologist is recommended to help determine eligibility for sports.

Cystic Fibrosis (CF)

Individual assessment is recommended. Generally, patients with CF can participate in sports as appropriate for the athlete's overall health status.
- Cardiopulmonary exercise testing can help a provider establish an individualized exercise and strengthening plan for an athlete with CF.
- Counsel on the increased risk of heat illness and dehydration in CF.
- Recommend salt-containing fluids during exercise.
- Evaluate for vitamin and nutrient deficiencies.
- Counsel on the control of diabetes mellitus with exercise.
- Consider additional risk factors for contact sports such as splenomegaly, hepatomegaly.

Eating Disorder

Athletes with an identified eating disorder should be connected with a multidisciplinary team, including sports nutrition and psychiatry. This multidisciplinary workup should be complete before determining eligibility for sport.
- Evaluate for other signs and symptoms of relative energy deficiency, such as low bone mineral density or menstrual dysfunction in females.

BOX 3.3 MEDICAL CONDITIONS AND SPORTS PARTICIPATION—cont'd

Heat Illness
In athletes with a history of heat illness, individual assessment is recommended to address any predisposing factors and to create an appropriate prevention strategy.
- Recommend a strategy that includes conditioning, optimization of hydration and salt intake, acclimatization, and sleep.

Hepatomegaly
Athletes with acute hepatomegaly may not return to sport until their hepatomegaly resolves and/or until workup for hepatomegaly is complete. For athletes with chronic hepatomegaly, individual assessment is recommended before permitting participation in contact sports.
- Consider associated conditions such as coagulopathy and nutritional deficiencies.

Hypertension
Athletes with persistent hypertension require individual assessment.
- Screen for family history of hypertension, as well as other risk factors such as caffeine, nicotine, anabolic steroid, or other drug use.
- Child and adolescent athletes diagnosed with hypertension should undergo workup for secondary causes of hypertension, as well as target organ disease. This evaluation should include a renal ultrasound.
- Athletes with stage 2 hypertension or findings of end-organ damage should not be cleared for sport until their workups are complete and their hypertension is under control.

Juvenile Idiopathic Arthritis (JIA)
Outside of disease flares, most athletes with well-controlled JIA and typical flexibility/strength may participate in all sports.
- In patients with systemic or polyarticular JIA with neck arthritis, obtain cervical spine imaging to assess the risk for spinal cord injury.
- Consider cardiovascular assessment in athletes with systemic or HLA-B27–associated arthritis for possible cardiac complications with exertion.
- Recommend ophthalmologic assessment in patients with uveitis and recommend eye protection during sports when appropriate.
- Recommend mouth guards, particularly in patients with jaw involvement.

Kidney, Solitary
In athletes with a single functioning kidney, the provider should engage the athlete in shared decision-making regarding participation in contact sports and other high-risk sports, such as off-road biking, extreme skiing, and horse racing.
- Counsel the athlete that a trauma to the functional kidney during sports, while uncommon, could lead to catastrophic outcomes, including the need for transplantation or dialysis.
- Counsel the athlete that protective gear may provide some protection for the functional kidney, but there are no published data to prove they reduce the risk of kidney injury.

Neurologic Trauma or Abnormality
In athletes with a history of cranial or spinal trauma (including epidural bleeding, subdural hematoma, intracerebral hemorrhage, second-impact syndrome, vascular malformation, neck fracture, etc.), individual assessment is recommended before allowing participation in sports.
- Refer to neurosurgery when appropriate.

Pregnancy/Postpartum
Individual assessment is recommended in collaboration with the athlete's obstetrician.
- Reassessment is necessary as the pregnancy progresses.
- Recommend avoiding sports with high risk of falling or blunt trauma.

Seizure Disorder, Poorly Controlled
Individual assessment is recommended.
- Counsel the athlete that a concussion may exacerbate their seizure disorder.
- Recommend avoiding noncontact sports that put the athlete and others at increased risk of injury. Such sports include archery, riflery, weightlifting, power lifting, water sports, strength training, and sports involving heights.

Sickle Cell Disease
Athletes with sickle cell disease may not participate in contact and collision sports.
- Counsel the athlete that they should also avoid highly strenuous activity, as well as chilling, overheating, and dehydration.

Skin Infections
Athletes with active skin infections or open wounds are not eligible for participation in certain sports until their wounds are healed.
- Common examples of such skin infections include herpes simplex virus, molluscum contagiosum, verrucae, *Staphylococcal* and *Streptococcal* infections, scabies, and tinea.
- Athletes with these skin conditions should avoid sports with high risk of transmission such as wrestling, martial arts, gymnastics or cheerleading on mats, or contact/collision sports.

Splenomegaly
Acute splenomegaly carries an increased risk of rupture, and participation in contact sports should be avoided.
- For athletes with chronic splenomegaly, individual assessment is recommended before permitting participation in contact sports.

Visual Disturbance (one-eyed, functionally one-eyed, detached retina, significant myopia, history of eye surgery, history of severe eye injury, connective tissue disorder)
Individual assessment and discussion are recommended.
- Recommend the use of eye guards or other protective gear with sports participation, but consider that protective eyewear is not permitted or practical in certain sports.
- Discuss the potential consequences of sustaining an injury to the athlete's functional or typical eye.

Athletes With the Following Diagnoses May Not Participate in Sports With Certain Caveats:

Acquired Heart Disease/Dysrhythmia
The following conditions place athletes at risk for sudden cardiac death (SCD). They require evaluation by a cardiologist with experience in treating athletes to determine medical eligibility. In some cases, athletes with milder conditions may still be able to participate in certain sports, depending on the intensity of activity, as directed by a cardiologist.
- Hypertrophic cardiomyopathy (HCM)
- Coronary artery anomalies
- Arrhythmogenic right ventricular cardiomyopathy (ARVC)

Continued

BOX 3.3 MEDICAL CONDITIONS AND SPORTS PARTICIPATION—cont'd

- Dilated cardiomyopathy
- Myocarditis
- Aortic rupture (Marfan syndrome)
- Aortic stenosis
- Atherosclerotic coronary artery disease (CAD)
- Long QT syndrome
- Wolff-Parkinson-White syndrome
- Brugada syndrome
- Short QT syndrome
- Postoperative congenital heart disease
- Primary pulmonary hypertension

Athletes With the Following Diagnoses May Not Participate in Sports:

Carditis

Athletes with carditis are at risk for sudden cardiac death with exertion.

Fever

Athletes with a fever are at higher risk of heat illness, dehydration, and orthostatic hypotension. Additionally, the fever may accompany infections and/or inflammatory conditions that put the athlete at further risk.

SIDELINE PREPAREDNESS AND EMERGENCIES 4

Robert J. Dimeff • Donald Kasitinon

GENERAL PRINCIPLES

- Sideline preparedness is the recognition and formation of medical services in order to promote athletic participation, provide exemplary medical care, and reduce risk of injury.
- It is achieved by having a unified system with qualified medical staff, pre-event planning, game-day preparation, and post-event evaluation.
- Many factors influence the type of injuries and emergencies that may occur, and it is critical that the director of medical services is knowledgeable about the competition.
- Medical services will vary widely when covering a multiday competition, a 1-day Ironman race, an American football game, or a gymnastics meet.
- During any sporting event, availability of medical services for participants, volunteers, and spectators is vital. The extent of services is often part of a signed contractual agreement.
- The medical team may consist of a single physician or athletic trainer or may include several different healthcare professionals with varying levels of knowledge, degrees, specialties, and experience. The medical staff may be paid for their services, provided in-kind services, or unpaid volunteers.
- Pre-event planning and practice are imperative to improve safety measures, reduce risks to athletes and spectators during the event, and provide appropriate medical care.
- Game-day preparation is essential, as it streamlines medical care for those injured on-site.
- Post-event evaluation is critical in order to provide continuing care for the injured and to provide strategic information for improvement in future events.

MEDICAL STAFF

- Director of medical services
  - Is usually a physician (a qualified MD or DO with an unrestricted medical license along with training and certification in sports medicine), but may be a certified athletic trainer or other healthcare provider.
  - Responsibilities include:
    - Making decisions regarding the health of all players.
    - Assembling medical staff.
    - Creating and rehearsing an emergency activation plan (EAP) and chain of command for practice and game environments.
    - Being available at all times and having back-up coverage when not available.
    - Coordinating care among others associated with the team.
    - Organizing medical transfers of injured and/or ill athletes.
    - Clearing athletes to play.
    - Safety assessment of the practice facility, event environment, and playing conditions.
    - Providing appropriate documentation of medical care.
    - Possible involvement in development of drug testing protocols, treatment, and prevention programs.
    - Communication with athletes, parents, administrators, coaches, athletic directors, general managers, owners, media, sports agents, legal experts, and others regarding any health issues related to sports participation.
- Associate physicians
  - May include orthopedic surgeons and primary care physicians with an interest and training in sports medicine.
- Additional physicians
  - May be required by league rules and can include trauma surgeons, neurologists, neurosurgeons, cardiologists, plastic surgeons, ophthalmologists, maxillofacial surgeons, dentists, dermatologists, and others.
- Head athletic trainer
  - Should be certified with an unrestricted license.
  - Works closely with the team physicians.
  - Provides all aspects of medical care.
- Other key members who may be included are assistant athletic trainers, exercise physiologists, strength and conditioning coaches, physical therapists, nurses, psychologists, dietitians, chiropractors, massage therapists, paramedics, and emergency medical technicians (EMTs).

MEDICAL EQUIPMENT

- Medical equipment needs are substantially variable and dependent on many factors, including the type of medical personnel in attendance; timing, duration, and location of the event; number of participants and spectators; access to medical facilities; and league policy.
- Pre-event communication among medical providers will better ensure that all equipment needs are met and unnecessary duplication of equipment is minimized.
- The medical director needs to know what supplies are available on-site and what is available at local medical facilities.
- On-site supplies may be provided by the physician, athletic trainer or physical therapist, organization or team, and/or paramedic or EMT squad.
- Required and/or essential and recommended and/or desirable supplies are listed in Table 4.1.

PRE-EVENT

- The medical staff should be aware of common injuries and illnesses that may occur during the planned sporting event. This may be accomplished by reviewing epidemiologic data, reports from previous similar events, published research, sports medicine textbooks and literature, and previous personal experiences. This knowledge will assist the medical staff in the creation of strategies and policies to promote athlete health, optimize medical care, and prevent injuries.
- The medical staff may need to clear athletes with medical disorders and identify those at risk of health issues related to participation.
- The medical staff should visit the course/venue to inspect for safety risks, location of training rooms and medical treatment facilities, optimum positioning of medical staff during the event, and ambulance/emergency access routes.
- The event EAP and injury protocols must be written, rehearsed, and practiced with all members of the healthcare team. Everyone should have a clear understanding of their roles and responsibilities in the event of a medical emergency.
- Successful care during a sideline emergency is achieved through regular practice drills of emergency situations.

DAY OF EVENT

- Game-day responsibilities will vary with the type of sporting event being covered and the venue where it is being held.
- The medical staff should arrive early, at least an hour before the start of the event. This will allow time to meet with other

Table 4.1 MEDICAL EQUIPMENT

	Required and/or Essential	Recommended and/or Desirable
Medical Bag	**General**	Benzoin
	Alcohol/betadine	Blister care
	Scissors	Contact lens solution
	Bandages	Cautery
	D50W/instant glucose	Postinjury instruction sheets
	Salt tabs	Emergency phone numbers
	Disinfectant	Mirror
	Gloves	Nail clippers
	Angiocatheters	Nasal tampons
	Local anesthetics	Paper bag
	Needles/syringes	Rx pad
	Pen and paper	Razor and cream
	Sharps box	Rectal thermometer
	Suture kit	Scalpel
	Surgical adhesive	Skin lubricant
	Wound irrigation	Skin stapler
	Thermometer	Tongue depressor
	Cardiopulmonary	Topical antibiotics
	Airway and mask	Preferred medications
	Blood pressure cuff	ACLS medications
	Stethoscope	IV fluids kit
	Cricothyrotomy kit	
	Epinephrine 1:1000	
	Beta-agonist inhaler	
	Head and Neck	
	Dental kit	
	Eye kit	
	Ophthalmoscope/otoscope	
	Pen light	
	Pin/sharp object	
	Reflex hammer	
Medical Supplies	AED/defibrillator	Blanket
	Extremity splints	Mylar sheets
	Cervical collar	Crutches
	Radio/phone access	Mouth guards
	Spine board	Sling psychrometer
	Sling and swathe	Tape cutter
	Ice	Concussion assessment tools
	Oral fluids	Glucometer
	Plastic bags	I-Stat
	Face mask removal equipment	
	Medical waste bags	

members of the medical staff, coaches, and administrators, opposing team's medical personnel and administrators, game officials, paramedics/EMTs, security and law enforcement members, and other volunteers.

- Dress appropriately for the event and ensure all staff have appropriate, all-access medical credentials. Standardized clothing will allow for easy identification of the medical team.
- Every member of the medical team must understand their roles in case of an emergency. Allow time to rehearse and review the EAP.
- The medical team should meet with the opposing team's medical staff to ensure that they have adequate medical coverage, know how to activate the EAP, and to review injury and illness scenarios.
- Determine who will be the first providers for an injured or ill athlete and the means of communicating with other staff to assist with care. Also determine who will be providing care to spectators, officials, coaches, volunteers, and others in attendance.
- Physician expertise and experience have an impact on game-day decisions on return to play. The physician must consider if the disorder may be worsened by participation, predispose the athlete to other health risks, or place others at an increased risk of injury or illness.

POST-EVENT

- Review injuries and illnesses that occurred during the event, follow-up with participants who required emergency transportation, replenish medical supplies, and determine and correct deficiencies.
- Communicate, if necessary, with appropriate nonmedical individuals and organizations such as parents, teachers, teammates, coaches, athletic directors, general managers, security staff, player agents, event sponsor, and the media.
- Health Insurance Portability and Accountability Act (HIPAA) rules must be followed with regard to athlete privacy. However, these are often superseded by collective bargaining agreements, player contracts, scholarship rules, and other legal positions. Nevertheless, it is critical to discuss medical issues and recommendations with the athlete first and foremost before communicating with others.

SIDELINE EMERGENCIES

- Perform a quick overall assessment to determine whether an injury or illness is life-threatening (e.g., cardiac event) or limb-threatening (e.g., joint dislocation with neurovascular compromise).
- Determine whether there are other injured or ill athletes that require triage.
- Ensure the safety of medical staff tending to injured or ill participants.
- Decide on the safest method to remove the athlete from the playing field, where the athlete will be further assessed (i.e., sideline, training room, or emergency room), and the best means and timing of transportation if necessary.
- If the athlete does not require emergent transportation, a decision must be made as to whether it is safe for the athlete to return to play.

Cardiopulmonary Arrest

- Check for responsiveness. If not responsive, then activate the EAP.
- Check airway for spontaneous breathing, ensure that athlete has a patent airway, and maintain cervical spine stability in neutral position, particularly if there is concern for head and neck injury.
- Remove face mask, if present, to gain access to and secure the oral airway.
- Check pulse; if absent, remove clothing and protective gear and start chest compressions at a depth of ≥2″ and a rate of 100–120 compressions/minute. If the patient is in ventricular fibrillation or unstable ventricular tachycardia, early defibrillation is necessary to restore normal electrical cardiac activity. Each minute of delay decreases the chance of survival by approximately 10%.
- Administer oxygen (O_2), secure intravenous (IV) access, and follow advanced cardiac life support (ACLS) protocols while awaiting ambulance transport to a medical facility.

Exercise-Associated Collapse (EAC)

- Defined as the inability to stand or walk unassisted during or after the completion of an exertional event.

- Collapse during or after exercise can be due to numerous disorders. The medical staff must be able to provide prompt and accurate on-site evaluation and treatment.
- Collapse before the finish line suggests a more serious disorder.
- The most common causes of EAC are postural hypotension, muscle cramps, dehydration, heat illness, hypoglycemia, hypothermia, and hyponatremia.

Postural Hypotension

- Occurs most commonly after completion of a running event and is due to venous pooling from gravity, dehydration, and loss of muscle pump.
- Treatment with elevation of legs and oral or IV fluids usually provides prompt recovery (see Fig. 97.3).
- Best method of prevention is to continue walking after event completion.

Muscle Cramps

- Often involves just the lower legs, but whole-body cramps may include thighs, abdomen, back, and upper extremities.
- Occurs in unacclimatized athletes, often in hot and humid environments.
- Likely due to a combination of dehydration, sodium or electrolyte depletion, muscle fatigue, and neural disturbance.
- Treatment includes stretching, oral salt and fluid intake, ice, massage, and possibly IV fluids.

Dehydration

- May impair performance and lead to collapse due to reduced blood volume.
- Occurs in hot and humid environments.
- Higher risk in those with acute illness and may increase the risk of hyperthermia.
- Treatment includes oral or IV fluids.
- Prevention includes ensuring adequate fluid, electrolyte, and carbohydrate intake before, during, and after exercise.

Heat Illness

- Ranges from heat cramps to heat exhaustion to life-threatening hyperthermia. It is critical to obtain a rectal (core) temperature if hyperthermia is suspected.
- Heat exhaustion: profuse sweating, muscle cramps, weakness, headache, vertigo, nausea and vomiting, hyperventilation, tachycardia, core temperature ≤104°F (40°C).
- Hyperthermia: diaphoretic, headache, hyperventilation, tachycardia, ataxia, significant altered mental status including seizure and coma, core temperature ≥104°F (40°C), often >108°F (42°C). The classic hyperthermia symptom of hot and dry skin is rare in athletes.
- Immediately cool athlete with cold water, fans, and/or cold towels; give fluids; and move to a cool, shady environment.
- Ice water immersion is the most effective means of lowering core temperature and should be started once hyperthermia is recognized.
- It should be discontinued to prevent overshoot and hypothermia when core temperature reaches ≤102°F (39°C).

Hypothermia

- Usually related to accidental prolonged exposure to cold, damp weather during long-distance races and during the swim portion of triathlons.
- Presents with mild confusion and shivering when core temperature is <95°F (35°C) and may progress to unconsciousness if core temperature continues to drop.
- Athlete should remove cold, wet clothes; be moved to a warm environment; change into dry clothes; and use warm blankets and heaters to increase body temperature.

Hypoglycemia

- More likely to occur during prolonged exercise bouts in athletes with diabetes, eating disorders, or poor carbohydrate intake.
- This life-threatening state is diagnosed by history, examination, and blood sugar level.
- Symptoms may include nausea, anxiety, weakness, diaphoresis, confusion, and coma.
- Corrected with oral or IV glucose.
- If blood sugar measurement is not possible, administration of IV glucose is recommended.

Hyponatremia

- Potentially fatal condition due to sodium losses in sweat, increased free water intake, or impaired urinary excretion due to persistent secretion of antidiuretic hormone (ADH).
- Risk factors: prolonged periods of exercise (>4 hours), female gender, body mass index (BMI) <20.
- Presents with bloating, headache, nausea, vomiting, mental status changes, seizures, and coma.
- If mild (sodium 125–134 mmol/L), restrict water and provide oral sodium (e.g., salt tabs, saltine crackers, or broth). Repeat sodium check every 20–30 minutes and consider IV normal saline if no improvement.
- If severe (sodium <125 mmol/L) or with mental status changes, consider 100 mL IV bolus of 3% NaCl every 10–15 minutes until symptoms improve or serum sodium ≥130 mmol/L. Transport urgently for further evaluation and treatment.

Asthma Exacerbations

- Assess severity by observing for increased respiratory rate, wheezing, cough, breathlessness, and use of accessory muscles.
- Initial sideline management includes two puffs of albuterol. This may be repeated in 15–20 minutes while assessing for improvement. Consider O_2 administration if needed.
- If athlete shows no change or worsening, transport to nearest medical facility for further care.

Anaphylaxis

- Severe, acute, life-threatening systemic reaction due to allergen exposure.
- Characterized by flushing, urticaria, angioedema, chest tightness, cough, wheezing, and stridor progressing to pulmonary failure and cardiac arrest.
- Inject epinephrine 0.3–0.5 mL of 1:1000 dilution into lateral thigh every 10–15 minutes (0.01 mg/kg in children; maximum 0.3 mg).
- Transport to emergency room. Administer supplemental O_2 and IV fluids. Consider beta-agonist inhalers, H_1 or H_2 blockers, and systemic corticosteroids if not improving.

Acute Hemorrhage

- Internal bleeding is difficult to diagnose at the athletic venue, requires a high index of suspicion, and necessitates urgent transportation for emergency evaluation and treatment. Depending on the source and severity of the bleeding, sign and symptoms may include anxiety, abdominal or chest pain, dyspnea, diaphoresis, dizziness, mental status changes, hypotension, and tachycardia.
- External bleeding is common in sports due to abrasions and lacerations. For bleeding injuries, clean with water or saline to remove any foreign bodies and apply direct pressure with gauze. After administration of a local anesthetic, thoroughly assess lacerations for possible muscle, tendon, and neurovascular injury before closing the wound with appropriate sutures, staples, or surgical adhesive.

- Combat Gauze® is a commercial product that may be used to control severe, potentially life-threatening bleeding due to major vessel injury.
- Lacerations of carotid, brachial, femoral, and popliteal arteries should be treated with constant direct pressure and tourniquet, when applicable, until a vascular or trauma surgeon is able to do emergency vessel repair or ligation.

Head and Neck Injuries

- Head and neck injuries are common in contact and collision sports. Most are benign and self-limited, but some are serious and life-threatening.
- Determine potential seriousness of the injuries, ruling out life-threatening ones such as intracranial hemorrhage and laryngotracheal fracture.
- Assume an unconscious athlete has a cervical spine injury until proven otherwise.
- Stabilize the head and neck, secure airway access, use a backboard, and transport athlete to designated medical facility. Helmet and shoulder pad removal can be deferred until the athlete has been transported to a medical facility, unless needed for airway access.
- The Glasgow Coma Scale (GCS) is a neurologic scale that provides an objective and reliable way to assess an athlete's consciousness (Fig. 4.1). GCS correlates with mild (13–15) (concussion), moderate (9–12), and severe (3–8) brain injury.
- Concussed athletes should never return to play the same day. Any deterioration in mental status or neurologic examination requires transportation to a medical facility for further evaluation. The Sport Concussion Assessment Tool 5 (SCAT5) has proven to be a reliable, standardized, diagnostic screening sideline test.

Facial Injuries

- Most common in contact and collision sports that do not require face masks or shields.
- Ensure adequate airway control and clear cervical spine.
- Inspect and palpate for swelling, crepitus, tenderness, or abnormal bony prominences and assess for normal range of motion of the jaw.
- Displaced nasal fractures should be reduced urgently. Monitor for uncontrolled bleeding and septal hematoma. Also observe for clear rhinorrhea suggestive of skull fracture and cerebrospinal fluid (CSF) leak.
- For ear trauma, check for lacerations, tympanic membrane rupture, and clear otorrhea suggestive of CSF leak.

Eye Injuries

- Type and severity of eye injuries depend on sport environment and mechanism of injury.
- Most sports-related eye injuries can be prevented with protective eyewear.
- Assess visual acuity and visual fields; palpate periorbital tissues and eye; examine conjunctiva, cornea, anterior chamber, pupil size and reaction to light, and iris shape and continuity. Check extraocular movements after ruling out perforation; then consider anesthetic and fluorescein stain to evaluate for corneal abrasion.
- Athletes with corneal irritation or abrasions; subconjunctival hemorrhage; or foreign bodies may return to play after evaluation, irrigation, and removal of offending substance.
- Corneal laceration, significant eyelid laceration, hyphema, orbital wall fracture, ruptured or penetrated globe, and posterior segment injuries (i.e., retinal tear, detachment, edema,

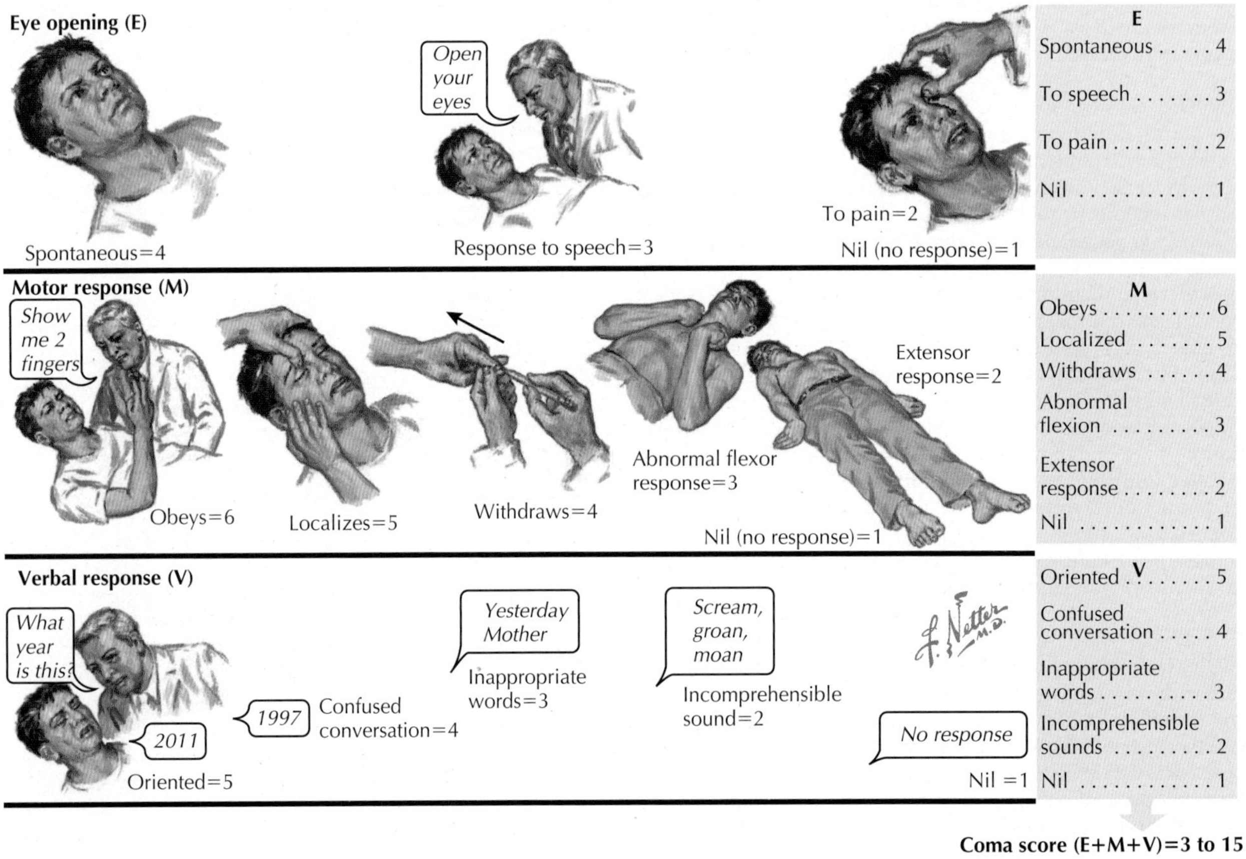
Eye opening (E)
Open your eyes
Spontaneous=4
Response to speech=3
To pain=2
Nil (no response)=1
E
Spontaneous 4
To speech 3
To pain 2
Nil 1
Motor response (M)
Show me 2 fingers
Obeys=6
Localizes=5
Withdraws=4
Abnormal flexor response=3
Extensor response=2
Nil (no response)=1
M
Obeys 6
Localized 5
Withdraws 4
Abnormal flexion 3
Extensor response 2
Nil 1
Verbal response (V)
What year is this?
2011
Oriented=5
1997
Confused conversation=4
Yesterday Mother
Inappropriate words=3
Scream, groan, moan
Incomprehensible sound=2
No response
Nil =1
V
Oriented 5
Confused conversation 4
Inappropriate words 3
Incomprehensible sounds 2
Nil 1
Coma score (E+M+V)=3 to 15

Figure 4.1 Glasgow Coma Scale.

or hemorrhage) should be protected with an eye shield and referred for emergent definitive ophthalmologic care.

Oral Injuries

- The most common injuries involving the oral cavity are abrasions and lacerations of the lips, tongue, and buccal mucosa, which are easily assessed, treated, and sutured on-site. Significant through-and-through oral lacerations may require transfer for appropriate and definitive treatment.
- Dental injuries include tooth fractures, subluxations, and avulsions.
- For bleeding around a tooth, use a simple finger pressure test to check for pain, numbness, and excess movement associated with fractures and subluxations.
- Type I fractures: involve only enamel and are painless, may continue to play, use delayed bonding for cosmesis.
- Type II fractures: involve dentin and are painful, may continue to play if tolerated, but require urgent bonding.
- Type III fractures: involve pulp and cause significant pain, usually cannot continue to play, require emergent treatment to preserve tooth and may require root canal.
- Avulsion is complete displacement of tooth from its base. Handle by crown, gently cleanse with water or saline, avoid disturbing the attached soft tissues, replace in socket, use clenched teeth to hold it in place. If unable to replace, transport in saline, water, saliva, or commercial tooth-saver solution. Saving the tooth is time dependent: 90% salvage rate if replaced within 30 minutes.

Chest Injuries

- Emergency chest injuries are rare and occur primarily because of direct blow by a fast-moving player or object.
- Life-threatening chest injuries include cardiac contusion, commotio cordis, tension pneumothorax, and damage to the great vessels or airway.
- Chest wall contusions and fractures may be complicated by brachial plexus injury, diaphragmatic rupture, pneumothorax, pulmonary contusion, and renal and hepatic injury.
- Assess vitals and O_2 saturation; observe for signs of respiratory distress and hemoptysis, tracheal deviation, distended neck veins, chest wall deformity, crepitus and tenderness, paradoxical chest movements, and abnormal breath sounds.
- If tension pneumothorax is suspected and the patient is unstable, perform emergent needle decompression by using a 14- to 16-gauge needle above the third rib along the midclavicular line of the affected side to release air. Administer O_2 and transfer to a medical facility for further imaging and care.
- Uncomplicated chest trauma may be treated with ice, analgesics, padding, and local anesthetic injection. Athlete may return to sport if tolerated, but will require frequent reassessment.

Abdominal Injuries

- Muscle strains and contusions are the most common abdominal sports injuries and can be treated with ice, analgesics, compression wraps, and participation as tolerated, with frequent reassessment.
- Severe abdominal injuries resulting in internal organ damage are uncommon in sports, with the spleen, kidney, and liver being the most frequently affected organs.
- Signs and symptoms of contusion, hematoma, and laceration of abdominal structures are often delayed; thus, frequent reassessment, including vital signs, is necessary.
- Liver injury produces right upper quadrant pain and tenderness, referred pain to the right shoulder, and ecchymosis around the umbilicus (Cullen's sign).
- Splenic injury causes left upper quadrant pain and referred pain to the left shoulder (Kerr's sign). Athletes with a history of recent infectious mononucleosis may be at a higher risk of splenic rupture.
- Kidney injury is often from back or flank trauma and may be associated with rib fractures, hematuria, flank ecchymosis (Grey-Turner's sign), and costovertebral angle tenderness.
- Potentially serious abdominal injuries can be difficult to assess on the sideline. If serious abdominal injury is suspected, athlete should be made NPO (nothing by mouth), have IV access established, and be transferred to a hospital for further evaluation and treatment.

Musculoskeletal Injuries

- The most common acute athletic injuries involve the musculoskeletal system.
- Return to play is predicated based on diagnosis, pain control, ability to protect the athlete from further injury or injuring others, and ability to perform sport-specific demands.
- Fractures may be difficult to diagnose without on-site imaging. Minor to obvious deformity, focal tenderness, crepitus, and ecchymosis may be present. Check neurovascular status, attempt reduction (particularly if there is neurovascular compromise), splint to include the joint proximal and distal to the injury site, use ice and analgesics, and arrange for definitive imaging and treatment.
- Cartilage injuries are difficult to diagnose without advanced imaging; joint swelling, decreased range of motion, and tenderness may be present. Athletes may attempt return to play if they are able to complete functional testing.
- Ligament sprains may be contact or noncontact and affect virtually any joint, leading to instability and possible joint subluxation or dislocation. Mechanism of injury and physical examination are usually sufficient to make a preliminary diagnosis. Sideline management will include attempted reduction of dislocated joints (particularly if there is neurovascular compromise), ice, analgesics, splinting, bracing, and taping, which may allow return to play in certain cases. Athletes should then be followed up for radiographic imaging and further definitive treatment. Hip and knee dislocations are acute emergencies due to potential neurovascular compromise (Fig. 4.2); immediate attempt at reduction should be considered with urgent transfer to the nearest medical facility.
- Acute muscle injuries include noncontact strains and direct contact contusions. On-site treatment includes ice, compression, elevation, and analgesics. Return to play may be possible. Athletes should be monitored for the development of acute compartment syndrome that may be associated with fractures and muscle injury (severe pain that worsens with stretching, paresthesias, paralysis, pulselessness, and pallor). Compartment pressures should be monitored, and emergency fasciotomy may be necessary.
- Tendon injuries range from minor strains to complete tears. Most are eccentric noncontact injuries and are diagnosed by history and physical examination and confirmed radiographically by advanced imaging such as musculoskeletal ultrasound (US) or magnetic resonance imaging. Acute treatment includes rest, ice, compression, immobilization, and analgesics; surgical treatment may be necessary. Same-day return to play is often difficult; athletes should not return to play until function is restored.
- Neurovascular injuries must be fully assessed by examination, advanced imaging, and neurodiagnostic testing. Athletes may return to play when pain is well-controlled and they have full range of motion, strength, power, and sensation.

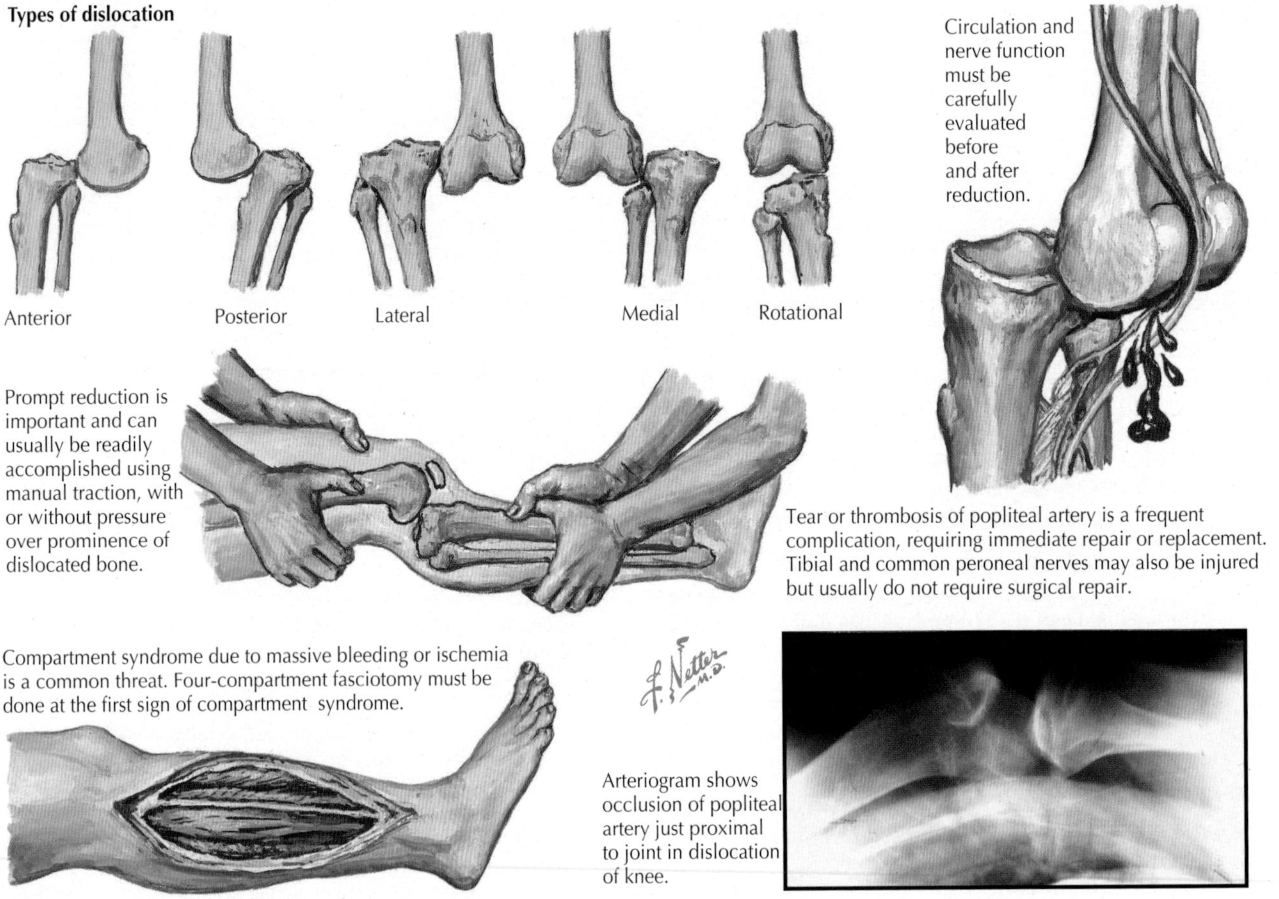
Types of dislocation
Anterior
Posterior
Lateral
Medial
Rotational
Circulation and nerve function must be carefully evaluated before and after reduction.
Prompt reduction is important and can usually be readily accomplished using manual traction, with or without pressure over prominence of dislocated bone.
Tear or thrombosis of popliteal artery is a frequent complication, requiring immediate repair or replacement. Tibial and common peroneal nerves may also be injured but usually do not require surgical repair.
Compartment syndrome due to massive bleeding or ischemia is a common threat. Four-compartment fasciotomy must be done at the first sign of compartment syndrome.
Arteriogram shows occlusion of popliteal artery just proximal to joint in dislocation of knee.

Figure 4.2 Dislocation of knee joint.

SIDELINE ULTRASOUND UTILIZATION

- US can be used on the sideline or in the training room for the focal assessment with sonography for trauma (FAST) (Table 4.2) and initial bone and soft tissue injury evaluation.
- FAST is specific but not sensitive for intraabdominal injuries. Thus, a positive FAST indicates a need for emergent intervention, but a negative FAST should be repeated and will ultimately require more definitive evaluation (such as a computed tomography [CT] of the abdomen) if clinical suspicion is high.
- An extended FAST (E-FAST) is the FAST plus US examination of the chest to evaluate for hemothorax and pneumothorax.

SUMMARY

- Sideline evaluation and treatment of injuries and illnesses, including safe return to play or transfer to a medical facility, requires extensive pre-event planning, game-day preparation, and post-event evaluation.
- It is essential to have well-trained medical personnel, appropriate equipment, and communication when providing medical coverage for a sporting event.
- Major life-threatening emergencies include cardiopulmonary arrest, hyperthermia, anaphylaxis, hypoglycemia, and hyponatremia.

Table 4.2 FOCUSED ASSESSMENT WITH SONOGRAPHY FOR TRAUMA (FAST)

Primary Views	Structures Evaluated
Subxiphoid	Heart
Right upper quadrant	Liver, kidney, Morrison's pouch (hepatorenal recess)
Left upper quadrant	Spleen, kidney
Suprapubic	Bladder

- Rapid assessment is critical to determine the need for life-saving or limb-saving treatments.
- Frequent sideline reassessment of athletes may be necessary to determine the need for transfer to a medical facility for further evaluation and treatment.
- Most injuries and medical disorders can be managed on-site by healthcare providers with appropriate training and equipment and can allow for rapid and safe return to play.

RECOMMENDED READINGS

Available online.

SPORTS NUTRITION 5

Erin Riley • Alexa Moriarty

ROLE OF NUTRITION IN ATHLETIC PERFORMANCE

- Exercise training and genetic makeup are major determinants of athletic performance.
- A healthy diet will not substitute for either factor, but making wise food choices will allow athletes to maximize their athletic potential by contributing to endurance, speed, and recovery of muscle tissue, as well as promoting optimal health and immune function.
- Athletes may lack nutrition knowledge regarding diet and performance. Additionally, athletes may be prone to the utilization of "fad" or "trendy" diet practices, which can often lead to impaired performance and health.
- To assess the dietary practices of athletes and provide general nutrition education, sports medicine professionals require an understanding of sports nutrition. In the case of an athlete requiring a more in-depth nutrition assessment or specific recommendations, such as when the athlete is seeking body composition changes, when disordered eating or low energy availability is suspected, or when an athlete requires medical nutrition therapy, he or she should be referred to a qualified sports dietitian.

ENERGY SOURCES FOR MUSCLES

- A basic understanding of how muscles use food as fuel is an important step in understanding an athlete's diet.
- The body cannot directly use the energy released from food; it must first convert the chemical energy found in food to adenosine triphosphate (ATP) (Fig. 5.1).
- A small amount of ATP can be found in resting muscle cells—just enough to keep the muscle working maximally for about 1–2 seconds.
- During extended periods of exercise, the body produces additional ATP by adding phosphocreatine to adenosine diphosphate (ADP), thereby producing more ATP for muscle contractions.
- Moreover, energy-yielding macronutrients such as carbohydrates, fats, and occasionally proteins are used as energy sources to produce more ATP (Table 5.1).

Carbohydrate: Major Fuel for Short-Term, High-Intensity Exercise

Anaerobic vs. Aerobic Metabolism

- The primary pathway to provide energy for sporting events where exercise intensity is near maximal for 30–90 seconds is glycolysis, or anaerobic metabolism.
  - During anaerobic glycolysis, lactate is produced; it accumulates in the muscles and increases acidity. As lactate increases, pH in the muscle lowers and is associated with the onset of fatigue. The muscle lactate produced from glycolysis is eventually released into the bloodstream and taken up by the liver, which resynthesizes the lactate into glucose. This pathway is called the *Cori cycle* and allows glucose to enter the bloodstream and be absorbed by cells to be used as energy.
- During anaerobic exercise, carbohydrate is the only substrate that can be used to resupply ATP.
- If oxygen is available to muscle cells and exercise is performed at a moderate or low intensity, then most of the pyruvate produced during glycolysis is shuttled into the mitochondria for ATP production via aerobic metabolism. Approximately 95% of ATP produced from carbohydrate metabolism is aerobically formed in the mitochondria.
- Aerobic metabolism supplies ATP more slowly than anaerobic pathways, but it releases greater energy and can be sustained for hours.

Glycogen

- Carbohydrates are stored in the form of glycogen in the body; it is stored both in the liver and the muscles.
- Through glycogenolysis, glycogen is broken down to glucose and metabolized via the anaerobic and aerobic pathways. Liver glycogen is used to maintain blood glucose, whereas muscle glycogen supplies glucose to working muscles.
- In events lasting <30 minutes, muscles primarily rely on muscle glycogen. As exercise time increases, muscle glycogen stores decline, and they begin to absorb glucose from the blood as an energy source (Fig. 5.2).
- Once glycogen stores are exhausted, exercise can continue, but the muscles can only work at 50% of maximal capacity; this state is often called "hitting the wall" or "bonking" because further exertion is hampered.
- In certain cases, before a competition, high-carbohydrate diets can be used to increase muscle glycogen stores to up to double the typical amount, thereby delaying the onset of fatigue and improving endurance.
- Maintenance of blood glucose becomes increasingly vital as exercise duration increases beyond 20–30 minutes. By maintaining blood glucose, the body saves muscle glycogen to use during sudden bursts of effort or for a second workout later in the day.
- A carbohydrate intake of 0.7 g/kg/h during strenuous endurance exercise that lasts for approximately ≥1 hour can help maintain adequate blood glucose, which, in turn, results in delayed fatigue.

Fat: Main Fuel Source for Prolonged, Low-Intensity Exercise

- At rest and during prolonged exercise at low to moderate intensity, fat becomes the predominant fuel source for exercising muscles. In fact, during very long activities such as ultramarathons, fat supplies approximately 50%–90% of the required energy.
- The rate of fatty acid oxidation in the muscle is affected by training level. The better trained a muscle is, the greater its ability to use fat as a fuel. The more unfit a muscle is, the greater its reliance on carbohydrate as opposed to fat. Training increases the size and number of mitochondria and the level of fatty oxidative enzymes, thus allowing athletes to use fat more readily as a fuel source, eventually conserving glycogen.

Protein: A Minor Fuel Source During Exercise

- Although protein can be used as fuel by muscles, its contribution is relatively small compared with that of carbohydrates and fat.
- Only approximately 5% of the body's energy needs is supplied by amino acid metabolism; however, proteins can contribute to energy needs during endurance exercise.
- If an athlete exhausts his or her muscle glycogen stores, proteins can contribute as much as 15% of the energy expenditure for exercise.

DIETARY RECOMMENDATIONS FOR ATHLETES

Energy Needs

- Athletes need varying amounts of energy depending on their body size, body composition, daily lifestyle, and type of training or competition.
- Monitoring body weight is an easy way to assess the adequacy of caloric intake; however, sport dietitians are now primarily using the concept of energy availability to monitor caloric requirements, as an athlete can in fact be weight stable while having a low energy availability.
  - Energy availability is the amount of energy left for bodily functions after the energy costs for training and competition have been calculated. Table 5.2 provides an example of how to calculate adequate energy availability for an athlete.
  - Typically, athletes with an energy availability of <30 kcal/kg of lean body mass have a greater risk of metabolic, hormonal, and performance disruptions, which could include reproductive functions as well. Physiologic functioning is optimized at energy availability amounts of greater than 45 kcal/kg. Inadequate intake of calories in relation to energy expenditure, also known as *low energy availability* or *relative energy deficiency in sports (RED-S)*, can result in fatigue, increased risk of injury, prolonged recovery period, and overall poor athletic performance, along with several other performance and health consequences, as noted in Figs. 5.3 and 5.4.

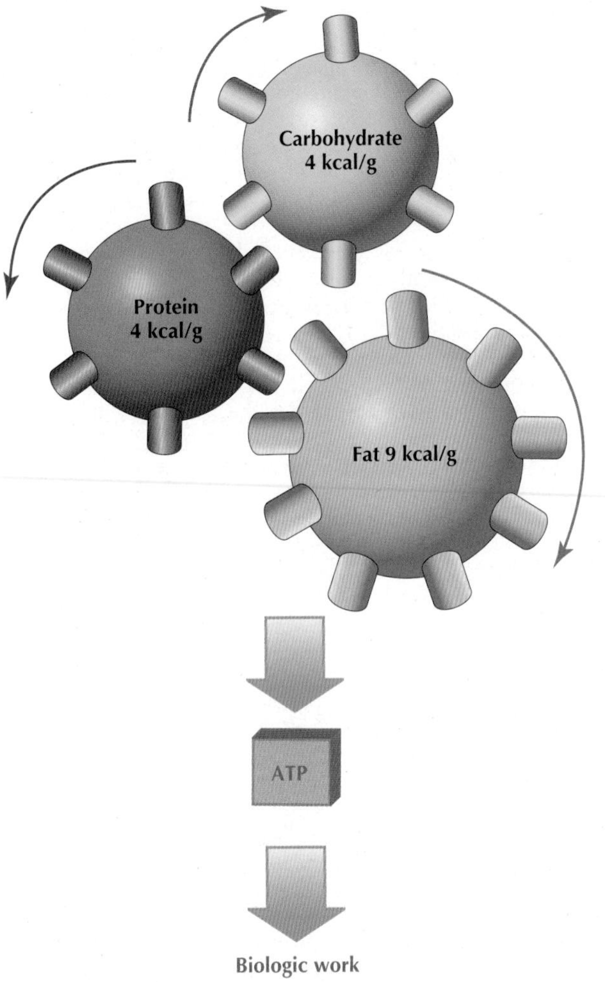
Carbohydrate
4 kcal/g
Protein
4 kcal/g
Fat 9 kcal/g
ATP
Biologic work

Figure 5.1 Sources of ATP for biologic work. ATP is harvested from macronutrients, carbohydrates, proteins, and fats to synthesize it for biologic work.

Carbohydrates

- Carbohydrates are the primary source of energy for exercising muscle, particularly when exercise intensity reaches 65% or greater of the maximum oxygen consumption (VO_2 max).
- In the past, carbohydrate recommendations have often been expressed as a percentage of total calories; however, this percentage is poorly correlated to both the amount of carbohydrate actually consumed and the required fuel needed to support an athlete's training and competition; thus, the concept of carbohydrate availability is now being used.
  - Carbohydrate availability matches the athlete's carbohydrate intake to his or her fuel needs for training and competition.
  - If athletes fail to consume adequate carbohydrates and energy during daily training, then muscle glycogen levels decrease, and training and competition performance becomes impaired.
  - If athletes consistently overconsume carbohydrates, just like any macronutrient, the excess energy can potentially be stored as fat in the body. It is important to note, however, that many athletes consume insufficient amounts of carbohydrate to meet fueling needs because of fear that carbohydrate consumption will lead to weight gain—a misconception that must also be addressed.
- In general, a wide variety of whole grains such as pasta, breads, and rice, along with fruits, vegetables, and dairy provide carbohydrates in addition to essential vitamins, trace minerals, and fiber that athletes need.

Carbohydrate Recommendations

- **Low-intensity exercise:** Carbohydrate intake ranges 3–5 g/kg of body weight
- **Moderate-intensity exercise:** Carbohydrate intake ranges 5–7 g/kg of body weight
- **Endurance exercise for several hours:** Carbohydrate intake ranges 6–10 g/kg of body weight
- **Extreme exercise lasting 4–5 hours:** Carbohydrate intake ranges 8–12 g/kg of body weight

Table 5.1 ENERGY SOURCES IN THE BODY

Energy Source	Storage Area	When Used	Activity
ATP	All tissues	All the time	Sprinting (0–3 seconds)
Phosphocreatine	All tissues	Short bursts	Shot put, high jump, bench press
Carbohydrate (anaerobic)	Muscles	High intensity lasting 30 seconds to 2 minutes	200-meter sprint, 50-meter swim
Carbohydrate (aerobic)	Muscles and liver	Exercise lasting 2 minutes to ≥3 hours	Jogging, soccer, basketball, swimming
Fat (aerobic)	Muscles and fat cells	Exercise lasting more than a few minutes; greater amounts are used at lower exercise intensities	Long-distance running, marathons, ultramarathons, day-long hikes

ATP, Adenosine triphosphate.

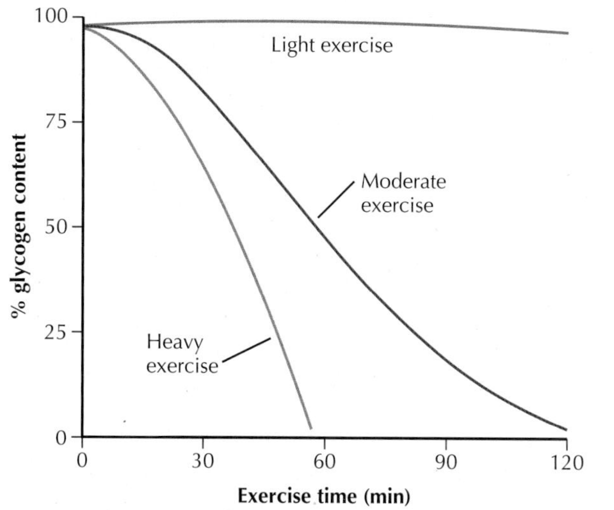
100
75
50
25
0
% glycogen content
Light exercise
Moderate exercise
Heavy exercise
0
30
60
90
120
Exercise time (min)

Figure 5.2 Rate of glycogen utilization in exercising muscle. (Data from Grisham CM, Garrett RG. *Biochemistry,* 3rd ed. Belmont, CA: Brooks/Cole Publishing Company; 2006.)

Table 5.2 SAMPLE CALCULATIONS TO DETERMINE ENERGY AVAILABILITY

Athlete's weight (kg)	68 kg
Workout expenditure (kcal/d)	900 kcal/d
Energy intake (kcal/d)	3200 kcal/d
Percent body fat (%)	13
Lean body mass (kg)	68 kg × 0.13 = 8.84 kg; 68 kg – 8.84 kg = 59.16 kg
Energy availability (kcal/lean mass)	3200 kcal – 900 kcal = 1900 kcal/59 kg lean mass = 32.2 kcal/lean mass

Application

- Carbohydrate intake is important for all athletes on a daily basis, but is especially important when performing multiple training bouts in 1 day, such as swimming practice or track and field events, or in tournament play when multiple games may be played in 1 day. Consumption of multiple meals and snacks that contain carbohydrates throughout the day will ensure a fuel source for exercising muscles.

Protein

- Protein consumption facilitates muscle synthesis and repair.
- Athletes need to consume more than double the protein amount required by a sedentary adult.
  - Most athletes can easily meet their protein requirements through a well-planned diet that includes high-quality proteins that are spread throughout the day rather than consumed in large amounts in one single meal.
  - Researchers have found that consuming >40 g of protein in a single meal has no additional benefits in stimulating more muscle protein synthesis (MPS), and any excess over this amount is simply oxidized by the body. Moreover, they have suggested that multiple meals containing 20–30 g of protein must be consumed throughout the day to stimulate MPS.
- Although the amount of protein an athlete needs is important, so is the quality of the protein because it influences the body's ability to synthesize MPS.
  - Protein quality depends on its essential amino acid profile, which includes both the specific amount and the proportion of essential amino acids (EAAs).
    - EAAs are ones that the body cannot make and must therefore be consumed in the diet.
    - There are nine EAAs, including three branched-chain amino acids (BCAAs).
- BCAAs are absorbed faster than small amino acids, and EAAs are absorbed faster than nonessential amino acids, with the essential BCAAs leucine, isoleucine, and valine being absorbed

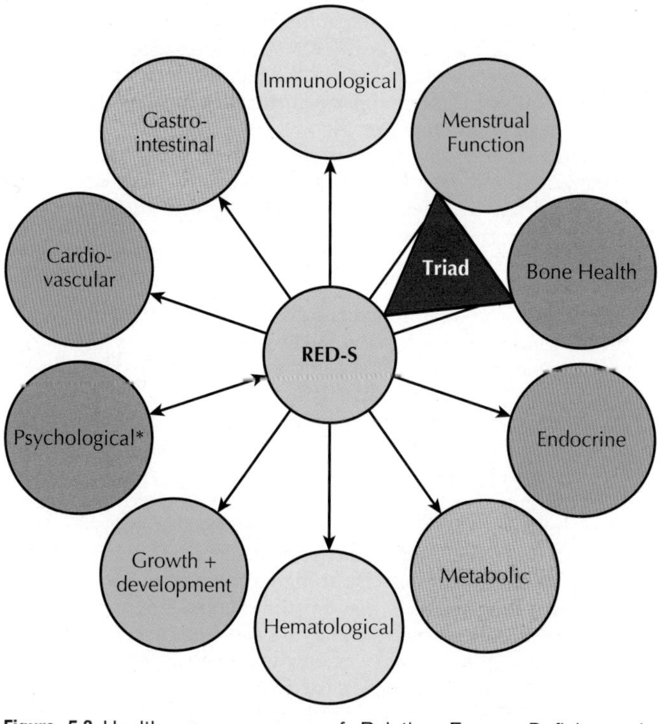
Immunological
Gastro-intestinal
Menstrual Function
Triad
Bone Health
Cardio-vascular
RED-S
Psychological*
Endocrine
Growth + development
Hematological
Metabolic

Figure 5.3 Health consequences of Relative Energy Deficiency in Sport (RED-S). (Adapted from Constantini NW. Medical concerns of the dancer. Book of Abstracts, XXVII FIMS World Congress of Sports Medicine, Budapest, Hungary, 2002:151.)

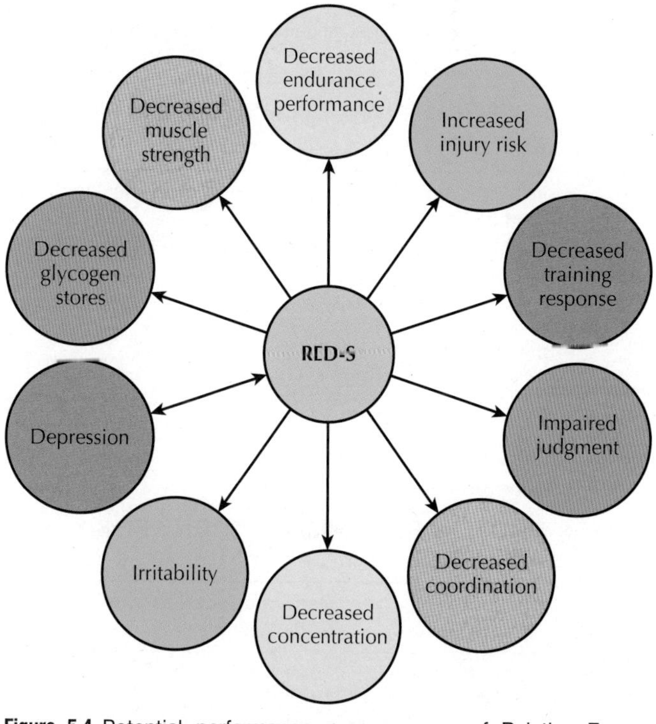
Decreased endurance performance
Decreased muscle strength
Increased injury risk
Decreased glycogen stores
Decreased training response
RED-S
Depression
Impaired judgment
Irritability
Decreased concentration
Decreased coordination

Figure 5.4 Potential performance consequences of Relative Energy Deficiency in Sport (RED-S). (Adapted from Constantini NW. Medical concerns of the dancer. Book of Abstracts, XXVII FIMS World Congress of Sports Medicine, Budapest, Hungary, 2002:151.)

the fastest. These physiologic properties give BCAAs the ability to stimulate the pathway that accelerates MPS.
- Research has shown that the amino acid leucine in combination with other BCAAs is critically important in stimulating MPS. Leucine is a key signaling protein of the mammalian target of rapamycin (mTOR) pathway, which is the pathway for stimulating MPS (Fig. 5.5). An effective dose of leucine is about 2–3 g/day. Box 5.1 lists food items that have a high leucine content.

Protein Recommendations

- Ideally, a mix of animal and plant protein sources should be included in the diet of an athlete.
- Protein recommendations for athletes are lined out in Table 5.3.
- Protein recommendations for athletes are higher than for the general population. However, it is common for some athletes to exceed their protein requirements by consuming additional protein in the form of shakes, powders, and protein bars, which can be detrimental to performance and health by crowding out other essential nutrients, like carbohydrates and fats, and potentially harmful in individuals with renal impairment. Table 5.3 lists the protein recommendations for athletes.

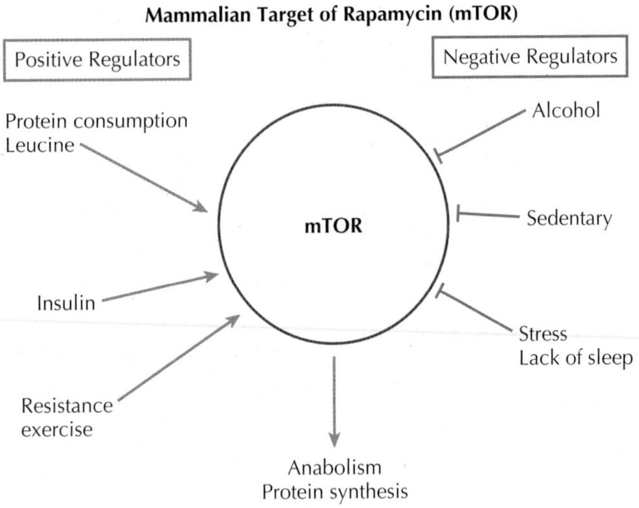
Mammalian Target of Rapamycin (mTOR)
Positive Regulators
Negative Regulators
Protein consumption
Leucine
Alcohol
mTOR
Sedentary
Insulin
Stress
Lack of sleep
Resistance exercise
Anabolism
Protein synthesis

Figure 5.5 Regulators that influence the mTOR pathway.

BOX 5.1 CONCENTRATION OF LEUCINE IN FOOD AND DAIRY PRODUCTS

- Meats, fish, chicken, turkey, eggs, and dairy products contain leucine and the other BCAAs
- Effective dose of leucine is approximately 2–3 g/day
  - 12 ounces of milk = 2000 mg leucine
  - 3 egg whites = 990 mg leucine
  - 1 cup of 1% cottage cheese = 2880 mg leucine
  - 3 oz tuna = 1740 mg leucine
  - 3 oz chicken breast = 3690 mg leucine
  - 3 oz beef = 3005 mg leucine

BCAA, Branched-chain amino acid.

Table 5.3 PROTEIN RECOMMENDATIONS FOR ATHLETES

Specific Athlete Group	Recommendation in g/kg of Body Weight
Endurance athletes	1.2–1.4
Strength athletes	1.6–1.8
Vegetarian athletes	1.3–1.8
Energy-restricted athletes	1.7–2.2

Application for Vegetarian Athletes

- Vegetarian athletes appear to meet or exceed their protein requirements; however, because plant proteins have less bioavailability, vegetarian athletes should increase their protein intake by approximately 10%.
- A disadvantage of being a vegetarian athlete is low levels of muscle creatine, a nitrogenous compound found in muscles, which phosphorylates and produces phosphocreatine. Phosphocreatine then donates a phosphate group to ADP to become ATP.
- Several studies have found that vegetarian athletes tend to have lower levels of muscle creatine compared with their omnivore counterparts; in addition, vegetarian athletes who consume creatine supplements had a greater potential for resistance training and greater lean tissue mass compared with a placebo group.
- Vegetarianism has several benefits for athletes, as vegetarian athletes gain a greater proportion of their energy needs from carbohydrates, including more fruits and vegetables, which may minimize their potential for free-radical damage, which may be advantageous to an athlete's training and health.
- However, there is the potential for nutritional concerns for vegetarian athletes, including vitamin B_{12}, iron, zinc, and calcium deficiencies; deficiencies in any of these nutrients can result in poor athletic performance.
- A sports dietitian can play a key role in educating vegetarian and vegan athletes, especially regarding menu planning, cooking, and food preparation, in order to maximize their athletic potential.

Fat

- The role of fats in the body is to supply a source of energy in addition to essential fatty acids and fat-soluble vitamins that play important roles in an athlete's diet. Most athletes often meet and/or exceed their recommendations of dietary fat usually because of increased caloric intake.
- High-fat diets are not recommended for athletes primarily because of their adverse health effects. Conversely, athletes who consume very low-fat diets (<15% of total calories from fat) do not exhibit any additional performance benefits and may in fact suffer health consequences.
- Athletes should aim to consume more healthy fats such as monounsaturated and polyunsaturated fatty acids and lesser saturated fatty acids and trans fats, along with the addition of more whole grains, fruits, and vegetables.

Fat Recommendations

- In general, fat recommendations for athletes follow public health guidelines, such as the Dietary Guidelines for Americans, which recommends fat intake in the range of 20%–35% of total caloric intake, with less than 10% coming from saturated fats; however, similar to carbohydrates, fat intake should be customized based on training levels and body composition.
- Some athletes believe that following a high-fat, low-carbohydrate diet can enhance rates of fat oxidation and improve endurance performance. Available literature suggests that high-fat, low-carbohydrate diets may match exercise capacity at moderate intensity but impair exercise at higher intensities.
- Although high-fat diets may impair exercise intensity, low-fat diets (<20% of calories from fat) are not recommended because they tend to restrict intake of nutrients such as fat-soluble vitamins and essential fatty acids, particularly *omega-3* fatty acids. In addition, individuals who restrict their dietary intake of fats to <20% of their calories for weight-loss purposes found no advantage of further weight loss following a very low-fat diet.

Micronutrients

- Micronutrients play a specific role in facilitating the release of energy from food and in tissue synthesis.
- In general, if an athlete meets overall energy intake and incorporates a wide variety of nutrient-dense foods, vitamin and mineral recommendations can be met through the diet itself.
- Moreover, athletes tend to consume more calories because of their energy expenditure during competition and training; therefore, they can meet their nutrient requirements with wise food choices. In addition, they may consume highly fortified "sport" foods and drinks, which provide several micronutrients and macronutrients.
- Certain athlete populations may be at risk of low or marginal intake of micronutrients. Athletes who compete in lean (distance running, gymnastics, swimming, and diving) or weight-restricted sports (wrestling and crew) are often at risk of low or marginal intake of micronutrients because of their low-caloric diets.

Iron

Functions: Iron is a part of oxygen-carrying transport proteins such as hemoglobin and myoglobin. Iron is also a component of cytochromes that carry electrons to molecular oxygen in the electron transport chain.

Effects on performance: Iron deficiency, with or without anemia, can impair performance and limit work capacity. Some athletes at the start of training experience sports anemia, wherein blood volume expands before the synthesis of red blood cells increases. This expansion results in dilution of the blood and a decrease in hemoglobin. Sports anemia is not detrimental to performance but is hard to differentiate from true anemia.

Etiology: Potential causes of iron-deficiency anemia can vary; as observed in the general population, female athletes are most susceptible to low iron status because of monthly menstrual losses. Special diets followed by athletes, such as low-energy and vegetarian, particularly vegan, diets are likely to be low in dietary iron. Distance runners should pay special attention to iron intake because their intense workouts may lead to foot-strike hemolysis or increased iron loss in sweat, feces, and urine, which can negatively influence the iron status.

Important interventions:

- **Screening:** Distance runners, other endurance athletes, vegetarians, and all female athletes should consider having their iron status checked at the beginning of the season and midseason. Laboratory tests to consider include serum iron, ferritin, and iron-binding capacity. Because of certain limitations in interpreting laboratory values, such as ferritin being an acute-phase protein, screening should ideally be done in the morning, in a hydrated state, with only low to moderate activity in the previous day, when there are no signs of illness.
- **Serum ferritin:** Currently, there is no consensus on a specific serum ferritin level that corresponds to a possible level of iron depletion/deficiency in athletes. Suggested normal values range from >10 to <35 ng/mL.
- **Iron intake:** Athletes who are at risk should aim for an iron intake of greater than the Recommended Dietary Allowances (RDA) (>18 mg for women and >8 mg for men) (Table 5.4). Athletes at risk must follow dietary strategies that increase food sources of iron, such as eating iron-fortified breakfast cereals with a source of vitamin C to enhance iron absorption, cooking in iron skillets, and ensuring proper overall energy availability.
- **Supplements:** Decisions regarding iron supplementation are best made on an individual basis. It may take 3–6 months to reverse iron-deficiency anemia. Although there is some evidence suggesting that iron supplements can improve performance in athletes with iron depletion without anemia, indiscriminate use of iron supplements is not advised and may cause gastrointestinal distress and toxicity. This is especially true in male athletes, where the risk of iron overload must be considered.

Calcium

Function: Calcium plays a major role in the formation and maintenance of bone. Athletes, particularly women trying to maintain a lean profile, can have marginal or low intakes of dietary calcium, particularly if they restrict their caloric intake or avoid calcium-rich foods. Of still greater concern are female athletes who suffer from menstrual disturbances, low energy availability, and bone loss/osteopenia. Low calcium intake in such female athletes contributes to an increased risk of bone fractures during training and competition.

Important interventions:

- **Screening:** Female athletes should be asked about current and past intake of calcium-rich foods, calcium supplementation, and menstrual history.
- **Calcium intake:** The RDA for calcium is 1300 mg/day for female athletes aged 9–18 years and 1000 mg/day for athletes aged 19–50 years. Female athletes should be educated about highly bioavailable dietary sources of calcium and how to incorporate these sources in their daily diet (Table 5.5).
- **Supplements:** Calcium supplementation should be determined after a nutritional assessment of dietary calcium. In general, 1500 mg/day of calcium and 1500–2000 IU/day of vitamin D are recommended for athletes with compromised bone health because of low energy availability and/or menstrual dysfunction. To optimize calcium supplement absorption, athletes should be advised to take their recommended calcium supplement spread out and with meals.

Hydration Guidelines

- Fluid loss of >2% of total body weight can compromise athletic performance and cognitive function, particularly in hot environments. Fluid loss ranging from 3%–5% of body weight further disturbs athletic performance, particularly in sports that require specific skills. Additional fluid loss of 6%–10% of body weight has profound effects on physiologic functions, including cardiac output, blood flow, and sweat production, and increases the risk of exertional heat illness.
- Thirst is a late sign of dehydration and is not a reliable indicator of an athlete's need to replace fluid during exercise. An athlete who drinks only when thirsty is likely to take 48 hours to replenish fluid loss.

Table 5.4 COMMON FOOD SOURCES OF IRON

Food	Serving Size	Iron (mg)
Fortified ready-to-eat cereals	1 oz	23.8
Fortified instant cooked cereals	1 packet	4.9–8.1
Soybeans, mature, cooked	½ cup	4.4
Pumpkin and squash seed kernels, roasted	1 oz	4.2
Lentils, cooked	½ cup	3.3
Spinach, cooked from fresh	½ cup	3.2
Beef, cooked	3 oz	3.0
Kidney beans	½ cup	2.6
Chickpeas, cooked	½ cup	2.4
Lamb	3 oz	2.3
Prune juice	¾ cup	2.3
Refried beans	½ cup	2.1

Nutrient values from Agricultural Research Service (ARS) Nutrient Database for Standard Reference, Release 17.

Table 5.5 CALCIUM CONTENTS OF DAIRY AND NONDAIRY FOOD SOURCES

Dairy Food Sources			*Nondairy Food Sources*		
Food	**Serving Size**	**Calcium (mg)**	**Food**	**Serving Size**	**Calcium (mg)**
Plain yogurt	8 oz	452	Fortified cereals	1 oz	236–1043
Romano cheese	1.5 oz	452	Soy beverage	1 cup	368
Fruit yogurt	8 oz	345	Sardines	3 oz	325
Swiss cheese	1.5 oz	336	Tofu, firm	½ cup	253
Ricotta cheese, part skim	½ cup	335	Spinach	½ cup	146
American cheese, processed	2 oz	323	Soybeans, cooked	½ cup	130
Cheddar cheese	1.5 oz	307	Oatmeal, instant, fortified	1 packet	99–110
Skim milk	1 cup	306	Cowpeas	½ cup	106
2% reduced-fat milk	1 cup	285	White beans, canned	½ cup	96
Chocolate milk	1 cup	280	Rainbow trout, cooked	3 oz	73

Nutrient values from Agricultural Research Service (ARS) Nutrient Database for Standard Reference, Release 17.

BOX 5.2 CALCULATING SWEAT RATE IN ATHLETES

An athlete can calculate sweat rate by using this equation:
Sweat Rate = (pre-exercise weight – postexercise weight) + (fluid intake – urine volume)/exercise time in hours. This equation will determine an hourly sweat rate. Two examples are listed here:

$$(71\ \text{kg} - 70\ \text{kg}) + (4\ \text{L} - 1\ \text{L})/2\ \text{h} = 1.5\ \text{L/h}$$

$$(125\ \text{kg} - 121\ \text{kg}) + (5\ \text{L} - 1.5\ \text{L})/3\ \text{h} = 1.2\ \text{L/h}$$

- To identify optimal fluid replacement strategies, athletes should know their individual sweat rates (Box 5.2); athletes should weigh themselves before and after exercise to identify sweat loss from exercise. The rule of thumb is for every pound lost during exercise, 2–3 cups of fluid should be consumed. Athletes should aim for a fluid intake that prevents weight loss during exercise and that avoids consuming too much fluid, resulting in weight gain during exercise.

Fluid type: Fluid from both food and beverages contributes to the overall hydration status. Water is an appropriate choice for most athletes; however, athletes who compete in multiple competitions, such as tournament play, or those who have restricted dietary intake or skipped pre-event meals, may benefit from consuming a sport drink with a carbohydrate concentration of 6%–8%. In addition, the sodium found in sports drinks may help with fluid retention. For exercise bouts that last >60 minutes, sports drinks can help maintain hydration and performance by maintaining blood glucose and by sparing muscle glycogen.

NUTRIENT TIMING

Pre-event Nutrition

- The pre-exercise meal should be primarily composed of carbohydrates and be moderate in protein and low in fiber and fat; this recommendation is based on the digestion rates of these macronutrients. Carbohydrate is digested most rapidly, followed by protein and fat.
- The meal or snack consumed before exercise should be sufficient enough so that the athlete is not hungry during exercise but not so large as to leave undigested food in the stomach. The selection of food, water, or a sports drink to be consumed 1–4 hours before exercise should be based on the athlete's preference and competitive situation.
  - Consume smaller meals closer to the event to allow the stomach to empty and nutrients to be absorbed, whereas larger meals can be consumed after exercise. In general, a carbohydrate feeding of 1.0 g/kg (0.5 g/lb) is appropriate 1 hour before exercise, whereas 3.0–4.0 g/kg (1.5–1.8 g/lb) can be consumed 3–4 hours before exercise.
- Athletes' individual differences must be identified and needs met. Certain athletes can consume large amounts of food just before exercise, whereas others may need the full 4 hours before exercise to digest their meal and feel ready for performance. Athletes usually know what works or what does not work for them. If they want to try new foods, they should first experiment in training before using the strategies during competition.

During Exercise

- For optimal hydration during exercise, athletes should drink enough fluids to replace fluids that are lost in sweat (see Box 5.2). Fluids lost in sweat should not exceed >2% of body weight so as to not affect performance.
- Consumption of colder fluids may reduce core temperature and improve performance in hot environments.
- Depending on the length of the exercise or training bout, drinking a sports drink with 6%–8% carbohydrates can provide a source of fuel for the exercising muscles during exercise. For exercise, including stop-and-start sports lasting 1–2.5 hours, the recommended carbohydrate intake is 30–60 g/h, which can be consumed in the form of sports drinks or food based on the nature of the sport.
- For ultraendurance exercise that lasts >3 hours, the recommended carbohydrate intake is up to 90 g/h. Research has found that a mixture of different sugars, such as glucose, sucrose, fructose, maltodextrins, or dextrose, may be most effective for carbohydrate oxidation.
- During brief exercise bouts lasting <45 minutes, no carbohydrates must be consumed.

Recovery Nutrition

- The goal of postexercise recovery is to restore fluids and nutrients used during exercise and restore the body back to its pre-exercise status.
- Recovery of glycogen levels is a priority after exercise. To refill muscle glycogen, time and adequate carbohydrates are required. The glycogen resynthesis rate is the highest within the initial 4–6 hours after exercise; approximately 1–1.2 g of carbohydrates/kg/h should be consumed to maximize glycogen.
- Postexercise protein consumption, particularly after strength and endurance sports, has been shown to be beneficial in stimulating MPS.

Table 5.6 FOODS THAT DECREASE INFLAMMATION

Animals	Fruits/Vegetables	Oils	Nuts	Herbs/Spices	Others
Salmon Mackerel Tuna Sardines	Tomatoes Spinach Kale Collards Beets Blueberries Strawberries Tart cherries	Olive oil Omega-3 fatty acids	Almonds Walnuts Pistachios	Ginger Turmeric	Dark chocolate Wine and alcohol Garlic Onions

- For practical purposes, combining carbohydrates and protein in a postexercise recovery snack will benefit both muscle glycogen restoration and MPS.

Nutrition and the Injured Athlete

- Injury results in inflammation in an athlete. Although inflammation is a necessary response for the healing process, chronic inflammation slows healing and may be damaging.
- Modifications to an injured athlete's diet may include adjustments of both calorie and macronutrient intakes. Baseline energy demands can actually increase after an acute injury or surgery, and it is therefore important that an athlete consume adequate calories to support the increased demand and healing process. Although carbohydrate consumption may decrease because of a change in physical activity, it is important to ensure the athlete continues to consume adequate carbohydrates to meet daily needs. Furthermore, protein needs after acute injury or surgery may increase to support tissue repair.
- An injured athlete needs to eat a variety of foods that focus on antioxidant-rich fruits and vegetables in addition to foods high in omega-3 fatty acids. Table 5.6 lists the foods that reduce inflammation.

SUPPLEMENTS

- The use of dietary and sports nutrition supplements by athletes with the goal of improving performance has been on the rise in recent years.
- Some commonly used sports performance supplements with strong research backing them include caffeine, creatine, beta alanine, nitrate (often in the form of beetroot juice or extract), sodium bicarbonate, and tart cherry juice. Other dietary supplements are often marketed to athletes with unsupported claims, such as improving body composition or boosting energy levels.
- Unfortunately, dietary supplements are not well regulated and can often contain mislabeled ingredients and contaminants. Athletes should be questioned regarding supplement usage and educated on the appropriate use of these products. It is important to encourage athletes to use only supplements that are third-party tested for ingredient accuracy and quality by organizations such as the National Sanitation Foundation (NSF) or Informed Choice.
- Any athlete using or intending to use any sports performance or general dietary supplement should be referred to a sports dietitian.

SUMMARY

- Food and fuel recommendations for athletes have moved into the era of evidence-based science and the employment or consulting services of registered dietitians (RDs) who are board certified in sports nutrition (CSSD).
- All sports medicine teams should include a sports dietitian (RD, CSSD) where possible to educate athletes about what foods to eat and how much to eat and to provide recommendations regarding the timing of food for pregame and postgame meals, which are of prime importance for athletic performance.

ACKNOWLEDGMENT

The authors would like to acknowledge the work of **Jacqueline R. Berning, MD,** on the previous edition chapter.

RECOMMENDED READINGS

Available online.

6 SPORTS SUPPLEMENTS

Stephanie Chu • Benjamin Krainin

PRODUCT OVERSIGHT AND MARKETING

Dietary Supplement Health and Education Act of 1994 (DSHEA)

Food and Drug Administration (FDA)

- Regulates dietary supplements under separate regulations from those that cover "conventional" foods and drug products (prescription and over the counter).
- Considers "dietary ingredients" a vitamin, mineral, herb, or botanical; amino acid; substance to increase total dietary intake; or a concentrate, metabolite, constituent, or various combinations or derivatives of the aforementioned categories.
- Under the DSHEA, a dietary supplement manufacturer is responsible for ensuring that the product is safe before it is marketed.
- Is responsible for taking action against any unsafe product after it reaches the market. They are not authorized to review supplements for safety and effectiveness before hitting the market.
- Unlike other drugs, manufacturers need not register or get approval from the FDA before producing or selling dietary supplements.
- It is the manufacturer's responsibility to make sure that product label information is truthful and not misleading; manufacturer also dictates product purity.
- Established a Dietary Supplements guideline in 2007 to require Current Good Manufacturing Practices (CGMP) for dietary supplements. Established guidelines require that dietary supplements be produced in a quality manner, not contain contaminants or impurities, and have accurate labeling.
- Postmarketing responsibilities of the FDA include monitoring safety (voluntary dietary supplement adverse event reporting) and inspecting product information (claims, labeling, package inserts, and accompanying literature). These guidelines do not address the underlying safety of the supplement itself and remain nonbinding to the manufacturer.
- The Federal Food, Drug, and Cosmetic Act (1997), with updated draft guidance published in 2016, requires manufactures to notify the FDA of marketing supplements with New Dietary Ingredients (NDIs). The NDI term applies to dietary ingredients not marketed in the United States before October 15, 1994. The company must provide information at least 75 days before hitting the market with supplemental information demonstrating why they feel this new ingredient will be reasonably safe. Between 1995 and 2014, the FDA has evaluated over 750 NDI notifications.

Federal Trade Commission (FTC)

- Responsible for overseeing truth in dietary supplement advertising.
- Requires that claims on products be symptom specific, not disease oriented. For example, statements such as "supplement X can stimulate the immune system" are acceptable. Even then, these supplements must additionally include: "This statement has not been evaluated by the Food and Drug Administration. This product is not intended to diagnose, treat, cure or prevent disease."
- Despite FTC requirement that claims on products be symptom specific, not disease oriented, one study that analyzed websites to assess the nature of marketing claims for the eight best-selling herbal products found that this rule is not always followed. The study revealed that most available information derives from vendor sites and half of these sites claim that these products can treat, prevent, diagnose, or cure specific diseases. Physicians should be aware that these claims were on the first page of the most commonly used Internet search engines.

Center for Food Safety and Applied Nutrition Adverse Event Reporting System (CAERS)

- The Center for Food Safety and Applied Nutrition (CFSAN) maintains an adverse event (AE) monitoring system known as CAERS (CFSAN Adverse Events Reporting System).
- Primary reporting system established by the FDA is a voluntary reporting system; less than 1% of all AEs are reported through CAERS per a report by the Office of the Inspector General.
- Dietary supplements are not evaluated for safety, and manufacturers are not required to prove safety. Is FDA's responsibility to prove harmful consequences.
- In 2006, the Dietary Supplement and Nonprescription Act mandated reporting of serious AEs by supplement manufacturers (deaths or life-threatening events, initial hospitalizations or prolongations of stay, disabilities or permanent impairments, congenital anomalies or birth defects), requiring supplement labels to include the manufacturer's contact information.
- Between January 2018 and March 2020, the FDA received over 14,000 reported AEs related to a wide variety of supplements. Though there was broad heterogeneity in the types of AEs reported, clinicians and consumers alike should closely scrutinize dietary supplements prior to consumption. Particularly at-risk populations include those who are pregnant or breastfeeding, and in children, unless specifically noted.
- Consumers and providers are encouraged to additionally report adverse reactions on the FDA Safety Reporting Portal (www.safetyreporting.hhs.gov).

Other Oversight

- The US Pharmacopoeia (USP) has set standards for natural product potency ranges. Their goal is "to improve global health through public standards and related programs that help ensure the quality, safety, and benefit of medicines and foods."
- Currently only 18 brands of dietary supplements are verified by the USP.
- ConsumerLab (www.consumerlab.com) is a helpful site that tests the supplements of various companies and reports their potencies.

Marketing

- In a 2018 survey, at least 70% of the population in every age group stated they used dietary supplements, with usage increasing with age.
- Dietary supplements are estimated to be a US$349 billion industry worldwide by 2026 (US$62 billion in the United States).
- Supplements are marketed to athletes' fears. Many athletes believe that they have to use supplements to stay equal to competitors or to gain a "competitive edge." They frequently fear that competitors are using supplements. More than 50% of Olympic-caliber athletes stated that they would take a banned substance if it meant they would win every competition for the next 5 years, even if they would then die from adverse effects of the substance. Among elite athletes, performance differences are minuscule between first-place and fourth-place winners; even minor enhancements may mean the difference between victory and defeat.

- Marketing companies rely heavily on testimonials of personal experiences, especially from famous people and athletes. Many companies successfully sell unproven products. Supplement manufacturers often sponsor supplement studies, and negative findings may not be published. Word of mouth and hopes to gain a "competitive edge" help fuel sales.
- Sports supplements frequently have no "instant" effects, so companies often add stimulants to give an "energy boost." Despite a new FDA label law to ensure accuracy in labeling of dietary supplements, there continues to be inaccurate labeling. In one FDA analysis of ephedra supplements, between 6 and 20 other ingredients were found. Cases have been reported of legal supplements containing trace amounts of illegal supplements. Is truly a "buyer beware" market (Box 6.1).

COMMONLY USED ATHLETIC PERFORMANCE SUPPLEMENTS

- Optimal dose and long-term side effects of most supplements are not known.
- Manufacturers recommend doses and durations that have been tested, and claimed side effects apply to these instructions.
- Many athletes may use higher doses than recommended and/or use them for longer periods, which raises concern for unknown effects.
- Most supplements try to enhance the normal effects of exercise on the body.

Arginine

- **Claims:**
  - Acutely improve exercise capacity; chronic effect results from stimulation of muscle protein synthesis and anabolism of muscle protein.
  - Soy, sesame, and peanut proteins are an excellent source of arginine.
- **Mechanism:**
  - May promote secretion of endogenous growth hormone (GH). Precursor in the synthesis of creatine.
  - Augments the production of nitric oxide.
  - Increased vasodilation can speed up removal of metabolic waste products, such as ammonia and lactate.
- **Efficacy:**
  - Little scientific evidence available to support claims of promoting and increasing functional capacity in healthy, athletic participants.
  - A 2016 systematic review did not support using arginine, either on its own or with creatine or caffeine, for enhanced recovery or athletic performance.
  - Particularly in well-trained athletes, no effect on nitric oxide concentration, blood flow, or exercise metabolites.
  - Significantly increases muscle blood volume but does not affect strength performance.
  - Effects on muscle protein synthesis are likely a net effect in combination with nitric oxide, as well as concurrent elevation of other amino acids.
- **Side effects:**
  - May result in gastrointestinal (GI) distress (bloating, anorexia, diarrhea) or cardiovascular effects (lowering of blood pressure).
  - Flushing reported occasionally with intravenous (IV) administration.
- **Dosage:** 2–20 g daily is used in studies.

BOX 6.1 "BUYER-BEWARE" INFORMATION ABOUT SUPPLEMENTATION

Most ergogenic aids lack scientific proof.
Most supplements have not been tested adequately for efficacy, purity, or safety.
Be careful of misleading product information.
"Natural" does not mean safe.
"More" is seldom better.
Nothing replaces a well-balanced diet that includes a variety of high-quality foods.
Athletes use supplements at their own risk.

Bovine Colostrum (BC)

- **Claims:**
  - BC supplementation may increase insulin-like growth factor-1 (IGF-1) levels.
  - May positively influence exercise performance characterized by short bursts of activity.
  - Improvement in body composition (e.g., gaining fat-free mass) shown in nonelite athletes, not found in elite athletes.
  - Claims include increased immune function after exercise.
- **Mechanism:**
  - Stimulates growth factors, including structurally identical IGF-1, which has an anabolic effect and is involved in the regulatory feedback of GH.
  - GH stimulates hepatic production of IGF-1, which provides negative feedback to reduce pituitary production of GH.
- **Efficacy:**
  - Limited studies show consistent beneficial effects on recovery and exercise performance and improved immune function in special athletic populations.
  - Mixed results on improvements in lean body-mass gains and no evidence of changes in either GH or testosterone levels were noted in a 2014 systematic review.
- **Side effects:**
  - Occasional minor GI complaints, including flatulence and nausea.
  - High percentage of participants complained about the "unattractive" taste of the beverage.
- **Dosage:** 20–60 g daily.

Branched-Chain Amino Acids (BCAAs)

- **Claims:**
  - Important source of energy in prolonged endurance exercise.
  - Proposed to increase endurance in long tennis matches, soccer, marathons, long-distance swimming, and cycling activities.
  - May contribute to increased body fat loss and maintenance of a high level of exercise performance.
  - Claims to decrease chronic fatigue/overtraining symptoms.
- **Mechanism:**
  - Replenishes loss of BCAAs (leucine, isoleucine, and valine) used as fuel, increases protein synthesis and GH secretion, shifts leucine metabolism to fat metabolism, stimulates fat metabolism over glycogen in hypocaloric diets, and prevents decrease in plasma glutamine.
  - Inhibits dietary tryptophan transport across blood-brain barrier, leading to decreased brain serotonin (associated with several brain regions that control central fatigue).
- **Efficacy:**
  - Most studies show neither beneficial nor detrimental effect of BCAAs.
  - A 2019 meta-analysis indicated that there was a large decrease in delayed onset of muscle soreness when utilizing BCAAs compared with placebo.
  - Studies of effect of BCAAs in hypocaloric states are limited.

- Have not been shown to reduce chronic fatigue/overtraining symptoms, and preworkout/event BCAA loading has no effect on performance.
- **Side effects:** Fatigue and ergolytic effects have been reported.
- **Dosage:**
  - Usually combined with other amino acids.
  - Range: 5–20 g daily or before exercise. May be safe to take a total of 40 grams daily.

Caffeine

- **Claims:**
  - Most widely used stimulant in the world and is present in beverages such as coffee, teas, colas, some energy drinks, foods containing chocolate, energy bars, and over-the-counter medications sold to increase alertness.
  - Central nervous system (CNS) stimulant that increases alertness and can make intense exercise feel easier.
  - Preworkout formulas usually contain caffeine.
  - Mildly elevates fat-burning and metabolic rate.
  - Some claims state that mild caffeine consumption may decrease risk for diabetes.
- **Mechanism:**
  - Lipid-soluble compound metabolized by the liver and through enzymatic action results in three metabolites: paraxanthine, theophylline, and theobromine.
  - Due to its lipid solubility, crosses the blood-brain barrier.
  - Acts on the CNS as an adenosine antagonist but may also have an effect peripherally on substrate metabolism and neuromuscular function.
- **Efficacy:**
  - Potential improvement in endurance exercise, high-intensity team sports, and strength-power performance.
  - Studied in special force operations where military personnel routinely undergo training and real-life operations in sleep-deprived conditions. Vigilance maintained or enhanced with caffeine in addition to run times and completion of an obstacle course.
  - May also be ergogenic by enhancing lipolysis and decreasing reliance on glycogen utilization.
  - Most likely to help with endurance events but not with shorter events like sprinting or weightlifting.
  - The American College of Sports Medicine (ACSM) in 2018 specifically recommended against consuming energy drinks before, during, or after strenuous exercise due to the lack of safety and efficacy data.
- **Side effects:**
  - Lethal dose in adult humans is estimated to be 10 g.
  - Higher doses of caffeine may induce mild tremor, tachycardia, insomnia, GI upset, chest pain, arrhythmias, and nervousness at doses over 600 mg/day.
- **Dosage:**
  - Single doses of ~200 mg improve cognitive function and 2–6 mg/kg body weight doses 15–60 minutes before exercise.
  - The National Collegiate Athletic Association (NCAA) limits athletes to 15 mcg/mL appearing in their urine, which is equal to consuming 6–8 cups of coffee 2–3 hours before competition. The International Olympic Committee (IOC) limits athletes to 12 mcg/mL.

Carbohydrate Supplements

- **Claims:**
  - Used to restore muscle glycogen after exercise, maintain plasma glucose during endurance events (especially those lasting more than 90 minutes), and maximize muscle glycogen before significant glycogen-depleting exercise (e.g., marathon, long-course triathlon).
  - Various sugars are used, including sucrose, glucose, fructose, and maltodextrin (popular among ultraendurance athletes).
- **Mechanism:**
  - Increased blood glucose stimulates insulin production and GLUT-4 translocation in muscle, which results in increased glucose uptake and glycogen storage in muscle.
  - Carbohydrates with high glycemic index increase plasma glucose quickly and serve as a fuel source in sustained exercise.
- **Efficacy:**
  - Reviews are mixed for pre-exercise supplementation and carbohydrate loading.
  - Benefits of supplementation after exercise and during long events (more than 90 minutes) are well supported.
- **Side effects:** Individual GI tolerance varies with different types of carbohydrate supplements, and some athletes may experience dyspepsia and GI upset.
- **Dosage:**
  - The ACSM released their latest position statement in 2016 regarding nutrition and athletic performance, which includes guidance for daily needs and acute fueling strategies.
  - Low-intensity athletes should aim for 3–5 g/kg daily, and those with very high-intensity demands lasting 4–5 hours per day should take in 8–12 g/kg daily.
  - Before exercise: 1–4 g/kg 1–4 hours pre-exercise; carbohydrate loading for events of greater than 90 minutes of sustained activity requires 10 g/kg/day of carbohydrates for 1.5–2 days before the event. For multiple sessions with fewer than 8 hours to recover, can consume 1–1.2 g/kg/h for 4 hours, then resume daily needs.
  - During exercise: 30–60 g/h for events lasting 1–2.5 hours. Exercise lasting longer than 2.5 hours may require up to 90 g/h. Sources include sports drinks (5–10 oz/15 min), sports gels or candies (2 gels with water), or gummy candy (a handful per hour with water).
  - Though not addressed in the ACSM position statement, recommendations after exercise: 0.7–1 g/kg every 2 hours for the first 4 hours after exercise (first 90 minutes postexercise is most important). Best if started within 30 minutes of stopping exercise. Use a food source with a high glycemic index. Addition of protein to carbohydrate supplement increases glycogen production.

Chromium

- **Claims:**
  - Trace mineral used for weight loss and for enhancement of glycemic control in the treatment of diabetes.
  - Proposed for the treatment of hyperlipidemia and hypercholesterolemia.
  - Used by athletes in attempts to gain muscle and lose fat.
- **Mechanism:**
  - Functions in carbohydrate, protein, and fat metabolism as a cofactor that enhances action of insulin and uptake of amino acids into muscles.
  - Food sources include broccoli, grape juice, and English muffins.
  - Improves lipid profile and is theorized to sensitize insulin receptors in the brain, resulting in appetite suppression and downregulation of insulin secretion.
  - Glycogen synthesis increases in chromium-deficient individuals.
  - Exercise may result in loss of chromium, but athletes conserve chromium and probably do not become deficient.
- **Efficacy:**
  - Possibly effective when used to reduce cholesterol, but probably ineffective for weight loss.
  - Mild hypoglycemic effect caused by a mechanism similar to metformin.

- Considerable scientific evidence indicates that chromium has no effect on body composition when taken in supplement form.
- **Side effects:**
  - Chromium interferes with iron metabolism and zinc absorption.
  - Though there are theoretical adverse effects with long-term use, the Institute of Medicine determined there is no upper intake limit for chromium. This does not mean that no toxic effects might be associated with high intake.
  - Commercial preparations containing ephedrine are restricted; low doses of the combined preparation have been found to cause hypertension, stroke, and death.
- **Dosage:**
  - Chromium picolinate is more easily absorbed than other forms of chromium; chromium is complexed to picolinate to facilitate absorption.
  - Dietary recommendation is 35 mcg/day for adult males and 25 mcg/day for adult females, with supplements generally containing 200–600 mcg.

Creatine

- Probably most frequently used and most researched supplement taken by athletes.
- **Claims:**
  - Creatine may increase exercise performance in short repetitive bouts of high-intensity exercise offset by brief rest periods (30–120 seconds).
  - Increase in exercise performance and work capacity probably leads to increased muscle mass in some athletes.
- **Postulated mechanism:**
  - Creatine is a low-molecular-weight, complex amino acid produced endogenously primarily in the liver and stored primarily in skeletal muscle.
  - Hydrolysis of creatine phosphate results in rapid production of adenosine triphosphate (ATP), which is needed for muscle contraction.
  - Maximal muscle stores of total creatine may enhance ATP turnover rate and increase phosphocreatine resynthesis, resulting in shorter recovery periods and overall increased training load (volume/intensity).
  - Creatine depletion is the limiting factor in anaerobic exercise.
  - Free creatine may stimulate protein synthesis and cause muscle hydration, which results in increased muscle mass and strength.
- **Efficacy:**
  - The International Society of Sports Nutrition (ISSN), the American Dietetic Association, Dieticians of Canada, and the ACSM have all concluded in position stands that creatine is the most effective ergogenic nutritional supplement currently available to athletes for increasing high-intensity exercise capacity and lean body mass during training.
  - Does not benefit aerobic training or performance and does not alter maximal force production.
  - Can aid in recovery from intense training by maintaining optimal glycogen levels, preventing overtraining during intensified training periods.
  - May reduce muscle damage and/or enhance recovery from intense exercise, experience less inflammation and/or muscle enzyme efflux after intense exercise.
  - Reported to increase muscle phosphocreatine content up to 20%, but this does not mimic physiologic changes related to training. Appear to be responders and nonresponders to creatine. Specifically, vegetarians who do not ingest primary exogenous sources of creatine (meat and fish) may benefit more from creatine supplementation.
- **Side effects:**
  - Since becoming popular in the early 1990s, over 1000 studies have been conducted; the only consistently reported side effect has been weight gain.
  - Short- and long-term studies in healthy and diseased populations, from infants to the elderly, at doses ranging from 0.3–0.8 g/kg/day for up to 5 years have consistently shown no adverse health risks.
  - Numerous well-controlled clinical studies have shown creatine supplementation does NOT increase the incidence of musculoskeletal injuries, dehydration, muscle cramping, GI upset, or promotion of renal dysfunction.
  - Areas of unsubstantiated anecdotal claims include the following:
    - **Renal:** Athletes with a history of renal dysfunction or disease that may lead to renal dysfunction should use creatine with caution. Using potentially nephrotoxic drugs (e.g., nonsteroidal anti-inflammatory drugs [NSAIDs]) may increase risk of renal dysfunction.
    - **GI:** Nausea, bloating, cramping, and diarrhea described in users, but effects are not supported by studies. No hepatic dysfunction reported.
    - **Dehydration:** Anecdotal reports of dehydration, especially in hot, humid conditions; adequate hydration in creatine users is encouraged.
    - **Muscular:** Anecdotal reports mention increased muscle cramping and strains but remain unproven.
- **Dosage:**
  - Normal diets that contain 1–2 g/day of creatine saturates 60%–80% of muscle creatine stores.
  - Most effective loading dose is to ingest 5 g (~0.3 g/kg body weight) four times daily for 5–7 days.
  - Maintenance dosing 3–5 g/day, with some studies suggesting 5–10 g/day in larger athletes.
  - Alternative dosing protocol of 3 g/day of creatine monohydrate for 28 days results in a gradual increase in muscle creatine content and takes longer to attain the desired intramuscular creatine levels.
  - Once creatine stores are fully elevated, 4–6 weeks are needed for creatine stores to return to baseline, and there is no evidence muscle creatine levels will fall below baseline after cessation of supplementation; therefore, long-term suppression of endogenous creatine synthesis does not appear to occur.

Fluid Replacement Beverages

- **Claims:** Used to prevent and treat dehydration. Dehydration greater than 3% decreases maximal aerobic power by 5%.
- **Mechanism:** Prevent dehydration/hypohydration and associated effects; prevent heat intolerance, maintain stroke volume, cognitive functioning, strength, and work capacity.
- **Efficacy:**
  - Numerous studies have shown decreased performance in “hypohydrated” athletes.
  - Recent studies demonstrate that hypohydration decreases strength.
- **Side effects:**
  - Overhydration may cause hyponatremia and is more commonly seen in recreational athletes with lower sweat rates or in ultraendurance athletes.
  - GI upset may occur, especially with fructose-containing fluid replacement drinks.
- **Dosage:**
  - The ACSM recommends consumption of 5–10 mL/kg of water 2–4 hours before exercise and 0.4–0.8 L/h during exercise; more is needed in climates associated with high sweat rates.
  - Drinking for thirst is important; can also monitor urine color and volume, along with body weight.

- Addition of carbohydrates is recommended for activities greater than 90 minutes.
- Hydration after exercise is also important. For individuals needing rapid recovery from dehydration, it is recommended to drink 1.25–1.5 L/kg of body weight lost during exercise.

HMB (Beta-Hydroxy Beta-Methylbutyrate)

- **Claims:**
  - Claims to regulate protein metabolism, thereby decreasing catabolism and increasing lean muscle mass and strength
  - Often used to enhance aesthetic physical appearance in bodybuilding.
- **Mechanism:**
  - Metabolite of leucine, a BCAA, and may regulate enzymes responsible for protein breakdown, inhibiting breakdown of muscle during and after vigorous activity.
  - HMB in liver and muscle cells is metabolized to HMG-CoA, which is then used in the synthesis of cholesterol. This increases the availability of cholesterol for cell wall synthesis. Localized deficiency of cholesterol for cell wall synthesis is postulated as one restriction to muscle hypertrophy, and increased local cholesterol stores could theoretically relieve this restriction.
  - HMB may also undergo polymerization, stabilizing the cell membrane, as it may be used as a structural component.
  - Also proposed to increase muscle cell fatty-acid oxidation by unknown mechanisms and lead to a decrease in fat mass.
- **Efficacy:**
  - Few scientific investigations are published. One poorly rated meta-analysis of HMB supplementation reported a statistically significant net increase of 1.4% in strength per week.
  - May have additive effects when combined with creatine.
  - May speed recovery from prolonged, intense exercise but probably not helpful for trained athletes.
- **Side effects:** No reported side effects in study protocols up to 8 weeks when participants took 3 g/day.
- **Dosage:** 1.5 g one to three times daily (2–3 g/day) in clinical trials.

Carnitine

- **Claims:** Claims to increase aerobic and anaerobic capacity and promote fat loss.
- **Mechanism:** Increases long-chain fatty acid oxidation in skeletal muscle during exercise.
- **Efficacy:**
  - Clinical trials inconclusive and suffer from design limitations.
  - Small studies show that L-carnitine levels in muscle do not change after supplementation or after single prolonged exercise session.
  - Twenty years of research finds no consistent evidence that carnitine supplements can improve exercise or physical performance in healthy individuals.
- **Side effects:**
  - Nausea, vomiting, abdominal cramps, diarrhea, and a "fishy" body odor.
  - Muscle weakness in uremic patients and seizures in individuals with known seizure disorder are rare side effects.
- **Dosage:** 2–6 g/day in two to three doses with meals.

L-Glutamine

- **Claims:**
  - L-Glutamine is the most abundant amino acid in the body.
  - Is used in treatment of wound healing, immune function, and chemotherapy-induced stomatitis.
  - Athletes use it to prevent impaired immune response after prolonged exercise.
- **Mechanism:**
  - Originally classified as a nonessential amino acid, glutamine is now considered essential for maintaining intestinal function, immune response, and amino acid homeostasis during times of stress.
  - Is an important fuel for cells of the immune system (lymphocytes and macrophages).
  - During prolonged exercise, as in other forms of chronic stress, plasma glutamine may decrease.
  - Muscle glutamine may drop in effort to sustain an anabolic state; if glutamine drops below critical levels, athletes may revert to a catabolic state.
- **Efficacy:**
  - Human and animal studies have shown conflicting data; reliable data lacking for most proposed uses.
  - Preliminary data suggest that glutamine supplementation may enhance immune function.
  - Glutamine has been shown to reduce upper respiratory infections in athletes after vigorous exercise, but more data are needed to confirm this finding.
- **Side effects:**
  - No significant adverse reactions reported; may be safe at appropriate doses.
  - Occasional GI upset reported.
- **Dosage:**
  - Typical dose: 20–30 g/day
  - Tolerated without side effects in doses up to 45 g/day for several weeks.

Nitric Oxide (NO)

- **Claims:**
  - NO thought to increase muscular strength and endurance.
  - Has been shown to be beneficial in patients with cardiac disease and endothelial dysfunction.
  - Marketed to athletes with claim that vasodilation associated with NO improves muscular vascular perfusion and that increase in blood flow improves muscular gains with resistance training.
- **Mechanism:**
  - NO is produced in the body by an enzyme called *nitric oxide synthase*, which converts the amino acid L-arginine to nitric oxide and L-citrulline.
  - Acts through vasodilatation, facilitating blood flow to muscle cells. Also, bactericidal, released by macrophages. Combination of these two effects is seen in septic shock.
- **Efficacy:** Supported in the 2016 ACSM Position Statement and a 2017 systematic review of beetroot juice for improving exercise tolerance and economy.
- **Side effects:**
  - When obtained from concentrated food sources, commonly beetroot juice, can cause GI discomfort.
  - Effects of beetroot juice undermined when combined with caffeine.
- **Dosage:**
  - Supplements rely on the conversion of an intermediate to NO, most often arginine.
  - 3–9 g of arginine daily typically used.
  - Two cups of beet juice 2–3 hours before exercise.

Protein Supplements

- **Claims:**
  - Protein supplementation above American Dietetic Association (ADA) recommendations (0.8 g/kg/day) is used to prevent negative nitrogen balance in sedentary individuals,

but in athletes the primary aim is for performance improvement and adaptation to training.
  - Many athletes, especially weightlifters, use protein supplements to "bulk up" or to add muscle mass. Most frequently used varieties include whey, soy, or egg whites.
- **Mechanism:**
  - Protein supplements aid synthesis of new muscle proteins.
  - Whey protein is a good source of BCAAs, which were discussed previously.
- **Efficacy:**
  - A 2018 systematic review and meta-analysis demonstrated statistically significant muscle mass and strength gains when augmenting resistance training.
  - No benefit observed above 1.6 g/kg/day of protein. The effect of protein supplementation also decreased with age.
  - Athletes require more protein then nonathletes (see Chapter 5: "Sports Nutrition"), and protein supplements may be used as adjuncts to diet.
- **Side effects:**
  - None documented at doses up to 2 g/kg/day in healthy individuals, but sustained use at this level is concerning.
  - Caution recommended in athletes with renal insufficiency or failure, as well as in individuals with lactose or dairy protein allergies.
  - Excessive protein intake stored as fat.
- **Dosage:**
  - Recommended dose for recreational athletes is 0.8–1.0 g/kg/day, for endurance athletes is 1.2–1.4 g/kg/day, and for strength-trained individuals, 1.6 g/kg/day.
  - The ACSM noted Grade I (Good) evidence to support consuming approximately 20–30 g of protein either during or after exercise, with the remainder distributed every 3–5 hours throughout the rest of the day for muscle adaptation.

Ribose

- **Claim:**
  - Many roles in human physiology.
  - Necessary substrate for synthesis of nucleotides and is part of the building blocks that form DNA and RNA molecules.
  - Claims to increase synthesis and reformation of ATP, improves high-power performance, improves recovery and muscle growth, and quickly restores energy levels in heart and skeletal muscles.
- **Mechanism:**
  - Structural component of ATP, which is primary energy source for exercising muscle.
  - During intense muscular activity, total amount of ATP available is quickly depleted.
  - Estimated to take approximately 3 days to restore ATP levels to baseline.
  - Ribose helps restore the level of adenosine nucleotides, and supplementation has been shown to increase the rate of ATP resynthesis after intense exercise.
- **Efficacy:**
  - Most evaluate effects on anaerobic cycle sprints with limited studies on strength and endurance.
  - Consistent ergogenic benefit not identified.
- **Side effects:**
  - Headache, nausea, hyperuricemia, and hyperuricosuria.
  - Doses greater than 200 mg/kg/h may cause diarrhea.
  - Precautions should be taken with ribose and diabetes because all simple sugars increase insulin levels; supplementation may cause hypoglycemia in a diabetic.
- **Dosage:**
  - 5–10 g/day, but markedly different ribose dosages used in studies.
  - Consensus on recommended dose of ribose lacking.

Tribulus Terrestris

- **Claim:** Herb claimed to "naturally" increase testosterone levels.
- **Mechanism:** Postulated to increase release of luteinizing hormone (LH), indirectly stimulating testosterone release.
- **Efficacy:**
  - Studies do not support claims of improved body composition or athletic performance.
  - One study with 30 infertile males taking 750 mg daily for 3 months showed no statistically significant difference in testosterone, LH, and semen parameters after treatment.
- **Side effects:**
  - No reported side effects in humans.
  - Animal studies in high doses include heart, liver, and kidney damage.
- **Dosage:**
  - 500- to 750-mg tablets for once-daily dosing frequently recommended.
  - Often combined with other "prohormones."

LESS COMMONLY USED ATHLETIC SUPPLEMENTS

Ginseng

- **Claims:**
  - The Chinese have used ginseng for thousands of years as a stimulant, a diuretic, to promote menstruation, and to fight infection.
  - Other claims address treatment of adrenal and thyroid dysfunction and aphrodisiac qualities.
  - Athletes use to enhance aerobic performance, energy level, and body resistance to stress.
- **Mechanism:**
  - Hypothesized to stimulate the hypothalamic-pituitary-adrenal axis, which may result in increased resistance to various types of stress.
  - May enhance myocardial metabolism, increase oxygen extraction by muscles, and optimize mitochondrial metabolism in muscle.
  - During strenuous exercise, ginseng may mitigate the catabolic effects of the stress hormone cortisol and enhance the body's ability to sustain muscle creatine phosphate levels, thus decreasing lactic acid production.
- **Efficacy:** No quality evidence supports the claim that ginseng supplementation enhances physical performance or reduces fatigue.
- **Side effects:**
  - The most common side effects are nervousness and excitability that may lead to insomnia, with a decrease in this effect after the first few days.
  - Many people find the taste unpleasant.
  - Hypoglycemia and difficulty concentrating reported.
  - Because of estrogen-like effect, women who are pregnant or breastfeeding should not take it.
  - Occasional reports of more serious side effects, such as asthma attacks, increased blood pressure, palpitations, and in postmenopausal women, uterine bleeding.
- **Dosage:**
  - Doses ranging from 300–6000 mg daily studied.
  - Most commonly used dosages 100–200 mg three times daily.
  - Study of 50 commercial products revealed a level of active ingredient ranging from 1.9%–9%, with 6 showing no evidence of ginseng.

Glutathione

- **Claims:** Stimulation effects of glutathione may counteract the free radical production resulting from extreme physical training.

- **Mechanism:**
  - Hepatic glutathione production increases with exercise duration.
  - Liver uses glutathione to remove vitamin E radicals and maintains vitamins C and E in their reduced (active) forms.
- **Efficacy:**
  - Effectiveness of aerosolized, intramuscular, or IV glutathione not well established.
  - Randomized control trials, meta-analyses, and systematic reviews are lacking in assessing the efficacy of glutathione to enhance athletic performance.
- **Side effects:**
  - Not well studied.
  - Long-term glutathione linked to low zinc levels.
- **Dosage:** Most supplement companies market 500-mg capsules taken daily.

Glycerol

- **Claims:** Oral ingestion may induce state of "hyperhydration," which may result in superior athletic performance.
- **Mechanism:** Simple polyol (sugar alcohol) that acts as an osmotic agent and increases water retention.
- **Efficacy:**
  - Randomized control trials, meta-analyses, and systematic reviews are lacking to assess the efficacy of glutathione to enhance athletic performance.
  - Results equivocal regarding the benefits of glycerol-induced hyperhydration on core temperature, plasma volume, and exercise tolerance.
  - Hyperhydration does not appear to offer benefit compared with euhydration.
  - Hyperhydrated athletes may be less likely to become dehydrated, especially during exercise in extreme environmental conditions of high heat and humidity.
  - Adverse effects of hyperhydration are concerning (e.g., electrolyte shifts), and practice should be to never replace proper oral hydration, proper acclimatization, and good sense during exercise in extreme conditions.
- **Side effects:** Isolated reports of headache, bloating, and nausea after oral ingestion; otherwise, data are limited.
- **Dosage:** Typically, 1–1.2 g/kg mixed with 1.5 L of fluid 1–2 hours before competition.

Lysine

- **Claims:** Used for prevention and treatment of recurrent herpes simplex labialis and improved athletic performance as a protein supplement.
- **Mechanism:**
  - Essential amino acid that inhibits the growth of herpes simplex virus (HSV) in vitro.
  - Important in collagen synthesis and bone formation.
  - Proposed that lysine, arginine, and ornithine increase human growth hormone (HGH).
- **Efficacy:**
  - Lysine reduces healing time, severity, and recurrence of HSV labialis.
  - Essential amino acids, such as lysine and ornithine, have shown no ergogenic benefit in resistance or aerobic exercise.
- **Side effects:**
  - Lysine contraindicated with renal disease or hepatic impairment because of inability to eliminate large amounts of nitrogen produced from supplemented amino acid breakdown.
  - Hypercalcemia may result from increased gastric absorption and decreased excretion.
  - No data support use in children or pregnant or breastfeeding women.
- **Dosage:**
  - For recurrent herpes: 1000 mg/day for 1 year or 1000 mg three times daily for 6 months.
  - No ergogenic dose established. Generally marketed in 500- to 1000-mg tablets for daily use.

Pyruvate

- **Claims:** Used to increase exercise endurance, facilitate weight loss, and reduce body fat content.
- **Mechanism:**
  - BCAAs transfer an amine group to pyruvate to form alanine.
  - Alanine has a role in increasing lipid oxidation and decreasing carbohydrate oxidation.
  - Pyruvate may also reduce free-radical production.
  - Enhances leg exercise endurance capacity by increasing glucose extraction by muscle.
- **Efficacy:**
  - Pyruvate not well absorbed orally, and studies fail to note increase in blood pyruvate in response to supplementation.
  - Evidence from randomized clinical trials, generally with weak methodologies, and a 2014 meta-analysis ultimately do not support weight-loss claims.
  - Increased time to exhaustion with endurance exercise noted in untrained participants. Further studies are needed before a recommendation can be made.
- **Side effects:**
  - GI upset, including gas, bloating, and diarrhea.
  - Appears to be safe for 30 g daily for 6 weeks.
- **Dosage:** Typical dosing 22–44 g/day.

Sodium Bicarbonate

- **Claims:** Claims to increase time to exhaustion and decreases sprint time for 400- to 1500-meter races.
- **Mechanism:** Buffers blood, which leads to metabolic alkalosis, decreasing the effects of lactic acid.
- **Efficacy:**
  - Mixed reviews published. In some studies, positive effects seen regarding power output for events lasting more than 1 minute and less than 7 minutes.
  - Endorsed in the 2016 ACSM Nutrition & Athletic Performance Position Statement for short, high-intensity events associated with anaerobic glycolysis.
  - Some athletes will see no benefit, whereas others may experience reduced performance.
- **Side effects:**
  - GI symptoms of belching, bloating, and flatulence.
  - Overdose a risk because of concern for electrolyte shifts associated with a large sodium intake.
- **Dosage:** Dosage used in studies is 200–300 mg/kg (~4–5 teaspoons of baking soda, often dissolved in liquid) 60–90 minutes before exercise.

GENERAL HEALTH SUPPLEMENTS

Apple Cider Vinegar

- **Claims:** Weight loss, glycemic control, appetite control, lowers blood pressure, decreased cancer risk, antibacterial.
- **Mechanism:**
  - Acetic acid is the main active ingredient of apple cider vinegar.
  - Proposed that acetic acid lowers blood sugar by suppression of hepatic glucose production, increased glucose utilization, and improved insulin secretion.
- **Efficacy:**
  - A 2020 systematic review looked at human and animal trials for the effects of vinegar for weight loss and

metabolic parameters. Concluded there is a lack of high-quality evidence and subsequently inadequate proof of its benefits.
  - Antibacterial claims are in vitro.
- **Side effects:** GI upset, erosion of tooth enamel, lower potassium levels, delayed gastric emptying.
- **Dosage:** Commonly 15–30 mL/day.

Chondroitin Sulfate

- **Claims:** Used as a chondroprotective against progressive osteoarthritis, a non-cyclooxygenase inhibitor, and an anti-inflammatory agent.
- **Mechanism:** Unknown. In animal models reduces inflammatory response and experimental cartilage destruction. In vitro studies show stimulation of chondrocytes to replace or repair damaged proteoglycans in the joint.
- **Efficacy:**
  - A 2015 Cochrane review concluded that few low-quality, randomized trials have shown that chondroitin alone or with glucosamine reduces osteoarthritis-related pain.
  - May slow progression of osteoarthritis when taken with glucosamine.
  - Large chondroitin sulfate molecules poorly absorbed, with approximately 10% bioavailability.
- **Side effects:**
  - Generally safe for long-term use with some mild stomach pain and nausea reported.
  - Supplements are made from bovine and calf cartilage; possible but unlikely risk of exposure to bovine spongiform encephalopathy.
- **Dosage:** 800–2000 mg/day in single or divided doses.

Glucosamine

- **Claims:**
  - Chondroprotective against progression of osteoarthritis.
  - May have anti-inflammatory effects.
- **Mechanism:**
  - In vitro, glucosamine stimulates cartilage cells to produce proteoglycans and glycosaminoglycans on dose-dependent basis.
  - Increases messenger RNA (mRNA) production.
  - Anti-inflammatory effect poorly understood.
  - Glucosamine is produced in the body by attachment of an amino group to glucose, acetylated to acetyl glucosamine.
- **Efficacy:**
  - Glucosamine sulfate is the preferred form.
  - Absorption rates approaches 80%–90%.
  - Some studies show decreased pain and stiffness associated with osteoarthritis, but results of randomized trials are variable.
  - A 2018 meta-analysis showed that glucosamine alone only improved stiffness scores, rather than pain, for those with knee or hip osteoarthritis.
- **Side effects:**
  - Glucosamine preparations may cause mild GI problems, including nausea, heartburn, diarrhea, and constipation.
  - People with shellfish allergy may have allergic reaction because glucosamine is made from marine exoskeleton.
  - Early findings that glucosamine increases serum glucose levels in diabetes have been refuted in later studies.
- **Dosage:**
  - 1500 mg/day of glucosamine sulfate in single or divided doses.
  - Inaccurate labeling, whether related to amount actually present or if it is even the right version of glucosamine (e.g., sulfate vs. hydrochloride) is a common problem.

Melatonin

- **Claims:**
  - Sedative/hypnotic effects; assists recovery from jet lag; improves sleep in blind patents and patients with other disorders that alter the sleep-wake cycle (e.g., shift workers).
  - Adjunct to chemotherapy and in treatment of depression.
  - Other claims include use as an antioxidant, prevention of aging effects, increase in energy, boost immune system, adjunct in treatment of epilepsy, contraception, and prevention of cancer.
- **Mechanism:**
  - Naturally produced in pineal gland and promotes sleep.
  - Secreted in diurnal fashion; release inhibited by light and stimulated by darkness.
  - Lowers alertness and body temperature.
  - Low levels of melatonin reported with insomnia.
- **Efficacy:**
  - Some systematic reviews show reduced jet lag, improved sleep, and improved circadian rhythm disturbances in blind, mentally retarded, and autistic patients.
  - A randomized control trial in 2020 of 99 children with post-concussive symptoms does not support the use of melatonin in this clinical scenario.
  - Insufficient data to support other claims in humans.
- **Side effects:**
  - Drowsiness; users should not operate motor vehicles or heavy machinery within 4 hours of oral ingestion.
  - Theoretical concern about interference with gonadal development in children and adolescents.
  - Can also cause irritability, dysphoria, dizziness, and abdominal cramping.
  - Data concerning long-term use are insufficient.
- **Dosage:**
  - Typical dosing for sleep disturbance is 0.5–6 mg at bedtime, with recommendations to start at lower physiologic doses of 0.1–0.5 mg.
  - Typical dosing for jet lag: 5 mg at nighttime for 3 days before flight.

Niacin (Vitamin B_3)

- **Claims:**
  - Claimed to augment energy during exercise.
  - Used by bodybuilders to increase superficial vascularity (causes vasodilation "flush") before bodybuilding contests.
  - Used with diet therapy to treat hypertriglyceridemia (>500), adjunct in treatment of peripheral vascular disease/coronary artery disease (PVD/CAD), and in prevention and treatment of niacin deficiency.
- **Mechanism:**
  - May increase homocysteine levels and modify abnormal coagulation factors that accompany PVD/CAD.
  - B-complex vitamins such as niacin are involved in energy production during exercise via oxidative phosphorylation and the Krebs cycle.
- **Efficacy:** Effective in lowering triglycerides and increasing high-density lipoproteins and may be effective for secondary prevention of heart attack or stroke.
- **Side effects:**
  - Low-dose dietary supplementation can cause minor effects such as flushing, which may be accompanied by pruritus, rash, headache, and occasionally muscle pain. Nicotinamide form of vitamin B_3 does not result in flushing.
  - Higher doses associated with headache, dizziness, nausea, and vomiting.
  - Doses above 1500 mg/day can raise blood sugar levels, even in those without diabetes.

- **Dosage:**
  - Dietary supplement dosage is 100 mg/day, though frequently marketed in 500-mg tablets; for hypertriglyceridemia 1000–2000 mg nightly of extended-release formulas.
  - Recommended Dietary Allowance (RDA) is 14–16 mg/day; 18 mg/day for pregnant women.

St. John's Wort

- **Claims:**
  - Used in the treatment of mild to moderate depression and obsessive-compulsive disorder.
  - Other claims include use for muscle spasms, ulcer, menstrual cramps, and as an expectorant.
- **Mechanism:**
  - Reported as a weak inhibitor of monoamine oxidase-A and -B activity.
  - Inhibits reuptake of serotonin, dopamine, and noradrenaline (norepinephrine) with approximately equal affinity.
  - 5-HT3 and 5-HT4 receptor antagonism.
  - May act as a receptor antagonist at GABA-A, GABA-B, glutamate, and adenosine receptors.
- **Efficacy:**
  - Effective compared with placebo in short-term treatment of mild to moderate depression.
  - Possibly as effective as low-dose tricyclics and some selective serotonin reuptake inhibitors (SSRIs; sertraline and fluoxetine).
  - Data insufficient for treatment of obsessive-compulsive disorder.
  - Other claims lack sufficient supporting evidence.
- **Side effects:**
  - Well tolerated and probably safe when used appropriately for short periods.
  - Most common side effect is insomnia, which can be alleviated by taking it in the morning or by decreasing the dose.
  - Other minor side effects include dry mouth, restlessness, agitation, headache, vivid dreams, dizziness, and paresthesias.
  - Important concerns arise from drug-drug interactions, especially involving other antidepressants.
  - Use with SSRIs may be synergistic and increase the risk of serotonin syndrome.
  - Addictive effects with monoamine oxidase inhibitors (MAOIs) include hypertension, hyperthermia, confusion, and coma.
  - Should not be used if MAOI was used in the past 14 days.
- **Dosage:**
  - Most trials have used St. John's wort with a hypericin content of 0.3% at a dose of 300 mg three times daily.
  - Doses up to 1200 mg/day have been reported.

Valerian

- **Claims:**
  - Purported sedative and anxiolytic effects, elevates mood, and improves concentration.
  - Other claims (from various websites) include beneficial use for treatment of tremors, epilepsy, attention deficit hyperactivity disorder, rheumatic pain, muscle spasm, menstrual cramps, ulcers, and hypertension.
- **Mechanism:**
  - Precise mechanism by which valerian root may cause sedation is not known.
  - Some data suggest that interference with catabolism of gamma aminobutyric acid (GABA) concentrations may result in its elevation.
- **Efficacy:**
  - Small studies indicate may be beneficial in elevating mood and improving concentration and as a sedative.
  - A 2006 systematic review showed valerian might improve sleep quality; however, there were significant methodological problems and widely variable treatment doses and durations.
  - Insufficient data to support other claims.
- **Side effects:**
  - Safe use has been documented in trials lasting up to 28 days.
  - Longer use associated with benzodiazepine-like withdrawal response.
  - Several reports of hepatotoxicity with longer-term use.
  - Potential side effects include drowsiness, headache, excitability, and cardiac disturbances.
- **Dosage:**
  - Numerous doses and formulations have been studied and marketed, typically ranging from 300–900 mg of extract (or 2–3 g dried root soaked for tea).
  - Tea, tincture, or extract in pill form.

Vanadyl Sulfate

- **Claims:** Used for diabetes, hypoglycemia, and heart disease and to increase muscle bulk with weight training.
- **Mechanism:**
  - Vanadyl sulfate contains ~30% elemental vanadium, which is a cofactor for various essential enzymatic reactions.
  - May mimic the effects of insulin or potentiate its actions.
- **Efficacy:**
  - Possibly effective in treatment of diabetes; however, systemic reviews have found no rigorous evidence that oral vanadium improves glycemic control.
  - No ergogenic effect in weightlifters compared with placebo.
  - Insufficient scientific evidence to support other claims.
- **Side effects:**
  - Possibly safe in small doses for short-term use.
  - Minor side effects include green discoloration of tongue and GI upset.
  - Serious effects have been reported with high doses, including leukocytosis and manic-depressive disorder.
  - Potentiates warfarin and digoxin.
- **Dosage:**
  - 10–60 mg/day vanadyl sulfate but marketed as high as 7.5 g per capsule.
  - Average diet provides 15–30 mcg/day of elemental vanadium.

Vitamin C

- **Claims:**
  - Claims to prevent or reduce the duration of upper respiratory infections but lacks evidence.
  - Antioxidant properties claimed to prevent cardiovascular disease and cancer.
  - Vitamin C used to treat exercise-induced asthma and osteoporosis.
  - Claims also include that it speeds recovery from injury and improves absorption of iron from the GI tract.
- **Mechanism:**
  - Water-soluble vitamin naturally found in citrus fruits and vegetables.
  - Plays a role in collagen formation and bone health.
  - Antioxidant properties led to speculation about a role in treating diseases in which oxidative stress may play a part.
  - Increases glucose and free fatty acid mobilization through epinephrine synthesis.
  - Enhances iron absorption.
- **Efficacy:**
  - Little evidence to support performance improvement for those with adequate dietary intake.
  - Promotes iron absorption from the GI tract and may have a role in preventing cancer when obtained directly from fruit

and vegetable sources. Same benefit not shown with supplement use.
    - Some evidence showing modest decrease in duration of common cold symptoms, especially in those exposed to vigorous activity in cold conditions. A 2013 Cochrane review reached a similar conclusion.
    - 2013 and 2014 Cochrane reviews could not support the use of vitamin C for managing asthma or exercise-induced bronchoconstriction.
    - A 2018 meta-analysis demonstrated in those with "higher" dietary intake of vitamin C that there was a statistically significant decrease in the risk of osteoporosis and increased bone mineral density of the femoral neck and lumbar spine. There was also a trend towards reduction in risk of hip fractures.
    - Decreases risk of complex regional pain syndrome 1 year post-wrist fracture when 500 mg given daily for 50 days.
    - Does not appear to prevent the common cold or aid treatment of cancer.
- **Side effects:**
    - Uncommon and dose related.
    - Hyperoxaluria, hematuria, crystalluria, hyperuricosuria, and predisposition to urinary stone formation may be related to intake greater than 1 g/day.
    - Other side effects include intestinal obstruction, other GI distress, headache, insomnia, fatigue, and flushing.
- **Dosage:**
    - RDA ranges from 75–120 mg/day.
    - Tobacco use increases daily requirements by 35 mg.
    - As a dietary supplement, typically taken at doses of 75–90 mg/day, with breastfeeding women requiring up to 120 mg/day.
    - Some common foods (guava, kiwifruit, broccoli, loganberry, brussel sprouts) can supply 80–100 mg of vitamin C/100 g of food.
    - Frequently marketed in 500- to 1000-mg capsules.
    - Doses of 1–3 g have been described for prevention and treatment of the common cold.

Vitamin D

- **Claims:**
    - Important in bone metabolism; without sufficient vitamin D, bones can become brittle or misshapen.
    - Prevents rickets in children and osteomalacia in adults while protecting older adults from osteoporosis.
    - Other roles include modulation of cell growth, neuromuscular and immune function, and reduction of inflammation.
- **Mechanism:**
    - Fat-soluble vitamin naturally found in very few foods, so fortified foods generally provide individual needs in American diets.
    - Flesh of fatty fish (salmon, tuna, and mackerel) and fish liver oils are best sources.
    - Produced endogenously when ultraviolet rays from sunlight trigger vitamin D synthesis through the skin, but impaired by sunscreen.
    - Must undergo two hydroxylations in the body for activation through the liver, where it is converted to 25-hydroxyvitamin D (calcidiol) and then in the kidney, where it forms 1,25-dihydroxyvitamin D (calcitriol).
    - Promotes calcium absorption and maintains calcium and phosphate concentrations to facilitate normal bone mineralization.
    - Necessary for bone growth and remodeling by osteoblasts and osteoclasts.
- **Efficacy:**
    - Most trials studying the effects on bone health include calcium, so isolating the effects of vitamin D is difficult.
    - Postmenopausal women and older men show a small increase in bone mineral density throughout the skeleton with supplementation of vitamin D and calcium.
    - A 2017 meta-analysis showed no risk reduction of fractures in the elderly for those taking vitamin D, whether alone or with calcium.
    - The ACSM does not recognize vitamin D as an ergogenic aid. Those with a history of stress fractures, signs of overtraining, and low exposure to ultraviolet B (UVB) may require supplementation with goals between 32 and 50 ng/mL.
- **Side effects:**
    - Toxicity threshold for vitamin D dosage is 10,000–40,000 IU/day and serum 25-hydroxyvitamin D levels of 500–600 nmol/L.
    - Toxic doses may cause nonspecific symptoms (anorexia, weight loss, polyuria, and heart arrhythmias) and more serious side effects from hypercalcemia leading to vascular and tissue calcification and subsequent damage to the heart, blood vessels, and kidneys.
- **Dosage:**
    - RDA for vitamin D is 400–800 IU/day.
    - Tolerable upper limits of intake levels for vitamin D are 5000–7000 IU/day, which is generally only recommended in those with serum levels <20 ng/mL.

Vitamin E

- **Claims:**
    - Antioxidant and similar claims to vitamin C concerning prevention of cardiovascular disease and cancer.
    - May be useful in treating diabetes and associated complications and Alzheimer disease and other dementias.
    - Numerous other claims include treatment of asthma and various neuromuscular disorders, prevention of allergies, negative side effects of air pollution, signs of aging, and cataracts.
    - Claims to reduce delayed onset of muscle soreness in extreme exercise.
- **Mechanism:**
    - Fat-soluble vitamin found naturally in grains, meats, poultry, eggs, fruits, and vegetables.
    - Widely distributed in different foods, so true vitamin E deficiency is rare.
    - Deficiency may occur with fat malabsorption syndromes or eating disorders.
    - Primary function is as antioxidant, protecting cell membranes from oxidation and destruction; proposed benefits are mostly related to this function.
    - May have anti-inflammatory, immune enhancement, and inhibition of platelet aggregation.
- **Efficacy:**
    - No evidence that supplementation improves health outcomes or athletic performance in healthy children or adults otherwise.
    - Role in the prevention of cardiovascular disease controversial. Controlled, blinded, multicenter trials have shown no benefit, whereas other studies have shown benefit from vitamin E supplementation.
    - May be efficacious for a large number of different problems, including treatment of dementia, liver disease, and normalizing retinal blood flow in diabetics.
- **Side effects:**
    - Dose-dependent but generally safe, even at doses exceeding RDA.
    - High-dose or long-term supplementation may cause vitamin E toxicity.
        - Data suggest a possible increase in mortality and in the incidence of heart failure with long-term use of vitamin E (400 IU or more), especially in patients with chronic diseases.

- May increase risk of bleeding.
- Reported side effects include GI distress, fatigue, weakness, rash, gonadal dysfunction, and creatinuria.
- **Dosage:**
  - Recommendations confusing expressed in mg, but most products labeled in IUs.
  - Convert to IU of natural vitamin E, multiply # mg by 0.67.
  - Convert to IU of synthetic vitamin E, multiply # mg by 0.45.
  - RDA for older children and adults is 15 mg/day; with lactation, 19 mg/day.
  - Doses vary for other claimed uses.

RECOMMENDED READINGS

Available online.

SPORTS PHARMACOLOGY OF PAIN AND INFLAMMATION CONTROL IN ATHLETES

7

Sourav K. Poddar • Kartik Sidhar

OVERVIEW

The pharmacology of pain management in the athletic arena can be a critical component in returning an athlete to play. Several options exist, and choosing an appropriate intervention should involve careful consideration of treatment goals and potential adverse reactions. In addition to selecting the appropriate pharmacologic therapy, it is crucial to determine the etiology of pain and incorporate a multidisciplinary approach to addressing pain in the athlete.

Types of Pain

The International Olympic Committee released a consensus on pain management that highlights the different types of pain.

- Nociceptive pain: associated with tissue damage or inflammation
- Neuropathic pain: lesion in the somatosensory nervous system
- Nociplastic/algopathic/nocipathic: neither nociceptive nor neuropathic; thought to be hypersensitivity secondary to altered nociceptive functioning

Management of Pain Principles From the International Olympic Committee Consensus Statement

- Early nonpharmacologic management, including implementation of biopsychosocial model for management
- Physical therapy, including modalities such as ultrasound, dry needling, iontophoresis, electric stimulation, and massage
- Psychological strategies should be encouraged, including muscle relaxation, guided imagery, and behavioral health therapy
- Medication management principles
  - Acute pain
    - Limit opioid or nonsteroidal anti-inflammatory drug (NSAID) prescriptions to 5 days and lowest effective dose
  - Subacute/chronic pain
    - Avoid chronic NSAID, acetaminophen, or opioid use
    - Consider a shift in focus from relieving pain to improving function
    - Multidisciplinary approach, including addressing the mental health burden of chronic pain
    - Consider adjunct medications

NONSTEROIDAL ANTI-INFLAMMATORY DRUGS

NSAIDs are frequently prescribed to athletes by sports medicine providers as a way to limit inflammation and pain and to subsequently facilitate return to play. Research regarding the effects of these widely used medications has brought into question the role of these drugs in treating athletic injuries.

Prevalence

- NSAIDs are one of the most commonly used medications. In the US population, >29 million adults are estimated to be regular users of NSAIDs.

Mechanism of Action

- NSAIDs work by primarily inhibiting the cyclooxygenase (COX) pathway and, to a lesser extent, the lipoxygenase pathway, thereby blocking the conversion of arachidonic acid to prostacyclins, prostaglandins, and thromboxanes.
- Through this mechanism, NSAIDs exert antipyretic, analgesic, and anti-inflammatory actions.
- Blocking the production of certain prostaglandins causes NSAIDs to exert an inhibitory effect on neutrophil aggregation and lysosomal enzyme release.
- NSAIDs are also thought to have nonprostaglandin effects on limiting leukotriene synthesis via inhibition of membrane-related processes.
- The two main forms of COX, COX-1 and COX-2, are thought to have different functions (Fig. 7.1).
  - COX-1 is presumably a constitutive enzyme involved in the synthesis of prostaglandins that regulate physiologic processes; it plays an important role in the function of the gastric mucosa, kidneys, vascular endothelium, and platelets.
  - COX-2, on the other hand, is primarily considered an inducible isoform (although data show that it may have a role in certain constitutive processes), involved in the synthesis of prostaglandins that mediate inflammation, pain, and fever in response to tissue injury.
  - The concept behind the development of COX-2–specific inhibitors was to theoretically preserve the physiologic function of COX-1 while limiting the effects of COX-2 on tissue injury.
  - Nonselective NSAIDs block both isoforms and subsequently may have more side effects than selective COX-2 inhibitors.

Alternative Mode of Delivery

Topical

- Pharmaceutical compounding of NSAIDs is readily available in the United States. These formulations are prescribed in the form of a gel, foam, spray, cream, or patch.
- Purported benefits of topical delivery of NSAIDs lie in the decrease in adverse systemic effects on the gastric mucosa, kidneys, and vascular endothelium.
- Serum concentrations of topical NSAIDs appear to be considerably lower than the levels measured after oral intake or intramuscular (IM) administration; this may result in fewer drug–drug interactions.
- Older adults report a higher incidence of adverse effects than younger individuals.
- The most common side effect is local irritation at the application site, although this is uncommon.
- Several trials have demonstrated the efficacy of topical NSAIDs with improvement in subjective pain symptoms. A Cochrane review showed the number needed to treat was less than 4 for several preparations of topical NSAIDs.
- Topical NSAIDs provide an alternative mode of use in the setting of acute superficial soft tissue injury with limited side effects.

Injectable

- Few NSAIDs are available for use as IM injections, and their use is controversial.
- IM ketorolac (Toradol) is widely used before athletic competitions in college and professional sports; however, there are limited data, and actual prevalence of use remains unknown.
- Ketorolac reaches its peak plasma concentration within 45 minutes when administered via an IM route compared with 20 minutes via the oral route.

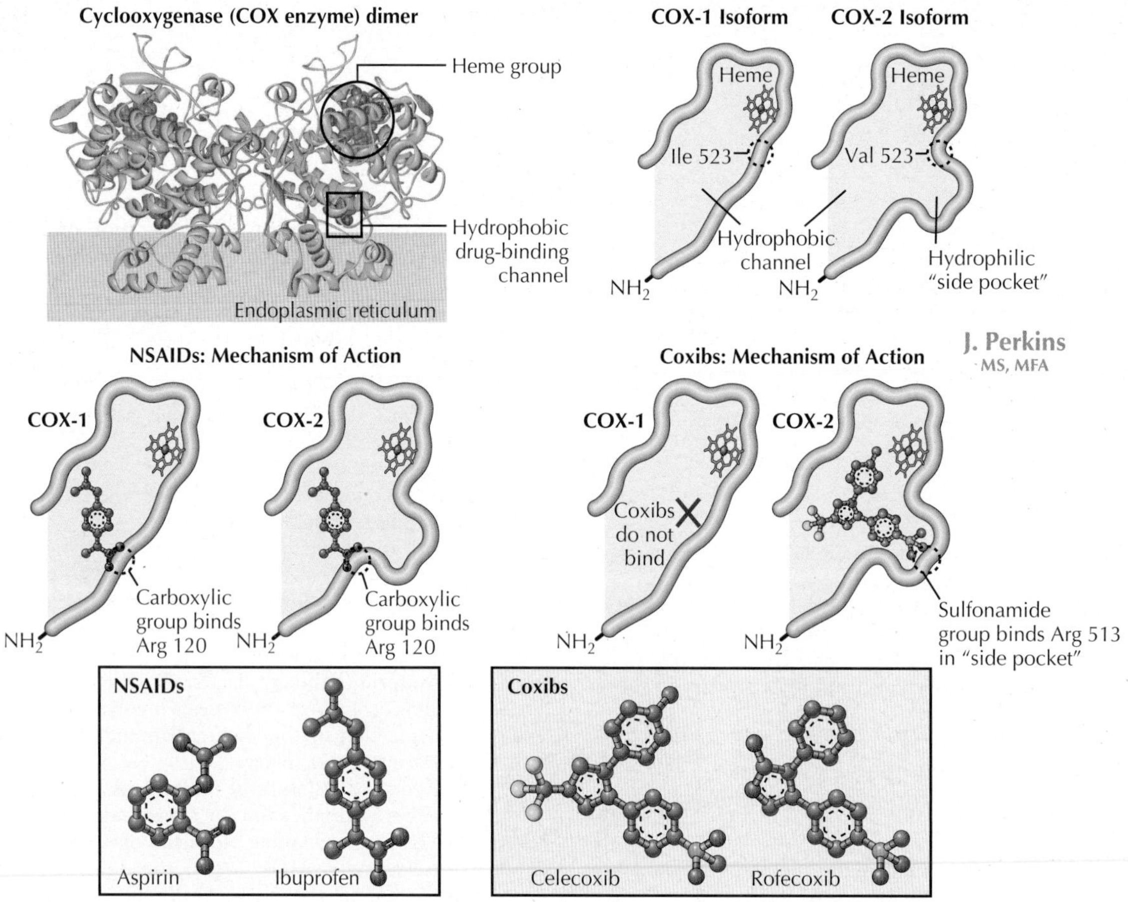

Cyclooxygenase (COX enzyme) dimer
Heme group
Hydrophobic drug-binding channel
Endoplasmic reticulum
COX-1 Isoform
COX-2 Isoform
Heme
Heme
Ile 523
Val 523
Hydrophobic channel
Hydrophilic "side pocket"
NH2
NH2
J. Perkins MS, MFA
NSAIDs: Mechanism of Action
COX-1
COX-2
Carboxylic group binds Arg 120
Carboxylic group binds Arg 120
Coxibs: Mechanism of Action
COX-1
COX-2
Coxibs do not bind
Sulfonamide group binds Arg 513 in "side pocket"
NSAIDs
Aspirin
Ibuprofen
Coxibs
Celecoxib
Rofecoxib

Figure 7.1 Nonopioids: NSAIDs, selective cyclooxygenase-2 inhibitors, and acetaminophen.

- In general, it is recommended that ketorolac not be used prophylactically as a means of reducing anticipated pain during practices or games.
- It should be given in the lowest effective therapeutic dose and should not be used in any form for >5 days, as the side effect profile is nearly equivalent to oral administration.
- General caution and discussion of risks and benefits with the athlete should be considered before administration of an IM NSAID such as ketorolac.

Types

Within the NSAIDs family, there are several subclasses that may provide subtle differences in metabolism and therapeutic effects (Box 7.1).

Adverse Reactions

- Considering the significant side effect profile of NSAIDs, physicians should be cautious when prescribing them.
- Long-term use of NSAIDs may increase the risk of stroke, myocardial infarction, and thrombotic events.
  - Previously, COX-2 inhibitors have been linked to increased risk of myocardial infarction, but studies have suggested an increased risk of myocardial infarction with nonselective NSAIDs as well.
  - Shown to have a negative impact on blood pressure, increasing both systolic and diastolic pressures.
- A common side effect associated with NSAID use is gastritis and gastrointestinal (GI) bleeding:
  - Development of COX-2 inhibitors was supposed to ameliorate this problem, but data regarding an overall decrease in GI side effects are conflicting.
  - Use of prophylactic medications such as H_2-receptor antagonists and proton pump inhibitors is common, but outcomes addressing risk reduction of stomach ulceration and GI bleeding are variable.
  - *Helicobacter pylori* eradication is recommended if long-term use of NSAIDs or antiplatelet therapy is implemented.
  - Increased risk of GI bleed, ulceration, and stomach or intestinal perforation may occur at any time without warning symptoms with both acute and chronic use.
  - Dosing for shorter intervals and consumption with food may reduce side effects.
- Effects of NSAID use on various musculoskeletal variables have also been studied:
  - A meta-analysis showed chronic NSAID use was associated with delayed healing or nonunion in adult patients.
  - Studies on NSAID use for ligament sprains and muscle strains have reported early improvement in symptoms and subsequent return to activity, but effects of long-term use on soft tissue healing remain unknown.
- NSAIDs block constitutive prostaglandins necessary for optimal kidney function.
  - Decrease sodium excretion and increase free water retention, particularly with long-term use
  - Avoid during endurance events due to potential renal morbidity and increased risk of hyponatremia
  - May also cause interstitial nephritis, regardless of duration of use

BOX 7.1 SUBCLASSES OF NSAIDs

Salicylic Acid Derivatives

- ASA
- Salicyl salicylate
- Diflunisal

Heteroaryl Acetic Acids

- Diclofenac
- Ketorolac
- Tolmetin

Fenamates

- Mefenamic acid
- Meclofenamic acid

Alkanones

- Nabumetone

Indole Acetic Acids

- Indomethacin
- Sulindac
- Etodolac

Arylpropionic Acids

- Ibuprofen
- Naproxen
- Ketoprofen

Enolic Acids

- Piroxicam
- Phenylbutazone

COX-2 Inhibitors

- Celecoxib

Pharmacokinetics

- Rapidly and completely absorbed in the GI tract
- Although most NSAIDs are metabolized via the cytochrome P450 system through the enterohepatic circulation, excretion occurs through the kidneys.
- Half-lives of different NSAIDs vary considerably, ranging from a few to several hours.

Therapeutic Recommendations

- Despite their significant side effect profiles, judicious short-term use of NSAIDs in the athletic arena is justifiable. In settings of sprains, acute muscle strains, eccentric load injury to muscle, and acute tenosynovitis or tendonitis, a 3- to 5-day course may help decrease pain and facilitate quicker return to activity.
- Caution should be exercised regarding use of NSAIDs with acute fractures or stress fractures of areas at a high risk for nonunion.

OTHER TOPICAL ANALGESICS

Lidocaine: Available in cream, ointment, spray, or patch preparations. Can provide local delivery of topical anesthetic to help alleviate pain.

Counterirritants: Include products that contain menthol, camphor, or mint products to create a cooling sensation to assist in distracting from and alleviating pain.

Capsaicin: Made from hot peppers and can initially result in a warm, burning sensation. This ultimately results in decreased skin hypersensitivity resulting in pain relief.

OTHER ANALGESICS

Opioids

- Opioid analgesics should be judiciously used.
- Significant side effects, such as sedation and subsequent deficits in coordination, cognition, and reaction time, make this medication class a poor choice for pain control before or during competition, and use during a sporting event cannot be justified (Fig. 7.2).
- Most opioids are banned by governing bodies of major sports unless prescribed for use by a physician with appropriate cause.
- Certain situations, such as a broken bone or severe acute trauma, may warrant the use of opioids; however, care must be taken to avoid extended use because of the risk of dependency or addiction.

Acetaminophen

- One of the most common over-the-counter medications recommended by physicians, acetaminophen is considered a first-line pain reliever according to numerous current guidelines.
- Exact analgesic mechanism is not known, but has inhibitory effects on the COX-1 and COX-2 pathways of the body.
- Exerts antipyretic effects via direct action on the hypothalamic heat-regulating center.
- Metabolism occurs via the cytochrome P450 system in the liver, and potentially toxic metabolites are then excreted in the urine.
- The maximal acetaminophen dosages should be reduced in athletes with renal or hepatic impairment, considering the potential accumulation of these toxic metabolites.
- The maximum recommended dose in healthy adolescents and adults is 3 g/day.

Tramadol

- Central opioid agonist: revised to a class IV controlled substance in 2014
- Produces its analgesic effect by binding to μ-opioid receptors and by weakly inhibiting norepinephrine and serotonin reuptake
- Extensively metabolized in the liver by the cytochrome P450 system, has the potential for several drug interactions, and has an active metabolite that increases the half-life of the drug in the body (Fig. 7.3)
- Short-term use in athletes for moderate to severe pain associated with injury
- Risk of dependency and abuse if prescribed for long-term use

ADJUNCT MEDICATIONS

Selective Norepinephrine Reuptake Inhibitors (SNRIs)

- Duloxetine and venlafaxine can be used as an adjunct for management of neuropathic pain.
- Mechanism of action: inhibition of serotonin and noradrenaline reuptake.
- Efficacy: systematic review of venlafaxine showed clinically significant reduction in neuropathic pain compared with placebo, specifically at higher doses. Duloxetine has also been shown to be efficacious in treating neuropathic pain.
- Adverse effects: SNRIs can cause nausea, dry mouth, constipation, headaches, and sexual side effects. More severe side effects

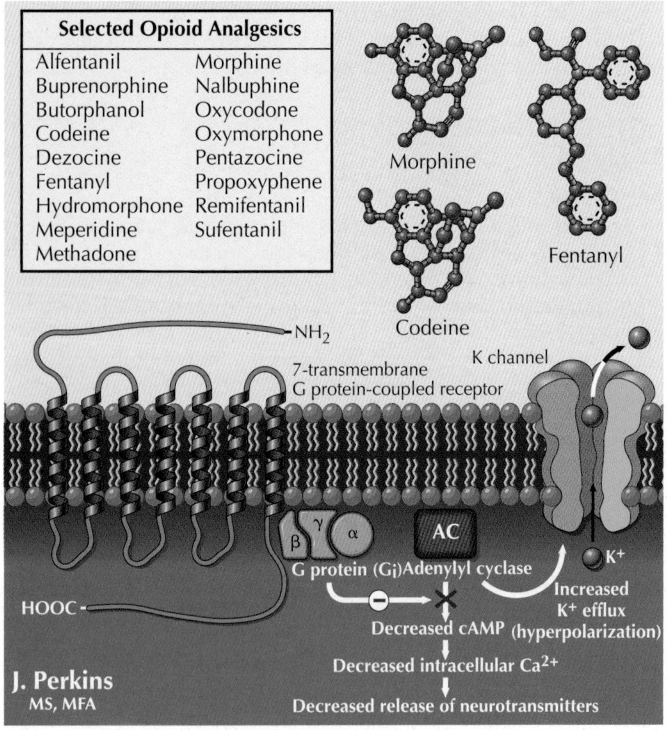
Selected Opioid Analgesics
Alfentanil
Buprenorphine
Butorphanol
Codeine
Dezocine
Fentanyl
Hydromorphone
Meperidine
Methadone
Morphine
Nalbuphine
Oxycodone
Oxymorphone
Pentazocine
Propoxyphene
Remifentanil
Sufentanil
Morphine
Fentanyl
Codeine
NH_2
7-transmembrane
G protein-coupled receptor
K channel
β
γ
α
AC
G protein (Gi)Adenylyl cyclase
K^+
Increased
K^+ efflux
(hyperpolarization)
HOOC
Decreased cAMP
Decreased intracellular Ca^{2+}
Decreased release of neurotransmitters
J. Perkins
MS, MFA

Figure 7.2 Opioids: receptor-transduction mechanisms.

are reported with venlafaxine compared with duloxetine and include cardiac conduction abnormality and increased risk of hyponatremia.

Tricyclic Antidepressants (TCAs)

- Amitriptyline and nortriptyline may be used as an adjunct for neuropathic pain, usually prescribed at lower doses than when used for treating depression
- Mechanism of action: pain management properties thought to be secondary to sodium channel blockade
- Greater side effect profile compared with SNRIs, which includes drowsiness, dizziness, dry mouth, constipation, and QT prolongation
- Risk for lethal overdose with TCAs; use with caution in athletes with suicidal ideation

Antiepileptics

- Gabapentin and pregabalin: initially used as antiepileptic medications, but were found to have neuropathic pain management properties
- Mechanism of action thought to be secondary to binding voltage-gated calcium channels, subsequently inhibiting excitatory neurotransmitter release
- Efficacy: both gabapentin and pregabalin were found to be efficacious in managing neuropathic pain. Gabapentin was found to have fewer side effects.

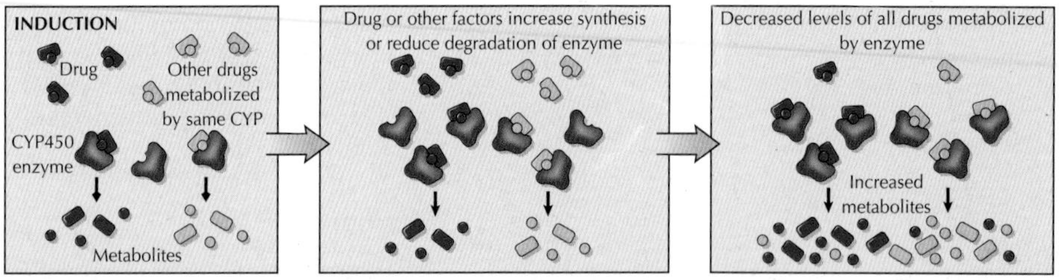
INDUCTION
Drug
Other drugs metabolized by same CYP
CYP450 enzyme
Metabolites
Drug or other factors increase synthesis or reduce degradation of enzyme
Decreased levels of all drugs metabolized by enzyme
Increased metabolites

CYP	Inducers	Inhibitors
1A2	Smoking, charbroiled foods, cruciferous vegetables, insulin, modafinil, nafcillin, omeprazole, phenobarbital, primidone, rifampin	Amiodarone, anastrozole, cimetidine, ciprofloxacin, diltiazem, enoxacin, erythromycin, fluoroquinolones, fluvoxamine, grapefruit (juice), mexiletine, norfloxacin, ritonavir, tacrine, ticlopidine
2A6	Dexamethasone, phenobarbital	Methoxsalen, ritonavir, tranylcypromine
2B6	Cyclophosphamide, dexamethasone, phenobarbital, phenytoin, primidone, rifampin	Efavirenz, nelfinavir, orphenadrine, ritonavir, thiotepa, ticlopidine
2C8/9	Dexamethasone, primidone, rifampin, secobarbital	Anastrozole, amiodarone, cimetidine, diclofenac, disulfiram, fluconazole, fluvoxamine, flurbiprofen, fluvastatin, isoniazid, ketoprofen, lovastatin, metronidazole, omeprazole, paroxetine, phenylbutazone, ritonavir, sertraline, sulfinpyrazone, sulfonamides, sulfamethoxazole, trimethoprim, troglitazone, zafirlukast
2C19	Barbituates, rifampin	Cimetidine, ketonconazole, modafinil, omeprazole, oxcarbazepine, ticlopidine
2D6	Dexamethasone, quinidine, rifampin	Amiodarone, bupropion, celecoxib, chlorpromazine, chlorpheniramine, cimetidine, clomipramine, cocaine, doxorubicin, fluoxetine, fluphenazine, fluvoxamine, haloperidol, lomustine, metoclopramide, methadone, norfluoxetine, paroxetine, perphenazine, propafenone, quinidine, ranitidine, ritonavir, sertindole, sertraline, terbinafine, thioridazine, venlafaxine, vinblastine, vinorelbine
2E1	Acetone, ethanol, isoniazid	Disulfiram, ritonavir
3A4	Barbituates, carbamazepine, dexamethasone, efavirenz, macrolides, glucocorticoids, modafinil, nevirapine, oxcarbazepine, phenobarbital, phenylbutazone, pioglitazone, phenytoin, primidone, rifabutin, rifampin, St. John's wort, sulfinpyrazone, troglitazone	Amiodarone, anastrozole, chloramphenicol, cimetidine, ciprofloxacin, clarithromycin, clotrimazole, danazol, delavirdine, diltiazem, erythromycin, fluconazole, fluoxetine, fluvoxamine, grapefruit juice, indinavir, itraconazole, ketoconazole, metronidazole, mibefradil, miconazole, nefazodone, nelfinavir, nevirapine, norfloxacin, norfluoxetine, omeprazole, paroxetine, propoxyphene, quinidine, ranitidine, ritonavir, saquinavir, sertindole, troglitazone, troleandomycin, verapamil, zafirlukast, zileuton

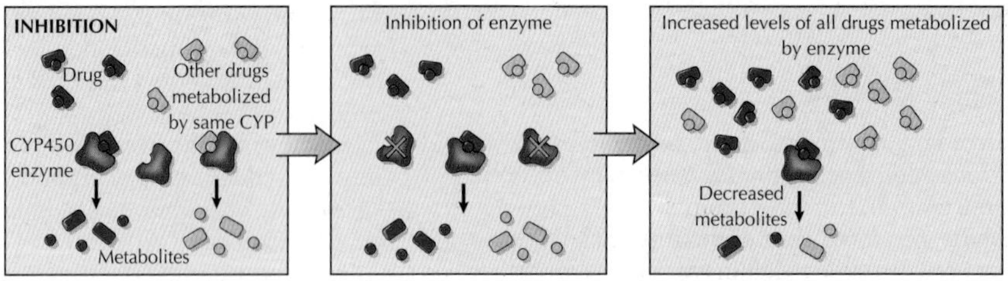
INHIBITION
Drug
Other drugs metabolized by same CYP
CYP450 enzyme
Metabolites
Inhibition of enzyme
Increased levels of all drugs metabolized by enzyme
Decreased metabolites

J. Perkins
MS, MFA

Figure 7.3 Metabolic enzyme induction and inhibition.

- Side effects: drowsiness, dizziness, decreased coordination, sedation, especially when used in conjunction with other sedative medications.

Low-Dose Naltrexone (LDN)

- Initially marketed to treat opioid use disorder and alcohol use disorder.
- Low doses, 1–4.5 mg, were found to affect pain pathways and are being studied for use in the management of chronic pain.
- Mechanism of action: at low doses, naltrexone acts as a glial modulator and binds to TLR-4, resulting in antagonistic properties on downstream inflammatory pathways. It also exhibits partial agonist properties against μ-opioid receptors and upregulates the endogenous opioid system.
- Efficacy: though still in early clinical use, LDN has shown efficacy in the management of fibromyalgia and complex regional pain syndrome.
- Adverse effects: at usual doses, side effects of naltrexone include nausea, vomiting, abdominal pain, decreased appetite, and very rarely, hepatotoxicity. However, side effects are minimal for LDN and usually are limited to vivid dreams. Though clinically unlikely to occur at low doses, ensure the patient is not on opioids before initiation, as this can theoretically precipitate withdrawal.

CORTICOSTEROIDS

- Potent anti-inflammatory agents that produce multiple glucocorticoid and mineralocorticoid effects
- Use in athletes should be judicious because of numerous systemic effects and drug interactions
- Available in oral formulations or administered as intra-articular injections for inflammation
- Consider tapering oral doses if used for >5–7 days
- Appropriate activity modification recommended with use of corticosteroids during the athletic season

Mechanism of Action

- Corticosteroids are lipid-soluble molecules that work by binding to intranuclear receptors. They inhibit the chemotaxis of inflammatory cells and decrease lysosomal enzyme release and production of inflammatory mediators.
- Intra-articularly, corticosteroids decrease migration of neutrophils into arthritic joints that are inflamed; in addition, they reduce prostaglandin synthesis and decrease interleukin-1 secretion and subsequent leukocyte aggregation by the synovium.
- Studies have demonstrated the indirect increase of synovial fluid viscosity in a joint injected with corticosteroid preparation via an increased concentration of hyaluronic acid (HA) in the joint.

Types

The original corticosteroid used for intra-articular injection was hydrocortisone (which explains the familiarity of several patients with the term "cortisone" injections). Subsequent research helped develop formulations with longer durations of effect, primarily mediated by solubility (Table 7.1).

Uses

- Uses of corticosteroids in athletes include as intra-articular injections for chronic and acute inflammation; pain relief in small joints is greater than that in larger joints.
- Lack of inflammatory markers in tendinopathy make the use of corticosteroids of controversial value in treatment. However, tendon sheath injections have proven beneficial in the treatment of tenosynovitis of the wrist and proximal biceps. Some studies have demonstrated its role in the treatment of inflamed bursae, with recommendations to avoid superficial locations, including the olecranon and prepatellar.
- Single injection for adhesive capsulitis of the shoulder joint provides faster pain relief and earlier improvement of shoulder function and motion when compared with NSAIDs.

Adverse Reactions

- Potential side effects of corticosteroids can be significant. Local effects include increased risk of tendon and ligament rupture secondary to inhibition of collagen synthesis. Injection into sites such as the Achilles or patellar tendon is contraindicated.
- Other potential adverse effects include skin atrophy at the injection site, fat atrophy, flare reaction, infection of the joint injected or injection site, and synovial calcification.
- Systemic effects of both oral and intra-articular administration of corticosteroids include inhibition of the hypothalamic-pituitary-adrenal axis at higher doses. Dose tapering is recommended to minimize the risk of adrenal insufficiency with prolonged or repetitive use.
- In individuals with diabetes, corticosteroids may result in short-term worsening of glycemic control (up to few weeks).
- Low-dose intra-articular injection of corticosteroids may have beneficial anti-inflammatory effects on distant joints.

VISCOSUPPLEMENTATION

Background

- HA is diminished in arthritic knees, which reduces the viscoelastic property of the synovial fluid; this increases stress and shear forces of the articular surface and may lead to further damage.
- Thus, the use of intra-articular viscosupplementation or HA injections in pain management in knee osteoarthritis has been established.

Mechanism of Action

- The exact mechanism of action of intra-articular viscosupplementation is unknown.
- At low shear forces in the joint, HA exhibits high viscosity and low elastic properties. Conversely, at high shear forces, the properties of HA are the opposite, demonstrating low viscosity and high elasticity.
- In addition, HA has both anti-inflammatory and analgesic properties:
  - Inhibits macrophage phagocytosis and neutrophil adherence
  - Reduces release of arachidonic acid (a precursor of inflammatory mediators) from fibroblasts in the synovium

Table 7.1 DURATION OF EFFECT OF COMMONLY USED CORTICOSTEROIDS

Generic Name	Average Duration of Effect (Days)
Methylprednisolone sodium succinate	4
Dexamethasone sodium phosphate	6
Triamcinolone diacetate	7
Methylprednisolone acetate	8
Dexamethasone acetate	8
Hydrocortisone acetate	8
Betamethasone acetate	9
Prednisolone tebutate	10–14
Triamcinolone acetonide	14
Triamcinolone hexacetonide	21

Adapted from Snibbe JC, Gambardella RA. *Clin Sports Med*. 2005;24:1-3.

- Analgesic effects include possible direct inhibition of pain receptors
- Moreover, HA purportedly and indirectly binds substance P, decreasing pain signals

Properties

- Several properties contribute to its effectiveness and tolerability.
- Lack of immunogenicity limits the chances of local reaction after intra-articular injection.
- HA exhibits passive diffusion into the synovial fluid and a prolonged half-life within the synovium.

Types

- Several different brands of viscosupplementation are available in the United States (Table 7.2); the number of injection series ranges from one to five.
- Each has a different molecular weight and preparation of purified sodium hyaluronate.
- Molecular weight ranges from 500–10,000 kDa.
- May be produced through bacterial processes of biologic fermentation or extraction of avian-derived molecules.
- All have relative contraindications for use in patients with avian or avian-derived product allergies, except Euflexxa, which is a bioengineered, fermentation-derived product.

Adverse Reactions

- Two to four percent per injection.
- Local reactions such as warmth, swelling, and pain can last for 1–2 days.
- Granulomatous inflammation arising within 48 hours after injection has been reported with hylan G-F 20, which usually resolves within 1–2 weeks.

Clinical Results

- Clinical efficacy well studied
- A systematic review of HA in knee arthritis shows improvement in pain and function scores without increasing adverse effects
- Improvement in pain and functionality versus placebo demonstrated in several studies
- Salutary effects may be similar to or better than intra-articular corticosteroid injections in the intermediate term
- A review of studies did not show clinical efficacy in hip joint compared with placebo or corticosteroid
- Currently, no Food and Drug Administration (FDA) approval for use in hip or shoulder
- In vitro and animal model studies suggest that early use of HA viscosupplementation in low-grade osteoarthritis may slow disease progression, suggesting additional studies on chondroprotective effects on use in younger patients could be valuable.

BIOLOGICS

Advent of autologous growth factor therapies holds the potential to use the body's own healing ability to accelerate and improve tissue repair.

Platelet-Rich Plasma Therapy

The concept of enhancing healing and accelerating an athlete's "return to sport" ability remains an elusive goal in sports medicine. Orthobiologics, including lipoaspirate, bone marrow aspirate concentrate (BMAC), and platelet-rich plasma (PRP), are increasingly utilized because of the presence of growth factors and the potential to induce additional release of local factors to enhance healing. BMAC and lipoaspirate remain outside of the scope of this chapter.

Background

- Growth factors mediate the repair process, and higher concentrations of growth factors in injured tissues are theorized to enhance or accelerate the healing process.

Table 7.2 BRANDS OF HYALURONIC ACID (HA) VISCOSUPPLEMENTS

Brand Name	Molecular Weight (kDa)	Comments
Hyalgan	500–730	Studies with 5 weekly injections show decrease in visual analog scale (VAS) pain scores at 26 weeks Additional studies with 3 weekly injections show benefit over placebo at 60 days
Synvisc	6000	Cross-linked mixture of gel and fluid formulation of HA Studies with 3 weekly injections show benefit versus placebo out to 26 weeks
Supartz	620–1170	Improvement in Lequesne index and VAS pain scale with 5 weekly injections followed up to 13 weeks
Euflexxa	2400–3600	Bioengineered HA that is not derived from purified rooster comb Series of 3 weekly injections showed improvement of VAS WOMAC index similar to that of Synvisc at 12 weeks
Orthovisc	1000–2900	Improvement in WOMAC pain scores observed up to 22 weeks after 3 weekly injections
Synvisc One	6000	Combines the 3 Synvisc injections into a single 6-mL injection Studies with a single injection show benefit versus placebo followed up to 26 weeks
Monovisc	1000–2900	Combines Orthovisc into a single 4-mL injection Improvement in WOMAC pain scores observed up to 22 weeks after 3 weekly injections
Gel-One	Unknown	Single 3-mL injection of cross-linked hyaluronate Improvement in WOMAC pain and function scores observed up to 13 weeks
Durolane	10,000	Single injection series Higher molecular weight is thought to result in longer-lasting pain relief
Hymovis	500–730	Pilot study showed enhanced type II collagen turnover with possible increase in lateral compartment cartilage volume

WOMAC, Western Ontario and McMaster Universities Osteoarthritis Index.

- PRP is prepared by taking the patient's own whole blood and centrifuging it to extract plasma, which contains concentrated platelets and growth factors.

Mechanism of Action

- PRP contains several nutrients and factors that are thought to promote healing.
- Platelets are one of the first cells to arrive on-site after injury; they play an instrumental role in the normal healing response via local secretion of growth factors and recruitment of reparative cells.
- Platelet alpha-granules are activated to release bioactive molecules, which include adhesive proteins, clotting factors, membrane proteins, and growth factors.
- Growth factors, including TGF-β, VEGF, PDGF, FGF, HGF, IGF, and EGF, are released.
- Literature supports the concept that PRP regulates the local production of growth factors and alters the environmental milieu.

Uses

- PRP is used in a variety of musculoskeletal injuries, which include muscle and ligament injuries, tendinosis, enthesopathy, osteoarthritis, and as an adjunct in orthopedic surgeries.

Considerations and Outcomes

- PRP can be prepared in either leukocyte-rich or leukocyte-poor forms.
- Data show trends toward better clinical outcomes with leukocyte-poor PRP (LP-PRP) preparations are used in the treatment of osteoarthritis.
- Leukocyte-rich PRP (LR-PRP) shows promise in the treatment of chronic tendinopathy resulting from a more robust inflammatory response.
- A wide variety of platelet concentrations are used; the optimum platelet concentration are not yet known, and each PRP system has different platelet capture efficiency.
- In vitro lidocaine is toxic to platelets and tenocytes so PRP preparations cannot be mixed with local anesthetic.
- Substantial evidence supports the use of PRP in chronic tendinopathy unresponsive to other conservative treatments.
- Soft tissue indications for use:
  - High-quality evidence supports LR-PRP for lateral epicondylitis
  - Moderate high-quality evidence for use of LR-PRP for patellar tendinopathy and plantar fasciitis
  - Insufficient evidence to recommend use for rotator cuff tendinopathy, high ankle sprain, Achilles tendinopathy, or muscle injuries
- Osteoarthritis:
  - High-quality evidence to support use in knee osteoarthritis
  - Insufficient evidence to recommend use in osteoarthritis of hip

SUMMARY

- Management of pain and inflammation in athletes can be a challenging task. Employ a multidisciplinary approach to pain management that includes understanding the underlying type of pain. Pharmacologic therapy is one component to comprehensive pain management.
- Side effects (both adverse and beneficial), drug interactions, and possible contraindications should be carefully considered.
- Although NSAIDs have long been a favorite in the armamentarium of the sports medicine practitioner, limiting its use to appropriate situations and shorter duration of therapy is prudent.
- Biologic therapy, including PRP, continues to be a developing treatment option with high-quality evidence to support use in knee osteoarthritis and lateral epicondylitis.

RECOMMENDED READINGS

Available online.

8 SPORTS PHARMACOLOGY OF CHRONIC DISEASE

Amy P. Powell • Kyle Goerl

INTRODUCTION

Adults are encouraged to engage in 150 minutes of moderate-intensity exercise weekly to maintain overall health and fitness. As the US population ages, many people are actively taking or have previously taken medications that may affect exercise performance. Managing athletes and patients on medications for chronic illnesses is an important skill for sports medicine physicians to master.

LIPID-LOWERING AGENTS

Statins

- Statins are some of the most commonly prescribed drugs worldwide.
- Statin drugs are widely used to prevent and treat coronary artery disease and cerebrovascular disease in adult patients.
- Fifty-six million Americans aged 40–75 years are now considered candidates for statin use and 87% of men aged over 60 years meet the eligibility criteria for statin treatment based on application of current guidelines.

Mechanism of Action

- Inhibitor of HMG-CoA reductase, an enzyme important for cholesterol synthesis

Musculoskeletal Adverse Effects

- Muscle-related complaints are reported in 1.5% of patients in randomized controlled trials on statin and 10% of patients in observational studies.
- Statin-induced myopathy exists on a spectrum. The mildest presentation is myalgia without elevation of creatine kinase. True myositis (defined as elevation of creatine kinase >10 times the upper limit of normal laboratory values) leading to rhabdomyolysis; death is the most severe presentation but very rare.
- Symptoms typically begin within 6 months of treatment initiation and resolve 2–3 months after statin discontinuation.
- Risk factors for statin-induced myopathy include higher medication dose, female gender, older age, low body mass index (BMI), untreated hypothyroidism, and lipophilic statin use (lovastatin, simvastatin, and atorvastatin are the most lipophilic). Concomitant treatment with other medications metabolized through or genetic alterations of the cytochrome p450 system may also increase the risk of myopathy (e.g., fibrates, calcium-channel blockers, and azole antifungal agents).
- Proximal muscles are preferentially affected.
- Symptoms include muscle pain, stiffness, muscle fatigue, tendon pain, and nocturnal cramping. Symptoms tend to be worse with exertion and after exercise.

Impact on Exercise Performance

- Conflicting reports exist regarding exercise performance while on statins.
- Certain investigators have found decreased muscle strength and reduced aerobic exercise performance in patients treated with statins, but available literature in this area has mixed results.

Alternative Lipid-Lowering Medications

- Two pro-protein convertase subtilisin/kexin type 9 (PCSK9) inhibitors were approved for use in 2015: evolocumab and alirocumab.
- PCSK9 is an enzyme that binds to the low-density lipoprotein (LDL) receptor and prevents the LDL receptor from appropriately removing LDL cholesterol.
- Inhibition of PCSK9 has been shown to be a powerful method of reducing LDL cholesterol, with initial trials showing 60% reduction in LDL levels after 12 months of treatment.
- PCSK9 inhibitors are administered by subcutaneous injection every 2–4 weeks.
- Annual treatment cost is $7000–$12,000, which may limit its regular use.
- Neurocognitive side effects (e.g., confusion and inattention) have been reported in several clinical trials. Myalgias, although reported, were rare.
- PCSK9 inhibitors are likely to be considered for athletes at high risk for coronary artery disease (e.g., familial hypercholesterolemia) who cannot tolerate statin drugs because of their adverse effects.

ANTIHYPERTENSIVE DRUGS

Background

- Hypertension (HTN) is the most common cardiovascular condition affecting adults in the United States. It is common in athletes of all ages and is a leading risk factor for cardiovascular morbidity and chronic kidney disease (CKD).
- HTN is associated with decreased exercise capacity in elite athletes.
- Systolic blood pressures continue to rise throughout life because of arterial stiffening, whereas diastolic pressures plateau in the sixth decade of life and subsequently decline.
- Approximately 55% of men and 65% of women will have HTN by the age of 60.

Mechanism of Action and Side Effects

Multiple medication classes can be utilized to treat HTN. More typical medication classes are reviewed here:

- **Angiotensin-converting enzyme (ACE) inhibitors** (lisinopril, enalapril, and captopril) primarily act by suppressing the renin-angiotensin-aldosterone system via inhibition of conversion of angiotensin I to angiotensin II; this blocks the breakdown of bradykinin, which can lead to side effects such as cough and angioedema. Other side effects include hyperkalemia and elevated creatinine associated with renal artery stenosis.
- **Angiotensin receptor blockers** (ARBs; losartan, valsartan, and olmesartan) block binding of angiotensin II to angiotensin type I receptors, thereby effectively reducing the ability of angiotensin II to cause vasoconstriction, sodium retention, and aldosterone release. Side effects are similar to ACE inhibitors, but cough is rare.
- **Beta-blockers:** Beta-1 receptor blockers (metoprolol and propranolol) inhibit sympathetic stimulation of the heart, thereby reducing heart rate. Others (labetalol and carvedilol) work by blocking alpha-1 receptor activity to cause peripheral vasodilation, and others have intrinsic sympathomimetic activity

(acebutolol), which reduces systemic vascular resistance while maintaining heart rate and cardiac output.
- **Calcium-channel blockers (CCBs):** Dihydropyridine CCBs (amlodipine and nifedipine) bind calcium channels in vascular smooth muscles, leading to vasodilation. Nondihydropyridine CCBs (verapamil and diltiazem) bind to calcium channels in the sinoatrial and atrioventricular nodes, leading to negative inotropic effects. Side effects may include lightheadedness, hypotension, and lower extremity swelling.
- **Diuretics:** Thiazide diuretics (hydrochlorothiazide and chlorthalidone) inhibit reabsorption of sodium and chloride, primarily in the distal tubules, which can lead to hyponatremia. Potassium-sparing diuretics (triamterene and spironolactone) inhibit sodium reabsorption in the distal tubules but are rarely used in monotherapy. Loop diuretics (furosemide, torsemide, and bumetanide) inhibit the reabsorption of sodium and chloride at the ascending loop of Henle and may commonly lead to hypokalemia.

Treatment of Hypertension

- The eighth Joint National Committee (JNC8) recommends initiation of treatment for blood pressures >150/90 mmHg in adults aged ≥60 years and at 140/90 mmHg in anyone aged <60 years and patients with CKD and diabetes.
- Athletes should begin treatment with nonpharmacologic options, including lifestyle modifications, such as decreased sodium intake, decreased fat intake, weight loss, decreased alcohol consumption, stimulant avoidance, limited nonsteroidal anti-inflammatory drug (NSAID) use, smoking cessation, relaxation techniques, and aerobic exercise.
- Choosing HTN medications in athletes can be challenging: the best choice of drug is one that reliably lowers blood pressure, has limited negative effects on exercise hemodynamics, and is legal for the athlete to use.
- Other existing medical comorbidities, drug–drug interactions, and response to previous medications must also be considered.
- ACE inhibitors, ARBs, and CCBs are typical first-line agents in athletes because they are well tolerated and have no major effects on energy metabolism or cardiovascular adaptation to exercise.
- Thiazide diuretics are also considered first-line agents but have certain negative effects that makes them less desirable choices in athletes.
- In patients with CKD, ACE inhibitors and ARBs should be the initial or first add-on choice of therapy.
- ACE inhibitors and ARBs should be cautiously used in women of reproductive age, as they are contraindicated during pregnancy.
- African Americans typically respond better to CCBs and thiazide diuretics.

Considerations in Athletes

- The prevalence of HTN in athletes is unknown but is thought to be half of that in the general population. However, in preparticipation cardiac screening, HTN is the most common abnormal finding. Among adolescent athletes with HTN, the blood pressure continues to remain elevated at the 1-year follow-up in approximately 80% of cases.
- Athletes at a greater risk for HTN include male athletes, strength-trained athletes, African Americans, obese individuals, athletes with diabetes, those with renal disease, and those with a family history of HTN. Collegiate and professional football players have higher rates of HTN compared with nonfootball athletes (19.2% vs. 7% and 13.8% vs. 5.5%, respectively).

Doping

- Certain medications are considered doping substances and may be banned by particular sport-governing bodies.
- Diuretics have been used as masking agents to dilute illegal substances; in addition, they have been used for rapid weight loss, making them popular in sports such as wrestling and boxing.
- Beta-blockers are banned in precision sports such as archery, shooting, diving, and figure skating, where steadiness may give an athlete an unfair advantage.
- As with any medication, consultation with the banned substance list of an athlete's sport governing body should precede a prescription for an antihypertensive medication to ensure compliance.

Negative Effects on Performance

- Diuretics can decrease plasma volume and lead to electrolyte disturbances, which can ultimately result in muscle cramping, dehydration, and cardiac arrhythmias.
- Beta-blockers decrease aerobic output by reducing the athlete's maximal heart rate; moreover, they can reduce the amount of time athletes can spend at submaximal exercise intensity by approximately 20% when used with cardioselective medications (e.g., atenolol, metoprolol, and nebivolol) and by approximately 40% with nonselective medications (e.g., propranolol, nadolol, carvedilol, and sotalol).

CHRONIC OBSTRUCTIVE PULMONARY DISEASE MEDICATIONS

Background

- Chronic obstructive pulmonary disease (COPD) affects approximately 7% of US adults and 10% of US adults aged ≥65 years; however, it is estimated to be actually higher because of underdiagnosis.
- COPD is the third leading cause of death in the United States.
  - The Global Initiative for Chronic Obstructive Lung Disease (GOLD) emphasizes both pharmacologic and nonpharmacologic treatments to control COPD.
  - Nonpharmacologic therapies include (1) smoking cessation, (2) reduction of other risk factors, (3) pneumococcal and influenza vaccinations for eligible patients, (4) oxygen therapy, and (5) pulmonary rehabilitation.
  - Pharmacologic therapy is typically added in a stepwise fashion based on the severity of the disease and may include anticholinergics, beta-2 agonists, and glucocorticoids.
- Goals for pharmacologic treatment:
  - Bronchodilation is necessary to increase exercise tolerance and decrease exertional dyspnea.
  - Long-term use of daily inhaled anticholinergic medication leads to improved inspiratory capacity, decreased thoracic gas volume, and improved health outcomes.

COPD Exacerbation Management

- Antibiotics are well supported for the treatment of acute infections and are indicated for increasing dyspnea, sputum production, or sputum purulence.
- Common pathogens in acute exacerbations include *Streptococcus pneumoniae*, *Haemophilus influenzae*, and *Moraxella catarrhalis*. Antibiotic selection may include amoxicillin, doxycycline, trimethoprim/sulfa methoxazole, cefuroxime, azithromycin, and clarithromycin.
- Macrolides and fluoroquinolones combined with statins increase the risk of QT prolongation; hence, it is recommended to hold statin treatment while taking these antibiotics.

Implications for Athletes

- Several medications used for COPD management have been defined as banned substances by governing bodies such as the World Anti-Doping Agency (WADA), the United States Anti-Doping Agency (USADA), the United States Olympics Committee (USOC), and the National Collegiate Athletic Association (NCAA). These include beta-2 agonists and glucocorticoids. Always check for in-season and out-of-season restrictions before initiating treatment with these medications.

ANTICOAGULANTS

Common Uses

- Venous thromboembolism (VTE) is a major cause of morbidity and mortality. Treatment for VTE is the same for athletes as for nonathletes, typically with anticoagulation and early mobilization.
- Athletes may have multiple risk factors for the development of a VTE, including orthopedic trauma, postinjury immobilization, frequent and prolonged travel, hemoconcentration after exercise, and polycythemia from altitude training or exogenous erythropoietin (EPO) use.
- Upper extremity deep venous thrombosis (UEDVT) has been well documented in overhead athletes, such as pitchers, and after heavy upper-body workouts.
- Other conditions requiring anticoagulation treatment include atrial fibrillation and pulmonary embolism.

Treatment

- Anticoagulation is the mainstay for VTE treatment. Use helps maintain collateral patency, reduces further thrombus growth, and reduces the risk of embolization.
- Common medications used to initiate treatment include subcutaneous low-molecular-weight heparin (LMWH), fondaparinux, or intravenous unfractionated heparin (UFH) and simultaneous initiation of a vitamin K antagonist (VKA) such as warfarin.
- Typically, LMWH, fondaparinux, or UFH is used for about 5 days and then discontinued when the patient's international normalized ratio (INR) is in the therapeutic range of 2.0–3.0 (target, 2.5) for 24 hours.
- Monotherapy with factor Xa inhibitors are an alternative for patients who wish to avoid monitoring; those proven effective in monotherapy include rivaroxaban and apixaban.
- Monotherapy with a direct thrombin inhibitor (e.g., dabigatran) also eliminates the need for specific INR monitoring.
- Treatment duration for a first-time provoked or unprovoked proximal DVT with a VKA or factor Xa/thrombin inhibitor should be at least 3 months. If the risk factor(s) for the DVT is transient but persistent at the end of 3 months, then anticoagulation should be continued until the risk factor(s) is resolved.
- For a first-time provoked or unprovoked distal DVT, 3 months of anticoagulation is typically adequate. Consultation with a thrombosis expert is recommended for athletes with recurrent DVT.

Return to Sport

- Athletes participating in contact/collision sports should be restricted from participation until their anticoagulation treatment is complete, or they are cleared for participation by a hematologist knowledgeable about anticoagulation in sport.
- Athletes participating in noncontact sports may return to sports after an informed discussion and an appropriate return-to-play protocol for their respective sports, unless that sport is suspected to be the cause of the VTE.
- Athletes should be instructed to report any recurrent symptoms consistent with a VTE and signs of internal bleeding, blood loss, or bruising.

Considerations in Athletes

- Combined use of anticoagulants and NSAID medications should be avoided. Athletes should be educated to avoid ibuprofen, naproxen, and other NSAIDs while actively using anticoagulant medications to reduce bleeding complications.

FLUOROQUINOLONE ANTIBIOTICS

Background

- Fluoroquinolones (FQs) are some of the most commonly prescribed antibiotics, and they are used to treat a broad spectrum of infections affecting the urinary, gastrointestinal (GI), and respiratory systems, bone, joints, and skin.
- FQs are used for their excellent GI absorption, tissue diffusion, and long half-life.

Mechanism of Action

- First- and second-generation FQs act by inhibiting DNA gyrase, and the newer-generation FQs inhibit topoisomerase IV, making it effective against anaerobes.

Medical Adverse Effects

- Most adverse effects from FQs are mild to moderate in severity and self-limiting.
- More serious adverse effects include *Clostridium difficile*–associated diarrhea, hemolytic uremic syndrome, hepatotoxicity, hypoglycemia, phototoxicity, and QT prolongation.

Musculoskeletal Adverse Effects

- FQs are known to negatively affect tendon, bone, muscle, and cartilage.
- In pediatric patients, FQs are typically avoided except in life-threatening situations because of irreversible cartilage damage reported in growing animals, as demonstrated by previous studies.
- Most commonly implicated second-generation medications in the descending order are pefloxacin, ofloxacin, norfloxacin, and ciprofloxacin.
- Over 100 cases of FQ-associated tendonitis and tendon rupture have been reported in the literature. Incidence of FQ tendinopathy is estimated as 0.14%–0.4%.
- The US Food and Drug Administration (FDA) issued a warning for FQ causing possible tendonitis in 1996 and then placed a boxed warning on FQs in 2008 for associated tendonitis.
- The risk of tendon rupture appears to be within the first month after FQ use in patients older than 60 years and in patients taking oral corticosteroids.
- Proposed mechanisms by which FQs negatively affect tendons are as follows:
  - FQs are shown to stimulate matrix-degrading protease activity in fibroblasts, thereby inhibiting cell proliferation and matrix ground substance synthesis.
  - FQs chelate cations like magnesium. Cations are used by integrins and transmembrane proteins for structural stability; hence, chelation of cations may weaken the cell and thus the tendon.
  - FQs stimulate oxygen radical production.

Recommendations for Use in Athletes

- Hall et al. (2011) proposed guidelines for the use of FQs in athletes:
  - Avoid FQs if possible.
  - Inform the athlete's care team if FQs are prescribed.
  - Do not prescribe oral or injectable corticosteroids simultaneously.
  - Consider prescribing magnesium with FQs.
  - Alter training regimens while on FQs, followed by a graded return to activity.
  - Stop athletic activity at the onset of symptoms.
  - Monitor the athlete closely for 1 month after completion of treatment.

CHEMOTHERAPEUTIC AGENTS

Background

- Some athletes are survivors of various types of adult or childhood cancers.

- Several chemotherapeutic agents have unfavorable side effect profiles that affect the ability to exercise after a malignancy is treated.

Drugs With Potential to Cause Peripheral Neuropathy

- Vincristine
- Vinblastine
- Cisplatin
- Paclitaxel
- Thalidomide
- These drugs are used to treat breast cancer, multiple myeloma, rhabdomyosarcoma, leukemia, lymphomas, ovarian cancer, non–small cell lung cancer, bladder cancer, and testicular cancer.
- Signs and symptoms include peripheral numbness, tingling, pain, and loss of reflexes.
- Dose reduction at the time of symptom onset (if possible) may prevent progression.
- Risk factors for the development of peripheral neuropathy include higher medication doses and co-treatment with other chemotherapeutic agents known to cause neuropathy.

Drugs With Potential to Cause Pulmonary Toxicity

- Bleomycin
- Carmustine
- Methotrexate
- Cyclophosphamide
- These medications are used to treat a variety of cancers, including head and neck squamous cell cancers; leukemia; lymphoma; brain tumor; multiple myeloma; and testicular, lung, breast, and ovarian cancers.
- Pneumonitis progressing to pulmonary fibrosis is a known complication with these drugs. Late-onset symptoms (>6 months after treatment onset) have a poorer prognosis than early-onset symptoms.
- Signs and symptoms of pulmonary toxicity include fatigue, exercise intolerance, dry cough, dyspnea, and wheezing.
- Risk factors for the development of pulmonary toxicity related to chemotherapeutic agents include older age (>70 years), combination treatments, radiation therapy to the chest wall, and history of lung disease.

Drugs With Potential to Cause Cardiac Toxicity

- Anthracycline drugs, including doxorubicin, daunorubicin, epirubicin, idarubicin, and mitoxantrone
  - Used to treat multiple cancers, including leukemia; lymphoma; bone sarcomas; and breast, ovarian, and prostate cancers
  - The most severe myocardial toxicity associated with anthracycline drugs is potentially fatal congestive heart failure, which can manifest either during therapy or months to years after treatment discontinuation.
  - Before initiating anthracycline drugs, guidelines recommend completing a full history and physical examination, obtaining baseline electrocardiogram (ECG), and evaluating baseline left ventricular ejection fraction (LVEF) with echocardiogram, multigated acquisition scan (MUGA), or cardiac magnetic resonance imaging (MRI).
- Cyclophosphamide
  - Various cardiac toxicities have been reported, including myocarditis, pericardial effusion resulting in tamponade, and potentially fatal congestive heart failure. Cardiotoxicity appears to be dose dependent.
  - Risk factors for chemotherapy-related cardiotoxicity include older age, combination therapy, history of cardiac disease, and history of radiation therapy to the chest wall.
  - Presenting symptoms include exercise intolerance, palpitations, tachycardia, dyspnea, fatigue, cough, and edema.

HIV MEDICATIONS

Significant advances in antiretroviral therapy have led to improved life expectancy among those infected with HIV; thus, more chronic diseases are presenting in an aging HIV population. Sports medicine physicians need to be aware of interactions with antiretroviral medications and commonly used drugs in sports medicine.

Cobicistat

- A pharmacokinetic booster; increases the action of other antiretroviral medications; and is a powerful inhibitor of cytochrome P450 3A enzymes, including CYP3A4.

Protease Inhibitors

- Commonly used protease inhibitors (PIs) include atazanavir, darunavir, fosamprenavir, indinavir, lopinavir/ritonavir, nelfinavir, saquinavir, and tipranavir, and these are frequently included in combination preparations.
- Mechanism of action: prevent viral replication by selectively binding to viral proteases.
- Metabolism of PIs is through the cytochrome P450 system, particularly CYP3A4. Co-administration of drugs also metabolized through CYP3A4 increases serum concentration of both substances.
- Side effects:
  - GI symptoms: nausea, vomiting, and diarrhea
  - Metabolic complications: dyslipidemia, hyperglycemia, glucose intolerance, and type 2 diabetes mellitus
  - Co-administration of PIs or cobicistat with steroid medications, even injections, can cause steroid excess, adrenal insufficiency, and adrenal crisis. Disruption of the hypothalamic-pituitary-adrenal (HPA) axis has been shown with oral, inhaled, intranasal, and injected corticosteroids.
  - Risk of HPA dysfunction has been shown to be higher in cobicistat or PI-treated patients who are older and who have received more than one steroid injection in a 6-month period.
  - Onset of symptoms is typically 30–90 days after steroid administration.
  - Recommendations:
    - Avoid corticosteroid injections in HIV patients on cobicistat or PIs in favor of alternative management strategies where possible.
    - Consult the patient's HIV specialist before administering corticosteroids.
    - After steroid administration, monitor the patient for signs/symptoms of steroid excess for up to 90 days.

RECOMMENDED READINGS

Available online.

9 SPORTS PHARMACOLOGY OF PSYCHIATRY AND BEHAVIORAL MEDICINE

Stephen R. Paul • Bevila John-Daniel • Bruce Helming

INTRODUCTION

- Optimal treatment is determined through a collaborative approach, including team physicians, psychologists, psychiatrists, athletic trainers, academic advisors, coaches, teammates, parents, and administrative staff. More institutions are promoting an integrative approach to mental health and well-being using a wide variety of interventions:
  - Self-care: exercise, sleep, nutrition
  - Social connections: informal groups, team activities, interest-based communities
  - Online or self-directed tools: mental health apps, life hacks, relaxation, mindfulness
  - Group or support sessions: peer- or mentor-based, group counseling, life coaching
  - Individualized mental healthcare: counseling, medications, intensive outpatient or inpatient programs and reassess care plans frequently
- Nonprescription therapies shown to be helpful:
  - Psychotherapy
  - Over-the-counter herbal and dietary supplements
  - Light therapy (seasonal affective disorder)
  - Electroconvulsive therapy (ECT) (treatment-resistant depression, mania, or psychosis)
- Athletes often self-treat their conditions with:
  - Overtraining
  - Avoidance
  - Self-help information
  - Self-medication with over-the-counter medications, alcohol, and illicit drugs
- Treatment with medications requires evaluation and monitoring:
  - Accurate diagnosis and identifying existing comorbidities
  - Suicidal ideation, self-harm, risk of harm to others, other safety concerns
  - Side effects and both positive and negative effects on school/work/sport performance
  - Efficacy and compliance
  - Attention to potential side effects that may affect athletic performance:
    - Daytime sedation
    - Orthostasis
    - Tremors
    - Arrhythmias
    - Nausea
    - Weight or appetite changes
- Table 9.1 lists syndromes associated with the medications reviewed:
  - Neuroleptic malignant syndrome (NMS), serotonin syndrome (SS), and extrapyramidal symptoms (EPS)
- Use caution with medication selection in athletes, pediatric, pregnant, potentially pregnant, or geriatric patients

TREATMENT FOR MAJOR DEPRESSIVE DISORDER (MDD)

- Table 9.2 summarizes antidepressant classifications and adverse effects.
- Psychotherapy alone is effective for mild depression. For moderate to severe mood disorders, a combination of psychotherapy and pharmacologic treatment provides a better outcome.
- Second-generation antidepressants include selective serotonin reuptake inhibitors (SSRIs), serotonin–norepinephrine reuptake inhibitors (SNRIs), and other medications that target neurotransmitters with similar mechanisms of action.
- Pharmacologic treatment is better than placebo in primary care practice settings (53% vs. 40%).
- Second-generation antidepressants have similar efficacy and response rates (60%), with primary differences in their respective side-effect profiles.
- Insufficient evidence to evaluate the comparative risk of suicidal thoughts and behaviors or rare but severe adverse events, such as seizures, cardiovascular events, hyponatremia, hepatotoxicity, and SS.
- Treatment is administered in phases:
  - Acute phase: 4–8 weeks needed for initial therapy with close monitoring.
  - Continuation phase: continue to monitor, treat for 4–9 months for an acute episode.
  - Maintenance phase: continue to reduce the risk of relapse (greater if history of MDD or chronic MDD).
  - Discontinuation of treatment: taper over several days to weeks, choose optimal time of low stressors/risks or high outside support. Some patients experience discontinuation symptoms that mimic a depressive episode, and adjustment of the taper may be necessary.
- If family history of previous successful antidepressant, consider that agent first.
- Start with an SSRI or bupropion.
- If failure with one SSRI agent occurs, consider another SSRI.
- If failure with two SSRIs, try an SNRI or another class of antidepressant.
- If partial response, optimize or augment treatment with a different class of antidepressant.
- Patients with associated insomnia, SSRIs have similar effectiveness (trazodone as an adjunct is beneficial with insomnia).
- Fluoxetine and bupropion are well tolerated in athletes.
- Tricyclic antidepressants (TCAs), particularly imipramine and clomipramine, have reasonable efficacy, but adverse effects limit their use.
- The only US Food and Drug Administration (FDA)–approved medications for adolescents are fluoxetine and escitalopram.

The Black Box Warning

- Use of antidepressants in young patients under the age of 25 years should balance the risk of suicidal behavior and attempts along with the clinical need. Important considerations with the black box warning are:
  - Mental health disease without treatment carries inherent risks of suicide
  - It is important to monitor the patient frequently for their symptoms and response to medication in the first weeks of treatment

TREATMENT FOR BIPOLAR DISORDER

- Table 9.3 lists common medications used in bipolar disorder.
- Bipolar disorder is often managed by or in consultation with a psychiatrist. Knowledge of treatment modalities may be helpful for the primary care physician, particularly to help stabilize patients waiting to consult with a psychiatrist.

Table 9.1 SYNDROMES ASSOCIATED WITH MEDICATIONS USED FOR PSYCHIATRIC DISORDERS

Serotonin Syndrome (SS)	
(Italics distinguish from neuroleptic malignant syndrome)	Potentially fatal, caused by a net increase in serotonin Occurs *rapidly* after medication change (usually within 24 hours) **Symptoms:** anxiety, agitation, disorientation, and delirium; autonomic (dilated pupils, tachycardia, hypertension, hyperthermia, diaphoresis, vomiting, and diarrhea); and neuromuscular (*hyperrigidity*, *myoclonus*, *hyperreflexia*, *tremor*, akathisia, *ataxia*, and *shivering*) **Treatment:** discontinue serotonergic drugs; supportive management with intravenous fluids, oxygen, blood pressure control, benzodiazepine to control agitation, and cyproheptadine (if other treatments fail)
Neuroleptic Malignant Syndrome (NMS) (Italics distinguish from serotonin syndrome)	May be a life-threatening emergency *Often develops over days* **Symptoms:** mental status changes (confusion, agitated delirium, mutism, and catatonic); muscular *rigidity (lead-pipe rigidity/cogwheeling), bradyreflexia*, hyperthermia, tremor, diaphoresis, tachycardia, and labile blood pressure **Treatment:** hospitalization; discontinue offending agent; consider benzodiazepines, dantrolene, bromocriptine, or amantadine and supportive care
Extrapyramidal Symptoms (EPS)	**Range of movement disorders:** dystonia (muscular spasms of neck, jaw, and back), akathisia (restlessness, nervousness, and anxiety), parkinsonism (rigidity, tremor, bradykinesia, shuffling gait, and masked facies), and tardive dyskinesia (involuntary muscle movements of distal extremities and face) **Treatment:** consider anticholinergic drugs, beta-blockers, benzodiazepines, and pramipexole

- Treatment guidelines include:
  - Adjunct therapies (e.g., cognitive behavioral therapy [CBT], dialectical behavior therapy [DBT])
  - Educate caregivers about early warning signs and support
- Treatment protocol depends on presenting symptoms (mania, hypomania, mixed state, depression, or maintenance), comorbidities, adverse effects, whether the patient (or a family member) has successfully been treated for bipolar disorder before, and the cost of medication
- Recovery rates improved with a combination of pharmacology and psychotherapy

Mania/Hypomania/Mixed States

- Acute mania with risk of harm to self or others initially treated with hospitalization and psychiatric consultation
- Severe mania is often treated with lithium/valproate and augmentation with an antipsychotic (haloperidol, olanzapine, quetiapine, or risperidone)
- Severe mania may not respond to single-drug therapy
- ECT is considered for severe mania nonresponsive to multidrug therapy
- If abrupt mood elevation with antidepressants, taper and discontinue and adjust the dose of the mood stabilizer/antipsychotic
- Avoid alcohol and drug abuse, caffeine, and nicotine

Bipolar Depression

- Use of antidepressants as monotherapy increases the risk of activating a manic spell
- Consider lithium or lamotrigine as first-line therapy; other options include lurasidone, quetiapine, aripiprazole, or olanzapine-fluoxetine combination
- New-onset, untreated bipolar depression: consider lurasidone, quetiapine, or lamotrigine as monotherapy or start with olanzapine combined with fluoxetine
- With a sleep disturbance, avoid using trazodone, which can induce mania (consider using benzodiazepines)
- If associated psychosis, add an antipsychotic

TREATMENT OF ANXIETY DISORDERS

- Treatment approach for anxiety is similar to depression (see Table 9.2)
- Obsessive-compulsive disorder (OCD) may need higher doses of SSRIs
- Athletes with anxiety disorders often welcome treatment; their symptoms may affect their athletic performance and participation
- Several anxiety disorders will respond to counseling, but this may take time
- CBT is the primary nonpharmacologic approach
- Initiate treatment with SSRI
- Second-generation antidepressants have similar efficacy (60%) in the treatment of anxiety and depression
- A small study of sport psychiatrists found buspirone was preferred for treatment in athletes but was considered second-line therapy when compared with SSRIs
- Consider benzodiazepines as a "short bridge" during acute onset pending treatment with SSRI; avoid or minimize benzodiazepine use in season due to side effects: sleepiness, balance and coordination problems, and potential for abuse

TREATMENT OF ATTENTION DEFICIT/ HYPERACTIVITY DISORDER

- Stimulant medications are used as first-line therapy for attention deficit/hyperactivity disorder (ADD/ADHD) in most cases and are similarly effective and safe in both children and adults (Table 9.4 provides information on stimulant medications).
- **Stimulant medications may be banned, prohibited in competition, or require specific documentation or formal permission from governing bodies; therefore, review the rules for athletic participation.**
- Before initiating treatment, assess for the presence of cardiac disease and risk of abuse.
- Dosing should be titrated (can be done quickly) to maximize response; increase the dose over 3- to 7-day intervals.
- Consider the goal of maximum tolerable dose rather than minimum effective dose (an increased dose may yield additional benefits).

Table 9.2 MEDICATIONS USED FOR DEPRESSION AND/OR ANXIETY

Name (Brand)	Mechanism, Adverse Effects (AEs), and Comments
Selective Serotonin Reuptake Inhibitor (SSRI)	Sexual dysfunction, drowsiness, weight gain, insomnia, anxiety, dizziness, headache, dry mouth, blurred vision, rash, itching, tremor, constipation, and stomach upset Caution with NSAIDs: gastrointestinal bleeding and serotonin syndrome
Citalopram (Celexa)	Some antihistamine effect
Escitalopram (Lexapro)	Best tolerated, fewest drug interactions
Fluoxetine (Prozac)	Activating properties (avoid with insomnia, anxiety) Lowest rate of withdrawal symptoms Long half-life
Paroxetine (Paxil)	Calming, good for anxiety
Paroxetine CR (Paxil CR)	Highest rate of withdrawal symptoms Highest rate of sexual AEs (16%)
Sertraline (Zoloft)	Activating properties Diarrhea
Serotonin Noradrenergic Reuptake Inhibitor (SNRI)	Not interchangeable, have different levels of NE and 5HT action Common: nausea, somnolence, dry mouth; dizziness, constipation, weakness; blurred vision, sweating
Desvenlafaxine (Pristiq)	Hypertension may occur during titration Withdrawal reaction Headache, anxiety, insomnia, and diarrhea
Duloxetine (Cymbalta)	Good for depression with chronic pain Less risk of hypertension 67% higher discontinuation due to AEs Start twice daily then switch to daily
Levomilnacipran (Fetzima)	Enantiomer of milnacipran Most noradrenergic action of SNRIs
Venlafaxine (Effexor)	First-line SNRI, most often prescribed Hypertension may occur during titration AE: 52% higher (nausea, vomiting), causing 40% higher risk of discontinuation, high rate of withdrawal symptoms XR form lower in AE
Serotonin Antagonist and Reuptake Inhibitor (SARI)	Mechanism: antagonize serotonin receptor and inhibit reuptake of serotonin, norepinephrine, or dopamine
Trazodone (Desyrel, Oleptro)	Priapism Lower dose increases somnolence (may improve sleep)
Vilazodone (Viibryd)	SSRI and 5HT1A partial agonist action Taken with food improves therapeutic level
Other	
Mirtazapine (Remeron, Remeron SolTab)	Mechanism: noradrenergic and specific serotonergic antidepressant (NaSSA), some alpha-adrenergic and serotonergic properties Weight gain (after 6–8 weeks), sedation Faster onset of action Sedation decreases with increased dose
Bupropion (Wellbutrin)	Mechanism: norepinephrine and dopamine reuptake inhibitor (NDRI), is both an active drug and precursor Not associated with weight gain or sexual dysfunction Activating and energizing properties Regular, SR, and XL preparations available
Buspirone	Mechanism: selective serotonin 5HT1A receptor agonist and dopamine agonist/antagonist May help treat anxiety if unable to tolerate SSRIs or SNRIs Decreased efficacy if on long-term benzodiazepine Multiple dosing may be a drawback
Vortioxetine (Trintellix)	SSRI; 5HT1A agonist; 5HT1B partial agonist action; and antagonistic action on 5HT3A, 5HT1D, and 5HT7 receptors
Brexanolone (Zulresso)	GABA-A modulator for postpartum depression Used as an infusion in hospital settings
Esketamine (Spravato)	NMDA receptor antagonist delivered IV and intranasally For treatment-resistant depression
Tricyclic Antidepressants (TCAs) (e.g., amitriptyline, nortriptyline, and clomipramine)	Dangerous and lethal in overdose (QT prolongation leading to arrhythmias) Inhibits reuptake of primarily serotonin and norepinephrine Rarely used because of side effects
Monoamine Oxidase Inhibitors (MAOI)	Mild anticholinergic Sedation, agitation, GI effects, weight gain, and suppressed REM sleep Rarely used because of dietary restrictions, drug interactions, and AEs Risk of SS

Table 9.2 MEDICATIONS USED FOR DEPRESSION AND/OR ANXIETY—cont'd

Name (Brand)	Mechanism, Adverse Effects (AEs), and Comments
Benzodiazepines (e.g., alprazolam, lorazepam, clonazepam, and diazepam)	Sedation, nausea, syndrome of inappropriate antidiuretic hormone secretion, blood dyscrasia, hyponatremia, anterograde amnesia, agitation, depression, cognitive impairment, hyponatremia, and extrapyramidal syndrome Used in combination in acute settings of mania/hypomania, particularly to reduce agitation in patients with acute mania Risk of tolerance and addiction Monitor complete blood count and liver function for long-term use Contraindicated in patients with myasthenia gravis or acute narrow-angle glaucoma Caution in patients with substance abuse

Anticholinergic: orthostatic hypotension, blurred vision, dizziness, urinary retention, constipation, dryness, abnormal heart rhythm.

- Short- and long-acting medications are similarly effective; consider once-daily dosing for convenience and cost-effectiveness.
- Flexibility in dose/formulations allows individualization to symptoms and schedule.
- No need for tapering to discontinue.
- In children, approximately 75% will respond to the first medication and 90%–95% will respond to the second, although the response can be idiosyncratic.
- Monitor: medication use, side effects, response to medication, mood, weight, heart rate, and blood pressure.
- Frequent side effects include appetite loss, weight loss, anxiety, irritability, and insomnia. May induce or exacerbate mania or psychosis in affected individuals.
- In children, abdominal symptoms and a small reduction in height velocity may occur (total height loss of 1–2 cm).
- Medications also benefit sports and daily life, as well as academic/work environments; assess function in all realms.
- One-third will have a comorbid psychological diagnosis; screen for medical conditions causing similar symptoms (including substance abuse) and cardiac conditions.
- For coexisting depression, a combination of SSRIs and stimulants is safe and effective; consider single-agent treatment with bupropion.
- For coexisting anxiety, stimulants are indicated; consider in combination with SSRIs and/or CBT.
- Incidence of substance abuse not increased with use of stimulant medications.
- Diversion and abuse may be less likely with longer-acting agents.

PHARMACOLOGIC TREATMENT OF EATING DISORDERS

- Eating disorders are commonly associated with other psychiatric disorders such as anxiety, depression, obsessive-compulsive and impulse control disorders, substance abuse, and trauma.
- Treatment is challenging and involves a multidisciplinary approach with psychosocial intervention and medications.
- Overall, a combination of CBT and medication was found to be superior to medication alone.

Anorexia Nervosa

- Individuals who are severely underweight and medically compromised are best served in a more intensive program, including hospitalization or an intensive outpatient program, where the focus is on weight restoration, psychotherapy, and nutritional counseling.
- Medications may be used as an adjunct (no clear consensus of efficacy); address comorbidities such as depression and anxiety.
- SSRIs (see Table 9.2) may help manage comorbid psychiatric disorders.

Bulimia Nervosa

- SSRIs (see Table 9.2) are the first-line treatment.
- Fluoxetine is the only FDA-approved medication.
- Lisdexamfetamine is helpful for binge eating disorder (note: a stimulant may need a therapeutic use exemption [TUE] with restricted stimulants in some sports).

TREATMENT OF INSOMNIA

- Seven to nine hours of sleep is ideal for adolescents and young adults; less than 7 hours is considered insufficient.
- Benefits of good sleep include improved memory and performance.
- Disturbed sleep can lower life expectancy and contribute to other conditions, such as obesity, diabetes, metabolic syndrome, cancer, heart disease, stroke, dementia, depression, substance abuse, and increased rates of suicide.
- Poor sleep adversely affects the immune system, causing weight gain and premature aging of the skin.
- Many conditions, diseases, and environments can cause insomnia (Table 9.5; see Chapter 24: "Travel Considerations for the Athlete and Sports Medical Team").
- Rule out and treat obstructive sleep apnea.
- Treatment includes psychological and behavioral treatments.
- Sleep hygiene education (Box 9.1) and relaxation therapy are preferred over medications.
- CBT is effective in treating insomnia (treatment of choice), especially in complex conditions.
- If nonpharmacologic treatments fail to improve insomnia, medications could be considered after medical evaluation, ruling out other contributing conditions and to ensure there are no contraindications for use due to side effects, which can impair performance and safety.
- Medications are considered a temporary bridge to long-term behavioral and psychological treatments (Table 9.6).
- First-line drugs (especially in the elderly) include control-release melatonin and doxepin. Second-line therapy includes zolpidem, zaleplon, and eszopiclone.
- **Benzodiazepines are no longer recommended because of their potential for abuse.**
- Antihistamines, antidepressants, and atypical antipsychotics should be reserved for treating insomnia associated with other conditions (e.g., depression).

RECOMMENDED READINGS

Available online.

Table 9.3 MEDICATIONS USED FOR BIPOLAR DISORDER

Medication	Adverse Effects (AEs) and Comments
Antidepressants (see Table 9.2)	Concern with using antidepressants as monotherapy for the risk of converting to manic state
Other (Mood Stabilizer) Lithium	Excessive thirst, polyuria, sedation, tremor, nausea, loose stools, cognitive effects, weight gain, hypothyroidism, and diabetes insipidus, renal disease, (avoid NSAIDs, ACE inhibitors and maintain hydration status) Use: mania, depression Before initiation, check/monitor: BMI, electrolytes, estimated glomerular filtration rate, thyroid, complete blood count, and consider ECG if risk factors for cardiovascular disease present Monitor serum lithium levels 1–2 times in the first week and 1 week after dose change Toxicity is dose dependent **Compared with valproate or carbamazepine, lithium lowers the risk of suicide** Protective against dementia
Typical Antipsychotics (First-Generation Antipsychotics) (e.g., haloperidol and Thorazine)	**Increased risk of dry mouth, sedation, EPS, NMS and tardive dyskinesia, restlessness, anxiety, headache, weight gain, insomnia, and depression** **Use: psychosis, mania** **Increase risk of cerebrovascular accident in older patients with dementia** **Rarely used since emergence of second-generation antipsychotics**
Atypical Antipsychotics (Second-Generation Antipsychotics)	EPS and tardive dyskinesia (but lower risk than typical antipsychotics), anticholinergic symptoms, sedation, metabolic effects (weight gain, hyperglycemia, dyslipidemia, and hyperprolactinemia), cardiac effects, hypotension, cataracts, and sexual dysfunction Rare: NMS, seizures, agranulocytosis, and hypersensitivity reactions Before initiation: document, then monitor weight/BMI, vitals, lipid profile, fasting glucose, complete blood count, and consider ECG if cardiovascular risk factors are noted Target doses often achieved within first week Caution in obese patients
Aripiprazole (Abilify)	Use: mania, mixed, psychosis, augmentation for bipolar depression Used as monotherapy or combination with lithium or valproate Used in adults and adolescents (aged 10–17 years)
Olanzapine (Zyprexa)	Increased risk: weight gain, glucose intolerance, and diabetes more than other agents Used in adults and adolescents (aged 13–17 years) for mania/mixed, in adults only for depression Used for agitation in bipolar mania
Olanzapine With Fluoxetine Combination (Symbyax)	Used in adults with depressive symptoms Effective in preventing manic relapse
Quetiapine (Seroquel)	Use: mania, mixed, depression, psychosis Used in adult and adolescents (aged 10–17 years) for acute mania Superior to monotherapy for maintenance if used with lithium or valproate
Risperidone (Risperdal)	Monitor prolactin levels Adults and adolescents (aged 10–17 years) can be used as short-term therapy for acute manic or mixed states
Asenapine (Saphris)	D2 and 5HT2A receptor antagonist with low anticholinergic activity Do not swallow. Avoid food or drink for 10 min after taking
Iloperidone (Fanapt)	D2 and 5HT2a receptor antagonist Twice-daily dosing with need for titration
Cariprazine (Vraylar)	D2, D3 and 5HT1A receptor partial agonist, 5HT2A receptor antagonist
Lumateperone (Caplyta)	Lumateperone is a serotonin, dopamine, and glutamate modulator with the potential to treat schizophrenia with few adverse effects
Paliperidone (Invega)	D2 and 5HT2A receptor antagonist Patients may see intact capsules in stools but are empty pills (OROS delivery system)
Brexpiprazole (Rexulti)	D2 and 5HT1A receptor partial agonist and serotonin 5HT2A receptor antagonist Used also as an adjunct for depression
Anticonvulsants	Monitor levels, check complete blood count and liver function
Valproic Acid (Depakene, Divalproex, Depakote, Stavzor)	Tremor, sedation, weight gain, nausea, diarrhea, alopecia, leukopenia, increase in liver enzymes, liver failure, pancreatitis, and PCOS, caution with liver disease Use: mania, depression, mixed Not recommended for women of childbearing potential More effective than lithium for mixed states
Lamotrigine (Lamictal)	Anticholinergic, tremor, somnolence, headache, nausea, rash, (reduced risk slow titration), toxic epidermal necrolysis, leukopenia, thrombocytopenia, pancytopenia, aseptic meningitis Use: mania, depression Acceptable for pregnancy with monitoring **Black box warning for increased risk of Stevens–Johnson syndrome**

EPS, Extrapyramidal symptoms; *NMS,* neuroleptic malignant syndrome.

Table 9.4 MEDICATIONS USED FOR ADHD

Stimulant Medications	Onset (Minutes)
Long-Acting	
Methylphenidate (Adhansia XR, Aptensio XR, Concerta, Cotempla XR-ODT, Daytrana, Jornay PM (Metadate CD, QuilliChew ER, Quillivant XR, Ritalin LA)	30–90 minutes: capsule, tablet 60–270 minutes: patch
Dextroamphetamine/amphetamine (Adderall XR, Mydayis)	20–60 minutes
Dexmethylphenidate (Focalin XR)	30–60 minutes
Lisdexamfetamine (Vyvanse)	60–120 minutes
Intermediate-Acting	
Methylphenidate (Ritalin, Metadate ER, Methylin ER)	60–180 minutes
Dextroamphetamine (Dexedrine)	60–90 minutes
Short-Acting	
Methylphenidate (Ritalin, Methylin) Dexmethylphenidate (Focalin) Dextroamphetamine/amphetamine (Adderall) Dextroamphetamine (Zenzedi, ProCentra)	20–60 minutes
Selective Norepinephrine Reuptake Inhibitor	Nonstimulant, not restricted for athletes and not subject to controlled substance restrictions Effect size smaller and onset of clinical response may be delayed (up to 4–8 weeks) Drowsiness, nausea, GI upset, decreased appetite
Atomoxetine (Strattera)	1–2 hours
Alpha-Adrenergic Agonists	Nonstimulant, used in pediatric patients 1–2 weeks to achieve clinical effect Somnolence and dry mouth
Guanfacine ER (Intuniv)	30–45 minutes
Clonidine (Kapvay)	30–60 minutes

Table 9.5 COMMON CAUSES OF INSOMNIA

Medical	Medications	Mood Disorders	Stimulants	Other
Chronic pain	Inhaled steroids	Anxiety	Alcohol	Circadian rhythm changes
Asthma	Antihistamines	Depression	Nicotine/tobacco	Poor sleeping environment
GERD	Beta-blockers	Stress	Caffeine	Erratic schedules
Obstructive sleep apnea	Alpha-blockers			Restless partner/child/pet in bed
Restless leg syndrome	Stimulants			Light, screens in bed

BOX 9.1 TEN WAYS TO IMPROVE SLEEP (SLEEP HYGIENE)

1. Keep a regular schedule
2. Get natural daylight during the day, and avoid light at night
3. Exercise regularly, but not too late at night
4. Nap during the day, keep less than 30 minutes and not late in the day
5. Avoid going to bed worried, upset, preoccupied, or angry
6. Limit excessive liquids or food late in the evening
7. Avoid caffeine, nicotine, or alcohol at night
8. Put away screens/electronic devices before going to bed and do not take them to bed
9. Keep your bedroom cool, dark, and comfortable
10. Turn away the clock (preset the alarm) do not look at it when in bed

Table 9.6 MEDICATIONS USED FOR INSOMNIA

Medication	Class Notes	Dose	Potential Side Effects
Melatonin	Supplement/hormone OTC First-line in elderly	2–3 mg before bedtime	Hypotension, gastrointestinal distress, insulin insensitivity
Ramelteon (prescribed, melatonin-like synthetic)	Melatonin receptor agonist	8 mg within 30 min of bedtime	N, D, F
Zaleplon (Sonata)	Nonbenzodiazepine hypnotic Second-line therapy	10 mg immediately before bedtime	Complex sleep-related behaviors (parasomnia), headache, N, D, risk for falls-elderly, *habit forming*
Zolpidem (Ambien, Intermezzo, Edluar)	Nonbenzodiazepine hypnotic Second-line therapy	Women 5 mg at bedtime Men 5–10 mg at bedtime	Same as above
Zolpidem (oral spray Zolpimist)	Nonbenzodiazepine hypnotic Second-line therapy	10 mg immediately before bedtime	Same as above
Eszopiclone (Lunesta)	Nonbenzodiazepine hypnotic Helps maintain sleep Second line therapy	1 mg immediately before bedtime	Same as above
Belsomra (Suvorexant)	Orexin (wakefulness neurotransmitter) receptor antagonist	10 mg within 30 min of bedtime	Daytime drowsiness, may have abnormal behavior and thinking, may worsen depression and suicidal ideation, parasomnia, hypnagogic hallucinations, headache
Doxepin (Silenor)	Antidepressant, tricyclic First-line in elderly	3–6 mg before bedtime	Dry mouth, constipation, N, D, confusion, hypotension, headache, sexual dysfunction, blurred vision, increased heart rate, urinary retention, confusion. Can exacerbate glaucoma, lower seizure threshold and is associated with arrhythmias in heart failure. Can be fatal in overdose.
*The following are **not** considered first-line therapy for insomnia*			
Antihistamines Diphenhydramine (Benadryl) 25–50 mg 30 min before bedtime Hydroxyzine (Atarax) 50–100 mg 30 min before bedtime Doxylamine (Unisom) 25 mg 30 min before bedtime			Dry mouth, constipation, urinary retention, increased heart rate, confusion
Antidepressant, Tricyclic (TCA) Amitriptyline (Elavil) 25–100 mg at bedtime Nortriptyline (Pamelor) 25–50 mg at bedtime Trimipramine (Surmontil) 50 mg at bedtime			Dry mouth, constipation, N, D, confusion, hypotension, headache, vision changes, priapism, sexual dysfunction, blurred vision, increased heart rate, urinary retention, confusion. Can exacerbate glaucoma, lower seizure threshold and is associated with arrhythmias in heart failure. Can be fatal in overdose.
Antidepressant, serotonin modulator Trazodone (Desyrel) 25–200 mg at bedtime			Same as above
The following are rarely used and if used should be used with caution			
Mirtazapine (Remeron)			Antidepressant, atypical, (unknown mechanism of action), used for insomnia with depression
Gabapentin (Neurontin)			Anticonvulsant (and neuropathic pain), GABA analog
Quetiapine (Seroquel)			Atypical antipsychotic
Benzodiazepines			No longer recommended for insomnia

D, Dizziness; *F*, fatigue; *N*, nausea.

SECTION II

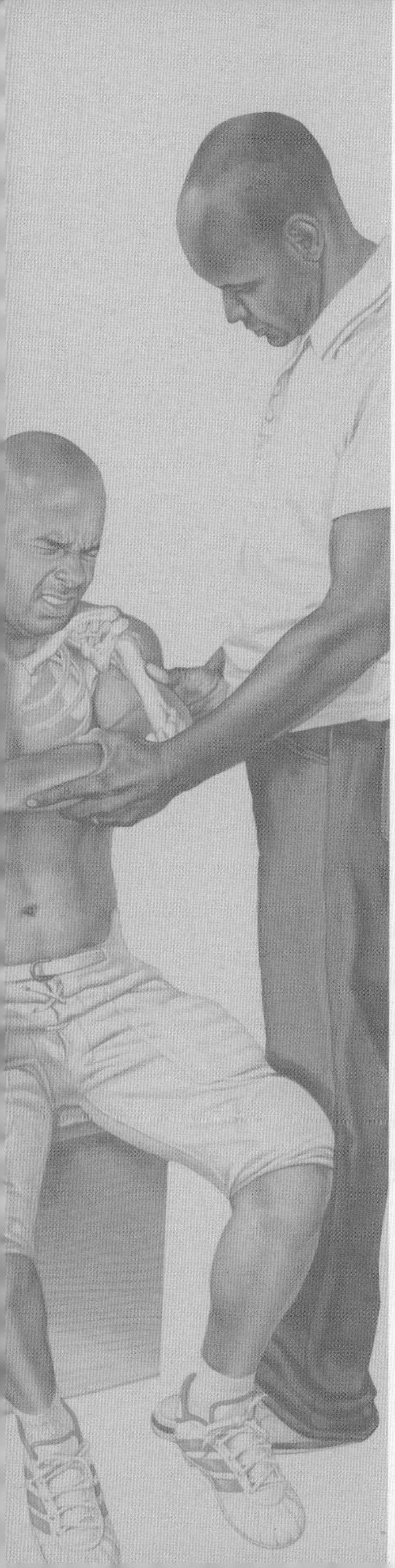

Special Considerations for Athlete Populations

THE PEDIATRIC ATHLETE

10

Holly J. Benjamin • David J. Jewison

GENERAL PRINCIPLES

- A pediatric athlete can be any child or adolescent usually under the age of 18 years who participates regularly in sports activities.
- Understanding physical and physiologic differences between pediatric and adult patients aids in the prompt recognition and management of most medical and orthopedic conditions affecting a pediatric athlete.
- Activity type, skill level, and motivation for sports participation greatly vary at different ages and levels of maturity; therefore, it is best to understand young athletes in the context of their chronologic age, developmental stage, and physical maturity, coupled with an assessment of the nature and level of sports participation.
- It is important to understand both the child's and parent's motivation for sports participation and to capitalize on opportunities to educate parents, athletes, and coaches on healthy athletic participation and sports safety.
- Sports specialization is defined as intense activity in only one sport throughout the year. Avoiding early sports specialization may decrease the risk of injury, overtraining, and burnout.
- The ultimate goal of youth sports participation should be the promotion of lifelong physical activity, pursuit of recreation, and enjoying the challenge of competition.
- Healthcare professionals face challenges at both ends of the physical activity spectrum: the sedentary obese child, who faces a lifetime of morbidity related to physical inactivity, and the highly competitive, overzealous, often anxious, and potentially undernourished young athlete are both at risk for a myriad of injuries associated with sedentary behaviors or excessive exercise. A successful pediatric athlete will lead a healthy, balanced lifestyle and integrate exercise, nutrition, and recreational pursuits with an adequate amount of rest and recovery.

MEDICAL CONCERNS OF THE PEDIATRIC ATHLETE

- Several conditions that affect pediatric athletes are similar to those that affect adult athletes. Examples include cardiac conditions (e.g., cardiac arrhythmias), pulmonary conditions (e.g., asthma), mental health conditions (e.g., eating disorders and stress/anxiety/depression), endocrine disorders (e.g., diabetes and obesity), renal conditions (e.g., polycystic kidney disease), and infectious diseases (e.g., community-acquired methicillin-resistant *Staphylococcus aureus* [CA-MRSA], HIV, mononucleosis, and coronavirus-19 [COVID-19]).
- Prompt recognition and management of these conditions may lead to safe and early return to sports.
- A preparticipation physical examination (PPPE) (refer to Chapter 3) is recommended for pediatric athletes before organized sports participation. It is usually a state-mandated legal requirement for participation in high school interscholastic athletics.
- The PPPE is a helpful tool for physicians to identify medical conditions that may affect participation in sports and physical activity.

EXERCISE AND THE PEDIATRIC ATHLETE

- According to 2018 guidelines from the US Department of Health and Human Services, children ages 6 to 17 years should engage in 60 minutes of physical activity every day, which should include 3 days per week of vigorous-intensity, muscle- and bone-strengthening activities. These guidelines also suggest that children ages 3 to 5 years should try to obtain 180 minutes of physical activity throughout each day.
- Suggestions to encourage physical activity:
  - Limit or reduce sedentary time (television, computer, video games, and phone) to 30 minutes/day outside of mandatory school computer time.
  - Find fun activities that children enjoy.
  - Incorporate parent role models.
  - Emphasize the social aspect of participating in team sports.
  - Promote the use of activity trackers (step counters, wireless trackers, wearables, etc.).
- There are numerous benefits of exercise in pediatric patients (Box 10.1).

Physicians, Patients, and Exercise

- The 2017 Youth Risk Behavior Survey from the Centers for Disease Control and Prevention (CDC) revealed that only 26.1% of high school–aged students reported levels of physical activity consistent with current guidelines for physical activity.
- Additionally, recent research has shown that only 23% of family physicians and only 33% of pediatricians were able to correctly identify physical activity guidelines for children aged 6–18.
- The activity prescription "MD FITT" is a useful tool for guiding and tracking physical activity (Table 10.1).

CHILDHOOD OBESITY

- Obesity is the most important health concern among children in the United States.
- The prevalence rate of obesity in children is 11%–22%, and it has doubled in the past 20 years.
- Childhood obesity is increasing at an epidemic rate, particularly in economically disadvantaged areas and minority populations.

Age Range: Preschool Through High School

- Preschoolers spend approximately 11% of their time in vigorous activities, 60% in sedentary activities, and an average of 3–5 hours/day watching television.
- Every hour of television is associated with a 2% increase in obesity risk.

Risks of Adult Obesity

- Fifty percent of children who are obese at the age of 6 years are likely to remain obese in adulthood.
- Seventy to 80% of children who are obese at the age of 10 years are likely to remain obese in adulthood.

BOX 10.1 COMMON BENEFITS OF PHYSICAL ACTIVITY IN CHILDREN AND ADOLESCENTS

Weight control
Lowers blood pressure
Raises high-density lipoprotein (HDL) or "good" cholesterol
Reduces risk of diabetes
Improves self-esteem

Table 10.1 DESCRIPTION OF "MD FITT" EXERCISE PRESCRIPTION

M–MODE	What type of activity (e.g., walking or biking)
D–DURATION	For how long does the patient exercise daily?
F–FREQUENCY	How often does the patient exercise (days/week)?
I–INTENSITY	How intense is the exercise (e.g., moderate)?
T–TIMELY FOLLOW-UP	How often the patient revisits the clinician
T–THERAPY	Are there any concerns of injury or side effects?

- Additional risk is associated with concurrent parental obesity: 23% of all deaths in the United States are associated with sedentary lifestyles that begin in childhood.

Body Mass Index (BMI) in Children

- BMI = [weight (kg)]/[height (m)^2]
- A child with a BMI in the 85th to 95th percentile is considered overweight and at risk of obesity.
- A child with a BMI in the 95th percentile and above is considered obese.
- Annual BMI calculation is recommended for children during routine and sports physical examinations and can be followed longitudinally. Pediatric growth charts based on age and gender include BMI and are available online (www.cdc.gov/growthcharts). Numerous electronic medical record (EMR) systems calculate BMI when height and weight measurements are entered.

Causes of Childhood Obesity

- Energy intake is routinely greater than energy expenditure.
- Endocrine, hormonal, and genetic syndromes can each cause or contribute to obesity in children.

Complications of Childhood Obesity

- Any and all organ systems in the body can be affected by childhood obesity: cardiac, orthopedic, endocrine, gastrointestinal, respiratory, and neurologic systems are among those most often affected.

Treatment Recommendations

- Assessment of energy intake and output, physical examination, and laboratory evaluation to exclude other causes of obesity, as well as providing nutritional and exercise education.
- Nutritional interventions include changes in advertising, healthy school lunches, and adequate and varied healthy food choices in the home environment.
- Exercise recommendations include increased recreational activities, organized sports participation, preservation of adequate physical education time in school, and decreased sedentary screen time (e.g., computer and television).
- A meta-analysis of 30 randomized controlled trials in children aged 5–17 years found that low-intensity, long-duration exercise coupled with resistance training was highly effective in altering and improving body composition.

GROWTH AND MATURATION AND THE YOUNG ATHLETE

- Concerns regarding potential negative effects of athletic competition on growth and maturation have existed for many years, particularly attributable to the trend of intense competition at younger ages.
  - The demands of sports require a certain level of physical and psychological maturity in order to participate. Feelings of insecurity, frustration, and failure may cause young athletes to quit because of burnout or inability to perform up to expectations.
  - While young athletes are struggling to master advanced sports-specific skills, their coaches may be less experienced and less educated in appropriate training techniques; these barriers can negatively affect a young athlete's enjoyment and participation in his or her sport(s).
- **A significant challenge for sports medicine healthcare providers** is the consideration of the development of the neurologic, cognitive, somatic, and psychological interdependent processes and the effects of each of these on the health and well-being of pediatric athletes.
  - An understanding of fundamental principles of normal child and adolescent growth and development is essential in providing quality healthcare for young athletes.
- Growth and maturation is a natural, fundamental, continuous process, with achievement of the same milestones in the same order.
  - The rate of progression varies greatly and seems predominantly genetically regulated.
  - Neuropsychological development often does not parallel physical development.
  - Growth refers to an increase in size of the body and its parts, including stature, body systems, and body composition.
  - Maturation refers to a biologically mature state of skeletal, sexual, and somatic development with variable timing and tempo.
  - Neurodevelopment is culturally mediated and is the acquisition and mastery of behavioral competence.
  - Quantitative milestones are easy to measure by the number of skills performed.
  - Qualitative milestones are harder to measure because they reflect mastery of specific skills.

Neurodevelopmental Domains

Motor: fine and gross motor, strength, and endurance
Visual: acuity, discrimination, and tracking
Cognitive: attention, alertness, memory, comprehension, and solving complex problems or simultaneously performing multiple tasks
Language: receptive and expressive
Auditory: hearing acuity and processing, sound discrimination, and auditory cues
Emotional and psychological: relationships with teammates and coaches and regulation of emotions
Motor: fine and gross, visual-spatial discrimination, temporal sequencing, proprioception, sports-specific motor adaptive skills, muscular strength and endurance, and reaction time

Motor Developmental Milestones in Various Age Groups

- Understanding developmental milestones from infancy through young adulthood is essential in successfully caring for the constantly growing pediatric athlete.
- It is difficult to "skip" major neuromuscular milestones during periods of growth; however, the rate at which young athletes progress is sometimes accelerated.
- Accelerated motor development can be problematic if the young athlete is not psychologically or emotionally ready to fully function at this new level of expectation and skill.
- Healthcare professionals should be familiar with the sequence of skill acquisition that is predictable among various young athletes.

- **Preschoolers (4–6 years)**
  - Ride bike without training wheels
  - Hop six times on one foot
  - Catch a small ball thrown from 10 feet
  - Run, gallop, and skip using alternating feet
  - Broad jump up to 3 feet
  - Throw a ball with a shift of their bodies at a target
  - Move from parallel play to interactive play with others
- **Middle childhood (6–11 years)**
  - Gender differences can be observed.
  - Girls excel at hopping, skipping, catching, and balance.
  - Boys excel at striking objects, jumping (vertical and long), kicking, and throwing and can run faster.

Implications for Sports Participation in Young Athletes

- Coach and parent reaction with appropriate feedback is crucial in sports development.
- Confidence, self-esteem, and body awareness are all developing.
- Young athletes should be taught to think "I'm learning and improving" rather than "I can or can't."

Gender Differences

- In preadolescents, there is little difference in strength, power, and endurance between boys and girls.
  - Girls are consistently more flexible.
  - Boys are consistently better throwers.
- Power and maximal oxygen uptake (VO_2 max) increase linearly with age until adolescence, when it accelerates. However, in adolescent boys, accelerated rate gains far exceed those seen in adolescent girls and are partly a result of increased muscle mass in such boys.

Neuropsychological and Emotional Readiness

- Peer relationships with teammates involve the ability to take turns, attend to the game, focus, and participate in teamwork.
- The coach–athlete relationship requires the ability to follow rules, understand strategies, and control emotions.

Implications for Organized Sports Participation

- Physical maturation is necessary to master sports-specific skills.
- Neurodevelopmental maturation allows simultaneous functional integration of multiple skills to meet the demands of the competition.
  - **Motor:** for example, a soccer player needs to simultaneously run and kick in a coordinated fashion
  - **Visual:** monitor for position of teammates and defenders
  - **Auditory:** process instructions from coaches
  - **Language:** communicate with teammates and coaches
  - **Cognitive:** problem-solving and implementing sports strategies
  - **Emotional:** possess the ability to process various emotions such as excitement, anxiety, elation of winning, and frustration of losing
- Athletes that are competing in sports at levels above their neurodevelopmental abilities will be more likely to experience negative feelings such as frustration, anger, and lower confidence and self-esteem. Moreover, they will be less likely to have fun and to enjoy the overall sports participation experience. Dropout as well as injury rates may be higher in these situations.

Psychological Concerns

- Following are the common mistakes made by parents that negatively influence young athletes:
  - Choosing sports participation based on what the parent wants and not what the child wants
  - Push their children to "overtrain"
  - Criticize the performance of the young athlete
  - Promote a "win-at-all-costs mentality"
  - Allow early sports specialization, often in the parent's sport of choice
  - Serve as parent-coaches who either favor or disfavor their own children
  - Lack of knowledge about common overuse injuries

Sports Safety

- The following modifications are appropriate for young, elementary school–aged participants:
  - Use smaller fields and courts and small-sided games (e.g., 6 vs. 6 instead of 11 vs. 11) to encourage participation, activity, and skill acquisition
  - Use size- and weight-appropriate equipment
  - Shorten duration of games and practice sessions
  - Adequate number and length of breaks with opportunities for hydration
  - Monitor environmental conditions
  - Establish emergency action plans (EAPs) that must be implemented for emergencies related to injury, illness, or environmental conditions
  - Additional time during sports participation dedicated for teaching and enforcing rules and safety
  - Promote equal playing time and rotate positions
  - Avoid score keeping and win-loss records; reinforce "fun" as the goal of sports participation

YOUTH STRENGTH TRAINING (ALSO SEE CHAPTER 15)

- Muscle strength development is an important topic with limited evidence-based information.
- Strength training is an important component of a young athlete's exercise regimen and should be included to increase performance, reduce obesity, and possibly reduce injury.
- Further research is needed to address the role of strength training in pediatric athletes.

Definitions

- *Strength training* is a broad term that is defined as the use of resistance methods to increase one's ability to exert or resist force. Machines, free weights, and/or a person's body weight can be used.
- Olympic-style *weightlifting* and *powerlifting* are competitive sports that contest maximum lifting ability.
  - Olympic-style *weightlifting* involves the clean-and-jerk and the snatch.
  - *Powerlifting* involves the squat, the bench press, and the dead lift.
- *Bodybuilding* is an esthetic sport that involves weight training but not competitive lifting.

How Much, How Soon?

- Following appropriate resistance techniques and safety can be safe and effective for preadolescents and adolescents.
- Children and adolescents should refrain from Olympic-style weightlifting, powerlifting, and bodybuilding until skeletally mature.
- It is important to note that several sports use intrinsic strength techniques to perform sports-specific exercises, such as the young gymnast who tumbles and vaults bearing his or her entire body weight on the hands and wrists.

Anatomy and Physiology: Training Effects on Strength

- Strength gains are a result of neuromuscular adaptation in preadolescents. Muscle hypertrophy is not seen in preadolescents but is evident during puberty.
- Effects of strength training on body composition can be evident at all ages and exert favorable effects on improving lean body mass, particularly in obese children.
- Increases in neuronal activation and intrinsic muscular adaptations and improvements in motor coordination (learning) seem to play vital roles in strength development during childhood.
- No long-term studies have been conducted on the effects of preseason resistance training on improved sports performance in children.
- It appears that strength gains made during training can be lost during periods of rest or "detraining." These must always be evaluated in the context of naturally occurring strength gains that are associated with normal growth and development.
- Good nutrition and age-specific activity guidelines should be followed. Strength training has no known negative effects on growth.

Risk Factors for Injury

- The greatest injury risk to children who perform strength training is lack of appropriate supervision.
- Other risks include inappropriate technique, inappropriately sized equipment, or inappropriate amounts of weight and repetitions.
  - Common acute injuries in weight training include fractures and muscle–tendon injuries.
  - Overuse injuries include sprains, strains, and growth plate injuries. Injuries to the spine and shoulders are most common.
  - No cases of growth plate fractures have been reported under appropriately supervised settings.

Guidelines for Strength-Training Programs

- Program design considerations should include education on appropriate techniques, progression, function, and fun.
- Strength training should be incorporated into the child's exercise program with aerobic conditioning, flexibility, and sports participation.
- The following should be kept in mind when creating a strength-training program:
  - Body weight exercises should be done first.
  - Perform two to three sessions per week, including two to three sets of 10–15 repetitions of each exercise.
  - Implement variations in a program and gradually add weight in 10% increments.
  - Use child-sized equipment for preadolescents, such as smaller, 1-pound plates; small dumbbells; and/or resistance bands.
  - Appropriate supervision at all times is essential.
  - Emphasize correct form and technique.
  - Use single- and multiple-joint activities and train antagonistic muscle groups equally.
  - Design an individualized program, vary it regularly, and maintain workout logs to monitor progress.

CHANGING TRENDS IN EXERCISE PATTERNS

As an increasing number of children are participating in organized athletics at younger ages, the incidence of overuse injuries is increasing. It is estimated that 30–45 million youngsters aged 6–18 years participate in athletics (two-thirds in organized and one-third in recreational sports). Many children participate in year-round same-sports activities or simultaneously on multiple sports teams.

EFFECTS OF EARLY SPORTS SPECIALIZATION

- Early sports specialization has become more common.
- Participation in one sport and year-round participation can be both physically and mentally detrimental to children, leading to burnout and overuse injuries. Newer research has shown that this is due to the overall higher volume of physical activity. Additionally, when activity volume is accounted for, sports specialization increased the risk of injury in female adolescents by 30% and does not increase the risk of overuse injuries of male adolescents.
- There has also been a significant increase in anterior cruciate ligament (ACL) and ulnar collateral ligament (UCL) reconstruction surgeries in adolescents overall in the past 15 years.
- It is important to assess the nature and level of sports participation in young athletes in context of their chronologic age, developmental stage, and physical maturity.
- Recent research has revealed decreased rates of injury and less psychological stress by avoiding sports specialization before puberty.
- Early sports specialization is most often adult driven.
- There is an assumption that practicing only one sport will lead to better abilities and achievements in that sport.
- There is evidence that specialization in a sport before puberty is not necessary to become an "elite athlete" (e.g., earning a college scholarship, making it to professional status).
- Although some degree of sports specialization is necessary to improve skills within a field of sport, this should, in most cases, occur after the athlete reaches puberty. This can lead to a wider range of developed physical and mental skills within a sport that are gained from playing other sports before specialization. In addition, athlete burnout and the risk of quitting sports can potentially be decreased.
- Recent research has revealed that pediatric athletes who did not start intense training and specialized competition until after puberty were more likely to achieve an elite status within their sport, with the exception of women's gymnastics. However, gymnasts are at a significant risk of burnout and overuse injuries.
- Overtraining can lead to burnout and/or increased injuries, which can eventually cause a young athlete to stop participating in athletic activities, sometimes permanently. Parental influence is a critical confounding factor that affects a young athlete's participation in sports and must be addressed by physicians who care for pediatric athletes.

Risks of Overuse Injuries

- There are both intrinsic and extrinsic risk factors for overuse injuries (Table 10.2).
- Recommendations for overuse injury prevention include the following:
  - Limit one sporting activity to 5 days per week
  - Provide 1 day of rest from organized activity
  - Take 2–3 months off per year from a single sport
  - Alter workout routines to maintain interest and fun
  - Educate athletes and parents about wellness, nutrition, sleep, hygiene, and stress management
  - Monitor for warning signs of injury
  - When returning to sport participation following injury or periods of interruption in sports, a slow, steady progression is recommended rather than an abrupt resumption of full activity
  - Monitor special events such as tournaments and showcases for signs of fatigue, pain, and alterations in sports performance

ORGANIZED SPORTS FOR CHILDREN AND PREADOLESCENTS

- Changing trends include a movement away from spontaneous, unstructured activity that allows imagination, enjoyment, and motor skill development.
- Organized sports participation is greatly influenced by goals and expectations of parents and coaches.
- Reactions and feedback from parents and coaches have a strong influence on the attitudes and confidence of preadolescent athletes.
- If the focus is placed on skill development, cooperative play, and having fun, then athletes seem to have greater enjoyment of sports participation.
- Advantages of organization include establishment of rules for participation, equity in matching competitors at similar skill levels, definition of readiness-to-play criteria, and fairness in the establishment of teams to promote safe participation.

Sports-Specific Issues: Endurance Event Competitions

- Endurance events such as marathons and triathlons are increasing in popularity among youth athletes.
- The American Academy of Pediatrics has stated that "triathlons for children and adolescents are reasonably safe as long as the events are modified to be age appropriate."
- Modifications include shorter duration of activities and following conservative guidelines for safety and environmental conditions (e.g., EAPs and exercising in heat and humidity).

Table 10.2 FACTORS AFFECTING THE RISK OF OVERUSE INJURIES

Extrinsic Factors	Intrinsic Factors
Training errors	Growth
Schedules	Anatomic alignment
Workload	Muscle–tendon imbalance
Environment	Flexibility
Psychological factors	Prior injury and conditioning
Equipment	Menstrual dysfunction

- Training regimens are often altered from traditional plans, including lower weekly mileage, gradual increases in training, and extra attention to hydration and nutrition.

COMMON PEDIATRIC SPORTS INJURIES RELATED TO GROWTH AND DEVELOPMENT

Physeal Fractures

Overview: Injuries unique to young athletes are growth plate fractures. An injury at the end of a long bone in a skeletally immature athlete is a physeal (growth plate) fracture until proven otherwise. The physis, made of bone and cartilage, is relatively weaker than the surrounding ligaments, tendons, joint capsule, and other soft tissue structures; thus, application of excessive force to the musculoskeletal system will likely result in a physeal fracture.

Presentation: The highest rates of physeal fractures are seen during the growth spurt of adolescence and are usually associated with concentric, eccentric, or shear forces applied on the physis at the time of injury. The Salter–Harris (SH) classification is based on the pathoanatomy of fractures and the radiographic appearance of the bone itself (Fig. 10.1):

- Type I: transphyseal injury
- Type II: transphyseal injury with metaphyseal extension
- Type III: transphyseal injury with epiphyseal extension into the joint space
- Type IV: extension from the epiphysis through the physis and into the metaphysis
- Type V: rare and involves a crush injury to the physis itself

Physical examination: Most common finding on examination is tenderness at the ends of long bones over the physis. Swelling, ecchymosis, bony deformities, inability to bear weight, or decreased resistance on strength testing may be present.

Diagnosis: Requires a high index of suspicion and a basic knowledge of growth plate anatomy.

- Radiographs are required.
- A bone scan, magnetic resonance imaging (MRI), or computed tomography (CT) scan may be necessary if the diagnosis is in question or the patient is not responding to clinical treatment as expected.

Treatment: Treatment depends on the location and classification of the injury, as well as the degree of displacement of the fractured fragment.

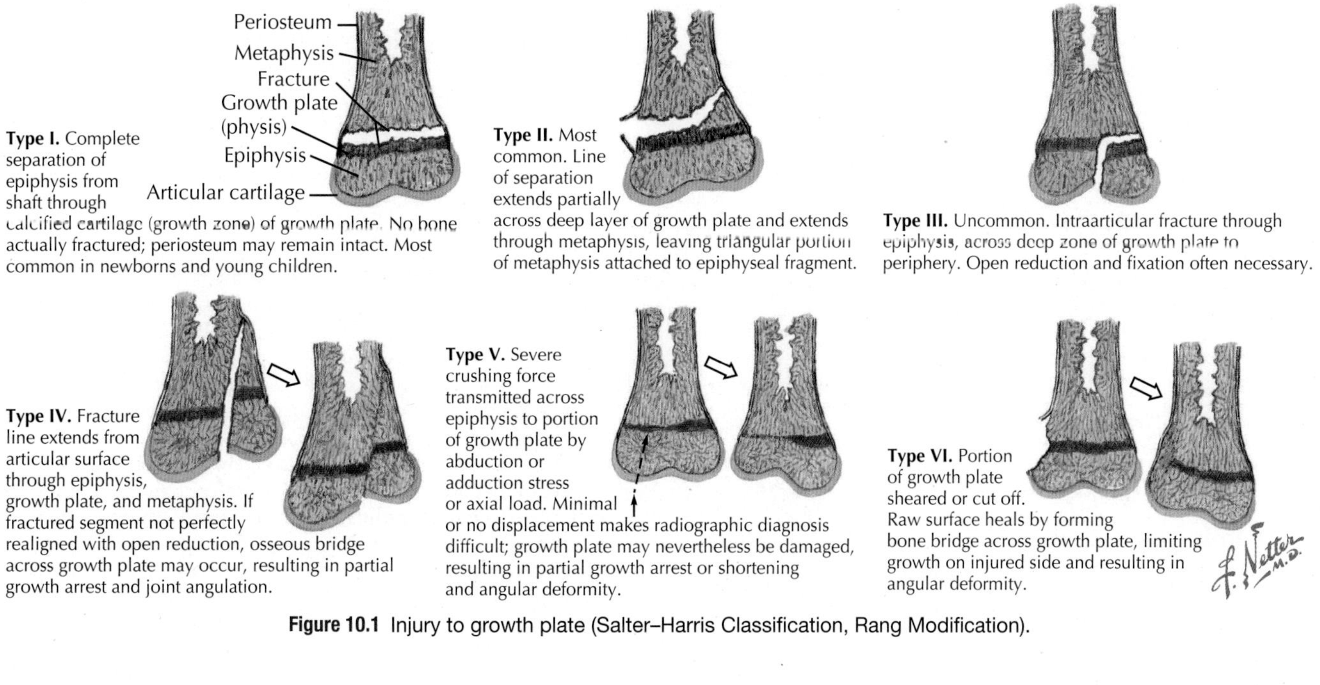
Periosteum
Metaphysis
Fracture
Growth plate (physis)
Epiphysis
Articular cartilage
Type I. Complete separation of epiphysis from shaft through calcified cartilage (growth zone) of growth plate. No bone actually fractured; periosteum may remain intact. Most common in newborns and young children.
Type II. Most common. Line of separation extends partially across deep layer of growth plate and extends through metaphysis, leaving triangular portion of metaphysis attached to epiphyseal fragment.
Type III. Uncommon. Intraarticular fracture through epiphysis, across deep zone of growth plate to periphery. Open reduction and fixation often necessary.
Type IV. Fracture line extends from articular surface through epiphysis, growth plate, and metaphysis. If fractured segment not perfectly realigned with open reduction, osseous bridge across growth plate may occur, resulting in partial growth arrest and joint angulation.
Type V. Severe crushing force transmitted across epiphysis to portion of growth plate by abduction or adduction stress or axial load. Minimal or no displacement makes radiographic diagnosis difficult; growth plate may nevertheless be damaged, resulting in partial growth arrest or shortening and angular deformity.
Type VI. Portion of growth plate sheared or cut off. Raw surface heals by forming bone bridge across growth plate, limiting growth on injured side and resulting in angular deformity.
F. Netter M.D.

Figure 10.1 Injury to growth plate (Salter–Harris Classification, Rang Modification).

- Most cases require casting with or without a closed reduction for minimally displaced fractures.
- Other fractures with significant displacement and/or instability of fractured fragments will require an open reduction-internal fixation (ORIF).
- Certain SH-I fractures, such as SH-I distal radius and fibular fractures, can be treated with splints.

Prognosis and return to play (RTP): Prognosis of SH-I to SH-III fractures varies but in general is good. Partial or complete growth arrest with malalignment is the greatest risk factor.

- Monitoring for 6–12 months after injury is typically required to assess continued long bone growth.
- RTP varies from approximately 3–12 weeks; immobilization is usually 3–6 weeks, as physeal injuries heal quickly.
- General RTP criteria should apply, including an assessment of range of motion, strength, and ability to perform sports-specific exercises with or without the use of a brace or other assistive device.

Apophyseal Injuries

Overview: Apophyseal injuries include both acute and overuse injuries and represent a stress injury to growth plates. Acute injuries are avulsion fractures at the apophyseal growth plate where a muscle–tendon unit attaches. Overuse injuries are far more common and typically present in a similar fashion as tendonitis with growth plate involvement.

Presentation: Concentric, eccentric, and shear forces create excessive biomechanical force at the apophysis that can initially result in a painful acute inflammatory condition (apophysitis). Excessive workload of repetitions of a sports-specific maneuver can lead to a chronic overuse tendinopathy presentation. Certain injuries are predictable in certain types of sports based on the stresses to the body in that sport. Common types of apophyseal injuries have been summarized in Table 10.3.

Table 10.3 COMMON APOPHYSEAL INJURIES IN THE PEDIATRIC ATHLETE

Injury	Location
Little League Elbow	Medial epicondyle at flexor-pronator attachment
Little League Shoulder	Proximal humerus epiphysis
Gymnast's Wrist	Distal radius epiphysis
Sinding–Larsen–Johansson Syndrome	Inferior pole of patella
Osgood-Schlatter Disease	Tibial tuberosity
Iselin Disease	Base of fifth metatarsal
Sever Disease	Calcaneus at Achilles tendon attachment
Pelvis Apophysitis	Anterior superior iliac spine, anterior inferior iliac spine, iliac crest
Hip Apophysitis	Ischial tuberosity, greater and lesser trochanter

Physical examination: Tenderness on palpation at the tendon and the apophysis is common. Perform a general assessment of biomechanical and genetic predisposition (e.g., check for severe pes planovalgus feet, genu valgum, or benign hypermobility).

Diagnosis: Diagnosis is often clinical, based on a high index of suspicion. Radiographs are helpful to evaluate acute injuries, malalignment, and growth disturbances but are frequently normal. Additional imaging studies are useful adjuncts for more chronic, severe, and persistent cases.

Treatment: Acute injuries may require a brief period (2–4 weeks) of immobilization, but more severe injuries can require ORIF to correct significant displacement (e.g., avulsion of the tibial tuberosity in the knee). Overuse injuries are treated similarly as tendonitis/tendinosis with relative rest and guided rehabilitation. Rehabilitation focuses on stretching to minimize forces at the apophysis, as well as to improve strength and proprioception. An assessment of sports-specific biomechanics may aid in the prevention of recurrences if errors in technique are corrected.

RTP: RTP is allowed when pain has resolved and the athlete can perform the necessary sports-specific maneuvers. A guided gradual resumption of normal sports activities is usually necessary to prevent frequent recurrence of symptoms.

Osteochondritis Dissecans

Overview: The term *osteochondritis dissecans* (OCD) is attributed to Konig in 1883 and is based on the theory that inflammation contributes to subchondral necrosis of bone and cartilage (Fig. 10.2). Trauma, ischemia, ossification defects, and genetic abnormalities are all likely to contribute to the pathophysiology. OCD has a juvenile and an adult form, distinguished by closure of the physes. The role of subchondral bone in providing cellular and humoral factors for healing contributes to the multilayered organization of articular cartilage and affects its ability to heal with conservative management. Although OCDs can occur in other joints, the three most common areas in pediatric athletes are the knee (femur), elbow (capitellum), and ankle (talus).

Presentation: Juvenile OCDs (JOCDs) are more common in athletes, and 40%–60% of JOCDs have a preceding history of trauma. Vague symptoms such as recurrent pain, crepitus, decreased range of motion, joint tenderness, and/or joint effusions may be present. More severe or advanced cases may include mechanical symptoms such as catching or locking.

Physical examination: Tenderness may be reproduced at the site of the OCD lesion, so the medial femoral condyle, the capitellum, or the talar dome should be palpated as clinically indicated. The presence of a nontraumatic joint effusion in an athlete is highly suspicious for an OCD lesion, as is the presence of mechanical symptoms. Gait abnormalities may be observed in the knees of OCD patients and include walking with the tibia externally rotated to decrease pressure on the lesion.

Diagnosis: Often made based on plain radiographs

- **Knee:** Anteroposterior (AP), notch or skier's, lateral, and sunrise views should be obtained. Often, the lesion in the posterior aspect of the medial femoral condyle is evident only on the notch or skier's view.
- **Elbow:** AP, lateral, and oblique views should be obtained with consideration of comparison views.
- **Ankle:** AP, lateral, and mortise views are necessary. The anterolateral talar dome and the posteromedial talus are common areas of occurrence in the ankle.
- In general, up to 50% of OCD lesions can be missed on plain radiographs. MRIs substantially improve the ability to image the lesion and allow for staging of joints with OCDs, with 92% sensitivity and 90% specificity. See Table 10.4 for MRI staging of OCD lesions.

Treatment: Varies, depending on the age of the patient, skeletal maturity, and location and size of the lesion. Conservative treatment with rest and decreased mechanical forces is often effective in 50%–91% of stage I–II lesions that are stable in skeletally immature patients. Indications for surgical referral to an orthopedic surgeon include persistent symptoms such as recurrent effusions, instability, chronic pain, ongoing mechanical symptoms, concomitant injury, loose bodies, and skeletally mature patients.

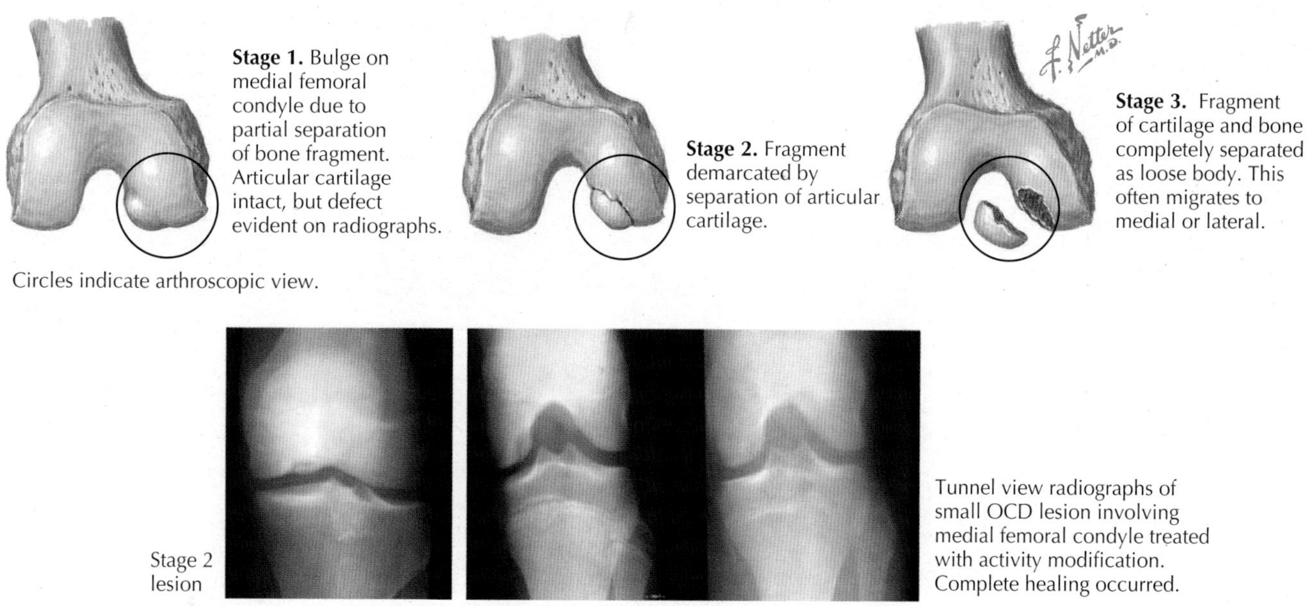
f. Netter M.D.
Stage 1. Bulge on medial femoral condyle due to partial separation of bone fragment. Articular cartilage intact, but defect evident on radiographs.
Stage 2. Fragment demarcated by separation of articular cartilage.
Stage 3. Fragment of cartilage and bone completely separated as loose body. This often migrates to medial or lateral.
Circles indicate arthroscopic view.
Stage 2 lesion
Tunnel view radiographs of small OCD lesion involving medial femoral condyle treated with activity modification. Complete healing occurred.

Figure 10.2 Osteochondritis dissecans.

Table 10.4 ANDERSON MRI STAGING OF OCD LESIONS

Stage	Findings on MRI
I	Thickening of articular cartilage and low signal changes
II	Articular cartilage is disrupted with low signal rim behind the fragment
III	Articular cartilage is widened with high signal changes behind the fragment
IV	Loose body: displaced intraarticular fragment

Spondylolysis

Overview: Studies indicate that 10%–30% of adolescent athletes suffer from low back pain. In young athletes, back pain that persists for >3 weeks should be evaluated for the presence of spondylolysis (Fig. 10.3). Spondylolysis can be acute (pars stress fracture) or chronic. *Spondylolisthesis* refers to subluxation or anterior displacement of a vertebral body. Patients with congenital spondylolysis have radiologic evidence by the age of 5–6 years, but symptoms are often delayed until adolescence, with athletes presenting at the age of 12–18 years. Both unilateral and bilateral pars defects are seen. In general, bilateral defects have a higher complication rate, have slower healing times, and are associated with a risk of slippage resulting in a concurrent spondylolisthesis.

Presentation: Typically, an athlete presents with activity-related back pain that is worse with extension. Neurologic and nighttime symptoms are rare.

Physical examination: There may be tenderness to palpation at the level of the fractured pars. Paraspinal muscle tenderness may be present. A "stork" test is a single-leg balance, spine-extension test that produces back pain when positive.

Diagnosis: Standard radiographs are AP, lateral, and right and left oblique views. A "Scottie dog" sign is a fracture of the pars seen best on oblique views. The lateral view will demonstrate the presence or absence of a "slip," or spondylolisthesis.

- Radiographs have a low sensitivity for detection of spondylolysis.
- Single-photon emission computed tomography (SPECT) bone scans are highly sensitive for pars injuries.
- MRIs are currently the gold standard in the evaluation of both pars defects and disc pathology with relatively good sensitivity and specificity. The sagittal stir sequences are particularly sensitive for spondylolysis.
- A reverse-angle thin-cut CT scan is best at evaluating healing or sclerosis versus nonunion of pars defects. If symptoms are localized, CT may be useful in diagnosis.
- A clinician should use his or her knowledge of the clinical situation, including physical examination, RTP concerns, and cost, along with other factors in the decision to utilize the different available imaging modalities.

Treatment: Activity modification with decreased sports participation until pain free, and guided rehabilitation that emphasizes core strength, posture, and hamstring/hip flexor flexibility. Sports participation is usually restricted for a minimum of 6 weeks. Bracing, although controversial, can be an important part of the treatment for pars defects, particularly if athletes are not pain free with rest from activities. Bracing type is also controversial, as is the length of time required (12–23 hours/day for 6 weeks to 6 months is the most common):

- The Boston brace is the traditional gold standard. It is a rigid lumbosacral orthosis (LSO).
- Semirigid orthoses (e.g., Warm-N-Form) are useful, cheaper, and increasingly popular because of improved compliance and similar outcomes when compared with use of a Boston brace.
- Soft lumbar orthoses are occasionally useful for less severe unilateral cases and when compliance is poor with the Boston brace or Warm-N-Form.
- Braces are unlikely to significantly limit extension; in fact, efficacy may be achieved through a proprioceptive mechanism.

Prognosis: Unilateral pars defects have a better prognosis for healing without long-term complications than do bilateral defects. Nevertheless, there is a relatively low rate of bone healing (50%): 25% cases show fibrous union or partial bone healing and 25% result in nonunions, as observed on follow-up CT scans.

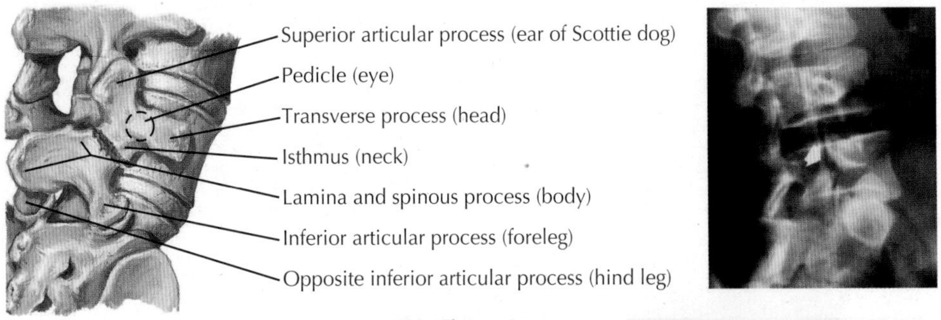
Superior articular process (ear of Scottie dog)
Pedicle (eye)
Transverse process (head)
Isthmus (neck)
Lamina and spinous process (body)
Inferior articular process (foreleg)
Opposite inferior articular process (hind leg)

Spondylolysis without spondylolisthesis Posterolateral view demonstrates formation of radiographic Scottie dog. On lateral radiograph, dog appears to be wearing a collar.

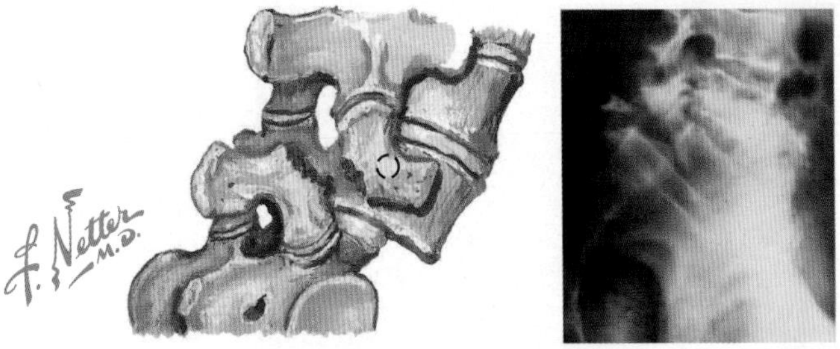
F. Netter M.D.

Isthmic-type spondylolisthesis Anterior luxation of L5 on sacrum due to fracture of isthmus. Note that gap is wider and dog appears decapitated.

Figure 10.3 Spondylolysis and spondylolisthesis.

RTP: Most athletes return to their previous level of sports participation. Athletes should be pain free. Some can return to participation in a brace after the initial period of rest (usually 6 weeks). High-risk back-extension activities such as gymnastics and weightlifting should not be performed for a minimum of 6 weeks and then only if athletes are pain free during activity. Recurrent symptoms are common. Treatment should include an evaluation of sports biomechanics and workload. Adjustments in amount and frequency of training, as well as changes in technique, should be made as part of a comprehensive treatment plan.

Hip Disorders in Young Athletes

Overview: Hip injuries in young athletes can be among the most serious injuries to occur. Hip trauma may be epiphyseal, apophyseal, or diaphyseal. Moreover, numerous soft tissue injuries are seen, but growth plate injuries are still the most common. Skeletal and vascular growth affects the development of immature bone, appearance of ossification centers, and blood supply to the femoral head.

Presentation: Acute injuries to the hip are common; they are usually the result of an injury during sports participation and require urgent evaluation. Overuse injuries to the hip may have a more insidious presentation and require a high index of suspicion and a thorough evaluation for accurate diagnosis. Athletes with hip disorders may not always experience hip pain. They may have referred pain to the thigh or knee alone, with or without stiffness, muscle weakness, and/or a limp.

- **Slipped capital femoral epiphysis (SCFE)** usually presents in an overweight or obese, rapidly growing male, aged 10–14 years. It is bilateral in 50% of cases (Fig. 10.4).
- **Legg–Calvé–Perthes disease (LCP)** is a condition of unknown etiology that appears as avascular necrosis of the femoral head. It is commonly seen in children age 4–10 years, with a 4:1 male predilection and a 20% occurrence of bilateral cases (Fig. 10.5).

Physical examination: A patient with SCFE or LCP typically presents with hip or groin pain or knee/thigh pain and a limp. A Trendelenburg gait is characteristic (see Fig. 10.5). Chronic cases may present with a limp or stiffness in the absence of pain. There may or may not be tenderness on palpation over the anterior hip joint. More typically, particularly in an SCFE case, when the hip is flexed, the leg rides into external rotation with considerable limitation of internal rotation.

Diagnosis: Radiographs should always include a lateral and frog-leg AP pelvis view. Comparison of both sides allows easier identification of pediatric hip pathology. In SCFE, subtle blurring or widening of the femoral physis is often noted in early cases. In more severe cases, there is an obvious deformity of the femoral neck. In Perthes cases, radiographs reveal a characteristic cessation in the growth of the bony epiphysis accompanied by sclerosis, fragmentation, collapse, and/or advanced avascular necrosis. LCP is staged based on radiographic appearance, as well as the percentage of femoral head involvement and alignment. Once the diagnosis is made, both SCFE and LCP patients should be immediately referred to a pediatric orthopedist for definitive care.

Treatment: Definitive treatment for SCFE is internal fixation or pinning of the epiphysis to stabilize it and prevent further slippage. Realignment is not routinely attempted because of the risk of disruption of vasculature to the femoral head. The **treatment of LCP** is complicated. Initial treatment involves rest with crutches and physical therapy to preserve range of motion and joint stability. For advanced cases, various surgical containment procedures may be performed by a pediatric orthopedist.

Blount Disease (Tibia Vara)

Overview: Tibia vara is a condition that involves a growth disturbance of the medial tibial physis (Fig. 10.6). It is most commonly seen in obese boys aged 10–14 years but can be seen in children as young as 2–3 years old and is more common in African Americans. Blount disease should be included in the differential diagnosis for any child presenting with a limp or bowlegs (genu varum) at any age.

Presentation: Typical presentation is of an obese child with a chronic progressive limp and either a unilateral or bilateral bowing of the tibia. Knee pain may be present and often localizes to the medial tibia.

Physical examination: Findings often include a leg length discrepancy, tenderness at the medial tibial physis, and tibial

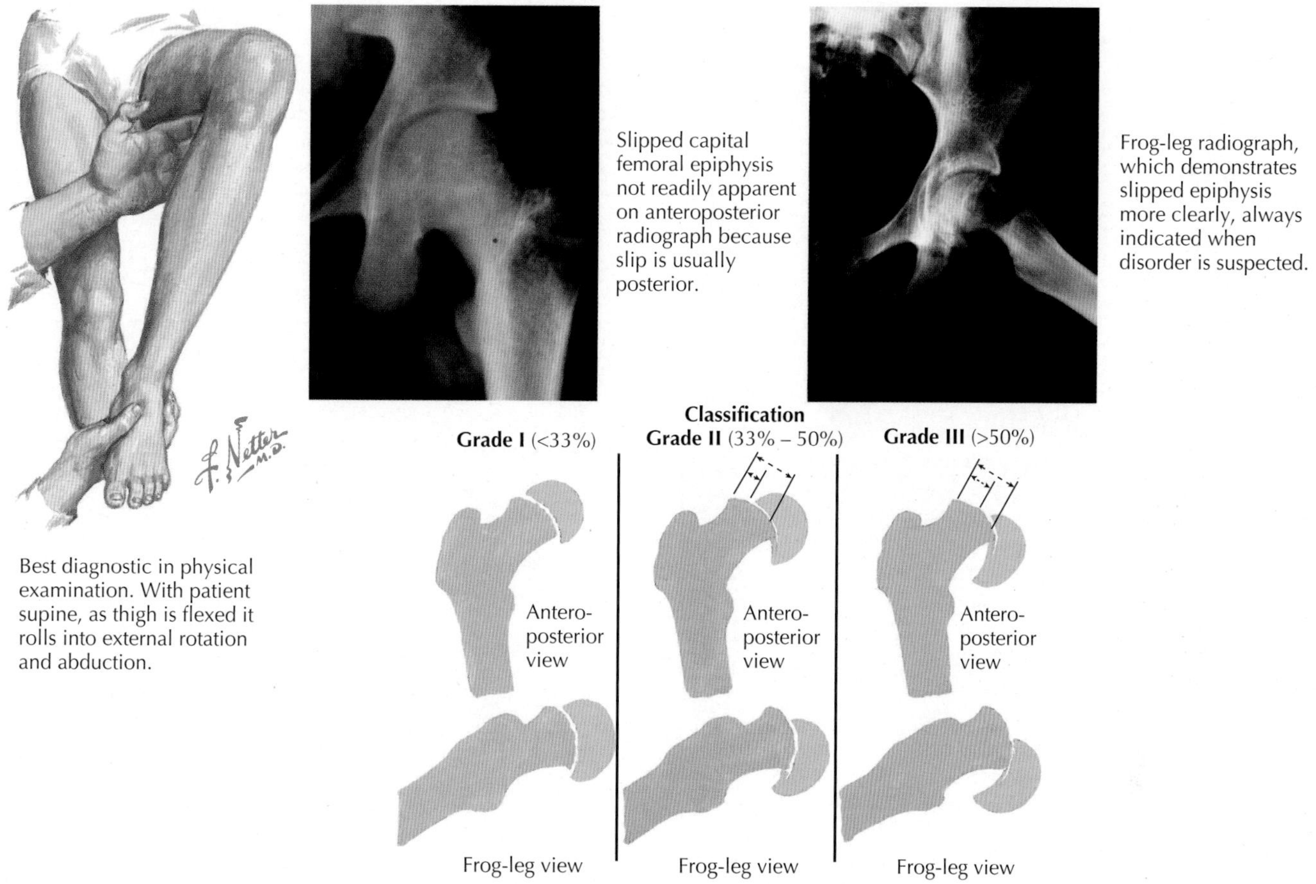
Slipped capital femoral epiphysis not readily apparent on anteroposterior radiograph because slip is usually posterior.
Frog-leg radiograph, which demonstrates slipped epiphysis more clearly, always indicated when disorder is suspected.
Best diagnostic in physical examination. With patient supine, as thigh is flexed it rolls into external rotation and abduction.
Classification
Grade I (<33%)
Grade II (33% – 50%)
Grade III (>50%)
Antero-posterior view
Antero-posterior view
Antero-posterior view
Frog-leg view
Frog-leg view
Frog-leg view

Figure 10.4 Slipped capital femoral epiphysis.

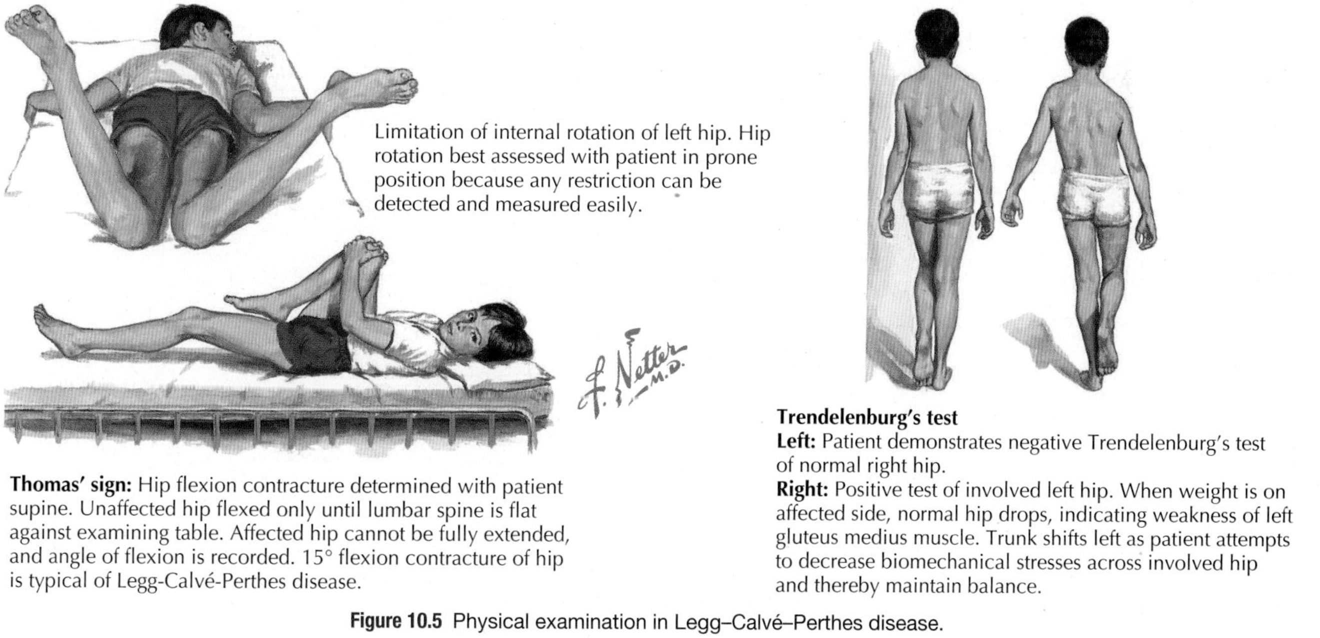
Limitation of internal rotation of left hip. Hip rotation best assessed with patient in prone position because any restriction can be detected and measured easily.
Thomas' sign: Hip flexion contracture determined with patient supine. Unaffected hip flexed only until lumbar spine is flat against examining table. Affected hip cannot be fully extended, and angle of flexion is recorded. 15° flexion contracture of hip is typical of Legg-Calvé-Perthes disease.
Trendelenburg's test
Left: Patient demonstrates negative Trendelenburg's test of normal right hip.
Right: Positive test of involved left hip. When weight is on affected side, normal hip drops, indicating weakness of left gluteus medius muscle. Trunk shifts left as patient attempts to decrease biomechanical stresses across involved hip and thereby maintain balance.

Figure 10.5 Physical examination in Legg–Calvé–Perthes disease.

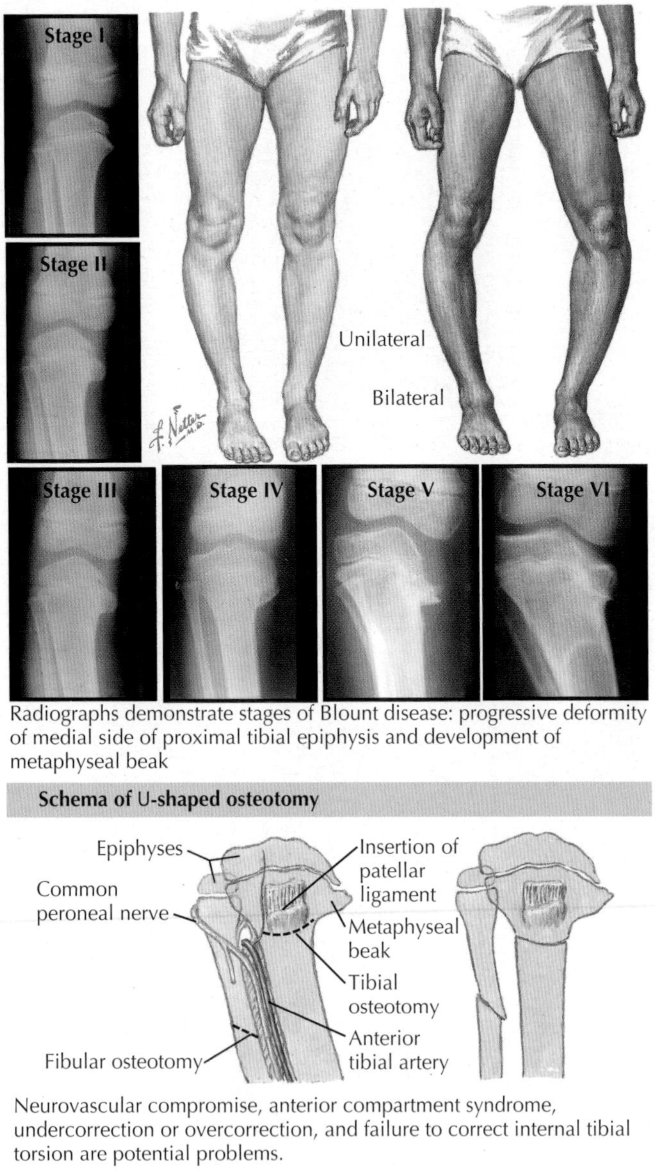
Stage I
Stage II
Unilateral
Bilateral
Stage III
Stage IV
Stage V
Stage VI
Radiographs demonstrate stages of Blount disease: progressive deformity of medial side of proximal tibial epiphysis and development of metaphyseal beak
Schema of U-shaped osteotomy
Epiphyses
Common peroneal nerve
Insertion of patellar ligament
Metaphyseal beak
Tibial osteotomy
Anterior tibial artery
Fibular osteotomy
Neurovascular compromise, anterior compartment syndrome, undercorrection or overcorrection, and failure to correct internal tibial torsion are potential problems.

Figure 10.6 Blount disease.

torsion associated with tibia vara. Instability to valgus stress testing may be present. Gait is usually antalgic and is notable with a varus thrust.

Diagnosis: Radiographs of the knee often reveal tibia vara and demonstrate growth arrest of the medial tibial physis with acute medial angulation of the proximal tibia. A standing bilateral lower extremity AP view showing pelvis to foot is the standard orthopedic view, but it is often not obtained until after diagnosis is made based on standard knee radiographs.

Treatment: Patients with Blount disease should be referred to a pediatric orthopedic surgeon for definitive care. Surgical treatment includes an osteotomy to realign the tibia into slight valgus, thus eliminating the leg length discrepancy and bowing. Other options include a stapling procedure of the lateral tibial physis to stop growth throughout the proximal tibia; this can result in a considerable leg length discrepancy compared with the contralateral side and may lead to further complications. Moreover, weight management as part of the comprehensive treatment for obesity must be emphasized in such patients.

Tarsal Coalition

Overview: Tarsal coalition involves a congenital bony or fibrocartilaginous fusion of tarsal bones (Fig. 10.7). It is seen in 1%–3% of the general population and may be autosomal dominant with variable penetrance. Bilateral occurrence is seen in 50%–60% of cases. Two types are commonly seen: calcaneonavicular and talocalcaneal.

Presentation: Symptoms usually develop in the second decade of life as increased bony ossification occurs. Progressive stiffness and limping may be seen. Pain is initially activity related.

Physical examination: A rigid flatfoot is seen with hindfoot valgus, along with decreased subtalar joint motion and limited inversion. Tenderness may be present along the lateral aspect of the subtalar joint and/or sinus tarsi.

Diagnosis: Bilateral weight-bearing AP, lateral, oblique, and Harris radiographs of the feet should be obtained; however, these are often nondiagnostic, particularly in the setting of a fibrocartilaginous coalition. Calcaneonavicular tarsal coalition is more likely to be seen on plain films. Secondary findings may include beaking of the talar neck and widening of the talonavicular joint. A bilateral noncontrast CT of the feet is the gold standard.

Treatment: A referral to a pediatric orthopedic surgeon is recommended. Initial treatment is conservative and includes observation, physical therapy, gait training, and orthotics. Immobilization may be performed for 4–6 weeks for a more painful condition. Definitive treatment may include surgical excision to decrease pain, improve mobility, and limit progressive degenerative changes. Surgical intervention is most effective if performed before the age of 14 years.

RECOMMENDED READINGS

Available online.

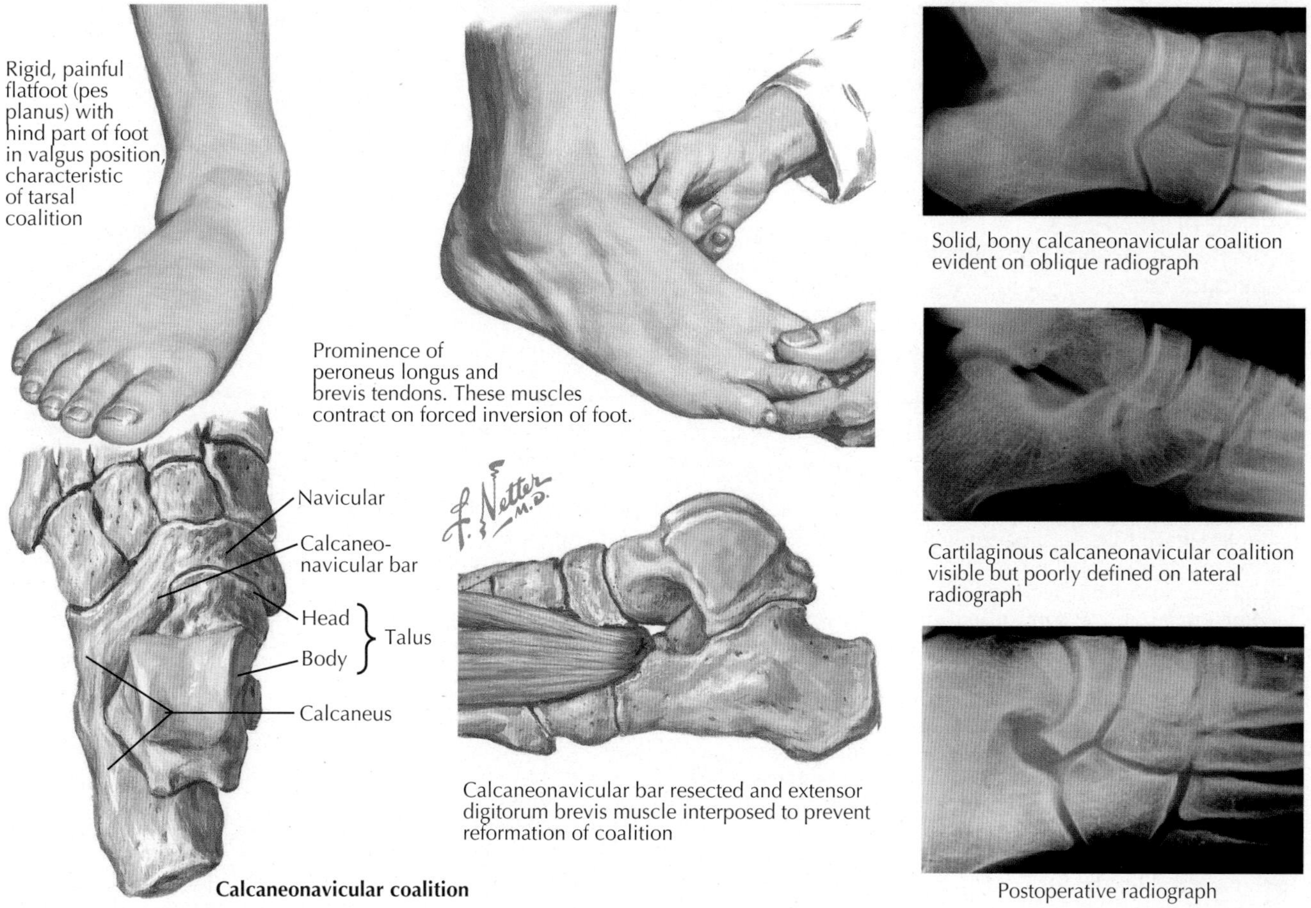
Rigid, painful flatfoot (pes planus) with hind part of foot in valgus position, characteristic of tarsal coalition
Prominence of peroneus longus and brevis tendons. These muscles contract on forced inversion of foot.
Solid, bony calcaneonavicular coalition evident on oblique radiograph
Navicular
Calcaneo-navicular bar
Head
Body
Talus
Calcaneus
Cartilaginous calcaneonavicular coalition visible but poorly defined on lateral radiograph
Calcaneonavicular bar resected and extensor digitorum brevis muscle interposed to prevent reformation of coalition
Calcaneonavicular coalition
Postoperative radiograph

Figure 10.7 Tarsal coalition.

11 THE HIGH SCHOOL ATHLETE: SETTING UP A HIGH SCHOOL SPORTS MEDICINE PROGRAM

Shayne D. Fehr • Kevin D. Walter

GENERAL PRINCIPLES

Athletic Healthcare in High-Level Collegiate and Professional Sports

- At the highest levels of sports, organizations are much like corporations; they function to increase success of shareholders by providing a product (i.e., winning team) linked to profitability.
- Although there are ethical concerns with this model, it provides an environment of highly established care because the athlete's health is linked to the team's success.
- The characteristics of such models include:
  - Remarkable financial resources
  - Well-defined roles and responsibilities
  - Risk management and loss control
  - Optimization of athletes' health for on-field performance
  - High organizational control and attention to detail
  - Professional personnel secured in adequate quantity
    - Certified athletic trainers (ATCs)
    - Qualified team physicians (sports medicine fellowship-trained primary care physicians, and orthopaedic surgeons)
    - Other allied healthcare professionals, including certified strength and conditioning coaches, nutritionists, psychologists, optometrists, dentists, exercise physiologists, and physical therapists (PTs)
- Compliance with *Team Physician Consensus Statement* (see Recommended Readings)
- Policies delineated and enforced routinely

Differences in Athletic Healthcare for the High School Athlete

- The effect of high-profile professional and collegiate sports has trickled down into secondary schools, with many school administrators, coaches, and parents looking for the same type of on-demand medical care
- However, most schools have the following concerns:
  - Lack of financial resources
  - Lack of leadership—just maintain status quo
    - Turnover of personnel (school board, superintendent, principal, athletic directors [ADs], and coaches)
    - Not a priority—too many other issues
  - Lack of medical resources
    - No ATC or team physician
    - Inadequate medical knowledge among coaches and ADs
    - Inadequate communication within the medical community
    - Results in incorrect or delayed care
  - Lack of consistent policies/standards
    - No overall single system of care at a school—each coach does his or her own thing
    - Each school may be different within a district
    - Assumed to be met by minimal standards and effort by external personnel or agencies, such as state-required preparticipation physical evaluations (PPPEs), volunteer team physicians, or presence of an ambulance

Solution: Goals and Requirements

- Goals: appropriate healthcare for athletes and minimal liability through a risk management (loss control) policy
- Requirements: knowledge, organization, and commitment toward detailed planning

Approach to Optimal High School Athletic Healthcare

Key Elements

Four key elements of the approach: family, school, medical community, and ATCs

FAMILY INVOLVEMENT

- Most high school athletes are minors and are dependent on their parent(s) or guardian(s)
- School, ATC, and physician must focus on communication with parents/guardians of injured athletes because parents/guardians:
  - Know the athlete's medical history
  - Are often more concerned with their children's health and academics than sport
  - Are important resources regarding psychosocial dynamics
- Financial concerns may prevent seeking appropriate care

SCHOOL COMMITMENT

- School should assume responsibility for operating safe programs
  - Obligations toward students and their families; commitment to meeting them; solutions must be internal as well as external
  - Qualifications and backgrounds of ADs and coaches
  - Should work as a unit, operating a single interscholastic athletic program and single athletic healthcare program
    - Institution of policies, guidelines, and procedures for daily use
    - Record-keeping system
    - Emergency action planning (EAP) and first-aid/cardiopulmonary resuscitation (CPR) training
- Seek assistance from the medical community for all sports: PPPEs as well as preseason fitness screening, weekly school visits, event coverage, therapies and treatments
  - Know what is desired from physicians, PTs, and clinicians
  - Designate team physician(s)
- Hire National Athletic Trainers' Association (NATA)–certified ATCs (state licensed if applicable), as they are the most suitable professionals to coordinate and operate the athletic healthcare program
  - Cannot be present simultaneously at all athletic venues
    - Use of student athletic trainers and educated coaches for assistance
  - Requires a support system
    - Policies and procedures, including record-keeping, accountability, and quality assurance systems
- Requires wireless communication and golf cart to meet obligations of daily coverage and emergency response
- Should insist on medical supervision and quality assurance system
- Should have an adequate budget
- Reasonable schedule demands
  - Known high turnover rate for ATCs due to heavy workload
  - Consider second ATC in large high schools

MEDICAL INVOLVEMENT (TEAM PHYSICIANS)

- A written contract is best
  - Delineates responsibilities and expectations
  - Helps ensure that the school has given careful thought to its obligations
  - Good communication leads to good working relationships

- Monetary compensation—yes or no?
  - Compensation may nullify "Good Samaritan" immunity
  - Amount offered is frequently meager compared with earnings in office
    - True value of assistance provided?
- Responsibilities (enumerated in Team Physician Consensus Statement)
- Jurisdiction: Are your decisions final?
- Medicolegal (liability) concerns
  - Good Samaritan law immunity may cover team physician in certain states
    - Team physician may not qualify as a Good Samaritan under strict definition—"someone without obligation who steps forward to render emergency care"
    - Has clearly defined responsibilities toward athletes, school, and athletic program
    - Event coverage is evidence of that responsibility
    - May be covered by "good intent, no compensation" concern
    - Good Samaritan immunity extends only to "emergency care" rendered during event coverage; protection does not extend to PPPEs, weekly injury clinics at school, and return-to-play (RTP) clearance evaluations
  - Potential responsibility and liability for ATC's actions
    - Need to clarify issue with school district
    - ATCs generally function "under direct medical supervision of a physician"
    - In states that have not specifically defined the "scope of practice" for ATCs through licensure, certification, or registration:
      - Team physician needs to assess implications and responsibilities of "direct medical supervision"
      - Analogous supervisory situation may be the physician–physician assistant relationship
  - Written standing orders for ATC and EAPs are essential for limiting any liability risks
  - Malpractice insurance and liability coverage
    - Incorporated into your personal or clinic policy (already existing or a new rider clause to be added)
    - Through school district insurance policy
- Medical privacy concerns (HIPAA and FERPA)
  - Health Insurance Portability and Accountability Act (HIPAA) of 1996 and Family Education Rights and Privacy Act (FERPA) in 1974 were developed to regulate "protected health information" (PHI)
  - FERPA regulations prevail within domain of public schools, including school nurses, school physicians, coaches, and ATCs
  - HIPAA Privacy Rule allows release of medical information without authorization for "treatment, consulting with other providers, referring the patient to other providers, and notifying a patient's family"
    - Athletes who consult at medical facilities outside of school will most likely fall under purview of HIPAA
  - Eligibility decisions regarding "cleared" or "not cleared" on PPPEs can be provided to coaches and school administrators (without inclusion of other medical information) without signed consent
  - For group PPPEs conducted at the school, must ensure confidential storage of forms, with PHI pertaining to restrictions shared only with those who have "need to know"
    - Need to know—always includes ATC, school nurse, and team physician
      - Variable for coach and administration depending on circumstances because the athlete's well-being may require one to understand his or her limitations or signs and symptoms
  - Coaches and administrators, as well as school nurses and ATCs, must be made aware of FERPA and HIPAA regulations and constraints regarding privacy of PHI
- Degree of involvement
  - Set overall medical policy with AD and ATC
  - Strongly consider forming a medical advisory board with school district
  - Provide medical advice to interscholastic athletic program
  - Provide medical coverage at games. Ideal goal—to see every team member at least once during the season—may require division of coverage among several physicians, possibly by sport or on a rotational basis
    - Football team: home varsity coverage (mandatory); away varsity and home subvarsity coverage (recommended)
    - Wrestling team: preseason weight class recommendations, midseason weight certification, assessment of skin for communicable diseases, and coverage of home matches (recommended)
    - Coverage of all tournaments at home school
    - Soccer team (boys and girls): coverage of events as schedule permits
    - Basketball team (boys and girls): coverage of events as schedule permits
    - Other sports as schedule permits with attention to contact or collision sports
  - Develop an emergency contacts list and EAP, including use of automated external defibrillator (AED) for sudden cardiac arrest
  - Develop a concussion action plan, including return to academics and sport
  - Conduct PPPEs
  - Visit school/athletes regularly
  - Educate coaches and ATCs
  - Provide support for ATC's authority
    - Medicolegal supervisor of the ATC
    - Assess knowledge, skills, and experience of the ATC and mutually develop an appropriate set of standing orders with cumulative working relationship and legal scope of practice for ATCs in their jurisdiction
    - Role in creating a job description, interviewing, and hiring
    - Role in job evaluation
    - Role in quality assurance of care rendered by ATC
      - Frequent and regular communication
      - Chart review and case studies as needed
- Role of a team physician in school without an ATC
  - Understand history and culture of the school
  - Assess strengths and weaknesses of how athletic care is and was provided
  - Greater challenge to meet responsibilities
  - Possible institution of athletic healthcare system (AHCS; see the following section)
  - Encourage school to recognize need for ATC
- Role of a new team physician in school with established ATC
  - The team physician should understand the methods and culture of the existing system.
  - ATC may welcome an active, involved, "hands-on" team physician or prefer a more distant consultant model if he or she is comfortable as the central focus of the AHCS and confident of his or her abilities and skills.
  - Team physician should develop an appropriate relationship with ATC.

ATHLETIC TRAINER

- Hiring considerations and working conditions (team physician should help school in the hiring process)
- Funding is a factor—ATC often low-paying, entry-level job
- If ATC is hired, under what conditions?
  - Full- or part-time ATC?
  - Teacher and ATC? How many classes?
  - How many working hours per week, including games?
  - How many working days per year?
    - ATC needs more days than regular school calendar

- If general contract calls for same number of days as teachers, it must account for preseason football days, weekends, and holiday tournament days
- Possible solution: part-time substitute ATC, who works 1 day per week throughout school year (40 days); this schedule decreases the risk of burnout for full-time ATC (from not having time off) and allows ATC to work same number of days as teachers
- Part-time ATC can service several schools each week, if more work is desired

- Medical backup and supervision
  - Head team physician should be specifically recognized as the medical supervisor of the ATC
  - Degree and frequency of communication should be clearly established
  - Whose decision is final regarding RTP?
- Adequate budget for equipment and supplies, professional fees, books, and continuing education
- Quality of training room
- Written job description
- Job performance (accountability and quality assurance)
  - Evaluated by team physician and others (e.g., AD, school nurse, coaches, principal, and athletes)
- Potential for career advancement

ATHLETIC HEALTHCARE SYSTEM

Generic Model System

- The AHCS was initially developed by adapting college and professional sports medicine programs to high school level
- This can be installed at any school, large or small, and at any school location, rural or urban
- The AHCS should be tailored to each school and adhere to accepted standards of practice
  - Effectiveness of the AHCS is greatly improved with an ATC and a sports medicine–trained team physician

Model System

- The AHCS was developed under strict guidelines of the US Department of Education from 1978 to 1982 and validated in 1982, 1987, and 1995
- The AHCS was nationally disseminated in the 1980s and 1990s by grants through the National Diffusion Network
  - This consortium was well known by schools with a track record for proven, cost-effective programs that worked
- In 2002, NATA developed a consensus statement with recommendations and guidelines for secondary school sports
  - In 2004, the consensus statement was augmented by an updated, science-based document

Key Elements of the Athletic Healthcare System

Assessment

- Complete evaluation of existing programs
- Standards for care delineated
- Areas of assessment
  - Identify AHCS team members that have a diverse skill set
  - Athletic facilities—safe practice and competition venues
  - Athletic equipment—selection, fit, and maintenance
  - EAP—development and implementation
  - Treatment facilities/athletic training room
  - Provision of athletic healthcare services
  - Documentation strategies and injury surveillance
- Self-assessment initially, followed by external evaluation
  - Concept and methodology similar to assessments by the Joint Commission on Accreditation of Health Organizations and educational assessments
  - Formal written report issued
  - Develop action plan based on weaknesses and deficiencies
  - Assessment frequency—every 3–5 years

Education

COACHES

- Know rules and expectations for coach education in your state or league
- Coaching education and standards provided by the National Federation of State High School Associations (NFHS), the National Association for Sport and Physical Education, and various other groups
  - Basic life support (BLS)
  - First aid, health, and safety
  - Concussion education
  - Nutrition and hydration
  - Mental health and sport psychology
  - Behavior and engagement of athletes and parents
  - Sports injury prevention and management
- Education on the culture of sport
  - Encourage an environment of honesty in reporting injuries without repercussions
  - Recognize injury; treat and completely rehabilitate to allow pain-free participation
    - No longer fall back on "no pain, no gain" philosophy
- Education on how to most effectively partner with ATCs and team physicians
  - Share responsibilities
  - Defer to knowledge of objective healthcare providers
  - Work with AHCS team to install injury reduction programs

STUDENT ATHLETIC TRAINING ASSISTANTS

- Assist coaches and ATCs in daily tasks
- Courses in summer and/or during school year
- May be funded through vocational education monies
- Provides career opportunities in the healthcare field

ATHLETIC DIRECTORS AND OTHER ADMINISTRATIVE PERSONNEL

- Athletic administration courses through national associations like the NFHS and the National Interscholastic Athletic Administrators Association
- Regional and state conferences
  - Focus on organizational management and implementation of a safe athletic program
  - Safety and liability issues
  - Strategies to interact with coaches, sports medicine team, and state associations

Athletic Training Room/Treatment Facilities

- Recommendations:
  - Should have privacy for evaluation of student-athletes
  - Should be accessible for both male and female athletes
  - Should not be a conditioning center or a weight room
  - Often used as a rehabilitation room
  - Ensure appropriate disposal of biohazard waste
  - Have a plan for equipment and supply inventory, stocking, and storage
  - Location: ideally close to locker rooms and athletic fields
  - Adequate plumbing and drainage for ice machine and tubs
  - Ensure appropriate heating, ventilation, and lighting
  - Ensure layout of room allows smooth flow of traffic
  - Educational resources for student-athletes: books, posters, and manuals
  - Ensure safety and security is assessed

Standard Procedures

PREPARTICIPATION EVALUATION

- Coordinate with medical community, ATC, and coaches
  - See Chapter 3: "The Preparticipation Physical Evaluation"

- Identify athletes with medical conditions (e.g., diabetes, asthma, seizures, or anaphylaxis) and develop EAPs and preventive management plans

PRESEASON SCREENING

- Create off-season fitness plan for athletes of every sport
  - Develop injury and illness prevention plans
  - Provide sound nutritional counseling and education
- Physical assessment
  - Flexibility
  - Strength and endurance
  - Aerobic capacity
  - Body composition
- Education and culture
  - Create an environment for appropriate reporting of injuries
  - Develop "mental toughness"—psychological and emotional makeup
  - Educate on playing within rules
  - Emphasize sportsmanship
  - Educate on appropriate nutrition and hydration
    - Discussion on safe weight gain and weight loss
    - Educate on avoiding supplements and performance-enhancing substances
  - Review common adolescent high-risk behaviors (e.g., substance abuse, use of seat belts and bike helmets, Internet and social media safety, or bullying)

TREATMENT PROTOCOLS AND GUIDELINES

- Share with athletes, coaches, and parents
- Create in conjunction with the team physician
- Identify local experts for referral of injuries, psychosocial pathology (e.g., eating disorders or depression), and medical illness
- PRICES
  - **P**rotection—brace/splint use
  - **R**est
  - **I**ce
  - **C**ompression
  - **E**levation
  - **S**upport—crutch use
- Use of over-the-counter (OTC) medications—if allowed
- Educational handouts for athletes and families on injuries
- Steps of rehabilitation
  - Control pain and swelling
  - Restore range of motion
  - Restore strength
  - Restore stability
    - Taping, bracing, and rehabilitation exercises
  - Restore general functioning
    - Aerobic capacity
    - Core stability
    - Neuromuscular function
    - Balance
  - Restore sport-specific functioning

RETURN-TO-PLAY POLICY

- Create in conjunction with AHCS team, particularly the team physician
  - To reduce the risk of inappropriate clearance by an external physician, establish which provider has the final say on medical clearance—should ideally be the team physician
- Share with parents, coaches, and athletes during preseason meetings
  - Set expectations for when an injured athlete can resume play
- Concussion-specific
  - Comply with state legislation
    - Written medical clearance
  - Follow a stepwise RTP progression
    - Concussion in Sport Group, Berlin Guidelines, 2016
  - Before beginning the program, an injured athlete should have fully resumed academics and must be asymptomatic and off the medications used for symptomatic treatment.
- Musculoskeletal injury
  - Little to no swelling
  - Little to no tenderness on palpation
  - Full, pain-free range of motion
  - Full, pain-free strength through range of motion
  - Pain-free joint stability—through rehabilitation, taping, bracing, or surgery
  - Full, pain-free general functional activities
  - Full, pain-free or minimal discomfort during sport-specific activities
- Medical disorders/issues
  - Should have written medical clearance delineating activities allowed and any follow-up care or considerations necessary

COMMUNICATION

- List of key people and contact information disseminated among the AHCS
  - Should include hospitals, clinics, and physicians
- All AHCS personnel should possess individual cell phones in case of emergency
  - If cell phones do not have reception, alternative modes of communication should be established (e.g., walkie talkies)
- Information cards for every athlete
  - Medical conditions
  - Emergency contacts

Emergency Preparedness

EMERGENCY ACTION PLAN

- Emergency information cards for every athlete
- Written EAP should be designed for every practice and competition location to include:
  - Annual training at every location with the staff and the team
  - Attention to location of AEDs
  - Checklist for first-aid kits
  - Procedure for alerting emergency medical services (EMS)/911
    - Map for route to athletic facility and fields
    - Sports medicine staff can call ahead to inform the hospital facility
  - Procedure for transfer of care from AHCS to EMS team
  - Procedure to notify parents, guardians, and caregivers of the injured athlete

PRACTICE AND PLAYING FIELD/FACILITY SAFETY

- Safety inspections at the start of the year and the season
- Daily inspection of playing surface and surroundings

EVALUATION PROCEDURE FOR ACUTE "ON-THE-FIELD" INJURIES

- Triage severity of injury to first rule out "worst-case injuries"
  - Life-threatening injuries/unresponsive or unconscious athletes
    - Begin BLS with focus on airway, breathing, and circulation (ABC)
    - Activate EMS
  - Unstable athlete—if left unattended, would athlete deteriorate?
    - Begin BLS and activate EMS
  - Examples of potentially life-threatening, limb-threatening, or unstable injuries
    - Airway obstruction
    - Acute bleeding (internal or external hemorrhage)
    - Anaphylaxis
    - Cardiovascular collapse

- Heat illness
- Neurologic impairment/head injury
- Severe fractures
- Dislocations
- Eye trauma
- Have a plan to address common athletic injuries that may not require activation of EMS
  - Initial triage and determination if it is safe to move the athlete off the playing surface
  - Evaluation of injury on the sideline
  - Follow-up injury evaluation to ensure the athlete is not decompensating
  - Communication with coaches regarding the athlete's status
  - Communication with the athlete's parent or guardian

Documentation and Injury Surveillance

- Always document every evaluation and care provided
- Reduces liability
- Allows review for quality improvement and accountability

RECORD-KEEPING

- Paper or electronic
- Athlete emergency information card
- Daily report of attendance and injuries
  - Note absent athletes to assess injuries or illnesses before RTP
- Keep athletic training room treatment log
  - Documentation on all treated athletes should include diagnosis, treatment(s), progress, and limitations
  - May need to pass on treatment notes of the injured athletes to families or medical care providers
- Maintain a file for correspondence from medical care providers
- Maintain a master list of injured athletes for each team
  - Daily review with coaches to determine full, limited, or no participation

INJURY SURVEILLANCE

- Follow injury trends in a sport from year to year
- NFHS partners with High School Reporting Injuries Online (High School RIO) to compile comprehensive high school injury data (Tables 11.1 and 11.2)
  - Random and convenient sampling at high schools by ATCs
- School-specific injury surveillance is helpful to determine any increase in injury rates that can provide AHCS and coaches information regarding potential risks
  - Example: communicable skin disease outbreaks in wrestling

Adoption and Implementation Process

- Goal is quality and outcome/athletic safety improvements
- Identify local resources to maintain excellence and establish "ownership"
- Promote awareness among athletes, parents, coaches, boosters, school board members, school teachers and administrators, and local healthcare providers
- Networking can improve quality
  - Other schools or sports clubs
  - State athletic association
  - NFHS
  - Medical community

Review of Components

- Identify members of the AHCS team
- Identify roles and responsibilities of each AHCS team member
- Create, review, and update policies and procedures
- Establish and maintain physical space and equipment
- Establish documentation standards and injury surveillance system

Table 11.1 INJURY RATES BY SPORT AND TYPE OF EXPOSURE: HIGH SCHOOL SPORTS-RELATED INJURY SURVEILLANCE STUDY, UNITED STATES, 2018–2019 SCHOOL YEAR[a]

	#Injuries	#Exposures	Injury Rate (per 1000 AEs)
Overall Total	**7253**	**4,003,991**	**1.81**
Competition	3904	1,002,942	3.89
Practice	3331	2,962,253	1.12
Performance	18	38,796	0.46
Boys' Football Total	**2328**	**621,653**	**3.74**
Competition	1360	111,867	12.16
Practice	968	509,786	1.90
Boys' Soccer Total	**519**	**278,500**	**1.86**
Competition	335	85,490	3.92
Practice	184	193,010	0.95
Girls' Soccer Total	**591**	**235,653**	**2.51**
Competition	400	73,106	5.47
Practice	191	162,547	1.18
Girls' Volleyball Total	**323**	**252,227**	**1.28**
Competition	127	84,717	1.50
Practice	196	167,510	1.17
Boys' Basketball Total	**567**	**312,149**	**1.82**
Competition	316	93,688	3.37
Practice	251	218,461	1.15
Girls' Basketball Total	**442**	**230,514**	**1.92**
Competition	255	69,942	3.65
Practice	187	160,572	1.16
Boys' Wrestling Total	**528**	**213,076**	**2.48**
Competition	239	55,326	4.32
Practice	289	157,750	1.83
Boys' Baseball Total	**244**	**241,993**	**1.01**
Competition	140	86,762	1.61
Practice	104	155,231	0.67
Girls' Softball Total	**243**	**172,851**	**1.41**
Competition	140	62,593	2.24
Practice	103	110,258	0.93
Girls' Field Hockey Total	**120**	**71,442**	**1.68**
Competition	61	23,496	2.60
Practice	59	47,946	1.23
Boys' Ice Hockey Total	**126**	**52,032**	**2.42**
Competition	105	17,745	5.92
Practice	21	34,287	0.61
Boys' Lacrosse Total	**275**	**132,645**	**2.07**
Competition	167	38,333	4.36
Practice	108	94,312	1.15
Girls' Lacrosse Total	**177**	**105,532**	**1.68**
Competition	101	32,319	3.13
Practice	76	73,213	1.04

Table 11.1 INJURY RATES BY SPORT AND TYPE OF EXPOSURE: HIGH SCHOOL SPORTS-RELATED INJURY SURVEILLANCE STUDY, UNITED STATES, 2018–2019 SCHOOL YEAR[a]—cont'd

	#Injuries	#Exposures	Injury Rate (per 1000 AEs)
Boys' Swimming Total	**14**	**85,434**	**0.16**
Competition	4	15,444	0.26
Practice	10	69,990	0.14
Girls' Swimming Total	**28**	**106,201**	**0.26**
Competition	2	20,500	0.10
Practice	26	85,701	0.30
Boys' Track Total	**164**	**260,689**	**0.63**
Competition	53	46,570	1.14
Practice	111	214,119	0.52
Girls' Track Total	**230**	**220,562**	**1.04**
Competition	57	39,358	1.45
Practice	173	181,204	0.95
Cheerleading Total	**119**	**178,077**	**0.67**
Competition	4	8689	0.46
Practice	97	130,592	0.74
Performance	18	38,796	0.46
Boys' Cross-Country Total	**101**	**126,692**	**0.80**
Competition	19	20,394	0.93
Practice	82	106,298	0.77
Girls' Cross-Country Total	**114**	**106,069**	**1.07**
Competition	19	16,603	1.14
Practice	95	89,466	1.06

[a]Only includes injuries resulting in time loss of ≥1 days.
AE, Athletic exposures.
From R. Dawn Comstock, PhD, National High School Sports-Related Injury Surveillance Study, available at https://coloradosph.cuanschutz.edu/docs/librariesprovider204/default-document-library/2018-19-convenience-sample.pdf?sfvrsn=e46300b9_2, Table 2.1, Page 26–27.

CHALLENGES RESULTING FROM THE SARS-2 NOVEL CORONAVIRUS (COVID-19) PANDEMIC

- The COVID-19 pandemic has severely affected sports participation at all levels of competition
- Participation rates have varied widely based on infection rates and state/local mandates
- Cycle of stopping/starting is expected with resurgences of COVID-19
- Should work with state and local health department, as well as state athletic associations, to help determine the risk and safety of allowing athletic participation: training, full practice, competition, and traveling for competition
- AD, head ATC, and team physician have a responsibility to develop protocols to protect their athletes, staff, and their families
- Strategies to combat the spread of infection are continually evolving
- Recommendations and guidelines to prevent and contain outbreaks have been provided by the Centers for Disease Control and Prevention (CDC), NFHS, and individual state associations, among others

Table 11.2 METHODS OF INJURY EVALUATION AND ASSESSMENT: HIGH SCHOOL SPORTS-RELATED INJURY SURVEILLANCE STUDY, UNITED STATES, 2018–2019 SCHOOL YEAR

	n	%[a]
% of Injuries Evaluated by[b]:		
Certified athletic trainer	6681	92.1%
General physician	1517	20.9%
Orthopedic physician/sports medicine	1399	19.3%
Physician's assistant	90	1.2%
Chiropractor	61	0.8%
Neurologist	49	0.7%
Nurse practitioner	30	0.4%
Dentist/oral surgeon	12	0.2%
Other	139	1.9%
Total	**7253**	
% of Injuries Assessed by[b]:		
Evaluation	7128	98.2%
X-ray	2438	33.6%
MRI	681	9.4%
CT scan	139	1.9%
Blood work/laboratory test	67	0.9%
Other	45	0.6%
Total	**7253**	**100.0%**

[a]Totals and n's are not always equal because of slight rounding or missing responses.
[b]Multiple responses allowed per injury report.
CT, Computed tomography; *MRI,* magnetic resonance imaging.
From R. Dawn Comstock, PhD, National High School Sports-Related Injury Surveillance Study, available at https://coloradosph.cuanschutz.edu/docs/librariesprovider204/default-document-library/2018-19-convenience-sample.pdf?sfvrsn=e46300b9_2, Table 2.11, Page 34.

COVID-19 Points of Emphasis

- Face coverings
  - Cloth face coverings have been shown to decrease transmission
- Social distancing
  - Adequate distancing may decrease infection risk
  - Symptomatic individuals should stay home, contact a medical provider, and follow treatment recommendations
- Hygiene
  - Avoid contact (e.g., handshakes), avoid touching face, and sneeze or cough into a tissue or inside of the arm/elbow
  - Disinfect frequently used items and surfaces as much as possible
  - Avoid sharing food or hydration (individual water bottles are best)

COVID-19 Illness Reporting

- Notification process for all event participants, staff and personnel, and spectators if a case of COVID-19 is suspected or confirmed
- Vulnerable individuals (as defined by the CDC) should be cautioned or restricted regarding participation in any practices/activities, contests, or events

RTP Considerations After COVID-19 Infection

- RTP guidelines after confirmed/possible infection have been developed by the CDC
  - Basic principles: individual should be asymptomatic and afebrile with at least 10–14 days from the onset of symptoms or a positive test before RTP

  - Additional guidelines have been suggested to address the risk of cardiac concerns identified in adults and for athletes diagnosed with multisystem inflammatory syndrome in children (MIS-C)
  - Some state associations have developed an RTP protocol
  - Some state associations have required cardiac screening and/or cardiology evaluation for athletes with moderate to severe illness or MIS-C
- Research on the long-term effects continues and will inform RTP decision-making

ACKNOWLEDGMENT

We would like to acknowledge **Dr. Stephen G. Rice** for his contributions to prior versions of this chapter.

RECOMMENDED READINGS

Available online.

THE FEMALE ATHLETE 12

Giselle A. Aerni

HISTORY OF WOMEN IN SPORTS

- Throughout history, women have participated in sports at much lower rates than men.
- Still, Egyptian temple wall illustrations depict women playing ball games in 2000 BCE. The first recorded women's athletic competition was the Heraean Games in the sixth century BCE held in the original Olympic stadium. The women of indigenous tribes in the Americas participated in multiple sports until European colonization and forced assimilation into Western culture. And the first women's professional sports team was the black women's baseball team, the Dolly Vardens, established in 1867.
- Title IX was passed in 1972, which stated that no person in the United States shall, on the basis of sex, be excluded from participation in, be denied the benefits of, or be subjected to discrimination under any educational program or activity receiving federal funding.
- US high school sport participation has improved since the introduction of Title IX. In 1971–1972, 7.4% of athletes were girls, compared with 42.9% in 2018–2019.
- Centers for Disease Control and Prevention (CDC) data from 2019 showed that 54.6% of high school girls played one or more sports in the previous year compared with 60.2% of boys. Racial disparities in sport participation also exist, with the following breakdown of self-identified race and percent participating in one or more sports: Asian 46.5%, Hispanic or Latino 51.6%, Black or African American 56.1%, and White 62%.
- Women's participation in the modern Olympic games has improved from 2.2% of athletes in the 1900 Paris games to 45.2% of athletes in the 2016 Rio games.
- Sociocultural determinants that improve female sports participation include parental support (may take form of verbal support, a rule to participate in sport, or role modeling), higher socioeconomic status, higher rates of sibling sports activity, and higher parental education level.
- Female participation in sports increased when the sport was perceived to be fun, involved friends, and had familial and school support through feedback and role modeling.
- Guidelines regarding transgender women participating in sport have varied depending on the sport governing body and may include duration of hormone therapy, legal recognition of their gender and time lived as their gender, and testosterone levels. Ultimately these guidelines do not always agree and may not always be rooted in evidence-based medicine. This presents a significant barrier to transgender women being able to participate in many competitive sports.
- There remains a significant gender disparity in coaching, with only 11% of accredited coaches at the Rio 2016 Olympic games being women. Women's coaches at the collegiate level have actually declined since the introduction of Title IX.
- Gender disparity in sports persists across multiple streams, including percentage of athletic directors and administrators, team physicians, head athletic trainers, professional sports pay, and media representation of women in sports, among others.
- Racial disparities for women of color in sports are essentially multiplied in addition to the gender disparities faced. These issues can significantly affect the role modeling and support that are necessary to encourage young female athletes in their sport participation.

BENEFITS AND RISKS OF SPORTS PARTICIPATION FOR WOMEN

- Studies show that women who participate in sports as adolescents enjoy an overall reduction in all-cause mortality and a significant reduction in cancer rates continuing into adulthood.
- Adolescent sports participation correlates with increased bone density, which extends into middle-age for women who previously participated in sports in comparison with those who did not.
- High school and collegiate girls who participate in sports every day have a decreased body mass index (BMI) and increased cardiorespiratory fitness compared with female nonathletes.
- Measures of mental health and well-being in terms of self-esteem, depression, and suicidality are all positively affected by sports participation in high school and college athletes in general, but this is not correlated with gender, race, or ethnicity.
- Studies have found overwhelming positive benefits to cognitive abilities, academic performance, and education levels relating to participation in high school and collegiate athletes. And in older adults, regular physical activity lowers rates of cognitive decline.
- Even controlling for race, mother's education, age, number of relationships, and alcohol consumption, risk of bullying, property violence, sexual abuse, rape, and violent contact is lower among female athletes than among nonathletes.
- Nonaccidental harms such as bullying and physical and sexual abuse have higher rates among para-athletes when compared with able-bodied athletes. Female para-athletes may have higher rates of sexual violence than their male counterparts.
- Noting that sexual behavior in female athletes is complex, overall, most studies suggest that there are positive effects from sports participation. This includes lower rates of sexual activity, pregnancy, and sexual risk-taking in high school and collegiate girls who participate in sports than in boys and nonathletes.
- High school and collegiate female athletes exhibit lower rates of smoking, marijuana use, and other illicit substance use than nonathletes. However, they may have increased rates of smokeless or chewing tobacco use and nonprescription opioid use.
- Alcohol use is much higher in the adolescent athlete population regardless of gender or race.

PHYSIOLOGY

- Girls achieve physiologic maturity quicker than boys, thus achieving earlier peak height velocity (11.5 years [y] vs. 13.5 y) and skeletal maturity (13.5 y vs. 14.3 y). Along with hormonal changes at the time of puberty, there are many physiologic differences between male and female athletes.
- Tables 12.1 and 12.2 outline the effects of estrogen and progesterone.

Cardiology

- Female athletes typically have a slightly higher resting heart rate (HR) and a lower systolic blood pressure (BP) than male athletes. With exercise, female athletes exhibit a lower absolute change in their systolic BP.
- Although males typically have larger hearts at baseline, both male and female athletes demonstrate physiologic cardiac hypertrophy in response to training. Of note, exercise in black female athletes is associated with greater left ventricular hypertrophy and repolarization changes than comparative white female athletes.

Table 12.1 EFFECTS OF ESTROGEN

System	Effect
Cardiovascular	↑ in thrombosis ↓ total cholesterol ↓ low-density lipoprotein (LDL) levels ↑ high-density lipoprotein (HDL) levels Vasodilates vascular smooth muscle ↑ blood pressure
Endocrine	↑ intramuscular and hepatic glycogen storage and update Glycogen sparing (↑ lipid synthesis, ↑ lipolysis in muscle, and ↑ utilization of free fatty acids) ↑ insulin resistance and ↓ glucose tolerance Deposition of fat in the breasts, buttocks, and thighs
Bone Metabolism	Facilitates uptake of calcium into bone
Neurologic	Cognitive function and verbal memory in postmenopausal women

Table 12.2 EFFECTS OF PROGESTERONE

System	Effect
Thermoregulation	↑ core body temperature of 0.3°C–0.5°C
Respiratory	↑ minute ventilation ↑ ventilatory response to hypoxia and hypercapnia
Metabolic	Fluid retention ↑ dependence on fat as a substrate Induce peripheral insulin resistance

- The mechanism for hypertrophy may be different in females compared with testosterone-driven muscle hypertrophy in males. Females have a higher Ca^{2+}/calmodulin-dependent kinase (CaMK) and protein kinase B/glycogen synthase kinase-3-beta (AKT/GSK-3) pathway signaling, as well as increased fatty acid metabolism, which may contribute more to female-specific physiologic cardiac hypertrophy.
- Pathologic cardiac hypertrophy and arrhythmias are less common in female athletes and considered secondary to estrogen's protective cardiac effects against harmful remodeling.
- Gender differences in cardiac functioning and contribution to maximal oxygen consumption (VO_2 max) may be more related to the larger size of male hearts that have greater stroke volume compared with smaller female hearts.

Pulmonology

- Beginning at around 2 years of age, male lungs are larger than female lungs even when normalized to height and length.
- In addition, females have considerably smaller airways, which can contribute to expiratory flow limitations.
- On approaching maximal exercise, females increase their end expiratory lung volumes back toward resting, hyperinflating their lungs in response to these expiratory flow limitations. Simultaneously, higher end inspiratory lung volumes are required to maintain tidal volume. Ultimately, the intensity of breathing is greater in females—approximately twice as high at maximal exercise.
- The prevalence of arterial oxyhemoglobin desaturation is higher in females than in males because of smaller lung volumes, smaller airways, lower resting diffusion capacity, and lower maximal expiratory flow rates.
- Interestingly, females experience less exercise-induced diaphragmatic fatigue than males.

Metabolism, Nutrition, and Hydration

- 17 β-Estradiol promotes lipid oxidation during endurance exercise, and female athletes have been shown to have a greater dependence on lipid oxidation during endurance events. In addition, 17 β-estradiol promotes hepatic glycogen sparing.
- This enhanced capacity of lipid oxidation, as well as a greater ability to maintain plasma glucose, may account for the ability of female athletes to outperform male athletes at very high distances.
- Females have a lower leucine oxidation rate at rest and during exercise, which accounts for their lower protein requirements.
- There is some evidence that female athletes do not obtain the same benefits from traditional carbohydrate loading compared with male athletes, and in fact need to ingest a proportionally higher amount of carbohydrates in order to gain the same effects.
- Lower ferritin and total body iron tend to be associated with higher oxidative stress. Female athletes are frequently shown to have higher levels of reactive oxygen metabolites and lower iron stores than their male counterparts.
- Throughout the menstrual cycle, from early follicular phase to luteal phase, total body water in females can increase by as much as 2 L. Females have been shown to have lower urine osmolality than do males at rest, with daily activities and with exercise, most likely because of differences in arginine vasopressin (AVP) concentrations.
- Female athletes do not sweat as much as male athletes do, although they do sweat over a greater proportion of their body. In addition, studies have shown that females tend to overconsume water in relation to their body size and metabolic rate.
- A study evaluating the relationship between blood lactate and cortical excitability during exercise revealed that females exhibited a significantly greater improvement in excitability of the primary motor cortex in response to increased lactate levels; this was attributed to the excitatory role of estrogens on the cerebral cortex.

Muscles/Ligaments/Tendons

- Female athletes have been shown to have a similar composition of muscle fibers and enzymatic activity as their male counterparts do when involved with similar sports and activities; however, female muscle fibers are smaller.
- Female athletes are able to achieve significant strength gains with training, but they cannot achieve the same strength levels or hypertrophy as a similarly sized and trained male athlete because of the difference in testosterone.
- Before puberty, both boys and girls have similar strength and joint laxity. At puberty, estrogen contributes to increased joint laxity and possibly increased muscle strength in girls, whereas testosterone contributes to increased muscle strength and hypertrophy in boys.
- Some of the increased injury risk seen in female athletes after the age of puberty is attributed to lax joints and strength imbalance caused by this hormonal change.
- Certain studies have shown lower collagen synthesis in tendons of combined oral contraceptive users, although not all studies have reported differences in tendon properties across the menstrual cycle.

Gastrointestinal Symptoms

- The incidence of gastrointestinal symptoms and complaints is higher in female endurance athletes.
- In addition, studies have revealed a higher incidence of gastrointestinal ischemia in female athletes than in male athletes; however, the underlying pathophysiology remains unknown.

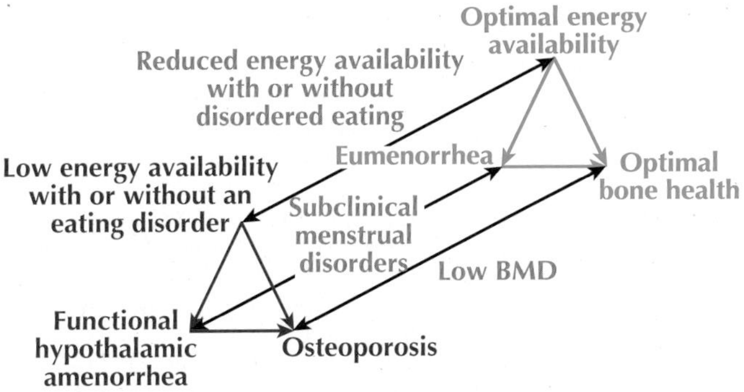
Optimal energy availability
Reduced energy availability with or without disordered eating
Low energy availability with or without an eating disorder
Eumenorrhea
Optimal bone health
Subclinical menstrual disorders
Low BMD
Functional hypothalamic amenorrhea
Osteoporosis

Figure 12.1 Female athlete triad continuum. (From Nattiv A, Loucks AB, Manore MM, et al. American College of Sports Medicine position stand. The female athlete triad. *Med Sci Sports Exerc*. 2007;39[10]:1867–1882.)

FEMALE ATHLETE TRIAD AND RELATIVE ENERGY DEFICIENCY IN SPORT

- The female athlete triad was initially identified in 1992, and over several decades of research has come to represent a spectrum of three components: low energy availability (EA), menstrual dysfunction, and low bone mineral density (BMD). Female athletes may have one or more of these components. Each component is on a spectrum of worsening intensity, ending with low EA with or without an eating disorder, functional hypothalamic amenorrhea, and osteoporosis (Fig. 12.1).
- The Female Athlete Triad Coalition maintains guidelines on screening, risk assessment, and return to play. In 2019 the coalition renamed the organization to The Female and Male Athlete Triad Coalition.
- In 2014, the International Olympic Committee (IOC) first published on Relative Energy Deficiency in Sport (RED-S), aiming to have an expanded focus on issues in all athletes that can be related to low energy availability (see Figs. 5.3 and 5.4).
- Similar to the Triad Coalition, the IOC RED-S group also has published on screening, risk assessment, and return to play. The differences and overlaps will be discussed in the appropriate sections that follow.

Energy Availability

- Low EA is the common etiology for both the triad and RED-S, with prolonged low EA leading to negative health and sport performance consequences. Low EA occurs when caloric intake does not meet the caloric expenditure needs of a female athlete.
- Optimal EA is typically seen at 45 kcal/kg*FFM/day, whereas negative health consequences have been seen to occur at an EA below 30 kcal/kg*FFM/day.
- Unfortunately, methods to quantify exact EA remain imprecise, and therefore there are no diagnostic criteria or standardized measurement in these clinical situations.
- Reduced EA may be unintentional or intentional, and may also fall into the realm of eating disorder concerns (for more information on eating disorders, see Chapter 27: "Eating Disorders in Athletes").
- Low EA is seen more frequently in female athletes than in male athletes and may have different hormonal/physiologic responses.
- Low EA in para-athletes requires more research. Wheelchair athletes likely have decreased energy needs, whereas amputee athletes have increased caloric needs with prosthetic use.
- Prolonged low EA may affect menstrual function and bone health (traditionally described in the triad and with more details later) and may also negatively affect other endocrine, metabolic, and physiologic processes (Box 12.1).

BOX 12.1 HEALTH CONSEQUENCES OF LOW ENERGY AVAILABILITY

- Fatigue
- Decreased recovery time
- Decreased training response
- Impaired performance
- Increased risk for heat illness
- Impaired endothelial-dependent arterial vasodilation
- Gastrointestinal (GI) changes
- Nutrient deficiencies
- Elevated low-density lipoprotein (LDL)
- Vaginal dryness
- Impaired skeletal muscle oxidative metabolism
- Cardiovascular consequences
- Increased risk osteoporosis and fractures
- Reproductive dysfunction
- Two to four times increase in stress fractures

Menstrual Dysfunction

- Low EA can lead to a functional hypothalamic amenorrhea: disruption in gonadotropin-releasing hormone pulsatility, which leads to decreased follicle-stimulating hormone (FSH) and luteinizing hormone (LH) levels and ultimately suppression of estrogen levels, which leads to menstrual dysfunction.
- Menstrual dysfunction begins with suppression of progesterone levels, resulting in a luteal phase that is <11 days.
- Menstrual dysfunction resulting from low EA has been studied and can be reversed with restoration of appropriate energy balance.

Low Bone Mineral Density

- Female athletes with either oligomenorrhea/amenorrhea or low EA have shown decreased BMD, altered bone microarchitecture, and bone turnover markers.
- Suppression of menstrual hormones causes low BMD because of a decrease in estrogen, androgens, insulin-like growth factor 1 (IGF-1), and growth hormone, which affects bone deposition.
- Low EA can also directly reduce BMD by restricting available nutritional resources to build new bone.
- Ninety percent of peak BMD is achieved by the age of 18 years. Adolescence is a critical age for achieving optimum BMD. Disruptions in bone mass accrual during this critical period can have lasting consequences.
- The American College of Sports Medicine (ACSM) defines low BMD as a Z score of <–1.0 in female athletes playing weight-bearing sports.
- Low BMD places the athlete at a higher risk of stress injury.
- Low BMD has been shown to be reversible with restoration of EA.

Screening

- Although screening for elements of the female athlete triad or RED-S is important, there is no clear consensus on the best method.
- As low EA is key to both the triad and RED-S, several screens have been developed in female athletes that focus on low EA and eating disorders: Low Energy Availability in Females Questionnaire (LEAF-Q), Female Athlete Screening Tool (FAST), Brief Eating Disorders in Athletes Questionnaire (BEDA-Q), and Athletic Milieu Direct Questionnaire (AMDQ). Unfortunately, these were all validated using DSM-IV criteria for eating disorders and have not yet been updated to the DSM-V criteria.

- Preparticipation screening is encouraged, and both the Triad Coalition and RED-S group have proposed screening tools and risk assessments that incorporate questions regarding dietary and weight concerns, history of eating disorders, menstrual irregularities, and bone health concerns.

Evaluation

- If an athlete has a positive screen or presents with health conditions concerning for low EA and its negative consequences, evaluation by a sports medicine physician should be performed and involvement of an interdisciplinary team should be considered.
- Assessing EA needs and deficits may be done in conjunction with a sport nutritionist, with the reminder that EA calculation is imprecise.
- In athletes with menstrual dysfunction, low EA/triad/RED-S should be a diagnosis of exclusion. It is important to first rule out pregnancy. Additional workup may include testing LH, FSH, prolactin, thyroid-stimulating hormone (TSH), free T_4, estradiol, testosterone, and Dehydroepiandrosterone-sulfate (DHEA-S) ± 8 am 17(OH) progesterone, a progesterone challenge test, and possibly a pelvic ultrasound.
- Dual energy x-ray absorptiometry (DXA or DEXA) screening is recommended to evaluate bone density in certain situations (Box 12.2).
- The Female Athlete Triad Coalition and IOC RED-S group both have risk assessments that can be used to categorize risk magnitude and aid in clearance and return-to-play decisions.

Treatment

- Treatment of the triad should be best undertaken by a multidisciplinary treatment team that includes a sport medicine physician, a licensed mental health professional, a sport nutritionist, and possibly others as the situation warrants.
- Inadvertent undereating may simply require nutrition education. In cases involving disordered eating, treatment can be difficult, more complicated, and require more resources. In rare situations, hospitalization may be necessary for athletes with eating disorders (see Chapter 27: "Eating Disorders in Athletes").
- Treatment focuses on increasing EA through changes in diet and exercise.
  - Caloric intake should be gradually increased, beginning with a 20%–30% increase over baseline energy needs, if known, or adding approximately 300–600 kcal/day.
  - Reduction in exercise may be difficult for the athlete. Decreasing training volumes, instituting rest days, or time off may be considerations.
- If a female athlete is underweight and amenorrheic, increased body weight by 5%–10% has been associated with resumed menstruation. Even with improvements in EA, recovery of normal menses can take months to over 1 year.
- Low BMD should be addressed with first optimizing EA, as well as calcium and 25-OH vitamin D intake. Transdermal estrogen replacement, but not combined oral contraceptives, has been shown to improve BMD in oligo-amenorrheic athletes. However, this is not yet standard practice and should be prescribed in consultation with a bone health expert.

Return to Play

- Athletes that are significantly underweight or with concomitant health issues may require activity restriction. In these situations, involving the multidisciplinary team and the use of an athlete contract with specific goals for resumption of activity may be useful (see Chapter 27: "Eating Disorders in Athletes").

BOX 12.2 INDICATIONS FOR DXA SCREENING

1. ≥1 "High-Risk" Triad Risk Factors:
   - History of DSM-V–diagnosed eating disorder
   - BMI ≤17.5 kg/m², <85% estimated weight, OR recent weight loss of ≥10% in 1 month
   - Menarche ≥16 years of age
   - Current or history of <6 menses over past 12 months
   - Two prior stress fractures, one high-risk stress fracture, or one low-energy nontraumatic fracture
   - Prior Z score of <−2.0 (after at least 1 year from baseline DXA)

OR

2. ≥2 "Moderate-Risk" Triad Risk Factors:
   - Current or history of DE for ≥6 months
   - BMI 17.5–18.5 kg/m², <90% estimated weight, OR recent weight loss of 5%–10% in 1 month
   - Menarche between 15 and 16 years of age
   - Current or history of 6–8 menses over past 12 months
   - One prior stress reaction/fracture
   - Prior Z score between −1.0 and −2.0 (after at least a 1-year interval from baseline DXA)
3. In addition, an athlete with a history of ≥1 nonperipheral or ≥2 peripheral long bone traumatic fractures (nonstress) should be considered for DXA testing if there are ≥1 moderate- or high-risk factors for the triad. This will depend on the likelihood of fracture, given the magnitude of trauma (low/high impact) and age at which the fracture occurred. Moreover, athletes on medication for ≥6 months that may affect the bone should be considered for DXA testing.

BMI, Body mass index; *DE,* disordered eating; *DXA,* dual-energy x-ray absorptiometry.
From De Souza MJ, Nattiv A, Joy E, et al. 2014 Female Athlete Triad Coalition Consensus Statement on treatment and return to play of the Female Athlete Triad. *Clin J Sport Med.* 2014;24:96–119.

- Recovery takes time to increase energy levels, improve hormone levels, and increase BMD.
- The return-to-play decision should be individualized and should include a comprehensive analysis of the individual athlete's situation and risk factors.
- Based on the severity of the athlete's presenting concerns, prolonged monitoring may be required in order to ensure that optimal health is maintained.

EATING DISORDERS AND BODY IMAGE IN SPORTS

- Female athletes are at a higher risk of disordered eating than the general population. The risks are typically worse in sports with weight classes, aesthetic sports, and sports where a low BMI is considered advantageous.
- Most validated screening tools to evaluate for eating disorders in female athletes were validated using DSM-IV criteria. One recently validated tool using DSM-V criteria is the six-item Eating Disorders Screen for Athletes (EDSA): a brief screening tool for male and female athletes.
- In sports, there is often an ideal body image that suggests improved performance because the body could be considered a tool for athletic performance by the athlete.
- Desires for a certain body image include a drive for thinness, muscularity, and/or leanness.
- Drive for thinness is often linked to disordered eating, whereas drive for muscularity is linked to disordered eating in male athletes but not in female athletes.
- Athletes with eating disorders will need evaluation, treatment, and monitoring from a multidisciplinary team that includes a sports medicine physician, licensed mental health practitioner, and sport nutritionist, among others.

CONCUSSION

- Female athletes have a greater reported incidence of concussions than do male athletes.
- Additionally, female athletes have higher postconcussion symptom scores, slower reaction times compared with baseline, greater cognitive decline, and prolonged time to recovery and return to sport than males in comparable sports.
- No definitive etiologies have been identified to explain this increased incidence. Proposed factors affecting incidence and severity include decreased neck strength in female athletes, greater reporting of symptoms, and possible impact of varied hormone concentrations at the time of concussion during the menstrual cycle.
- In general, female brains have greater metabolic requirements than male brains, but this has not yet been clearly linked with the incidence of concussion.
- Baseline neurocognitive evaluations have shown some gender differences. In general, females perform better with verbal scores, whereas males perform better with visual tests. In addition, males have been shown to have faster speeds or reaction times, whereas females tend to be slower but more accurate. Differences in baselines could affect the interpretation of post-concussion testing and the ability to create standardized norms.
- Further research is needed to explore the explanations for the higher rate of reported concussions in female athletes.
- See Chapter 45: "Head Injuries."

ASTHMA

- The overall prevalence, severity, morbidity, and mortality associated with asthma are worse in females; however, before puberty, it is actually males who have a higher incidence of asthma.
- This gender switch at puberty is possibly related to the difference in lung development between young males and females. Prepubertal males have an increased number of bronchioles, which are individually smaller in size and thus more susceptible to inflammation and constriction.
- Over time, the incidence and severity of asthma improve with puberty in males, whereas it worsens in females. The incidence evens out in older age, as postmenopausal females have a similar disease prevalence as do age-matched males.
- It is frequently noted that symptoms and severity of asthma can worsen with pregnancy.
- Because of the changing incidence with puberty and menopause, studies have investigated the role of estrogen and progesterone on the respiratory system. For example, progesterone has been shown to decrease the beat frequency of cilia, which may contribute to the worsening of asthma symptoms during the premenstrual phase.
- In addition, studies have revealed that women with mild-to-moderate asthma may benefit from taking oral contraceptive pills (OCPs), which limit premenstrual exacerbations of asthma.
- Females have been shown to report greater symptoms than males, with similar diagnostic disease severity and lung function test results.
- Interestingly, a recent meta-analysis demonstrated no difference in the prevalence of exercise-induced bronchospasm between male and female athletes, whereas male athletes had higher rates of atopy.

ANTERIOR CRUCIATE LIGAMENT

- The incidence of anterior cruciate ligament (ACL) tear is 2–10 times higher in females than in males.
- Anatomic predisposing factors include greater Q angles, increased tibial and meniscal slopes, narrower femoral notches, and smaller ACL size.

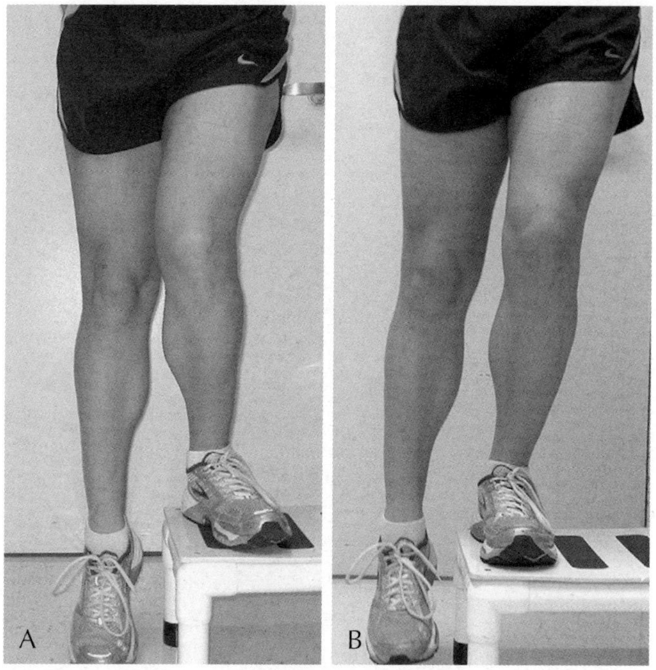
A
B

Figure 12.2 ACL injury biomechanics. **A,** "Position of no return" that places the ACL at risk during landing or cutting. The left leg has adduction and internal rotation of the hip. The knee is in valgus with external rotation of the tibia and the foot pronated with weight on the ball of the foot. **B,** A safer landing position has flexion at the hip with less or no adduction. The knee is flexed without tibial rotation and the foot balanced. (From Boles CA, Ferguson C. The female athlete. *Radiol Clin N Am*. 2010;48:1249–1266.)

- The relationship between hormonal fluctuations during menses and ACL injuries remains controversial. Both ACL and skeletal muscles have estrogen receptors, and studies have shown alterations in ligament laxity and neuromuscular control patterns in relationship to fluctuations in estrogen levels, although no consistent relationship has been elucidated.
- Females have been shown to exhibit biomechanical and neuromuscular activation patterns that are associated with increased risk of ACL injury, including landing with greater knee valgus and a greater quadriceps-to-hamstring ratio activation and recruitment (Fig. 12.2).
- During growth and development, male and female children have been shown to have a similar risk of ACL injury before puberty. It appears that the anatomic, hormonal, and biomechanical patterns that place females at a higher risk of ACL injury do not develop until puberty.
- Meta-analysis has shown poorer subjective pain and activity scores after reconstruction despite similar objective measures between males and females.
- Recent research has shown differences in genetic variation within matrix metalloproteinase 3 in the extracellular matrix of the ACL between males and females with noncontact ACL injuries.

PATELLOFEMORAL PAIN SYNDROME

- Patellofemoral pain is one of the most common presenting musculoskeletal complaints. Females are two to three times more likely than males to experience patellofemoral pain, with no difference seen in terms of age or athletic participation.
- Anatomic factors that probably contribute to the higher incidence of patellofemoral pain syndrome (PFPS) in females include wider pelvis, greater hip varus, increased femoral

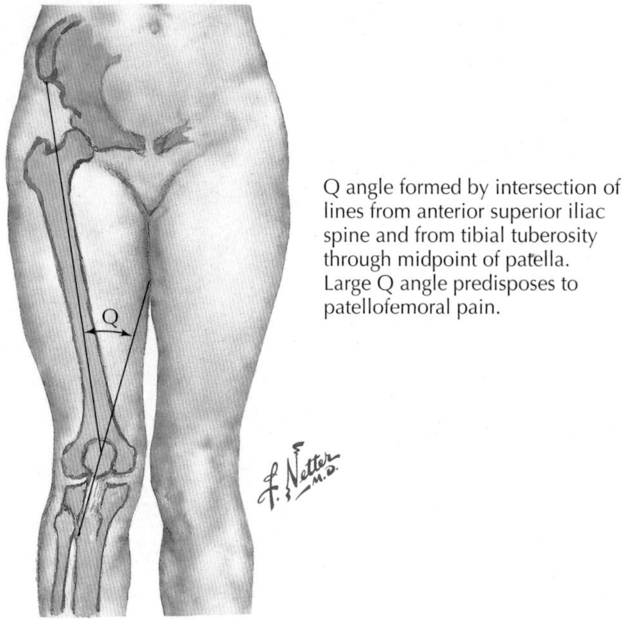
Q angle formed by intersection of lines from anterior superior iliac spine and from tibial tuberosity through midpoint of patella. Large Q angle predisposes to patellofemoral pain.
Q

Figure 12.3 Quadriceps angle.

anteversion, increased knee valgus, and increased external tibia rotation. Taken together, these factors contribute to a greater Q angle in female athletes (Fig. 12.3).

- Females also have a higher incidence of patellar instability and dislocation. Anatomically, females have a higher incidence of patella alta and trochlear dysplasia and an increased tibial tuberosity-to-trochlear groove distance, which, in general, may contribute toward both instability and patellofemoral pain.
- Dynamic or kinematic factors that may contribute to the increased incidence of patellofemoral pain in females include excessive contralateral pelvic drop, more upright landing, less hip and knee flexion with landing, more weight on the forefoot, and ultimately, greater dynamic knee valgus.
  - Increased knee valgus can cause lateral patellar tracking, which leads to increased loading forces on the lateral patellofemoral joint.
  - Certain studies have suggested that weak hip abductors may contribute to PFPS. However, studies evaluating the gluteus medius have conflicted with this finding, demonstrating that normalized gluteus medius activation is greater in females than in males at baseline, whereas other studies have shown no difference in gluteus medius activation in females with and without PFPS.
  - Other studies have shown that males with patellofemoral pain may have a different biomechanical mechanism. Male athletes with PFPS run and squat with less hip adduction, putting their knee into greater knee varum; such males were shown to have a more lateral center of pressure and an increased external knee adduction moment.
  - With an overly small Q angle, males may be overloading on their medial facet (as opposed to the lateral facet for females with PFPS), which may have implications in diagnosis, as well as treatment/management considerations for males versus females with PFPS.
- Significant research has shown that pain in PFPS may have a greater relation to kinesiophobia than joint-loading variables. Additionally, individuals with patellofemoral pain have been found to have widespread reduced pain thresholds to pressure such that mechanically induced pain is likely amplified.
- Gender has not been shown to be a predictive factor in short- or long-term outcomes for patients with PFPS.

STRESS FRACTURES

- Female athletes have a greater risk and rates of stress fracture.
- Bones in females are smaller and less dense than in males at peak bone mass. Additionally, bone microarchitecture and bone strength are more favorable in black women than in white women.
- Estrogen is believed to play a significant role in bone metabolism: it is important for bone mineral deposition in females during puberty and peak bone mass accrual.
- Several studies have reported conflicting results regarding whether estrogen or mechanical loading is more important in female bone accrual. Certain studies have found that estrogen inhibits bone deposition in response to mechanical loading, whereas others have found that estrogen is necessary for females to exhibit any response to mechanical loading.
- A study that prospectively evaluated physical activity levels during childhood and obtained DXA scans at the age of 17 years found that the females who had been most active during their early childhood had significantly greater bone densities.
- In addition, women with menstrual irregularities, amenorrhea, or delayed menarche are shown to have lower bone density. If amenorrhea or delayed menarche occurs during adolescence, which is the period of peak bone mass accrual, these females may never achieve normal peak bone mass.
- Athletes who participate in weight-bearing sports and are eumenorrheic have higher BMD than do similar athletes who are amenorrheic/oligomenorrheic. Additionally, athletes participating in weight-bearing sports should have a higher BMD compared with their nonathletic peers.
- Finally, females also experience a considerable decrease in bone mass at menopause when there is a substantial decline in endogenous estrogen levels.
  - Bone loss at the microstructure level displays a loss of connectivity between trabeculae in females, whereas in males, bone loss is a product of trabecular thinning and decreased bone formation. This may also contribute toward the increased risk of fracture in females.
- The role of estrogen and peak bone density is extremely vital for female athletes, particularly during adolescence and at or after menopause. Females with a prolonged history of amenorrhea, eating disorder, or the triad or RED-S may be at an increased risk of stress injuries even if they resume normal menses and body weight.
- IGF-1 stimulates osteoblast proliferation, bone matrix protein synthesis, alkaline phosphatase activity, and differentiation. Elevated levels of IGF-1 are associated with increased BMD in women and vice versa. Studies have shown that alterations in IGF-binding proteins 2 and 5 are associated with an increased risk of stress fractures.
- Bone-specific tartrate-resistant acid phosphatase 5b (TRAP-5b) is a bone resorption biomarker that has been shown to be significantly elevated in female athletes with stress fractures.
- See Chapter 59: "Stress Fractures" for additional information regarding the diagnosis and management of stress injuries.

EXERCISE DURING AND AFTER PREGNANCY

- The beneficial effects of exercise in pregnancy mean most women should be encouraged to achieve 150 minutes of moderate-intensity aerobic exercise per week and participate in resistance training.
  - Benefits include higher incidence of vaginal delivery and lower incidence of excessive weight gain, gestational diabetes, gestational hypertension or preeclampsia, preterm birth, cesarean birth, and lower birth weight.
- Physiologic changes during pregnancy include increased blood volume with decreased vascular resistance, compression of venous return, increased tidal volume, increased oxygen demand,

BOX 12.3 CONTRAINDICATIONS TO EXERCISE DURING PREGNANCY

- Significant heart disease
- Restrictive lung disease
- Incompetent cervix (including those who are status-post cerclage)
- Severe preeclampsia
- Uncontrolled type 1 diabetes
- Placental abruption, placenta previa, vasa previa
- Active preterm labor
- Intrauterine growth restriction

shifted center of gravity, ligamentous laxity, and increased metabolism resulting in increased body temperature.

- Because of physiologic changes, the rate of perceived exertion may be more effective than heart rate parameters to determine exercise intensity.
- See Box 12.3 for contraindications to exercise during pregnancy.
- Pregnant female athletes should avoid scuba diving, maintained supine position after 20 weeks' gestation, and training at higher altitudes.
- Caution should be taken with high-impact sports, particularly after the first trimester, when the gravid uterus exceeds the protection of the bony pelvis.
- Women should be mindful of caloric and hydration needs throughout pregnancy and the postpartum period and adjust intake to meet those needs.
- Postpartum exercise helps improve energy, sleep, stress levels, and abdominal toning and may help prevent postpartum depression.
- Consensus expert opinion recommends that exercise can and should be resumed gradually after pregnancy, with early resumption after vaginal delivery compared with cesarean.
- Regular postpartum exercise has been shown to have no impact on milk production or composition. Women who are breastfeeding may consider feeding or expressing milk before exercise to avoid discomfort of engorged breasts.
- Team physicians taking care of high school, collegiate, or professional athletes should consider both the American College of Obstetricians and Gynecologists guidelines and the policies of specific sports organizations in balance with the goals and circumstances of each individual athlete when making recommendations.

PELVIC FLOOR DYSFUNCTION

- Pelvic floor dysfunction (PFD) refers to a variety of disorders of the pelvic floor muscles. PFD can be divided into two broad categories: relaxing PFD (includes stress urinary incontinence, fecal incontinence, and pelvic organ prolapse) and nonrelaxing PFD (symptoms of impaired urination/defecation, sexual dysfunction, and pelvic pain).
- More is known regarding relaxing PFD, with 30%–80% of elite female athletes reporting stress urinary incontinence (SUI).
- Females in higher-impact sports demonstrate higher rates of SUI. Studies conflict whether SUI resolves or continues after cessation of sport.
- Urinary incontinence is distressing to female athletes, is underreported, and can affect sport participation.
- Female athletes who have delivered vaginally have higher rates of SUI.
- Pelvic floor therapy can reduce episodes of urinary incontinence.

RECOMMENDED READINGS

Available online.

13 THE SENIOR ATHLETE

Zach D. Bowers • Jeffrey T. Abildgaard • John M. Tokish

GENERAL CONSIDERATIONS

Demographics

- It is widely accepted that the average life expectancy continues to increase; as it does, the proportion of older adults in the population also increases.
  - In Western industrialized countries, the average life expectancy increased from 47 years in 1900 to 78 years in 2007.
  - The number of individuals older than 85 years has increased by 232% from 1960 to 1990, along with a total population growth of 39% during the same period.
  - By 2030, 20% of the US population will be older than 65 years.
- It is important to maintain a working knowledge of the anatomic and physiologic changes associated with normal aging and to be able to differentiate them from pathologic entities.

Physical Activity and Health Promotion

- Numerous athletes are able to maintain a high level of participation and performance into their middle age and well beyond.
- Cumulative recommendations from the American College of Sports Medicine (ACSM), the American Academy of Orthopaedic Surgeons (AAOS), and the American Heart Association (AHA) encourage older adults to maintain a physically active lifestyle with an emphasis on moderate-intensity aerobic and muscle-strengthening activities, as well as activities that promote increased flexibility and balance for older adults who are at a risk of falls.
- Evidence over the years has demonstrated that senior athletes are not only able to participate in more endurance activities and competitive sports but also able to compete longer than ever and outperform historical comparisons.
- This growth is demonstrated by the increasing number of athletes participating in the National Senior Games, marathons, and triathlon competitions.
  - Participation in the National Senior Games, which is a biennial competition for men and women aged ≥50 years, has increased from 2500 competitors in 1987 to >12,000 athletes in 2007.
  - Almost half of all US participants in marathons are aged over 40 years. One-fourth of marathon runners in their 60s are able to outperform half of the runners aged 20–54 years.
  - The overall participation in triathlons has increased by almost 60% since 2008, and now, an estimated 850,000 adults aged over 40 years compete in triathlons in the United States.
- Despite increased rates of participation, older adults remain the least active group in the United States. Healthcare providers need to continue to counsel older adults regarding health benefits that coincide with an active lifestyle.
- Several changes associated with aging can be limited, prevented, or even reversed with sustained exercise.

PHYSIOLOGIC CHANGES ASSOCIATED WITH AGING

General Considerations

- Aging is an individual process that is influenced by a multitude of factors, including genetics, ethnicity, culture, diet, illness, environmental exposure, occupation, and physical activity.
- Age-related structural and functional changes occur at the molecular level and result in a gradual decline in the physiologic performance of virtually every organ system.
- At the cellular level, multiple changes are observed:
  - Decreased capacity for division and cellular repair
  - Impaired exchange of nutrition, cellular waste, and oxygen
  - Intracellular accumulation of lipids and pigments
  - Lipofuscin—“aging pigment” breakdown product of erythrocytes that collects in multiple tissues, particularly smooth muscles and myocardium

Effects of Aging on Specific Physiologic Systems

Cardiovascular

- An age-associated decline in cardiac output may be attributed to reductions in maximal heart rate, myocardial contractility, and stroke volume; these changes can result in an age-related drop in myocardial oxygen consumption/utilization (mVO_2).
- Regular cardiovascular exercise and endurance training have been shown to increase mVO_2 in individuals aged up to 70 years.
- Fatty and fibrous tissue deposits may occur in the myocardium that can interrupt normal conduction pathways, contributing to the occurrence of arrhythmias.
- Cardiac valves may thicken and lose compliance, contributing to the formation of valvular regurgitation, clinically manifesting as a murmur.
- Vascular physiology is affected by age-related changes in vascular compliance, microcirculation, and baroreceptor function; these changes, combined with atherosclerosis, can produce an increased peripheral vascular resistance, resulting in increased cardiac effort to maintain cardiac output.
  - Increased blood pressure and orthostatic hypotension are commonly observed as consequences of vascular changes.
  - Decreased capillary density and impaired vascular proliferation have also been implicated in reducing the exercise capacity of aging individuals.

Pulmonary

- Reduction in pulmonary microvasculature and alveoli number results in limitations in oxygen exchange and an increased sense of respiratory effort exerted during exercise.
- Decreased lung compliance results from weakness of respiratory and accessory muscles, decreased alveolar tissue elasticity, and stiffening of costovertebral and sternocostal cartilages.
- Overall, these changes contribute to a decrease in total lung capacity; vital lung capacity; inspiratory and expiratory air flows; and an increase in residual volume, respiratory frequency, and work of breathing.

Renal

- A progressive loss in the number of glomeruli, along with increased vascular rigidity and atherosclerosis, results in a decreased glomerular filtration rate with aging. Coexisting renal disease and nephrotoxic medications can exacerbate this age-related decline.
- In addition, the ability of the kidneys to concentrate urine decreases with age, resulting in a greater relative water output; this can negatively affect a senior athlete's ability to remain adequately hydrated.

Neurologic

- Progressive central nervous system deterioration has been shown to result in impaired hearing, short-term memory, balance, fine motor skills, and cognition. In addition, extrapyramidal dysfunction can result in impaired coordination and rapidity of motions and with a resultant increase in motor response time.
- Even in the absence of any known neurologic disease, peripheral nerve conduction velocities are known to decrease with age, affecting vibration and proprioception nerve fibers first.

Vision

- Progressive vision impairment is common with age. Typical changes include decreased visual acuity, accommodation, contrast sensitivity, peripheral vision, and ability to adapt to low-light situations.

Endocrinal

- As part of a normal consequence of aging, hormone levels gradually decline. Effects of this decline are noted in multiple organ systems:
  - With age, basal metabolic rate decreases, along with increased rates of metabolic syndrome, diabetes mellitus type 2, and obesity.
  - Adrenal function is reduced, resulting in decreased aldosterone and reduced ability to regulate fluid/electrolyte balance, as well as decreased stress response by cortisol.
  - Moreover, decreased rates of trophic hormones such as testosterone and insulin-like growth factor are associated with a decrease in skeletal muscle mass with age.

Musculoskeletal

- Senile sarcopenia is the age-related decrease in skeletal muscle mass. Between the ages of 50 and 80 years, an average person will lose one-third of their muscle mass. At the cellular level, decreased cell numbers and proliferative capacity of satellite cells leads to decreased muscle regeneration and response to injury. Extracellularly, dysfunction of actin-myosin cross-linking causes muscle units to become stiffer and more susceptible to injury, particularly muscular strains.
- The structure of both ligaments and tendons changes with aging. Aging ligaments exhibit fewer fibroblasts and mechanoreceptors, which may contribute to decreased ultimate failure load and mechanical stiffness. On the other hand, aging tendons exhibit fewer fibroblasts and increased degenerative changes; this, along with a less robust blood supply (watershed areas), helps explain the epidemic of tendon injuries in senior athletes.
- Articular cartilage is particularly susceptible to injury and degeneration with aging (Fig. 13.1). Few, if any, chondrocytes are produced after skeletal maturity. Production of extracellular matrix proteoglycans is more variable with time, rendering them less effective. Response to mechanical loading is impaired by decreasing cartilage water content and more rigid collagen fibrils, secondary to increased cross-linking, which increases the risk of fissuring or shear injury.
- With age, a progressive loss of bone mineral density results in compensatory widening of the diaphysis. Consequently, the susceptibility to fragility fractures and stress injuries increases.
- Men exhibit a 0.5%–0.75% annual loss of bone mass after the age of 40 years. In women, bone mass decreases much more

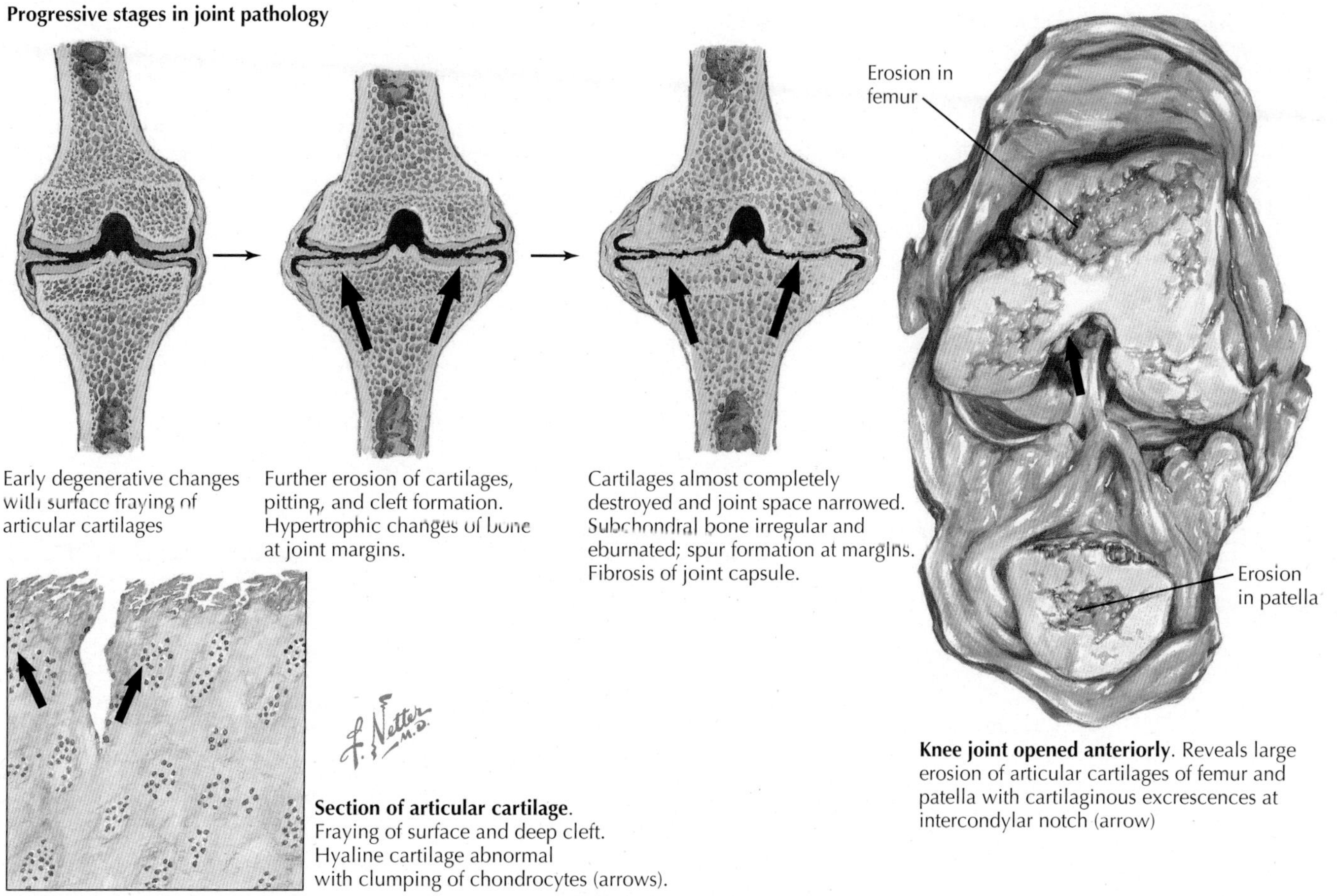
Progressive stages in joint pathology
Erosion in femur
Early degenerative changes with surface fraying of articular cartilages
Further erosion of cartilages, pitting, and cleft formation. Hypertrophic changes of bone at joint margins.
Cartilages almost completely destroyed and joint space narrowed. Subchondral bone irregular and eburnated; spur formation at margins. Fibrosis of joint capsule.
Erosion in patella
Knee joint opened anteriorly. Reveals large erosion of articular cartilages of femur and patella with cartilaginous excrescences at intercondylar notch (arrow)
Section of articular cartilage. Fraying of surface and deep cleft. Hyaline cartilage abnormal with clumping of chondrocytes (arrows).
F. Netter M.D.

Figure 13.1 Osteoarthritis

rapidly, at a pace of 1.5%–2.0% before menopause and accelerating further after menopause to up to 3% per year.

DECLINE IN ATHLETIC PERFORMANCE WITH AGING

General Considerations

- Successful care of aging athletes depends on understanding the differences between normal and pathologic aging.
- It is well recognized that sedentary older adults exhibit more significant changes in functional capacity and body composition than adults who remain physically active as they age.

Factors Affecting Performance

Decreased Muscle Strength

- Decrease in lean muscle mass (senile sarcopenia) is paralleled by an equal or greater decrease in strength and power. Senior athletes also experience an increase in muscle fatigability.
- Muscle power is lost at a greater rate than endurance capacity.
- Muscle cross-sectional area in men declines by 14.7% over a 12-year period, beginning at the age of 65 years.

Loss of Endurance Capacity

- Decreased maximal aerobic capacity (VO_2 max) is a primary contributor to decreased endurance capacity.
- VO_2 max is dependent on heart rate, cardiac output, and tissue oxygen uptake.
- Peak blood lactate concentration is an indirect measure of anaerobic glycolytic activity. Peak lactate concentrations after maximal activity have been shown to be lower in men aged >60 years.

Loss of Exercise Economy

- Decreased flexibility, joint motion, and coordination contribute to a decline in exercise economy.

Effects of Age and Gender on Athletic Performance

- A slow progressive decline in athletic performance is seen in most athletes, starting after 35–40 years of age. Aging athletes remain capable of high levels of physical performance into their 70s.
  - Significant loss of function observed before the age of 70 years can likely be attributed to disuse, sedentary lifestyle behaviors, and genetic predisposition. Between 70 and 75 years of age, most athletes reach a tipping point, and athletic performance typically plunges.
- Analysis of running and sprinting records of master athletes in the Senior Olympics shows a <2% decline in performance per year among both men and women aged 50–75 years.
  - Age-associated decline in performance is typically greater in women. Examples in peer-reviewed literature have shown these differences to be greatest in endurance running and sprint-type swimming events.

BENEFITS OF EXERCISE IN OLDER ADULTS

General Considerations

- A continually growing body of evidence establishes the benefits of exercise in aging athletes. Recommendations from the ACSM advocate for a combined physical activity regimen for all adults, including resistance, endurance, flexibility, and balance training (Table 13.1).
- The prevalence of various diseases, including diabetes, cardiovascular disorders, mental disorders, and certain types of cancer, are lower in people who engage in consistent physical activity.
- The incidence of mortality and amount of functional disability are also lower in active aging populations.

Musculoskeletal Benefits of Exercise

- Impact exercise can help to counteract age-related changes in bone mineral density.
  - Considerably increased bone mineral density has been observed in Senior Olympic runners aged >65 years compared with control subjects.
- Participation in resistance activities is the most effective method to offset sarcopenia.
  - Resistance training in elderly adults has been shown to increase muscle strength and cross-sectional area, increase joint range of motion, and improve dynamic balance.
- Although structural alterations in tendon and ligament tissues are observed with aging, mechanical properties can be improved with regular physical activity.
  - Physical activity has been shown to result in increased tensile strength, ultimate load, and mechanical stiffness of ligaments and preserve the size and mechanical properties of tendons.
- A decrease in age-related cartilage volume loss has been demonstrated with exercise.
  - Senior athletes participating in moderate- to high-intensity activities that load the knee and strengthen knee extensors exhibit decreased patellar and tibial cartilage volume loss.

Systemic Benefits of Exercise

- Participation in sustained, moderately intense, aerobic activity has cardioprotective benefits (Fig. 13.2).
- Stroke volume, which is a major determinant of cardiac output, can decline with age. Sustained exercise can reduce this decline by 50%.
  - Additional cardiovascular benefits include increased vascular compliance, lower blood pressure, and decreased formation of atherosclerotic plaques.

Table 13.1 RECOMMENDED MINIMUM EXERCISE FOR SENIOR ATHLETES

Factor	Duration	Intensity (0–10)[a]	Comments
Endurance	150–300 min/week	5–8	At least 10- to 30-min episodes
Resistance	8–10 exercises of 8–12 repetitions	5–8	≥2 days/week
Flexibility	≥2 days/week	5–6	Sustained stretches, static/nonballistic movements
Balance	No specific recommendations	As tolerable	Progressively difficult postures, stressing postural muscle groups (particularly for frequent fallers)

Adults who are unable to tolerate the aforementioned recommendations should be encouraged to maintain the highest possible activity level and avoid a completely sedentary lifestyle.

[a]On a scale of 0–10 for level of physical exertion, 5–6 for moderate intensity, and 7–8 for vigorous intensity.

From Chodzko-Zajko WJ, Proctor DN, Fiatarone Singh MA, et al. American College of Sports Medicine: American College of Sports Medicine position stand: Exercise and physical activity for older adults. *Med Sci Sports Exerc*. 2009;41:1510–1530.

- VO_2 max is frequently increased with moderately intense aerobic activity, which is beneficial for other organ systems: improved pulmonary gas exchange, renal function (resulting from better blood flow), and lactate threshold.
- Maintenance of flexibility with regular stretching activities has been demonstrated to decrease the risk of musculotendinous strains in senior athletes.
- Balance training can decrease the rate of falls in older adults at a higher risk of fall injuries.

PREPARTICIPATION MEDICAL EVALUATION (PPPE)

- In general, exercise does not provoke cardiovascular events in healthy individuals with a normal cardiovascular system. Individuals with atherosclerosis or decreased cardiac performance are at an increased risk of an acute myocardial event with moderate- to high-intensity physical activity; moreover, this risk is compounded in individuals with a previous sedentary lifestyle who abruptly begin intensive training regimens.

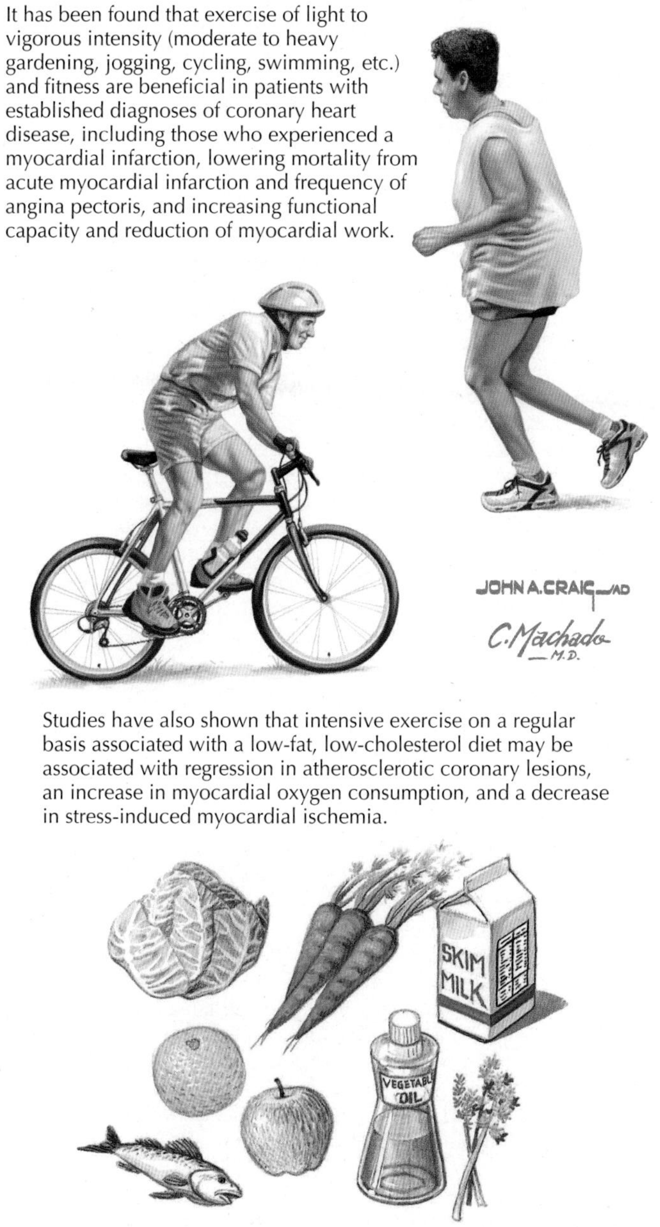
It has been found that exercise of light to vigorous intensity (moderate to heavy gardening, jogging, cycling, swimming, etc.) and fitness are beneficial in patients with established diagnoses of coronary heart disease, including those who experienced a myocardial infarction, lowering mortality from acute myocardial infarction and frequency of angina pectoris, and increasing functional capacity and reduction of myocardial work.
Studies have also shown that intensive exercise on a regular basis associated with a low-fat, low-cholesterol diet may be associated with regression in atherosclerotic coronary lesions, an increase in myocardial oxygen consumption, and a decrease in stress-induced myocardial ischemia.
SKIM MILK
VEGETABLE OIL

Figure 13.2 Effects of exercise on cardiovascular physiology.

- The risk of sudden cardiac arrest or myocardial infarction is very low in healthy individuals who perform moderate-intensity activities. The ACSM cautions that vigorous exercise confers an acute increased risk of sudden cardiac death and/or myocardial infarction in individuals with either diagnosed or occult cardiovascular disease.
- Cardiac assessment is not required before initiating moderate-intensity exercise programs in a majority of senior athletes. Older adults with more than two risk factors are considered to be at a moderate risk of adverse responses to exercise and are advised to undergo medical examination and exercise testing before initiating high-intensity/vigorous exercise (Table 13.2).
- The American Heart Association Committee on Exercise endorses preparticipation exercise testing for all master athletes of any age with symptoms suggestive of underlying coronary disease and for those aged ≥65 years even in the absence of risk factors and symptoms.

TREATMENT OF MUSCULOSKELETAL INJURIES IN OLDER ATHLETES

General Considerations

- Senior athletes are often victims of two types of injuries: those that occurred in their youth and continue to be symptomatic and those that result from current athletic activity.

Table 13.2 RISK FACTOR THRESHOLDS OF CORONARY ARTERY DISEASE FOR ACSM RISK STRATIFICATION

Positive Risk Factor	Defining Criteria
Age	Men ≥45 years; women ≥55 years
Family history	Myocardial infarction, coronary revascularization, or sudden death before 55 years of age in father or any other first-degree male relative or before 65 years of age in mother or any other first-degree female relative.
Cigarette smoking	Current smoker or smoker who quit within previous 6 months or exposure to environmental tobacco smoke.
Hypertension	Systolic blood pressure (BP) ≥140 mmHg or diastolic BP ≥90 mmHg confirmed by measurements on at least two occasions or prescription for antihypertensive medication.
Hypercholesterolemia	Low-density lipoprotein (LDL) cholesterol >130 mg/dL, high-density lipoprotein (HDL) cholesterol <40 mg/dL, or on lipid-lowering medications. If only total serum cholesterol is known, use >200 mg/dL.
Impaired fasting glucose	Fasting blood glucose >100 mg/dL confirmed by measurements on at least two separate occasions.
Obesity	Body mass index >30 kg/m² or waist circumference >102 cm for men and >88 cm for women.
Sedentary lifestyle	Individuals not participating in a regular exercise program or accumulating ≥30 minutes of moderate-intensity physical activity most days of week for at least 3 months.
Negative	
High serum HDL cholesterol	>60 mg/dL

- Younger athletes have a higher incidence of acute traumatic injury to their ligaments and tendons than do older athletes, partly because of their participation in higher-velocity/higher-impact sports.
- A senior athlete is not immune to high-velocity injuries; however, injuries are far more likely to occur due to degenerative tissue problems that result from wear and tear from chronic overuse or trauma experienced over years of athletic stress.
  - For example, postural malalignment of the knee, such as genu varus, can lead to overloading of the medial compartment with an increased risk of meniscal tears and degenerative chondral changes.
- Senior athletes are particularly prone to acute muscle strains and injuries at the myotendinous junction because of age-related changes in biomechanical properties of the tendon and subsequent decrease in flexibility and tensile strength.
  - Age-related decrease in blood supply to the so-called watershed areas in tendons helps to contribute to increased pathology.
  - Ruptures of quadriceps and Achilles tendon occur more frequently in middle-aged and senior athletes.
- Tendinosis is common in older athletes and results from repetitive loading and cumulative microtrauma to tendons.
  - Common tendinopathies seen in older golfers include rotator cuff tendinopathy, medial and lateral epicondylitis, and inflammation of wrist tendons, including the extensor capri ulnaris tendinosis.
  - Lateral epicondylitis, or tennis elbow, occurs most commonly in middle-aged persons and is related to overuse of wrist extensors (Fig. 13.3).
  - Older joggers are particularly prone to development of Achilles tendinitis, along with posterior tibialis tendon insufficiency.
- The rotator cuff is particularly susceptible to age-related changes and pathology in aging athletes (Fig. 13.4). Rotator cuff dysfunction can range from tendinitis to massive rotator cuff tears. Partial-thickness tears are common in aging athletes and can represent a frequent source of disability.

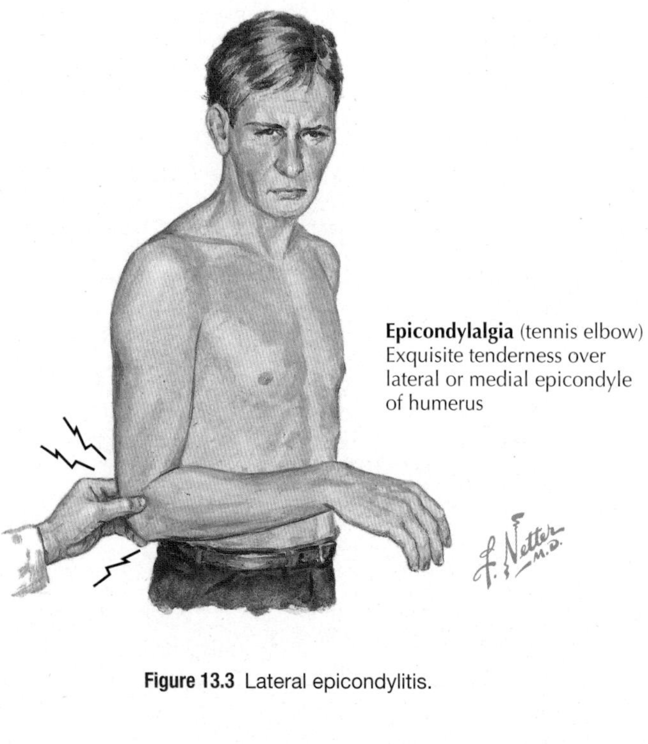
Epicondylalgia (tennis elbow)
Exquisite tenderness over lateral or medial epicondyle of humerus
F. Netter M.D.

Figure 13.3 Lateral epicondylitis.

  - Senior athletes who sustain a traumatic shoulder dislocation are more prone to rotator cuff injuries compared with younger athletes, who are more likely to sustain labral injuries.
- The proximal biceps tendon can be a frequent source of pain in aging athletes and is particularly susceptible to degenerative tearing. Ruptures of this tendon can often relieve biceps-related pain; however, such ruptures frequently occur in association with rotator cuff pathology (Fig. 13.5). Distal biceps tendon ruptures are more frequently seen in aging male athletes; the risk of such ruptures is greater among athletes who participate in weightlifting activities with eccentric loading of the biceps tendon.
- Repetitive, high-impact loading of joints seen in athletics can result in microtrauma to cartilage and subsequent degeneration.

Treatment Principles

- Some reports have indicated that senior athletes are more likely to wait longer to seek medical treatment for athletic injuries. In addition, some healthcare professionals may be more inclined to develop a negative attitude toward aging athletes and simply attribute injuries to expected effects of aging.
- Conflicting reports exist regarding healing rates in older athletes. Age alone does not appear to prolong healing periods; however, degenerative changes in tissues at the time of the injury can adversely affect treatment outcomes.
- Initial management should include careful history and physical examination. Care should be taken to understand not only specific injury details and pathophysiology but also patients' desires and expectations regarding continued athletic activity.
- A vast majority of injuries in senior athletes are responsive to nonoperative treatment measures.
- Principles of relative rest and activity modification can be effective.
  - For example, conversion of tennis athletes from an overhead stroke to a side-arm stroke can allow continued participation in the setting of activity but limit overhead discomfort.
- Physical therapy or home exercise regimens should be encouraged to minimize potential complications such as range-of-motion loss, cardiovascular deconditioning, or accelerated loss of bone mineral density. In addition, alternative methods of training should be discussed to avoid negative sequela from inactivity.

Pharmacotherapy

Nonsteroidal Anti-inflammatory Drugs

- Nonsteroidal anti-inflammatory drugs (NSAIDs) represent a common treatment modality for musculoskeletal injuries.
- Use of nonselective NSAIDs in patients aged >60 years has been associated with a fourfold to fivefold increased risk of gastrointestinal ulceration.
  - Individuals considered to be at a high risk (those with history of peptic ulcer disease and concurrent corticosteroid use and those who are anticipated to use NSAIDs for >3 months) should be placed on either misoprostol and/or a proton pump inhibitor. In addition, a COX-2 selective inhibitor can be effective in patients with prior gastrointestinal irritation.
- Moreover, NSAIDs may negatively affect bone and soft tissue healing. Multiple reports have documented impaired fracture healing with concurrent use of COX-2 inhibitors during the postfracture or postoperative period. Healthcare providers may choose to discontinue use in settings of fracture or soft tissue repair.

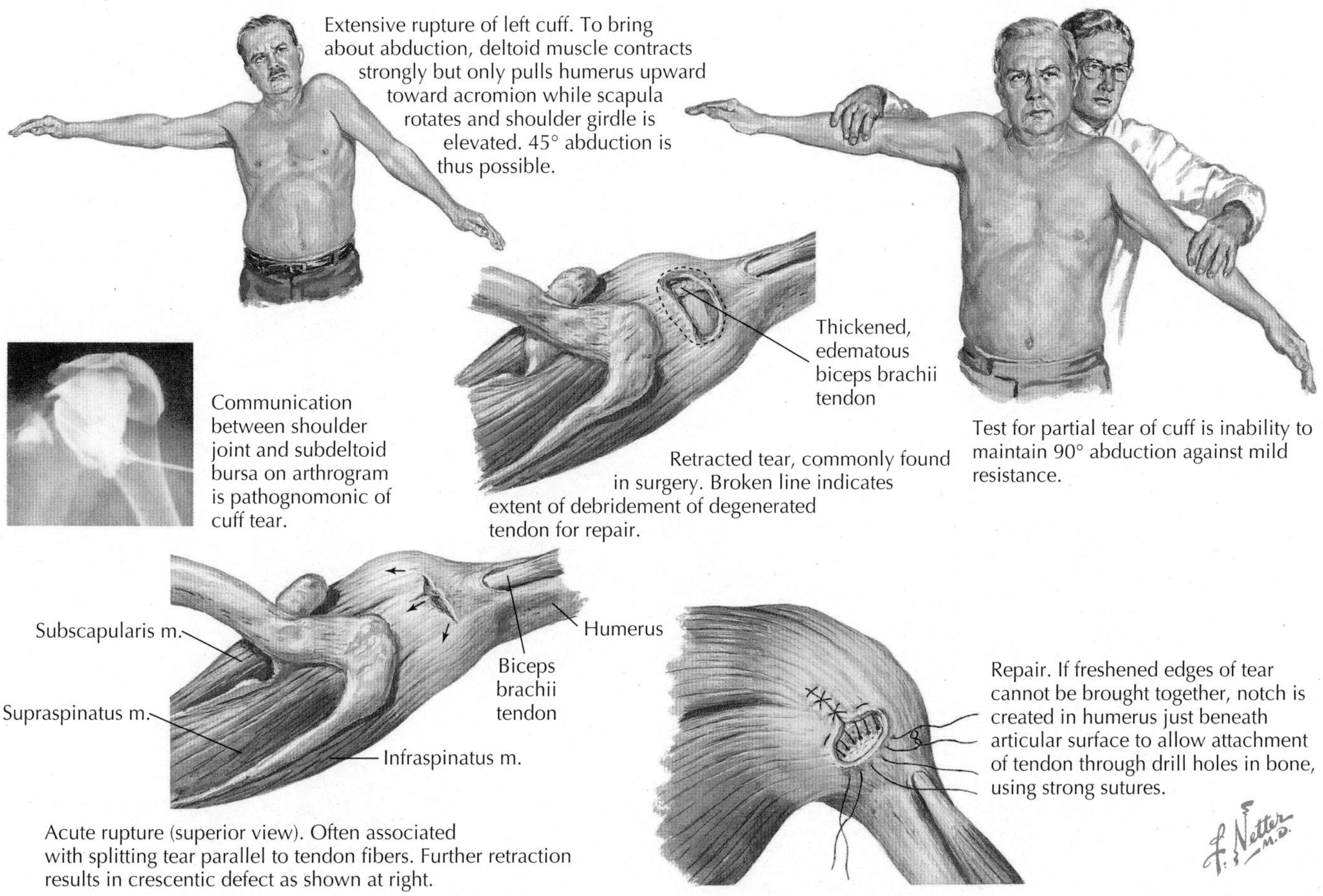
Extensive rupture of left cuff. To bring about abduction, deltoid muscle contracts strongly but only pulls humerus upward toward acromion while scapula rotates and shoulder girdle is elevated. 45° abduction is thus possible.
Communication between shoulder joint and subdeltoid bursa on arthrogram is pathognomonic of cuff tear.
Thickened, edematous biceps brachii tendon
Retracted tear, commonly found in surgery. Broken line indicates extent of debridement of degenerated tendon for repair.
Test for partial tear of cuff is inability to maintain 90° abduction against mild resistance.
Subscapularis m.
Supraspinatus m.
Humerus
Biceps brachii tendon
Infraspinatus m.
Acute rupture (superior view). Often associated with splitting tear parallel to tendon fibers. Further retraction results in crescentic defect as shown at right.
Repair. If freshened edges of tear cannot be brought together, notch is created in humerus just beneath articular surface to allow attachment of tendon through drill holes in bone, using strong sutures.
F. Netter M.D.

Figure 13.4 Aging athletes are prone to rotator cuff pathology. Patients with rotator cuff pathology can present with symptoms of pain and weakness. Patients with massive rotator cuff tears can demonstrate pseudoparalysis, or the inability to actively elevate the shoulder along with anterior superior escape of the humeral head.

Antiaging/Ergogenic Aids

- Testosterone: It is well understood that testosterone levels decrease with normal aging. Approximately 20% of 60-year-olds and 50% of 80-year-olds exhibit levels below the normal range observed in younger men. Testosterone replacement, designed to restore levels to those normal for younger men, have been shown to lead to increased lean body mass, muscle strength, bone density, and decreased body fat. Testosterone therapy is contraindicated in individuals with a history of prostate cancer and should be reserved for individuals with symptomatic hypogonadism rather than as an athletic performance aid.
- Human growth hormone (hGH): Currently, there is very little evidence to suggest that hGH supplementation offers any significant ergogenic advantage. Studies have shown that in a healthy elderly population, a minimal improvement in body composition leads to a considerable improvement in strength. At present, hGH supplementation is illegal for antiaging purposes in the United States and cannot be recommended in the healthy elderly population.

MUSCULOSKELETAL INJURY PREVENTION IN OLDER ATHLETES

- A primary goal of the PPPE is prevention of musculoskeletal injuries.
- Few studies exist on the prevention of injuries in older athletes; hence, evidence-based recommendations are difficult to provide. The typical assumption is that preventive guidelines for younger athletes can also be applicable to aging athletes.
- Appropriate warm-up before activity and adequate cool-down after activity are important.
- Abrupt changes in frequency, duration, or intensity of activity should be avoided.
- Days of intense physical activity should be alternated with less strenuous days to allow adequate recovery time.
- Soft playing surfaces can reduce ground reaction forces on lower limbs; however, uneven surfaces should be avoided, particularly in athletes with balance issues.
- Aging athletes should attempt to optimize environmental factors:
  - Athletes with deteriorating vision should optimize lighting conditions if possible.
  - Avoidance of extreme temperatures and humidity can aid hydration and thermoregulation.
- Activities that may exacerbate an underlying condition should be avoided; for example, athletes with osteoarthritis of the lower limb should restrict high-impact activities.
- Adequate nutrition should be maintained.

EXERCISE AND OSTEOARTHRITIS

- It is estimated that 50% of the population aged >65 years has osteoarthritis in at least one joint. Osteoarthritis is the second leading cause of work disability in men aged over 50 years, behind only cardiovascular disease.
- Repetitive, high-impact loading of joints seen with a lifetime of athletic participation can result in microtrauma to cartilage and subsequent degeneration.

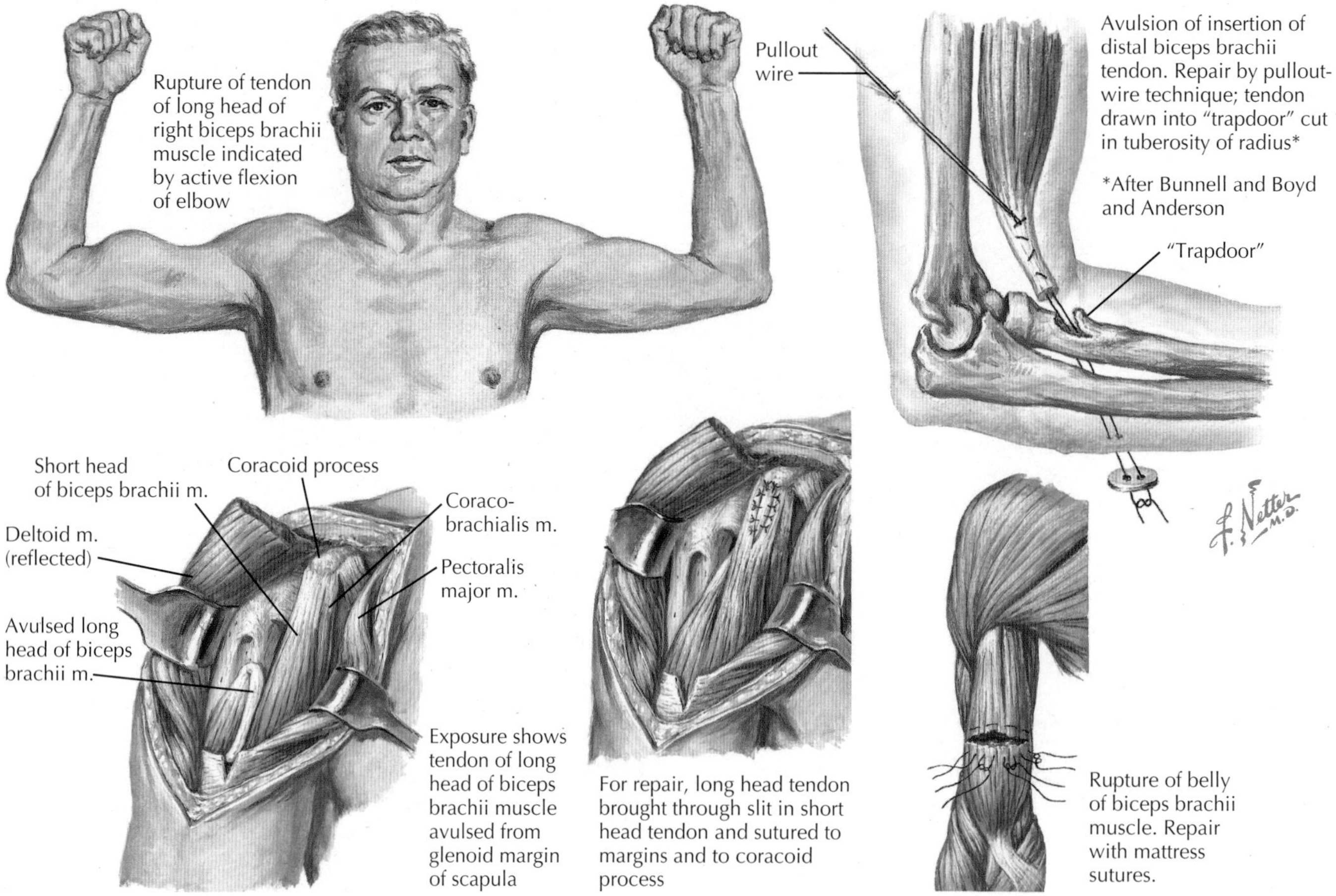
Rupture of tendon of long head of right biceps brachii muscle indicated by active flexion of elbow
Pullout wire
Avulsion of insertion of distal biceps brachii tendon. Repair by pullout-wire technique; tendon drawn into "trapdoor" cut in tuberosity of radius*
*After Bunnell and Boyd and Anderson
"Trapdoor"
Short head of biceps brachii m.
Coracoid process
Coraco-brachialis m.
Deltoid m. (reflected)
Pectoralis major m.
Avulsed long head of biceps brachii m.
Exposure shows tendon of long head of biceps brachii muscle avulsed from glenoid margin of scapula
For repair, long head tendon brought through slit in short head tendon and sutured to margins and to coracoid process
Rupture of belly of biceps brachii muscle. Repair with mattress sutures.
F. Netter M.D.

Figure 13.5 Rupture of the proximal and distal biceps brachii tendons.

- Several risk factors have been identified for the development of osteoarthritis, including increased age, obesity, female gender, joint trauma, prolonged occupational or sports stress, joint hypermobility or instability, malalignment, and genetic predisposition.

Management of Osteoarthritis

- Priorities in the management of osteoarthritis are to (1) reduce pain; (2) maintain mobility; (3) minimize disability; and (4) slow, halt, or reverse arthritis progression.
- Exercise programs with muscle strengthening for individuals with osteoarthritis have demonstrated improvements in strength, pain, function, and quality of life.
- Low-impact aerobic exercises can reduce pain and improve joint function.
- Participation in regular, low-impact exercise programs such as walking, aquatic exercise, and resistance training has not been shown to accelerate progression or exacerbate osteoarthritis in those who are already suffering from the disease.
- Over-the-counter supplements such as glucosamine and chondroitin sulfate have gained popularity in recent years. Although these supplements contain properties that could aid in restoring cartilage, clinical trials have failed to demonstrate a clinically meaningful benefit despite an excellent safety profile.
- Corticosteroid injections can be rapidly effective, offering short-term pain relief and often functional improvement. Corticosteroid injections are ideal for acute flares of pain.
- Viscosupplementation with hyaluronic acid injections may be considered for osteoarthritis management. Early clinical results suggested a benefit of up to 6 months of pain relief, and several studies have demonstrated sustained relief beyond placebo injections with saline. However, a recent meta-analysis has demonstrated limited benefits, with results that did not affect the clinically minimal difference and noted a risk of adverse events that was not negligible. Currently, the American Academy of Orthopaedic Surgery clinical practice guidelines on the management of knee osteoarthritis does not recommend the use of hyaluronic acid injections.
- Injections of biologics such as platelet-rich plasma (PRP) and stem cells are interventions that have spawned much interest in recent years.
  - Randomized clinical trials have demonstrated superior reduction in pain and functional improvement with PRP compared with viscosupplementation at 6 months in patients with early osteoarthritis aged <50 years. Additional studies have revealed that the benefit duration can vary widely.
- Mesenchymal stem cells from bone marrow and adipose tissues have demonstrated the ability to differentiate into chondrocytes. Use of these cells to treat osteoarthritis is under development and lacks randomized clinical trials at this time to demonstrate efficacy. However, early animal studies have shown the ability of stem cells to incorporate into areas of damaged articular cartilage and improve clinical, radiographic, and histologic features of joints compared with controls.
- Surgical options for the management of osteoarthritis in athletes can be divided into two strategies: joint preservation and joint replacement. For example, in the knee, joint preservation strategies can include arthroscopic debridement and meniscectomy, chondroplasty, cartilage restoration procedures such as microfracture, or high tibial osteotomy in patients with mechanical axis malalignment.

ATHLETIC ACTIVITY AFTER ARTHROPLASTY

General Considerations

- As the population of adults aged >65 years increases, the number of total joint replacements performed each year has steadily increased as well. Currently, over 500,000 hip and knee arthroplasties and approximately 50,000 shoulder arthroplasties are performed annually in the United States.
- Patient expectations after arthroplasty are changing beyond the traditional goals of pain relief and restoration of basic function, with some patients choosing to pursue participation in athletic activity. Maintaining sports participation constitutes an important aspect of patients' quality of life.
- Patients should be encouraged to maintain a physically active lifestyle to not only promote joint health but also general health.
- Patient and sports-related factors must be considered when recommending return to athletic activity after arthroplasty.
  - Participant experience level: Prior experience and proficiency in a sporting activity increase the likelihood of safely resuming activity after arthroplasty.
  - Athletic activity and extent of participation: Higher activity levels have been implicated in early implant loosening, bearing surface wear, and decreased implant survivorship. Limiting activities to sports that demonstrate low joint loads (e.g., walking or swimming) can decrease excessive wear and may allow a more predictable long-term outcome.
- There is a lack of high evidence level studies to support recommendations for athletic activity after arthroplasty; therefore, it should be noted that a majority of recommendations are based on expert opinion.

General Health Benefits

- Total joint arthroplasty has been shown to improve general and cardiovascular health.
- Marked improvements were observed in maximum oxygen consumption and Arthritis Impact Measurement Scales for mobility, walking, and range of motion after total knee arthroplasty when compared with a nonarthroplasty group.
- Increased ability to ambulate >60 minutes. Although patients are still at a risk of gaining weight after joint arthroplasty, they should be encouraged to take advantage of their potentially increased function.

Total Hip Arthroplasty

- Osteoarthritis of the hip is commonly seen in senior athletes; total hip arthroplasty often provides excellent pain relief and restoration of joint function but is accompanied by concerns regarding implant durability and survivorship.
- Stem design can play an important role in the durability of hip arthroplasty. Proximally porous-coated stems offer the advantage of loading the proximal femur, which can lead to less thigh pain and decreased proximal stress shielding.
- Although the surgical approach is often determined by surgeon preference and experience, use of different approaches can be guided by patient-related factors. The anterior and anterolateral approaches offer decreased disruption of posterior tissues and have demonstrated dislocation rates of <1% without the use of hip precautions. The posterior approach may place individuals who participate in deep flexion activities involving the hip at an increased risk of dislocation.
  - Appropriate component positioning, appropriate soft tissue tensioning, and use of implants with a larger head diameter can decrease the risk of dislocation.
  - Wear-related osteolysis is a major cause of failure in hip arthroplasty, making the choice of bearing surface material of critical importance in the athletic population.
- Conventional ultra-high-molecular-weight polyethylene (UHMWPE) demonstrates a wear rate of 0.1–0.2 mm/year. Wear rates >0.1 mm/year have been associated with osteolysis and eventual component loosening.
- Highly cross-linked UHMWPE is more resistant to wear and generates smaller wear particles. Wear rates with modern metal on highly cross-linked polyethylene are less than half of that observed with conventional polyethylene.
- Ceramic bearings demonstrate excellent wear properties but have been associated with component squeaking and fracture. Although these issues have been largely resolved with newer-generation materials, ceramic components are limited to femoral heads of a smaller size, thus potentially increasing the risk of dislocation.
- Metal-on-metal bearing surfaces were originally deemed advantageous because of the large femoral head size; however, high serum metal ion levels and adverse tissue reactions have been well documented, leading to a drastic decline in their use.
- High rates of return to athletic activity after total hip arthroplasty have been well documented. Recommendations for athletic activity are sport specific and should be thoroughly discussed with the operating surgeon (Table 13.3).
- In general, rehabilitation after total hip arthroplasty lasts 4–5 months, and certain patients are able to return to sports within 3–6 months.

Hip Resurfacing

- Hip resurfacing has several theoretical benefits over total hip arthroplasty, including increased head size and range of motion, decreased femoral bone resection, and a decreased wear rate with metal-on-metal articulation.
- Findings of variable outcomes in the literature regarding implant survival and return to sports.
- Prospective studies with short-term follow-ups have suggested that return to sports can be >90%. Age at the time of surgery and preoperative activity level are common predictors of postoperative level of function.
- Implant-associated risk of femoral neck fractures, increased levels of metal ions in blood and urine—which carry an unknown

Table 13.3 ACTIVITY RECOMMENDATIONS AFTER TOTAL HIP ARTHROPLASTY

Recommended	Recommended With Experience	Not Recommended
Golf	Weight lifting	Singles tennis
Swimming	Cross-country skiing	Racquetball/squash
Double tennis	Downhill skiing	Jogging/running
Stair climber	Ice skating/roller blading	Snowboarding
Walking/speed walking	Pilates	Contact sports (football, hockey, or soccer)
Hiking		High-impact aerobics
Stationary skiing		Martial arts
Bowling		Waterskiing
Cycling		Handball
Elliptical		
Low-impact aerobics		
Dancing		
Rowing		
Weight machines		
Treadmill (walking)		

From Vogel LA, Cartenuto G, Basti JJ, Levine WN. Physical activity after total joint arthroplasty. *Sports Health*. 2011;3:441–450.

risk—and risk of developing pseudotumors should be discussed with patients before surgery.

Total Knee Arthroplasty

- Knee osteoarthritis is a common source of disability and is frequently encountered in the athletic population because of either a posttraumatic etiology or age-related degenerative changes.
- Total knee arthroplasty has demonstrated considerable success in patients with end-stage tricompartmental arthritis (Fig. 13.6).
- Studies regarding levels of return to activity after total knee arthroplasty have reported an average return to sports of 63%–77% for athletes returning to low-impact activities.
  - Patients should avoid athletic activities until their quadriceps and hamstrings are adequately rehabilitated to decrease the risk of postoperative injuries.
  - On average, patients returning to golf demonstrate an increase in their handicap rate and decrease in the driving distance.
  - Most patients can expect a return to walking, cycling, and other low-impact activities in 3–6 months.
- Surgical implants that allow knee flexion beyond 125 degrees have demonstrated greater patient-subjective outcomes and carry the potential for decreased bearing surface wear for individuals participating in deep knee flexion activities.
- General consensus by most orthopedic surgeons is to avoid high-impact activities (Table 13.4). Despite these recommendations, there are reports of patients participating in higher-impact activities with excellent midterm results and no increased risk of revision surgery.

Unicompartmental Knee Arthroplasty

- Unicompartmental knee arthroplasty has several advantages over total knee arthroplasty, including decreased recovery time, preserved bone stock, improved quadriceps function, increased knee flexion, and more normal gait kinematics.
- Unicompartmental knee arthroplasty is contraindicated in patients with concurrent anterior cruciate ligament (ACL) insufficiency, tricompartmental arthritis, fixed varus/valgus deformity >10 degrees, inflammatory arthritis, and <90 degrees of motion or a significant flexion contracture.
- Several studies have examined return to sports after unicompartmental knee arthroplasty, with approximately 90% of patients returning to sport at any level and up to 60% returning to the same level of play.

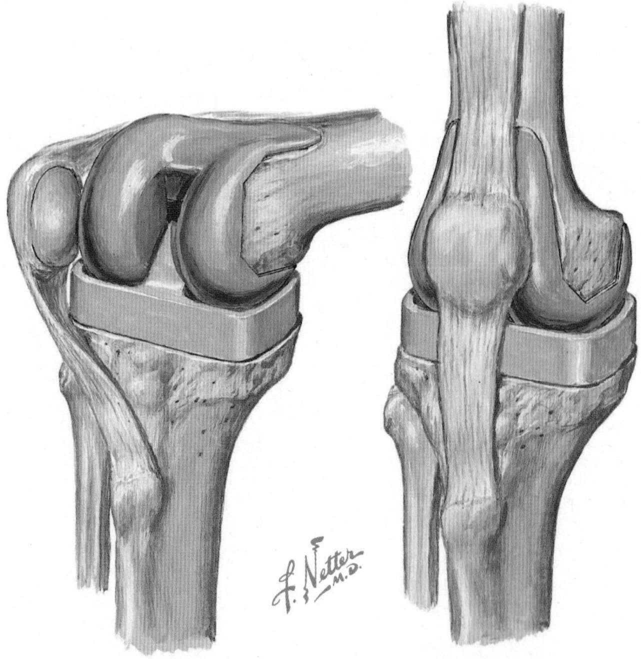
F. Netter M.D.
All components in place
Knee extended

Figure 13.6 Total knee arthroplasty.

Total Shoulder Arthroplasty

- A recent study examining athletic activity after shoulder arthroplasty revealed that 64% of patients who underwent surgery listed their desire to continue to play sports as a factor in their decision to undergo surgery. In addition, 50% of patients were able to increase their level of participation and 71% exhibited improvement in their ability to play.
  - Most patients were able to partially return to sports at 3.6 months and completely return to sports by 5.8 months after surgery.
- Historically, reverse shoulder arthroplasty has been performed in low-demand patients with rotator cuff arthropathy and massive irreparable rotator cuff tears. As the procedure has evolved, patients' expectations have risen as well. Literature regarding return to sports is limited; however, a 2015 study revealed that 60% of patients were able to return to sports after reverse shoulder arthroplasty; of these patients, 95% were able to play at the same level as they did before surgery.
- None of the previous studies have demonstrated an increased risk of implant loosening with activities such as golf; nevertheless, recommendations for athletic activities after shoulder arthroplasty are based on limited evidence and expert recommendation (Table 13.5).

METABOLISM AND NUTRITION IN OLDER ATHLETES

General Considerations

- Age-related decline in resting metabolic rate can contribute to a change in body composition.
  - Resting metabolic rate, which is estimated to constitute 75% of daily energy expenditure, decreases by 10% from childhood to adulthood and an additional 10% by the sixth decade of life.
  - Recent studies have suggested that age-related decline in resting metabolic rate can be attenuated with regular exercise.
- Typically, aging athletes attempting to lose weight combine physical activity with a decrease in caloric intake, which can lead to a negative energy balance. A deficiency of 1000 calories per

Table 13.4 ACTIVITY RECOMMENDATIONS AFTER TOTAL KNEE ARTHROPLASTY

Recommended	Recommended With Experience	Not Recommended
Low-impact aerobics	Cycling	Racquetball/squash
Bowling	Hiking	Contact sports (football, hockey, or soccer)
Golf	Rowing	Rock climbing
Dancing	Cross-country skiing	Jogging/running
Walking	Stationary skiing	Singles tennis
Swimming	Speed walking	Waterskiing
	Doubles tennis	Baseball/softball
	Ice skating	Handball
		Martial arts

From Vogel LA, Cartenuto G, Basti JJ, Levine WN. Physical activity after total joint arthroplasty. *Sports Health*. 2011;3:441–450.

Table 13.5 ACTIVITY RECOMMENDATIONS AFTER TOTAL SHOULDER ARTHROPLASTY

Recommended	Recommended With Experience	Not Recommended
Jogging/running	Racquetball/ squash	Contact sports (football, hockey, or soccer)
Aerobics	Baseball/softball	Martial arts
Tennis	Downhill skiing	Weight lifting
Basketball	Snowboarding	Volleyball
Stair climber		Waterskiing
Hiking		Handball
Cross-country skiing		Gymnastics
Ice skating/roller blading		Rock climbing
Bowling		
Cycling		
Rowing		
Walking/speed walking		
Dancing		
Pilates		
Golf		
Swimming		
Elliptical		
Fencing		

From Vogel LA, Cartenuto G, Basti JJ, Levine WN. Physical activity after total joint arthroplasty. *Sports Health*. 2011;3:441–450.

day results in muscle catabolism and decreased metabolic efficiency. A chronic negative energy balance has been associated with decrease in bone mass and an eightfold increase in the risk of stress fracture.

Macronutrients

- In general, older adults need fewer calories to maintain body weight, which indicates an increased emphasis on the quality of calories consumed.
- Training volume is the key factor for predicting energy needs and nutrient requirements.
- Carbohydrate intake should be in the range of 45%–65% of total daily caloric intake. For older athletes, calculating carbohydrate needs based on grams per kilogram of body weight is more likely to be appropriate for energy needs of athletes. Typically, 5–7 g/kg/day is sufficient for general training needs; requirements of endurance athletes are often higher and may necessitate 7–10 g/kg/day.
- Protein recommendations for senior athletes have not been established; however, a diet with sufficient protein is important to help offset age-induced sarcopenia. Protein intake of 1.2–1.7 g/kg/day should provide adequate amino acids to help maintain a positive balance for muscle synthesis and repair.
- The recommended daily intake of fat should be 20%–30% of total daily calories. Low-fat diets have not been shown to increase athletic performance.

Micronutrients

- To help offset age-related changes, adults over the age of 50 years have increased needs for vitamin D, vitamin B_6, and calcium. Currently, there is lack of evidence to suggest the exact requirements in older individuals who participate in sports.
- Recent reports state that 77% of the US population have a vitamin D deficiency. Vitamin D has been considered essential for maintaining bone health. In addition, vitamin D receptors have been identified in almost every cell type in the human body and are thought to play important roles in skeletal muscle maintenance.
  - Multiple performance studies in older adults have related low vitamin D levels to decreased reaction time, poor balance, and an increased risk of fall injuries. Supplementation has demonstrated improvement with strength, walking distance, and decrease in general discomfort.
  - Previous studies have established the optimal vitamin D level as >40 ng/mL. Supplementation in younger athletes to obtain optimal levels has demonstrated improvements with short-distance sprinting and jumping compared with individuals on placebo.
  - Current recommendations for adults include daily vitamin D intake of approximately 1000 IU. To optimize performance, athletes may consider supplementation to obtain levels >40 ng/mL.
  - In addition, vitamin D can be synthesized from exposure to the sun. Athletes living at latitudes above 35–37 degrees should not rely on sun exposure alone for vitamin D production.
- Calcium is equally important in appropriate maintenance of bone health. A minimum intake of 1200 mg of calcium per day is necessary.
- Vitamin B_6 is necessary for the breakdown of glycogen stores in muscle and helps convert lactic acid to glucose in the liver. Requirements for B_6 increase with age. Men and women older than 50 years should consume at least 1.7 and 1.5 mg of vitamin B_6 per day, respectively.
- Iron is the only micronutrient that is needed in smaller amounts for women with age. After menopause, the recommended dietary allowance (RDA) for iron decreases from 15 mg/day to 8 mg/day. For men, the value does not change with age. For athletes participating in endurance exercise, additional iron supplementation of approximately 30% is needed to offset losses observed with exercise.
- Antioxidant vitamins such as vitamins A, C, and E have been proposed to help reduce exercise-related tissue damage and even promote repair.
- Deficiency of most micronutrients is rare if athletes consume a balanced diet that includes fresh fruits and vegetables.

Fluids

- Adequate hydration during athletic activity is vital to compensate for fluid loss. Older athletes are susceptible to dehydration because of a diminished thirst sensation, decreased renal function and urine concentration capacity, and greater insensible fluid losses compared with younger individuals.
- Adequate hydration during exercise can help maintain performance level, lower submaximal heart rate, and control core body temperature.
- Athletes should not rely on thirst to decide when to drink and should consume fluids on a regular schedule during activity. For optimal recovery, it is recommended that 150% of weight lost acutely during activity should be replaced with fluid.

RECOMMENDED READINGS

Available online.

14 THE ATHLETE WITH PHYSICAL DISABILITY

Katherine L. Dec • James A. Underwood

GENERAL CONSIDERATIONS

Definitions

Physically challenged, physically disabled, and "disabled" athletes are terms often used to collectively refer to all groups of athletes competing in international competitions such as Paralympics and have an impairment that limits their ability to participate in athletic arenas within a manner considered "normal" for regulated sport. The impairment is not a "disability" in their selected sport, as these athletes have tremendous ability yet require adaptions to the sport regulations to compete with their impairment.

Impairment: any loss or abnormality of psychological, physical, or anatomic structure or function

Disability: any restriction imposed from an impairment that limits an individual's ability to perform an activity within a manner considered "normal" for an able-bodied individual

Handicap (as defined by the World Health Organization): a disadvantage resulting from an impairment or disability that interferes with a person's efforts to fulfill a role that is normal for that person; handicap is a *social concept*, representing social and environmental consequences of a person's impairments.

Statistics

- Over 61 million disabled people in the United States.
- Over 250,000 people in the United States with spinal cord injury (SCI).
  - Includes traumatic and nontraumatic.
  - A reported 17,000 new injuries per year; average age at injury is 43 years.
  - Sixty percent tetraplegia, 40% paraplegia.
- Over 1,540,000 million people in the United States with limb loss.
  - Incidence of congenital limb deficiency is 60 per 100,000 live births.
  - People older than 65 years account for 19.4 per 1000 of those with limb loss.
  - Common comorbidities: diabetes, vascular, and malignancy.
  - Incidence:
    - Lower extremity amputation (LEA), diabetes, and younger than 30 years: 7.2%.
    - LEA, diabetes, and older than 30 years: 9.9%.
    - Dysvascular disease: 46.2 per 100,000 with limb loss.
- Multiple sclerosis: 400,000 cases diagnosed in the United States each year.
- Muscular dystrophies: new cases estimated at 250,000 each year in the United States; Duchenne muscular dystrophy (DMD) is one of nine types of muscular dystrophy.

History

- First sports event for disabled athletes: 1888, Sport Club for the Deaf; Berlin, Germany.
- First international competition: International Silent Games, 1924.
- First international sports competition for people with various physical impairments: Stoke Mandeville Games for the Paralyzed, 1948.
- Youth divisions, in addition to adult, for athletes with physical impairment: 1950s.

Competition

- Physical impairment cannot require changes in rules of a sport, lowering of standards for achievement, or modification of a defined sport to accommodate athletes at the interscholastic, collegiate, or professional level.
- Neither adaptive equipment nor physical impairment can impart danger or an advantage to athletes or others competing in that sport.
- Football:
  - Since 1978, athletes with below-knee amputation (BKA) may participate in high school football with prosthesis.
  - Upper extremity amputation (UEA) is also allowed: if a UEA is a ball carrier and the prosthesis comes loose, the play is stopped immediately.
  - Check for final rules, as variance in application and competition governance.
  - National Federation of State High School Associations' rules concerning contact sports:
    - Metal hinges restricted to lateral and medial; require covering.
    - No metal in front of knee unless appropriately padded.
    - Prosthesis wrapped with minimum of half-inch foam rubber or appropriate polyurethane.
    - Approval of physician associated with amputee care recommended.
- Wrestling
  - Athletes with hearing loss have successfully competed with normal-hearing athletes; if hearing loss is >55 decibels in the better ear, qualifies for physically challenged.
  - Those with limb loss must weigh in with prosthesis, if used.
- Paralympics
  - Includes athletes with 10 eligible impairment types: impaired muscle power, impaired passive range of motion, limb deficiency, leg length difference, short stature, hypertonia, ataxia, athetosis, vision impairment, and intellectual impairment.
  - Each Paralympic sport defines which impairment groups they allow for participation.
  - Athletes must meet minimum disability criteria to compete.

Classification Systems

- Systems used for athlete evaluation to allow for equitable competition using objective methods.
- Sport-specific and may differ at international and local competitions.
  - May be through medical diagnosis or functional measurements.
  - Sport class: Paralympic classification system unique to each sport, with determination of impact of disability on their sport.
  - Athletes may reclassify during their career if disability progresses.

GENERAL CONSIDERATIONS FOR THE TREATMENT OF ATHLETES

- Adult: management of comorbid medical conditions, social isolation, functional status, and independence.
- Youth: peer interaction, relationships, cognitive and coping skills, school accommodations.
  - Missed social/peer opportunities.

- Constant change in size/fit of adaptive equipment.
- Resource limitations: insurance benefits and Medicaid limits.
- Counseling: assist athlete in redesigning athletic or career goals.
- Financial needs: insurance coverage, equipment needs, cost of accessibility, changes to home.
- Physical office facilities: Americans With Disabilities Act (ADA) criteria for accessibility.
  - Adjustable-height examination table.
- Collaboration with other healthcare professionals (e.g., neurosurgeon, physiatrist, therapist, vocational rehab, psychologist, primary care physician, prosthetist, or orthotist).

ORGANIZATIONS

- Several US and international organizations address the needs of physically challenged athletes, for example, Move United (https://www.moveunitedsport.org/).
  - Joint effort of Disabled Sports USA and Adaptive Sports USA with over 150 local chapters.
- In addition, many cities have local organizations that provide athletic opportunities for disabled athletes.

SPINAL CORD INJURY

Definitions

- The American Spinal Injury Association (ASIA) has developed the ASIA Impairment Scale (AIS) assessment used to classify the severity of SCI (Fig. 14.1).
  - Based upon the Frankel scale, ranging from A (complete) to E (return of normal function) measuring motor and sensory function at each neurologic level.

Physiologic Changes in Exercise

- Cardiovascular changes:
  - Possible blunting of heart rate in response to exercise.
  - Cardiac repolarization abnormalities.
  - Decreased total peripheral resistance (increased vasodilation).
  - Decreased venous return, consequent decreased ability to respond to exercise stress.
  - Decreased reflexive regulation of blood flow.
  - Increased peripheral pooling.
  - Decreased oxygenated blood to exercising muscle.
    - Fatigue, limited aerobic endurance.
- Pulmonary changes:
  - Limited pulmonary capacity, generally restrictive type (because of respiratory muscle weakness).
  - Paraplegics and people with high-level SCI can increase VO_2 max with exercise.
    - Dependent on intensity, frequency, and duration.
- Musculoskeletal changes:
  - Kinetic chain disruption: loss of ground reactive force from lower extremity.
  - Stabilizing muscles become prime movers.

Medical Concerns in SCI

History

- SCI level and completeness; chronicity, type, and etiology.
- Medical history:
  - Concurrent with injury (e.g., traumatic brain injury [TBI], amputation, polytrauma).
  - Related to impairment (e.g., pressure sores, neurogenic bowel/bladder, neuropathic pain, spasticity, recurring urinary tract infection [UTI]).
  - Comorbid conditions: individuals with SCI have lower levels of physical activity and earlier onset of many chronic diseases (e.g., diabetes, hyperlipidemia, cardiovascular disease).

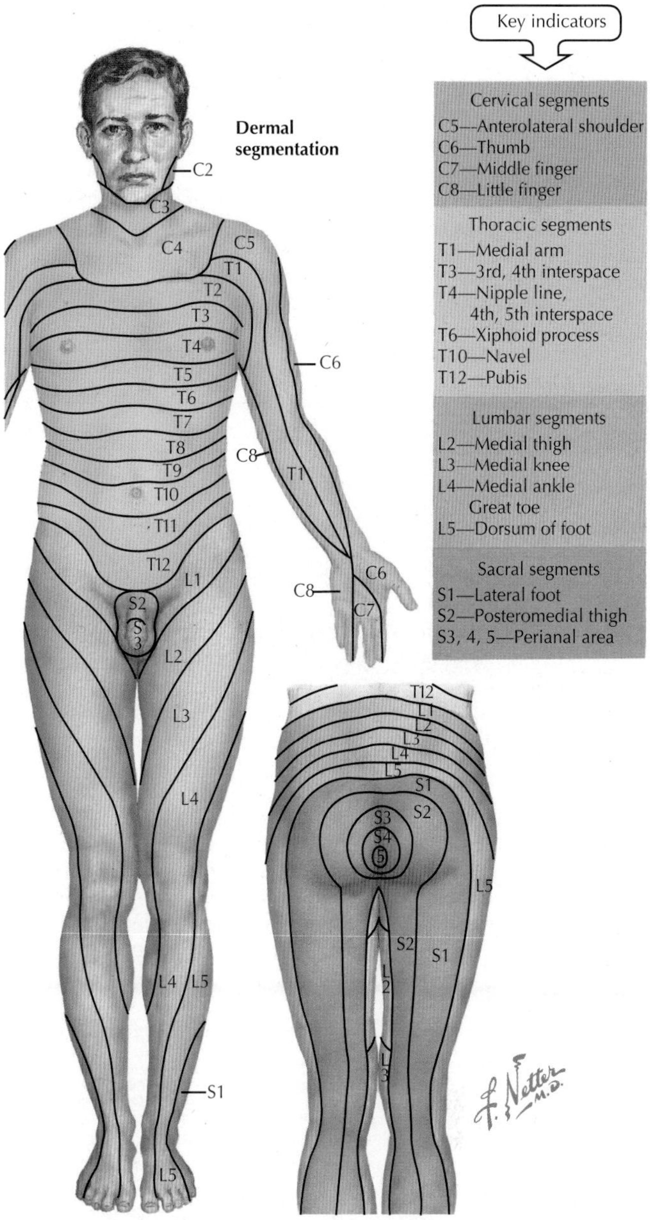
Key indicators
Dermal segmentation
Cervical segments
C5—Anterolateral shoulder
C6—Thumb
C7—Middle finger
C8—Little finger
Thoracic segments
T1—Medial arm
T3—3rd, 4th interspace
T4—Nipple line, 4th, 5th interspace
T6—Xiphoid process
T10—Navel
T12—Pubis
Lumbar segments
L2—Medial thigh
L3—Medial knee
L4—Medial ankle Great toe
L5—Dorsum of foot
Sacral segments
S1—Lateral foot
S2—Posteromedial thigh
S3, 4, 5—Perianal area
C2
C3
C4
C5
T1
T2
T3
T4
T5
T6
T7
T8
T9
T10
T11
T12
C6
C7
C8
L1
L2
L3
L4
L5
S1
S2
S3
S4
S5

Figure 14.1 Sensory impairment related to level of SCI.

- Surgical history: spinal fusion, muscle, tendon, or nerve transfers, surgically implanted medical devices.
- Medications: antispasmodics, antiepileptics, tricyclic antidepressants, anticholinergics, baclofen pumps, pain medications, and bowel medications.
- Level of functional independence: transfers, mobility, personal hygiene, bowel/bladder programs.
- Equipment needs: sport-specific or general mobility.

Conditions to Consider in Athletes With SCI

Autonomic Dysreflexia

- Defined by uncontrolled hypertension with a systolic increase of greater than 20 mmHg, can be associated with bradycardia, flushing of the face, sweating, and/or nasal congestion.
  - May also be asymptomatic.
- Medical emergency; typically occurs in patients with AIS level of injury at the sixth thoracic level (T6) and above.
- No supraspinal inhibition.

BOX 14.1 TREATMENT STEPS FOR AUTONOMIC DYSREFLEXIA

- Sit person up, lower legs
- Loosen clothing or constrictive devices
- Check for and remove offending stimulus—bladder distension is most common
- Bladder catheterization: 2% topical lidocaine jelly helpful
- Check blood pressure every few minutes until patient stabilizes
- 1–2 inches of topical Nitropaste or immediate-release nifedipine 10 mg, bite and swallow
- Repeat medicine in 15 minutes if no improvement
- Continue to monitor blood pressure and symptoms for 2 hours after episode
- If offending stimulus still present, recurrence of autonomic dysreflexia possible

    - Common causes include distended bowel or bladder, UTI, skin injury, fracture, tight clothes, or heterotopic ossification.
- Treatment: sit patient up, treat blood pressure with fast-acting agent, and evaluate for and remove offending stimulus (Box 14.1).
- Boosting: dangerous performance-enhancing technique used to purposefully induce autonomic dysreflexia (AD) during competition.
    - Performance enhancement through increased release of catecholamines.

Deep Venous Thrombosis

- Resulting from venous pooling in lower limbs.
- Risk factors: recent SCI, obesity, trauma to pelvis and lower extremities, congestive heart failure, malignancy, tight garments below level of the lesion, and previous thromboembolism.
- Prevention: passive stretching of limbs, graded pressure stockings, pharmacologic methods.

Thermoregulation

- SCI patients at risk of both hyperthermia and hypothermia.
- Hyperthermia:
    - Sweating impaired below level of SCI and decreased evaporative cooling.
    - Treatment: decrease clothing, give fluids, and douse the skin with water.
- Hypothermia:
    - Resulting from decreased muscle mass below level of the lesion, loss of vasomotor control, and possible decreased input to hypothalamic thermoregulatory centers.
    - Risk increased by impaired sensation: unaware of clothing dampness, which augments heat loss.

Pulmonary Complications

- Restrictive lung disease is most common form; SCI results in decreased total lung capacity, vital capacity, and forced expiratory volume in 1 second (FEV_1) and an increase in residual volume.
- Atelectasis, pneumonia, and mucous plugging are the most common causes of morbidity in high-thoracic SCI and tetraplegia.

Neurogenic Bowel

- Categorized as spastic (reflexic) vs. flaccid (areflexic) bowel.
- Successful bowel program: desired frequency and avoidance of incontinent bowel movements; utilize nutritional plan, positioning, gastrocolic reflex, and medications.
    - Nutrition to include adequate fluid and fiber intake.
    - Medications: stool softeners, prokinetics, rectal suppositories, and enemas.

Neurogenic Bladder

- Categorized as spastic (reflexic) vs. flaccid (areflexic).
    - Reflexic (increased tone, low postvoid residuals, involuntary voiding).
    - Areflexic (decreased tone, high postvoid residuals).
- Treatment includes monitored fluid intake, bladder program, and medications.
    - Bladder programs:
        - Intermittent urinary catheterization: insert catheter into urethra and bladder to drain urine into a disposable bag; performed on a strict schedule, often preferred method because of lower infection risk
        - Continuous (indwelling) urinary catheter: long-standing indwelling catheters contribute to recurrent UTIs
        - Suprapubic catheter: least common in athletes
- Medications:
    - Anticholinergics (e.g., oxybutynin, tolterodine, imipramine, and propantheline) for detrusor hyperreflexia
    - Alpha-adrenergic antagonists (e.g., terazosin, prazosin, and phenoxybenzamine) reduce internal sphincter tone
    - Antispasticity drugs (e.g., baclofen, diazepam, tizanidine, and dantrolene) for those with severe spasticity of perineal muscles
    - Medications for both types of neurogenic bladder can have side effects related to medication class

Urinary Tract Infection

- Common in SCI due to neurogenic bladder; long-term use of indwelling catheters increases risk of UTI
- Symptoms in SCI include increased spasticity, malaise, sweating, hematuria, or AD; traditional symptoms (dysuria, frequency, flank pain) often not present because of impaired sensation
- Prevention: rigorous personal hygiene and intermittent catheterization for bladder program
- Treatment: defined as complicated UTI, important to determine bacterial sensitivities because of high frequency of resistance; asymptomatic bacteriuria usually managed without antibiotics

Pressure Sores

- SCI patients at risk because of impaired sensation below level of the SCI; concern for progression to osteomyelitis
- Other factors: inappropriately fitting prosthetics, poor seat position/posture in wheelchair, skin shear with transfers, prolonged sitting
- In athletes, sport wheelchairs increase pressure over the sacrum and ischium because of positioning (Fig. 14.2)
- Prevention:
    - Appropriate wheelchair positioning; accurate fit of prosthetics/orthotics
    - Adequate cushioning, seat system
    - Patient education: instruction on regular pressure reliefs and weight shifts
    - Reducing skin moisture (wearing absorbent fabric)
    - Minimizing skin shear
    - Close monitoring and frequent skin checks
- Treatment:
    - Early wound management is key
    - Progressive sitting program
    - Topical medications, debridement

Spasticity

- See "Spasticity" subsection in the "Cerebral Palsy" section
- Medications are more successful in SCI than in brain-mediated injuries; monitor for negative effects of medications on athletic performance

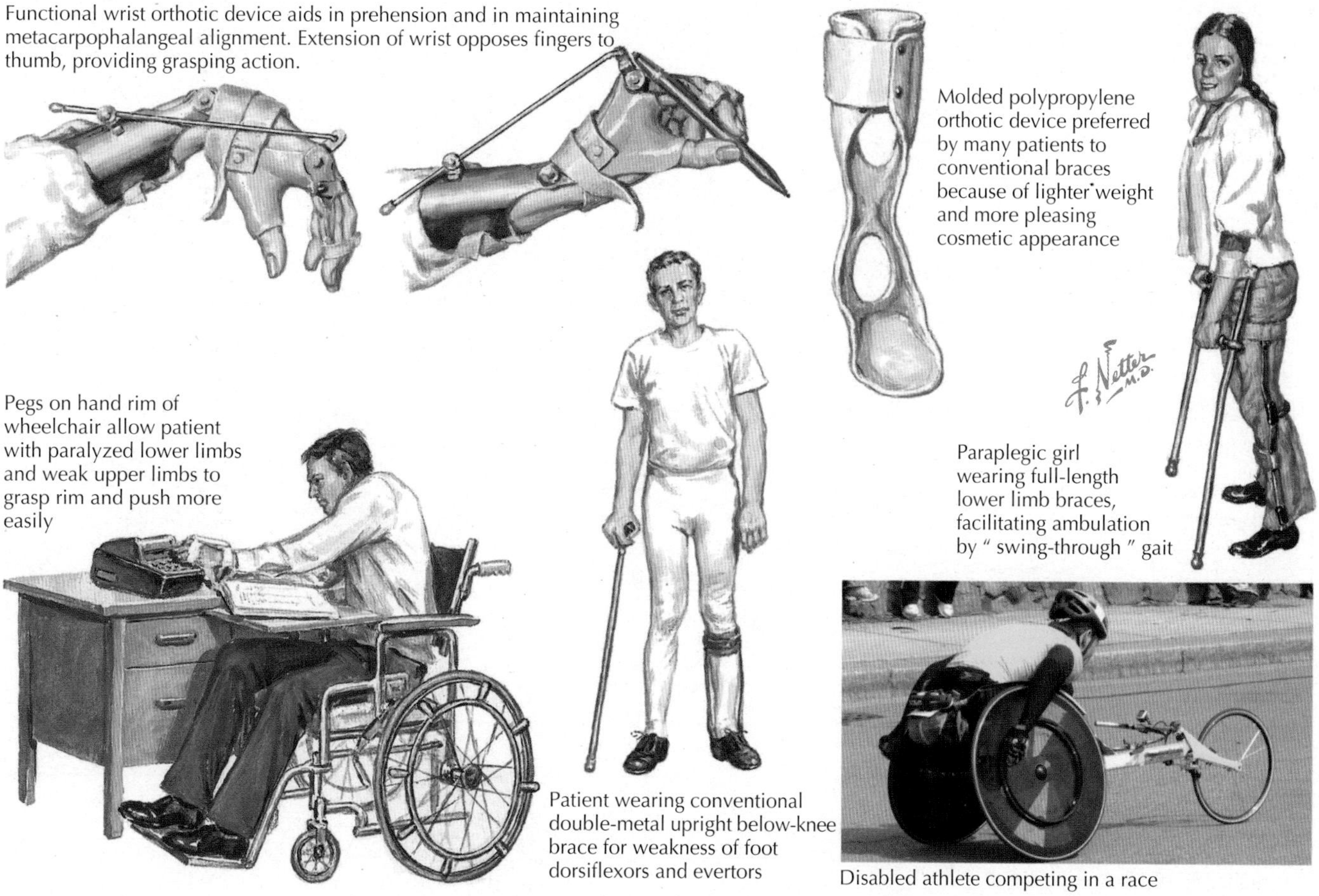
Functional wrist orthotic device aids in prehension and in maintaining metacarpophalangeal alignment. Extension of wrist opposes fingers to thumb, providing grasping action.
Molded polypropylene orthotic device preferred by many patients to conventional braces because of lighter weight and more pleasing cosmetic appearance
Pegs on hand rim of wheelchair allow patient with paralyzed lower limbs and weak upper limbs to grasp rim and push more easily
Paraplegic girl wearing full-length lower limb braces, facilitating ambulation by " swing-through " gait
Patient wearing conventional double-metal upright below-knee brace for weakness of foot dorsiflexors and evertors
Disabled athlete competing in a race
F. Netter M.D.

Figure 14.2 Medical issues in SCI.

Osteoporosis

- More common in SCI, with up to 50% decline in total bone content 10 years after SCI
- Unique pattern of involvement in SCI population; lower extremity bones more affected than upper extremity
- Causes: immobilization, imbalance of osteoclast and osteoblast activity, parathyroid hormone suppression, reduced absorption of calcium from gastrointestinal tract, vitamin D deficiency, and loss of active muscle traction effect (Wolff law)
- Treatment: range of motion (ROM), weight-bearing exercises, lower extremity orthoses, treadmill walking, functional electrical stimulation, and medications (e.g., bisphosphonates, Fig. 14.3)

Heterotopic Ossification

- Defined as formation of bone outside of the skeleton
  - Incidence in SCI: 16%–53%
  - Common locations: hip, followed by knee, shoulder, and elbow
- Prevention:
  - Nonsteroidal anti-inflammatory drugs (NSAIDs) in acute phase after SCI and passive ROM/mobilization
  - Risk decreases two to three times with appropriate prevention
- Diagnosis:
  - Symptoms: fevers, joint pain, warmth, swelling, and decreased ROM
  - Imaging: triple-phase bone scan; radiographs often negative for first month of symptom presentation
  - Laboratory findings: fractionated alkaline phosphatase significantly elevated
- Treatment:
  - First-line: stretching and passive ROM exercises
  - Medications: NSAIDs (e.g., indomethacin) and bisphosphonates (e.g., etidronate)
  - Surgical excision: high recurrence rate; lesser if delayed until skeletal maturity/low bone turnover rate
  - Radiation: used for both treatment and prevention, most frequently to the hip joint

LIMB DEFICIENCY

History

- Chronicity, type, and etiology of limb deficiency
- Medical history:
  - Concurrent with illness (e.g., TBI, diabetes, vascular disease, and cardiac disease)
  - Related to impairment (e.g., skin breakdown from prosthesis, low back pain)
- Surgical history: related to type of amputation or limb difference (Figs. 14.4 and 14.5), surgical muscle transfers for functional improvement, or surgically implanted medical devices
- Medications: antispasmodics, tricyclic antidepressants, analgesics (may affect cognition), and other medications for comorbidities
- Presence of phantom limb pain or sensation
- Level of functional independence: if multiple limb loss or difference, adaptive equipment needs for mobility, independence donning adaptive equipment or prosthesis
- Adaptive equipment for sports-specific needs: prosthesis, orthosis, or sports equipment

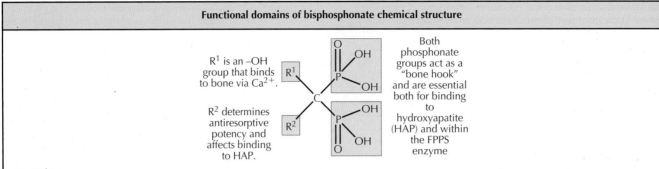

Functional domains of bisphosphonate chemical structure

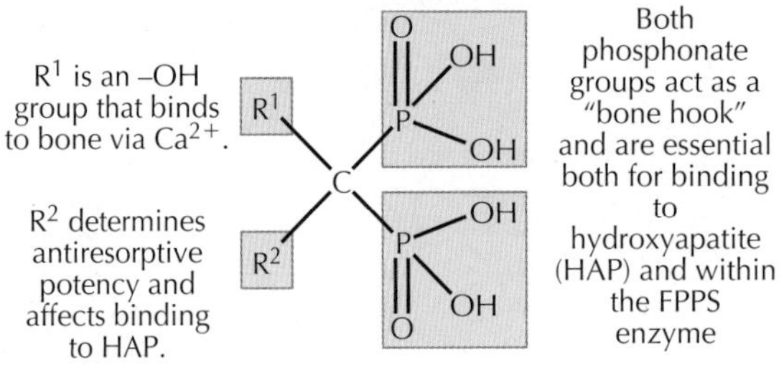
R[1] is an –OH group that binds to bone via Ca^{2+}.
R[2] determines antiresorptive potency and affects binding to HAP.
R[1]
R[2]
C
P
O
OH
OH
Both phosphonate groups act as a "bone hook" and are essential both for binding to hydroxyapatite (HAP) and within the FPPS enzyme

Key Points

- The P–C–P moiety is common to all. The P–C–P backbone is sometime referred to as the "bone hook" and is essential for binding to calcium in hydroxyapatite.
- The R^1 group is important for binding to hydroxyapatite. R^1 is a hydroxyl (–OH) group for nearly all bisphosphonates currently used in osteoporosis.
- The R^2 group is what differentiates the actions of the bisphosphonates. The R^2 group is critically involved in both FPPS enzyme inhibition and additional mineral binding effects. The R^2 group is different for each BP and contributes to the unique chemical and pharmacologic properties of each drug.

Background

- Phosphonate: or phosphonic acid, an organic compound containing one or more C–PO(OH)$_2$ or C–PO(OR)$_2$ (with R=alkyl, aryl) groups (the phosphorous is bound to carbon)
- Phosphate: an inorganic salt of phosphoric acid, H_3PO_4 (phosphorus is not bound to carbon)
- Phosphorus: the chemical element that has the symbol P and atomic number 15
- Pyrophosphate: the anion, the salts, and the esters of pyrophosphoric acid, $H_4P_2O_7$

From Russell RGG. *Bisphosphonates: from bench to bedside. Annals of the New York Academy of Sciences.* 2006;1068:367-401.

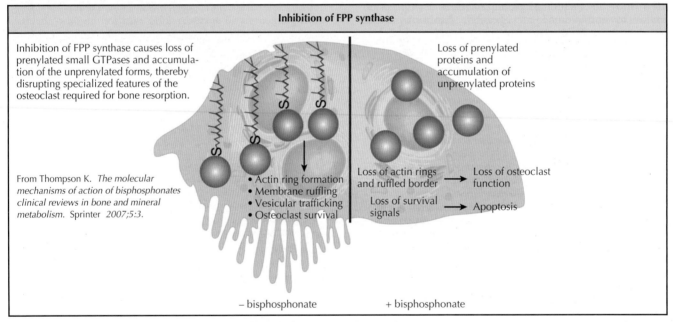

Inhibition of FPP synthase

Inhibition of FPP synthase causes loss of prenylated small GTPases and accumulation of the unprenylated forms, thereby disrupting specialized features of the osteoclast required for bone resorption.

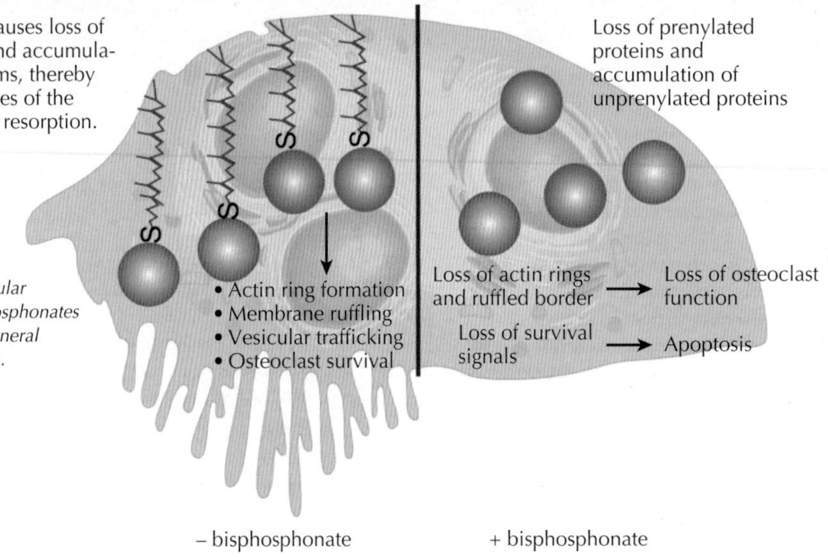
S
S
S
S
• Actin ring formation
• Membrane ruffling
• Vesicular trafficking
• Osteoclast survival
Loss of prenylated proteins and accumulation of unprenylated proteins
Loss of actin rings and ruffled border
Loss of osteoclast function
Loss of survival signals
Apoptosis
– bisphosphonate
+ bisphosphonate

From Thompson K. *The molecular mechanisms of action of bisphosphonates clinical reviews in bone and mineral metabolism.* Sprinter *2007;5:3.*

Figure 14.3 Treatment of osteoporosis.

Conditions to Consider

Skin Breakdown

- Related to inappropriately fitting prosthesis, impact type of the sport at prosthesis-skin interface and weight-bearing surfaces
- Treatment: achieving accurate fit (see "Pressure Sores")

Phantom Pain

- Phantom limb sensations: occur within first few weeks after amputation in approximately 70% of individuals; about 20% of individuals have painful sensations that persist
- Medications: antidepressant and anticonvulsant medications, acupuncture and biofeedback (e.g., mirror therapy), desensitization therapy (e.g., transcutaneous electrical stimulation [TENS], scrambler therapy, contrast baths)

LEA Secondary Issues

- Energy expenditure during ambulation is greatly increased in LEA compared with normal ambulation without amputation:
  - BKA: additional 16%–25%
  - Above-knee amputation (AKA): additional 56%–65%
- Challenges to ambulation: increased balance and strength requirements, lack of proprioceptive and tactile feedback, prosthesis fit
- Low back pain: >50% of individuals with LEA

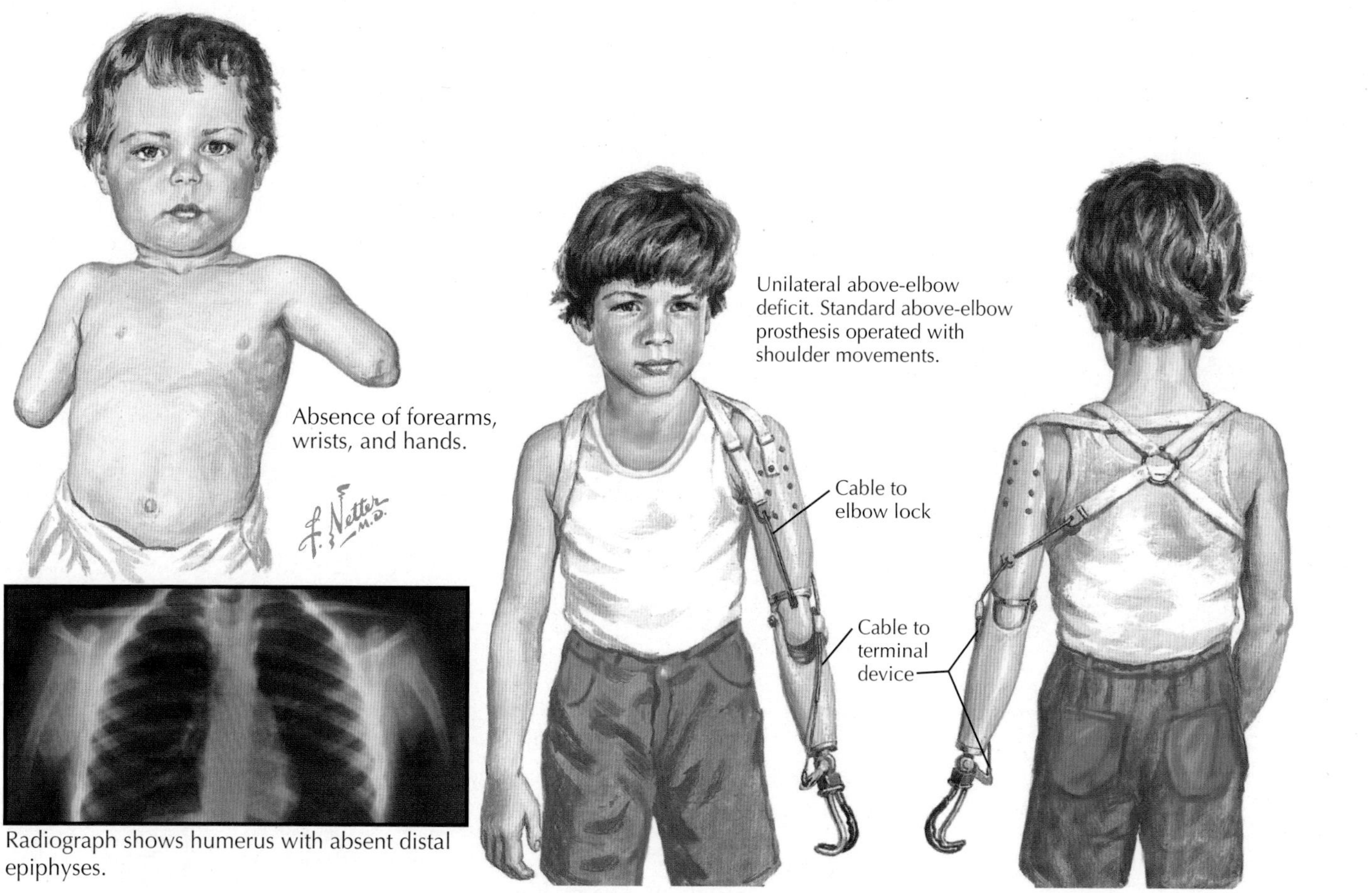
Absence of forearms, wrists, and hands.
Radiograph shows humerus with absent distal epiphyses.
Unilateral above-elbow deficit. Standard above-elbow prosthesis operated with shoulder movements.
Cable to elbow lock
Cable to terminal device

Figure 14.4 Amputation of the forearm and hand.

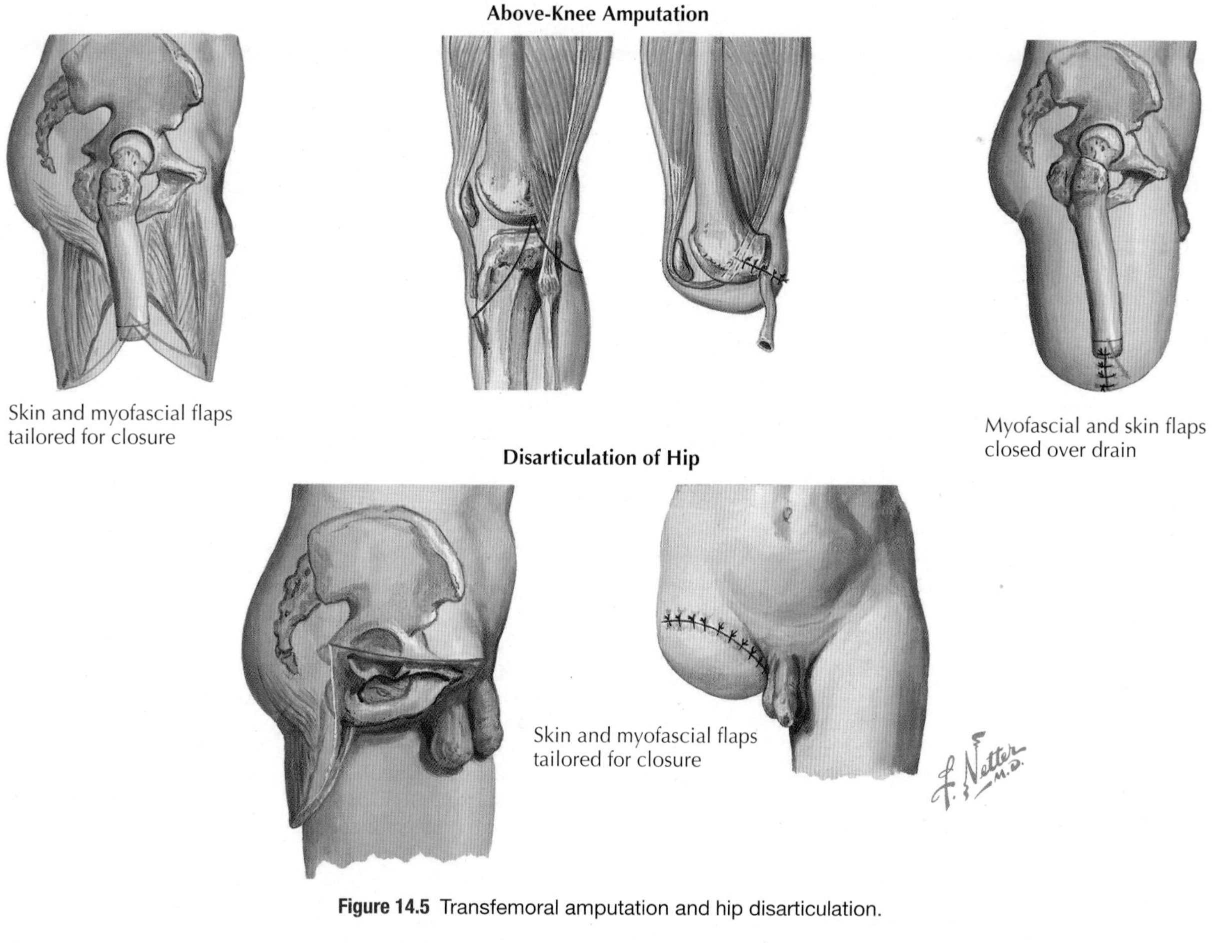
Above-Knee Amputation
Skin and myofascial flaps tailored for closure
Myofascial and skin flaps closed over drain
Disarticulation of Hip
Skin and myofascial flaps tailored for closure

Figure 14.5 Transfemoral amputation and hip disarticulation.

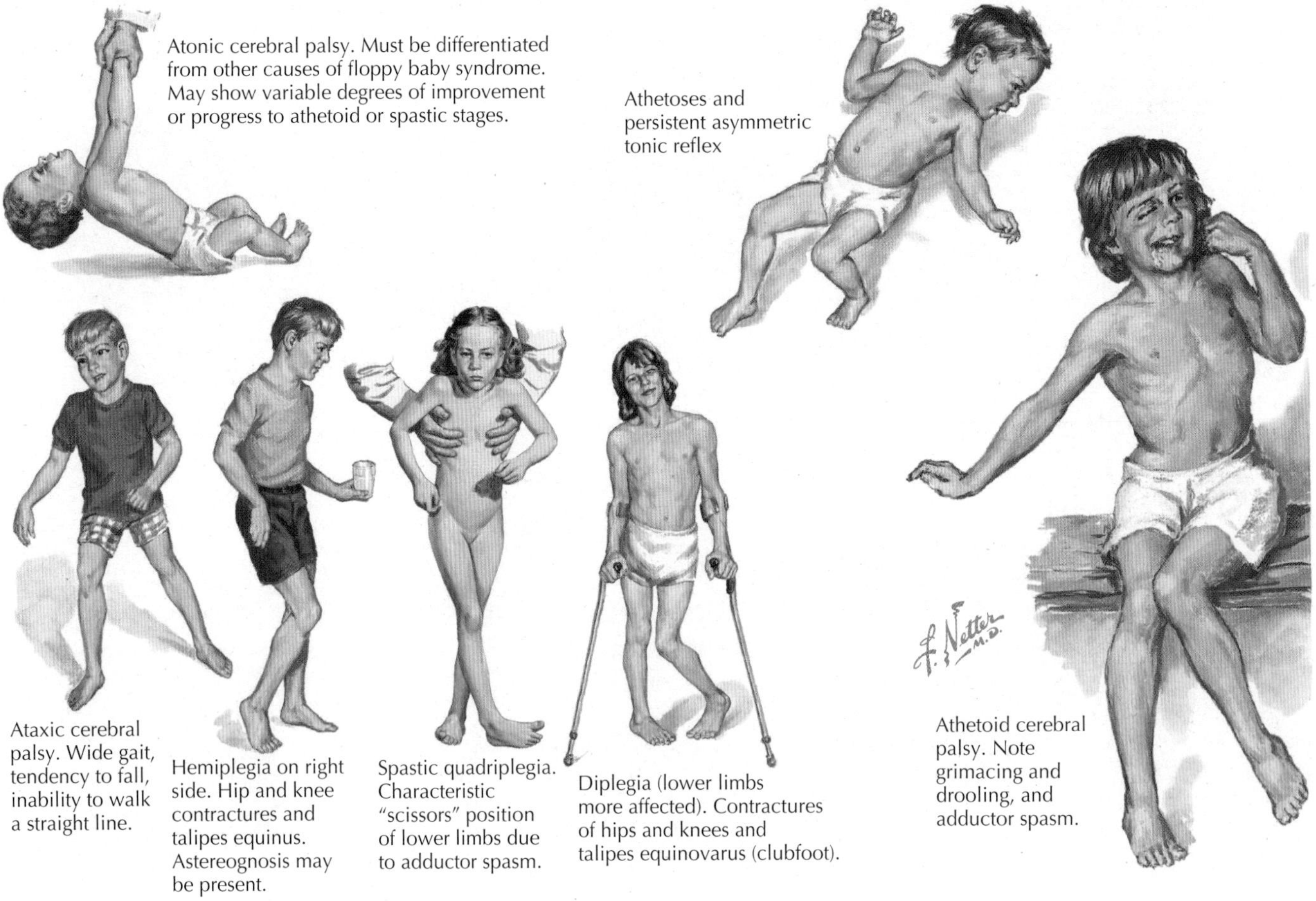
Atonic cerebral palsy. Must be differentiated from other causes of floppy baby syndrome. May show variable degrees of improvement or progress to athetoid or spastic stages.
Athetoses and persistent asymmetric tonic reflex
Ataxic cerebral palsy. Wide gait, tendency to fall, inability to walk a straight line.
Hemiplegia on right side. Hip and knee contractures and talipes equinus. Astereognosis may be present.
Spastic quadriplegia. Characteristic "scissors" position of lower limbs due to adductor spasm.
Diplegia (lower limbs more affected). Contractures of hips and knees and talipes equinovarus (clubfoot).
Athetoid cerebral palsy. Note grimacing and drooling, and adductor spasm.

Figure 14.6 Glossary in cerebral palsy.

- Knee pain: three times greater risk on the side contralateral to the side with AKA, twice greater risk with intact limb in BKA, five times *reduced* risk in prosthetic limb of the side with BKA

CEREBRAL PALSY

- Impaired neurologic function typically caused by a nonprogressive injury to the brain before birth
  - May result in persistence of primitive reflexes and posture-mediated movement patterns

Glossary in Cerebral Palsy (Fig. 14.6)

Spastic cerebral palsy (CP): most common form; affects 70%–80%; increased muscle tone and stiffness; spasticity increases with excessive fatigue or anxiety

Athetoid CP: four limbs, trunk, and occasionally face; athetonia is slow, writhing involuntary muscle movement; muscle tone can be mixed: increased or decreased

Ataxic CP: four limbs and trunk, primarily decreased coordination of movement, also hypotonia; intention tremor present

Diplegia: lower limbs involved more than upper limbs

Hemiplegia: upper and lower limbs on one side more involved

Triplegia: three limbs, usually both lower limbs and one upper limb involved

Quadriplegia: both upper and lower limbs involved

History

- Medical history:
  - Comorbidities related to impairment: spasticity, nutritional support (e.g., gastrostomy tube) and seizures
  - Concurrent illness: diabetes, visual impairment, hearing impairment, and cardiac disease
  - Cognitive impairment (e.g., memory, calculation/organizational aspects)
    - Intellectual disability *atypical* for athletes at international-level competitions
    - Impulsivity or risk-taking behavior may be present
- Surgeries related to injury: muscle transfers, surgically implanted medical devices, gastrostomy tube placement, and tendon-lengthening procedures
- Medications: antispasmodics, antiepileptics, tricyclic antidepressants, analgesics, medications for comorbid conditions such as cardiac disease
- Level of functional independence: donning adaptive equipment, personal hygiene
  - Children with CP evaluated by Gross Motor Classification System (GMFCS), a five-level scale predicting functional outcomes (Table 14.1)
- Level of independence in mobility: GMFCS 1–3 likely need orthoses, GMFCS 4–5 typically rely on wheelchair for mobility
- Adaptive equipment: necessary for mobility or sports-specific equipment

Table 14.1 GROSS MOTOR FUNCTION CLASSIFICATION SYSTEM (GMFCS) IN CEREBRAL PALSY

GMFCS Level	Functional Ability (Age 6–12 Years)
I	Can ambulate independently in community, can climb stairs without use of handrail, can run and jump, but there are limitations in balance and coordination.
II	Can ambulate in most settings and climb stairs with assistance of handrail; may have difficulty ambulating long distances, which may require use of assistive device; minimal ability to perform gross motor skills such as running or jumping.
III	Can ambulate with use of handheld assistive device, may require wheelchair for longer distances, can self-propel wheelchair for shorter distances.
IV	Use assisted mobility or powered mobility in most settings, may be able to ambulate short distances with assistive device in home setting.
V	Use assisted mobility or powered mobility in all settings, limited ability to maintain posture and control limb movement.

Spasticity

- Pathophysiology unclear; theory is velocity-dependent increase in tonic stretch reflexes (muscle tone) with exaggerated tendon jerks, resulting from hyperexcitability of stretch reflex; increased with nociceptive stimulus, such as UTI, distended viscera, and bowel obstruction (Fig. 14.7)
- Decision to treat spasticity depends on help (ability to ambulate) or hindrance (impedes independence with mobility and self-care; pain; pressure ulcers)

Treatment

- ROM and positioning are mainstays of treatment
- Oral medications:
  - Baclofen: GABA-B receptor; must monitor patient for sedation and, if stopped, must be weaned to avoid withdrawal
  - Tizanidine: alpha-2a receptor; monitor for dizziness, dry mouth, and sedation; also causes hypotension, which can be limiting for treatment
  - Dantrolene: works peripherally on sarcoplasmic reticulum of skeletal muscle; must monitor liver function at treatment initiation and every 3–6 months during treatment; most likely to cause weakness
  - Diazepam: GABA-B receptor; works with similar effect to baclofen
- Intrathecal baclofen via an implanted pump in the abdomen able to produce more effect with lower dose and fewer systemic effects
- Injections: botulinum toxin A or phenol into key spastic muscles (e.g., thigh adductors)
  - Risks: chronic dysesthesia (phenol), pain, skin sloughing, peripheral edema, wound infection
- Surgery: tendon lengthening, muscle-release procedures for joint position issues
- Intention tremor (subset): medication options include primidone, propranolol, buspirone, and benzodiazepines and localized botulinum toxin A injections; cooling extremities with circulating cold wrap also reduces tremors 30 minutes after cooling

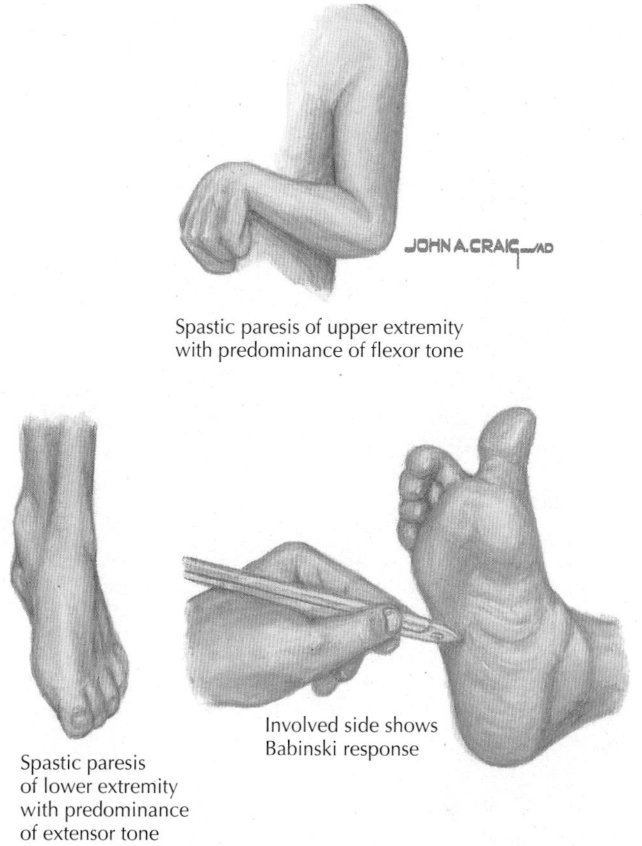
JOHN A.CRAIG—AD
Spastic paresis of upper extremity with predominance of flexor tone
Involved side shows Babinski response
Spastic paresis of lower extremity with predominance of extensor tone

Figure 14.7 Characteristic pattern in spastic limbs.

- Heterotopic bone formation: see "Conditions to Consider in Athletes With SCI" and "Heterotopic Ossification"

LOCOMOTOR DISORDERS

History

- Comorbidities related to:
  - Impairment: spasticity, type and success of bowel/bladder management program, restrictive lung disease (muscular dystrophy or neuromuscular condition), nutritional support (e.g., gastrostomy tube), seizures, and skeletal deformity (Fig. 14.8)
  - Concurrent illness (e.g., TBI, diabetes, visual impairment, low back pain, cardiac disease, and respiratory illness)
- Surgeries and medications similar to those used in CP (see "Cerebral Palsy")
- Adaptive equipment, level of functional and ambulatory independence, and training (see "Cerebral Palsy")

Conditions to Consider

- Spasticity, neurogenic bowel or bladder, seizure, joint contracture, pulmonary issues caused by muscle weakness

Short Stature Syndrome

Disproportionate

- Average-size torsos, unusually short limbs
- Causes: skeletal dysplasia or chondrodystrophy, caused by inherited or spontaneous gene mutations
- Spondyloepiphyseal dysplasia (SED) and diastrophic dysplasia: progressive kyphosis and/or scoliosis are typical (Fig. 14.9); eye complications can be present in SED
- Can involve joint defects, limited ROM, and high incidence of joint dislocation

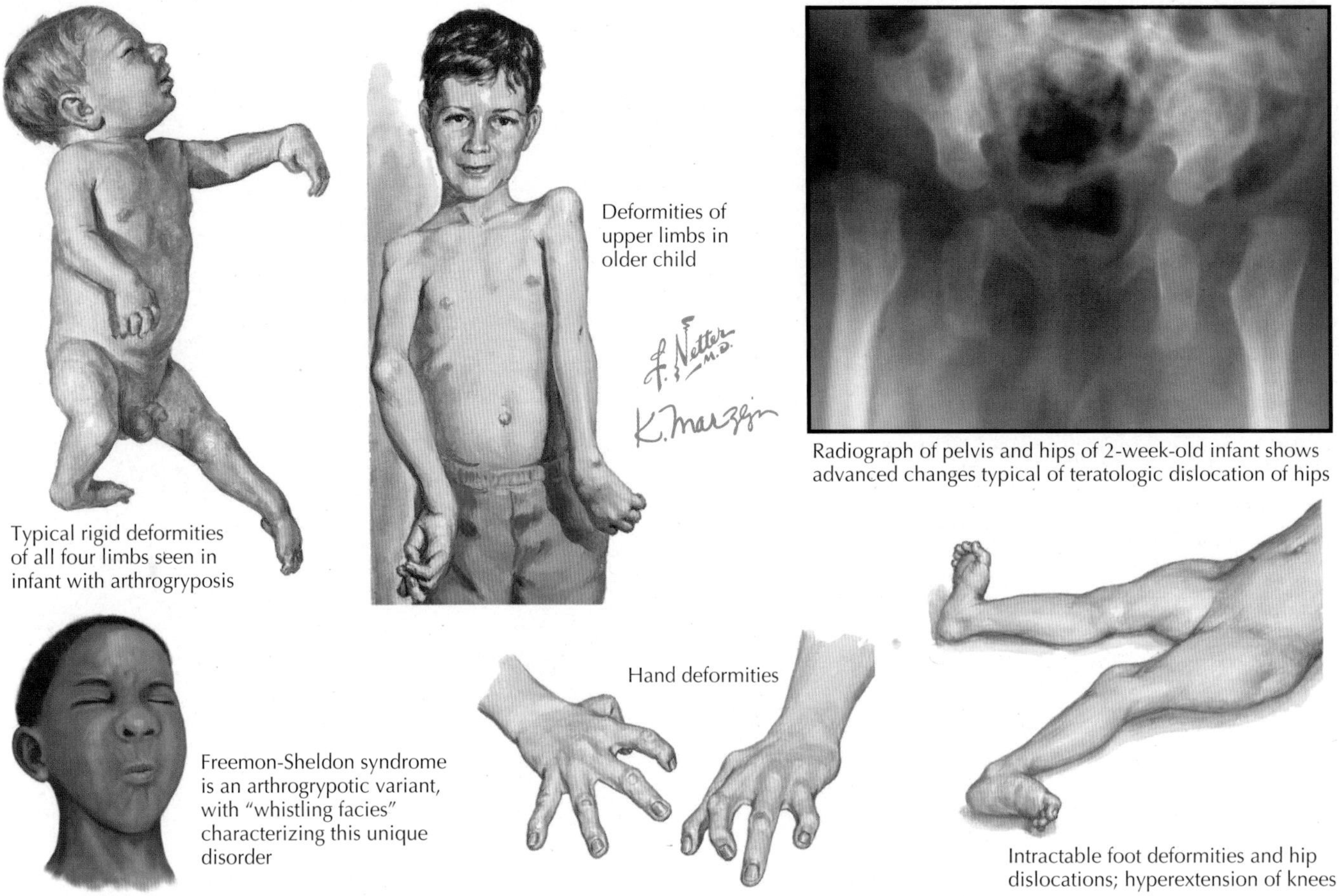
Typical rigid deformities of all four limbs seen in infant with arthrogryposis
Deformities of upper limbs in older child
Radiograph of pelvis and hips of 2-week-old infant shows advanced changes typical of teratologic dislocation of hips
Freemon-Sheldon syndrome is an arthrogrypotic variant, with "whistling facies" characterizing this unique disorder
Hand deformities
Intractable foot deformities and hip dislocations; hyperextension of knees

Figure 14.8 Arthrogryposis multiplex congenita.

Proportionate

- Overall unusually small size for age
- Causes: endocrine or growth hormone deficiency are most likely

Muscular Dystrophy and Genetic Myopathies

Overview

- Collection of progressive genetic muscle diseases
- DMD and Becker muscular dystrophy (BMD) most common types; DMD more severe in involvement; males more affected than females (Fig. 14.10)
- Others include myotonic muscular dystrophy and facioscapulohumeral muscular dystrophy
  - Variation in muscle involvement and concurrent medical issues

Diagnosis

- Muscle biopsy (for histologic features)
- Electromyography (EMG)
- Genetic/DNA testing (for dystrophinopathy) and laboratory tests (elevated creatine kinase)

Management

- Multidisciplinary therapies (physical therapy [PT] or occupational therapy [OT]) address specific functional deficits
  - Mild, noncontact physical activity
  - Resistance training should be performed only in muscles with at least antigravity strength
  - Monitoring of physical and physiologic status: nutritional status, cardiac function (routine electrocardiogram [ECG], echocardiogram), and ventilatory function (pulmonary function tests—obtain before exercise prescription)
- Corticosteroids may help improve muscle strength and overall energy in DMD
- Angiotensin-converting enzyme (ACE) inhibitors and angiotensin receptor blockers (ARBs) may slow the progression of cardiomyopathy in DMD/BMD
- Noninvasive (positive airway pressure) ventilator support and cough assist devices to help manage respiratory secretions—improve life expectancy and quality of life in DMD

VISUAL IMPAIRMENT

- Classification assists fair competition by grouping athletes and determining eligibility (see "Classification Systems" earlier)
- Visual class: based on eye with better visual acuity and/or fields while wearing best optical correction
  - International Blind Sports Federation (IBSF) has developed the B1-4 classification system (Table 14.2)

JUVENILE RHEUMATOID ARTHRITIS

- Joint impairment: *if* significant, an athlete with juvenile rheumatoid arthritis (JRA) may qualify for competitions in the "les autres" category (Fig. 14.11)

FRIEDREICH ATAXIA

- Progressive autosomal recessive disorder with ataxia, visual changes, weakness, and loss of sensation in limbs; onset typically age 5–15 years

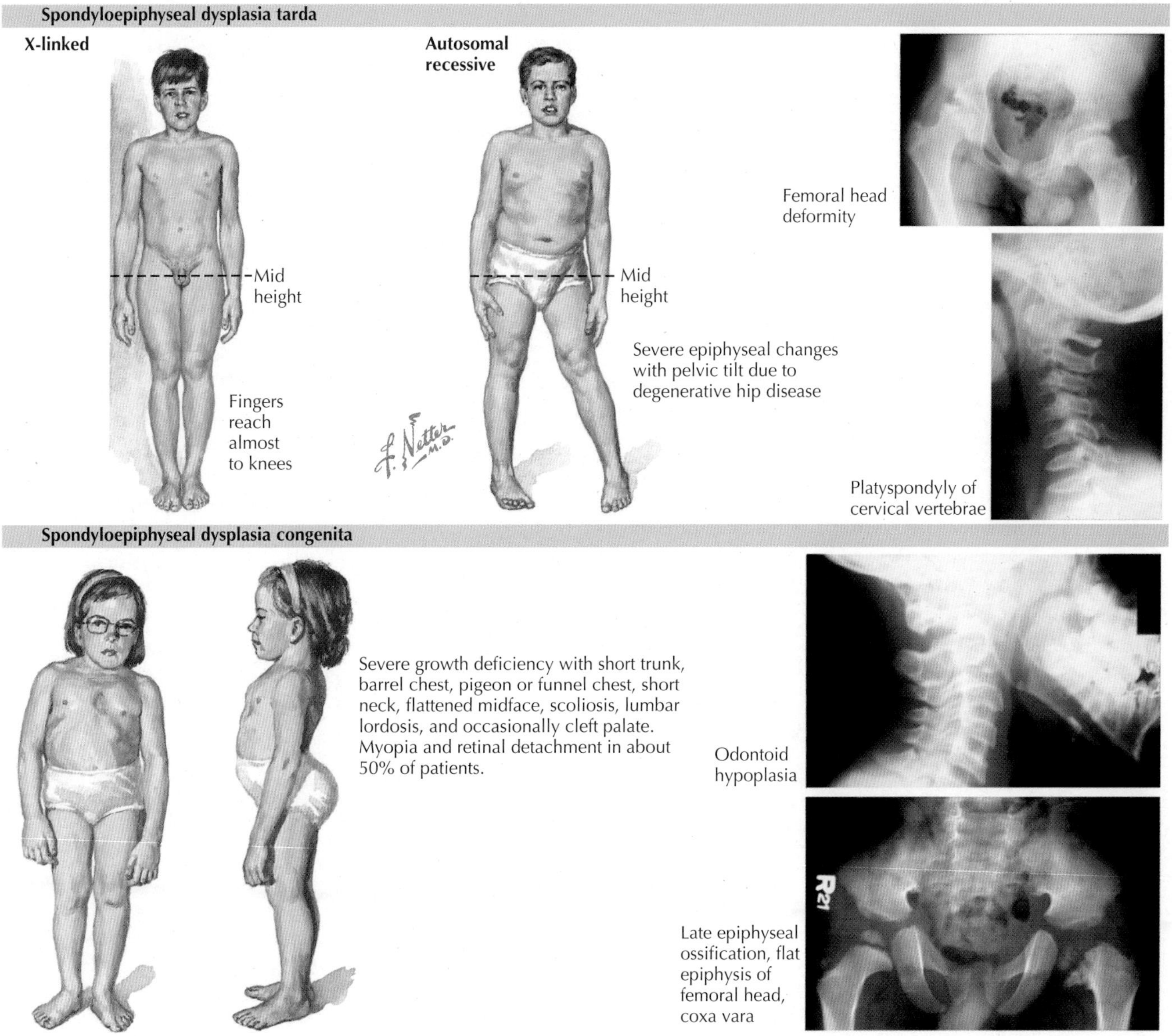

Spondyloepiphyseal dysplasia tarda
X-linked
Mid height
Fingers reach almost to knees
Autosomal recessive
Mid height
Severe epiphyseal changes with pelvic tilt due to degenerative hip disease
Femoral head deformity
Platyspondyly of cervical vertebrae
Spondyloepiphyseal dysplasia congenita
Severe growth deficiency with short trunk, barrel chest, pigeon or funnel chest, short neck, flattened midface, scoliosis, lumbar lordosis, and occasionally cleft palate. Myopia and retinal detachment in about 50% of patients.
Odontoid hypoplasia
Late epiphyseal ossification, flat epiphysis of femoral head, coxa vara

Figure 14.9 Spondyloepiphyseal dysplasia.

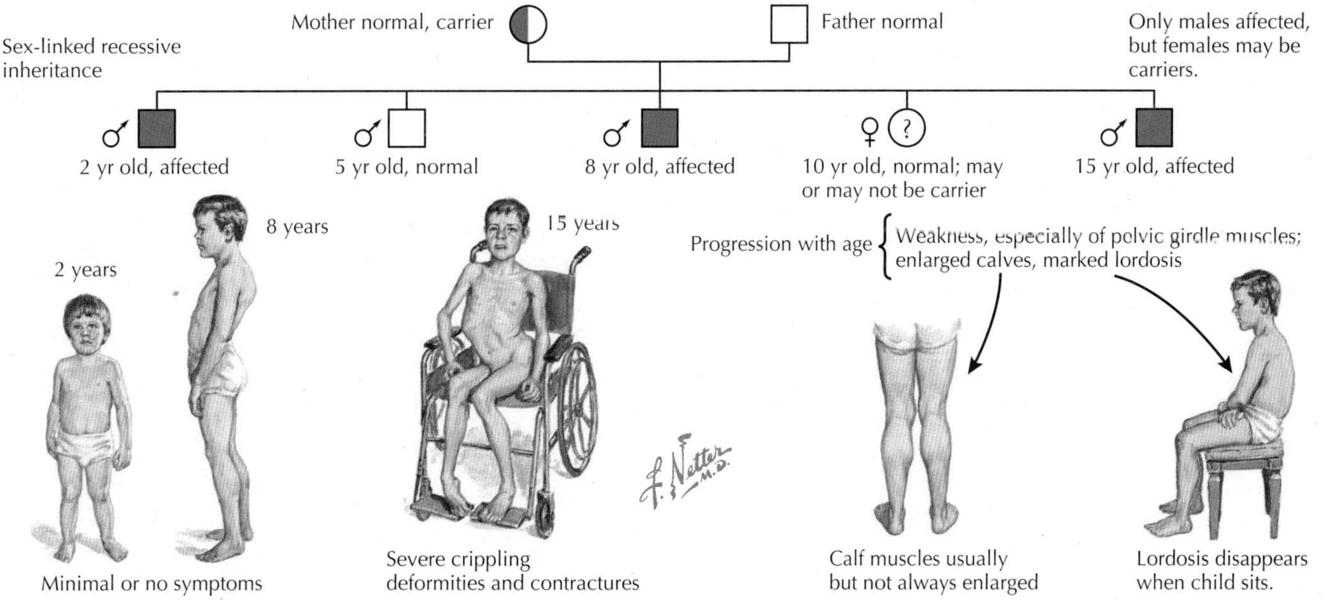

Sex-linked recessive inheritance
Mother normal, carrier
Father normal
Only males affected, but females may be carriers.
2 yr old, affected
5 yr old, normal
8 yr old, affected
10 yr old, normal; may or may not be carrier
15 yr old, affected
2 years
8 years
15 years
Progression with age
Weakness, especially of pelvic girdle muscles; enlarged calves, marked lordosis
Minimal or no symptoms
Severe crippling deformities and contractures
Calf muscles usually but not always enlarged
Lordosis disappears when child sits.

Figure 14.10 Duchenne muscular dystrophy.

Table 14.2 VISUAL IMPAIRMENT RATINGS ACCORDING TO THE INTERNATIONAL BLIND SPORTS ASSOCIATION (IBSA)

B1	Visual acuity < Logarithm of minimum angle of resolution (LogMAR) 2.6
B2	Visual acuity ranging LogMAR 1.5–2.6 and/or visual field constricted to diameter <10 degrees
B3	Visual acuity ranging from LogMAR 1.4–1.0 and/or visual field constricted to diameter <40 degrees
B4	National only—Visual acuity above 6/60 up to and including visual acuity of 6/24 (up to 25%); no visual field considered

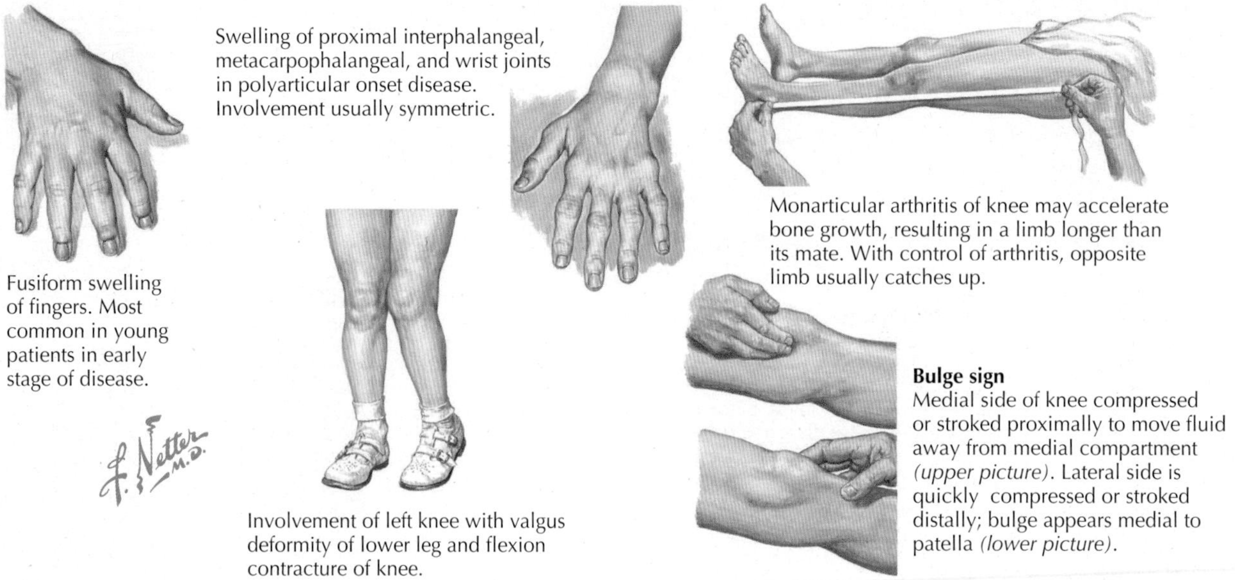
Swelling of proximal interphalangeal, metacarpophalangeal, and wrist joints in polyarticular onset disease. Involvement usually symmetric.
Monarticular arthritis of knee may accelerate bone growth, resulting in a limb longer than its mate. With control of arthritis, opposite limb usually catches up.
Fusiform swelling of fingers. Most common in young patients in early stage of disease.
F. Netter M.D.
Bulge sign
Medial side of knee compressed or stroked proximally to move fluid away from medial compartment (upper picture). Lateral side is quickly compressed or stroked distally; bulge appears medial to patella (lower picture).
Involvement of left knee with valgus deformity of lower leg and flexion contracture of knee.

Figure 14.11 Joint issues in juvenile arthritis.

- Issues in balance, coordination, and vision can affect function in competition
- Additionally, often have cardiac abnormalities such as dilated cardiomyopathy or arrhythmia, which may require additional screening before athletic participation

RECOMMENDED READINGS

Available online.

CARE OF ATHLETES AT DIFFERENT LEVELS: FROM PEE-WEE TO PROFESSIONAL

15

Ashraf M. Elbanna • Kurt P. Spindler • Mark Schickendantz

GENERAL CONSIDERATIONS (BOX 15.1)

Availability

- Being a team physician requires a tremendous time commitment.
- Must have a sincere desire to care for athletes and allow their expedient return to play.

Ability

- Possess the necessary skills to accurately diagnose and appropriately treat the athlete.
- In addition to the team physician's *actual* ability, their *perceived* ability is important. One must portray a certain level of confidence when examining, treating, and discussing treatment options with an athlete.
- A certain level of comfort and familiarity comes with time; the more experience team physicians gain by covering sporting events and communicating with athletes, the more confident and competent they will become.

Affability

- Possess the necessary social skills required to interact with not only athletes but also parents, coaches, and other staff members.
- Nurturing a professional relationship with athletes will not only increase their confidence in their own ability but also increase their adherence to treatment guidelines, particularly if it conflicts with their personal desire to return to play at any cost.
- A team physician should not try to become best friends with an athlete and should maintain a professional relationship.

Advocacy

- View the individual as a patient first and then as an athlete
- Always uphold your Hippocratic oath to do no harm to the patient

Affiliation

- Surround yourself with those who have more experience, and learn from their prior experience

DIFFERENCES FOUND AT EACH LEVEL OF PLAY

Athletic Trainers

- **Pro** teams will have multiple certified athletic trainers (ATCs) on staff; most also employ a medical director, who oversees the athletic training staff. The team physician must understand the organizational hierarchy and establish appropriate communication so that decision-making is performed by necessary individuals.
- **College** teams will typically have multiple ATCs, depending on the size of the school and available resources.
- **High school/grade school** teams may not have an ATC at all, depending on available resources.
  - Responsibilities typically relegated to an ATC may fall upon the team physician's shoulders.
  - Must arrange appropriate follow-up for athletes who need to be supervised during the week if no ATC is available to do so

BOX 15.1 THE FIVE A'S OF BEING AN EXCELLENT TEAM PHYSICIAN

- Availability
- Ability
- Affability
- Advocacy
- Affiliation

Team Physicians

- **Professional** teams typically have a medical team structure that includes a head team physician and several assistant team physicians.
  - Most will also have a list of consultants who provide specialty care, such as ophthalmology and cardiology.
  - With such a large staff, communication is critical. Ideally, the head team physician is kept in the loop regarding the complete medical care of athletes, even if he or she is not the primary caregiver.
- **College** teams will also typically have multiple physicians responsible for the care of athletes; as mentioned earlier, collaboration and communication are paramount.
- At the **high school/grade school** level, having only one physician is the most likely scenario.
  - Impossible to cover every single practice, training room, and game, try to coordinate coverage with opposing team physician, if available.

Compensation

- At the **pro** or **college** level, there may be some financial remuneration for your services. This typically is not substantial.
  - In several cases, your practice or the institution you are affiliated with pays for a marketing contract for the title of "official medical provider."
  - You may experience an increased case volume based on either your presence on the sidelines as a team physician or the advertising associated with being the official medical provider.
- **High school/grade school**–level teams most often do not include any formal salary.
  - You may see an increase in surgical/clinical volume based on athletes operated on, as well as friend and family referrals through word of mouth from those affiliated with the team.
  - Do not expect this increased patient referral or surgical volume to be proportionate to the time and effort invested on your part to care for the team.
  - Even if you do not receive compensation, the team physician typically is not covered by a state's Good Samaritan laws. You must continue to uphold your ethical duty and provide the highest level of care possible irrespective of compensation.

Public Scrutiny

- **Pro:** Team physicians may often face public pressure to try the latest fads in the medical field. They may also face this same pressure from the organization, coach, or player. The physician has the autonomy to refuse to provide care that he or she does not deem medically appropriate. However, physicians should

counsel the athlete regarding potential risks and benefits and encourage them to make an informed decision.
  - The outcome of the athlete, whether positive or negative, may have a huge impact on public perception of the physician's abilities. Although it is normal for physicians to be cognizant of the fact that their decisions will face public scrutiny, they should not be so overly concerned with this fact that it alters their decision-making process.
- **College:** May be similar to the pros depending on the prestige or ranking of the school. Division I schools in large power conferences will be more like the professional level, whereas Division II and III schools are more similar to high school.
- **High school/grade school:** Typically, physicians will not experience the public scrutiny that is commonplace at the college/professional level.

Medical Resources

- **Pro:** Very low threshold for obtaining advanced imaging (typically magnetic resonance imaging [MRI]); no need to deal with insurance before authorizations typically needed for MRI or surgery; no shortage of supplies in the training room; adequate space available for examinations/treatment.
- **College:** Depending on resources/funding of the program, this may vary considerably. Athletes will need to go through their insurance provider to obtain imaging or to schedule surgery; advanced imaging is ordered with more discretion than at the pro level. Some schools may have insurance plans available for athletes who do not have prior coverage or are coming from overseas.
- **High school/grade school:** Again, may vary considerably depending on school funding/resources or public versus private; not atypical for several inner-city schools to have a shortage of supplies. Athletes often purchase their own tape and other medical supplies for use.

Patient Autonomy/Decision-Makers

- **Pro:** At the professional level, the team physician is responsible for providing team management with accurate medical information about the athlete. With regard to the athlete, it is imperative that the team physician clearly outline the risks, benefits, and alternatives to treatment so that the athlete can make an informed decision. Often, an athlete will ask for specific recommendations, wanting the physician to simply "do what you think is best." It is the responsibility of the team physician to always do what is in the best interest of the player and not the team. It is not uncommon for athletes to seek second opinions outside of the team physician, especially for surgery.
- **College:** Physicians have the authority to clear for participation or bench a player. Athletes themselves have the legal right and authority to make their own treatment decisions. They should be given all the information necessary to make an informed decision and should be counseled regarding potential conflicts between short- and long-term gains (i.e., if diagnosed with a potentially repairable meniscal tear, they should be told about short- and long-term outcomes, risks, and length of convalescence with both meniscectomy and repair).
- **High school/grade school:** Team physicians have the ability to clear or bench a player. If under the age of 18 years, an athlete's parents have the final say regarding medical decisions and treatment options.

Immediate Return to Play

- **Pro:**
  - At the professional level, judicious use of local anesthetic to allow immediate and safe return to play is indicated for selected conditions, such as low-grade acromioclavicular (AC) sprain. It is important that the team physician understand the league rules regarding use of other injectable agents such as Toradol.
- **College:**
  - May consider local anesthetic injections (not in knee, ankle, hip, or shoulder [i.e., glenohumeral]) to allow short-term participation with relatively minor injuries (e.g., AC separation or back spasms)
  - If the athlete has a suspected concussion and passes sideline testing, they may be able to return to play once concussion is ruled out.
- **High school/grade school:**
  - Rarely appropriate to administer injections of local anesthetic agents.
  - Even the suspicion of a concussion warrants immediate removal, with no potential for return to play.

Drugs in Sports Appropriate at All Levels

- Physicians must discourage the use of illegal substances at all levels of play. Moreover, they should be familiar with the list of banned substances at each level of play: pro, college, or high school/grade school.
- The physician should obtain a thorough history of all substances being used by an athlete, including natural supplements, and should encourage athletes to be honest and forthcoming regarding their use of all substances.
- The physician must encourage compliance with governing bodies at each respective level in terms of participation and requirements for drug testing and enforcement of all policies.

Confidentiality

- Team physicians should be familiar with the Health Insurance Portability and Accountability Act (HIPAA) and Federal Educational Rights and Privacy Act (FERPA); the latter pertains to the privacy of educational records/medical information that is part of a student athlete's health record.
- **Pro:** Professional sports teams have HIPAA forms that clearly outline who the athletes' job-related medical information will be shared with. All athletes are required to sign this document.
  - There is a distinction made between personal and team-related medical information at the professional level. The physician has a duty to communicate any relevant team-related medical information with the organization that may have an impact on an athlete's participation.
- **College:** If the physician is employed by the school, medical information is not considered protected health information (PHI); however, if the school directly receives any federal funding, the medical information is governed by FERPA. Technically, medical information that is not electronically stored is not governed by HIPAA; this would then allow physicians to communicate with coaches and trainers on the sideline regarding a player's assessment. Several schools now require athletes to sign a waiver before season play, which permits sharing of their medical information with coaches or ATCs.
- **High school/grade school:** Parental consent must be obtained before sharing medical information of athletes aged <18 years. However, a physician also has an obligation to prevent harm to other players on the team, which may arise with certain infectious diseases.

Second Opinions

- **Pro:** Rules related to second opinions vary from league to league. Level of play may also be a factor. For instance, Minor League professional baseball players are considered employed

at will and as such have less autonomy than their Major League counterparts regarding medical care outside of the organization.
  - One should not take offense if an athlete chooses to pursue surgery or seek other forms of treatment from a different provider. Particularly at the professional level, several athletes may have preexisting relationships with orthopedic surgeons, and they may choose to continue their care with them. If the athlete so desires, the team physician should facilitate second opinions and share medical information with other healthcare professionals.
- **College** or **high school/grade school:** Typically, an athlete will only seek external care in the form of surgery or imaging if their insurance provider does not allow care at their own institution.

Team Travel/Cross-Coverage

- **Pro:** Depending on the sport, physicians may or may not travel with the team. Note that for sports in which physicians do not travel, you may also be responsible for providing coverage to the opposing team. In such situations, do not directly approach players (except in cases of medical emergency). Always interact with the ATC of the opposing team, who will make the decision regarding whether they would like you to evaluate a player.
- **College:** May or may not travel; may share responsibilities with other physicians; important to develop a schedule before the season starts so that any lapses in coverage can be promptly remedied; be cognizant of laws when crossing state lines. A study conducted in 2012 revealed that 18 of the 54 medical boards (that responded) allowed physicians traveling with their team to practice medicine with their home-state license. The remaining 36 states (67%) do not provide a legal pathway for the practice of medicine without their state license. This may come into consideration if an unfortunate circumstance of malpractice claim arises.
- Controlled substances should not be distributed outside of the physician's local jurisdiction, where their Drug Enforcement Agency (DEA) permit is valid. Arrangements can be made with the host's team physician to provide controlled substances, if needed.
- When traveling to an outside venue, discuss emergency planning, including the location of automated external defibrillators (AEDs) or the nearest emergency room (ER), with the host team.
- **High school/grade school:** Typically, travel is limited to within state borders; similar understanding of local on-the-field and medical care in the community should be assessed.

Factors to Consider Regarding Timing of Surgery or Return to Play

- **Pro:** What position does the athlete play? In season or off season? At what point in the season are you, nearing playoffs, etc.? What is the team record? At what point in their career is the athlete?
- **College:** Does the athlete play more than one sport? More than one position? Do they have aspirations to turn pro? Is it possible or wise for them to red-shirt this season because of an injury or surgery?
- **High school/grade school:** Does the athlete play multiple sports, multiple positions? Are they in club teams year-round? What year in school are they? Do they plan on playing in college? Is a scholarship at stake? Will they be cleared to play at the next game that may have college scouts present?

SUMMARY

- Team physicians will often be faced with ethical dilemmas regardless of the level of participation.
- These conflicts frequently revolve around return to play, confidentiality, patient (athlete) autonomy, and informed consent.
- The team physician must, at all times, act upon their ethical duty to provide the highest level of care possible to the athlete.
- In situations where the physician's obligation lies to a team or organization, they must at no time pursue a course of action that they reasonably believe could lead to any harm to the athlete, either in the near or distant future.

RECOMMENDED READINGS

Available online.

16 THE WILDERNESS ATHLETE AND ADVENTURER

Aaron D. Campbell

INTRODUCTION

- Wilderness sports differ from traditional sports in several ways.
- Participation levels of athletes may vary: professional, sponsored, and paid athletes; athletic individuals and adventurers; and intermittent recreational participants.
- The setting of wilderness sports is often austere, remote, and not regulated by organized bodies as traditional sports are.
- Participants range in age from children to older adults and seniors.
- Typically, there is no distinction in participation between male and female participants in wilderness sports.
- Competition does occur but is often an individual endeavor to achieve a personal best.
- It is probable that 90% or greater of athletes are not professional.
- Other important distinctions are that wilderness sports are typically not team sports, except for certain exceptions such as team-based overland adventure races and the team concept that applies to accomplishing common goals such as in climbing sports and events.
- Participants may be those with disabilities, pregnant females, or individuals who may have chronic health conditions, particularly older adults, who may be affected by conditions or environments where they occur (e.g., wilderness sports/adventures occurring at high altitudes).
- Although it is difficult to quantify participation in wilderness sports participation, primarily because of lack of tracking data, overall participation has increased in recent years.
- Approximately half of all Americans participated in at least one outdoor activity in 2014, which equates to over 141 million individuals collectively participating in approximately 12 billion outdoor outings.
- Increase in ski and snowboard sales, including backcountry equipment, as well increase in the sales and development of companies in the climbing and mountain biking industries support the increasing participation in wilderness and adventure activities.
- Accordingly, providers must understand how wilderness sports differ from traditional sports, particularly to evaluate and advise participants in the setting of a preparticipation evaluation (PPE) and to understand and manage injuries and illnesses occurring as a result of the activities.
- International travel or remote domestic travel is common in wilderness sports/adventures and calls for unique considerations:
  - Travel insurance is available for international travel.
  - Insurance is also available, as are global positioning system (GPS)–locating devices, in the event search and rescue services are warranted.
  - Travel-specific disease prevention utilizing preventive practices, vaccines, and occasionally medications (Traveler's Health at www.cdc.gov) is helpful.
- Although it is difficult to comprehensively enlist all wilderness and adventure activities, examples of general categories of wilderness sports are illustrated in Table 16.1.

TERMINOLOGY

Wilderness: A wild and uncultivated region such as a forest or desert, which is generally uninhabited or inhabited only by wild animals, and in which travel by land or water by humans can be considered a sport or adventure.

Backcountry: Refers to areas outside of controlled borders in wilderness regions, such as out of bounds at ski resorts for skiing/snowboarding or, perhaps, areas that could be out of cell phone or Internet range; can be applied to any wilderness sport.

PREPARTICIPATION EVALUATION FOR THE WILDERNESS ATHLETE AND ADVENTURER

Overview

- The PPE is an evaluation of athletes or sports participants before participation in a sport, an event, or an adventure.
- PPE is common in traditional and organized sports, specifically high school or collegiate sports, where it is often required despite limited supporting evidence.
- PPE for wilderness sports is performed less frequently compared with that for traditional sports, but recent literature offers guidance and methodology for clinicians who perform PPEs for wilderness sports.
- Common reasons an athlete or adventurer may request a PPE may include a requirement from an agency or a guide service, a training course in outdoor education or wilderness skills, or individually requested based on personal goals and/or medical conditions.
- Examples of important considerations for the PPE for the wilderness athlete/adventurer are outlined in Table 16.2.
- Laboratory data may be desired to ensure stability and optimization of chronic health conditions.
- Moreover, specialty consultation may be helpful in assessment of cardiovascular health (e.g., exercise treadmill stress test), pulmonary function and capacity, and gastrointestinal or musculoskeletal health.

Setting, Timing, and Structure of a Wilderness Sports/Adventure PPE

- Can be office-based or conducted in a private setting; sometimes Internet or phone consultation.
- Virtual appointments are reasonable and becoming more common.
- Ample duration should be allowed before the event for completion of immunizations and additional evaluation, which may include further diagnostic testing. A minimum of 6 weeks is mostly sufficient.
- Providers should be prepared to perform a wilderness PPE, borrowing principles from traditional sports PPE and modifying with variables such as unique preparticipation planning, prolonged physical and mental demands, and other extrinsic challenges such as environment, regional location, and remoteness.
- As in most health evaluations, medical history is the most important factor during the PPE for wilderness sports.
- Physical examinations may be more important in the presence of chronic health conditions and previous illness or injury associated with wilderness adventures.

Ethical, Legal, and Administrative Considerations of a Wilderness Sports/Adventure PPE

- Should follow typical Health Insurance Portability and Accountability Act (HIPAA) procedures
- Utilized as an evaluation for a planned event but should also incorporate typical features of a wellness visit, including immunizations, status of chronic conditions, and assessment of medications

- Literature is available to guide inexperienced providers, but referral to a trained provider may be valuable in more challenging medical and environmental scenarios.
- Specialty consultation may be pertinent to further evaluate chronic health conditions such as heart disease (may need an electrocardiogram [ECG] or stress test), pulmonary disease (may need pulmonary function tests, including provocative examinations), and gastrointestinal disease (may need updated colonoscopy or unique dietary plans).
- See e-Fig. 16.A for an example of a health history form that could be used by a provider performing a PPE for wilderness sports or adventures.

Table 16.1 EXAMPLES OF GENERAL CATEGORIES OF WILDERNESS SPORTS[a]

Wilderness Event Category	Sport/Adventure
Climbing sports	Rock
	Ice
	Mixed rock and ice
	Mountaineering/alpinism
Snow sports	Backcountry skiing
	Backcountry snowboarding
	Glacier travel
Water sports	River running (kayaking or rafting)
	Surfing
	Open water swimming
Cycling sports	Mountain biking
Endurance/trekking events	Hiking
	Backpacking
	Trekking
	Trail running (ultra-marathons)
	Overland adventure racing

[a]Note: This is not an inclusive list.

CHRONIC HEALTH CONDITIONS AND WILDERNESS SPORTS AND ADVENTURES

Overview

- In general, key principles involve optimization and/or stabilization of chronic conditions before wilderness travel, sports, or adventures.
- Ensure access to medications used regularly or for disease exacerbations and include adequate supply for the same number of days of sojourn and an additional 2–3 days of supply (or more) depending on potential travel itinerary changes, possibility of event prolongation, or loss of medication.
- Certain conditions may be affected more by specific environments, such as cold or hot temperatures or high altitudes, and others are more generalized.
- Some individuals with chronic health conditions or unexplained signs and symptoms may require more advanced diagnostic evaluation depending on the activity, duration of event, or required intensity (see the section "Preparticipation Evaluation for the Wilderness Athlete and Adventurer" earlier).
- Table 16.3 illustrates a simplified list of chronic conditions and rationales for related issues experienced in wilderness sports/adventures.

Table 16.2 SIMPLIFIED LIST OF IMPORTANT CONSIDERATIONS FOR PPE OF A WILDERNESS ATHLETE OR ADVENTURER

Consideration	Rationale for Consideration
Travel	• Domestic vs. international will yield different health concerns • Insurance policies for health and emergency issues abroad are available
Immunizations	• Important for international travel in endemic areas, as well as in certain domestic areas
Chronic medications	• Additional supplies or pharmacy refills before travel depending on location and event demands

Prophylactic medications	• Helpful in both endemic international areas and certain domestic remote backcountry areas
	  • Antibiotics
	  • Pain management
	  • Wound care
	  • General illness (e.g., diarrhea, nausea/vomiting, respiratory symptoms, and rashes)

General physical conditioning	• Fitness and conditioning base vs. need for specific activities in a healthy athlete/adventurer
Nutrition	• Adequate caloric replacement for the desired activity, considering lightweight, easily tolerated foods that include elements of healthy fats, carbohydrates, and proteins • Other nutritional supplementation (e.g., vitamins) may be considered, given the nature of prepared or dehydrated foods and inability to carry perishables or heavy meat products
Altitude	• Acclimatization, history of altitude illness, weather, and elemental exposure

Hot environments	• Heat exposure issues
	  • History of heat illness
	  • Cooling abilities
	  • Sun protection
	  • Hydration

Cold environments	• Cold exposure issues
	  • History of cold illness
	  • Frostbite
	  • Layered clothing
	  • Prevention of heat loss and sweating

Presence of chronic disease	• Stabilization/optimization of health conditions • May need medical specialty consultation • Diagnostic data during PPEs may be helpful in certain cases, such as evaluation of iron levels, before travel to altitude and assessment of chronic disease stability (e.g., diabetes; CAD; valvular heart disease; COPD; and thyroid, hepatic, or renal disease)

CAD, Coronary artery disease; *COPD,* chronic obstructive pulmonary disease; *PPE,* preparticipation evaluation.

Table 16.3 SIMPLIFIED LIST OF CHRONIC CONDITIONS AND RATIONALE FOR ISSUES IN WILDERNESS SPORTS/ADVENTURES

Organ System	Rationale for Health Issue
Pulmonary	• Airway is the primary organ system to sustain life. • Multiple risk factors and health conditions affect airways. • Allergens and air quality can lead to exacerbation of chronic conditions or trigger new acute symptoms. • Asthma, COPD, and/or emphysema should be stable with available medications, along with instructions for management of acute exacerbations.
Cardiovascular	• Stress on the heart: conditions such as altitude, temperature extremes, and physical exertion can trigger chronic cardiac conditions such as ischemic heart disease, occult vessel lesions, arrhythmias, and pump deficits.
Hematologic	• Patients with injuries sustained in wilderness areas may be at an increased risk if participants are using blood-thinning agents such as warfarin. • Genetic bleeding disorders can pose issues for hemostasis in the event of lacerations, abrasions, or cuts. • Blood clotting disorders may go unrecognized, and possible delay in obtaining imaging results or in initiation of anticoagulation could be life threatening.
Gastrointestinal	• Infectious or foodborne issues leading to fluid loss through diarrhea or vomiting or the inability to eat can lead to dehydration or nutritional deficiencies. • Counseling on food and toilet hygiene should be emphasized to prevent acute issues. • Chronic conditions should be stable and medications must be available for exacerbations.
Musculoskeletal	• Use of the musculoskeletal system is inherent in physical movement. Injuries can lead to difficulties with ambulation or in performing essential tasks for completion of the sport or event or self-extrication. • Joint laxities such as recurrent shoulder dislocations should be evaluated and managed with physical therapy and possible surgical intervention. • Conditions such as arthritis (any kind) could pose issues if pain or systemic exacerbations occur.
Central nervous	• Head injuries or spinal compromise can be life threatening or require prompt recognition for early and appropriate management to allow either resolution or immobilization for transport or extrication. • Concussion management should be discussed in terms of recognition and management to avoid long-term complications. • Disorders such as multiple sclerosis or Parkinson disease could be exacerbated by heat or altitude; thus, thermoregulation is an important consideration.
Ophthalmologic	• Visual disturbances can compromise abilities to navigate and care for oneself during wilderness sports/adventures. • History of refractive surgeries (LASIK, radial keratotomy) or glaucoma: vision may be affected by altitude or other barometric pressure changes. • Corrective eyewear should be available in multiple forms to avoid loss of visual acuity.
Psychiatric	• Psychotic episodes can be triggered in unfamiliar terrain or when threats are perceived from the environment and can compromise personal or expedition member safety. • Coping skill mechanisms, response to stress, and stress management are essential. • Concerns regarding substance abuse or medication withdrawal can be life threatening or lead to issues with other participants.

COPD, Chronic obstructive pulmonary disease; *LASIK,* laser-assisted in situ keratomileusis.

ALTITUDE-RELATED ISSUES

High-Altitude Illness

- Spectrum of illnesses that are specifically caused by rapid ascent to high altitude.
- Includes acute mountain sickness (AMS), high-altitude cerebral edema (HACE), and high-altitude pulmonary edema (HAPE).
- The Wilderness Medical Society (WMS) organized an expert panel to produce evidence-based, comprehensive consensus guidelines for the prevention and treatment of acute altitude illness. Most information presented in this section is adopted from these guidelines, which are regularly updated.
- High-altitude illness (HAI) can be ameliorated by low-risk ascent profiles or a well-planned and appropriately controlled ascent.
- Ascent profiles describe the number of days planned to achieve a particular altitude, where the sleeping altitude is most important, and several days may be required to achieve a maximum altitude, with scheduled camps for sleeping along the way in order to avoid complications of HAI.
- Common signs and symptoms of HAI are listed in Table 16.4.
- Risk categories established for HAI are outlined in Table 16.5.
- Medications available for the prevention of HAI are outlined in Table 16.6.
- For treatment of all HAIs, considerations include rest, medications (see Table 16.6), descent, and oxygen.

Acute Mountain Sickness (See Tables 16.4, 16.5, and 16.6)

- Symptoms can be mild, moderate, or severe.
- All symptoms include headache plus one or more additional symptoms ranging in severity.
- Prevention is based on a low-risk ascent profile, possibly a moderate-risk ascent profile if no history of AMS.
- In case of history of AMS, an individual with altitude experience and known elevations of symptom presentation can slow his or her ascent to altitude and/or increase the number of sleeping nights during ascent.
- Consider medications for prophylaxis in moderate- to high-risk situations.

High-Altitude Cerebral Edema (See Tables 16.4, 16.5, and 16.6)

- Considered to be a severe form of AMS.
- Signs of central nervous system (CNS) disturbance accompanied with severe symptoms of AMS.
- Consider medications for prophylaxis in moderate- to high-risk situations.

High-Altitude Pulmonary Edema (See Tables 16.4, 16.5, and 16.6)

- Hypoxia of altitude can lead to constriction of certain pulmonary blood vessels, shunting blood to fewer other blood vessels,

Table 16.4 SIGNS AND SYMPTOMS OF HIGH-ALTITUDE ILLNESSES

High-Altitude Illness	Symptoms	Signs
Acute mountain sickness (AMS)	Headache plus one or more of the following signs varying from mild or moderate to severe: • Nausea or vomiting • Fatigue • Lassitude • Dizziness • Sleep difficulty	Nothing specific
High-altitude cerebral edema (HACE)	Worsening symptoms of AMS, considered upper end of severe AMS • Severe lassitude	• Ataxia • Altered mental status • Encephalopathy
High-altitude pulmonary edema (HAPE)	• Extreme fatigue • Breathlessness at rest • Chest tightness, fullness, or congestion • Drowsiness	• Fast, shallow breathing • Cough with possible pink, frothy sputum • Gurgling and rattling breath sounds • Blue or gray lips or fingertips

Modified from Luks AM, Auerbach P, Freer L, et al. Wilderness Medical Society consensus guidelines for the prevention and treatment of acute altitude illness: 2019 update. *Wilderness Environ Med*. 2019;30(4S):S3–18, Table 3.

Table 16.5 RISK CATEGORIES FOR HIGH-ALTITUDE ILLNESSES

Risk Level	Ascent Vignette
Low risk	• No previous history of altitude illness and plans to ascend no more than 2800 m (9186 ft) as the maximum altitude for sleeping • Plans to ascend to 2500–3000 m (8202–9842 ft) in no less than 2 days with increases in sleeping altitude afterward of no more than 500 m/day (1640 ft)
Moderate risk	• Past history of AMS and plans to ascend to altitudes of 2500–2800 m (8202–9186 ft) in a single day • No past history of AMS but plans to ascend to >2800 m (9186 ft) in a single day • Any individual with plans to increase their sleeping altitude by >500 m (1640 ft) in a single day at altitudes >3000 m (9842 ft); add an extra day of acclimatization every 1000 m
High risk	• Previous history of AMS and plans to ascend to >2800 m (9186 ft) in a single day • An individual who has experienced HAPE or HACE previously • An individual planning to ascend to >3500 m (11,482 ft) in a single day for the first sleeping elevation • An individual who increases their sleeping altitude by >500 m (1640 ft) while over 300 m (9842 ft) • Very rapid ascents of high-altitude peaks (e.g., Mt. Kilimanjaro in <7 days, >3500 m)

Modified from Luks AM, Auerbach P, Freer L, et al. Wilderness Medical Society consensus guidelines for the prevention and treatment of acute altitude illness: 2019 update. *Wilderness Environ Med*. 2019;30(4S):S3–18, Table 2.

Table 16.6 MEDICATIONS COMMONLY USED FOR THE PREVENTION AND TREATMENT OF HIGH-ALTITUDE ILLNESSES IN ADDITION TO A GRADUAL ASCENT RATE

High-Altitude Illness	Prevention in Moderate- to High-Risk Situations[a]	Treatment[d]
Acute mountain sickness (AMS)	• Acetazolamide 125 mg oral twice daily[b] Pediatrics: 2.5 mg/kg oral every 12 hours • Dexamethasone 2 mg oral every 6 hours or 4 mg oral every 12 hours[c] Pediatrics: not recommended • Ibuprofen: 600 mg every 6–8 hours	• Acetazolamide 250 mg oral twice daily Pediatrics: 2.5 mg/kg oral every 12 hours • Dexamethasone 4 mg (oral, IV, or IM) every 6 hours Pediatrics: 0.15 mg/kg/dose every 6 hours until symptoms subside
High-altitude cerebral edema (HACE)	• Acetazolamide 125 mg oral twice daily Pediatrics: 2.5 mg/kg every 12 hours • Dexamethasone 2 mg (oral, IV, or IM) every 6 hours, or 4 mg every 12 hours Pediatrics: not recommended	• Dexamethasone 8 mg (oral, IV, or IM) loading dose, then 4 mg every 6 hours Pediatrics: 0.15 mg/kg/dose every 6 hours
High-altitude pulmonary edema (HAPE)	• Nifedipine SR 30 mg oral every 12 hours or SR 20 mg oral every 8 hours • Tadalafil 10 mg oral twice daily • Sildenafil 50 mg every 8 hours • Salmeterol 125 mcg inhaled twice daily	• Nifedipine SR 30 mg oral every 12 hours or SR 20 mg oral every 8 hours

[a]For the general population, prophylactic medications should not be used in place of a gradual ascent rate, and such medications are not typically needed in low-risk situations (refer to Table 16.6). In addition, prophylactic medications can be discontinued upon initiation of descent.

[b]Acetazolamide is a sulfonamide derivative; however, cross-reactivity to sulfonamides is rare, and individuals reporting an allergy to sulfonamide medications should consider a trial of acetazolamide before the expedition. Anaphylaxis from sulfonamide medications is an absolute contraindication to the use of acetazolamide.

[c]Dexamethasone should be limited to no more than 10 days to prevent glucocorticoid toxicity and adrenal suppression.

[d]Continue until definitive care is reached at lower altitudes.

Modified from Luks AM, Auerbach P, Freer L, et al. Wilderness Medical Society consensus guidelines for the prevention and treatment of acute altitude illness: 2019 update. *Wilderness Environ Med*. 2019;30(4S):S3–18, Table 1.

which leads to increased pulmonary pressure and subsequent leakage of fluid to lung parenchyma.
- Contributing factors beyond the hypoxic environment at high altitudes are increased exertion and cold temperatures.
- Consider medications for prophylaxis for moderate- to high-risk situations.

Health Conditions Affected by Altitude

Lung Disease and Altitude

- See Chapter 23: "Altitude Training and Competition" for discussion of the physiology of high altitude and definitions of elevation levels.
- Chronic lung disease may be worsened at high altitudes.
- Etiology may include increased alveolar hypoxia, hypoxemia, increased pulmonary vascular resistance, and sleep-disordered breathing issues.
- Work of breathing increases because of increase in ventilation at high altitudes.
- If individuals are using supplemental oxygen at low altitudes, it is recommended they discuss how to use supplemental oxygen at high altitudes with their healthcare provider during a PPE because it may be different from their baseline use.

ASTHMA

- Unique environmental factors at high altitude affect individuals with asthma.
  - Hypoxia: Decreased barometric pressure leads to lower alveolar and arterial oxygen tensions.
  - Hypocapnia: Hypoxia stimulates chemoreceptors and carotid bodies leading to an increase in minute ventilation (hypoxic ventilatory response). Increased inspiratory flow resistance and work of breathing from decreased arterial carbon dioxide tension affects airway function.
  - Decreased air density: Theoretically can decrease airway obstructions, but there is a paucity of high-quality studies to demonstrate the effect.
- Travel to altitude often requires travel to countries with traffic and other industrial pollution, which can affect asthmatics.
- Asthmatics should be as well-controlled as possible before travel and ensure they are properly using bronchodilator inhalers plus or minus inhaled glucocorticoids depending on their asthma status. Additionally, they should carry plenty of extra inhalers to ensure they do not run out and can treat exacerbations appropriately.
- In general, remaining at lower altitudes (500–2000 m) vs. traveling to high altitude has a beneficial effect because of lower airway inflammation and decreased benefit of bronchoconstrictor stimuli occurring at higher altitudes.
- There are conflicting and limited data for moderate altitude (2000–3000 m).
- At high altitudes (3000–5000+ m), well-controlled asthmatics may theoretically do better because of a decrease in allergens and air pollution, but the factors of hypoxia, hypercapnia, and lower air density have been shown to affect well-controlled mild asthmatics similarly to non-asthmatics in field studies from the standpoint of symptoms.
- Intense exercise should be avoided at high altitude.
- Respiratory infections are common at high altitude and can lead to exacerbations; exposures should be avoided using social distancing, personal hygiene, and possibly the use of a face mask (that does not inhibit breathing) whenever possible.
- Asthma management principles are the same at all altitudes.
- Acute exacerbations with respiratory distress can be treated with a combination of interventions.
  - Oral prednisone (or equivalent corticosteroid) 60 mg daily for a 5- to 7-day burst.
  - Inhaled beta-2 agonist (albuterol or equivalent) repeatedly, 2–4 puffs, every 15 minutes scheduled until steroids take effect, which may be one or several days.
  - Supplemental oxygen (if available) per nasal canula or face mask to achieve O_2 saturation level >90%.
  - Epinephrine 0.3 mL subcutaneous 1:1000 mix should be considered.
  - Plans for evacuation should ensue.
- Many wilderness expedition companies operate under protocols similar to these interventions.
- Inhalers should be kept warm and individuals made aware that cold temperatures can decrease the delivery of medication, thus possibly decreasing the number of doses available in a multidose inhaler.
- Exercise-induced bronchospasm (EIB) may worsen at elevations over 2500 m (~8200 ft) because of large-volume ventilation of dry cold air and subsequent heat loss.
- Participants should be advised to use inhalers and medications consistent with their routine asthma treatment regimen, although long-acting beta-agonists may be considered for EIB and prolonged event duration at high altitudes.

CHRONIC OBSTRUCTIVE PULMONARY DISEASE

- Chronic obstructive pulmonary disease (COPD) should be optimized and stabilized before altitude sojourns, with instructions to continue scheduled inhaled medications and monitor oxygen saturation levels by using a pulse oximeter.
- Exercise tolerance and capacity should be determined for individuals with COPD participating in adventure and wilderness events requiring exertion that exceeds baseline activities.
- Patients with severe forced expiratory volume at 1 second (FEV_1 30%–50% predicted) or very severe disease (FEV_1 <30% predicted) or those with carbon dioxide retention or right heart failure should be advised against exceeding baseline activity tolerance and ascending to an altitude higher than that of their current residence.
- Access to corticosteroids in addition to inhalers and counseling on how to manage COPD exacerbations is essential.
- Descent will always be an intricate part of the initial management in any COPD exacerbation.

SLEEP-DISORDERED BREATHING

- Sleep-disordered breathing at altitude refers to both obstructive sleep apnea (OSA) and central sleep apnea (CSA).
- In general, OSA may improve at altitude because of increased muscle tone in the upper airways.
- Individuals with OSA can develop CSA, or CSA can be worsened by altitude.
- Acetazolamide, a diuretic, is a favorable medication for preventing exacerbations of both OSA and CSA, whether or not continuous positive airway pressure (CPAP) is used.
- Participants with moderate to severe OSA should plan to bring and use their CPAP machines while at altitude, and battery/power will have to be considered.

Cardiovascular Conditions

HYPERTENSION

- A mild increase in blood pressure normally occurs with ascent to higher altitudes.
- Individuals with hypertension can observe considerable variability in systolic blood pressure increases at altitude (usually >3000 m or 9840 ft), with increases as high as 30–40 mmHg.
- Altitude-induced changes are transient and will resolve soon after descent to lower elevations.
- Because of the transient nature of these changes, frequent monitoring of blood pressure is neither advised nor does it need to be treated in asymptomatic individuals.
- If symptoms develop while at altitude, no ideal treatment plan has been established except for continuation of routine dosing of regular medications and descent or perhaps extrication (depending on severity).

- Certain clinicians may recommend medications for pro re nata (PRN) use for significant blood pressure increases, but this should be individualized, and an action plan should be discussed with the healthcare provider during a PPE.
- For individuals with labile hypertension (HTN), monitoring with a reliable, portable wrist cuff may be helpful, and use of nocturnal supplemental oxygen can improve the variation in blood pressures.

ATHEROSCLEROTIC HEART DISEASE

- Atherosclerotic heart disease (ASHD) is a common cause of sudden cardiac death in older athletes.
- These individuals will most likely self-select their participation in altitude activities based on exercise capacity and the presence of symptoms.
- Important considerations for risk assessment include identifying cardiovascular risk factors and known disease status and stability, baseline exercise capacity, and anticipated exercise and event intensity.
- Exercise stress testing should be considered if there is a large discrepancy between the actual fitness level of the patient and the expected exercise/event demands (may be predicted using metabolic equivalent of tasks [METs]).
- Defining exercise capacity and disease stability will guide the development of a graduated training program to help accommodate the anticipated demands.
- Additional risk stratification should include symptoms noted at present; recent ischemic events; other comorbidities; and past results of ECG, exercise stress tests, and echocardiograms.
- All individuals with heart disease should be encouraged to achieve and maintain good cardiovascular fitness, whether at low elevations or when they intend to travel to higher altitudes.

CARDIAC ARRHYTHMIAS

- Ascent to altitude causes a release of catecholamines, which may trigger cardiac arrhythmias.
- Premature atrial and ventricular contractions are common at high altitudes and are usually benign.
- An individual experiencing arrhythmia symptoms that have not been appropriately evaluated or are unstable should not participate in wilderness and adventure activities.
- Individuals with poorly controlled, dangerous arrhythmias should be advised not to travel to high altitudes.
- Stable chronic atrial fibrillation may be managed with appropriate rate-control medication and symptomatic paroxysmal atrial fibrillation with PRN rescue medications (e.g., beta-blockers or calcium channel blockers).
- Patients taking anticoagulant and antiplatelet medications should be counseled about the risk of bleeding if there is a high risk of fall injuries.

CONGESTIVE HEART FAILURE

- Congestive heart failure (CHF) must be well controlled before any ascent to altitude, and participants should be made aware of the associated risks during PPE.
- It is important to determine American College of Cardiology/American Heart Association (ACC/AHA) classification (A–D) of heart failure.
- Class A and B patients with normal exercise capacity established by formal exercise testing usually tolerate wilderness activity well if exercise capacity does not exceed beyond wilderness activity demands.
- Class C patients are at a considerable risk of decompensation if activity demands exceed exercise capacity; thus, it is safest to advise against participation in wilderness events that are likely to stress the cardiovascular system to that degree.
- Ascent to altitude is associated with the risk of HAPE even in healthy individuals.
- Class D patients are typically incapable of participating in wilderness events.

RECOMMENDED READINGS

Available online.

SECTION III

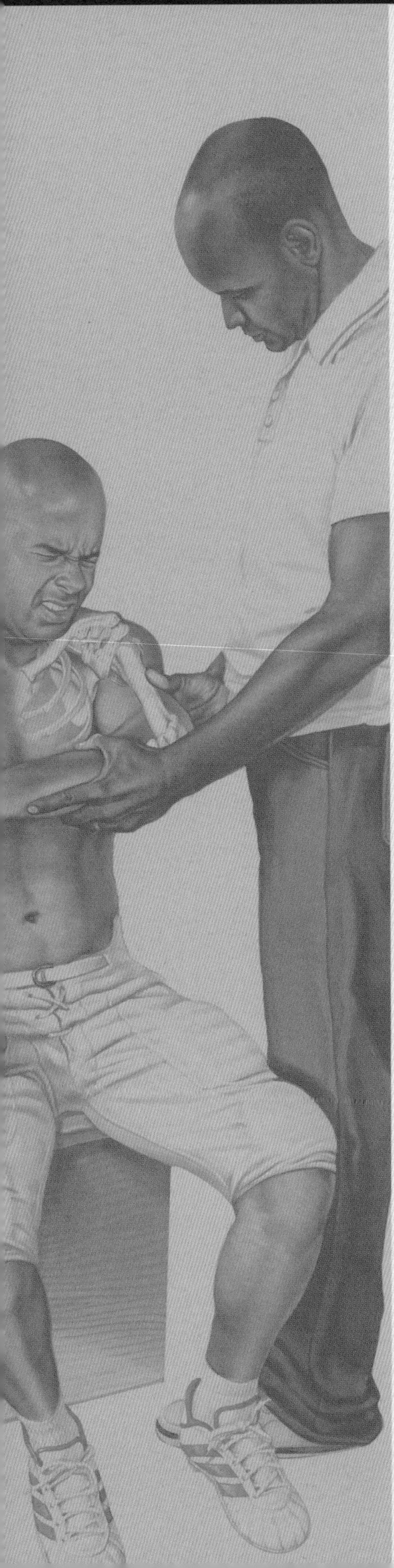

Conditioning

EXERCISE PRESCRIPTION AND PHYSIOLOGY 17

O. Josh Bloom • Karl B. Fields • Todd M. McGrath • Timothy R. Draper

EXERCISE PHYSIOLOGY

- Science of processes and mechanisms of skeletal muscle contraction and the corresponding interaction of other body systems that facilitate and respond to skeletal muscle contraction.
- Skeletal muscle contraction that exceeds physiologic limits, is inappropriate in duration or intensity, or for which the musculoskeletal system has been inadequately prepared can lead to injury or poor performance and adaptation to training.
- Clinical relevance lies in identification of the pathology; what triggered it; and how to correct, alleviate, and/or prevent this in both individuals and populations of active people.

Terminology

- Metabolic equivalents (METs): expression of metabolic cost of exercise in terms of oxygen consumption
  - Rest defined as 1 MET, which is an oxygenation of 3.5 mL O_2/kg/min
  - MET chart (Table 17.1)
- VO_2 max: maximal oxygen utilization
  - Gold standard for evaluating cardiorespiratory fitness
  - Measured in mL O_2/kg/min
- Anaerobic threshold: point at which oxygen demand exceeds oxygen availability
- Workload: amount of energy required to complete a specific task (Table 17.2)

Basic Science

- The sarcomere, which is the basic unit of muscle, is composed of actin and myosin filaments (Fig. 17.1).
- This linkage between actin and myosin is facilitated via acetylcholine release at the motor endplate, which triggers depolarization and subsequent release of calcium from the sarcoplasmic reticulum; this is followed by a series of reactions, causes formation of an adenosine triphosphate (ATP)–myosin complex, a subsequent change in myosin unit conformation, and ultimately, traction on the actin filament. This pulls on the sarcomere's connective tissue components, resulting in muscle contraction (Fig. 17.2) and movement.
- The motor nerve center directs the timing and sequencing of motor unit recruitment and firing, which facilitates coordinated movement.
- Continued muscle contraction relies on an adequate supply of ATP in each sarcomere.
- ATP is provided by three interlinked, overlapping energy systems that synthesize ATP for both short periods of intense vigorous activity and longer periods of lower-level sustained activity.
- Exercise results in increases in protein synthesis within muscle, with long-term/cumulative changes to the steady-state level of protein synthesis with repetitive exercise.
- Body weight and glucose control are influenced by the energy requirements of muscle contraction.

Energy Systems

PHOSPHAGENS (ATP–CREATINE PHOSPHATE SYSTEM)

- Anaerobic system used in maximum-intensity exercise lasting only seconds
- Composed of ATP and creatine phosphate stored in the cytoplasm of each sarcomere
- Phosphagens provide rapid resynthesis of ATP on myosin heads, facilitating brief, high-intensity bursts of muscle activity.
- Particularly important during very high-intensity exercise and at the beginning of exercise

GLYCOGEN TO PYRUVATE ("LACTIC ACID SYSTEM")

- Anaerobic process that degrades muscle glycogen to pyruvate
  - Pyruvate is an essential substrate that can be oxidized to ATP via the aerobic energy system (see "Oxidative System").
- Also directly provides some ATP, which becomes part of the phosphagen pool.
- Energy source in high-intensity, short-burst exercise (typically ≤3 minutes).
- Pyruvate can be reversibly converted to lactate, which can be transported out of the cell for use by other tissues.
  - Also serves as a negative feedback loop because increased lactate causes metabolic acidosis, which increases the rate of ventilation and causes muscle discomfort; these reactions will eventually encourage the individual to reduce the intensity of exercise.

OXIDATIVE SYSTEM (RESPIRATORY RESPONSE TO EXERCISE)

- The aerobic energy system
- Quantitatively the most important system
- Typically used in activities lasting >3 minutes
- Dependent on oxygen availability at the cellular level
- The body's physiology is structured to facilitate the transport of O_2 to tissues via the cardiorespiratory system
- Dependent on oxidation of *pyruvate*, *acetyl-CoA* (formed directly from glucose), or *free fatty acids*
- A low-power but extremely high-capacity energy system

Adaptations to Chronic Exercise ("Training")

- Mitochondrial volume and density may increase up to 40% to accommodate increase in aerobic exercise.
- Musculoskeletal and cardiorespiratory systems are highly adaptable to regularly performed exercise.
- Adaptation to repetitive exercise can be understood in terms of several factors, which can be represented by the mnemonic **P-ROIDS.**
  - **P**rogression: Gradual increase in intensity, duration, and difficulty of physical activity to improve strength, endurance, and sport-specific skills
  - **R**eversibility: Training is generally continuous or cyclic in nature, because of the rapid loss of benefits from conditioning when people stop exercising
    - Inactivity for as little as several days can lead to reduction in work capacity secondary to a decrease in protein synthesis from baseline with loss of exercise stimulus

Table 17.1 METS IN COMMON COMPETITIVE AND RECREATIONAL SPORTS

Sport	METs
Basketball (comp)	7–12
Biking (rec)	3–8
Dancing	3–7
Football	6–10
Golf (cart)	2–3
Jogging (5–6 mph)	7–15
Skiing (downhill)	5–8
Soccer	5–12
Tennis	4–9
Volleyball	3–6

Modified from Mead WF, Hartwig R. Fitness evaluation and exercise prescription. *J Fam Pract*. 1981;13(7):1039–1050.

Table 17.2 METS IN WALKING

Workload	Miles	Minutes
5 METs	1	15–18
6 METs	1.5	21–25
8 METs	2	24–29
10 METs	4	50–54
12 METs	5	70–80

Modified from Mead WF, Hartwig R. Fitness evaluation and exercise prescription. *J Fam Pract*. 1981;13(7):1039–1050.

- **O**verload: Exercising above normal levels through combinations of type of activity, intensity, duration, and/or frequency
- **I**ndividual **D**ifferences
- **S**pecificity: Specific training develops specific adaptations beneficial to a particular sport/activity
- Training should focus on energy system that is most important to that sport (e.g., distance runners spend more time working on oxidative system)
- Modern training programs typically incorporate cross-training because training focused on optimizing all energy systems can improve sport-specific performance (e.g., dry-land and weight training can improve the performance of skiers)
- Concurrent training: integration of both aerobic/endurance and resistance training into the training plan
- Lower-volume, high-intensity interval training can improve aerobic fitness in sedentary subjects
- Ratio of acute to chronic training load can be used to monitor response to exercise and mitigate injury risk
  - Acute training load: workload performed over 7 days
  - Chronic training load: 28-day average of acute training load

Types of Exercise

- Aerobic/endurance exercise: fueled by an oxidative energy system and in place when oxygen supply/delivery to tissues is adequate for sustained low- to moderate-intensity exercise
  - Increased lipid mobilization and oxidation by skeletal muscle
  - Increased number of mitochondria with adaptation
- Anaerobic exercise: typically high-intensity, shorter-duration exercise that exceeds capacity of oxidative system and is fueled primarily by phosphagens and glycogen to pyruvate energy systems

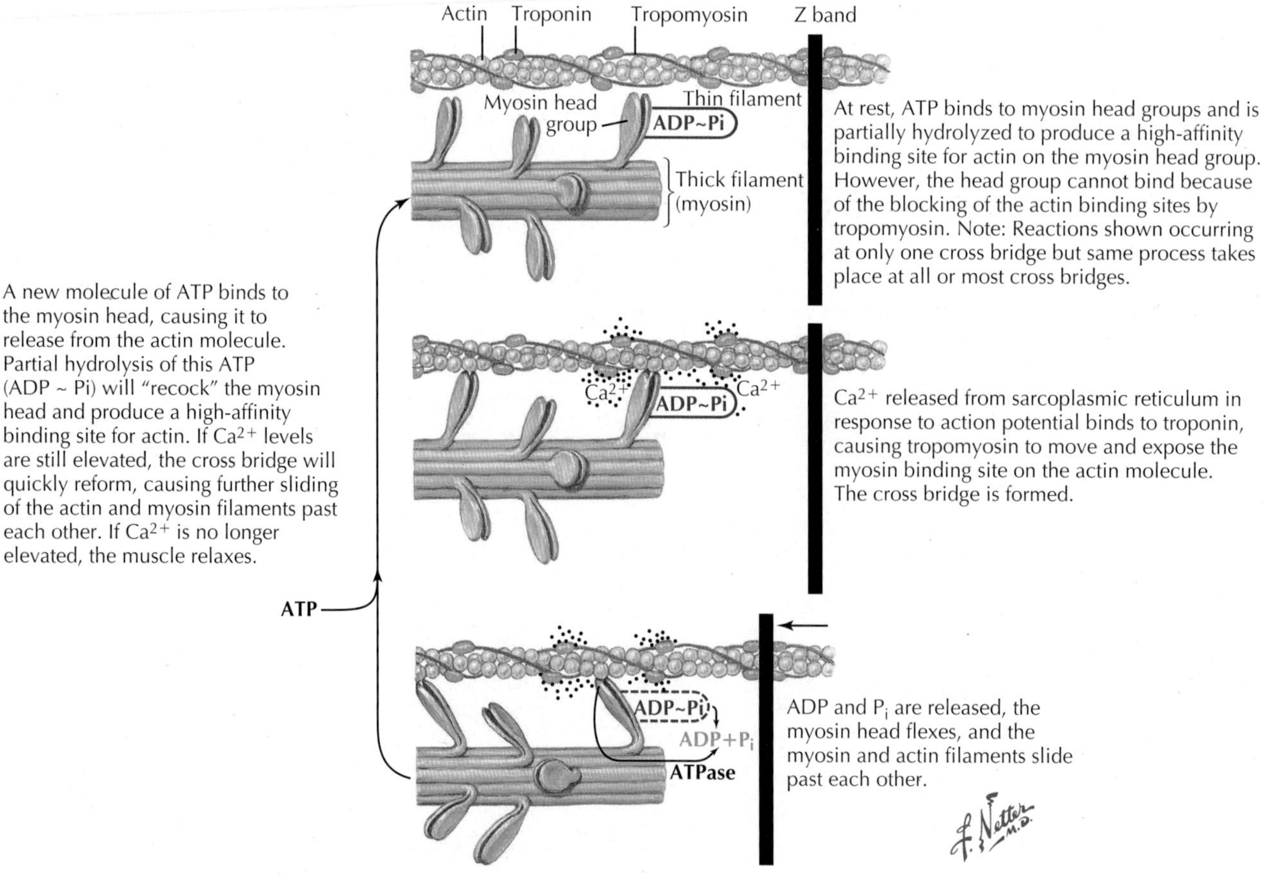

Actin
Troponin
Tropomyosin
Z band
Myosin head group
Thin filament
ADP~Pi
Thick filament (myosin)
At rest, ATP binds to myosin head groups and is partially hydrolyzed to produce a high-affinity binding site for actin on the myosin head group. However, the head group cannot bind because of the blocking of the actin binding sites by tropomyosin. Note: Reactions shown occurring at only one cross bridge but same process takes place at all or most cross bridges.
A new molecule of ATP binds to the myosin head, causing it to release from the actin molecule. Partial hydrolysis of this ATP (ADP ~ Pi) will "recock" the myosin head and produce a high-affinity binding site for actin. If Ca2+ levels are still elevated, the cross bridge will quickly reform, causing further sliding of the actin and myosin filaments past each other. If Ca2+ is no longer elevated, the muscle relaxes.
Ca2+
ADP~Pi
Ca2+
Ca2+ released from sarcoplasmic reticulum in response to action potential binds to troponin, causing tropomyosin to move and expose the myosin binding site on the actin molecule. The cross bridge is formed.
ATP
ADP~Pi
ADP+Pi
ATPase
ADP and Pi are released, the myosin head flexes, and the myosin and actin filaments slide past each other.

Figure 17.1 Biochemical mechanics of muscle contraction.

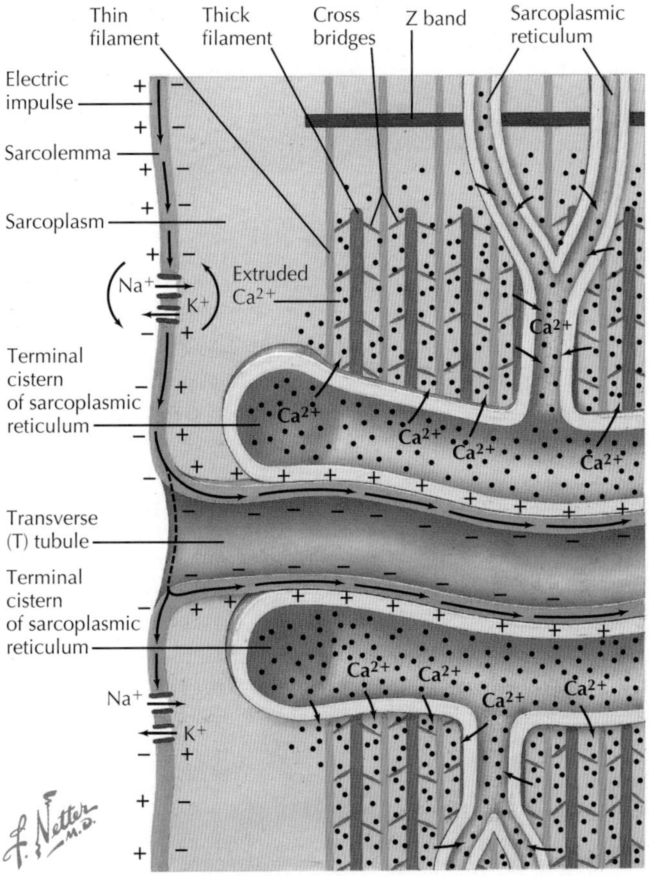
Thin filament
Thick filament
Cross bridges
Z band
Sarcoplasmic reticulum
Electric impulse
Sarcolemma
Sarcoplasm
Na+
K+
Extruded Ca2+
Terminal cistern of sarcoplasmic reticulum
Ca2+
Transverse (T) tubule
Terminal cistern of sarcoplasmic reticulum
Na+
K+

Electric impulse traveling along muscle cell membrane (sarcolemma) from motor endplate (neuromuscular junction) and then along transverse tubules affects sarcoplasmic reticulum, causing extrusion of Ca^{2+} to initiate contraction by "rowing" action of cross bridges, sliding filaments past one another.

Figure 17.2 Initiation of muscle contraction by electric impulse and calcium movement.

- Resistance exercise: training for maximal contractile force and muscle hypertrophy
- Range of motion/stretching/warm-up/cool-down exercises (Fig. 17.3)
- Flexibility exercise: increases ability to lengthen muscle–tendon units and improve motion around specific joints
- "Lifestyle activity": cumulative, nonstructured, moderate-intensity physical activities that individuals do during a typical day (e.g., taking stairs and walking from parking lot)
  - Ten minutes of moderate-intensity exercise three times a day facilitates changes comparable to health benefits of 30 minutes of continuous exercise
  - Increasing lifestyle activity is as effective as structured activity for improving cardiorespiratory fitness and reducing cardiovascular disease (CVD) risk factors.

EXERCISE PRESCRIPTION

General Considerations

- A tool to teach, coach, and educate patients regarding opportunities to improve overall health and well-being
  - Can also enhance exercise and sport-specific performance
- Exercise is safe for a majority of patients and has numerous health/fitness benefits
- Written exercise prescription has been demonstrated to increase activity levels more compared with verbal advice alone
- Prescription should include exercises to improve aerobic fitness, strength, and mobility

Implement as Part of Clinical Practice

- Identify those who would benefit from exercise prescription
- Identify conditions amenable to exercise therapy
- Assess patient's activity level
- Educate patient about the benefits of exercise
- Assess patient interest, motivation, and goals
- Strive to find activities that are sustainable
- Monitor progress; assess barriers
- Encourage use of measurement tools such as pedometers, accelerometers, and smart phone applications

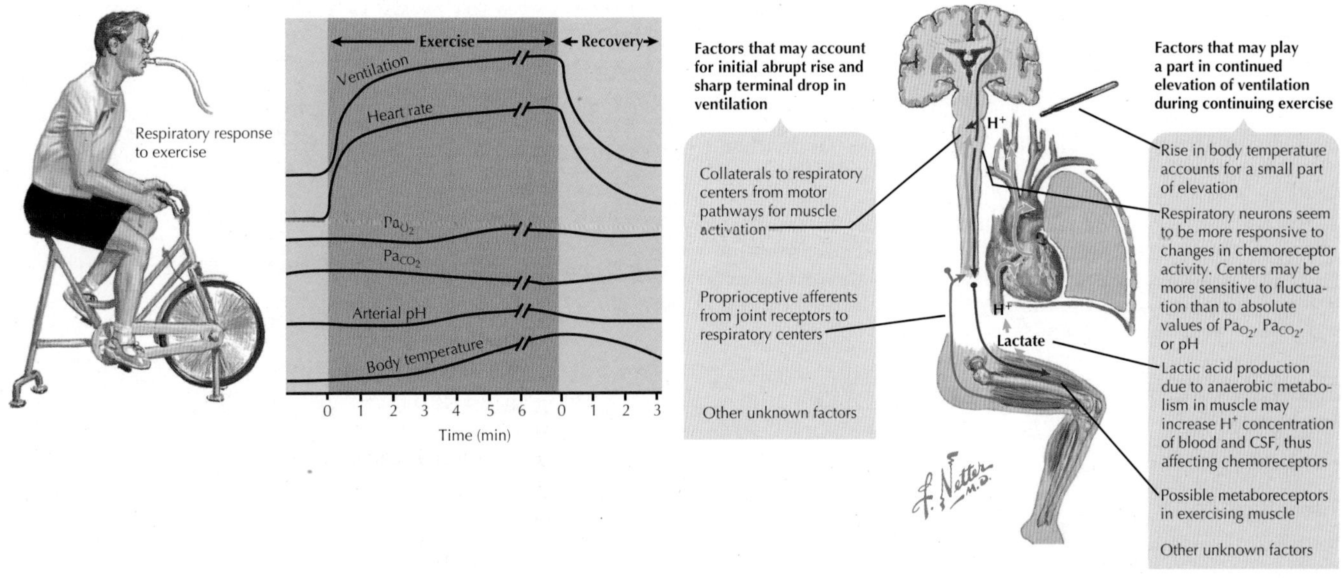
Respiratory response to exercise
Exercise
Recovery
Ventilation
Heart rate
PaO2
PaCO2
Arterial pH
Body temperature
0 1 2 3 4 5 6 0 1 2 3
Time (min)
Factors that may account for initial abrupt rise and sharp terminal drop in ventilation
Collaterals to respiratory centers from motor pathways for muscle activation
Proprioceptive afferents from joint receptors to respiratory centers
Other unknown factors
H+
Lactate
Factors that may play a part in continued elevation of ventilation during continuing exercise
Rise in body temperature accounts for a small part of elevation
Respiratory neurons seem to be more responsive to changes in chemoreceptor activity. Centers may be more sensitive to fluctuation than to absolute values of PaO2, PaCO2, or pH
Lactic acid production due to anaerobic metabolism in muscle may increase H+ concentration of blood and CSF, thus affecting chemoreceptors
Possible metaboreceptors in exercising muscle
Other unknown factors

Figure 17.3 Physiologic response to exercise and cool-down.

BOX 17.1 MAJOR CARDIAC RISK FACTORS (AMERICAN HEART ASSOCIATION)

Nonmodifiable Factors

- Male gender
- Increasing age
- Heredity

Modifiable Factors

- Smoking
- Hyperlipidemia
- Hypertension
- Diabetes mellitus
- Physical inactivity
- Obesity and overweight

Modified from American Heart Association. *Risk Factors and Coronary Heart Disease,* AHA Position Statement.

BOX 17.2 LINEAR 6–20 BORG SCALE OF PERCEIVED EXERTION OF PAIN

6
7 Very, very light
8
9 Very light
10
11 Fairly light
12
13 Somewhat hard
14
15 Hard
16
17 Very hard
18
19 Extremely hard
20

From Morrison C, Norenberg R. Using exercise test to create the exercise prescription. *Prim Care.* 2001;28(1):137–158.

Initiation of an Exercise Program

- Start slowly and allow fitness level to improve
- Goal is long-term lifestyle change
- Initially, prescribe shorter periods of light- to moderate-intensity exercise and build in duration, frequency, and intensity over time

Safety

- Data are reassuring
  - An overwhelming majority of medical-related problems are soft tissue and overuse injuries
  - Encourage appropriate warm-up and cool-down
  - Stretching should be done when muscles are warm
  - Scientific evidence to support that stretching prevents injuries is limited
- Sudden death during exercise is rare
  - A majority (approximately 80%) of instances are caused by coronary heart disease
  - The risk is greater in sedentary people who start vigorous activity
  - The relative risk of sudden death during vigorous activity is 2.1 times that of the risk during less strenuous activity
- Regular activity is protective
  - Exercise-associated cardiovascular (CV) risks lessen as individuals become more active/fit
  - Exercise-related CV events are uncommon and frequently preceded by warning signs and symptoms
  - Encourage slow start, consistency, and progress over time

Basic Principles of Exercise Prescription

- Tailor prescription to individuals based on goals, physical/financial/time considerations, medical conditions, and motivation
- Prescreen as indicated:
  - History and physical examination is the most important tool
  - Exertional chest pain, syncope, near-syncope, disproportionate dyspnea on exertion, and marked decrease in exercise capacity are red flags warranting further evaluation (Box 17.1)
- Conduct functional/orthopedic evaluations as needed.

Elements of Exercise Prescription (FITT-VP)

Frequency

- Ideally three or more times per week

Intensity

- Instruct on methods to assess exercise intensity:
  - Rating of perceived exertion
  - Borg scale (Box 17.2)
  - VO_2 max
- Maximum predicted heart rates can be calculated by subtracting age from 220
- "Talk test": ability to talk without significant breathlessness; rough marker of moderate- or low-intensity exercise
  - Moderate intensity: Can talk but not sing
  - Vigorous intensity: Difficulty talking

Time/Duration

- Current guidelines recommend 150 min/week of moderate-intensity activity or 75 min/week of vigorous activity. Patients will need to gradually work up to this goal.
- Regular walking is highly beneficial for most inactive, unfit subjects.
- Cycling, water aerobics, ballroom dancing, or gardening also provide excellent exercise.
- Strength training should be twice weekly, exercising all major muscle groups.

Type

- Evidence supports benefits of cross-training in terms of injury prevention, improved function, fitness level, and compliance.
- Dynamic flexibility exercises and disciplines (e.g., yoga or Pilates) may be useful in individuals who pursue activities that require excellent flexibility and in older individuals who tend to lose mobility around joints with aging (Fig. 17.4).

Volume

- Gradually increase volume of activity

Progression

- Progress from lighter levels of exertion to more vigorous and more complex exercise over time as patient improves fitness level, tolerance, and functional capacity
  - Initial stage: start at 40% of maximum heart rate (MHR) and progress to 70% of MHR over 4 weeks
  - Improvement stage: increase intensity to 60%–85% MHR and continue for 4–5 months
  - Maintenance stage: starts after 6 months of training with a target heart rate (HR) of 50%–85% MHR

Screening/Exercise Testing

- Current evidence-informed model for pre-exercise screening is based on three factors:
  1. Individual's current level of physical activity
  2. Presence of signs or symptoms and/or known CV, metabolic, or renal disease
  3. Desired exercise intensity

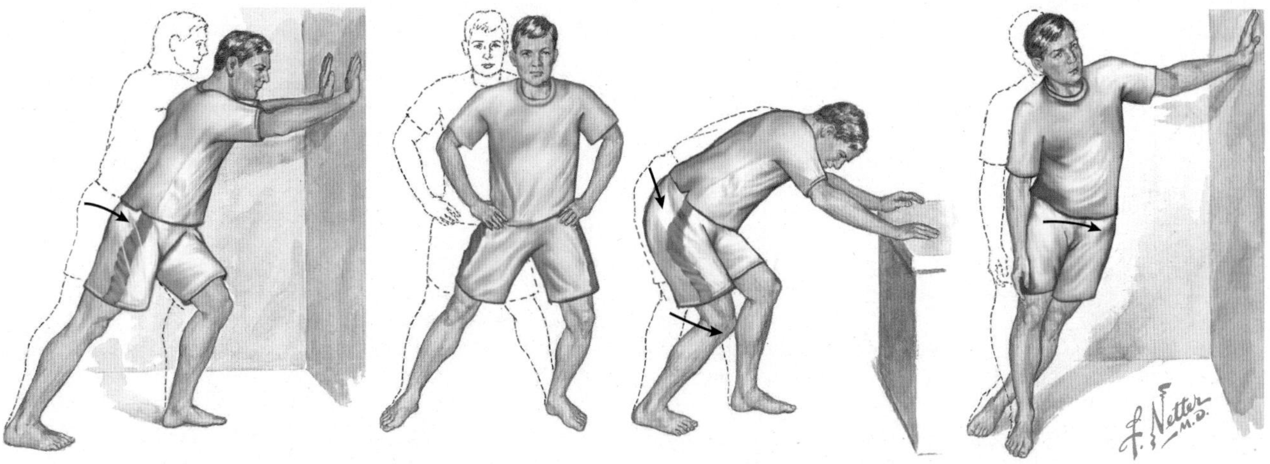
F. Netter M.D.

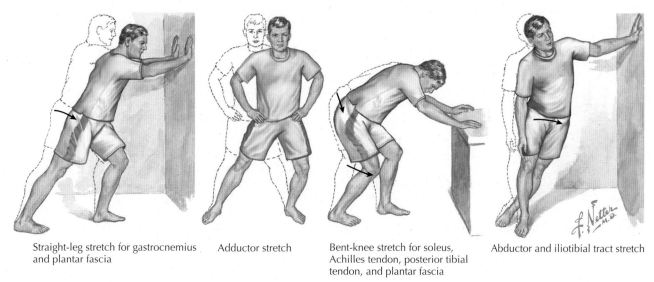

Straight-leg stretch for gastrocnemius and plantar fascia

Adductor stretch

Bent-knee stretch for soleus, Achilles tendon, posterior tibial tendon, and plantar fascia

Abductor and iliotibial tract stretch

Figure 17.4 Stretching exercises.

- Current recommendations no longer endorse *low-/moderate-/high*-risk classification or use of CVD risk profile as indication for referral to a medical care provider before initiating moderate- to vigorous-intensity exercise programs.
  - High prevalence of CVD risk factors in adults combined with rarity of exercise-related sudden cardiac death and acute myocardial infarction argues that ability to predict these rare events by assessing CVD risk factors is relatively poor.
- Current recommendations advocate *medical clearance* versus specific recommendations for *medical examinations* or *exercise stress tests (ESTs).*
  - Manner of clearance left to discretion of medical provider
  - Decisions about referral to a healthcare provider for *medical clearance* before initiation of an exercise program should be made on an individual basis based on clinical judgment
- *2015 ACSM algorithm: see "Recommended Readings"*

Mortality Data

- Sedentary behavior is strongly associated with increased all-cause mortality and with many chronic diseases.
- Sedentary behavior is increasing and is a worldwide issue, with one in four adults physically inactive.
- Exercise capacity (fitness level) is an independent powerful predictor of clinical outcomes.
- In healthy patients and those with known CVD, peak exercise capacity is a stronger predictor for all-cause mortality than hypertension, diabetes, smoking, obesity, or hypercholesterolemia. All-cause mortality in patients who achieve <5 METs is double the all-cause mortality in those who achieve >8 METs.
- There is an inverse relationship between fitness level and mortality (i.e., higher fitness level correlates with lower mortality).
- Those with low fitness levels have a fourfold increased relative risk (RR) of CV death and an eightfold increased RR of cancer death compared with peers with high fitness levels.
- Those who are unable to achieve 5–6 METs on EST are at increased risk of coronary events and all-cause mortality.
- Inability to achieve 6 METs on EST increases the risk of triple-vessel or left main coronary artery disease and at least quadruples the age-adjusted risk of a cardiac event.
- Poor fitness level is a modifiable risk factor.
- Every 1 MET increase in exercise capacity confers increased survival rates of 8%–18%.
- Performing any amount of exercise is better than being sedentary.
- Greatest improvements in survival rates are typically between the least and the next-to-least fit quintiles.

Special Populations

Diabetes Mellitus

EXERCISE PRECAUTIONS

- Individualized approach to CV screening before initiating exercise. No randomized, controlled trials support EST for asymptomatic individuals with diabetes mellitus (DM) before starting exercise program.
- Consider baseline EST if higher risk:
  - Known or suspected coronary artery disease (CAD), cerebrovascular disease, or peripheral artery disease
  - Additional CVD risk factors other than diabetes:
    - Type 1 or 2 diabetes >10 years
    - Hypertension
    - Cigarette smoking
    - Dyslipidemia
    - Proliferative or preproliferative retinopathy
    - Nephropathy, including microalbuminuria
    - Autonomic neuropathy
    - Advanced nephropathy with renal failure
- Retinopathy—avoid strenuous exercise and weight training (increased risk of vitreous hemorrhage and retinal detachment)
- Significant peripheral neuropathy—risk of ulcerations/skin breakdown and fracture
  - Appropriate socks/footwear important
- Caution during extremes of weather
- Adequate hydration before, during, and after exercise is core principle for all people with diabetes
- Skin issues and trauma around insulin pump site
- Caution regarding hypoglycemia and hyperglycemia
  - Type 2 diabetes not treated with insulin or insulin secretagogues confers low risk for exercise-induced hypoglycemia

- Type 1 diabetes confers higher risk for hypoglycemia with exercise; patients should monitor glucose regularly to understand their individual response to levels of exercise, as well as carbohydrate intake.
- Higher-intensity aerobic exercise increases the risk of hypoglycemia.
- Exercise induces a spike in endogenous insulin secretion; hence, individuals may develop hypoglycemia relatively early during exercise.
- Delay vigorous exercise if glucose is >250 mg/dL or ketosis. More modest hyperglycemia (<250) is NOT contraindication to exercise if the individual feels well and has no ketosis.
- Increased availability of continuous glucose monitoring tools enables real-time monitoring and allows for modification of exercise and hypoglycemic agents (including insulin).

EXERCISE IMPROVES INSULIN SENSITIVITY

- Improvements decline rapidly (typically ≤48 hours after exercise).
- Accordingly, patients with diabetes are recommended to exercise daily and not skip exercise for >1 day.

IMPROVES GLYCEMIC CONTROL

- Meta-analysis (of 14 studies, 12 aerobic exercise and 2 resistance exercise, at moderate intensity, performed only 2.5–3.4 times/week) shows a 0.66% drop in hemoglobin A1C (irrespective of weight or body mass index [BMI] change).

PREVENTS PROGRESSION

- Exercise prevents progression of glucose intolerance from "prediabetes" to diabetes.
  - Inverse relationship between level of physical activity and risk of type 2 diabetes.
  - Each 500 kcal expended in exercise per week is associated with a 6% decline in the risk of diabetes.
- Improved fitness level decreases mortality at each level of glycemic control.

GENERAL EXERCISE RECOMMENDATIONS

- Regular exercise is roughly comparable to taking one oral hypoglycemic medication.
- Encourage 150 minutes/week of moderate (brisk walking) to vigorous aerobic exercise (more if obese) spread across the week (at least 3 days).
- Similar benefits may be achieved with 75 minutes per week of more vigorous aerobic exercise (jogging 9.6 km/hour).
- In addition to aerobic activity, encourage moderate- to vigorous-resistance training at least 2–3 days/week.
- Milder exercise (e.g., yoga) has shown mixed results.
- Avoid exercise if blood glucose is >250 with ketosis or >300.

Hypertension (See Also Chapter 36: "The Hypertensive Athlete")

- Higher fitness level correlates with lower current and subsequent risk of hypertension independent of other risk factors.
- Studies have demonstrated exercise to be effective in lowering blood pressure (BP) independent of weight changes.
  - Meta-analysis of 127 randomized controlled trials (RCTs) irrespective of baseline showed systolic BP reductions of 3.4–4.7 and diastolic BP reductions of 2.4–3.1 mmHg.
  - Higher initial BPs confer larger reductions (average BP reduction in hypertensive patients is 7.4 mmHg in systolic BP and 5.8 mmHg in diastolic BP).
  - Meta-analysis of 54 RCTs conducted in hypertensive and normotensive patients revealed that all frequencies, intensities, and types of aerobic exercise lowered BP for everyone.
- Hypertensive physically fit men and women had a 60% lower mortality rate than physically unfit normotensive men and women.
- As little as 4 months of an exercise program positively affects left ventricular remodeling, along with other benefits, typically being achieved by 3 months.
- BP benefit is lost with cessation of exercise.
- Moderate-intensity exercise performed for >150 minutes per week showed the best results.
- Vigorous exercise for at least 75 minutes per week also shows substantial benefit.
- In sedentary adults, "lifestyle activity" was as effective as a structured exercise program for BP reduction.
- Consistent aerobic exercise:
  - Effective in lowering BP, resting and exercise HR, and myocardial oxygen demand
  - Increases vagal tone and decreases plasma norepinephrine
  - Decreases resting sympathetic tone
  - BP has been shown to be reduced for up to 22 hours after endurance exercise—this phenomenon is known as *postexercise hypotension* (PEH)
- Regular resistance training lowers BP by an average of up to 5 mmHg.
  - Circuit training at 30%–50% maximum HR, with 15–30 seconds of rest
  - Regular resistance training decreases BP and HR response to any given workload (may be cardioprotective).
- High-intensity lifting can considerably transiently increase BP (systolic BP >300 mmHg documented in power lifters).
  - Much milder increases in BP with less intensity
  - No documented clinical evidence of increased risk from BP increase during static exercise
- Consistently, circuit-type low- to moderate-resistance strength training appears most beneficial in hypertensive individuals.

PRECAUTIONS/RECOMMENDATIONS/MEDICATIONS

- Exercise testing is not indicated in most patients who start an exercise program. It should be considered in sedentary patients with suspected CVD and in those who are currently exercising but develop new signs or symptoms of CVD.
- Exercise programs are ideally tailored to the individual based on their baseline activity level, physical limitations, and interests. The goal is sustained implementation of regular exercise as part of their lifestyle.
- BP should be <180/105 before initiating an exercise program.
- Exercise is safe in patients with uncomplicated mild hypertension and who are not on any antihypertensive medications.
- Angiotensin-converting enzyme inhibitors (ACEIs) and angiotensin receptor blockers (ARBs) are the least likely to affect exercise tolerance.
- Beta-blockers will impede the heart rate response and can decrease exercise tolerance.
- Calcium channel blockers (CCBs) are generally well tolerated but can cause postexercise orthostasis (cool-down period helps). CCBs may be preferred in African-American patients.
- Exaggerated BP response to exercise occurs even in well-conditioned athletes; this may help identify athletes who are at a greater risk of developing CV complications in the future.
- Caution should be exercised with regard to heat and dehydration, particularly in patients who are on diuretics.

Osteoarthritis

- Aerobic exercise, resistance training, and physical therapy can reduce pain and disability in people with osteoarthritis (OA).
- Improvements observed in strength, symptoms, function, and balance.
- Benefits on pain, self-reported disability, walking speed, function, and overall patient global assessment.
  - Walking, biking, swimming, and low-weight/high-repetition resistance training have demonstrated beneficial effects.
  - Isometric exercises are particularly helpful in lower-extremity OA.

  - Range-of-motion exercises have not been shown to be beneficial.
- Moderate-intensity exercise is safe (including in the elderly).
- Increases in exercise intensity should be kept to a minimum during flare-ups of OA.
- High-intensity versus low-intensity exercise for hip or knee OA remains unclear.
- Exercise does *not* cause OA in previously normal joints.
  - Runners and walkers have a lower risk of developing hip OA and total hip replacement (THR), with lower BMI playing a role.
- Known benefits of exercise in OA include all of the following: decreased pain, increased strength, mobility and fitness, improved functional capacity, and reduced anxiety and depression.

Chronic Obstructive Pulmonary Disease

- Although exercise has not been shown to reverse physiologic changes of chronic obstructive pulmonary disease (COPD), studies have shown exercise improves dyspnea by reducing the rate of ventilation and improving exercise tolerance.
- Studies confirm that pulmonary rehabilitation improves symptoms, quality of life, pulmonary function, and healthcare utilization in patients with COPD. This likely occurs with consistent home-based exercise programs as well.
- Regular (daily) moderate-intensity exercise is most beneficial in improving functional capacity.
- Strong evidence demonstrates that in COPD patients, supervised physical exercise training improves exercise capacity when combined with aerobic and strength exercises, showing greater benefits than when either are performed alone.
- Quadriceps strength plays a key role in maintaining function for activities of daily living (ADLs) in patients with COPD.
- Athletes with COPD from sarcoidosis and cystic fibrosis have competed at elite international levels in basketball and other demanding sports, underscoring that mild to moderate pulmonary limitation rarely prevents participation.
  - Cardiopulmonary testing and periodic pulmonary function tests can be used to assess if athletes with alpha-1 antitrypsin deficiency, cystic fibrosis, or other chronic pulmonary diseases can achieve the MET level required for a particular sports activity without developing acidosis, hypoxia, or other complications that would limit participation.
  - Functional tests like the "get up and go," "6-minute walk," and "1-minute sit to stand test" correlate well with formal exercise testing of patients with COPD.

Obesity

- Exercise is key to the primary prevention of obesity, and continuing physical activity lessens the risk of weight gain.
- Negative caloric balance (less caloric intake than caloric expenditure) is required for weight loss. Increasing physical activity is crucial to establish this negative caloric balance.
- In obese patients, a diet is necessary for weight loss because physical activity without control of caloric intake will not control weight gain.
- Studies have demonstrated that physical activity is critical to maintaining weight loss.
- Regardless of weight loss, improvements in body composition (loss of body fat and increase of muscle mass) can be expected with increased physical activity.
- Increasing lean muscle mass will increase the basal metabolic rate, allowing increased baseline calorie utilization. Because resistance training has been demonstrated to substantially improve lean muscle mass, it should be considered as part of an exercise prescription for overweight and obese individuals.
- Obese but fit men have considerably lower all-cause mortality than unfit, normal-weight men.
- Longer duration of exercise (60–90 minutes/day) is necessary for sustainable weight loss.
- Increased lifestyle activity has been shown to be as efficacious as formal exercise for weight control.
- Meta-analysis shows that individuals with a genetic risk of obesity (*FTO* gene) can lessen this risk with physical activity.
- Specific weight-related considerations for overweight and obese patients:
  - Overweight and obesity are major risk factors for CAD. Accordingly, appropriate medical evaluation is warranted before initiating an exercise prescription.
  - Low-impact or non–weight-bearing exercises (e.g., swimming, water aerobics, biking, and circuit-type weight programs) should be considered for some overweight and obese individuals because of the increased risk and prevalence of orthopedic problems.
- Thermoregulation can be an issue.
  - Exercising during cooler periods of the day, wearing loose-fitting clothing, and ensuring adequate hydration may reduce the risk of heat-related problems.

KEY CONSIDERATIONS

- A basic understanding of exercise physiology guides the physician in preparing a safe exercise prescription.
- Written exercise prescriptions appear to improve compliance with exercise recommendations.
- An exercise prescription should incorporate frequency, intensity, time, type, volume, and progression (FITT-VP).
- Most patients even with chronic disease can begin an exercise program without an EST. Physicians should individually assess patients to decide who merits an EST before initiating an exercise program.
- Patients with chronic disease greatly benefit from exercise, but their exercise prescription and medications must be individualized to maximize their health outcomes.
- Specific benefits for exercise have been demonstrated for most chronic diseases.

RECOMMENDED READINGS

Available online.

18 AEROBIC TRAINING

John C. Hill • Inigo San-Millan

INTRODUCTION

- In the early days of sporting events, coaches and athletes learned through trial and error that they could not simultaneously develop maximal endurance and maximal power. They found that by first establishing an aerobic endurance base and later adding faster training, they could peak at appropriate times.
- It was not until the 1960s that the study of exercise as a science became widespread, and gradual changes in training methods occurred in the 1970s. By the 1980s, exercise science grew by quantum leaps, and the explosion in scientific information continued even during the 1990s. Now, we can use evidence gleaned from studies involving top cyclists, runners, swimmers, rowers, and triathletes to better understand which physiologic components can be pushed to allow performance at a higher and more economic aerobic potential than ever thought possible.
- Aerobic physical fitness is measured in two basic components: cardiorespiratory adaptations (central) and muscle metabolic adaptations (local).
- Elite endurance athletes have excellent values for these two physiologic traits; however, this is not true for recreational athletes. A very high measure of maximal cardiorespiratory capacity may be a genetic phenomenon that only few individuals possess, but muscle metabolic adaptations can be significantly improved with appropriate training techniques (Fig. 18.1; see also Fig. 18.3).

CENTRAL VS. LOCAL ADAPTATIONS TO EXERCISE

- Skeletal muscles possess a very high demand for oxygen during exercise.
- Both the cardiovascular and respiratory systems must work together to achieve the delivery of oxygen to muscles.
- This cardiorespiratory response to exercise reflects central adaptations to exercise. However, other elements in muscles are crucial for athletic performance.
- Once oxygen is delivered to muscles, it must be appropriately utilized.

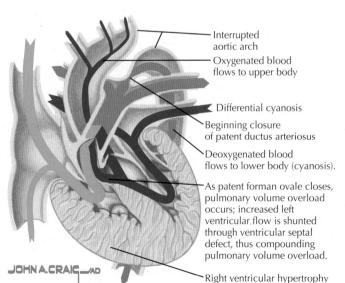

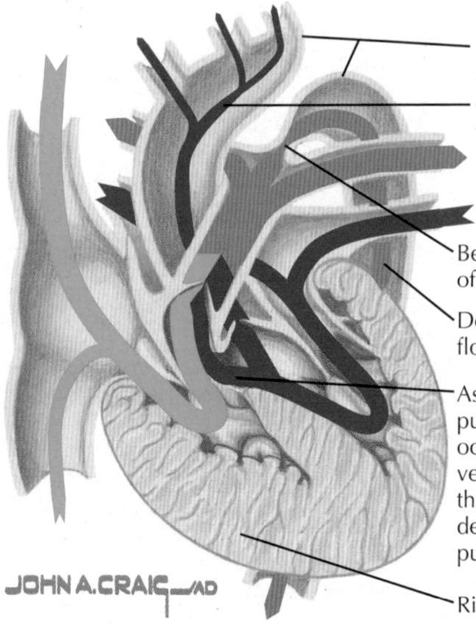
Interrupted aortic arch
Oxygenated blood flows to upper body
Differential cyanosis
Beginning closure of patent ductus arteriosus
Deoxygenated blood flows to lower body (cyanosis).
As patent forman ovale closes, pulmonary volume overload occurs; increased left ventricular flow is shunted through ventricular septal defect, thus compounding pulmonary volume overload.
Right ventricular hypertrophy
JOHN A.CRAIG_AD

Figure 18.1 Physiologic adaptation to exercise.

- Moreover, muscles must synthesize adenosine triphosphate (ATP) to produce muscle contraction and function. ATP is synthesized from carbohydrates (carbon–hydrogen–oxygen [CHO]), fats, and proteins in the mitochondria.
- Muscle metabolism during exercise elicits different byproducts, such as lactate, that need to be efficiently metabolized; these metabolic responses in skeletal muscles represent local adaptations to exercise.
- Over the past decade, there has been substantial research regarding and improvement in understanding muscle metabolism, and local adaptations during exercise may be most important when it comes to athletic performance.

Cardiorespiratory Adaptations—Central

- The cardiovascular system has central and peripheral components (Fig. 18.2):
  - **Central components** include heart rate (HR), stroke volume (SV), and cardiac output (CO = HR × SV).
  - **Peripheral components**
    - Arterial–mixed venous oxygen difference (a $-\dot{V}O_2$ difference).
    - Ability of tissues to extract and use oxygen for ATP resynthesis is another primary component of the cardiovascular system during physical activity.
- Maximal oxygen consumption ($\dot{V}O_2$ max)
  - $\dot{V}O_2$ max is the maximum capacity that the body has to transport and use oxygen during exercise, and it represents cardiorespiratory adaptations to exercise, as well as the **aerobic capacity** of an individual.
  - $\dot{V}O_2$ max measurement is considered the "gold standard" for aerobic capacity in athletes.
  - In general, it is expressed in milliliters of O_2 consumed per kilogram of body mass per minute (mL/kg/min) and may also be expressed in liters per minute (L/min).
- French chemist Antoine Lavoisier measured the first oxygen consumption in humans in 1873. Ever since then, $\dot{V}O_2$ max measurement has been of great interest by physiologists and considered the "gold standard" for aerobic capacity in athletes.
- Largely determined by genetics and is limited by certain structural components such as heart size, SV, and lung capacity.
- Because oxygen is used by mitochondria, a direct relationship exists between mitochondrial capacity and mitochondrial oxidative enzymes, which are part of local components of an athlete's physiology.
- Although considerable attention has been paid to $\dot{V}O_2$ max over the years, more recent knowledge and insights in muscle metabolism indicate that $\dot{V}O_2$ max is a poor indicator of performance, particularly in competitive athletes.
- In addition, it has been documented that numerous elite athletes greatly improve their performances throughout their careers without improving their $\dot{V}O_2$ max.
- It is well documented that local changes at the metabolic level in skeletal muscles are largely responsible and are crucial for improving athletic performance.

Muscle Metabolic Adaptations—Local Adaptations

- The ability of humans to exercise ultimately depends on the ability to transform chemical energy into mechanical energy, which ultimately takes place in the mitochondria of skeletal muscles. Thus, mitochondria (Fig. 18.3) are one of the most

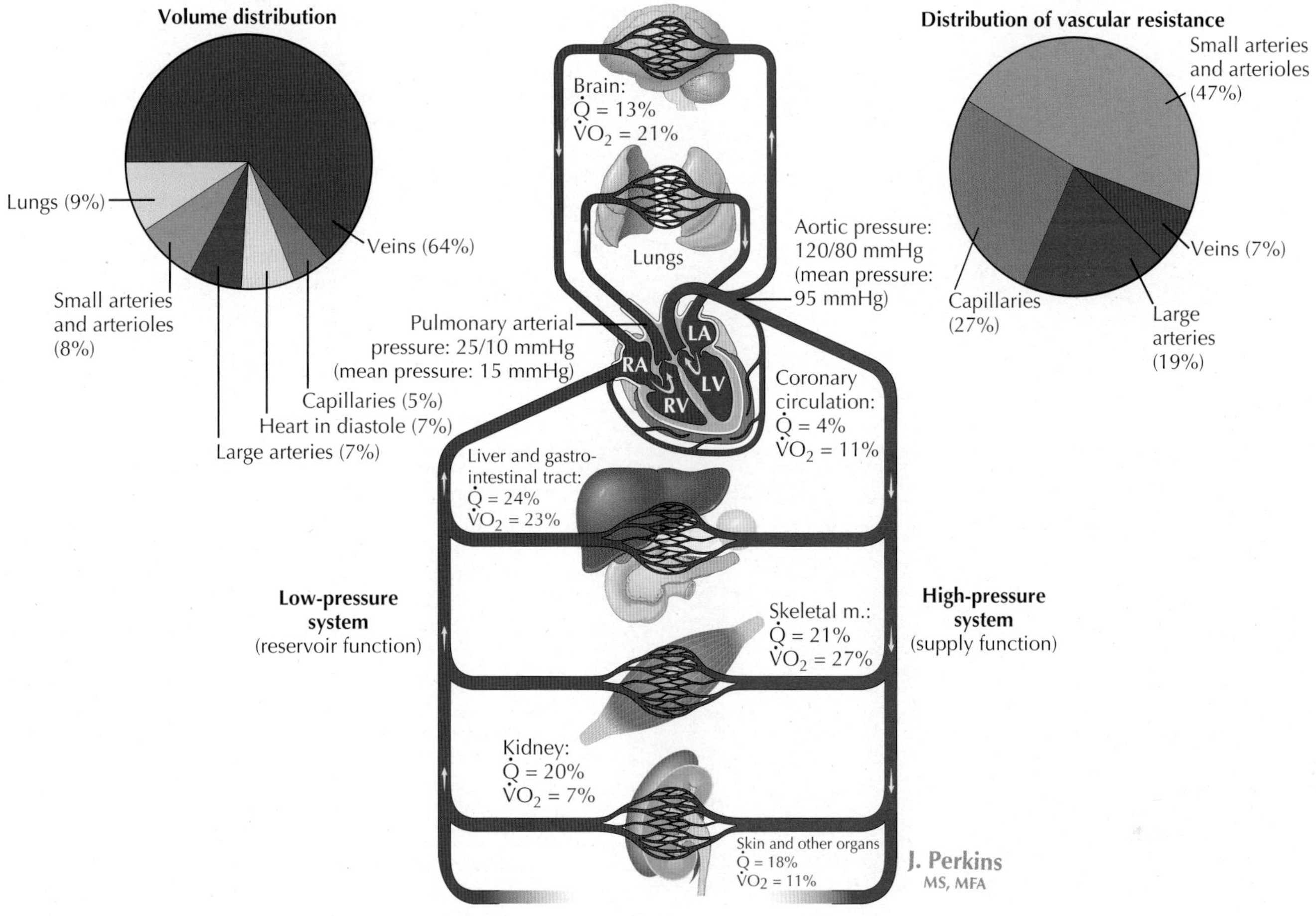
Volume distribution
Lungs (9%)
Veins (64%)
Small arteries and arterioles (8%)
Capillaries (5%)
Heart in diastole (7%)
Large arteries (7%)
Brain: Q̇ = 13% V̇O2 = 21%
Lungs
Pulmonary arterial pressure: 25/10 mmHg (mean pressure: 15 mmHg)
Aortic pressure: 120/80 mmHg (mean pressure: 95 mmHg)
RA
LA
RV
LV
Coronary circulation: Q̇ = 4% V̇O2 = 11%
Liver and gastro-intestinal tract: Q̇ = 24% V̇O2 = 23%
Low-pressure system (reservoir function)
High-pressure system (supply function)
Skeletal m.: Q̇ = 21% V̇O2 = 27%
Kidney: Q̇ = 20% V̇O2 = 7%
Skin and other organs Q̇ = 18% V̇O2 = 11%
Distribution of vascular resistance
Small arteries and arterioles (47%)
Veins (7%)
Capillaries (27%)
Large arteries (19%)
J. Perkins MS, MFA

Figure 18.2 Components of the cardiovascular system.

important players in skeletal muscle metabolism and athletic performance.

- Fats, CHOs, and proteins are oxidized in mitochondria for ATP synthesis. At very high rates of cellular glycolytic flux and under anaerobic conditions, glucose is oxidized into cytosol, synthesizing two ATPs and producing lactate.
- Moreover, characteristics of skeletal muscle fibers play a vital role in muscle metabolism, substrate utilization, and ATP synthesis.
- Skeletal muscle is composed of three kinds of muscle fibers:
  - Slow twitch/red/oxidative muscle fibers, also called *type I*
  - Fast twitch/white/glycolytic muscle fibers, also called *type II*, that are divided in two subgroups called *types IIa and IIb*
- Muscle fiber contraction obeys a sequential recruitment pattern related to exercise intensity, wherein type I muscle fibers are the first to be recruited at lower intensities.
- As exercise intensity increases, type IIa and finally type IIb fibers are recruited.
- Each muscle fiber has different biochemical properties and thus different metabolic behaviors during exercise (Fig. 18.4).

Type I Muscle Fibers

- Small motor neuron and fiber diameter, high mitochondrial and capillary density, and high content of myoglobin and oxidative enzymes.
- Possess a high capacity to oxidize free fatty tissue from subcutaneous adipose tissue and from intramuscular triglycerides.
- Although they have the slowest contraction time and force production of all fibers, they have the highest resistance to fatigue.
- Type I muscle fibers are mainly contracted during endurance events.

Type IIa Muscle Fibers

- Possess a larger motor neuron and fiber diameter, high glycolytic capacity, and a good or intermediate oxidative capacity, although not as much as type I muscle fibers do.
- Mitochondrial density and fat oxidation capacity are lower than that of type I muscle fibers.
- Have a higher content of glycogen and glycolytic enzymes; thus, glucose oxidation is higher.
- Contraction time is longer and resistance to fatigue is lower than that of type I muscle fibers.
- Because most competitions are performed at high intensities, in the glycolytic state, type IIa muscle fibers play an important role in most athletes, including endurance athletes.

Type IIb Muscle Fibers

- Also called fast glycolytic or fast white.
- Have the fastest contraction time and greatest force among all fibers.
- Mitochondrial density is very low, and most ATP synthesis in these fibers comes from anaerobic glycolysis and from stored ATP and phosphocreatine (PC), which binds to adenosine diphosphate (ADP) hydrolyzed from ATP to regenerate ATP.
- Type IIb muscle fibers are pure anaerobic fibers and are extremely crucial in athletic events of very short duration and high intensity, such as sprinting a 400-m race.

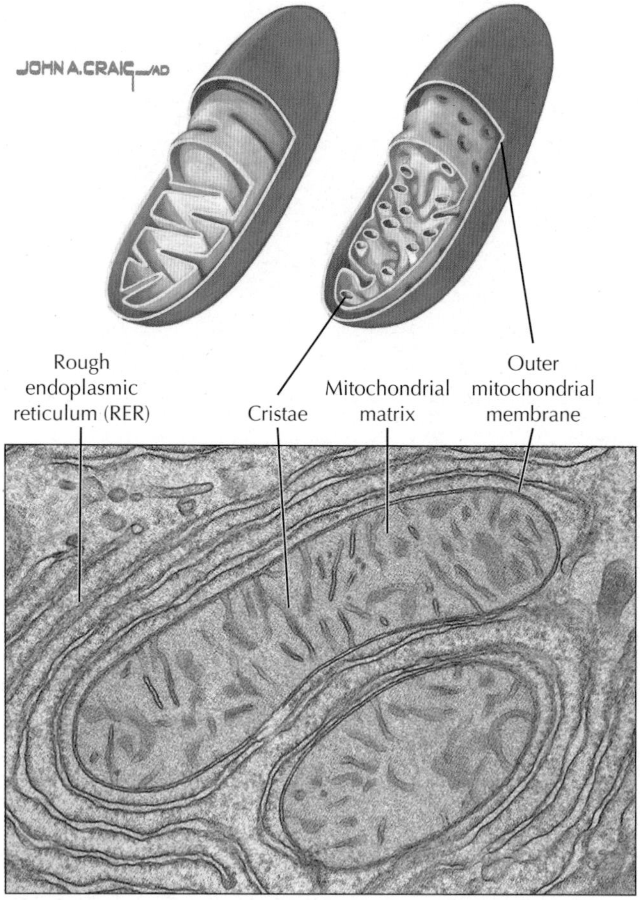
JOHN A.CRAIG—AD
Rough endoplasmic reticulum (RER)
Cristae
Mitochondrial matrix
Outer mitochondrial membrane

Reprinted with permission from Ovalle W, Nahirney P. *Netter's Essential Histology*. 2nd ed. 2013.

Figure 18.3 Schematic presentation of mitochondria and electron microscope image (EM) of mitochondria in a hepatocyte.

MUSCLE METABOLISM AND BIOENERGETICS

- ATP synthesis is generated by anaerobic and aerobic metabolism, primarily from fats and CHOs, with some contribution from amino acids derived from proteins.
- Fat is primarily stored in adipose tissue but is also stored in small amounts in skeletal muscles.
- CHOs are stored in the form of glycogen in skeletal muscles (approximately 80%) and in the liver (approximately 15%).
- Exercise intensity, physiologic stress, and muscle fiber recruitment patterns dictate the energy system and the substrates utilized.

THE ROLE OF MITOCHONDRIA IN EXERCISE METABOLISM

- Mitochondria (singular: mitochondrion) are the key cellular organelles necessary for exercise bioenergetics. Mitochondria are found in eukaryotic organisms and are the "powerhouses of cells" where CHOs, fat, and protein are oxidized for ATP generation. Skeletal muscle is one of the tissues in the body with the highest mitochondria due to the high metabolic activity of skeletal muscle. Mitochondrial function is key for metabolic health. People suffering from metabolic syndrome, as well as prediabetes and type 2 diabetes, are characterized by mitochondrial dysfunction, which is a key hallmark of the pathogenesis of these diseases. Furthermore, mitochondrial dysfunction has also been implicated in other diseases such as Alzheimer disease and cancer.
- The vast majority of CHOs (~80%) after a meal are oxidized in skeletal muscles, mainly in the mitochondria. Therefore, mitochondrial dysfunction will pose significant challenges to metabolizing CHOs and fats correctly, leading to a term called *metabolic inflexibility*. In the long term, the difficulty metabolizing CHOs and fats in skeletal muscle mitochondria during rest will lead to severe metabolic complications, giving rise to diseases like type 2 diabetes. Regular exercise is the only known mechanism to stimulate and maintain proper mitochondrial function.

FAT METABOLISM DURING EXERCISE

- Fats or lipids are the preferred energy source during endurance exercise.
- Most utilization occurs in type I muscle fibers.
- Highly orchestrated process, which starts with adipose tissue and ends with mitochondria in skeletal muscles.
- Fat stored in adipose tissue is broken down by lipolysis into free fatty acids (FFAs), which must subsequently travel through the blood to skeletal muscles.
- Once in the skeletal muscles, FFAs are attached to coenzyme A (CoA) to form fatty acyl-CoA, which is then transported across the outer mitochondrial membrane by carnitine–palmitoyl transferase I (CPT-I) and finally transported to the mitochondrial matrix by carnitine.
- Once inside the mitochondrial matrix, FFAs undergo β-oxidation where fatty acyl-CoA is degraded to acetyl-CoA, which can then enter the citric acid cycle for ATP synthesis.
- Moreover, skeletal muscle cytoplasm stores some fat called *intramuscular triglycerides* (IMTGs), which are stored close to the mitochondria and can contribute to energy generation. Based on the level of physical condition, IMTGs can contribute up to 15%–30% of all fat oxidation through exercise.
- The advantage of fat metabolism is that fat stores are unlimited, and even the leanest individual will never run out of fat stores.
- Therefore, fat is the preferred substrate for endurance activity during lower-intensity exercises.
- However, as exercise intensity increases, ATP must be synthesized faster, and fat cannot be oxidized fast enough to meet high ATP demands. At this point, the body starts utilizing a faster type of substrate: CHOs.

CARBOHYDRATE METABOLISM DURING EXERCISE

- As exercise intensity increases, CHOs are mobilized and eventually become the preferred source of fuel by skeletal muscle.
- CHOs are stored in skeletal muscles (~80%), liver (~15%), and in the form of glycogen (~5% in the form of glucose in the blood).
- Glycogen storage is limited (300–600 g) depending on the size and weight of an athlete.
- Glycogen cannot be directly utilized by skeletal muscles to obtain energy and needs to be broken down to glucose through a process called *glycogenolysis*.
- In muscles, glucose is oxidized to ATP through a multistep process called *glycolysis* that results in the formation of pyruvate, which is then further oxidized to acetyl-CoA for ATP synthesis through the citric cycle in mitochondria.
- At higher intensities, fat cannot synthesize ATP quickly enough, and all ATP synthesis is achieved through glycolysis.
- Considering the importance of CHOs for ATP synthesis during high-intensity exercise, appropriate glycogen stores are key for athletic performance.

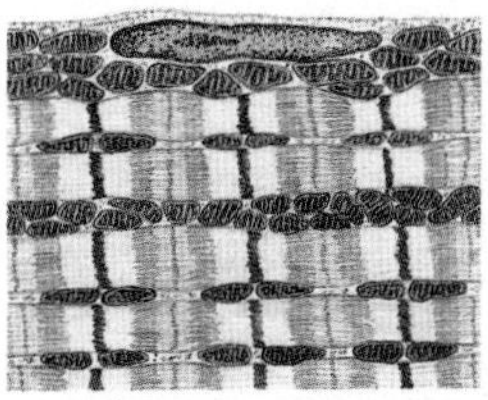

Type I: Dark or red fiber. Large profuse mitochondria beneath sarcolemma and in rows as well as paired in interfibrillar regions. Z lines wider than in type II.

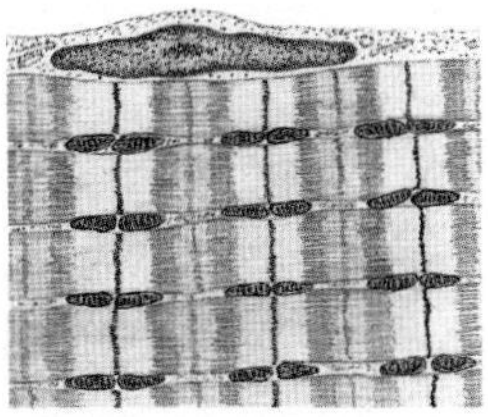

Type II: Light or white skeletal muscle fiber in longitudinal section on electron microscopy. Small, relatively sparse mitochondria, chiefly paired in interfibrillar spaces at Z lines.

Histochemical classification

Fiber type | **ATPase stain** | **SDH stain**

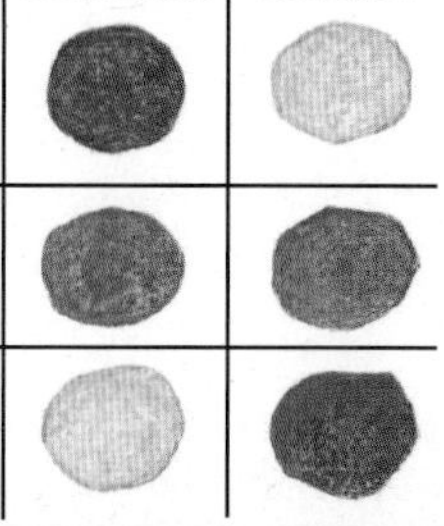

1. Fast-twitch, fatigable (IIb)
Stain deeply for ATPase, poorly for succinic acid dehydrogenase (SDH), a mitochondrial enzyme active in citric acid cycle. Therefore fibers rapidly release energy from ATP but poorly regenerate it, thus becoming fatigued.

2. Fast-twitch, fatigue-resistant (IIa)
Stain deeply for both ATPase and SDH. Therefore fibers rapidly release energy from ATP and also rapidly regenerate ATP in citric acid cycle, thus resisting fatigue.

3. Slow-twitch, fatigue-resistant (I)
Stain poorly for ATPase but deeply for SDH. Therefore fibers only slowly release energy from ATP but regenerate ATP rapidly, thus resisting fatigue.

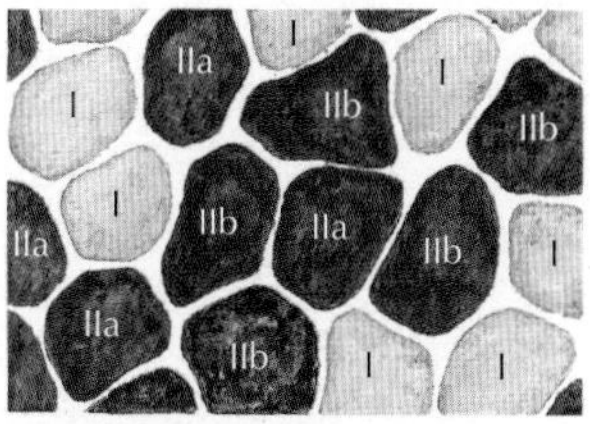

IIa
I
IIb

Cross section of skeletal muscle fibers stained for ATPase

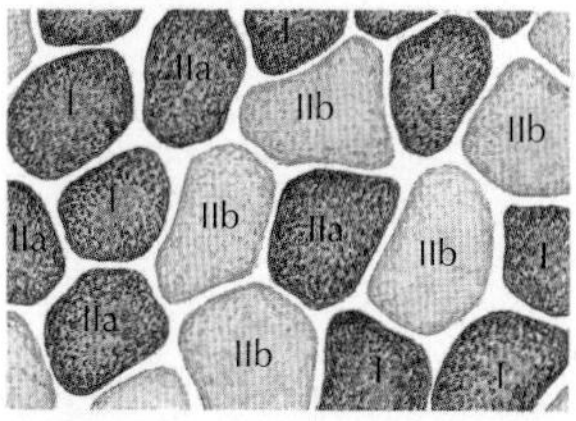

IIa
I
IIb

Identical section stained for SDH

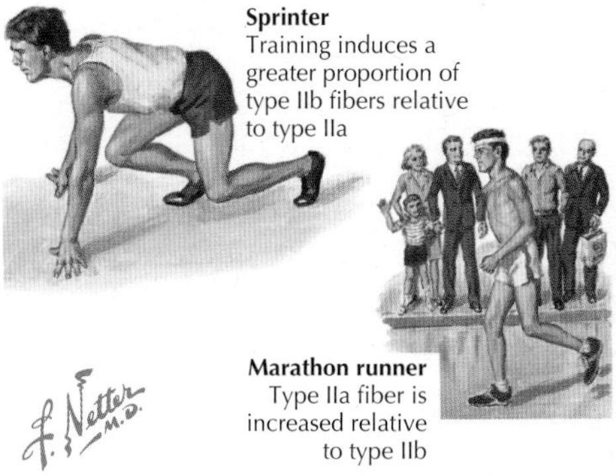

F. Netter M.D.

Sprinter
Training induces a greater proportion of type IIb fibers relative to type IIa

Marathon runner
Type IIa fiber is increased relative to type IIb

Characteristics of the Three Muscle Fiber Types

Fiber Type	Type I	Type IIa	Type IIb
	Slow Twitch (ST)	Fast Twitch (FTIIa)	Fast Twitch (FTIIb)
Contraction time	Slow	Fast	Very fast
Resistance to fatigue	High	Intermediate	Low
Metabolism	Oxidative Aerobic	Oxidative Aerobic	Anaerobic
Force production	Low	High	Very high
Mitochondrial density	High	High	Low
Capillary density	High	Intermediate	Low
Oxidative capacity	High	High	Low
Glycolytic capacity	Low	High	High
Major fuel used	FAT	CHO	CHO+ATP+CP

Figure 18.4 Muscle fiber types.

- Fat is the preferred fuel up until exercise intensities of approximately 55%–75% of $\dot{V}O_2$ max, although CHO is also used at a low rate.
- At higher-intensity exercise beyond 75% of $\dot{V}O_2$ max, ATP must be synthesized at a faster rate to meet muscle contractile demands.
- Fat cannot synthesize ATP quickly enough, and thus, CHO becomes the major energy source used by skeletal muscles up to 100% of $\dot{V}O_2$ max.
- When exercise intensities are close to maximal, ATP cannot be generated by either fat or CHO, and anaerobic metabolism takes over through the PC system, mobilizing ATP stored in skeletal muscles (Fig. 18.5).

PROTEIN METABOLISM

- Protein contributes minimally to energy generation during exercise.
- Total energy produced could range from 3% to 10% depending on exercise intensity and duration.
- Protein (mainly skeletal muscle protein) is degraded to amino acids for oxidation.
  - Branched-chain amino acids (BCAAs) play an important role during exercise.
  - Leucine, isoleucine, and valine make up BCAAs and can play vital roles during exercise, particularly under low glycogen stores, where BCAA utilization for ATP synthesis increases.
  - Another important amino acid is alanine, which is synthesized in skeletal muscles and then exported to the liver to be converted to glucose through the glucose–alanine cycle in a process called *gluconeogenesis*.

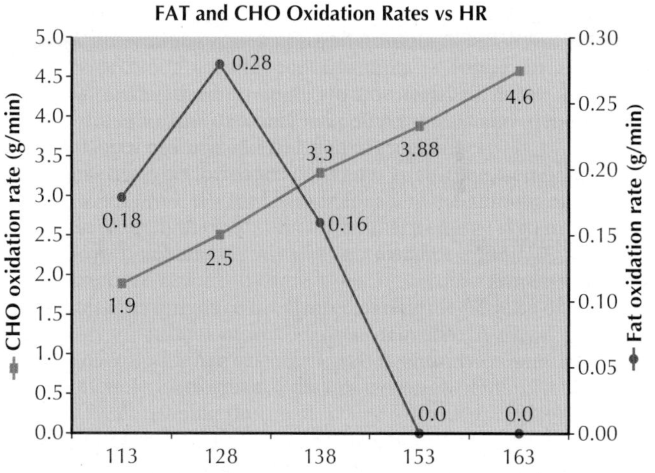

FAT and CHO Oxidation Rates vs HR
CHO oxidation rate (g/min)
Fat oxidation rate (g/min)
5.0
4.5
4.0
3.5
3.0
2.5
2.0
1.5
1.0
0.5
0.0
0.30
0.25
0.20
0.15
0.10
0.05
0.00
0.28
0.18
0.16
0.0
0.0
1.9
2.5
3.3
3.88
4.6
113
128
138
153
163

Figure 18.5 Fat and carbohydrate utilization during exercise. As exercise intensity increases, fat utilization decreases and eventually disappears, and carbohydrate utilization increases.

LACTATE METABOLISM

- Lactate is the byproduct of glucose utilization by muscle cells.
- The higher the glucose flux into the cell, the higher the lactate production, independent of oxygen availability.
- Historically, lactate was simply understood to be a waste product of anaerobic exercise, a waste product that may even crystallize and cause muscle soreness.

Table 18.1 DIFFERENCES IN BLOOD LACTATE BETWEEN COMPETITIVE CYCLISTS OF DIFFERENT LEVELS[a]

Workload	*Junior Cyclist*	*Top Amateurs*	*Avg. Pro-Tour*	*World Class*
w/kg	**Blood La (mmol/L)**	**Blood La (mmol/L)**	**Blood La (mmol/L)**	**Blood La (mmol/L)**
3	1.3	1.1	1.1	0.8
3.5	1.8	1.3	1.2	0.8
4	3	2.3	2	0.96
4.5	6.6	3.5	3.2	1.8
5	10	7.6	5.8	3.1
5.5		9.2	8.2	5.2
6				8.9

[a]As observed, the lactate clearance capacity in world-class athletes is remarkable compared with even their professional peers.
Modified from San Millán I, González-Haro C, Sagasti M. Physiological differences between road cyclists of different categories. A new approach. *Med Sci Sports Exerc.* 2009;41(5):64–65.

- Lactate studies date back from the 19th century when in 1863, a Nobel Laureate, Louis Pasteur, proposed that lactate was produced by lack of oxygen during muscle contraction.
- It was not until late in the 20th century when the importance of lactate and its key role in exercise and metabolism became clear, largely because of Dr. George Brooks, from the University of California at Berkeley, who extensively studied lactate for over 40 years. His work illustrates that lactate formation occurs under aerobic conditions, that lactate is not a waste product, and that lactate is the most crucial gluconeogenic precursor (new glucose generator) in the body. Approximately 30% of all the glucose used during exercise is derived from lactate "recycling" to glucose.
- High-intensity exercise is associated with high glycolytic activity in type II muscle fibers, which results in the production of large amounts of lactate, even under aerobic conditions.
- During intense exercise, lactate production is manifold higher than resting levels, buildup exceeds clearance, and the release of hydrogen ions (H^+) associated with lactate can cause an important reduction of contractile muscle pH, resulting in acidosis.
- This excessive accumulation of H^+, not only from lactate but also from ATP breakdown for muscle contraction (ATP hydrolysis), may interfere with muscle contraction at different sites competing with calcium (Ca^{++}) for troponin C binding site (a protein involved in muscle contraction regulation).
- In addition, H^+ may inhibit Ca^{++} release and reuptake from the sarcoplasmic reticulum, which is involved in muscle contraction.
- These effects can result in decreased muscle contraction capacity, which can cause a considerable decrease in peak twitch force, as well as maximum muscle shortening velocity and performance.
- Lactate is oxidized through a highly developed complex called the *mitochondrial lactate oxidation complex (mLOC)* that comprises monocarboxylate transporter-1 (MCT1), its chaperone (CD147), a mitochondrial lactate dehydrogenase (mLDH), and cytochrome oxidase (Cox).
- The ability to clear lactate is probably the most important capacity in endurance athletes and the physiologic parameter that discriminates most athletes (Table 18.1).

LACTATE THRESHOLD

- **Lactate threshold (LT)** is probably the most used training term by coaches and athletes worldwide.
- Commonly known as the *exercise intensity* or *blood lactate concentration* an athlete can sustain during a high-intensity effort for a specific period.
- **Is sometimes referred to as *aerobic threshold*, which is inaccurate because lactate is constantly produced under aerobic conditions.**

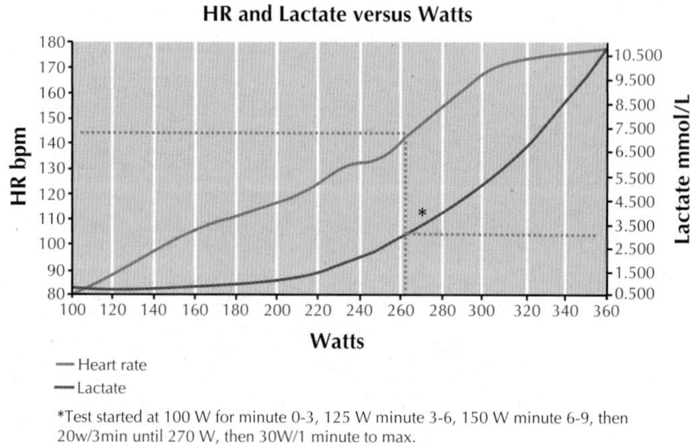
HR and Lactate versus Watts
HR bpm
180
170
160
150
140
130
120
110
100
90
80
100 120 140 160 180 200 220 240 260 280 300 320 340 360
Watts
10.500
9.500
8.500
7.500
6.500
5.500
4.500
3.500
2.500
1.500
0.500
Lactate mmol/L
*
— Heart rate
— Lactate
*Test started at 100 W for minute 0-3, 125 W minute 3-6, 150 W minute 6-9, then 20w/3min until 270 W, then 30W/1 minute to max.

Figure 18.6 Physiologic characteristics and lactate threshold of a road cyclist. As the effort increases, the heart rate increases, but serum lactate levels remain stable until at an effort of 264 watts and a heart rate of 145, when lactic acid levels begin to exponentially rise. This indicates the lactate threshold.

- LT is the point at which the rate of lactate production exceeds clearance and begins to accumulate in skeletal muscle, resulting in exportation to the circulatory system. At this point, energy production is dependent on glucose and glycogen.
- Higher LT as a percentage of $\dot{V}O_2$ max allows athletes to generate more power and sustain longer efforts.
- LT may be as low as 40%–50% $\dot{V}O_2$ max in sedentary individuals and may be 80%–90% $\dot{V}O_2$ max in highly trained aerobic athletes, who also achieve higher $\dot{V}O_2$ max.
- If two cyclists have identical maximal aerobic capacity, but one has LT at 70% $\dot{V}O_2$ max and the other has LT at 90% $\dot{V}O_2$ max, the latter has a significant physiologic advantage in a head-to-head endurance test.
- Compared with aerobic capacity, which is relatively fixed and related to genetic capabilities, LT is highly trainable. **Exercise physiologists have proven in multiple studies and in highly trained athletes that programs based on improving lactate thresholds are highly effective.**

Determining the Lactate Threshold

- An exercise test can determine an athlete's LT.
- Lactate accumulates in the blood when the requirements of energy production are so high that the body can no longer effectively clear the lactate from skeletal muscles.
- When LT is crossed, lactic acid builds in muscles and fatigue ensues. **The level of exercise intensity at which contractile forces in muscle begin to shut down is LT** (Fig. 18.6).

- The best way to determine LT for a cyclist is to ride a stationary bike at a given intensity for 45 minutes in the laboratory. The same type of test can be conducted for a runner using a treadmill. A small sample of blood is collected from the finger or earlobe and analyzed for lactic acid. The workload is then slightly increased. The sampling process is repeated every few minutes after the workload is increased (Fig. 18.7). Lactic acid concentration values are plotted against oxygen consumption and HR. When lactic acid levels precipitously rise, it is noted as the lactate threshold. Rise in respiratory rate corresponds to increasing lactate levels. Exercise is continued to a point of absolute exhaustion, which indicates $\dot{V}O_2$ max. Subsequently, a range of HRs or power outputs is calculated to guide the cyclist in their training intensity (Table 18.2).

Training Lactate Clearance Capacity and Lactate Threshold

- Lactate primarily produced in fast twitch muscle fibers as the byproduct of excessive glucose utilization is preferably cleared by mitochondria of slow twitch muscle fibers in the mLOC.
- Robust mitochondrial capacity in type I muscle fibers is critical for optimal performance.

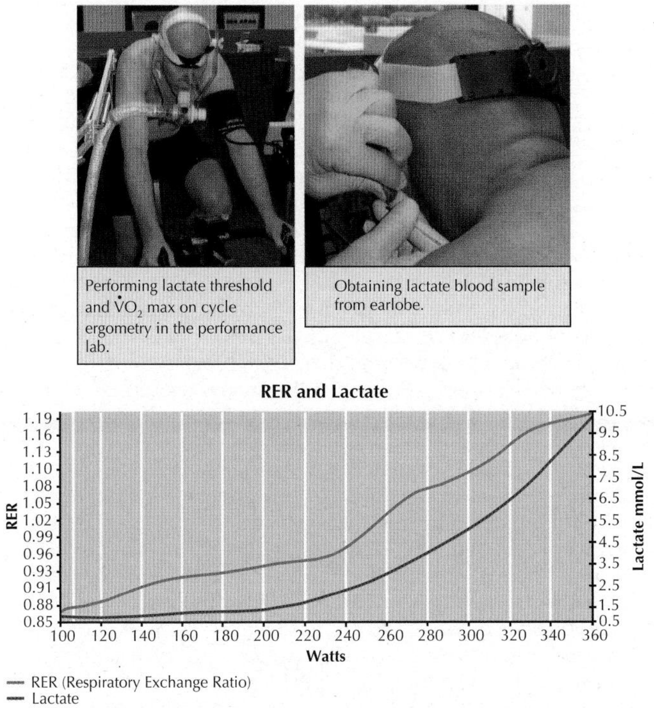
Performing lactate threshold and $\dot{V}O_2$ max on cycle ergometry in the performance lab.
Obtaining lactate blood sample from earlobe.
RER and Lactate
RER
1.19
1.16
1.13
1.10
1.08
1.05
1.02
0.99
0.96
0.93
0.91
0.88
0.85
Lactate mmol/L
10.5
9.5
8.5
7.5
6.5
5.5
4.5
3.5
2.5
1.5
0.5
100 120 140 160 180 200 220 240 260 280 300 320 340 360
Watts
RER (Respiratory Exchange Ratio)
Lactate

Rise in respiratory rate corresponds to a rise in lactate. As lactic acid builds in bloodstream, you must increase breath more rapidly to neutralize its effects.

Figure 18.7 Determining lactate threshold for a cyclist.

- Typical training mistake involves training at the LT to improve lactate clearance capacity. This is not quite accurate because mitochondria in slow twitch muscle fibers clear lactate through mLOC. Accordingly, it is important to train slow twitch muscle fibers to increase mLOC.
- Endurance training, in particular Z2 (see Table 18.2), is essential to improve type I muscle fiber function, mitochondrial capacity, and mLOC.
- Training at LT is essential to improve glycolytic fibers (type IIa) and their machinery ("turbo"). LT training should be a key part of any comprehensive and competitive training program.

Field Estimate of Lactate Threshold Heart Rate

- To determine the lactate threshold heart rate (LTHR) for either cycling or running, complete a 30-minute time trial as follows. Find a course that is relatively flat. Warm up as you would before a short race and then begin the time trial. Start the HR monitor immediately, preferably a monitor with an average HR mode. The effort of this time trial should be racelike—maximum intensity. Ten minutes into the time trial (20 minutes to go), press the "lap" button on the HR monitor so you have the average HR for the last 20 minutes when finished. This value is an approximation of LTHR.
- Pay attention to the HR whenever a burning sensation is experience in the legs with onset of heavy breathing. LTHR refinement will occur with test repetitions, particularly by observing HR relative to breathing during workouts.

ECONOMY

- Compared with recreational runners and cyclists, elite runners and cyclists use less oxygen to hold a steady submaximal pace.
- World-class runners appear to move effortlessly, and elite athletes use less energy to produce the same power output as nonelite athletes.
- Economy refers to lower oxygen and caloric use to perform the same amount of work.
- Becomes more significant in long endurance events and racing (Fig. 18.8).
- **Fatigue can also negatively affect economy.** The longer the race, the more critical economy becomes in determining the eventual winner.
- **Just as with LT, economy is highly trainable.** Economy will increase with all aspects of endurance training, but sport-specific activity is critical: the only way to train swimming economy is by swimming, and the only way to train cycling economy is by riding a bicycle; cycling economy cannot be improved by rollerblading.

Perspective

A word of caution relative to the aforementioned discussion: it implies that fitness and race results can be easily quantified and

Table 18.2 EXAMPLES OF HEART RATE AND POWER TRAINING ZONES

RPE	Zone	Zone Description	HR	Power	% of LTHR
<10	1	Active recovery	<102	<150	65%–81%
10–12	2	Endurance	103–125	151–200	82%–88%
13–14	3	Tempo	126–141	201–245	89%–93%
15–16	4	Lactate threshold	142–159	246–286	94%–100%
17–18	5	$\dot{V}O_2$ max	160–165	286–350	101%–105%
19–20	6	Anaerobic capacity	165+	350+	106%+

Heart rate and power meter zones as percentage of lactate threshold for an athlete (see Fig. 18.7) whose lactate threshold occurred at HR of 145 and power of 264 watts.
RPE, Borg Relative Perceived Exertion.

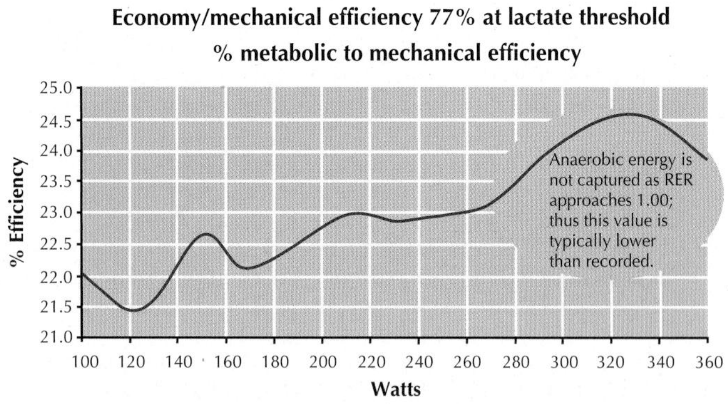
Economy/mechanical efficiency 77% at lactate threshold
% metabolic to mechanical efficiency
% Efficiency
Watts
Anaerobic energy is not captured as RER approaches 1.00; thus this value is typically lower than recorded.
25.0
24.5
24.0
23.5
23.0
22.5
22.0
21.5
21.0
100 120 140 160 180 200 220 240 260 280 300 320 340 360

Figure 18.8 Mechanical efficiency. Mechanical efficiency reached a steady state of 23% before the lactate threshold. This indicates that overall economy is 77%.

predicted. You might think that scientists can take a group of athletes, predict who has elite potential, train them in a state-of-the-art facility, prod, probe, and analyze their performance. At the end of the day, they should be able to predict outcomes of all major sporting events. This could not be further from the truth. Although information about LT training is effective, it does not represent the "real world" of racing. Several variables are beyond scientific explanation. The incredible drive of certain athletes allows them to perform far beyond their abilities, whereas other genetically gifted individuals never seem to win any races.

TRAINING GUIDELINES AND STRESS

- The *American College of Sports Medicine's Guidelines for Exercise Testing and Prescription* takes abstract concepts of aerobic training and puts them into practical guidelines that can be easily followed.
- **All successful training programs require a balance in frequency, duration, and intensity, also described as *volume* or *workload*.**
- Improvement of fitness never occurs in an unbroken continuum, and fatigue is the principal reason why. We will define each of these terms and discuss the interaction each has with the other.

Frequency

- Refers to how often training sessions are conducted. Studies have revealed that training three to five times per week provides the greatest aerobic gains for time invested, but as your overall fitness improves, so must your training frequency. When training begins, three to five workouts per week will produce rapid improvements in fitness. Aerobic conditioning frequently improves by 10%–20% within a few weeks. If the same novice athlete were to train more frequently, instead of more rapid improvements, his or her fitness would decrease due to overtraining. Elite athletes training for a spot on the Olympic team may need to schedule 12–15 workouts each week and may only improve their fitness by 1% because they are so close to achieving their full potential.
- The ideal frequency of workouts is dependent on current adaptations of the body. For example, an experienced cyclist who has not trained for 3 weeks should restart his or her training regimen at a lower frequency than where he or she left off 3 weeks back to avoid the risk of overtraining.

Duration

- Individual training sessions may vary considerably in length. Some may last several hours with a goal of improving aerobic fitness, whereas others are short in length and will promote either speed or recovery. As with frequency, the duration of a training session is dependent on an athlete's conditioning. As fitness improves, the athlete's body will be able to tolerate longer training sessions.
- The appropriate length of a workout is directed by the length of a race. If a runner never competes in a race longer than 5000 m, there is no real benefit of 4-hour runs. However, if the runner competes in ultra-marathons, which last 12–30 hours, he or she may train less frequently but will need to train for a much longer duration.

Intensity

- Frequency and duration are much easier to quantify than intensity. Intensity is often referred to as *volume* or *workload* or simply, "*hardness*" of a workout. **Poor understanding of intensity is the primary reason that training programs are ineffective.** If you are performing your workouts with precise frequency and duration, but you allow them to become too hard, your aerobic fitness will suffer due to overtraining. If the training sessions are too easy, again your aerobic fitness will suffer due to inadequate stress.
- Athletes often describe their training in terms of volume. For example, if they rode 5 days last week for 1 hour each day, then they would relate that they trained for 5 hours. This actually describes the volume of training (frequency × duration) but does not quantify intensity. **A better summary of your training is workload, defined as a combination of volume and intensity.** Understanding how much effort or power went into each workout gives you a better understanding of training stress. Table 18.2 presents three individual ways to assess intensity. For example, if your goal is to ride at a tempo pace (zone 3), at 90% of your LT for 30 minutes, then you could quantify this by using an HR monitor, a power meter, or the Borg Relative Perceived Exertion scale. Planning your workload around one of these scales is critical.
- Athletes need to determine their systematic training objectives to be able to appropriately plan for intensity training. Optimal endurance adaptations take place with long workouts at lower intensities. Numerous seasoned athletes use an easy "over-distance" pace ("Active Recovery" in Table 18.2) for endurance training, whereas a majority of less intense athletes train at a slightly higher intensity ("Endurance" in Table 18.2), which can preclude optimal adaptations that occur at the slightly lower level. At least half, and usually more, of most training regimens should be spent at these lower intensities for most of the training cycle. A smaller proportion of training occurs at higher intensity levels, and the amount of time spent training at these higher levels increases as the training cycle moves toward peaking for competition. Tempo pace, hill workouts, and intervals are examples of higher-intensity workouts. Race pace and racing occur at and above LT; hence, very little time is spent here until nearing peak performance, where 5%–15% of training may be performed at this level, with adequate recovery.
- Training intensity is the stressor that most athletes get wrong. Many athletes overtrain or train without appropriately varying intensity levels. If you exercise too intensively when you should be taking it easy, you will be tired on days when you should perform high-intensity training. All training days begin to look alike and shift toward mediocrity as easy runs become too hard and hard runs become too easy.

Fatigue

- Fatigue is the reason we are all not world champions. When and to what extent we experience weariness is an optimal predictor of our fitness level. **Delaying the onset of fatigue is the**

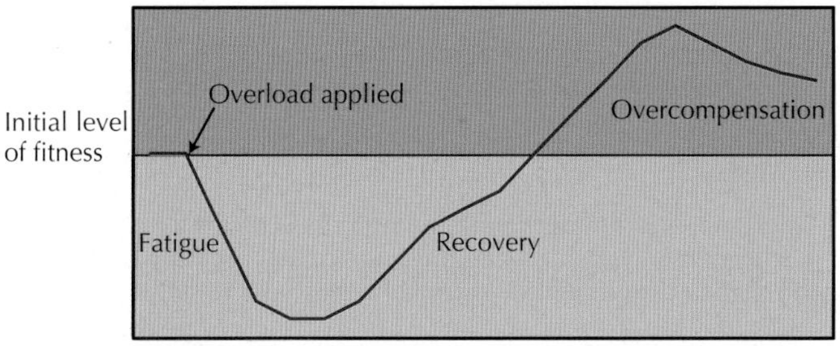
Initial level of fitness
Overload applied
Overcompensation
Fatigue
Recovery

Figure 18.9 Overcompensation and improved fitness resulting from training workload.

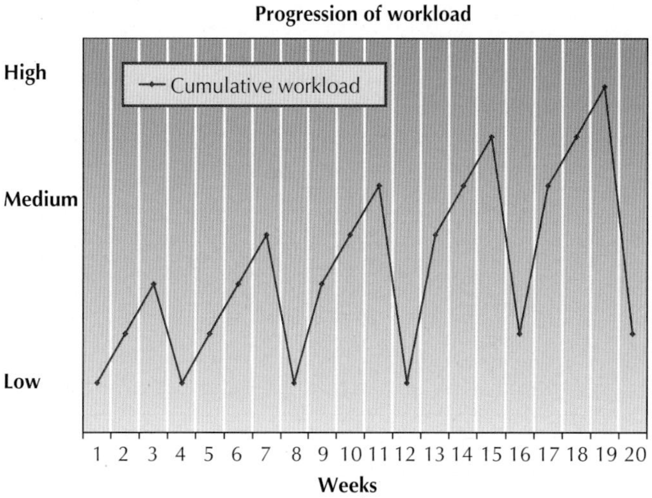
Progression of workload
High
Medium
Low
Cumulative workload
1 2 3 4 5 6 7 8 9 10 11 12 13 14 15 16 17 18 19 20
Weeks

Figure 18.10 Example of weekly cumulative workload progression.

primary reason for training. The fittest athletes are those who can best resist the crippling effects of fatigue. As previously discussed, the causes of fatigue are lactate accumulation, glycogen depletion, and muscle failure; each of these causes of fatigue can be addressed by understanding the principles of LT training.

TRAINING PRINCIPLES

Overload

- Overload is to impose work stresses that are greater than those normally encountered. The purpose of training is to cause your body to positively change to better manage physiologic stresses of competition. **To stress your body, you must present a load that challenges its current level of fitness.** This load will initially cause fatigue, followed by recovery, and eventually an increased level of fitness or overcompensation. If workouts are of the right magnitude (i.e., slightly more than the body can handle), adaptation occurs and fitness steadily progresses (Fig. 18.9).
- **It is important to remember that overload occurs during workouts, but adaptation and overcompensation occur at rest. In other words, the potential for fitness is produced during training sessions, but the realization of fitness occurs during rest.** If you repeatedly deprive your body of rest, you will not continually improve, and you will also lose fitness—this is called *overtraining*. The biggest mistake most athletes make is disregarding their need to rest or reduce the intensity of training. Smart athletes will know when to back off in training or rest. However, when the load of training is reduced for prolonged periods, your body will adapt to this as well; this is called "being out of shape."

Progression

- Progression involves a gradual and systematic increase in training intensity or volume as improvement occurs. If you have ever performed a workout or a race so intense that for days afterward you were too sore to even walk, much less run, then you have slowed your training progression. Such workouts violate the progression principle. Your body does not get stronger; rather, you lose fitness and waste time and energy.
- You must gradually increase workloads with intermittent periods of rest and recovery. The stresses must be greater than your body is accustomed to handling. As the intensity of the workload is increased by small increments, usually 5%–15% every week to week and a half, you can avoid overtraining and injury and provide enough stress for adaptation to occur. The cumulative training volume should not exceed 5%–15% per year, and athletes training over 600 hours/year should probably not increase the volume by more than 10% per year. Workload increases are primarily based on individual needs, particularly in terms of intensity (Fig. 18.10).

Periodization

- **Periodization** is the structuring of training hours for a given cycle to produce a progressive increase of training stress and performance. Several athletes use training cycles, frequently dividing the competition year into 4-week cycles (meso- or microcycles), although experienced athletes may individualize the lengths. Each cycle is planned to stimulate the appropriate training response for that part of the year relative to peak performance and competition. Many athletes will increase intensity in a stepwise manner over the first 3 weeks of a microcycle, then scale back hours and intensity during the final week of the cycle. Alternatively, experienced athletes individualize this pattern. On the other hand, a training year may be divided into different stages or cycles (macrocycles) such as base, building or intensity, and peak and/or race (Fig. 18.11). Periodization takes place from cycle to cycle (micro and macro).
- The basic premise of all periodization programs is that training should progress from general to specific. Early in the season, training is focused on maintaining weight, strength training, and general aerobic fitness. Later in the season, more time is spent focusing on a specific sport. The reason for dividing the year into specific periods is to emphasize specific aspects of fitness while maintaining others developed during earlier periods (see Fig. 18.11). Trying to simultaneously improve all aspects of training is impossible for an athlete to handle. Periodization of training helps reduce injury, maintain flexibility, and limit burnout. Scientific evidence to support such training programs is limited, but logically, it does make sense. In addition to the logic, a majority of the world's elite aerobic athletes follow these principles.

Individualization

- Many factors contribute toward an athlete's capacity to handle a given workload. These factors are not purely physiologic but are psychological, socioeconomic, environmental, and genetic. Each of these factors has the ability to improve or impede fitness. Periodization of training addresses many of these individual variables. Several books have been written on the subject of periodization. Simply put, two athletes should not perform exactly the same workouts. Also, an athlete should not perform the same training each day, or each week, or each month. Constantly varying workouts during the week and over the year is the key to progressing in your aerobic fitness.

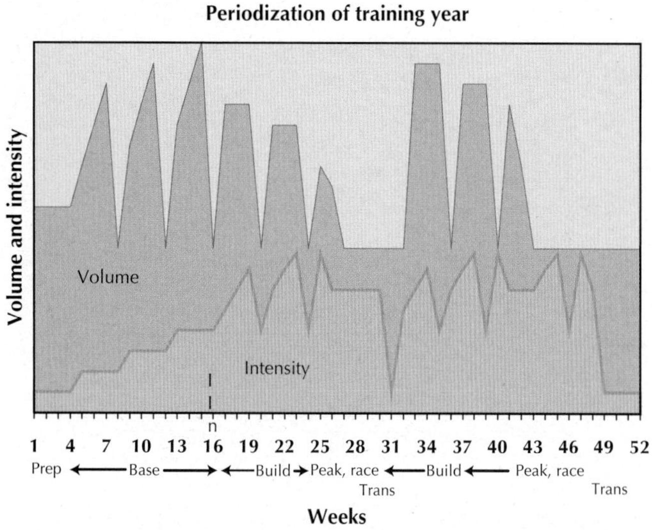
Periodization of training year
Volume and intensity
Volume
Intensity
1 4 7 10 13 16 19 22 25 28 31 34 37 40 43 46 49 52
Prep Base Build Peak, race Build Peak, race
Trans
Trans
Weeks

Figure 18.11 Hypothetical training year divided into periods showing the interplay between volume and intensity. Prepare to train. Base is to establish speed, strength, and endurance; Build is to increase intensity and improve weaknesses; Peak is to taper for race readiness; Race is for priority races; and Transition is the recovery period.

Principle of Specificity

- Training specificity is best accomplished through a training program that involves movement patterns and speeds similar to a given exercise task or competition goal (e.g., bikers must bike and runners must run). It contributes to exercise economy, has both neuromuscular and metabolic components, and is one of the most important conditioning principles.

SUMMARY

- Fatigue is a significant determining factor of our fitness level. The primary reason for training is to delay the onset of fatigue. The fittest athletes are those who can best resist its crippling effects. We know that lactic acid is always being produced, even at rest. A consistently low level of lactic acid in the serum during moderate exercise implies that the body can clear it from the blood as fast as it is generated. The point at which lactic acid levels begin to rise in the serum depends on $\dot{V}O_2$ max and LT; this is the point at which lactic acid production is greater than the body's ability to clear it and when effort becomes disabling.
- $\dot{V}O_2$ max alone is not a good predictor of performance. It is the person who can maintain the highest value of $\dot{V}O_2$ max for an extended period who stands the best chance of winning a race. This sustainable high value is equivalent to LT. The purpose of aerobic conditioning is to cause your body to positively change to better manage the physiologic stresses of competition. To appropriately stress your body, you must present a load that challenges its current level of fitness. This load will initially cause fatigue, followed by recovery, and will eventually lead to an increased level of fitness or overcompensation. If the workouts are of the right magnitude, slightly more than the body can handle, adaptation occurs and fitness steadily progresses.

RECOMMENDED READINGS

Available online.

RESISTANCE TRAINING 19

William J. Kraemer • Gwendolyn A. Thomas • Disa L. Hatfield • Tunde K. Szivak

GENERAL PRINCIPLES

- Resistance training is the most potent form of exercise to strengthen tissues and help prevent injury and improve sports performance. Appropriately prescribed and implemented resistance training programs are necessary to achieve these goals.
- The size principle of motor unit recruitment demonstrates that the recruitment of motor units and their associated muscle fibers occurs in an orderly manner from low- to higher-threshold motor units, and as one climbs the recruitment ladder, greater amounts of force can be produced.
- Strength (maximal force production) is a key factor in highly trained athletes; however, other trainable variables (e.g., power [force ÷ time] or rate of force development, local muscular endurance, and hypertrophy of muscle) are equally important.
- For athletes, a total conditioning program (i.e., resistance training, aerobic conditioning, flexibility, speed and agility, plyometrics, nutritional components, body composition, and psychological aspects) is needed; however, such a program must be appropriately designed, or else, it could result in incompatibility (e.g., too much endurance training can interfere with power development).

The Needs Analysis

- The development of a resistance training program depends on matching individual needs of an athlete with demands of the sport.
- A sport must be analyzed by its biomechanical movements (e.g., isometric or dynamic; concentric or eccentric) that have to be reflected in the resistance training program. If a range of motion is not trained, then the tissues become more susceptible to injury because of a lack of adaptation.
- The metabolic profile of a sport can vary and differ from a cross-country runner to a wrestler. What is the basic metabolism that predominates? Most sports played at high school and collegiate levels rely on a high adenosine triphosphate–phosphocreatine (ATP–PC) and glycolysis involvement supported by a basic aerobic endurance component.
- Understanding the injury profile of a sport is important to strengthen tissues and movements of the affected joint.
- Testing is needed for informed decisions regarding the needs of an exercise prescription.

Specificity of Training

- The specificity of training is related to the recruitment of muscle tissues reflected in the "size principle." Considering the need for greater force and power demands, more motor units must be recruited. The recruitment of motor units always occurs in an orderly manner from lower-threshold motor units composed of type I slow twitch muscle fibers to higher-threshold motor units (i.e., type II muscle fibers, fast twitch).
- The amount of force or power needed determines how much of the muscle is activated and thus trained in a given exercise. Heavier resistances in a program ensure that all muscles have been trained.
- It is important to use resistances and velocities across the entire force–velocity spectrum (i.e., light to heavy, reflecting high to low velocities). Training for maximal power should be performed with no deceleration except for gravity in the exercises performed (e.g., Olympic-type lifts).
- Ultimately, the specificity of training is related to the physiologic systems that are used to support the motor unit recruitment demands of an exercise.

DEVELOPMENT OF A WORKOUT

- A key factor in the prescription of exercises in resistance training is the acute program variable and choices made because these determine the exercise stimuli.

Choice of Exercise

- Exercise choice involves the type of weight-training equipment and type of muscle action that will be used in a workout.
- Exercises are classified as structural (i.e., involving multiple joints) or body part (i.e., involving an isolated joint).
- **Structural exercises** include whole-body lifts that require coordinated actions of muscle groups and joint movements (e.g., closed kinetic chain exercises). Most primary or core exercises are structural (e.g., squats or power cleans). These should be included in the training program of every athlete.
- **Body-part exercises** attempt to isolate a particular muscle group or joint (e.g., bicep curl). Most assistance exercises can also be classified as body-part or single-joint exercises.

Order of Exercise

- Larger muscle group exercises should be performed first to allow higher resistances to be lifted.
- New or complex exercises should be performed first in a workout to allow development of better exercise techniques because of less fatigue.
- When creating a circuit weight-training workout, one has to decide whether the order and choices are going from arm to arm or leg to leg exercises or arm to leg exercises or upper to lower body exercises.
- The fitness level of an athlete and exercise tolerance are important considerations when designing a workout or training program.

Number of Sets

- The number of sets in a workout is part of a volume calculation (e.g., sets × rep × resistance = total kg) and is related to the training goals of a program (e.g., low or high workout volume for different workouts or training cycles).
- Three to six sets are used to achieve optimal adaptations. Not every exercise in the workout must have the same number of sets.
- To date, no single-set system has been shown to be superior to multiple-set programs and should only be used to reduce the volume of a workout or training cycle.
- Training for muscular power is accomplished with more sets and fewer repetitions (e.g., six sets of three repetitions each) to optimize the power output of each set.
- During needs analysis, the practitioner will evaluate the athlete and decide the primary goal of the resistance training program; this training goal will be used to determine specific loads, rest, and repetition arrangements.

Length of Rest Periods

- The length of rest periods between sets and exercises is crucial for all exercise prescriptions.
- Rest periods determine how much of the ATP–PC energy source is recovered.
- Lactate is a buffer and not responsible for the acid–base disruption or fatigue and does not play any role in muscle soreness; in fact, lactate is essentially just a good marker of metabolic demands. Nausea and dizziness caused by excessive physiologic stress should not be equated with a "good workout."
- Short rest periods can lead to greater psychological anxiety and fatigue and higher metabolic demands (e.g., high lactate production, pH decreases, and H^+ increases). As a result, certified strength and conditioning specialists (CSCSs) may have to gradually expose athletes to such workouts and use no more than two per week.
- Rest periods of <1 minute are classified as being very short, 1.5–2 minutes as short to moderate, 3–5 minutes as long, and >5 minutes as very long rest periods. As the resistance gets heavier, longer rest periods are needed.
- Popular extreme commercial programs have a tendency to repeat too many of such short rest periods per week, and this can promote overreaching/overtraining.

Amount of Resistance

- The amount of resistance used for each specific exercise is the most important variable (i.e., size principle).
- Resistance is a major stimulus related to changes in measures of strength, power, and local muscular endurance.
- The amount of resistance must be selected for each exercise in a given resistance training program.
- A repetition maximum training zone **(RM zone)** allows only a specified number of repetitions to be performed targeting a three-repetition range (i.e., zone) for loading. Changes can be made for each set in a workout. If an RM zone is 3–5 RM and the athlete can only perform 2, the resistance is lowered; similarly, if she or he can perform 6, the resistance is increased to stay within the zone. It is a way to set a resistance load for an exercise.
  - Six or fewer very heavy RM resistances appear to have the greatest effect on strength, which contributes to the force component of a power equation. In addition, it recruits the maximum number of motor units and thus stimulates hypertrophy of the entire motor unit array of a muscle.
  - Resistances in the 8–10 RM range contribute to both strength and hypertrophy.
  - Twenty or more RM resistances improve local muscular endurance measures (e.g., repetitions at 75% of 1 RM).
  - This RM zone continuum makes it possible to develop a specific feature of muscular performance to varying degrees over a range of RM resistances.
  - The RM zone cues loading and should not be done to failure as a target end point because this can cause increased compression on joints and fosters overreaching.
- Another standard method of determining resistance for specific exercises is to use **percentages of 1 RM** (e.g., calculating 70% or 85% of 1 RM tested to determine the training load). This method requires regular testing of maximal strength in various lifts used in the training program or prediction of 1 RM by using an equation (e.g., Epley Eq. 1 Repetition Maximum Prediction = 0.033 (reps) × [repetition weight] + [repetition weight]; used for major muscle group exercises).
- The relationship between possible RM and percentages of 1 RM varies with the amount of muscle mass needed to perform an exercise (e.g., leg presses require more muscle mass than do knee extensions).
- When athletes use machine resistances with 80% of 1 RM (previously thought to be primarily for strength-related prescriptions), the number of repetitions that can be performed is >10, particularly for large muscle group exercises such as leg presses.
- Percentages were developed for free-weight exercises and do not translate very well to machine exercises, particularly as the muscle mass used increases.

Frequency of Training

- The frequency of training can range from 1 to 6 days per week and is related to the required volume of work or recovery time.
- Elite athletes may require periodized training frequencies of 4–5 days to achieve gains over short periods.
- Athletes may train twice daily with 4–6 hours of rest between workouts to reduce volume within a single workout so that the quality (intensity) of the workout can be maintained at the highest level.
- Training frequencies of more than twice a week typically involve different training programs and do not repeat the same program during each workout.
- A minimal frequency of two sessions per week for a given exercise is needed for any improvement.
- Certain types of variations (i.e., periodization) must be employed when consecutive training days are used.
- Progression in frequency depends on the phase of the training cycle, fitness of the athlete, goals of the program, training history, exercise selection, training volume, intensity, recovery ability, and nutrition.
- Excessive soreness indicates a lack of recovery, and subsequent workouts must be adjusted to reduce this stress.
- Training with heavy loads increases the required recovery time before subsequent exercise sessions.

Considerations for Women

- The same general principles apply to the training of women and men. By understanding specific gender differences (e.g., weaker upper body in women), the required elements can be added to a training program. The maximal mean total body strength of an average woman is 63.5% of that of an average man; moreover, the isometric upper body strength of an average woman is 55.8% of that of an average man, and the isometric lower body strength of an average woman is 71.9% of that of an average man.
- Some initial evidence indicates that strength gains in women may plateau after 3–5 months of training. This plateau may be more pronounced in the upper body, where the absolute muscle mass is less than that in men. Thus, emphasis on development of upper lean body mass in women may be warranted for sports wherein upper body strength is a limiting factor of performance.
- In certain cases, women may need much more maximal strength to optimize power development.
- Body somatotype can have a dramatic influence on muscle strength and size gains, which is reflective of the number of muscle fibers in various muscles. Target goals should be set by accounting for not only muscle but also the importance of strengthening other tissues such as connective tissues, as well as training other physiologic systems and their organ structures (e.g., cardiovascular and endocrine systems).

Training Cycles

- In classic program time frames, most sport coaches consider training as comprising three basic time frames: off-season, preseason, and in-season. Certified strength and conditioning specialists (e.g., National Strength and Conditioning Association [NSCA]-CSCS) view such older forms of training delineations

to be defied by a periodized training schedule. It consists of a macrocycle (the annual cycle or training phase), a mesocycle (3- to 6-month phases), and a microcycle (1 day to 4 weeks). Each of these depend on the periodization model used, which is based on the need for quality training and the required rest and recovery times to mitigate any overreaching or overtraining syndromes.
- Sport and practices can induce physical and mental trauma that can be problematic to optimal training. For targeted goals in a strength and conditioning program, this can contribute to the development of nonfunctional overreaching, and in extreme cases, overtraining, which can last for over a year and can permanently diminish a competitive career.
- Quality of training is vital for effective use of time and variation in the training stimulus (e.g., resistance used or volume of workouts) along with rest days allow effective adaptations and resilience. It is important to educate coaches regarding the value of rest days in improving performance.

Variation in Training

- The principle of variation relates to changes in the characteristics of a training program to match the changing program goals, as well as to provide a changing target for the body's adaptation. For experienced lifters, it is prudent to design resistance training program cycles that vary as often as every 2–4 weeks (linear microcycles).
- New terminology: overreaching—an intentional hard training phase to push an athlete's performance for a short period, followed by a remarkable reduction in stress, which produces an increase rebound (supercompensation).
- Nonfunctional overreaching—mistakes are made in training that diminish an athlete's performance, but the exact cause is not known, and recovery is possible in days or weeks only if rest is allowed.
- Overtraining is less common than previously claimed and most of the time is due to nonfunctional overreaching that can be caused by mistakes in exercise prescription and/or a medical issue causing excessive stress (maladaptive state); performance remains decreased for a few weeks to a few months.
- Certain variables do meet a genetic maximum for development, and not all plateaus in training are a sign of overreaching or overtraining because there is a limit to training progress; this underscores the importance of realistic training goals and targets for improvements.

GENERAL PREPARATORY CONDITIONING

- Acute program variables must be carefully used to design a workout by using the program concepts outlined next. Effective strength and conditioning programs must be designed, implemented, and monitored by experienced NSCA-CSCSs, who work closely with the sports medicine team.
- A general preparatory conditioning phase (2–4 weeks) is typical of linear periodization programs (crucial at the start of a training program for beginners); it can also be helpful for beginners who are using a nonlinear program.
- Appropriate progression considers progressive overload, specificity, and variation to match dynamic training goals and fitness levels of an athlete.
- A major issue is doing "too much, too soon" in a strength and conditioning program and overshooting an athlete's ability to recover from a workout or to mentally cope with a training program.
- Educational aspects of resistance training, appropriate exercise techniques, aerobics, and nutrition should be stressed. Resistance loads should be light to moderate because the ability to concentrate with less fatigue helps learning.

Periodization of Training

- Over the past 25 years, the concept of periodization of training has taken several different forms, and each of them has been effective in its own way by meeting the needs for variation, rest, and recovery. Each individual adapts and recovers differently to a resistance training program. The most effective programs monitor progress with testing and develop individualized programs.
- Regular monitoring and testing are needed to evaluate day-to-day progress and progress over each training cycle. If testing is performed, one has to adhere to the credo "if you test or monitor it, you have to manage it," indicating that the program must be altered or not based on testing results.
- This requires integration of sports medical teams (physicians, dieticians, athletic trainer, physical therapists, and sport psychologists) and strength and conditioning teams, along with the use of evidence-based practices. Integration with sports medicine elements is vital for full program connections.
- Again, periodized training programs are bracketed by time, as noted by a macrocycle (1–4 years), mesocycle (3–6 months), and microcycle (1 day to 1–4 weeks depending on the periodization model used).

Classic "Linear" Format

- Decreases training volume and increases training intensity as a program progresses.
- Used in athletes who are peaking for a single performance in a strength/power sport (e.g., weightlifting or field events such as shot and discus) in a major competition (e.g., World Championships or Olympic Games).
- Classic periodization methods use progressive increases in intensity with a small variation in each 2–4-week microcycle. To move through a microcycle faster to get to other stimuli, linear periodization now has also cut the length of the microcycle down to 2-week segments and some even to 1 week. This allows even more variation that is typical of what can be noted in nonlinear programs. A classic 2-week microcycle linear periodized program is outlined in Box 19.1. Certain variations can be observed within each microcycle, considering the repetition range of each cycle, but the general trend noted in these programs is a steady linear increase in intensity of a training program.
- In addition, resistance loading can take the form of a percentage of the 1 RM. However, this is typically used in exercises and in athletes who are very familiar with their maximal 1 RM limits, as with competitive weightlifters and powerlifters. Otherwise, an RM zone can be used.

Special Consideration for Athlete Populations

- Each 8- to 16-week program is called a *mesocycle* (composed of microcycles), and a 1-year training program is typically composed of several mesocycles. Each mesocycle attempts to increase muscle hypertrophy, strength, local muscular endurance, and/or power toward an athlete's theoretical genetic

BOX 19.1 GENERAL EXAMPLE OF A LINEAR PERIODIZED PROGRAM WITH 2-WEEK MICROCYCLES

Microcycle 1: 3–5 sets of 12–15 RM zone
Microcycle 2: 4–5 sets of 8–10 RM zone
Microcycle 3: 3–4 sets of 4–6 RM zone
Microcycle 4: 2–3 sets of 1–3 RM zone
ACTIVE REST CYCLE of approximately 1–2 weeks before the start of a new mesocycle of training

RM, Repetition maximum.

maximum. Thus, the linear method of periodization is theoretically based on the development of muscle hypertrophy and improved nerve function and strength and power. This process is repeated with each mesocycle to make progress in training programs.

- Training volume starts with a higher initial volume, and as the intensity of the program increases, volume gradually decreases. Drop-off between intensity and volume of exercise can decrease as the training status of an athlete advances. Advanced athletes can tolerate higher starting intensities and volumes of exercise during heavy and very heavy microcycles.
- Increases in the intensity of periodized programs begin the development of required adaptations in the nervous system for enhanced motor unit recruitment. Adaptations develop as a program progresses, and heavier resistances or velocities of movement are used. Heavier weights demand involvement of high-threshold motor units in the process of force production. Moreover, exercises with higher power output and training velocities use specialized motor unit recruitment patterns.
- Athletes must be careful to not progress too quickly to high volumes using high intensities. Pushing too hard can lead to serious overreaching or, at the worst, overtraining syndromes. Although it takes a great deal of excessive work to produce true overtraining effects, highly motivated athletes can easily make mistakes out of sheer desire to achieve gains and see what is called *nonfunctional overreaching*, where performance diminishes but can be recovered within days if discovered by a strength and conditioning professional. However, in the case of true overtraining, it may take weeks to recover performance levels from mistakes made during an exercise prescription program and see any progress in training and performance. It is important to monitor the stress of workouts. Rest between training cycles (active rest phases) allows time for required recovery so that overreaching to overtraining issues are reduced, if not eliminated; 1–2 days of complete rest during a training week has been shown to reduce the chance of overtraining.
- High-volume exercise in early microcycles marks the initiation of a linear periodized program; thus, late cycles of training are linked to early cycles by changing the stimulus of the training. Once basic strength has been developed, specialized power training programs allow separate development of power capabilities in muscles.
- Maintenance or continued improvement in strength is needed for power development as loading is reduced. A major error in certain training programs, particularly in those for women, is to drop off the high-resistance loading that is required for strength development for prolonged periods while focusing on power by using lighter and more ballistic loading schemes. This has led to the use of 2-week microcycles for power development and different linear progression strategies.

"Nonlinear" or Undulating Format

- Developed out of the need to periodize throughout multiple competition sports wherein one peak does not necessarily produce success; shown to be very effective in college and high school settings wherein schedule influences are dramatic.
- Useful in sports with long seasons wherein success during the season and qualification for major tournaments and competitions are important.
- Varying training volumes and intensity so that fitness gains are achieved over long training periods.
- Training volume and intensity are varied using different workouts for each day to address a specific trainable feature (e.g., strength, power, muscle size, and local muscular endurance); this is achieved by using percentages of 1 RM or near RM training zones, varying volumes of work, varying rest periods, in varying orders, and varying supplemental exercises.
- Nonlinear or undulating periodized programs are designed to maintain variation in training stimuli without holding an athlete to strict phasing of linear periodized programs.
- Nonlinear programs facilitate easier implementation of a program when schedule or competitive demands over long periods limit sequential variation in a linear manner. In addition, they allow variation in intensity and volume within each 7- to 14-day cycle over the course of a training program (e.g., 16 weeks).
- Typically, changes in intensity and volume of training vary within each 7- to 14-day cycle. For example, in 12- to 16-week programs, an active rest phase of 1–2 weeks may be followed by another nonlinear cycle or even by a linear program, if desired. Box 19.2 offers an example of loading or intensity variation over a 5-day rotation during a 12- to 16-week mesocycle.
- Important to this concept is the fact that one can also have a different priority for each mesocycle, thereby allowing additional workouts to emphasize one style and at the same time, keeping a lot of variation in the program (e.g., a power mesocycle or a strength mesocycle, wherein additional workouts will be directed toward such types of workouts over 16 weeks).
- Variation in training is much greater within each 5-day workout over 10 days. Intensity spans a maximal range of 15 RM (possible 1-RM sets vs. 15-RM sets). In addition, workout cycles may include other types of training protocols (e.g., plyometric protocols or 6–10 sets of 2–3 repetitions at 30% of 1 RM for power and velocity training days). The key element is variation during an acute 1- to 2-week cycle within a 12- to 16-week mesocycle.
- An athlete trains different components of muscle within each microcycle. Although nonlinear programs attempt to train various components of the neuromuscular system within the same cycle, only one feature (e.g., power or strength) is trained during a single workout.
- The mesocycle is completed within a certain number of workouts (e.g., 48) instead of a certain number of training weeks. Workouts rotate between different styles for each training session. If an athlete misses a Monday workout, the rotation order is simply pushed forward. In this way, no workout stimulus is missed during a training program.
- Primary exercises are typically periodized. Similarly, supplemental exercise movements (e.g., hamstring curls or abdominal exercises) can be periodized as well.
- Nonlinear programs accomplish the same effects and are superior to linear programs in certain situations. The key to success in all training programs appears to be variation. Different approaches can be used over the year to reach the training goals of an individual athlete in his or her specific sport.
- The concept of "flexible" nonlinear periodization was created to individually optimize the quality of each workout and not just go through the paces. Not all athletes are ready to perform a scheduled workout during a training program because of a lack of recovery from the previous day, sport demands of practice or competition, illness, or injury, and therefore, the workout to be used is decided on each single day to determine if a scheduled

BOX 19.2 GENERAL EXAMPLE OF A NONLINEAR PERIODIZED PROGRAM PROGRESSION

This program uses a 5-day rotation:
Monday: 2 sets of 12–15 RM zone
Wednesday: 6 sets of 1–3 RM zone
Friday: 3 sets of 4–6 RM zone
Monday: Power day: 10 sets of 2–3 repetitions at 30% of 1 RM
Wednesday: 4 sets of 8–10 RM zone

RM, Repetition maximum.

workout will work in a nonlinear periodized schedule. This can involve preworkout testing (e.g., vertical jump to see if one can train power) or progression of a workout log to see if the number of reps for each set with a prescribed resistance can be performed and, if not, the workout must be typically changed to a lower volume or lighter resistance or a rest day. This places additional responsibility on the strength and conditioning professional to develop a system to accomplish a more effective "quality" workout program.

Training Adaptations

- Different programs result in different training adaptations and physiologic responses. Specificity of training applies to all features of each exercise used in the conditioning program (e.g., each specific workout has varying effects on various physiologic systems, signaling molecules, and gene expression).
- Development of muscle size is dependent on the number and type of muscle fibers. Moreover, body somatotypes (ectomorph, mesomorph, and endomorph) influence the gain potential for strength and size, whereas limb lengths and body dimensions affect several performance outcomes.
- Heavier weights have a higher neuroelectric Hz stimulus to all muscle fibers that form different motor units and promote greater hypertrophic responses across the fiber array in a muscle and thus support the need for heavier loadings as part of a periodized program for both men and women.
- Strength increases are specific to the mode of muscle action used during training.
- Most sport skills develop in <0.2 milliseconds (rate of force development), which makes the ability to produce force in short periods vital to performance, which requires power training.
- Speed repetitions, wherein an athlete holds on to weight (e.g., bench press or military press), should not be used to train for muscular power because an athlete's body tries to decelerate mass by activating antagonist muscles and reducing activation of agonist muscles. Instead, power exercises such as Olympic high pulls, power cleans, isokinetic exercises, pneumatic exercises, and medicine ball exercises should be used to promote power development.
- Typically, velocity of movement is associated with the type of resistance used, choice of exercise, and exercise modality. Terms such as *speed*, *strength*, and *power* relate to rapid development of force at high speeds of movement. Continuum of velocities is used in conventional resistance training, from very slow concentric movements (e.g., 1 RM lift) to higher-speed power movements (e.g., 30%–50% of 1 RM). Slower, high-resistance training enhances development of high force but has little carryover to faster velocities or rate of force development; conversely, high-speed training has little carryover to development of slower speed force.

PHYSIOLOGIC COMPATIBILITY OF EXERCISE TRAINING MODES

- Aerobic endurance exercise (e.g., running and cycling), when concurrently performed with resistance training at a substantially high intensity and volume, has the potential to compromise increases in strength and power and limit type I muscle fiber size increases.
- For example, training incompatibility for strength and power is noted with extremely high-intensity long-distance running.
- For most sports, the phenomenon of interference can be accommodated by prioritization of goals. Prioritization involves working on the most important training goals first and maintaining others. For example, one training phase may focus on power development, but high levels of strength also must be maintained to optimize power.

RECOMMENDED READINGS

Available online.

20 FLEXIBILITY

Ian Shrier

GENERAL PRINCIPLES

- The term *flexibility* is often used as a synonym for range of motion (ROM) around a joint.
- Both muscles and ligaments can limit ROM.
- *Mobility* refers to a limited ROM because of ligaments; *flexibility* is usually reserved to refer to limited ROM caused by the muscle–tendon unit.
- Flexibility depends on both muscle stiffness (force required to stretch a muscle) and the stretch tolerance of an individual (amount of discomfort felt when a muscle is stretched).

Definitions of Related Terms

Stretching: an activity wherein a person purposefully attempts to increase ROM by applying a longitudinal force to a muscle

Elastic effects: increase in tissue length that immediately returns to the original length when stress is removed

Viscous effects: increase in tissue length that is dependent on time and returns to the original length at a slow rate (i.e., it is reversible); viscous effects occur because molecules move when force is applied over time, and thus, the return to original length is not immediate

Viscoelastic effects: a combination of viscous and elastic effects

Plastic effects: a permanent change in the molecular structure of a tissue, as that which occurs when force is applied to a plastic sheet without completely tearing it. Plastic deformation indicates that damage has occurred to a tissue—it does not occur with appropriate stretching (i.e., the ROM returns to normal within a reasonable time frame after appropriate stretching)

Flexibility training: program of stretching exercises designed to increase ROM of targeted joints to a desired level or to maintain that level once it is attained

Specificity of Flexibility Training

- The immediate gain in ROM with stretching is mostly limited to the muscle being stretched, with some increase in the contralateral limb as well. This suggests that a neurologic reflex is one of the mechanisms for the effects of an acute stretch.
- If one stops moving a joint, one loses flexibility. It is unknown how much or how often movement is necessary to maintain flexibility.

Effects of Temperature on Flexibility Training

- Most studies have suggested that the effectiveness of stretching increases when the tissue is warmer.
- The most effective way to increase muscle temperature is with muscle activity, although deep heating methods (e.g., ultrasound) can be effective.
- Superficial heat is not an effective method to warm deep muscles.

Age and Gender Differences

- Changes in flexibility appear to coincide with changes in levels of activity, but whether or not this relationship is causal remains to be determined. For example, one begins to walk at approximately 1 year (flexibility begins to increase). When one starts school around 5–8 years of age, which is associated with increased sitting, flexibility begins to decrease. Flexibility increases again at the age of 12–14 years, which coincides with increases in general activity such as walking to secondary school and social relationships. Flexibility decreases again after age of 20–24 years, which coincides with people entering the workforce and again becoming less active.
- Although females are generally more flexible than males, differences within the general population are small. The general perception that females are much more flexible may occur because females participate in activities and sports that include a large amount of flexibility training (e.g., dancing or gymnastics). There are two additional reasons why the increased flexibility in females may not be caused by sex hormones: (1) it is seen before puberty and (2) the increase in flexibility that occurs around the time of adolescence occurs earlier in boys than in girls (but girls enter puberty earlier than boys).

Stretch Reflex

- The stretch reflex is mediated by muscle spindles; it causes stretched muscles to contract and thus prevents excessive ROM.
- The stretch reflex is the primary reason certain people advise against ballistic stretching (bounce stretching). As stretch is released during the bounce, muscles contract and then subsequent stretch occurs against an eccentrically contracting muscle. This theoretically increases the risk of injury, but there are no studies that actually compare rates of injury with ballistic stretching versus other types of stretching. An alternative view is that a force involved with appropriate ballistic stretching is very small and much less than what occurs during regular sport. Therefore, if an injury occurs during a ballistic stretch, some argue that it would likely have occurred during the sport as well.

ROLE OF FLEXIBILITY IN INJURY PREVENTION

Optimal Flexibility

- A graph of the relationship between flexibility and injury risk would be U-shaped. Both individuals who are inflexible and those who are extremely flexible are at a higher risk of injury than are those with an intermediate level of flexibility. Individuals with increased flexibility may be representative of a hypermobility group (because of their ligaments) rather than a hyperflexible group (because of their muscle–tendon unit) because these two features are sometimes difficult to differentiate.
- The U-shaped curve is based on cross-sectional data and does not mean that inflexible individuals would reduce their risk of injury if they begin to stretch before exercise. First, some other factor may be associated with inflexibility that is responsible for the risk of injury, and this other factor might not be affected by stretching. Second, the *immediate effects of stretching are opposite to the long-term effects of stretching* (see the following text). In general, cross-sectional data on flexibility refer to long-term effects and thus provide minimal information on the effects of stretching immediately before exercise.
- Stretching immediately before exercise: Immediately after an acute bout of weightlifting, muscles are fatigued and weaker. Similarly, but perhaps through a different mechanism, muscles are also weaker after stretching. This would not be expected to reduce the risk of injury, and most studies have shown no change in the risk of injury when a pre-exercise stretching intervention is initiated.

- Regular stretching: If a person does weightlifting over weeks to months, muscles become stronger. Similarly, but perhaps through a different mechanism, muscles are also stronger after weeks to months of stretching. This is expected to reduce the risk of injury. Three studies examining the effects of regular stretching on the risk of injury have reported beneficial effects, but only one was statistically significant. The beneficial effects of yoga may work through this mechanism, although certain types of yoga include strengthening and balancing exercises in addition to stretching exercises. The potential psychological benefits of yoga (and stretching in general) could be explained through other possible mechanisms.
- This area warrants more research. For example, most studies examined lower-intensity activities such as jogging, and their generalizability to higher-intensity sports such as basketball remains to be determined.

ROLE OF FLEXIBILITY IN PERFORMANCE ENHANCEMENT

- As one must differentiate the effects of different types of stretching on the risk of injury, one must differentiate the effects of an acute stretch with those of regular stretching.
- An acute stretch reduces the maximal force of the muscle and its ability to contract rapidly.
- If one stretches regularly over weeks, both force and velocity of contraction increase.
- Different sports have different requirements, and performance does not solely depend on force and velocity of contraction.
- In the running gait, energy is lost with each step; however, the energy lost is less when the gastrocnemius complex is stiff.
- Some recent studies have examined the effect of stretching on reaction time, but results at this time are inconclusive.
- The performance of a ballerina depends much more on esthetics than on the height of a jump. If stretching improves esthetics, the performance is improved, even if the jump height is ≤2 cm. In addition, if a hurdler cannot get the leg over a hurdle without immediately stretching before the race, then stretching will improve performance, even if "running speed" is reduced.

ROLE OF STRETCHING IN REHABILITATION AFTER INJURY

- Postinjury weakness occurs with almost every injury. There are no studies suggesting that delaying strengthening exercises until full ROM is achieved is beneficial.
- To our knowledge, no studies have compared a rehabilitation program with stretching to a rehabilitation program without stretching after an acute injury, unless they also included additional cointerventions thought to be effective such as warm-up or strengthening. Because stretching affects type III and IV fibers that transmit pain, stretching should have an analgesic effect just as it does for other conditions. Moreover, if stretch-induced hypertrophy occurs, as it does in healthy tissue, stretching should increase the strength of the tissue and improve healing.
- If the purpose of stretching is to increase strength, then it would be more logical to use a strengthening program. Additional studies are needed in this regard for acute injuries. With regard to chronic injuries, two studies that compared a strengthening program to a stretching program without strengthening have suggested that strengthening is much more important (see Recommended Readings).
  - For chronic groin pain (Holmich and colleagues), the strengthening group exhibited 23 excellent results versus 4 excellent results in the static stretching group.
  - For lateral epicondylitis (Svernlov and colleagues), the eccentric strengthening program had a 71% success rate at 1 year compared with only 39% for the proprioceptive neuromuscular facilitation (PNF) stretch group.
- Strengthening exercises to restore tissue strength are the foundation of most rehabilitation programs. Therefore, the most relevant clinical studies would be those that compare stretching plus strengthening with strengthening alone to determine whether there is a clinically meaningful benefit in adding stretching exercises.

TECHNIQUES FOR IMPROVING FLEXIBILITY

- Daily stretching improves flexibility; however, the minimum frequency required remains to be determined.
- The optimal way to stretch likely depends on each individual person, the muscle (e.g., muscle pennation), and the baseline stiffness of a muscle. This hypothesis is based on studies showing the optimal duration of a stretch is different for different muscles of the same person and different for different individuals.
- Considering the interindividual variability, one proposed but unstudied method individualizes the treatment. A person begins by stretching the muscle to an acceptable length and holding the stretch. Once the sensation of force decreases, the stretch is increased so that the sensation felt during initial stages of the stretch is resumed. As long as ROM increases over time, the technique is effective.
- Some examples of types of stretching are as follows:
  - **Static stretching:** One holds a stretch for a given period. It is important to feel the sensation of the stretch but not pain.
  - **Active stretching:** One performs a stretch by contracting the antagonist muscle. For example, one may contract the quadriceps to stretch the hamstring, with no other passive force being applied to the hamstring. Although this technique gained a lot of popularity several years ago, it is no more effective at increasing ROM than static stretching.
  - **PNF stretching:** One uses a combination of muscle contraction and passive force to improve the effectiveness of the stretch. Certain forms of PNF contract the muscle being stretched, and other forms contract the antagonist muscle. PNF stretching is the most effective type of stretch. The original hypothesis that PNF stretching would decrease muscle activity/tone has been disproved in several studies, and the effect is more likely an increase in stretch tolerance (because there is also an effect on the contralateral limb).
  - **Ballistic stretching:** One moves to the end ROM, then relaxes and returns to the end ROM using a bouncing technique. The amount of force used and how much movement occurs during the relaxation phase vary according to various recommendations. Certain authors advocate a full return to the neutral position, whereas others advocate small oscillations at the end ROM. In general, traditional ballistic stretching is not superior to static stretching. There are theoretical reasons why ballistic stretching might be more dangerous and other reasons why it would be less dangerous. There are no published studies.
  - **Dynamic stretching:** Different authors use this term differently. One common use refers to moving the joint through a regular ROM without applying force at the end of the motion (i.e., a form of ballistic stretching). Because muscle contractions are involved and can increase the temperature, force, and aerobic capacity of the muscle, one expects this technique to be superior to a stretching technique that does not include these other performance-enhancing components. Because there are no studies comparing its effectiveness with other forms of stretching in terms of risk of injury or performance, all claims should be interpreted with great caution.

OBJECTIVES IN PERSONALIZING A STRETCHING PROGRAM

- As with any intervention, one must clearly understand the objectives. Is the objective to reduce injury, improve performance tests, improve performance, or something else? Do not confuse performance tests (e.g., force achieved on a maximal voluntary contraction test) with performance (e.g., vault in gymnastics). Performance requires a more sophisticated level of muscle coordination, often has an esthetic value, and is greatly influenced by an athlete's psychological state of mind. The effect of a stretching program on performance is a combination of multiple factors.
- Different sports require different ROMs for different joints. Any stretching program should target the specific muscles that require flexibility for that specific sport.
- Most sports require an increase in ROM with increasing velocity of contraction. For example, jogging *generally* requires greater ROM than walking (more specifically, increased knee flexion but decreased knee extension), and running requires greater ROM than jogging.
- Because different muscles have different optimal stretching times, and different individuals have different optimal stretching times, it is important to evaluate the effectiveness of any program shortly after it is initiated. Regardless of the program, a person should improve his or her ROM for the muscles being stretched. If this does not occur within 2 weeks (or sooner), the program should be modified. This may mean changing how long the stretch is held, how many times the stretch is applied in one session, how many sessions are conducted per day or week, and how much force is applied with each stretch. As a starting point, I ask patients to stretch a muscle so that they feel a slight pulling or tension. I ask them to hold this position until they no longer feel the stretch, and then to stretch the muscle a little farther so that the sensation of tension is felt again. During the second time, the stretch is held for approximately the same amount of time as the first stretch. In general, most people will end up stretching each muscle for approximately 20–40 seconds using this method. It should be acceptable if patients wish to stretch more than once a day.
- Several stretch positions have been deemed "dangerous" by the sport medicine community:
  - As with any exercise, injury will occur when the stress applied to a tissue exceeds the stress it can withstand.
  - A stretch should not place stress on tissues that are not targeted for increased ROM. For example, the target muscle for the hurdler's stretch is the hamstring muscle when leaning forward and the quadriceps muscle when leaning backward; however, there is also an increased stress to the medial aspect of the knee that appears unnecessary. Therefore, this stretch should be replaced using positions that do not stress the medial aspect of the knee, unless stressing the medial aspect of the knee is a specific objective for that person.

RECOMMENDED READINGS

Available online.

SECTION IV

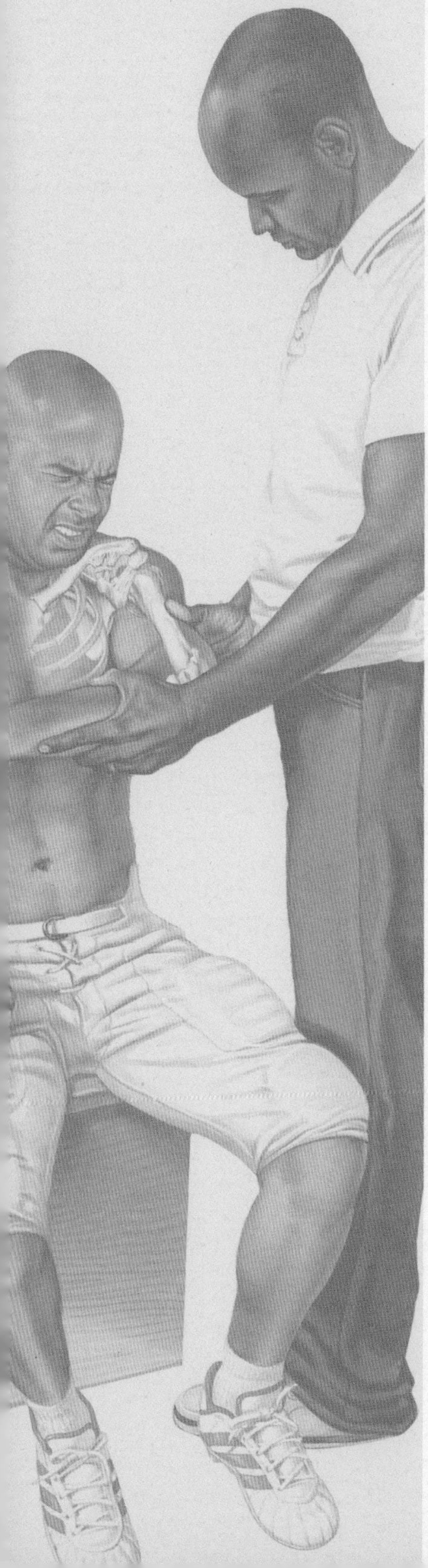

Environment

EXERCISE IN THE HEAT AND HEAT ILLNESS 21

Jon Divine • Stephen Dailey, Jr. • Bret E. Betz

HEAT PRODUCTION

Exercise: The Body's Furnace Caused by the Inefficiency of Work

- The body utilizes energy in the form of energy-rich chemical compounds to maintain normal function (Fig. 21.1) and is inefficient; most reactions produce heat.

Resting Heat Production

- Sources of nonexercising heat production include involuntary smooth muscle contraction, myocardial contraction, muscle group contraction to maintain posture, shivering, digestion, and cellular metabolism.

Heat Production During Exercise

- Increases to 15–20 times the resting rate because of increased muscular contraction and cellular metabolism.
- At maximum exercise, the body's work efficiency is only 15%–30%; thus, 70%–85% of muscle energy consumption is converted to heat and must be dissipated.
- The thermoregulatory system cannot maintain a homeostatic environment when heat production is increased beyond the body's ability to transfer heat, resulting in an elevated core temperature.

HEAT DISSIPATION AND HEAT TRANSFER

Thermoregulation

- Even at rest, thermoregulation requires complex interactions among the central nervous system (CNS), cardiovascular system, and integumentary system to maintain a core body temperature of approximately 98.6°F (37°C).
- The CNS temperature regulatory center is located in the hypothalamus.
- Increases in core temperature are sensed and centrally regulated by thermal detectors in the hypothalamus, which then provide stimulus via the sympathetic nervous system to initiate sweating and increased peripheral blood flow (Fig. 21.2).
- Core body temperature is determined by the net balance of metabolic heat production and heat exchange to and from the surrounding environment. Core temperature change can be defined in the heat balance equation described here (Eq. 21.1).

$$S = M\ (\pm \text{work}) - E \pm R \pm C \pm K \qquad \text{(Eq. 21.1)}$$

  S = amount of stored heat
  M = metabolic heat production
  E = evaporative heat loss
  R = radiant heat loss or gain
  C = convection heat loss or gain
  K = conductive heat loss or gain
- Heat loss can be divided into:
  - Nonevaporative heat loss
  - Evaporative heat loss

Nonevaporative Heat Loss by Conduction, Convection, and Radiation

- Nonevaporative heat loss dissipates most body heat when the ambient temperature is below 68°F (20°C).

Conduction Heat Loss

- A warmer body in direct contact with a colder body will result in heat transfer to the colder body.
- *Fourier's law:* the rate of conductive heat loss is directly dependent on the size of the contact area, thermal conductivity of materials, and temperature difference between materials and is indirectly related to material thickness.

Convection Heat Loss

- Convection heat loss is heat transfer resulting from forced fluid flow across a warmer, relatively stationary surface.
- *Newton's law of cooling:* the rate of heat transferred is directly related to the difference between an object's temperature and that of its surroundings.
- Every object has a **convective heat transfer coefficient (k)**
  - The heat transfer coefficient (k) of water is 50–100 times greater than that of air.
  - Blood has a slightly higher k than water (i.e., relatively large amount of heat energy is transported with only a moderate increase in temperature of blood).
- When the difference between the temperature of blood and that of the tissue through which it flows is significant, convective heat transfer will occur, altering the temperature of both the tissue and blood and follows *Pennes's model* (1948).
- Convective heat transfer depends on the rate of tissue perfusion of blood and the "local" vascular anatomy.
- Convective heat loss is directly related to:
  - Amount of body surface exposed to circulating air
  - Speed of circulating air in contact with skin
  - Cutaneous blood flow (transferring heat) rate through dilated peripheral vessels at the skin surface
  - Convective *heat loss is inversely related to the skin's thickness* between the peripheral veins and skin surface.
- Convective heat loss is the primary principle guiding the use of **cold-water immersion (CWI)** for individuals being treated for hyperthermia.

Radiation Heat Loss

- Radiation heat loss occurs via the transfer of electromagnetic waves when energy (heat) flows from high temperature to low temperature.

Evaporative Heat Loss

- Evaporation accounts for most heat loss when the temperature is above 68°F (20°C).
- Heat is transferred through the evaporation of sweat and respiratory moisture.
  - Insensate respiratory loss of moisture equals 600 mL per day.

Sweating

- Sweating usually begins when the body temperature is above 98.6°F (37°C).
- Amount is proportional to body surface area (BSA).
- Sweat rate is dependent on acclimatization and level of conditioning.
- Sweat rates vary between 600 and 3500 mL/h.
- **Heat of vaporization** of water governs the cooling effect of perspiration.

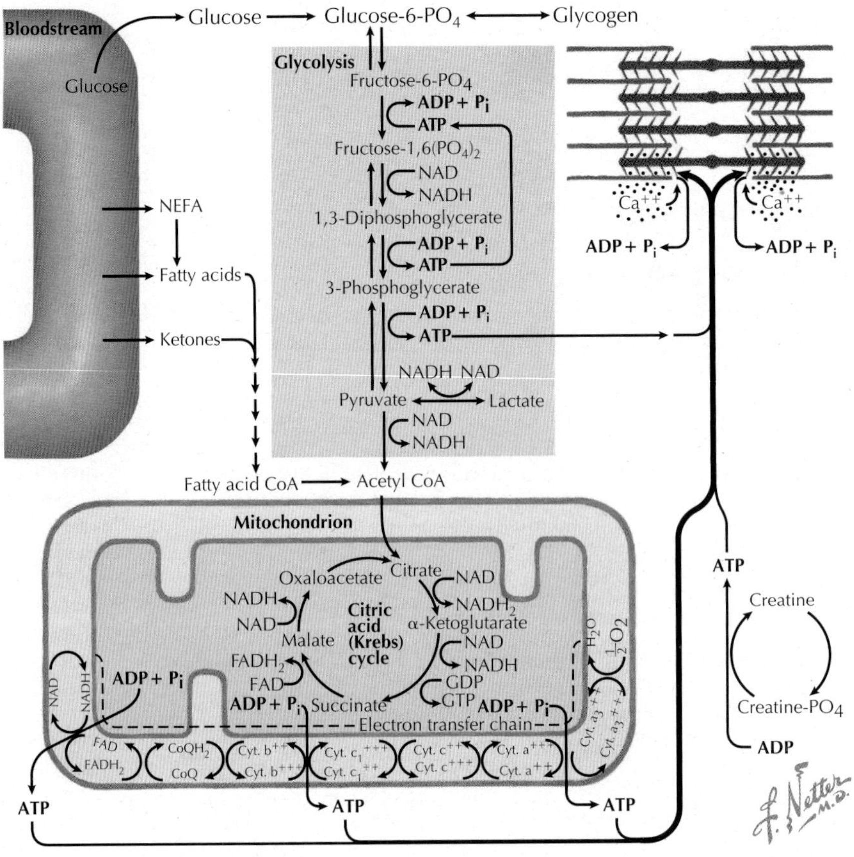
Bloodstream
Glucose
Glucose
Glucose-6-PO4
Glycogen
Glycolysis
Fructose-6-PO4
ADP + Pi
ATP
Fructose-1,6(PO4)2
NAD
NADH
NEFA
1,3-Diphosphoglycerate
ADP + Pi
ATP
Fatty acids
3-Phosphoglycerate
ADP + Pi
ATP
Ketones
NADH NAD
Pyruvate
Lactate
NAD
NADH
Fatty acid CoA
Acetyl CoA
Ca++
Ca++
ADP + Pi
ADP + Pi
Mitochondrion
Oxaloacetate
Citrate
NAD
NADH2
NADH
NAD
Citric acid (Krebs) cycle
α-Ketoglutarate
Malate
NAD
NADH
FADH2
FAD
GDP
GTP
ADP + Pi
Succinate
ADP + Pi
ADP + Pi
Electron transfer chain
NAD
NADH
FAD
FADH2
CoQH2
CoQ
Cyt. b++
Cyt. b+++
Cyt. c1+++
Cyt. c1++
Cyt. c++
Cyt. c+++
Cyt. a++
Cyt. a+++
Cyt. a3++
Cyt. a3+++
H2O
½O2
ATP
ATP
ATP
ATP
Creatine
Creatine-PO4
ADP
F. Netter M.D.

Figure 21.1 Regeneration of ATP for a source of energy in muscle contraction. The body utilizes energy in the form of energy-rich chemical compounds to perform the required work to maintain normal body function.

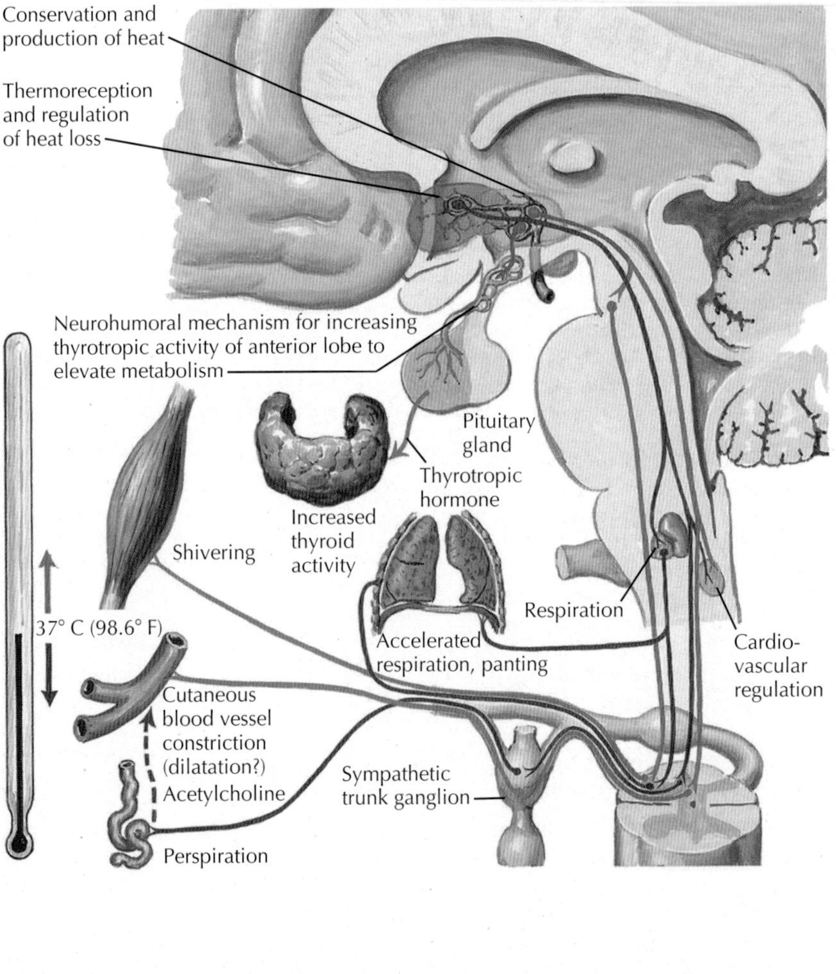
Conservation and production of heat
Thermoreception and regulation of heat loss
Neurohumoral mechanism for increasing thyrotropic activity of anterior lobe to elevate metabolism
Pituitary gland
Thyrotropic hormone
Increased thyroid activity
Shivering
Respiration
Cardio-vascular regulation
37° C (98.6° F)
Accelerated respiration, panting
Cutaneous blood vessel constriction (dilatation?)
Acetylcholine
Sympathetic trunk ganglion
Perspiration
F. Netter M.D.

Figure 21.2 Temperature regulation. Increases in core temperature are sensed and centrally regulated by thermodetectors in the hypothalamus, which then provide stimulus via the sympathetic nervous system to initiate sweating and increase peripheral blood flow.

- Cooling as a result of the evaporation of sweating is directly related to:
  - Sweat rate (L/h): multiplied by 580 calories per gram (heat of vaporization of water on skin)
  - Total BSA
  - Velocity of air crossing the skin surface area
- **Heat dissipation in a hot and humid environment:**
  - Evaporative cooling is *indirectly* related to humidity.
  - Evaporation can account for 98% of heat loss in a hot, dry environment.
    - At temperatures above 95°F (35°C), convection and radiation do not contribute to heat loss.
  - Sun radiation causes heat gain.
    - In heat-acclimated athletes, equilibrium between heat production and heat dissipation results in core temperatures during exercise ranging between 98.6°F (37°C) and 104°F (40°C) without diminished performance.
    - If heat-dissipating mechanisms fail or overwhelming heat stress is present, the core temperature will continue to rise to dangerous levels.

Cardiac Output and Plasma Volume for Heat Dissipation

- Specific demands for cardiac output (CO) and plasma volume are utilized for efficient heat dissipation
- Fifteen percent of CO is shunted to working muscles early during exercise.
- Fifteen to twenty-five percent of CO is shunted from the central circulation to the skin for cooling, which effectively lowers the central plasma volume.
- A single bout of exercise decreases plasma volume (sweat rate 500–2000 mL/h), venous return, and stroke volume.
- Conversely, a known training effect of regular exercise is a gradual increase in plasma volume, venous return, and stroke volume—resulting in improved heat regulation.
- To maintain the necessary CO at a given exercise intensity and core temperature, heart rate must increase to compensate for the reduced stroke volume.
- The cooling process can be favorably changed by reducing exercise intensity, building plasma volume (hydration), and improving nonevaporative heat loss mechanisms (e.g., improving convection by increasing skin surface exposure or circulating local wind/water speed and reducing radiation exposure).

EXERTIONAL HEAT ILLNESS

Exercise-Associated Muscle Cramps

Signs and symptoms: Progressive, painful involuntary muscle contraction of skeletal muscles during or after intense, prolonged exercise; large lower limb muscles are commonly affected, but any muscle may be involved, including abdominal and intercostal muscles.

Etiology: Exercise-associated muscle cramps (EAMCs) can occur in warm, cold, or temperature-controlled environmental conditions and are not directly related to an elevated core body temperature. EAMCs often begin with early muscle fasciculation in an affected muscle group and may progress to severe and diffuse muscle spasm. Although the exact mechanism is unknown, muscle fatigue, dehydration, high sweat rates, high sodium sweat concentration, electrolyte imbalance, and altered neuromuscular control have been implicated in the development of EAMCs.

Predisposing factors: Lack of acclimatization and conditioning, ongoing negative sodium balance ("salty sweaters"), history of EAMCs, faster competition performance times, and prior local muscle or tendon injury.

Treatment:
- Rest and cooling
- Passive, static muscle stretching
- Ice and muscle massage
- Oral hydration with an electrolyte and carbohydrate solution
- Oral intake of salt-containing foods
- Intravenous (IV) normal saline bolus may be indicated if oral hydration is ineffective
- Refractory muscle cramps may require IV medications
  - Diazepam 1–5 mg IV
  - Midazolam 1–2 mg IV
  - Magnesium sulfate 2 g intravenous piggyback (IVPB)

Prevention: Conditioning and heat acclimatization, maintaining fluid and salt balance.

Complications: Rare, but may be a warning sign for impending heat exhaustion. Rhabdomyolysis may develop after prolonged episodes involving multiple muscle groups.

Heat Syncope

Signs and symptoms: Syncope or near-syncope is often seen in unfit or nonheat-acclimatized individuals who stand for extended periods in a warm environment.

Etiology: Often associated with dehydration, venous pooling in peripheral-dependent extremities, decreased preload, and reduced CO with resultant decreased cerebral blood flow leading to syncope; is generally a self-limited condition.

General treatment of heat illness:
- Assess airway, breathing, circulation (ABCs)
- Lie down and elevate legs (Trendelenburg position)
- Rest in a cooler, shaded environment
- Oral hydration

Exercise-Associated Collapse (EAC)

Signs and symptoms: Faintness, dizziness, or syncope after the completion of prolonged, strenuous activity; accounts for approximately 85% of medical visits after marathons, ultramarathons, or triathlon events.

Etiology: During exercise, repetitive contraction of skeletal muscles helps maintain venous return to the heart (i.e., the "second heart" mechanism). As the intensity of muscle contraction decreases at the end of the event, vasodilatation persists, leading to blood pooling in the peripheral circulation and decreased preload. Combined with inadequate sympathetic tone and decreased cerebral perfusion pressure, this results in syncope.

Predisposing factors: Abruptly ending exercise without cooldown, dehydration, lack of acclimatization, and advanced age.

Evaluation and treatment:
- General treatment of heat illness (see earlier)
- Rest in a cooler, shaded environment with air movement
- Initiate oral hydration
- ***Before confirming the EAC diagnosis, exertional heat stroke (EHS) and exercise-associated hyponatremia (EAH) must be ruled out.***
  - Core temperature <104°F (40°C), normal mental status, and normal sodium levels are consistent with EAC.
- With treatment, symptoms should resolve in <30 minutes.
- Follow vital signs closely

Complications: Rare, but may be a warning sign for a more ominous cause of syncope or heat illness.

Exercise-Associated Hyponatremia

EAH (serum sodium ≤135 mEq/L) is observed in athletes usually associated with endurance/ultraendurance exercise.

Incidence: Observed in 5%–13% of marathon participants and 0.3%–27% of ultraendurance participants, most of whom are minimally symptomatic or asymptomatic.

Symptoms: Complaints of "not feeling right," nausea, lightheadedness, malaise, lethargy, and cramps; vomiting is extremely common.

Signs of fluid overload: Edema (e.g., ring or wrist band fitting more tightly), weight gain, and emesis; more ominous signs of fluid overload are indicative of early pulmonary and cerebral edema and include tachypnea and mental status changes (confusion, seizure, coma, and death).

Etiology: Thought to be a combination of excessive hypotonic fluid intake, loss of sodium in sweat, and inappropriate exercise-elevation of antidiuretic hormone (ADH).

Predisposing factors:

- Endurance activity lasting >4 hours; hot and humid environment
- Body mass index (BMI) <20 kg/m^2
- Weight gain during endurance event: Runners who fail to lose 0.75 kg of body weight during a marathon are seven times more likely to develop hyponatremia than are those who lose >0.75 kg.
- Female gender (likely secondary to lower BMI): Women in the postluteal phase of their menstrual cycle have also been at an increased risk of EAH because progesterone-influenced fluid retention and increased sensitivity to ADH during this phase.
- Use of nonsteroidal anti-inflammatory medications (NSAIDs) and selective serotonin reuptake inhibitors (SSRIs): Etiology remains controversial; may result from decreased glomerular filtration rate.

Prevention:

- Prerace assessments and education:
  - Stress importance of measuring prerace and postrace weights
  - Teach athletes how to calculate their sweat rate (see "Calculating Sweat Loss Under Similar Conditions" section at the end of the chapter)
  - Educate athletes not to drink more than their sweat rate (usually 600–1200 mL/h)
  - Prerace questionnaire to self-assess the risk of hyponatremia
  - List of postrace symptoms associated with hyponatremia
  - Encourage salty food and fluid intake in a cool environment
  - Dilute urine production offers a favorable prognosis
  - Hypotonic carbohydrate (6%–8%) fluids *may* be more beneficial for preventing EAH than water in high salt sweaters
  - Event organizers can increase the distance between drinking stations for endurance events

Evaluation and treatment:

- Postrace symptomatic assessment of milder EAH (serum sodium <135 mEq/L with few or no symptoms):
  - Participant presents with weight gain or postevent symptoms of hyponatremia and no mental status changes
  - Obtain vital signs, weight, serum electrolytes, and glucose
  - Observe for symptomatic changes while encouraging oral fluid intake
  - IV fluids are typically not needed unless oral fluids cannot be tolerated
  - Production of dilute urine indicates progress toward normal sodium levels
- Postrace assessment of more serious EAH (serum sodium <135 mEq/L with markedly mental status changes—seizures, coma, or increasing delirium):
  - Usually not seen unless sodium levels are <128 mEq/L
  - Usually, worsening mental status is followed by rapid deterioration of respiratory status because of the pathophysiologic link between cerebral and pulmonary edema
  - Establish and monitor airway
  - Establish IV access and use hypertonic saline: 3% NS, 100 mL for over 10 minutes, and follow with 1 mL/min/kg, up to 70 mL/h, until symptoms improve
  - Arrange for immediate transport to a medical facility
  - In intensive care unit (ICU) setting with central pressure monitoring, loop diuretics and mannitol may be used to reduce pulmonary and cerebral edema

Heat Exhaustion

Overview: Heat exhaustion is the most common exertional heat-related illness. It is characterized by an inability to effectively exercise in heat secondary to a combination of cardiovascular insufficiency, hypotension, energy depletion, and central fatigue.

Signs:

- Elevated core temperature usually ≤105°F (40.5°C)
- Decreased CO (tachycardia, orthostatic hypotension, tachypnea, and syncope)
- **If *any* mental status changes are present, proceed to heat stroke evaluation and management**

Symptoms:

- Fatigue/inability to continue exercise
- Headaches
- Nausea and vomiting
- Muscle cramps
- Chills or piloerection

Etiology: Failure of cardiovascular system's response to workload. Usually, a combination of exertional heat stress and dehydration, resulting in the inability to dissipate heat adequately; occurs most frequently in hot and humid conditions, but can occur in normal environmental conditions with intense physical activity; most commonly affects unacclimatized or dehydrated individuals with a BMI of >27 kg/m^2.

Evaluation and treatment:

- General treatment of heat illness (see "Heat Syncope")
- Obtain vital signs and core body temperature
- If core body temperature *is <104°F (40°C):*
  - Remove clothing and equipment that restrict heat dissipation
  - Use ice towels and ice bags to assist in cooling
  - Initiate oral hydration with electrolyte-containing solution
  - If unable to tolerate oral fluids, IV fluids may be necessary
  - Closely monitor vital signs, core temperature, and mental status
  - **Initiate rapid cooling protocol if status deteriorates**
- Symptoms usually resolve within 2–3 hours. Slow recovery should prompt transfer to a medical facility for further evaluation.

Complications: No long-term sequelae of heat exhaustion have been reported; however, evidence suggests that one episode of marked heat illness *may increase the risk of future episodes of heat illness*

Exertional Heat Stroke

EHS is a life-threatening condition characterized by extreme hyperthermia **(core temperature >104°F [40.0°C])** with eminent thermoregulatory failure, multiorgan failure, and profound CNS dysfunction.

Signs and symptoms:

- Core temperature >104°F (40.0°C); may be as high as 107°F–110°F (41.7°C–43.3°C)
- Markedly impaired CO (hypotension, tachycardia, and tachypnea)
- Pronounced mental status changes (irritability, ataxia, confusion, disorientation, syncope, hysterical or psychotic behavior, seizures, or coma)
- Diminished peripheral cooling ability
- Unlike classic heat stroke, which generally affects children and elderly, athletes with EHS will usually have hot and wet skin
- Life-threatening conditions such as disseminated intravascular coagulation (DIC), acute renal failure (ARF), and neurologic sequelae are associated with prolonged elevated core body temperature
- Morbidity and mortality increase as duration of critically elevated core body temperature (>105°F [40.5°C]) is prolonged.

- ***Prompt and accurate diagnosis of EHS and rapid cooling using CWI (see later) have a marked impact on the survivability of critically ill individuals.***

Etiology: Total thermoregulatory failure that will not spontaneously reverse itself; the risk of EHS is most significant when the wet bulb globe temperature (WBGT) is >28°C (82°F) during higher-intensity exercises and when strenuous exercise lasts for >1 hour. The WBGT index is calculated using the following formula (Eq. 21.2):

$$\text{WBGT} = 0.7\,(\text{WB}) + 0.2\,(\text{BB}) + 0.1\,(\text{DB}) \quad \text{(Eq. 21.2)}$$

WB = wet bulb temperature: humidity indicator
BB = black bulb temperature: measures radiant heat
DB = dry bulb temperature: average air temperature

Pathophysiology:
- Occurs when core body temperature exceeds a critical level; results in a cascade of cellular and systemic responses.
- An increase of inflammatory cytokines and alteration of heat shock proteins decreases the body's ability to prevent thermal denaturation of structural proteins and enzymes and results in early circulatory collapse and systemic damage.
- Activation of the coagulation (clotting) pathway occurs as a result of vascular endothelial damage.
- At critical hyperthermia levels, the degree of tissue injury and death is related to thermal stress levels and duration, resulting in thermoregulatory failure, heat stroke, and circulatory shock.

Predisposing factors:
- Dehydration (acute or chronic)
- Lack of acclimatization to heat
- Approximately 25% of patients have preexisting gastrointestinal or respiratory illness, and many experience warning signs of impending illness.
- Frequently occurs near race finish line when an already hot, dehydrated athlete increases speed, causing increased muscle heat production, increased muscle blood flow, secondarily decreased skin blood flow, and an increase in core temperature.

Evaluation and treatment:
- **Event medical staff preparation:** Medical staff should prepare for heat illness by monitoring weather, educating athletes, and having a CWI tank prepared before practice or event. CWI tank should be nearby, in a cooler or shaded environment, and half-filled with an ice layer on top of the water.
- **Critical intervention: CWI up to the neck is the most effective cooling modality for patients with EHS. Once the diagnosis is confirmed, the CWI protocol should begin. (See: NATA 2015 Position Statement: Exertional Heat Illness. Strength of Recommendation Level A.)**
- **CWI protocol: Initial response:**
  1. Once EHS is suspected, **prepare to cool the patient** and contact emergency medical services (EMS).
     - Move the athlete safely to the CWI: ice water bath is most ideal, however, if not available, then a cold whirl pool or cold shower may be used
  2. Determine vital signs immediately before immersion.
  3. **Core body temperature by using a rectal thermometer**
     - Oral, tympanic membrane, aural canal, and axillary temperatures do not correlate with core temperature in heat-injured patients and may measure temperature >33.8°F (1°C) lower than actual core temperature.
  4. Airway, breathing, pulse, and blood pressure
     - Level of CNS dysfunction
  5. **Cover as much of the body as possible with ice water while cooling**
     - If full-body coverage is not possible because of the container's dimensions, cover the torso as much as possible.
     - Keep the athlete's head and neck above water.
     - Place an ice/wet towel over the head and neck while the body is being cooled in the tub.
  6. **Circulating water:** Water temperature should be approximately 35°F–59°F (1.7°C–15°C). During cooling, *water should be continuously circulated to optimize cooling: using a short paddle or oar is ideal.*
  7. **Continued medical assessment:**
     - Vital signs should be monitored at regular intervals.
     - Continuous rectal temperature monitoring is preferred.
  8. **Fluid administration:** An IV fluid line can be placed for hydration and support cardiovascular function; however, *this should not delay ice-water immersion.*
  9. **Cooling duration:** Continue cooling until the patient's rectal temperature reduces to 102°F (39°C).
     - If rectal temperature cannot be measured and CWI is indicated, cool for 10–17 minutes and then transport to a medical facility.
     - An approximate estimate of cooling via CWI is 1°C for every 3 minutes if water is aggressively stirred.
  10. **Patient transfer:** Remove the patient from the immersion tub only after rectal temperature reaches 102°F (39°C) and then transfer to the nearest medical facility via EMS.
     - ***Cooling to <102°F (39°C) must be achieved before transport.***

EHS complications extend to all major organ systems:
- CNS injury—may be permanent in up to 20% of cases
- Rhabdomyolysis—results in myoglobinuria, which may lead to acute tubular necrosis (ATN) and renal failure
- ARF—approximately 25% of EHS patients develop it
- DIC—may lead to circulatory collapse
- Hepatic failure
- Myocardial injury—may lead to arrhythmias, myocardial infarction, and cardiac arrest
- Pulmonary injury—may lead to pulmonary edema, pulmonary infarction, or acute respiratory distress syndrome (ARDS)
- Metabolic/laboratory abnormalities—hypokalemia (early), hyperkalemia (later), hypernatremia, hyponatremia, hypocalcemia, hyperphosphatemia, hypoglycemia, lactic acidosis, uremia, elevated creatine phosphokinase, elevated transaminase, leukocytosis, elevated coagulation studies, myoglobinuria, anemia, hemoconcentration

Morbidity and mortality: Rates vary directly with the time elapsed between core temperature elevation and cooling therapy initiation. **Mortality rates increase significantly if >30 minutes before cooling is initiated.**

Return to play (RTP) after EHS: Evidence suggests that an episode of EHS may reset thermoregulatory adaptations, which may lead to an increased risk of subsequent heat injury months after the initial event. A graduated RTP protocol should be followed (Box 21.1). Although RTP guidelines vary, the primary considerations after EHS are treating associated sequelae and identifying the cause of EHS to aid prevention techniques. Exercise heat tolerance testing (EHTT) has helped determine the appropriate time for an athlete to RTP. Much like a graded exercise test used to monitor cardiovascular responses to an increased workload, in EHTT, an exercise protocol that monitors the physiologic response to a series of challenging exercise heat exposures has been utilized by both the US and Israeli military and the Korey Stringer Institute.

RISK FACTORS AND POPULATIONS AT INCREASED RISK OF HEAT-RELATED ILLNESS

Normally Healthy Adults

- Poorly acclimated or conditioned to heat or humidity
- Inexperienced
- Salt or water depleted

BOX 21.1 A GRADUATED RETURN-TO-PLAY PROTOCOL AFTER HEAT ILLNESS

REST: Before returning to activity, an athlete should rest for 7–21 days, allowing recuperation and all blood work to return to normal.
LOW AND COOL PROGRESSION: Once an athlete has returned to baseline, he or she may begin with low-intensity exercise in a cooler environment and gradually increase the intensity, duration, and level of heat exposure over 2 weeks.
CONSIDER TESTING: If return to pre-EHS activity levels seems challenging, consider a laboratory-based exercise-heat tolerance test at 1 month after an EHS event.
COMPETITION: An athlete may be cleared for full competition if heat tolerance exists after 2–4 weeks of training.

EHS, Exertional heat stroke.

Large or Obese Adults

- Generate more heat for the same level of activity; adipose tissue has lower specific heat than does lean tissue
- Dissipate heat less efficiently
  - Lower body surface-to-mass ratio
  - Fewer heat-activated sweat glands
  - Poorer fitness levels

Children

- Produce more metabolic heat per mass unit compared with adults
- Sweat less and require more significant core temperature increases to trigger sweating
- Acclimatize slower
- Lower CO at any given workload
- May lack adequate blood flow for both muscle and cooling needs
- Transition to adult thermoregulation begins after puberty

Elderly Individuals

- Generally less efficient at cooling
- Reduced vasodilator response, which may begin as early as 50 years of age
- Lowered maximum heart rate leads to decreased maximum CO
- Reduced thirst response
- Often have reduced fitness levels

Others

- **Having a history of heat injury:**
  - Unknown mechanism: CNS-controlled cooling mechanism may be irreversibly damaged, resulting in higher threshold requirement to begin diaphoresis
- **Women during the postovulatory phase of the menstrual cycle:**
  - Heat dissipation may be reduced because of an increased temperature threshold to begin sweating or possibly a smaller plasma volume
- **Acute infectious or inflammatory illnesses:**
  - Increased metabolic demand for blood flow throughout the body; specifically, gastrointestinal illness:
    - Increased risk because increased splanchnic circulation competes with skin blood flow for CO
    - Often associated with dehydration and electrolyte disturbances
- **Chronic illnesses associated with heat illness:**
  - Cystic fibrosis, diabetes mellitus (uncontrolled), and history of malignant hyperthermia
  - Attention-deficit disease (ADD)
  - Presence of sickle-cell trait (SCT): See Chapter 31: "Hematologic Problems in the Athlete"
  - Alcoholism and other substance abuse:
    - Alcohol has residual effects on thermoregulation capacity, predisposing athletes to dehydration and reduced cooling efficiency.
    - Acute stimulant intoxication (cocaine or methamphetamine) may be challenging to differentiate from heat stroke because of increased metabolic activity.
- **Use of certain medications:**
  - Anticholinergic agents, antihistamines, beta-blockers, diuretics, tricyclic antidepressants, monoamine oxidase inhibitors, and stimulant agents for ADD or attention-deficit/hyperactivity disorder (ADHD)

PREVENTION OF HEAT-RELATED ILLNESS

- Preparticipation medical history and evaluation to identify athletes who are at risk of sustaining heat-related illness.
- Gradual exposure to continuous daily aerobic exercise of 90–100 minutes in higher heat/humidity conditions is optimal.
- Ensure adequate physiologic acclimation and conditioning
  - Physiologic effects of acclimation to exercise in heat require 7–10 days of exposure and include:
    - **Improved cooling efficiency from sweating:** earlier initiation of sweating, *increased rate* of sweating, increased maximum sweating capacity, and lower sweat sodium concentration
    - **Increased cardiovascular efficiency:** increased basal plasma volume, stroke volume, and decreased heart rate at a given workload
    - **Thermal adaptive effects:** increased exercise capacity in heat, lower core and skin temperature at a given workload and heat stress, reduced perceived intensity of exercise, and increased subjective thermal comfort
- Approximately 75% of the effects occur in the initial 4–6 days.
- Acclimation effect persists for 1–4 weeks.

General Points for Improving Heat Acclimation

- Preseason conditioning should include strength, endurance, and skills acquisition drills in a warm environment.
- Delay full participation until minimum conditioning levels are met.
- Heat acclimation generally requires 10–14 days.
- Avoid supramaximal efforts, such as performance testing, in heat—particularly those involving athletes with SCT.
- Historical practice of fluid restriction to improve heat adaptability or conditioning is hazardous and should never be done.
- Provide education regarding heat-related illness to all athletes and their coaches; content should include:
- Awareness and counseling regarding signs and symptoms of early heat stress, dangers and sequelae of heat-related illness, and strategies to minimize the risk of developing these illnesses
- Importance of staying hydrated, adequate sleep, avoiding drugs and alcohol, knowing each athlete's limitations, and avoiding exercise in dangerous environmental conditions.

Monitor Atmospheric and Environmental Conditions

- The American College of Sports Medicine (ACSM) and several high school athletic federations have guidelines on when to restrict activity during periods of high temperatures.
- Monitor weather reports for local "heat index."
- Simple and convenient sources of approximate temperature and humidity readings are helpful to calculate heat stress (Fig. 21.3), but may not allow for local variations of sun exposure, wind velocity, or local airflow.

- ACSM endorses the use of color-coded warning flags along the course of an endurance event, which is used to alert runners/participants regarding relative risks of continuing a given race based on relative heat stress (Fig. 21.4).

Adjust Workout Schedule Based on Environmental Conditions

- Reschedule workouts, practices, and competitions to a cooler time of day or cancel altogether.

Air temperatures (°F)

Relative humidity (%)	70	75	80	85	90	95	100	105	110	115	120
0%	64	69	73	78	83	87	91	95	99	103	107
10%	65	70	75	80	85	90	95	100	105	111	116
20%	66	72	77	82	87	93	99	105	112	120	130
30%	67	73	78	84	90	96	104	113	123	135	148
40%	68	74	79	86	93	101	110	123	137	151	
50%	69	75	81	88	96	107	120	135	150		
60%	70	76	82	90	100	114	132	149			
70%	70	77	85	93	106	124	144				
80%	71	78	86	97	113	136					
90%	71	79	88	102	122						
100%	72	80	91	108							

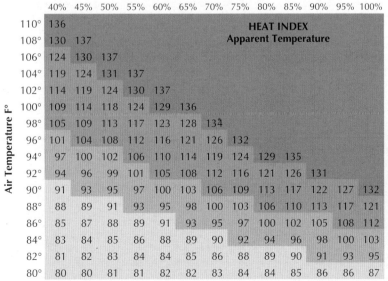

Figure 21.3 Heat stress (apparent temperatures in °F): calculation of heat stress and heat stress risk. (Modified from National Weather Service: Heat Wave and US Department of Commerce, National Oceanic and Atmospheric Administration, PA 85001, 1985. Color code adapted from ACSM Position Statement [1975] on preventing heat injuries during distance running.)

- Alter practices and workouts by (Table 21.1):
  - Decreasing their intensity and duration
  - Providing more frequent breaks
  - Modifying clothing to increase evaporative cooling
  - Moving to a more shaded or breezy area

APPROPRIATE CLOTHING FOR EXERCISE IN THE HEAT

- Short-sleeved, loose-fitting, open-weave or mesh jerseys improve skin exposure and evaporation.
- Evidence to support or discourage the wearing of newer, "sweat-wicking" shirts (made of fabric that absorbs sweat away from the skin to the outer surface to promote evaporative cooling) to reduce the risk of heat illness is lacking.
- Wearing no shirt has both benefits (better heat loss from evaporation and convection) and risks (more radiant heat gain).
- Athletes should practice or play in shorts when possible.
- Light-colored uniforms reflect sunlight and thus reduce radiation absorption.
- As they become sweat-soaked, uniforms or clothing should be changed to allow efficient evaporation.
- Avoid restrictive clothing and bulky protective equipment such as poorly aerated helmets, heavy long-sleeved uniforms, protective pads, and rubberized workout suits, which block skin surface area and reduce cooling by radiation, convection, and evaporation.
- Using water-based sunscreen, applied frequently, is the ideal means to provide adequate sun protection without adversely affecting heat dissipation; oil- or gel-based sunscreens may block evaporative cooling.

Close Monitoring of Athletes

- Observe athletes who are at an increased risk for heat-related illness.

Prevent Athletes With Fevers and Acute Illnesses From Participating

- Core temperature elevations caused by fever and illness are additive to those caused by activity; therefore, both CO and

Relative Humidity

HEAT INDEX
Apparent Temperature

Air Temperature F°	40%	45%	50%	55%	60%	65%	70%	75%	80%	85%	90%	95%	100%
110°	136												
108°	130	137											
106°	124	130	137										
104°	119	124	131	137									
102°	114	119	124	130	137								
100°	109	114	118	124	129	136							
98°	105	109	113	117	123	128	134						
96°	101	104	108	112	116	121	126	132					
94°	97	100	102	106	110	114	119	124	129	135			
92°	94	96	99	101	105	108	112	116	121	126	131		
90°	91	93	95	97	100	103	106	109	113	117	122	127	132
88°	88	89	91	93	95	98	100	103	106	110	113	117	121
86°	85	87	88	89	91	93	95	97	100	102	105	108	112
84°	83	84	85	86	88	89	90	92	94	96	98	100	103
82°	81	82	83	84	84	85	86	88	89	90	91	93	95
80°	80	80	81	81	82	82	83	84	84	85	86	86	87

EXTREME DANGER
Heat stroke or sunstroke highly likely

DANGER
Sunstroke, muscle cramps, and/or heat exhaustion likely

EXTREME CAUTION
Sunstroke, muscle cramps, and/or heat exhaustion possible

CAUTION
Fatigue possible

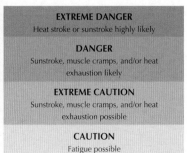

Figure 21.4 Color-coded warning flags were used during an endurance event to alert runners and participants regarding relative risks of continuing the event based on relative heat stress. (From National Oceanic and Atmospheric Administration, National Weather Service. http://www.nws.noaa.gov/om/heat/heat_index.shtml).

Table 21.1 ALTERATION OF PRACTICES AND WORKOUTS BASED ON HIGH HEAT AND HUMIDITY

WBGT		
°F	°C	Restraints on Activities
<75.0	<24.0	All activities allowed, but decrease intensity and be alert for symptoms of heat-related illness
75.0–78.6	24.0–25.9	Shorten practice duration and provide more frequent rest periods in the shade Enforce drinking of fluids every 15 minutes Maximize sweat evaporation with appropriate clothing choices and maximize wind exposure
79.0–84.0	26.0–29.0	Stop activity for unacclimatized and high-risk athletes and shorten activity duration for all others Consider cancellation of long-distance races
>85.0	>29.0	Cancel all athletic activities

WBGT, Wet-bulb globe temperature.

aerobic capacity are reduced in febrile athletes. Exercise with fever may be dangerous, particularly in the heat.

- Aspirin, NSAIDs, acetaminophen, or other antipyretics cannot reduce core temperature elevations caused by exercise.
- When in doubt regarding participation, apply "neck check" rule: no participation if symptoms (e.g., cough, abdominal pain, nausea, vomiting, and diarrhea) are present below the neck or if fever is present.

Prevent Dehydration

- Dehydration reduces endurance exercise performance, decreases time to exhaustion, and increases heat storage.
- When fluid deficits exceed:
  - 2% of body weight, work capacity decreases by 15%–20%, and thermoregulatory function is impaired
  - >3%–5% of body weight, sweat production and blood flow to the skin begin to decrease
  - >6%–10% of body weight, CO decreases considerably, resulting in lower sweat production and reduced blood flow to both skin and working muscles
- Dehydration plus heat stress of exercise cause:
  - Greater reduction in central volume, venous return, and consequently stroke volume and CO, compared with either factor alone
  - Performance reduction is proportional to the level of dehydration and intensity of exertional heat stress
  - Reduced heat dissipation resulting from decreased skin flow and diminished sweating
- Monitoring body weight helps assess dehydration
  - Acute weight loss implies dehydration.
  - Caution is indicated when an athlete has a workout weight loss of >3% of body weight or fails to regain the previous day's weight loss by the next day's workout. During summer workouts, dehydration can be cumulative over several days, such as during two-a-day football workouts.
  - Athletes with large or persistent acute weight loss should be restricted from activity until rehydrated.
- For prolonged or repetitive endurance exercise in the heat, carbohydrate–electrolyte solutions (6%–8% carbohydrates) may limit dehydration, accelerate rehydration, and have been reported to maintain performance.
- Thirst is not an adequate guide for humans' fluid consumption: Calculation of individual fluid replacement rates should be encouraged for all athletes.
  - Athletes may not feel thirsty until they have depleted >5% of the volume in the euvolemic state.
  - Inexperienced athletes may automatically associate heat illness symptoms with being dehydrated and drink excessively, resulting in overhydration, which increases the risk of hyponatremia.
  - For optimal individual hydration, individuals should drink at regular intervals (every 15–20 minutes) and replace what they sweat. Fluid loss from sweat usually occurs at a rate of 600–1200 mL/h, but can be higher or lower in certain athletes and varies based on weather conditions, exercise intensity, BSA, and genetics.

Calculating Sweat Loss Under Similar Conditions

- Calculating sweat loss under similar conditions is the ideal method to determine fluid replacement. The most accurate method involves:
  - Weigh nude before an activity.
  - Perform the activity at a competitive level for 1 hour.
  - Track fluid intake (in mL) during the activity.
  - Record nude weight after activity, subtract from starting weight, and convert the difference in body weight to mL.
  - To determine hourly sweat rate, add the difference in body weight (in mL) to the volume of fluid consumed.
  - To determine how much to drink every 15 minutes, divide the hourly sweat rate by 4. This amount becomes the guideline for fluid intake every 15 minutes of the activity.
- Note the environmental conditions on this day and repeat measurements on another day when the environmental conditions are different. This difference in weather will give the athlete an idea of how different conditions affect his or her sweat rate.

RECOMMENDED READINGS

Available online.

EXERCISE IN THE COLD AND COLD INJURIES 22

Jessie R. Fudge • Christopher C. Madden

GENERAL PRINCIPLES

Physiology of Cold Exposure

Mechanisms of Heat Loss

RADIATION

- Radiation involves the direct emission or absorption of heat energy from the body (mostly infrared radiation).
- Radiation is the largest source of heat loss from the body.
- Clothed, sedentary individuals in a calm, temperate climate lose more body heat (approximately 60%) by radiation than active individuals (approximately 45%) in a thermoneutral environment where heat production equals heat loss.
- The human body constantly radiates heat to nearby solid objects with a cooler temperature, and the rate of heat loss increases with the difference in temperature between the body and the object.
- Radiant heat loss increases as temperature decreases but only becomes a significant concern in extremely cold environments.
- Clothing does not markedly affect radiant heat loss.

EVAPORATION

- Evaporation occurs when water or moisture is transformed into vapor.
- Evaporation occurs with perspiration on the body's surface and in respiratory passages as inspired air is warmed and moistened.
- High altitude increases heat and water losses from the lungs because breathing deepens and the respiratory rate increases.
- A small amount of "insensible" perspiration occurs at cold temperatures but may become significant in active individuals who are not appropriately dressed for that temperature.
- Vigorous exercise with increased sweating leads to greater evaporative heat loss than with normal evaporative loss in sedentary individuals in a temperate climate (a difference of approximately 20%–30%).
- Vapor barrier systems meant to decrease evaporative water loss are ineffective in physically active individuals because they trap perspiration between the barrier and the skin and lead to increased heat loss by convection when the sweat rate exceeds the rate of permeability (Fig. 22.1).
- Wet clothing combined with wind leads to significant evaporative heat losses.

CONVECTION

- Convection involves the transfer of heat from the body to cold air or water in contact with the body surface.
- Ongoing heat loss occurs when warmed air or water is continually displaced from the body surface and is replaced by air and water of colder temperatures.
- The amount of heat loss that occurs by convection is determined by the temperature difference between the air and the body surface and by the speed of the air moving over the body.
- Convective heat loss increases greatly with **wind** moving over the body surface, particularly with submersion in cold water.
- **"Wind chill"** is wind combined with cold that causes a lower "equivalent" temperature (Fig. 22.2) than current environmental temperature and greatly accelerates heat loss by convection; wind chill is most significant with the first 20-mph increase in wind speed, with some additional effects at higher wind speeds.
- In addition to **natural wind, wind moving over the body surface** created by cycling, skiing, running, windsurfing, or other activities that increase air flow over the body can cause marked heat loss, particularly at cold temperatures sustained over prolonged periods.
- Cold-water swimmers lose significant heat by convection because continuous motion prompts the ongoing displacement of water away from the body, resulting in constant exposure of a "warm" body to cold water.
- Windproof clothing, particularly combined with appropriate insulation layers, can greatly reduce convective heat loss in most environments by trapping warm air and minimizing air displacement.

CONDUCTION

- Conduction involves the direct transfer of heat from the body when it is in contact with a surface colder than the body's temperature (e.g., fuel, water, snow, ice, or rocks).
- Water is an excellent conductor, and it has an exponentially greater volumetric heat capacity than air, which can lead to significant heat losses for anyone immersed in cold water, particularly without protective clothing.
- Wet clothing increases conductive heat losses.

Mechanisms of Heat Production

- Metabolic and biochemical reactions (slight increase)
- Muscular activity
  - Involuntary shivering (increases heat production 2–6 times the basal levels; subsides after several hours when core temperature drops below 86°F [30°C])
  - Voluntary exercise (increases heat production up to 10 times the basal levels)
- Nonshivering thermogenesis
  - Increases thyroxine, epinephrine, and norepinephrine and a subsequent slight increase in overall tissue metabolism
  - Relatively ineffective in preventing cold injury; may increase heat production by 10%–15% in adults

Thermoregulation and Physiologic Adaptations

- The hypothalamus is the thermoregulatory center for maintenance of body temperature and physiologic response to cold.
- The body needs to stay between 95°F and 105°F (34°C and 40.5°C) to maintain normal organ function; core temperature normally ranges between 97.7°F and 99.5°F (36.5°C and 37.5°C).
- The body dissipates heat relatively efficiently but is less effective at compensating for cold.
- The body initially responds to cold by regulating the **core** (brain and other major organs) and **shell** (skin, muscle, and extremities).
  - Exposure to cold stimulates thermoreceptors in the skin that signal the hypothalamus to activate shivering and nonshivering thermogenesis, constrict peripheral or "shell" circulation, and decrease sweating in an effort to increase heat production and maintain core temperature.
  - The body shell acts as an interface between the body and environmental stresses—shell temperature may vary widely in contrast to core temperature.
  - Athletic performance may be decreased with shell cooling as cold weakens and slows muscle contractions, decreases tissue elasticity, and slows nerve conduction.

- Prolonged cooling causes body core temperature to drop and results in several physiologic changes:
  - When core temperature falls below 95°F (35°C), rates of essential biochemical reactions decelerate.
  - Shivering gradually ceases at approximately 88°F–90°F (31°C–32°C) as muscles become cooler and stiffer.
  - Severe cold may affect all organ systems, particularly the central nervous system (CNS) and the cardiovascular system (Table 22.1).
  - As temperature decreases, heart rate and cardiac output reduce, and arrhythmias may occur secondary to myocardial irritability.
  - Cerebral blood flow decreases, leading to dilated pupils, obtundation, stupor, and eventually coma.
  - Respiratory rate reduces and so does oxygen consumption.
  - Diuresis occurs secondary to shunting of blood volume to the body core from the periphery.
  - Lactic acidosis develops secondary to decreased shell tissue perfusion (decreased tissue oxygenation) and subsequent anaerobic glycolysis combined with carbon dioxide retention that occurs with reduced respiratory rate.
  - Insulin activity reduces and hyperglycemia develops.

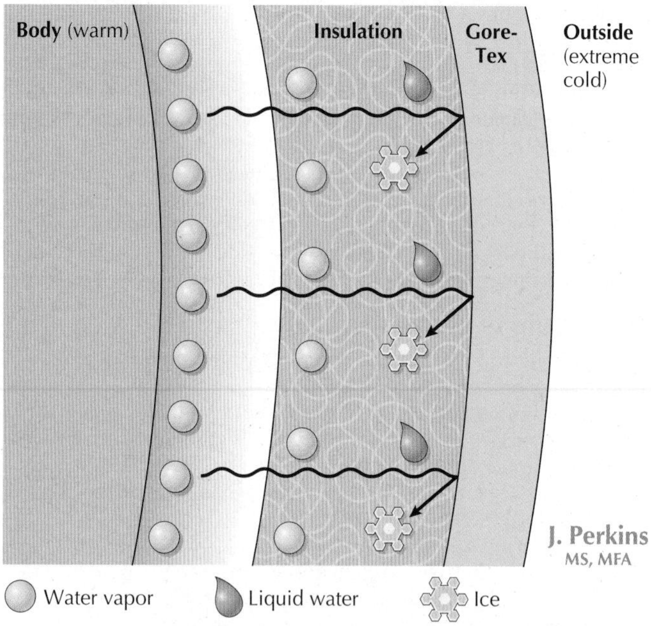
Body (warm)
Insulation
Gore-Tex
Outside (extreme cold)
J. Perkins MS, MFA
Water vapor
Liquid water
Ice

Figure 22.1 Vapor barrier systems.

Exercise in the Cold

Sports Associated With Cold Injury

- Any cold-weather or cold-water sport can be associated with cold injury.
- Risk of cold injury corresponds with level of cold exposure, wind, precipitation, and the athlete's preparation for cold exposure and individual risk factors.
- Specific sports may include skiing (all types), snowshoeing, mountaineering and rock climbing, snowmobiling, canoeing, kayaking, white-water rafting, open-water swimming, and skating. Windsurfing and small-boat sailing may result in cold injury after unexpected capsizing. Moreover, unprepared runners, hikers, backpackers, and cyclists may experience significant cold injuries, particularly with prolonged and inadequate exposure combined with unexpected weather (e.g., blizzard, cold rain, high winds, dropping temperature, and wind chill).

Prevention

Almost all cold illness is caused by exposure to cold, often unexpected, without adequate protection. **Appropriate planning is imperative to prevent cold illness and injury.**

INCREASE HEAT PRODUCTION

- Increasing heat production is the least effective way to prevent cold illness.
- Exercise: voluntary muscular activity will produce heat
- Shivering: involuntary muscular activity will also produce heat
- Eating: frequent meals or snacks are needed to replenish glycogen and fat stores, particularly with prolonged exercise in cold environments
- Hydration: consume adequate fluids to prevent dehydration and subsequent impairment in circulating blood volume

DECREASE HEAT LOSS

- Decreasing heat loss is the most effective way to prevent cold illness.

Temperature (°F)

Wind (mph) / Calm	40	35	30	25	20	15	10	5	0	–5	–10	–15	–20	–25	–30	–35	–40	–45
5	36	31	25	19	13	7	1	–5	–11	–16	–22	–28	–34	–40	–46	–52	–57	–63
10	34	27	21	15	9	3	–4	–10	–16	–22	–28	–35	–41	–47	–53	–59	–66	–72
15	32	25	19	13	6	0	–7	–13	–19	–26	–32	–39	–45	–51	–58	–64	–71	–77
20	30	24	17	11	4	–2	–9	–15	–22	–29	–35	–42	–48	–55	–61	–68	–74	–81
25	29	23	16	9	3	–4	–11	–17	–24	–31	–37	–44	–51	–58	–64	–71	–78	–84
30	28	22	15	8	1	–5	–12	–19	–26	–33	–39	–46	–53	–60	–67	–73	–80	–87
35	28	21	14	7	0	–7	–14	–21	–27	–34	–41	–48	–55	–62	–69	–76	–82	–89
40	27	20	13	6	–1	–8	–15	–22	–29	–36	–43	–50	–57	–64	–71	–78	–84	–91
45	26	19	12	5	–2	–9	–16	–23	–30	–37	–44	–51	–58	–65	–72	–79	–86	–93
50	26	19	12	4	–3	–10	–17	–24	–31	–38	–45	–52	–60	–67	–74	–81	–88	–95
55	25	18	11	4	–3	–11	–18	–25	–32	–39	–46	–54	–61	–68	–75	–82	–89	–97
60	25	17	10	3	–4	–11	–19	–26	–33	–40	–48	–55	–62	–69	–76	–84	–91	–98

Frostbite Times: 30 minutes; 10 minutes; 5 minutes

$$\text{Wind Chill } (^\circ F) = 35.74 + 0.6215T - 35.75(V^{0.16}) + 0.4275T(V^{0.16})$$

Where, T= Air Temperature (°F) V= Wind Speed (mph)

Effective 11/01/01

Figure 22.2 Wind chill chart. (From National Oceanic and Atmospheric Administration, National Weather Service. http://www.nws.noaa.gov/om/winter/windchill.shtml.)

Table 22.1 CLINICAL MANIFESTATIONS OF HYPOTHERMIA

System	Mild Hypothermia (95°F–90°F [35°C–32°C])	Moderate Hypothermia (90°F–82.4°F [32.2°C–28°C])	Severe Hypothermia (<82.4°F [28°C])
Central nervous system	Confusion, slurred speech, impaired judgment, amnesia	Lethargy, hallucinations, loss of papillary reflex, EEG abnormalities	Loss of cerebrovascular regulation, decline in EEG activity, coma, loss of ocular reflex
Cardiovascular system	Tachycardia, increased cardiac output, and systemic vascular resistance	Progressive bradycardia (unresponsiveness), decreased cardiac output, BP, atrial and ventricular arrhythmias, J (Osborn) wave on ECG	Decline in BP and cardiac output, ventricular fibrillation (82.4°F [28°C]) and asystole (68°F [20°C])
Respiratory system	Tachypnea, bronchorrhea	Hypoventilation (decreased RR and tidal volume), decreased oxygen consumption and CO_2 production, loss of cough reflex	Pulmonary edema, apnea
Renal	Cold diuresis	Cold diuresis	Decreased renal perfusion and GFR, oliguria
Hematologic	Increase in hematocrit, decreased platelet and white blood cell counts, coagulopathy, and DIC		
Gastrointestinal		Ileus, pancreatitis, gastric stress ulcers, hepatic dysfunction	
Metabolic/endocrine	Increased metabolic rate, hyperglycemia	Decreased metabolic rate, hyperglycemia or hypoglycemia	
Musculoskeletal	Increased shivering	Decreased shivering (89.6°F [32°C])	Patient appears dead "pseudorigor mortis"

BP, Blood pressure; *DIC,* disseminated intravascular coagulation; *ECG,* electrocardiogram; *EEG,* electroencephalogram; *GFR,* glomerular filtration rate; *RR,* respiratory rate.
From Mellion M. *Sports Medicine Secrets.* 3rd ed. Philadelphia, PA: Hanley & Belfus; 2002.

- Physiologic mechanisms for increasing heat production are much less effective than strategies applied to decrease heat loss.
- Heat loss is primarily prevented with adequate **layering** of clothing.
- Insulation and permeability are important properties of cold weather clothing.
- Most versatile cold weather clothing systems are usually composed of three layers:
  - Inner hydrophobic polyester fabric (e.g., Capilene, Coolmax, Thermax, Thermolite, or Thermostat) that allows wicking of moisture away from the body. Avoid cotton.
  - Middle insulating material can be a second light layer (similar to inner layer fabric) or a heavier layer such as wool and wool/synthetic blends (heavy when wet but excellent insulator even then), pile and fleece (varying weights offer versatility for exercising athletes, fleece replacing pile), synthetic fillers (e.g., Primaloft, Liteloft, Dacron, Hollofill, Quallofil, or Thinsulate), or down (good in cold dry conditions, loses insulating properties when wet); the middle layer can lead to overheating.
  - Outer protective shell that is windproof and water repellant (e.g., newer treated nylons):
    - Newer treated nylons are best because they offer the highest breathability: fibers are tightly woven, and sprays are used to increase water repellency.
    - Laminates such as Gore-Tex and other brand-specific materials designed to mimic Gore-Tex are advertised as "waterproof" and breathable, but the amount of sweat produced during exercise can exceed the capability of the laminate to transmit water vapor.
    - Breathability of the outer layer is inversely proportional to the degree of water repellency and waterproofing; adequate breathability is important during exercise.
- Middle and outer layers should each be slightly larger than the direct inner layer to allow a narrow space for warm air trapping; avoid "tight" layering.
- The primary goal with layering is to stay relatively warm without excessively sweating or overheating, and layers must be shed or added depending on current activity levels and environmental conditions.
- Ventilation ports in certain outer garments may be opened for adequate breathing and are particularly important when using laminates.
- Excessive sweating causes heat loss through increased evaporation and conduction and may affect the insulating property of certain fabrics. This can be avoided with proper layer adjustments during the activity.
- Wind chill can cause dangerously large amounts of heat loss through convection without windproof garments and appropriate insulation adjusted to activity levels.

SPECIAL PROTECTION

- Special protection and other measures to minimize heat loss and injury should be implemented.
- Prevent significant conductive loss by placing a "barrier" between the body and colder objects (e.g., foam or other sleeping pads such as Therma-Rest, wet or dry suits with cold-water exposure, or leather or plastic boots with an inner insulating layer).
- Maintain adequate trunk warmth to minimize vasoconstriction in hands and feet that may result in subsequent cold injury.
- Wear mittens instead of gloves, preferably with a protective and windproof outer shell and an inner insulating layer.
- Prevent radiant heat loss from the head (blood supply to the head is maintained in cold conditions) by wearing an insulating cap or balaclava and by using a hood when needed (high wind or wet weather).
- Protect the exposed skin of the face and ears by using a balaclava or neck gaiter pulled up over the face (neck gaiters also decrease heat loss from relatively superficial, large vessels of the neck).
- Prevent genital injury by wearing undershorts with a windproof front panel.
- Protect eyes (corneal freezing) by using ski goggles.
- Avoid excessive wetness at all times, and if immersed in cold water, minimize movement and pull the body into a "tight" position (assume the HELP posture—**h**eat **e**scape **l**essening

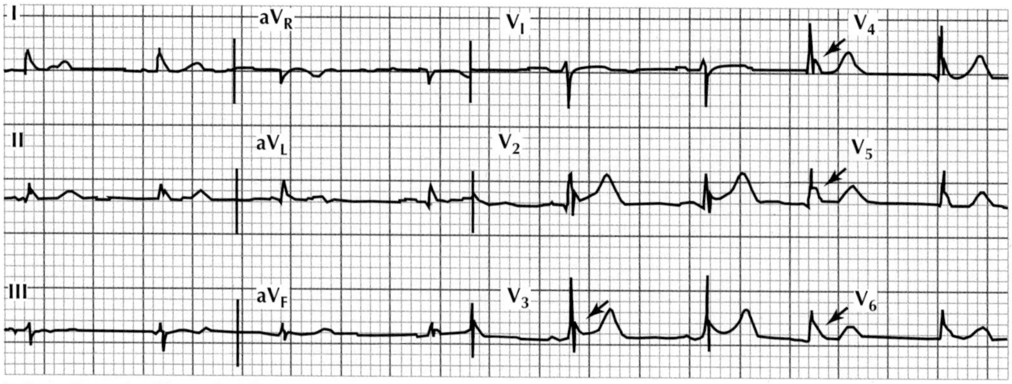
I
aVR
V1
V4
II
aVL
V2
V5
III
aVF
V3
V6

Figure 22.3 Systemic hypothermia. (From Goldberger A. *Clinical Electrocardiography: A Simplified Approach*. 7th ed. Philadelphia: Mosby; 2006.)

posture—which is similar to an "upright fetal" position) to decrease exposed surface area unless close to shore or a boat.
- Adequately warm up before exercising in cold conditions (may warm up indoors or use insulated protective clothing if outdoors).
- Avoid the use of emollients on the face because these have been shown to increase the incidence of frostbite and other cold injuries.

EXTERNAL WARMING SOURCES

See treatment discussion in the "Accidental Hypothermia" section.

SPECIFIC INJURIES

Systemic Cold Injury

Accidental Hypothermia

Definition: Unintentional decline in core body temperature below 95°F (35°C) not the result of organic disease
- **Mild** (95°F–90°F [35°C–32°C])
- **Moderate** (90°F–82°F [<32°C–28°C])
- **Severe** (82°F [<28°C])
- Certain authorities define these values more conservatively. The advanced cardiac life support (ACLS) algorithm for the treatment of hypothermia classifies severe hypothermia as below 86°F (30°C).

Risk factors: Extremes of age, alcohol, CNS depressants, hypothyroidism, hypopituitarism, hypoadrenalism, diabetes mellitus, sepsis, CNS insult (e.g., cerebrovascular accident or trauma), malnutrition, and hypoglycemia

Presentation: Assume hypothermia until proven otherwise when evaluating an athlete with confusion, dysarthria, and ataxia who has been exposed to cold (see Table 22.1). Rectal temperature (estimation of core temperature) and clinical findings establish the definitive diagnosis, but low-reading rectal thermometers are frequently not available. **Low-reading rectal thermometers should be available in first-aid kits during cold-weather athletic events.** The degree of hypothermia can be estimated using clinical observation: quickly note the **level of consciousness** and **presence of shivering.** A conscious individual who is shivering likely has a core temperature above 88°F–90°F (31°C–32°C), whereas a severely confused or obtunded individual who is not shivering likely has a core temperature below 88°F–90°F (31°C–32°C).
- **Mild hypothermia:** Confusion, poor judgment, dysarthria, amnesia, dizziness, apathy and fatigue, mood lability, ataxia, increased shivering, tachycardia, tachypnea, elevated blood pressure, increased urinary frequency (cold diuresis), hyperreflexia, and hyperglycemia
- **Moderate hypothermia:** Lethargy, stupor, occasional unconsciousness; shivering slows, becomes intermittent, and then ceases; hallucinations, loss of pupillary reflex, bradycardia, atrial fibrillation and other arrhythmias, decreased ventricular fibrillation threshold, hypotension, decreased rate and volume of breathing, hyporeflexia or areflexia, muscle rigidity and decreased or absent voluntary motion, paradoxical undressing, and electrocardiographic changes (prolonged P-R, QRS, and Q-Tc intervals, and J [Osborn] wave) (Fig. 22.3).
- **Severe hypothermia:** May appear dead, profound coma, hypotension, respiratory depression, pupils fixed and dilated, severe muscular rigidity, areflexia (even to painful stimuli), atrial arrhythmias common, ventricular fibrillation easily induced with minimal patient movement, asystole, pulseless electrical activity and other arrhythmias, pulmonary edema, oliguria, and coagulopathy
- **Paradoxical undressing:** A conscious, profoundly hypothermic patient undresses, usually when near or just before death. Perception of warmth and cold relies on temperature receptors near the skin surface. When core temperature drops significantly, vasoconstricted vessels in the periphery may suddenly dilate, "fooling" the body into thinking it is warm. Combined with severely impaired consciousness and judgment, the feeling of warmth causes the affected individual to shed clothing. This is a poor prognostic sign.

Treatment:

General principles (all degrees of hypothermia)
- **Preventing further heat loss** is the highest priority.
- Gently *remove* hypothermic individual *from the cold* to a shelter (tent, snow cave, or other natural or constructed shelter), remove wet clothing and *insulate* against further heat loss.
- Insulate using sleeping bags or by using a combination of sleeping bags and a vapor barrier such as a tarp, parka, or plastic bag.
- Minimize conductive heat loss by placing blankets or a sleeping pad between the patient and the ground.
- Affected individual should be kept in a horizontal position to minimize potential orthostatic worsening of hypotension.
- Remove all wet clothes by gently cutting them off.
- Hypothermia should always be treated before frostbite.

Mild hypothermia
- Patients without impaired consciousness or severe confusion and dysarthria should be encouraged to eat warm food and to drink warm sugar- or calorie-containing noncaffeinated fluids to boost morale, supply calories, and curb dehydration.
- Once adequately protected from the cold and well insulated, the affected individual should be allowed to "shiver back to normal" (passive rewarming).
- Exercise is occasionally recommended in individualized circumstances.
- Active external warming measures (see the following discussion) in mild hypothermia with intact shivering response are not likely to significantly increase the core body temperature and are controversial because they may hinder the shivering mechanism.

Moderate and severe hypothermia

- Field management
  - Such patients are **unable to rewarm themselves.**
  - Field management involves preventing further heat loss, stabilizing the patient, and arranging for emergent transport to a medical facility for definitive care.
  - Basic life support principles should be applied. Cautious endotracheal intubation is indicated in patients with significantly impaired consciousness, coma, or respiratory distress.
  - Moderately to severely hypothermic patients should be handled extremely gently because minimal motions may trigger ventricular fibrillation, which is often fatal.
  - When **shivering is absent** in moderately to severely hypothermic patients, some form of **active external rewarming** in addition to **noninvasive active internal rewarming** (e.g., heated humidified oxygen) is probably safe in the field.
  - Humidified warmed oxygen is not likely to have a significant effect on the core temperature but may prevent further heat loss through the airways.
  - Slow administration of warmed intravenous D5 normal saline provides only a small amount of heat, but it may slowly correct intravascular volume depletion and may help stabilize the conduction system of the heart.
  - **Active external rewarming** involves the application of heat directly to the skin. External rewarming requires effective circulation to return peripherally rewarmed blood to the core.
    - Forced heated air devices (e.g., Bair Hugger)
    - Hot packs or bottles placed over high-flow areas such as the neck, axilla, and groin
    - Hot pads or blankets
    - Radiant heat using heat lamps
    - Body-to-body contact
  - Active external rewarming techniques are relatively ineffective for core rewarming compared with active internal rewarming techniques. If used, care must be taken to avoid thermal burns with certain techniques.
  - Minimal warming of the cardiovascular and respiratory systems may help stabilize cardiorespiratory parameters even if the core temperature cannot be significantly increased.
  - Because the core temperature is essentially unaffected or, at best, minimally elevated, complications resulting from rapid rewarming do not usually occur. The amount of core rewarming, if any, achieved using these methods is controversial, but certain studies have claimed this as beneficial.
  - In conclusion, exogenous rewarming may be cautiously instituted in moderately to severely hypothermic patients, particularly if active internal core rewarming is not immediately available.
  - **Afterdrop considerations:**
    - The central perception of warmth caused by warm objects in contact with the body causes decreased vasoconstriction in cold extremities and movement of peripheral blood to the core.
    - Active external rewarming can contribute to **"afterdrop"** in core body temperature in moderately to severely hypothermic patients when blood from the periphery moves to the core and contributes to a further drop in core temperature.
    - There is no strong evidence that supports theoretical massive peripheral vasodilation and subsequent hypotension and shock resulting from exogenous rewarming. Recent studies have suggested that the "afterdrop" observed in temperature is not a true temperature drop and is related to differences in core temperature measuring techniques. The exception may be with whole-body immersion in hot water, which must be avoided in all settings.
- Cardiopulmonary resuscitation (CPR)
  - **CPR is indicated if there is no sign of pulse or breathing after assessing for 30–45 seconds.** It may be extremely difficult to detect pulse or respiration in profoundly hypothermic individuals.
  - **Do not withhold basic life support (BLS) until the victim is rewarmed.** A cardiac monitor should be used if available. Start rescue breaths immediately if respirations are not detected. Begin compressions if there is no pulse or if there is any doubt about whether a pulse is present.
  - If ventricular tachycardia (VT) or ventricular fibrillation (VF) is present, attempt defibrillation. Treat with one shock followed by resumption of CPR. If VT/VF persists, defer further defibrillation attempts, as successful conversion to sinus rhythm may not be possible until patient is rewarmed. Focus on CPR and rewarming.
  - Intravenous (IV) medications should be held at temperatures <86°F (30°C) due to reduced drug metabolism and risk of accumulation of toxic levels in peripheral circulation. Once temperature is 86°F (30°C) or above, medication may be administered (at longer-than-standard intervals), and defibrillation can be repeated as indicated.
  - CPR should not delay transfer to a medical facility for definitive management and should ideally be performed simultaneously with transfer, even if intermittent.
  - No patient should be pronounced dead until he or she is "warm and dead," with a normal core body temperature. The exception to this rule is an injury not compatible with life in a wilderness situation.
- Hospital management
  - Serious cardiovascular, CNS, and acid–base complications may occur with rewarming.
  - All patients should be placed on a cardiac monitor, given warm humidified oxygen, and have intravascular access. Warm D5 normal saline (104°F [40°C]) is administered as indicated to correct dehydration and volume depletion (minimally elevates core temperature, <1°C per hour). Endotracheal and nasogastric tubes and bladder catheters are used in appropriate clinical situations.
  - Appropriate laboratory tests (complete blood count, comprehensive metabolic profile, coagulation studies, consider uncorrected arterial blood gas) must be performed, and close serial monitoring is required. Serum potassium >10 mEq/L in the presence of hypothermia is a strong indicator of death. Electrocardiogram (ECG) and chest radiograph should be performed.
  - Heated humidified oxygen raises the core temperature by 1°C–2°C per hour and may be a useful adjunct to other rewarming methods. Passive external rewarming alone in a warm environment will raise the core temperature by approximately 1.5°C per hour.
  - Active core rewarming techniques deliver direct heat to the body core and are the procedures of choice in severely hypothermic patients and in those with cardiovascular instability or poor perfusion. Temperature monitoring is best accomplished with an esophageal temperature probe.
    - Extracorporeal blood rewarming is the most effective method for active core rewarming and increases core temperature by 1°C–2°C every 3–5 minutes. This can be done by cardiopulmonary bypass, arteriovenous rewarming, venovenous rewarming, or hemodialysis.
    - Other effective methods include peritoneal lavage and closed thoracic lavage (both raise the temperature by 2°C–3°C per hour) if extracorporeal blood rewarming is not available.
    - Less effective methods include gastric, colonic, and bladder irrigation secondary to limited area for heat exchange.

COLD-WATER IMMERSION

- Drowning or fatal cardiac arrhythmia may cause death earlier than hypothermia after cold-water immersion.
- Hypothermia usually requires a significant duration of immersion (30 minutes to 2 hours) to kill a victim. On the other hand, drowning may occur relatively quickly as a result of the cold shock response.
- Sudden exposure to cold water causes an immediate and involuntary gasp that may result in aspiration of water and/or laryngospasm; this is followed by profound hyperventilation that results in respiratory alkalosis and subsequent muscle tetany and cerebral hypoperfusion.
- Breath-holding duration is significantly reduced (kayakers who roll may even have a hard time holding their breath for the duration of the roll).
- Severe tachycardia, increase in blood pressure, and vagal overload may induce lethal cardiac arrhythmias.
- Cold water–induced peripheral vasoconstriction facilitates rapid cooling of extremities and greatly decreases neuromuscular activity, making it almost impossible to tread water (without a flotation device), hold onto a flotation device, signal, or grasp anything (e.g., rescue line or hoist).
- If an arrhythmia does not occur, immersed individuals often drown because of excessive inhalation of water (particularly under turbulent conditions) and failure to initiate or maintain survival performance.

Local Injury

Frostnip

Description: Occurs before tissue freezing when cold induces local vessel constriction

Symptoms: Ice crystals may form on the skin surface, and the skin may appear whitish or pale.

Physical examination: Deeper tissues are soft and pliable, and affected skin is easily thawed by covering the face (with mittens or neck gaiter) or by placing affected hands in armpits or under other garments.

Treatment: Almost instant thawing may be followed by redness, pain, hypersensitivity, and occasionally swelling. Skin often peels a few days later. **Frostnip indicates inadequate protection** and **risky environmental conditions,** and attention should be directed toward preventing frostbite and further cold injury.

Frostbite

Definition: Localized cold injury produced by freezing of tissues. Hands, feet, face (particularly nose), and ears are most frequently affected. Frostbite may occur in any environment where the temperature is below freezing (32°F [0°C]) and is frequently associated with hypothermia.

Risk factors: Environmental risk factors may include cold temperature, wind chill (wind velocity plus temperature), high altitude, high humidity, prolonged exposure, and direct skin contact with conductors such as cold metal, gas, or other liquids. Other risk factors may include previous frostbite, wet or inadequate clothing, dehydration, diminished mental capacity (e.g., drug-induced or other), associated trauma, alcohol use, tobacco use, use of drugs that cause vasoconstriction or alter thermoregulation, and comorbid medical conditions, particularly those that compromise circulation (e.g., atherosclerosis or diabetes mellitus).

Athletes at risk: Any athlete exercising or competing in cold weather, particularly without adequate protection, may sustain frostbite. Alpine and Nordic skiers, mountaineers and climbers, snowshoers, snowboarders, cold-weather distance runners and cyclists, speed skaters, snowmobilers, and players on almost any outdoor (cold weather) team sport (e.g., football, soccer) may suffer from frostbite.

Pathophysiology: Frostbite occurs with tissue freezing, subsequent tissue ischemia and release of inflammatory mediators, and eventual healing or tissue necrosis. The net result of frostbite involves varying degrees of direct cell damage and progressive tissue ischemia. Inflammatory mediators such as prostaglandins, thromboxanes, bradykinin, and histamine likely play critical roles in endothelial injury, edema formation, and arrest of dermal blood flow during all phases.

Pathophysiologic classification: prefreeze, freeze–thaw, vascular stasis, and late ischemic phases

- *Prefreeze:* tissue chilling, alternating vasoconstriction and vasodilation, capillary membrane instability, plasma leakage, and early edema
- *Freeze–thaw:* cyclic vasodilation and vasoconstriction at cold temperatures lead to tissue freezing and partial thawing (causes significant damage); extracellular ice crystal formation is followed by fluid shifts that cause intracellular dehydration and intracellular ice crystal formation; vascular endothelium may encounter microemboli, and arteriovenous shunting bypasses obstruction (leads to severe hypoxia of the affected tissue)
- *Vascular stasis phase:* continued plasma leakage, formation of ice crystals, vasospasm and vasodilation, and shunting; stasis coagulation may be more pronounced than that observed during the earlier stages
- *Late ischemic phase:* characterized by continued tissue ischemia, vascular thrombosis, arteriovenous shunting, autonomic dysfunction, denaturation of tissue proteins, and tissue necrosis and gangrene

Clinical classification: Historically, frostbite is classified into four categories: first-, second-, third-, and fourth-degree frostbite. A more clinically practical classification of **superficial** (previously first- and second-degree) and **deep** (previously third- and fourth-degree) frostbite is now more frequently used by clinicians.

- *Superficial frostbite injuries* involve only the skin, and permanent tissue loss almost never occurs.
- *Deep frostbite injuries* involve the skin and underlying tissues, which may include muscles, nerves, vessels, bone, and cartilage, and it is almost always associated with permanent tissue loss.
- It is important to realize that most frostbite injuries appear the same at initial evaluation (unless thawing is initiated) and that the *classification of frostbite is applied when tissue changes become evident after rewarming.*

Presentation:

- Frostnip is a mild form of frostbite before tissue freezing. Appropriate management of frostnip decreases the risk of a more severe injury.
- **Initial freezing:** coldness, numbness, clumsiness, and pain in affected extremity.
- As freezing progresses, pain disappears, and the affected body part turns stiff and hard.
- Typically, all degrees of frostbite initially present with paleness, coldness, and firmness of affected tissue.
- The affected body part may also appear yellowish, mottled blue, and waxy.
- Initial tissue pliability may indicate superficial frostbite, whereas frozen solid tissue without pliability usually indicates deep frostbite.
- As tissue thaws with **rewarming,** signs and symptoms follow a relatively predictable pattern that illustrates the severity of tissue injury.
- Numbness and throbbing pain occur with tissue thawing.
- *Superficial frostbite:* hyperemia, increased sensation, and subsequent edema and blisters filled with clear or yellow fluid (Fig. 22.4A).

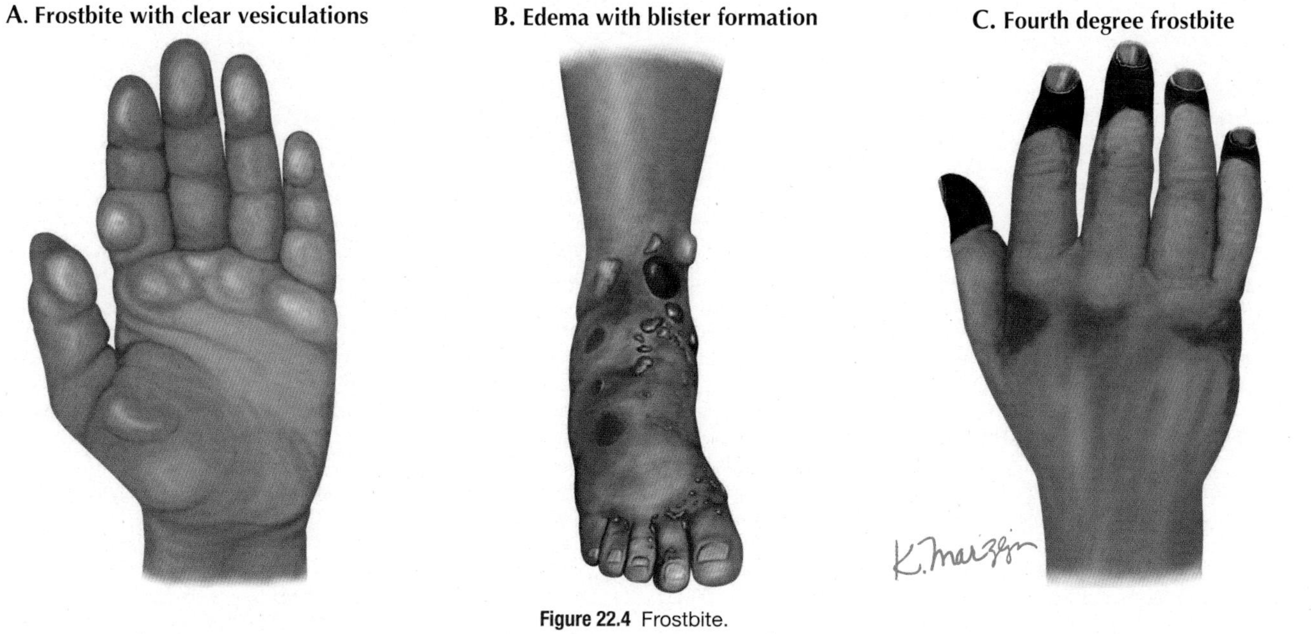
A. Frostbite with clear vesiculations
B. Edema with blister formation
C. Fourth degree frostbite
K. Marzen

Figure 22.4 Frostbite.

- *Less severe deep frostbite:* hemorrhagic blisters form and eschars form after blisters desquamate (Fig. 22.4B).
- *Severe deep frostbite:* no blebs or blisters form, edema is minimal (particularly proximal to injury), the affected body part lacks sensation, skin initially turns dark reddish and purple and eventually black, and mummification and autoamputation may occur weeks after injury (Fig. 22.4C).
- Mummification is the formation of a line of demarcation between viable and necrotic tissue.
- Progression of events: edema usually develops a few hours after thawing, blisters form within 24 hours, eschars may form over affected tissue after 1–2 weeks, and mummification may occur in 3–6 weeks.

Treatment:

General considerations: In-field treatment of frostbite should be balanced against time for evacuation and available treatment facilities. Frostbite is best rewarmed in an appropriate medical facility under strictly controlled conditions. The longer the tissue stays frozen, the greater the tissue damage. Therefore, certain experts recommend rapid in-field rewarming (provided appropriate equipment is available) if evacuation is not imminent (within a few hours) and if the affected body part can be absolutely protected from refreezing (more significant tissue damage may occur with refreezing after thawing). Spontaneous thawing may be allowed under the aforementioned circumstances if equipment is not available for rapid rewarming. As a last resort, individuals with frostbitten feet may walk to safety, but they must realize that there is an increased risk of fracture and soft tissue damage.

In-field treatment

- The *best treatment is prevention.* Adequate protection and appropriate planning minimize exposure of skin to cold environmental conditions.
- Continuously monitor tissue status in cold conditions, particularly if numbness is present, and seek safe conditions with any warning signs of frostbite.
- Individuals exposed to cold should:
  - Wear mittens instead of gloves
  - Ensure adequate trunk insulation and layering (prevents peripheral vasoconstriction)
  - Keep head, face, and neck covered
  - Avoid getting/staying wet (via exposure or perspiration)
  - Avoid tight footwear and clothing
  - Avoid prolonged exposure to cold
  - Avoid using tobacco, alcohol, and vasoconstrictive drugs
  - Maintain adequate hydration and caloric intake
  - Avoid direct skin contact with cold conductive substances such as metal or gasoline
- Avoid cold-protecting ointments or emollients
  - Application of ointments or emollients, particularly to the face and ears, is a traditional technique believed by many to protect against frostbite. Use of ointments is particularly common in women and children of Finland, where the incidence of frostbite is high.
  - The use of ointments may be a considerable risk factor for developing frostbite, particularly of the face and ears. Ointments at best provide a negligible thermal insulation effect. They create a subjective skin-warming perception during acute cold exposure that may contribute to a false sense of safety. The net result is an increased incidence of frostbite, probably resulting from neglect of effective protective measures.
- All frostbitten individuals should be evacuated to an appropriate medical setting as soon as possible.
- Ibuprofen or other anti-inflammatory medications should be administered (inhibits inflammatory mediators involved in tissue injury).
- Tight and/or wet garments should be removed and replaced with dry insulating garments that protect the affected body part from further exposure.
- Affected extremities should be adequately padded.
- Oral hydration should be encouraged.
- If equipment is available, certain experts feel that rapid rewarming may be performed during transport if transport time to a definitive treatment facility is minimal.
- Avoid tissue massage and use of dry or radiant heat.

Definitive treatment: Rapid rewarming of frozen tissue

- Rapid rewarming protocols are based on the work of McCauley and colleagues.
- Frostbite patients should be admitted to a specialized unit, if available. Affected body parts should be rapidly rewarmed in warm water (104°F–108°F [40°C–42°C]) for 15–30 minutes or until thawing is complete.
- Active motion during rewarming is helpful, but massage should be avoided.

- White blisters may be selectively debrided at the discretion of the treatment provider; hemorrhagic blisters should be left intact.
- Affected body parts should be elevated, and splinting may be used as indicated.
- Antitetanus prophylaxis, ibuprofen or other anti-inflammatory medicines, and narcotic analgesics are administered as indicated.
- Empiric antibiotics are not routinely recommended
- Adequate intravascular hydration should be maintained.
- The saying "Frostbite in January, amputate in July" illustrates that surgical debridement of severely frostbitten tissue is normally reserved as late treatment of frostbite, after the demarcation line between viable and necrotic or gangrenous tissue is clear. Complete injury demarcation may take 1–3 months.
- Early surgical intervention is reserved for escharotomy and fasciotomy, as indicated for circulatory compromise and compartment syndrome.
- Tissue plasminogen activator (TPA) can decrease amputation rates. Intravenous or intraarterial TPA should be considered within 24 hours of rewarming for severe injuries without contraindications.
- The use of technetium bone scanning (scintigraphy) within the first few days after injury may help predict eventual tissue demarcation by identifying deep tissue and bone infarction but fails to identify the condition of surrounding, potentially viable tissues. Magnetic resonance imaging (MRI) and magnetic resonance angiography (MRA) show promise because they allow direct visualization of surrounding tissue and may thus facilitate a more accurate early assessment of the line of demarcation between viable and ischemic tissue.

Long-term sequelae: Significant tissue and limb loss may occur with deep frostbites. Other morbidities may include permanent cold sensitivity and susceptibility to cold injury, sensory loss, tingling and paresthesias, hyperhidrosis, chronic pain, growth plate disturbances (most common, phalanges in children), osteoarthritis, and heterotopic calcification.

Chilblains

Description: Also referred to as *pernio*, chilblains ("cold sores") are characterized by tissue injury that may involve localized erythema, cyanosis, plaques, nodules, and occasionally in more severe cases, vesicles, bullae, and ulceration after *pronounced nonfreezing cold-induced vasoconstriction.*

Pathophysiology: May be related to vascular hypersensitivity, sympathetic instability, and subsequent lymphocytic vasculitis.

Symptoms: Symptoms of intense pruritis, burning paresthesias, and skin changes may occur 12–14 hours after cold exposure.

Treatment: Includes anti-inflammatory medication, gentle rewarming, dry bandaging, and elevation to minimize swelling

Trench Foot

Description: Otherwise known as *immersion foot*, trench foot involves tissue (e.g., muscles, nerves, and/or vessels) injury secondary to prolonged vasoconstriction and subsequent ischemia from *prolonged exposure to nonfreezing cold* and *wet conditions.*

Pathophysiology: May share a common pathophysiology with chilblains; progresses through prehyperemic, hyperemic, and posthyperemic phases.

Symptoms: Occur after days of exposure to cold and wet conditions and include painful paresthesias, numbness, and initial erythema, followed by pallor, mottling, and swelling.

Complications: Vesiculation, ulceration, and gangrene may occur.

Treatment: Includes anti-inflammatory medications and keeping affected extremity dry, warm, protected, and elevated.

Prognosis: Lifelong cold sensitivity, and occasionally pain, is common after injury.

Miscellaneous Cold Injuries

COLD-INDUCED BRONCHOSPASM

Description: Cold may induce *bronchospasm*, particularly in asthmatics.

Risk factors: Most frequently affects athletes who exercise or compete in cold, dry conditions such as ice hockey and winter outdoor aerobic activities (e.g., running, cycling, and cross country skiing)

Treatment: May include pre-exercise warm-up in a warm environment and/or pretreatment with beta-agonists, mast cell stabilizers, or leukotriene modifiers

COLD-INDUCED URTICARIA AND/OR ANAPHYLAXIS

Description: Most frequently affects athletes during pre-exercise warm-up in cold conditions.

Presentation: Athletes present with wheals, hives, or pruritis; angioedema may be present, but true anaphylaxis involving laryngeal edema and hypotension is rare.

Prevention: Achieved with appropriate clothing and avoidance of cold-water activities.

Treatment: Acute treatment may include antihistamines, and epinephrine administration may be required if anaphylaxis occurs. Prophylaxis using antihistamines (both H1 and H2 blockers may be used), the tricyclic antidepressant doxepin, and/or leukotriene modifiers is occasionally effective.

RAYNAUD PHENOMENON

Description: Vasospastic disorder characterized by initial pallor (ischemia secondary to vasoconstriction) followed by hyperemia (rebound vasodilation) of the digits (fingers most common) after cold exposure and/or emotional stress

Pathophysiology: May be primary idiopathic (Raynaud disease) or secondary (Raynaud phenomenon or syndrome) to various disorders

Presentation: The initial "white" ischemic phase may be followed by a "blue" cyanotic phase before the "red" hyperemic phase begins.

Treatment: Acute treatment includes warming the affected extremity and addressing the underlying disorders.

Prevention: May be achieved by avoiding direct cold exposure, ensuring adequate trunk insulation (minimizes peripheral vasoconstriction), wearing mittens instead of gloves, and using appropriate footwear; prophylaxis using vasodilating medications (e.g., calcium channel blockers and phosphodiesterase inhibitors) may be attempted if other primary preventive measures fail

COLD AGGLUTININ DISEASE

Pathophysiology: Usually develops after an infection and may follow *Mycoplasma* infections or infectious mononucleosis in athletes; may also be idiopathic or associated with various other disorders

Symptoms: Symptoms of cyanosis, mottling, numbness, and pain in exposed body parts may occur when cold-activated IgM antibodies agglutinate red blood cells.

Treatment: Initially includes warming the affected body part and protecting from further exposure to cold

COLD-INDUCED RHINITIS

Description: Occurs in athletes exposed to cold air (e.g., skiers); it is a form of nonallergic, occasionally referred to as vasomotor, rhinitis that has minimal clinical significance and resolves after removal from the cold environment

Treatment: Ipratropium nasal spray may be administered if an athlete prefers treatment.

RECOMMENDED READINGS

Available online.

ALTITUDE TRAINING AND COMPETITION 23

Benjamin D. Levine • Robert F. Chapman • Mikaela C. Gabler

ALTITUDE ENVIRONMENT

- Barometric pressure is reduced at high altitudes, with a parallel decrease in inspired partial pressure of oxygen (P_IO_2); thus, **hypobaric hypoxia is the most prominent physiologic manifestation at high altitudes.** Fig. 23.1 shows the accepted terminology for the range of terrestrial altitudes, as well as the magnitude of effects on selected outcome variables.
- Temperature decreases at a rate of approximately 6.5°C per 1000 m.
- Other features include dry air (increasing the risk of dehydration), decrease in air density and therefore air resistance (marked effects in high-velocity sports such as cycling or speed skating and flight characteristics of objects; i.e., golf, baseball, archery, or soccer; or people; i.e., ski jumping, or even ice skating), and increase in the amount of ultraviolet light (4% per 300 m), which increases the risk of sunburn.
  - Therefore, athletes must cope with hypoxia, cold, and dehydration and yet maintain maximal performance.
  - Timing of altitude exposure and degree of acclimatization are critical to successful outcomes.
  - Physiologic adaptation to high altitude may be beneficial. Altitude training is frequently used by elite athletes in an attempt to improve sea-level performance, but the manner in which it is completed will considerably affect the outcomes.
- In a laboratory or home-based setting at or near sea level, hypoxia can be simulated by reducing the fraction of inspired O_2 by adding exogenous N_2 (termed *normobaric hypoxia* [NH]). This exposure is in contrast to terrestrial altitude, or hypobaric hypoxia (HH), where the ambient pressure is reduced.
- The method of hypoxia utilized (NH or HH) is relevant to consider, as some physiologic responses that affect performance or adaptive function may differ between methods, despite the partial pressure of O_2 being the same (e.g., oxygen saturation is lower and oxidative stress is higher in HH; acute mountain sickness [AMS] is more severe in HH; plasma volume decline and diuresis are greater in NH). It must be emphasized, though, that most of these differences between HH and NH are small and of questionable physiologic significance; the most prominent and physiologic important stressor at altitude is the reduction in partial pressure of oxygen. Athletes who choose to use home-based methods of NH versus travel to terrestrial altitude will need to carefully consider exposure time and level of hypoxia if the goal is to achieve equivalent erythropoietic and performance improvements (see "Altitude Dose Recommendation" section later).

EFFECT OF ALTITUDE ON EXERCISE

- *Oxygen cascade* is the term used to describe the physiologic effects of altitude on exercise: Oxygen moves from the **environment** (determined by the altitude achieved) to the **alveoli** (function of ventilation and hypoxic ventilatory response) across the **pulmonary capillary bed** (limited by diffusion) to be transported by the **cardiovascular system** (function of cardiac output and hemoglobin concentration) and diffused into **skeletal muscles** (depends on capillarity and biochemical state of muscles) to be used by muscle **mitochondria** (influenced by oxidative enzyme activity) for aerobic respiration and adenosine triphosphate (ATP) production.
- **Altitude-induced hypoxia reduces the amount of oxygen available to perform physical activity.**
  - Maximal aerobic power ($\dot{V}O_2$ max) is reduced by approximately 1% for every 100 m above 1500 m in nonathletic but healthy individuals.
  - For endurance-trained athletes, this effect is even greater—reductions in $\dot{V}O_2$ max and performance can be identified at altitudes as low as 500 m and are linear (decrease of approximately 0.5%–1.5% for every 100-m increase in altitude) at altitudes ranging from 300 m to 3000 m.
    - Occurs because of diffusion limitation in both lung and skeletal muscles exacerbated by high pulmonary and systemic blood flow (cardiac output) in endurance athletes; severe hypoxemia can develop even during submaximal exercise (e.g., oxyhemoglobin saturation [SaO_2] <80% in an elite male runner at a pace of 6 min/mile at 2700 m).
    - This magnitude of $\dot{V}O_2$ max and performance decline at altitude, particularly in endurance-trained athletes, shows substantial interindividual variability. Data from several studies and other reports indicate the ability to maintain SaO_2 as a primary factor.
  - **During submaximal exercise at altitude, ventilation, lactate, and heart rate are greater for the same absolute work rate, which increases the sensations of dyspnea and fatigue.**
    - As a result of this increased rate of perceived exertion and dyspnea, training velocity (runners), training power output (e.g., cyclists), and $\dot{V}O_2$ max are lower during training at altitude.
    - Heart rate and lactate responses to training at altitude are the same as training at sea level at the same relative effort, which complicates the determination of appropriate training zones/paces at altitude.
  - **Peak** blood lactate concentration is **lower** in individuals acclimatized to high altitude (termed *lactate paradox*), although this outcome is controversial and depends on nuances of workload and training altitude.
- Competitive performance outcomes at altitude, compared with that at sea level, is strongly influenced by the amount of aerodynamic drag on the body and the primary energy system utilized.
  - **Lower-velocity events** (e.g., distance running): in event distances requiring high levels of aerobic power (>2 minutes), performance is impaired at altitude because of a reduction in skeletal muscle oxygen delivery. In event distances requiring higher sustained power outputs (30 seconds to 2 minutes), performance may or may not be impaired at altitude, depending on the interplay of oxidative and glycolytic energy pathways.
  - **Higher-velocity events** (i.e., sprint running, cycling, or speed skating): the reduced air resistance at altitude actually results in an improvement in performance, despite systemic hypoxemia. In sprint events requiring short bursts of high-intensity activity (≤30 seconds), ATP production is not primarily dependent on oxygen transport. In high-velocity events lasting >2 minutes, the decline in aerobic power with reduced skeletal muscle oxygen delivery is effectively smaller than the influence of reduced air resistance. For example, as of October 2020, every world record in speed skating events from 500 m to 10,000 m in length was set at altitudes >1200 m, despite an expected reduction in $\dot{V}O_2$ max at these altitudes.

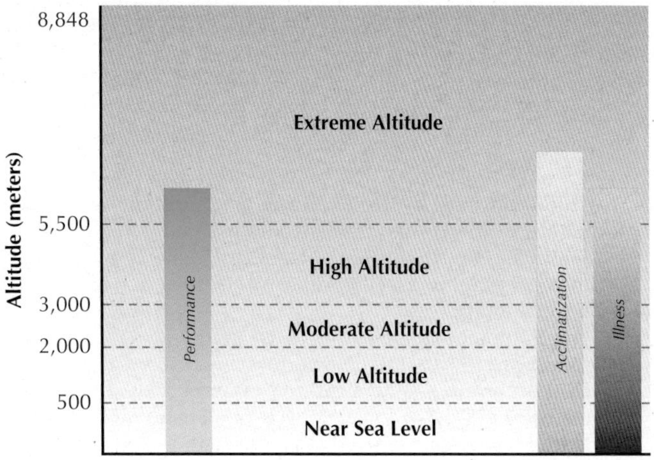
8,848
Extreme Altitude
Altitude (meters)
5,500
High Altitude
3,000
Moderate Altitude
2,000
Low Altitude
500
Near Sea Level
Performance
Acclimatization
Illness

Figure 23.1 Accepted altitude definitions and ranges, from 2007 FIFA Consensus Conference. The amount of shading in the vertical bars represents the magnitude of variable (as influenced by altitude), with darker shading indicating a high level. (Data from Bärtsch P, Saltin B, Dvorak J. Federation Internationale de Football Association. Consensus statement on playing football at different altitude. *Scand J Med Sci Sports.* 2008;18[S1]:96–99.)

ACCLIMATIZATION PROCESS

- Chronic exposure to altitude stimulates acclimatization, which includes adaptations that improve **submaximal** work performance at altitude. Individual physiologic components of acclimatization have unique time frames of response, ranging from minutes to hours, days, months, or even generations. In addition, the rate and completeness of acclimatization are dependent on the altitude of residence (i.e., the hypoxic dose). For example, at high and extreme altitudes (≥4000 m), $\dot{V}O_2$ max never returns to sea-level values despite prolonged acclimatization. At low altitudes (<2000 m), the maximal oxygen uptake may approach sea-level values after 1–2 weeks in nonathletic individuals.
  - Increases in alveolar ventilation and reductions in mixed venous oxygen content minimize the decline in exercise capacity at altitude—**this begins immediately on ascent.**
  - Hyperventilation causes respiratory alkalosis, which stimulates renal excretion of bicarbonate and loss of plasma volume **over the first week** to normalize acid–base balance.
  - Ventilation at rest (and to some extent during exercise) at altitude is influenced by the sensitivity of peripheral chemoreceptors; this hypoxic ventilatory response (HVR) is highly individualistic, with elite endurance athletes commonly showing blunted HVRs in comparison with untrained individuals. At low and moderate altitudes, a high HVR may affect the magnitude of dyspnea; at high and extreme altitudes, a high HVR may be critical for maintenance of even basic levels of physical activity and even survival.
  - Sympathetic activation acutely (minutes to hours) increases heart rate and cardiac output so that oxygen delivery to tissues remains close to sea-level values at rest and during submaximal activity. By **2–3 weeks,** systemic and regional blood flow return to sea-level values as oxygenation improves. However, sympathetic activity continues to increase and may reach extraordinary levels, particularly at higher altitudes (>4000 m).
  - The oxygen-carrying capacity of blood increases as a result of the increase in hemoglobin and hematocrit: **early** (1–2 days) increases result from plasma volume reduction; **later** (weeks to months) increases result from increases in red cell mass. **This critical adaptation offsets the reduction in atmospheric oxygen availability, thereby restoring oxygen transport to normal sea-level values.**
  - Peripheral uptake of oxygen by skeletal muscles is facilitated by increased capillary density, mitochondrial number, myoglobin concentration, and 2,3-diphosphoglycerate (2,3-DPG), although these local changes may take weeks or months to manifest and are not universally observed.
  - The buffering capacity of skeletal muscles may be increased as well.

FAILURE OF ACCLIMATIZATION: HIGH-ALTITUDE ILLNESS AND OVERTRAINING

Acute Mountain Sickness

- With moderate or higher altitudes (>2000 m) and rapid ascent rates (>300 m sleeping altitude per day above 3000 m), a maladaptive state called AMS may develop.
- Symptoms include headache, nausea, anorexia, fatigue, and difficulty sleeping.
- Symptoms are usually mild and self-limited; rest and analgesics are sufficiently effective treatment.
- There is no evidence that competitive athletes are at any greater risk of developing AMS than nonathletes, although exercise may exacerbate the development of AMS, and physical activity should be appropriately reduced in symptomatic individuals.
- For patients who do not improve with rest, supplemental oxygen or descent to lower altitude virtually always results in prompt symptom relief.
- Other effective treatments include acetazolamide, dexamethasone, and simulated descent with a portable hyperbaric bag.
- AMS is best prevented by limiting the rate of ascent, allowing for rest or acclimatization days, maintaining adequate hydration, avoiding alcohol or sedatives during the early acclimatization phase, and limiting training volume and intensity during the first few days at altitude.
- Use of drugs to prevent AMS is discouraged in endurance athletes who are going to moderate altitude (<3000 m) unless a clear history of recurrent AMS is reported.
- The most frequently used drug is acetazolamide, which may be effective at low doses (125 mg at night or twice daily). However, diuretics, including acetazolamide, are on the World Anti-Doping Agency banned list as masking agents. Dexamethasone is probably more potent but is also banned as a steroid.

Severe High-Altitude Illness

- In some individuals, AMS may progress to or be associated with more severe and life-threatening forms, including high-altitude pulmonary edema (HAPE) or high-altitude cerebral edema (HACE).
- **HAPE** is characterized by **dyspnea at rest,** cyanosis, severe hypoxemia, and noncardiogenic pulmonary edema.
- **HACE** is characterized by vomiting, **ataxia,** reduction in level of consciousness, and, in some cases, frank coma.
- Both of these syndromes can quickly result in death. **Immediate descent is mandatory.** High-flow supplemental oxygen or a portable hyperbaric bag, if available, may be useful adjunctive therapy while descending or if descent is delayed.
- Both HAPE and HACE are rare at moderate altitudes to which most athletes are exposed (<0.1%), although occurrence in athletes at low to moderate altitude (<2000 m) should initiate a search for congenital abnormalities of the pulmonary circulation.
- Medications that lower pulmonary arterial pressure may be used for adjunctive treatment of HAPE (this is less effective than descent and oxygen). Nifedipine has been most extensively studied and is effective both for treatment and prophylaxis. Phosphodiesterase inhibitors (e.g., sildenafil or tadalafil) are also beneficial, but they may exacerbate AMS. Very recent studies suggest that dexamethasone is effective at preventing both

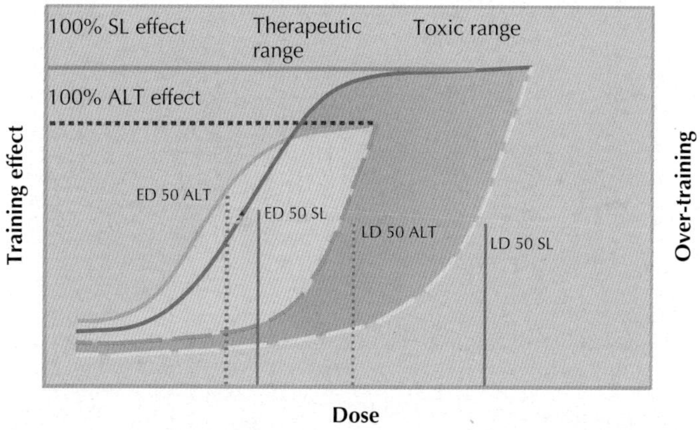
100% SL effect
Therapeutic range
Toxic range
100% ALT effect
ED 50 ALT
ED 50 SL
LD 50 ALT
LD 50 SL
Training effect
Over-training
Dose

Figure 23.2 Toxic/therapeutic range of exercise training: The effect of high altitude. Although the mechanical stress of exercise is likely to be less at high altitudes because of the reduction in training speed, the metabolic stress may well be greater, at least with regard to the effect of hypoxia on the central nervous system. Thus, exercise training at high altitudes narrows the toxic/therapeutic range of exercise, possibly enhancing the training effect, but also increasing the risk of toxicity. *ALT,* Altitude; *ED,* effective dose at which 50% of the maximal response is achieved; *LD,* lethal dose at which 50% of the maximal toxicity is achieved; *SL,* sea level.

AMS and HAPE and is the most effective adjunctive therapy for HACE. Drug treatment should be considered in athletes only if oxygen is unavailable or descent/evacuation is delayed. A staged slow ascent is the most effective preventive strategy, and it sidesteps the need to use banned substances for prevention.

Overtraining

- Another potentially serious problem with training at altitude is the increased risk of overtraining.
- A comparison between exercise training and administration of medication, as shown in Fig. 23.2, is helpful. Every medication has a specific dose–response relationship, accompanied by a toxic/therapeutic range. These parameters define the optimal dose and frequency of administration to maximize benefits but minimize side effects and toxicity. Exercise can be conceived as medication (so-called "exercise is medicine"): training response is proportional to volume and intensity (ED 50), but too much exercise results in clear toxic effects of musculoskeletal injury and systemic effects of overtraining (LD 50).
- **Overtraining may be precipitated by:**
  - **Inappropriately hard workouts:** Training at too high of a workload because of narrowed training zones and/or athlete inexperience; recovery training sessions/gentle workouts completed at too high of a workload
  - **Inadequate recovery:** Dehydration, sleep disturbances, and too short recovery times (either between workouts or between intervals within a hard workout)

PRACTICAL STRATEGIES FOR IMPLEMENTING ALTITUDE TRAINING

From a practical perspective, critical issues for athletes and coaches are **"indications"** for altitude training, and if indicated, use of an appropriate training model and application of an appropriate "dose" of both altitude exposure and training

Indications

Which Athletes Should Use Altitude Training?

- Athletes in events where $\dot{V}O_2$ max is important for performance (i.e., endurance athletes in events lasting >2–3 minutes); sprint athletes may benefit from (1) neuromuscular/kinesthetic training because of faster speeds allowed by reduced air resistance and (2) improvements in aerobic capacity, which may enhance overall training volumes and quality upon return to sea level because of enhanced recovery between efforts in interval training.
- Athletes who compete at altitude because appropriate acclimatization will mitigate performance declines at altitude.
- Because a supervised training camp is a powerful stimulus for training, even in elite athletes, already well-trained athletes with general and competition-specific fitness are most likely to obtain benefits from altitude.
- **Altitude training is no substitute for a focused, well-designed training program with appropriate rest and nutrition.**
- Athletes who respond best to altitude training exhibit a robust and sustained increase in erythropoietin (EPO) concentrations at altitude and a strong ability to maintain velocity and oxygen flux during training. These responses may be genetically determined.

Which Athletes Should Not Use Altitude Training?

- Team sports that depend more on strategy and technique for success (e.g., water polo, baseball, field hockey, or handball) are unlikely to derive much benefit from altitude training for sea-level performance. However, recent data suggest that repeated sprint training in hypoxia may be beneficial in improving fitness and performance in certain team sports like soccer.
- Sports that depend on normal air resistance for fine motor skills (e.g., basketball, archery, tennis, or soccer) are likely to be impaired by altitude training; such sports may require an adjustment period both at altitude and on return to sea level to compensate for differences in projectile movement through air at altitude.
- Swimming is most controversial. Recent data suggest a performance benefit with the live high–train low model of altitude training (see the "Altitude Training Models" section later), even during shorter events that are not traditionally thought to be limited by oxygen delivery. Because of extremely low mechanical efficiency, performance in swimming is more strongly tied to **biomechanics** than **physiology.**
- Iron-deficient athletes should not engage in altitude training (see the "Nutritional Factors" section later).
- Athletes with a small and brief increase in EPO at altitude and those who cannot maintain training speeds even at low altitudes are least likely to respond well.
- Inflammatory cytokines have been suggested to impair EPO production, so athletes with injury or infection may need to reconsider altitude training or delay until recovered.

Altitude Training Models/Best-Practice Recommendations

- For competitions at altitude:
  - **Acclimatization** is critical and clearly improves performance **at altitude.**
  - Adequate time should be allowed for acclimatization to minimize altitude-mediated performance decrements. Evidence suggests that performance is worst on arrival, improves incrementally over a period of approximately 14–19 days, and does not significantly improve beyond that time point (out to 28 days).
  - If adequate time for acclimatization is not possible, anecdotal experience among athletes suggests that competing immediately (i.e., within 2–4 hours of arrival) at altitude may be best because it may minimize negative effects of plasma volume loss or poor sleep at altitude. Recent laboratory data utilizing simulated altitude (NH) indicate mean cycling performance

is not different between arriving at altitude 2 hours before a race and overnight (14 hours before the race). However, there were clear individual responses that suggest *some* individuals may see an outsized benefit dependent on the timing of altitude arrival.

- Recent studies have suggested that for low-altitude competitions (500–2000 m), living at altitudes higher than that of the competition may be worse for competitive performance than living at competition altitude, unless acclimatization for at least 19 days is possible.

- For competitions at sea level:
  - Concurrent living **and** training at altitude has not been shown to improve performance at sea level; this is likely because of a reduced training effect at altitude (i.e., training slower at a lower oxygen flux).
  - **Living at altitude and training as close to sea level as possible (known as *living high–training low*) does improve sea-level performance.** Additional iterations and improvements of this model have shown that only completing high-intensity workouts at low altitude (i.e., remaining at moderate altitude for gentle/recovery workouts) produces the same performance outcomes as completing all workouts at low altitude.
  - A recent meta-analysis reported mean increases in aerobic power of approximately 4.0% following application of the live high–train low model of altitude training, while classical altitude training (live high–train high) produced a nonsignificant change in aerobic power of 0.9% in subelite and 1.6% in elite athletes.

Altitude Dose Recommendations (for Improving Performance at Sea Level)

- The variables that influence the "dose" at altitudes are critical in the amount of sea-level performance enhancement experienced with live high–train low altitude training.
- **How high to live:** Locations that are 2200–2700 m above sea level will maximize acclimatization and minimize complications. Living lower may not provide an adequate erythropoietic stimulus, whereas living higher adds components of acclimatization that negatively affect performance (e.g., poor sleep, AMS, and greater ventilatory work during exercise). Simulated altitude techniques, such as sleeping in a nitrogen-enriched environment to simulate hypoxia of high altitude, may promote similar benefits of terrestrial altitude living; **however, hypoxic exposure of >12–14 hours/day may be required** in most individuals to significantly increase hemoglobin mass, and excessive bedrest must be avoided.
- **How long to reside at altitude:** EPO levels increase acutely, are clearly still elevated after 2 weeks, and return to sea-level values by 4 weeks. Thus, a minimum of 3–4 weeks appears necessary to develop sufficient acclimatization and augmented red cell mass, particularly for competition at sea level. "Intermittent" hypoxic exposures ranging from a few minutes, on and off, to up to 3 hours at extremely high altitudes have no benefits for sea-level performance.
- **How high to train: High-intensity training:** For workouts that are faster than lactate threshold/maximal steady-state pace, best practice is to complete the workout at as low an altitude as possible, preferably <1500 m. **Low-intensity training:** Can be performed at an altitude that minimizes the logistical travel burden to low altitude; however, **low-intensity training must be performed at a relatively easy pace to prevent overtraining. Careful monitoring of heart rate and/or blood lactate during training may help ensure the correct training pace.**
- **When to compete on return to sea level:** Emerging scientific and anecdotal data suggest competing either immediately on return (<72 hours after return to sea level) or after 2–3 weeks of sea-level training. Competing immediately allows the athlete to take advantage of the highest levels of hemoglobin mass but does include the potential negative effects of higher amounts of respiratory muscle activity from ventilatory acclimatization effects. On the other hand, competing after 2–3 weeks of sea-level training may facilitate enhanced chronic training effects, secondary to increased oxygen delivery to skeletal muscles at sea level. Athletes anecdotally report feeling "flat" or "off" when competing during a window of approximately 3–14 days after return, but there is no clear evidence to support this.

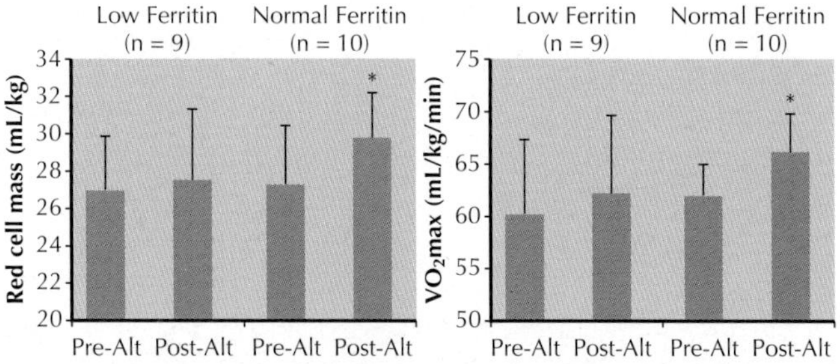
Low Ferritin (n = 9)
Normal Ferritin (n = 10)
Red cell mass (mL/kg)
34
32
30
28
26
24
22
20
Pre-Alt
Post-Alt
Pre-Alt
Post-Alt
*
Low Ferritin (n = 9)
Normal Ferritin (n = 10)
VO2max (mL/kg/min)
75
70
65
60
55
50
Pre-Alt
Post-Alt
Pre-Alt
Post-Alt
*

Figure 23.3 Red cell mass *(left)* and maximal oxygen uptake *(right)* measured before and after altitude training camp (4 weeks at 2500 m) in groups of athletes with low serum ferritin (women, <20 ng/mL; men, <30 ng/mL) and normal serum ferritin upon departure for altitude* significantly different from prealtitude measurement; $P < 0.05$. (Data from Okazaki K, Stray-Gundersen J, Chapman RF, Levine BD. Iron insufficiency diminishes the erythropoietic response to moderate altitude exposure. *J Appl Physiol.* 2019;127:1569–1578.)

Nutritional Factors

- Nutritional factors, particularly iron stores, play a critical role in the ability to respond to altitude training.
- Numerous athletes (both male and female) exhibit reduced iron stores based on low serum ferritin. Such athletes are unable to increase their $\dot{V}O_2$ max and the volume of red cell mass (blood volume – plasma volume), despite an acute and sustained increase in EPO; thus, they are unable to obtain the primary potential benefits of altitude acclimatization (Fig. 23.3).
- Simple measurement of hemoglobin concentration is inadequate for determining iron stores because of the outsized effect of hydration status on this measure. Similarly, measurement of serum iron is inadequate because it does not reflect bone marrow iron stores. Moreover, because iron is a critical moiety in myoglobin and in mitochondrial cytochromes, iron deficiency may not only compromise oxygen-carrying capacity but also inhibit oxygen extraction (arteriovenous O_2 difference) and reduce O_2 flux, thereby limiting $\dot{V}O_2$ max and performance even in nonanemic athletes. Before initiation altitude training of any duration, iron stores (measured as serum ferritin) must be normal (women, minimally >20 ng/mL; men, >30 ng/mL; though a goal of >50 ng/mL for all would be reasonable).
- High doses of oral iron (150–400 mg elemental iron daily) are usually required to maintain ferritin levels during altitude training. Even athletes with normal iron stores at the start of an altitude training program experience a rapid decline in serum ferritin levels at altitude and must be supplemented and closely monitored.
- Athletes should have serum ferritin measured and commence iron supplementation 2–3 weeks before altitude exposure to have adequate time to normalize iron stores, if deficient, and maximize the erythropoietic benefits of altitude training.
- Smaller, more frequent doses of oral iron (e.g., multiple doses per day) will likely minimize gastrointestinal distress. However, iron intake causes a sustained rise in hepcidin levels, which

impairs iron bioavailability with subsequent doses in the same day. For example, taking a single oral dose of 200 mg of iron is superior for optimizing changes in hemoglobin mass with chronic altitude exposure compared with split doses of 100 mg twice a day. Every-other-day dosing may maximize this benefit, especially for those athletes who are not clearly iron deficient to begin with.

- Intravenous (IV) iron can be considered with severely iron-deficient athletes or in iron-deficient athletes who cannot tolerate oral iron preparations. It is important for the clinician to be aware of the current World Anti-Doping Association (WADA) code regarding allowed volumes of infusion. A therapeutic use exemption (TUE) from WADA may be necessary.
- Other dietary supplements may have positive effects on performance or acclimatization outcomes at altitude. For example, beetroot juice (BRJ) is an emerging supplement utilized for its high inorganic nitrate (NO_3^-) content that is eventually catabolized into nitric oxide (NO). In hypoxia, where tissue O_2 delivery is compromised, NO provides mediation through vasodilation and its resultant increase in blood flow.
- In hypoxic conditions, BRJ has been shown to enhance exercise economy by 5%–10% and may also reduce resting blood pressure, improve oxygen saturation, prolong time to exhaustion, and improve performance time. However, compared with the average individual, elite athletes commonly consume more foods high in nitrate; therefore, the effects on performance in this population are equivocal.
- Due to hypoxia-induced appetite suppression coupled with increased basal metabolic rate (BMR), weight loss is commonly experienced at high and extreme altitudes. Therefore, energy and fluid requirements are greater. Athletes should be informed their appetite may not reflect their actual nutritional needs.
- Current evidence suggests carbohydrate (CHO) intake levels of 10–12 g of CHO/kg/day, in addition to 30–70 g CHO/hr of exercise, depending on intensity and duration. Ultraendurance athletes may require over 90 g/CHO/hr during competition.
- Athletes are at a higher risk of dehydration in the first few days after arrival at altitude primarily because of increased urinary water loss, but also from exacerbated respiratory water loss by augmented ventilation. Consistent monitoring of body mass and (if practical) urine osmolality is recommended to ensure adequate hydration.

ACKNOWLEDGMENT

The authors would like to acknowledge **James Stray-Gundersen, MD,** for his major contributions to the previous editions of this chapter.

RECOMMENDED READINGS

Available online.

24 TRAVEL CONSIDERATIONS FOR THE ATHLETE AND SPORTS MEDICAL TEAM

Craig C. Young • Nicolai Esala

GENERAL PRINCIPLES

Modern transportation systems facilitate easy access to most regions of the world. Although this has allowed for the rapid growth of international competition, it also creates unique physiologic and psychological challenges for athletes as well as the sports medicine team.

JET LAG AND CHRONOBIOLOGY

- The American Academy of Sleep Medicine defines jet lag as a syndrome involving insomnia or excessive daytime sleepiness after travel across at least two time zones. Jet lag is a syndrome of symptoms manifested by physiologic adaptations that occur when the body is shifted to a new time zone.
- Travel fatigue is a more complex combination of physiologic, psychological, and environmental factors that develop during travel; it may accumulate over the course of a season and reduce an athlete's capacity to recover and perform.
- Chronobiology is the field that examines cyclic phenomena in living organisms and their adaptation to solar- and lunar-related rhythms; these cycles are known as *circadian rhythms*.

Physiology of Jet Lag

- An average human experiences endogenous cycles of energy, mood, and activity that last approximately 25 hours.
- The primary pacemaker is the suprachiasmatic nuclei of the hypothalamus. When a traveler changes time zones, this pacemaker must undergo entrainment, which is the process of resynchronization with the new environmental light–dark cycle. Physiologic mechanisms involved in this process include:
  - Melatonin, which is a hormone that is typically secreted at dusk by the pineal gland, helps the body anticipate the daily onset of darkness.
  - Adenosine accumulates when a person is awake and causes progressive sleepiness.
    - Adenosine accumulation is blocked by caffeine.
  - Direct neural pathway from the retina
    - Blue wavelength light, in particular, can interfere with the sleep cycle.
  - Arginine vasopressin
- Zeitgebers are environmental cues that help reset the pacemaker; these include light, temperature, exercise, social interactions, and eating and drinking patterns.
- Disorders of circadian rhythm are most commonly experienced in the setting of a jet lag when a new sleep–wake cycle is required on entering a new time zone.
  - Signs and symptoms of jet lag include changes in mood, headaches, digestive difficulties, and increased susceptibility to illness. Typically, athletes suffer decreases in cognition, concentration, visual acuity, and memory, which may have adverse effects on physical and athletic performance.
- The rate of adjustment to a new time zone is typically a day for each time zone crossed.

Prevention of Jet Lag and Travel Fatigue

- A structured athlete travel program that encompasses preflight, inflight, and postflight periods is the first step in establishing an effective approach to travel fatigue and jet lag.
- Because there is no physiologic adaptation with repetitive time zone transitions, each long-distance journey is unique and requires its own specific travel strategy based on the direction of travel, duration, and times of arrival/departure.
- By adopting a structured program and fatigue monitoring system, athletes and medical staff can help minimize travel-related physiologic and psychological issues, limit symptoms, and improve overall performance.
- **Preflight component:**
  - Although it may be difficult because of schedule restrictions, introducing a schedule within 7 days of travel is generally optimal.
  - Consider gradually changing the sleep–wake cycle and meals to the new time zone by shifting an hour a day.
  - Consider adjusting training to the destination time zone
  - Avoid bright light for 2–3 hours before bedtime
  - An emphasis should be placed on getting enough sleep before travel to reduce sleep debt.
- **Inflight component:**
  - If they have not already done so, advise athletes to adjust their schedule to be in sync with the destination time zone as soon as they board the plane to assist them in preparing for the destination (e.g., watches, meals, and sleep schedules).
  - Maintaining appropriate hydration should be a priority.
  - Avoid light-projecting devices, such as computers, tablets, and movies.
- **Postflight component:**
  - The postflight period stretches 2–4 days or more beyond arrival. During this time, the activities of an athlete (including meals, sleep, rest, and recovery) should be strategically planned by the staff to accommodate rapid circadian adjustment.
  - The most effective intervention in such situations is a combination of scheduled light therapy, light avoidance, and melatonin.
  - Additional fatigue countermeasures include the judicious use of napping and caffeine, both of which can synergistically improve alertness and reduce symptoms of fatigue.

Pharmacologic Measures

- **Melatonin:** Melatonin supplements can aid in managing jet lag symptoms, both preflight and postflight.
  - Preflight low doses (0.5–1.5 mg) of melatonin are most effective, whereas higher doses (3–5 mg) are recommended after flight.
  - Pretravel melatonin may be used to gradually shift the feeling of dusk and bedtime to the anticipated time zone.
  - Doses should be taken 30 minutes before bedtime on the night of travel and the initial 2–3 nights after arriving at the destination. This will mitigate sleep disturbances associated with jet lag while enhancing circadian adaptation.
- **Sedatives:** Athletes who do not suffer from jet lag or who do not respond to melatonin and experience 1–2 days of insomnia on arrival will likely benefit from the use of a traditional medium-acting (20–30 minutes) or medium half-life (6 hours) sedative (e.g., eszopiclone or temazepam). Very-short-acting (<15 minutes) and short half-life (4 hours) sedatives (e.g., zaleplon or zolpidem) can be useful for sleep during the flight. However, caution must be exercised with inflight use of sedatives because this may increase the risk of deep vein thrombosis

(DVT) and decrease responsiveness in the event of an inflight emergency. Use of sedatives may be considered illegal in certain sports without a therapeutic use exemption waiver.

- **Stimulants:** Caffeine and other stimulants (e.g., modafinil) may be useful in combating fatigue. However, use of stimulants may be illegal for some athletes without a therapeutic use exemption waiver.
  - Caffeine: The strategic use of caffeine (e.g., a 50–200-mg pill or beverage) in combination with a 15- to 30-minute nap has been shown to be effective in improving cognitive function in sleep-deprived states and at the lowest point of the circadian cycle. Athletes should be cautioned that caffeine above certain levels is often considered illegal by doping codes and may result in suspension, loss of medals, and vacation of victories.

Nonpharmacologic Measures

Preadaptation and light therapy: Light exposure is the primary cue for circadian rhythms. Exposure to bright light of adequate intensity and duration can advance or delay circadian rhythms based on the timing of exposure. Bright light exposure in the morning will help advance the body clock, whereas exposure in the late evening will help delay it. Attempts to shift circadian rhythms with preflight exposure to bright light before departure have been successful during both eastward and westward travel. Exposure to natural bright light promotes circadian shifts. Avoidance of bright light, particularly short-wavelength blue light in the evening, may help with shift for eastward travel. Use of blue blocking glasses, such as amber safety glasses, may diminish this exposure. Athletes should be cautioned to avoid evening use of tablets, computers, televisions, and mobile phones to minimize blue light exposure.

Sleep: Sleep can be used to acclimate or adjust an athlete's circadian rhythm before travel or decrease symptoms of sleepiness upon arrival. Shifting the sleep schedule 1–2 hours toward the destination time zone in the days preceding departure may shorten the duration of jet lag. In addition, strategic napping has been discussed as a potential method to mitigate the symptoms of jet lag. The best time to nap (inflight or postflight) is nighttime in the destination time zone. "Power naps" (20 minutes) do not result in sleep inertia and may decrease daytime sleepiness in individuals experiencing jet lag. However, naps of >20 minutes may delay sleep adaptation and slow resynchronization.

DEEP VEIN THROMBOSIS AND TRAVEL

- DVT is a condition wherein a blood clot develops in the deep veins, most commonly in the lower extremities. A part of the clot has the potential to break off and travel to the lungs, causing a potentially life-threatening pulmonary embolism (PE).
  - Prolonged periods of inactivity caused by space limitations may diminish circulation and produce lower extremity edema. Prolonged sitting with bent knees compresses the popliteal veins, which is another potential risk factor for clot formation.
- "Economy class syndrome": Long-distance air travel has been associated with a two- to fourfold increased risk of venous thromboembolism (VTE), including DVT.
  - Environmental factors in flight, such as low oxygen, low humidity, and low cabin pressure, contribute to dehydration, which concentrates the blood; this effect is worsened when passengers consume alcohol or do not adequately replenish fluids lost as a result of dehydration. However, there is no evidence that dehydration is directly associated with VTE.
  - Reports have suggested that flights of ≥8 hours increase the risk of VTE in the presence of additional risk factors in a patient.
  - Other risk factors include age over 40 years, obesity, and estrogen use.
  - Athletes and individuals in general good health are at a lower risk of VTE.
- A DVT most often originates in the calf, with persistent cramping, or "charley horse," that intensifies over several days. This pain may be accompanied by leg swelling and discoloration.
- In most cases, travel-related VTE occurs in the first 1–2 weeks after travel. The risk returns to baseline after 8 weeks.
- **Treatment:** Early detection and anticoagulant drugs (e.g., heparin, low-molecular-weight heparin, warfarin; see Chapter 31: "Hematologic Problems in the Athlete" for additional details)
- **Prevention:** Maintaining hydration, exercise, and wearing support stockings may help decrease the overall risk. Periodic activity, approximately every 2 hours, can include isometric exercises, walks along the aisles, or stretching exercises. Below-the-knee graduated compression stockings that provide 15–30 mmHg of pressure have been advocated as a preventive measure. Drugs such as aspirin have antithrombotic properties but are not recommended as a prophylactic measure in otherwise healthy individuals.

INFECTIOUS DISEASES

- Infectious diseases are common among travelers. Travel to developing countries results in approximately 8% of travelers requiring medical treatment. Although preventing athletes from acquiring infections may be challenging, use of commonsense approaches can minimize the risks. Team physicians should investigate which infectious agents are common at the destination, educate the athlete on appropriate preventive measures, and have treatment available.
- Transportation issues:
  - Airplanes: Because modern commercial aircraft use high-efficiency particulate air (HEPA) filters, the risk of transmission for respiratory illness is primarily from the time the particulate/virus is exhaled until it is collected for filtering and recycling or dumped overboard. Therefore, it is primarily the two rows in front of and behind seat that are considered the higher-risk area for transmission or respiratory illness. Having an infected person wearing a mask substantially decreases transmission risks. Having an uninfected person wearing a mask slightly decreases transmission risk. Having both infected and uninfected persons wearing masks leads to maximal decrease in transmission.
  - Surfaces in public transportation may be contaminated with pathogens; therefore it is important that travelers use hand sanitizer or wash their hands frequently and avoid touching their face with their hands.
- **Traveler's diarrhea (TD):** Approximately 50% of travelers, even in low-risk industrialized countries, will develop at least one diarrheal episode per short-term trip (Fig. 24.1). Besides the discomfort and time lost to bowel movements, fluid and electrolyte imbalances have the potential to adversely affect athletic performance.
  - Preventive dietary measures include avoidance of tap water, ice, unpasteurized dairy products, raw vegetables, salads, undercooked meat, and seafood.
  - In 2012, the British Olympic Medical team was successful in reducing illness by educating athletes regarding hygiene, including the importance of lowering the toilet seat lid before flushing to minimize risk of aerosolization of fecal bacteria.
  - Bismuth subsalicylate (Two tablets [262 mg each] four times/day) may be used for prophylaxis and decreases the risk of TD by 50%.
  - Prophylactic antibiotics were considered an effective measure in the past but are no longer recommended because of the developing antimicrobial resistance; nevertheless, short-term use for critical trips or in high-risk patients may be considered.
    - Parasites, not bacteria, are the most common cause of diarrhea in developing countries.

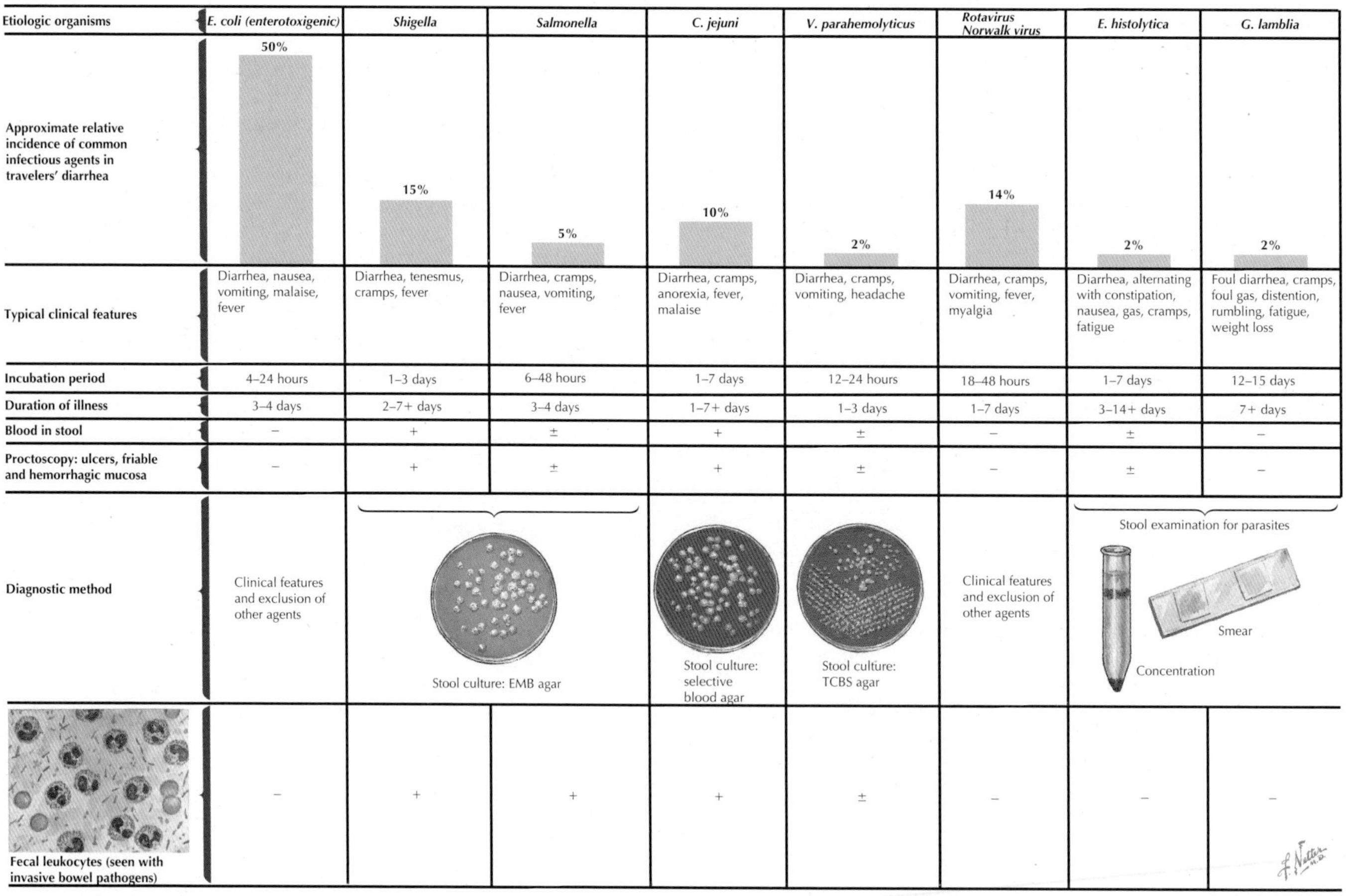
Etiologic organisms
E. coli (enterotoxigenic)
Shigella
Salmonella
C. jejuni
V. parahemolyticus
Rotavirus Norwalk virus
E. histolytica
G. lamblia
Approximate relative incidence of common infectious agents in travelers' diarrhea
50%
15%
5%
10%
2%
14%
2%
2%
Typical clinical features
Diarrhea, nausea, vomiting, malaise, fever
Diarrhea, tenesmus, cramps, fever
Diarrhea, cramps, nausea, vomiting, fever
Diarrhea, cramps, anorexia, fever, malaise
Diarrhea, cramps, vomiting, headache
Diarrhea, cramps, vomiting, fever, myalgia
Diarrhea, alternating with constipation, nausea, gas, cramps, fatigue
Foul diarrhea, cramps, foul gas, distention, rumbling, fatigue, weight loss
Incubation period
4–24 hours
1–3 days
6–48 hours
1–7 days
12–24 hours
18–48 hours
1–7 days
12–15 days
Duration of illness
3–4 days
2–7+ days
3–4 days
1–7+ days
1–3 days
1–7 days
3–14+ days
7+ days
Blood in stool
– + ± + ± – ± –
Proctoscopy: ulcers, friable and hemorrhagic mucosa
– + ± + ± – ± –
Diagnostic method
Clinical features and exclusion of other agents
Stool culture: EMB agar
Stool culture: selective blood agar
Stool culture: TCBS agar
Clinical features and exclusion of other agents
Stool examination for parasites
Smear
Concentration
Fecal leukocytes (seen with invasive bowel pathogens)
– + + + ± – – –

Figure 24.1 Traveler's diarrhea: Incidence and differential features.

   - Antimotility agents, such as loperamide and diphenoxylate–atropine, may be used in cases of nonfebrile, nonbloody diarrhea.
- Mosquito-borne illnesses, including malaria, dengue fever, and chikungunya, are common causes of febrile illness in travelers and should be considered even if symptoms do not occur until after travelers return home.
   - Prevention measures include wearing loose-fitting, long-sleeve shirts and long pants treated with permethrin; use of bed netting; and limiting evening outdoor activities.
   - Sprays to prevent bites include 20%–30% N,N-diethyl-meta-toluamide (DEET), 20% picaridin, or 30% oil of lemon eucalyptus.
- Parasites are a potential concern, particularly in extreme sport athletes in tropical and subtropical climates, who are at a particularly high risk of contracting nematode and protozoan infections (Fig. 24.2).
- **Vaccinations:** The Centers for Disease Control and Prevention's online Yellow Book contains recommendations of vaccinations for most destinations; these should be offered to all athletes well in advance of departure.

INFLIGHT MEDICAL EMERGENCIES

- Occasionally, physicians will find themselves called upon by a flight crew to evaluate a passenger who has developed a medical issue. A physician may determine that he or she can treat and stabilize that patient or that an emergency landing will be needed.
- Typical airline first-aid supplies will include stethoscope, blood pressure cuff, oral airways, bag masks, cardiopulmonary resuscitation (CPR) masks, intravenous (IV) supplies, gloves, needles, syringes, antihistamines (oral and injectable), atropine injection, albuterol inhaler, aspirin, 50% dextrose injection, epinephrine injection, lidocaine injection, nitroglycerin tablets, and automated external defibrillator (AED).

PREPARING A MEDICAL PLAN FOR TRAVEL

- Determination of contents of a medical kit (Table 24.1) will depend on numerous factors, including quality and availability of healthcare at the destination, the sport being covered, and potential injuries. In more remote locations, as well as in developing countries, inclusion of sterile equipment should also be considered because these may not be readily available. For international travel, physicians should carry the following documents:
   - Letter from the team requesting medical coverage
   - List of medical supplies, including medications being transported
   - Check with the destination to ensure that all medications are legal (e.g., stimulant medications such as ***Adderall***, lisdexamfetamine, and modafinil are illegal in Japan. Possession of this type of medication, even with a valid prescription from the athlete's home country, may result in arrest and jail time)
   - Larger volumes of medications intended for the team (e.g., stock bottles of ibuprofen or acetaminophen), in addition to personal medications prescribed for quantities beyond specific amounts (typically 30 days), may need special permission or customs declarations and forms for international travel
   - Medical license and passport
   - List of local medical contacts

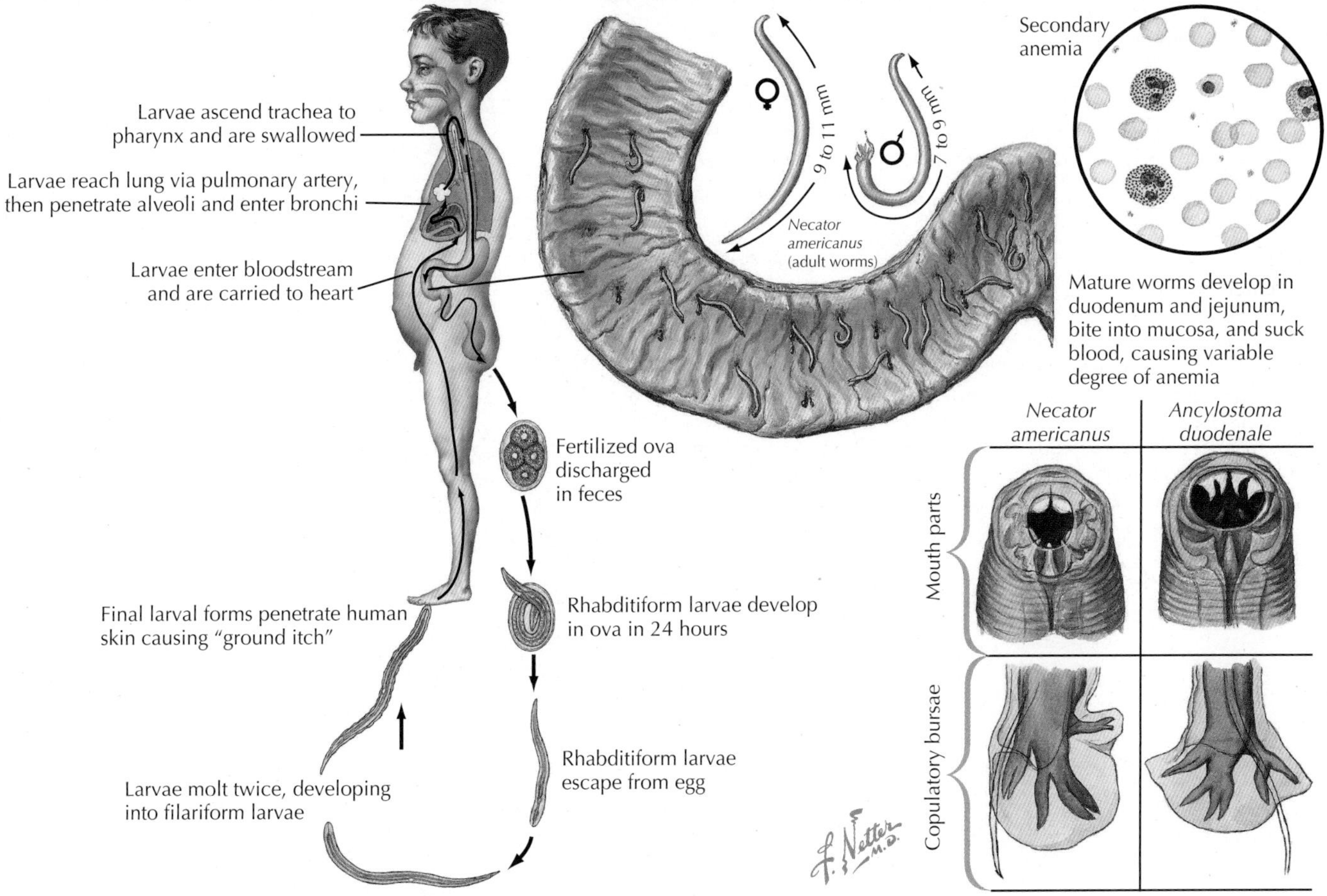

Larvae ascend trachea to pharynx and are swallowed
Larvae reach lung via pulmonary artery, then penetrate alveoli and enter bronchi
Larvae enter bloodstream and are carried to heart
Fertilized ova discharged in feces
Rhabditiform larvae develop in ova in 24 hours
Rhabditiform larvae escape from egg
Larvae molt twice, developing into filariform larvae
Final larval forms penetrate human skin causing "ground itch"
9 to 11 mm
7 to 9 mm
Necator americanus (adult worms)
Secondary anemia
Mature worms develop in duodenum and jejunum, bite into mucosa, and suck blood, causing variable degree of anemia
Necator americanus
Ancylostoma duodenale
Mouth parts
Copulatory bursae

Figure 24.2 Parasitic diseases: Necatoriasis and ancylostomiasis.

Table 24.1 SAMPLE INVENTORY LIST FOR TRAVEL MEDICAL SUPPLIES

Documents	• Inventory list • Medical license • Hospital ID • Business cards • Passport[a] • Copy of prescriptions for personal medications[a] • Letter describing team responsibilities[a] • Medical evacuation contact numbers[a] • World Anti-Doping Agency (WADA) prohibited substance list or online access or sports equivalent[b]		• Povidone iodine • Bandages • Triangular bandage • Elastic bandages • Sterile contact solution • Penlight • Fluorescein strips • Tampons • Cotton applicators • Laceration kit • Butterfly bandages/adhesive skin closures • Scalpel • Forceps • Hemostats • Needles (18G and 25G) • Syringes • Sharps container • Splints • Mylar blanket • Plastic zipper storage bags • Rubber bands • Pen • Electric plug converters[a] • Voltage converter[a] • International (GSM [Global System for Mobiles]-capable) cell phone[a]
Medications	• Acetaminophen • Anti-inflammatory agents • Antibiotics • Gastrointestinal medications (for nausea, diarrhea, and heartburn) • Corticosteroid (topical) • Antihistamines (e.g., diphenhydramine; plus a nonsedating variety) • Anesthetic (injectable) • Albuterol inhaler[c] • Glucose tablets		
Supplies	• Gloves (examination and sterile) • Cardiopulmonary resuscitation (CPR) mask • Thermometer (and covers) • Stethoscope • Blood pressure (BP) cuff • Bandage scissors • Alcohol prep pads	**May Be Considered If Athletes Are Not Drug Tested**	• Corticosteroids (injectable)[c] • Decongestants[c] • Jet lag medications[c]

Note: Do not carry any pain medication. All pain medications should be carried only by the individual for whom it was prescribed: Transportation by any other individual or as "team supplies" is against US Drug Enforcement Agency (DEA) regulations and may result in loss of DEA certificate, medical license, or prosecution.

[a]For international trips.

[b]For coverage of athletes subject to drug testing.

[c]Carry and use with caution—may be restricted by WADA or other sports governing bodies.

- **Travel medical insurance coverage:** consideration should be given to the following issues:
  - 24-hour physician-backed support center
  - Network of referral providers
  - Guarantee of medical payments abroad
  - Direct pay to foreign hospitals and physicians
  - Preauthorizations or second-opinion requirements before emergency treatment or surgery
  - Coverage of higher-risk activities (e.g., parasailing, mountain climbing, or scuba diving)
  - Coverage for preexisting conditions
- **Medical evacuation:** Medical evacuation is very expensive, particularly if not contracted in advance. For international travels, planners should strongly consider having both medical and medical evacuation (back to the home country) insurance coverage for each member of the traveling party.

MEDICOLEGAL CONCERNS

Traveling with a team may create additional issues, particularly if state or national borders are crossed. The passage of the Sports Medicine Licensure Clarity Act of 2017 allows team physicians to practice medicine when traveling with their teams within the United States, but it does not specifically allow teams to travel with medications, nor does it cover international sports coverage. The Good Samaritan Act should not be counted on to cover team physicians because this varies from state to state. In addition, physicians should check with their malpractice insurers to ensure that their activities are covered while traveling.

RECOMMENDED READINGS

Available online.

SECTION V

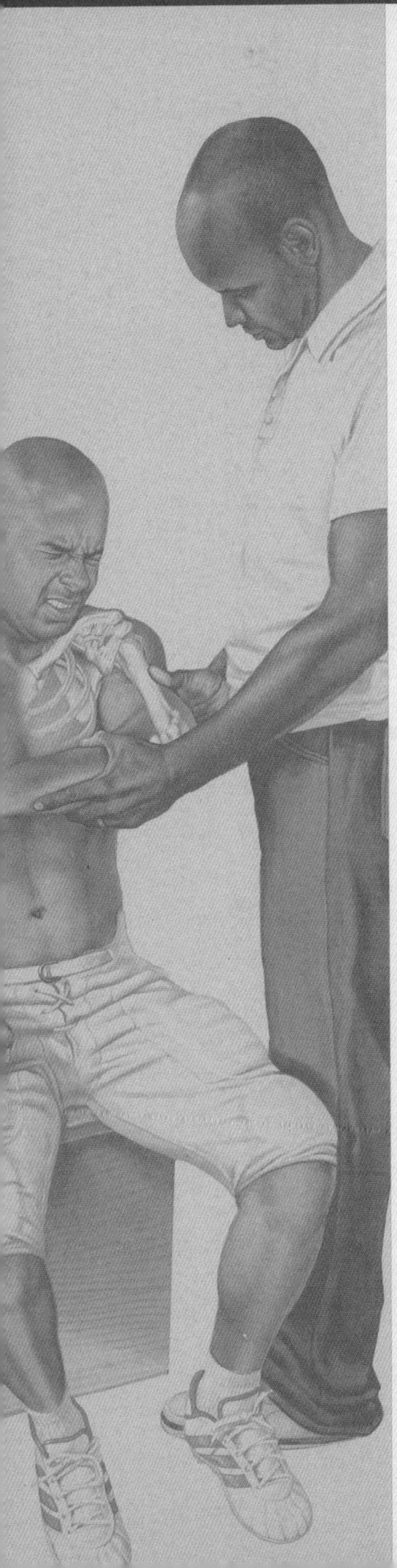

Behavioral and Psychological Problems

THE ROLE OF SPORT PSYCHOLOGY AND SPORTS PSYCHIATRY

25

David B. Coppel • Claudia L. Reardon

INTRODUCTION

Athlete mental health (MH) symptoms and disorders have emerged as a major focus within athletic/sports organizations, international and national sport governing bodies, and the sports medicine environment. This focus has resulted in the development of multiple consensus statements and guidelines regarding MH issues in athletes and articles aimed at increasing awareness and reducing stigma. The sport psychology and sports psychiatry fields have been leaders in this effort. The inclusion of sport psychologists and sports psychiatrists within the sports medicine team can provide athletes with additional support in dealing with MH issues and psychological factors that affect their functioning in both sports and life.

WHAT IS SPORT PSYCHOLOGY?

Definitions

- The American Psychological Association (APA) and APA Division 47 (Society for Sport, Exercise and Performance Psychology) defined sport psychology (SP) as including:
  - Helping athletes apply psychological principles to achieve improved or optimal sport performance and MH.
  - Increasing knowledge regarding the impact of sport/exercise and physical activity on psychological development, health, and well-being over the lifespan.
- SP is seen as a proficiency that uses psychological knowledge and skills to address the well-being of athletes, developmental aspects of sports participation, and systemic issues within sports settings and organizations.
- **In a multidisciplinary context, SP is increasingly seen as a strong component of the sports medicine team.**
- Psychology has played a well-established and vital role in physical medicine and rehabilitation (PMR) programs; hence, its application in sports medicine is natural.
- There are increasing references to psychological factors or the influence of emotional/MH factors on physical health and sports injury recovery and performance.
- Although it is clear that physical injuries, illness, or disease can directly affect athletic performance and/or participation, psychological factors (broadly defined to include behavioral, emotional, or cognitive patterns; personality variables; developmental or adjustment issues; or diagnosable clinical issues) are also critically important to optimal athletic performance and injury recovery.
- Within the sports medicine team, sport psychologists can be involved in psychological care and consultation with athletes at all levels of competition.
- Sport psychologists use their training and experience to provide a unique contribution to the sports medicine team in dealing with injuries. They can address factors (e.g., stress) that may influence the risk of injuries and the psychological factors related to recovering from injury. Sport psychologists can help in the management of concussion patients with prolonged/persistent symptoms, many of which are often associated with emotional or psychological or psychiatric factors.

QUALIFICATIONS OF A SPORT PSYCHOLOGIST

Influence of history: SP has emerged from its roots in motor learning and kinesiology research and applications of clinical and counseling psychology principles to athletic settings. As a result, there are a range of SP practitioners, from academicians and researchers in exercise and sport science to applied/clinical or counseling psychologists.

US Olympic and Paralympic Committee (USOPC): In the early 1980s, the USOC created a registry of sport psychologists. Over the years there have been ongoing efforts to expand the registry to include only those practitioners who meet the standards and certain criteria in their educational training and supervised practice in SP. **USOPC Registry** members are often involved in consulting with elite/Olympic athletes or teams or serve as regional referrals to athletes or teams.

Association for Applied Sport Psychology (AASP)—Certified Mental Performance Consultant (CMPC) status: AASP reviews and approves individual credentials, coursework, and experience, certifying that these consultants meet the standards in their educational training in sport science and psychology. Consultants can teach athletes specific mental, behavioral, psychosocial, and emotional control skills for sports and physical activity. Consultants with clinical or counseling training are qualified to work with athletes who have MH symptoms or disorders.

Importance of licensure: For clinical issues and/or emotional disorders in athletes, a referral to a licensed mental healthcare provider is essential; a referral to a provider who has experience in working with athletes is optimal. Other providers/practitioners may offer "sport psychology consultation," focusing on mental skills training or performance enhancement. Qualified clinical or counseling psychologists may also provide performance enhancement consultation. The title of "psychologist" is typically one that requires licensure by states; therefore, practitioners identifying themselves as "sport psychologists" should be licensed **and** have competency (education and training) in the field of sport and performance psychology.

SPORT PSYCHOLOGIST ROLES

- **A psychological skills training consultant** typically educates athletes or teams about mental skills that enhance performance. These skills include goal setting, relaxation, imagery or visualization, positive self-talk, arousal regulation, increased concentration/focus, precompetitive routine/mental preparation, adaptability/handling pressure, time management, and general communication skills. Team consultation can enhance communication and cohesion among athletes.
- **A licensed clinical or counseling sport psychologist** may provide the same services that a psychological skills training consultant can, but they can also provide assessment and interventions to athletes dealing with MH symptoms and disorders. Assessments can include the following:
  - Assessment or diagnosis of a presenting issue and identifying etiology and/or contributing factors, which may include acquiring a detailed understanding of personal and sport-specific issues or problems.
  - Interview, behavioral observation, psychological testing, neuropsychological testing, and completion of inventories or questionnaires.
  - Integration of an athlete's predisposing factors, precipitating factors, and current maintenance factors.

- **A specialized role for a clinical sport psychologist** with training and experience as a neuropsychologist involves evaluation and consultation regarding sport concussion. This role involves evaluation of neurocognitive, emotional, and reported physical symptoms after a concussion. Sport neuropsychologists may use neuropsychological testing to assess cognitive status and provide inputs to team physicians and/or the sports medicine team (see Chapter 45: "Head Injuries"). In addition, sport neuropsychologists can evaluate, and in certain cases treat, the often overlooked emotional symptoms of concussion.

WHAT IS SPORTS PSYCHIATRY?

Definition and Qualifications

- A sports psychiatrist is a licensed physician who has completed medical school and residency training in an accredited psychiatry residency training program. They may have completed additional fellowship training in a variety of accredited subspecialty areas (e.g., addiction psychiatry/medicine, child and adolescent psychiatry, psychosomatic medicine, etc.), noting that sports psychiatry is not an accredited subspecialty of psychiatry.
- Their area of clinical focus is most commonly the diagnosis and treatment of MH symptoms and disorders in athletes. They may also work with athletes on psychological performance enhancement and may work with nonathletes and athletes on the use of exercise as a preventive measure and treatment for MH symptoms and disorders.
- Sports psychiatrists ideally will have furthered their education and training in the field of sport and MH, such as through obtaining the International Society for Sports Psychiatry Certificate of Additional Training in Sports Psychiatry, through the International Olympic Committee's Diploma Program on MH in Elite Sport, and/or through mentored clinical experiences with experienced sports psychiatrists in the field.

SPORTS PSYCHIATRIST ROLES

A sports psychiatrist is positioned to do the following:

- Provide comprehensive diagnostic evaluations of athletes with complex MH symptoms and disorders or complex management needs
- Consider and evaluate for various diagnostic possibilities, including all MH disorders, substance use disorders, concussion, overtraining, and other medical factors, that could explain psychiatric symptoms
- Offer psychiatric medication prescribing and monitoring
- Order and evaluate laboratory and vital sign monitoring if needed for MH symptoms and disorders or for psychiatric medications prescribed
- Provide needed elements of physical examination if certain psychiatric medications are prescribed (e.g., Abnormal Involuntary Movement Scale [AIMS] examination if antipsychotic medications are prescribed)
- Provide needed elements of the physical examination if substance intoxication or withdrawal is suspected
- Complete therapeutic use exemption (TUE) paperwork if needed (e.g., for stimulant medication at international levels of competition) and help to ensure that requisite paperwork is on file for collegiate athletes who may need to use prohibited psychiatric medications such as stimulants
- Provide support and guidance to the sports medicine team regarding individual athletes with significant MH symptoms and disorders
- Provide support and guidance to the sports medicine team regarding the development of systemic interventions such as treatment guidelines (e.g., for eating disorders, attention-deficit/hyperactivity disorder [ADHD], etc.), prevention protocols (e.g., for eating disorders or substance use disorders in relatively higher-risk teams/sports), or emergency MH action plans
- Help to ensure that all the necessary members of a multidisciplinary treatment team are in place for athletes with complex or severe MH symptoms and disorders (e.g., early psychosis programs for athletes with first-break psychosis, registered dieticians for athletes with eating disorders, etc.).
- Facilitate MH "commitment" proceedings (i.e., involuntary treatment orders) in athletes with imminent dangerousness to self or others or grave inability to care for self (depending on exact state statutes)
- In some settings, provide psychological performance enhancement strategies, especially within the context of overt MH symptoms and disorders
- In some settings, provide psychotherapy (individual, couple, and/or group) for MH symptoms and disorders in athletes
- Evaluate for and monitor MH symptoms and disorders (e.g., depression, anxiety, eating disorders, substance use disorders, etc.) as athletes are retiring from sport
- Help with assessment of when retirement or short-term breaks from sport might be prudent

MH SYMPTOMS AND DISORDERS IN ATHLETES

General Information

- Clinical concerns include all of the MH symptoms and disorders that can affect nonathletes.
- Prospective studies report that MH disorders occur in 5%–35% of elite (including collegiate, professional, and Olympic) athletes over a period of up to 12 months.
- Evidence suggests that these symptoms/disorders relevant to MH may be *more common* in some athletes relative to nonathletes: eating disorders, some substance use disorders, ADHD, gambling disorder, and some sleep disorders (e.g., sleep apnea in American football players).
- Evidence suggests that these symptoms/disorders relevant to MH are probably *at least as common* in athletes relative to nonathletes: certain sleep problems (insufficient sleep, circadian dysregulation, insomnia disorder), depression, generalized anxiety disorder, social anxiety disorder, obsessive-compulsive disorder (OCD), panic disorder, posttraumatic stress disorder (PTSD).
- MH symptoms and disorders can be associated with increased injury risk and performance decrements.
- Sport-specific risk factors for MH symptoms and disorders in athletes include severe musculoskeletal injuries, multiple surgeries, decreased sport performance, maladaptive perfectionism in sport, and times of peak training loads.

Sleep Concerns

- Sleep concerns are common in athletes.
  - Fifty percent of US collegiate athletes get less than 7 hours of sleep per night.
  - Sixty-four percent of Olympic athletes report **insomnia** symptoms.
  - **Sleep apnea** is especially common among American football players.
  - **Circadian dysregulation** is defined as misalignment between the individual's sleep–wake pattern and the desired pattern and is relevant for athletes for many reasons. These reasons include frequent travel across time zones and timing of sport training, especially in the early morning, leading to impaired sleep. Because of an athlete's chronotype (degree to which they are naturally a "morning" or "evening" person), the timing of their training or competition may not align with their personal time of peak performance.
- **Management**
  - Screen for primary sleep disorders (e.g., insomnia disorder, sleep apnea, and circadian dysregulation).
  - Encourage healthy sleep as part of the training protocol.

BOX 25.1 SYMPTOMS OF DEPRESSION

- Depressed mood
- Loss of pleasure or interest
- Feelings of excessive or inappropriate guilt
- Thoughts of death or suicidal ideation
- Feelings of worthlessness
- Low self-esteem
- Hopelessness
- Helplessness
- Indecisiveness
- Insomnia or hypersomnia
- Change in appetite or weight
- Fatigue
- Decreased concentration
- Restlessness or psychomotor slowing

- Use nonpharmacologic treatments first (e.g., sleep hygiene, cognitive behavioral therapy for insomnia, etc.).
- Athletes taking any sleep aids should be advised of the importance of allowing a full night of sleep.
- Many sleep aids can cause next-day sedation that is problematic for athletes; melatonin appears least likely to do so among those sleep aids that have been studied in athletes.

Depression

- **Major depressive disorder** has diagnostic criteria (*Diagnostic and Statistical Manual of Mental Disorders*, 5th ed. [DSM-5]) that require 2 weeks of symptoms that affect a person's capacity to function (Box 25.1, Fig. 25.1).
- **Persistent depressive disorder (dysthymic disorder)** has diagnostic criteria that require at least 2 years of symptoms,

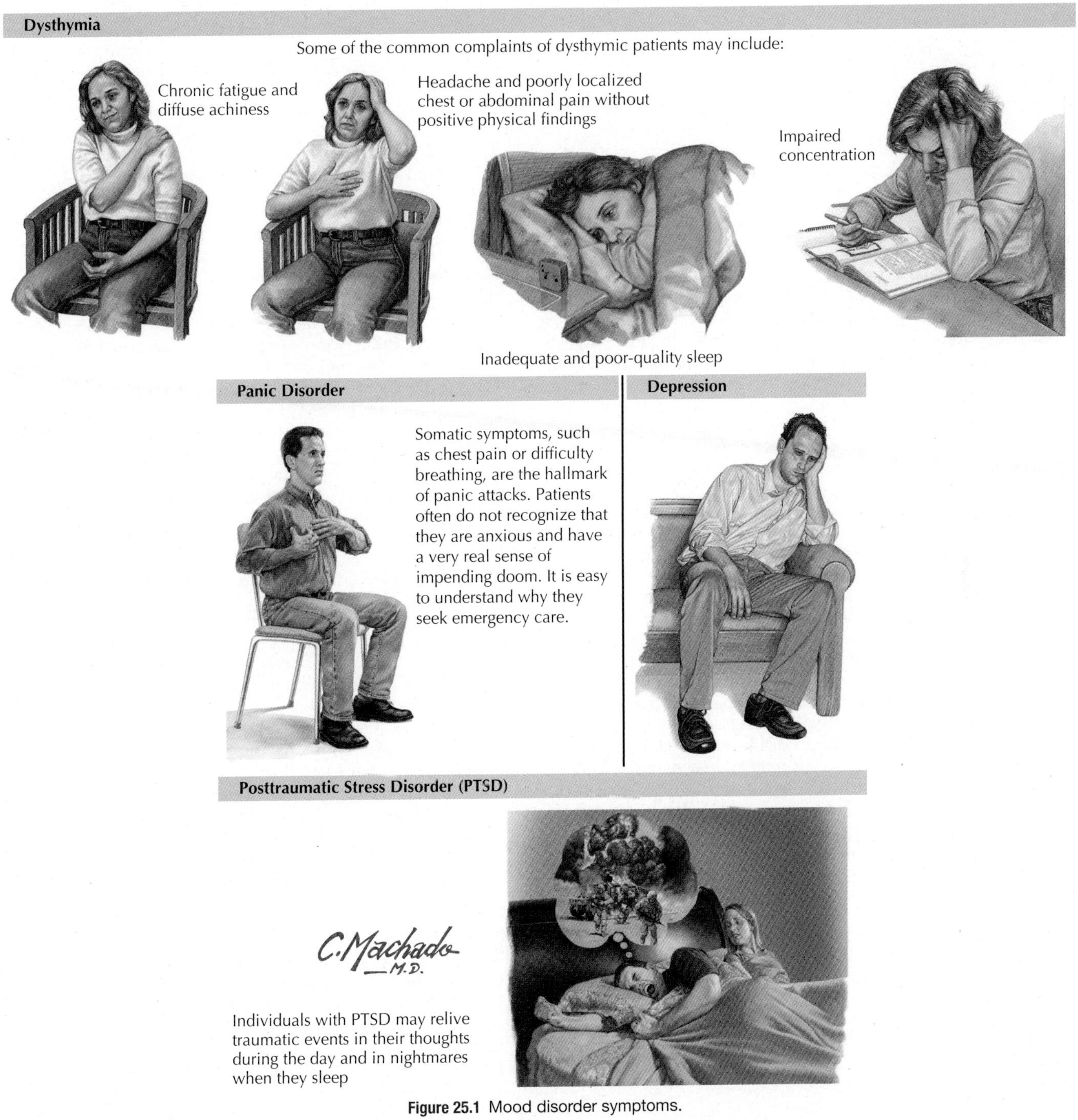
Dysthymia
Some of the common complaints of dysthymic patients may include:
Chronic fatigue and diffuse achiness
Headache and poorly localized chest or abdominal pain without positive physical findings
Impaired concentration
Inadequate and poor-quality sleep
Panic Disorder
Somatic symptoms, such as chest pain or difficulty breathing, are the hallmark of panic attacks. Patients often do not recognize that they are anxious and have a very real sense of impending doom. It is easy to understand why they seek emergency care.
Depression
Posttraumatic Stress Disorder (PTSD)
C.Machado M.D.
Individuals with PTSD may relive traumatic events in their thoughts during the day and in nightmares when they sleep

Figure 25.1 Mood disorder symptoms.

with individuals often seen as chronically unhappy, irritable, and pessimistic. Athletes with dysthymia may not self-report depression but may be ruminative, pessimistic, and not seem to be enjoying their athletic involvement.
- The prevalence of depressive symptoms in elite athletes approximates that in the general population.
- Relatively greater risk is seen in some athlete populations:
  - Female athletes are twice as likely to report depressive symptoms.
  - Individual sport athletes are at greater risk than team athletes.
  - Among National Collegiate Athletic Association (NCAA) athletes, track and field athletes are at relatively greater risk than other sports studied.
- Nonfunctional overreaching (NFO) and overtraining should be considered as possible relevant factors in athletes who present with depressive symptoms.
  - Decreased training in NFO or overtraining often improves mood and associated symptoms, whereas depressed athletes without an element of NFO/overtraining who do not exercise may experience worsened mood as they lose the antidepressant effects of exercise.
- **Management**
  - Treatment usually consists of psychotherapy with or without medications.
  - Providers usually aim for antidepressants that are relatively more energizing or at least relatively less likely to cause sedation.

Anxiety Disorders

- Anxiety disorders, which include panic disorder, generalized anxiety disorder, and social anxiety disorder, commonly involve intense apprehension; general fearfulness; fear of losing control; avoidance of anxiety-provoking situations; and associated physical symptoms such as palpitations, tremors, or nausea.
- Avoidance ultimately perpetuates the anxiety symptoms and causes life disruption but is consciously or subconsciously intended to reduce the anxiety.
- Rates of panic disorder, generalized anxiety disorder, and social anxiety disorder appear similar to those in the general population.
- Subpopulations of athletes at greater risk for anxiety are those who are: dissatisfied with their career; female; younger; and those suffering from musculoskeletal injury.
- **Panic disorder** involves acute periods of severe fear or discomfort with significant concomitant physical symptoms such as palpitations, dizziness, nausea, lightheadedness, fear of losing control or going crazy, numbness, or tingling. These experiences may result in emergency room visits for suspected cardiac or other general medical issues; subsequently, individuals focus on panic sensations or the possibility of having a panic attack and become anxious about being anxious (see Fig. 25.1).
- **Generalized anxiety disorder** usually involves long-standing anxiety symptoms, such as excessive worry about multiple things (e.g., sports, school, work, health, family, relationships) that can result in symptoms such as insomnia, restlessness, low energy, trouble concentrating, irritability, and muscle tension. The athlete perceives that vigilance to threats in the environment reduces threat or bad things from happening to the individual; any perceived "success" (no occurrence of bad things) reinforces the approach.
- **Social anxiety disorder** (social phobia) involves fear of evaluation in social situations. Individuals are concerned about and fear poor or inadequate performance or embarrassment in front of others. This can include athletic competitive situations, social interactions, public speaking, or other performance/outcome situations. This fear of negative outcome/evaluation can lead to avoidance behavior, which, in turn, reduces general functioning and reinforces negative self-perceptions.
  - Athletes may describe anxiety before a competition, but this does not typically rise to the intensity of symptoms found in social anxiety disorder. These athletes may have a greater negative response to real or perceived performance failures, and increased social media use before or during competitions is associated with increased performance anxiety.
- **Management**
  - Psychotherapy is effective and most commonly incorporates elements of cognitive behavioral therapy (e.g., exposure therapy, response prevention, arousal reduction).
  - Medications, if used, commonly include the selective serotonin reuptake inhibitors, which are reasonable choices for athletes. Short-acting medications, such as benzodiazepines and beta-blockers, are not typically used because of side effects and prohibitions in sport, respectively.

Obsessive-Compulsive Disorder

- OCD involves recurrent obsessions (thoughts, ideas, images, or impulses) and/or compulsions (behaviors, which may be physical or mental, that are often repetitive and serve to reduce anxiety and distress, typically done in response to obsessions) that create significant distress and/or dysfunction.
- Athletes will often have precompetitive routines or rituals, which generally do not rise to the level of OCD; however, if athletes associate successful performance with only a narrow set of behaviors, and if these behaviors become increasingly time-consuming and rigid, OCD may develop.
- **Management**
  - Same as anxiety disorders discussed earlier

Posttraumatic Stress Disorder

- PTSD involves a group of symptoms emerging as an intense emotional response to an event that involved actual or possible death or injury (or involved witnessing an event or learning about it occurring to a close friend or family member or being exposed to aversive details on a repeated basis) (see Fig. 25.1).
- Symptoms include re-experiencing aspects of the trauma, such as via flashbacks or nightmares; avoidance of cues associated with the trauma; physiologic hyperarousal (vigilance, extreme startle response, and decreased attention and concentration); and negative alterations in cognitions and mood.
- Athletes may encounter traumatic experiences that range from sports injuries to life events outside of sport.
- There is increasing awareness that sport-related injury (with musculoskeletal injury and concussion the most studied) is associated with PTSD symptoms.
- PTSD can result in avoidance of rehabilitation exercises or other sport circumstances reminiscent of the traumatic injury. Inhibited sport effort associated with PTSD may paradoxically increase the risk of reinjury.
- **Acute stress disorder (ASD)** consists of similar symptoms as in PTSD, but symptoms are of shorter duration, lasting between 3 days and 1 month.
- **Management**
  - Psychotherapy is effective, with evidence-based modalities including cognitive behavioral therapy, cognitive processing therapy, cognitive therapy, and prolonged exposure therapy.
  - If medications are needed, selective serotonin reuptake inhibitors are generally the agents of choice.

Bipolar and Psychotic Disorders

- Bipolar disorder involves manic (in the case of bipolar disorder type I) and/or hypomanic (in the case of bipolar disorder type II) episodes and usually also major depressive episodes. **Manic symptoms** are listed in Box 25.2, and **hypomanic episodes** are milder versions of manic episodes. Manic/hypomanic episodes last days to weeks or more on end and cause distinct changes in functioning and behavior.

BOX 25.2 SYMPTOMS OF HYPOMANIA OR MANIA (AS IN BIPOLAR DISORDER)

- Abnormal and persistently elevated, expansive, or irritable mood and abnormally and persistently increased activity or energy lasting several days to weeks
- Decreased need for sleep
- Grandiose notions
- Increased talking
- Racing thoughts
- Distractibility
- Increase in goal-directed activity or psychomotor agitation
- Excessive involvement in activities that have a high potential for painful consequences (e.g., excessive spending, sexual indiscretions, or business investments)

- Psychotic disorders such as schizophrenia and related conditions are usually characterized by hallucinations and delusions. Schizophrenia may also involve disturbed speech, thought, behavior, affect, and cognition and significantly impaired functioning.
- Bipolar and psychotic disorders show a peak age of onset coincident with the usual age of peak sporting performance; thus, it is important for clinicians and other key professionals in the world of sport to be aware of relevant symptoms.
- Substances used by athletes, including stimulants, cannabinoids, and glucocorticoids, may be associated with mood (including hypomanic and manic) and psychotic episodes.
- Some evidence suggests that vigorous exercise may exacerbate mania in patients with bipolar disorder. Thus, it may be prudent to monitor amounts of exercise in athletes with bipolar disorder to ascertain any patterns that suggest markedly increased exercise concomitant with times of hypo/mania.
- **Management**
  - Medication evaluation and management by a psychiatrist is recommended. Medications to treat bipolar disorder and psychosis may cause performance-limiting side effects such as sedation, weight gain, tremor, and cardiac side effects. Lithium can become toxic if hydration is not maintained. Care must be taken to balance efficacy, safety, and tolerability.
  - Psychotherapy can be helpful, with modalities including family therapy, cognitive behavioral therapy, and (in bipolar disorder) social rhythms therapy.

Eating Disorders

- Common eating disorders include anorexia nervosa, bulimia nervosa, and binge-eating disorder (see Chapter 27: "Eating Disorders in Athletes").
- Eating disorders are prevalent in athletes, and disordered eating (i.e., symptoms that are problematic and may be possible warning signs of future progression to eating disorders but do not currently meet the full criteria for eating disorders) is even more common in athletes than are full eating disorders.
  - Warning signs of disordered eating include:
    - Pathogenic behaviors (e.g., occasional restricting, use of diet pills, bingeing, purging, or use of saunas or sweat runs) used to control weight but not with regularity.
    - Preoccupation with "healthy eating" or significant attention to nutritional parameters of most foods eaten.
    - Cognitive focus on burning calories when exercising.
- There are several known risk factors for eating disorders:
  - General: low self-esteem; depression; anxiety; family history of eating disorder; perfectionistic personality style.
  - Sport-specific: weight-sensitive sports (e.g., weight class sports, sports that may be aesthetically judged, or gravitational sports in which lower body fat may be advantageous); team weigh-ins; sport-specific training before the body is fully mature (which may hinder an athlete from choosing a suitable sport for their adult body type); performance pressure; injury.
- **Management**
  - Multidisciplinary treatment is recommended for athletes with eating disorders, with the treatment team commonly including a sports medicine physician, psychiatrist, psychotherapist such as psychologist, athletic trainer, and registered dietician.
  - Evaluation of medical stability (e.g., through monitoring of laboratory values and physical examination parameters such as vital signs and possibly electrocardiography and bone mineral density testing) is recommended.
  - An important management consideration is the level of care that is required (e.g., inpatient hospitalization, residential, partial hospitalization program, intensive outpatient program, or standard outpatient treatment)
  - Psychotherapy is an important aspect of care
  - Medications are most evidence-based for bulimia nervosa (fluoxetine) and binge eating disorder (lisdexamfetamine—but this is a stimulant and thus requires the requisite paperwork just as when used for ADHD, as explained next). Medications may also be used to treat comorbid mental health symptoms and disorders such as depression and anxiety.

Attention-Deficit/Hyperactivity Disorder

- ADHD involves symptoms related to two clusters: inattention and hyperactivity/impulsivity. An athlete needs to have several symptoms in one or both of these clusters in order to receive an ADHD diagnosis.
- Impairment must occur before the age of 12 years in multiple settings (e.g., school, work, and home).
- ADHD is commonly comorbid with other MH symptoms and disorders, including mood, anxiety, and substance use disorders, and as such, a diagnosis of ADHD should be made only after a thorough assessment. Symptoms are often treated in a hierarchical approach such that mood, anxiety, and substance use concerns may be treated first to see if any inattention as a possible part of ADHD remains.
  - Assessment should include a detailed clinical interview addressing psychiatric symptoms, substance use, other medical symptoms/disorders including concussion history, academic record, and family history. Certain interview protocols include use of standardized rating scales completed by the athlete, parents, and/or teachers, depending on the age of the athlete. Formal psychological and/or neuropsychological testing may provide additional data regarding the cognitive status of an individual and help in the differential diagnosis.
- Although many individuals experience a decline in ADHD symptoms as they enter adulthood, a significant number of adults describe ongoing symptoms and resulting dysfunction.
- ADHD may be more common in athletes than in the general population, as individuals with ADHD may be drawn to sport because of the positive reinforcing effects of physical activity.
- Attentional difficulties or problems with impulsivity, focus, and follow-through may create problems within the competitive sports environment. Such athletes may respond positively to a structured sports environment, which helps reduce distraction.
- **Management**
  - Primary treatment options for ADHD include psychosocial/behavioral interventions (often tried first) and medications.
  - Psychosocial interventions include, depending on the age of the athlete, behavior therapy or cognitive behavioral therapy; individual education plans; parent teaching/training and caregiver support; and education for athletes, families, and coaches.

- Nonstimulant medication options should be considered and include atomoxetine (commonly takes weeks to months to take effect), bupropion (not approved for use in ADHD), clonidine, and guanfacine.
- Stimulant medication options include medications within the methylphenidate and mixed amphetamine salts classes. Stimulants are prohibited by the NCAA and *in competition* by the World Anti-Doping Agency (WADA), except as medically indicated. In the case of the NCAA, the requisite paperwork must be maintained on file to justify and document the proper use of a stimulant. In the case of WADA (for athletes competing at potentially international levels of competition), an athlete and their care team must apply for and be approved for a TUE in advance of any relevant competitions.
  - Athletes have different perceptions of the impact of stimulant medications on sports performance. Although various lines of evidence suggest performance enhancement, some athletes perceive performance impairment and thus prefer to avoid having these medications in their systems during practices or competition.

Substance Use and Behavioral Addictions

- Athletes may use substances from various classes for social/recreational purposes, self-treatment, or to boost performance.
- Alcohol, cannabis, nicotine, and prescribed opioids and stimulants appear to be the most commonly used substances in elite athletes, but generally at rates that are lower than nonathletes.
- In contrast, use/misuse rates for *binge* alcohol, *oral* tobacco, *nonprescription* opioids, and anabolic-androgenic steroids are higher in athletes, especially in power and collision sports, compared with the general population.
- Gambling disorder is a "hidden addiction" that affects many athletes.
  - Between 1.8% and 4.0% of male NCAA athletes have serious gambling-related problems, despite prohibition by the NCAA against gambling.
  - Among professional athletes, 56.6% participated in some form of gambling during the past year and 8.2% had a gambling problem (either current or in the past).
- **Management**
  - Psychosocial modalities (e.g., psychotherapy) are first-line treatments for most substance use disorders and gambling disorder.
  - Brief individual or group interventions delivered by clinicians may prevent or diminish binge drinking or other substance use in athletes.
  - Medications may be used to manage withdrawal and cravings and to treat comorbid MH symptoms and disorders.

Personality Disorders

- Personality disorders involve personality or behavioral traits that endure over time and are maladaptive, causing significant subjective distress and/or observable functional impairment in major areas of life (school, work, or family) (see Fig. 25.1).
- Individuals are not usually diagnosed with personality disorder until the age of 18 years.
- Disorders are grouped into three clusters:
  - **Cluster A** includes schizoid, paranoid, and schizotypal personality disorders, which are characterized by atypical interpersonal behavior, odd interaction styles, and perceptions of the world.
  - **Cluster B** includes histrionic, borderline, narcissistic, and antisocial personality disorders, which are characterized by affective and behavioral deregulation.
  - **Cluster C** includes avoidant, obsessive-compulsive, and dependent personality disorders, which are characterized by symptoms of anxiety and avoidant behavior.
- These disorders or their subclinical variants (traits or features that are present but do not meet diagnostic criteria) may be present in athletes who have repeated interpersonal difficulties with teammates or staff, problems with authority or complying with rules, disciplinary issues, aggression or emotional dyscontrol, or issues with accepting responsibilities. Comorbid issues may include substance misuse, eating disorders, and mood/anxiety disorders.
- **Management**
  - Psychotherapy can be helpful and may need to be longer-term. Cognitive behavioral approaches have been helpful in reducing symptoms and enhancing functional levels. Dialectical behavioral therapy is helpful for borderline personality disorder.

PSYCHOLOGICAL ASPECTS OF INJURY

- Injury can trigger psychological responses, and the sports medicine team should be aware of the cognitive, emotional, and behavioral responses to being injured in addition to responses to the recovery/rehabilitation process.
- **There may be certain stages of physical recovery**; however, there are also psychological stages of coping with injury, which are individualized and influenced by psychosocial factors (e.g., social support, impact on team or career, or general personality traits).
- **The sports medicine team should consider referral for MH consultation because it can enhance physical recovery.**
- Psychological components of injury and recovery can include shock and emotional disorganization immediately after injury; general anxiety and uncertainty regarding the future during evaluation and treatment decision-making; and impatience, anger, frustration, lack of control, and depression during recovery.
- Psychological issues can develop during the return-to-play phase and may involve the fear of reinjury or of not being able to perform at the preinjury level. In addition, self-doubt and rumination can emerge, producing decreased confidence.
- Moreover, psychological factors such as stressful life events may contribute to the risk of athletic injuries. Personality factors have not been found to reliably relate to the risk of athletic injury, but athletes with high levels of stress, low or ineffective coping skills, low social support, and low self-esteem may be at particular risk of injury; such athletes may also be at risk of a challenging injury response and recovery course. Other potential risk factors include social/organization-based stress or pressure, lifetime history of sexual or physical abuse, and poor athlete–coach communication.
- Athletes make efforts to deal with being injured in individualized ways and time frames. Emotional responses can include sadness and feelings of isolation, irritation, frustration, and anger in addition to changes in sleep, appetite, and energy (fatigue). These symptoms can worsen and emerge as issues during the recovery/rehabilitation process. Depression is the most common response: it can progress from sadness to a more clinical level of depression.
- Of note, athletes often use their training/exercise and general physical activity as a coping mechanism and outlet for dealing with stress; thus, an injury can reduce access to this coping strategy, which, in turn, adds to the emotional stress. In some instances, a stressful injury and recovery may trigger behaviors involving substance use/misuse, gambling, and disordered eating or eating disorders.
- Signs of poor adjustment to injury include exaggerated or generalized fear of reinjury, general impatience or irritability, mood swings, withdrawal from significant others or the social network, rumination about guilt for being injured and letting others down, increased somatic focus, obsession with return to play, general pessimism about the future in sports and other areas (demoralization), or apathy.

- Injured athletes who are strongly identified with their sport may experience a greater sense of identity loss. Separation and loneliness (from the team) are experiences that can increase the probability of problematic emotional responses to injury. Maintaining contact with teammates reduces the sense of isolation and gives the athlete opportunities for support.
- Return-to-play issues include physical and psychological readiness and clearance. Assessment of psychological readiness is crucial to successful return to play and should be considered by the athletic trainer, team physician, team psychologist (if available), and other members of the athlete's support network.

HARASSMENT AND ABUSE IN SPORT

- The athletic culture and environment provide opportunities for positive growth and experiences but also have been the setting for harassment and abusive behaviors through multiple mechanisms.
- These mechanisms include physical and/or sexual abuse/contact, verbal abuse, cyber abuse, negligence, and more generally, bullying and hazing. Unfortunately, these abusive behaviors have been noted to occur across all sports and at all levels of sport, with higher risk at elite levels. Child athletes, LGBTQ athletes, and disabled athletes can be at higher risk.
- These abusive experiences can have a devastating impact on an individual's development, resulting in loss of self-esteem, reduced academic performance, distorted body image, eating disorders, self-harm and suicidal behaviors, depression, anxiety, and substance use.
- Victims are at greater risk for developing physical and MH symptoms and disorders. In addition, abusive behaviors can be connected to poorer athletic performance and early sport dropout.
- Witnessing abusive events may also have significant negative psychological and MH consequences.
- **Within the sports medicine context, inquiry regarding the history of these experiences may be important in treatment planning and referral to appropriate providers such as a sports psychiatrist and/or sport psychologist.**

SUMMARY

- Sport psychologists and sports psychiatrists provide a range of educative and consultative services to individual athletes and teams for various MH symptoms and disorders; in addition, they can provide psychological skill training related to performance enhancement and team building.
- Inclusion of licensed MH professionals on the sports medicine team is thought to provide an excellent opportunity to address psychological aspects of performance, adjustment, and injuries, in addition to responding to MH symptoms and disorders.
- Sports psychiatrists can provide comprehensive assessment of significant and/or complex psychiatric presentations, review the need for psychiatric medications, and contribute to the development of protocols for emergency response plans and treatment planning for these patients.
- SP and sports psychiatry can make particularly useful contributions to the team physician and sports medicine team in dealing with injured athletes and providing support related to MH symptoms and disorders that can be triggered.

RECOMMENDED READINGS

Available online.

26 DRUGS AND DOPING IN ATHLETES

Gary A. Green • Daniel Eichner • Amy Eichner

DEFINITION

According to the World Anti-Doping Agency (WADA) Code, doping is defined as the occurrence of one or more of the following antidoping rule violations:

- The presence of a prohibited substance or its metabolites or markers in an athlete's bodily specimen.
- Use or attempted use of a prohibited substance or prohibited method.
- Refusing, or failing without compelling justification, to submit to sample collection after notification as authorized in applicable antidoping rules or otherwise evading sample collection.
- Violation of applicable requirements regarding athlete availability regarding out-of-competition testing, including failure to provide required whereabouts information and missed tests that are declared based on reasonable rules.
- Tampering, or attempting to tamper, with any part of doping control.
- Possession of prohibited substances and methods.
- Trafficking in any prohibited substance or prohibited method.
- Administration or attempted administration of a prohibited substance or prohibited method to any athlete, or assisting, encouraging, aiding, abetting, covering up, or any other type of complicity involving an antidoping rule violation or any attempted violation.
- Association by an athlete with someone currently sanctioned under WADA rules (e.g., working with or receiving coaching by someone who is sanctioned).
- Acts by an athlete or other person to discourage or retaliate against people reporting doping to authorities (whistleblowers), newly adopted in the WADA 2021 Code.

HISTORICAL EVENTS IN MODERN SPORTS DOPING

- 1964: Drug testing begins at the Olympics.
- 1968: Formal drug testing adopted for Summer and Winter Olympic Games. Drug testing has been used at every Olympiad since.
- East German swimmers admit to systematic doping in the 1970s that was sanctioned by their National Olympic Committee.
- Widespread use of blood doping by US cyclists participating in the 1984 Summer Olympic Games discovered.
- In 1985, the National Collegiate Athletic Association (NCAA) began a series of quadrennial surveys that documented substance use and abuse patterns by intercollegiate athletes. The methodology changed significantly in 1997 and increased the number of participating schools and subjects. The ninth iteration in 2017 measured the substance use patterns in 23,028 men and women athletes. Periodic surveys are helpful in assessing usage patterns of recreational and ergogenic substances in order to allocate resources for overall deterrence.
- Following a series of doping scandals, the International Olympic Committee (IOC) convened the World Conference on Doping and Sport in February 1999 that led to the creation of the WADA. WADA was charged with developing standards and a consistent, worldwide doping-control program. WADA develops criteria for inclusion on a prohibited substances list that is provided in Box 26.1 along with a clinical guide to those substances in Table 26.1.
- In 2003 the investigation into the Bay Area Lab Co-Operative (BALCO) revealed a sophisticated conspiracy involving professional athletes as well as US and international Olympic athletes. In addition to developing designer anabolic steroids, the BALCO records were used to discipline athletes based on "nonanalytic" positives (i.e., athletes were suspended based on doping records rather than an adverse analytical finding on a drug test). The use of nonanalytical positives and forensic investigations has increased since 2003 as another antidoping tool.
- 2007: Major League Baseball (MLB) commissions the Mitchell Report that details past and current anabolic steroid use that leads the MLB to implement a comprehensive drug testing program.
- 2012: Lance Armstrong stripped of his seven Tour de France titles and banned for life from competitive cycling. Highlights the extent of doping in cycling. An example of a typical doping regimen from the Tour de France is listed in Box 26.2.
- Biogenesis investigation in 2013 leads to criminal prosecution and suspensions of multiple professional athletes.
- 2014: Sochi Olympics reveals systematic doping under the aegis of the Russian Sports Federation. Extensive investigation by WADA culminates in the Maclaren Report with hundreds of athletes involved in 30 sports (Fig. 26.1).
- 2020: Rodchenkov Anti-Doping Act is signed into law imposing criminal sanctions on international doping fraud conspiracies. Similar legislation has been passed in several European countries.

SCOPE OF THE PROBLEM

- The prevalence of doping in sport has always been difficult to ascertain because of limitations on testing data, surveys, and defining who is an "athlete" and which substances are considered "doping."
- Reliance on testing data to determine the extent of doping underestimates depending on the program and the use of no-notice testing vs. announced testing. The positive test rates for various organizations are listed in Table 26.2.
- Research using surveys has revealed a relatively low prevalence of doping in athletes. One of the largest is the NCAA quadrennial survey of athletes from the three NCAA divisions. The most recent iteration was conducted in 2017 involving 23,000 student-athletes. For ergogenic drugs, they reported that amphetamines and anabolic steroids were used 1.5% and 0.4%, respectively, in the previous year. Interestingly, there was little difference in usage rates between the three divisions. Among men's sports, the highest reported use of these substances was 6.7% amphetamine use for lacrosse and 1.9% anabolic steroid use for wrestling. Interestingly, although the reported use of amphetamines and anabolic steroids was quite low, 11% admitted to using various other performance-enhancing drugs (PEDs) in the past year. These included human growth hormone (hGH), clenbuterol, erythropoietin (EPO), and other ergogenic substances. The use of testosterone boosters was reported as 0.7%, higher than the use of anabolic steroids.
- Because of the limitations of test results and surveys, it is difficult to obtain an accurate extent of the use of PEDs in sport. As was demonstrated from both the Maclaren Report on Russia (see Fig. 26.1) and the NCAA 2017 survey, doping is not limited to high-profile sports or sports that generate the most revenue or attention.

Sports Pharmacology

- One method for classifying substance use in athletes depends on their reason for use, rather than the chemical structure, mechanism of action, or pharmacologic effects. Under this nomenclature, a drug is classified as ergogenic, recreational, or therapeutic depending on the main reason for use, which can influence prevention, identification, treatment, and in some cases, sanctions.
  - Ergogenic drugs are substances that are taken specifically to increase performance.
  - Nonperformance ("recreational" drugs or "substances of abuse") are used by athletes for the same reasons as nonathletes and carry the risk for addiction and adverse events. These drugs often have adverse effects on performance.
  - Therapeutic drugs are taken to treat an underlying condition.
- The problem is that there can be significant overlap whereby a therapeutic drug can be ergogenic and might still be subject to antidoping restrictions, even if legitimately prescribed to treat a condition.

BOX 26.1 SUMMARY OF INCLUSION CRITERIA FOR WADA PROHIBITED LIST (FROM WADA CODE 2021)

At least two of the three following criteria must apply:
1. The substance has the potential to enhance performance
2. Use of the substance poses an actual or potential health risk
3. Use of the substance violates the spirit of sport[a]

Substances or methods that mask the effect or detection of prohibited substances are also prohibited. In addition, a substance that has not been approved for human use is likely to be prohibited.

The Prohibited List is reviewed annually in consultation with scientific, medical, and antidoping experts to ensure it reflects current medical and scientific evidence and doping practices. The Prohibited List comes into effect on January 1 of each year and is published by WADA three months before coming into force; however, in exceptional circumstances, a substance or method may be added to the Prohibited List at any time.

[a]Spirit of Sport is defined in the WADA Code as the celebration of the human spirit, body, and mind. It is the essence of Olympism and is reflected in the values we find in and through sport, including health, ethics, fair play, respect for rules and laws, and many others.

Data from World Anti-Doping Code International Standard Prohibited List, 2021 at https://www.wada-ama.org/en/content/what-is-prohibited.

The Physician's Role

- Often complicated relationship between physicians and drugs in sport has a long historical legacy.
  - Since the ancient Greek Olympics, athletes have sought out physicians to provide performance aids.
  - 2012 NCAA study: 20.9% of anabolic steroid users named an athletic staff member as a source of their drugs.
- Physicians play a central role in the use and abuse of drugs by athletes.
  - Physicians are asked to provide education, act as medical directors or medical review officers for drug testing, and provide therapeutic use exemptions (TUEs). It is imperative that physicians who serve as team physicians are familiar with PEDs used by athletes and with the procedures used to determine a positive test result.
  - It is important to remember that the majority of high-profile doping scandals could not have been possible without the active participation of physicians.
  - Although it is ultimately an athlete's responsibility for what they ingest, physicians who are treating athletes subject to drug testing need to be aware of the prohibited list for that particular sport before prescribing any medication.

DETERRENCE

The overall measure of effectiveness of any antidoping program is in the deterrent effect. This can be achieved by a combination of education, testing, and discipline. As an example, MLB developed a stepwise

Table 26.1 CLINICAL GUIDE TO THE WADA PROHIBITED LIST

WADA Prohibited List Category	Examples of Medications Subject to Restrictions
S0. Unapproved Substances	Investigational drugs or drugs in clinical trials. Athletes participating in drug clinical trials may need a therapeutic use exemption.
S1. Anabolic Agents	Testosterone creams, patches, or injections, Prasterone/DHEA, HRT with androgens, SARMs (Enobosarm) and others
S2. Peptide Hormones, Growth Factors and Related Substances	Erythropoietin (EPO) and agonists, CG and LH (in males) and their releasing factors, corticotrophins, growth hormone (GH) and growth factors (e.g., platelet-derived growth factors, thymosin beta$_2$ and TB-500), and others
S3. Beta$_2$-agonists	All inhaled or oral beta$_2$-agonists are prohibited except for albuterol, formoterol, salmeterol, and vilanterol, which have routes of administration and dosage restrictions.
S4. Hormone and Metabolic Modulators	Aromatase inhibitors, SERMs (tamoxifen), clomiphene, insulin, meldonium, and others
S5. Diuretics and Masking Agents	Hydrochlorothiazide, acetazolamide, canrenone, spironolactone, and others
M1. Manipulation of Blood M2. Chemical Physical Manipulation M3. Gene and Cell Doping	Introduction of any type of red blood cell products, or any form of intravascular manipulation (including plasmapheresis/plasma donation, IV infusions of any type, use of nucleic acids, gene editing)
S6. Stimulants	Adrafinil/modafinil, amphetamine and most ADHD medications, cocaine, pseudoephedrine, epinephrine (Epi-Pen), strychnine, and others
S7. Narcotics	Oxycodone, methadone, heroin, pethidine, morphine
S8. Cannabinoids	THC, and other natural cannabinoids, synthetic cannabinoids
S9. Glucocorticoids	Prednisone, methylprednisolone (Medrol-Dose pack), triamcinolone and others
P1. Beta-Blocker (prohibited in certain sports)	Atenolol, timolol, and others

The WADA Prohibited List changes every year. Check the website for the most up-to-date information. This is not an exhaustive list. Medications listed here might require a therapeutic use exemption, have restrictions on dosage or on when the substance is used relative to competition, how it is delivered (route of administration), whether it is used in combination with other medications, or it may be restricted in certain sports.

Data from World Anti-Doping Code International Standard Prohibited List, 2021. https://www.wada-ama.org/en/content/what-is-prohibited.

BOX 26.2 EXAMPLE OF DRUG USE BY A TOUR DE FRANCE CYCLIST IN 2008

Recombinant erythropoietin (r-HuEPO)
Continuous erythrocyte receptor activator (CERA)
Recombinant human growth hormone (rhGH)
Thyroid hormone
Blood transfusions
Albumin
Insulin
Testosterone
Designer anabolic steroids
Injectable cortisone

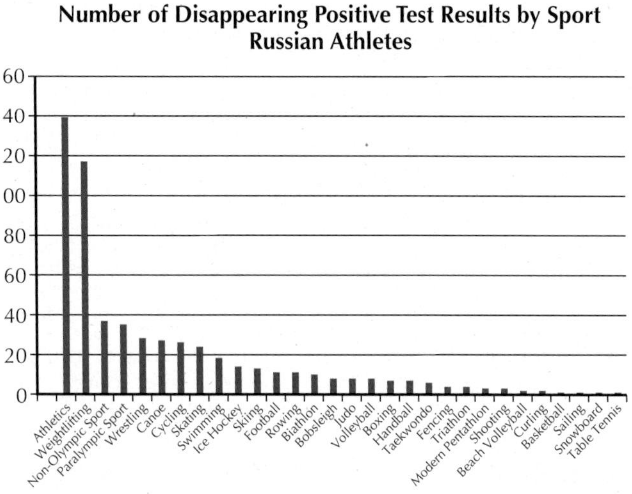
Number of Disappearing Positive Test Results by Sport
Russian Athletes
160
140
120
100
80
60
40
20
0
Athletics
Weightlifting
Non-Olympic Sport
Paralympic Sport
Wrestling
Canoe
Cycling
Skating
Swimming
Ice Hockey
Skiing
Football
Rowing
Biathlon
Bobsleigh
Judo
Volleyball
Boxing
Handball
Taekwondo
Fencing
Triathlon
Modern Pentathlon
Shooting
Beach Volleyball
Curling
Basketball
Sailing
Snowboard
Table Tennis

Figure 26.1 Number of disappearing positive test results by sport Russian athletes. (Data from McLaren Independent Investigation Report—Parts I and II [2016]. World Anti-Doping Agency. https://www.wada-ama.org/en/resources/search?f%5B0%5D=field_topic%3A23&f%5B1%5D=field_resource_type%3A115.)

Table 26.2 POSITIVE TEST RATES IN OLYMPIC SPORT AND MAJOR LEAGUE BASEBALL IN 2018

Sport	Analyzed Samples	Positive Tests
Olympic/Paralympic (WADA/Global)	228,560	1519 (0.66%)
Olympic/Paralympic (USADA/USA)	6,607	66 (0.9%)
MLB (US)	11,526	11 (0.09%)

Data from test rates for Olympic sport were taken from the 2018 Anti-Doping Testing Figures published by the World Anti-Doping Agency. https://www.wada-ama.org/sites/default/files/resources/files/2018_testing_figures_report.pdf; Major League Baseball testing stats: https://www.mlb.com/news/mlb-players-union-release-annual-testing-results-summary/c-40478624.

deterrence program for their player-development academies beginning in 2005 when the positive test rate for anabolic steroids was over 5%. Because of Dominican law at the time, the only available option for players who tested positive was education. This was in place from 2005 to 2008 and saw a mild reduction in positive tests. Beginning in 2008, suspensions were allowed under the law, and the positive rate began to decrease. In 2011 a series of financial disincentives were added, leading to a further reduction to a rate below 1%. This demonstrates that in a population with a high prevalence of PED use, deterrence can be accomplished with a multipronged approach. These interventions are summarized in Fig. 26.2.

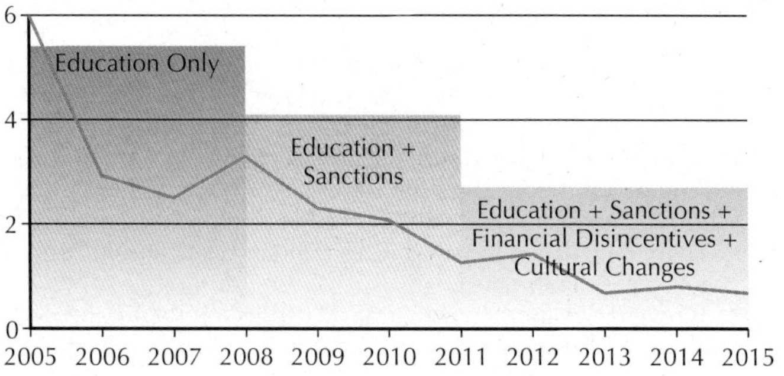
6
4
2
0
Education Only
Education + Sanctions
Education + Sanctions + Financial Disincentives + Cultural Changes
2005
2006
2007
2008
2009
2010
2011
2012
2013
2014
2015

Figure 26.2 Effect of interventions in MLB-affiliated players in the Dominican Republic.

ANABOLIC-ANDROGENIC STEROIDS

Definition: Testosterone or testosterone-like synthetic drugs that result in both anabolic and androgenic effects, for example, increase protein synthesis (anabolism) and enhance the development of male secondary sexual characteristics (androgenic).

Prevalence:

- Since 1988 surveys have sought to assess usage rates in athletes and nonathletes, with conflicting results. However, it is clear that the use of anabolic-androgenic steroids (AAS) is no longer confined to athletes participating in organized sports, but is also used in the general population for nonathletic enhancement.
- 2019: Monitoring the Future Study reported that 1.0% of 12th graders had used AAS in the previous 12 months, with a lifetime prevalence of 1.6%.
- A 2014 global meta-analysis of 271 studies by Sagoe et al. determined a lifetime prevalence of AAS use of 6.4% for men and 1.6% for women.
- Androgenization program developed by the former German Democratic Republic (GDR) provided anecdotal information supporting the efficacy of AAS, as well as adverse effects.
- Current estimates indicate that there are as many as 3 million AAS users in the United States and that 2.7%–2.9% of young American adults have taken AAS at least once in their lives.
- Recent estimates are that 1.5 million teenagers have tried AAS and that teenage girls may be the fastest-growing demographic for AAS use.

Mechanism of action:

- AAS are bound by cytoplasmic proteins and transported to the nucleus. Activation of DNA-dependent RNA polymerase results in production of messenger RNA for protein synthesis.
- Muscle size increases in AAS users through hypertrophy and formation of new muscle fibers. As reported by Kadi et al., muscle biopsies suggest that use of AAS enhances activation of satellite cells and contributes to muscle fiber growth.
- AAS also may have an anticatabolic effect by attenuating effects of cortisol. Haupt proposed that AAS displace cortisol from receptors, allowing athletes to train at a high level. He also suggested that AAS increase motivation through heightened aggressiveness.

In vivo studies of athletes and anabolic steroids:

- Numerous studies of anabolic steroid use by male athletes have produced conflicting results. Some support improvement in strength, whereas others found no significant improvement in strength. The American College of Sports Medicine's (ACSM's) official position statement, as well as many other systematic reviews, support the following position on AAS:
  - Use of steroids by athletes is contrary to the rules and ethical principles of athletic competition.

- With adequate diet, AAS can contribute to increases in body weight and lean mass.
- Gains in muscular strength achieved through steroid use at doses beyond those utilized in clinical medicine improve performance and seem to increase aerobic power or capacity for muscular exercise, giving an unfair advantage to those who are willing to risk the potential side effects to achieve gains in athletic performance.
- AAS have been associated with adverse side effects in therapeutic trials and in limited research on athletes.

- Well-conducted study by Bhasin et al. in 1996 demonstrated increase in fat-free mass and muscle size and strength in weightlifters using weekly injections of 600 mg testosterone enanthate for 10 weeks. First study to demonstrate that supraphysiologic doses of testosterone in trained weightlifters, combined with resistance training, can increase strength.

AAS: Chemical alternations to existing synthetic AAS in order to avoid detection by drug testing:

- **Norbolethone**
  - Originally documented 30 years ago; isolated in two urine samples from a female athlete in 2002 who later received a lifetime ban.
  - Never commercially marketed because of possible toxic effects in animal studies and/or reports of menstrual irregularities.
  - Anabolic activity 20 times higher than its androgenic activity; thus, very attractive to athletes looking to gain a competitive edge.
- **Tetrahydrogestrinone (THG)**
  - Unlike norbolethone, THG is a new chemical entity and would have remained undetectable if a syringe containing it had not been anonymously sent to the United States Anti-Doping Agency (USADA) in 2003.
  - Closely related to gestrinone, a progestin, and to trenbolone, a veterinary androgen.
  - Little information about the safety and anabolic effects of THG; has been found to be a potent androgen.
  - Several Olympics labs have reported positive results for THG.
  - Additional designer AAS have appeared as increasing sophistication of drug testing continues.

Over-the-counter steroids:

- 1994 Dietary Supplement and Health Act made supplements available over the counter, including testosterone (androstenedione, androstenediol, dehydroepiandrosterone [DHEA]) and nandrolone precursors (19-norandrostenedione, 19-norandrostenediol).
- Athletes use these short-acting compounds to increase muscle mass, despite lack of definitive studies of benefits and adverse effects.
- Some have been found to increase testosterone and nandrolone metabolites. Assumed to have similar profile to AAS.

Governmental regulation:

- 1990 Anabolic Steroid Control Act: AAS were added to Schedule III of the Controlled Substances Act.
- 2004 Anabolic Steroid Control Act: added steroid precursors such as androstenedione to the list of controlled substances. DHEA was not included in the act and is still legally available as a dietary supplement despite being banned by many sports organizations. Also increased the penalties for trafficking.
- Designer Anabolic Steroid Control Act of 2014: further defined designer AAS and increased penalties.

Potential therapeutic uses:

- True medical indications for AAS probably account for <3 million prescriptions/year. **Indications** include refractory anemias, hereditary angioedema, palliation therapy in advanced breast carcinoma, replacement therapy in hypogonadal males, and muscle-wasting states associated with HIV infection. AAS also may be useful in patients with constitutional delay of growth (as an adjunct to growth hormone [GH] therapy) and osteoporosis and has potential use as a male contraceptive.
- Acquired hypogonadism: A major marketing effort by pharmaceutical companies and "antiaging" clinics has increased the number of prescriptions for testosterone amid the liberalization of the diagnosis of hypogonadism. The Endocrine Society has published guidelines for the legitimate prescribing of testosterone in men with androgen deficiency. These include:
- The diagnosis of hypogonadism should only be made in men with symptoms and signs consistent with testosterone deficiency.
- The use of accurate assays for measurement of total and free testosterone that should be confirmed by repeated measurements of fasting, morning specimens.
- If androgen deficiency is determined, diagnostic evaluation should be done to ascertain the cause.

Dosage

- **Doses taken by athletes may be 10–40 times higher than therapeutic doses.**
- Athletes frequently use combinations of anabolic steroids **(stacking)** or cycling in a pyramidal fashion to achieve maximum effect.

Adverse reactions:

- **Gastrointestinal:** hepatocellular dysfunction, peliosis hepatis, and case reports of hepatocellular carcinoma. Hepatic effects are increased with 17-α-alkylated compounds consumed orally. Serum liver function tests should be checked in athletes with suspected history of AAS use.
- **Cardiovascular:** increase in total cholesterol and low-density lipoprotein (LDL) cholesterol; decrease in high-density lipoprotein (HDL) cholesterol; hypertension; increased risk of deep vein thrombosis; compartment syndromes; reported cases of myocardial infarction (MI), atrial fibrillation, and cerebrovascular accident. The Food and Drug Administration (FDA) has released a warning to reflect the potential increased risk of MI and stroke with testosterone use. However, although retrospective reports have suggested that testosterone therapy increases cardiovascular risk, randomized controlled trials have been insufficiently powered to evaluate risk for cardiovascular events in men who have undergone testosterone replacement therapy. A 2017 study by Baggish et al. found 71% of current AAS users had a depressed left ventricular ejection fraction.
- **Psychological effects:** changes in libido, mood swings, aggressive behavior, exacerbation of underlying mental illness, delirium, addiction to the appearance on AAS, and suicide attempts. Dependence pattern with opioid medications, as well as conduct disorder, has been reported. Pope and Katz interviewed 41 bodybuilders and football players who had used AAS and found that, according to DSM III-R criteria, 9 (22%) displayed full affective syndrome and 5 (12%) had psychotic symptoms in association with AAS use. However, a well-designed study by Bahrke et al. of current AAS users, previous users, and nonusers demonstrated that although perceived or actual psychological changes may occur, they were not demonstrated on several standardized inventories.
- **Male reproductive effects:** oligospermia, azoospermia, decreased testicular size, and gynecomastia. Case of adenocarcinoma of prostate also has been reported. In addition, a case with a young male using high doses of oral turinabol suggests a potential causal relationship to intratesticular leiomyosarcoma.
- **Female effects:** reduced luteinizing hormone (LH), follicle-stimulating hormone (FSH), estrogens, and progesterone;

menstrual irregularities; male pattern alopecia; hirsutism; clitoromegaly; and deepening of voice. Last three are probably irreversible.

- **Youths:** irreversible, premature closure of the epiphyses. Several highly publicized cases of suicide in high school athletes related to steroid use (e.g., Taylor Hooton).
- **Additional drug use:** AAS users are likely to use other drugs. A 2007 study by Elliot of high school female students revealed that AAS users were more likely to use alcohol, cigarettes, marijuana, and cocaine. In 2009, Ip conducted the Anabolic 500 survey that demonstrated AAS-dependent users were significantly more likely to report heroin use within the past 12 months and endorse a history of physical and sexual abuse.

Miscellaneous:

- Spontaneous tendon rupture.
- Increase in sebaceous glands and acne.
- Infectious complications, including HIV (due to sharing of contaminated needles), hepatitis B and C, and intramuscular abscess.
- A case report described bilateral deltoid myositis ossificans in a patient who repeatedly injected anabolic steroids in his bilateral deltoids in the past.
- Worsening of tic symptoms in patients with Tourette syndrome.
- Suppression of humoral immunity and immunoglobulin levels.
- Anecdotal reports of an association with compartment syndromes after trauma and/or surgical procedures.
- Reduction in glomerular filtration rate with supraphysiologic usage of AAS.
- Polycythemia requiring phlebotomy.

Side effects: Documented in secret AAS program for elite athletes sponsored by GDR: liver damage, gynecomastia, polycystic ovarian syndrome, arrested body growth, and three deaths.

Prevention: Programs designed to reduce AAS use have been developed (e.g., by Goldberg and the ATLAS program) for use at the high school level.

Detection: Clinical suspicion should be aroused by the presence of the aforementioned adverse effects. Drug testing (discussed later) can detect AAS with high degree of accuracy.

SELECTIVE ANDROGEN RECEPTOR MODULATORS (SARMs)

Definition: Nonsteroidal ligands for the androgen receptor. Some of the common ones are Ostarine, Andarine, LGD-4033 (Ligandrol), and RAD140 (Testolone).

Prevalence: According to WADA 2018 testing figures, SARMs accounted for 4% of positive tests involving anabolic substances globally Actual usage rates are unknown; a 2017 Internet search by Van Wagoner et al. yielded 210 products from 51 supplier sites advertising SARMs.

Mechanism of action: Ligands bind to the androgen receptor and exert tissue-selective effects such as muscle growth. They have been shown to have anabolic properties in rodents, and early clinical trials demonstrated anabolic activity in older individuals.

Therapeutic use: They have not received FDA approval, and clinical trials have investigated its use in the treatment of cachexia, cancer, osteoporosis, male contraception, prostate enlargement and cancer, and muscular dystrophy.

Adverse reactions: Trials using therapeutic doses have demonstrated testosterone suppression, decreases in HDL cholesterol, increases in LDL cholesterol, and liver function abnormalities. Users of Andarine have reported visual disturbance (yellowing of vision) in various blogs. It remains to be seen if the higher doses typically consumed by athletes would result in more significant adverse reactions as seen with traditional AAS.

Detection: These substances are readily detectable in urine through gas chromatography–mass spectrometry (GC/MS).

Related compounds: Peroxisome proliferator-activator δ are part of a family of hormone and lipid-activated nuclear receptors that are involved in the metabolism of long-chain fatty acids, cholesterol, and sphingolipids and can act as transcription factors. They have been involved in research studies in the treatment of metabolic syndrome, dyslipidemia, carcinogenesis, and diabetes. They are frequently found in dietary supplements labeled as SARMs, with GW501516 (Cardarine) being one of the more common ones. Because these substances theoretically may trigger transcriptional remodeling of muscle, they have become attractive to the sports community. These are not approved for human use, and safety has not been determined.

GROWTH FACTORS

Human Growth Hormone

Definition: Polypeptide hormone composed of 191 amino acids with molecular weight of 21,500 and contains many different isoforms, the predominant one being a 22 kD isomer and about 10% 20 kD. Normally, 5–10 mg is stored in the anterior pituitary. Men have a production rate of 0.4–1.0 mg/day. The production of recombinant hGH (rhGH) in the 1980s dramatically increased the potential supply. As opposed to natural GH, rhGH contains only the 22 kD isomer.

Prevalence: With the growing effectiveness of GC/MS detecting AAS and testosterone, many athletes have turned to hGH. Prevalence is difficult to estimate, but is thought to be widely used by many types of professional athletes.

Mechanism: hGH stimulates the production of various markers, the most prominent being insulin-like growth factor (IGF-1) or somatomedin-C. Although there is some debate about whether substances such as hepatic-produced IGF-1 are markers or mediators, hGH exerts most of its effects through receptors at target cells. There is little evidence that the commercially available IGF-1 products have any ability to increase IGF-1 levels or strength. It is also clear that although some controlled, albeit limited, studies of hGH have revealed increases in IGF-1 and changes in lean body mass, none have definitively demonstrated increases in strength or athletic performance with hGH alone.

- **Function:** Administration of hGH to GH-deficient children results in positive nitrogen balance and stimulation of skeletal and soft tissue growth.
- **Metabolic effects:** GH reduces glucose and protein metabolism and has a net anti-insulin effect by inhibiting cellular uptake of glucose. It also stimulates mobilization of lipids from adipose tissue, and protein synthesis is greatly increased in hypophysectomized animals.
- **Effects on muscle:** Several studies report conflicting data about the effect of hGH on muscle. Animal experiments by Goldberg concluded that hGH increased basal metabolic rate of protein synthesis but that this effect was also determined by the amount of muscular work. It is difficult to predict the ability of hGH to increase contractile elements and improve performance of normal muscle in normal humans. Deyssig showed in studies of hGH that although there may be increases in IGF-1 and changes in lean body mass, there is no definitive demonstration of increases in strength or athletic performance. Studies have demonstrated increases in muscle mass in the setting of current or past use of AAS.
- hGH treatment of adults with acquired GH deficiency increased lean body mass, decreased fat mass, and increased basal metabolic rate. Study concluded that hGH can regulate body composition through anabolic and lipolytic actions.

Therapeutic uses: The FDA under USC 33(e) has established guidelines for the legitimate use of hGH, and it cannot be used for "off-label" use (Box 26.3). The FDA

BOX 26.3 FDA-APPROVED INDICATIONS OF HUMAN GROWTH HORMONE

Children, Poor Growth Because of

- Turner syndrome
- Prader-Willi syndrome
- Chronic renal insufficiency
- hGH insufficiency/deficiency
- Children born small for gestational age who fail to manifest catch-up growth by age 2
- Idiopathic short stature or growth failure associated with short stature homeobox gene *(SHOX)* deficiency
- Noonan syndrome

Adults

- Wasting syndrome of HIV/AIDS
- hGH deficiency
- Short bowel syndrome

Data from Department of Justice Drug Enforcement Administration Office of Diversion Control: "Human Growth Hormone."

has established the use of the GH stimulation test to diagnose adult GH deficiency. **Low serum IGF-1 levels alone are not considered evidence of GH deficiency.**

Dosage: FDA-approved dose is 0.003–0.004 mg/kg/day via subcutaneous injection, although some recommend 0.15–0.3 mg/day, regardless of body weight.

Adverse reactions:

- **Acromegaly** is a potentially serious side effect of megadoses of hGH. It is estimated that acromegalic patients with hGH concentrations of 5–30 ng/mL have production rates of 1.5–9 mg/day. **As little as a twofold increase in the recommended dose may result in acromegaly, leaving a narrow therapeutic window.** With athletes consuming up to 20 mg/day, the risk of acromegaly is significant. Complications of acromegaly include diabetes; arthritis; myopathies; and characteristic coarsening of bones of the face, hands, and feet.
- Side effects using physiologic replacement doses in GH-deficient patients are generally low. Reported adverse reactions include intracranial hypertension, hyperglycemia, and glycosuria. However, in 2012 the FDA reported that the long-term epidemiologic French study, SAGhE, demonstrated a 30% increased risk of death when using rhGH. Data suggested mortality was associated with bone tumors and cardiovascular events (mainly subarachnoid or intracerebral hemorrhage). Risk is higher when higher-than-normal doses were prescribed. The FDA maintained that when appropriately used, benefits outweigh risks.
- Adult patients using hGH have described fluid retention, arthralgia, myalgia, gynecomastia, hypoesthesia, and paresthesia (e.g., carpal tunnel syndrome via median nerve edema).
- **The use of hGH by "antiaging" clinics without the establishment of GH deficiency constitutes illegal prescribing.**
- Creutzfeldt-Jakob disease has resulted from the use of hGH derived from cadaveric pituitary glands. Although use of synthetic hGH obviates this problem, athletes often obtain substances from black market sources, thereby increasing risk for this catastrophic neurologic disorder.

Detection: hGH is banned by WADA, and there are two established serum methods of detection.

- **Isoform test:** Immunoassays are used to estimate the amounts of the various GH isomers in serum. Although the majority of circulating GH is 20 kD and 22 kD, many other isomers naturally exist. When rhGH (22 kD) is given, natural production of all GH isomers is suppressed, thus the ratio of 22k D to non-22 kD isomers will increase, indicating use of synthetic GH. The test can detect the use of hGH for up to 72 hours, and there have been several positive tests worldwide. Recent research has established decision limits for this test, and the Court of Arbitration for Sport (CAS) has upheld it. The current detection threshold is 1.45 for males and 1.8 for females.
- **Biomarker test:** Measures the serum markers IGF-1 (from liver) and procollagen type III (P-III-NP, from bone) that can discriminate hGH users from nonusers up to 2 weeks after use. The test was first used at the 2012 London Olympic Games and revealed positive tests in two Russian Paralympian weightlifters who admitted use. The test protocols were adopted for use worldwide in 2016 by WADA labs.

IGF-1

- hGH stimulates the production of IGF-1 by the liver.
- There is little evidence that the commercially available IGF-1 products have any ability to increase IGF-1 levels or strength.
- Limited controlled studies of rhGH have revealed increases in IGF-1 and changes in lean body mass, but none have definitively demonstrated increases in strength or athletic performance.
- The use of supplements containing deer antler velvet have been advertised to contain IGF-1. Although these products do contain IGF-1, research has demonstrated that it is actually human IGF-1 that was added postproduction and thus illegal.
- Adverse effects related to IGF-1 use include hypoglycemia; decreased hGH secretion; carbohydrate oxidation preferentially over lipids; interference in the insulin–glucagon axis; and an association with carcinoma of the prostate, colon, and lung.
- Mechano growth factors are a new form of IGF-1 that are produced in response to mechanical loads and have been described by Goldspink.

Growth Hormone–Releasing Peptides (GHRPs)

- Synthetic peptides with small fraction of GH that are potent stimulants of GH secretion.
- GH peaks in 15–30 minutes with return to baseline in 2–3 hours.
- Ghrelin analogs GHRP 1, 2, 4, 5, 6, ipamorelin, etc.
- Oral, intravenous (IV), and nasal routes with metabolites detectable for 20 hours by liquid chromatography–mass spectrometry (LC-MS).
- Multiple positives in professional and Olympic sports.
- Has been detected in nutritional supplements and in injectable products available online that are marketed for "research purposes only" with the disclaimer that they are "not for human consumption." Numerous blogs and videos depict people describing how to use and dose the products, however. Because they are not labeled as a food, drug, or dietary supplement, they largely evade scrutiny by the FDA
- These are not approved for human use, and thus adverse effects are difficult to determine. There is a fatal case report of GHRP activating Hodgkin lymphoma in an athlete that had been in remission. There have been anecdotal reports of increased cortisol levels and prolactin production (GHRP2).

Insulin

- Physicians are trained to view insulin as a solely therapeutic drug, but increasing anecdotal information associates AAS use with insulin, and a study by Parkinson and Evans found 25% of AAS users also used insulin.

- It is speculated that insulin might enhance strength through its inhibitory functions (deters lipolysis, glycolysis, gluconeogenesis, proteolysis, and ketogenesis); when combined with an anabolic agent such as hGH or AAS, the protein-sparing effects of insulin produce larger anabolic results and significantly increase lean body mass.
- Risks of insulin use in normoglycemic athletes include lethal hypoglycemia, lipodystrophy, lipoatrophy, insulin allergy/resistance, and the production of insulin autoantibodies.
- Insulin is prohibited by WADA, although there is no approved test for its detection.

AMPHETAMINES

Definition: Stimulants classified as indirect-acting sympathomimetic amines with central and peripheral effects. Amphetamine use in athletes is complicated by the fact that they can be used for ergogenic, recreational, or therapeutic uses.

Prevalence:
- 2017 NCAA study reported 1.5% use of amphetamines in the past 12 months. Additionally, the use of methylene-n-methylamphetamine (Ecstasy or Molly) as a recreational stimulant has caused concern, with 2.4% of male NCAA athletes admitting to its use in the previous year.
- **The 2017 NCAA study revealed that 14% of NCAA athletes had used attention-deficit/hyperactivity disorder (ADHD) medications, but 7.5% reported using those medications without a prescription, indicating that the 1.5% usage rate for amphetamines likely underestimates actual use.**
- Estimating the use of amphetamines in sports is difficult, as athletes can use amphetamines for recreational, ergogenic, or therapeutic reasons.
- Commonly found on the black market ("greenies") and often found to contain clobenzorex.

Mechanism of action: Several theories have been proposed to explain central and peripheral effects of amphetamines: increased liberation of endogenous catecholamines, displacement of bound catecholamines, inhibition of monoamine oxidase, interference with catecholamine reuptake, and production of false neurotransmitters. All probably contribute to observed physiologic responses, including increases in blood pressure and heart rate, bronchodilation, increased metabolic rate, and increased free fatty acid production.

Relationship to athletic performance: Literature contains contradicting data.
- Smith and Beecher reported that 75% of trained swimmers, weight throwers, and runners had improved performance after taking amphetamines.
- Chandler and Blair demonstrated no substantial improvement in athletic performance.
- Explanation may be that amphetamine enhances performance of simple, repetitive tasks but not of more complicated maneuvers.

Therapeutic uses: Amphetamines have been used legitimately to treat many conditions, including refractory obesity, narcolepsy, ADHD, and severe depression. High abuse potential has limited their utility in these conditions. The estimated incidence of ADHD in the young adult male population is difficult to accurately determine, but has been estimated at 4%–5% with some studies up to 13%. This is difficult to determine, as it depends on the criteria used, and there are large variations by race. MLB reported about 8% of players in 2020 were granted TUEs for treatment with ADHD stimulant medications.

Dosage: Taken orally, amphetamines exert effects within 30 minutes of ingestion; their actions can last 12–24 hours. Dosages vary depending on athlete and type of preparation.

Adverse reactions:
- Central nervous system: restlessness, insomnia, psychological addiction, psychosis, tremor, anxiety, dizziness, headache, and cerebral hemorrhage.
- Cardiovascular: lowered threshold for arrhythmias and provocation of angina.
- Miscellaneous: disruptions in thermoregulation, predisposition to heat illness.

Detection: Amphetamines are readily detected by urine tests because both unchanged amphetamines and metabolites appear in urine.

TUEs: Amphetamines present a difficult challenge for sports to address in terms of TUEs for ADHD. It is a clinical diagnosis with limited objective criteria and varying standards. The NCAA requires that student-athletes have a diagnosis, have a medication dosage, have considered nonbanned alternatives, have checked the blood pressure and pulse, and must submit a written evaluation of a comprehensive clinical evaluation. The NCAA does not specify qualifications for conducting the examination, except that it should be completed by a clinician capable of meeting these requirements. MLB requires that the examination be done by a board-certified psychiatrist who has been certified by the league. In order for a TUE to be accepted, the player undergoes an Adult ADHD Clinical Diagnosis Scale, neuropsychological testing, and full evaluation and history. The information is then submitted to a three-person independent expert panel for review. If the TUE is accepted, the prescribing physician cannot have involvement with a team (e.g., be a team physician). When a stimulant medication is prescribed, preference is given to long-acting preparations to reduce the possibility of abuse. Finally, these TUEs must be renewed yearly to confirm the ongoing need for the medication, compliance, and necessary follow-up. These renewals are again reviewed by the independent expert panel. These procedures are helpful to ensure the medications are being used for a legitimate purpose.

COCAINE

See online.

CAFFEINE

Definition: Naturally occurring plant alkaloid derived from aqueous extracts of *Coffea arabica* and *Cola acuminata*. Caffeine is classified as a central nervous system stimulant and is found in coffee, tea, and cola drinks. It is a methylxanthine and chemically related to theobromine and theophylline. It has been used by athletes for its stimulant properties and potential for increased work and power.

Prevalence:
- Sixty percent of Americans over age 18 years drink coffee daily and average three cups per day.
- Energy drinks for the US market have continued to grow at 10% per year. Worldwide sales of energy drinks topped $55 billion in 2002. Alcohol intake appears significantly higher when energy drinks are mixed with alcohol.

Mechanism of action: Rapidly absorbed, and peak levels in 30–60 minutes, with half-life of 3.5 hours. Competitive antagonist of adenosine and causes vasoconstriction (except in renal afferent artery), increased diuresis and natriuresis, central nervous system stimulation, increased lipolysis in adipocytes, and increased gastric secretion. **Dietary supplements may contain high levels of caffeine. Anhydrous caffeine, a highly concentrated form of caffeine, has been associated with several deaths. Companies have also marketed oral pouches containing caffeine to use as substitutes for spit tobacco.**

Performance:

- Increased work and power probably result from increased mobilization of free fatty acids, increased rate of lipid metabolism, and direct effects on muscle contraction.
- Overall, ability of caffeine to enhance or prolong work output has been controversial. Any benefits in athletic performance are likely limited to endurance activities.

Therapeutic uses: Caffeine has been used as a stimulant in fatigue states, in combination with analgesic compounds, and in diet pills.

Adverse reactions:

- Central nervous system: anxiety, hypochondriasis, insomnia, headache, tremors, depression, scotomata, and addiction with withdrawal states.
- Cardiovascular: tachyarrhythmias, especially paroxysmal atrial tachycardia.
- Renal: diuretic effect, which is of significance in athletes at risk of dehydration.

Detection and dosage: WADA no longer bans caffeine but maintains monitoring. The NCAA has set the maximum urinary concentration of caffeine at 15 μg/mL. One study found that to exceed that threshold, the athlete needed to consume almost 1000 mg of caffeine within 3 hours of testing. This is above the average daily consumption of 200 mg of caffeine. Athletes concerned about testing should be aware that caffeine excretion is variable and can be affected by many factors, including exercise and the concomitant use of selective serotonin reuptake inhibitors (SSRIs) (e.g., fluoxetine) and cimetidine.

SYMPATHOMIMETIC AMINES

Definition: Synthetic congeners of naturally occurring catecholamines. In addition to amphetamines, several other weaker sympathomimetic amines have the potential to be abused by athletes, including phenylpropanolamine, phenylephrine, ephedrine, and pseudoephedrine.

Prevalence: Sympathomimetic amines appear in various cold remedies, common nasal and ophthalmologic decongestants, and most asthma preparations. After passage of the Dietary Supplement Health and Education Act in 1994, ephedrine appeared in various over-the-counter dietary supplements for weight loss and energy and was often listed as ephedra and ma huang. However, after at least 150 deaths, including several high-profile athletes purportedly linked to ephedrine use (Steve Bechler of the Baltimore Orioles, Korey Stringer of the Minnesota Vikings, and Rashidi Wheeler of Northwestern University), the FDA in 2004 banned dietary supplements containing ephedrine. Despite the ban, ephedrine-containing products are still available on the Internet, and 0.9% of NCAA athletes in 2012 still reported using ephedrine in the previous 12 months.

Mechanism: Response of sympathomimetic amines depends on relative selectivity of specific drug. Although earlier scientific studies demonstrated that ephedrine improved athletic performance, three studies have shown no significant increases in performance.

- Alpha effects: smooth muscle contraction, primarily vasoconstriction.
- $Beta_1$ effects: production of intracellular cyclic adenosine monophosphate (cAMP), increased heart rate, and strength of contraction.
- $Beta_2$ effects: smooth muscle relaxation, bronchodilation, stimulation of skeletal muscle.

Therapeutic uses: Nonemergent treatment of allergic reactions, asthma, hypotension during spinal anesthesia, atrioventricular block, and nasal congestion.

Dosage: Many types of drugs in this category have varying potencies and durations of action.

Adverse reactions with increasing doses: Anxiety, epigastric distress, palpitations. tremulousness, insomnia, drowsiness, hypertension, stroke, seizures.

Detection: Sympathomimetic amines are banned by WADA and can be detected by drug testing. WADA allows the use of inhaled selective $beta_2$-agonists, terbutaline, albuterol, bitolterol, orciprenaline, and rimiterol. Sympathomimetic amines such as ephedrine and synephrine are banned by the NCAA; however, phenylephrine and pseudoephedrine are not.

Clenbuterol Has Garnered Attention for Potential as an Anabolic Substance

Definition: $Beta_2$-agonist, similar to albuterol, used as a bronchodilator. It has recently been considered an anabolic or "repartitioning" agent. Anabolic effects have been purported to occur only with oral forms, not via the inhalation route.

Prevalence: Limited information about prevalence is derived mostly from increasing numbers of athletes who are disqualified by positive drug tests. Between 2016 and 2018, clenbuterol accounted for 963 positive tests globally, according to WADA testing statistics. Six Olympians were disqualified in 1992: two Americans, two Germans, and two British. Parkinson and Evans reported clenbuterol use for fat loss by AAS users. A 2007 report found that clenbuterol was illegally present in some dietary supplements available on the Internet. Clenbuterol is used in livestock for meat production in some countries, and there have been antidoping cases reportedly resulting from athletes consuming contaminated meat.

Mechanism: Most data about anabolic effects of clenbuterol are derived from animal studies. No studies to date have examined effects of oral clenbuterol on nonasthmatic athletes. Livestock treated with clenbuterol demonstrated increased muscle mass and decreased fatty deposits. Denervated rat hindlimbs demonstrated reduced muscle wasting when treated with clenbuterol, as well as a decreased net bone loss. Clenbuterol produced no changes in muscle cross-sectional area in a randomized study by Maltin et al. of patients undergoing medial meniscectomy. Although the finding was not statistically significant, the authors asserted that the clenbuterol group regained strength more rapidly. The exact mechanism of clenbuterol's anabolic effects has not been determined, but it has been previously shown that catecholamines attenuate amino acid release from muscle by beta-mediated depression of protein catabolism. Clenbuterol may also act by increasing contractile tension.

Therapeutic uses: Clenbuterol is used as a bronchodilator for the treatment of asthma; however, it is not legally available in the United States.

Dosage: Recommended dosage for asthma is 0.02–0.03 mg twice daily. The anabolic dosage is not known, but extrapolation from animal data translates into 0.001–0.01 mg/kg or 0.07–0.7 mg in a 70-kg person. Maltin and associates used the lower asthma dose, 0.02 mg twice daily, in their study of orthopedic patients.

Adverse reactions (typical $beta_2$ effects): Muscle tremor, palpitations, muscle cramps, tachycardia, tenseness, headaches, and peripheral vasodilation. There has been a case report of clenbuterol potentiating the effects of AAS that resulted in MI, as well as multiple other cases associating its use with MIs.

Detection: Clenbuterol is prohibited by WADA and NCAA. It is also banned by the Association of Official Racing Chemists for its ergogenic effects on thoroughbred racehorses. It can be detected in urine by GC/MS.

Other $beta_2$-agonists: Debate about clenbuterol has raised questions about anabolic effects and possible banning of other $beta_2$-agonists. This is controversial because most studies of athletes reveal that 10% suffer from exercise-induced asthma and depend on $beta_2$-agonists to compete. Whereas most studies have been inconclusive about ergogenic effects of other inhaled beta$_2$-agonists, a recent randomized, double-blind cross-over study demonstrated increased power output associated with increased rates of glycolysis and glycogenolysis in skeletal muscle of sprinters who had been given inhaled terbutaline. Additionally, the counteraction of reduction of adenosine triphosphate (ATP) in type II fibers with the use of terbutaline demonstrated in this study may argue for delay in the development of fatigue in these fibers. Although further research is warranted, it would be extremely difficult to deny asthmatics the use of inhaled beta$_2$-agonists.

Designer stimulants: Many new stimulants have appeared in recent years in order to circumvent regulations regarding dietary supplements and potentially avoid drug testing. These include heptaminol, methylhexanamine (dimethylamylamine [DMAA]), dimethlybutylamine (DMBA), oxilofrine, higenamine (norcoclaurine), and others. Many of these have never been studied in humans and have been associated with significant adverse effects.

NONSTEROIDAL ANTI-INFLAMMATORY DRUGS

See online.

ALCOHOL

Definition: Ethanol, the most abused recreational drug in the United States, is classified as a depressant.

Prevalence: Approximately 70% of adult Americans drink alcohol, and per capita consumption is estimated at 2.23 gallons/year. Perhaps 5%–10% of drinkers are, or will become, alcoholics. There are 75,000 annual alcohol-related deaths. 2017 NCAA study revealed that 77% of student-athletes consume alcohol. Moreover, 36% consumed alcohol weekly and 42% engaged in binge drinking. It has been suggested that athletes are a high-risk group for such behaviors.

Mechanism: Physiologic effects of alcohol are well known and not reviewed here.

Therapeutic uses: None.

Adverse reactions: Physicians are familiar with many adverse consequences of alcohol abuse. With respect to athletes:

- **After literature review, ACSM issued a current comment about use of alcohol in relation to athletic performance:** Acute ingestion of alcohol has a deleterious effect on many psychomotor skills, including reaction times, hand–eye coordination, accuracy, balance, and complex coordination. Alcohol consumption does not substantially influence physiologic functions crucial to physical performance (VO_2 max, respiratory dynamics, cardiac function). It does not improve muscular work capacity and may decrease performance levels, as well as impair temperature regulation during prolonged exercise in cold environments.
- Study by Urbano-Marquez et al. concluded that alcohol is toxic to striated muscle in a dose-dependent manner.
- Arrests for driving while impaired substantially increase the risk of eventual death in alcohol-related crash.

Detection: Alcohol is prohibited on a sport-by-sport basis, particularly in motor sports. It is not prohibited by WADA and is not tested for in WADA-style tests. Alcohol is banned in the NCAA in rifle sport only.

Identification:

- The American Medical Association defines **alcoholism** as "illness characterized by significant impairment that is directly associated with persistent and excessive use of alcohol. Impairment may involve physiologic, psychological, or social dysfunction."
- Because effects of alcoholism may take 5–20 years to develop and usually occur after age 30, early identification of athletes with alcohol problems is imperative. Several measures are designed to help assess alcohol problems, including Perceived Benefit of Drinking Scale (PBDS), Children of Alcoholics Test (CAST), Michigan Alcoholism Screening Test (MAST), and **CAGE questionnaire.**
- Education and identification are keys to prevention in athletes.

NICOTINE

Definition: Volatile alkaloid derived from tobacco and responsible for many effects of tobacco. It first stimulates (small doses) then depresses (large doses) autonomic ganglia and myoneural junctions. Methods of consumption include cigarettes and smokeless tobacco (loose leaf tobacco [chewing], moist or dry powdered tobacco [snuff or "dipping"], compressed tobacco ["plug"], electronic cigarettes [e-cigs]).

Prevalence: According to the 2017 NCAA study, the number of athletes who had consumed cigarettes in the past year decreased to 10.5%, with spit tobacco also decreasing to 13.4%. In addition, 8.2% admitted to using e-cigarettes in the past 12 months. Furthermore, cigar use in the past year was at 17%, with hookah use at 10%. This demonstrates that tobacco is consumed in a variety of ways, and in surveying athletes, it is important to ask questions in multiple ways. This has been compounded by advertising for e-cigarettes and vaping implying that these are "safer" forms of consuming tobacco products. The addition of flavoring is clearly aimed at inducing younger people to consume these products.

Mechanism: Nicotine has various actions, depending on receptor binding and dose, and readily crosses the blood-brain barrier. It binds to acetylcholine receptors at autonomic ganglia, the adrenal medulla, neuromuscular junction, and in the central nervous system. Stimulation of central nicotinic receptors activates central nervous system neurohumoral pathways to release acetylcholine, norepinephrine, dopamine, serotonin, vasopressin, growth hormone, and adrenocorticotropic hormone (ACTH). Nicotine affects sympathetic nerves by release of catecholamines. At low doses, ganglionic stimulation and sympathetic discharge lead to increase in heart rate and blood pressure mediated through the central nervous system. At moderate doses, direct peripheral nervous system effects lead to ganglionic stimulation and adrenal catecholamine release. At high doses, ganglionic blockade leads to hypotension and bradycardia. Pharmacodynamic tolerance develops to subjective and hemodynamic effects.

Therapeutic uses: As an aid to smoking cessation, nicotine gum and transdermal patches have been somewhat effective in reducing withdrawal symptoms of physical nicotine dependence in smokers trying to quit. Bupropion has been used to reduce cravings, and varenicline may assist quitting by blocking alpha-4-beta-2 nicotinic acetylcholine receptors. There are conflicting reports about the use of e-cigarettes as adjuncts to smoking cessation and at this point cannot be recommended as a safe alternative.

Dosage: Smokeless tobacco users have blood nicotine levels equivalent to nicotine-dependent smokers. Normal single dose of snuff contains 1.5–2.5 g of tobacco; each gram has 14 mg of nicotine. Ten percent of nicotine is absorbed, leading to 2.0–3.5 mg nicotine in bloodstream (2–3 times higher than dose of standard 1-mg cigarette). Average single dose of chewing tobacco contains 7 g, with nicotine content of 7.8 mg/g; 8% is available to be absorbed. Eight to ten chews/day result in nicotine dose equivalent to 30–40 cigarettes/day.

Adverse reactions: Long-term effects of cigarette smoking are well known and are not reviewed here. Studies on the effects of smokeless tobacco have demonstrated:

- **Oropharynx:** 50-fold increase in oral carcinomas, 2.4 times higher incidence of dental caries, increases in gingival disease and leukoplakia.

- **Hemodynamics** (cigarette smoking compared with smokeless tobacco): similar levels of nicotine throughout the day, equivalent increases in heart rate and myocardial oxygen demand. Increased sodium (added for flavoring) absorption from smokeless tobacco may lead to increases in blood pressure.
- **Reaction time and concentration:** Smokeless tobacco has long been touted for its ability to improve reaction time and concentration. Study of athletes and nonathletes by Edwards et al. demonstrated no neuromuscular performance enhancement; no changes in reaction time, movement time, or total response time; and significant elevation in heart rate. Survey by Connolly et al. of MLB players who used smokeless tobacco found that only 10% believed that it improved concentration, and none felt it sharpened reflexes.
- **Addiction:** Smokeless tobacco can be as addictive as cigarette smoking. The National Cancer Institute, in conjunction with MLB, has prepared "Beat the Smokeless Habit: Game Plan for Success" to give readers the facts about smokeless tobacco. It includes a "9-inning game plan" to help athletes quit smokeless tobacco. An additional program, "Knock Tobacco Out of the Park," can be found at tobaccofreebaseball.org.
- Vaping and e-cigarettes: In addition to the previously noted effects of nicotine, inhaling volatile chemicals has been shown to cause significant lung injury leading to hypoxia and possible severe respiratory failure. Although the nicotine dose may be reduced compared with traditional cigarettes, acute lung damage may be a serious adverse effect and should not be encouraged as a safe alternative. Lastly, the use of tobacco either by vaping or combustion would be expected to exacerbate respiratory infections such as COVID-19.

Detection: Nicotine is not currently tested for by international organizations or NCAA, but NCAA bans the use of tobacco products by players, coaches, and officials during competition. MLB bans the use of spit tobacco in the Minor Leagues and open displays in the Major Leagues. Players who began their Major League service after 2017 are prohibited from using tobacco products in the stadium. Many stadiums now ban the use of any tobacco products by spectators or participants.

THC AND OTHER CANNABINOIDS

Definition: THC (δ9-tetrahydrocannabinol) is the psychoactive compound in the cannabis plant that most drug testing agencies test for. However, WADA prohibits all cannabinoids except for cannabidiol.

Prevalence: It is estimated that over 50% of Americans have tried marijuana at some point in their lives, with about 35 million regular users. In the 2017 NCAA study, 77% of marijuana users cited social reasons as the main reason for use and 19% for pain management. The availability of THC and CBD in smoked, vaped, and edible products has proliferated enormously in the last 10 years. The 2017 NCAA study revealed that 24% of student-athletes had inhaled marijuana in the past year, with 11% having consumed edibles.

Mechanism: THC exerts its effects on various tissues, with the central nervous system and cardiovascular system being the most prominent. Effects depend on route, dose, setting, and prior experience of user.

- **Cardiovascular:** Tachycardia is dose-related and can be blocked by propranolol. Systolic blood pressure increases in supine position and decreases in standing position.
- **Central nervous system:** Impaired motor coordination, decreased short-term memory, difficulty in concentrating, decline in work performance.
- **Male reproductive system:** Decreased plasma testosterone, gynecomastia, oligospermia.

Therapeutic uses: THC has been used as antiemetic agent in conjunction with chemotherapy for cancer patients and lowering intraocular pressure in glaucoma. Cannabidiol is also approved for use in treating two rare, severe forms of epilepsy. Many states now allow the medicinal use of marijuana, and others have legalized its nonmedicinal use. It is important for athletes to remember, especially for interstate travel, that regardless of state law, marijuana use is still a violation of federal law and banned by most drug testing programs.

Dosage: THC content of marijuana in the United States ranges from 0.5%–11%; serum concentration depends on method of ingestion.

Adverse reactions: Renaud and Cormier found the following effects on exercise performance: reduction of maximal exercise performance with premature achievement of VO_2 max; no effects on tidal volume, arterial blood pressure, or carboxyhemoglobin compared with controls. Marijuana causes inhibition of sweating that can lead to increase in core body temperature.

Detection: Marijuana is banned by WADA in competition above a level of 150 ng/mL, whereas it is considered a street drug by NCAA and is prohibited at a level of 5 ng/mL. Because of its high lipid solubility, marijuana can be detected for as long as 2–4 weeks by drug testing. Although many CBD products claim to be free of THC, in actuality most are likely to contain small amounts of THC. Athletes subject to drug testing should be cautious in using CBD products, as they could lead to a positive test result.

Synthetic cannabinoids: First developed for research purposes in the 1980s by John W. Huffman (JWH) and not for human consumption. Products are usually herbal mixtures sprayed with synthetic cannabinoids and are classified as Schedule I by the Drug Enforcement Agency (DEA). They can cause lethargy, hypotension, seizures, hallucinations, and paranoia. There should be a high index of suspicion in an impaired individual with a negative toxicology screen for THC. These are banned by most sports organizations and can be detected in urine.

BLOOD DOPING

Definition: Blood is infused into a nonanemic athlete for the purposed of increasing red blood cell mass. Blood doping can be autologous (from the same person) or heterologous (donated from another person).

Prevalence: Extent of blood doping is unknown. In 1984, the United States Olympics Committee (USOC) admitted that seven US cyclists had engaged in blood doping at the Summer Olympic Games. In 1990, a study by Scarpino et al. of 1018 Italian athletes revealed that 7% had tried blood doping. The advent of better testing for EPO has led athletes back to blood doping. Cyclist Tyler Hamilton tested positive for blood transfusions after winning the gold medal at the Athens 2004 Olympics.

Mechanism: Transfusion increases oxygen delivery to exercising muscle, and studies confirm that red cell mass and VO_2 max are well correlated. Studies of blood doping in elite runners compared with controls demonstrated improvement in maximal oxygen consumption, increased total exercise time, and increased hemoglobin concentration.

Therapeutic uses: Red cell transfusions are limited to patients with symptomatic anemia.

Dosage: Most studies have used 2000 mL of homologous blood or 900–1800 mL of cryopreserved autologous blood.

Adverse reactions: Improperly matched donor blood can result in transfusion reactions that may be fatal. Immune side effects are reported in 3% of all transfusions. Using donor blood has attendant risks of infectious complications. Risk is substantially lower with use of autologous blood.

Detection: WADA bans blood doping, but enforcement is limited by lack of effective technique for its detection. A test for heterologous blood transfusions was implemented at the 2004 Summer Olympic Games in Athens. This test can show that doping took place by providing evidence of different cell populations. WADA and the Partnership for Clean Competition are funding research projects aimed at developing a test for autologous transfusions through various methods, including microRNA and other potential markers. WADA has also implemented the Athlete Hematological Passport to detect subtle changes in hematologic parameters that may be indicative of hemoglobin manipulation.

ERYTHROPOIETIN AND RELATED COMPOUNDS

Definition: Sialic acid–containing hormone that enhances erythropoiesis by stimulating formation of proerythroblasts and release of reticulocytes from bone marrow. It is mainly secreted by the kidneys, and the level of EPO is inversely related to the number of circulating red cells. In 1986, a recombinant form of EPO (called r-HuEPO) was discovered that is identical to natural EPO except for the addition of sialic acid residues. In 2002, a long-acting form called darbepoetin was introduced. In 2008 a large (60 kDa) polyethylene glycol compound called continuous erythropoietin receptor activator (CERA or trade name Micera) was approved with a half-life 20 times greater than h-HuEPO with very little urinary excretion.

Prevalence: With increased attention (and attendant risks) to blood doping, r-HuEPO has become a potential avenue of abuse for athletes.

- Unexplained deaths of 18 Dutch and Belgian cyclists between 1987 and 1990 raised the specter of r-HuEPO abuse.
- The Festina cycling team was expelled in the first week of the 1998 Tour de France after a team car was found loaded with PEDs, including r-HuEPO.
- Several cyclists, including Bernard Kohl and members of Lance Armstrong's cycling team, have admitted to the use of EPO products.

Mechanism: Subcutaneous injection of r-HuEPO stimulates red cell production within days, and effects can be seen for as long as 3–4 weeks. Based on data from red cell reinfusion studies, r-HuEPO can theoretically increase VO_2 max by 10%. An uncontrolled study demonstrated an increase in mean maximal oxygen uptake and run time to exhaustion using r-HuEPO.

Therapeutic uses:

- In patients suffering from anemia secondary to end-stage renal disease, studies demonstrate that r-HuEPO eliminates the need for transfusions and restores hematocrit to normal in many patients; can partially correct renal anemia and results in significant increase of both exercise capacity and maximum work and can maintain normal hemoglobin concentration in uremic patients over time.
- r-HuEPO was found to be useful in the treatment of anemias secondary to prematurity, multiple myeloma, and cancer and in patients with AIDS treated with zidovudine.
- r-HuEPO increases the yield of autologous blood donors safely and effectively over a 21-day period and can reduce the need for transfusions in patients undergoing hip replacement.

Dosage: In a study of autologous blood donors with initially normal hemoglobin levels, 600 U/kg of r-HuEPO was given IV six times over 21 days. Doses in chronic renal patients have ranged between 15 and 500 U/kg three times/week. R-HuEPO is usually given subcutaneously, but improved detection methods have led athletes to begin IV microdosing to avoid detection.

Adverse reactions:

- Observed side effects in patients with renal anemia:
  - Hypertensive patients required additional antihypertensive medication.
  - Serum levels of potassium and bilirubin increased.
  - Twenty percent of patients developed flulike syndrome.
  - Fourteen percent of patients developed thrombosis of arteriovenous fistulas and veins.
  - Eleven patients reported visual hallucinations.
- Potential risks of r-HuEPO in athletes with normal hemoglobin:
  - Increases in hemoglobin and blood viscosity accentuated with dehydration may lead to cerebral or cardiovascular ischemia, vascular thrombosis, hypotension, hyperkalemia, and iron deficiency.
  - Attendant risks of IV medication (e.g., infection with hepatitis, HIV, endocarditis)

Detection: Direct test for the presence of r-HuEPO in the urine. The test shows the isoform patterns of r-HuEPO in urine by separation in an electrical field and detection with a very sensitive and selective method. The isoform pattern of r-HuEPO is distinctively different from native EPO. The isoelectric focusing urine test also yields a pattern for darbepoetin alfa that is distinct from both EPO and r-HuEPO. Testing for CERA with standard urinary isoelectric focusing is difficult because of low urinary excretion, but a related serum test using the SARCOSYL-PAGE method has proved adept at its detection.

AGENTS WITH ANTIESTROGENIC ACTIVITY

Definition: These are substances that oppose estrogens and include:

- Aromatase inhibitors such as anastrozole and letrozole.
- Selective estrogen receptor modifiers such as tamoxifen and raloxifene.
- Other antiestrogen substances such as clomiphene.

Prevalence: Unknown, but multiple anecdotal reports among users of anabolic steroids.

Mechanism: High doses of androgens will overwhelm hepatic capacity, and some of the excess is aromatized to estrogenic compounds, creating unwanted adverse effects in males. These drugs are used to counteract the effects, although they are not technically performance-enhancing themselves in men. AAS users have also used clomiphene to help the testes resume testosterone production, but there is little data on the efficacy, although they it improve fertility.

Potential therapeutic uses: These drugs are used for a variety of legitimate uses, mainly in women, including adjuvant therapy in breast cancer and ovulation induction.

Adverse reactions: These drugs are rarely used therapeutically in males, and as such, the adverse reactions are limited to women. It is likely that interfering with the hypothalamic–pituitary–gonadal axis will have major adverse effects in males.

Detection: These drugs are banned by WADA and can be detected using LC-MS technology.

GENETIC DOPING

Definition: The nontherapeutic use of genes, genetic elements, and/or cells that have the capability to enhance athletic performance.

Mechanism: May be achieved through several methods:

- Viral vector, such as modified adenovirus.
- Gene transfer that produces a specific message, or "switch," to turn on production of a desired substance.

Potential therapeutic uses: Genetic manipulation has the potential to cure a wide assortment of diseases, such as muscular dystrophy, and has been used in congenital immunodeficiency states.

Adverse reactions: Use of gene therapy has resulted in some severe effects, including the development of cancer. Primate studies with the insertion of an EPO-producing gene resulted in the animals requiring regular phlebotomies due to uncontrolled red cell production. Immune reactions are a major concern.

Specific drugs: It has been speculated, but unconfirmed, that the patented drug Repoxygen may have been used by athletes. The drug alters EPO production in response to low oxygen tension.

Detection: Although the practice is banned by WADA, there are no tests for detection. In 2004, WADA also created an Expert Group on Gene Doping to study the latest advances in the field of gene therapy, the methods for detecting doping, and the research projects funded by WADA in this area.

Possible deterrents include:

- Detection of the viral genome, but may be difficult if a common virus is used.
- Detection of the identifying switch.
- Testing serial biomarkers or pharmacodynamic tests.
- Manufacturer "labeling" of genetic material to allow detection.
- Control over the production and supply of materials.

Miscellaneous: In addition to genetic doping, the practice of genetically identifying sport-specific genes in children has begun in order to promote athletic success. Some of these markers include creatine kinase, angiotensin-converting enzyme, and mitochondrial enzymes.

Summary: Genetic doping and genetic identification of athletic traits is on the horizon and likely very difficult to harness once unleashed. It raises ethical issues and threatens the very definition of "sport."

DRUG TESTING

Purpose: Drug testing has been the major means of attempting to enforce compliance with the banned substance list. Public awareness has been heightened by positive tests in elite athletes. To date, most drug testing has been of the "announced" variety at championship or Olympic events, although there are attempts to increase unannounced testing.

Antidoping authorities: In the United States, Olympic, Paralympic, and Pan-American Sports are all WADA Code signatories. The USADA is the antidoping agency for these sports. The NCAA is the antidoping authority for college sports. Most professional sports have their own antidoping programs as a part of an employee/employer contract and an athlete/employee union.

Cost: USADA's testing and results management expenses were $21 million in 2019 to conduct approximately 10,000 blood and urine tests both in and out of competition.

Reliability: Tests vary in specificity, sensitivity, and expense.

- **Radioimmunoassay and enzyme-multiplied immunoassay:** Two most commonly used screening methods. Although manufacturers claim a 97%–99% accuracy rate, such is not usually the case. To avoid false-positive tests when an athlete's career may be at stake, a second highly sensitive and specific test is often required.
- **GC/MS:** Gold standard and only drug test legally admissible in court. All state-of-the-art laboratories must use GC/MS as a confirmatory test because it provides a "fingerprint" of the detected substance. Unfortunately, the high cost of both the equipment and test prohibits smaller laboratories from using GC/MS.
- **Gas chromatography-combustion isotope ratio mass spectrometer (IRMS):** IRMS is based on the finding that 98.9% of the carbon atoms in nature are ^{12}C, with 1.1% being ^{13}C (an isotope that contains an additional neutron). The ratio of $^{13}C/^{12}C$ can be measured with high accuracy and precision by an IRMS. Very small differences in the abundance of ^{13}C can be detected to allow differentiation of carbon sources. The IRMS values for steroids are expressed as delta values: $\delta^{13}C\%$. The more negative a delta value, the less ^{13}C the compound contains. Pharmaceutical testosterone is manufactured from a soy compound that contains relatively less ^{13}C content compared with endogenously produced testosterone, thus yielding significantly different results on IRMS analysis. However, analysis of seized illegal testosterone has revealed the presence of ^{13}C-enriched testosterone products that could potentially reduce the effectiveness of the test.
- **Athlete Biological Passport (ABP):** Comparing multiple tests on the same athlete over time reduces intraindividual variation of hormone levels, allowing for the detection of smaller changes.

Testing for anabolic steroids/testosterone:

- To combat use of exogenous testosterone, the ratio of testosterone to its isomer epitestosterone (T:E) has been quantified. The normal T:E ratio is 1:1. When exogenous testosterone is administered, serum testosterone is elevated out of proportion to epitestosterone. A ratio >6:1 is considered a positive test by the NCAA; however, USADA and the National Football League (NFL) consider a ratio >4:1 to be positive. The test is limited because of genetic variations in testosterone metabolism that can result in T:E ratios >4:1. Because of improved accuracy of high-resolution GC/MS in detecting synthetic AAS, use of exogenous testosterone has increased. Athletes have used epitestosterone in conjunction with testosterone ("the cream") to maintain "normal" T:E ratio. To combat this practice, epitestosterone is prohibited by WADA in concentrations >200 ng/mL.
- **GC-IRMS as noted earlier.**
- Athlete Steroid Profile: Similar to the ABP, this longitudinal test can detect perturbations in an athlete's endogenous steroid profile, suggesting androgen use.

Circumvention by athletes: Although GC/MS may approach 100% accuracy, athletes have attempted numerous methods of avoiding detection.

- **Masking agents:** Diuretics and tubular blocking agents such as probenecid have been used to mask or dilute banned substances or in urine. Drug tests now use minimum urinary specific gravity to combat this practice and ban these drugs. IV infusions and use of plasma expanders are also prohibited methods to make sure athletes cannot disrupt the detection of the drug.
- **Determination of drug half-life:** With announced drug testing, athletes can determine how long drug can be detected in urine. This problem can be addressed with random, unannounced testing.
- "Microdosing" with multiple small quantities of prohibited substances so that the amount in the athlete's sample is below the detection level. The ABP helps to address this.
- **Use of short-lived substances:** Athletes might try novel peptide agents that exert their actions quickly and are then metabolized and excreted. New detection methods and the use of new matrices can help combat this problem in the future.
- **Substitution of urine:** Athletes have developed numerous methods to substitute "clean" urine, including self-catheterization and innovative "delivery systems." To eliminate this problem, collection is conducted under constant supervision and direct observation.

Extent of testing: Most athletic organizations, professional and amateur, have developed drug testing programs. These policies are subject to frequent change depending on law, collective bargaining, and contemporary issues. It is best to check with respective organizations when specific questions arise.

- Olympic level: USADA conducts drug testing in all Olympic, Paralympic, and Pan-American sports and for other sporting agencies by contract. International and national "testing pool" (e.g., elite) athletes are required to provide their whereabouts to USADA (e.g., their schedule and location 24 hours a day, 365 days per year) to allow for unannounced testing at any time. Sanctions for antidoping rule violations can range from a public warning to a permanent (lifetime) ban. Antidoping sanctions are not limited to athletes, as coaches, team physicians, and other support personnel can also be sanctioned.
- Collegiate level: NCAA began testing in 1986 at postseason football games and championship events at Division I, II, and III levels. The NCAA conducts year-round drug testing on the campuses of NCAA Division I and Division II member schools and on the campuses of Division III schools that sponsor Division I or Division II sports. The first positive test results in a 1-year suspension and a second positive test for PEDs results in permanent loss of eligibility.
- MLB: Separate programs for the Minor and Major Leagues, with both programs testing in and out of season. First positive test for a PED results in an 80-game suspension, second positive test is 162 games (e.g., one full season), and a third positive test results in a permanent suspension.
- National Basketball Association: Amphetamine and its analogs, cocaine, lysergic acid diethylamide (LSD), opiates, phencyclidine (PCP), marijuana, and steroids, are prohibited. Individual players can be tested with "reasonable cause" for prohibited substances without prior notice, and rookies are tested on a random basis throughout the season.
- NFL: Currently tests both in and out of season in an unannounced fashion. The first positive test for stimulants, diuretics, or masking agents is two games; for anabolic agents, it is six games; and for violations such as attempts to substitute, adulterate, or manipulate test results, it is eight games. Second violations receive a 16-game suspension, except second violations for stimulants, diuretics, or masking agents, which are 5 games. A third offense receives a minimum 2-year ban. All suspensions are without pay.
- Beta-blockers are prohibited in competition in specified sports, particularly target shooting sports.

Effectiveness: The current consensus is the effectiveness of antidoping relies on the perception that there is a high likelihood of getting caught and there are significant punishments (e.g., financial losses, loss of medals and results, embarrassment/shame; "perceptual deterrence model"). A 2017 survey conducted by USADA of US athletes found that 80% of athletes support drug testing to keep sports clean, but almost half of US athletes do not feel their international competitors are tested to the same standard.

Announced vs. unannounced testing: Limitations of testing only at competitions are obvious, and sports organizations have moved to unannounced testing to deter drug use.

Legal issues: This evolving aspect of law varies according to state, and many issues have yet to be fully resolved. It is prudent to consult local legal experts before embarking on a testing program. Several landmark cases have involved drug testing:

- 1987: As a result of a suit by Stanford athletes, the court ruled that drug testing violates student-athletes' right to privacy. Overturned in 1994 by US Supreme Court.
- 1994: US Supreme Court rules that random drug tests violate privacy rights of University of Colorado athletes, trainers, and cheerleaders.
- 1995: US Supreme Court rules that urine drug screening of junior high and high school student-athletes is allowable. Court states that minors are not protected by Fourth Amendment rights to privacy like adults, and "individualized suspicion" is not necessary to conduct drug testing of athletes.
- 2002: US Supreme Court ruled in the Earls case that students possess limited privacy rights, the intrusion of drug testing was not significant, and the government had a legitimate interest in deterring drug use.

Guidelines for drug testing: The WADA publishes the International Standards for Testing and Investigations, which is mandatory for all WADA Code signatories. The NCAA also has their own guidelines for college sport drug testing.

Alternative matrices: Drug testing has traditionally involved urine testing, but the need for witnessed urination and the possibility of substitution and adulteration have led to the exploration of other methods. Blood testing is now used for the ABP, hGH testing, and some EPO testing, and some surveys have suggested that athletes prefer blood tests to observed urine collection. In addition, there is work being done with oral fluids, sweat testing, exhaled breath, and hair analysis. All of these have limitations and would have to withstand forensic scrutiny.

Nonanalytical rule violations have allowed antidoping organizations to apply sanctions in cases where there is no positive doping sample but where there is evidence that a doping violation has occurred (e.g., through a combination of three missed tests, whereabouts failures, longitudinal testing, evidence brought forward through an investigation).

THERAPEUTIC USE EXEMPTIONS

TUEs involve approval given to an athlete to use a medication that is normally prohibited in their sport by the restrictions of a doping control program. Key components of a successful TUE program include:

- Many substances that can be abused as PEDs also have legitimate therapeutic uses. Healthcare providers that treat athletes should be familiar with these prohibited medications (Table 26.3) that might require a TUE.
- The TUE process should be applied for, and approved, before the athlete uses the medication.
- Retroactive approval is considered only in case of emergency treatment of an acute condition or exceptional circumstances.
- Athlete must have a documented need for the prohibited substance or method and would experience serious adverse consequences if the use of the medication or method was not allowed.
- There must be no reasonable alternatives to the use of the prohibited substance or method.
- The necessity for the use of a medication cannot be the result of prior use of a prohibited substance (e.g., the use of testosterone replacement therapy because of chronic suppression of the pituitary-gonadal axis from chronic steroid use).
- The approval of the TUE would not allow use of a prohibited substance or method to enhance performance above what would be found if the athlete returned to normal health.

DRUG EDUCATION

- **Education of athletes** is essential for compliance with antidoping rules.
- Although education may alert athletes to risks of **performance-enhancing substances**, positive benefits of improved performance make drug testing a necessary component of deterrence.

Table 26.3 COMMONLY DIAGNOSED CONDITIONS OFTEN REQUIRING THE THERAPEUTIC USE OF PROHIBITED MEDICATIONS

Condition/Diagnosis	Prohibited Medications Requiring a TUE	Permitted Medications (2021)
Acne	Spironolactone, canrenone	Topical benzoyl peroxide, salicylic acid
Addiction	Methadone	
ADHD	Amphetamines, methylphenidate	Guanfacine, atomoxetine
Adrenal insufficiency, Addison disease	Oral corticosteroids, DHEA	NA
Allergies	OTC preparations that contain pseudoephedrine	Cetirizine
Anaphylaxis	Epinephrine (Epi-Pen), systemic corticosteroids	NA
Asthma	$Beta_2$-agonists	Inhaled corticosteroids, and a few inhaled $beta_2$-agonists used under a certain dosage
Blood pressure	Beta-blockers (e.g., atenolol, timolol)	NA
Cancer, estrogen dependent	Tamoxifen	NA
Cardiovascular conditions	Beta-blockers, diuretics	Salicylic acid, ACE inhibitors, angiotensin II receptor blockers, lipid-lowering agents, nitrates
Dehydration	Intravenous infusions of anything, including saline	Oral rehydration
Diabetes	Insulin and insulin mimetics	Alogliptin, metformin, exenatide
Growth hormone deficiency	Growth hormone	NA
Heart medications	Hydrochlorothiazide	Aspirin, atorvastatin
Hemorrhoids	Rectally inserted corticosteroids	Topical/perianal corticosteroids
Hormone replacement therapy	Testosterone, DHEA, other androgens	Estrogen, progesterone
Hypogonadism	Testosterone or other androgens, hCG	NA
Infertility (female) or polycystic ovarian syndrome	Clomiphene, letrozole	Follicle-stimulating hormone, cyproterone acetate, drospirenone
Inflammatory bowel disease, colitis	Corticosteroids	Anti-TNF alpha agents
Musculoskeletal injuries	Intramuscular or oral corticosteroids, narcotics, Tramadol in some sports	NSAIDs
Narcolepsy/intrinsic sleep disorders	Modafinil, amphetamine derivatives	Caffeine, certain antidepressants
Nondrowsy cold and flu medications	Pseudoephedrine, ephedrine, lisdexamfetamine	Phenylephrine, guaifenesin, NSAIDs
Pain	Oxycodone (narcotics), cannabinoids	Topical lidocaine, Novocain, NSAIDs
Rash	Oral corticosteroids	Topical corticosteroids, hydrocortisone
Renal disease or transplant	Erythropoietin (EPO), diuretics, corticosteroids, beta-blockers, hypoxia-inducible factor (HIF), prolyl-hydroxylase inhibitors	
Sinusitis/rhinosinusitis	Oral glucocorticosteroids, pseudoephedrine	Saline or corticosteroid nasal sprays, guaifenesin
Transgender athletes	Spironolactone, testosterone	
Vitamin or iron deficiency	Vitamin or iron infusions of more than 100 mL	Oral vitamins, oral iron, or small-volume injections (less than 100 mL)

- The use of PEDs violates the rules of most sports and thus is considered "cheating." Most athletes conform to the rules of sport, and reminding athletes about the consequences of cheating (e.g., social, family, public repercussions) can be an effective educational tool for deterrence.
- **Substance abuse patterns of athletes are constantly changing,** depending on current social practices and technologic advances. Sports medicine professionals have an obligation to keep abreast of such changes.

RECOMMENDED READINGS

Available online.

27 EATING DISORDERS IN ATHLETES

Sasha Steinlight

OVERVIEW

- The American Psychiatric Association's Diagnostic and Statistical Manual of Mental Disorders (DMS-V), updated in 2013, and the World Health Organization's (WHO's) International Statistical Classification of Diseases and Related Health Problems, updated in 2019, identifies and defines the following eating disorders (EDs): anorexia nervosa (AN), bulimia nervosa (BN), binge eating disorder (BED), other specified feeding or eating disorder (OSFED), unspecified feeding or eating disorder (UFED), and avoidant/restrictive food intake disorder (ARFID).
- Disordered eating (DE) behaviors such as binging, purging, excessive exercise, calorie restriction, laxative, or diuretic use may be present without a formal diagnosis of ED.
- EDs are thought to be the result of a combination of biologic, psychological, and social factors.
- Male and female athletes are at higher risk for developing an ED than the general population.
- Screening and early intervention of ED/DE are vital to reducing possible serious consequences.

ANOREXIA NERVOSA

Diagnostic Criteria

- Essential features and diagnostic criteria (Fig. 27.1):
  - Restriction of calorie intake relative to requirements, leading to a significantly low body weight in the context of the age, sex, developmental trajectory, and physical health.
  - Intense, pathologic fear of gaining weight or becoming fat or persistent behavior that interferes with weight gain.
  - Individuals are often disturbed by their body weight or shape, their self-worth is influenced by body weight or shape, or there is a persistent lack of recognition of the seriousness of their low body weight.
- The WHO uses a threshold of body mass index (BMI) less than 18.5 kg/m^2 in adults and BMI for age under fifth percentile in children and adolescents.
  - Severity of AN (based on BMI):
    - Mild: ≥17 kg/m^2
    - Moderate: 16–16.99 kg/m^2
    - Severe: 15–15.99 kg/m^2
    - Extreme: <15 kg/m^2

Emotional and behavioral characteristics: Intense fear of weight gain, preoccupation with weight/food, overvaluation of body image, inflexible thinking, limited social spontaneity, restrained emotion, strong need for control

Common comorbidities: Anxiety, depressive disorders, obsessive-compulsive disorders

Complications of Anorexia Nervosa

Medical complications: due to malnutrition

Endocrine/metabolic (Fig. 27.2):

- A result of the body's attempt to conserve energy for more vital processes.
- Amenorrhea/anovulation/infertility: A decrease of pulsatile hypothalamic gonadotropin-releasing hormone secretion causes low levels of follicle-stimulating hormone (FSH) and luteinizing hormone (LH), known as *functional hypothalamic amenorrhea (FHA)*.
- Reduced testosterone in males (hypogonadotropic hypogonadism) can result in low libido and infertility.
- Decreased leptin and oxytocin and increased ghrelin, protein YY, and adiponectin, which are appetite-regulating hormones.
- Increased growth hormone.
- Increased cortisol level because of increased adrenal production and reduced renal clearance.
- Low insulin growth factor-1 (IGF-1).
- Hypothermia.
- Euthyroid sick syndrome: thyroid function abnormalities; resolves with weight gain.
- Hypokalemia, hyponatremia, hypoglycemia.
- Low bone density: The result of low estrogen; low testosterone; and increases in stress hormones, catecholamines, and cortisol. This results in reduction of bone formation and calcium absorption. Low energy availability leads to decreased IgF-1 and bone formation marker levels. There is also an increase in bone resorption. Changes in bone structure result in an increased risk of stress fractures. Fracture risk persists for years after diagnosis and may be irreversible.

Cardiovascular:

- Hypotension.
- Arrhythmias.
  - Sinus bradycardia (heightened vagal tone due to profound weight loss). Resting heart rate (RHR) is often seen below 60 beats per minute (bmp). If RHR is <40 bpm, hospitalization is often required.
  - Prolonged QTc: Increased risk of sudden death.
  - Heart block.
- Endothelial dysfunction increasing cardiovascular risk.
- Structural changes: Left ventricular atrophy, pericardial effusion.

Gastrointestinal: Elevated liver function tests, gastroesophageal reflux disease (GERD), bleeding, ulceration, dysphagia, gastroparesis leading to early satiety and bloating, constipation, dental/gingival issues.

Neurologic: Brain atrophy, memory loss, poor concentration, insomnia.

Integumentary: Lanugo, hair loss, acrocyanosis, carotenoderma, dry hair and nails, poor wound healing.

Hematologic: Anemia, leukopenia, thrombocytopenia.

Other: Increased injury risk and decreased athletic performance because of dehydration, reduced glycogen stores, or loss of muscle mass. Impaired cognition and mood can also negatively affect performance.

BULIMIA NERVOSA

Diagnostic Criteria

- Recurrent episodes of binge eating: These episodes consist of eating significantly more food in a defined period (e.g., within 2 hours) than others would eat under the same circumstances
- Episodes are marked by feeling out of control
- Binge eating episodes are followed by inappropriate compensatory behaviors (purging, fasting, excessive exercise, inappropriate laxative, or diuretic use)
- Must occur once weekly for 3 months
- Self-evaluation is unjustifiably influenced by body and shape
- Severity scale
  - Mild: 1–3 episodes of inappropriate compensatory behaviors per week
  - Moderate: 4–7 episodes per week
  - Severe: 8–13 episodes per week
  - Extreme: 14 or more episodes per week

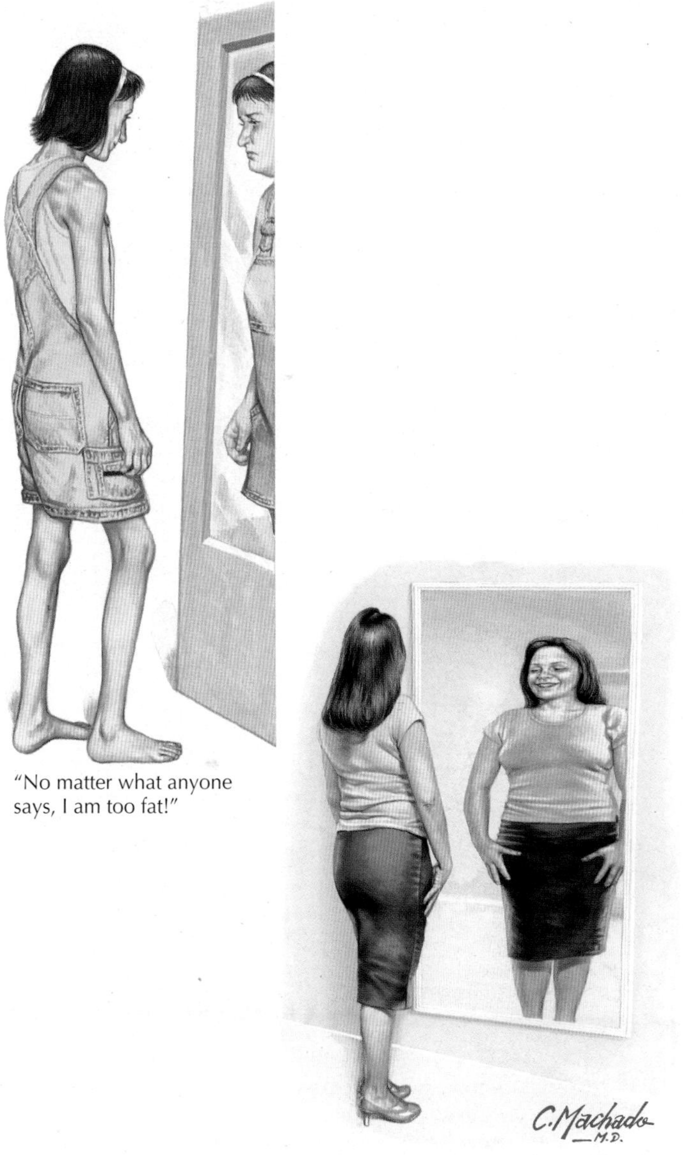
"No matter what anyone says, I am too fat!"
C. Machado M.D.

Two Forms	Restrictive anorexia nervosa. Bulimia nervosa; binge eating
Common Findings	Body image distortion @ ages 14-18; women > men Amenorrhea at least 3 months, and often precedes Weight loss >15% of ideal body weight Preserved secondary sex characteristics
Psychiatric Associated Disorders	Affective Anxiety OCD Personality Substance abuse
Differential Diagnosis	Adrenal insufficiency Inflammatory bowel and other GI disease Diabetes mellitus recent onset CNS posterior fossa lesions Primary depression
Endocrine Findings	Serum cortisol and growth hormone increased Serum LH & FSH low Insulin-like growth factor IGF-I low

Figure 27.1 Eating disorders.

- Weight is often within normal range but may be overweight

Emotional and behavior characteristics: Uncomfortable eating around others, food rituals, hoarding food, fear of eating in public, disappearing after eating, withdrawing from friends and activities

Common comorbidities: Anxiety, depression, obsessive-compulsive disorder, self-injury, impulsivity, suicidal ideation, substance abuse

Complications of Bulimia Nervosa

Medical complications of purging or diuretic use:
- **Gastrointestinal:** GERD, dysphagia, dyspepsia, hematemesis due to Mallory-Weiss tear.
- **Oral/dental:** Erosion of tooth enamel, mucositis, cheilitis, sialadenosis.
- **Electrolyte abnormalities:** Metabolic alkalosis, hypokalemia. These abnormalities can lead to cardiac arrhythmias. Increased aldosterone as a result of volume depletion may result in edema. This may require treatment with spironolactone.
- **Integumentary:** Russel sign: calluses on the back of the hand and fingers from self-induced purging.

Medical complications of laxative use:
- **Electrolyte abnormalities:** Hyperchloremic metabolic acidosis
- **Gastrointestinal:** Diarrhea, hemorrhoids, hematochezia

BINGE EATING DISORDER

- Recurrent episodes of binge eating as described for BN
- Episodes marked by feeling out of control as with BN
- Associated with three or more of the following:
  - Eating too quickly
  - Eating large quantities of food even if not feeling hungry
  - Eating until uncomfortably full
  - Feeling guilty, embarrassed, or disgusted
  - Eating alone to hide the behavior
- Occurs at least once weekly over 3 months
- BED differs from BN in that there are no compensatory behaviors after a binge

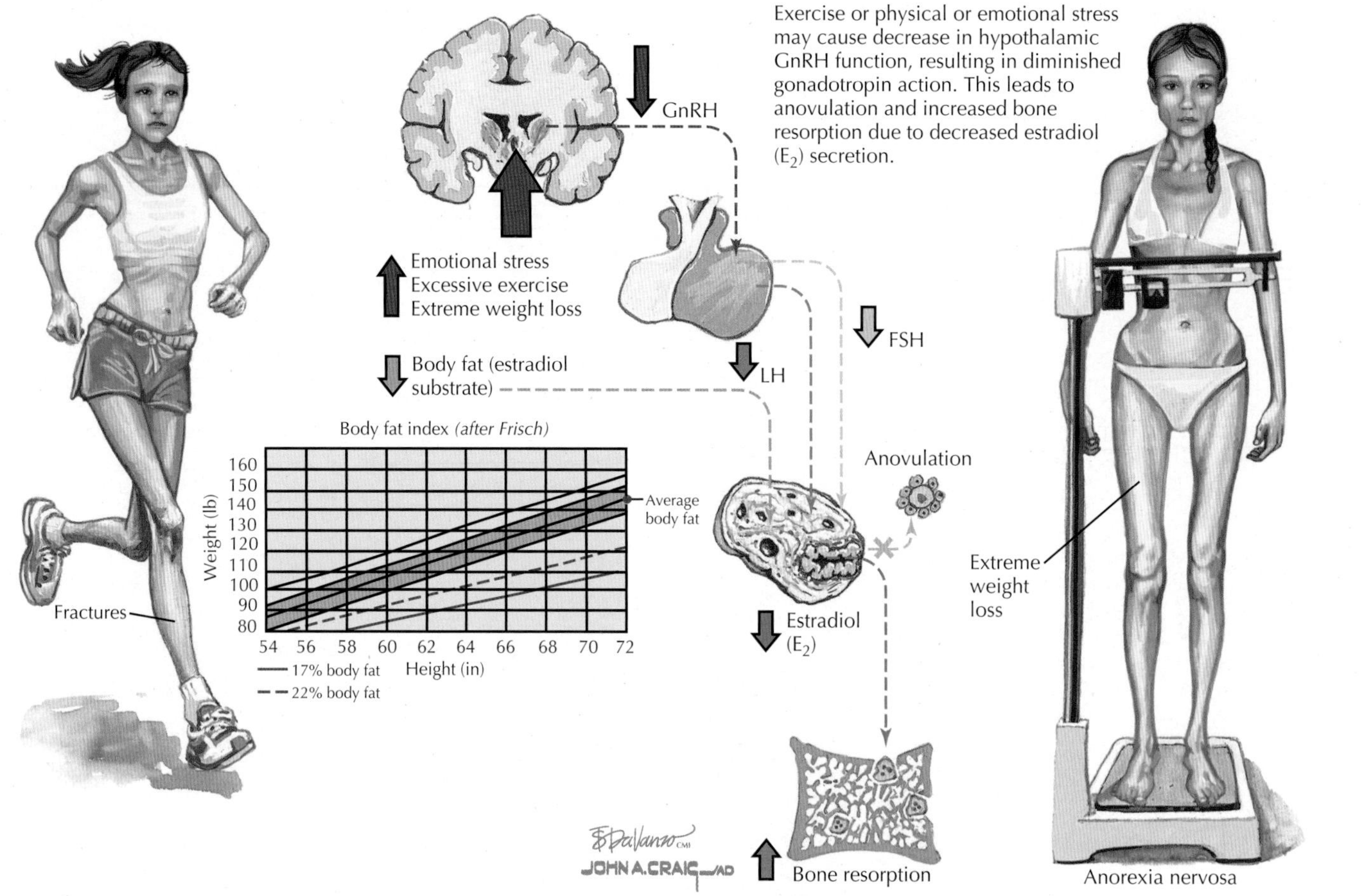
Exercise or physical or emotional stress may cause decrease in hypothalamic GnRH function, resulting in diminished gonadotropin action. This leads to anovulation and increased bone resorption due to decreased estradiol (E_2) secretion.
GnRH
Emotional stress
Excessive exercise
Extreme weight loss
Body fat (estradiol substrate)
FSH
LH
Body fat index (after Frisch)
Weight (lb)
Height (in)
Average body fat
17% body fat
22% body fat
Anovulation
Fractures
Extreme weight loss
Estradiol (E_2)
Bone resorption
Anorexia nervosa

Figure 27.2 Osteoporosis associated with amenorrhea.

- May occur with depression, anxiety, bipolar disorder, kleptomania, body dysmorphic disorder

OTHER SPECIFIED EATING OR FEEDING DISORDERS

- **Atypical anorexia:** meet criteria for AN without being underweight
- BED or BN at lower frequency than stated by DSM-V
- **Purging disorder:** purging without binging
- **Night eating syndrome:** recurrent eating after awakening from sleep or excessive eating at nighttime

UFED

- Symptoms of a feeding or eating disorder without meeting full criteria of diagnosed EDs

ARFID

- Lack of interest in eating food or avoiding foods based on sensory consequences of food
- Persistent failure to meet nutritional or energy needs with one or more of the following:
  - Significant weight loss
  - Nutritional deficiency
  - Dependence on nutritional supplements
  - Interference with psychosocial functioning
- Disturbance is not caused by other medical or psychological condition, lack of food availability, or cultural practice
- It does not occur during AN or BN and does not involve perception of body weight or shape

Rumination Disorder

- Repeated regurgitation of previously swallowed food or repeated chewing and then spitting out food
- Regurgitation behavior occurs several times per week
- Not due to a medical condition
- Does not occur exclusively during AN, BN, BED, or ARFID
- Severe enough to warrant individual attention if in the context of another mental health disorder

Orthorexia

- Not recognized by the DSM-V
- Individuals are fixated on "healthy" or "clean" eating
- Often occurs with obsessive-compulsive disorder
- Individuals often cut out multiple food groups, compulsively check nutrition labels, or feel distressed when "safe" or "healthy" foods are unavailable

RISK FACTORS FOR ED/DE

- **General:** Low self-esteem, depression, anxiety, perfectionism.
- **In athletes:** early sport specialization, external performance pressure or body shaming, competing at an elite level, injury. Poor body image is a strong predictor of EDs in athletes. Athletes are also more inclined to follow a rigid diet and strenuous exercise program.
- Endurance sports (i.e., distance running and cycling), aesthetic-based sports (i.e., gymnastics, figure skating), and weight-based sports (i.e., wrestling, horse jockeys) are at increased risk for ED or DE.
- Risk factors in males also include gender role expectations and ideals of muscularity and masculinity. Following traditional

BOX 27.1 DIAGNOSTIC TESTING FOR INDIVIDUALS WITH SUSPECTED EATING DISORDER/DISORDERED EATING

CBC
Comprehensive metabolic panel
Thyroid-stimulating hormone
ESR
Gonadotropins (LH/FSH)
Sex steroids (estradiol/testosterone)
Prolactin
HCG
Urinalysis
Amylase (if purging)
ECG, if indicated
DEXA, if indicated

CBC, Complete blood count; *DEXA,* dual energy x-ray absorptiometry; *ECG,* electrocardiogram; *ESR,* erythrocyte sedimentation rate; *FSH,* follicle-stimulating hormone; *HCG,* human chorionic gonadotropin; *LH,* luteinizing hormone.

male gender norms may increase the dissatisfaction with an individual's own muscularity. Males may also be less likely to pursue help because of gender norms, shame, and thinking EDs are a female problem. Men may be more likely to control weight through overexercising.

- Individuals with type 1 diabetes mellitus are also at increased risk

PREVALENCE

- Lifetime prevalence of AN reported as approximately 0.3%–1% in females; 0.1%–0.3% in males
- Males may account for up to approximately 25% of individuals with AN
- There is an increased risk of premature death (6–12 times higher) in women with AN compared with the general population
- Individuals 15–24 years old with AN have a 10 times higher risk of mortality compared with their peers
- Lifetime prevalence of BN is reported as 0.3%–4% in women and 0.1%–1% in men
- Lifetime prevalence of BED reported as 0.6%–5.8% in women and 0.3%–2% in men
- Prevalence of ED/DE in athletes reported ranges from 6% to 45% in females and from 0% to 19% in males
- Prevalence also varies by sport
- Athletes may be more likely to underreport DE than nonathletes

DIAGNOSIS AND EVALUATION

- A thorough history, physical examination, and laboratory studies are required. An electrocardiogram (ECG) may also be indicated (Box 27.1).
- Dual energy x-ray absorptiometry (DEXA) scan may be required to assess bone health in individuals who have been symptomatic for more than 6 months.
- Screening can be performed during the preparticipation evaluation. The American Medical Society for Sports Medicine (AMSSM) and American College of Sports Medicine (ACSM) include four questions regarding eating behaviors in the *Preparticipation Physical Examination* monograph, fourth edition. The Female Athlete Triad Coalition also published an 11-question screening tool that includes questions on menstrual history, hormone replacement, bone density, and stress fractures.
- The Athletic Milieu Direct Questionnaire (AMDQ), Female Athlete Screening Tool (FAST), and Brief Eating Disorders in Athletes Questionnaire (BEDA-Q) are screening tools that have been validated for female athletes.

BOX 27.2 BEDA-Q SCREENING TOOL ADAPTED FROM THE INTERNATIONAL OLYMPIC COMMITTEE (IOC) SPORT MENTAL HEALTH ASSESSMENT TOOL 1 (SMHAT-1)

Rated on a scale of Never, Rarely, Sometimes, Often, Usually, Always over the previous 2 weeks (first six questions only):

1. I feel extremely guilty after overeating
2. I am preoccupied with the desire to be thinner
3. I think that my stomach is too big
4. I feel satisfied with the shape of my body
5. My parents have expected excellence of me
6. As a child, I tried very hard to avoid disappointing my parents and teachers
7. Are you trying to lose weight now? (yes/no)
8. Have you tried to lose weight? (yes/no)
9. If yes, how many times have you tried to lose weight? (1–2 times, 3–5 times, or >5 times)

- The International Olympic Committee (IOC) released its Sport Mental Health Assessment Tool 1 (SMHAT-1) and accompanying Sport Mental Health Recognition Tool 1 (SMHRT-1) in 2020, which include a triage tool and screening tools. The BEDA-Q is used as one of the screening tools to identify athletes who require further evaluation for ED/DE. Each response in the BEDA-Q assessment is given a point value of 0–3. The authors of the SMHAT-1 identified a result of 4 or more points as a cutoff where further clinical evaluation is required (Box 27.2).
- The SCOFF is a five-question screening tool that is not validated in athletes but may be better at identifying males with ED/DE.
  - **The SCOFF questions*:**
    - Do you make yourself **S**ick because you feel uncomfortably full?
    - Do you worry you have lost **C**ontrol over how much you eat?
    - Have you recently lost more than **O**ne stone in a 3 month period?
    - Do you believe yourself to be **F**at when others say you are too thin?
    - Would you say that **F**ood dominates your life?
- An in-person interview may be more valuable as a screening tool in athletes. Athletic trainers, who interact with the athletes on a regular basis, are vital resources for identifying individuals at risk.
- Screening tools are not diagnostic and are meant to prompt the need for further evaluation.
- The female athlete triad is a recognized condition that includes the spectrum of EDs and DE relating to energy availability, menstrual function, and bone health. It is important to recognize the components of the triad, as they may include the initial presenting concern such as poor performance, stress fractures, or menstrual irregularities.
- In 2016, the IOC developed a comprehensive term, Relative Energy Deficiency in Sport (RED-S), which describes the relationship of energy deficiency and its impairment on physiologic function, including but not limited to metabolic rate, menstrual function, bone health, immunity, protein synthesis, and cardiovascular health. RED-S is also more inclusive of male athletes.

TREATMENT

- Early identification and intervention can shorten recovery time. Initially the appropriate level of care must be determined.

*One point for every "yes"; a score of ≥2 indicates a likely case of anorexia nervosa or bulimia.

Treatment can occur on an outpatient basis, partial (day) program, residential program, or inpatient hospital program. Hospitalization may be required for acute medical stabilization (i.e., severe electrolyte disturbances, ECG abnormalities, or hemodynamic instability) or acute psychiatric stabilization (i.e., food refusal, suicidal ideation).

- A multidisciplinary healthcare team made up of mental health professional, physician, registered dietitian, and certified athletic trainer has been shown to be most effective.
- Psychotherapy is an essential part of the treatment plan. Cognitive behavioral therapy (CBT) has been shown to be an effective treatment and is often first-line therapy. Family-based therapy (FBT) is also used in children and adolescents.
- Psychotropic medications may be useful to treat comorbid conditions. However, there is limited evidence that they improve clinical outcomes. Selective serotonin reuptake inhibitors (SSRIs) may help during weight maintenance of AN. Fluoxetine is Food and Drug Administration (FDA) approved for use in BN. Lisdexamfetamine can be used for management of BED; however, it is a stimulant and is banned by the World Anti-Doping Agency and the National Collegiate Athletics Association (NCAA) and requires a therapeutic use exemption.
- For individuals who are underweight, a goal of treatment is to restore approximately 90% of ideal body weight or a BMI of greater than or equal to 18.5 kg/m^2.
- Severely malnourished patients should begin refeeding under the guidance of a physician with expertise in management of EDs in consultation with a nutritionist. In these cases, refeeding must be monitored closely to avoid refeeding syndrome, which can result in severe electrolyte abnormalities such as hypophosphatemia, hypokalemia, and hypomagnesemia. Newer evidence shows that early weight restoration may improve outcomes, and a more aggressive approach to refeeding earlier on in EDs may be preferred. This can be accomplished by close medical monitoring and nutritional supplementation when necessary.
- Routine outpatient follow-ups should include monitoring of vital signs, including a blinded weight, assessing daily function and physical symptoms.
- Weight restoration and return of menses are key to improving low bone mineral density. Optimal bone health may never be reached. There is no strong supporting evidence that hormone replacement therapy improves bone mineral density. Transdermal estrogen patches with cyclic oral progestin have shown some improvement in adolescents. Otherwise, estrogen therapy is not useful in AN. Calcium and vitamin D alone do not restore bone density; however, supplementation of 1500 mg/day (calcium) and 1500–2000 IU daily (vitamin D) are often recommended. Bisphosphonates may be effective after 1 year of treatment; however, there is a known risk of teratogenicity, so these are not generally used, especially during the reproductive years. Testosterone therapy can be considered for men; however, there are not enough data available to determine its benefit.
- Recent studies show that recovery may take approximately 9 years for BN and longer for some with AN. Poorer outcomes are associated with lower BMI, binging/purging behaviors, high body image concerns, depressed mood, or other comorbidities.

RETURN TO PLAY

- The Female Athlete Triad Coalition Consensus Statement on Treatment and Return to Play of the Female Athlete Triad (2014): Cumulative Risk Assessment is a tool that can be used to guide return-to-play decisions. There are six risk factors identified that each carry a point value based on magnitude of risk. A cumulative risk score can then be correlated to low risk, moderate risk, or high risk.
- The IOC developed the RED-S risk assessment model for sport participation using a red light, yellow light, and green light system. Individuals with a more severe presentation are placed in the "red light" category and are not cleared to participate. Individuals in the moderate or "yellow light" category are given provisional clearance with close follow-up. Individuals who are identified as low risk are given the "green light" for full sport participation.
- If an individual has a BMI <16.5 or is purging four or more times per day, it is advised that they be restricted from sport participation.
- Ideally, an athlete will be able to participate during their treatment, which can be a strong motivating factor. Activity participation may also aid in managing comorbid conditions.
- Some athletes may benefit from a verbal or written treatment contract with their providers, which identifies treatment requirements and level of sport participation. These contracts can be altered to allow more participation as the individual's weight improves or can be more restrictive if no improvements are being made (E-Fig. 27.A).

PREVENTION

- Provide accurate information on nutrition and weight control to athletes
- Promote healthy body image among teammates and coaching staff
- Educate athletes, coaches, and the athlete's entourage on pathologic eating behaviors and consequences
- Utilize peer-led groups to discuss eating habits and body image

RECOMMENDED READINGS

Available online.

OVERTRAINING

28

Thomas M. Howard • Francis G. O'Connor

INTRODUCTION

- Overtraining syndrome (OTS) is among the most challenging medical disorders that confronts the sports medicine provider. OTS, although most commonly associated with endurance athletes (e.g., runners, swimmers), can also be identified in strength athletes. At present, OTS is complicated by multiple diagnostic and therapeutic challenges, as current research in this area is limited by a small number of studies and inconsistent results.
- Researchers have concluded the following: there are poorly established diagnostic criteria; there are significant confounding influencers, including illness, injury, menstruation, and unique training methods for different sports; and it is difficult, if not impossible, to establish controls and/or laboratory models to study the illness.
- Recent consensus statements reflect that there are currently no conclusive data on the causes, pathophysiology, early identification, and prevention of OTS.
- This chapter will review the epidemiology and key terminology of this disorder and describe the proposed pathophysiology of OTS. Importantly, we will discuss current guidance on the clinical presentation, diagnosis, management, and prevention of this complex disorder.

EPIDEMIOLOGY

- OTS is an issue that has plagued athletes, trainers, coaches, and clinicians for generations. As evidenced by this quote from Dr. D. C. Parmenter in 1923, this ailment is not new to the medical literature:

"Overtraining or staleness is the bug-a-boo of every experienced trainer…a condition difficult to detect and still more difficult to describe…evaluation should focus on training load, nutrition, sleep and rest, competition stress and psychological state."

- The current literature on OTS has limited insight into the incidence and prevalence of this disorder. However, observational data and clinical experience suggest that OTS is not rare, with some authors postulating that the prevalence of the disorder may be increasing and spreading to nonelite athlete populations. An early study reported that 65% of elite competitive swimmers had experienced staleness at some time in their career. A subsequent survey study of endurance runners described a prevalence rate of 10% during one training cycle and a lifetime risk of 64% and 60% among male and female runners, respectively. A recent systematic review of the literature evaluating overtraining in strength athletes identified an urgent need for practical tools for diagnosis in this population.
- Athletes who have experienced OTS also appear more likely to relapse: a study of college swimmers reported that 91% of swimmers who experienced OTS in their freshman year suffered a repeat episode during the subsequent year as opposed to 34% of those who did not experience an initial episode.

TERMINOLOGY

Training: A series of stimuli used to stress or displace homeostasis to provide stimulation for adaptation. Training involves progressive load in an effort to improve performance in a sport or activity. Training for success involves a balance between achieving peak performance and avoiding negative consequences of overtraining.

Load: Training results in a stimulus that is identified as the load. Load is further defined as external, which is the actual work completed by the athlete, and internal, which represents the individual physical, physiologic, and psychological characteristics that respond to the load. Athletes respond individually to internal and external loads.

Adaptation: Physiologic response to stress that results in an adjustment in function or dimension of an organism.

Recovery: The period after a training stimulus when work capacity returns to prestimulus levels. If recovery time is optimal, supercompensation results, whereas excessive training, without rest, can result in a decline in performance (Fig. 28.1). The available literature describes four components of recovery: hydration and nutrition; sleep and rest; relaxation and emotional support; and stretching and active rest. Recovery that is inadequate results in fatigue. Fatigue may be classified as either pathologic or physiologic.

- Physiologic fatigue includes categories such as insufficient sleep, nutritional, jet lag, pregnancy, and training-induced (from either excessive competition or overreaching).
- Pathologic fatigue includes the following categories: medical, including infectious; neoplastic, hematologic, endocrine, toxic, iatrogenic, and psychiatric; chronic fatigue syndrome; and OTS.

Periodization: Planned sequencing of increased training loads and recovery periods within a training program.

Overload: Overload occurs when the balance between external and internal loads is dysfunctional so that the body's adaptive response and capacity are exceeded with resultant decreased performance.

Acute fatigue (AF): The immediate response to overload training; although fatigued, the athlete experiences no perceivable decline in performance.

Recovery–fatigue continuum: Recovery and fatigue are on a continuum and jointly affected by both physiologic and psychological determinants. An imbalance of accumulated long-term fatigue and inadequate recovery create an unfavorable environment for nonfunctional overreaching, OTS, and decreased performance.

Functional overreaching (FOR): Short-term decrement in performance after a period of overload training usually lasting <2 weeks after a period of overload training.

Nonfunctional overreaching (NFOR): A longer period of performance decline (2 weeks to 2 months) after a period of overload training.

OTS: Maladaptive response to training from an extended period of overload (usually 2 months or more); the result of too severe or a prolonged period of overreaching (see Fig. 28.1). Overtraining is manifested by decreased sport-specific performance and enhanced fatigability, pronounced vegetative complaints, sleep disorder, emotional instability, organ-related complaints without organic disease, overuse injuries, blood chemistry changes, and immune dysfunction.

PATHOPHYSIOLOGY

Overview

- The pathophysiology of OTS has not been fully elucidated. Multiple models and hypotheses attempt to explain the signs and symptoms of this disorder, including the autonomic imbalance hypothesis, the central fatigue hypothesis, the glycogen depletion hypotheses, and the cytokine hypothesis.
- Fig. 28.2 summarizes the various hypotheses to explain the complexity of this disorder.

Autonomic Imbalance Hypothesis

The autonomic imbalance hypothesis proposes that underlying imbalances in the autonomic nervous system cause OTS. The initial stage of this proposed mechanism involves negative feedback caused by a surge of catecholamine release during periods of heavy training. This causes a decrease in baseline catecholamine secretion. Second, an increase in metabolism during exercise causes an imbalance among plasma amino acids and alterations in brain neurotransmitter metabolism, leading to an increase in the concentrations of aromatic amino acids (phenylalanine, tryptophan, and tyrosine). The resulting increases in hypothalamic tryptophan and cerebral dopamine concentrations cause "metabolic error signals" with inhibitory effects on the sympathetic nervous system. In addition, the increase in core temperature associated with high-intensity training (HIT) may exert inhibitory effects on the sympathetic centers of the hypothalamus. Third, a neuronal negative feedback system results in down-regulation of catecholamine receptors in the exercising muscles.

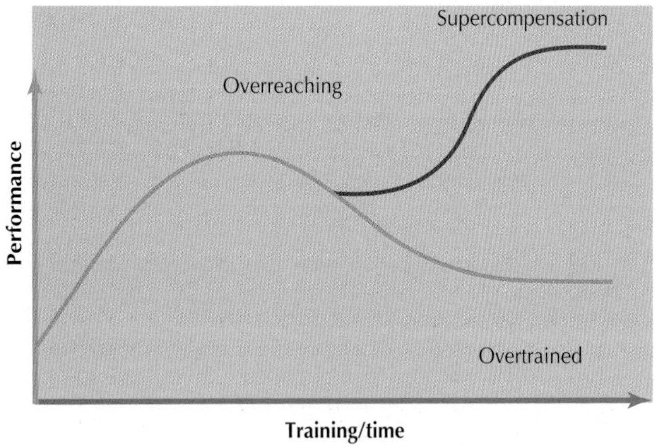
Supercompensation
Overreaching
Performance
Overtrained
Training/time

Figure 28.1 Hypothetical overtraining syndrome model.

Central Fatigue Theory

The central fatigue theory hypothesizes that OTS is caused by an increase in the synthesis of 5-hydroxytryptomine (5-HT) in the central nervous system (CNS). Extensive exercise results in glycogen depletion in muscles, leading to the use of secondary energy sources by these muscles. The branched-chain amino acids (BCAAs: leucine, isoleucine, and valine) are oxidized to glucose. Concurrently, levels of fatty acids increase as well. Fatty acids compete with tryptophan for albumin-binding sites, leading to an increase in plasma tryptophan. Because both BCAAs and tryptophan use the same transporter to pass through the blood-brain barrier, a decrease in plasma BCAAs and an increase in plasma tryptophan lead to an increase in tryptophan passing through into the CNS. In the brain, tryptophan is converted into the neurotransmitter 5-HT. 5-HT is known to play a role in various neuroendocrine and emotional functions, all of which can be seen with OTS. This connection between OTS and an increase in the free tryptophan/BCAA ratio form the basis for this hypothesis.

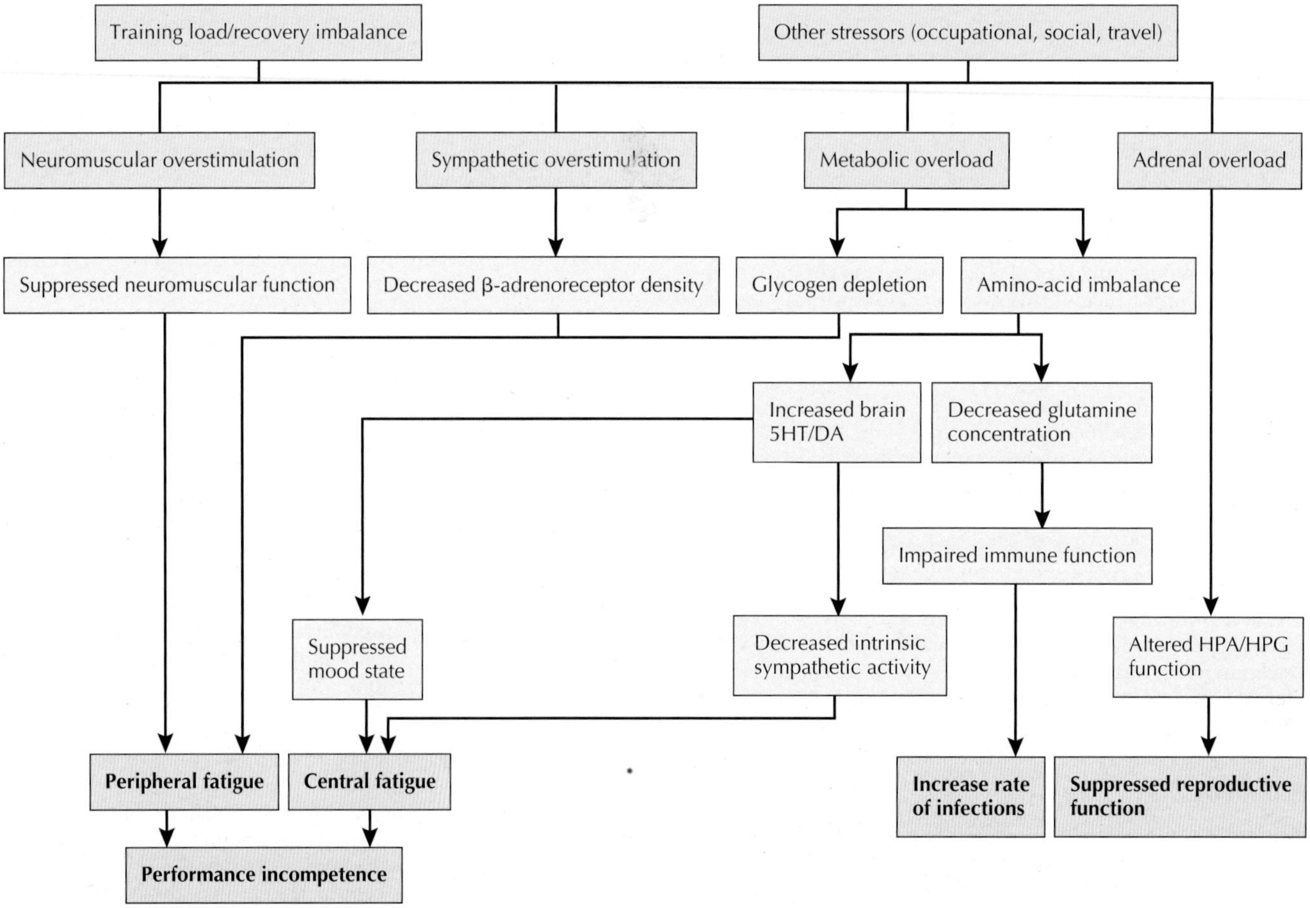
Training load/recovery imbalance
Other stressors (occupational, social, travel)
Neuromuscular overstimulation
Sympathetic overstimulation
Metabolic overload
Adrenal overload
Suppressed neuromuscular function
Decreased β-adrenoreceptor density
Glycogen depletion
Amino-acid imbalance
Increased brain 5HT/DA
Decreased glutamine concentration
Impaired immune function
Suppressed mood state
Decreased intrinsic sympathetic activity
Altered HPA/HPG function
Peripheral fatigue
Central fatigue
Increase rate of infections
Suppressed reproductive function
Performance incompetence

Figure 28.2 Genesis of overtraining syndrome. *5-HT,* Serotonin; *DA,* dopamine. (Modified from Foster C, Lehmann M. Overtraining syndrome. In: Guten GN, ed., *Running Injuries*. Philadelphia: WB Saunders; 1997.)

Glycogen Depletion Hypothesis

- Glycogen is the predominant energy source for moderate to intense exercise.
- According to the glycogen hypothesis, glycogen depletion may lead to overtraining through the following three mechanisms:
- Direct effects of glycogen depletion: low levels of muscle glycogen stores may cause muscular fatigue and poor performance.
- Glycogen depletion may also cause increased oxidation of BCAAs, which eventually leads to central fatigue.
- Glycogen depletion may lead to a net negative caloric state, which induces a catabolic state and multiple neuroendocrine changes.

Cytokine Hypothesis

- The cytokine hypothesis theorizes that chronic tissue injury without regenerative healing leads to a systemic inflammatory and immune response. This systemic inflammatory response leads to increased concentrations of interleukins, interferons, tumor necrosis factor, and other proinflammatory factors.
- These factors are thought to act centrally, promoting central fatigue, anorexia, depression, a catabolic state, and changes in the hypothalamic–pituitary–adrenal and hypothalamic–pituitary–gonadal axes.

PARADOXICAL DECONDITIONING

- Caldegiani and Kater proposed a new paradigm of OTS as a result of their Endocrine and Metabolic Response on Overtraining (EROS) study. In their study of 51 overtrained athletes and assessment of 67 parameters, they opined that the pattern of findings in overtraining was more akin to that of deconditioned individuals. The onset of this syndrome is multifactorial and not just related to excessive training.

CLINICAL PRESENTATION

Overview

- Although a universal feature of OTS is decreased performance, it may include a broad array of psychiatric, musculoskeletal, cardiovascular, and immunologic symptoms (Table 28.1).

Table 28.1 CLINICAL PRESENTATION OF OVERTRAINING SYNDROME

Sport-Specific Performance Complaints	• Inability to meet prior performance standards • Prolonged recovery time • Decreased coordination • Decreased muscular strength
Physiologic Findings	• Blood pressure changes • Increased resting heart rate • Weight loss • Increased incidence of injuries • Increased incidence of infections • Amenorrhea
Subjective Complaints	• Fatigue • Feeling of depression • Anorexia • Hypersomnia/disturbed sleep • Myalgias • Gastrointestinal disturbances • Headaches • Increased irritability • Concentration difficulties • Apathy

However, on account of individual variation, few (if any) athletes exhibit all features of overtraining.

- Training volume, training intensity, or lack of rest alone may not explain many, or even most, cases of OTS. Rather, OTS commonly develops when the cumulative stress imposed on an individual outstrips his or her ability to cope with that stress. Contributing factors can include the training regimen, rest status, nutritional state, concurrent infectious disease, allergic reactions, and issues outside of sports to include school and work stressors and financial and relationship stress.

Psychological Features

- Fatigue
- Loss of appetite or libido
- Anxiety, irritability, or anger
- Insomnia or hypersomnolence
- Depression

Cardiovascular Features

- Increased first-morning resting heart rate (increase of 5–10 beats per minute over baseline is suggestive)
- Reduced maximum heart rate and VO_2 max
- Decreased stroke volume and altered contractility
- Possible relative decrease in plasma volume

Musculoskeletal Features

- Muscular fatigue at previously tolerated exercise levels
- Decreased performance
- Persistent soreness

Immunologic Features

- Demonstrated increase in the rate of upper respiratory tract infections in endurance athletes during periods of intense training that are not followed by adequate rest
- Decreased serum and secretory immunoglobulin A (IgA)
- Decreased natural killer cell function

DIAGNOSIS

Differential Diagnosis

- The diagnosis of OTS is clinically confirmed—there is no currently available confirmatory laboratory test. Accordingly, OTS **is considered a diagnosis of exclusion.**
- The differential diagnosis of overtraining is extremely broad and should be considered before a diagnosis of OTS is established. Infectious, inflammatory, malignant, endocrine, cardiopulmonary disease, renal disease, hematologic disease, myopathies, and psychiatric disease, as well as substance abuse, should be considered (Table 28.2 and Figs. 28.3 and 28.4).
- A broad laboratory evaluation is not initially recommended but may be necessary over the course of several visits to exclude many of the aforementioned conditions. Fig. 28.5 presents a possible evaluation strategy.

Laboratory Analysis

- Although various hormonal and hematologic abnormalities have been elucidated in OTS, there is no one characteristic set of abnormalities, and many changes may represent points along a continuum.
- Clinical and laboratory markers that have been proven to have poor sensitivity and specificity in evaluating OTS include body mass, resting heart rate and blood pressure, hematocrit, ferritin, creatinine kinase, and hormonal markers.

Table 28.2 DIFFERENTIAL DIAGNOSIS OF OVERTRAINING SYNDROME

Infectious Etiologies	• Postviral syndrome • Infectious mononucleosis • Lyme disease • Viral hepatitis • Myocarditis
Collagen Vascular Disorders	• Polymyalgia rheumatica • Systemic lupus erythematosus • Fibromyalgia • Chronic fatigue syndrome
Metabolic	• Nutritional deficiency • Hypothyroidism or hyperthyroidism • Anemia • Electrolyte disorders
Pharmacologic	• Alcohol • Caffeine • Illegal or performance-enhancing drugs
Psychiatric	• Depression • Physical abuse • Sexual abuse • Emotional abuse • Posttraumatic stress disorder • Malingering
Other	• Cancer • Myopathy • Pregnancy • Sleep deprivation

- Glutamine has recently been a frequent subject of study as a possible marker of overtraining. Glutamine is an amino acid that is depleted in catabolic states such as overtraining, infection, surgery, and acidosis. Moreover, several studies have demonstrated a decline in glutamine levels in overtrained states; however, there are multiple confounding factors, as discussed earlier, and glutamine testing is not yet widely available for practical use.

Neuropsychological Testing

- Many of the earliest symptoms of overtraining are psychological, and a number of screening questionnaires have been developed to evaluate these. A commonly used questionnaire that has been validated for OTS screening and risk assessment is the Profile of Mood States (POMS).
- POMS is a survey wherein patients rate 65 adjectives on a 5-point scale in accordance with how well the adjective describes their feelings over the past week. POMS is designed to assess tension/anxiety, depression/dejection, anger/hostility, vigor/activity, fatigue/inertia, and confusion/bewilderment. The test is summarized in one global score, which subtracts the sum of points assessed for positive mood states from that of negative mood states.
- Other commonly used standardized tests include the Total Quality Recovery Score by Kentta and Hassmen; the Daily Analyses of Life Demands for Athletes, which is used by Australian Olympic teams; and the Psycho-Behavioral Overtraining Scale, which has been used by certain British athletes.

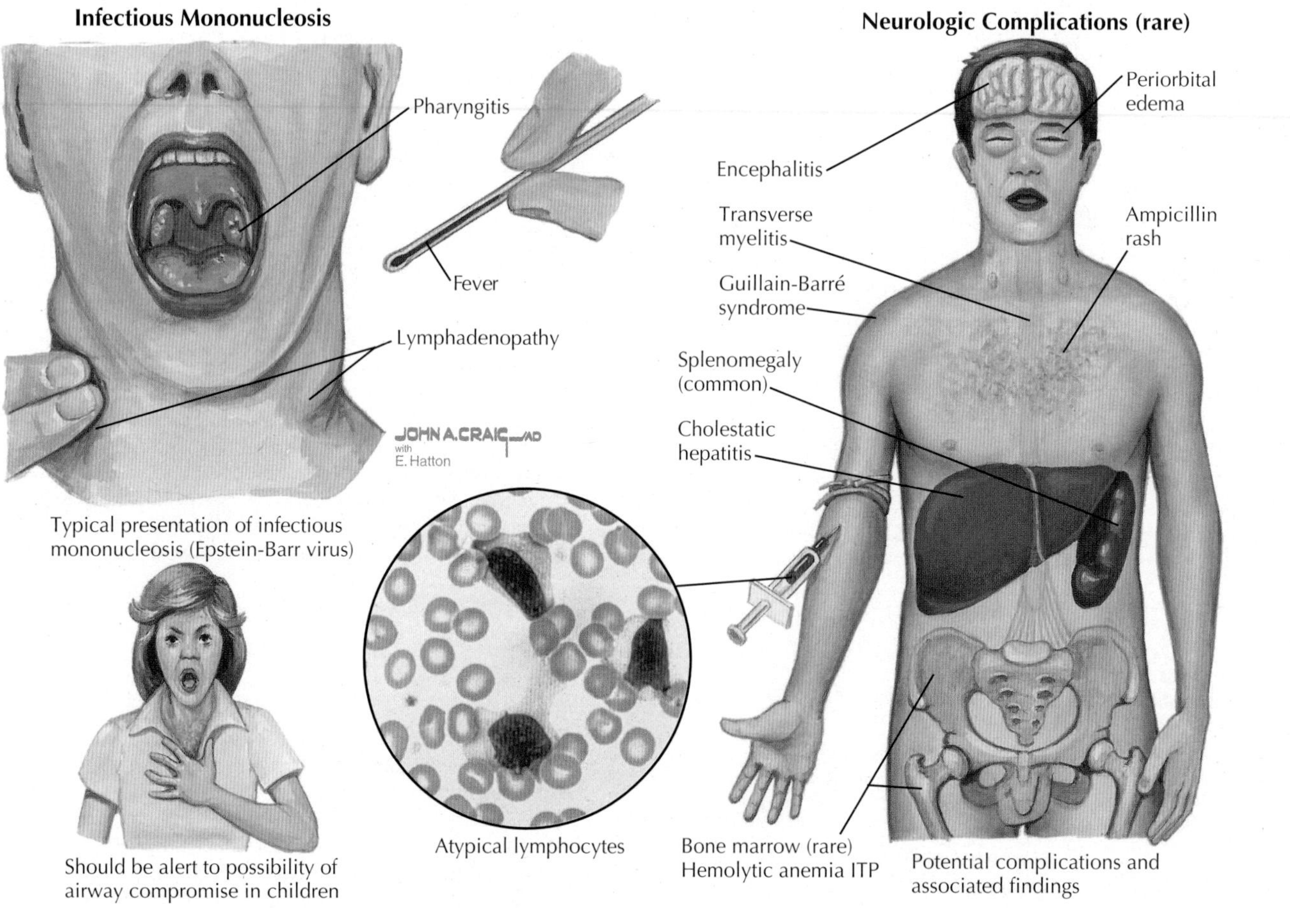

Infectious Mononucleosis
Pharyngitis
Fever
Lymphadenopathy
JOHN A.CRAIG_AD
with
E. Hatton
Typical presentation of infectious mononucleosis (Epstein-Barr virus)
Should be alert to possibility of airway compromise in children
Atypical lymphocytes
Neurologic Complications (rare)
Periorbital edema
Encephalitis
Transverse myelitis
Ampicillin rash
Guillain-Barré syndrome
Splenomegaly (common)
Cholestatic hepatitis
Bone marrow (rare) Hemolytic anemia ITP
Potential complications and associated findings

Figure 28.3 Infectious mononucleosis.

Performance Testing

- Preliminary research suggests that a diminished serum lactate concentration after performance testing is a consistent finding in overtrained athletes. However, lactate studies are often limited by the availability of prior baseline data.
- A previous study reported the diagnosis of OTS in athletes by using a two-bout exercise test protocol. The study included 10 underperforming athletes, 5 of whom were ultimately diagnosed with OTS and 5 with NFOR. After performing the two-bout maximal exercise protocol (two maximal exercise tests separated by a 4-hour interval), athletes with OTS exhibited reduced maximal lactate concentrations (concentrations ≤8 mmol/L) along with higher serum prolactin and adrenocorticotropic hormone (ACTH) concentrations. This two-bout exercise protocol may be a useful test for diagnosing OTS, but additional studies are warranted for validation.

MANAGEMENT

- Because OTS is considered a diagnosis of exclusion and because assessing response to therapy requires time, the initial workup should be divided into two appointments, separated by a 2- to 3-week interval. The first appointment includes history and physical examination, dietary evaluation, and review of training diaries. At this time, a screening hematologic panel may be obtained to investigate other causes of decreased performance (see Fig. 28.5).
- The mainstay of treatment in OTS is **rest.** The athlete's response to imposed rest is also critical in achieving an accurate diagnosis. After the initial visit, a period of 2–3 weeks of rest from training is recommended. Athletes may remain active, but not in their chosen sport, and training volume should generally be decreased by at least 50%.
- At the 2- to 3-week follow-up visit, the athlete may resume training if symptoms have resolved and the laboratory workup is within normal limits, but the training regimen should be closely assessed for appropriate periods of recovery. If the athlete's symptoms have not resolved at the follow-up visit and the laboratory workup reveals no explanation, longer periods of imposed rest are necessary while tracking symptoms and mood scores.
- A multidisciplinary treatment approach is often useful and may include sports psychology and nutrition consultations. All four components of recovery must be considered: hydration and nutrition, sleep and rest, relaxation and emotional support, and stretching and active rest.
- **Glutamine:** There may be a role in the future for enteral or parenteral glutamine supplementation. To date, no study has demonstrated improved immune function or recovery with glutamine supplementation in healthy athletes.
- **BCAAs:** BCAA supplementation may improve subjective reporting of mood and energy and positively affect POMS scores. However, no definitive improvement in athletic performance has been demonstrated with BCAA supplementation. Supplementation with BCAAs is often limited by gastrointestinal side effects, with possible poor tolerance of doses >7–10 g/day.
- **Selective serotonin reuptake inhibitors (SSRIs) and tricyclic antidepressants (TCAs):** Numerous studies have demonstrated that dramatic increases in training volume lead

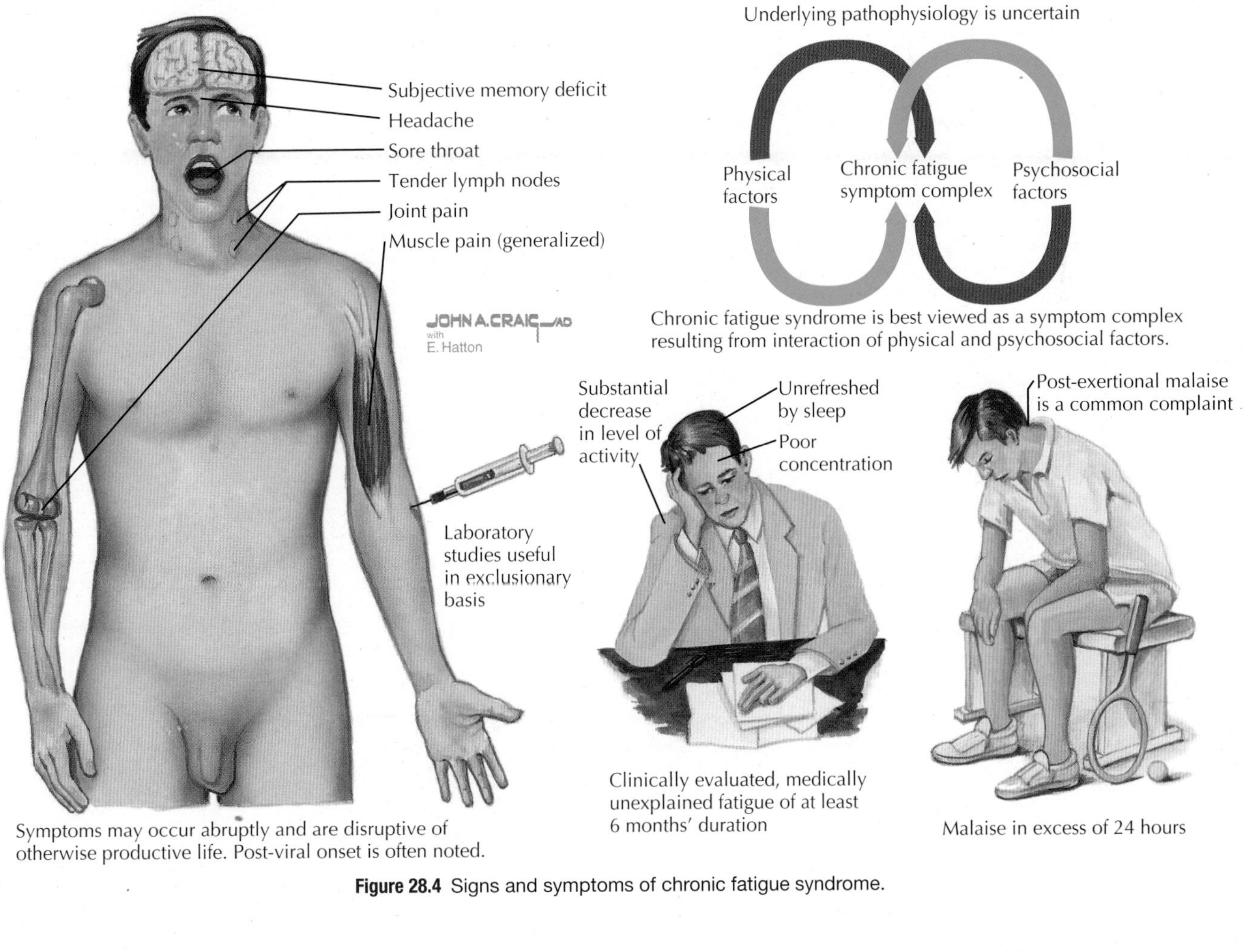

Underlying pathophysiology is uncertain
Physical factors
Chronic fatigue symptom complex
Psychosocial factors
Chronic fatigue syndrome is best viewed as a symptom complex resulting from interaction of physical and psychosocial factors.
Subjective memory deficit
Headache
Sore throat
Tender lymph nodes
Joint pain
Muscle pain (generalized)
JOHN A.CRAIG_AD
with
E. Hatton
Laboratory studies useful in exclusionary basis
Substantial decrease in level of activity
Unrefreshed by sleep
Poor concentration
Post-exertional malaise is a common complaint
Symptoms may occur abruptly and are disruptive of otherwise productive life. Post-viral onset is often noted.
Clinically evaluated, medically unexplained fatigue of at least 6 months' duration
Malaise in excess of 24 hours

Figure 28.4 Signs and symptoms of chronic fatigue syndrome.

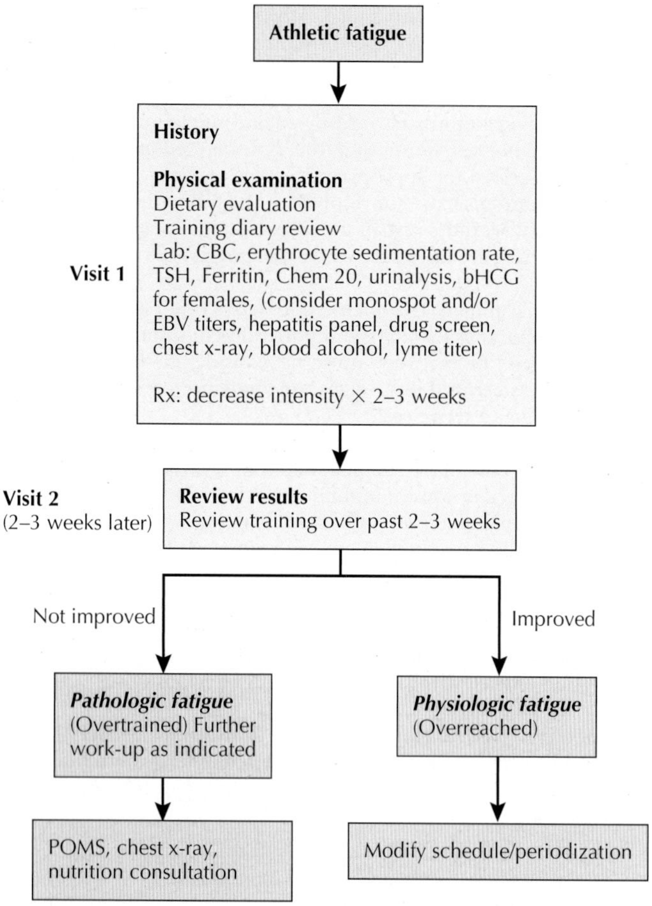
Athletic fatigue
Visit 1
History
Physical examination
Dietary evaluation
Training diary review
Lab: CBC, erythrocyte sedimentation rate, TSH, Ferritin, Chem 20, urinalysis, bHCG for females, (consider monospot and/or EBV titers, hepatitis panel, drug screen, chest x-ray, blood alcohol, lyme titer)
Rx: decrease intensity × 2–3 weeks
Visit 2
(2–3 weeks later)
Review results
Review training over past 2–3 weeks
Not improved
Improved
Pathologic fatigue
(Overtrained) Further work-up as indicated
Physiologic fatigue
(Overreached)
POMS, chest x-ray, nutrition consultation
Modify schedule/periodization

Figure 28.5 Proposed clinical evaluation of athletic fatigue.

to undesirable mood changes. Increases in fatigue, depression, anger, and global mood disturbances are common and may lead to clinical depression. Care should be taken before initiating an SSRI or TCA if symptoms of fatigue predominate, because increased central serotonin has been hypothesized to cause central fatigue early in OTS. As symptoms progress, particularly if the patient meets or is close to meeting diagnostic criteria for a mood disorder, a TCA or SSRI may be helpful.

PREVENTION

- Once OTS has developed, there is no treatment other than rest, which indicates prevention as the best strategy. Coaches, athletes, physicians, and trainers should closely monitor athletes for early signs of overtraining. Careful attention to the recovery process is paramount. **Mood and sleep disturbances and resting heart rate elevation may be the earliest signs.** Athletes at a high risk of developing OTS may be monitored with daily training logs, frequent screening tests (POMS), and first-morning basal heart rate monitoring. The normal resting heart rate of an athlete should be determined when he or she is healthy. Consistent elevation of >10 beats per minute above the baseline should raise concern for OTS. Periodic assessment of athletic performance, such as time trials in a runner or swimmer, may also be performed to screen for decrease in performance associated with OTS.
- Care should be taken to maintain adequate sleep, nutrition, and hydration and to minimize external stressors. Training regimens should be individualized and flexible, with periodization of training and adequate recovery time. A decrease in training volume at the first sign of overtraining may facilitate a quicker recovery. Counsel athletes to avoid the tendency to *panic train*, or train harder after a decline in their performance. Care must be taken to not allow the development and progression of OTS because the required prolonged recovery time may significantly interfere with an athlete's preparation and participation.
- There has been tremendous recent interest in the role of HIT in the sports-conditioning community. A recent study in swimmers concluded that selective utilization of periodic HIT may, in fact, be a means to improve performance while decreasing training volumes that may lead to OTS. In this study, 41 elite swimmers were randomly assigned to either an HIT or a control group (CON). For 12 weeks, both groups trained for approximately 12 hours/week. The amount of HIT was approximately 5 and 1 hour, and the total distance was approximately 17 and 35 km/week in the HIT and CON groups, respectively. After the 12-week intervention, compared with the CON group, general stress levels were 16.6% (2.6%–30.7%; mean and 95% confidence interval [CI]) lower and general recovery levels were 6.5% (0.7%–12.4%) higher in the HIT group. These promising results indicate that increasing training intensity and reducing training volume can reduce general stress and increase general recovery levels and may be a strategy to assist in preventing OTS.
- Adolescent athletes may be particularly vulnerable to OTS and burnout with predictable short- and long-term consequences. The American Academy of Pediatrics has published consensus recommendations to assist in preventing OTS in this population. Commonsense recommendations include encouraging athletes to strive to have 1–2 days off per week from competitive athletics, sport-specific training, and competitive practice to allow them to recover both physically and psychologically and encouraging athletes to take at least 2–3 months away from a specific sport during the year.

RECOMMENDED READINGS

Available online.

SECTION VI

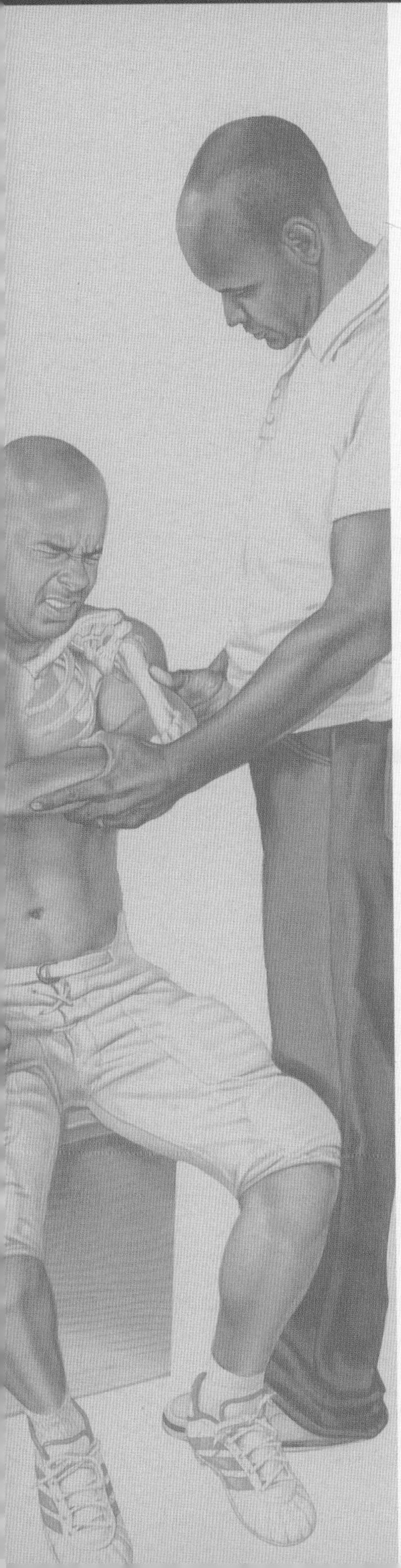

General Medical Problems in Athletes

INFECTIONS IN ATHLETES

29

Mark Stovak • Kyle Goerl • Leslie Greenberg

GENERAL PRINCIPLES

- Athletes may be immunosuppressed due to a variety of psychological, environmental, and physiologic stressors, especially when combined with inadequate diet and sleep.
- Infectious outbreaks affect sports participation and performance and can easily spread to team staff, spectators, and other contacts.
- Appropriate diagnosis may help decrease sports disruption, return the patient to health, foster sports success, and quell a regional epidemic.
- An athlete's increased risk of contracting infections is attributed to the following:
  - Contact with surfaces like a mat or artificial turf may cause skin breaks
  - Athlete-to-athlete contact
  - Athletes may be more apt to be risk-takers, which can increase infections such as sexually transmitted infections
  - Sharing personal toiletries and congregating in dormitories, locker rooms, or showers
  - Sports equipment, gloves, pads, and protective gear may be contaminated and difficult to sanitize

Exercise Immunology

- In 1994, Nieman demonstrated a relationship between exercise and susceptibility to infections in the form of a J-shaped curve.
  - The model suggested that whereas engaging in moderate activity enhances immune function above sedentary levels, excessive amounts of prolonged high-intensity exercise have detrimental effects on immune function.
- Gleeson found postexercise immune function depression was most pronounced when exercise is moderate to high intensity, continuous, and prolonged.
- Leukocyte function may continue to remain depressed at 24 hours after the last exercise bout.
- If the recovery time between consecutive bouts of intense exercise is insufficient, chronic immunosuppression can occur, which is often observed in overtrained athletes.

COMMON RESPIRATORY INFECTIONS

Febrile Illness

- Fever is a normal physiologic response to infection, with the intent to increase host survival and decrease the length of illness.
- The Centers for Disease Control and Prevention (CDC) defines fever as an internal temperature of >100.4°F (38°C).
- Fever can cause undesirable effects in the body, including increased insensible fluid losses, dehydration, increased metabolic demands, and body temperature dysregulation.
- Hyperthermia with dehydration leads to a reduction in both cardiac output and blood pressure. This concerning combination can lead to reduced exercise tolerance, endurance, and muscle strength.
- Exercising during a febrile illness can further potentiate negative effects from the disease process and can evolve into potentially lethal myocarditis from viral illnesses.
- Athletes should be withheld from physical activity until their fever has resolved, and return to participation should be gradual.
- To decrease the spread of infections, hand washing is the most common and effective method. Separating an athlete from the team also helps.

Upper Respiratory Tract Infections

Etiology: An upper respiratory tract infection (URTI) is a common cold. It is caused by respiratory viruses, usually **rhinoviruses.** Transmission is through nasal secretions by sneezing, coughing, and nose blowing.

Epidemiology: Cough is the 3rd, whereas nasal congestion is the 15th most common presenting symptom in all office visits. URTIs are the 3rd most common primary care diagnosis.

Symptoms: URTIs are self-limited, lasting up to 10 days with symptoms of fever, cough, rhinorrhea, nasal congestion, sore throat, headache, and myalgias.

Examination and diagnosis: Fever, rhinorrhea, erythema, cobblestoning or swelling of the posterior oropharynx, fluid level behind the tympanic membrane, and cervical lymphadenopathy; diagnostic testing is only necessary to diagnose group A streptococcal or mononucleosis infections. Influenza and COVID-19 are discussed separately.

Treatment: Treatment is symptomatic and supportive and includes antipyretic and nonsteroidal anti-inflammatory drugs (NSAIDs), decongestants, nasal saline irrigation, intranasal ipratropium, and zinc. Antibiotics are ineffective.

Return to play (RTP): The **"neck check"** is a helpful tool when considering whether physical activity is appropriate. An afebrile athlete with URTI symptoms "above the neck," without systemic signs or symptoms, may attempt 10–15 minutes of mild to moderate exercise and, if tolerated, may participate as tolerated.

Prevention: Encourage hand washing. No sharing of water bottles.

Infectious Mononucleosis (Fig. 29.1)

Etiology: Infectious mononucleosis (IM), or "mono," is an **Epstein–Barr virus** (EBV) infection. EBV is the primary cause in 90% of cases, but cytomegalovirus and toxoplasmosis can cause a similar syndrome as well. The oral transmission of the virus has caused IM to be nicknamed the "kissing disease." The incubation period is 30–50 days. It causes a cell-mediated immune response, leading to T-lymphocyte proliferation, lymphoid hyperplasia, lymphocytosis, and **atypical lymphocytes** on a peripheral blood smear.

Epidemiology: EBV is very common; 90%–95% of adults display immunity to EBV, indicating prior infection. There are approximately 500 new cases per 100,000 persons per year in the United States. Adults aged 15–24 are most at risk, with no increased risk to athletes compared with nonathletes.

Symptoms: An EBV infection can be clinically insignificant in children but symptomatic in adolescent and adult patients. Usually, a 3- to 5-day prodrome of malaise, fatigue, and anorexia progresses to the classic "triad" of IM with **pharyngitis, fever, and lymphadenopathy.** Rarely, laryngeal edema occurs, potentially leading to airway obstruction.

Examination and diagnosis: The reactive lymphadenopathy classically leads to enlargement of **posterior cervical lymph nodes**, but axillary and inguinal nodes may also be enlarged. Posterior palatine petechiae, jaundice, exudative pharyngitis, rash (commonly seen in a patient who started penicillin for a suspected group A streptococcal infection), and splenomegaly are also possible. Jaundice is uncommon, but 90% of patients have mildly elevated aspartate transaminase (AST) and alanine transaminase (ALT). Exudative pharyngitis can be mistaken for streptococcal pharyngitis, but concomitant infections do occur in up to 30% of patients. Splenomegaly and increased

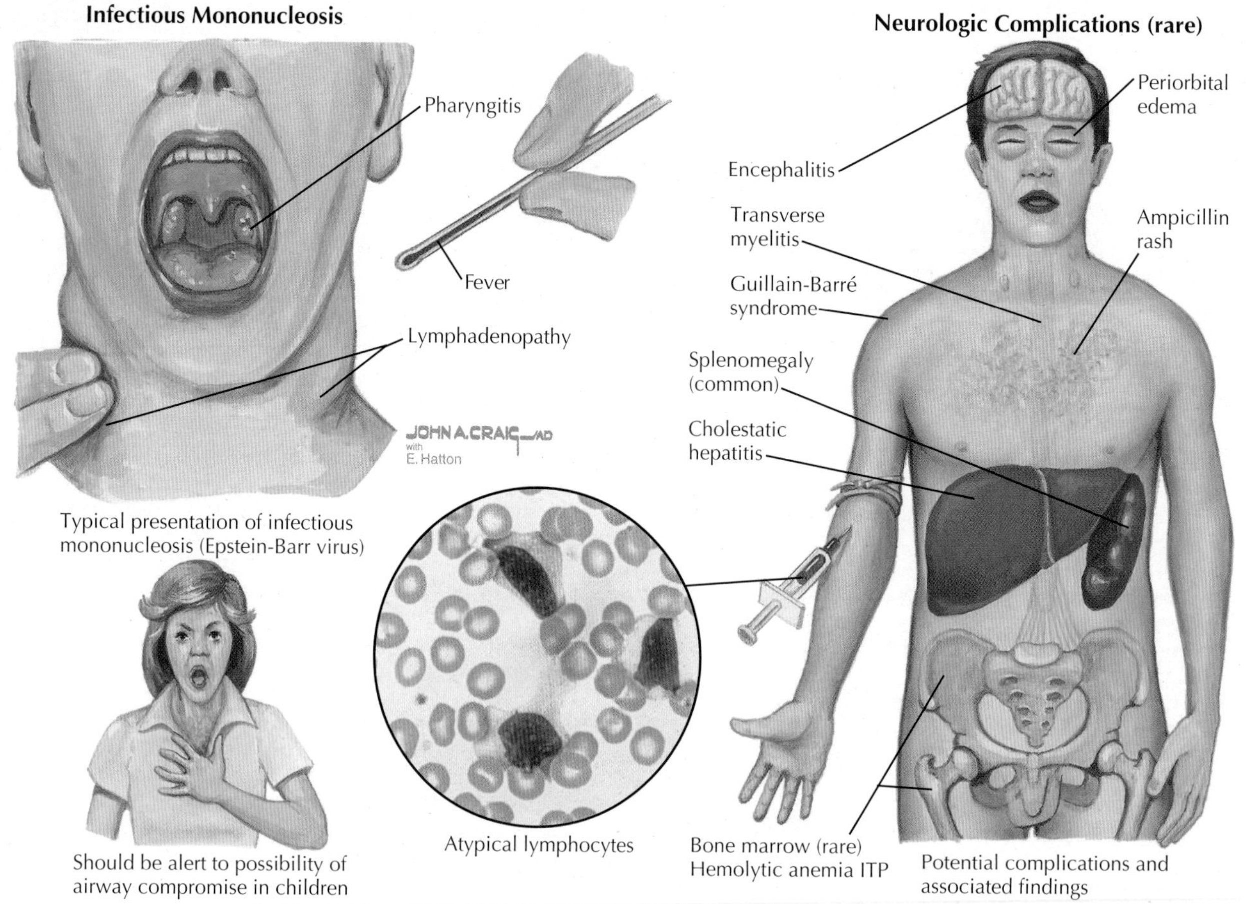
Infectious Mononucleosis
Pharyngitis
Fever
Lymphadenopathy
JOHN A.CRAIG_AD
with
E. Hatton
Typical presentation of infectious mononucleosis (Epstein-Barr virus)
Should be alert to possibility of airway compromise in children
Atypical lymphocytes
Neurologic Complications (rare)
Periorbital edema
Encephalitis
Transverse myelitis
Ampicillin rash
Guillain-Barré syndrome
Splenomegaly (common)
Cholestatic hepatitis
Bone marrow (rare)
Hemolytic anemia ITP
Potential complications and associated findings

Figure 29.1 Infectious mononucleosis.

risk of rupture resulting from splenic friability is concerning for athletes, but routine imaging is not regarded as useful in RTP decisions. Splenic size can be normal with increased friability and risk of rupture. Splenomegaly alone does not predict the risk of rupture. A **Monospot** test, which detects the presence of heterophile antibodies, is clinically used, but has a false-negative rate of 25% in the first week of illness in adults and may remain negative in children. Testing for EBV viral capsid antigen (VCA) immunoglobulin M (IgM) and immunoglobulin G (IgG) in addition to EBV nuclear antigen (EBNA) may be useful if Monospot is negative. The CDC states that Monospot is not recommended for general use, as heterophile antibodies can be caused by other conditions such as HIV, toxoplasmosis, leukemia, lymphoma, pancreatic cancer, rubella, and systemic lupus erythematosus and may lead to a false-positive result. Atypical lymphocytes have a sensitivity of 75% and a specificity of 92%. A lymphocyte count of less than 4000 has a 99% negative predictive value.

Treatment: Treatment is supportive, including rest, hydration, and NSAIDs. In addition, given the negative effects IM may have on the liver, acetaminophen should be used with caution. Avoid aspirin because of bleeding risk and an association of IM with Reye syndrome in pediatric patients. Corticosteroids are not needed but may be considered if laryngeal edema or painful swallowing interferes with oral intake.

Return to play: Splenic rupture is the most concerning issue while making RTP decisions. All athletes should be withheld from competition until their symptoms have resolved. Follow-up laboratory and splenic imaging results demonstrating normalization are not necessary. Published guidelines (expert opinion) recommend athletes **not participate for 3–4 weeks.** A recent study by Sylvester et al. concluded that symptom level could not be used to allow early RTP, as 88% of the patients in this study were diagnosed with mono after the splenic rupture occurred. Also, 73.8% of the splenic ruptures occurred by day 21 and 90.5% occurred by day 31. In severe cases, recovery may take up to 3 months.

Prevention: Encourage hand washing and refrain from the sharing of water bottles.

Influenza (Fig. 29.2)

Etiology: Influenza is an airborne viral illness infecting the respiratory tract. It is a single-stranded RNA virus in the Orthomyxovirus family. **Influenza A** causes most influenza illnesses. The incubation period is 18–72 hours, with viral shedding occurring anywhere from 24 hours before symptoms to up to 5–10 days thereafter.

Epidemiology: The World Health Organization (WHO) estimates 3–5 million severe influenza cases with 250,000–500,000 deaths annually worldwide. Older adults, young children (<5 years), persons with chronic medical conditions, and pregnant women are at the highest risk of complications.

Symptoms: Classic symptoms include sudden onset of **fever, myalgias, headache**, malaise, rhinitis, sore throat, and cough. Severe complications are rare in healthy children and adults but can include pneumonia, encephalitis, respiratory failure, multiorgan failure, and death.

Examination and diagnosis: Influenza is typically **clinically diagnosed based on the sudden onset of the aforementioned symptoms.** Patients may have fever, rhinorrhea, erythema, cobblestoning or swelling of the posterior oropharynx,

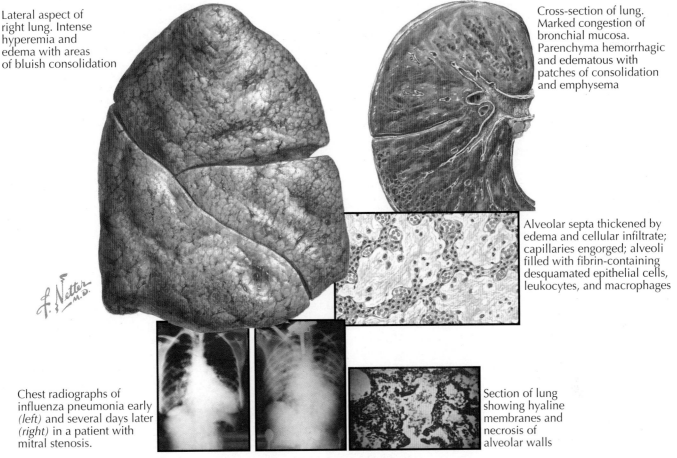

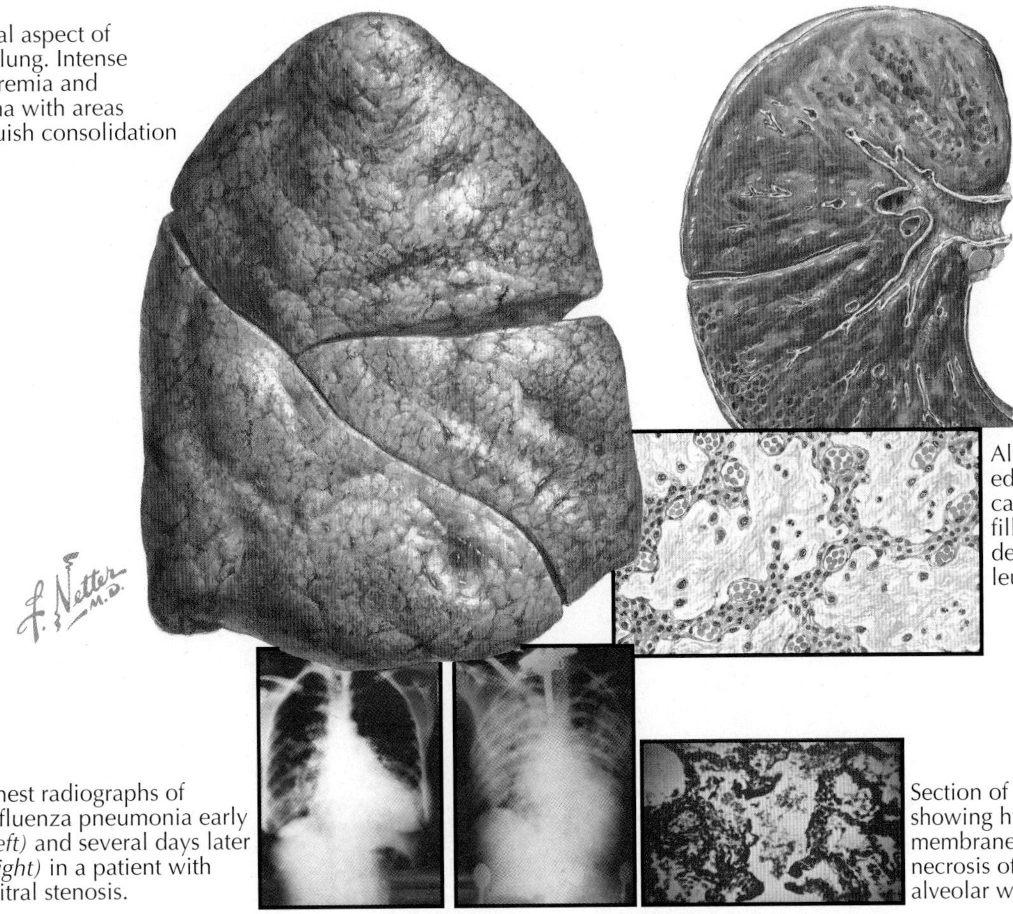
Lateral aspect of right lung. Intense hyperemia and edema with areas of bluish consolidation
Cross-section of lung. Marked congestion of bronchial mucosa. Parenchyma hemorrhagic and edematous with patches of consolidation and emphysema
Alveolar septa thickened by edema and cellular infiltrate; capillaries engorged; alveoli filled with fibrin-containing desquamated epithelial cells, leukocytes, and macrophages
F. Netter M.D.
Chest radiographs of influenza pneumonia early (left) and several days later (right) in a patient with mitral stenosis.
Section of lung showing hyaline membranes and necrosis of alveolar walls

Figure 29.2 Influenza pneumonia.

a fluid level behind the tympanic membrane, and cervical lymphadenopathy. Cardiac and pulmonary auscultation is typically normal unless there is associated pneumonia or cardiac complications such as pericardial effusion. Rapid tests have variable sensitivities (10%–70%); hence, a negative test does not rule out infection, but the tests are highly specific (95%).

Treatment: Symptomatic treatment includes NSAIDs and antipyretic medications, decongestants, and cough suppressants. Encourage hydration. **Antiviral medications such as oseltamivir (Tamiflu), zanamivir (Relenza), and baloxavir marboxil (Xofluza) are not typically recommended in healthy children and adults without complications.** Consider antivirals if symptoms are present for <48 hours. Antivirals may shorten the duration of illness and decrease the risk of complications. Influenza is very contagious, so exposed teammates may benefit from prophylactic antiviral treatment.

Return to play: When athletes are afebrile (without antipyretics) and symptoms are well controlled, they can RTP.

Prevention: The CDC recommends **all people over 6 months of age receive influenza vaccination.** Encourage hand washing. Affected athletes should isolate from teammates until asymptomatic and afebrile to avoid transmission.

COVID-19

Etiology: COVID-19 is the disease caused by the novel coronavirus, SARS-CoV-2.

Epidemiology: It was first identified in late 2019 in Wuhan, China, and was declared a pandemic by early 2020. Much of our knowledge regarding this disease process is currently being developed.

Symptoms: Range from none, to a mild URTI, to severe acute respiratory distress syndrome (ARDS) and death. Eighty-five percent of patients will present with one of these three symptoms: cough, fever, and/or shortness of breath. Loss of taste and smell, especially with other URTI symptoms, should raise suspicion for infection. Many patients are asymptomatic and spread the virus unknowingly to others. Of particular importance in athletes, COVID-19 can cause myocarditis. Clinical presentation is variable. Recommendations at the time of this publication, which are still evolving, are based on expert opinion and revolve around varying symptom classifications (e.g., asymptomatic, mild, moderate, severe, significant, hospitalized vs. nonhospitalized). Signs and symptoms may include fatigue, dyspnea on exertion, decreased exercise tolerance, chest pain, tachycardia, and heart failure.

Examination and diagnosis: Testing for COVID is typically by a reverse transcriptase polymerase chain reaction (PCR), but antibody and antigen testing are in rapid development. Tests are more accurate when symptoms are present.

- Evaluation of myocarditis includes a careful cardiovascular examination.
- Asymptomatic positive athletes and athletes with mild and/or brief noncardiac symptoms are primarily evaluated clinically with physical examination, and electrocardiogram (ECG) should be considered because subclinical cardiac injury is possible.
- Further cardiac evaluation and cardiac referral should be considered for all athletes with ongoing moderate symptoms and all athletes with severe symptoms.
- Evaluation of athletes with "significant" moderate to severe symptoms should include ECG (insensitive; changes may or

may not be present and can include ST elevation or depression, PR depression, new bundle branch block [BBB], prolonged QT, premature ventricular contractions [PVCs], atrioventricular [AV] block, and others) and may also include cardiac biomarkers (high-sensitivity troponins; normal does not exclude myocarditis); echocardiogram (ECHO); and cardiac magnetic resonance imaging (MRI) if high suspicion or any of the ECG, troponins, or ECHO are abnormal.

Treatment: Symptomatic treatment for milder COVID cases. Complicated infections, especially resulting in respiratory distress, may require hospitalization, respiratory support, steroids, and other interventions; antiviral medication; and other supportive treatments that are being studied. Treatment of myocarditis should involve a cardiologist and is primarily supportive, with attention to arrhythmias.

Return to play: There is evidence for cardiac, pulmonary, neurologic, renal, and other complications, and return to play/activity (RTP/A) should be made based on individual complications and published guidance available at the time. Asymptomatic positive athletes and athletes with mild and/or brief noncardiac symptoms may return to activity after being asymptomatic for at least 2 weeks and a normal ECG is reassuring. For myocarditis associated with COVID, RTP guidance at the time of this publication is evolving. Because intense exercise can promote virulence and inflammation with myocarditis, which can result in arrhythmias and sudden death, RTP/A for all athletes with myocarditis should be based on current myocarditis guidelines, where RTP/A may be delayed for 3–6 months or more.

COMMON SKIN AND SOFT TISSUE INFECTIONS

Herpes Simplex Virus Infection

Etiology: Herpes simplex virus (HSV) on the skin is called "herpes gladiatorum" in wrestlers and "herpes rubeiorum" or "scrumpox" in rugby players. HSV-1 on the lips, or "herpes labialis," is usually referred to as *cold sores.* Time from virus exposure to vesicle appearance is 4–11 days.

Epidemiology: Most prevalent in sports with frequent, direct contact between players, such as rugby and wrestling; most common infection sites are head, face, and neck, followed by the extremities and trunk. Transmission is usually via direct contact with open wounds and skin tears. HSV is uncommon in the lower extremities.

Symptoms: Mild flulike prodromal symptoms of burning, tingling, or stinging may occur, followed by development of small clusters of painful papules or vesicles. Fatigue, weight loss, pharyngitis, and lymphadenopathy occur in severe cases.

Examination and diagnosis: Small clusters of painful papules or vesicles (may follow a dermatomal pattern in the case of shingles). Testing is unnecessary, but Tzanck preparation can be confirmatory, revealing large, multinucleated giant cells. Culture and PCR testing have a high specificity as well.

Treatment: Oral antiviral medications (acyclovir, valacyclovir, or famciclovir) and covering lesions decrease contagious spread.

Return to play: The National Federation of High School (NFHS) guidelines for herpetic lesions (simplex, fever blisters/cold sores, zoster, or gladiatorum): To be considered "noncontagious" all lesions must be scabbed over with no oozing or discharge and no new lesions in the preceding 72 hours. For primary (first episode of herpes gladiatorum), wrestlers should be treated and not allowed to compete for a minimum of 10 days. If general physical signs and symptoms such as fever and swollen lymph nodes are observed, the minimum period of treatment is extended to 14 days. Recurrent outbreaks require a minimum of 120 hours or 5 full days of oral antiviral treatment as long as no new lesions have developed and all lesions are scabbed over with no swollen lymph nodes in the affected area. **The National Collegiate Athletic Association (NCAA) guidelines for herpetic lesions (simplex, fever blisters/cold sores, zoster, gladiatorum)** require skin lesions to have a firm, adherent crust at the time of competition and have no evidence of secondary bacterial infection. For primary (first episode of herpes gladiatorum) infection, a wrestler must have developed no new blisters for 72 hours before the examination; be free of signs and symptoms such as fever, malaise, and swollen lymph nodes; and have been on an appropriate dosage of systemic antiviral therapy for at least 120 hours before and at the time of the competition. Recurrent outbreaks require a minimum of 120 hours of oral antiviral treatment as long as no new lesions have developed and all lesions are scabbed over. Active herpetic infections should not be covered to allow participation.

Prevention: Daily suppressive therapy is an option for recurrent infections. Valacyclovir (Valtrex) provides the easiest dosing of 500 mg BID during the sports "season," which may increase compliance and decrease the spread of infection. HSV can survive for several hours on inanimate objects or shared equipment. Thorough cleaning of water bottles, fomites, and clothing is recommended. Nonabrasive uniforms may reduce skin abrasions and tears and therefore reduce transmission of infection. Wrestling mats have not been shown to be a mode of transmission, but regular cleaning of mats is still recommended. Prepractice and match athlete screening for active lesions helps prevent contact with known vectors.

Verrucae (Warts)

Etiology: Papillomaviruses

Epidemiology: Transmission is via direct contact, shared showers, or locker room floors

Symptoms: Plantar warts are well-defined hyperkeratotic lesions, singular or in clusters, with a smooth collar of thickened keratin. Plantar warts are painful as they grow inward because they exist on the plantar weight-bearing surface of the feet. Verrucae vulgaris are firm, rough papules or nodules, 2–10 mm in diameter with punctate black dots within the lesion that appear on the rest of the body.

Treatment: Plantar warts may be treated with 30%–70% trichloroacetic acid, 40% salicylic acid, or taping with salicylic tape or duct tape for several days. Verrucae vulgaris may be treated with repeated cryotherapy with liquid nitrogen, 1% salicylic acid or lactic acid, or curettage with electrodesiccation.

Return to play: No NFHS limitations, as are not considered highly contagious, but should be covered if prone to bleeding; NCAA guidelines for wrestlers with multiple digitate verrucae of their face will be disqualified if infected areas cannot be covered with a mask. Solitary or scattered lesions can be curetted off before a meet or tournament. Wrestlers with multiple verruca plana or verrucae vulgaris lesions must have the lesions adequately covered.

Prevention: Wear flip-flops in public showers or locker rooms.

Molluscum Contagiosum

Etiology: Poxvirus

Epidemiology: Transmission is via direct skin contact or fomites. Incubation period is 2–6 weeks.

Symptoms: Single or multiple small, flesh-colored papules with central umbilication.

Treatment: Cryotherapy, curettage, cantharidin, or podophyllotoxin.

Return to play: NFHS/NCAA: Curettage or hyfrecation of all lesions before the meet

Prevention: Avoid direct contact with lesions or fomites

Tinea Infections (Fig. 29.3)

Etiology: Most commonly *Trichophyton rubrum* and *T. tonsurans*. Specific fungal infections are *tinea pedis* (athlete's foot), *tinea cruris* (jock itch), *tinea corporis* (ringworm), *tinea capitis* (cradle cap), and *tinea versicolor* caused by *Malassezia furfur*.

Epidemiology: Sweat-soaked clothing, suntan beds, communal showers, infrequently washed/sanitized clothing, occlusive clothing, and local skin trauma associated with form-fitting equipment puts athletes at risk of developing tinea infections.

Symptoms: Local pruritus, erythema, and burning.

Examination and diagnosis: Potassium hydroxide (KOH) preparation and microscopic examination of skin scrapings can be confirmatory quite quickly, whereas culture takes longer.

- **Tinea pedis:** Malodorous maceration of the skin of interdigital spaces with associated peeling, cracking, scaling, and pruritus.
- **Tinea cruris:** Itchy, red, often ring-shaped rashes on the skin of buttocks, genitals, and inner thighs.
- **Tinea corporis:** Circular or ring-shaped, scaly, raised plaque with irregular erythematous borders with central clearing.
- **Tinea capitis:** Patchy scale with erythema leading to hair breaking off flush with the scalp, leaving patches of alopecia with follicular plugs that create a characteristic "black dot" appearance.
- **Tinea versicolor:** Hypopigmented, scaly patches in a diffuse pattern.

Treatment: Topical or oral antifungal medications with continuation of treatment 2 weeks after clinical resolution for tinea pedis, tinea cruris, and tinea corporis. Tinea capitis requires only oral medication. Tinea versicolor can be treated with topical or oral antifungals.

Suppression and prophylactic doses have been successful and include fluconazole (100–200 mg once/week) or itraconazole (400 mg every other week). Daily sterilization of the sports environment, including the locker room, equipment, and clothing, is recommended.

Return to play: NFHS and NCAA guidelines for tinea lesions (ringworm on scalp or skin): Oral or topical treatment for 72 hours for skin infections. Oral treatment for 14 days for scalp infections before RTP, but continued treatment with 1% ketoconazole shampoo until scalp lesion resolution.

NCAA guidelines state that wrestlers with solitary or closely clustered localized lesions will be disqualified if lesions are in a body location that cannot be adequately covered. **There are no NFHS or NCAA restrictions on RTP for tinea versicolor because it has a very low transmission rate.**

Prevention: Appropriate clothing barriers; laundering of towels, uniforms, padding, and equipment; use of shower footwear; and routine showering in addition to prompt identification and treatment of all cases.

A condition that can mimic tinea infection is **erythrasma** (caused by *Corynebacterium minutissimum*). Coinfections with dermatophytes are also common. Symptoms include erythematous brown patches or plaques in the axilla, inframammary areas, umbilicus, groin, or interdigital area that reveal coral-red fluorescence with a Wood's lamp. Treatment consists of topical clindamycin or erythromycin twice daily for 2 weeks.

Community-Acquired Methicillin-Resistant *Staphylococcus aureus* (CA-MRSA)

Etiology: Colonization of the skin or exposure to MRSA through an open skin lesion.

Epidemiology: Originally a hospital-acquired infection starting in the 1960s, MRSA may cause substantial morbidity and mortality in athletes. Often believed to be spider or insect bites, identification and treatment can be delayed. High-risk sports for MRSA infection are those with frequent, repetitive, and direct skin contact. Transmission also occurs with shared equipment, towels, and whirlpools.

Symptoms: Tender lesion on the skin usually rapidly progressing from cellulitis to an abscess.

Testing: Consensus guidelines recommend cultures in the presence of a purulent lesion and at least one of the following features: treatment with antibiotics, signs of systemic toxicity, multiple or large lesions, bite as the cause, association with water exposure, lack of response to initial treatment, or occurrence during a suspected outbreak. Culturing when antibiotics are used allows determination of sensitivities, which can guide antibiotic choices in the case of a poor response to the initial antibiotic.

Treatment: Lesion incision and drainage (I&D); culture samples from the wound. Infectious Disease Society of America guidelines recommend antibiotic treatment after I&D of suspected MRSA lesions for patients with severe or extensive disease, rapid progression of associated cellulitis, signs of systemic toxicity,

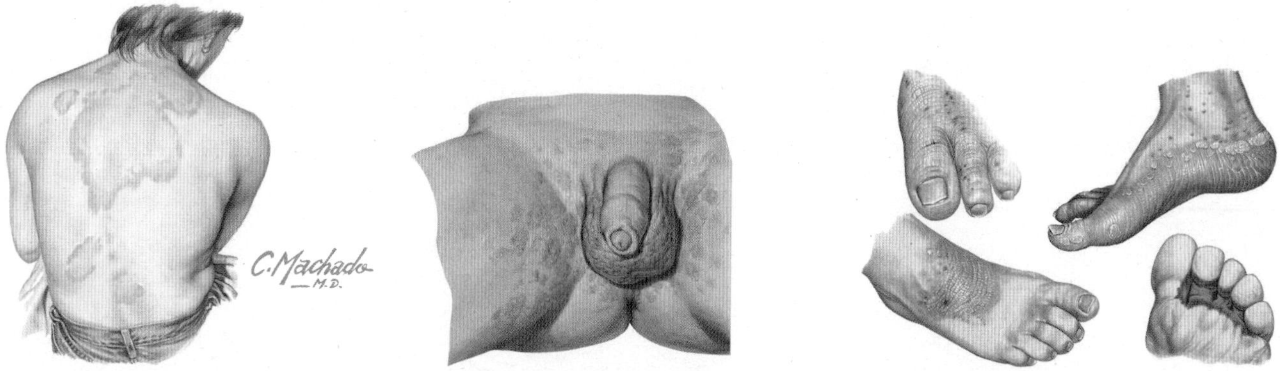
C.Machado
—M.D.

Tinea corporis ("ringworm") - causes a ring-shaped rash, usually on the legs or trunk of the body.

Tinea cruris ("jock itch") - affects the inner thighs and groin. It causes pain and severe itching and usually a rash of red, ring-like patches that grow outward in the crease of the thighs. The patches usually have bumps and a different color than nearby skin.

Tinea pedis ("athlete's foot") - causes severe itching and a rash on bottoms of the feet and between the toes. Itching is often worst between the toes.

Figure 29.3 Tinea infections.

lesions that are difficult to drain (e.g., in the groin or axilla), and a lack of response to I&D alone. Oral antibiotics effective against CA-MRSA include trimethoprim-sulfamethoxazole, tetracycline, clindamycin (perform D-test if erythromycin-resistant strain is suspected), and linezolid. Decolonization of MRSA carriers has a limited role. Protocols typically involve topical antimicrobial scrubs and nasal mupirocin with limited evidence for the overall utility for these protocols. Consider decolonization for patients with recurrent MRSA infection, for close contacts of culture-confirmed carriers, and in training room outbreaks. Decolonization can be achieved through a daily body wash with 4% chlorhexidine solution and 2% mupirocin ointment applied to each nostril two times per day for 5 days.

Return to play: NFHS guidelines for bacterial diseases (impetigo, boils): To be considered "noncontagious," all lesions must be scabbed over with no oozing or discharge. If new lesions develop or drain, consider MRSA, and I&D is recommended (with or without antibiotics) with no further lesion development or drainage for 72 hours. **NCAA guidelines for bacterial infections (furuncles, carbuncles, folliculitis, impetigo, cellulitis or erysipelas, staphylococcal infection, and CA-MRSA):** Wrestlers must not have any new skin lesion development for 48 hours before the event; must have completed 72 hours of antibiotic therapy; and have no moist, exudative, or draining lesions at the time of the meet or tournament. Gram stain of exudate from questionable lesions (if available). Active bacterial infections should not be covered to allow participation.

Prevention: Screen athletes regularly and teach them to report all skin injuries. Keep skin injuries clean and covered until healed. Encourage hand washing by all athletes and staff, as contaminated hands are the primary mode of MRSA transmission. Routine showering immediately after activity, cleaning of facilities and showers, and using liquid antibacterial soap and clean towels help. Discourage sharing of fomites, equipment, and razors.

ATHLETIC PARTICIPATION AND OTHER INFECTIONS

Human immunodeficiency virus (HIV) infection: No evidence supports moderate-intensity exercise is harmful to an HIV-infected athlete. Exercise may be beneficial to HIV-infected athletes by reducing anxiety and depression. HIV-infected athletes should be allowed to participate in sports if they are asymptomatic and show no evidence of deficiencies in immunologic function. There are no well-documented, confirmed reports of HIV transmission during sport.

Hepatitis B virus (HBV) infection: Participation should be determined based on signs or symptoms such as fever, fatigue, or hepatomegaly. There is no evidence that intense, competitive training is harmful to an asymptomatic HBV carrier (acute or chronic) without evidence of organ impairment. HBV transmission has been documented in Japan in five members of a high school sumo wrestling club.

Hepatitis C virus (HCV) infection: There are no current CDC recommendations regarding athletic participation for athletes who have an HCV infection, but participation based on signs and symptoms, similar to HBV, is probably safe. No studies have found evidence of HCV transmission during sport.

Pericarditis (2015 American Heart Association/American College of Cardiology [AHA/ACC] Scientific Statement): No exercise or sports during the acute phase; return to full activity with resolution of active disease (no effusion on ECHO and serum markers of inflammation normalized). Chronic constrictive pericarditis is a contraindication to participation in sports.

Myocarditis (2015 AHA/ACC Scientific Statement): Athletes with probable or definite myocarditis should not participate in competitive sports while active inflammation is present. Recovery may take several months. There is a risk of lethal arrhythmias until recovery is complete. Current recommendations include evaluation using resting ECHO, 24-hour Holter monitor, and exercise stress test 3–6 months after initial illness before returning to competitive sport. May return to sport if:

- Ventricular systolic function has returned to normal.
- Serum markers of myocardial injury, inflammation, and heart failure have normalized.
- Arrhythmias such as frequent or complex repetitive forms of ventricular or supraventricular ectopic activity are absent on Holter monitor and graded exercise ECGs.

REPORTABLE DISEASES

- Reportable diseases are infections of great public importance that must be reported when they are diagnosed by doctors or laboratories.
- Reporting allows researchers to identify disease trends and track disease outbreaks. Every state has a reportable disease list.
- Is the responsibility of the healthcare provider, not the patient, to report disease cases. It is very important to be aware of how and when to report reportable diseases.
- Common reportable diseases are chickenpox, tuberculosis, HIV, hepatitis A, hepatitis B, hepatitis C, meningitis, gonorrhea, and chlamydia.
- County or state health departments will try to identify the source of several of these illnesses, and for sexually transmitted diseases, the county or state will try to locate sexual contacts of infected people.
- Cooperation with state health workers can facilitate locating the source of infection and help quell the spread of an epidemic.

RECOMMENDED READINGS

Available online.

GASTROINTESTINAL PROBLEMS 30

Travis Miller • Michael K. Neilson • Joshua Baker • Anthony Beutler

GENERAL PRINCIPLES

The gastrointestinal (GI) system and its processes are a secondary priority for the body during exercise. As a result, GI dysfunction and disease can often impede maximal athletic potential. During exercise, blood flow is diverted from the splanchnic circulation and preferentially distributed to demanding peripheral muscles. Additionally, sustained movement created during athletic activity can cause disruption to physiologic GI functioning. These factors are thought to be the most common source of various GI problems experienced by athletes. Fortunately, despite almost 90% of some populations reporting some exercise-associated GI symptoms, the severity of illness is typically mild.

APPROACH TO GI PROBLEMS IN ATHLETES

History

- Red-flag symptoms include weight loss, dysphagia, black or bloody stools, and abdominal masses.
- Differentiate upper GI from lower GI symptoms: nausea, cramping, bloating, and diarrhea
- Determine severity of disease: hematochezia vs. melena
- Consider effects of foods and beverages, anxiety/stress, caffeine, tobacco, alcohol, nonsteroidal anti-inflammatory drugs (NSAIDs) or other medications, drugs of abuse, or other supplements
- Assess possibility of undiagnosed systemic disease (e.g., celiac or inflammatory bowel disease)

Physical Examination

- Signs of abnormal palpatory examination: localized or generalized abdominal tenderness, organomegaly, mass, hernia, and peritoneal signs
- Signs of volume depletion: orthostatic hypotension and tachycardia
- Signs of inflammatory bowel disease: oral ulcers, dermatologic and ocular signs, and joint manifestations
- Signs of thyroid disease: thyromegaly, altered reflexes, and dermatologic and ocular manifestations
- Signs of systemic wasting: temporal wasting, lymphadenopathy, hepatomegaly, and splenomegaly

Differential Diagnosis (Table 30.1)

- Infectious: gastroenteritis and hepatitis
- Neoplastic: GI tract cancer and lymphoma
- Endocrine: hyperthyroidism, hypothyroidism, and pancreatic disease
- Autoimmune: Crohn disease, ulcerative colitis, and celiac disease
- Trauma: GI and genitourinary organs
- Vascular: cardiac and mesenteric ischemia
- Other: peptic ulcer disease, irritable bowel syndrome (IBS), constipation, medication- or supplement-induced disorder, food allergy, and other problems related to food or beverage intake

Laboratory Data

- Determine the necessity of tests based on the severity of symptoms. Tests may include cell blood count, iron studies, hepatic function panel, *Helicobacter pylori* testing, electrolytes, thyroid studies, erythrocyte sedimentation rate/C-reactive protein (ESR/CRP), and **occult blood in stool** and other stool studies

UPPER GI PROBLEMS

- Upper GI pain related to training and competition often presents a diagnostic dilemma, as both serious and benign etiologies often have similar presentations. Common symptoms include epigastric pain, dysphagia, dyspepsia, nausea, vomiting, and heartburn.
- During exercise, central blood volume is maintained by redirecting blood away from internal organs, particularly the splanchnic bed. Studies have revealed that splanchnic blood flow declines from 1.56 L/min at rest to 0.3 L/min at maximal exercise.
- **Possible negative effects of exercise-induced shunting:** Decreased esophageal motility, erosive hemorrhagic gastritis, delayed gastric emptying, diarrhea, and intestinal bleeding.
- **Angina or cardiac ischemia:** Epigastric pain referred from the heart is a "Can't Miss" diagnosis that should always be seriously considered in patients, especially in older athletes.
- **Gastroesophageal reflux (GER)**
  - Vigorous exercise causes GER in healthy subjects, notably in runners, bicyclists, and weightlifters, and those just initiating exercise programs.
  - Frequency, amplitude, and duration of esophageal contractions decline with increasing exercise intensity.
  - Hypoperfusion resulting from exercise-induced arterial shunting to muscles and skin may cause reduced esophageal motility.
  - Treatment: H_2 blockers for acute episodes. For persistent occurrence, consider proton pump inhibitors (PPIs) daily for 1–2 weeks. Taking PPIs on an "as needed" basis may not provide optimal acid reduction. Otherwise, may adhere to standard medical management for GER, alteration of oral intake (avoid symptom-triggering foods and beverages, no food for 3 hours before exercise).
- **Gastritis:** Erosive gastritis may be induced by exercise-related hypoperfusion, mechanical forces, or NSAIDs: often hemorrhagic. If hemorrhagic, typically self-limited within 72 hours, but can resolve acutely with medication. Treat with H_2 blockers, PPIs, and antacids (Fig. 30.1).
- **Peptic ulcer disease** is as common in runners as in the general population; use standard medical management (Fig. 30.2).
- **Delayed gastric emptying** may be related to bloating, reflux, or both; likely only at severe exercise; may be caused by hypoperfusion, resulting from arterial shunting away from the splanchnic bed.
- **Upper GI bleeding:** May be related to hemorrhagic gastritis or peptic ulcer disease (see the "Gastritis" section); mechanical cause is proposed in some cases. Gastric fundus is the most common site for gastric bleeding because the shearing force from the adjacent diaphragm may be the source.
  - Evaluate and treat using standard upper GI methodologies.
  - Improve hydration before and during performance. Increased plasma volume may reduce ischemia.
- **Exercise-associated transient abdominal pain (ETAP):** Often referred to as a "side-stitch"; presents as pain, most often in the lateral aspect of the midabdomen. Incidences decline with age and fitness level. It is a benign condition with proposed mechanisms including diaphragm spasm, exertional irritation of parietal peritoneum, compression of thoracic intercostal nerves, and trapped gas in hepatic or splenic flexure. Avoid solid

Table 30.1 GASTROINTESTINAL PROBLEMS

Upper GI Problems	Lower GI Problems	General GI Problems
Angina/Cardiac Ischemia Gastroesophageal Reflux Gastritis Peptic Ulcer Disease Delayed Gastric Emptying Upper GI Bleed Exercise-Associated Transient Abdominal Pain	Runner's Diarrhea Lower GI Bleed Ischemic Colitis Cecal Slap Syndrome Celiac Artery Compression Syndrome	Anxiety/Stress Acute Gastroenteritis Traveler's Diarrhea Celiac Disease/Nonceliac Gluten Sensitivity Irritable Bowel Syndrome Inflammatory Bowel Disease

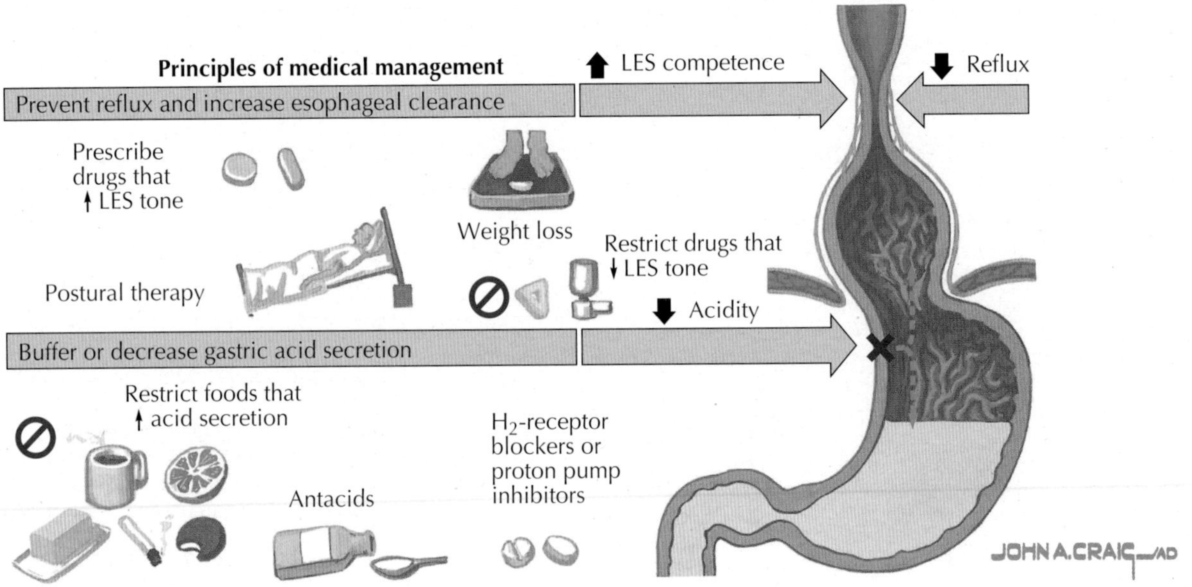
Principles of medical management
↑ LES competence
↓ Reflux
Prevent reflux and increase esophageal clearance
Prescribe drugs that ↑ LES tone
Weight loss
Postural therapy
Restrict drugs that ↓ LES tone
↓ Acidity
Buffer or decrease gastric acid secretion
Restrict foods that ↑ acid secretion
Antacids
H_2-receptor blockers or proton pump inhibitors
JOHN A.CRAIG_AD

Figure 30.1 Gastroesophageal reflux.

meals 2–3 hours before exercise for prevention; may consider liquid meals. Acute treatment strategies include deep breathing, decreasing exercise intensity, pressing on the area, and stretching. Typically symptoms resolve within minutes once exercise is stopped.

LOWER GI PROBLEMS

Runner's Diarrhea ("Runner's Trots")

- Characterized by looser stools stimulated by intense endurance running, with or without accompanying GI bleeding.
- Up to 62% of runners have urge to defecate during training and is the leading cause for runs to be halted.
- More vigorous running increases susceptibility, and women appear to be more affected than men.
- See Box 30.1 for general recommendations for prevention/treatment.

Proposed Etiologies

- Anxiety-induced diarrhea (see "Anxiety and Stress Reaction" section)
- Increased GI motility: Exercise increases the secretion of gastrin, motilin, and other hormones that affect motility; IBS
- Mechanical turbulence and emulsification: Runners see much greater incidence than cyclists.
- Dietary factors: High-fiber diet may cause exercise-induced diarrhea in a small subset of runners; a higher incidence of lactose intolerance in patients with exercise-induced diarrhea than in general population; symptoms may occur only during exercise; sorbitol or fructose intolerance with fruit-intensive diets; large doses of caffeine or vitamin C; osmotic effects of high-fructose sports drinks or gels.
- Possible immune system etiology: Variant of exercise-induced anaphylaxis; generalized urticaria, including urticarial lesions in intestines
- Endotoxins have been proposed as a cause of GI symptoms.

Treatment

- Once other diarrheal etiologies are ruled out, training regimen changes and symptomatic treatment with loperamide can be initiated.
- Oral rehydration strategies should focus on GI losses in addition to sweat loss.
- NSAIDs should be avoided.
- Future prerace diets should limit calories and osmotically active components.

Lower GI Bleeding

- Grossly bloody diarrhea stimulated by intense performance: large amounts of red, maroon, or clotted blood may be seen; severe abdominal pain
- More common after competition than training, suggesting degree of effort plays a role
- Microscopic increases in fecal hemoglobin after intense running are more common than gross blood and have been noted in endurance bicyclists; may be caused by upper or lower GI bleeding; transient in endoscopic studies

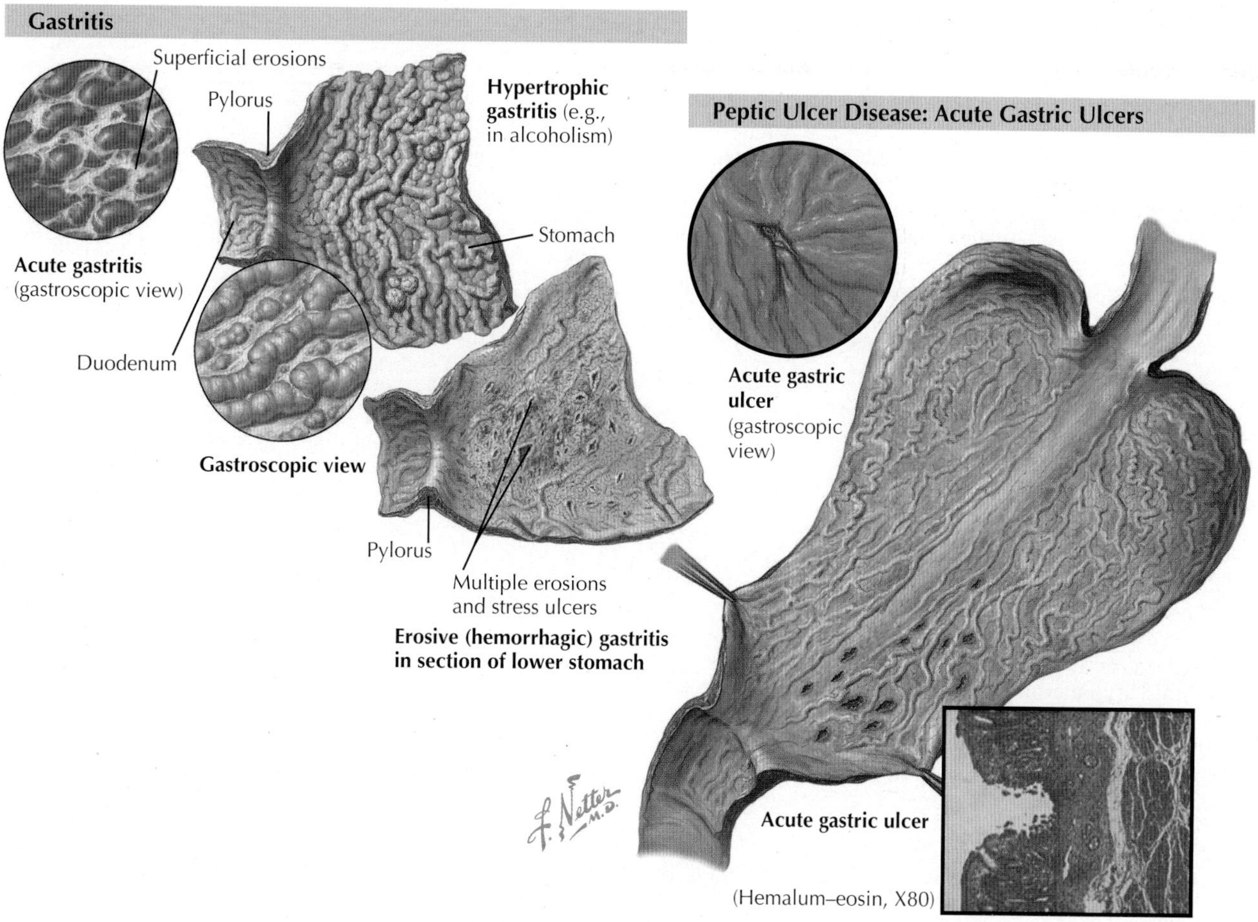
Gastritis
Superficial erosions
Pylorus
Hypertrophic gastritis (e.g., in alcoholism)
Stomach
Acute gastritis (gastroscopic view)
Duodenum
Gastroscopic view
Pylorus
Multiple erosions and stress ulcers
Erosive (hemorrhagic) gastritis in section of lower stomach
Peptic Ulcer Disease: Acute Gastric Ulcers
Acute gastric ulcer (gastroscopic view)
Acute gastric ulcer
(Hemalum–eosin, X80)

Figure 30.2 Upper gastrointestinal (GI) problems.

BOX 30.1 GENERAL RECOMMENDATIONS FOR PREVENTION AND TREATMENT OF DIARRHEA

- Encourage bowel movement. Have a light meal a few hours before competition and then jog to stimulate gastrocolic reflex.
- Improve hydration before and during performance: increased plasma volume may decrease ischemia (with or without diarrhea).
- Dietary manipulations:
  - Athletes on low-fiber diet may improve by adding fiber to absorb intraluminal fluid.
  - Athletes on high-fiber diet may improve by reducing fiber to decrease stimulation of intestinal motility. Several athletes prefer a high-fiber diet because it stimulates intestinal motility, thus reducing intraluminal contents.
  - Eliminate foods that trigger bowel symptoms in individual athletes—lactose, fructose, sorbitol, and caffeine.
- Antimotility medications may be helpful in cases of diarrhea that appear to be a form of functional bowel syndrome and in those that remain undiagnosed: Imodium (risk of hyperthermia) and Lomotil.
- Decrease training and competition level by 20%–40% in both mileage and intensity, then build back up slowly. May be able to cross-train.
- Surgery involving division of obstructing diaphragmatic fibers and denervation of celiac ganglion may benefit patients with celiac compression syndrome but remains controversial.

Proposed Etiologies

- Crampy abdominal pain combined with frank blood in stool (likely loose) should be an indication to stop exercise and rest and likely seek further medical attention.
- **Ischemic colitis:** Heralded with abdominal pain and diarrhea, it is caused by hypoperfusion shunting blood flow from mesentery to muscles and skin; strenuous exercise may decrease flow by up to 80% (may be magnified by dehydration). Relative gut ischemia, particularly in watershed areas of colon, causes focal areas of necrosis and ulceration. In addition, ischemia may cause intestinal malabsorption, thereby precipitating diarrhea; this condition is most often seen in endurance athletes, especially in oppressive heat. Key factor for recovery is knowing when to stop, as prolonged ischemia can lead to colectomy.
- **Cecal slap syndrome:** Mechanical trauma from running reported to cause hemorrhagic cecal lesions and diarrhea.
- **Celiac artery compression syndrome** (median arcuate ligament syndrome): Rare and controversial cause of chronic recurrent abdominal pain reported in nonathletes.
  - External compression of celiac and occasionally superior mesenteric artery (SMA) by the median arcuate ligament of the diaphragm (left crus or fibrous band connecting left and right crus), particularly during exhalation (Fig. 30.3).
  - Diagnosis of exclusion: All other GI pathology must be ruled out, with a high index of clinical suspicion.
  - No clear diagnostic criteria, and no imaging modality predicts response to surgery.
  - Most common in young individuals, those with recent weight loss, and women.

- Pain may be sharp, dull, steady, or crampy and may worsen after meals, weight loss, or position changes.
- **Loud systolic bruit** may be appreciated in the epigastrium.
- **Four proposed mechanisms for pain:** Compression of celiac and SMA, resulting in mesenteric ischemia; extensive collateral circulation "steals" from primary distribution of SMA in the fed state; inadequate collateral circulation, resulting in nonocclusive ischemia during hypotension or decreased perfusion; irritation of celiac plexus or overstimulation of sympathetic nerve fibers.
- **Arteriography** confirms clinical diagnosis of celiac artery compression syndrome; duplex ultrasonography recently used to measure flow velocities in SMA and celiac arteries

GENERAL GI PROBLEMS IN ATHLETES

Anxiety and Stress Reaction

- Performance anxiety
- Inhibitory effects on upper GI function: decreased acid secretion in the stomach, diminished motor activity, and reduced blood flow
- Continued anxiety may result in acid hypersecretion
- Stimulant effect on lower GI activity: increased motility and decreased transit time
- **Symptoms:** dry mouth, dyspepsia ("knot in stomach"), heartburn, reflux, abdominal cramping, and diarrhea
- **Treatment:** reassurance and education, behavior modification, and relaxation exercises

Acute Gastroenteritis

- Incidence second only to that of upper respiratory tract infections in adolescents and young adults

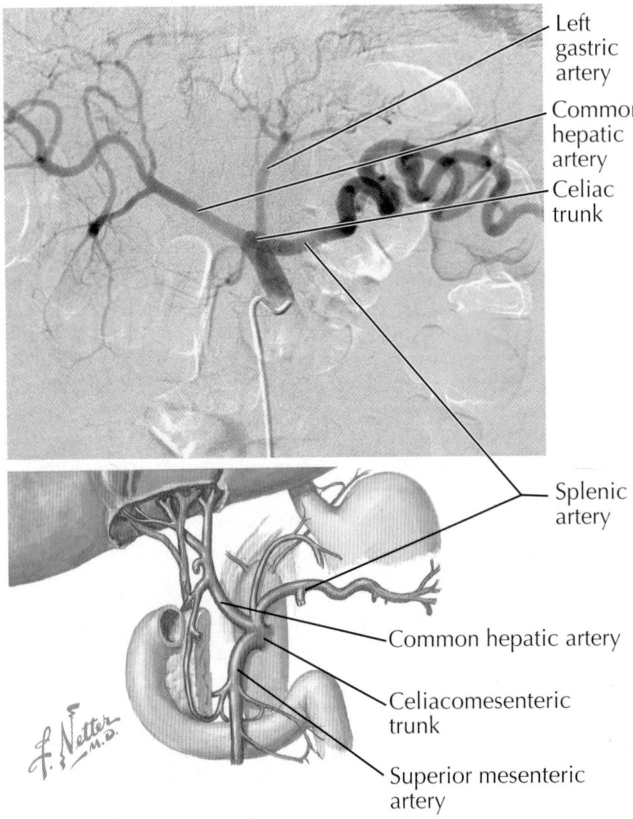

Left gastric artery
Common hepatic artery
Celiac trunk
Splenic artery
Common hepatic artery
Celiacomesenteric trunk
Superior mesenteric artery
F. Netter M.D.

Figure 30.3 Celiac trunk: Normal and variant.

- Etiologic agents: viral (most common, including rotavirus, Norwalk, and norovirus), bacterial, and protozoan *(Giardia lamblia)*
- Peak incidence: winter in cities and summer in rural or outdoor sports
- **Symptoms:** nausea, vomiting, abdominal cramps, diarrhea, fever, and myalgia

Treatment

- Usually self-limited (2–3 days)
- Clear and electrolyte-containing fluids (e.g., sport drinks) are cornerstone; replace fluid loss liter for liter
- Assess the severity of dehydration (body weight, urine output, and blood pressure) before strenuous practice or game
- Antimotility drugs may be effective for abdominal cramps but may also prolong the carrier state of certain organisms: loperamide (Imodium) and diphenoxylate hydrochloride with atropine (Lomotil).

"Traveler's Diarrhea"

- Ninety percent caused by bacteria, with *Escherichia coli* being the predominant organism; Viruses comprise 5%–10% (noro-, rota-, and astroviruses), and parasites comprise a small percentage (*Giardia* being most common).

Treatment

- Depends on severity of illness. Adequate fluid replacement essential for any severity of diarrhea, and most cases are self-limiting and resolve within 3–7 days. Voluminous consumption of overly sweet drinks may cause worsening of symptoms with osmotic diarrhea.
- Antibiotics may be warranted in moderate cases and are always warranted in severe cases for nonbloody diarrhea. Antibiotics shorten disease course and severity but may carry side effects.
- First-line antibiotic therapy is azithromycin. Fluoroquinolones are now recommended as alternative agents because of fluoroquinolone-associated tendinopathy and tendon rupture. Loperamide (Imodium) may be combined with antibiotic administration for symptomatic relief. Loperamide should be avoided in cases with bloody diarrhea or if fever is present.
- Bloody diarrhea can reflect an enterohemorrhagic *E. coli* infection, an uncommon cause of traveler's diarrhea, for which antibiotic treatment has been associated with an increased risk of hemolytic-uremic syndrome. In addition, *Salmonella*, *Shigella*, and *Campylobacter* may cause bloody diarrhea but are uncommon with traveler's diarrhea and are typically self-limiting. Antibiotic therapy should be cautioned in this situation.
- Stool studies are recommended before antibiotic administration. Afterwards, monitor for persistent symptoms (antibiotic resistance) or worsening colitis (*Clostridium difficile* infection).

Prevention

- Controlled studies show prophylactic antibiotics can reduce diarrhea rates by 90% or more. However, prophylactic antibiotics are not recommended for most travelers. Prompt treatment at first sign of symptoms without prophylaxis typically resolves cases in 6–24 hours. Symptomatic therapy also saves the patient from unnecessary medication side effects, disturbances of protective digestive microflora, and preventing antibiotic resistance.
- If prophylaxis is desired, rifaximin is recommended over bismuth salicylate. The large doses of bismuth salicylate required for prevention can increase the risk of salicylate toxicity. Moreover, bismuth may reduce the absorption of antibiotics. Optimal dose of rifaximin is uncertain, but most experts favor 200 mg PO TID during time of exposure (for a period of <2 weeks).

- Return to competition limited only by hydration status, infective nature of problems (norovirus), symptom complex (i.e., frequent diarrhea), and reconditioning.
- Probiotics have shown potential in small-scale studies to reduce GI symptoms caused by intraluminal floral shifts that occur 1–2 weeks after antibiotic use.

Celiac Disease

- Hereditary autoimmune disorder to gluten or gliadin that damages small intestinal mucosa, which results in villous atrophy and decreased nutrient absorption; includes a wide variety of symptoms: diarrhea, bloating, vomiting, fatigue, anemia, arthralgia, and myalgia (Fig. 30.4).
- Approximately 30% of the population have genetic markers for celiac disease; however, only about 1% have active disease. Women are 2.5 times more likely than men to have active disease.
- Initial workup should include tissue transglutaminase antibody level. The gold standard for diagnosis is a biopsy of the small intestine that demonstrates blunted villi.
- Avoidance of gluten is the only known treatment.

Nonceliac Gluten Sensitivity

- The diagnosis of nonceliac gluten sensitivity remains elusive because of poor understanding of the underlying mechanism, unavailability of testable biomarkers, and considerable overlap with other allergy and functional syndromes. Differential diagnosis should be excluded first before trial of removing gluten-containing foods.
- Gluten-free diets are often endorsed for athletic performance in modern social media. There are no studies available to back up this claim. One 2016 study by Lis et al. demonstrated no performance impact or reduction in GI symptoms in a 4-week double-blind study comparing gluten-free and gluten-fed cyclist groups. As diet is not "blind" in real life, it is possible any gains may be attributed to placebo or a "belief effect."
- The new target for avoidance may be the more specific FODMAPs (fermentable oligosaccharides, disaccharides, monosaccharides, and polyols). FODMAPs are a family of short-chain fermentable carbohydrates that are slowly or poorly absorbed in the upper intestinal tract and rapidly fermented by colonic bacteria (Table 30.2). Research in this area is in its infancy, and more study is needed before definite guidance can be given.
- Because of a lack of strong evidence, excluding gluten-containing foods from a diet should be heavily cautioned, as dietary exclusion could affect caloric and macronutrient intake. However, low-FODMAP intake may be considered as a tool for susceptible individuals.

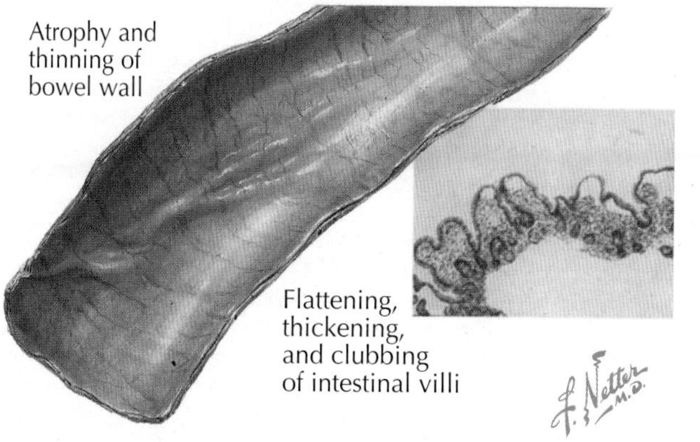
Atrophy and thinning of bowel wall
Flattening, thickening, and clubbing of intestinal villi
F. Netter M.D.

Figure 30.4 Celiac disease enteropathy.

Irritable Bowel Syndrome

- Characterized by abdominal pain with a change in defecation patterns. Defecation often relieves the abdominal pain.
- Exercise has a known benefit on regulation of IBS.
- Divided into various types based on predominance of symptoms: constipation predominant, diarrhea predominant, or mixed.
- Constipation predominant: consider fiber or polyethylene glycol. Diarrhea predominant: consider loperamide as first-line treatment. For significant pain: consider dicyclomine or hyoscyamine. Be wary of side effects of anticholinergic medications.
- Depression and anxiety are often associated with IBS. Tricyclic antidepressants (TCAs) (diarrhea) and selective serotonin reuptake inhibitors (SSRIs) (constipation) may be considered, as they have shown benefit for refractory cases.

RECOMMENDED READINGS

Available online.

TABLE 30.2 LOW FODMAP DIET NAVIGATION CHART

Types of Foods	May Cause Symptoms[a]	Alternatives to Try Instead
Dairy	Cow's milk, cottage cheese, custard, ice cream, mascarpone, pudding, ricotta cheese, yogurt	Almond milk, coconut milk, hard cheeses (feta, brie, etc), lactose-free milk, lactose-free yogurt, rice milk
Fruits	Apples, apricots, blackberries, cherries, mangoes, nectarines, pears, peaches, plums, watermelon	Bananas, blueberries, cantaloupe, grapefruit, honeydew, kiwi, lemon, lime, oranges, strawberries
Vegetables	Artichokes, asparagus, beetroot, brussels sprouts, broccoli, cabbage, cauliflower, celery, garlic, mushroom, onions, snow peas	Bamboo shoots, bell peppers, bean sprouts, carrots, chives, cucumbers, eggplant, ginger, lettuce, olives, parsnips, potatoes, turnips, zucchini
Protein		Chicken, fish, pork, beef, eggs, tofu
Nuts/seeds	Cashews, pistachios	Almonds, macadamia, peanuts, pine nuts, pumpkin seeds, walnuts
Grain	Rye, wheat	Corn, corn flour, gluten-free pasta, oats, oat bran, rice, rice bran, quinoa, sourdough breads
Legumes	Chickpeas, kidney beans, lentils, soy products	
Sweeteners	Agave nectar, high fructose corn syrup, honey, sugar-free gum, mints, and cough medicines/drops	

[a]Only limit problematic foods.

31 HEMATOLOGIC PROBLEMS IN THE ATHLETE

Jennifer S. Harvey • Anthony S. Ceraulo • Tracy R. Ray

RED BLOOD CELL DISORDERS AND INHERITED HEMOGLOBINOPATHIES

Sickle Cell Syndromes

Description: Sickle cell warrants special consideration for athletes. Inheritance of a gene from one parent results in sickle cell trait (SCT), and inheritance from both results in sickle cell disease (SCD). Other allele formations that lead to sickling include hemoglobin SC and sickle cell beta-thalassemia. Whereas SCD is a contraindication for competitive sports because of the high risk of life-threatening crisis, those with SCT are able to participate with activity modifications.

Epidemiology: SCT is present in 6%–9% of African Americans and 0.05% in the remaining US population. There have been 18 documented collegiate football–related deaths attributed to SCT (daSCT) from 1974 to 2010. After National Collegiate Athletic Association (NCAA) legislation mandating SCT screening in 2010, only one daSCT was recorded from 2010 to 2019.

Pathophysiology: Sickle cell gene causes mutation of the red blood cell (RBC) B globin molecule. When an RBC is under stress, it enters an oxidative crisis, leading to polymerization, which in turn leads to sickling. Sickled cells form vaso-occlusive clots causing ischemic insults. The vast majority of those with SCT will be asymptomatic throughout life, but there is a risk of sickling with extreme physical activity. The exact causes of sudden death because of SCT is unknown and highly debated. The end result is sickling, vascular occlusion, and perhaps exertional collapse associated with sickle cell trait (ECSAT). Factors thought to increase this risk include fatigue, poor conditioning, altitude changes, heat, and concurrent febrile illness.

Laboratory testing: Hemoglobin (Hgb) electrophoresis, high-performance liquid chromatography (HLPC), or an Hgb solubility test are the methods most often used for sickle cell identification. Sickle cell testing is included in the newborn screen for every child born in the United States. Since 2010, the NCAA has mandated sickle cell testing for all incoming athletes after a lawsuit regarding the death of a football player suffering a daSCT.

Clinical presentation: Exertional sickling (ES) is similar to heat-related illness and exertional cardiac illness and can be difficult to distinguish. In ES, muscular symptoms are typically sudden with more weakness but less pain than heat illness cramping. The legs slowly become weak, leading to collapse. Mentation is typically normal, and temperature is normal to only slightly elevated.

Evaluation and treatment: If ES is suspected, the athlete should be immediately evaluated with a complete set of vital signs. If temperature measurements are consistent with heat-related illness, they should be immediately treated as such. If that is not the case, an automated external defibrillator (AED) should be placed, intravenous (IV) fluids may be started depending on ambulance wait time, and the athlete should be closely monitored until emergency services arrive.

Prevention: For ES, it begins with determining at-risk individuals by laboratory testing. If an athlete is identified as having SCT, special attention should be paid during athletic participation. Athletes should have an individualized training program that allows for a slower build of strength and conditioning with increased frequency of rest and hydration. Education should emphasize appropriate water intake. If the athlete will be participating at higher altitude or warmer climate, a proper, gradual acclimatization program should be implemented. Coaches and staff should be aware of the athlete's sickle cell status and be instructed to stop training immediately and have the athlete evaluated if symptoms arise.

Return to play: Athletes who collapse during exercise should be thoroughly evaluated to rule out cardiac, electrolyte, respiratory, or other metabolic etiologies of collapse. Risks and benefits to continued athletic participation should be discussed. Once the athlete has clinically recovered and laboratory work has normalized, he or she may choose to return to sport.

Thalassemia

Description: Thalassemia is an inherited disease that is a risk factor for poor outcomes in athletes. Like sickle cell, thalassemia has a spectrum of disease presentations ranging from asymptomatic to outcomes that are not compatible with life. There are both alpha- and beta-thalassemias. Disease severity depends on how many of the four alleles are inherited and the specific alleles inherited.

Epidemiology: Roughly 5% of the world's population has at least one thalassemia allele. These alleles initially arose in populations where malaria was endemic as a protective factor.

Pathophysiology: The disrupted ratio of alpha- and beta-globin production leads to unpaired alpha- and beta-chains that then precipitate, causing destruction of RBC precursors.

Clinical presentation: Thalassemia trait is the most common condition and is largely asymptomatic with a normal complete blood count (CBC), mild microcytosis, or mild anemia.

Laboratory testing: Includes CBC, peripheral smear, and iron panel.

Treatment: No recommended treatment for thalassemia trait. It is important to differentiate thalassemia and iron deficiency, which can have a similar clinical presentation because iron is not advised in patients with thalassemia because of the risk of iron overload. This risk contributes to the recommendation against universal iron supplementation.

Iron Deficiency

Description: Iron plays an important role in both overall health and peak sport performance. Iron is important in oxygen transport to skeletal muscles and in in aerobic metabolism via adenosine triphosphate (ATP) production in the electron transport chain. Decreased iron stores may result in effects ranging from minimal to anemia (i.e., drop in Hgb below standard value). Patients with iron-deficiency anemia (IDA) require treatment. Iron deficiency without anemia (IDNA) seems to play a role in both subjective and objective markers relating to athletic performance. Specifics regarding evaluation and treatment of IDNA athletes is much more controversial.

Epidemiology: Prevalence of iron deficiency in athletic females and males ranges from 15% to 50% and 3% to 11%, respectively. The prevalence of athletes with true IDA is much lower, at about 2% for females and 0.1% for males. Endurance athletes are at greatest risk.

Risk factors and causes for iron deficiency in the athletic population: Once IDNA or IDA is diagnosed, the cause should be identified, if possible. Blood loss (e.g., gastrointestinal [GI], gastrourinary [GU], and menstrual losses) is the major cause of iron deficiency. Menstruating females comprise the highest percentage of those with iron deficiency. In addition to typical blood loss risk factors of the general population, there are mechanisms specific to athletes that may contribute to iron deficiency. During periods of intense and prolonged exercise, blood may be shunted from the gut to working skeletal muscles, leading to GI tract microischemia. Reports have shown that up to 85% of athletes have a positive fecal occult blood test after prolonged vigorous exercises. Hematuria caused by mechanical forces on the bladder during intense exercise and iron loss through excessive sweating have also been postulated. Lastly, hepcidin, a regulator of iron absorption, has been shown to play a part. Exercise causes an inflammatory response, which upregulates hepcidin, which then downregulates iron absorption and transfer of iron along metabolic pathways. The level of hepcidin typically peaks 3–6 hours after strenuous exercise. Additionally, relative energy deficiency in sport (RED-S) is very likely linked to iron deficiency, either by decreased amounts of iron intake through restrictive diets or by diminished iron absorption.

Clinical presentation: The severity of symptoms often correlates to the degree and acuity of iron deficiency. Some cases are asymptomatic, whereas mild to moderate cases may present with fatigue, decreased exercise tolerance, or depressed mood. Severe cases classified as IDA have symptoms that may include palpitations, shortness of breath, dizziness, or syncope and physical examination findings that may include tachycardia, increased respiratory rate, pale conjunctiva, generalized paleness, and systolic murmurs (Fig. 31.1).

Laboratory studies: Initial laboratory work includes CBC, serum ferritin, plasma iron, total iron binding capacity (TIBC), and transferrin; fecal occult blood test or urinalysis if history suggests. The laboratory tests should be drawn in the morning, not within 48–72 hours of vigorous exercise, and not in the time of sickness or infection. This is important, as increased levels of inflammation may affect the results and make it difficult to assess. There are no guidelines regarding screening of asymptomatic individuals, but many institutions do screen those at higher risk.

Diagnosis: Iron deficiency is divided into three stages:

1. Stage I: Low ferritin
2. Stage II: Low iron and/or low transferrin and increased TIBC + low ferritin
3. Stage III: Low hemoglobin (female Hgb <12, males Hgb <14) + stage II findings

The World Health Organization defines iron depletion at a serum ferritin <15 for adults. The ferritin cutoff for iron deficiency in the athletic population remains controversial. Studies show a decrease in athletic performance when serum ferritin <20 and perhaps a subjective decrease in fatigue and mood when ferritin <30. Stage III iron deficiency is related to decreased oxygen transport on hemoglobin, which certainly affects athletic performance. It is thought that with stage I and II, there may be impaired function of oxidative enzymes and respiratory proteins that results in decreased aerobic power and diminished exercise performance.

Treatment: Indicated in IDA and considered in IDNA. The literature suggests treating iron deficiency to keep serum ferritin >20. If a diagnosis is made, repeat testing should be done in 6- to 8-week intervals until adequate iron status is achieved. Typically 100% of iron is obtained through digestion. The two sources of iron are free iron and heme iron (found in animal products). Heme iron is much more readily absorbed by the gut; thus, vegetarians should take care in monitoring their iron consumption. As iron becomes deficient in the body, the body

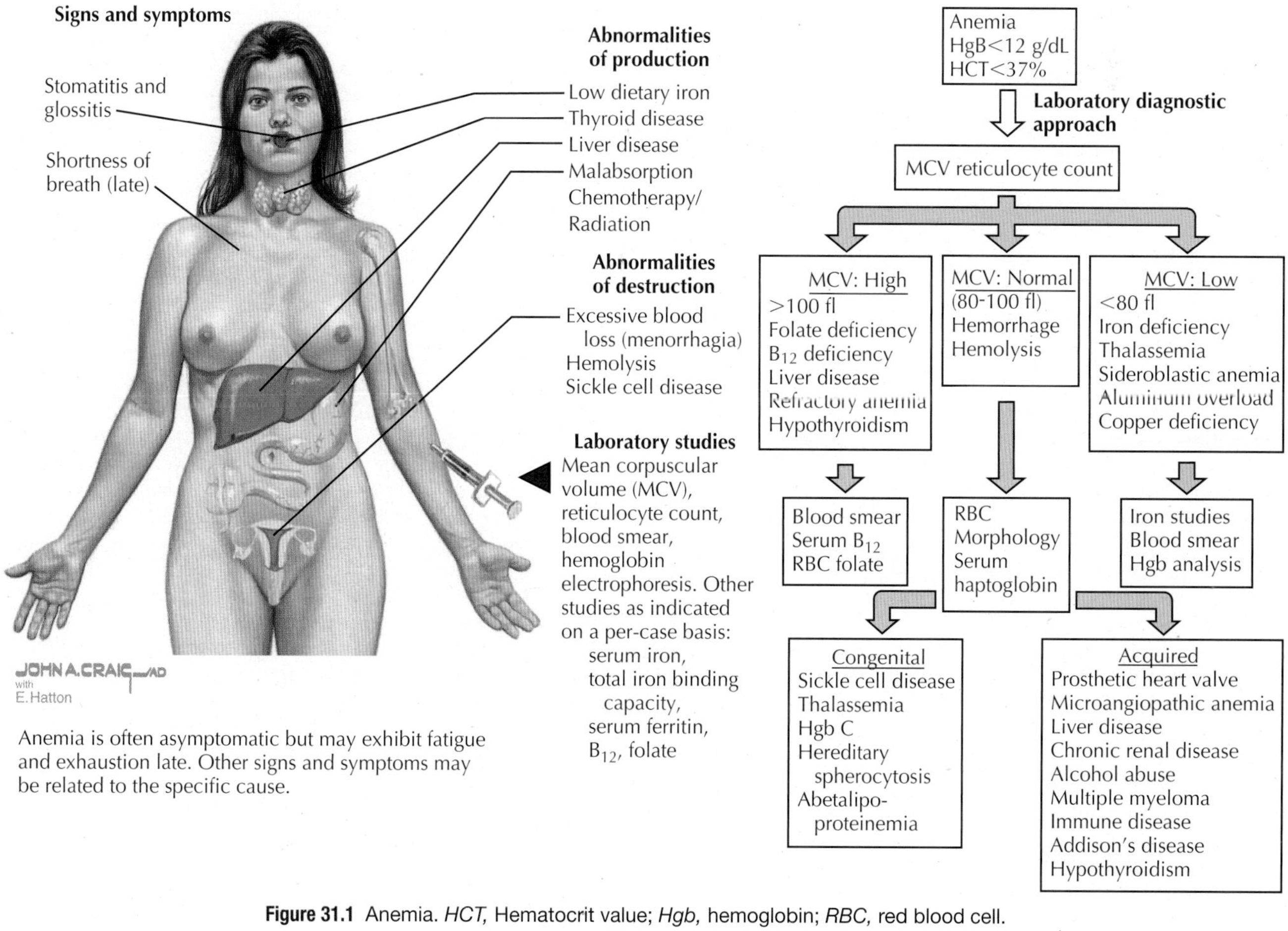
Signs and symptoms
Stomatitis and glossitis
Shortness of breath (late)
Abnormalities of production
Low dietary iron
Thyroid disease
Liver disease
Malabsorption
Chemotherapy/Radiation
Abnormalities of destruction
Excessive blood loss (menorrhagia)
Hemolysis
Sickle cell disease
Laboratory studies
Mean corpuscular volume (MCV), reticulocyte count, blood smear, hemoglobin electrophoresis. Other studies as indicated on a per-case basis: serum iron, total iron binding capacity, serum ferritin, B12, folate
JOHN A.CRAIG_AD
with E.Hatton
Anemia is often asymptomatic but may exhibit fatigue and exhaustion late. Other signs and symptoms may be related to the specific cause.
Anemia
HgB<12 g/dL
HCT<37%
Laboratory diagnostic approach
MCV reticulocyte count
MCV: High
>100 fl
Folate deficiency
B12 deficiency
Liver disease
Refractory anemia
Hypothyroidism
MCV: Normal
(80-100 fl)
Hemorrhage
Hemolysis
MCV: Low
<80 fl
Iron deficiency
Thalassemia
Sideroblastic anemia
Aluminum overload
Copper deficiency
Blood smear
Serum B12
RBC folate
RBC
Morphology
Serum
haptoglobin
Iron studies
Blood smear
Hgb analysis
Congenital
Sickle cell disease
Thalassemia
Hgb C
Hereditary spherocytosis
Abetalipoproteinemia
Acquired
Prosthetic heart valve
Microangiopathic anemia
Liver disease
Chronic renal disease
Alcohol abuse
Multiple myeloma
Immune disease
Addison's disease
Hypothyroidism

Figure 31.1 Anemia. *HCT,* Hematocrit value; *Hgb,* hemoglobin; *RBC,* red blood cell.

upregulates absorptive pathways to increase iron bioavailability. Recommended dietary iron intake is around 14 mg/day.

Supplementation: For those who require it, 40–80 mg of elemental iron is recommended once daily. Consider every-other-day dosing, addition of vitamin C, and the avoidance of coffee and calcium at the time of dosing to aid in absorption. In more extreme or refractory cases, IV iron can be considered. The major side effect is GI symptoms, which occur in up to 70% of people. It may be reasonable to discontinue supplementation once iron stores have normalized; however, if the athlete's cause of iron deficiency is chronic, continued supplementation may be considered. Universal iron supplementation, although often performed, is not recommended.

Dilutional Anemia

Description: Dilutional anemia (aka sports anemia or pseudoanemia) is the phenomenon where conditioned athletes have an increase in their overall plasma volume, which causes an apparent drop in hemoglobin. This is not a true anemia.

Epidemiology: Most common cause of mild hemoglobin drop in the athletic population.

Pathophysiology: Dilutional anemia is an adaptive response in well-trained athletes. During exercise, the plasma volume generally drops. Within 3–5 hours after exercise, plasma volumes return to baseline before volume expansion occurs secondary to increases in regulating factors. This mechanism leads to less viscous blood, which is thought to improve oxygen delivery by improving stroke volume and thus cardiac output.

Clinical presentation: This is an asymptomatic finding.

Laboratory tests: Mild anemia with a hemoglobin drop of up to 1 g/dL in men and 0.5 g/dL in women, which normalizes within 3–5 days of discontinuing exercise.

Treatment: None required.

Exercise-Induced Hemolysis

Description: Exercise-induced hemolysis refers to intravascular destruction of RBCs secondary to consequences of exercise. It was previously referred to as *foot strike hemolysis*, but it has become clear there must be other mechanisms of hemolysis given its presence in swimmers and cyclists.

Pathophysiology: The three main pathways are foot strike hemolysis, increased muscle contractility, and vasoconstriction of internal organs as blood is shunted to working skeletal muscles. Once hemolysis occurs by one of these pathways, Hgb is released into the intravascular space. Haptoglobin, an intravascular protein, then binds to free Hgb. Once haptoglobin becomes saturated, the excess Hgb spills into the urine, producing hemoglobinuria.

Clinical presentation: Most often with the discovery of hemoglobinuria.

Laboratory testing: Urinalysis will reveal hemoglobinuria that should resolve within 3–5 days of exercise cessation. Haptoglobin levels will be decreased. Hemolysis is not typically severe enough to cause anemia, but macrocytosis and increased reticulocyte count are possible.

Treatment: If the etiology of hemoglobinuria is uncertain, 3–5 days of rest followed by repeat urinalysis is reasonable. For runners, consider alterations in gait, running shoes, running surfaces, and the training regimen.

Return to play: The athlete may continue to participate.

CLOTTING DISORDERS

Venous Thromboembolism

Description: Venous thromboembolism (VTE) includes both deep vein thrombosis (DVT) and pulmonary embolism (PE). Relevant factors regarding VTE in the athlete include both unique risk factors for clotting and return-to-play decisions.

Epidemiology: VTE may affect up to 1 in 1000 athletes, which is similar to the general population.

Pathophysiology and risk factors: Although there are several risk factors that are unique to athletes, it is important to remain aware of inherited hypercoagulable states. Common inherited hypercoagulable states in the United States include factor V Leiden and prothrombin gene mutation. Protein C deficiency, protein S deficiency, and antithrombin deficiency are also important, as they are less prevalent but carry a higher probability of developing thrombosis. The Virchow triad of venous stasis, endothelial injury, and hypercoagulability contributes to VTE. Athletes are at risk of venous stasis because of bradycardia, lower blood pressure, and overdevelopment of major musculature, as well as during long-distance travel and immobilization after injury. Hypercoagulability risk factors include exercise, dehydration, hemoconcentration after exercise, altitude changes, hypoxia, some performance-enhancing drugs, and oral contraceptives. Endothelial injury may be caused by repetitive microtrauma of long and vigorous exercise.

Clinical presentation: DVT presentation includes unilateral extremity pain, swelling, and erythema. When subtle, symptoms can be similar to muscular injury. A PE may present with any combination of chest pain, shortness of breath, palpitations, tachycardia, or hypoxia.

Evaluation: Venous duplex ultrasound is recommended for evaluation of DVT, and computed tomography (CT) angiogram is recommended for PE. Consider genetic testing depending on occurrence and severity of disease.

Treatment: Depends on location. Peripheral lower extremity DVTs may not require anticoagulation if asymptomatic or may require a shorter duration of anticoagulation (6–12 weeks). Upper extremity DVTs may have better outcomes with catheter-directed thrombolysis in addition to anticoagulation. Surgical treatment is also discussed in refractory cases of upper extremity DVTs. Proximal DVTs and PEs require uninterrupted anticoagulation for at least 3 months if the VTE was provoked, followed by intermittent prophylaxis for periods of long travel or immobilization. If the VTE is unprovoked, treatment should continue for 6 months. There are several possible treatment strategies; however, a direct oral anticoagulant (DOAC) is preferred, particularly rivaroxaban or apixaban. Consider compression stockings with lower extremity DVTs to decrease postthrombotic syndrome.

Return to play: With appropriate counseling and initiation of treatment, an athlete may begin noncontact exercise at 2–3 weeks after initiation of treatment and once symptomatically improved. The decision of when to return to contact or collision sports is controversial. Traditionally, an athlete may return to contact sports after completion of anticoagulation and normalization of blood work. For contact sport athletes that require an anticoagulation period of greater than 3 months, there is a suggested protocol for interrupted dosing after the mandatory and uninterrupted 3-month period. The basis of this protocol allows the plasma drug levels to decrease to a level that the risk of bleeding is minimal during competition. After competition is complete, a dose is given to promptly restart therapeutic anticoagulation. The same concept may be used for athletes who require indefinite anticoagulation. This individualized approach is only considered for elite athletes with substantial resources and under the direction of a specialist, given the risk and monitoring involved.

Effort-Induced Thrombosis

Description: Effort-induced thrombosis is also known as *Paget-Schroetter syndrome.* It represents a subset of venous thoracic outlet syndrome (vTOS). This is most commonly seen in the dominant arm of athletes involved in strenuous upper extremity activities.

Epidemiology: vTOS occurs in about 2 per 100,000 people per year with 10%–20% composed of those with exercise-induced thrombosis. Typically presents in adults 18–30 years of age.

Pathophysiology: Thrombus origin is secondary to repetitive subclavian vein (SCV) compression in the supraclavicular space, which is bordered by the clavicle, anterior scalene, and first rib. Repetitive compression leads to venous scarring, venous stenosis, and turbulent blood flow, which leads to thrombosis.

Clinical presentation: Athletes typically present with sudden swelling, pain, heaviness, and cyanosis of the affected arm. There may also be swelling of collateral veins. This full clinical picture may not be apparent until complete venous occlusion occurs.

Testing: Ultrasonography is the initial test of choice. If clinical suspicion continues, a catheter-based upper extremity venography will provide a definitive answer.

Treatment: In the young, athletic population, pharmacomechanical thrombolysis provides the most rapid results. A slower, catheter-directed infusion of a thrombolytic agent may also be considered. Once the thrombosed veins are patent, anticoagulation is often initiated to prevent recurrent thrombosis. Additionally, surgical treatment aimed at thoracic outlet decompression and management of SCV stenosis is often required in order to prevent repeat episodes.

Return to play: There is no universal answer. Consider return to play in 12 weeks after definitive treatment, assuming that the course of recommended anticoagulation is complete and blood work has normalized.

BLEEDING DISORDERS

Hemophilias

Description: Hemophilia A and hemophilia B are some of the most common bleeding disorders and pose a very real bleeding risk to the normal population and even more so to athletes. Although exercise and athletic participation are beneficial to an individual's overall health, the main risk to participation is of excessive and dangerous bleeding after an injury.

Epidemiology: The hemophilias are sex linked; thus, the majority of cases occur in men. Hemophilia A is by far the most common, occurring in 1 in 5000 men. Hemophilia B occurs in 1 in 20,000 men.

Pathophysiology: Hemophilias occur because of an X-linked gene that results in a deficiency of clotting factors. Disease severity corresponds to factor deficiency severity. Those with mild disease have excessive bleeding risks only after significant trauma or surgery. Those with more severe disease typically have more significant bleeding problems, including into muscles and joints. In addition to the general benefits of exercise, individuals who participate in regular physical activity have more circulating factor than those who are more sedentary.

Risk with sports participation: Decisions regarding sports participation should begin at a very early age so that all parties have a clear understanding of the potential risks involved. The National Hemophilia Foundation (NHF) has categorized different activities based on their risk for injury. These discussions should include the expertise of a hematologist.

Treatment: All athletes who have hemophilia should be comanaged by a hematologist and sports medicine physician. If indicated, the athlete may require dosing of his or her factor before competition. All parties should be educated on early signs of bleeding so that prompt evaluation may occur.

Von Willebrand Disease

Description: Von Willebrand disease (vWD) affects the clotting mechanism by decreasing the amount of Von Willebrand factor (vWF). Most commonly, the disease is split into three categories ranging from mild to severe symptoms that correspond to the amount of normal vWF present. Although much more common than hemophilia, the clinical presentation is often milder with vWD, thus posing less of a risk with sports participation.

Epidemiology: Most common inherited disorder of bleeding; roughly 1.0% of the population is affected.

Clinical presentation: Varying levels of mucosal bleeding is the typical presentation of vWD. Menorrhagia, epistaxis, and easy bruising may be seen in mild to moderate cases. Severe cases of vWD are often diagnosed in infancy because of more significant mucosal bleeding.

Diagnosis: Made after a careful history, including family history and physical. There are specific blood tests that evaluate the activity of vWF.

Sports participation: Similar to hemophilia; the higher the injury risk, the higher the risk for mucosal bleeding.

Treatment: Athletes with vWD must be comanaged with a hematologist. Treatment options include desmopressin (increases release of vWF), vWF, and agents that stabilize clots after acute injuries. The treatment of choice depends on the severity and nature of vWD.

Idiopathic Thrombocytopenic Purpura

Description: Idiopathic thrombocytopenic purpura (ITP) is an autoimmune disease affecting platelets. A significantly decreased number of platelets can lead to excessive bleeding after injury or trauma.

Epidemiology: The prevalence of ITP in the United States is about 9.5 in 100,000 adults and 5.3 in 100,000 children. Athletes with ITP should be comanaged with a hematologist.

Sports participation: Although there is no consensus regarding sports participation with ITP, it is commonly accepted that participation is restricted when platelet levels fall below 50,000.

RECOMMENDED READINGS

Available online.

32 RENAL AND GENITOURINARY PROBLEMS

Jack Spittler • Kartik Sidhar

ANATOMY

Genitourinary system: Composed of internal and external organs of the urinary system and genital/reproductive system. Both systems are contained in the abdomen and pelvic region.

Urinary system: Composed of kidneys, ureters, bladder, and urethra

Reproductive system: Male (penis, testicles), female (ovaries, Fallopian tubes, uterus, vagina, vulva)

Female genitourinary system: Situated within the pelvis, except for the vulva, which is external (Fig. 32.1)

Male genitourinary system: Prostate and internal portion of male urethra located within the pelvis. Penis, scrotum, and testes are located externally and are most vulnerable in men (see Fig. 32.1).

Kidneys: Located in the retroperitoneal region from T12 through L3 vertebral level (Fig. 32.2). The right kidney lies slightly lower than the left because of the liver. The kidneys are contained in a cushion of pericapsular fat and protected by the posterior abdominal wall musculature (erector spinae muscles, latissimus dorsi).

Ureters: Run along the posterior peritoneal wall from the kidneys to bladder. Also protected by the muscles of posterior abdominal wall. Most vulnerable where they cross the brim of the pelvis.

Bladder: When empty, lies completely within the pelvis and protected anteriorly by the pubic rami. Therefore, it is most vulnerable to trauma when full.

PHYSIOLOGY

- The major function of the kidneys is to keep the composition of the blood stable via regulation of fluid and electrolytes
- Renal blood flow at rest is approximately 1100 mL per minute and is approximately 20% of cardiac output
  - Oxygen consumption of kidneys at rest is 26 mL per minute and is approximately 10% of resting metabolism
  - Daily urine volume may vary from 500 mL to 15 L
- Volume of urine determined primarily by antidiuretic hormone (ADH)
  - ADH regulates water reabsorption by increasing permeability of distal tubule of the nephron and collecting duct
  - ADH is released from posterior pituitary in response to signals from hypothalamus
  - The main stimuli for release of ADH:
    - Increased plasma osmolality
    - Decreased blood volume
    - Decreased blood pressure
  - ADH release may increase threefold in heavy exercise, helping to prevent free water loss and dehydration
- At rest, 15%–20% of renal plasma flow is continuously filtered by glomeruli
  - Results in about 170 L of filtrate per day
  - Ninety-nine percent is reabsorbed in tubular system
- Exercise results in a reduction of renal blood flow proportional to the intensity of the activity due to shunting of blood to exercising muscle
  - Mechanism is via constriction of afferent and efferent arterioles because of increased circulating levels of epinephrine and norepinephrine
  - Moderate exercise (50% $\dot{V}O_2$ max) results in a 30% reduction; strenuous exercise leads to a 40%–50% decrease in both renal blood flow and glomerular filtration rate (GFR)
  - During maximal exercise (65% $\dot{V}O_2$ max), there is a 75% reduction in renal blood flow, which is approximately 1% of the cardiac exercise output
  - Renal blood flow decreases even more if the individual is dehydrated
  - Renal blood flow usually returns to pre-exercise levels within 60 minutes

HEMATURIA

- Can be gross or microscopic (Fig. 32.3)
- Microscopic hematuria generally defined as more than three red blood cells (RBCs) per high-power field
- In athletes, rates of microscopic hematuria can be as high as 75%–80% and often asymptomatic; can occur in both contact and noncontact sports
- Although hematuria typically resolves within 48–72 hours, in ultraendurance athletes resolution may take up to 7 days

Etiology

Overview: Etiologic factors can be categorized by location (kidney vs. bladder).

Nontraumatic renal: Decreased renal blood flow (700 mL per minute to 200 mL per minute, with decrease proportional to intensity) leads to ischemia in the nephron, increased permeability, and subsequent passage of RBCs. Also increased glomerular filtration pressure, secondary to efferent vasoconstriction, leads to passage of RBCs at the glomerulus. Clots are usually not renal in etiology; dysmorphic cells are suggestive of renal source.

Traumatic renal: Direct contact (helmet, ski pole, balance beam, etc.) vs. indirect trauma ("jarring" during running, jumping, etc.).

Bladder: Sports hematuria of bladder origin is almost always traumatic. This can be the result of single, large blunt trauma or multiple lesser forces. Repetitive contact of flaccid posterior bladder wall against anterior wall (trigone) is known as "bladder slap." It can occur in athletes participating in intense physical activity such as long-distance running, track, swimming, lacrosse, and football. Cystoscopy shows damage of the superficial urothelium or contusion. Incidence can be decreased if bladder is partially filled and adequate hydration maintained.

Prostate/urethra: Usually traumatic, most often seen in cyclists because of repetitive jarring. May be the result of improper seat height and pitch.

Other causes of hematuria:
- Nephrolithiasis
- Urinary tract infection
- Sickle cell anemia or other blood disorder
- Malignancy
- Drug or medication use (including penicillin, cephalexin, thiazides, allopurinol, nonsteroidal anti-inflammatory drugs [NSAIDs], aspirin, furosemide, and oral contraceptives)
- "Foot strike hemolysis": possible phenomenon where trauma occurs to RBCs circulating in the feet during running, leading to hemolysis. As a result, haptoglobin binds free hemoglobin, and if haptoglobin binding becomes saturated, then hemoglobin is excreted in urine.
- Rhabdomyolysis (hematuria on urinalysis [UA] with absent RBCs on microscopy).
- Red-colored (without hematuria or RBCs on microscopy) urine attributed to beets, berries, food coloring, phenazopyridine, phenytoin, ibuprofen, nitrofurantoin, sulfamethoxazole, and rifampin.

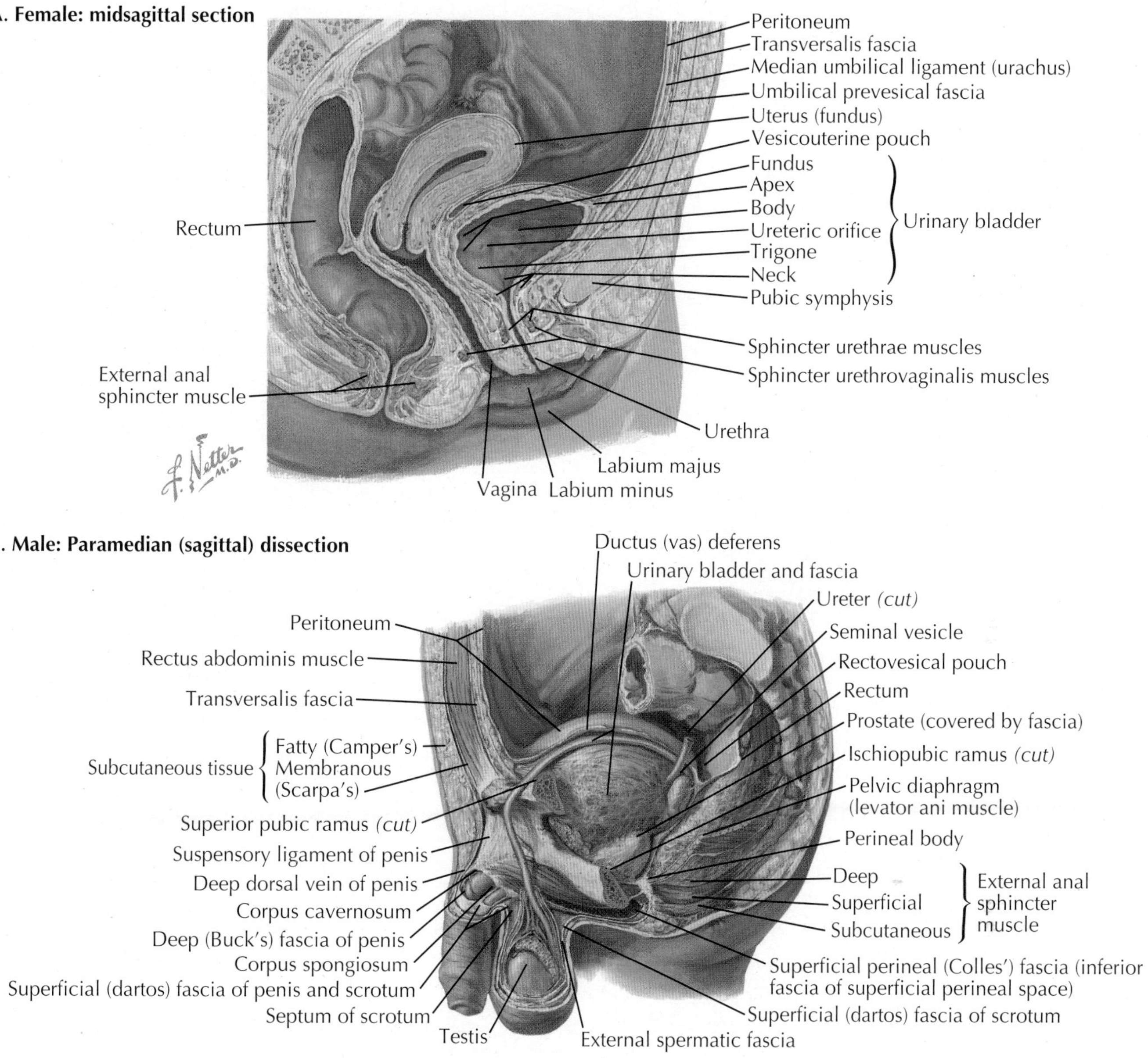
A. Female: midsagittal section
Peritoneum
Transversalis fascia
Median umbilical ligament (urachus)
Umbilical prevesical fascia
Uterus (fundus)
Vesicouterine pouch
Fundus
Apex
Body
Ureteric orifice
Trigone
Neck
Urinary bladder
Pubic symphysis
Rectum
Sphincter urethrae muscles
Sphincter urethrovaginalis muscles
External anal sphincter muscle
Urethra
Labium majus
Vagina
Labium minus
F. Netter M.D.
B. Male: Paramedian (sagittal) dissection
Ductus (vas) deferens
Urinary bladder and fascia
Ureter (cut)
Seminal vesicle
Rectovesical pouch
Rectum
Prostate (covered by fascia)
Ischiopubic ramus (cut)
Pelvic diaphragm (levator ani muscle)
Perineal body
Peritoneum
Rectus abdominis muscle
Transversalis fascia
Subcutaneous tissue
Fatty (Camper's)
Membranous (Scarpa's)
Superior pubic ramus (cut)
Suspensory ligament of penis
Deep dorsal vein of penis
Corpus cavernosum
Deep (Buck's) fascia of penis
Corpus spongiosum
Superficial (dartos) fascia of penis and scrotum
Septum of scrotum
Testis
External spermatic fascia
Deep
Superficial
Subcutaneous
External anal sphincter muscle
Superficial perineal (Colles') fascia (inferior fascia of superficial perineal space)
Superficial (dartos) fascia of scrotum

Figure 32.1 Genitourinary system.

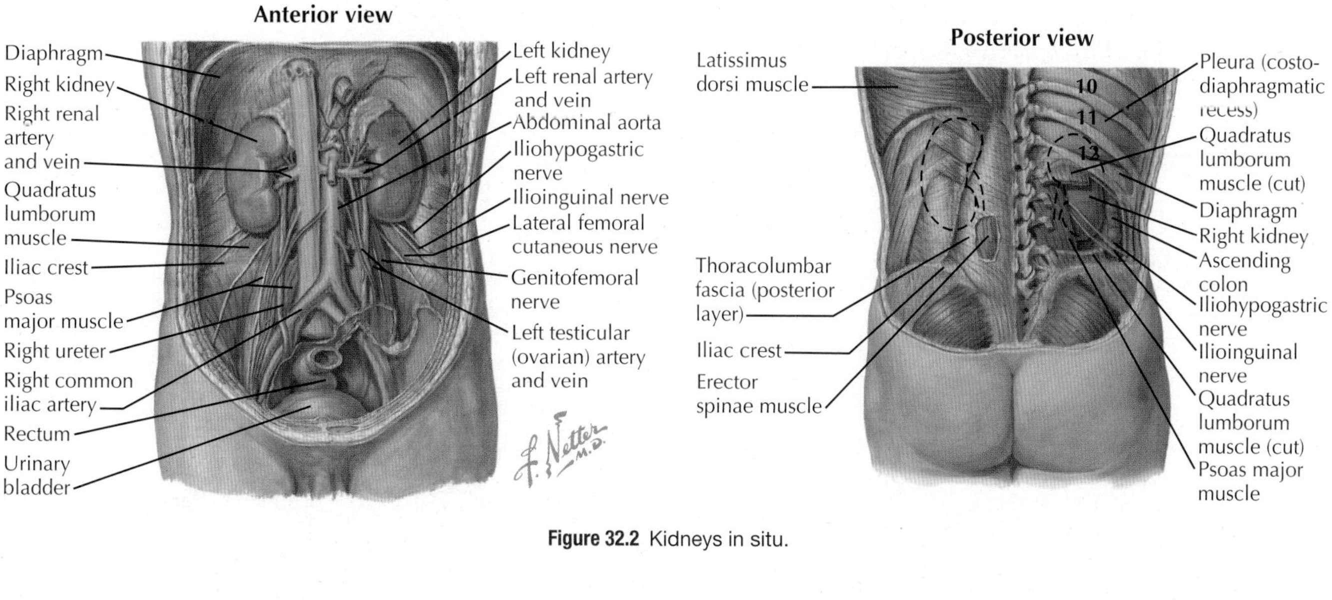
Anterior view
Diaphragm
Right kidney
Right renal artery and vein
Quadratus lumborum muscle
Iliac crest
Psoas major muscle
Right ureter
Right common iliac artery
Rectum
Urinary bladder
Left kidney
Left renal artery and vein
Abdominal aorta
Iliohypogastric nerve
Ilioinguinal nerve
Lateral femoral cutaneous nerve
Genitofemoral nerve
Left testicular (ovarian) artery and vein
F. Netter M.D.
Posterior view
Latissimus dorsi muscle
Thoracolumbar fascia (posterior layer)
Iliac crest
Erector spinae muscle
10
11
12
Pleura (costo-diaphragmatic recess)
Quadratus lumborum muscle (cut)
Diaphragm
Right kidney
Ascending colon
Iliohypogastric nerve
Ilioinguinal nerve
Quadratus lumborum muscle (cut)
Psoas major muscle

Figure 32.2 Kidneys in situ.

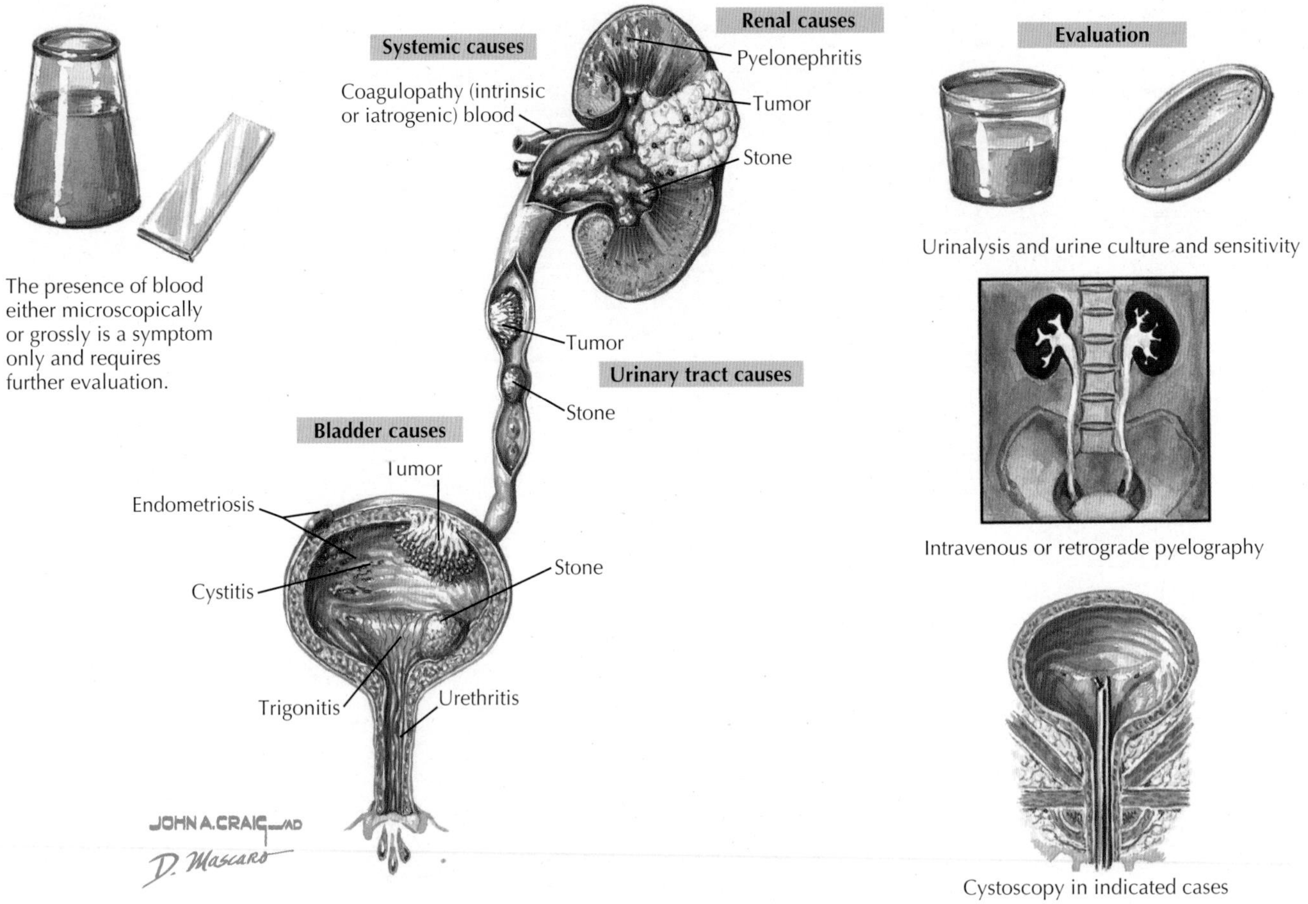

Systemic causes
Coagulopathy (intrinsic or iatrogenic) blood
Renal causes
Pyelonephritis
Tumor
Stone
Evaluation
Urinalysis and urine culture and sensitivity
The presence of blood either microscopically or grossly is a symptom only and requires further evaluation.
Tumor
Urinary tract causes
Stone
Bladder causes
Tumor
Endometriosis
Cystitis
Stone
Trigonitis
Urethritis
Intravenous or retrograde pyelography
Cystoscopy in indicated cases
JOHN A.CRAIG_AD
D. Mascaro

Figure 32.3 Hematuria.

Diagnostic Considerations

- Diagnosis made by urine dipstick and confirmed with microscopy
- Timing of hematuria during urination is important to consider:
  - Initial hematuria (beginning of urination) often urethral in origin
  - Terminal hematuria (end of urination) may originate in bladder or prostate (men)
  - Continuous hematuria suggests renal origin
- Some have advocated using mean corpuscular volume (MCV) and RBC morphology to help establish the origin of hematuria:
  - MCV less than 72 fL considered to be of glomerular origin
  - MCV more than 72 fL considered to be of nonglomerular origin
  - Casts or dysmorphic appearance of cells consistent with glomerular origin

Treatment

- If no concerning history, physical examination, or diagnosis, stop exercise and/or suspected medications and repeat UA after 24–72 hours.
  - If urine clears after 24–72 hours and the patient is under 40 years old, can diagnose exercise-induced hematuria (benign)
  - If gross or microscopic hematuria persists or patient is over 40 years old, consider further workup:
    - Urine: culture, cytology
    - Blood: creatinine, prothrombin time/partial thromboplastin time (PT/PTT), blood urea nitrogen (BUN), complete blood count (CBC), sickle cell (in high-risk populations)
    - Imaging: renal ultrasound, computed tomography (CT) urography, and/or direct visualization with cystoscopy
- If testing remains normal and hematuria persists, must consider intrinsic renal disease:
  - Creatinine clearance and protein excretion should be measured
  - Renal ultrasound, retrograde pyelography, and CT scan may be useful
  - Indications for renal angiography and renal biopsy are controversial

Return to Play

- Athletes with benign hematuria secondary to exercise may return to activity once hematuria resolves
- Return to play for other causes of hematuria is diagnosis-dependent

Prevention

- Athletes, especially those with prior episodes of hematuria, should be encouraged to drink fluids before and during exercise to avoid dehydration
- Keeping a slightly distended bladder during exercise can help prevent "bladder slap"

PROTEINURIA

- May be present in up to 70% of athletes after exertion and usually asymptomatic

- Exercise-induced proteinuria is a function of the intensity of exercise
  - Strenuous exercise can cause protein excretion to reach 1.5 mg/min, but usually does not rise beyond 1–2 g/day (normal: 150–200 mg/day)
  - Usually occurs within 30 minutes of exercise and clears in 24–48 hours

Etiology

- Root cause unknown, but renin–angiotensin system (RAS) and prostaglandins play a major role:
  - Plasma concentration of angiotensin II increases during exercise, resulting in increased protein filtration through the glomerular membrane
  - Strenuous exercise also activates the sympathetic nervous system, which releases catecholamines, also increasing glomerular membrane permeability
- Creatine supplements do not increase proteinuria
- In patients with underlying chronic kidney disease (CKD), low-intensity exercise does not increase proteinuria or lead to rapid progression of CKD

Diagnostic Considerations

- Urine dipstick is generally a good tool for initial evaluation
  - Screening for proteinuria at sports preparticipation examinations is not recommended, as the diagnostic utility is low
  - If a routine UA shows protein and was collected within 24 hours of intense exercise, repeat testing in absence of prior exercise to determine transient vs. persistent proteinuria
- Other causes for false-positive proteinuria on UA:
  - Highly concentrated urine (specific gravity >1.030)
  - Contamination with antiseptics
  - Pyridium (phenazopyridine HCl) use
    - Highly alkaline urine (pH >8)
- Thorough history should be taken, including personal and family history of:
  - Renal disease
  - Anemia
  - Hypertension—make sure to get accurate, manual blood pressure reading
  - Diabetes
  - Medication use (e.g., NSAIDs, antibiotics)
- Further workup may include:
  - Serum tests for renal function (BUN, creatinine)
  - Twenty-four-hour urine for total protein, creatinine, and creatinine clearance
  - Fasting blood glucose or hemoglobin A1c
  - CBC or other tests as medically indicated
    - Imaging: renal ultrasound, CT
    - Renal biopsy

Treatment

- If proteinuria is transient and exercise-induced, no treatment is indicated
- If proteinuria is persistent and medically related, treatment depends on underlying cause

Return to Play

- If proteinuria clears within 24–72 hours, OK for return to play
- If proteinuria persists, further workup is needed before clearance

Prevention

- As exercise-induced proteinuria is likely a normal physiologic process during exercise, there are no known prevention strategies

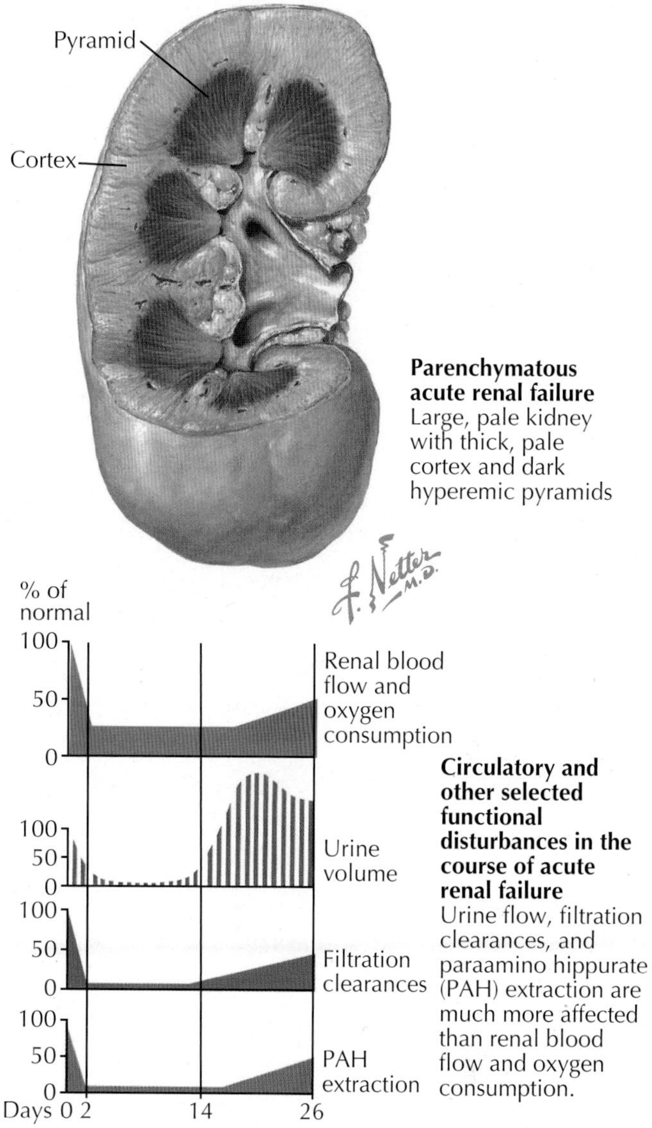
Pyramid
Cortex
Parenchymatous acute renal failure
Large, pale kidney with thick, pale cortex and dark hyperemic pyramids
F. Netter M.D.
% of normal
100
50
0
Renal blood flow and oxygen consumption
Circulatory and other selected functional disturbances in the course of acute renal failure
Urine flow, filtration clearances, and paraamino hippurate (PAH) extraction are much more affected than renal blood flow and oxygen consumption.
Urine volume
Filtration clearances
PAH extraction
Days 0 2 14 26

Figure 32.4 Acute renal failure.

- Exercise-induced proteinuria does not decrease with regular physical training, even in high-level athletes
- Adequate hydration with exercise can help avoid overly concentrated urine and subsequent false-positive proteinuria on urinalysis

ACUTE KIDNEY INJURY

- Acute kidney injury (AKI) is uncommon in sports, but occurrence is well documented
- Criteria for meeting AKI is becoming more prevalent in athletes with rise of ultraendurance events

Etiology

- Combined effects of exercise to exhaustion, dehydration, hyperpyrexia, and rhabdomyolysis culminate in renal dysfunction by release of muscle enzymes and myoglobin that precipitates in renal tubules (Fig. 32.4)
  - Over 25% of participants in ultraendurance races have evidence of AKI (at least 1.5–2× normal creatinine)
- Underlying renal disease, dehydration, heat stress, genetic predisposition (i.e., sickle cell trait), and NSAID use are risk factors

Diagnostic Considerations

- AKI defined as an increase in serum creatinine by ≥0.3 mg/dL or an increase to ≥1.5 times the baseline value
- Creatine kinase (CK) levels correlate well with myoglobin concentrations in the blood and can be associated with AKI in rhabdomyolysis
- Although CK levels of 20,000 IU per liter is the typical threshold for treatment and hospitalization, levels over 100,000 have been reported in asymptomatic individuals during and after exercise
- AKI with rhabdomyolysis may also be associated with:
  - Disseminated intravascular coagulation (DIC)
  - Hyponatremia, hyperkalemia, hyperphosphatemia, hyperuricemia
  - Hypocalcemia—caused by precipitation of calcium phosphate in muscle from hyperphosphatemia

Treatment

- An athlete with AKI should be treated according to standard treatment guidelines—crystalloid solution, electrolyte replacement, etc.
- Hypertonic saline should be used in the case of acute neurologic deterioration with concurrent exercise-associated hyponatremia

Return to Play

- Serum creatinine, CK, and electrolyte levels should return to baseline before return to play initiated
- There is only theoretical risk, but no proven evidence, that repetitive AKI in athletes leads to development of CKD

Prevention

- Prevention is primarily related to proper hydration before and during exercise
- Adequate training, heat acclimatization, and avoidance of NSAIDs may help as well

MEDICATION SIDE EFFECTS

NSAIDs

- NSAIDs may have deleterious effects because of their ability to inhibit cyclooxygenase within the kidney (Fig. 32.5)
- Cyclooxygenase is the rate-limiting enzyme for synthesis of prostaglandins (PGs)
- Vasodilatory PGE_2 and PGI_2 play a protective role in the kidney by modulating renal vasoconstriction caused by:
  - Increased renal sympathetic activity
  - Renin-angiotensin II
  - Circulating catecholamines
- Under stress conditions (salt restriction, dehydration, and heat), ibuprofen decreases GFR after 45 minutes of exercise at 65% $\dot{V}O_2$ max, compared with placebo or acetaminophen
- Both indomethacin and celecoxib showed decreases in free water clearance, which in certain environments or conditions can predispose to hyponatremia

Creatine

- Creatine monohydrate is widely used as an ergogenic aid for muscle performance
- Increases muscle stores of creatine, leading to greater adenosine triphosphate (ATP) synthesis
- In healthy individuals, there is no known link between creatine ingestion and renal dysfunction if used over the short term in typical doses (loading dose 20 g/day × 5 days and then 3–5 g/day maintenance dose)
- There have been case reports of acute renal failure in individuals who were long-term, high-dose users
- Those with established renal disease should avoid supplementation
- End product of creatine is creatinine, which is filtered in the glomeruli and excreted; this can be a false indicator of renal dysfunction
- In those using creatine, renal function can be evaluating by measuring, under resting conditions, the albumin excretion rate (normal: <20 mcg/min)

STRESS INCONTINENCE

- Defined as involuntary loss of urine during physical exertion
- Women twice as likely to be affected as men
- Twenty-eight percent to 47% of regularly exercising women report some degree of incontinence
- Stress incontinence also occurs in premenopausal women and can limit involvement in practice and sports
- Important to screen for stress incontinence, as this can be a barrier to exercise

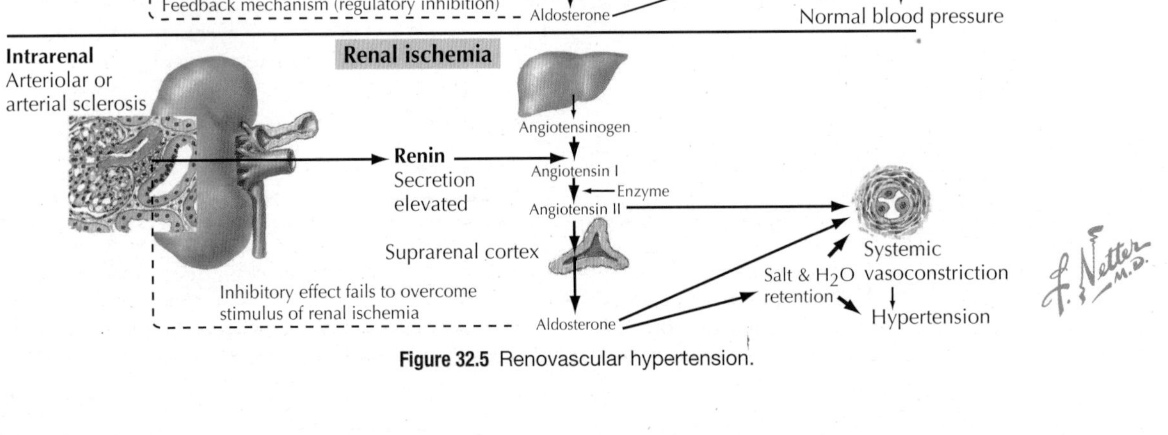
Normal
JG apparatus
Renin
Angiotensinogen
Angiotensin I
Enzyme
Angiotensin II
Suprarenal cortex
Normal vascular tone
Normal blood pressure
Feedback mechanism (regulatory inhibition)
Aldosterone
Intrarenal
Arteriolar or arterial sclerosis
Renal ischemia
Angiotensinogen
Renin
Secretion elevated
Angiotensin I
Enzyme
Angiotensin II
Suprarenal cortex
Systemic vasoconstriction
Salt & H_2O retention
Hypertension
Inhibitory effect fails to overcome stimulus of renal ischemia
Aldosterone
F. Netter M.D.

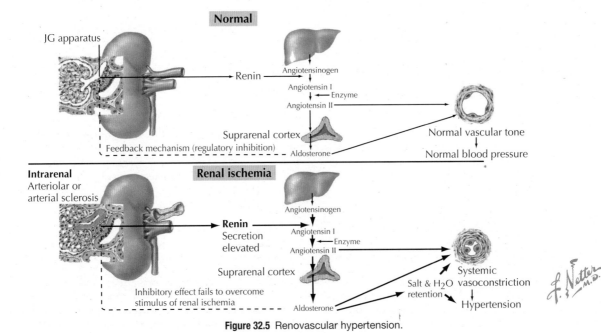

Figure 32.5 Renovascular hypertension.

Etiology

- Bladder outlet incompetence
- Urethral sphincters:
  - Internal sphincter composed of smooth muscle and under *involuntary* control
    - Prevents urine leakage via contraction under sympathetic stimulation
  - External urethral sphincter composed of skeletal muscle and under *voluntary* control
    - Prevents urine leakage via contraction under somatic nervous system stimulation
- Sports requiring jumping, running, or prolonged Valsalva maneuver may exacerbate incontinence

Diagnostic Considerations

- Usually this is a clinical diagnosis that does not require further testing
- Important to rule out urinary tract infection (UTI)
- Consider postvoid residual (PVR) bladder volume if history is suspicious for bladder outlet obstruction or overflow incontinence

Treatment

- **Behavioral:** emphasis on establishing proper pelvic muscle function:
  - Kegel exercises; other pelvic floor exercises
  - Vaginal pessary is associated with good outcomes
  - Vaginal cones (or vaginal weights)
  - Smoking cessation
  - Use of pads
  - Decrease caffeine and alcohol consumption
  - Bladder training, timed voids, and manage constipation
- **Pharmacologic:** generally not recommended because of limited efficacy and side effects
  - Topical estrogen for postmenopausal women to treat genitourinary atrophy
  - Alpha-adrenergic agents (i.e., phenylpropanolamine) can be considered to help control internal urethral sphincter
- **Surgical:** effective treatment, but should be considered only if other measures fail

INGUINAL HERNIA

- Protrusion of abdominal contents through the inguinal canal
- More likely to occur in men than women because of residual space left from descent of testicles into scrotum from abdomen

Etiology

- Caused by weakness in the abdominal wall in conjunction with elevated abdominal pressure
- Most contain only soft tissue; however, can be dangerous if contains omentum or intestines

Diagnostic Considerations

- May be symptomatic or asymptomatic
- Males often have a swollen scrotum, and females may have a bulge in the labia
- Palpable mass felt in inguinal canal, often more prominent with Valsalva maneuver
- Red flag signs for strangulated hernia: sudden pain, nausea, vomiting, bowel obstruction

Treatment

- Symptomatic hernias often require surgical treatment; can be delayed if not significantly limiting participation and hernia not strangulated
- A randomized control trial found 60%–70% of asymptomatic hernias required surgical intervention within 7–10 years because of progression of symptoms
- Emergent treatment indicated for strangulated hernia

Return to Play

- Athletes with asymptomatic inguinal hernias may participate in all sports
- If symptomatic, may return to play based on severity of symptoms

RENAL/URINARY TRACT INJURY

Renal

- Most common traumatic genitourinary injury
- Exact incidence in athletics unknown, but approximately 245,000 cases of traumatic renal injury occur worldwide/year
  - One systematic review estimated approximately 11% of renal injuries occurred from sports

Etiology

- Most cases in sports caused by a direct blow to the flank
- In athletics, these are often isolated injuries as opposed to motor vehicle accidents or falls, which often result in multiple traumatic injuries

Diagnostic Considerations/Treatment/Return to Play

- May have flank pain, costovertebral angle (CVA) tenderness, ecchymosis, and hematuria (Fig. 32.6)
- No correlation between amount of hematuria and degree of injury
- Hypovolemic shock may result from extensive bleeding, so it is important to check and monitor vital signs
- Ultrasound (US) can detect renal lacerations, but cannot definitively assess depth or extent
- US helpful in identifying patients that require more aggressive radiologic investigation
- CT abdomen with IV contrast (gold standard) or intravenous pyelogram (IVP) needed for definitive diagnosis
- Examining physician should also check for injury to other abdominal organs
- Focused assessment with sonography for trauma (FAST) is a rapid bedside ultrasound examination that can evaluate the abdominal organs and heart for bleeding:
  - Positive FAST will show a dark ("anechoic") collection of fluid
  - FAST examination is over 90% sensitive and specific

Five Classes of Renal Injury

Graded from 1 to 5 based on severity by the American Association for the Surgery of Trauma (AAST) (Fig. 32.7):

Grade 1: Contusion or subcapsular hematoma without parenchymal laceration. Majority of sports-related renal injuries. Hematuria (microscopic or gross) and flank pain may be present. Treatment usually consists of observation, rest, and repeat urinalysis. No sports until hematuria clears and no contact sports for 6 weeks.

Grade 2: Nonexpanding perirenal hematoma (confined to renal retroperitoneum) or renal or cortical laceration less than 1 cm deep without urinary extravasation. IVP shows extravasation of dye. X-ray may have loss of psoas shadow. Treatment is often observation, rest, and repeat UA. No sports until hematuria clears and no contact sports for 6 weeks.

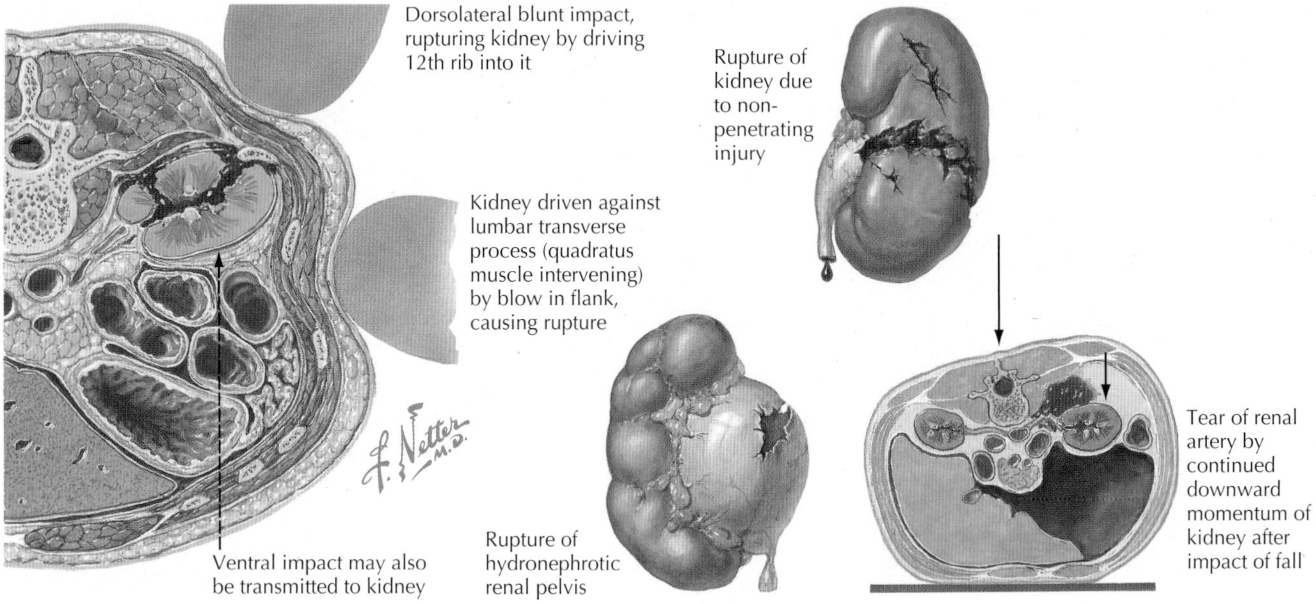
Dorsolateral blunt impact, rupturing kidney by driving 12th rib into it
Rupture of kidney due to non-penetrating injury
Kidney driven against lumbar transverse process (quadratus muscle intervening) by blow in flank, causing rupture
Tear of renal artery by continued downward momentum of kidney after impact of fall
Ventral impact may also be transmitted to kidney
Rupture of hydronephrotic renal pelvis
F. Netter M.D.

Figure 32.6 Renal trauma: Nonpenetrating trauma of kidney.

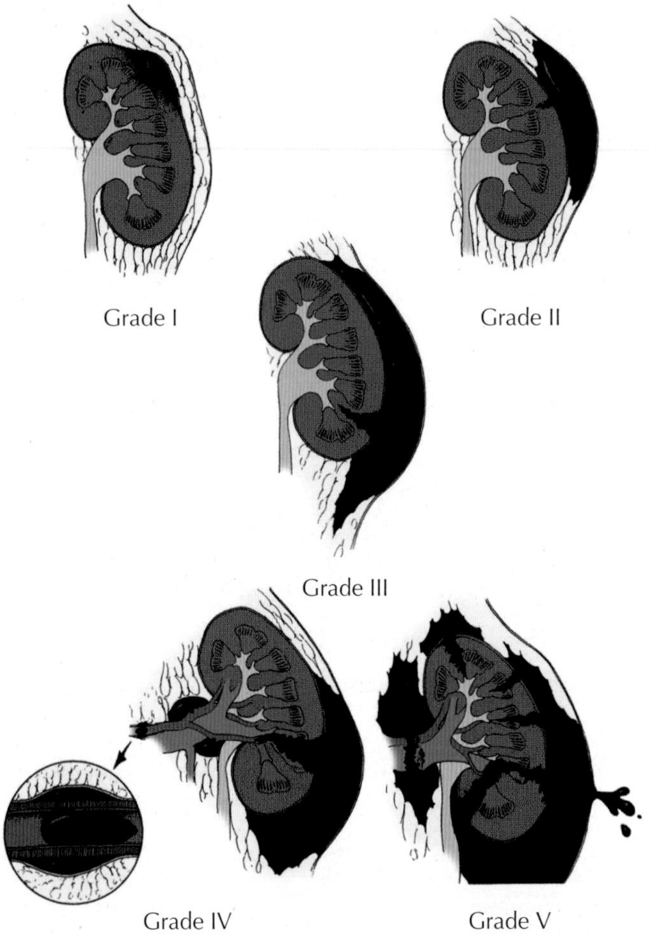
Grade I
Grade II
Grade III
Grade IV
Grade V

Figure 32.7 Classification of renal injuries by grade. Based on the organ injury scale of the American Association for the Surgery of Trauma. (Reprinted with permission from McAninch JW, Santucci RA. Genitourinary trauma. In: Walsh PC, Retik AB, Vaughan ED Jr, et al., eds. *Campbell's Urology*. 8th ed. Philadelphia: Elsevier; 2002.)

Grade 3: Parenchymal laceration deeper than 1 cm into the cortex without collecting system rupture or urinary extravasation. Imaging shows intact capsule with intrarenal extravasation and disruption of pelvicaliceal system. Angiography may be used to further delineate surgical versus nonsurgical cases. Treatment involves observation or surgery in more severe cases.

Grade 4: Major parenchymal laceration extending through the corticomedullary junction and into the collecting system (complete renal fracture), injury to main renal artery or vein with contained hemorrhage. Rare in sports. Imaging shows separation of pelvicaliceal system with intrarenal and extrarenal dye extravasation. Management is usually nonoperative, especially with advancements in angioembolization.

Grade 5: Multiple major lacerations resulting in a shattered kidney or renal pedicle injury. Will present in hypovolemic shock. Rare in sports. Kidneys usually not visualized on IVP. Selective renal arteriogram shows renal vascular damage. Treatment almost always involves surgery.

Athlete With One Kidney

- Incidence of unilateral renal agenesis is 1:500 to 1:1800, so likely that many athletes are unaware of having one kidney; most found incidentally. Nephrectomy can be another reason for an athlete to have one kidney.
- To develop participation recommendations consider age of athlete, type of sport, and motivation for participation, as well as position, size, and function of remaining kidney.
- Most physicians agree the athlete should be excluded from contact/collision sports if the remaining kidney is ectopic, is multicystic, or has any degree of obstruction or impairment of function.

Prevention

- Though not well supported by evidence, padding and other protective equipment over flanks in contact sports may be implemented to reduce risk of injury.

Ureter

- Ureteral injuries rare in sports and represent only 1% of overall genitourinary trauma

Etiology

- Usually a result of blunt trauma in sports
- Most often associated with major renal damage
- Must also consider pelvic and lumbar vertebrae fracture

Diagnostic Considerations

- No typical signs or symptoms, but hematuria is present in half of patients
- Diagnosed by CT urography (preferred) or IVP showing extravasation of contrast dye

Treatment

- Almost always requires surgery
- May involve nephrectomy if associated with severe renal injury

Return to Play

- As this injury is very rare in sports, there are no standard return-to-play guidelines

Bladder

- Significant bladder injury is rare in sports. Major bladder injury is present in less than 5%–10% of pelvic fractures.

Etiology

- Bladder injuries most often related to blunt trauma on a distended bladder
- Two types of bladder trauma are common: contusion and rupture
- Repetitive contact of flaccid posterior bladder wall against anterior wall (trigone) is known as "bladder slap"
- Can occur in athletes participating in intense physical activity such as long-distance running, track, swimming, lacrosse, and football

Diagnostic Considerations

- Most patients with significant bladder trauma will present with suprapubic tenderness and hematuria
- May also have inability to void, suprapubic bruising, and abdominal distention
- CT urography or retrograde pyelogram used for definitive diagnosis
- Contusion:
  - May have suprapubic pain and guarding
  - May pass small clots and have dysuria and hematuria
  - Degree of hematuria does not correlate well with severity of injury
- Bladder rupture:
  - Rare in sports
  - Usually associated with pelvic fracture

Treatment

- Severe contusions may require use of indwelling catheter for 7–10 days with concurrent antibiotics
- Intraperitoneal bladder ruptures usually require surgery
- Extraperitoneal bladder rupture (most common) may be managed with indwelling catheter

Return to Play

- Return to play from contusion only after symptoms and hematuria resolve
- Return to play from rupture dependent on outcomes

Prevention

- Keeping bladder partially full (but not overdistended) can help protect against bladder slap or bladder contusion/rupture

GENITAL INJURY

- More common in males compared with females because of anatomic differences with prominence of external genitalia

Male Injuries

Testicles/Scrotum

- Testicles are paired organs that are contained within the scrotum
- Significant testicular trauma can lead to subfertility and atrophic testes

ETIOLOGY

- Direct trauma to scrotum may cause testicular contusion/rupture or scrotal hematoma
- May also get testicular torsion due to twisting of spermatic cord

DIAGNOSTIC CONSIDERATIONS

- May present with testicular pain, pallor, nausea, anxiety, and syncope
- If pain persists more than 1 hour or is severe, acute-onset pain, must rule out testicular torsion or rupture
  - Cremasteric reflex usually absent with torsion
- Ultrasonography with Doppler can evaluate for intra-/extratesticular hematoma, contusion, rupture, or torsion

TREATMENT

- Ice and elevation should be used to control bleeding and swelling for scrotal hematoma or testicular contusion
- Urgent surgical intervention is needed for testicular rupture, tense hematoma, or testicular torsion

RETURN TO PLAY

- For scrotal hematoma or testicular contusion, once symptoms resolve
- Depends on surgical intervention for more severe injuries
- Participation in contact sports with one testicle (either congenital or after trauma/orchiectomy) is controversial because of risk of infertility with damage to remaining testicle

PREVENTION

- Use of an athletic protective cup in contact sports may reduce risk of injury

Penis

- Penile injuries are not common in sports

ETIOLOGY

- Trauma caused by straddle injuries or direct blow to pubis
- Mechanism could lead to partial or complete urethral rupture, although complete rupture has not been described during sports

DIAGNOSTIC CONSIDERATIONS

- May present with immediate pain, swelling, and perineal ecchymosis
- Diagnostic retrograde urethrogram may be needed to assess for significant injury
- Erect penis susceptible to fracture of tunica albuginea:
  - Area of fracture swollen and ecchymotic
  - Penis bent to affected side
- Penile frostbite described in runners wearing inadequate clothing in cold weather
- Traumatic irritation of pudendal nerve, causing penile issues, is not uncommon:
  - Especially common in bicycle racers or touring cyclists
  - May cause priapism, impotence, paresthesia, or ischemic neuropathy

TREATMENT

- Complete urethral rupture is a urologic emergency that requires repair
- Penile facture is also an emergency requiring hematoma evacuation and tunica albuginea repair

PREVENTION

- Use of an athletic protective cup in contact sports may reduce risk of penile injury
- Proper bike fit may help reduce risk of repetitive pudendal trauma in cyclists

Female Injuries

- The vulva is highly vascular, and trauma can result in hematoma formation
- May require evacuation if large, which can cause urethral outflow obstruction
- Fall while water skiing may force water into vagina, resulting in water-related vaginal injury
- Though rare, this may lead to significant vaginal laceration and bleeding

SPECIAL POPULATIONS

Athletes Who Use a Wheelchair

- Neurologic control of the urinary tract is often lost after spinal cord injury (Fig. 32.8)
- Athletes who are paraplegic or quadriplegic are at significant risk for:
  - Bladder and kidney infections
  - Kidney stones
  - Bladder distention
  - Urethral fistula
- Renal failure secondary to infection is a main cause of death in people with spinal cord injury
- Athletes who are wheelchair users have demonstrated lower incidence and frequency of urinary tract complications when compared with sedentary wheelchair users
- Can decrease risk of urinary tract complications with adequate perineal hygiene, regular bladder emptying, and appropriate use of catheters
- Autonomic dysreflexia:
  - Athletes with spinal cord injury above T6 level are at risk; autonomic dysreflexia is an uncontrolled sympathetic response from noxious stimuli below the lesion level
  - Common symptoms include headache, hypertension, flushing, diaphoresis, and bradycardia
  - Despite the danger associated with autonomic dysreflexia, some athletes attempt to induce it for a competitive advantage, referred to as "boosting"
  - An athlete may self-induce autonomic dysreflexia by overdistending the bladder, by sitting on sharp objects, or by the use of tight leg straps
  - The use of noxious stimuli results in vasoconstriction below the level of neurologic lesion, thus theoretically increasing blood flow to active muscles

Cyclists

Pudendal Neuropathy

- Prevalence of perineal and penile/labial numbness is 50%–91% in competitive cyclists

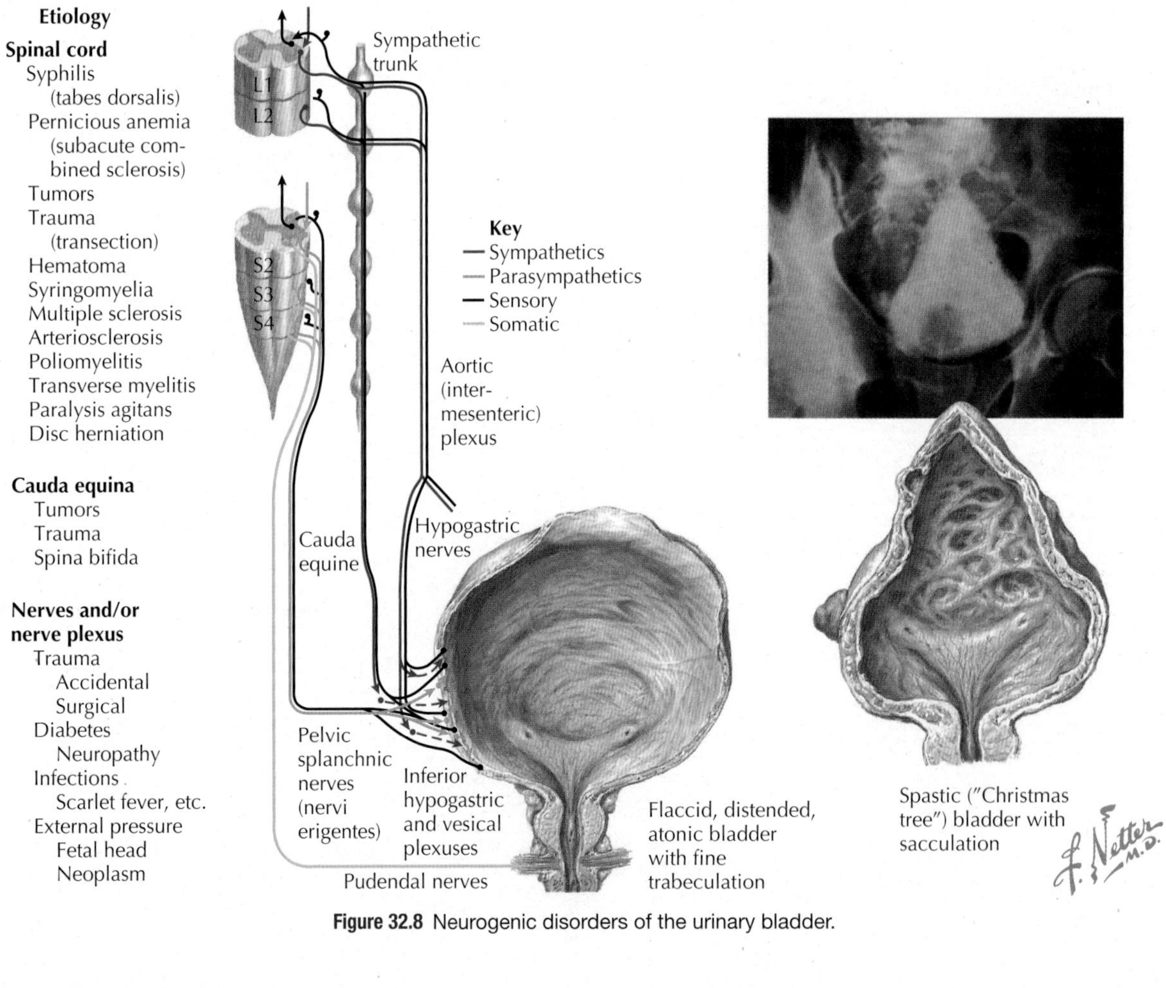
Etiology
Spinal cord
Syphilis (tabes dorsalis)
Pernicious anemia (subacute combined sclerosis)
Tumors
Trauma (transection)
Hematoma
Syringomyelia
Multiple sclerosis
Arteriosclerosis
Poliomyelitis
Transverse myelitis
Paralysis agitans
Disc herniation
Cauda equina
Tumors
Trauma
Spina bifida
Nerves and/or nerve plexus
Trauma
Accidental
Surgical
Diabetes
Neuropathy
Infections
Scarlet fever, etc.
External pressure
Fetal head
Neoplasm
L1
L2
S2
S3
S4
Sympathetic trunk
Key
Sympathetics
Parasympathetics
Sensory
Somatic
Aortic (intermesenteric) plexus
Hypogastric nerves
Cauda equine
Pelvic splanchnic nerves (nervi erigentes)
Inferior hypogastric and vesical plexuses
Pudendal nerves
Flaccid, distended, atonic bladder with fine trabeculation
Spastic ("Christmas tree") bladder with sacculation
F. Netter M.D.

Figure 32.8 Neurogenic disorders of the urinary bladder.

- Risk factors are age above 50, high body weight, increased cycling time (>10 years, >3 hours per week)
- Treatment is cessation until numbness resolves:
  - Upon return to riding, rising from saddle intermittently during rides may decrease recurrence of symptoms
  - Proper bike fit is important—appropriate seat height, seat tilt, etc.
  - Wider rear saddle in upright riders or a more narrow rear saddle in riders using the forward racing position may help

Erectile Dysfunction

- Prevalence of erectile dysfunction, either transient or chronic, in cyclist is 13%–24%
- Risk factors are similar to pudendal neuropathy, and etiology is thought to be neurovascular
- Central saddle cutouts have not proven to decrease incidence
- Consider adjustments in handlebar height and saddle position

Athletes Missing a Paired Organ

- There is not an absolute contraindication to sports for those athletes with a solitary kidney, ovary, or testicle
- The American Academy of Pediatrics Council on Sports Medicine and Fitness makes some recommendations with regard to participation for athletes with solitary organs:
  - Solitary kidney—"qualified yes"
    - Individual assessment for contact, collision, and limited-contact sports
    - Protective equipment may reduce risk of injury to remaining kidney
  - Solitary ovary—"yes"
    - Risk of severe injury to remaining ovary is minimal
  - Solitary testicle—"yes"
    - Certain sports may require use of a protective athletic cup
    - Participation is best decided on a case-by-case basis after discussion with the athlete, the family, the coach, and physicians

RECOMMENDED READINGS

Available online.

33 THE ATHLETE WITH DIABETES

George D. Harris

GENERAL PRINCIPLES

- Diabetes mellitus (DM) is a chronic group of metabolic diseases characterized by hyperglycemia resulting from defects in insulin secretion leading to an absolute insulin deficiency due to beta-cell destruction (type 1), by defects in insulin action because of progressive insulin secretory loss along with increasing insulin resistance (type 2), or by other causes such as pregnancy (gestational), neonatal diabetes or maturity-onset diabetes of the young (monogenic diabetes), diseases of the exocrine pancreas, or drug- or chemical-induced causes.
- A majority of patients with DM have type 2 (90%–95%). Athletes with DM range in sports participation from youth to competitive Olympics and professionals.
- Of the 210,000 individuals 19 years of age and younger diagnosed with diabetes in the United States, about 187,000 have mainly type 1 diabetes (T1DM) and 23,000 have type 2 diabetes (T2DM) or other types. The ratio of T1DM and T2DM changes with age in the general population.
- Each sport and the type of exercise have their own effects on DM management. Numerous factors affect glucose levels, including stress, level of hydration, rate of glycogenolysis and gluconeogenesis, and secretion of counter-regulatory hormones.
- Management includes excellent clinical care, continuous patient self-management, patient education, and longitudinal support to prevent long-term complications (renal failure, blindness, peripheral vascular disease, and peripheral neuropathy).

Anatomy and Pathophysiology

- **T1DM** has two subtypes: type 1A and type 1B. Each type can occur at any age, but typical onset is before the age of 30 years, with peak incidence during adolescence.
- Type 1A is an autoimmune disease characterized by cellular antibodies that may form against islet cells (ICA), insulin (IAA), and glutamic acid decarboxylase (GAD65). Type 1B is an idiopathic, nonautoimmune disease state with loss of beta-cell function and is not human leukocyte antigen (HLA)–associated but is an inherited form of diabetes.
- Both types are caused by loss of insulin secretion because of progressive loss of insulin production.
- These physiologic changes lead to increased hyperglycemia, weight loss, possible ketoacidosis, and possible death if insulin is not administered.
- **T2DM** occurs in most patients older than 40 years and is characterized by defects in both insulin secretion and resistance to insulin action.
- Type 2 patients may present with diabetic ketoacidosis (DKA), especially in certain ethnic minorities (Latino or African Americans).
- Impaired insulin secretion, increased hepatic glucose production, and decreased muscle glucose uptake lead to increased levels of insulin production and eventual insulin resistance.
- Both genetic (family history or familial hyperlipidemia) and environmental (sedentary lifestyle or inappropriate diet with increased caloric intake) factors are involved in the development of insulin resistance. Insulin resistance is associated with obesity, hypertension, and hyperlipidemia and may precede the onset of diagnosed DM by 10–20 years.
- T2DM occurs in athletes with an increased body mass for their particular sport (football lineman or rugby players) or those who do not remain fit (e.g., certain baseball players).
- Patients with T1DM and T2DM benefit from regular exercise:
  - Exercise decreases the insulin resistance of peripheral tissues and alleviates the defect of insulin-stimulated glycogen metabolism in skeletal muscles.
  - It improves postprandial hyperglycemia and possibly postprandial insulin secretion.
- For patients with T2DM, both aerobic and resistance exercises can benefit glycemic control.

Epidemiology

- The incidence of DM is increasing worldwide. It is estimated that 463 million people are living with diabetes in the world. It is predicted this figure will increase to 642 million people by 2040.
- Currently, in the United States, approximately 30 million patients have DM, with about 23 million diagnosed with T2DM.

GENERAL MEDICAL CONCERNS

- In comparison with inactive individuals, the additional demands of training and competition affect glucose homeostasis in athletes with DM, thus creating additional challenges.
- Challenges include the athlete's safety during athletic participation, adequate glucose monitoring, and diet and insulin adjustments for safe and effective athletic performance.
- The most significant concern for athletes using insulin or insulin secretagogues (sulfonylureas and meglitinides) is the potential for exercise-related hypoglycemia; it can occur during, immediately after, 6–15 hours after exercise, or up to 48 hours after exercise.
- Most competitive athletes learn to manage their DM during training and competition by trial and error while sharing personal experiences with other athletes.
- Medical concerns include unsafe dietary patterns, using nutritional supplements with no benefit or even detrimental effects, and using illegal drugs.
- Other concerns include the female athlete triad (amenorrhea, osteoporosis, and eating disorder), rapid weight loss to "make weight" in the respective wrestling or gymnastic competition, and excessive consumption of a single macronutrient (carbohydrate, protein, or fat) in certain athletes such as football players.
- In sports with weight categories (wrestling, boxing, and weightlifting), insulin is often omitted so that athletes can lose weight before weigh-ins; the consequence is poor glucose control and the risk of ketoacidosis.
- All athletes with a diagnosis of type 1 or type 2 diabetes should have a personalized diabetic care plan for their exercise, practices, and games that is supported by the team physician and athletic trainer.
- SGLT2 inhibitors promote glucosuria and a have a modest diuretic effect. Dehydration is a potential concern, but no dose adjustments are recommended before initiating an exercise routine.

Athletes With Type 1 Diabetes Mellitus

- Appropriate hydration and maintenance of glucose levels can maximize performance. The excitement of competition can increase catecholamine release, resulting in hyperglycemia, but adjustment of insulin dosing is usually unnecessary.

- For these athletes, hypoglycemia usually occurs within 45 minutes of starting aerobic exercise unless treatment regimen adjustments are made to prevent it.
- Athletes with T1DM learn their personal requirements from training and recognize that they always require a certain amount of insulin supplementation.
- Glucose monitoring before, during, and after exercise can establish an athlete's usual glycemic responses and allow for maintaining euglycemia with appropriate adjustments in insulin dosing and carbohydrate ingestion.
- When an athlete with T1DM is insulin deficient, hyperglycemia occurs with a risk of further elevation in glucose levels, which may exacerbate or precipitate ketoacidosis. Moreover, osmotic diuresis with relative dehydration occurs as well.
- Morning endurance sports are less likely to cause hypoglycemia because of the physiologically elevated diurnal cortisol and growth hormone levels. Events that occur later in the day require adjustments in food and insulin.
- Certain athletes with T1DM intentionally avoid achieving good blood glucose (BG) control before their competitive event to have increased lipid utilization, which prevents exercise-induced hypoglycemia.

Athletes With Type 2 Diabetes Mellitus

- The duration the athlete has been diagnosed with T2DM and the specific sport will determine management. Endogenous insulin production or secretion early in the disease requires little, if any, exogenous insulin. These athletes maintain the ability to physiologically decrease or increase endogenous insulin secretion and are generally able to achieve optimal glucose levels in the desired range.
- With progression of the disease, endogenous insulin secretion diminishes and exogenous insulin administration becomes necessary and must be adjusted to prevent hypoglycemia.
- It is not uncommon for such athletes to decrease exogenous insulin requirement by ≥50% with competition.
- Athletes with T2DM who use oral insulin secretagogues and sensitizers may need to decrease their dosing as training and insulin sensitivity increase and body fat decreases, resulting in an overall increase in lean body mass.

SPORT-SPECIFIC ISSUES

Endurance Athletes (Distance Cyclists and Runners)

- Appropriate glucose management before, during, and after exercise is crucial to care of an athlete with DM.
- Endurance runners often strive for optimal prerun BG levels of 120–180 mg/dL, use minimal insulin, and estimate a glucose reduction of 10–15 mg/dL/mile.
- When running for 30–60 minutes, self-monitoring of BG or continuous glucose monitoring (CGM) during the training period will delineate the athlete's predicted response.
- Distance cyclists and runners may choose to set the basal rate of insulin infusion via continuous subcutaneous insulin infusion (CSII) or insulin pump at a lower rate or may select a decreased long-acting basal insulin dosage (not uncommon to have to decrease by 50%). Carbohydrates are then gradually ingested to match energy utilization with exercise. By creating a steady-state balance between exercise requirements, basal insulin infusion, and ingestion of energy (carbohydrates), glucose levels are held constant (e.g., 130–150 mg/dL) over several hours.
- When a cyclist or runner with T1DM encounters a demanding section of a course, they will either adjust the basal rate of insulin downward or ingest additional carbohydrates to maintain optimal glucose levels.
- For runners and cyclists who are prone to hypoglycemia, performing a series of anaerobic sprints or resistance exercise before the aerobic endurance event may help prevent subsequent hypoglycemia.
- Running sports pose special problems for athletes with DM and include skin breakdown or other lesions because of vascular compromise or neuropathy.
- Athletes should travel with at least two pairs of well-fitting shoes that (1) are well broken in, (2) have no areas of material weakness or breakdown, and (3) cause no discomfort with exercise. In addition, (4) athletes should have their feet examined by the certified athletic trainer (ATC)/healthcare provider on a weekly basis, (5) avoid switching to a new pair of shoes on competition day, and (6) avoid using any alcohol-based lotion on the feet that may cause skin drying.

Altitude Sports

- BG regulation is affected by altitude exposure in people with and without diabetes.
- Glycemic control decreases in athletes with T1DM and may affect certain patients with T2DM at high altitudes. Hyperglycemia is the result of (1) increased sympathetic tone with subsequent increased hepatic glucose production, (2) increased insulin resistance, (3) loss of appetite at high altitude, and (4) the increased energy expenditure at higher altitudes.
- Other problems encountered include variation in reliability of glucose monitors and adequate insulin protection from temperature extremes or at high altitudes. As insulin temperature approaches freezing temperatures, it becomes less active.
- Acute mountain sickness may mimic the signs of hypoglycemia, necessitating frequent monitoring of BG levels.
- High-altitude athletes should maintain insulin close to their body to maintain optimal insulin temperature.

Water Sports, Swimming, or Scuba

- Water sports limit the use of insulin pumps and continuous glucose monitors depending on the specific device and company model. Although insulin pumps are water resistant and one model is waterproof to 12 feet for up to 24 hours, other models do not withstand pressure.
- Insulin pumps usually are removed before showering or bathing, whereas implanted glucose monitor skin sensors can remain in place; however, separate external glucose monitor devices are not waterproof.
- Scuba diving is discouraged for athletes with T1DM, although several accomplished divers dive with partners who are aware of their condition. Because recreational dives usually last 30–45 minutes, glucose monitoring can be accomplished on an interval basis at the surface level.

Ice Hockey, Wrestling, or Football

- Use of external devices is discouraged in these sports. Wrestling and football competitions can cause damage to insulin pumps or external glucose monitors. Hockey players cannot wear any equipment that would be harmful to another player. A letter from a healthcare provider is required for any special medical equipment.
- Athletes often resort to intermittent insulin injections and glucose monitoring outside the competition area.

Baseball or Softball

- These sports are ideal for athletes with DM because they require bursts of anaerobic energy without prolonged exercise periods.
- In the dugout, during each inning, athletes should test their glucose levels, ingest carbohydrates, and maintain hydration as needed.
- There has been some success in using insulin pumps with these sports.

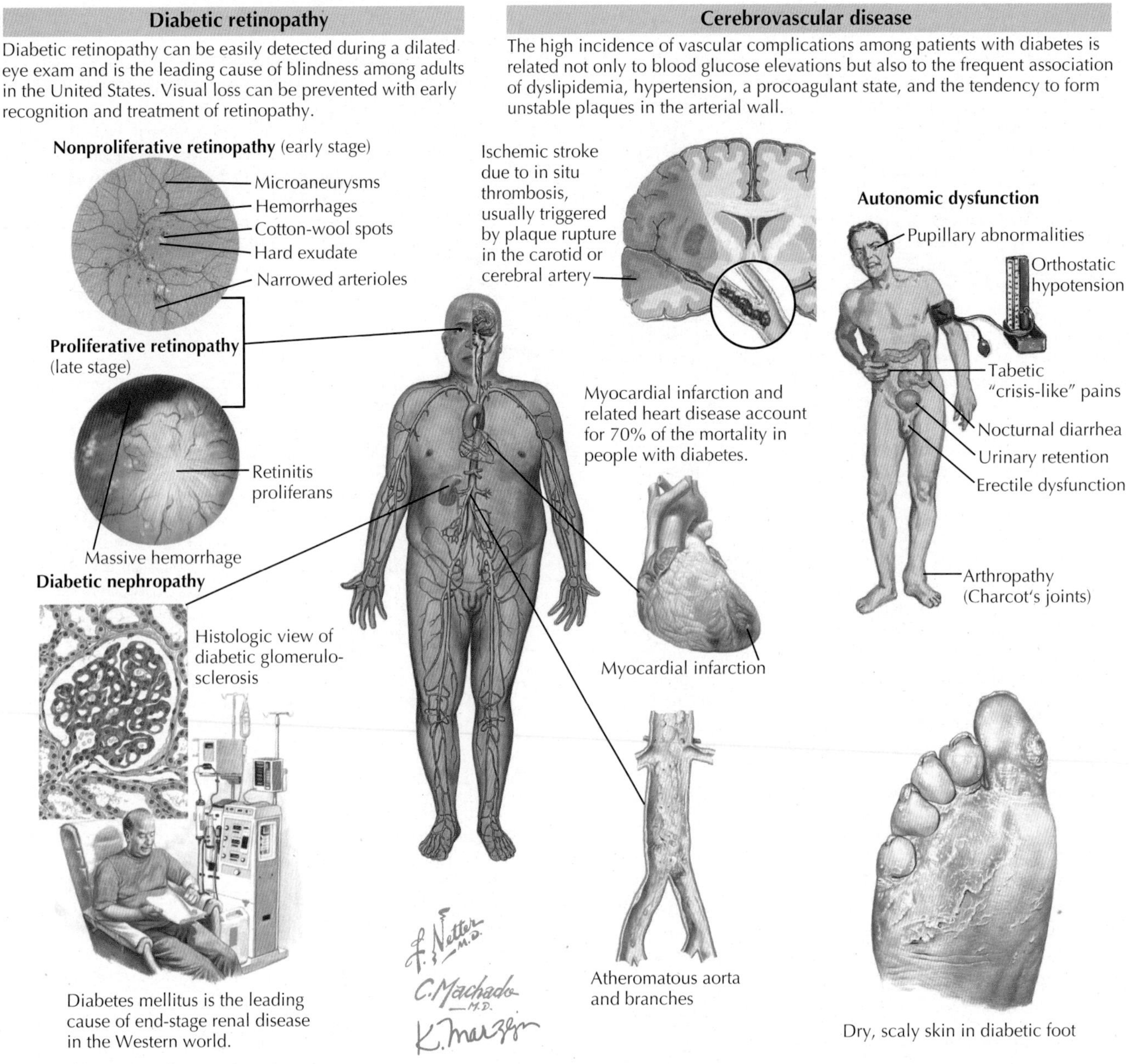
Diabetic retinopathy
Diabetic retinopathy can be easily detected during a dilated eye exam and is the leading cause of blindness among adults in the United States. Visual loss can be prevented with early recognition and treatment of retinopathy.
Nonproliferative retinopathy (early stage)
Microaneurysms
Hemorrhages
Cotton-wool spots
Hard exudate
Narrowed arterioles
Proliferative retinopathy (late stage)
Retinitis proliferans
Massive hemorrhage
Diabetic nephropathy
Histologic view of diabetic glomerulo-sclerosis
Diabetes mellitus is the leading cause of end-stage renal disease in the Western world.
Cerebrovascular disease
The high incidence of vascular complications among patients with diabetes is related not only to blood glucose elevations but also to the frequent association of dyslipidemia, hypertension, a procoagulant state, and the tendency to form unstable plaques in the arterial wall.
Ischemic stroke due to in situ thrombosis, usually triggered by plaque rupture in the carotid or cerebral artery
Myocardial infarction and related heart disease account for 70% of the mortality in people with diabetes.
Myocardial infarction
Atheromatous aorta and branches
Autonomic dysfunction
Pupillary abnormalities
Orthostatic hypotension
Tabetic "crisis-like" pains
Nocturnal diarrhea
Urinary retention
Erectile dysfunction
Arthropathy (Charcot's joints)
Dry, scaly skin in diabetic foot
F. Netter M.D.
C. Machado M.D.

Figure 33.1 Signs of neuropathic joint disease and peripheral vascular disease.

Triathlons

- Most diabetic triathletes have T1DM and, through their training, have learned to satisfactorily manage their insulin and glucose levels, making insulin adjustments on competition days based on training experiences.
- During the swimming element, either a waterproof pump is worn or the insulin pump and glucose monitor are removed.
- After exiting the water, athletes may attach an external glucose monitor and insulin pump. The process requires ≤10 seconds.
- Athletes may suspend, continue, or increase the same infusion based on glucose monitor readings without ceasing activity.
- With special permission from race officials, along the course route, athletes may be provided with glucose supplements.

RISK OF EXERCISE

- Hypoglycemia is a major risk in athletes with T1DM, with additional risks of exacerbation of hyperglycemia and ketoacidosis. All diabetics are at an increased risk of coronary artery and peripheral vascular disease.
- Other associated risks include retinopathy, injury from neuropathy (ankle and foot injuries), and autonomic dysfunction (abnormal sweating mechanisms affecting heat dissipation or abnormal heart rate response to exercise) (Fig. 33.1).
- Running is prohibited in patients with active proliferative retinopathy, which must be treated, stabilized, and cleared by an ophthalmologist before resuming activity.

SPECIAL EQUIPMENT

- The CSII is a device that contains a reservoir of rapid-acting insulin within a pump along with a small computer and catheter connected to a quick-release device inserted into the subcutaneous tissue of the athlete (abdomen). Basal insulin is provided in the form of a continuous slow infusion. A bolus of insulin can be administered to cover carbohydrate intake. The device

can be interrupted or suspended for short periods (<60 minutes) without any adverse effects.
- In addition, CGM can be used to monitor glucose levels. A small sensor is implanted in the subcutaneous tissue, which analyzes glucose levels in the interstitial fluid. Severe low or high levels are signaled, allowing the athlete to have more control over his or her DM management and exercise programs.

TREATMENT

Principles of Glucose Management in Diabetes Mellitus

- The American Diabetes Association recommends the following glycemic goals:
  - Fasting glucose of 90–130 mg/dL
  - Two-hour postprandial glucose <180 mg/dL
  - Limit postprandial glucose versus premeal glucose to ≤50 mg/dL
- The total daily dose (TDD) of insulin = 0.7 × weight in kg
  - Basal insulin dose per 24 hours = 50% of TDD
  - Bolus insulin dose per 24 hours = 50% of TDD
  - Percentages vary from individual to individual based on glucose measurements and activity, work, and exercise schedule.
  - Prandial insulin can be determined by weight (0.1 units/kg/meal, see Example 1) or can be determined by premeal glucose measurements and calculated grams of carbohydrate in the upcoming meal (1 unit for each 30 g of glucose in the meal, see Example 2).
    - Example 1: 70 kg male × 0.1 units/meal = 7 units with that meal
    - Example 2: Premeal glucose = 150 mg% (target level is 120 mg%)
    - For BG levels above a described target number, that is, one unit for each 15 g of glucose (150 − 120 = 30 mg%/15 = 2 units)
      PLUS
      60 g glucose meal (60 g/30 = 2 × 1 unit for each 30 g of glucose in meal = 2 units)
      Total units given premeal = 4 units.
- Patients with T1DM require bolus insulin before meals (Table 33.1) and basal insulin (Table 33.2) throughout the day.
- CSII (insulin pump therapy) is very effective in distance events. Several athletes wear a CGM system that renders current glucose levels and a trend graph. Distance athletes learn how to balance ingested carbohydrates and administered insulin with exercise and competition demands.
- Patients with T2DM *may* require insulin to achieve initial glycemic control but are typically managed with oral agents alone such as metformin (Table 33.3 and Fig. 33.2). Exercise and appropriate diet are beneficial to disease management and may lead to decreased medication doses with progressive training.

Management of Hypoglycemia

- Hypoglycemia should be treated with 15–20 g of fast-acting carbohydrates, preferably glucose tablets designed to treat hypoglycemia or a sugar-sweetened beverage or juice.
- Repeat treatment if no improvement in symptoms or glucose levels after 15 minutes.
- If there is a concern for recurrent hypoglycemia once the athlete resumes play, additional complex carbohydrates should be consumed before returning to activity.
- Hypoglycemia provokes a counter-regulatory hormonal response; thus, excessive carbohydrate intake should be avoided to prevent a significant hyperglycemic rebound.
- Severe hypoglycemia with cardiac arrhythmias, unconsciousness, or seizures is a life-threatening condition that requires an emergency response and parenteral glucagon or intravenous (IV) dextrose 50%, give 20–50 mL over 1 to 3 minutes.

PREVENTION

The best approach in the management of hypoglycemia during exercise is to prevent its occurrence.

Hypoglycemia

- Exercise, stress, level of hydration, rate of glycogenolysis and gluconeogenesis, and secretion of counter-regulatory hormones can affect glucose levels.
- Hypoglycemia in diabetic athletes can be either immediate or delayed.
- Immediate hypoglycemia occurs during or shortly after exercise and is most common in patients with T1DM because of inadequate caloric intake to meet metabolic demands.
- Other causes include excessive exogenous insulin administration or injection of insulin into the site of an exercising muscle or overlying subcutaneous tissue, resulting in increased rate of absorption.
- Symptoms and signs are primarily because of adrenergic causes (from the release of sympathomimetic mediators) and neuroglycopenic causes (from an inadequate amount of glucose being available to support brain activity).
- Adrenergic signs and symptoms consist of hunger, anxiety, sweating, tremor, tachycardia, palpitations, and/or a feeling of impending doom.
- Neuroglycopenic symptoms and signs include weakness or fatigue, slow or slurred speech, impaired performance of tasks, lack of coordination, blurred vision, odd behavior, confusion, vertigo, paresthesias, stupor, seizures, and loss of consciousness.
- To prevent immediate hypoglycemia, avoid injection of insulin into an exercising muscle (e.g., use of anterior thigh in a runner) and instead inject into the abdominal area.
- Calories should be continually replaced during periods of prolonged activity.
- Careful glucose monitoring during activities allows athletes to determine individual caloric requirements and make appropriate adjustments.

Delayed Hypoglycemia (Nocturnal Hypoglycemia)

- Usually occurs 6–12 hours after exercise and has been reported to sustain for up to 28 hours after exercise.
- Pathophysiology involves vigorous exercise that severely depletes body glycogen stores, followed by inadequate replacement of glycogen stores in the postexercise interval ("golden replenishment period").
- Athletes either underestimate caloric requirements or ingest limited calories and defer eating until later. Over ensuing hours, liver and muscle tissues extract circulating BG to replenish depleted glycogen stores, and glycogen synthetase is activated.
- Peripheral muscle tissues are more sensitive to any available insulin after exercise.
- Subsequent severe and persistent delayed hypoglycemia often requires parenteral glucagon and continuous caloric intake over several hours to correct and replenish the depleted glycogen stores.
- Adequate replenishment of glycogen stores (1.5 g of carbohydrates per kg of body weight) immediately after exercise; it is critical to replace glycogen stores during the "golden recovery period" in order to avoid the risk of delayed hypoglycemia

GUIDELINES FOR AVOIDING EXERCISE-ASSOCIATED HYPOGLYCEMIA

- These guidelines are only estimates that must be modified for a given person.
- Measure BG before exercise and ingest carbohydrates using the following criteria if the intensity is low to moderate. Realize

Table 33.1 BOLUS INSULIN PREPARATIONS

	Chemical	Onset of Action	Peak (Hours)	Duration (Hours)
Rapid-Acting Class				
Aspart (NovoLog)	Insulin analog	5–15 minutes	1–2	3–4
Glulisine (Apidra)	Insulin analog	5–15 minutes	1–2	3–4
Lispro (Humalog)	Insulin analog	5–15 minutes	1–2	3–4
Short-Acting				
Regular Humulin R Novolin R	Human insulin	30–60 minutes	2–4	6–8
Intermediate-Acting				
NPH (Neutral Protamine Hagedorn) Humulin N Novolin N	Human insulin	1–4 hours	6–10	10–16
Premixed				
70/30 (70% NPH/30% Reg)	Human insulin	0.5–1.0 hour	0.5–1.0 hour 1st peak-2–3 2nd peak hours later	10–16
50/50 (50% NPH/50% Reg)	Human insulin	0.5–1.0 hour	0.5–1.0 hour 1st peak-2–3 2nd peak hours later	10–16

Table 33.2 BASAL INSULIN PREPARATIONS

	Chemical	Onset of Action	Peak	Duration (Hours)
Basal Insulin Class				
Insulin glargine (Lantus or Basaglar)	Human insulin	1–4 hours	None	24
Insulin detemir (Levemir)	Human insulin	1–4 hours	None	20–24
Insulin degludec (Tresiba)[a]	Human insulin	30–90 minutes	None	>24
Premixed				
Humalog mix 75/25 (75% protamine lispro/25% insulin lispro)	Insulin analog	15 minutes	0.5–1.2	10–16 hours
Insulin degludec/Aspart (Ryzodeg) (70% insulin degludec/30% aspart)	Insulin analog	10 minutes	None	>24 hours
BiAsp 70/30 (70% NPH/30% aspart)	Insulin analog	15 minutes	0.5–1.2	10–16 hours
Lispro mix 50/50 (50% NPH/50% aspart)	Insulin analog	15 minutes	0.5–1.2	10–16 hours

[a]Ultra-long-acting.

that high-intensity exercise leads to increased BG levels and hence, lesser carbohydrates, not more, are needed.

- If BG is <90 mg/dL, initially consume 10–20 g of carbohydrate before starting exercise and delay exercise until BG >90 mg/dL. Monitor glucose levels during exercise. Consume 30 g of carbohydrate per 60 minutes of light to moderate exercise (60% $\dot{V}O_2$ max).
- If BG is 90–120 mg/dL, consume 10 g of carbohydrate before starting exercise and then consume 30 g of carbohydrate per 60 minutes of light to moderate exercise.
- If BG is 120–180 mg/dL, start exercise and consume 30 g of carbohydrate per 60 minutes of light to moderate exercise.
- If BG is 180–250 mg/dL, do not consume food before exercise. If the exercise is heavy and the duration exceeds 30 minutes, take a second BG reading and use the criteria stated in the first three items of this list.
- If BG is ≥250 mg/dL, check urine for ketones. Exercise is permissible if no ketones are present, but do not exercise if ketones are present or BG levels are >300 mg/dL because the action of counter-regulatory hormones may cause BG to rise during exercise and increase ketone levels as well. Perform frequent (every 15 minutes) checks of BG levels.
- **Easily digested carbohydrates should be readily available for supplemental feeding** with the athletic trainer or coach and on the athlete's person (e.g., pocket of running shorts or pack on bicycle). Glucose gel or tablets elicit faster rise in BG than do fruit or fruit juices.
- **Decrease the dosage of insulin that peaks during exercise.** Rapid-acting analog insulin normally taken before meals might be decreased or deleted.

BENEFITS OF EXERCISE

Available online.

EXERCISE GUIDELINES

Available online.

Table 33.3 PHARMACEUTICAL AGENTS AND MECHANISM OF ACTION FOR TYPE 2 DIABETES MELLITUS (SEE FIG. 33.2)

Agents (Generic Name)	Mode of Action	Side Effects
1. Sulfonylureas (SU) Glyburide (DiaBeta, Micronase) Glipizide (Glucotrol) Glipizide-GITS (Glucotrol XL) Glyburide (Micronized glynase) Glimepiride (Amaryl) Glipizide/metformin (Metaglip) Glyburide/metformin (Glucovance) Pioglitazone/glimepiride (Duetact)	Insulin secretagogues Stimulate insulin release, reduce glucose output from the liver, and increase insulin sensitivity at peripheral sites	Hypoglycemia in elderly; renal insufficiency; weight gain
2. Biguanides Metformin (MF) (Glucophage) Metformin XL (Fortamet) Metformin XR (Glucophage XR) Glumetza (Metformin oral suspension)	Decreases hepatic glucose production and glucose absorption from GI tract Increases peripheral glucose utilization	Caution in elderly and in renal failure. Withhold for contrast studies. Improves fertility in PCOS Can cause diarrhea, weight loss, and vitamin B_{12} deficiency Have low risk of hypoglycemia
3. Alpha-glucosidase inhibitors[a] Acarbose (Precose) Miglitol (Glyset)	Slows gut absorption of CHOs by inhibiting alpha-glucosidase enzymes	Hypoglycemia Cause flatulence and diarrhea Avoid in malabsorption syndromes; inflammatory bowel disease, bowel obstruction
4. Thiazolidinediones (TZDs) Pioglitazone (Actos) Rosiglitazone (Avandia)	Increases tissue sensitivity to insulin in skeletal muscles by activation of intracellular peroxisome proliferator-activated receptors	Weight gain, resumption of ovulation, avoid in patients with stage III/IV CHF; increased fracture risk in women
5. Meglitinides[a] Repaglinide (Prandin) Nateglinide (Starlix)	Rapid-acting insulin secretagogue with short-acting sulfonylureas (same mechanisms but different binding site on pancreatic cells)	More effective in reducing postprandial glucose when compared with MF, SU, and TZDs Caution use in renal and liver impairment
6. DPP-4 inhibitors Sitagliptin (Januvia) Sitagliptin + metformin (Janumet/ Janumet XR) Linagliptin (Tradjenta) Linagliptin + metformin (Jentadueto) Alogliptin (Nesina) Alogliptin + metformin (Kazano) Alogliptin + pioglitazone (Oseni) Saxagliptin (Onglyza) Saxagliptin + metformin (Kombliglyze XR)	Block the action of DPP-4 enzymes, resulting in a two- to threefold increase in plasma endogenous GLP-1 levels	Skin rash and rhinitis; doses are based on renal status with the exception of linagliptin. Does NOT increase risk of CAD, HF, hospitalization for CHF
7. GLP-1 receptor agonists Exenatide (Byetta) Exenatide QW (Bydureon) Duralutide (Trulicity) Semaglutide (Ozempic) (Oral formulation—Rybelsus) Liraglutide (Saxenda, Victoza) Lixisenatide (Adlyxin) Lixisenatide + insulin glargine (Soliqua)	Enhance nutrient-stimulated secretion biomarkers. Exenatide is injected BID with meals Exenatide QW is injected once weekly Liraglutide is injected once daily without regard to meals; marketed for chronic weight management Semaglutide is injected once weekly	Weight loss; favorable effect on CV; preserve B-cell function via activation of GLP-1 receptors on B cells; inhibit glucagon secretion. Positive effect on endothelial cell function in humans; no cause of pancreatitis; delay gastric emptying; nausea is common side effect; lower risk of hypoglycemia when used with insulin/insulin secretagogues
8. Synthetic amylin analog Pramlintide (Symlin)	Exogenous replacement with insulin deficiency. Injected pre-prandially; caution in patients with hypoglycemic unawareness	Adjunct therapy in amylin, which is deficient in proportion. T1DM or T2DM who have not achieved glucose control despite optimal insulin therapy
9. SGLT2 inhibitors Canagliflozin (Invokana) Dapagliflozin (Farxiga) Empagliflozin (Jardiance) Empagliflozin + linagliptin (Glyxambi) Empagliflozin + metformin (Synjardy) Dapagliflozin + metformin (Xigduo XR)	Reduces renal threshold of glucose. Inhibits sodium-glucose transporter 2 in tubules of glomeruli. Glucose is not absorbed into the plasma producing a decrease in FPG and postprandial glucose	Urinary frequency, glycosuria, UTIs, decreases urine absorption from the SGL2 co-transporter GU tract; agents require dose adjustment if co-administered with other medications or in renal failure

BID, Twice daily; *CAD*, coronary artery disease; *CHF*, congestive heart failure; *CHO*, carbohydrate; *CV*, cardiovascular; *FPG*, fasting plasma glucose; *GI*, gastrointestinal; *GU*, gastrourinary; *HF*, heart failure; *PCOS*, polycystic ovarian syndrome; *UTI*, urinary tract infection.

[a]American Diabetes Association (ADA) does not list them as part of their algorithm any longer.

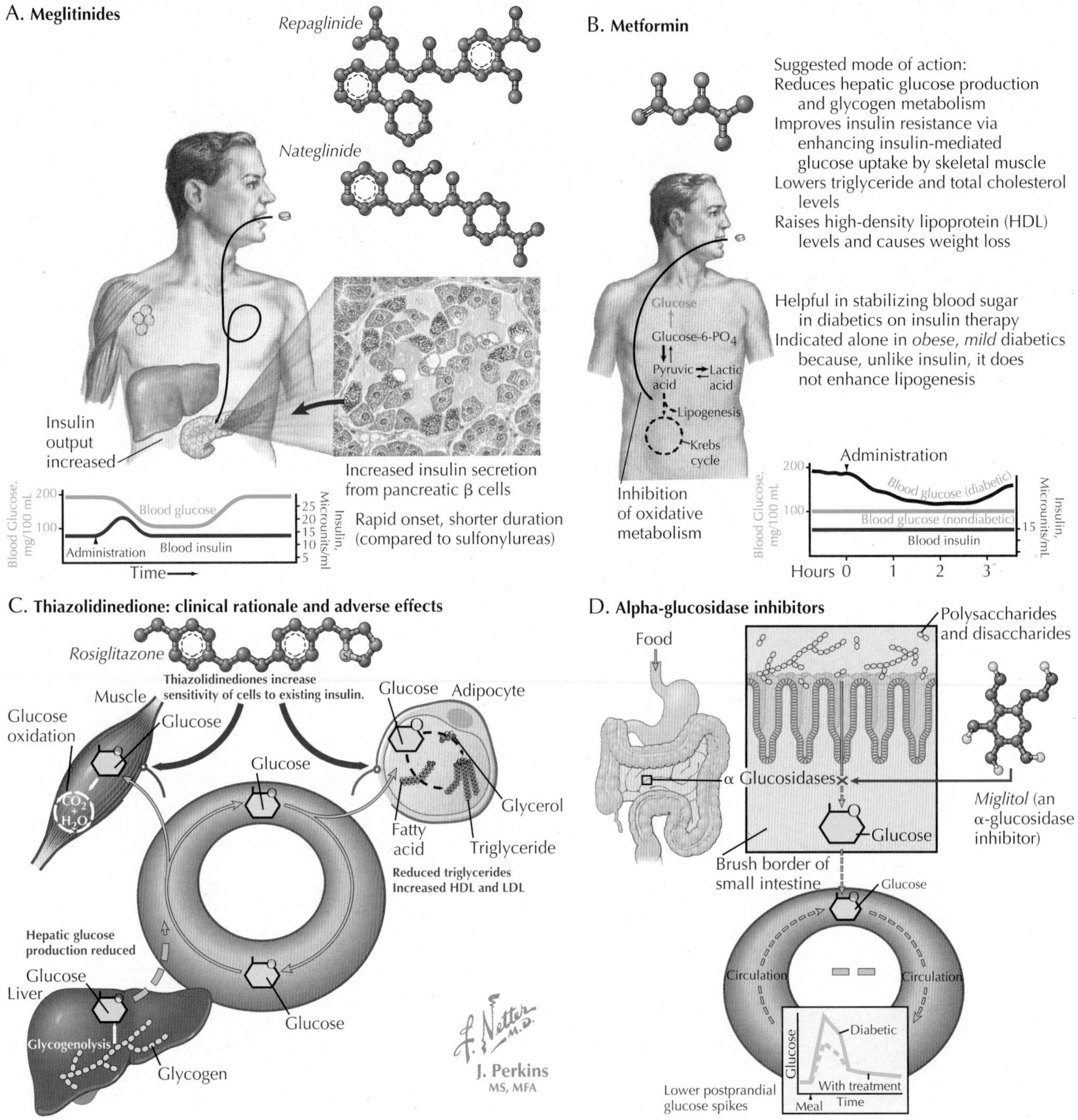
A. Meglitinides
Repaglinide
Nateglinide
Insulin
output
increased
Increased insulin secretion
from pancreatic β cells
Rapid onset, shorter duration
(compared to sulfonylureas)
Blood Glucose, mg/100 mL
200
100
Blood glucose
Blood insulin
Administration
Time
Insulin, Microunits/ml
25
20
15
10
5
B. Metformin
Suggested mode of action:
Reduces hepatic glucose production
and glycogen metabolism
Improves insulin resistance via
enhancing insulin-mediated
glucose uptake by skeletal muscle
Lowers triglyceride and total cholesterol
levels
Raises high-density lipoprotein (HDL)
levels and causes weight loss
Glucose
Glucose-6-PO4
Pyruvic acid
Lactic acid
Lipogenesis
Krebs cycle
Inhibition
of oxidative
metabolism
Helpful in stabilizing blood sugar
in diabetics on insulin therapy
Indicated alone in obese, mild diabetics
because, unlike insulin, it does
not enhance lipogenesis
Administration
Blood Glucose, mg/100 mL
200
100
Blood glucose (diabetic)
Blood glucose (nondiabetic)
Blood insulin
Insulin, Microunits/mL
15
Hours 0 1 2 3
C. Thiazolidinedione: clinical rationale and adverse effects
Rosiglitazone
Thiazolidinediones increase
sensitivity of cells to existing insulin.
Muscle
Glucose
oxidation
Glucose
CO2 + H2O
Glucose
Glucose
Adipocyte
Glycerol
Fatty
acid
Triglyceride
Reduced triglycerides
Increased HDL and LDL
Hepatic glucose
production reduced
Glucose
Liver
Glycogenolysis
Glycogen
Glucose
J. Perkins
MS, MFA
D. Alpha-glucosidase inhibitors
Food
Polysaccharides
and disaccharides
α Glucosidases
Glucose
Miglitol (an
α-glucosidase
inhibitor)
Brush border of
small intestine
Glucose
Circulation
Circulation
Glucose
Diabetic
With treatment
Meal
Time
Lower postprandial
glucose spikes

Figure 33.2 Medications that may contribute to hypoglycemia.

CONTRAINDICATIONS TO EXERCISE

Available online.

RECOMMENDED READINGS

Available online.

ECG INTERPRETATION IN ATHLETES

34

Mustafa Husaini • Bradley J. Petek • Jonathan A. Drezner

INTRODUCTION

- Sudden death related to cardiovascular disorders is the most common cause of death among athletes during sports and exercise.
- Genetic cardiovascular disorders, such as cardiomyopathies and ion channelopathies, are the primary causes of sudden cardiac death (SCD) in athletes.
- Acquired cardiac conditions, such as myocarditis, also represent an important cause of SCD in young athletes.
- Most of these disorders can be identified through characteristic changes on a resting 12-lead electrocardiogram (ECG).

APPROACH TO ECG INTERPRETATION

- Analyzing the ECG of an athlete requires careful interpretation to distinguish normal physiologic changes related to regular exercise from pathologic patterns suggestive of underlying disease.
- The most current ECG interpretation guideline, the "International Criteria," were published in 2017 and provide a framework of three different categories of ECG findings consisting of normal physiologic changes ("green zone"), borderline ECG abnormalities ("yellow zone"), and potential pathologic ECG findings ("red zone") (Fig. 34.1).
- The International Criteria have greatly improved the specificity (i.e., lowered the false-positive rate) while maintaining sensitivity to detect cardiovascular conditions that are associated with an increased risk for SCD.
- Utilization of the International Criteria by centers with experience in ECG interpretation in athletes has decreased the false-positive rate to as low as 1.3% in college athletes and 1.5% in elite adolescent soccer players.
- The secondary investigation of an abnormal ECG requires additional cardiac testing directed at the specific ECG abnormality, as recommended in the International Criteria.
- Informed decisions regarding sports participation after the diagnosis of a pathologic cardiac disorder should include a multidisciplinary team consisting of the patient, their family/support network, a cardiologist, the sports medicine physician, and others at the discretion of the patient.

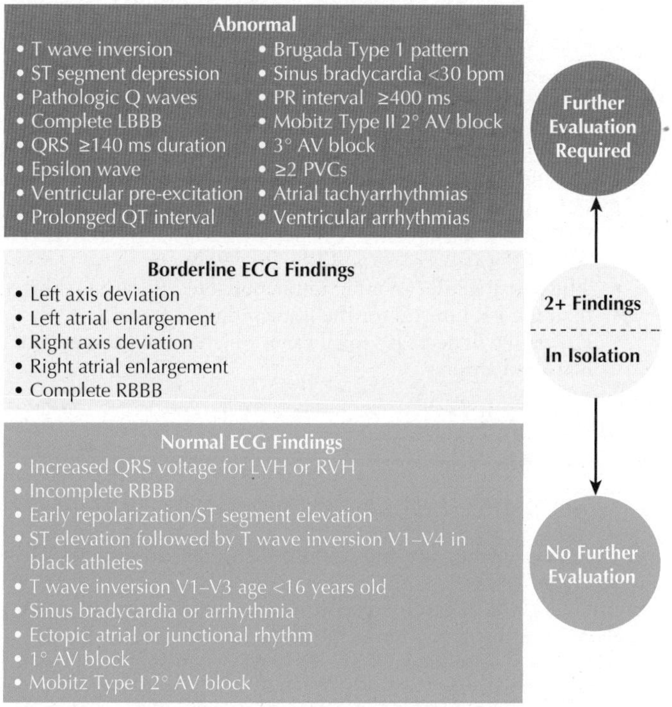
Abnormal
• T wave inversion
• ST segment depression
• Pathologic Q waves
• Complete LBBB
• QRS ≥140 ms duration
• Epsilon wave
• Ventricular pre-excitation
• Prolonged QT interval
• Brugada Type 1 pattern
• Sinus bradycardia <30 bpm
• PR interval ≥400 ms
• Mobitz Type II 2° AV block
• 3° AV block
• ≥2 PVCs
• Atrial tachyarrhythmias
• Ventricular arrhythmias
Further Evaluation Required
Borderline ECG Findings
• Left axis deviation
• Left atrial enlargement
• Right axis deviation
• Right atrial enlargement
• Complete RBBB
2+ Findings
In Isolation
Normal ECG Findings
• Increased QRS voltage for LVH or RVH
• Incomplete RBBB
• Early repolarization/ST segment elevation
• ST elevation followed by T wave inversion V1–V4 in black athletes
• T wave inversion V1–V3 age <16 years old
• Sinus bradycardia or arrhythmia
• Ectopic atrial or junctional rhythm
• 1° AV block
• Mobitz Type I 2° AV block
No Further Evaluation

Figure 34.1 Normal ECG findings represent physiologic adaptations and do not require additional evaluation. Abnormal ECG findings may represent an underlying pathologic cardiac disorder and warrant further evaluation. Presence of two or more borderline findings warrants further evaluation, whereas a single borderline finding found in isolation and without other clinical markers of concern does not require additional testing.

NORMAL CARDIAC ADAPTATIONS IN ATHLETES

Introduction

- The heart undergoes physiologic changes in response to regular exercise, termed *exercise-induced cardiac remodeling (EICR)*, or the "athlete's heart."
- EICR can consist of increased cardiac chamber size, wall thickness, and/or vagal tone, all of which can lead to unique ECG changes.
- ECG findings related to increased cardiac chamber size or thickness include voltage criteria for left ventricular hypertrophy (LVH), right ventricular hypertrophy (RVH), and incomplete right bundle branch block (RBBB), all of which are considered normal findings on an athlete's ECG.
- Findings consistent with increased vagal tone include early repolarization, sinus bradycardia, sinus arrhythmia, first-degree atrioventricular (AV) block, Mobitz type I second-degree AV block, and junctional and ectopic atrial rhythms.

Specific Findings Related to Physiologic Adaptations to Exercise

- **QRS voltage criteria for LVH:**
  - Definition: Sokolow–Lyon criteria: sum of the S wave in V_1 and the R wave in V_5 or V_6 (using the largest R wave) as >3.5 mV.
  - Present in up to 55% of male and 10% of female athletes.
  - When pathologic LVH is present, such as in hypertrophic cardiomyopathy (HCM), the voltage criteria for LVH are usually associated with other abnormal ECG findings (i.e., T-wave inversion, ST-segment depression, and/or pathologic Q waves).
- **QRS voltage criteria for RVH:**
  - Definition: Sokolow–Lyon criteria: R wave in V_1 + largest S wave in V_5 or V_6 >10.5 mV.
  - Up to 13% of athletes meet these criteria.
  - Very poor correlation with arrhythmogenic cardiomyopathy (AC), pulmonary hypertension, or other right ventricle (RV) disorders.
- **Incomplete RBBB:**
  - Definition: QRS duration 100–120 ms with terminal R wave in lead V_1 (commonly characterized as an rSR′ pattern) and wide terminal S wave in leads I and V_6.
  - Present in up to 40% of highly trained athletes (particularly endurance and mixed-sport athletes).
  - Caused by delayed conduction given RV dilation from sustained exercise.

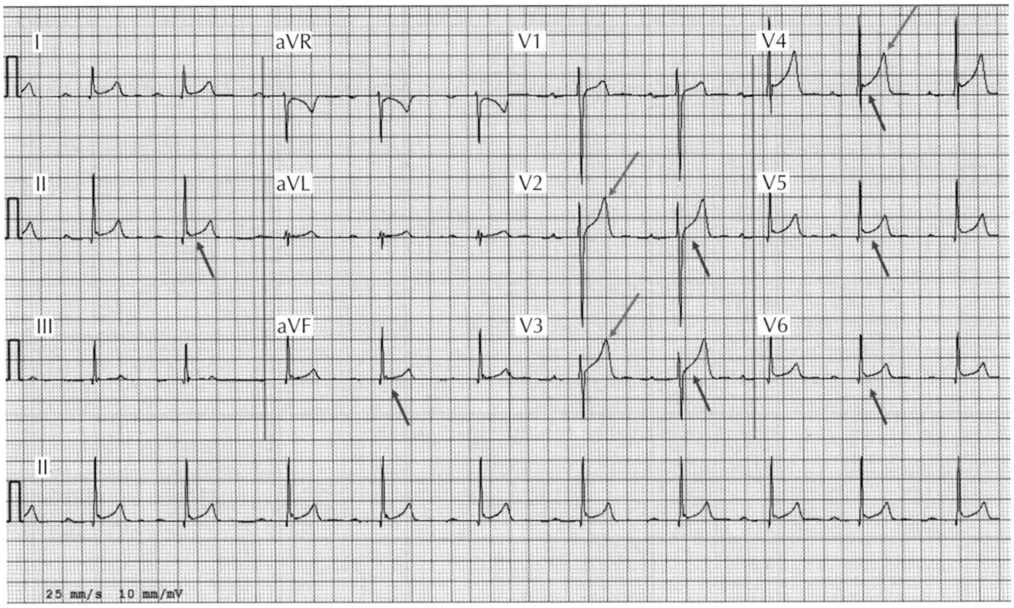
I
aVR
V1
V4
II
aVL
V2
V5
III
aVF
V3
V6
II
25 mm/s 10 mm/mV

Figure 34.2 ECG demonstrating early repolarization (J-point and ST-segment elevation) in II, aVF, and V_4–V_6 *(red arrows)* and tall, peaked T waves *(blue arrows)*. These are common training-related findings in athletes and do not require more evaluation.

- **Early repolarization:**
  - Definition: elevation of the QRS-ST junction (J-point) by ≥0.1 mV often associated with late QRS slurring or notching (J wave), most commonly found in the inferior (II, III, aVF) and/or lateral leads (V_5–V_6, I, aVL) (Fig. 34.2).
  - High prevalence in the general population and more common in young, male, and black individuals; seen in 45% of Caucasian athletes and 63%–91% of African-American athletes.
  - Available evidence suggests that all early repolarization patterns are normal in young athletes.
- **Early repolarization in black athletes**
  - Five percent to fifteen percent of black/African athletes demonstrate a specific repolarization variant: J-point elevation with convex ST segment followed by T-wave inversion in the anterior leads (V_1–V_4) (Fig. 34.3).
  - No association with cardiomyopathy with long-term follow-up.
  - T-wave inversion that extends to the lateral leads (V_5 or V_6) should always be considered abnormal and warrants careful evaluation to exclude cardiomyopathy.
- **"Juvenile" ECG pattern**
  - Definition: T-wave inversion in V_1–V_3 in asymptomatic athletes aged <16 years (or prepubertal) and independent of race.
  - T-wave inversion beyond V_2 is rare in Caucasian athletes age ≥16 or postpubertal athletes (0.1%), so warrants further investigation when seen.
- **Sinus bradycardia**
  - Definition: heart rate (HR) <60 beats per minute (bpm).
  - Present in up to 80% of highly trained athletes.
  - Sinus bradycardia should resolve with exertion.
  - HR ≥30 bpm is considered normal in trained athletes.
- **Sinus arrhythmia**
  - Definition: subtle oscillation in HR with breathing related to elevated vagal tone.
  - Should resolve with exertion and is not associated with symptoms.
- **Junctional escape rhythm**
  - Occurs when increased vagal tone decreases the resting sinus rate below the resting pacemaker cells within the AV junction.
  - Narrow complex QRS with QRS morphology similar as sinus rhythm but no preceding P waves.
  - HR <100 and regular RR interval.
  - Similar to other vagally mediated rhythms; will resolve with exercise.
- **Ectopic atrial rhythm**
  - P waves are present but different in morphology compared with normal sinus rhythm.
  - Inverted P waves in the inferior leads (II, III, aVF) suggest a "low atrial" ectopic rhythm.
  - Eight percent of athletes have ectopic atrial rhythm or junctional escape rhythm.
- **First-degree AV block**
  - Definition: PR interval >200 ms.
  - Occurs in 4.5%–7.5% of athletes.
  - Vagally mediated and should resolve with exertion.
- **Mobitz type I (Wenckebach) second-degree AV block**
  - Definition: progressive PR lengthening until a nonconducted P wave occurs (no QRS after P wave).
  - The first PR interval after a nonconducted P wave is shorter than the PR interval for the last conducted P wave.
  - Exertion will decrease vagal tone, which should resume normal conduction.

CARDIOMYOPATHIES

Introduction

- Cardiomyopathies are a heterogeneous group of heart muscle diseases.
- Collectively, they are the leading identified cause of SCD in young athletes.
- Individuals with cardiomyopathies may be asymptomatic, with the presenting sign often being SCD.
- The ECG is abnormal in 85%–95% of individuals with cardiomyopathies.
- Common ECG findings found in cardiomyopathies are listed in Table 34.1.

Hypertrophic Cardiomyopathy

- Unexplained, asymmetric LVH (≥16 mm) associated with nondilated ventricular chambers and the absence of another cardiac

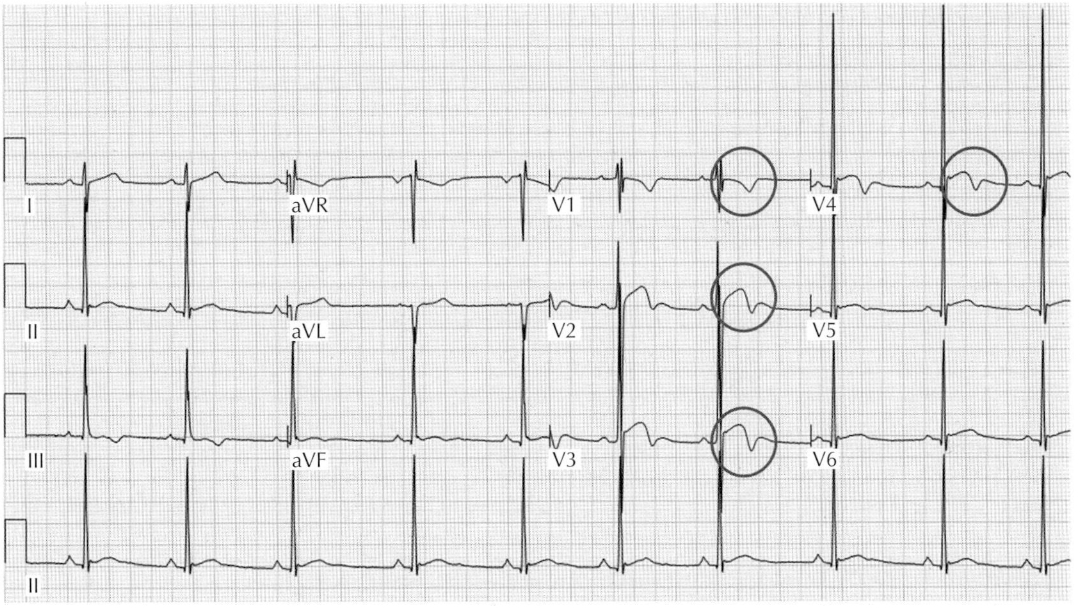
I
aVR
V1
V4
II
aVL
V2
V5
III
aVF
V3
V6
II

Figure 34.3 ECG from a 24-year-old asymptomatic black athlete. ECG demonstrates J-point elevation with a convex "domed" ST segment followed by T-wave inversion confined to leads V_1–V_4 *(blue circles)*. This is a normal repolarization variant in black athletes.

or systemic disease that could be responsible for the increase in wall thickness.
- Genetic disorder with autosomal-dominant inheritance pattern.
- Common associations include diastolic dysfunction, mitral regurgitation, myocyte disarray on histopathology, and LV outflow tract obstruction (at rest and increased with exercise).
- The most common site of asymmetric LVH is the intraventricular septum.
- Apical-variant HCM is a variation that accounts for one-third of HCM found in competitive athletes and presents with a markedly abnormal ECG pattern consisting of deep T-wave inversions (>2 mm) and ST-segment depression in the lateral or inferolateral leads (Fig. 34.4).
- Prevalence of approximately 1:200–1:500 in adults (1:800–2600 in young competitive athletes).

Arrhythmogenic Cardiomyopathy

- Genetic disorder related to abnormal desmosomes (cell adhesion proteins) leading to subsequent fibrofatty replacement of the myocardium.
- Predominately affects the RV free wall (Fig. 34.5), but equal (RV and LV) or predominant LV involvement can occur in some cases.
- Often manifests in the second to fourth decade of life with a progressive nature characterized by four phases (concealed, overt electrical disorder, RV failure, and biventricular pump failure).
- Athletic activity accelerates disease progression and arrhythmic triggers.

Dilated Cardiomyopathy (DCM)

- Heart muscle disorder wherein weakened contractile function leads to heart chamber enlargement without associated increase in wall thickness.
- Etiologies include viral, toxin mediated (drug/alcohol), tachycardia induced (atrial fibrillation, frequent premature ventricular contractions), and familial dilated cardiomyopathies.

Left Ventricular Noncompaction (LVNC)

- Heart muscle disorder characterized by failure of trabeculated structures to "compact" from spongy to solid myocardium. This noncompaction is phenotypically expressed as deep trabeculations and thinned compacted myocardium, often in a >2:1 ratio. Mutations in sarcomere genes are seen in ~32% of cases; however, the final common pathway leading to LVNC remains unknown.
- Evaluation requires multimodality imaging (e.g., echocardiogram and cardiac magnetic resonance imaging [MRI] and careful clinical evaluation for symptoms, as hypertrabeculation is more common in athletes and black individuals. Clinical correlation is important.
- A diagnosis of pathologic LVNC usually requires concurrent systolic dysfunction.

Myocarditis

- AC (often viral or inflammatory) where ECG abnormalities often overlap with findings found in other myocardial diseases.
- Acute presentation may include fever, chest pain, flulike viral syndrome, arrhythmias, syncope, and change in exercise tolerance.
- ECG manifestations of myocarditis include sinus tachycardia, T-wave inversion, ST-segment depression, diffuse ST-segment elevation, pathologic Q waves, and PR depression.
- In addition to the clinical history, other diagnostic considerations include reduction in left ventricular systolic function on echocardiography and/or supporting criteria on cardiac MRI. Other markers of inflammation (erythrocyte sedimentation rate [ESR], C-reactive protein [CRP]) and high-sensitivity cardiac troponin can also be used during the diagnostic process.

ECG Findings Suggestive of Cardiomyopathy

T-Wave Inversions

- >1 mm of depth in two or more anatomically contiguous leads V_2–V_6, II and aVF, or I and aVL (excludes leads III, aVR, and V_1); isolated T-wave inversion in V_5 or V_6 is also considered abnormal.

Table 34.1 ECG ABNORMALITIES IN CARDIOMYOPATHIES THAT PREDISPOSE TO SCD

	Pathologic Q Waves	ST-Segment Depression	T-Wave Inversion	Other Findings
HCM	32%–42% of individuals	~50% of individuals	Lateral (V_5–V_6, I, aVL) or inferior (II, aVF) (52%–64% of individuals)	Left atrial enlargement Voltage criteria for LVH Multiple PVCs Complete LBBB (~2% of individuals) Nonspecific IVCD Prolonged QTc
AC	Uncommon	Uncommon	Anterior (V_1–V_4) with a flat or depressed ST segment (85% of individuals)	Multiple PVCs Epsilon wave = small negative deflection just after QRS in leads V_1–V_3 Delayed S-wave upstroke ≥55 ms from nadir of S wave to the end of the QRS complex (in absence of RBBB) Low limb lead voltage (<5 mV)
DCM	10%–25% of individuals	Uncommon	Anterior, lateral, and inferolateral leads (25%–45% of individuals)	Complete LBBB (9%–25% of individuals) Nonspecific IVCD Goldberger triad (criteria suggestive of DCM) = deep S waves in the anterior precordial leads V_1–V_3, low limb lead voltage, and poor precordial R-wave progression
LVNC	Variable	~50% of individuals	Lateral, inferolateral (41% of individuals)	Complete LBBB Nonspecific IVCD
Myocarditis	Variable	Variable	Variable	Sinus tachycardia Diffuse ST-segment elevation PR depression Multiple PVCs

  - Directionality (i.e., positivity or negativity) refers to the direction of T-wave deflection with regard to the electrically neutral ECG baseline, conventionally defined as the PR segment.
  - Excludes T-wave inversion found in the repolarization variant in black athletes confined to V_1–V_4.
  - Excludes juvenile T-wave inversion in leads V_1–V_3 when age is <16 years.
- Recommended follow-up evaluation:
  - In lateral (V_5–V_6, I, aVL) or inferolateral leads: T-wave inversion in these territories is likely associated with quiescent cardiomyopathy and deserves full evaluation and follow-up.
    - Echocardiogram (if nondiagnostic, then cardiac MRI).
    - Cardiac MRI is indicated for any "markedly" abnormal ECG with >2 mm lateral or inferolateral T-wave inversion and ST-segment depression to exclude apical-variant HCM or other LV-dominant AC.
    - If imaging nondiagnostic or "gray-zone" hypertrophy (13–15 mm), then exercise ECG test and 24-hour ECG monitor to evaluate for nonsustained ventricular tachycardia.
  - Inferior leads (II and aVF) alone: T-wave inversion confined to the inferior leads is not a strong predictor of cardiomyopathy in the absence of other ECG criteria or clinical features, but has not been studied in detail.
    - Echocardiogram with additional evaluation based on abnormal echocardiographic findings or clinical suspicion.
  - Anterior leads (V_1–V_4): After exclusion of the black athlete repolarization variant or juvenile pattern in athletes age <16 years, anterior T-wave inversion in the absence of J-point elevation or with coexistent ST depression is concerning for RV-dominant AC.
    - Evaluation includes an echocardiogram, cardiac MRI, exercise ECG test, and 24-hour ECG monitor.
  - Because of variable phenotypic expression, patients with abnormal T-wave inversion and initial normal cardiac imaging require serial (i.e., annual) re-evaluation, as multiple studies have found that approximately 6% of patients develop clinical cardiomyopathy. Thus, the ECG manifestations of cardiomyopathy can occur before the morphologic changes.

ST-Segment Depression

- ≥0.5 mm in depth in two or more anatomically contiguous leads.
  - This finding is rare in healthy athletes, as it is not a feature of athletic training; thus, its presence requires the exclusion of cardiomyopathy.
- Recommended follow-up: Echocardiogram

Pathologic Q Waves

- Q/R ratio ≥0.25 or ≥40 ms in duration in two or more contiguous leads (except III and aVR)
  - Nonpathologic Q waves are commonly seen in young athletes, specifically long "skinny" Q waves related to overall increases in QRS amplitude
  - Pathologic Q waves are exaggerated (deep or wide) initial negative QRS deflections
- Could represent premature atherosclerotic coronary artery disease (CAD) in older athletes (≥30 years of age)
- Recommended follow-up:
  - Echocardiogram (and CAD risk factor assessment in older athletes)
  - Cardiac MRI if ST depressions, T-wave inversion, or other suspicious clinical findings are present.

Complete Left Bundle Branch Block (LBBB)

- QRS ≥120 ms, predominantly negative QRS complex in lead V_1 (QS or rS), and upright notched or slurred R wave in leads I and V_6.
- Rare finding in athletes.
- Recommended follow-up: A comprehensive evaluation to exclude cardiac pathology must be performed in the presence of LBBB. Start with echocardiogram and cardiac MRI.

PRIMARY ELECTRICAL DISEASES

Introduction

- Inherited arrhythmia syndromes are important causes of SCD in young individuals.
- Individuals may be asymptomatic or present with syncope, palpitations, or SCD.

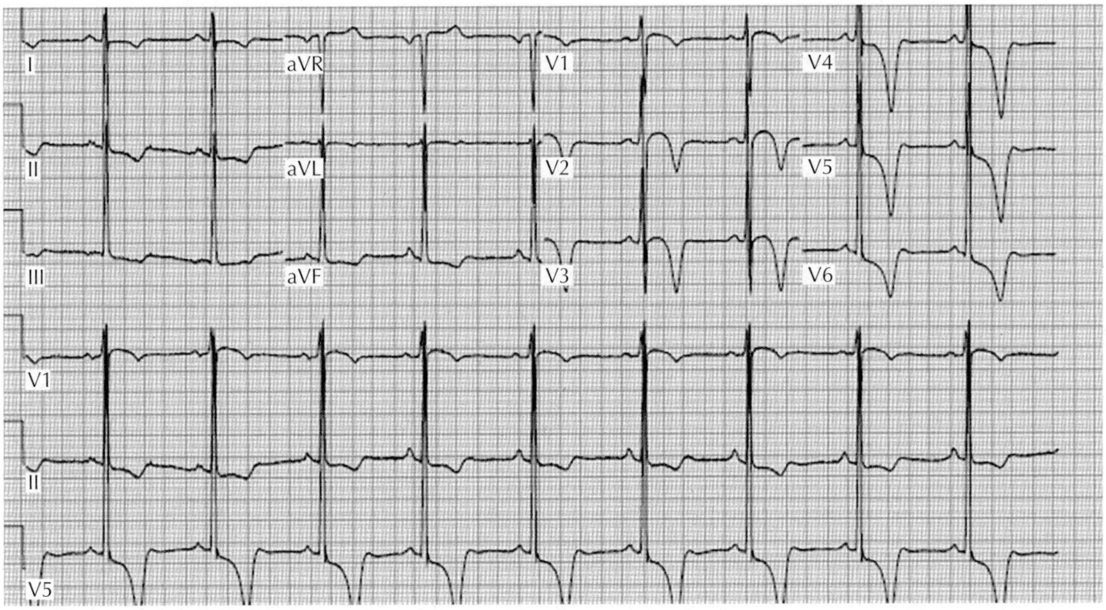
I
aVR
V1
V4
II
aVL
V2
V5
III
aVF
V3
V6
V1
II
V5

Figure 34.4 ECG from a patient with hypertrophic cardiomyopathy demonstrates deep T-wave inversion and ST-segment depression predominantly in the lateral precordial leads V_4–V_6.

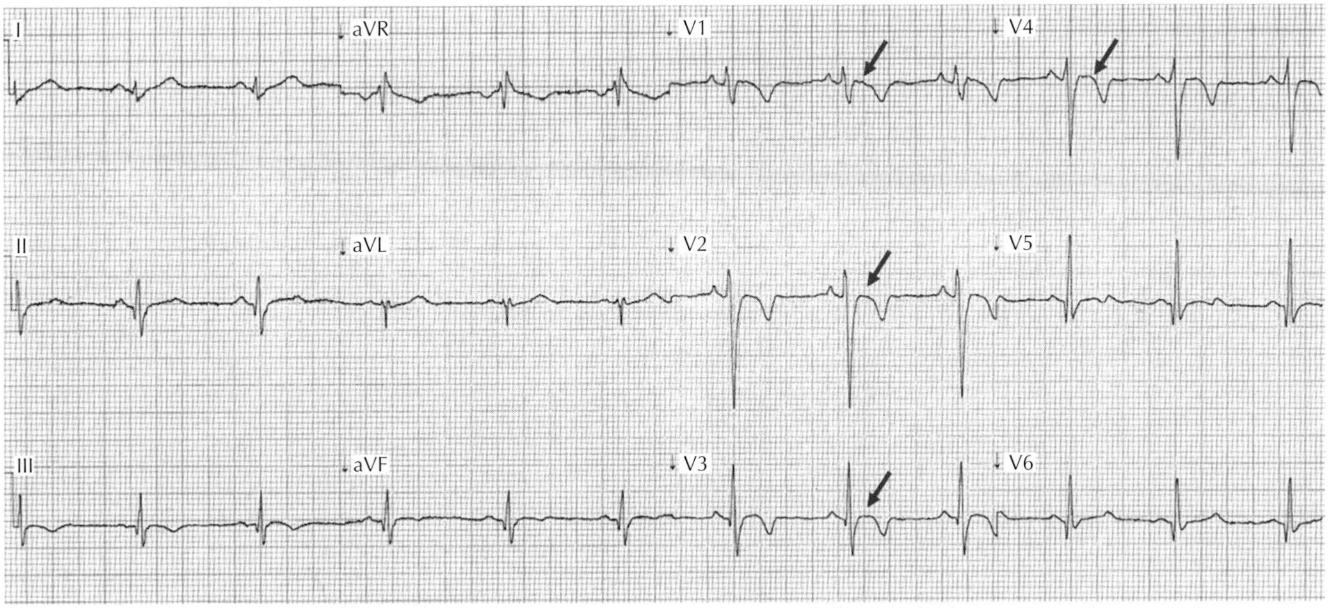
I
aVR
V1
V4
II
aVL
V2
V5
III
aVF
V3
V6

Figure 34.5 ECG with anterior T-wave inversions (V_1–V_4) preceded by a nonelevated J-point and ST segment *(red arrows)*, suggestive of AC.

- These primary electrical diseases usually exhibit detectable ECG abnormalities.

Congenital Long QT Syndrome (LQTS)

- A genetic cardiac channelopathy characterized by a prolonged QT segment, indicating a delay in ventricular repolarization, which can lead to ventricular fibrillation *(torsades de pointes)* and/or SCD.
- The three most common genotypes include:
  - LQT1 = broad T wave, triggered by exercise or emotional stress, high prevalence of SCD during swimming (Fig. 34.6).
  - LQT2 = bifid or notched T wave (i.e., V_4 or V_5), triggered by emotional stress, startling, or sudden loud sounds; also associated with pregnancy or the postpartum state.
  - LQT3 = late T wave, majority of SCD during rest or sleep.
- Significant overlap in QTc duration exists between individuals with and without LQTS.
  - Thus, a single prolonged QTc on an ECG does not equate with a diagnosis of LQTS; subsequent evaluation is needed (see later).

Catecholaminergic Polymorphic Ventricular Tachycardia (CPVT)

- An inheritable cardiac channelopathy associated with ventricular arrhythmias triggered by exercise or emotional stress.
- Arrhythmias may present as syncope or SCD.
- Resting ECG is typically normal in CPVT, so a graded exercise stress test is used for the diagnosis; should be considered in

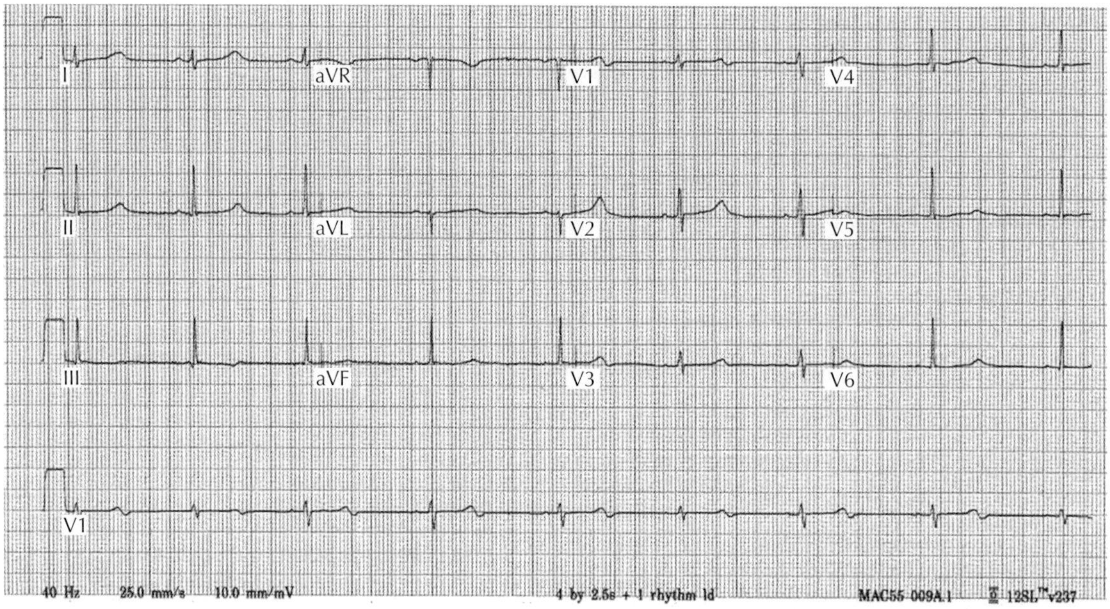
I
aVR
V1
V4
II
aVL
V2
V5
III
aVF
V3
V6
V1
40 Hz
25.0 mm/s
10.0 mm/mV

Figure 34.6 ECG from a 17-year-old female with a QTc of 525 ms and subsequently diagnosed with LQT1 syndrome.

children and adolescents who develop syncope during exercise or from emotional stress.

- Polymorphic ventricular ectopy increasing in frequency with higher-intensity activity and leading to bidirectional polymorphic ventricular tachycardia is diagnostic.
- A negative stress test does not exclude the diagnosis, and other testing, including epinephrine drug challenge or extended ambulatory ECG monitoring, should be considered when clinically suspected.

Brugada Syndrome (BrS)

- A genetic cardiac arrhythmia syndrome that predisposes to ventricular fibrillation, most commonly during rest or sleep.
- Brugada pattern is the associated ECG findings (see later) without clinical characteristics such as sustained ventricular arrhythmias, family history of SCD <45 years of age, Brugada-pattern ECG findings in first-degree relatives, and/or syncope.

Ventricular Pre-excitation/Wolff–Parkinson–White (WPW) Pattern

- Cardiac conduction abnormality wherein an accessory pathway bypasses the AV node leading to abnormal electrical conduction between the atria and the ventricle (Fig. 34.7).
- High-risk pathways allow for rapidly conducted beats to bypass the AV node, which can lead to ventricular fibrillation from 1:1 conduction in the presence of atrial tachyarrhythmias (i.e., atrial fibrillation, atrial flutter).

ECG Findings Suggestive of Primary Electrical Disease

Long QTc interval

- QTc cutoff values suggestive of LQTS: ≥470 ms in males; ≥480 ms in females (Fig. 34.6)
  - A QTc ≥500 ms is markedly prolonged and carries a greater risk of ventricular arrhythmias.
- The QT interval is affected by HR; thus, measured QT intervals are corrected to an HR of 60 bpm (QTc) using validated formulas (most commonly Bazett)
  - Bazett HR correction formula is $QTc = QT/\sqrt{RR}$ (where RR interval is measured in seconds).
  - This formula will underestimate QTc at an HR <50 bpm and overestimate at an HR >90 bpm.
- Care should be used when measuring the QT segment.
  - Lead II or V_5 usually provides the best demarcation of the end of the T wave and thus allows the most accurate measurement of the QT interval.
  - U waves should not be included in the QT measurement.
  - A straight line drawn on the downslope of the T wave to the isoelectric line should mark the end of the T wave for measurement purposes.
- Recommended follow-up:
  - Repeat ECG testing on a separate day and review for QT-prolonging medications. If repeat ECG is still abnormal, referral to a cardiologist or electrophysiologist is indicated.
    - Consider laboratory tests to exclude electrolyte abnormalities, family screening, an exercise ECG test (QT prolongation in the recovery phase), and genetic testing.

Ventricular Pre-excitation/WPW Pattern

- Short PR interval <120 ms with a delta wave (slurred upstroke in the QRS complex) and QRS ≥120 ms (Fig. 34.7).
- Additional findings associated with WPW pattern include a large Q wave in lead III, the absence of a Q wave in V_6, and ST segment depression.
- Recommended follow-up:
  - Echocardiogram to rule out associated structural conditions (Epstein anomaly, HCM).
  - Exercise ECG test for risk stratification of the accessory pathway.
    - Abrupt cessation of pre-excitation (loss of delta wave) at higher HRs suggests a low-risk pathway.
    - If pre-excitation does not resolve on a stress test, an electrophysiologic study should be considered to assess the characteristics of the bypass pathway, with possible ablation of high-risk pathways.
    - Recent evidence suggests that risk stratification by exercise stress testing can be inaccurate; thus, an electrophysiologic study can be considered in any young athlete detected with WPW.

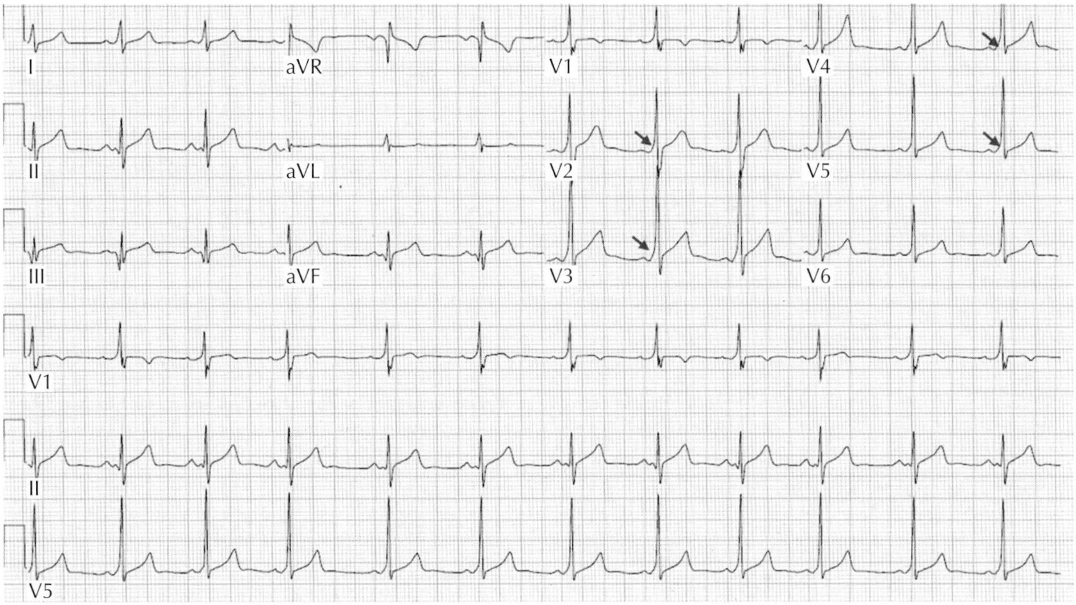
I
aVR
V1
V4
II
aVL
V2
V5
III
aVF
V3
V6
V1
II
V5

Figure 34.7 ECG demonstrating the classic findings of Wolff–Parkinson–White pattern with a short PR interval (<120 ms), delta wave with slurred QRS upstroke *(red arrows)*, and prolonged QRS (>120 ms).

Brugada Type 1 Pattern

- In the anterior precordial leads (V_1–V_3), high take-off (≥2 mm) and downsloping ST-segment elevation, followed by a negative symmetric T wave in ≥1 lead.
- Placement of the right precordial leads (V_1 and V_2) in more cranial positions (second or third intercostal spaces) can increase sensitivity in some patients because of differing anatomy of the RV outflow tract.
- Recommended follow-up: Referral to a heart rhythm specialist/electrophysiologist.

Other ECG Abnormalities

Profound Nonspecific Intraventricular Conduction Delay (IVCD)

- QRS ≥140 ms
- Disease-specific findings: Concerning for myocardial disease.
- Recommended follow-up: Echocardiogram.

Profound Sinus Bradycardia

- Resting HR <30 bpm
- Disease-specific findings: Concerning for primary sinoatrial node disease if heart rate does not appropriately respond to exercise.
- Recommended follow-up: Repeat ECG after mild aerobic activity.

Profound First-Degree Heart Block

- PR interval ≥400 ms
- Disease-specific findings: If PR does not shorten with exercise, there is a concern for primarily electrical disease or cardiomyopathy.
- Recommended follow-up: Repeat ECG after mild aerobic activity or exercise ECG test.

High-Grade AV Block

- Defined as Mobitz type II second-degree AV block or third-degree heart block.
  - Mobitz type II second-degree AV block: intermittently non-conducted P wave with a fixed PR interval.
  - Third-degree AV block (complete heart block): more P waves than QRS complexes and no association between the two; QRS complexes are regular.
- 2:1 second-degree AV block is a special category where every other P wave is not conducted and could be either of the following conditions:
  - Mobitz type I AV block (normal ECG finding in athletes).
  - Mobitz type II AV block (abnormal ECG finding in athletes).
  - To differentiate, exercise will affect AV nodal conduction, resulting in either:
    - Normal 1:1 conduction (Mobitz type I AV block).
    - Worsening conduction with 3:1, 4:1, etc., block (Mobitz type II AV block).
- Disease-specific findings: Concern for primary electrical disease or cardiomyopathy.
- Recommended follow-up: Once documented, cardiology consultation is recommended, as high-grade AV block denotes conduction disease below the AV node and often signifies the need for a permanent pacemaker. Cardiac imaging (echocardiogram ± cardiac MRI) should also be performed.

Multiple Premature Ventricular Contractions (PVCs)

- More than two PVCs per 10 seconds of ECG tracing indicates the potential for a high 24-hour PVC burden.
- Disease-specific findings
  - In athletes with >2000 PVCs in 24 hours, up to 30% have structural heart disease.
  - PVCs that suppress with exercise are usually benign.
  - It is vital to assess QRS morphology for PVCs, as certain patterns are associated with a higher risk of myocardial disease (atypical RBBB and QRS ≥130 ms or LBBB with superior-to-intermediate axis).
  - In high-dynamic athletes (e.g., cyclists, triathletes, and rowers), pathologic remodeling of the right ventricle may occur with high training volumes over a long period, leading to PVCs associated with exercise-induced AC.
- Recommended follow-up:
  - Echocardiogram, 24-hour ECG monitor, exercise ECG test.

- If >2000 PVCs on ambulatory ECG monitor, a cardiac MRI is also recommended.

Atrial Tachyarrhythmias

- Heterogeneous group of tachycardic conditions (HR >100 bpm) wherein the electrical impulse originates from the sinoatrial node, atrium, or AV node.
- Includes sinus tachycardia, supraventricular tachycardia (SVT), atrial fibrillation, and atrial flutter.
- Disease-specific findings: Can be associated with myocarditis, congenital heart disease, and any cardiomyopathy.
- Recommended follow-up: Echocardiogram, 24-hour ECG monitor, exercise ECG test, and cardiology consultation.

Ventricular Arrhythmias

- Defined as any heart rhythm originating from a ventricular focus.
- Ventricular couplets, triplets, and nonsustained ventricular tachycardia (a run of ≥3 PVCs lasting <30 seconds) do not independently predispose to SCD.
- Disease-specific findings: Can be associated with myocarditis, HCM, AC, DCM, CPVT, and myocardial infarction.
- Recommended follow-up: Initial evaluation includes an echocardiogram and 24-hour ECG monitor. Cardiac MRI should be considered.

BORDERLINE ECG FINDINGS IN ATHLETES

Introduction

- Emerging data suggest that several ECG findings previously thought to be abnormal may represent physiologic changes in athletes and are not predictive of diseases predisposing to SCD.
- These changes include complete RBBB, left and right axis deviation, and left and right atrial enlargement.
  - When these findings are found in isolation with no other ECG abnormalities or clinical markers of concern, no further evaluation is warranted.
  - However, when these findings are found in combination (≥2 borderline findings) or with other compelling personal or family history, further evaluation is warranted.
- The recommended follow-up for two or more borderline findings is an echocardiogram.

Borderline ECG Findings

- Complete RBBB: rSR′ pattern in lead V_1 and S wave wider than R wave in lead V_6 with a QRS duration of ≥120 ms
- Left axis deviation: –30 to –90 degrees
- Left atrial enlargement: Prolonged P-wave duration of >120 ms in leads I or II with the negative portion of the P wave ≥1 mm in depth and ≥40 ms in duration in lead V_1
- Right axis deviation: >120 degrees
- Right atrial enlargement: P-wave amplitude ≥2.5 mm in leads II, III, or aVF

ADDITIONAL CONSIDERATIONS

Athletes >30 Years of Age

- The most common cause of SCD in older athletes >30 years of age is atherosclerotic CAD.
- Multiple studies have demonstrated an exercise paradox where exercise can trigger SCD in individuals with occult heart disease while also illustrating that those who perform quantitatively more exercise have a lower risk of SCD.
- ECG findings that could indicate prior myocardial ischemia include:
  - Pathologic Q waves, ST-segment depression, T-wave inversion, LBBB, abnormal R-wave progression, left anterior hemiblock, and/or atrial fibrillation
- In addition to excluding the presence of cardiomyopathy for these findings, in athletes aged >30 years, stress testing or a coronary artery calcium score should be considered to evaluate for occult CAD.

Shared Decision-Making

- Current guidelines emphasize the importance of shared decision-making regarding risks of exercise and competitive sport for specific cardiac conditions and no longer support uniform and mandatory disqualification from competitive sport.
- Central to this process is patient and family education; exploring the preferences and values of the athlete; a discussion of the evidence, knowledge gaps, and risk assessment; and the risk tolerance of relevant stakeholders.
- Shared decision-making often requires multiple visits and is facilitated by building a trusting patient–physician relationship through longitudinal follow-up.

SUMMARY

- SCD is the most common cause of death in young athletes during sports and exercise.
- ECG changes are present in approximately 60% of disorders that predispose athletes to SCD.
- It is critical to accurately differentiate pathologic ECG changes from those caused by physiologic adaptations and cardiac remodeling from regular training.
- Once an ECG abnormality is identified, the appropriate further evaluation should be performed to exclude relevant cardiac pathology.
- Collaboration with a cardiologist knowledgeable about the physiologic cardiac adaptations secondary to exercise and the diseases associated with SCD in athletes is a critical component to comprehensive sports cardiology care. Shared decision-making should be employed for athletes identified with conditions predisposing to SCD.

RECOMMENDED READINGS

Available online.

CARDIAC DISEASE IN ATHLETES 35

Katie M. Edenfield • Kimberly G. Harmon

THE ATHLETE'S HEART

Definition

Intense regular physical exercise can induce physiologic and morphologic cardiac changes known as "athlete's heart." These adaptations are a normal response to repetitive exercise and training.

Physiologic Changes

- Increased vagal tone
- Morphologic changes, including left ventricular (LV) enlargement, increases in LV wall thickness, and LV mass

Pathologic vs. Physiologic Hypertrophy

- Physiologic changes that occur in response to training can be difficult to differentiate from the pathologic processes that occur in hypertrophic cardiomyopathy (HCM) (Table 35.1).
- Magnetic resonance imaging (MRI) can detect atypical patterns of hypertrophy and late gadolinium enhancement, which may be suggestive of HCM.
- If the distinction between pathologic and physiologic hypertrophy cannot be established, a period of deconditioning should be considered.

Participation Recommendations

- Athlete's heart describes normal physiologic adaptations to regular intense exercise, and thus, no treatment or limits on sports participation are required.

SUDDEN CARDIAC DEATH

Epidemiology

- Sudden cardiac death (SCD) is the leading medical cause of death in young athletes.
- Actual incidence of SCD in athletes is difficult to estimate because of the lack of a mandatory national reporting system.
- High-quality studies suggest the incidence of SCD is around 1 in 50,000 athlete-years (AY) in college and 1 in 80,000 AY in high school athletes, with some higher-risk subgroups (Table 35.2).
- Males and African Americans are at a higher risk, with men's basketball appearing to be at a disproportionately higher risk: 1 in 9000 AY.

Presentation

- The prevalence of cardiovascular disorders in young people that can lead to SCD is approximately 1 in 300.
- Most individuals with cardiovascular disorders will not experience sudden cardiac arrest (SCA) or SCD; however, athletes may be at a higher risk because increased physical activity can trigger some arrhythmias.
- SCD is the presenting symptom of underlying cardiovascular pathology in 50%–90% of athletes.
- Warning symptoms of underlying cardiovascular disease include a history of exertional chest pain, exertional syncope or presyncope, dyspnea or fatigue disproportionate to the degree of exertion, and palpitations or irregular heartbeats. Athletes with any of these symptoms require a careful workup before returning to exercise.
- A family history (FH) of sudden unexplained death or SCD before the age of 50 years or an FH of cardiac disorders known to cause SCD also warrant further diagnostic investigation before participation.

Etiology of SCD in Athletes

- Older studies in US athletes suggested HCM as the leading cause of SCD in athletes; however, these data were subject to ascertainment bias. More recent studies in National Collegiate Athletic Association (NCAA) athletes and European athletes suggest that autopsy-negative sudden unexplained death (AN-SUD) is the most common cause of death, believed to be secondary to arrhythmias or electrical disease.
- Studies in other countries and a recent meta-analysis suggest HCM may be less common as a cause of SCD (Table 35.3).
- Specialized autopsy by a cardiovascular pathologist and molecular autopsy should clarify etiologies in the future.

CAUSES OF SUDDEN CARDIAC DEATH

Structural

Hypertrophic Cardiomyopathy

Epidemiology: Reported prevalence of 1 per 500 in the general US population; however, in larger-scale screening studies of athletes, prevalence ranges between 1 in 1000 and 1 in 5000. Reported to cause 2%–36% of SCD cases in athletes (see Table 35.3).

Table 35.1 DISTINGUISHING HCM FROM ATHLETE'S HEART

HCM	Athlete's Heart
Unusual pattern of LVH, may be heterogeneous	Symmetric LVH or uniform distribution of hypertrophy
Wall thickness >16 mm	Wall thickness <12 mm
LV cavity <45 mm (small)	LV cavity >55 mm (not small)
Left atrial enlargement	No left atrial enlargement
Abnormal LV filling	Normal LV filling
ECG abnormalities (see Chapter 34: "ECG Interpretation in Athletes")	ECG with high voltage, but no Q-wave changes (see Chapter 34: "ECG Interpretation in Athletes")
Thickness does not decrease with deconditioning	LVH decreases with deconditioning
Family history of HCM	No family history of HCM
Positive genetic testing for HCM	Negative genetic testing for HCM

ECG, Electrocardiogram; *HCM,* hypertrophic cardiomyopathy; *LV,* left ventricle; *LVH,* left ventricular hypertrophy.

Table 35.2 INCIDENCE OF SUDDEN CARDIAC DEATH AND ARREST IN ATHLETES

Study	Study Design and Population	Case Identification	Denominator	Sports-Related SCD or All SCD?	SCD or All SCA/D?	Study Years	Age Range; Number of Cases	Annual Incidence
Van Camp 1996	Retrospective cohort; high school and college athletes	National Center for Catastrophic Sports Injury Research and media reports	Data from NCAA, NFHS, NAIA, and NJCAA, added together with conversion factor (1.9 for high school and 1.2 for college) used to account for multisport athletes "based on discussions with representatives from the national organizations."	Sports-related	SCD	1983–1993	13–24; N = 160	**College + High School:** Overall 1:188,000 Male 1:134,000 Female 1:752,000 **High School:** Overall 1:213,000 Male 1:152,000 Female 1:861,000 **College:** Overall 1:94,000 Male 1:69,000 Female 1:356,000
Maron 1998	Retrospective cohort; Minnesota high school athletes	Catastrophic insurance claims	Minnesota State High School League (Estimated using conversion factor of 2.3 to account for multisport athletes)	Sports-related (school-sponsored only)	SCD	1985–1997	16–17; N = 3	**High School:** Overall 1:217,000 Male 1:129,000 Female 0
Corrado 2003	Prospective cohort; athletes and nonathletes in the Veneto Region of Italy	Mandatory reporting of sudden death	Registered athletes in the Sports Medicine Database of the Veneto Region of Italy and the Italian Census Bureau	All	SCD	1979–1999	12–35; N = 51 12–35; N = 208	**Athletes:** Overall 1:47,000 Male 1:41,000 Female 1:93,000 **Nonathletes:** Overall 1:143,000
Drezner 2005	Retrospective survey; college athletes	Survey of NCAA Division I institutions (244/326 responded)	Reported number of athletes	All	SCD	2003	N = 5	**College:** Overall 1:67,000
Corrado 2006	Prospective cohort; athletes and nonathletes in the Veneto Region of Italy	Mandatory reporting to the Registry on Juvenile Sudden Death	Registered athletes in the Sports Medicine Database of the Veneto Region of Italy and the Italian Census Bureau	All	SCD	1979–2004	12–35; N = 55 12–35; N = 265	**Athletes:** 1:24,000 (prescreen) 1:233,000 (postscreen) **Nonathletes:** 1:127,000 (unscreened)
Maron 2009	Retrospective cohort; amateur and competitive athletes	US Registry for Sudden Death in Athletes	An estimated 10.7 million participants per year ≤39 years of age in all organized amateur and competitive sports	All	SCA + SCD	1980–2006	8–39; N = 1046	**Athletes:** 1:164,000
Drezner 2009	Cross-sectional survey; high school athletes	Survey of 1710 high schools with AEDs	Reported number of student athletes	All cases occurring on campus	SCA + SCD	2006–2007	14–17; N = 14	**High School:** 1:23,000 (SCA + SCD) 1:64,000 (SCD)

Holst 2010	Retrospective cohort; athletes and general population in Denmark	Review of death certificates, Cause of Death Registry, and National Patient Registry in Denmark	Interview data of people aged 16–35 years from the National Danish Health and Morbidity Study	Sports-related SCD in athletes vs. all SCD in the general population	SCD	2000–2006	12–35; N = 15 12–35; N = 428	**Athletes:** 1:83,000 **General Population:** 1:27,000
Marijon 2011	Prospective cohort; general population in France	Data from emergency medical system	General population statistics, data from the Minister of Health and Sport to estimate young competitive athlete population	Sports-related SCA or SCD with moderate or vigorous exercise	SCA + SCD	2005–2010	10–75; N = 820 10–35; N = 50	**General Population:** 1:217,000 **Young Competitive Athlete:** 1:102,000 **Young Noncompetitive Athlete:** 1:455,000
Steinvil 2011	Retrospective cohort; athletes in Israel	Retrospective review of two Israeli newspapers	Competitive athletes registered in the Israel Sport Authority in 2009; extrapolated this data for prior 24 years based on the growth of the Israeli population (age 10–40) from the Central Bureau of Statistics; allowed for a presumed doubling of the sporting population over 24 years	All	SCD	1985–2009	12–44; N = 24	**Athletes:** 1:38,000
Harmon 2011	Retrospective cohort; college athletes	Parent Heart Watch database, NCAA Resolutions list, catastrophic insurance claims	Participation data from the NCAA	All	SCD	2004–2008	18–26; N = 37	**College:** Overall 1:43,000 Male 1:33,000 Female 1:76,000 Black 1:17,000 White 1:58,000 Male, black 1: 13,000 Male, basketball 1: 7000 Male, Div. I basketball 1:3000
Maron 2013	Retrospective cohort; Minnesota high school athletes	US Registry for Sudden Death in Athletes	Minnesota State High School League statistics (Estimated using conversion factor of 2.3 to account for multisport athletes)	All	SCD	1986–2011	12–18; N = 13	**High School:** Overall 1:150,000 Male 1:83,000 Female 0
Roberts 2013	Retrospective cohort; Minnesota high school athletes	Catastrophic insurance claims	Minnesota State High School League statistics (Sum of unduplicated athletes 1993– 1994 through 2011– 2012 school years)	Sports-related (school-sponsored only)	SCD	1993–2012	12–19; N = 4	**High School:** 1:417,000 (1993–2012) 1:909,000 (2003–2012) Female 0

Continued

Table 35.2 INCIDENCE OF SUDDEN CARDIAC DEATH AND ARREST IN ATHLETES—cont'd

Study	Study Design and Population	Case Identification	Denominator	Sports-Related SCD or All SCD?	SCD or All SCA/D?	Study Years	Age Range; Number of Cases	Annual Incidence
Maron 2014	Retrospective cohort; college athletes	US Registry for Sudden Death in Athletes and NCAA resolutions list	Participation data from the NCAA	All	SCD	2002–2011	17–26; N = 64	**College:** Overall 1:63,000 Male 1:56,000 Female 1:333,000 Black 1:26,000 White 1:143,000
Toresdahl 2014	Prospective observational; high school students and student-athletes	2149 high schools monitored for SCA events on school campus	Reported number of students and student-athletes	All cases occurring on school campus	SCA + SCD	2009–2011	14–18; N = 44	**Student Athlete:** Overall 1:88,000 Male 1:58,000 Female 1:323,000 **Student Nonathlete:** Overall 1:326,000 Male 1:286,000 Female 1:357,000
Drezner 2014	Retrospective cohort; Minnesota high school athletes	Public media reports	Minnesota State High School League statistics (Sum of unduplicated athletes 2003– 2004 through 2011– 2012 school years)	All	SCA + SCD	2003–2012	14–18; N = 13	**High School:** Overall 1:71,000 Female 0 Male, basketball 1:21,000
Harmon 2014	Retrospective cohort; high school athletes from 7 states in the United States	Public media reports	Participation data from the NFHS	All	SCA + SCD	2007–2013	14–18; N = 109	**High School:** Overall 1:67,000 Male 1:45,000 Female 1:238,000 Male, basketball 1:37,000
Risgaard 2014	Retrospective cohort; competitive and noncompetitive athletes in Denmark	Review of death certificates and the Danish National Patient Registry	Competitive and noncompetitive athlete populations in Denmark estimated based on survey data from the Danish National Institute of Public Health	Sports-related SCD in competitive vs. noncompetitive athletes	SCD	2007–2009	12–35; N = 44	**Competitive Athlete:** 1:213,000 **Noncompetitive Athlete:** 1:233,000
Harmon 2015	Retrospective cohort; college athletes	Parent Heart Watch database, NCAA Resolutions list, catastrophic insurance claims	Participation data from the NCAA	All	SCD	2003–2013	17–26; N = 79	**College:** Overall 1:53,000 Male 1:38,000 Female 1:122,000 Black 1:21,000 White 1:68,000 Football 1:36,000 Male, soccer 1: 24,000 Male, black 1: 16,000 Male, basketball 1: 9000 Male, black, basketball 1: 5300 Male, Div. I basketball 1:5200

Bohm 2016	Prospective cohort; sports-related SCD in all persons in Germany	Voluntary reporting to German National Registry, web-based media search, regional institutes	Physical activity estimated from the German Health Update study and extrapolated to population data from the German Federal Statistical Office	Sports-related SCD	SCD	2012–2014	10–79; N = 144	**Sports Participants:** 1:1,200,000
Grani 2016	Retrospective; sports-related SCD in all persons in German-speaking Switzerland	Forensic reports	Physical activity estimated from survey on sports participation by the Swiss Federal Office of Sports	Sports-related SCD	SCD	1999–2010	10–39; N = 69	**Sports Participants:** Competitive: 1:90,000 Recreational: 1:192,000
Maron 2016	Retrospective cohort	Records of the Medical Examiner	Data from the Minnesota Department of Education, National Center for Education Statistics, and the Minnesota State High School League for Hennepin County, Minnesota	All	SCD	2000–2014	14–23; N = 27	**Nonathlete:** 1:39,000 **Athlete:** 1:121,000
Harmon 2016	Retrospective cohort, US high school athletes	Media reports	NFHS participation statistics	All	SCA/SCD	2007–2013	14–18; N = 104	**High School:** Overall 1:67,000 Male 1:45,00 Female 1:237,000 Male, basketball 1:37,000
Chatard 2018	Prospective, Pacific Island athletes who were screened	Prospectively followed	Defined cohort of 1450 athletes		SCD	2012–2015	10–40; N = 3	**Pacific Island Athletes:** 1:2416
Malhotra 2018	Prospective	Followed from time of screen to 2016	Defined cohort of 11,168 elite soccer athletes	All	SCD	1996–2016	15–17; N = 8	**Elite Male Soccer Athletes:** 1:14,794

Table 35.3 STUDIES OF THE ETIOLOGIES OF SUDDEN CARDIAC DEATH IN YOUNG PEOPLE

Study	Years of Study	Methods	Autopsy	Country	"Sports-Related" or All Deaths	Age Range	Cases	HCM
Corrado	1979–1999	Prospective, mandatory reporting, all deaths in Veneto region	Standard procedure at referral center	Italy	All	12–35	46	2%
De Noronha	1996–2008	All cases SCD referred to CRY	Standard procedure at referral center	UK	All	6–34	88	13%
Maron	1980–2006	Retrospective, registry, media reports	Review of available autopsy, 359 had either pathologically normal heart or autopsy unavailable	US	All—includes SCA	8–39	1049	24%
Holst	2000–2006	Retrospective, death certificates	Autopsy reports, hospital records	Denmark	Sports-related	12–35	14	0%
Suarez-Mier	1995–2010	All cases of SCD referred to National Institute of Forensic Sciences of Madrid	Standard procedure at referral center	Spain	Sports-related	9–35	81	10%
Harmon	2003–2013	Retrospective, media reports, NCAA database	Autopsy reports, ancillary reports	US	All	18–26	64	8%
Finochiaro	1994–2014	All cases SCD referred to CRY	Standard procedure at referral center	UK	All	18–35	179	8%
Bohm	2012–2014	Retrospective	Media reports, registry	Germany	Sports-related	10–34	29	7%
Harmon	2007–2013	Retrospective, media reports	Autopsy reports	US	All	14–18	50	14%
Peterson	2014–2016	Media reports, reports to NCCSIR	Autopsy reports	US	All	11–29	83	18%
Morentin	2010–2017	Retrospective	Standard procedure at referral center	Spain	Sports-related	15–24	14	14%
Thiene	1980–2015	Prospective	Standard procedure at referral center	Italy	All	<40	75	5%
Total							**1758**	**18%**

Idiopathic LVH/ Fibrosis	Coronary Artery Anomalies	ARVC	DCM	AN-SUD	CAD	Myocarditis Related	Aortic Dissection	LQTS	WPW	Other
0%	13%	26%	2%	2%	22%	11%	2%	2%	0%	17%
32%	7%	10%	0%	30%	0%	3%	0%	0%	0%	6%
5%	11%	3%	1%	34%	2%	4%	2%	2%	1%	10%
7%	7%	29%	0%	29%	14%	7%	0%	0%	0%	7%
9%	6%	15%	0%	23%	14%	5%	0%	0%	0%	19%
17%	11%	5%	3%	25%	9%	9%	5%	2%	3%	3%
14%	4%	14%	1%	44%	0%	2%	0%	0%	0%	13%
3%	10%	3%	3%	17%	21%	31%	0%	0%	0%	3%
28%	8%	2%	0%	18%	6%	14%	0%	0%	0%	12%
16%	16%	5%	5%	10%	2%	4%	6%	4%	2%	13%
21%	0%	36%	0%	0%	0%	21%	0%	0%	0%	7%
0%	16%	27%	0%	11%	23%	4%	0%	0%	0%	15%
9%	**10%**	**7%**	**1%**	**30%**	**5%**	**5%**	**2%**	**2%**	**1%**	**11%**

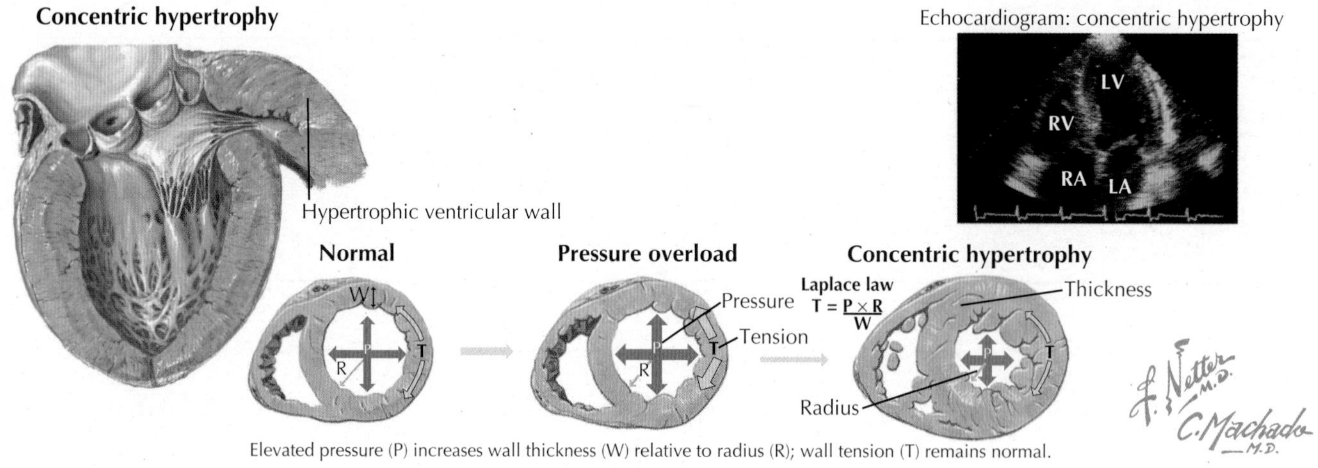

Concentric hypertrophy
Echocardiogram: concentric hypertrophy
LV
RV
RA
LA
Hypertrophic ventricular wall
Normal
Pressure overload
Concentric hypertrophy
Laplace law
T = P × R / W
Pressure
Tension
Thickness
Radius
W
R
T
P
Elevated pressure (P) increases wall thickness (W) relative to radius (R); wall tension (T) remains normal.

Figure 35.1 Left ventricular hypertrophy.

Pathologic features: Characteristic morphologic features include asymmetric LV hypertrophy (usually involving the ventricular septum), LV wall thickness of ≥16 mm (normal, ≤12 mm; borderline, 13–15 mm), septum to free wall ratio of ≥1.3, and a nondilated LV. Histologic analysis shows disorganized cellular architecture. Intramural tunneling (myocardial bridging), wherein a segment of coronary artery is completely surrounded by the myocardium, is present in approximately one-third of cases (Fig. 35.1).

Development: Genotype to phenotype positive conversion most commonly presents between 12 and 20 years of age, at the time of substantial LV remodeling during accelerated body growth, supporting interval cardiac screening in this age group.

Symptoms: SCA is the presenting symptom in 80% of cases. Symptoms may include exertional chest pain, dyspnea, lightheadedness, or syncope.

Physical examination (PE) findings: Frequently normal; but if an outflow tract obstruction exists, a systolic murmur may be heard best at the left lateral sternal border in positions that decrease preload (squat-to-stand or Valsalva maneuver). This emphasizes the importance of dynamic cardiac auscultation.

Diagnostic tests: Electrocardiogram (ECG) is *abnormal* in up to 95% of athletes with HCM. The most common finding is T-wave inversions (TWIs) in the lateral leads. ST-segment depression, pathologic Q waves, and left bundle branch block (LBBB) are also seen. MRI is the standard to confirm septal thickness (≥16 mm) and can identify segmental hypertrophy in the anterolateral LV free wall or at the apex. An MRI can also confirm myocardial fibrosis and late gadolinium enhancement, which may have prognostic value. Echocardiogram can identify septal thickness and diastolic dysfunction but is more difficult to assess the apex and right ventricle. If ECG is markedly abnormal, MRI should always be obtained. Seventy percent of mutations are in two genes: β-myosin heavy chain *(MYH7)* and myosin-binding protein C *(MYBPC3)*.

Return to play (RTP): Risk for sudden death in the genotype-positive/phenotype-negative HCM population appears very low, and participation in competitive athletics is reasonable for this population. Intense exertion increases the risk of ventricular tachycardia/fibrillation by acting as an arrhythmogenic substrate and is a modifiable risk factor in phenotype-positive HCM patients. Participation in athletics should involve a shared decision-making process with involved parties, including the athlete, their family, consulting cardiologist, and if applicable, team physicians and additional cardiologists.

Congenital Coronary Anomalies (CCAs)

Epidemiology: CCAs account for 6%–17% of cases of SCD in athletes (see Table 35.3).

Pathologic features: Most common CCA is an abnormal origin of the left main coronary artery arising from the right sinus of Valsalva. Other features that may contribute to ischemia during exercise include an acute angled take-off, hypoplastic ostium, or impingement of the anomalous artery as it traverses between the expanding great vessels during exercise (Fig. 35.2).

Symptoms: Chest pain, exertional syncope, and SCA

PE findings: None

Diagnostic tests: ECG does not typically identify CCAs. Echocardiogram can identify CCAs of coronary artery origin in 80%–97% of patients. Advanced cardiac imaging such as computed tomography angiography (CTA), magnetic resonance angiography (MRA), or coronary angiography may be necessary.

RTP: Detection should result in exclusion from all competitive sports, pending surgical repair. Participation may be considered 3 months after correction of the defect if patient remains symptom free and has a normal maximal exercise test.

Myocarditis

Epidemiology: Acute inflammatory process involving the myocardium associated with cardiac dysfunction; both infectious and noninfectious etiologies. Coxsackie B virus is implicated in more than 50% of cases, but echovirus, adenovirus, influenza, *Chlamydia pneumoniae*, and coronavirus, including COVID-19, have also been associated with myocarditis. Early studies examining the incidence of myocarditis in athletes after COVID-19 infection demonstrated a 0.7% and 0.6% incidence in a cohort of NCAA (n = 3018) and professional (n = 789) athletes, respectively. Myocarditis has been reported as the cause of death in 3%–13% in studies on SCD in athletes (see Table 35.3).

Pathologic features: Lymphocytic infiltrate of myocardium with necrosis or degeneration of adjacent myocytes. Acute phase presents with flulike illness, which may lead to dilated cardiomyopathy. SCD may occur in the presence of active or healed myocarditis (Fig. 35.3).

Symptoms: Characteristic symptoms include a prodromal viral illness, followed by angina-type chest pain or progressive exercise intolerance and heart failure symptoms of dyspnea, cough, and orthopnea.

PE findings: May be normal or have S_3 gallop and signs of heart failure (e.g., edema and pulmonary rales)

Diagnostic tests: ECG may show diffuse low voltage, ST and T wave changes, heart block, or ventricular arrhythmias (see Chapter 34:

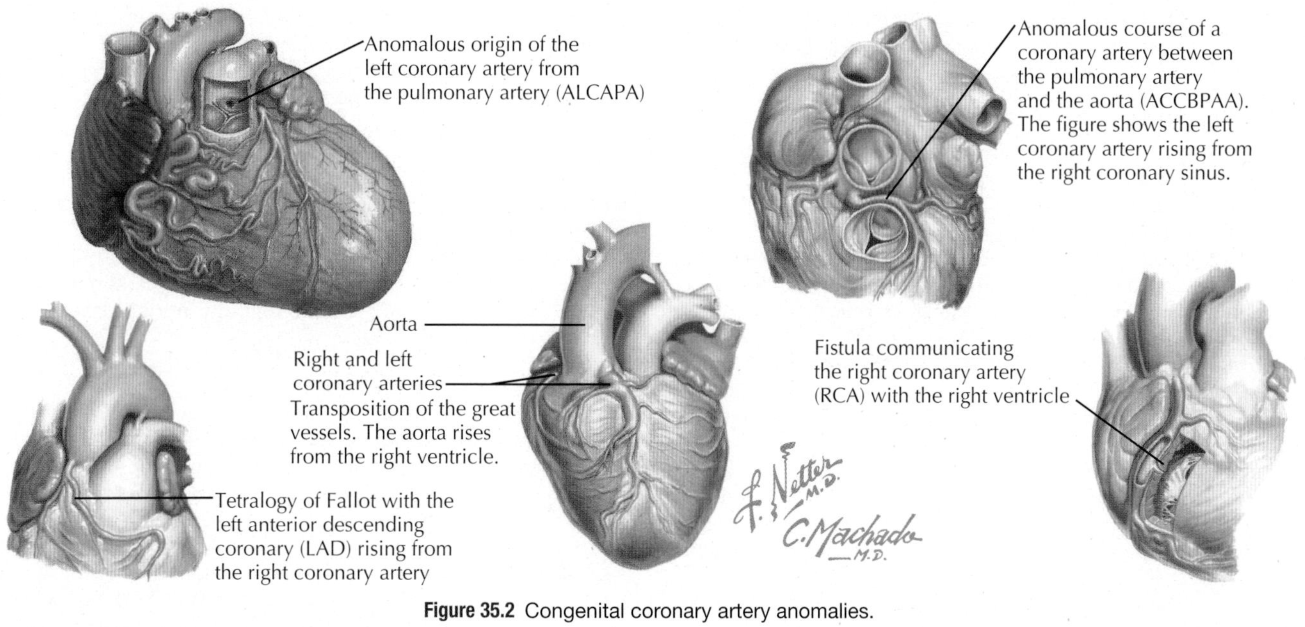

Anomalous origin of the left coronary artery from the pulmonary artery (ALCAPA)
Anomalous course of a coronary artery between the pulmonary artery and the aorta (ACCBPAA). The figure shows the left coronary artery rising from the right coronary sinus.
Aorta
Right and left coronary arteries
Transposition of the great vessels. The aorta rises from the right ventricle.
Fistula communicating the right coronary artery (RCA) with the right ventricle
Tetralogy of Fallot with the left anterior descending coronary (LAD) rising from the right coronary artery
F. Netter M.D.
C. Machado M.D.

Figure 35.2 Congenital coronary artery anomalies.

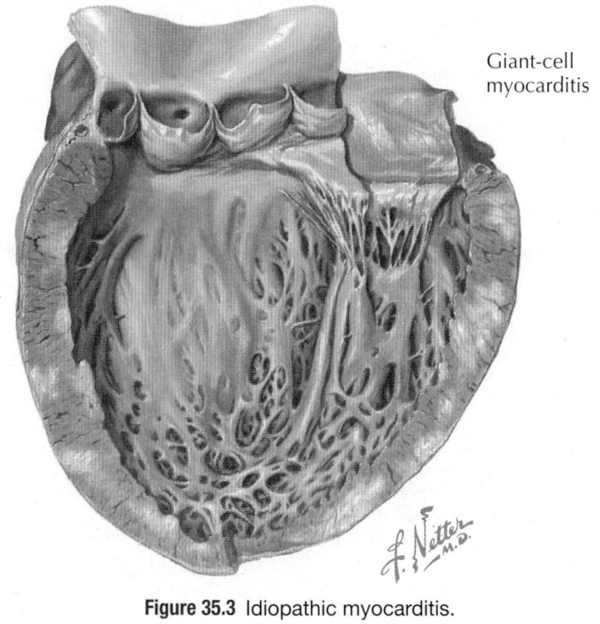

Giant-cell myocarditis
F. Netter M.D.

Figure 35.3 Idiopathic myocarditis.

"ECG Interpretation in Athletes"). Laboratory tests may show elevated myocardial enzymes (most commonly high-sensitivity troponins), a leukocytosis, eosinophilia, elevated sedimentation rate, or C-reactive protein. Echocardiography may show dilated LV, global hypokinesis, segmental wall abnormalities, decreased LV ejection fraction, and a pericardial effusion. Cardiac MRI may show regional increase in water content on T2 weighted images and epicardial or midmyocardial late gadolinium enhancement.

RTP: Athletes with definitive or probable myocarditis should not compete. Resolution is variable, but return to sport should not be considered before 3–6 months after the onset of the illness. The athlete may return to competitive sports if ventricular systolic function has returned to normal, serum markers of myocardial injury have normalized, and clinically relevant arrhythmias are absent.

Arrhythmogenic Right Ventricular Cardiomyopathy (ARVC)

Epidemiology: Estimated prevalence 1 case per 5000 population; based on previous studies, ARVC accounts for 3%–27% of SCD in athletes (see Table 35.3).

Pathologic features: Progressive fibrofatty replacement of the right ventricular myocardium causing wall thinning and right ventricular dilatation.

Symptoms: May present with syncope, chest pain, palpitations, or SCA.

PE findings: Normal

Diagnostic tests: Diagnosed by meeting a combination of "major" and "minor" criteria involving ECG abnormalities, including inverted T waves in the right precordial leads; echocardiogram or cardiac MRI abnormalities (e.g., right ventricular dilatation and wall thinning, reduced right ventricular ejection fraction, right ventricle wall motion abnormalities, or right ventricular aneurysms); abnormal myocardial biopsy; FH; and documented arrhythmias.

RTP: No competitive athletics because exercise contributes to disease progression and arrhythmogenic risk. SCD frequently occurs during exertion in ARVC. Although there is a trend toward shared decision-making in most other cardiac conditions, there is near-universal agreement that those with ARVC should not exercise.

Left Ventricular Noncompaction

Epidemiology: True prevalence not known in general population due to relatively recent recognition and lack of agreement on criteria for diagnosis; but has been observed at 0.014% to 1.3% of patients undergoing echocardiography and 3% to 4% of patients with heart failure.

Pathologic features: Prominent trabeculae and deep intertrabecular recesses, resulting in a thickened myocardium, with continuity between the left ventricular cavity and the deep intertrabecular recesses.

Symptoms: May present with dyspnea, heart failure, palpitations, chest pain, presyncope or syncope.

PE findings: May be normal, or could be signs of heart failure if present.

Diagnostic tests: Transthoracic echocardiography identifying specific morphologic diagnosis criteria, most often the Jenni criteria, which includes a ratio of noncompacted to compacted myocardium >2:1 at end-systole. Cardiac MRI also provides additional structural details.

RTP: Asymptomatic athletes with normal systolic function and without relevant tachyarrhythmias may be considered for competitive sports until more clinical information is available. Athletes with impaired systolic function, relevant tachyarrhythmias, should not participate in competitive sports with the possible exception of class 1A sports, unless further clinical information becomes available.

Dilated Cardiomyopathy (DCM)

Epidemiology: Estimated prevalence is 1 case per 2500 population. DCM is a less common cause of SCD in athletes, attributed to 0%–8% of cases (see Table 35.3).

Pathologic features: LV dilatation and systolic dysfunction with normal LV wall thickness; secondary DCM results from prolonged untreated systemic hypertension, ischemic heart disease, viral myocarditis, infiltrative diseases (e.g., sarcoidosis, amyloidosis, hemochromatosis), autoimmune illnesses, or toxins (e.g., ethanol).

Symptoms: Progressive exertional intolerance, dyspnea, orthopnea, fatigue, and edema

PE findings: S_3 or S_4 may occur; holosystolic murmur suggestive of mitral regurgitation

Diagnostic tests: ECG and Holter monitoring may show supraventricular and ventricular tachyarrhythmias in addition to major conduction delays (e.g., bundle branch block and atrioventricular [AV] block). Echocardiogram diagnostic, demonstrating a dilated LV with reduced ejection fraction.

RTP: Athletes with DCM should be excluded from all competitive sports, with possible exception of low-intensity sports.

Aortic Rupture/Marfan Syndrome

Epidemiology: Reported incidence for Marfan syndrome is 1 in 5000–10,000 individuals.

Pathologic features: Multisystem disorder of connective tissue, with cardiovascular manifestations as a major cause of morbidity and mortality. Progressive dilatation and weakness (cystic medial necrosis) of proximal aorta and myxomatous degeneration of mitral and aortic valves leading to valvular dysfunction and possible aortic dissection.

Symptoms: Aortic root dissection symptoms include chest and thoracic pain. Heart failure may also occur secondary to aortic valve incompetence.

PE findings: Highly variable clinical features usually manifested in adolescence and young adulthood; diagnosis of Marfan syndrome is most commonly based on the 2010 revised Ghent Criteria. These criteria rely on the presence or absence of family history, physical examination, imaging of the aorta, and in some cases, genetic testing (Table 35.4).

Diagnostic tests: Echocardiogram is diagnostic for aortic root dilatation and aortic regurgitation. Slit-light ophthalmologic examination for ectopia lentis and lumbosacral MRI or computed tomography (CT) for dural ectasia.

RTP: Based on aortic root dimension and pathologic features of the disease. RTP recommendations should be guided by risk assessment performed by a specialist familiar with aortic root pathology.

Atherosclerotic Coronary Artery Disease

Epidemiology: The most frequent cause of SCD in athletes over the age of 30 years. The incidence of exercise-related sudden death in adults is 1 in 15,000–18,000.

Pathologic features: Most often caused by atherosclerotic plaque disruption; exercise may be a stimulus for plaque disruption. Development is progressive and related to coronary risk factors (hypertension, diabetes, dyslipidemia, tobacco use, illicit drug use, and FH of premature atherosclerotic disease).

Symptoms: Exertional chest pain, angina, lightheadedness, palpitations, or SCD

PE findings: No specific cardiac findings

Diagnostic tests: ECG may show evidence of prior ischemia. Exercise stress testing may show ST-segment depression or U-wave inversion. Stress echo may show wall motion abnormality, and cardiac CT, MRI, or angiography will show extent of coronary artery narrowing.

RTP: Dependent on extent of disease, symptoms, and stability after medical management, percutaneous coronary interventions, or surgery; RTP recommendations often guided by risk assessment and management by a specialist.

Primary Electrical Disease

Channelopathies: Diseases predisposing to potentially lethal ventricular tachyarrhythmias characterized by mutations in ion-channel proteins leading to dysfunctional sodium, potassium, calcium, and other ion transport across cell membranes. Likely that many deaths with a pathologically normal heart are the result of channelopathies.

Long QT Syndrome (LQTS)

Epidemiology: The most common ion channelopathy.

Pathologic features: Characterized by prolongation of ventricular repolarization and QT interval corrected for heart rate (QT_c); there are six defined types, with three of them (LQTS-1, LQTS-2, and LQTS-3) occurring more frequently.

Symptoms: LQTS-1: syncope or presyncope related to physical exertion, especially swimming, or emotional stress; LQTS-2: syncope or presyncope triggered by emotional stressors, sleep, and auditory events (loud noises); LQTS-3: most susceptible to events during sleep.

Diagnostic tests: In an asymptomatic athlete without FH of SCD, current cutoff values for a prolonged QT_c is 470 ms in males and 480 ms in females. Must rule out other causes of QT prolongation (i.e., medications) and be demonstrated on repeat ECGs.

Table 35.4 REVISED GHENT CRITERIA FOR THE DIAGNOSIS OF MARFAN SYNDROME (MFS) AND RELATED CONDITIONS

In the Absence of Family History:
1. Aortic root diameter (Z-score 2) and ectopia lentis = MFS[a]
2. Aortic root diameter (Z-score 2) and causal FBN1 mutation = MFS
3. Aortic root diameter (Z-score 2) and systemic score 7 points = MFS[a]
4. Ectopia lentis and causal FBN1 mutation with known aortic root dilatation = MFS
In the Presence of Family History:
5. Ectopia lentis and family history of MFS = MFS
6. Systemic score 7 points and family history of MFS = MFS[a]
7. Aortic root diameter (Z-score 2 above 20 years old, 3 below 20 years) and family history of MFS = MFS[a]
Scoring of Systemic Features of MFS
1. Wrist AND thumb sign –3 points (wrist OR thumb sign –1 point)
2. Pectus carinatum deformity –2 points (pectus excavatum or chest asymmetry –1 point)
3. Hindfoot deformity –2 points (plain pes planus –1 point)
4. Protrusio acetabuli –2 points
5. Reduced upper segment/lower segment ratio AND increased arm/height AND no severe scoliosis –1 point
6. Scoliosis or thoracolumbar kyphosis –1 point
7. Reduced elbow extension –1 point
8. Facial features (3/5) –1 point (dolichocephaly, enophthalmos, downslanting palpebral fissures, malar hypoplasia, retrognathia)
9. Skin striae –1 point
10. Myopia > 3 diopters –1 point
11. Mitral valve prolapse (all types) –1 point
12. Pneumothorax –2 points
13. Dural ectasia –2 points

[a]Caveat: Without discriminating features of Shprintzen-Goldberg syndrome, Loeys-Dietz syndrome, or vascular form of Ehlers-Danlos syndrome AND after TGFBR1/2, collagen biochemistry, COL3A1 testing if indicated.

RTP and treatment: Guided by a heart rhythm specialist or a genetic cardiologist experienced in the care of athletes. Competitive sports participation may be considered after implementation of treatment for at least 3 months and appropriate precautionary measures with informed shared-decision making.

Short QT Syndrome (SQTS)

Epidemiology: SQTS recently described (in 2000)
Pathologic features: Hyperfunctioning of potassium channel
Symptoms: Palpitations, syncope, atrial fibrillation, and SCA/SCD
Diagnostic tests: ECG changes include a QT_c interval <340 ms and tall peaked T waves.
RTP and treatment: Sports participation may be considered, assuming appropriate precautionary measures and disease-specific treatments are in place and the athlete has been asymptomatic on treatment for at least 3 months.

Brugada Syndrome

Epidemiology: First described in 1992. It is a rare channelopathy that is more prevalent in males from Southeast Asia.
Pathologic features: Abnormalities of sodium channels
Symptoms: Syncope, SCA/SCD, and sudden death during sleep
Diagnostic tests: ECG shows a pattern of right bundle branch block and ST-segment elevation in leads V_1–V_3. ECG patterns may not be present unless "unmasked" with the administration of sodium-channel blockers (e.g., flecainide or procainamide) (see Chapter 34: "ECG Interpretation in Athletes").
RTP and treatment: Sports participation may be considered, assuming appropriate precautionary measures and disease-specific treatments are in place and the athlete has been asymptomatic on treatment for at least 3 months.

Catecholaminergic Polymorphic Ventricular Tachycardia (CPVT)

Epidemiology: A familial disorder characterized by stress-induced ventricular arrhythmias that result in SCD in children and young adults.
Pathologic features: Abnormalities in calcium channel function
Symptoms: Syncope, sudden death, and polymorphic ventricular tachycardia triggered by vigorous physical exertion or acute emotion
Diagnostic tests: Resting ECG is normal, although certain patients will have prominent U waves. Exertion or epinephrine challenge can induce ventricular tachycardia.
RTP: Athletes with CPVT should not participate in competitive sports.

Wolff–Parkinson–White (WPW) Syndrome

Epidemiology: Approximately 1% of ECGs will show changes consistent with WPW syndrome; however, only a small subset will go on to develop the associated arrhythmias that define the syndrome. Risk of SCD in WPW is estimated as 1 per 1000 patient-years.
Pathologic features: A tachyarrhythmia caused by an accessory pathway (the bundle of Kent) that directly connects the atria and ventricles and bypasses the AV node; the arrhythmia can be AV tachycardia (80%), atrial fibrillation (15%–20%), or atrial flutter (5%) (Fig. 35.4). SCD occurs when atrial fibrillation and atrial flutter are rapidly conducted to the ventricle by the accessory pathway, triggering ventricular fibrillation.
Symptoms: Palpitations, syncope, and near-syncope
Diagnostic tests: ECG shows characteristic changes (see Chapter 34: "ECG Interpretation in Athletes"); once diagnosed, exercise stress testing can be considered, as can electrophysiology studies.

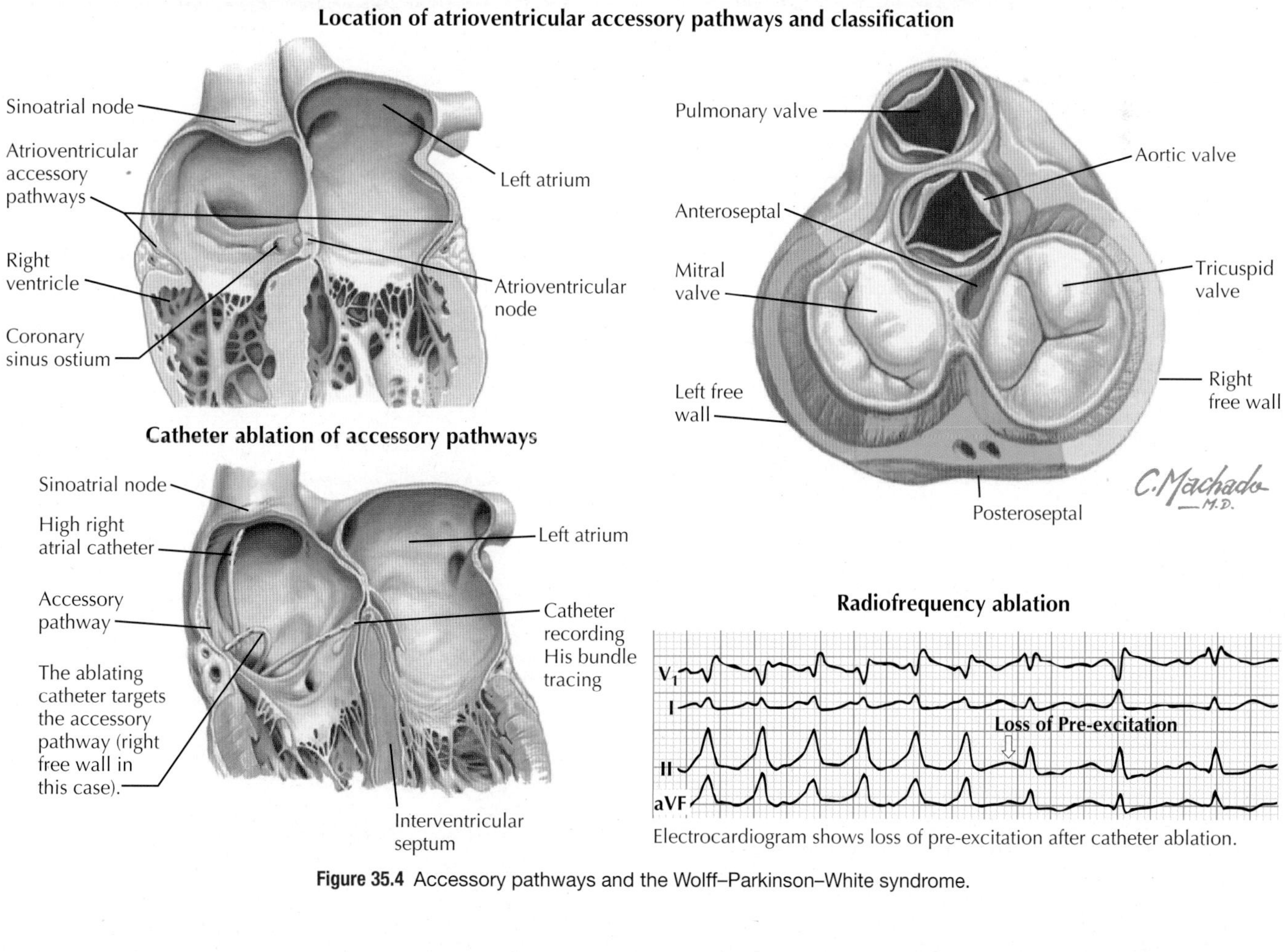
Location of atrioventricular accessory pathways and classification
Sinoatrial node
Atrioventricular accessory pathways
Right ventricle
Coronary sinus ostium
Left atrium
Atrioventricular node
Pulmonary valve
Aortic valve
Anteroseptal
Mitral valve
Tricuspid valve
Left free wall
Right free wall
Posteroseptal
C. Machado — M.D.
Catheter ablation of accessory pathways
Sinoatrial node
High right atrial catheter
Accessory pathway
The ablating catheter targets the accessory pathway (right free wall in this case).
Left atrium
Catheter recording His bundle tracing
Interventricular septum
Radiofrequency ablation
V1
I
II
aVF
Loss of Pre-excitation
Electrocardiogram shows loss of pre-excitation after catheter ablation.

Figure 35.4 Accessory pathways and the Wolff–Parkinson–White syndrome.

RTP and treatment: There is a trend toward ablation for all pathways, including in asymptomatic athletes and athletes who have pathways that would have previously been classified as "low risk." RTP after an ablation can usually occur within 1 week.

Traumatic

Commotio Cordis

Epidemiology: Commotio cordis occurs in a **structurally normal heart** after the chest wall is struck with a blunt object. If the blow is sustained at a vulnerable phase of ventricular repolarization (just before peak of T wave), it can lead to ventricular fibrillation. More than 80% of cases involve sports with a firm projectile (e.g., baseball, softball, hockey puck, and lacrosse ball). Attempts to prevent commotio cordis include the use of chest protectors and "safety balls." In animal model studies, chest protectors have not decreased the incidence of arrhythmia, whereas the use of "safety balls" has been associated with a lower incidence of arrhythmia. Other preventive measures include educating athletes, coaches, and caregivers regarding the presentation of commotio cordis, especially in sports that include projectiles; avoiding "shot blocking" in sports such as lacrosse and ice hockey; and an emergency action plan (EAP) that includes early access to defibrillation.

Pathologic features: Structurally normal heart

Symptoms: Collapse immediately after a blow to the chest. In approximately half of cases, a brief period (10 seconds) of consciousness occurs before the collapse.

RTP and treatment: Treatment is expedient defibrillation. Survival is possible with early defibrillation, with survival rates of 25% if resuscitation is initiated within 3 minutes from collapse, and only a 3% survival if resuscitation is initiated later than 3 minutes after collapse. No limits to RTP, as heart is otherwise normal.

ATHLETES WITH SUSPECTED OR KNOWN CARDIOVASCULAR DISEASE

Recognition and Evaluation of Worrisome Symptoms

- Twenty to fifty percent of athletes with SCD have had prior symptoms. Many consulted providers and were reassured.
- Exertional syncope is *always* alarming and should be thoroughly investigated.
  - ECG will detect HCM 95% of the time and also screens for LQTS, SQTS, Brugada syndrome, and pre-excitation syndromes. Other diseases that may cause changes in the ECG (myocarditis) can also be detected.
  - Echocardiogram is useful in evaluation of HCM, coronary artery anomalies, structural heart disease, and aortic root dilatation.
  - Exercise stress testing may uncover exertional arrhythmias, channelopathies, or ischemia secondary to coronary artery disease or anomalies.
  - Holter monitor or event monitor may also identify arrhythmias.
  - Cardiac MRI or CT may show structural abnormalities such as coronary artery anomalies, ARVC, or apical-variant HCM.
  - Electrophysiology studies may identify inducible arrhythmias or re-entrant pathways.
  - Tilt table testing may provide supporting evidence that syncope occurred because of hemodynamic changes (neurocardiogenic syncope).
- Consultation with a specialist is recommended if a cardiac abnormality is suspected or identified.
- Athletes should be restricted from sports participation until the diagnostic workup is complete.

Athletes With Cardiovascular Disease

- When athletes are identified with cardiac diseases that place them at a risk for SCA or disease progression, the question of advisable athletic activities is complex. Exercise is a known trigger for SCD because of increased catecholamine levels. Activity recommendations have evolved from strict disqualification decisions made by the treating physician to a model of shared decision-making by considering a myriad of factors.
- Detailed eligibility and disqualification recommendations have been published in a scientific statement from the American Heart Association and American College of Cardiology.

Legal Considerations

Restriction of participation: An institution has a right to restrict an individual from participation as long as that restriction is based on objective medical evidence and supported by the team physician and institutional medical consultants. Decision regarding medical eligibility to play may differ between institutions.

EMERGENCY PREPAREDNESS AND MANAGEMENT OF SCA

Emergency Action Plan

- Every school or institution that sponsors athletic activities should have a written and structured EAP that is reviewed and practiced at least annually by all potential responders to an SCA.
- The EAP should be developed in concert with local emergency medical services (EMS), school safety officials, likely first responders, and school administrators.
- The EAP should be specific to each individual athletic venue and provide plans for:
  - **Communication:** A system should be in place to activate the EMS system and to alert local/school responders and expedite transfer of emergency equipment (e.g., automated external defibrillator [AED]) to the scene.
  - **Personnel:** An identified team of targeted first responders (e.g., coaches and school health officials) should receive training in the recognition of SCA, cardiopulmonary resuscitation (CPR), and AED use.
  - **Equipment:** On-site AED programs are strongly encouraged and are likely the only means of achieving early defibrillation in the athletic setting.
  - **Transportation:** Routes for arriving EMS should be defined in addition to transport to an identified hospital with advanced cardiac life support services.
- The target time interval from collapse to first shock should be *less than 3 minutes.*

Management of SCA

- Initial management of SCA should include early activation of EMS, CPR, defibrillation, and transition to advanced cardiac life support.
- Approximately 50% of athletes with SCA have brief myoclonic or seizure-like activity that should not be mistaken for a seizure.
- Agonal respirations or gasping and inaccurate rescuer assessment of pulse can also delay recognition of SCA.
- **SCA should be suspected in any collapsed and unresponsive athlete,** and an AED should be applied as soon as possible.
- Commotio cordis should be suspected in any collapsed athlete who has been struck in the chest.
- CPR should be performed while waiting for an AED. "Hands-only" CPR is currently recommended for lay responders.

RECOMMENDED READINGS

Available online.

THE HYPERTENSIVE ATHLETE 36

Mark W. Niedfeldt • Leon Y. Cheng

GENERAL PRINCIPLES

- An estimated 108 million Americans over the age of 18 years have hypertension (HTN).
- HTN is the most common cardiovascular condition observed in competitive athletes.
- Athletes are usually considered to be free from cardiovascular disease because of their apparent high level of fitness.
  - The overall incidence of HTN in athletes is approximately 50% less than that in the general population.
- HTN begins in young adulthood; incidence increases with age
  - Almost 80% of adolescents with an elevated blood pressure (BP) (>142/92 mmHg) during preparticipation physical examinations have HTN.

DEFINITION AND STAGING OF HYPERTENSION (2017 ACC/AHA/AAPA/ABC/ACPM/AGS/APHA/ASH/ASPC/NMA/PCNA GUIDELINE)

- Normal BP: Systolic <120 mmHg and diastolic <80 mmHg
- Elevated BP: Systolic 120–129 mmHg and diastolic <80 mmHg
- HTN:
  - Stage 1: Systolic 130–139 mmHg or diastolic 80–89 mmHg
  - Stage 2: Systolic ≥140 mmHg or diastolic ≥90 mmHg
- If there is a disparity in category between systolic and diastolic pressures, the higher value determines stage (Table 36.1)
- **Stage 1: systolic 130–139 mmHg or diastolic 80–89 mmHg**
  - Associated with increased cardiac output (CO), which primarily increases systolic BP, along with "normal" vascular total peripheral resistance (TPR)
  - TPR is normal compared with resting levels in normotensives but inappropriately high when CO is elevated.
    - In nonhypertensive patient, TPR falls to compensate for rise in CO, thereby maintaining normal BP.
    - Lack of decrease in TPR is result of impaired baroreceptor function.
    - Baroreceptors are "reset" to maintain elevated rather than normal BP over time.
  - People with stage 1 HTN are hypersensitive to catecholamine secretion and mental stress and have a hyperkinetic circulatory state.
- **Stage 2:**
  - **Systolic BP 140–159 mmHg and diastolic BP 90–99 mmHg**
    - Increased heart rate (HR) and CO and decreased TPR
    - Decreased arterial lumen and disturbed autoregulation of peripheral blood flow
  - **Systolic BP >160 mmHg and diastolic BP >100 mmHg**
    - Normal HR and CO; increased TPR
      - Increased afterload leads to left ventricular hypertrophy (LVH) and increased diastolic BP. Severe and/or uncontrolled HTN may lead to development of diastolic dysfunction and congestive heart failure (CHF).
      - CO can no longer increase in response to exercise or other physiologic demands.
      - Loss of contractility and CHF may develop.
- Most active individuals with HTN will fall into stage 1 or lower stage 2 (<160 mmHg/<100 mmHg).
- Those with comorbidities, such as diabetes or renal disease, should be treated at stage 1 levels.
- Values for pediatric athletes under age 13 are adjusted for age, gender, and height (Table 36.2).
- Higher stages are associated with a higher risk of nonfatal and fatal cardiovascular disease in addition to progressive renal disease (Fig. 36.1).

CLINICAL PATHOPHYSIOLOGY OF HYPERTENSION

Primary Hypertension

- Ninety-five percent of cases
- Abnormal neuroreflexes and sympathetic control of peripheral resistance
- Abnormal renal and metabolic control of vascular volume and compliance
  - Abnormal local smooth muscle and endothelial control of vascular resistance
  - Sustained increases in systemic vascular resistance (SVR)

Secondary Hypertension

- Five percent of cases
- Younger patients or adults with rapid onset of HTN and no prior history of HTN
- BP is often poorly responsive to routine therapy.

Causes (Fig. 36.2)

- **Renal (most common)**
  - Renovascular disease
    - Increased renin stimulates conversion of angiotensin I to angiotensin II, which is a vasoconstrictor, in addition to release of aldosterone
    - Renal retention of sodium and water
    - Fibromuscular dysplasia in younger patients and atherosclerosis in older patients
  - Renal parenchymal disease
    - Inability of damaged kidneys to excrete sodium and water
- **Endocrine**
  - Adrenal
    - Pheochromocytoma
    - Cushing syndrome
    - Primary aldosteronism
  - Thyroid
    - Hyperthyroidism
    - Hypothyroidism
  - Acromegaly
  - Hyperparathyroidism
- **Other**
  - Coarctation of the aorta
  - Obstructive sleep apnea

RISK FACTORS FOR HYPERTENSION

- **Age**
  - Five to ten percent in adults aged 20–30 years
  - Twenty to thirty-five percent in middle-aged adults
  - More than 50% in adults aged over 60 years
  - Residual lifetime risk of 90%
- **Genetic factors**
  - Males more than females
  - African Americans more than Caucasians (2:1); Asians lowest risk

Table 36.1 CLASSIFICATION OF HYPERTENSION

	Systolic (mmHg)	Diastolic (mmHg)
Normal	<120	<80
Elevated blood pressure	120–129	<80
Hypertension		
Hypertension: Stage 1	130–139	80–89
Hypertension: Stage 2	≥140	≥90

Classification of blood pressure (BP) for adults aged ≥18 years. The classification is based on the mean of two or more appropriately measured seated BP readings on each of three or more office visits. In contrast with the classification provided in the JNC 7 report, a new category designated "elevated blood pressure" is combined with stage 1 hypertension to replace the prehypertension category. All blood pressures over 140 mmHg systolic or 90 mmHg diastolic are considered stage 2 hypertension. If there is a disparity in category between the systolic and diastolic pressures, the higher value determines the stage.

Whelton PK, Carey RM, Aronow WS, et al. 2017 ACC/AHA/AAPA/ABC/ACPM/AGS/APhA/ASH/ASPC/NMA/PCNA guideline for the prevention, detection, evaluation, and management of high blood pressure in adults: executive summary: a report of the American College of Cardiology/American Heart Association Task Force on clinical practice guidelines. *J Am Coll Cardiol*. 2018;71(19):2199–2269. Erratum in: *J Am Coll Cardiol*. 2018;71(19):2273–2275, Table 6, Page 2209.

Table 36.2 2017 AMERICAN ACADEMY OF PEDIATRICS UPDATED DEFINITIONS FOR PEDIATRIC BLOOD PRESSURE CATEGORIES

	For Children Aged 1 to <13 Years	For Children Aged ≥13 Years
Normal BP	Systolic and diastolic BP <90th percentile	Systolic BP <120 and diastolic BP <80 mmHg
Elevated BP	Systolic and diastolic BP ≥90th percentile to <95th percentile or 120/80 mmHg to <95th percentile (whichever is lower)	Systolic BP 120–129 and diastolic BP <80 mmHg
Stage 1 HTN	Systolic and diastolic BP ≥95th percentile to <95th percentile + 12 mmHg or 130/80—139/89 mmHg (whichever is lower)	130/80–139/89 mmHg
Stage 2 HTN	Systolic and diastolic BP ≥95th percentile + 12 mmHg or ≥140/90 mmHg (whichever is lower)	≥140/90 mmHg

Flynn JT, Kaelber DC, Baker-Smith CM, et al; Subcommittee on Screening and Management of High Blood Pressure in Children. Clinical practice guideline for screening and management of high blood pressure in children and adolescents. *Pediatrics*. 2017;140(3):e20171904, Table 3. Erratum in: *Pediatrics*. 2017; Erratum in: *Pediatrics*. 2018;142(3).

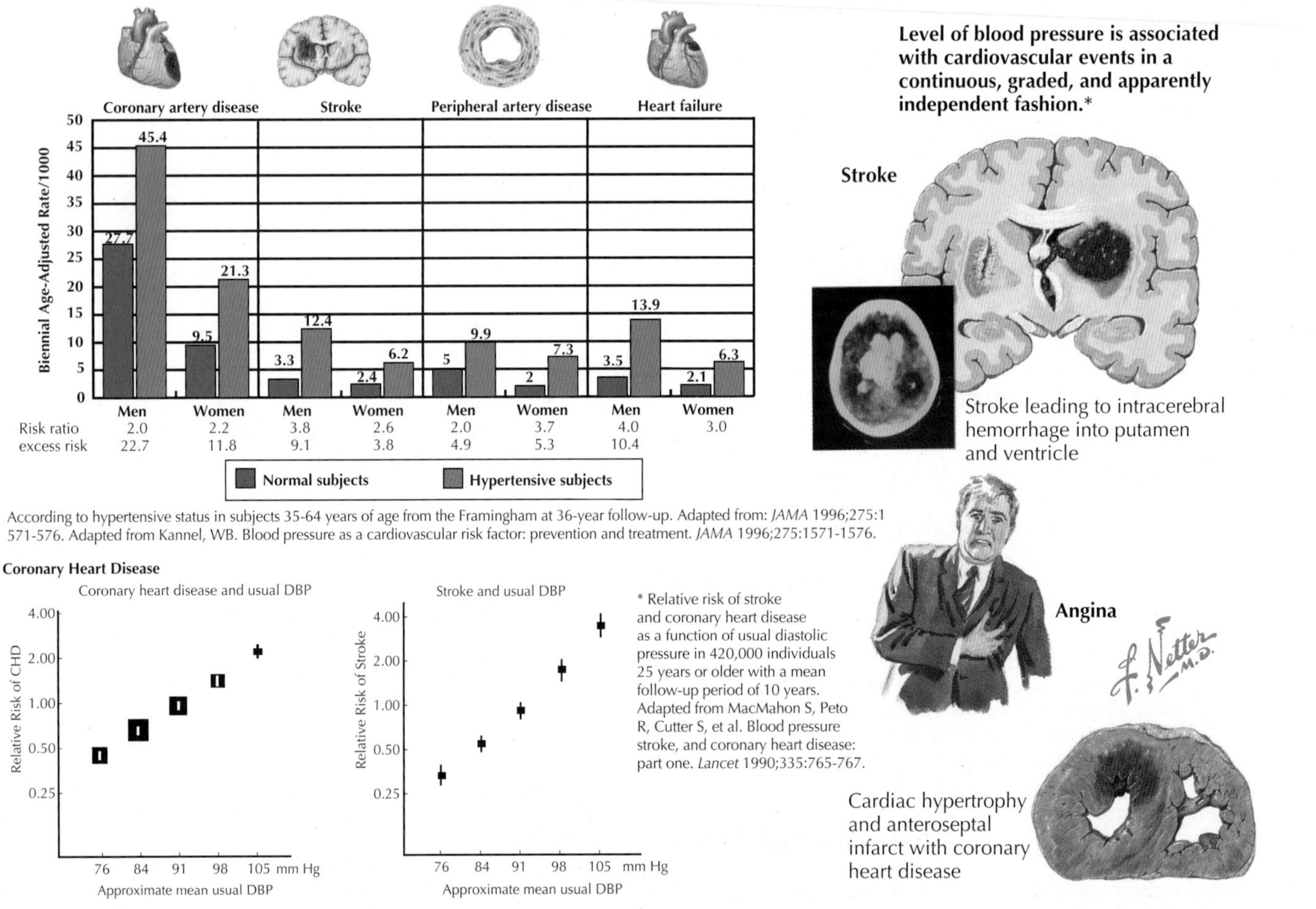
Coronary artery disease
Stroke
Peripheral artery disease
Heart failure
Biennial Age-Adjusted Rate/1000
Men
Women
Risk ratio
excess risk
Normal subjects
Hypertensive subjects
According to hypertensive status in subjects 35-64 years of age from the Framingham at 36-year follow-up. Adapted from: JAMA 1996;275:1 571-576. Adapted from Kannel, WB. Blood pressure as a cardiovascular risk factor: prevention and treatment. JAMA 1996;275:1571-1576.
Level of blood pressure is associated with cardiovascular events in a continuous, graded, and apparently independent fashion.*
Stroke
Stroke leading to intracerebral hemorrhage into putamen and ventricle
Coronary Heart Disease
Coronary heart disease and usual DBP
Relative Risk of CHD
Approximate mean usual DBP
Stroke and usual DBP
Relative Risk of Stroke
* Relative risk of stroke and coronary heart disease as a function of usual diastolic pressure in 420,000 individuals 25 years or older with a mean follow-up period of 10 years. Adapted from MacMahon S, Peto R, Cutter S, et al. Blood pressure stroke, and coronary heart disease: part one. Lancet 1990;335:765-767.
Angina
Cardiac hypertrophy and anteroseptal infarct with coronary heart disease
F. Netter M.D.

Figure 36.1 Hypertension as a risk factor for cardiovascular disease.

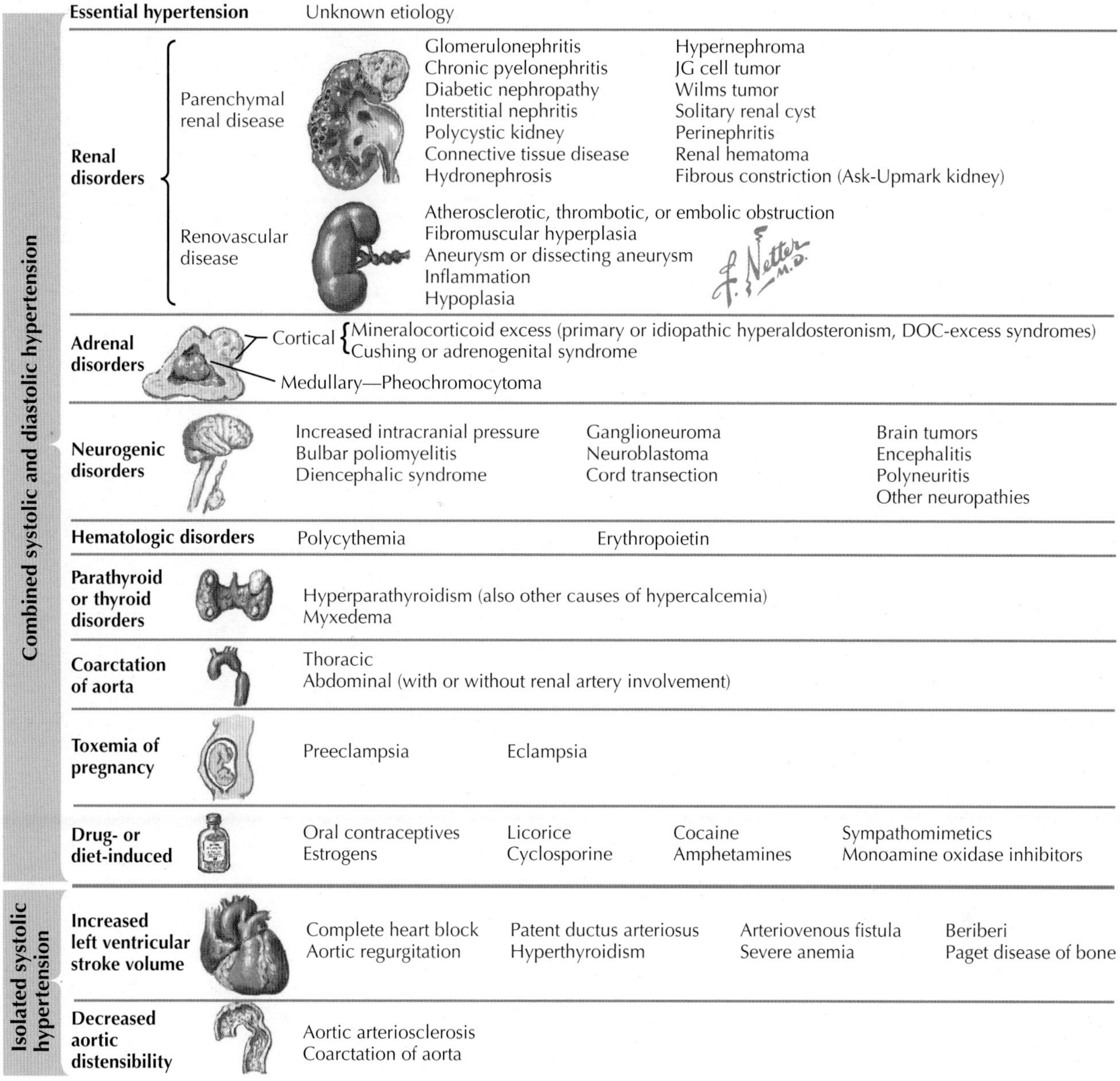
Essential hypertension
Unknown etiology
Combined systolic and diastolic hypertension
Renal disorders
Parenchymal renal disease
Glomerulonephritis
Chronic pyelonephritis
Diabetic nephropathy
Interstitial nephritis
Polycystic kidney
Connective tissue disease
Hydronephrosis
Hypernephroma
JG cell tumor
Wilms tumor
Solitary renal cyst
Perinephritis
Renal hematoma
Fibrous constriction (Ask-Upmark kidney)
Renovascular disease
Atherosclerotic, thrombotic, or embolic obstruction
Fibromuscular hyperplasia
Aneurysm or dissecting aneurysm
Inflammation
Hypoplasia
F. Netter M.D.
Adrenal disorders
Cortical
Mineralocorticoid excess (primary or idiopathic hyperaldosteronism, DOC-excess syndromes)
Cushing or adrenogenital syndrome
Medullary—Pheochromocytoma
Neurogenic disorders
Increased intracranial pressure
Bulbar poliomyelitis
Diencephalic syndrome
Ganglioneuroma
Neuroblastoma
Cord transection
Brain tumors
Encephalitis
Polyneuritis
Other neuropathies
Hematologic disorders
Polycythemia
Erythropoietin
Parathyroid or thyroid disorders
Hyperparathyroidism (also other causes of hypercalcemia)
Myxedema
Coarctation of aorta
Thoracic
Abdominal (with or without renal artery involvement)
Toxemia of pregnancy
Preeclampsia
Eclampsia
Drug- or diet-induced
Oral contraceptives
Estrogens
Licorice
Cyclosporine
Cocaine
Amphetamines
Sympathomimetics
Monoamine oxidase inhibitors
Isolated systolic hypertension
Increased left ventricular stroke volume
Complete heart block
Aortic regurgitation
Patent ductus arteriosus
Hyperthyroidism
Arteriovenous fistula
Severe anemia
Beriberi
Paget disease of bone
Decreased aortic distensibility
Aortic arteriosclerosis
Coarctation of aorta

Figure 36.2 Causes of hypertension.

- Family history (HTN twice as common if either parent has HTN)
- **Metabolic factors**
  - Obesity
  - Glucose intolerance
  - Endocrine disorders (see "Causes")
- **Stress**
  - Environmental
  - Social
  - Leads to chronic neurogenic activation of the sympathetic nervous system
- **Behavioral factors**
  - High sodium intake
  - Excessive alcohol consumption
  - Drug abuse (see later)
- **Medications**
  - Oral contraceptive pills (OCPs); 5% will develop HTN over 5 years
  - Nonsteroidal anti-inflammatory drugs (NSAIDs), particularly chronic use
  - Antidepressants, including tricyclic antidepressants, selective serotonin reuptake inhibitors, and monoamine oxidase inhibitors
  - Corticosteroids, including both glucocorticoids and mineralocorticoids
  - Decongestants, such as phenylephrine and pseudoephedrine
  - Some weight-loss medications
  - Attention-deficit/hyperactivity disorder (ADHD) medications such as methylphenidate and amphetamines
  - Illicit drug use
    - Recreational: cocaine, methamphetamines or tobacco (chew)
    - Ergogenic: stimulants, erythropoietin, human growth hormone, or anabolic steroids

DIAGNOSIS OF HYPERTENSION

Resting Blood Pressure

- Diagnosis of HTN can be confirmed by serial (at least three) office-based BP measurements with a mean of ≥130/≥80 mmHg spaced over a period of weeks to months (see Table 36.1).

- Should be confirmed with home BP monitoring or ambulatory blood pressure monitoring (ABPM) if possible.
- In children and early adolescents, HTN is defined as average systolic or diastolic BP ≥95th percentile for age, gender, and height, measured on three separate occasions. Adolescents over age 13 use the same measurements as adults (see Table 36.2).

Environment During Measurement

- Measurement of BP should be performed in a standard measurement situation, preferably a quiet area.
- Avoid exercise and caffeine for >30 minutes before measurement.
- Let the athlete sit in a chair with back supported and feet flat on the floor for a few minutes if possible.
- Choose the appropriate-size BP cuff. Many athletes will need a large cuff, and a thigh cuff should be available for very large athletes.
  - BP cuff's inflatable bag should cover approximately 80% of arm's circumference.
  - BP may be overestimated if the BP cuff is too small, whereas BP may be underestimated if the BP cuff is too big.
- Avoid rapid deflation of the cuff.
- Repeat BP measurements if elevated.
  - In younger athletes, if BP in arm is elevated, obtain BP measurement in leg to assess for aortic coarctation.

"White Coat" Hypertension and Other Stress Phenomena

- Anxiety provoked by medical examination or other sources of mental stress can lead to artificially elevated BP, known as *"white coat" HTN*.
- Average of several readings is a better estimate of true BP.
- If initial BP is high, have athlete rest for 5 minutes and repeat BP measurement.
- If BP remains elevated, check BP at least once per week for at least two additional visits.
- Averaged daily BP is a better predictor of later end-organ damage than random office BP.
- Twenty-four-hour ABPM may more accurately assess BP in people with variable readings in the office or at home but can be difficult and expensive.
- Home BP monitoring correlates well with ABPM.
- Athletes/exercisers can take their own BP, but must be well trained in measurement of BP.
- Emphasize importance of *accurate* readings.

CLINICAL EVALUATION

History

- **Family history of HTN**
- **Cardiovascular risk factors:**
  - Smoking
  - Family history of cardiac disease in men younger than 55 years and women younger than 65 years
  - Obesity
  - Physical inactivity
  - Diabetes
  - Dyslipidemia
- **Lifestyle factors:**
  - High sodium and saturated fat intake
  - Alcohol consumption
  - Herbs and supplements (particularly those for energy or weight loss)
  - Drug use
    - Over the counter (NSAIDs, decongestants, caffeine, and diet pills)
    - Prescription (glucocorticosteroids, erythropoietin, cyclosporine, methylphenidates, and amphetamines)

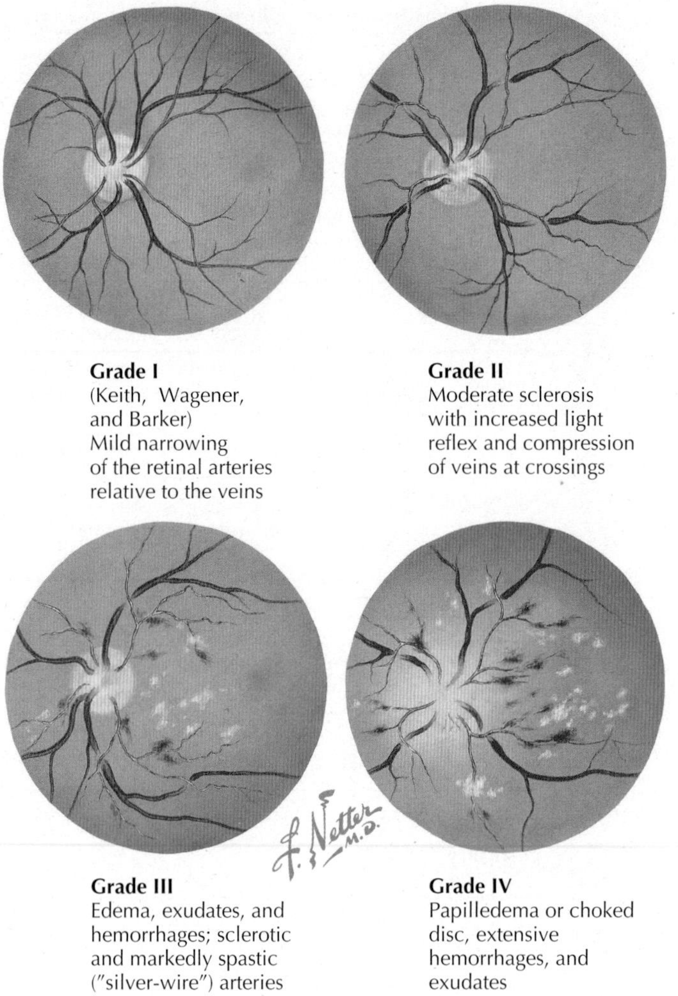
Grade I
(Keith, Wagener, and Barker)
Mild narrowing of the retinal arteries relative to the veins
Grade II
Moderate sclerosis with increased light reflex and compression of veins at crossings
Grade III
Edema, exudates, and hemorrhages; sclerotic and markedly spastic ("silver-wire") arteries
Grade IV
Papilledema or choked disc, extensive hemorrhages, and exudates
F. Netter M.D.

Figure 36.3 Eye grounds in hypertension.

    - Illicit (ergogenic aids, cocaine, and phencyclidine [PCP])
  - Stress (family, work, school)
  - Symptoms of sleep apnea
- **Review of systems to rule out secondary causes of HTN**

Physical Examination

- Evaluate for secondary causes of HTN, established cardiovascular disease, and end-organ damage
- Body mass index (BMI) often not useful in athletes because of higher levels of muscle mass
- Fundoscopic examination for retinopathy, as indicated by retinal hemorrhages or exudates, with or without papilledema (Fig. 36.3)
- Thyroid
- Cardiovascular (pulses, murmurs, and bruits)
- Abdominal masses
- Peripheral edema

Diagnostic Studies

- Complete blood count (CBC), electrolytes (including calcium), blood urea nitrogen (BUN), creatinine, fasting glucose, lipid panel, thyroid-stimulating hormone (TSH), urinalysis
- Electrocardiogram (ECG)
  - ECG should be interpreted by a clinician familiar with ECG changes commonly associated with athlete's heart, which

may suggest pathology in nonathletes but are normal variants in this population.
- Further workup if suspicious of secondary causes indicated by unusual presentation of HTN, drug-resistant HTN, or a clinical clue on examination or initial testing.
- Renal ultrasound recommended for pediatric athletes with established HTN.
- ECG is recommended in pediatric athletes with diabetes or renal disease associated with BP between 90th and 94th percentiles, all children with stage 2 HTN and BP in the ≥95th percentile, or if pharmacologic therapy is being considered.

APPROACHES TO MANAGEMENT OF HYPERTENSION

- Management of hypertensive athletes (or exercising adults with HTN) typically involves a combination of nonpharmacologic therapies, often with one or more antihypertensive medications.
- Goals:
  - Goal BP varies according to patient's age and comorbidities
  - BP <140/90 mmHg for most athletes
  - BP <130/80 mmHg if coexisting disease
    - Chronic kidney disease (CKD) with proteinuria
    - Diabetes mellitus
    - Secondary prevention of recurrent cardiovascular disease
    - Primary prevention in adults with an estimated 10-year atherosclerotic cardiovascular disease risk ≥10%
- Special considerations in athletes:
  - Potential influence of exercise and training on HTN
  - Potential side effects of antihypertensive medications on athletic performance
  - Certain therapies are banned by various sports governing bodies, including the International Olympic Committee (IOC) and National Collegiate Athletic Association (NCAA).

Nonpharmacologic Therapy

- Nonpharmacologic strategies provide safe and effective foundation for any good antihypertensive regimen with low to nonexistent risk of side effects
- Dependent on long-term compliance and lifestyle changes, which can be difficult because of deeply ingrained behaviors
- Most appropriate for elevated BP and stage 1 HTN
- Adjunct for stage 2 HTN and when pharmacologic therapy is initiated

Weight Reduction

- Obesity is defined as BMI >30 kg/m^2.
- Obesity increases preload and afterload, resulting in hypertensive effect, but mechanism not well understood.
- Hyperinsulinemia and insulin resistance may play a central role because obesity, glucose intolerance, and HTN are components of metabolic syndrome.
- Weight reduction is the most effective nonpharmacologic measure of BP reduction.
  - For each 1 lb of weight loss, the systolic and diastolic BP each fall by approximately 1 mmHg.
  - Weight reduction of 10 pounds reduces BP in overweight athletes with HTN and enhances BP-lowering effects of medications, possibly because of reductions in both preload and afterload.

DIETARY APPROACH TO STOP HYPERTENSION (DASH) DIET

- Reduced levels of total and saturated fat and cholesterol, sweets, sugar-sweetened beverages, and red meats
- Increased potassium, calcium, magnesium, fiber, and protein
- Emphasizes fruits, vegetables, low-fat dairy, whole grains, fish, poultry, and nuts
- Showed decreases in BP equivalent to medications (11.4/5.5 mmHg in hypertensive patients and 5.5/3.0 mmHg decrease in those with elevated BP) and is particularly effective in African Americans

ELECTROLYTES

- **Sodium (Na^+)**
  - Reduction can result in significant decrease in BP in all age groups.
  - Reduction is especially beneficial when combined with DASH diet.
  - Two to four g/day can reduce systolic BP by 2–8 mmHg.
  - Recommended intake is 2.4 g/day (6 g NaCl).
  - Salt-sensitive groups benefit most
    - Two-thirds of African Americans
    - Diabetics
    - Older people
- **Potassium (K^+)**
  - Increased potassium intake in hypertensives can lower BP by a mean of 5.3/3.1 mmHg.
  - Increasing K^+ decreases BP in hypokalemic patients (e.g., endurance athletes) and may protect from ventricular ectopy.
  - Effects of K^+ supplementation greatest in those with higher levels of sodium in diet because low K^+ intake may reduce sodium excretion.
  - Goal is 120 mEq/day.
  - Good sources are fruits and vegetables.
- **Calcium (Ca^{2+})**
  - An increase in **Ca^{2+}** intake slightly reduces both systolic and diastolic BP in normotensive people, particularly in young people, suggesting a role in prevention of HTN.
  - Adequate calcium intake should be encouraged; 1000–1500 mg/day through diet or supplementation is the goal.
- **Magnesium (Mg^{2+})**
  - Controversial, possible benefits
  - Important in patients who are deficient, particularly from diuretics
  - Supplementation not routinely recommended, but may be beneficial in those with insulin resistance, prediabetes, diabetes, or cardiovascular disease

Exercise

- Vigorous exercise correlates with lower risk of developing HTN.
  - Decrease in BP dependent more on intensity of exercise than frequency
  - Both aerobic exercise and resistance training (e.g., weightlifting) lower resting BP; combining aerobic activity and resistance training may have additive effects on lowering BP.
- Regular aerobic exercise regimen in people with essential HTN can lower BP by as much as 5–15 mmHg within 4 weeks.
- Certain clinical trials show that aerobic exercise conditioning lowers resting systolic BP by an average of 11 mmHg and diastolic BP by an average of 6 mmHg in hypertensives.
  - Benefits more marked in elevated BP and stage 1 HTN
  - Difficult to determine if benefit is a direct effect of exercise or secondary to weight loss
- Moderate-intensity resistance training lowers resting BP by 4/4 mmHg.
- High-intensity interval training (HIIT) significantly reduces BP up to 12/8 mmHg.

Lifestyle Changes

- Alcohol consumption should be limited to two drinks per day for men or one per day for women.
- Stimulants—caffeine acutely raises BP, but avoidance is unnecessary because of the rapid development of tolerance
- Avoidance of medications or illicit drugs that can raise BP (see "Risk Factors" earlier)

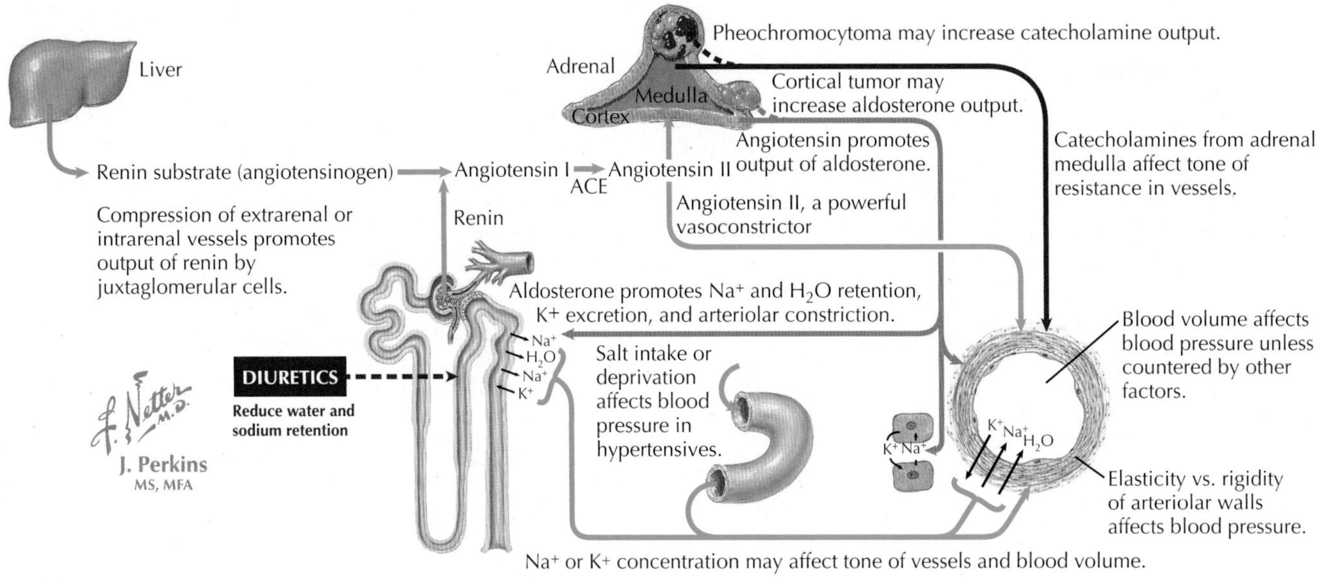

Pheochromocytoma may increase catecholamine output.
Liver
Adrenal
Medulla
Cortex
Cortical tumor may increase aldosterone output.
Angiotensin promotes output of aldosterone.
Catecholamines from adrenal medulla affect tone of resistance in vessels.
Renin substrate (angiotensinogen)
Angiotensin I
ACE
Angiotensin II
Angiotensin II, a powerful vasoconstrictor
Compression of extrarenal or intrarenal vessels promotes output of renin by juxtaglomerular cells.
Renin
Aldosterone promotes Na+ and H2O retention, K+ excretion, and arteriolar constriction.
Blood volume affects blood pressure unless countered by other factors.
DIURETICS
Reduce water and sodium retention
Salt intake or deprivation affects blood pressure in hypertensives.
J. Perkins
MS, MFA
Elasticity vs. rigidity of arteriolar walls affects blood pressure.
Na+ or K+ concentration may affect tone of vessels and blood volume.

Figure 36.4 Hypertension treatment: Diuretics.

- Stress management
  - Relaxation techniques such as biofeedback, muscle relaxation techniques, meditation, and yoga may be used as adjunctive therapies.

Fish Oil Supplementation

- Reduces systemic vascular resistance
- High doses may decrease BP by 6/4 mmHg, but long-term safety of fish oil at these doses is unknown

Pharmacologic Therapy

Basic Concepts

- Each antihypertensive agent is roughly equal in efficacy, but wide variability in response, as some athletes respond well to one drug but not another.
- Must be individualized and carefully monitored for potential side effects.
- In absence of "compelling" indications based upon comorbidities, initial therapy should be chosen from among the following four classes of medications.
  - Thiazide-like or thiazide diuretics
  - Angiotensin-converting enzyme (ACE) inhibitors
  - Angiotensin II receptor blockers (ARBs)
  - Long-acting calcium channel blockers
- Many individuals will require two or more medications to achieve goal BP.
- If initial BP is >20/10 mmHg over goal, consider initiating therapy with two agents.
- Monitor effects of therapy on athletic performance; ideal therapy controls BP without compromising exercise capacity.
- NSAIDs may decrease the activity of several antihypertensive medications.
  - Beta-blockers, ACE inhibitors, and diuretics may have their therapeutic activity inhibited.
  - Limited reports suggest possibility of acute increase in BP with use of cyclooxygenase-2 (COX-2) inhibitors.
- IOC and NCAA regulations ban use of certain medications such as diuretics and beta-blockers (in certain events).

Diuretics (Thiazide, Thiazide-Like, and Loop Inhibitors)

- Decrease plasma volume, CO, and SVR (Fig. 36.4)
  - Short-term use reduces maximal exercise capacity and submaximal endurance.
  - Attenuated increase in BP, decreased SV, but maintenance of normal HR response during exercise.
- Thiazide-like (e.g., chlorthalidone or indapamide) have shown decreased mortality and morbidity in the elderly and are superior in preventing one or more forms of cardiovascular disease
- Inexpensive
- Side effects:
  - Hypovolemia, orthostatic hypotension—not recommended for athletes prone to dehydration because of further reductions in intravascular volume.
  - Urinary loss of K^+ and Mg^{2+}, which can lead to muscle cramps, arrhythmias, and rhabdomyolysis, particularly when competing or exercising vigorously in warm weather. Cramping may occur despite normal serum potassium.
  - Increases in plasma cholesterol, glucose, and uric acid at higher doses.
  - Higher incidence of sexual dysfunction in males.
- Thiazide or thiazide-like diuretics can be first-step therapy for casual exercisers, active elderly, and African Americans.
- Loop diuretics are inappropriate for use in athletes.
- All diuretics are banned by athletic associations and cannot be used by athletes subject to drug testing because they dilute the concentration of steroids and performance-enhancing drugs in the urine.

Angiotensin-Converting Enzyme Inhibitors

- Benazepril, captopril, enalapril, fosinopril, lisinopril, moexipril, perindopril, quinapril, ramipril, and trandolapril (Fig. 36.5)
- Competitive inhibition of conversion of angiotensin I to angiotensin II by ACE in plasma and vascular smooth muscles
- Blocks vasoconstriction and Na^+ retention from angiotensin II
- Increases stroke volume, slight decrease in HR, and decreases TPR
- Beneficial effects in patients with heart failure, systolic dysfunction, ST elevation myocardial infarction (MI), or nephropathy; reverses ventricular hypertrophy and microalbuminuria and preserves renal function
- In exercise:
  - No major effect on energy metabolism
  - No impairment of $\dot{V}O_2$ max, training, or competition
  - Decreased "exaggerated" BP effects during exercise, including isometric exercise
  - Major side effect is dry, nonproductive cough

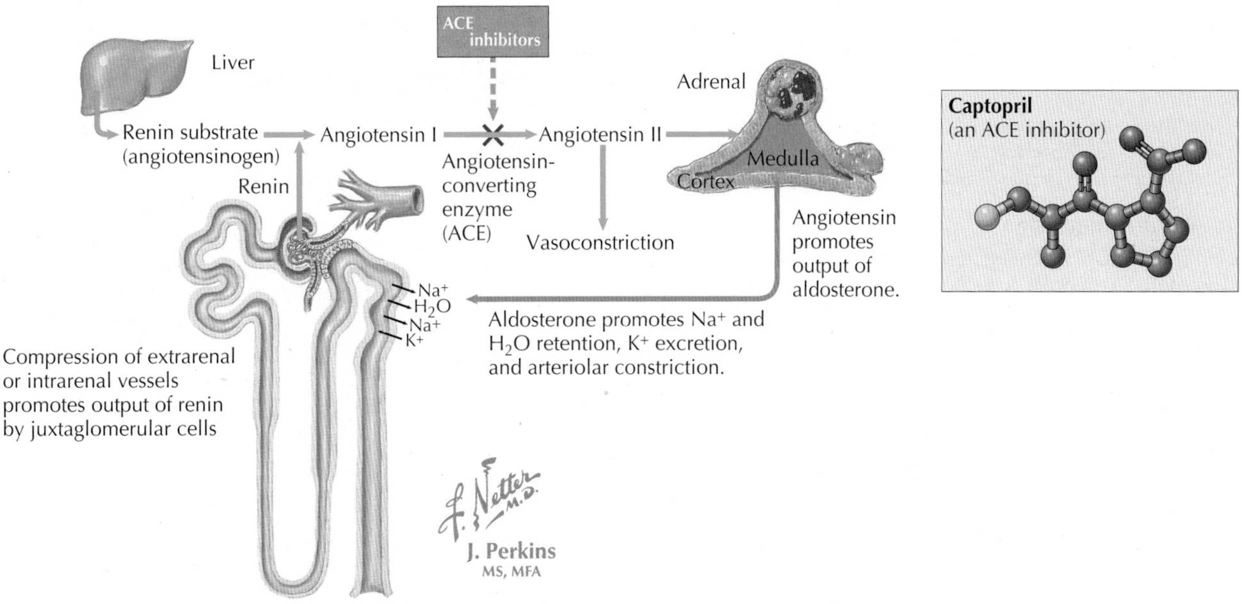
ACE inhibitors
Liver
Renin substrate (angiotensinogen)
Angiotensin I
Angiotensin II
Angiotensin-converting enzyme (ACE)
Renin
Adrenal
Medulla
Cortex
Vasoconstriction
Angiotensin promotes output of aldosterone.
Na+
H2O
Na+
K+
Aldosterone promotes Na+ and H2O retention, K+ excretion, and arteriolar constriction.
Compression of extrarenal or intrarenal vessels promotes output of renin by juxtaglomerular cells
Captopril
(an ACE inhibitor)
J. Perkins
MS, MFA

Figure 36.5 Hypertension treatment: Angiotensin-converting enzyme inhibitors.

- Anecdotal reports of postural hypotension when stopping abruptly after intense exercise (i.e., adequate cool-down needed)
- Excellent for mild to moderate HTN, and effectiveness may be improved with addition of low-dose thiazide or thiazide-like diuretics
- Often first-line agent for HTN in active athletes
- Concomitant use of NSAIDs may increase potassium-sparing effects and potentially cause hyperkalemia
- Women of childbearing age need contraception because this class is contraindicated in pregnancy

Angiotensin II Receptor Blockers

- Candesartan, eprosartan, irbesartan, losartan, olmesartan, telmisartan, and valsartan
- Block renin–angiotensin system by preventing angiotensin II from binding to its subtype 1 receptor
- Selective blockade prevents vasoconstriction and aldosterone secretion
- Effects similar to ACE inhibitors without dry cough side effect
- May improve exercise tolerance in hypertensives because angiotensin II levels increase during exercise
- May be beneficial in athletes with early diastolic dysfunction because of blocking effects during left ventricular (LV) relaxation
- Generally recommended for those who cannot tolerate ACE inhibitor because of cough
- Women of childbearing age need contraception because this class is contraindicated in pregnancy

Calcium Channel Blockers

- Include dihydropyridines (i.e., amlodipine, felodipine, isradipine, nicardipine, nifedipine, and nisoldipine) and nonhydropyridines (i.e., verapamil and diltiazem)
- Inhibit calcium slow-channel conduction, reducing calcium concentration in vascular smooth muscle cells and leading to decreased SVR (i.e., generalized vasodilatation)
- Effective in reversing ventricular hypertrophy
- Dihydropyridines (e.g., nifedipine and amlodipine)
  - More potent vasodilators
  - Reflex tachycardia
  - Fluid retention (i.e., pedal edema)
  - Vascular headaches
- Nondihydropyridines (e.g., verapamil and diltiazem)
  - HR suppression
  - Minor impairment of maximal HR
  - Decreased LV contractility and worsening cardiac output
  - Verapamil decreases pressor response during isometric exercise
  - Women show greater BP responsiveness to exercise with diltiazem than men
  - Constipation (e.g., verapamil)
- In exercise:
  - No major effect on energy metabolism
  - $\dot{V}O_2$ max generally preserved
  - Potential for competitive "steal" of muscle blood flow because of vasodilatation
  - Earlier onset of lactate threshold
  - Verapamil preferred over dihydropyridines for high-intensity exercise because of improved BP control
- This class of drugs can be used as first-line therapy in athletes
  - Generally well tolerated and effective in active patients, particularly young African Americans
  - May be particularly effective in hypertensive patients who are noncompliant with dietary salt restriction
  - May also be preferred in patients concurrently taking NSAIDs because antihypertensive efficacy is not blunted
  - Combining with ACE or ARB can reduce common side effect of peripheral edema

Alpha$_1$-Receptor Blockers

- Prazosin, terazosin, and doxazosin
- Competitively block postsynaptic alpha$_1$ arteriolar smooth muscle receptors
- Decrease SVR (i.e., no reflex increase in HR or CO)
- First-dose effect of syncope; hence, first dose must be administered at night
- During exercise
  - No major changes in energy metabolism
  - $\dot{V}O_2$ max preserved
  - No major effect on training or sports performance
- Not recommended for initial monotherapy
  - Possible exception for older men with symptoms of prostatism

- May be useful for diabetic athletes with HTN and hypercholesterolemia
- Antihypertensive and Lipid-Lowering Treatment to Prevent Heart Attack Trial (ALLHAT)
  - Discontinued doxazosin arm because of increased CHF compared with diuretics
  - Use with caution in master athletes aged over 55 years

Central Alpha-Antagonists

- Clonidine, guanabenz, guanfacine, and methyldopa
- Act on $alpha_2$ receptors in brainstem to block central sympathetic stimulation with decreased HR and TPR at rest
- Also block sympathetically mediated sodium retention
- During exercise:
  - No major changes in energy metabolism
  - $\dot{V}O_2$ max preserved
  - No major effect on training or sports performance
- Side effects:
  - Mild to moderate drowsiness and dry mouth
  - Impotence
  - Rebound HTN with abrupt discontinuation of oral clonidine
- Clonidine available in transdermal system (i.e., weekly patch)
- Not recommended for initial monotherapy
- Rarely used because of side effects

Beta-Blockers (Table 36.3)

- Noncardioselective
  - Decreases HR by 20%–30%
  - Decreases contractility
  - Increases SVR (muscle and skin)
  - Inhibition of lipolysis and glycogenolysis
  - Increased cholesterol (i.e., decreased high-density lipoprotein [HDL])
  - Increased perception of exertion
  - Bronchoconstriction in predisposed athletes
- Cardioselective
  - Fewer effects on $beta_2$ vasodilatation, lipolysis, and glycogenolysis
  - Impairment of CO and $\dot{V}O_2$ max is generally similar but may be less because of compensatory increase in systolic volume (SV)
- Beta-blockers with intrinsic sympathetic activity (ISA) may be less likely to impair myocardial function
- During exercise
  - Significant loss of $\dot{V}O_2$ max
    - Decreased CO and skeletal muscle flow
    - Well-trained athletes have a greater decrease in $\dot{V}O_2$ max than untrained subjects
  - Beta-blockers increase perceived exertion in working muscles, thus causing reduced endurance, probably as a result of metabolic effects with no increase in perceived cardiovascular exertion.
  - Beta-blockers decrease performance more in people with a high percentage of slow-twitch muscle fibers. This effect is more pronounced with propranolol (noncardioselective) than with atenolol (cardioselective).
  - Impairment of substrate mobilization results in earlier fatigue and lower lactate threshold.
    - Blocks lipolysis and glycogenolysis
    - Symptoms of hypoglycemia during or after intense exercise may be masked in diabetics
  - Exercise bronchospasm may be increased; thus, use with caution in athletes with asthma
  - Side effects less with cardioselective beta-blockers
- Not recommended for initial monotherapy in athletes unless underlying condition requires their use
  - Ischemic heart disease or heart failure with decreased ejection fraction where increased exercise tolerance may be noted

Table 36.3 BETA-BLOCKING AGENTS ARRANGED BY CARDIOSELECTIVITY AND INTRINSIC SYMPATHOMIMETIC ACTIVITY (ISA)

	No ISA	ISA
Cardioselective	Atenolol Metoprolol Betaxolol Bisoprolol Nebivolol	Acebutolol
Noncardioselective	Nadolol Propranolol Sotalol Timolol	Pindolol Carteolol Oxprenolol Penbutolol

  - Hypertensives with excessive rise in systolic BP during exercise
  - Rate control in atrial fibrillation
  - Performance anxiety in minimal-exertion sports
- Banned in precision sports (e.g., shooting sports and golf)

Combined Alpha- and Beta-Blockers

- Labetalol and carvedilol
- Three effects (Fig. 36.6)
  - Beta-blockade (i.e., decreased HR leading to decreased CO and renin)
  - $Alpha_1$-blockade (i.e., decreased vasoconstriction leading to decreased TPR)
  - $Beta_2$-agonist (i.e., decreased TPR)
- Beta effects greater than alpha effects (3:1 for oral formulations)
- Decreased SVR
- Less impairment of muscle blood flow and $\dot{V}O_2$ max
- May be the best choice if beta-blockade is necessary
  - CO decreased 10%–14% at rest and during exercise after 1 year of therapy
  - CO gradually returns to baseline over next 5 years because of increased SV
  - TPR remains decreased 15%–20%
  - Exercise hemodynamics return to normal

APPROACH TO ACTIVE PATIENTS

Elevated Blood Pressure and Stage 1 Hypertension

- Modify lifestyle

Stage 1 Hypertension With Preexisting Conditions or Stage 2 Hypertension

- Nonpharmacologic intervention:
  - Three to six months
  - Monitor frequently
  - If nonpharmacologic intervention fails to reduce BP, pharmacologic therapy is required
- Pharmacologic therapy:
  - Low dose
  - Observe for 4–6 weeks, monitor for efficacy and side effects
  - If inadequate response, titrate dose and recheck in 4–6 weeks
- Initial therapy:
  - Monotherapy based on age and race
  - ACE, ARB, or calcium channel blocker for most athletes
  - Thiazide diuretic initially if indicated or added if Na^+ sensitive
  - Combined beta-/alpha-blocker if beta-blockade needed
- Emphasize need for long-term follow-up care and management

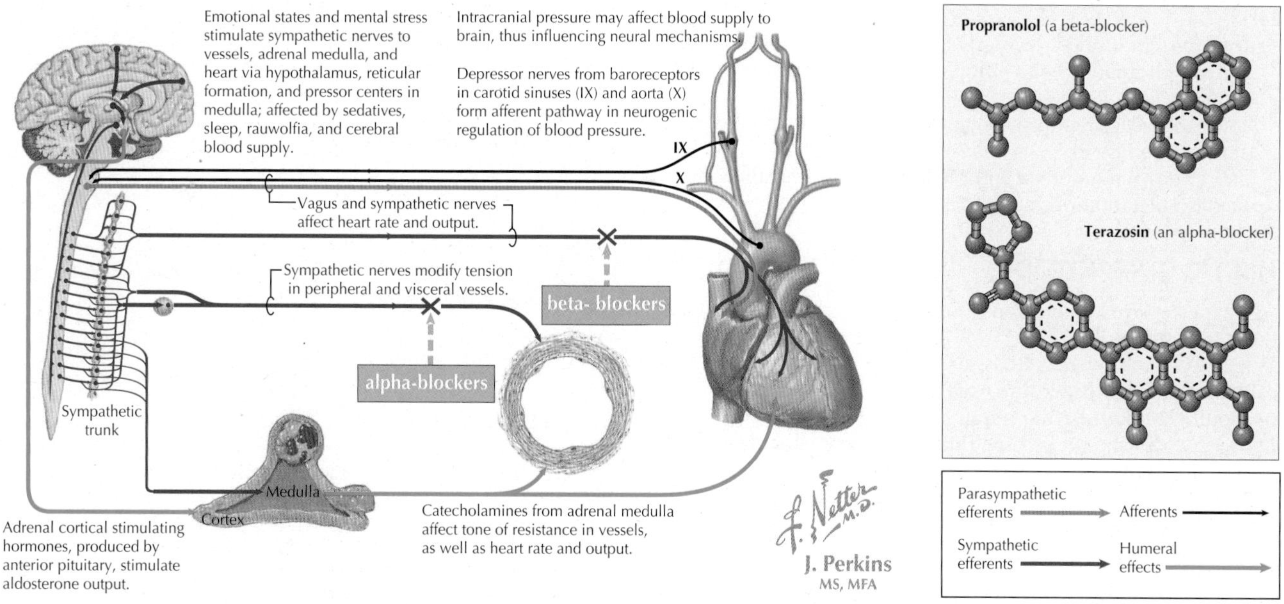

Emotional states and mental stress stimulate sympathetic nerves to vessels, adrenal medulla, and heart via hypothalamus, reticular formation, and pressor centers in medulla; affected by sedatives, sleep, rauwolfia, and cerebral blood supply.
Intracranial pressure may affect blood supply to brain, thus influencing neural mechanisms.
Depressor nerves from baroreceptors in carotid sinuses (IX) and aorta (X) form afferent pathway in neurogenic regulation of blood pressure.
IX
X
Vagus and sympathetic nerves affect heart rate and output.
Sympathetic nerves modify tension in peripheral and visceral vessels.
beta- blockers
alpha-blockers
Sympathetic trunk
Medulla
Cortex
Adrenal cortical stimulating hormones, produced by anterior pituitary, stimulate aldosterone output.
Catecholamines from adrenal medulla affect tone of resistance in vessels, as well as heart rate and output.
J. Perkins MS, MFA
Propranolol (a beta-blocker)
Terazosin (an alpha-blocker)
Parasympathetic efferents
Afferents
Sympathetic efferents
Humeral effects

Figure 36.6 Hypertension treatment: Beta-blockers and alpha-blockers.

EXERCISE PRESCRIPTION FOR HYPERTENSIVE PATIENTS

- The recommended mode, frequency, duration, and intensity of exercise are generally the same as those for nonhypertensive individuals (Fig. 36.7).
- Repetitive performance of both aerobic and resistance exercise lowers systolic and diastolic BP.
  - Each 30-minute period of aerobic exercise at 50% of maximal oxygen uptake lowers BP for 24 hours.
  - An even greater reduction is seen with exercise at 75% of maximal oxygen uptake.
- Monitor BP every 2–4 months to monitor the impact of exercise.
- Prescribing exercise—"FITT"
  - Frequency: 3 sessions/week initially with goal of 5–6 sessions/week
  - Intensity: 55%–70% of predicted maximum HR (MHR)
    - Moderate-intensity exercise (55%–70% MHR or 40%–70% $\dot{V}O_2$ max) lowers BP more effectively than higher-intensity exercise (80%–85% MHR). Higher-intensity exercise may actually increase resting BP.
    - Training at 20% and 60% of maximum work capacity results in similar resting BP reductions.
    - In older or less fit patients, start at 55%–60% MHR; in relatively more fit patients, start at 65%–70% MHR
    - Predicted MHR: 220 minus age
- Time (duration): Initially 15–20 minutes/session; eventually 30–40 minutes/session
  - Goal is to accumulate 150 minutes/week
  - Can accumulate in shorter blocks of time more frequently
- Type of exercise: "dynamic isotonic exercise," or moving body through space, is most effective (e.g., walking, jogging, swimming, cycling, cross-country skiing, and aerobic dance)
- Resistance training
  - Circuit weight training may reduce BP when performed at 30%–50% maximum resistance with intervals of 15–30 seconds between stations.
  - Progressive resistance exercise results in small reductions in resting BP.
  - Regular resistance training leads to attenuated BP and HR responses to any given load.

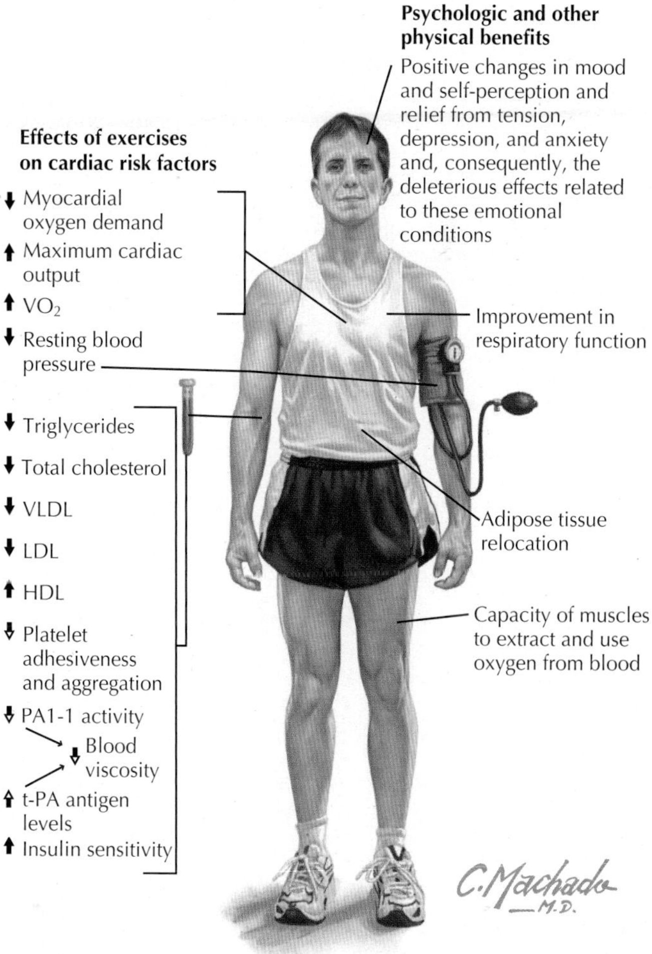

Psychologic and other physical benefits
Positive changes in mood and self-perception and relief from tension, depression, and anxiety and, consequently, the deleterious effects related to these emotional conditions
Effects of exercises on cardiac risk factors
↓ Myocardial oxygen demand
↑ Maximum cardiac output
↑ VO2
↓ Resting blood pressure
Improvement in respiratory function
↓ Triglycerides
↓ Total cholesterol
↓ VLDL
↓ LDL
↑ HDL
↓ Platelet adhesiveness and aggregation
↓ PA1-1 activity
↓ Blood viscosity
↑ t-PA antigen levels
↑ Insulin sensitivity
Adipose tissue relocation
Capacity of muscles to extract and use oxygen from blood
C. Machado M.D.

The physical activity guidelines are targeted to increase physical activity to promote health but will not necessarily result in physical fitness and should not diminish the importance of achieving physical fitness.

Figure 36.7 Effects of exercise on cardiovascular health.

- HIIT
  - Intermittent, usually regularly timed, bouts of high-intensity activity alternating with brief, often timed, periods of low-intensity activity or rest
  - HIIT had better improvement of $\dot{V}O_2$ max than moderate aerobic exercise
  - HIIT shown to improve endothelial function that allows better vasodilatation of the arteries

ATHLETIC COMPETITION

- Antihypertensive medications should generally be continued during competition
- When ACE inhibitors, ARBs, or long-acting dihydropyridine calcium channel blockers are used, there is no need to withhold or modify the dose during training or competition
- Diuretic doses should be timed to avoid maximal diuresis during competition
- Recommendations regarding athletic participation are based on the 36th Bethesda Guidelines and update from the American Heart Association and the American College of Cardiology (Table 36.4):
  - Elevated and stage 1 HTN should be encouraged to modify their lifestyles but should not be restricted from physical activity.
  - Presence of stage 2 HTN with systolic BP <160 mmHg and diastolic BP <100 mmHg in the absence of target organ damage, including LVH or concomitant heart disease, should not limit the eligibility for any competitive sport.
  - Athletes with systolic BP >160 mmHg or diastolic BP >100 mmHg, even without evidence of target organ damage, should be restricted, particularly from high static sports (i.e., activities that generate large intramuscular forces with little change in muscle length), such as weightlifting, boxing, and wrestling, until HTN is controlled by either lifestyle modification or drug therapy.
    - Low-intensity sports are recommended.
    - Should avoid "collision" sports that could lead to kidney damage.

Table 36.4 EXERCISE RECOMMENDATIONS FOR HYPERTENSIVE ATHLETES

Elevated blood pressure and stage 1 hypertension (120/80–139/89 mmHg)	No restrictions
Stage 2 hypertension (140/90–159/99 mmHg with no target organ damage)	No restrictions, monitor BP
Stage 2 hypertension (>60/>100 mmHg)	Restricted from high static sports until BP controlled
Controlled with end-organ damage	Low-intensity sports recommended
Controlled severe hypertension	Should avoid "collision" sports that could lead to kidney damage

Data from 36th Bethesda Conference. Recommendations for determining eligibility for competition in athletes with cardiovascular abnormalities. *JACC*. 2005;45(8):1318–1375; Maron BJ, Zipes DP, Kovacs RJ; on behalf of the American Heart Association Electrocardiography and Arrhythmias Committee of the Council on Clinical Cardiology, Council on Cardiovascular Disease in the Young, Council on Cardiovascular and Stroke Nursing, Council on Functional Genomics and Translational Biology, and the American College of Cardiology. Eligibility and disqualification recommendations for competitive athletes with cardiovascular abnormalities: preamble, principles, and general considerations: a scientific statement from the American Heart Association and American College of Cardiology. *Circulation*. 2015;132:e256–e261.

  - Athletes diagnosed with stage 1 or stage 2 HTN accompanied by signs of end-organ damage may not participate in sport until their BP is well-controlled.

RECOMMENDED READINGS

Available online.

EXERCISE-INDUCED BRONCHOCONSTRICTION, URTICARIA, AND ANAPHYLAXIS

37

Venkat Subramanyam • Marci A. Goolsby • Marc A. Molis • Whitney E. Molis

EXERCISE-INDUCED BRONCHOCONSTRICTION

Definitions: Exercise-induced bronchoconstriction (EIB) is defined as a transient narrowing of airways in response to exercise and can be classified as with asthma (EIBa) or without asthma (EIBwa). EIB can present with classic asthma symptoms or with more subtle fatigue or effects on performance. EIB was previously defined as exercise-induced bronchospasm, as opposed to bronchoconstriction, and exercise-induced asthma (EIA) described symptoms brought on by exercise in those with underlying asthma. The expert consensus is that EIB is now defined as noted earlier, with the two subtypes EIBa and EIBwa. Objective evidence of bronchial hyperresponsiveness in response to exercise should be included alongside symptoms when diagnosing EIB. In those without a confirmed diagnosis of asthma, measured decrease in forced expiratory volume in 1 second (FEV_1) of 10% or more in response to a bronchoprovocation challenge can be used to diagnose EIB.

Epidemiology: Approximately 5%–20% of the total population experiences EIB, but it is more common in athletes, particularly elite athletes. Forty-one percent of people with a history of allergic rhinitis experience EIB. Forty to ninety percent of asthmatics have exercise-related symptoms. EIB occurs equally between both genders and can develop at any age. The prevalence of EIB is highest among high-ventilation sports, particularly in cold-weather sports and swimming.

Risk factors: A history of asthma is the biggest risk factor for EIBa. Other EIB risk factors include allergic rhinitis, a family history of atopy, cold-weather sports, and sports that require a sustained high ventilation rate (e.g., Nordic skiing, soccer, and distance running). Swimming has a particularly high risk because of the high ventilation rate and exposure to chlorine by-products.

Mechanism: Current understanding of the pathophysiology of EIB is that dry air leads to osmotic changes at the airway surface. This hyperosmolar environment causes mast cell degranulation and the release of mediators that cause bronchoconstriction and airway inflammation. The release of neuropeptides from sensory nerves may also play a role.

Triggers:
- Oral breathing
- Dry, cold air
- Environmental pollutants and allergens
- Intense exercise
- Chemicals such as chlorine in pools, pesticides, and fertilizers

Clinical signs and symptoms: Symptoms usually develop within 15 minutes after 5–8 minutes of intense exercise and resolve within 30–90 minutes. There can be a late-phase response that occurs 4–8 hours after exercise. Symptoms can be brought on with all strenuous activity or only in certain environments like extreme cold. Those with EIBa may experience symptoms that extend into nighttime or early morning and symptoms brought on by other triggers outside of exercise such as upper respiratory infections (URIs) and seasonal environmental allergens
- Wheezing
- Shortness of breath
- Coughing
- Chest tightness
- Chest pain (usually reported in children)
- Increased mucus production
- Poor athletic performance
- Fatigue

Physical examination: May include the following on examination:
- Lungs: wheezing (particularly expiratory phase with wheezing at rest consistent with asthma); rales or rhonchi
- Skin: signs of atopic disease such as eczema
- Nose: enlarged and boggy turbinates
- Throat: cobblestoning and enlarged tonsils
- Sinus: tenderness on pressure

Testing: EIB should be diagnosed based on both signs and symptoms in addition to objective testing, but not one without the other. EIBa can be identified by spirometry with standard asthma testing protocols. Initial testing for EIB should be spirometry with assessment of bronchodilator response. In well-conditioned athletes, spirometry alone may appear normal, so checking response to a short-acting beta-agonist is a critical part of the test. Reversibility is defined as an increase in FEV_1 of more than 200 mL and ≥12% from baseline. This cutoff may not be appropriate to use in younger children. If spirometry is not diagnostic, then bronchoprovocation testing should be done (Table 37.1). This can be done using direct (methacholine or histamine challenge) or indirect challenges, including exercise challenge tests (ECTs), eucapnic voluntary hyperpnea (EVH) challenge, hypertonic saline challenge, inhaled adenosine monophosphate (AMP) challenge, and inhaled mannitol powder challenge. EVH is considered the gold-standard test for EIB and is advised by the International Olympic Committee (IOC) but is not widely available. Exercise challenge testing is another option but carries low sensitivity and can be unreliable. In children and adolescents, particularly in those without signs of asthma or response to EIB treatment, one should consider cardiopulmonary exercise testing to look for other causes of their symptoms.

Types of testing:
- **Exercise challenge test:** Testing should be ideally performed for 8 minutes, allowing the athlete to reach 85% of peak heart rate by 2 minutes and maintaining the same for another 6 minutes. Spirometry is done at baseline and specific time intervals after exercise. Sport-specific field testing

Table 37.1 WADA-APPROVED BRONCHIAL PROVOCATION TESTS FOR DIAGNOSING EIB

Bronchial Provocation Test	Decrease in FEV_1 for Positive Test Result
Eucapnic Voluntary Hyperpnea	>10%
Methacholine Aerosol Challenge	>20%
Mannitol Inhalation (not available in the United States)	>15%
Hypertonic Saline Aerosol Challenge	>15%
Exercise Challenge (field or laboratory)	>10% at any two consecutive time points
Histamine Challenge	>20% during graded test of 2 minutes

EIB, Exercise-induced bronchospasm; *FEV_1*, forced expiratory volume in 1 second; *WADA*, World Anti-Doping Agency.

may be needed, particularly in winter sports, especially if laboratory-based testing is not diagnostic and/or environmental factors need to be reproduced.

- Free running/skiing
  - Advantages—Cost-effective, requires minimal cardiovascular (CV) monitoring
  - Disadvantages—Depending on the season, difficult to control environmental factors such as temperature and humidity and may not trigger EIB in all patients
- Treadmill/cycle ergometer
  - Advantages—CV and pulmonary monitoring can be performed during the workout. Workload can be standardized.
  - Disadvantages—Expensive equipment needed; may not represent environment in which symptoms occur.
- Bronchial provocation testing
  - The patient inhales a substance designed to induce bronchoconstriction. Examples include EVH challenge, hypertonic saline challenge, inhaled AMP challenge, and inhaled mannitol powder challenge. It may be used as a primary diagnostic test or when exercise challenge is equivocal. EVH testing is performed by having the athlete ventilate 22–30 times per minute for 6 minutes using dry air containing 5% carbon dioxide.
- Other testing:
  - Skin testing: can be helpful if clinically indicated, as there is a strong correlation between allergies and EIB/EIA
  - Chest radiograph or computed tomography (CT) chest: may show signs of underlying lung disease
  - Echocardiogram/other cardiac testing: if a CV abnormality is a possible cause of the symptoms

Medications and testing: When performing tests, certain medications (e.g., inhalers, leukotriene receptor antagonists) must be avoided or stopped at least 8–24 hours before testing so as to not confound the testing and produce false-negative results.

Differential diagnosis:

- **Exercise-induced laryngeal dysfunction (EILD):**
  - EILD, also called *exercise-induced laryngeal obstruction (EILO)*, was previously known as *paradoxical vocal cord motion disorder (PVCM)* or *vocal cord dysfunction (VCD)* and describes the transient glottic closure associated with physical activity (Fig. 37.1).
  - EILD symptoms typically occur at maximal effort and resolve quickly with cessation of exercise. Subjects usually have inspiratory wheezing and/or stridor as opposed to EIB and asthma, which primarily produce expiratory wheezing. The stridor in EILO occurs because of paradoxical closure of the vocal cords. Patients complain of difficulty "getting air in" and difficulty in breathing. EILO is frequently misdiagnosed as asthma and warrants special consideration in the diagnosis of EIB. It can also exist alongside EIB. Symptoms of EILO usually do not respond to inhaled beta-agonists.
  - The diagnosis of EILO is often made based on clinical presentation with description or video of symptoms. A flow-volume loop obtained while the patient is symptomatic can show flattening of the inspiratory loop. Continuous laryngoscopy during exercise, which allows visualization of vocal cord adduction on inspiration, is considered the gold standard of diagnostic testing for

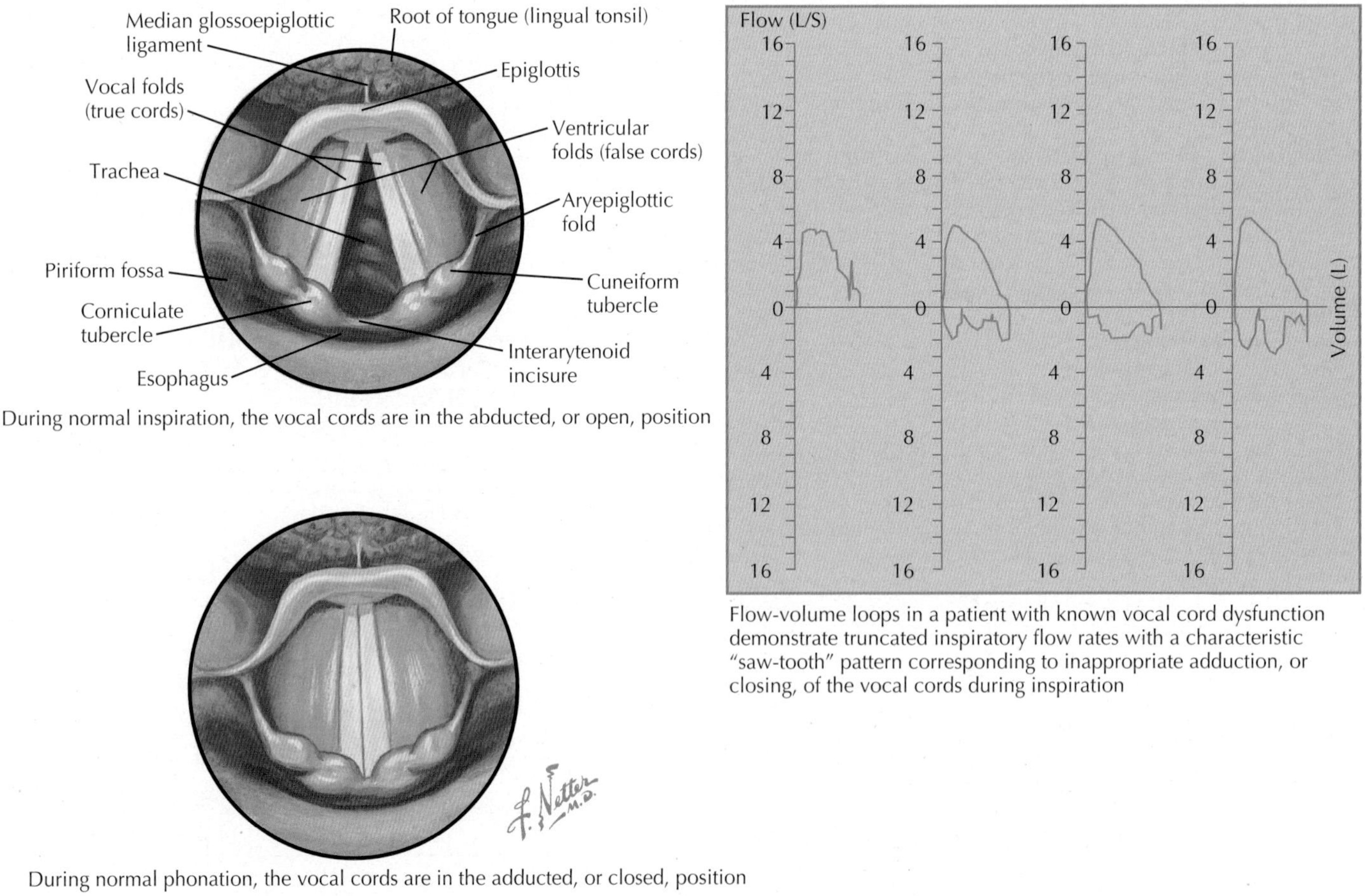
Median glossoepiglottic ligament
Root of tongue (lingual tonsil)
Epiglottis
Vocal folds (true cords)
Ventricular folds (false cords)
Trachea
Aryepiglottic fold
Piriform fossa
Cuneiform tubercle
Corniculate tubercle
Interarytenoid incisure
Esophagus
Flow (L/S)
16
12
8
4
0
4
8
12
16
Volume (L)
F. Netter M.D.

During normal inspiration, the vocal cords are in the abducted, or open, position

Flow-volume loops in a patient with known vocal cord dysfunction demonstrate truncated inspiratory flow rates with a characteristic "saw-tooth" pattern corresponding to inappropriate adduction, or closing, of the vocal cords during inspiration

During normal phonation, the vocal cords are in the adducted, or closed, position

Figure 37.1 Vocal cord dysfunction.

EILO. Treatment is reassurance, education, avoidance of triggers, and speech therapy for breathing techniques.
- **Gastroesophageal reflux disease (GERD):**
  - May present with atypical symptoms such as chronic cough and wheezing
  - Consider in athletes who have symptoms of GERD or worsening symptoms of EIB associated with regurgitation, large meals, or alcohol
- **Swimming-induced pulmonary edema (SIPE):**
  - SIPE presents with shortness of breath and cough during or immediately after swimming with associated evidence of pulmonary edema.
  - Spirometry reveals an acute restrictive pattern, with changes lasting up to 1 week.
- **Other:**
  - General deconditioning
  - Other obstructive or restrictive pulmonary disorders
  - Cardiovascular conditions
  - Exercise-induced anaphylaxis
  - Pulmonary embolism

Prevention and treatment:
- **Nonpharmacologic treatment and prevention**
  - Conditioning may help reduce symptoms and severity of EIB.
  - Short burst of vigorous exercise (e.g., 30-second bouts) may be used to treat EIB and induce short-term refractoriness, which is attributed to endogenous release of prostaglandins and depletion of constrictive mediators.
  - Warming up before activity induces bronchodilation and refractoriness to EIB.
  - Cooling down after strenuous exercise decreases EIB symptoms after exercise.
  - Avoid hyperventilation.
  - Cold weather may exacerbate EIB; hence, dressing appropriately may help. In addition, in cold weather, a buff or breath warming device may help retain warmer and more humid air, thereby reducing EIB symptoms.
  - Avoid exercising in areas that have high pollen counts or heavy pollution, as air quality inversely correlates with exercise-induced respiratory symptoms.
  - Avoid vigorous activity when the patient has a cold or when allergies are not well controlled.
  - Use nasal breathing (as opposed to mouth breathing) to help warm the air when exercising.
  - Dietary modifications, including low salt, and supplementing with omega-3 fatty acid intake and vitamin C, are thought to reduce symptom severity.
  - Caffeine has bronchodilatory properties and modulates respiratory dynamics by decreasing physiologic dead space and increasing tidal volume.
  - Breathing control training, such as yogic breathing, may also be considered.
- Pharmacologic
  - **Inhaled beta-adrenergic agonists:** Prevention and treatment can be achieved by using a short-acting beta$_2$-agonist (e.g., albuterol) inspired approximately 15–30 minutes before exercise; this can often prevent or reduce the symptoms of EIB. The typical dose of these medications is 90 to 180 mcg inhaled. Administration should ideally be performed using a spacer with the inhaler to maximize the concentration of the medicine; only albuterol in an aerosolized form has been shown to be effective in EIB and asthma (Fig. 37.2). Chronic administration of beta-agonists may lead to tolerance, decreased medication efficacy, or decreased broncho-protection during exercise.
  - **Leukotriene antagonists (e.g., montelukast):** Can be added as an adjunct to beta-agonists or occasionally as monotherapy. Recommended dosing is 1 to 2 hours before activity; less risk of developing tolerance compared with beta-agonists.
  - **Inhaled corticosteroids:** Not effective in EIBwa, but the mainstay of treatment of persistent asthma; all athletes who have persistent asthma and have symptoms with exercise should be on an inhaled steroid. The measured benefit of inhaled corticosteroids may not occur until weeks after initiation of therapy. Inhaled corticosteroids with a long-acting beta-agonist (e.g., formoterol or salmeterol) may benefit athletes participating in long-term activity, such as distance runners or multiple workouts per day. Long-acting beta-agonists are not recommended as monotherapy for EIB because of risks of severe exacerbation and sudden cardiac death and have the potential for creating tolerance to beta-agonists. However, they can be found in conjunction with inhaled steroids as so-called *combination therapy*, and this can be of use in certain athletes.
  - **Antihistamines/intranasal steroids:** Both will help athletes who have underlying allergic rhinitis. Treating allergic rhinitis symptoms is a critical part of the EIB treatment plan. Athletes who follow World Anti-Doping Agency (WADA) guidelines should avoid antihistamines combined with the banned decongestant, pseudoephedrine.
  - **Other medications:** Cromolyn, a mast cell–stabilizing agent, can be used as an adjunctive treatment for asthma. Muscarinic antagonists, both short-acting and long-acting, cause bronchial smooth muscle relaxation and can be effective for EIB. These agents are often used with beta-agonists for asthma control independent of exercise.
  - See Table 37.2 for a list of governing bodies and their rules for pharmacologic treatment of asthma.

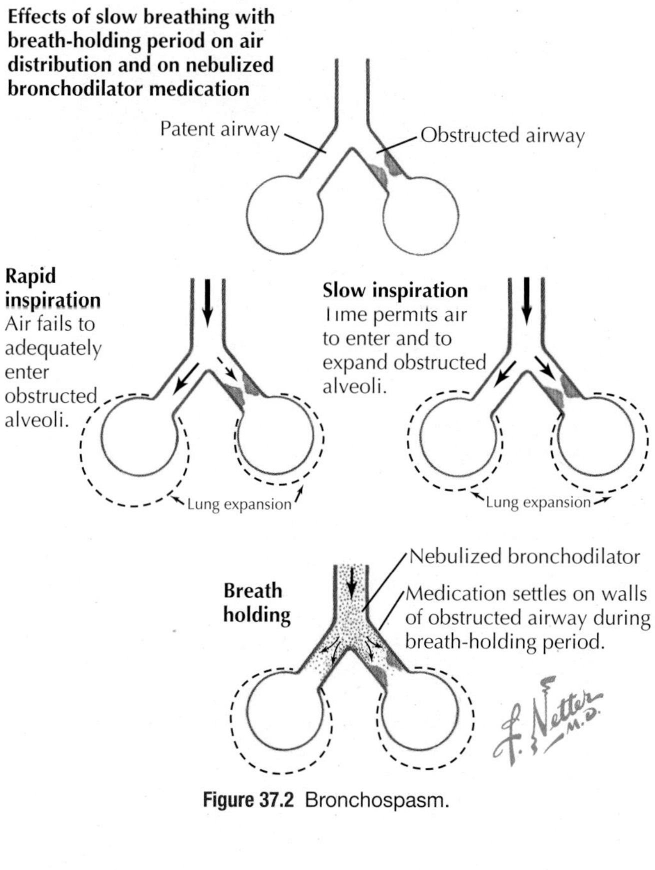
Effects of slow breathing with breath-holding period on air distribution and on nebulized bronchodilator medication
Patent airway
Obstructed airway
Rapid inspiration
Air fails to adequately enter obstructed alveoli.
Lung expansion
Slow inspiration
Time permits air to enter and to expand obstructed alveoli.
Lung expansion
Nebulized bronchodilator
Breath holding
Medication settles on walls of obstructed airway during breath-holding period.
F. Netter M.D.

Figure 37.2 Bronchospasm.

Table 37.2 GOVERNING BODIES FOR PHARMACOLOGIC TREATMENT OF ASTHMA

Governing Body	Policy on EIB	Medications
NCAA	Need documentation of diagnosis, medical history, and dosage information	Beta$_2$-agonists are prohibited, unless inhaled and with a valid prescription
World Anti-Doping Agency	It is recommended that all athletes who may be prescribed asthma medications seek a clear diagnosis from a respiratory specialist and undergo the appropriate tests to optimize management and to exclude other possible diagnoses. This is mandatory if a TUE is being sought to prescribe a systemic glucocorticoid in competition or a prohibited inhaled beta$_2$-agonist in and out of competition.	All selective and nonselective beta$_2$-agonists are prohibited, except inhaled salbutamol, formoterol, or salmeterol at allowable concentrations.

EIB, Exercise-induced bronchoconstriction; *NCAA,* National Collegiate Athletic Association; *TUE,* therapeutic use exemption.

CHOLINERGIC URTICARIA

Definition: Cholinergic urticaria is the name given to wheals with a surrounding flare reaction (hives) that are precipitated by an increase in core body temperature.

Epidemiology: Cholinergic urticaria is believed to account for 5% of all cases of chronic urticaria and approximately 30% of all physical urticaria. Approximately 15% of the general population will experience at least one episode in their lifetime. Typical onset is the second or third decade of life, and the condition affects both sexes equally. Familial cases have been reported but are rare (all affected patients in these cases were males with father-to-son transmission).

Triggers:
- Heat or cold
- Sunlight
- Physical or emotional stress
- Hot baths
- Heavy clothing
- Spicy foods
- Gluten
- Certain fruits, vegetables, and nuts
- Alcohol

Pathogenesis: Cholinergic urticaria is the result of a hypersensitivity to acetylcholine. The exact mechanism is unclear, but theories include impaired cholinesterase activity and the formation of antigen–antibody immune complexes. Studies have shown elevated plasma histamine in such patients, and studies postulate that sweat may contribute to the reaction.

Clinical signs and symptoms: Typical appearance is that of numerous punctate wheals (1–3 mm) surrounded by large flares after exercise with core temperature elevation. The response can be seen with a body temperature rise as little as 1°C. This is distinct from exercise-induced anaphylaxis, which features large wheals. As the response progresses, the flares may coalesce to form large areas of erythema. The wheals typically involve the trunk and extremities (Fig. 37.3). Patients will often experience various sensations including itching, burning, or tingling and can progress to systemic symptoms such as hypotension, angioedema, and bronchoconstriction (rare).

Testing: The presence of classic lesions in the context of a typical inciting trigger is often enough for diagnosis, but confirmatory testing can be attempted. Provocation testing:
- An intradermal injection of methacholine in saline produces hives around the injection site. However, this test is only positive in about one-third of patients who do have cholinergic urticaria.
- Can also conduct specific provocation testing to provoke a response; would include having the patient mimic the activity (e.g., exercising or eating certain foods) to try and produce a reaction, including exercising in a warm room.
- Can also try and raise the core body temperature by having the patient partially submerged in a hot water bath at 40°C until the body temperature has been raised by 0.7°C; the appearance of generalized urticaria confirms the diagnosis. Note: Aquagenic urticaria may be precipitated by this procedure, but the wheals should only occur in submerged portions of the skin.

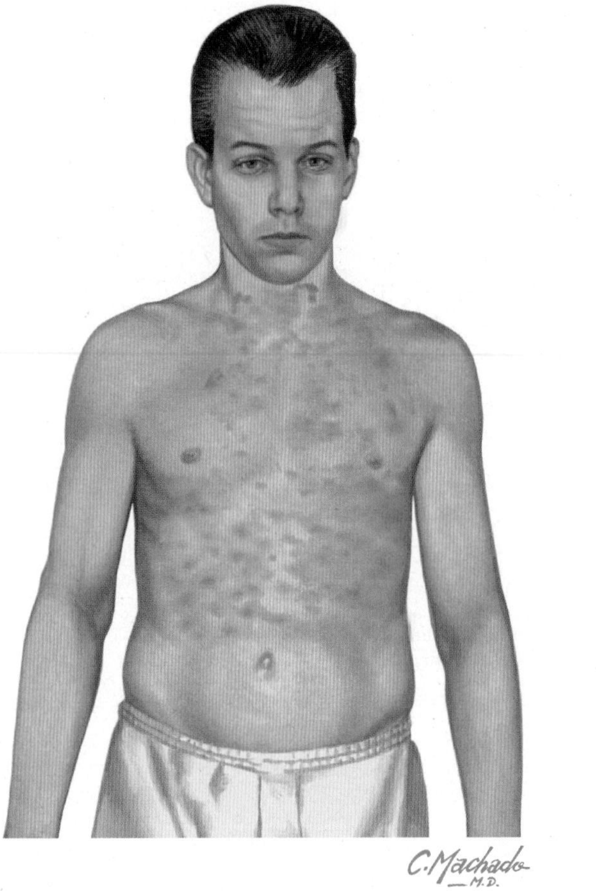
C. Machado M.D.

Figure 37.3 Urticaria.

Treatment:
- **Nonpharmacologic:** Identification and avoidance of known triggers is the first step in controlling cholinergic urticaria. Avoid strenuous exercise in hot weather and bathing in overly hot water. Physical desensitization may also benefit, such as efforts to gradually increase body temperature.
- **Pharmacologic:** H1-antihistamines are the treatment of choice, and among these, hydroxyzine is the agent of choice. A low dose should be initiated and gradually increased until the urticaria is controlled; the literature describes cases requiring as much as four times the licensed dose. Omalizumab, a monoclonal antibody, is reserved as second-line treatment for those who do not respond to antihistamines.

EXERCISE-INDUCED ANAPHYLAXIS

Definition: Exercise-induced anaphylaxis is a distinct form of allergic reaction wherein physical exertion can cause a spectrum of symptoms, including pruritus, urticaria, angioedema, wheezing, hypotension, syncope, and even death. Exercise-induced anaphylaxis can occur at any time during exercise, including postexertion.

Epidemiology: Age of onset ranges from early childhood through adulthood and seems to be more prevalent in females. Approximately 50% of patients have a history of atopy.

Triggers: Can be triggered by any physical activity but most commonly seen with aerobic sports and jogging; factors that have been associated with exercise-induced anaphylaxis include menstruation, use of aspirin or nonsteroidal anti-inflammatory drugs (NSAIDs), and exposure to cold weather. Certain patients have a food-dependent or drug-dependent variant where exercise after a certain food or medication can provoke an anaphylactic reaction. Common foods associated with these reactions are celery, shellfish, cheese, eggs, chicken, hazelnuts, oranges, apples, peaches, grapes, wheat, and cabbage. Other, less common, causes include dancing, sexual intercourse, or household activities such as gardening.

Pathogenesis: The exact mechanism remains unknown, but mast cells are known to be a crucial factor because of studies that have demonstrated elevation of serum histamine and tryptase levels during attacks. Modified enzyme or cytokine expression during exercise may prime an altered response and increase the immunogenicity of certain medications or foods. An additional theory suggests that blood flow during exercise is diverted to muscles and skin, which may cause cellular changes to pH or osmolality, favoring reaction to an allergen.

Clinical signs and symptoms: Patients experience a spectrum of symptoms, including flushing, urticaria, diffuse itching, warmth, malaise, nausea or vomiting, abdominal pain, hypotension, and breathing difficulty. The urticarial wheals are notably larger than in exercise-induced urticaria and may become confluent. Dermatologic symptoms may precede systemic symptoms and should prompt the athlete to stop exercising. Once an attack occurs, it lasts from 30 minutes to 4 hours. A late phase has been described, which can cause headache, fatigue, and warmth that lasts for 24–72 hours.

Testing: Exercise testing is the preferred diagnostic method. Testing must be performed in a controlled environment, with the appropriate medical personnel, epinephrine, and resuscitative equipment present. Vital signs and spirometry should be monitored. It is recommended that an intravenous (IV) line be in place to both draw serum markers and administer medications. False-negative challenges are common, so the testing may need to be repeated on multiple occasions.

Treatment:

- **Nonpharmacologic:** The first step in effective management is to identify and avoid any inducing foods, medicines, or other triggers. The patient may need to limit the intensity and/or frequency of exercise and avoid exercising 4–6 hours after eating or in extremely hot, humid, or cold weather. They should stop exercising at the first sign of symptoms.
- **Pharmacologic:** Patients should always carry self-injectable epinephrine at all times. The athlete also must exercise or train with a partner who is trained in the use of injectable epinephrine, if necessary. Antihistamine therapy has demonstrated only partial benefits in the prevention of anaphylaxis and may mask symptoms.

RECOMMENDED READINGS

Available online.

38 NEUROLOGIC PROBLEMS IN THE ATHLETE

David J. Petron • Steven A. Makovitch

EPILEPSY AND SEIZURE ACTIVITY IN ATHLETES

Definition

Seizure: A transient disruption of brain function from abnormal, excessive, synchronous neuronal activity in the brain; its clinical manifestation depends on the specific region and extent of the brain involved, which may include altered motor function, sensation, alertness, perception, and autonomic function.

Epilepsy: An enduring predisposition to generate recurrent, unprovoked epileptic seizures; worldwide prevalence is approximately 8.2 per 1000 individuals; 75% of epileptics experience their first seizure before the third decade of their life.

Classification

Seizures can be systematically classified as focal or generalized.

Generalized

Overview: Seizures involve both cerebral hemispheres, are of abrupt onset, and involve alteration in consciousness.

Tonic-clonic (grand mal): Occurs at all ages; may have a prodromal phase lasting hours to days. Typically starts with a tonic phase (rigid extension) lasting up to 20 seconds, followed by a clonic phase (synchronous muscle jerking) lasting 1–2 minutes; most last for <1 minute. Characteristics include loss of consciousness, convulsions, muscle rigidity, and urinary but not fecal incontinence; may progress to generalized status epilepticus; a postictal phase (confusion, headache, and fatigue) is common. May be followed by focal weakness or paralysis, including vision and speech function, reflecting postictal depression of the epileptogenic cortical area; this phenomenon, known as *Todd paralysis*, is reversible and usually resolves within 48 hours.

Absence (petit mal): Occurs generally in children; no prodromal or postictal phase reported.

- **Typical:** Onset is acute, as is recovery, with seizure activity lasting <10 seconds.
- **Atypical:** Lasts for >10 seconds, with more gradual onset and recovery; sudden loss of awareness with associated staring, rhythmic blinking, and possibly clonic jerks.

Generalized status epilepticus: Defined as a continuous seizure activity lasting 30 minutes or as two or more discrete seizures between which consciousness is not fully regained. Seizures lasting >5 minutes have a high likelihood of progressing to status epilepticus and should be treated aggressively. **This is a medical emergency. Activate emergency medical services (EMS).** Ensure adequate airway, breathing, and circulation. Attempt to obtain intravenous (IV) access and to prevent aspiration. Benzodiazepines are the drugs of choice for initial treatment because they are fast acting and effective. Lorazepam at a dose of 0.1 mg/kg IV over 2 minutes is considered first-line treatment. Consider metabolic etiologies. Complications include dysrhythmias, metabolic abnormalities, hyperthermia, pulmonary edema, rhabdomyolysis, and pulmonary aspiration.

Focal

Overview: Originate in a localized region of the brain and cause symptoms specific to the part of the cortex wherein they originate; partial seizures may become secondarily generalized.

BROAD TYPES

Simple focal: May include motor, sensory, autonomic, or psychic symptoms; no alteration of consciousness occurs; may be isolated or progress to complex focal or generalized seizures; associated with Todd paralysis (see "Tonic-Clonic Seizures").

Complex focal: Most common type of seizure in epileptic adults; characterized by focal repetitive, purposeless, and complex movements (e.g., chewing, gesturing, lip smacking, and finger snapping) with alteration of consciousness; associated with auras that represent sensory and psychoillusory phenomena; most originate in the temporal lobe; typically last for <90 seconds and are associated with the postictal phase; amnesia specific to the event is common.

Posttraumatic Seizures

Description: Provoked seizures after traumatic brain injury (TBI); classified by timing of the seizure activity

Immediate (concussive convulsions): Occurs within the first 24 hours after TBI; about one-half of seizures occur during the first 24 hours and one-quarter during the first hour; controversial classification, as they are not felt to represent a true seizure, but rather a fairly benign phenomenon that occurs immediately after a concussion; usually do not require anticonvulsant therapy

Early: Occurs within 1 week of TBI; risk factors include young age, severity of injury, alcoholism, and intracerebral or subdural hematoma. Incidence is approximately 6%–10% but higher in patients with marked head injury. Seizure activity is usually tonic-clonic within the first 24 hours, progressing to more focal symptoms thereafter. A computed tomography (CT) scan of the head is indicated, considering the higher incidence of intracranial bleeding; not felt to represent epilepsy but often treated with prophylactic antiepileptic medication to minimize the risk of status epilepticus and secondary injury; treatment with antiepileptic medications does not affect the risk of posttraumatic epilepsy.

Late: Occurs over 1 week after TBI, with most occurring before 2 years after injury.

- **Risk factors:** Early posttraumatic seizures, severity of injury, age >65 years, alcoholism, brain contusion, and intracerebral or subdural hematoma. Overall incidence is approximately 2% but is strongly correlated with severity of TBI. Seizures are also associated with underlying brain pathology. They may recur in up to 70% of cases and often require long-term anticonvulsant medication.

Precipitating Factors for Seizure

Idiopathic, new-onset epilepsy, stress, sleep deprivation, fatigue, prenatal or perinatal brain injury, hyperthermia, metabolic (dehydration, hypoglycemia, hyponatremia, etc.), infectious (e.g., meningitis), trauma, drugs/alcohol (intoxication and withdrawal), febrile (usually occur between 6 months and 5 years of age), and intracranial lesions (mass, hematoma, etc.)

Evaluation of Epileptic Athletes

Before participation, the physician should be familiar with certain aspects of seizure history, including seizure types (frequency, duration, and manifestations); precipitating factors; postictal recovery; any history of status epilepticus; current anticonvulsant use, including side effects and medication adherence; and head trauma history.

On-Field Treatment

- Standard guidelines for management of airway, breathing, and circulation should be followed.
- Assist the patient to the ground and clear the area of any potential hazards.
  - Do not restrain the athlete.
  - Rolling the athlete to his or her side while he or she is convulsing may lead to injury; wait until the seizure is over before attempting this.
- Do not place anything in the athlete's mouth, particularly fingers. The mouth guard may be removed if it can be performed safely.
- If there is any concern for status epilepticus, activate EMS for transport to a medical facility.
- If this was the patient's first onset of a seizure or if clinical presentation is different from baseline seizure history, additional workup, including imaging, is indicated.

Epilepsy and Sports

- Points to consider:
  - Does the specific type of seizure disorder place the athlete at an increased risk of injury (e.g., absence vs. simple focal)?
  - Will the athlete's condition place others at risk of injury?
  - How intent is the athlete on playing the sport?
- Sports participation is associated with factors that may alter the seizure threshold.
  - Stress: Known risk factor for seizures, and this should be addressed on an individual basis.
  - Hyperventilation: Resting hyperventilation may predispose to a decreased seizure threshold. Exercise-induced hyperventilation, however, is a physiologic response and does not seem to have a negative effect on the seizure threshold.
  - Alterations in drug metabolism: Studies have found no significant difference in metabolism during pre-exercise, exercise, and postexercise periods. However, if seizure activity increases, this should be considered.
  - Exercise-induced seizures:
    - Although there are certain cases of exercise lowering the seizure threshold, this seems to be the exception. Overall, the frequency of seizure is decreased by aerobic activity and is supported by electroencephalogram (EEG) findings.
    - Prolonged exercise, as seen in endurance athletes, may alter physiologic parameters associated with seizure activity (hyponatremia, hypoglycemia, etc.).
    - Consider diagnosis of seizures with episodes of exercise-induced syncope.
- People with epilepsy are less active, less physically fit, less likely to participate in sports, and are at a risk of social isolation.
- Exercise should be encouraged in people with epilepsy, as it has been shown to promote quality of life and well-being through socialization and physical conditioning.
  - In clinical studies exercise has been associated with reduced epileptiform discharges and an increased seizure threshold.
- There is currently no evidence that contact sports are harmful to most athletes with epilepsy.
  - There is evidence to suggest that severe head injury causes or exacerbates preexisting epilepsy, but this does not apply to repeated mild TBI.
- Contact sports should be evaluated on an individual basis based on the presumed danger an athlete may present to themselves or others.

Sport-Specific Guidelines

Contact sports: No restriction unless newly diagnosed or unclear course.

Water sports: Generally permitted with appropriate precautions (avoid open water, wear flotation device, and supervised by qualified personnel); scuba diving, competitive underwater swimming, and diving prohibited with active epilepsy, although may be considered after a prolonged seizure-free period (e.g., the UK Sport Diving Medical Committee suggests 5 years free of seizures without medication).

Motor sports: Discouraged with active epilepsy.

Aerobic sports: No restrictions; wear appropriate protective gear.

Sports at heights: Equestrian sports should be avoided with active epilepsy. Certain gymnastic events (e.g., high bar) should be discouraged. Skydiving, hang gliding, and free climbing should be discouraged. Pilot's license is prohibited.

Shooting sports: Specific consideration for type and frequency of seizures, pattern of occurrence, and type of weapon fired.

CERVICAL CORD NEURAPRAXIA (TRANSIENT QUADRIPARESIS)

Overview: Transient neurologic episodes characterized by a temporary loss of motor or sensory function, or both. This is likely secondary to central cord contusion with or without associated ischemia. Most common with contact sports. Prevalence is estimated at 7 per 10,000 football participants.

Mechanism of injury: Varied mechanisms (usually hyperflexion, hyperextension, or axial loading of the neck) resulting in cervical cord contusion and decreased blood flow; suspected to be associated with spinal stenosis and the shape of the spinal canal. Degree of stenosis may be estimated using the Torg ratio (ratio of spinal canal width to vertebral body diameter). A ratio of <0.80 is considered indicative of "significant cervical stenosis"; this ratio has been shown to be an unreliable measure in larger athletes because of the relative vertebral body width yielding poor positive predictive value, and it has been replaced by magnetic resonance imaging (MRI) evaluation.

Symptoms: Bilateral sensory changes, motor changes, or combined sensorimotor deficits. Total body numbness may occur. Neck pain is usually absent.

Physical examination:

- **On the field**
  - Assume cervical spine injury until proven otherwise. Follow cervical spine precautions and use cervical collar and spine board.
  - Athlete should be stabilized and transported to the nearest appropriate facility by EMS for further evaluation.
  - For football, remove the face mask, but helmet and shoulder pads should remain in place. According to the most recent position statement by the American College of Sports Medicine (ACSM), it is strongly advised to not remove an American football helmet and shoulder pads from an unconscious athlete or an athlete who has sustained a neck injury. If any of the following criteria are met, the helmet and the shoulder pads should be removed, maintaining cervical spine precautions:
    - If the helmet and chin strap do not securely hold the head, such that immobilization of the helmet does not also immobilize the head
    - If the design of the helmet and chin strap is such that even after removal of the face mask, the airway cannot be controlled or ventilation provided
    - If after a reasonable period, the face mask cannot be removed to gain access to the airway
    - If the helmet prevents immobilization for transportation in an appropriate position
    - Standard guidelines for management of airway, breathing, and circulation must be followed

Table 38.1 PERIPHERAL NERVE INJURY CLASSIFICATION

Seddon	Sunderland	Pathology	Electrodiagnostic Findings	Prognosis
Neuropraxia	I	Demyelination	Conduction block	Excellent, recovery typically 2–3 months
Axonotmesis	II	Demyelination and axon loss	Axon loss	Good, but limited by distance to muscle
Axonotmesis	III	II + endoneurium involvement	Axon loss	Fair, surgery may be required
Axonotmesis	IV	III + perineurium involvement	Axon loss	Poor, surgery usually required
Neurotmesis	V	IV + epineurium involvement	Axon loss	Poor, no spontaneous recovery and surgery required

- **Off the field**
  - Thorough cervical spine and neurologic evaluation is necessary.
  - Pain and tenderness over the cervical spine are not associated with transient quadriparesis and should prompt consideration of other injuries such as fracture.

Diagnostics: Plain cervical spine trauma radiograph series should be obtained to rule out fracture or dislocation. Once a fracture is definitively ruled out, flexion and extension views may be obtained to check for ligamentous instability. CT to rule out occult facture. MRI should be obtained to evaluate spinal stenosis, spinal cord, and associated injuries.

Treatment: Initial treatment should focus on cervical spine immobilization, medical stabilization, and transport via EMS. The most recent Cochrane review recommends high-dose methylprednisolone within 8 hours of spinal cord injury because it has been shown to improve recovery of motor functions. However, controversy still exists, and additional research is needed. There is no role for steroids in athletes with transient quadriparesis who show resolution of symptoms. Systemic hypothermia, which is thought to decrease tissue metabolism and limit secondary hypoxic injury, has also been used but is still experimental and not part of routine care.

Prognosis and return to play (RTP): Temporary condition by definition, but both extent and duration of neurologic dysfunction factor in the overall prognosis; average rate of recurrence for players who return to football is 56%. Repeat episodes may be associated with cervical radiculopathy and myelopathy. Predisposition to permanent neurologic injury after an episode of cervical cord neurapraxia is controversial, but there are published case reports regarding the same; RTP decisions are made on an individual basis, taking into account history of injuries, anatomic predisposition, and future risk of injury. Although discussing all possible scenarios is beyond the purpose of this text, we have enlisted a few examples here: If an athlete is asymptomatic without documented stenosis, it is generally accepted that he or she be allowed to RTP. If an athlete is asymptomatic with documented stenosis, significant controversy exists regarding RTP. Stenosis is more accurately defined by adequate cerebrospinal fluid around the cord as opposed to by absolute canal diameter. Opinions range from considering this as a relative contraindication to an absolute contraindication. Multiple episodes without documented stenosis should prompt serious consideration of discontinuing contact sports.

PERIPHERAL NERVE INJURY IN ATHLETES

Overview of anatomy: The peripheral nervous system includes cranial nerves, spinal nerves and their roots and branches, peripheral nerves, and neuromuscular junctions.

Classification of injury: There are two primary classification systems: Seddon and Sunderland. Descriptions of each type, prognosis, and associated electrodiagnostic findings are compared in Table 38.1 (Fig. 38.1). Neuropraxia (grade I) is typically a demyelinating injury with good recovery. Axonotmesis (grades II–IV) involves axon disruption but with preservation of some degree of supporting structures (endoneurium, perineurium, and epineurium). The more supporting structures involved, the worse the outcomes. Neurotmesis (grade V) is complete disruption of both axons and supporting structures, with limited scope of recovery without surgical intervention.

Mechanism of injury: Injuries can be subcategorized into acute, subacute, or chronic. Acute injuries may result from nerve compression, stretch/traction, or laceration and usually result from an unexpected fall or extrinsic force (e.g., tackle). Stretch/traction injuries are the most common; most nerves can tolerate 10%–20% lengthening before structural damage occurs. Subacute or chronic injuries are best classified as overuse injuries resulting from repetitive microtrauma or compression. This may occur from forced movement of a nerve through a fascial restriction, around a bony prominence, or from nearby tendinosis (e.g., sciatic neuritis from proximal hamstring tendinopathy).

Evaluation: History should elicit a specific time course and mechanism of injury. Symptoms may include a deep-seated, poorly localized pain described as soreness, numbness, electric shock, and burning sensation. A detailed physical examination is essential and includes muscle bulk inspection, strength testing, deep tendon reflexes, and sensory examination. Provocative maneuvers should be performed, including neural tension testing (i.e., straight leg raise) and direct nerve percussion (i.e., Tinel sign). Check for altered sensation in the specific peripheral nerve distribution, which may also be accompanied by hyperalgesia or allodynia. Equipment should be inspected for appropriate use and fit. In addition, a kinetic chain evaluation must be performed in search of a root cause for overuse injuries (i.e., a volleyball athlete with knee pain leading to shoulder overuse and subsequent suprascapular nerve injury).

Diagnostics:

- **Electrodiagnostic testing:** Used to assess the neurophysiologic function of the peripheral nervous system, including nerve roots, plexus, and peripheral nerves; testing includes nerve conduction studies (NCSs) and needle electromyography (EMG). Used as an extension of physical examination and can help clarify or confirm a suspected diagnosis; more specifically, it can help to define the location, duration, severity, and prognosis of neuromuscular disorders. NCSs are performed by placing electrodes on the skin and stimulating the nerve of interest with electrical impulses. NCSs are divided into motor and sensory nerve testing and help determine whether there is dysfunction of the myelin sheath (slowed electrical impulse), axons (reduced amplitude), or a combination of both. EMG involves a needle electrode that is inserted into a muscle of interest in order to analyze motor units and their recruitment. Moreover, EMG can detect muscle denervation and evidence of re-innervation after prior nerve injury, which can help guide prognosis.
- **MRI:** Useful as an adjunct in diagnosis and prognosis; may help with acute injuries in assessing soft tissue damage and deciding on surgical intervention. Normal peripheral nerves appear isointense compared with surrounding muscles, reveal a fascicular pattern, and are usually surrounded by a small rim of fat tissue. Nerve hyperintensity can be detected

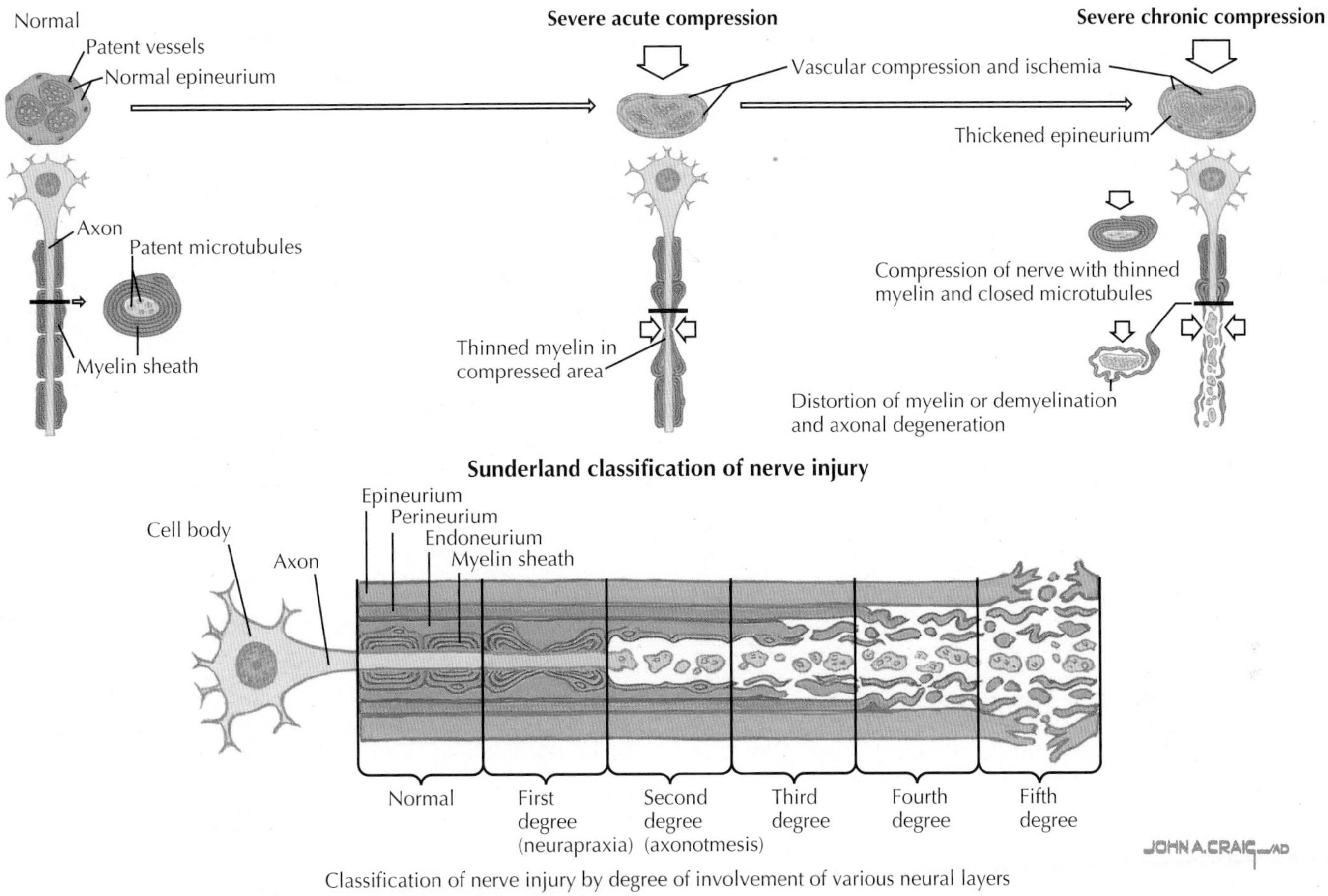
Normal
Patent vessels
Normal epineurium
Severe acute compression
Vascular compression and ischemia
Severe chronic compression
Thickened epineurium
Axon
Patent microtubules
Myelin sheath
Thinned myelin in compressed area
Compression of nerve with thinned myelin and closed microtubules
Distortion of myelin or demyelination and axonal degeneration
Sunderland classification of nerve injury
Cell body
Axon
Epineurium
Perineurium
Endoneurium
Myelin sheath
Normal
First degree (neurapraxia)
Second degree (axonotmesis)
Third degree
Fourth degree
Fifth degree
JOHN A.CRAIG_MD
Classification of nerve injury by degree of involvement of various neural layers

Figure 38.1 Peripheral nerve injury classification.

on T2-weighted MRI within 24 hours of a nerve injury. Focal demyelination reveals hyperintensity at the lesion site, whereas axonal injury with Wallerian degeneration reveals hyperintensity in the entire nerve segment distal to the lesion. Magnetic resonance neurography (MRN) refers to nerve-specific imaging using pulse sequences for optimal visualization. Axial T1-weighted and fluid-sensitive fat-suppressed T2-weighted images serve as the mainstay for interpreting peripheral nerve signal intensity, course, caliber, fascicular pattern, size, perineural fibrosis, and mass lesions. MRI can also identify masses that cause nerve compression.

- **Ultrasound:** Provides immediate, nonionizing, high-resolution, bedside assessment of peripheral nerves and surrounding tissues with ease of contralateral comparison; functional assessment is possible and can detect abnormal nerve motion and nerve entrapment with joint movement (subluxating ulnar nerve at the elbow). In addition, sonopalpation (transducer pressure) to the area of nerve dysfunction is useful for confirming typical symptoms. In long-axis view, peripheral nerves appear fascicular with hypoechoic fascicles surrounded by hyperechoic connective tissue. In short-axis view, peripheral nerves display a honeycomb or speckled appearance. With regard to nerve entrapment, ultrasound can demonstrate sudden flattening (notch sign) or gradual narrowing (dumbbell sign) at the compression site with proximal hypoechoic nerve swelling.

Treatment:

- **Surgical:** Open, sharp traumatic injuries should be immediately repaired through surgical intervention. For open, blunt injuries, delayed repair after 2–3 weeks is recommended to allow scar formation and demarcation of healthy nerve ends. Closed injuries are usually initially treated conservatively. Axonotmetic versus neurotmetic lesions should be differentiated using serial examinations and electrodiagnostic studies after 3 weeks. Surgical exploration using intraoperative electrophysiologic monitoring is suggested if no recovery is seen after 3–4 months. At that time, neurotmetic lesions are repaired and axonotmetic lesions are treated conservatively.
  - **"Rule of three":** Immediate surgery within 3 days for clean and sharp injuries; early surgery within 3 weeks for blunt injuries; delayed surgery at 3 months for closed injuries
- **Conservative management:** Includes a period of rest and avoidance of aggravating activities along with bracing and padding for protection of the injured region; a full kinetic chain evaluation should be performed to identify underlying faulty biomechanics predisposing to an overuse neuropathy. Physical therapy can aid in neuromuscular retraining and progressing back to appropriate sport-specific technique. Medications for symptomatic relief, including anti-inflammatory and neuromodulating agents (i.e., gabapentin), can be used for unpleasant dysesthesias. In cases of chronic nerve entrapment, ultrasound-guided hydrodissection may be considered. Hydrodissection uses fluid (saline, anesthetic, steroid, and 5% dextrose in water) to separate a nerve from surrounding compressive tissue. Relief of neuropathic pain may result from release of pressure on the nervi nervorum and vasa nervorum, which supply the affected peripheral nerve.

Prognosis and recovery: Largely dependent on the type of nerve injury; most traumatic injuries are a combination of axonal and demyelinating pathologies, and prognosis depends on the predominant injury. Mechanisms of recovery include resolution of conduction block (failure of nerve propagation beyond the demyelinated segment), distal axonal sprouting, and axonal regeneration. Resolution of conduction block is typically the first mechanism to promote strength recovery. Recovery after an ischemic injury is quick, whereas demyelinating injuries take up to several months. With an incomplete axonotmesis injury, distal sprouting of intact motor axons starts within 4 days after an injury. In minor axonotmesis injuries, axons can traverse the segment of injury in 8–15 days and then regenerate at a rate of 1–5 mm/day. The regeneration rate is faster for more proximal lesions and after a crush injury, whereas it is slower for distal lesions and after a laceration injury. Even if axons are unable to grow across the injury site, sprouting of motor axons can re-innervate about five times their original muscle fiber territory. Moreover, recovery depends on muscle integrity when the nerve reaches it. Muscle remains viable for re-innervation until about 18–24 months after an injury, after which fibrosis develops. Therefore, recovery, including surgical repair, is poor if denervation persists beyond 1–2 years.

Optimal timing of electrodiagnostic testing: NCS can help immediately localize a lesion, as conduction is absent across the injury site and is normal distally until Wallerian degeneration is complete as early as day 7. EMG in the first week can help determine whether an injury is complete or incomplete. Presence of even a single motor unit firing on EMG signifies at least partial axonal continuity of a nerve. Using NCS to achieve stimulation above and below an injury site can differentiate between neuropraxia and more severe axonotmesis and neurotmesis as early as day 7 for motor and day 11 for sensory nerves because of completion of Wallerian degeneration. However, the most useful diagnostic information can be obtained 3–4 weeks after an injury when needle EMG reveals denervation abnormalities. Findings of re-innervation are first seen proximally, progressing distally. Paraspinal re-innervation can be seen as early as 6–9 weeks after an injury, followed by proximal and then distal muscles between 2 and 6 months.

BRACHIAL PLEXUS AND CERVICAL ROOT INJURIES ("STINGERS/BURNERS")

Overview: Transient neurologic injury accompanied by burning pain in the upper extremity believed to be the result of unilateral nerve traction or compression, generally involving C5 or C6 levels or the superior trunk of the brachial plexus (Fig. 38.2); unclear if this results from brachial plexus or cervical root injury. One of the most common injuries in sports medicine; up to 65% of college football athletes have reported such an injury in their career.

Proposed mechanisms of injury: Neck extension with lateral bending, resulting in a compression injury; distraction of the shoulder from the head and neck causing nerve traction; or direct blow to the supraclavicular region at Erb point (where the brachial plexus is most superficial), causing compressive injury. Cervical stenosis predisposes to stingers and may contribute to more complicated mechanisms.

Presentation: Symptoms include unilateral, transient burning pain or numbness with or without weakness starting from the neck/shoulder and commonly radiating in a C5 or C6 distribution. A circumferential rather than dermatomal pattern may be present. Symptoms in lower extremity or bilateral upper extremities should prompt consideration of central cord injury. Care should be taken to distinguish this condition from transient quadriparesis, which may present with bilateral sensory changes, motor changes, or combined sensorimotor deficits. Typically not associated with neck pain or limited range of motion (ROM); symptoms generally last from seconds to minutes; if symptoms last longer or if there is cervical pain or limited ROM, cervical spine MRI should be strongly considered before RTP. Up to 10% have a neurologic deficit lasting from hours to weeks.

Physical examination: Athletes frequently leave the field shaking their arm and hand and may elevate the arm to decrease the neural tension. Initial evaluation should focus on the cervical spine for any evidence of fracture (bony tenderness [particularly midline], deformity, or swelling). If initial evaluation is normal, assess ROM. Conduct a complete neurologic examination, including strength, sensory, and muscle stretch reflex testing. The time of onset and severity of weakness may vary. C5 and C6 are the most common levels affected. Most common sites of weakness are deltoid, biceps, supraspinatus, and infraspinatus, resulting in weak shoulder abduction, elbow flexion, and external rotation of upper arm. Percussion of Erb point may elicit radiation of pain. A Spurling maneuver has been shown to recreate symptoms in 70% of cases—good specificity but variable sensitivity. Contralateral examination should be normal. If bilateral symptoms are present, full cervical precautions should be initiated, and the athlete must be transported to an appropriate medical facility for further evaluation and imaging. Shoulder examination must also be performed to rule out other injuries.

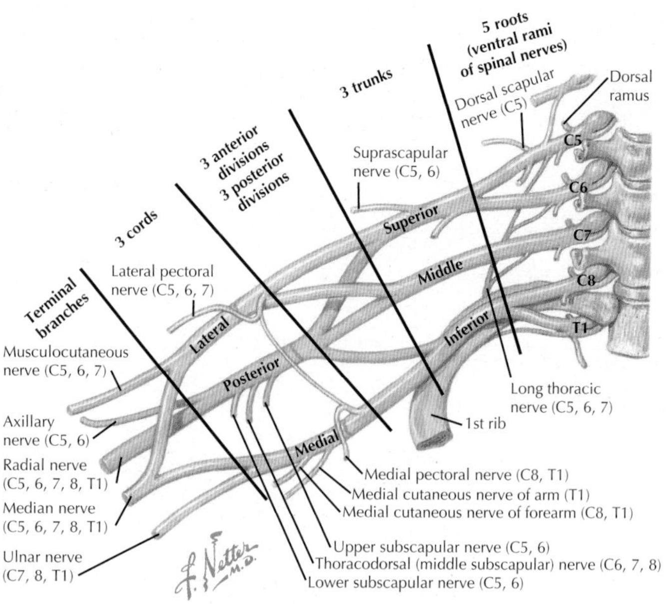
5 roots (ventral rami of spinal nerves)
3 trunks
Dorsal scapular nerve (C5)
Dorsal ramus
C5
C6
C7
C8
T1
3 anterior divisions
3 posterior divisions
Suprascapular nerve (C5, 6)
Superior
Middle
Inferior
3 cords
Lateral pectoral nerve (C5, 6, 7)
Terminal branches
Lateral
Posterior
Medial
Musculocutaneous nerve (C5, 6, 7)
Axillary nerve (C5, 6)
Radial nerve (C5, 6, 7, 8, T1)
Median nerve (C5, 6, 7, 8, T1)
Ulnar nerve (C7, 8, T1)
Long thoracic nerve (C5, 6, 7)
1st rib
Medial pectoral nerve (C8, T1)
Medial cutaneous nerve of arm (T1)
Medial cutaneous nerve of forearm (C8, T1)
Upper subscapular nerve (C5, 6)
Thoracodorsal (middle subscapular) nerve (C6, 7, 8)
Lower subscapular nerve (C5, 6)

Figure 38.2 Brachial plexus schema.

Diagnostics: Diagnosis based on physical examination. Radiographs usually normal; consider MRI for prolonged symptoms or recurrent stingers. EMG may be appropriate if symptoms persist beyond 3 weeks. The role of EMG in RTP decisions is controversial because EMG findings may remain abnormal long after clinical symptoms have resolved.

Treatment: Athletes should be removed from play until completely asymptomatic. Immediate supportive treatment includes rest and use of a sling. More chronic symptoms may necessitate anti-inflammatory medications, physical therapy, and occasionally, nerve root blocks. Prevention of recurrence is central to treatment. Rehabilitation should be instituted for neck and shoulder strengthening.

Preventive equipment: To limit excessive neck extension and lateral flexion, high-riding shoulder pads and neck rolls may be considered, but efficacy is debatable. Straps that connect the helmet and shoulder pads are not recommended. Evaluate tackling technique.

Prognosis and RTP: Decision is clinical. Athletes may return to full contact when they have pain-free, full ROM of the neck and shoulder and normal neurologic examination, including normal symmetric strength. Longer rest periods are indicated for symptoms lasting >15 minutes and for recurrent stingers in the same season. Continue to evaluate for delayed weakness during the same event and for the next 2 weeks. Repetitive or prolonged episodes warrant additional diagnostic testing. Chronic and recurrent stingers have been associated with cervical disk disease, spinal stenosis, and/or neural foraminal narrowing. Prolonged time to symptom resolution (particularly >3 weeks) and recurrent stingers over a short period have poorer prognosis. Some experts advocate that if cervical foraminal stenosis is discovered, the athlete should discontinue contact sports.

AXILLARY NERVE INJURY

Overview: The axillary nerve is derived from the posterior cord of the brachial plexus at the C5 or C6 level with occasional contribution from C4. It travels across the anteroinferior aspect of the subscapularis muscle before entering the quadrilateral space and dividing into two branches. The anterior branch passes around the surgical neck of the humerus, and the posterior branch travels adjacent to the inferior aspect of the glenoid rim before dividing into the upper lateral brachial cutaneous nerve and the nerve to the teres minor (Fig. 38.3). The quadrilateral space is bordered by the long head of the triceps medially, humerus laterally, teres minor superiorly, teres major and latissimus dorsi muscles inferiorly, and subscapularis anteriorly. Branches:

- Anterior branch: Motor innervation of the deltoid
- Posterior branch: Motor innervation of the teres minor
  - Superior lateral cutaneous nerve: sensory innervation over the inferior portion of the deltoid (upper and lateral arm)
- Uncommon nerve injury, representing <1% of all nerve injuries

Common sports for injury: Baseball, football, hiking, hockey, martial arts, rugby, volleyball, and wrestling

Mechanism of injury: Most commonly incurred with other brachial plexus injuries

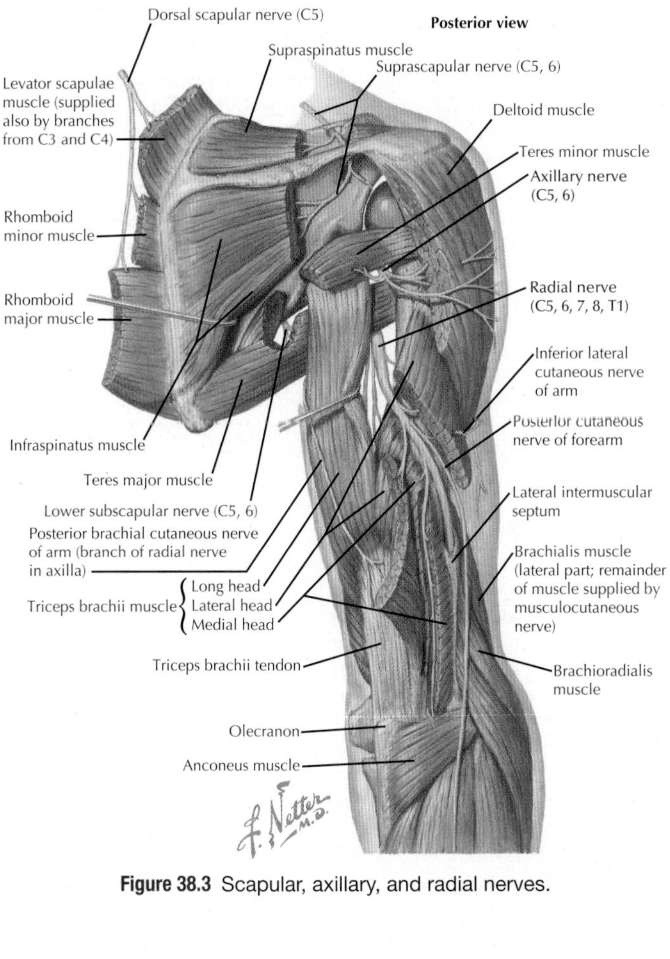
Posterior view
Dorsal scapular nerve (C5)
Supraspinatus muscle
Suprascapular nerve (C5, 6)
Levator scapulae muscle (supplied also by branches from C3 and C4)
Deltoid muscle
Teres minor muscle
Axillary nerve (C5, 6)
Rhomboid minor muscle
Rhomboid major muscle
Radial nerve (C5, 6, 7, 8, T1)
Inferior lateral cutaneous nerve of arm
Posterior cutaneous nerve of forearm
Infraspinatus muscle
Teres major muscle
Lower subscapular nerve (C5, 6)
Lateral intermuscular septum
Posterior brachial cutaneous nerve of arm (branch of radial nerve in axilla)
Brachialis muscle (lateral part; remainder of muscle supplied by musculocutaneous nerve)
Triceps brachii muscle
Long head
Lateral head
Medial head
Triceps brachii tendon
Brachioradialis muscle
Olecranon
Anconeus muscle

Figure 38.3 Scapular, axillary, and radial nerves.

- **Traumatic:** Direct (e.g., contusion to anterolateral deltoid or humeral fracture) or indirect (e.g., shoulder traction with dislocation).
- **Compression:** Quadrilateral space syndrome; this is a rare condition characterized by compression of the posterior humeral circumflex artery and axillary nerve as they pass though the quadrilateral space. Compression is believed to be caused by fibrotic bands within the space or by hypertrophy of the muscles that form the borders, but the exact etiology is unclear.
- **Iatrogenic** (e.g., rotator cuff surgery).

Symptoms: Variable. The athlete may not complain of frank weakness. Possible symptoms include early fatigue or weakness, particularly with overhead activities or abduction. The athlete may notice numbness in the lateral upper arm region. Night pain is frequently reported.

Differential diagnosis: Cervical pathology (typically C5/C6), rotator cuff injury, vascular compression, and suprascapular nerve injury.

Physical examination: Visual inspection may reveal deltoid or teres minor atrophy with late presentation. Examine the neck, shoulder, and arm. ROM and strength in all planes should be tested. Palpate the deltoid for contraction during the initiation of abduction. Be sure to evaluate all three heads of the deltoid because nerve injury may not be uniform throughout. Weakness may occur with external rotation, abduction, and/or forward flexion. Evaluate sensation in the upper lateral arm region.

Diagnostics: Radiographs should be obtained to check for fracture of the humerus. Cervical spine films assess bony cervical pathology. MRI and electrodiagnostics should be considered.

Treatment: Depends on the underlying etiology and injury to surrounding structures.

Address underlying shoulder dislocation and/or fracture. Conservative treatment includes rest and physical therapy for active and passive ROM and strengthening. Electrical stimulation of the deltoid is an optional treatment.

Prognosis and RTP: Full recovery with nonoperative treatment is expected in 85%–100% of cases within 12 months if they are associated with dislocation or fracture. Various case series describing injuries from direct contusion have shown poorer prognosis with respect to recovery of deltoid function, but a substantial proportion of these patients returned to contact sports despite deltoid paralysis. RTP decisions depend on the associated injuries involved, but full shoulder ROM and good strength are recommended.

SUPRASCAPULAR NERVE INJURY

Overview: The suprascapular nerve originates from the superior trunk of the brachial plexus (C5 and C6 with variable contribution from C4). It travels laterally across the posterior triangle of the neck through the suprascapular notch and under the superior transverse scapular ligament before sending off branches to the supraspinatus. The nerve then travels around the spinoglenoid notch to enter the infraspinatus fossa, where it divides to supply the infraspinatus (Fig. 38.4) and innervates the supraspinatus and infraspinatus with sensory branches to the acromioclavicular and glenohumeral joints. Sensory innervation of the proximal-lateral arm is reported in 15% of patients. The nerve is the most frequently injured peripheral branch of the brachial plexus in athletes.

Common sports for injury: Volleyball, baseball, basketball, tennis/racquetball, football, weightlifting, hiking, wrestling, cycling, and ballet dancing

Mechanism of injury:

- **Trauma:** Direct (e.g., scapular or clavicular fracture, shoulder dislocations, and penetrating trauma) and indirect (e.g., traction or repetitive overuse)

- **Compression:** Usually via surrounding ligaments or mass lesions (e.g., cyst, lipoma, and fibrous band); overhead activities such as throwing lead to greater degrees of friction, traction, and compression; external rotation, cross-body adduction, and forward flexion are also implicated; proposed "sling effect" refers to friction of the nerve against surrounding structures of the suprascapular notch with depression and retraction or hyperabduction of the shoulder.
- **Iatrogenic**

Symptoms: Include dull pain at the posterior aspect of the shoulder exacerbated by overhead maneuvers and/or weakness of the affected shoulder, particularly during rotation and abduction. Atrophy present in up to 80% of patients (see Fig. 38.4); onset is usually insidious but may follow an acute event. Lesions at the spinoglenoid notch often present with asymptomatic atrophy of the infraspinatus alone, whereas lesions at the suprascapular notch often reveal atrophy of both infraspinatus and supraspinatus.

Differential diagnosis: Cervical spine pathology, brachial plexopathy, biceps tendonitis, adhesive capsulitis, impingement syndrome, rotator cuff, and intra-articular glenohumeral pathology

Physical examination: Visual inspection may reveal atrophy of the infraspinatus or supraspinatus. Atrophy of the infraspinatus is better visualized from behind and above, but supraspinatus atrophy may be difficult to visualize. Physical examination may reveal tenderness at the injury site, and cross-arm adduction may increase pain. Physical examination findings are similar to those of impingement syndrome. Include thorough neurologic evaluation, including neck and upper extremity, specifically during external rotation and abduction.

Diagnostics: Often considered a diagnosis of exclusion; may try injection of a local anesthetic into the suprascapular notch for diagnostic purposes, but this is nonspecific. An anteroposterior radiograph directed caudally at 30 degrees or a Stryker notch view may be useful to assess the shape of the suprascapular notch. MRI is considered the optimal imaging modality for evaluating suprascapular nerve palsy because it should reveal both mass lesions and other rotator cuff or soft tissue pathology. Ganglion cysts causing suprascapular nerve compression are often associated with labral tears. Ultrasound may also be useful but is operator dependent. Electrodiagnostics may help localize the site of injury and rule out a C5 or C6 radiculopathy.

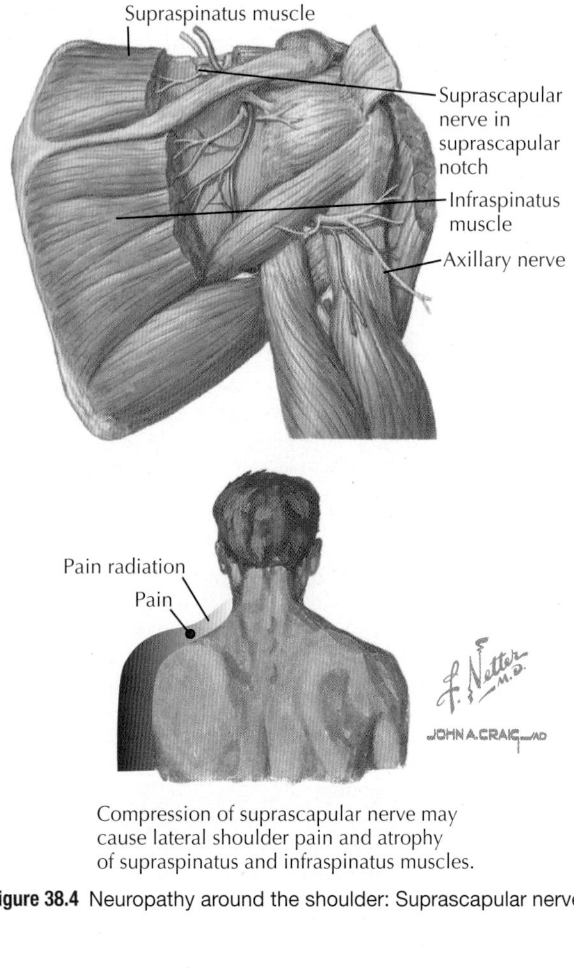
Supraspinatus muscle
Suprascapular nerve in suprascapular notch
Infraspinatus muscle
Axillary nerve
Pain radiation
Pain
F. Netter M.D.
JOHN A.CRAIG_AD
Compression of suprascapular nerve may cause lateral shoulder pain and atrophy of supraspinatus and infraspinatus muscles.

Figure 38.4 Neuropathy around the shoulder: Suprascapular nerve.

Treatment: Treatment and prognosis depend on the underlying etiology. Initial treatment is conservative and includes avoidance of aggravating activities, anti-inflammatory medications, and rehabilitation for stretching and strengthening of surrounding structures. Structural lesions (e.g., labral pathology) correlating with clinical symptoms should be surgically treated. Nonoperative treatment of ganglion cysts has a high failure rate, and cysts are frequently drained surgically. Occasionally, exploration and decompression of compressive lesions or bands may be required. If symptoms are not caused by known structural lesions or if atrophy continues to persist for >6 months, surgical exploration should be considered. Follow-up EMG may aid in the decision to proceed with surgical therapy.

Prognosis and RTP: Natural history of the injury varies greatly, but resolution of symptoms in the absence of a mass lesion is expected within 6–12 months of the diagnosis. The patient may continue his or her chosen sport at a competitive level despite muscle atrophy if appropriate strength permits safe participation. RTP decisions are individual and activity specific.

LONG THORACIC NERVE INJURY

Overview: The long thoracic nerve arises from the anterior branches of C5 through C7, with 20% of contributions from intercostal nerves. At 22–24 cm in length, it descends posteriorly to C8 and T1 rami, passes beneath the clavicle, and continues distally on the external surface of the serratus anterior (Fig. 38.5). This nerve innervates the serratus anterior, which protracts and rotates the scapula and stabilizes the scapula during abduction.

Common sports for injury: Tennis/racquetball, backpacking, archery, basketball, bodybuilding, football, golf, gymnastics, martial arts, hiking, shooting, volleyball, and wrestling

Mechanism of injury:

- **Traumatic:** Direct (e.g., contusion to shoulder or lateral thorax) and indirect (e.g., stretching of the nerve can occur with the neck turned to the contralateral direction and the arm raised overhead or shoulder depression in conjunction with contralateral neck bending)
- **Compression:** Multiple possible areas for compression by surrounding structures, crutches, or inflamed bursa
- **Iatrogenic** (e.g., postoperative)

Symptoms: Typical winging or popping of the scapula during movement secondary to compromised glenohumeral biomechanics; others may complain of pain in the shoulder, neck, and/or scapular area lasting up to a few weeks, followed by insidious weakness with overhead activities or forward elevation

Differential diagnosis: Cervical disc disease, rotator cuff pathology, brachial neuritis (Parsonage–Turner syndrome), adhesive capsulitis, glenohumeral instability or arthritis, acromioclavicular joint arthritis, thoracic outlet syndrome, and spinal accessory nerve injury

Physical examination: Visual inspection will reveal winging of the affected scapula exaggerated by forward elevation or pushing off a wall (see Fig. 38.5). Atrophy of the serratus anterior may be visible. Winging is associated with both long thoracic and spinal accessory nerve injuries. Winging associated with spinal accessory nerve injury is generally not exaggerated by forward

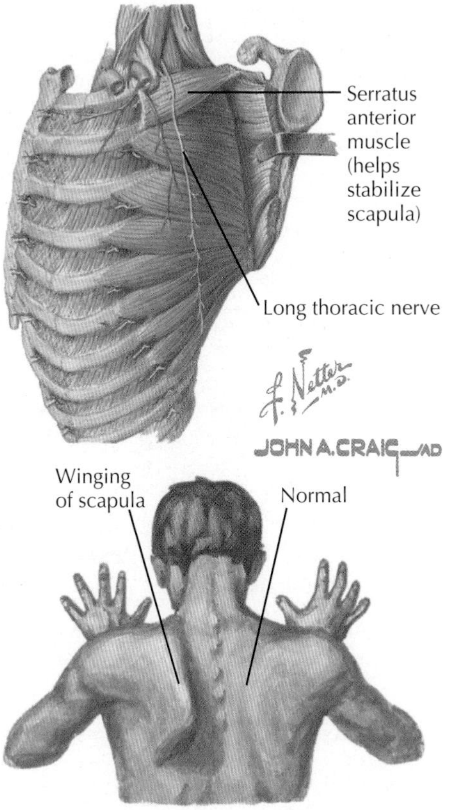
Serratus anterior muscle (helps stabilize scapula)
Long thoracic nerve
Winging of scapula
Normal
JOHN A.CRAIG_AD

Figure 38.5 Neuropathy around the shoulder: Long thoracic nerve.

elevation as is seen with long thoracic etiology. Physical examination reveals weakness with forward elevation, often limiting movement to 110 degrees. Altered scapulohumeral rhythm may be found.

Diagnostics: Considered a clinical diagnosis; plain radiographs are generally normal; CT and MRI generally not useful unless used to rule out other pathologies; electrodiagnostics help distinguish from other causes of scapular winging (dorsal scapular and spinal accessory nerve injury)

Treatment: Conservative treatment includes rest, reassurance, anti-inflammatory medications or medications for neurogenic pain, maintaining ROM, and strengthening of surrounding structures. Bracing may be considered for improved function or pain control but has not been highly effective. Indications for surgical consultation include symptoms persisting beyond 1 year with no improvement on EMG and iatrogenic injury.

Prognosis and RTP: Isolated atraumatic long thoracic nerve palsy generally resolves in 1–2 years. RTP decisions should be individualized and based on the athlete's strength and the demands of the sport.

SPINAL ACCESSORY NERVE INJURY

Overview: The spinal accessory nerve is a pure motor cranial nerve. It enters the foramen magnum and then exits the jugular foramen before passing through the upper third of the sternocleidomastoid (SCM). The nerve then assumes a subcutaneous course in the posterior cervical triangle to the trapezius. This nerve provides motor innervation to the trapezius and SCM.

Common sports for injury: Hockey, backpacking, lacrosse, wrestling, and martial arts

Mechanism of injury:

- **Traumatic:** Direct (e.g., penetrating or blunt trauma to the posterior neck) or indirect (e.g., traction)
- **Compression:** Mass lesions or external (e.g., backpack)
- **Iatrogenic:** Subject to insult during lymph node dissection, carotid endarterectomy, etc.

Symptoms: Pain around the shoulder, weakness, difficulty with abduction and overhead activities, and sagging of the shoulder; radicular pain caused by traction from the drooping shoulder may also occur

Differential diagnosis: Long thoracic nerve injury or cervical pathology

Physical examination: Visual inspection may reveal asymmetry of the neckline, drooping of the affected shoulder, loss of normal scapulohumeral rhythm, and "lateral" scapular winging. Atrophy of the trapezius and SCM with associated spasm of the levator scapulae and rhomboids may be present. Physical examination may reveal weakness with abduction and forward elevation and inability to shrug the affected shoulder. Winging of the scapula may occur but is generally not as severe as that seen with long thoracic nerve injury. Winging associated with spinal accessory nerve injury is not exaggerated by forward elevation as is seen with long thoracic nerve injury. Scapular stabilization against the back by the physician may relieve symptoms.

Diagnostics: Radiographs of the cervical spine, chest, and shoulder are indicated but are usually negative. MRI is useful only for ruling out mass lesions. Electrodiagnostics are usually warranted.

Treatment: Treatment and prognosis depend on the underlying etiology. Conservative treatment comprises anti-inflammatory drugs, electrical stimulation, limitation of overhead activities, and physical therapy focusing on shoulder girdle and scapular rehabilitation. A sling may be used as needed but be wary of frozen shoulder. Braces to stabilize the scapula have not been highly effective. Indications for surgical consultation include symptoms and persistent atrophy for >6 months, penetrating trauma, and iatrogenic injury.

Prognosis and RTP: Injuries caused by blunt trauma typically recover in <1 year with conservative treatment. With injury caused by penetrating trauma or laceration, prognosis is better if surgical intervention is not delayed for >6 months. RTP decisions are individual and activity specific.

RADIAL NERVE INJURY

Overview: The radial nerve originates from the posterior cord of the brachial plexus (C5–T1); it runs with the deep artery before passing into the cubital fossa and descending between the brachioradialis and brachialis. At the level of the lateral epicondyle, it branches into the superficial and deep branches (Fig. 38.6). The deep branch courses around the neck of the radius and enters the posterior compartment, terminating at the posterior interosseous, which continues under the supinator in the radial tunnel. The superficial branch passes anterior to the pronator teres, eventually entering the dorsum of the hand. Branches:

- **Forearm branches:** Motor innervation of triceps brachii, anconeus, brachioradialis, and extensor carpi radialis longus
- **Posterior interosseous nerve (PIN):** Motor innervation of the extensor carpi radialis brevis, extensor carpi ulnaris, extensor digiti minimi, extensor digitorum, supinator, extensor indicis proprius, abductor pollicis longus, and extensor pollicis longus and brevis
- **Posterior cutaneous nerve:** Sensory innervation of posterior arm and forearm
- **Inferior lateral cutaneous nerve:** Sensory innervation of lateral arm
- **Superficial branch:** Sensory innervation of proximal dorsal three and a half digits and dorsal hand

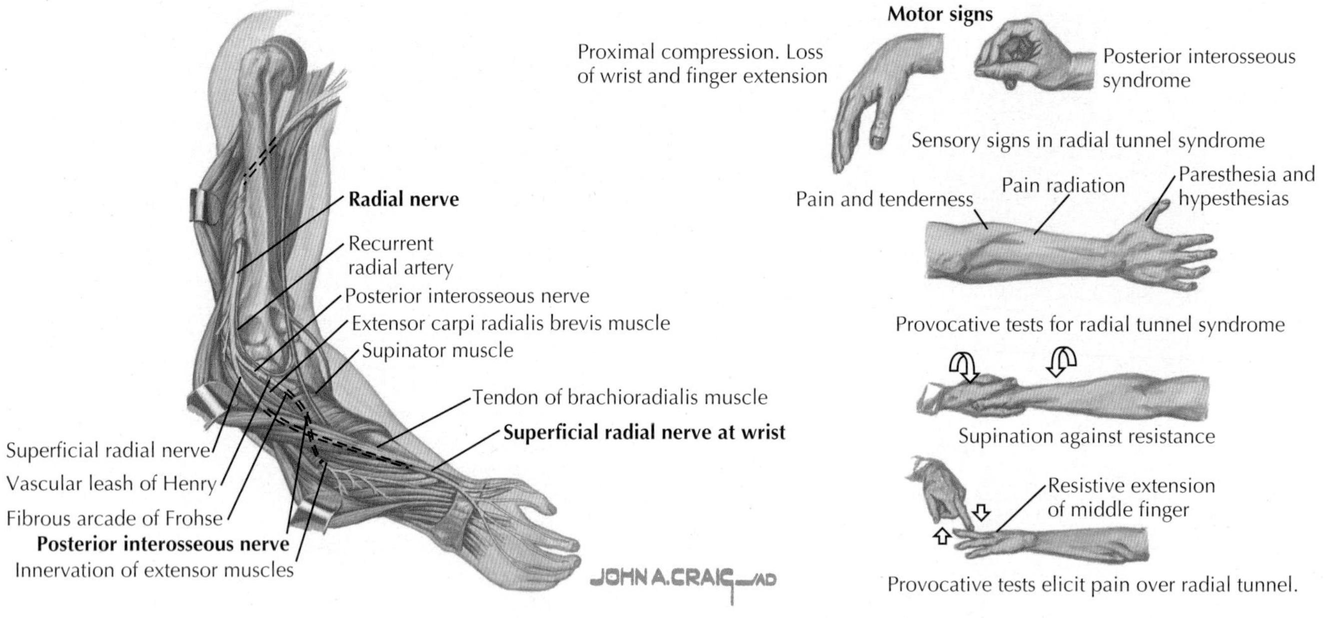
Radial nerve
Recurrent radial artery
Posterior interosseous nerve
Extensor carpi radialis brevis muscle
Supinator muscle
Tendon of brachioradialis muscle
Superficial radial nerve at wrist
Superficial radial nerve
Vascular leash of Henry
Fibrous arcade of Frohse
Posterior interosseous nerve
Innervation of extensor muscles
JOHN A.CRAIG_MD
Motor signs
Proximal compression. Loss of wrist and finger extension
Posterior interosseous syndrome
Sensory signs in radial tunnel syndrome
Pain and tenderness
Pain radiation
Paresthesia and hypesthesias
Provocative tests for radial tunnel syndrome
Supination against resistance
Resistive extension of middle finger
Provocative tests elicit pain over radial tunnel.

Figure 38.6 Radial nerve in forearm.

Common sports for injury: Arm wrestling, baseball, football, tennis/racquetball, weightlifting, frisbee/discus throw, rowing, and gymnastics

Mechanism of injury:
- **Traumatic:** Direct (e.g., humeral shaft fracture) or indirect (e.g., muscle strain)
- **Compression:** Multiple possible sites of compression; repetitive pronation/supination increases compressive forces. More proximal lesions may occur with tourniquet use, inappropriate use of axillary crutches, and "Saturday night compression palsy."
  - Radial tunnel syndrome (RTS)—compression at the elbow
  - Wartenberg syndrome—caused by direct trauma to or compression of the superficial branch in the forearm

Symptoms: Symptoms around the elbow may mimic lateral epicondylitis; of the patients with lateral epicondylitis, 5%–10% have associated radial nerve entrapment.
- **RTS:** Deep ache distal to the lateral epicondyle that is worse at night and after throwing; generally not associated with sensory loss or weakness. Syndrome is controversial; may occur with racquet sports because of repetitive supination/pronation.
  - The radial tunnel is the area between the lateral epicondyle and the supinator muscle, which exists as a potential space with numerous sites of compression.
- **PIN compression syndrome:** The same structures are compressed as with RTS, but symptoms are predominantly weakness of the purely motor PIN-supplied muscles after a prodrome of lateral forearm or elbow pain. Throwers may note decreased control and velocity.
- **Wartenberg syndrome:** May be caused by any tight-fitting strap or band around the wrist; symptoms include pain and decreased sensation over the dorsoradial hand, dorsal thumb, and index finger; not associated with throwing

Differential diagnosis: Varies depending on symptoms

Physical examination: Complete neurologic examination of the upper extremities is warranted. Specific tests (see Fig. 38.6):
- **RTS:** Resisted extension of the middle finger with the elbow extended, forearm pronation with the wrist flexed, elbow flexion and supination, or supination with the elbow extended may elicit pain. Certain tests will be positive with lateral epicondylitis. Certain studies support the use of diagnostic blocks.
- **PIN:** Same as earlier but with weakness on extension of the wrist, thumb, and index finger; forearm supination and grip are also weak. Symptoms may be reproduced by compression of three fingerbreadths below the lateral epicondyle and can also worsen if misdiagnosed as lateral epicondylitis with application of a counterforce brace over the site of entrapment.
- **Wartenberg syndrome:** Tinel sign should be positive; not associated with weakness. Pseudo-Finkelstein test can be positive with forced pronation and ulnar flexion of the wrist.
- Check for cervical radiculopathy and thoracic outlet syndrome.

Diagnostics: Plain radiographs are generally negative in the absence of trauma but may reveal calcifications. MRI is helpful only if a mass lesion is suspected. Electrodiagnostics are usually not helpful with RTS but may be diagnostic in PIN. Negative test does not rule out entrapment; consider testing if associated with trauma.

Treatment:
- RTS: Standard conservative treatment includes rest (may be assisted with splinting), avoidance of provocative movements, anti-inflammatory medications, physical therapy, and pain management.
- PIN: All of the items mentioned for RTS plus splinting to maintain function
- Wartenberg syndrome: Standard conservative treatment includes rest (may be assisted with splinting in supination) and anti-inflammatory medications.
- Surgical intervention for RTS is rare.

Prognosis and RTP: Generally responds to conservative treatment; limited case series show a good prognosis with surgical decompression.

MEDIAN NERVE INJURY

Overview: The median nerve arises from two cords of the brachial plexus, lateral (C6 and C7) and medial (C8 and T1), with occasional input from C5. It descends on the medial arm and enters the cubital fossa before passing between the heads of the pronator teres, where it gives off the anterior interosseous branch. It then descends between the flexor digitorum superficialis (FDS) and the flexor digitorum profundus (FDP), giving off the palmer cutaneous branch before passing within the carpal tunnel to reach the hand (Fig. 38.7). Branches:

- Forearm branches: motor innervation of the pronator teres, flexor carpi radialis, and palmaris longus
- Anterior interosseous nerve: motor innervation of the FDP (radial half), flexor pollicis longus (FPL), and pronator quadratus
- Terminal motor branches: motor innervation of the FDS, abductor pollicis brevis, opponens pollicis, flexor pollicis brevis, and lateral two lumbricals
- Palmer cutaneous nerve: sensory innervation of lateral palm
- Digital cutaneous branches: sensory innervation of volar and distal dorsal surfaces of the radial three and a half digits

Common sports for injury: Wrist: archery, basketball (wheelchair), bicycling, weightlifting, football, golf, and wrestling; palmer branch: cheerleading and golf; and pronator teres: archery and baseball

Mechanism of injury:

- **Traumatic:** Direct or indirect
- **Compression:** Most commonly within the carpal tunnel (carpal tunnel syndrome [CTS]) but occurs at multiple sites, including within the pronator teres (pronator syndrome [PS]) and along the anterior interosseous nerve (anterior interosseous syndrome [AIS]) (Fig. 38.8)

Symptoms:

- **CTS:** Paresthesias and weakness in the radial three and a half digits of the hand; increased symptoms with repetitive movements; pain may radiate proximally; nighttime symptoms are common
- **PS:** Pain in the proximal volar surface of the forearm often radiating distally, which generally increases with activity; often described as fatigue; more distal sensory symptoms may occur but are uncommon; not typically associated with nighttime symptoms
- **AIS:** Deep constant pain in the proximal volar forearm preceding gradual weakness of the FPL and FDP; no sensory loss noted

Differential diagnosis: Varies depending on symptoms

Physical examination: Thenar muscle wasting may be present in advanced cases, usually with CTS. Thorough neurologic examination, including two-point discrimination, should be performed. Specific tests:

- **CTS:** Tinel sign (tapping over the median nerve at the wrist reproduces index symptoms) and Phalen sign (wrist flexion for 60 seconds produces paresthesias in a median nerve distribution) are typical.
- **PS:** Pronator compression test wherein compression over the pronator teres reproduces symptoms; tenderness over the pronator is also common. Tinel sign over the cubital fossa and reproduction of symptoms with resisted pronation in the extended elbow support the diagnosis; may cause numbness in the thenar eminence in the distribution of the palmar cutaneous branch of the median nerve (spared with CTS).
- **AIS:** Weakness of the FDP and FPL, manifesting as inability to make an appropriate circle with the index finger and thumb.
- Check for cervical radiculopathy and thoracic outlet syndrome.

Diagnostics: Plain radiographs may reveal osteophytes or bony abnormalities causing compression. MRI should be obtained

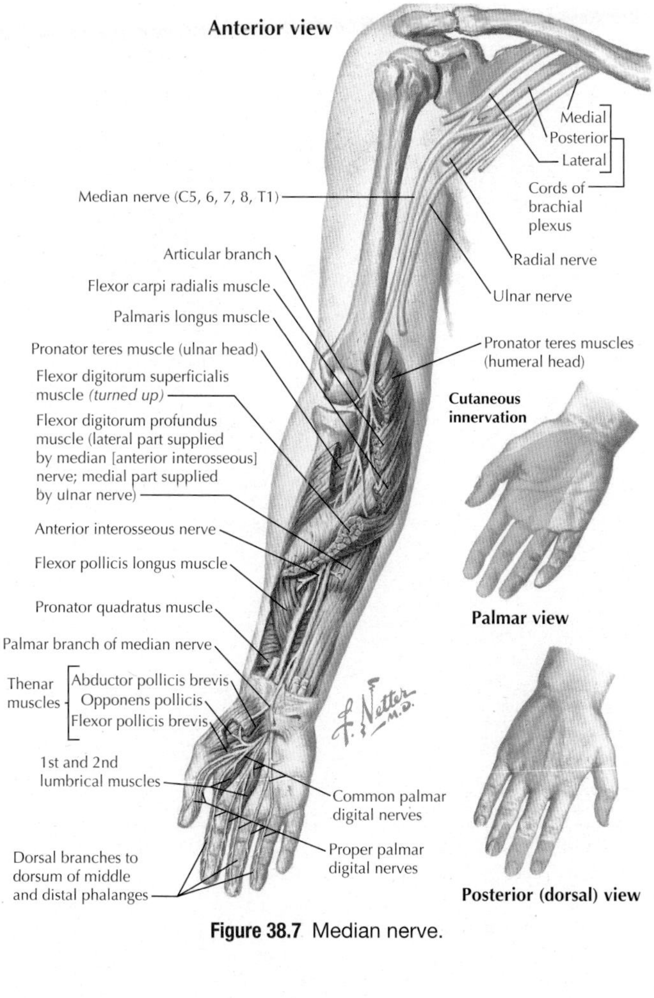

Anterior view
Medial
Posterior
Lateral
Cords of brachial plexus
Median nerve (C5, 6, 7, 8, T1)
Articular branch
Radial nerve
Flexor carpi radialis muscle
Ulnar nerve
Palmaris longus muscle
Pronator teres muscle (ulnar head)
Pronator teres muscles (humeral head)
Flexor digitorum superficialis muscle (turned up)
Cutaneous innervation
Flexor digitorum profundus muscle (lateral part supplied by median [anterior interosseous] nerve; medial part supplied by ulnar nerve)
Anterior interosseous nerve
Flexor pollicis longus muscle
Pronator quadratus muscle
Palmar view
Palmar branch of median nerve
Thenar muscles
Abductor pollicis brevis
Opponens pollicis
Flexor pollicis brevis
1st and 2nd lumbrical muscles
Common palmar digital nerves
Proper palmar digital nerves
Dorsal branches to dorsum of middle and distal phalanges
Posterior (dorsal) view

Figure 38.7 Median nerve.

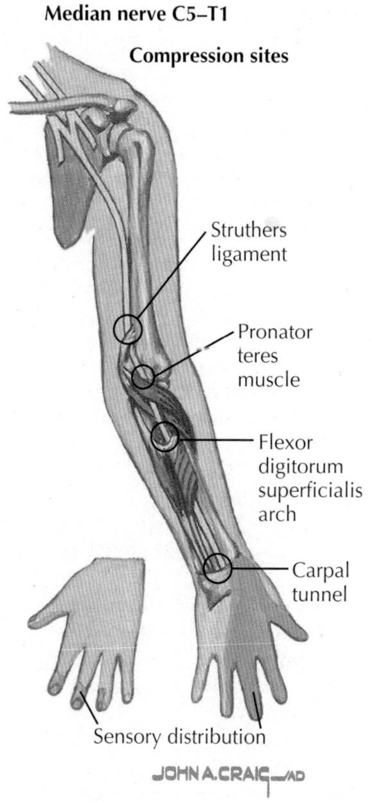

Median nerve C5–T1
Compression sites
Struthers ligament
Pronator teres muscle
Flexor digitorum superficialis arch
Carpal tunnel
Sensory distribution
JOHN A.CRAIG_AD

Figure 38.8 Common sites of upper extremity nerve entrapment.

if compressive masses are suspected. Electrodiagnostic studies are warranted with CTS and AIS but are unreliable with PS. Comparison studies on sensory nerve conduction in the hand using the Combined Sensory Index (CSI) improves the sensitivity of mild CTS detection. However, negative studies do not rule out CTS.

Treatment:
- **CTS:** Conservative treatment with splinting the wrist in neutral position, including at night, rest, physical therapy, and anti-inflammatory medications. Corticosteroid injections into the carpal tunnel may relieve symptoms.
- **PS:** Rest, anti-inflammatory medications, and immobilization with elbow flexion at 90 degrees and the forearm in neutral position for 3–6 weeks. Use of injectable corticosteroids is debatable.
- **AIS:** Same as PS.
- Indications for surgical consultation include failed conservative management and progressive symptoms. Specific periods for trial of conservative treatment are 6 months for CTS and 3–6 months for PS and AIS, but these vary according to available literature.

Prognosis and RTP:
- **CTS:** Prognosis is variable but generally responds well to conservative treatment within a few months with very good prognosis is expected if surgical treatment required
- **PS:** Fifty percent resolution in 6–8 weeks with conservative treatment; very good prognosis if surgical decompression required
- **AIS:** Frequently resolves with conservative management; good prognosis if surgical intervention required

ULNAR NERVE INJURY

Overview: The ulnar nerve arises from the C8 and T1 roots. Contribution from C7 is not uncommon. It descends distally, just medial to the axillary artery. After passing posterior to the medial epicondyle of the humerus within the cubital tunnel, it enters the anterior compartment of the forearm between the heads of the flexor carpi ulnaris (FCU). Descending between the FCU and FDP, the nerve gives off the palmar cutaneous branch and then the dorsal cutaneous nerve. After passing through Guyon canal, the nerve splits into superficial sensory and deep motor branches (Fig. 38.9). The nerve may move as much as 7 mm anteromedially and lengthen as much as 4.7 mm during flexion. Branches:
- Forearm branches: motor innervation of FCU and FDP (ulnar half)
- Superficial motor branch: motor innervation of the palmaris brevis
- Deep motor branch: motor innervation of the hypothenar muscles, adductor pollicis, all interossei, medial two lumbricals, and the deep head of flexor pollicis brevis
- Dorsal and palmar sensory branch: sensory innervation of medial palm/dorsal hand and volar and distal dorsal surfaces of ulnar one and a half digits

Common sports for injury:
- **Elbow:** baseball; tennis; bicycling; bodybuilding/weightlifting; judo, karate, and kickboxing; cross-country skiing; and wrestling
- **Wrist:** basketball (wheelchair), bicycling, football, cross-country skiing, and snowmobiling
- **Flexor carpi ulnaris:** weightlifting and golf
- **Deep motor branch:** weightlifting

Mechanism of injury:
- **Trauma:** Direct and indirect trauma (i.e., traction and friction)
- **Compression:** Common sites for compression at the elbow include the ulnar groove, below the medial epicondyle (also known as the *cubital tunnel*), and above the medial epicondyle (also known as the "arcade of Struthers"). Compression at the wrist usually occurs at Guyon canal (see Fig. 38.9); may also occur with muscular hypertrophy of the FCU, ulnar artery aneurysm, lipoma, etc.

Symptoms:
- **Cubital tunnel syndrome:** Common in baseball pitchers because of the large valgus stress at the elbow and repetitive flexion/extension (valgus overload syndrome); pain may occur at the medial joint line or paresthesias during late cocking or early acceleration; radiation to the hand is common. Snapping of the nerve may occur with flexion/extension. Symptoms may also be focused more distally, mimicking ulnar tunnel syndrome. Sleeping with elbows fully flexed can aggravate the symptoms.
- **Ulnar tunnel syndrome (Guyon canal syndrome):** Also known as *handlebar* or *cyclist's palsy* because of repetitive loads on the palmar aspect of the wrist during cycling; symptoms include paresthesias and pain in the fourth and fifth digits, decreased grip strength (40% of the grip strength is derived from ulnar nerve musculature), and pain at the volar wrist ulnar aspect; fourth and fifth digit abduction and adduction weakness imply poorer prognosis.

Differential diagnosis: C8 and/or T1 radiculopathy, brachial plexopathy, and polyneuropathy; other causes of wrist pain include hypothenar hammer syndrome, fracture of the hook of the hamate, ganglion cysts, ulnar carpal instability, and ulnar artery aneurysm

Physical examination: Visual inspection for flexion contractures or valgus deformity at the elbow, muscle hypertrophy or atrophy, and claw hand deformity; palpate for a subluxating ulnar

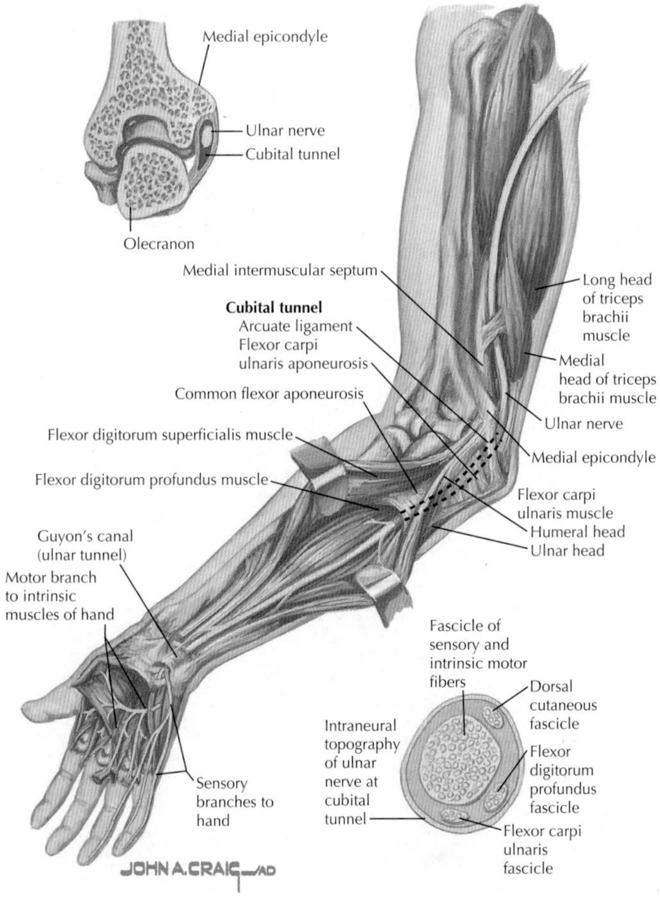
Medial epicondyle
Ulnar nerve
Cubital tunnel
Olecranon
Medial intermuscular septum
Cubital tunnel
Arcuate ligament
Flexor carpi ulnaris aponeurosis
Common flexor aponeurosis
Flexor digitorum superficialis muscle
Flexor digitorum profundus muscle
Guyon's canal (ulnar tunnel)
Motor branch to intrinsic muscles of hand
Long head of triceps brachii muscle
Medial head of triceps brachii muscle
Ulnar nerve
Medial epicondyle
Flexor carpi ulnaris muscle
Humeral head
Ulnar head
Fascicle of sensory and intrinsic motor fibers
Dorsal cutaneous fascicle
Intraneural topography of ulnar nerve at cubital tunnel
Flexor digitorum profundus fascicle
Flexor carpi ulnaris fascicle
Sensory branches to hand
JOHN A.CRAIG—AD
Figure 38.9 Compression of ulnar nerve.

nerve as the elbow is flexed. Stress the ulnar collateral ligament (UCL) for laxity; thorough neurologic examination, including intrinsic muscles of the hand. Dorsal symptoms rule out the possibility of ulnar nerve entrapment at the wrist. Specific tests:

- Elbow flexion test: holding elbow in maximal flexion with full wrist extension for 1 minute to test for symptom reproduction
- Tinel sign: palpation of the ulnar nerve reproducing symptoms at the cubital tunnel (particularly combined with elbow flexion) or Guyon canal
- Phalen sign: wrist flexion eliciting paresthesias in an ulnar distribution
- Froment sign: weakness of adduction of the thumb (Fig. 38.10)
- Evaluate for cervical radiculopathy and thoracic outlet syndrome

Diagnostics: Choice of imaging is based on location of the lesion. Plain radiographs may reveal bony changes or osteophytes around the elbow (ulnar sulcus or cubital tunnel view) or hamate fracture at the wrist (carpal tunnel view). MRI studies and angiograms may reveal occult hamate fracture and/or ulnar artery thrombosis. Electrodiagnostics help in localization of the lesion.

Treatment: Treatment and prognosis depend on the underlying etiology and injury to surrounding structures.

- Cubital tunnel syndrome: Rest, ice, anti-inflammatory medications, and physical therapy; splinting in mild flexion (elbow pad worn in "reverse" or fiberglass volar flexion "block" splint) or use of an elbow pad to avoid pressure on the cubital tunnel may help.
- Ulnar tunnel syndrome: Similar to CTS treatment, plus wrist splinting in functional position with slight dorsiflexion; corticosteroid injection into Guyon canal may be considered but often yields only transient relief.
  - In cases of cyclist's palsy, use of padded gloves, specialized grips, altering and frequently changing hand position, and appropriate bicycle fitting may decrease symptoms.
- Indications for surgical consultation include failure to respond to conservative treatment, persistent motor weakness, intrinsic paralysis, or progression of symptoms. Surgical intervention for cubital tunnel syndrome frequently includes decompression of the nerve and/or anterior transposition for neuropathy associated with elbow deformity or subluxation of the nerve.

Prognosis and RTP: RTP decisions depend on the associated injuries involved and treatment required.

TIBIAL NERVE INJURY

Overview: The tibial nerve derives from the L4–S3 roots as part of the sciatic nerve. It branches from the sciatic nerve in the distal thigh and continues through the popliteal fossa, entering the calf between the two heads of the gastrocnemius muscle. At the medial ankle, the nerve passes into the foot through the tarsal tunnel. The tarsal tunnel is a fibro-osseous tunnel inferior and posterior to the medial malleolus, formed by the bony floor and the flexor retinaculum. Within the tunnel, it splits into the medial and lateral plantar nerves (LPNs) (Fig. 38.11). The medial plantar nerve (MPN) passes distally between the abductor hallucis and flexor digitorum brevis. The LPN passes between the quadratus plantae and flexor digitorum brevis. Branches:

- **Direct branches:** motor innervation of the semimembranosus, semitendinosus, biceps femoris (long head), plantaris, popliteus, gastrocnemius, soleus, tibialis posterior, flexor hallucis longus, and flexor digitorum longus; sensory innervation of posterolateral calf via sural branches
- **MPN:** motor innervation of the abductor hallucis, flexor digitorum brevis, flexor hallucis brevis, and first lumbrical; sensory innervation of the medial sole and medial three and a half toes
- **LPN:** motor innervation of the quadratus plantae, flexor digiti minimi, adductor hallucis, interossei, abductor digiti

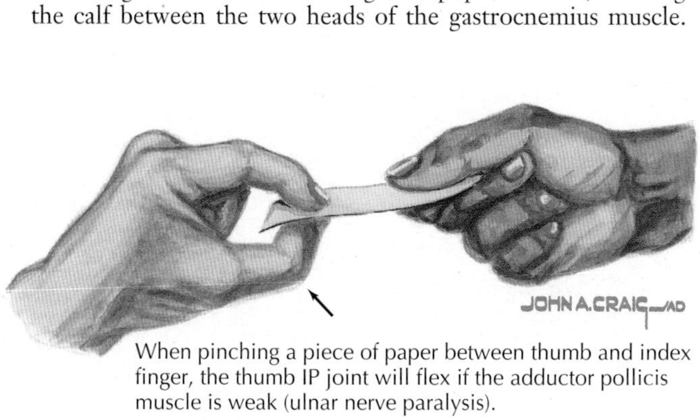
JOHN A.CRAIG—AD
When pinching a piece of paper between thumb and index finger, the thumb IP joint will flex if the adductor pollicis muscle is weak (ulnar nerve paralysis).

Figure 38.10 Positive Froment sign.

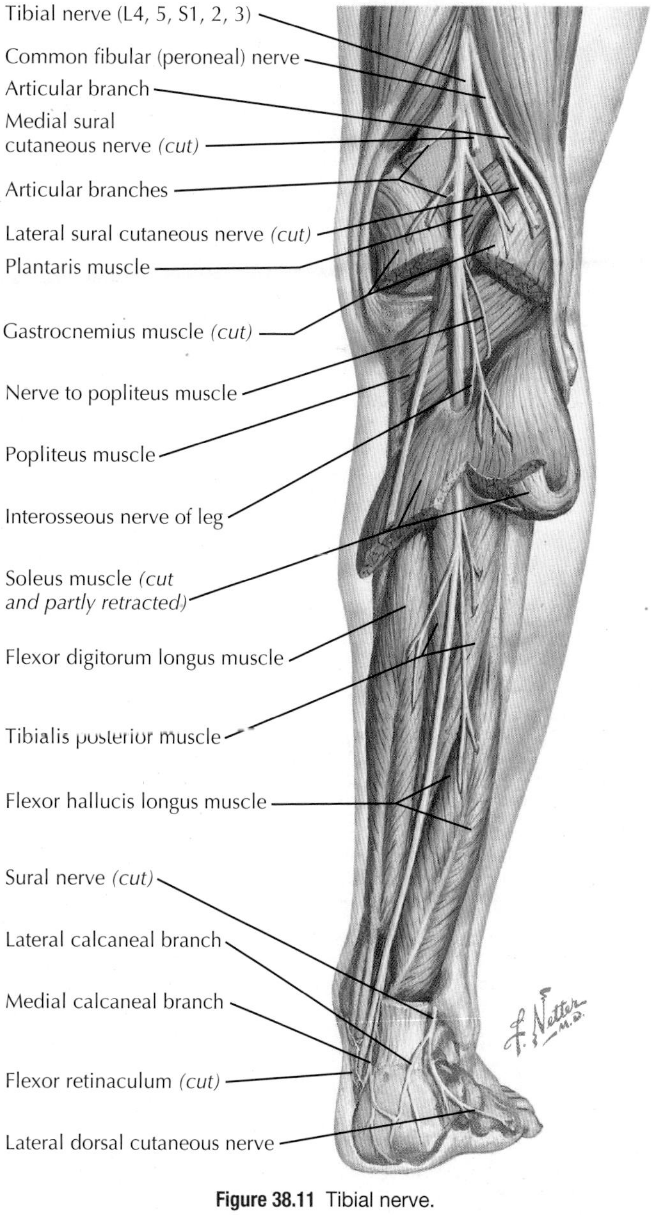
Tibial nerve (L4, 5, S1, 2, 3)
Common fibular (peroneal) nerve
Articular branch
Medial sural cutaneous nerve (cut)
Articular branches
Lateral sural cutaneous nerve (cut)
Plantaris muscle
Gastrocnemius muscle (cut)
Nerve to popliteus muscle
Popliteus muscle
Interosseous nerve of leg
Soleus muscle (cut and partly retracted)
Flexor digitorum longus muscle
Tibialis posterior muscle
Flexor hallucis longus muscle
Sural nerve (cut)
Lateral calcaneal branch
Medial calcaneal branch
Flexor retinaculum (cut)
Lateral dorsal cutaneous nerve
F. Netter M.D.

Figure 38.11 Tibial nerve.

minimi, and lateral three lumbricals; sensory innervation of the lateral sole and lateral one and a half toes
- **Medial calcaneal nerve:** sensory innervation of the plantar and medial heel

Common sports for injury: Running, hockey, hiking, skiing, ballet, and gymnastics

Mechanism of injury:
- Traumatic: direct or indirect trauma (most commonly to the distal tibia or ankle), overuse, and fractures
- Compression: mass lesion, exostosis, accessory flexor digitorum longus, varicose veins, overpronation, rearfoot valgus deformity, and muscular hypertrophy
- Systemic disorders: such as rheumatoid arthritis, diabetes, etc.

Symptoms: Posterior tibial nerve injury (tarsal tunnel syndrome) is the most common neuropathy involving this nerve. Compression occurs within the tarsal tunnel. Patients experience burning pain on the medial plantar foot, which is worse with prolonged standing or walking. Proximal radiation to the calf is not uncommon. Motor weakness is generally not reported, but weakness of toe flexion may occur. Occasional night pain may be reported.

Differential diagnosis: Varies depending on symptoms

Physical examination: Visual inspection in advanced cases may reveal atrophy of intrinsic foot muscles. Physical inspection should include thorough examination of soft tissues for evidence of mass lesion. Complete neurologic examination of bilateral lower extremities should be included. Inspect the lower back for signs of radiculopathy. Specific tests:
- Pain when the ankle is placed in extremes of dorsiflexion; Tinel sign behind medial malleolus at the tarsal tunnel or at various entrapment sites distal to the tunnel reproducing symptoms; decreased sensation along the plantar aspect of the foot; tenderness and/or mass or swelling at the tarsal tunnel; occasionally weakness with great toe plantarflexion
- A two-point discrimination test on medial and lateral sides of the foot may localize the lesions.

Diagnostics: Plain radiographs may reveal fracture or osteophytes. MRI rules out mass lesions. Nerve conduction studies of the medial and/or plantar nerves may be prolonged.

Treatment: Determined based on the underlying cause: conservative treatment includes rest, change in footwear or running posture, orthotic with medial support, splinting, anti-inflammatory medications, and corticosteroid injections. Indications for surgical intervention include mass lesions and failure of conservative treatment after 3–6 months.

Prognosis and RTP: Conservative treatment is successful in a majority of cases. If surgical intervention is required, approximately 80%–90% of patients will experience improvement or resolution of symptoms; this estimate drops to 75% if the specific cause is not known.

Less common tibial nerve injuries:
- MPN injury ("jogger's foot"): Symptoms include burning heel pain, aching in the arch, and decreased sensation in the plantar foot behind the great toe. Compression occurs distal to the tarsal tunnel, most commonly in the abductor tunnel behind the navicular tuberosity. There may also be tenderness of the MPN at the entrance of the abductor tunnel and weakness of intrinsic foot musculature; difficult to differentiate from plantar fasciitis.
- LPN injury: Symptoms may include decreased sensation at the lateral one third of the plantar foot. There may be weakness of the abductor digiti quinti, but this is difficult to determine.

COMMON FIBULAR (PERONEAL) NERVE INJURY

Overview: The common fibular (peroneal) nerve (CFN) derives from L4 to S2 roots as part of the sciatic nerve. The fibular nerve branches from the sciatic nerve in the upper popliteal fossa before giving off a lateral sural cutaneous branch, which becomes part of the sural nerve. Traveling posterior to the fibular head, the nerve enters the peroneal (fibular) tunnel and then splits into the superficial fibular nerve (SFN) and the deep fibular nerve (DFN) (Fig. 38.12). Traveling within the lateral compartment, the SFN continues distally along the anterior intermuscular septum, eventually piercing the deep fascia at the distal third of the leg to become subcutaneous. The DFN travels on the interosseous membrane in the anterior compartment before crossing the distal end of the tibia and continuing under the extensor retinaculum and through the anterior tarsal tunnel (a flattened space between the inferior extensor retinaculum and the fascia overlying the talus and navicular) to enter the foot. Branches:
- Direct branches: motor innervation of biceps femoris (short head) and sensory innervation of lateral leg
- Lateral sural cutaneous: sensory innervation of the lateral and posterior leg
- DFN: motor innervation of tibialis anterior, extensor hallucis longus and brevis, peroneus (fibularis) tertius, and extensor digitorum longus and brevis; sensory innervation of the first web space
- SFN: motor innervation of peroneus longus and brevis and sensory innervation of dorsum of foot and toes except lateral fifth toe and first web space

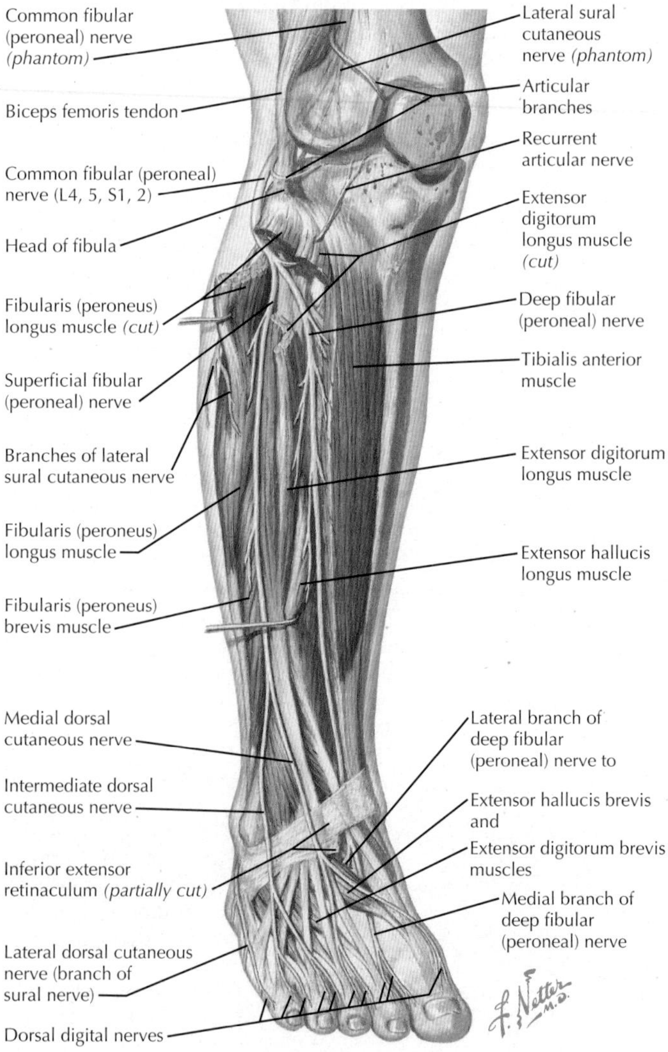

Common fibular (peroneal) nerve (phantom)
Biceps femoris tendon
Common fibular (peroneal) nerve (L4, 5, S1, 2)
Head of fibula
Fibularis (peroneus) longus muscle (cut)
Superficial fibular (peroneal) nerve
Branches of lateral sural cutaneous nerve
Fibularis (peroneus) longus muscle
Fibularis (peroneus) brevis muscle
Medial dorsal cutaneous nerve
Intermediate dorsal cutaneous nerve
Inferior extensor retinaculum (partially cut)
Lateral dorsal cutaneous nerve (branch of sural nerve)
Dorsal digital nerves
Lateral sural cutaneous nerve (phantom)
Articular branches
Recurrent articular nerve
Extensor digitorum longus muscle (cut)
Deep fibular (peroneal) nerve
Tibialis anterior muscle
Extensor digitorum longus muscle
Extensor hallucis longus muscle
Lateral branch of deep fibular (peroneal) nerve to
Extensor hallucis brevis and
Extensor digitorum brevis muscles
Medial branch of deep fibular (peroneal) nerve
F. Netter M.D.

Figure 38.12 Common fibular (peroneal) nerve.

Common sports for injury: Running, bicycling, soccer, auto racing, football, ballet dancing, hockey, martial arts, surfing, horse racing, and skiing

Mechanism of injury:

- Traumatic: Direct contusion, repetitive motion injury, or stretch injury; the latter mostly occurs where the nerve passes through the peroneus longus muscle; may occur with knee dislocations, fibular fracture, proximal tibiofibular instability, and severe ankle inversion
- Compression: Most common at the peroneal tunnel; also occurs with internal masses (e.g., fabella), casting, weight loss, and after prolonged bed rest or prolonged positions such as squatting, kneeling, or sitting cross-legged
- Iatrogenic: During a surgery (i.e., knee arthroscopy) or caused by positioning

Symptoms:

- **CFN injury:** Partial or complete foot drop; may be insidious or acute and may present as tripping or falls. Lateral lower leg and dorsal foot paresthesias are common; occurs with compression at the peroneal tunnel.
- **SFN injury:** Pain or paresthesia over the lateral calf, lower leg, and/or dorsum of the foot reproduced by resisted ankle dorsiflexion and eversion; etiology usually undetermined but may be associated with fascial defect(s); associated with lateral compartment syndrome
- **DFN injury** (anterior tarsal tunnel syndrome): Pain over the dorsomedial aspect of the foot with radiation into or numbness within the first web space; occurs with compression of the nerve at the ankle as it passes the talonavicular joint; associated with anterior compartment syndrome

Differential diagnosis: Varies depending on symptoms

Physical examination: Visual inspection in chronic cases may display atrophy in the anterior and lateral compartments of the leg. Observation of the patient while ambulating may reveal steppage gait or hip hiking. Physical inspection should include thorough examination of soft tissues around the knee for evidence of mass lesion or fascial hernia. Consistent neurologic findings include difficulty in heel walking, weakness with dorsiflexion, great toe extension, and weakness with foot inversion while in dorsiflexion but not plantarflexion. Forced inversion may increase pain. Sensory deficits are more common at the first web space (DFN) than over the SFN and CFN distribution. Reflexes should be normal. Specific tests:

- CFN: Weakness of ankle and toe dorsiflexors and ankle eversion; hypoesthesia to touch and pain in the lower two-thirds of the lateral leg and dorsum of the foot; Tinel sign may be positive at the CFN (fibular head)
- SFN: Worsening of symptoms with plantarflexion and inversion of the foot
- DFN: Weakness of the extensor digitorum brevis muscle; sensory deficit in the first web space; ankle eversion normal; Tinel sign may be positive at the DFN (anterior compartment, middistal tibia)
- Consider palpation of the muscular compartments after exercise to evaluate for compartment syndrome, particularly with DFN symptoms
- Inspect the lower back for signs of radiculopathy. Be sure to differentiate back pain secondary to abnormal gait from primary lower back pathology associated with radiculopathy.

Diagnostics: Plain radiographs to rule out fracture or compressive exostosis; MRI should rule out mass lesions. Electrodiagnostics are considered the gold standard for fibular nerve injuries. Compartment pressure testing may be warranted if clinically suspected.

Treatment: Conservative treatment includes avoidance of continued compression by any object or position (may include use of protective pads), rest, anti-inflammatory medications, and physical therapy. Wearing a looser shoe for DFN compression may help. Corticosteroid injections are also used. Based on the degree of weakness, bracing with an ankle–foot orthosis may be required for foot drop and prevention of contracture. Indications for surgical referral include nerve laceration, compression by a mass lesion, and lack of clinical improvement with conservative measures. Concurrent anterior compartment syndrome with DFN lesions may require decompression.

Prognosis and RTP: Resolution should be expected within 2–6 months depending on the etiology. SFN is less likely to respond to conservative treatment and usually requires surgery. If surgical intervention is necessary, typically, a good response is expected, but this may vary with site of compression and degree of palsy.

COMPLEX REGIONAL PAIN SYNDROME (CRPS)

Overview: An array of painful conditions characterized by continued regional pain that is disproportionate in time or degree to usual course of trauma/lesion. Pain is regional (not in a specific nerve territory), usually with distal predominance of abnormal sensory, motor, sudomotor, vasomotor, and/or trophic findings. Synonyms include reflex sympathetic dystrophy (CRPS I), causalgia (CRPS II), posttraumatic pain syndrome, Sudeck atrophy, and shoulder–hand syndrome. The diagnosis of CRPS is often missed. The average time between symptom onset and diagnosis in children has been reported to be 1 year. Two subtypes are recognized: Type I corresponds with no evidence of peripheral nerve injury (90% of presentations), and type II corresponds to the presence of peripheral nerve injury.

Diagnostic criteria: Multiple diagnostic criteria have been published. The Budapest Criteria became the official International Association for Study of Pain (IASP) diagnostic criteria for CRPS in 2012. **Budapest Criteria:** For clinical diagnosis of CRPS, the following must be met:

- Continuing pain disproportionate to inciting event
- At least one symptom in three of the four categories must be reported:
  - Sensory: Hyperesthesia and/or allodynia
  - Vasomotor: Temperature asymmetry and/or skin color changes and/or skin asymmetry
  - Sudomotor/edema: Edema and/or sweating changes and/or sweating asymmetry
  - Motor/trophic: Decreased ROM and/or motor dysfunction (weakness, tremor, or dystonia) and/or trophic changes (hair, skin, or nails)
- Must display at least one sign at time of evaluation in two or more of the following categories:
  - Sensory: Hyperalgesia (to pinprick) and/or allodynia (to light touch and/or temperature and/or deep somatic pressure and/or joint movement)
  - Vasomotor: Temperature asymmetry (>1°C) and/or skin color changes and/or asymmetry
  - Sudomotor/edema: Edema and/or sweating changes and/or sweating asymmetry
  - Motor/trophic: Decreased ROM and/or motor dysfunction (weakness, tremor, or dystonia) and/or trophic changes (hair, skin, or nail)
- No other diagnosis that better explains the signs and symptoms
- Mean age for adults is 36–46 years, with 60%–80% of patients being women
- Children aged 9–15 years are most commonly affected, with a girl-to-boy ratio of 3:1.

Presentation: Pathophysiology is unclear. Common associated precipitating conditions include immobilization, fracture, strains/sprains, minor trauma, postsurgical, and contusion or crush injury. In certain cases, no initiating event is identified. A deviation from the normal course of recovery may be the first indication of CRPS. Symptoms include neurogenic pain (particularly "burning pain"), allodynia (e.g., minimal stimulus such as bed sheets over affected area causes severe pain), hyperesthesia, asymmetry of color/temperature, increased sweating of the affected limb, edema, sensory deficits, stiffness, weakness, night pain, and skin mottling (particularly after showers). Stressors in the lives of pediatric patients with CRPS may play a greater role than in their adult counterparts. Lower extremity involvement is more common in children at a ratio of 5:1, whereas upper extremity involvement is more common in adults.

Physical examination: Pain assessment is critical. General examination should include ROM and a thorough neurologic examination. Specific testing for unilateral weakness, skin temperature changes, allodynia, edema, and sudomotor changes should be included. The key to the examination may be in comparing the affected and unaffected limbs.

Diagnostics: The diagnosis of CRPS is clinical, and no objective test is needed. Additional objective tests such as thermography, triple-phase bone scan, quantitative sudomotor axon reflex test, and sympathetic ganglion block have been described but are again not necessary. Other objective tests (MRI, electrodiagnostics, duplex ultrasound, etc.) may be needed to rule out conditions that could account for similar signs and symptoms.

Treatment: CRPS is a complex biopsychosocial condition that requires a multidisciplinary approach with a goal of improving function. If multidisciplinary resources are not available, sports physicians may design a home program consisting of desensitization exercises (rubbing affected body part with various stimuli such as washcloth, toothbrush, shaving cream, and hot and cold), stretching, and strengthening exercises. Initial exercises of a short duration (few seconds) and progressing through tolerated discomfort for increasing periods; serial follow-up is important, especially initially. Psychological support is recommended if pain lasts for >2 months. Rehabilitation is the core treatment. Additional therapeutics should be aimed at facilitating therapy. Several pharmacologic therapies have been incorporated into the standard treatment regimen of CRPS, including antidepressants, antiepileptic medications, opioids, topical analgesics, NMDA antagonists, bisphosphonates, etc.; rotating schedules should be employed. Interventional pain management (e.g., epidural anesthesia, sympathetic nerve blocks, and neurostimulation, etc.) is common.

Prognosis and RTP: Prognosis and RTP decisions are based on individual cases and vary widely; in general, a more prolonged course is associated with poor prognosis. RTP should not be the primary goal of treatment with pediatric athletes; rather, symptom management and activities of daily living should be prioritized. Studies have reported that 50% of pediatric athletes with CRPS will return to competitive sports. Be mindful of the fact that this presentation may offer the pediatric athlete a way out of competitive sports without parental disapproval.

RECOMMENDED READINGS

Available online.

HEADACHE IN THE ATHLETE

39

Kinshasa C. Morton

GENERAL PRINCIPLES

- **Headache is one of the most common disorders and symptoms reported to primary care, the emergency department, and team physicians.**
- Complaints of headache account for 1%–4% of primary care office and emergency department visits.
- In the general population, the prevalence of headache in a 1-year period is >90% and the lifetime prevalence is 93%–99%.
- Headaches are one of the most commonly reported pain complaints among children and adolescents.
  - In a population study of adolescents aged 11–21 years, >90% had experienced headaches, regardless of the type, over 1 year.
  - Among children aged 4–17 years in the United States, 6.7% had frequent headache pain over a 12-month period.
- Various studies on athletes have shown a headache prevalence of 35%–50% related to participation in their sport.

Causes of Headache

- The exact cause of many headaches is a source of much debate and likely differs for each specific type of headache. Physiologic changes in the head and brain that consist of, but are not limited to, changes in neurotransmitter regulation, vascular dilation and constriction, and cranial nerve irritation that cause activation of pain signals are all contributors to the development of headache. Cyclical hormonal changes and genetic predisposition are also thought to play an important role.
- Tension-type headache (TTH), migraine, and cluster headaches combine to make up >90% of headaches experienced by the general population.
- Adults mostly experience TTHs, whereas children are more likely to have migraine headaches.
  - Among children aged 3–18 years who visit pediatric neurologic clinics, vascular/migrainous headaches account for 52%, chronic headaches/TTHs for 21%, and unclassified headaches for 19%. Remainders are mixed tension-migraine, psychogenic, or posttraumatic.
- Of headache-caused emergency department visits:
  - Migraine and TTHs account for 25%–55% of visits.
  - Headache associated with systemic illness accounts for 33%–39% of visits.
  - Headache caused by a serious neurologic condition (subarachnoid hemorrhage, intracranial mass, meningitis, or hemorrhage) accounts for 1%–16% of visits.

Classification of Headache Disorders

- **In 1988, the International Headache Society (IHS) created its first classification of headache disorders. This *International Classification of Headache Disorders* (ICHD) has subsequently been updated and revised twice, with finalization of the third version (ICHD-3) occurring in 2018.**
- Headache has many causes. The IHS classification gives a physician a logical approach to make a rapid and accurate differential diagnosis.
- Headache disorders are classified as primary, secondary, or those caused by cranial neuralgias.
  - Primary headaches are those that have no underlying cause; there are three main types: migraine headache, TTH, and cluster headache (trigeminal autonomic cephalalgias).
  - Secondary headaches are those that may be attributed to certain underlying pathologic conditions (i.e., infectious, neoplastic, vascular, psychiatric, traumatic, drug-induced, or homeostatic changes).
  - Cranial neuralgia headaches are those that are initiated by compression, distortion, or irritation of specific cranial nerves and subsequently cause pain in the area that those nerves innervate.
- The athletic population suffers from the same headache disorders as the general population but may also have a predisposition to suffer from other headache disorders and subtypes because of the effects of exercise and because of participation in their specific sports.
  - Sports-/exercise-related primary headaches are exercise-/effort-induced migraine and primary exertional headaches.
  - Sports-/exercise-related secondary headaches are acute and chronic posttraumatic headache (PTH), cervicogenic headache, high-altitude headache, and diving headache.
  - Sports-/exercise-related cranial neuralgia headaches are external compression headache and cold-stimulus headache.

ASSESSING HEADACHE IN THE GENERAL AND ATHLETIC POPULATION

Like all other medical evaluations, the assessment of headache begins with a thorough history and physical examination. Most patients will have a completely normal general physical and neurologic examination, so obtaining a detailed history is critical. After history and physical examination have been completed, a further investigation may be warranted, depending on the history and physical findings. This investigation may include laboratory workup, imaging, and/or diagnostic procedures.

Headache History

- When was the first onset of headache?
- What is the frequency?
- Where is the location, and is there any radiation of pain?
- What is the character of the pain (dull, throbbing, sharp)?
- What is the intensity of the pain?
- Are there any associated symptoms?
  - Nausea/vomiting
  - Photophobia/phonophobia
  - Confusion
  - Blurry vision
  - Gait disturbances
- Were any medications taken?
- Are there any alleviating or exacerbating factors?
- Is there a prior history of headache?
- Is there a family history of headache?
- Has there been a change in the headache characteristics (if prior history is positive)?
- Is there a history of other medical issues?
- What medications is the athlete taking?

Physical Examination

- Assess for level of consciousness, orientation, alertness, minimental status, and overall affect.
- Check vital signs to rule out hypertension.
- Evaluate head, eyes, ears, nose, and throat to assess for papilledema. Check for central nervous system abnormalities, including cranial nerve testing, ptosis, pupil reactivity, and head trauma.
- Conduct musculoskeletal evaluation to assess for nuchal rigidity, temporomandibular joint problems, cervical spine range of motion, areas of scalp tenderness, and neck tenderness.
- Conduct neurologic examination to assess for motor, sensory, and reflex response; also include evaluation of gait.
- Check for evidence of systemic illness (assess abnormalities in the cardiovascular, respiratory, and gastrointestinal [GI] systems).

Additional Investigation

Laboratory evaluation: To rule out metabolic issues. Laboratory examinations that may aid in diagnosis are erythrocyte sedimentation rate, complete blood count, liver function tests, thyroid function tests, antinuclear antibodies, antiphospholipid antibodies, and drug screening. Appropriate tests must be conducted as indicated by the history and physical examination.

Imaging tests: Possibilities include cervical spine films, computed tomography (CT) (with or without contrast), magnetic resonance imaging (MRI), electroencephalogram (EEG), and magnetic resonance (MR) angiography. Selection of tests should be individualized.

- Cervical spine radiography (flexion/extension views) in patients with trauma/neck pain, possible fracture, and instability.
- CT scan with contrast for patients with new-onset exertional headache.
  - Some experts do not advocate CT unless neurologic examination is abnormal.
  - May not be helpful for suspected posterior fossa lesions
- CT better for acute bleeding and bony fractures; detects surgical lesions as well as MRI scan
- MRI has greater tissue contrast resolution than CT.
  - Better to perform MRI >48 hours after trauma and in patients with arteriovenous malformations (AVMs) or tumor
  - Study of choice when looking for lesions in the posterior fossa
  - Less radiation exposure compared with CT
- According to the Quality Standards Subcommittee of the American Academy of Neurology, routine use of brain imaging is not warranted for adults with recurrent headaches that have been defined as migraines with no recent change in pattern, no history of seizure, and no other focal neurologic signs or symptoms.

Diagnostic procedure: Lumbar puncture (LP) to rule out subarachnoid hemorrhage from aneurysm; detects minor leaks, which occur in 39% of patients who later have ruptures. CT scans are negative in 55% of patients with minor leaks.

General Considerations

- Consider the same diagnostic evaluation in athletes as in nonathletes, except in cases of trauma with an increased risk of intracranial bleed.
- Workup should be complete when diagnosis is in question. This may include, but is not limited to, evaluation for drug abuse, hypertension, vascular lesions, neoplasms, intracranial bleeding, and psychiatric issues.
- Be cognizant of "red flags" within the history or physical examination that should prompt further neurologic evaluation in the form of either imaging or other diagnostic procedures (Box 39.1).

BOX 39.1 RED FLAGS IN THE EVALUATION OF HEADACHE

1. Headache onset after the age of 50 years
2. Sudden onset of severe headache
3. Change in headache pattern
4. Headache associated with systemic illness and fever
5. Headache associated with neck stiffness
6. Headache with focal neurologic deficits
7. Presence of papilledema
8. Headache in the setting of moderate/severe trauma
9. Alteration of consciousness or amnesia
10. Early morning nausea and vomiting without headache
11. Occurrence of seizure(s) after headache

PRIMARY HEADACHE DISORDERS

See Table 39.1.

MIGRAINE HEADACHE

- **Definition:** Migraine is a chronic, idiopathic neurologic disorder characterized by episodic headaches of high intensity that may be preceded by, accompanied with, or followed by other associated symptoms (Figs. 39.1 and 39.2).
- Associated symptoms
  - **Premonitory (prodrome) symptoms:** Occur hours up to 1–2 days before development of migraine headache. These symptoms are often thought of as a warning of an impending migraine.
    - Fatigue
    - Difficulty concentrating
    - Yawning
    - Change in appetite
    - Change in sleep patterns
    - Change in mood
  - **Aura:** A set of reversible focal neurologic symptoms that occur at the beginning of a migraine headache or just before its onset. Auras typically last for <60 minutes. Visual symptoms are most common.
    - Visual changes (scintillating scotoma, visual field deficits, and blurry vision)
    - Sensory disturbances (pins and needles sensation and numbness)
    - Speech disturbances (dysphasia)
    - Motor deficits (rare)
  - **Resolution (postdrome) symptoms:** These are symptoms that follow the headache and may include certain premonitory symptoms.
    - Exhaustion
    - Exhilaration
    - Depression
    - Nausea
    - Scalp tenderness
- Migraine headache is divided into two major subtypes by the IHS.
  - Migraine without aura
  - Migraine with aura (10%–15% of migraines)
- Migraine headaches are typically unilateral but can be bilateral. Bilateral migraine is more likely to occur in children/adolescents than adults. They also tend to have a pulsating nature; moderate-to-severe intensity; exacerbation by activity; and an association with nausea, vomiting, photophobia, and phonophobia.
- IHS diagnostic criteria for migraine are listed in Box 39.2.

Table 39.1 CHARACTERISTICS OF MIGRAINE, CLUSTER, AND TENSION-TYPE HEADACHES

	Migraine	Cluster	Tension-Type
Onset	Peaks in adolescence	30′ s or 40′ s	Variable; ≥20′ s
Frequency	1–2 attacks/mo, often with menses	≥1 attacks/day for 6–8 wk	Episodic: <15 days/mo Chronic: >15 days/mo
Location	Unilateral more common than bilateral; frontotemporal or orbital	100% unilateral Generally orbitotemporal	Bifrontal, bioccipital, neck
Quality	Throbbing or intense pressure	Nonthrobbing, penetrating, boring	Squeezing, pressing, aching
Duration	4–72 hr, usually 12–24 hr	30 min–2 hr, usually 45–90 min	Episodic: several hours Chronic: all day
Prodrome	Changes in mood, energy, appetite	May include brief, mild burning in eye and internal nares	None
Aura	Up to 60 min, usually 20 min; "often" visual	None	None
Associated Symptoms	Nausea, vomiting, photophobia	Ipsilateral ptosis-miosis, conjunctival injection, tearing, stuffed and running nose	Episodic: loss of appetite, light or sound sensitivity Chronic: light or sound sensitivity, nausea
Behavior	Go to dark, quiet room	Frenetic pacing, rocking	Generally not affected or mild decrease in function

Modified from Marks DR, Rapoport AM. Practical evaluation and diagnosis of headache. *Semin Neurol*. 1997;17(4):307–312.

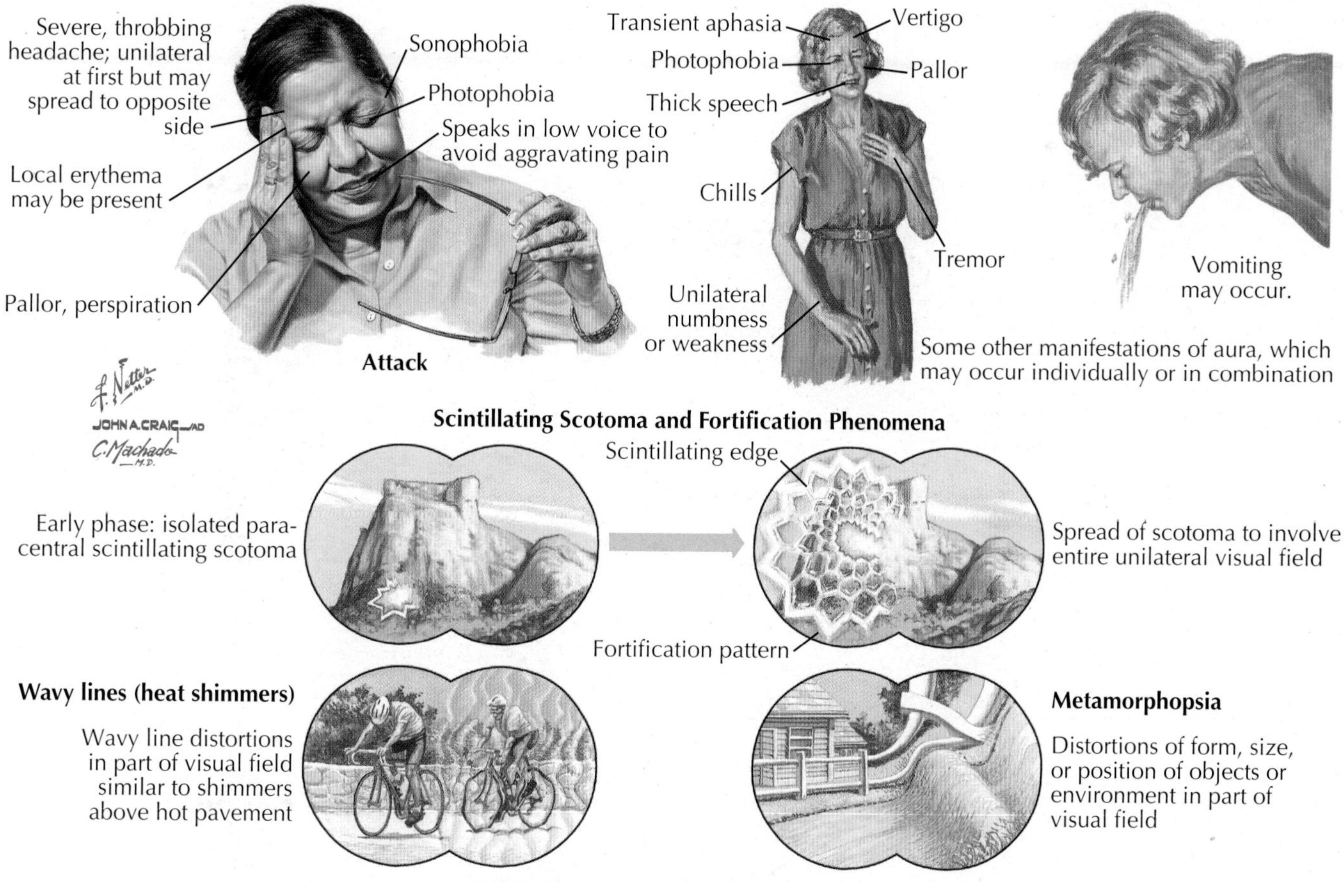
Severe, throbbing headache; unilateral at first but may spread to opposite side
Local erythema may be present
Pallor, perspiration
Sonophobia
Photophobia
Speaks in low voice to avoid aggravating pain
Attack
Transient aphasia
Photophobia
Thick speech
Vertigo
Pallor
Chills
Tremor
Unilateral numbness or weakness
Vomiting may occur.
Some other manifestations of aura, which may occur individually or in combination
Scintillating Scotoma and Fortification Phenomena
Scintillating edge
Early phase: isolated para-central scintillating scotoma
Spread of scotoma to involve entire unilateral visual field
Fortification pattern
Wavy lines (heat shimmers)
Wavy line distortions in part of visual field similar to shimmers above hot pavement
Metamorphopsia
Distortions of form, size, or position of objects or environment in part of visual field
JOHN A.CRAIG—AD
C.Machado M.D.

Figure 39.1 Mechanisms of migraine.

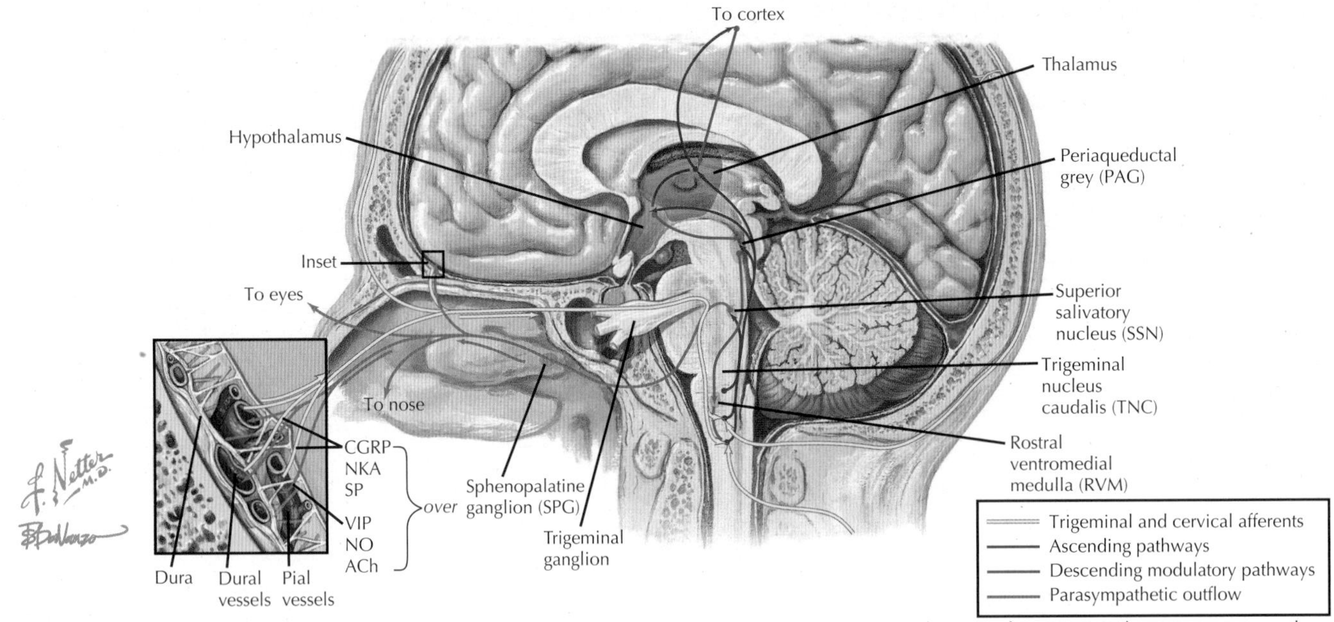
To cortex
Thalamus
Hypothalamus
Periaqueductal grey (PAG)
Inset
To eyes
Superior salivatory nucleus (SSN)
Trigeminal nucleus caudalis (TNC)
To nose
Rostral ventromedial medulla (RVM)
CGRP
NKA
SP
over
VIP
NO
ACh
Sphenopalatine ganglion (SPG)
Trigeminal ganglion
Dura
Dural vessels
Pial vessels
Trigeminal and cervical afferents
Ascending pathways
Descending modulatory pathways
Parasympathetic outflow

Pain-producing structures in the head send pain information via primary sensory afferent neurons through the trigeminal nerve and upper cervical roots to synapse on the second-order neurons in the trigeminal nucleus caudalis (TNC) as part of the trigeminocervical complex. Neurons in the TNC send projections to the thalamus (via the trigeminothalamic or quintothalamic tract, which decussates in the brainstem), which then projects to the cortex. The TNC is thought to project to other structures as well, including the periaqueductal gray (PAG), which also send signals to the thalamus and hypothalamus, with projections to the cortex. There are descending projections from the cortex back to the thalamus and hypothalamus. Descending modulation of the TNC takes place via nuclei in the hypothalamus, as well as direct projections from the PAG through the rostral ventromedial medulla (RVM).

Cranial parasympathetic outflow stems from a reflex connection from the TNC to the superior salivatory nucleus (SSN) in the pons. Efferents from the SSN (via the facial nerve) connect with neurons in the sphenopalatine ganglion (SPG; pterygopalatine). The SPG then projects to innervate intracranial vessels (vasodilation), as well as the nasal and lacrimal glands.

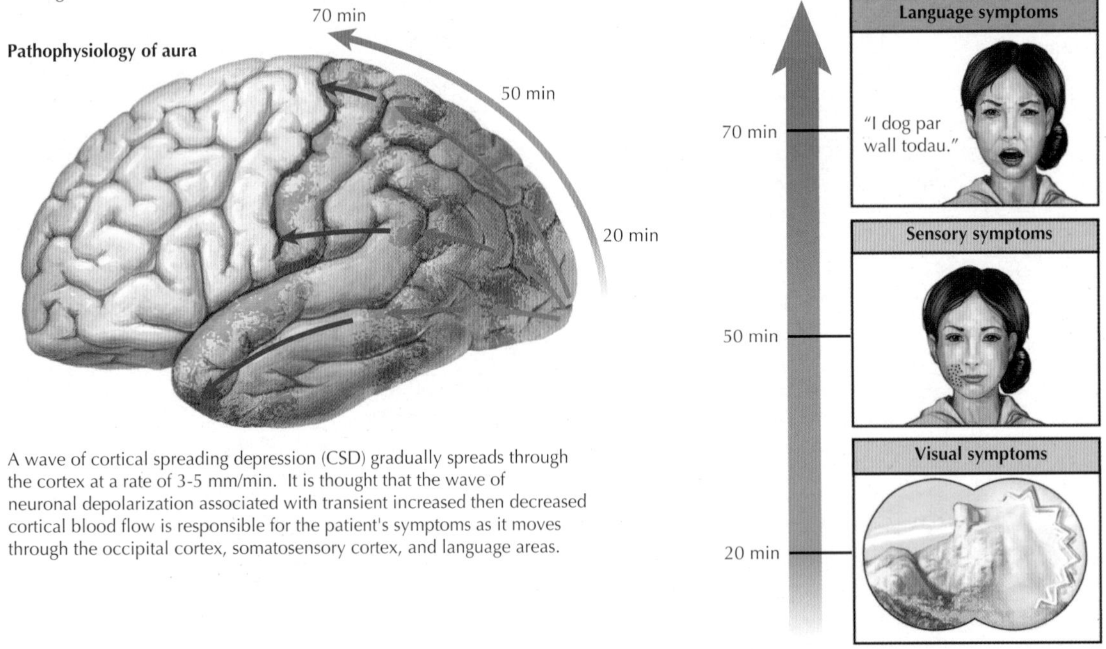
Pathophysiology of aura
70 min
50 min
20 min
Language symptoms
"I dog par wall todau."
Sensory symptoms
Visual symptoms
70 min
50 min
20 min

A wave of cortical spreading depression (CSD) gradually spreads through the cortex at a rate of 3-5 mm/min. It is thought that the wave of neuronal depolarization associated with transient increased then decreased cortical blood flow is responsible for the patient's symptoms as it moves through the occipital cortex, somatosensory cortex, and language areas.

Figure 39.2 Migraine pathophysiology.

- Typical age of onset is in adolescence.
- Eighteen percent of women and 6% of men report headaches that meet the definition of migraine. The female-to-male ratio is 3:1.
- A survey of 791 male and female National Collegiate Athletic Association (NCAA) Division I basketball players showed a total prevalence rate of 2.9% (0.9% of males, 4.4% of females).
- Seventy percent of females who suffer from migraines note a relationship between their menstrual cycles and migraine attacks.
  - Migraine without aura: highest incidence during first 3 days of menses
- Severe, debilitating forms of migraine include status migrainous, in which migraine lasts for >72 hours, and chronic migraine, in which migraines occur for ≥15 days per month.

BOX 39.2 IHS DIAGNOSTIC CRITERIA FOR MIGRAINE WITHOUT AURA

A. At least five attacks fulfilling criteria B–D
B. Headaches lasting for 4–72 hours
C. Headache has at least two of the following characteristics:
  1. unilateral location
  2. pulsating quality
  3. moderate or severe pain intensity
  4. aggravated by physical activity
D. During headache, at least one of the following is present:
  1. nausea and/or vomiting
  2. photophobia and phonophobia
E. Cannot be attributed to another disorder

Modified from Headache Classification Subcommittee of the International Headache Society (IHS). The International Classification of Headache Disorders, 3rd edition. *Cephalalgia*. 2018;38(1):1–211.

- Common migraine triggers include aspartame, caffeine (use or withdrawal), estrogens, monosodium glutamate, nicotine, nitrates, progesterone, alcohol, cheese, chocolate, menstruation, missed meals, perfume, red grapes, sleep (too much or too little), stress, changes in environment/weather, and exercise.

Treatment Options

Overview: Abortive treatment is appropriate if headaches occur once or twice per month, particularly if predicted by aura. It is more effective if used as early as possible, and a large single dose is more effective than multiple smaller doses.

Nonsteroidal anti-inflammatory drugs (NSAIDs): Chronic use should be avoided, particularly in those with a history of peptic ulcer disease, gastritis, and renal insufficiency. Soluble forms of ibuprofen and diclofenac are more rapidly absorbed, which may reduce the severity of migraines more quickly, but have shorter half-lives than other NSAIDs and usually require more frequent dosing. Specific medication examples and initial dosages:
- Ibuprofen: 800–1200 mg PO (peak effect at 1 hour)
- Diclofenac: 50 mg PO (peak effect at 1–2 hours)
- Naproxen: 500–825 mg PO (peak effect at 2 hours)
- Aspirin (ASA): 975 mg PO
- Indomethacin: 50 mg PO
- Ketorolac: 30–60 mg IM, with additional 30 mg in 8 hours if necessary

Dihydroergotamine (DHE-45): Is only available in parenteral form and is typically given with an antiemetic. DHE-45 is still an effective drug, but has largely been replaced by the use of triptans.
- **DHE-45:** 1.0 mg IV/IM/SQ, given 30 minutes after metoclopramide 5 mg or prochlorperazine 5 mg; may be repeated in 1 hour (90% effective)
- **DHE-45 (nasal):** 1.0 mg of intranasal puffs, repeating in 15 minutes
- Favorable side-effect profile when compared with ergotamine (minimal cardiovascular effects and nausea; no rebound headache; nausea/vomiting, GI upset, and muscle cramping have been reported)
- DHE-45 is a vasoconstrictor and is therefore contraindicated in patients with cerebrovascular, cardiovascular, or peripheral vascular disease. It is also contraindicated in patients with severe hypertension, ischemic heart disease, renal or hepatic disease, sepsis, recent infection, or those who may be pregnant.

Triptans: This class of medication causes vasoconstriction and blocks pain pathways within the brainstem. They are selective 5-hydroxytryptamine (5-HT) receptor agonists and are specifically used to treat migraines. All medications belonging to this class have similar side-effect profiles (nausea, dizziness, chest pressure, asthenia, and dry mouth). They also carry the same precautions in that they should be avoided if possible in those with cardiovascular disease, peripheral vascular disease, hypertension, and hepatic dysfunction.
- **Sumatriptan (Imitrex):** 5-HT1D receptor agonist; the first triptan developed, it is available in injectable, oral, and intranasal spray forms
  - Injectable dosage: 4–6 mg SC initially; may repeat in 1 hour (maximum of two 6-mg injections in 24 hours); recommended initial dose is 6 mg
  - Oral dosage: 25–100 mg initially; may repeat dosage in 2 hours (maximum of 200 mg in 24 hours). The recommended initial dose is 50 mg because it is more efficacious than 25 mg and has fewer side effects than 100 mg without loss in efficacy.
  - Nasal spray dosage: 5–20 mg initially; may repeat in 2 hours (maximum of 40 mg in 24 hours); recommended initial dose is 20 mg
  - Tfelt-Hanson showed that 6 mg of the injectable form was more efficacious than 100 mg of the oral form and had the fastest onset of action of all forms. The intranasal form has the same efficacy and a faster onset of action than the oral form, but limited therapeutic effects are seen for the first 30 minutes.
  - DHE versus SC sumatriptan: DHE less effective at 2 hours (73% vs. 85%), but no difference after 2 hours; headache recurred in 45% of sumatriptan-treated patients and 17.7% of DHE-treated patients.
  - Other efficacious triptans include **naratriptan (Amerge), frovatriptan (Frova), rizatriptan (Maxalt), eletriptan (Relpax), zolmitriptan (Zomig), and almotriptan (Axert)**

Others:
- **Triptan/NSAID combinations** may show greater efficacy than either class used alone. The combination of sumatriptan 85 mg/naproxen 500 mg has shown both a greater 2-hour headache relief rate and a higher 24-hour sustained relief response than either drug in monotherapy.
- **Acetaminophen** is more often used for migraines of mild severity. When used in combination with an antiemetic, it may reach headache relief rates similar to that of sumatriptan.
  Dosage: 1000 mg PO; may repeat in 4–6 hours (maximum 4000 mg in 24 hours)
- **Butalbital combinations** (butalbital/ASA/caffeine or butalbital/acetaminophen/caffeine) may also be used. Special concerns may arise regarding abuse potential and sedation.
  Dosage: 2 tablets PO; may repeat in 4 hours (maximum of 6 tablets in 24 hours).
- **Intranasal butorphanol:** Mixed agonist–antagonist opioid analgesic, used for severe attacks; one puff equals 5 mg morphine. Use should be stringent secondary to abuse potential.
  Dosage: 1 spray; may repeat in 1 hour.
- **Intranasal lidocaine 4% solution** provided rapid relief (within 5 minutes) of headache, nausea, and photophobia in a prospective, double-blind, placebo-controlled trial. Relapse was common.
- **Intravenous antiemetic medications** (chlorpromazine, prochlorperazine, and metoclopramide) have shown some efficacy as monotherapy in the treatment of migraine. Practical use of such medications outside of the emergency department setting is low.

First-Line Choice in Athletes

Overview: Because of the efficacy, ease of administration, and relatively quick onset of action, athletes should use triptans for first-line therapy of moderate to severe migraines. Nasal and injectable triptans may have faster action than oral. For mild migraines, NSAIDs or acetaminophen, with or without an antiemetic, should be tried initially. Nasal DHE may be another good option secondary to ease of administration.

Prophylactic treatment: Indicated in patients with ≥4 attacks per month or attacks lasting several days that cause severe disability

- **Beta-blockers** are agents of choice.
  - Only two are Food and Drug Administration (FDA) approved: propranolol and timolol, which lack intrinsic sympathomimetic activity (ISA)
  - Long-acting form of propranolol increases compliance and is useful in patients with coexisting hypertension, angina pectoris, or thyrotoxicosis.
  - Contraindicated in patients with asthma, chronic obstructive pulmonary disease, congestive heart failure, atrioventricular conduction problem, or prescription for monoamine oxidase inhibitors.
  - Other beta-blockers used despite lack of FDA approval: nadolol, metoprolol, and atenolol.
  - Metoprolol is a selective beta-blocker that can be used in patients with concomitant pulmonary disease.
  - **Beta-blockers and athletes:** Negative effects on aerobic performance cause some concern for use in athletes. Moreover, beta-blockers are banned in certain sports and by certain athletic rules committees because they may provide an unfair advantage.
- **Calcium channel blockers:** Nimodipine, a selective cerebrovascular vasoconstrictor, and verapamil have been shown to be useful in migraine prophylaxis.
- **NSAIDs:** Various NSAIDs may be used with varying degrees of efficacy. They are more efficacious for **menstrual migraines** and should be started 2–3 days before menses (see later discussion).
- **Antidepressants (tricyclic):** Amitriptyline and clomipramine are used most often. Efficacy is attributed to antidepressant and analgesic actions. They are particularly effective in patients with coexisting migraine and TTH. They are sedating and hence should be used at bedtime.
- **Antiepileptics:** Valproate, topiramate, and gabapentin are used most often. Only valproate and topiramate are FDA approved for this indication. They are category C and D drugs, respectively, so there should be a concern for use in premenopausal female athletes; ensure birth control. There are no known adverse effects on exercise, although certain antiepileptics are sedating.

Menstrual migraine treatment: **"Miniprophylaxis"** may be achieved with the use of NSAIDs or long-acting triptans (frovatriptan and naratriptan) when initiated 2–3 days before menstruation and continued until 3 days after. **Hormonal treatment** can be used to prevent estrogen withdrawal, which contributes to the development of menstrual migraine. Treatment strategies include the use of extended- and regular-cycle oral contraceptive pills with supplemental estrogen during the inactive pill week and the use of supplemental estrogen alone during menstruation.

Tension-Type Headache

- Definition: TTHs are headaches of mild to moderate intensity that can be either episodic with varying frequency or chronic, with episodic headaches being much more common. Pain is usually bilateral, and patients often report it being "vicelike." The most significant examination finding is pericranial tenderness to palpation (Fig. 39.3).
- IHS diagnostic criteria for episodic TTH are listed in Table 39.2.
- TTH is the most common type of primary headache, with prevalence reaching 80% in the general population.
- Both episodic and chronic TTHs may exhibit photophobia and phonophobia, but nausea is usually isolated to chronic TTH.
- Chronic TTH (CTTH): defined by IHS as headache present for >15 days per month for >3 months.
- CTTH prevalence in general population is 2% in men and 5% in women.

Treatment Options

Overview: TTHs are often responsive to nonpharmacologic therapy or over-the-counter headache medications. Those who suffer from frequent TTHs may benefit from stress reduction and relaxation techniques. For athletes, alteration of training regimens may be helpful. Counseling for patients with psychosocial issues, including but not limited to anxiety and depression, is also beneficial.

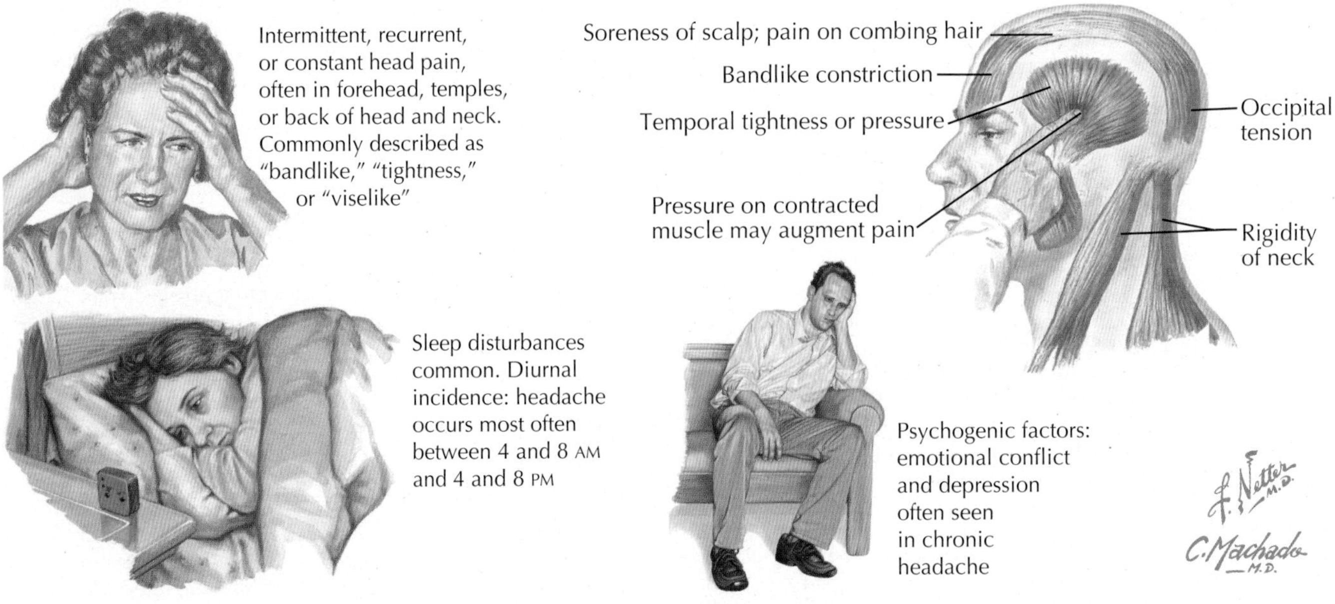
Intermittent, recurrent, or constant head pain, often in forehead, temples, or back of head and neck. Commonly described as "bandlike," "tightness," or "viselike"
Soreness of scalp; pain on combing hair
Bandlike constriction
Temporal tightness or pressure
Occipital tension
Pressure on contracted muscle may augment pain
Rigidity of neck
Sleep disturbances common. Diurnal incidence: headache occurs most often between 4 and 8 AM and 4 and 8 PM
Psychogenic factors: emotional conflict and depression often seen in chronic headache
F. Netter M.D.
C. Machado M.D.

Figure 39.3 Tension-type headache.

Table 39.2 IHS CRITERIA FOR EPISODIC TTH

Infrequent Episodic TTH	Frequent Episodic TTH
A. At least 10 episodes occurring on <12 days per year and fulfilling criteria B–D	A. At least 10 episodes occurring on >1, but <15 days of a month for 3 months and fulfilling criteria B–D
B. Headache lasts from 30 min to 7 days	
C. Headache has at least two of the following: 1. bilateral location 2. pressing/tightening (nonpulsating) nature 3. mild or moderate intensity 4. not worsened by physical activity	
D. Headache has both of the following: 1. no nausea or vomiting 2. only one of photophobia or phonophobia	
E. Cannot be attributed to another disorder	

Modified from Headache Classification Subcommittee of the International Headache Society (IHS). The International Classification of Headache Disorders, 3rd edition. *Cephalalgia*. 2018;38(1):1–211.

Abortive treatment:

- **NSAIDs:** Ibuprofen, naproxen, indomethacin, ketorolac, and others are used. Smaller dosages than used in migraine are typically effective for TTHs.
- **Acetaminophen:** Less effective than NSAIDs for TTHs, but still useful in those where NSAIDs may be contraindicated.
  Dosage: 1000 mg PO; may repeat in 4–6 hours (maximum 4000 mg in 24 hours)
- **Butalbital combinations** (butalbital/ASA/caffeine or butalbital/acetaminophen/caffeine) may be used as well; less frequent dosing intervals than those used for migraine are usual. Special concerns may arise regarding abuse potential and sedation.
  Dosage: 2 tablets PO; may repeat in 4 hours (maximum of 6 tablets in 24 hours)
- **Tramadol (Ultram):** An opioid analog; it may have some abuse potential
  Dosage: 100 mg PO four times daily (maximum of 400 mg in 24 hours)

Prophylactic treatment:

- **Tricyclic antidepressants: Amitriptyline is most commonly used.**
- **Beta-blockers:** Propranolol and timolol are used; not a great choice for athletes because they impair aerobic exercise. They act by reducing VO_2 max and maximum heart rate and increasing fatigue. They are banned by the International Olympic Committee in diving and shooting.

General TTH treatment considerations: Watch for headache secondary to analgesic use and "rebound pain." Concerns and side effects in athletes differ from those in the general population; individualize treatment if possible.

Cluster Headaches

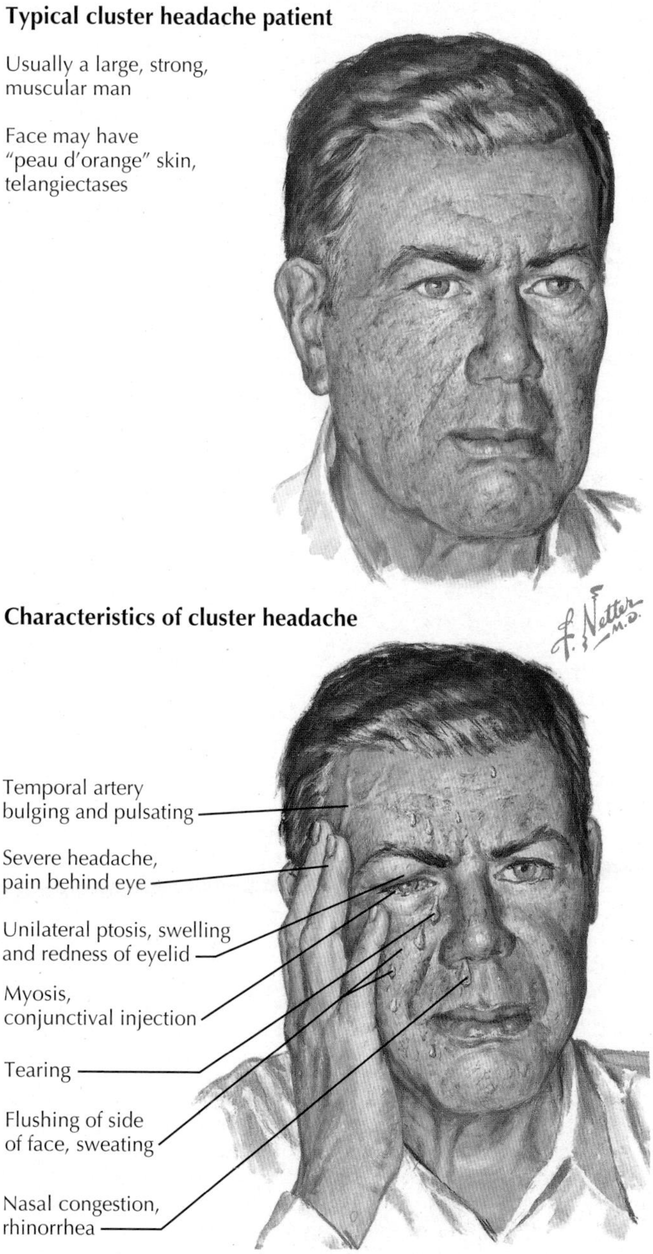
Typical cluster headache patient
Usually a large, strong, muscular man
Face may have "peau d'orange" skin, telangiectases
Characteristics of cluster headache
F. Netter M.D.
Temporal artery bulging and pulsating
Severe headache, pain behind eye
Unilateral ptosis, swelling and redness of eyelid
Myosis, conjunctival injection
Tearing
Flushing of side of face, sweating
Nasal congestion, rhinorrhea

Figure 39.4 Cluster headache.

- **Definition:** Cluster headaches present as a series of recurring headaches that persist from weeks to months at a time, followed by remission periods. Pain is always unilateral and is of a severe, penetrating, and stabbing nature. The location of these headaches is orbital, periorbital, or temporal (Fig. 39.4).
- Most important differentiating feature of cluster headaches is the presence of transient autonomic symptoms.
- Recur throughout the day and wake approximately 50% of patients from sleep
- IHS diagnostic criteria for cluster headaches are listed in Box 39.3.
- Occur more frequently in men than in women, with research showing male-to-female ratios that range from 2:1 to 6.7:1
- Typical age of onset is between the third and fifth decades.
- Alcohol, nitroglycerine, and histamine may trigger headaches.
- Patients pace, rock, or bang head against the wall (vs. patients with migraine, who sleep).
- Chronic cluster headache is a more severe form wherein headache attacks occur for >1 year either without remission or remission lasting for <1 month.

BOX 39.3 IHS CRITERIA FOR CLUSTER HEADACHES

A. At least five attacks fulfilling criteria B–D
B. Severe unilateral orbital, supraorbital, and/or temporal pain lasting for 15–180 minutes
C. Headache is accompanied by at least one of the following transient autonomic symptoms:
 1. ipsilateral conjunctival injection and/or lacrimation
 2. ipsilateral nasal congestion and/or rhinorrhea
 3. ipsilateral eyelid edema
 4. ipsilateral forehead and facial sweating
 5. ipsilateral miosis and/or ptosis
 6. sensation of fullness in the ear
 7. a sense of restlessness or agitation
D. Attacks have a frequency of one every other day to up to eight per day
E. Cannot be attributed to another disorder

Modified from Headache Classification Subcommittee of the International Headache Society (IHS). The International Classification of Headache Disorders, 3rd edition. *Cephalalgia*. 2018;38(1):1–211.

Treatment Options

ABORTIVE TREATMENT

- Limited duration of headache makes most abortive treatment ineffective.
- **DHE-45** as used with migraine; DHE (0.5–1.0 mg) IV, IM, or intranasal
- **Oxygen:** Inhalation with a nonrebreather mask; 8–12 L per minute over 10–15 minutes; 70% response
- **Sumatriptan** as used with migraine; because of its rapid onset, it is considered the most effective agent. Intranasal preparation is administered to the **contralateral** side of the cluster headache secondary to frequently present rhinorrhea on the affected side.
- **Intranasal lidocaine 4%:** Injected into sphenopalatine fossa, effective in certain cases.
- Oxygen and sumatriptan are abortive treatments of choice in athletes.

PROPHYLACTIC TREATMENT

- **Calcium channel blockers:** They inhibit the initial vasoconstrictive phase of cluster headaches. Verapamil is most often used and is the drug of choice for prophylaxis against cluster headaches in athletes. Verapamil 120–360 mg daily divided into two, three, or four doses; one-time daily dosing may be achieved with use of extended-release tablets.
- **Corticosteroids:** Used as a bridge between abortive and prophylactic therapy, they are effective in halting the cluster cycle. **Prednisone:** 40–60 mg PO daily for 5 days and tapered over 2–4 weeks.
- **Lithium carbonate:** One of the first drugs used for prophylactic treatment of chronic cluster headache. Blood levels must be monitored, and thyroid function tests must be followed; concern that in athletes, dehydration may cause increase in lithium levels; generally only used when other drugs are ineffective or contraindicated.
- **Anticonvulsants:** Valproate and topiramate may play a role in nonpharmacologic treatment of cluster headaches.

SPORTS-/EXERCISE-RELATED PRIMARY HEADACHES

Athletes make up a special subset of the headache-suffering population. This is because they may suffer from specific types of headaches that are the direct result of participation in their sport.

BOX 39.4 IHS CRITERIA FOR PRIMARY EXERCISE HEADACHES

A. At least two headache episodes fulfilling criteria B and C
B. Lasting for <48 hours
C. Brought on by and occurring only during or after physical exertion
D. Cannot be attributed to another disorder

Modified from Headache Classification Subcommittee of the International Headache Society (IHS). The International Classification of Headache Disorders, 3rd edition. *Cephalalgia*. 2018;38(1):1–211.

Exercise-/Effort-Induced Migraine

- **Definition:** Exercise-/effort-induced migraines are headaches that fit the criteria for migraine headache (primarily in that they are severe, unilateral, throbbing, and last for 4–72 hours) and are triggered by exercise. Those who experience exercise-/effort-induced migraines usually have a history of nonexercise–related migraines.
  - In a previous study, high-intensity bicycling for a duration of 30 seconds was shown to precipitate a typical migraine 4.5–5.5 hours after the cessation of the exercise in women with a previous history of migraine.
- Headache occurs after activity and may be with or without aura.
- Activities that usually trigger the migraines are aerobic, such as running and swimming.
- Dehydration, excessive heat, hypoglycemia, and hypomagnesemia are predisposing factors.
- Elevation of nitric oxide, which has been shown to increase during exercise and is responsible for causing central vasodilation and subsequent increased central nervous system sensitivity, has been proposed as a potential cause of these headaches.
- **Treatment:** Responds to the same prophylactic and abortive treatments as ordinary migraine. A slow warm-up regimen has been recommended as an adjunct in the prevention of exercise-/effort-induced migraines.

Primary Exercise Headache

- **Definition:** Primary exercise headaches (PEHs) are headaches that are precipitated by any form of exercise in the absence of any intracranial disorder. This IHS classification combines two headache entities that were previously well known to the sports medicine community as "benign exertional headache (BEH)" and "effort headache."
  - BEHs are thought to arise from brief, strenuous physical exercise that involved increasing intrathoracic pressure and performing Valsalva maneuvers (e.g., weightlifting, sprinting, and specific swimming events). These headaches are brief in duration.
  - Effort headaches are thought to arise from longer aerobic exercise activity common to a multitude of sports. These headaches typically have more migrainous features.
- This type of headache was first described by Tinel in 1932 and termed "la cephalee a l'effort."
- PEH is the most commonly diagnosed headache type in athletes.
- PEH occurs in trained athletes and in those who exercise infrequently.
- IHS diagnostic criteria for PEH are listed in Box 39.4.
- This type of headache often occurs with exercise in hot weather or higher altitude.
- Thorough evaluation should be conducted before diagnosing exertional headache because it may not always arise from primary causes.
  - An early study in 1968 followed 103 patients diagnosed with BEH; 10 eventually had underlying organic disease.

- In another series of 221 patients with brain tumor, 60% had headaches, and 22% of these had headaches that worsened with cough and exertion; in 18%, pain increased with stooping or bending over.
- There have also been case reports of spontaneous cerebrospinal fluid leaks causing headache with Valsalva being misdiagnosed as BEH.
- **Treatment:** May be prevented by limiting the amount of exercise and controlling the exercise environment; most primary exertional headaches respond to NSAID therapy. Indomethacin can be used prophylactically, taken in 25- to 50-mg doses 1–2 hours before exercise. Moreover, twice- or thrice-daily dosing of 50–150 mg of indomethacin may be used to abort such headaches in those who have begun to have frequent episodes.

SPORTS-/EXERCISE-RELATED PRIMARY HEADACHE PRETENDERS

- Several conditions may present as primary exercise-related headaches. An intuitive physician will at least be cognizant of this fact and will take into account all the differentials before making the final diagnosis.
- **Cardiac cephalalgia:** Case reports describe these as headaches that begin with vigorous exercise and are relieved by rest. The severity of the headache may increase as the intensity and duration of the exercise increase.
  - Headache is caused by cardiac ischemia.
  - Neurologic evaluation is normal.
  - Diagnosis is made using exercise stress testing. The onset of the patient's headache may correlate with electrocardiogram (ECG) changes indicative of myocardial ischemia.
  - Headache may improve with nitroglycerin treatment (vasodilator) and worsen with triptan treatment (vasoconstrictor), which is in marked contrast to primary exercise-related headaches such as exercise-induced migraine that will likely worsen with nitroglycerin and improve with triptan treatment.
  - **Treatment:** Myocardial revascularization has been shown to lead to complete resolution of such headaches.
- **Other differential diagnoses of exercise-related primary headaches:**
  - Intracranial: brain tumors, subacute and chronic subdural hematomas, and vascular malformations
  - Craniospinal abnormalities: platybasia, Arnold–Chiari malformation, and basilar impression
  - Metabolic disorders: pheochromocytoma, Cushing disease, myxedema, thyrotoxicosis, and hypoglycemia of any etiology
  - Neurologic diseases: hydrocephalus, chronic central nervous system infections, and multiple sclerosis

SPORTS-/EXERCISE-RELATED SECONDARY HEADACHES

Acute and Persistent Posttraumatic Headache

- **Definition:** PTH is any form of headache (migraine, TTH, or cluster) that occurs after a known head trauma. They are categorized by the IHS as either acute or persistent and as either occurring from mild or moderate/severe head trauma.
  - Acute PTH occurs within 7 days after the head trauma and resolves within 3 months.
  - Persistent PTH also occurs within 7 days after trauma to the head but persists for >3 months.
- When PTH does not occur in isolation, but instead is accompanied by additional symptoms including difficulty balancing, inability to concentrate, memory problems, fatigue, dizziness, emotional lability, and insomnia, the athlete may be suffering from postconcussion syndrome.
- Headache is the most common neurologic symptom after head trauma; it persists for >2 months in 60% of patients.
- Location, severity, and pain characteristics vary considerably. Most studies have shown that PTH is *less* common when the head trauma is *more* severe.
- TTH is the most common PTH.
- Women are at a higher risk of developing PTH.
- In a study of 443 high school and collegiate football players, 85% reported developing headache as the direct result of hitting.
- **Etiology** is controversial: both organic and psychogenic theories exist.
  - May be related to axonal injury or excitotoxic amino acid release, which results in neural injury
  - May be related to altered cerebral hemodynamics and/or slowed cerebral circulation
- **Posttraumatic migraine (footballer's migraine)** has been noted in sports such as boxing and soccer, where taking blows to the head or repetitively heading the ball causes migraine.
  - Does not require significant trauma; not associated with significant amnesia
  - After symptom-free interval of several minutes, visual, motor, sensory, or brainstem signs and symptoms begin (scintillating scotoma, flashing lights, blurred vision, or other sensory symptoms); last for 15–30 minutes
  - Subsequently, severe throbbing headache develops, associated with nausea and vomiting
  - Predisposing factors include history of nonsports-related migraine and family history of migraine (60% have a parent with migraine; 70% have a parent or sibling with migraine; 77% have a parent, sibling, or grandparent with migraine).
- **Important to rule out an organic basis for symptoms**
  - Do not return athlete to play if he or she remains symptomatic.
  - Immediate concerns include second-impact syndrome, vascular abnormalities, and other neurologic disorders.
  - **Intracranial bleeds that cause PTH** include epidural hematoma, subdural hematoma, and subarachnoid hemorrhage.
- **Treatment:** Once an organic cause is ruled out, treatment depends on the type of headache pattern (migraine, TTH, or cluster). Acute PTH that is nonmigrainous in nature and occurs within hours of a trauma should be treated in the short term with non-NSAID analgesics. This is done to prevent worsening of an intercranial bleed by the antiplatelet effect of the NSAID in the event an intercranial bleed has occurred.

Cervicogenic Headache

- **Definition:** A cervicogenic headache is a headache that is caused by abnormalities within structures of the cervical spine, including the muscular, ligamentous, nervous, vascular, articular, and discogenic elements. It is usually, but not always, accompanied by neck pain.
- Pain typically starts in the neck and spreads to the oculofrontotemporal area. Pain is "dull" or "boring" in nature and fluctuates in intensity.
- Headache is constant and may last from hours to weeks.
- Often accompanied by restricted range of motion of the neck and by ipsilateral, nonradicular, neck, shoulder, or arm pain
- Often seen in response to moderate/severe head trauma
- Affects women more than men with a female-to-male ratio of 4:1
- **Treatment:** Physical therapy has been shown to provide the most long-term relief of cervicogenic headache. This may include cervical traction, massage, and strengthening. Anesthetic blockade may provide temporary relief but is not a long-term solution. Those who are provided relief with blockade but are

not helped by physical therapy may benefit from radiofrequency neurotomy.

High-Altitude Headache

- **Definition:** Headache that occurs with ascent to altitudes above 2400–3000 meters and is caused by hypoxia. They are dull and are of mild to moderate intensity. They typically develop within 6–24 hours of ascent and resolve within 8 hours after descent.
- Headache is the primary symptom of acute mountain sickness (AMS).
- Twenty to fifty percent of skiers and mountaineers experience headache at altitudes of 3000–5000 meters.
- **Treatment:** Primary treatment is descent to a lower altitude. High-altitude headaches may be prevented by allowing appropriate acclimation to one altitude before climbing to a higher altitude. Pharmacologic treatments include:
  - **Pretreatment with aspirin:** Raises headache threshold; associated with less pronounced cardiorespiratory response to short-term exercise at altitude; can prevent headache.
  - **Ibuprofen:** More effective than placebo in altitude-related headache. In randomized, double-blind crossover study, ibuprofen 600 mg was effective in treating headache, whereas sumatriptan 100 mg was ineffective.
  - **Prophylaxis:** Acetazolamide 250 mg PO twice daily or 500 mg PO once daily with use of extended-release tablets; prophylaxis should be initiated on the day before the climb

Diving Headache

- **Definition:** Headache that is caused secondary to hypercapnia and most readily associated with deep-water diving; carbon dioxide builds up in divers who practice "skip breathing," which is the act of intentionally holding respiration to conserve air or affect buoyancy in the water.
  - Hypercapnia causes cerebrovascular vasodilation and elevated intracranial pressure, which leads to headache.
  - Diving headache is nonspecific in character, but migrainous-type headaches may occur.
  - Occurs at depths below 10 meters.
  - Worsens during resurfacing or decompression phase of the dive.
- **Treatment:** Taking deep, slow breaths may help prevent these headaches from occurring. Treatment with 100% oxygen will usually resolve these headaches within 1 hour.

SPORTS-/EXERCISE-RELATED CRANIAL NEURALGIA HEADACHES

External Compression Headache

- **Definition:** Headache that results from continuous stimulation of the cutaneous nerves of the head. The continuous nerve stimulation is caused by externally applied pressure. This pressure usually results from wearing tight headbands, swim goggles, or diving masks.
- Headache is dull and increases in intensity as duration of compression increases.
- May contribute to the development of diving headache.
- **Treatment:** Removal of the compressing device (headband, mask, or swim goggles) results in complete resolution of the headache.

Table 39.3 DRUGS OF CHOICE FOR HEADACHES IN ATHLETES

	Tension Headache	Migraine Headache	Cluster Headache
Abortive Treatment	Acetaminophen NSAIDs	Sumatriptan Other 5-HT agonists DHE-45 (nasal) Intranasal lidocaine	Oxygen Sumatriptan DHE-45
Prophylactic Treatment	NSAIDs TCAs at bedtime	Verapamil Valproate, topiramate TCAs at bedtime	Verapamil

DHE, Dihydroergotamine; *NSAIDs,* nonsteroidal anti-inflammatory drugs; *TCAs,* tricyclic antidepressants.

Cold-Stimulus Headache

- **Definition:** Headache that occurs after exposing unprotected head to cold temperatures (e.g., diving in cold water)
- Headache is dull and diffuse
- May contribute to the development of diving headache
- **Treatment:** Headache resolves with removal of the cold stimulus

CHARACTERISTICS OF PRIMARY HEADACHE DISORDERS

See Table 39.1.

DRUG CHOICES FOR HEADACHES IN ATHLETES

See Table 39.3.

RECOMMENDED READINGS

Available online.

SKIN PROBLEMS IN THE ATHLETE 40

R. Robert Franks, Jr.

GENERAL PRINCIPLES

- Skin infections account for 21% of illnesses and injuries reported in collegiate sports and 8.5% in high school sports.
- In collegiate sports, skin infections account for 1%–2% of all time-loss injuries. Twenty percent of National Collegiate Athletic Association (NCAA) wrestlers lose practice or competition time because of skin problems annually.
- Common dermatologic lesions and examples are listed in Table 40.1.

Pathophysiology

- Increase in methicillin-resistant *Staphylococcus aureus* (MRSA) transmission is of concern in the contact sports of wrestling, fencing, and football.
- Other etiologies for skin infections include other bacterial, viral, and fungal infections. Other skin issues apart from infections can occur in sports.
- Although the overall incidence of skin infections is low, prevention is possible.
- Skin lesions are most often transmitted from person to person but can also be from fomites.
- Risk factors for skin infections include:
  - Previous history of infection
  - Compromised host immunity
  - Close contact sports
  - Poor personal hygiene
  - Body shaving, waxing
  - Antibiotic overuse
  - Sharing of towels, razors, uniforms, and equipment
  - Facility and equipment cleanliness

Methods to Reduce Infection Transmission

- History of past infections and treatment should be noted.
- Routine skin checks are recommended in all sports, particularly in high-risk sports (e.g., wrestling, football, and rugby). The NCAA recommends skin checks several times a week, and the National Federation of High Schools (NFHS) also has published guidelines. Skin checks should be performed with the athlete in briefs, and sports bra if female, in room with good lighting with a chaperone. Athlete positioning should be feet shoulder-width apart with arms adducted at 90 degrees and thumbs pointed superiorly. Special attention should be given to hairline and scalp.
- Infection spread can be decreased by withholding infected athletes from practice and/or competition until completely treated.
- Good hygiene should be promoted with immediate bathing after practices/games and trimming of nails.
  - Wash uniforms, towels, and equipment immediately after their use.
  - Instruct athletes to dry the area of any skin lesion last and discard the towel.
  - Regularly wash hands with soap and water or an alcohol-based hand gel.
  - Avoid sharing of equipment, uniforms, towels, clothing, bedding, bar soap, razors, and toothbrushes.
- Wound coverage as the primary treatment or prevention of spread of a skin lesion is never appropriate.
- Skin lesions should be covered only after they are noninfectious to prevent secondary infection. Consider prophylactic medication for those with frequent outbreaks.
- Student-athletes should be encouraged to immediately report skin wounds and lesions.
- Equipment and other surfaces that multiple athletes have had contact with should be frequently cleaned.
- In wrestling specifically, cleaning techniques are critical to prevent disease transmission. Best practices should include:
  - Clean all mats with a residual disinfectant.
  - Encourage the backward-mopping technique for cleaning mats.
  - Encourage hand washing or hand gel by wrestlers immediately before each match.
  - Encourage annual influenza vaccination for all wrestlers.
- Education of coaches, officials, and healthcare practitioners regarding common skin lesions should be conducted at least annually.

VIRAL INFECTIONS

Herpes Gladiatorum (Traumatic Herpes)

Overview: Caused by the herpes simplex virus (HSV); HSV is common in the general population and among athletes, particularly wrestlers. Herpes consists of two types, HSV-1 or HSV-2, but can be mixed and found anywhere on the body. HSV-I is associated with cold sores and fever blisters. HSV-2 is associated with genital herpes. Ninety-four to ninety-seven percent of herpes gladiatorum (HG) is caused by HSV-1. In a typical season, 2.6% of high school wrestlers and 7.6% of college wrestlers will suffer from HG, and up to 87.4% of infections are subclinical and go undiagnosed. It spreads skin to skin via an active rash or rash fluid, from fomites to skin, or by respiratory droplets or saliva. Breaks in the skin barrier can increase the risk of infection. Stress, either physical or emotional, and sun exposure can increase the likelihood of infection. The virus incubation period is typically 2–14 days.

Presentation: One in four infected with primary HG will begin with flulike symptoms approximately 2–24 hours before appearance of rash. Rashes may have a prodrome of itching or burning. In wrestling, common appearance of the rash is usually on the right side of the wrestler's face, neck, or arm, which are points of most contact with the mat or site of dominant arm or dominant tie-up side. The rash disappears in 2 weeks without scarring. Recurrent HG usually involves fewer vesicles that are present for a shorter duration and systemic symptoms are much less common.

Physical examination: The rash begins as a burning or tingling sensation on the skin, which is already in its contagious phase. This area then becomes the site of red bumps that form clusters of tiny blisters filled with cloudy fluid on an erythematous base. The blisters collapse to form yellowish-brown scabs, which form in 2–4 days. Reactivation of the virus in ganglia, usually due to a stressor, including lack of sleep or poor nutrition, will cause the rash to occur in the individual in the same dermatomal or peripheral nerve pattern.

Diagnosis: The rash is usually characteristic; however, viral cultures and HSV polymerase chain reaction can also be performed to confirm diagnosis and type (HSV-1 vs. HSV-2). Tzank smear is no longer recommended.

Table 40.1 DESCRIPTION OF COMMON DERMATOLOGIC TERMS

Terminology	Definition	Example
Macule	Nonraised change of skin color <1 cm	Vitiligo Petechiae
Patch	Nonraised change of skin color >1 cm	Vitiligo Pityriasis
Papule	Raised skin change with defined borders <1 cm in diameter that comes in a variety of shapes (i.e., domed, umbilicated)	Measles Acne vulgaris
Nodule	Raised skin change >1 cm in diameter appearing in epidermis, dermis, or subcutaneous tissue	Warts Squamous or basal cell carcinoma
Tumor	Solid mass within skin or subcutaneous tissue greater than a nodule	Lipoma Seborrheic keratosis
Plaque	Raised, solid lesion >1 cm in diameter on skin surface	Psoriasis Mycosis fungoides
Vesicle	Raised fluid-filled lesions <1 cm in diameter appearing on skin surface	Herpes simplex Herpes zoster
Bulla	Larger fluid-filled lesion >1 cm on skin surface with true circumscribed border	Blisters Pemphigus
Pustule	Elevated lesion on skin surface containing pus with circumscribed border Vesicles can become pustules Fluid may be infectious or noninfectious	Acne vulgaris Impetigo
Wheal	Area of edema found in epidermis	Urticaria Bee or wasp sting
Burrow	Linear change in skin due to tunnel formation by skin infestation	Scabies
Telangiectasia	Prominent, permanent dilation of superficial blood vessels in skin	Osler–Weber–Rendu disease Ataxia-telangiectasia
Ulcer	Open, crater-like lesion of epidermis or mucous membranes	Decubitus ulcer Aphthous ulcer
Lichenification	Elevated lesion containing proliferation of keratinocytes and stratum corneum due to continued skin irritation	Eczematous dermatitis
Scales	Peeling or flaking skin areas due to abnormal formation of stratum corneum as a result of increased production of epidermal cells	Psoriasis Eczema
Crusts	Skin change resulting from dried serum, blood, or purulence	Impetigo Herpes simplex
Atrophy	Thinning or absence of epidermis or subcutaneous fat	Steroid-induced atrophy Scleroderma
Erosion	Depressed skin area where epidermis is partially or completely removed	Infection Trauma
Excoriation	Loss of skin from scratching, friction, or rubbing	Chronic hepatitis C Skin picking disorder
Fissure	Linear skin break that leads into the dermis	Dry skin Trauma (scratches)
Scar	Fibrotic changes to skin as a result of dermal damage Change of pigment is often associated with scars	Surgery Trauma
Eschar	Hard, darkened plaque covering ulcer with significant tissue necrosis	Burns Pressure wounds
Keloids	Extensive connective tissue response to skin injury that is larger than original wound	Surgery Trauma
Petechiae	Smaller bleeding skin lesion Does not blanch when pressed	Strep throat Vasculitis
Purpura, ecchymosis	Larger bleeding skin lesion Does not blanch when pressed Purpura may be palpable	Hemangiomas Senile purpura

Treatment: Treatment is with oral antivirals for 10–14 days for initial infections. Consider valacyclovir (Valtrex) 1 g BID. Treatment for recurrent infections should be valacyclovir 1 g BID for 5–7 days. Consider suppression dosing for those with chronic recurrent infections approximately six times per year. The drug of choice would be valacyclovir 500 mg PO daily if recent infection was longer than 2 years ago and valacyclovir 1 g PO daily if most recent infection was less than 2 years prior. Famciclovir can also be considered if there is resistance to valacyclovir. Topical antivirals are often not effective if used alone.

Return to play: Varies. Return for wrestling for the NCAA for primary or secondary HG is after a course of 5 days of oral antiviral treatment with no new lesions for 72 hours, all lesions must be dry and crusted, there is no apparent secondary bacterial infection, and in the case of primary HG, there are no systemic symptoms. Return for wrestling for the NFHS for primary HG is 10 days of antiviral treatment for cutaneous lesions only and 14 days if there are systemic symptoms, all lesions crusted over, and no new lesions for 48 hours. Return for wrestling for the NFHS for secondary HG is 5 days of antiviral therapy, all lesions crusted over, and no new lesions for 48 hours. In all cases of return, coverage of lesions alone is inappropriate to allow participation.

Herpes Labialis (Fever Blister, Oral Herpes, and Cold Sores)

Overview: Caused by HSV-1 and is spread skin to skin or by fomites (Fig. 40.1); the infection is seen around the lips, beginning as vesicles on an erythematous base that break and then crust over. The virus can express itself during times of physical or emotional stress or from environmental factors such as direct sunlight.

Presentation: Begins with prodrome of pain or pruritus at the site of lesion, followed by clear vesicles on an erythematous base that eventually break and crust over. The athlete becomes infectious during the prodrome and is infectious until the lesions crust. Infection course is generally 7–14 days.

Physical examination: Clear vesicles on an erythematous base around the lip and possibly between the nose and lip that evolve into areas of ruptured vesicles on an ulcerated base.

Diagnosis: Characteristic rash, but viral culture is definitive

Treatment: Treatment includes oral antivirals: consider valacyclovir 2 g BID for 1 day, which should be started as soon as the athlete experiences the viral prodrome.

Return to sport: Varies, but for specific NCAA and NFHS guidelines for wrestling, see "Herpes Gladiatorum" section.

Herpes Zoster (Shingles)

Available online.

Molluscum Contagiosum (Water Warts)

Overview: Viral lesion from Poxviridae family that spreads skin to skin or via fomites; characterized by single or multiple discreet, flesh-colored, dome-shaped papules with a central dimple. If ruptured, caseous material is released with high viral content inducting spread. The rash most often occurs in contact athletes, on the face, trunk, or hands.

Presentation: Athletes have these lesions, painless and nonpruritic, in clusters for several weeks to months and often only present when their spread is noticed.

Physical examination: Clustered, dimpled papules found on face, trunk, or hands

Diagnosis: Characteristic rash, but also identified by observation under microscope or biopsy

Treatment: Mechanical via curettage, electrotherapy, or cryotherapy; chemical and immunologic methods can also be used

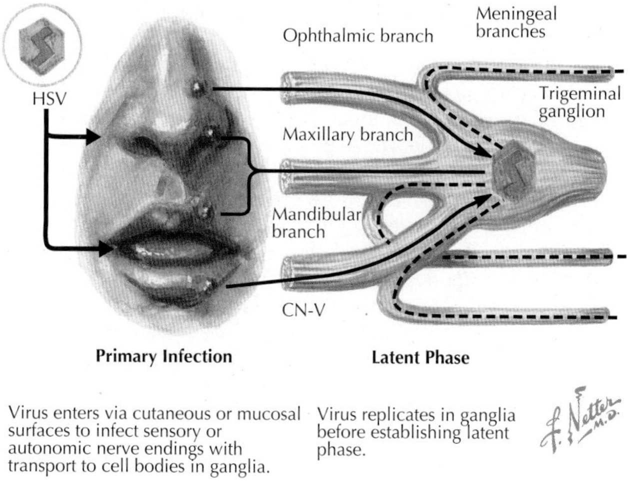

HSV
Ophthalmic branch
Meningeal branches
Trigeminal ganglion
Maxillary branch
Mandibular branch
CN-V
Primary Infection
Latent Phase
Virus enters via cutaneous or mucosal surfaces to infect sensory or autonomic nerve endings with transport to cell bodies in ganglia.
Virus replicates in ganglia before establishing latent phase.
F. Netter M.D.

Figure 40.1 Herpes simplex.

Return to sport: Data inconclusive; lesion removal and coverage with bio-occlusive dressing is suggested, but 48 hours of recovery to prevent secondary infection is often recommended.

Verruca Vulgaris/Plantaris (Common/Plantar Warts)

Overview: Verrucous plaques and papules found most often on the epidermis of the hands caused by the human papilloma virus. They can, however, be seen anywhere on the body. Warts on the plantar surface of the athlete's foot, most often the heel or ball, can cause a change in the athlete's ambulation.

Presentation: Painless papules or plaques most often on hands, present for weeks to months; athletes usually try self-removal before presentation via over-the-counter preparations, cutting, scraping, or picking. Can be painful with local trauma to area.

Physical examination: Seen anywhere, but usually on hands and feet; papules with a typical scaly "cauliflower" appearance

Diagnosis: Distinguished from calluses by the presence of hemorrhages seen when the wart is shaved; no normal skin lines in the wart

Treatment: Removed by curettage, cryotherapy, or use of salicylic acid; immunotherapy is also successful in wart resolution. Treatments may have to be repeated. Care must be taken not to permanently damage or destroy skin with continued attempts at removal. If a wart is present in a sensitive area, paring and covering may be used in-season with definitive treatment after the season. Warts should be covered; low risk of transmission. The wart can be protected by use of doughnut pads or moleskin until definitive treatment can be administered. Use of footwear in locker rooms and shower areas can prevent transmission.

Return to sport: No restrictions, but should cover area with bio-occlusive dressing

SARS-CoV-2 (Coronavirus-19)

Available online.

BACTERIAL INFECTIONS (FIG. 40.2)

MRSA

Overview: Rapidly spreading bacterial infection characterized by *S. aureus* that is resistant to several antibiotic classes; the most common strain seen in athletes is community-acquired (CA-MRSA) species. Spread is via skin-to-skin contact, fomites, crowding, poor hygiene, scratching, and compromised skin integrity. As many as 76% of college wrestlers are carriers of CA-MRSA.

Presentation: Most often confused with spider bites or simple pustules

Physical examination: Infection begins with a small pimple-like lesion that quickly progresses to a hot, erythematous, inflamed, painful indurated area much larger than the original lesion; can occur on any part of the body

Diagnosis: Challenging, as the infection looks like other common infections; Gram stain and bacterial culture are diagnostic

Treatment: Treatment should begin, if suspected, before the culture results are identified. Treatment is via incision and drainage, if applicable, and intravenous (IV) antibiotics such as vancomycin for serious lesions. Minor or less serious lesions are treated with oral antibiotics for 7 to 14 days. Consider trimethoprim with sulfamethoxazole (Bactrim) 2 DS BID or doxycycline 100 mg BID, unless the athlete will be spending time in direct sunlight, for 7–14 days. Clindamycin 400 mg PO TID or linezolid 600 mg PO BID can be used also for 7–14 days. It is recommended to add mupirocin 2% ointment TID to the noted antibiotic regimens; prevented by not sharing uniforms, towels, or equipment. Area of infection should be dried last after showering, and the towel must be immediately laundered. Treatment of chronic carriers is controversial.

Return to sport: After complete antibiotic course with wounds dried and crusted and formation of no new lesions. It is not enough just to cover active infectious lesions to allow competition by the athlete.

Prevention: The efficacy of treating potential MRSA carriers via decolonization in order to prevent spread of infection remains inconclusive. When attempted, the combination of chlorhexidine washes combined with 2% mupirocin ointment is recommended. Written policies for identification and treatment of skin infections and procedures for equipment cleaning may decrease CA-MRSA infections.

Impetigo

Overview: Caused by beta-hemolytic *Streptococcus* or *S. aureus*. Infection usually begins as small red blisters on erythematous skin. Blisters then break, forming characteristic honey-colored scabs that may be pruritic. If left untreated, impetigo can cause renal damage. Infection usually resolves within 2 weeks without scarring. Spread is either skin to skin or via fomites; can spread by scratching or drying after shower.

Presentation: Often begins as a small lesion; often, if initial rash begins around the mouth, it can be confused with herpes labialis

Physical examination: Most often seen on face or forehead, but can occur anywhere

Diagnosis: Characteristic rash, but Gram stain with bacterial culture is definitive

Treatment: Small areas may be treated with antibiotic creams or ointments

Consider 2% mupirocin (Bactroban) TID for 7–14 days. Oral antibiotics should be used for larger areas. Consider clindamycin 400 mg PO TID, cephalexin 250 mg PO QID, or dicloxacillin 250 mg PO QID 7–14 days combined with mupirocin 2% ointment TID. Consideration should be given to immediate treatment for MRSA, if suspected. Infection often prevented by not sharing uniforms, towels, or equipment. Area of infection should be dried last after showering and the towel immediately laundered.

Return to sport: Return is not advisable until all blisters have crusted and 3 days of antibiotic treatment have been completed without new lesions for 48 hours before competition. It is not enough just to cover active infectious lesions to allow competition by the athlete.

Cellulitis

Overview: Infection of the dermis and subcutaneous tissues usually by group A *Streptococcus* and/or *S. aureus*.

Cellulitis most often occurs after a break in the skin such as a laceration, abrasion, or puncture wound (see Fig. 40.2); can spread skin to skin or by fomites

Presentation: Often begins with a gradual onset of pain and swelling that may or may not be associated with a recent break in the skin

Physical examination: Presents initially as a painful, erythematous, swollen patch that spreads as the infection spreads; the infection can be associated with fever and chills

Diagnosis: Characteristic rash of an erythematous, edematous patch; Gram stain or bacterial culture and/or blood cultures are diagnostic

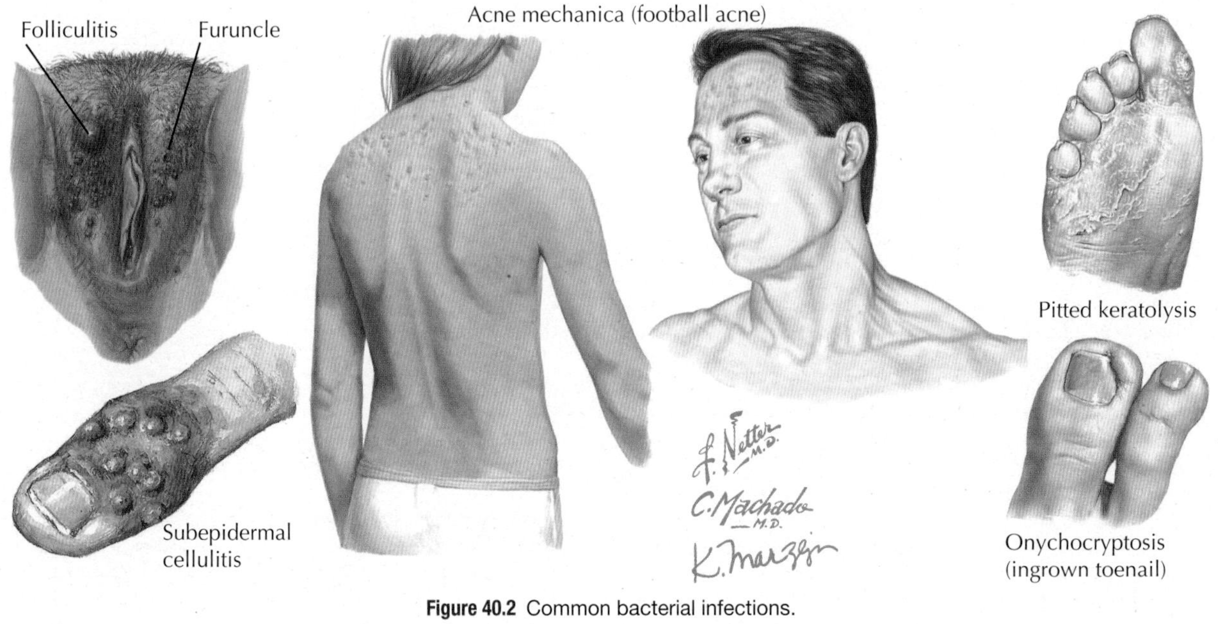
Folliculitis
Furuncle
Acne mechanica (football acne)
Pitted keratolysis
Subepidermal cellulitis
Onychocryptosis (ingrown toenail)
F. Netter M.D.
C. Machado M.D.
K. Marzen

Figure 40.2 Common bacterial infections.

Treatment: Oral antibiotics, and if severe, IV antibiotics. Oral antibiotics can include cephalexin 250 mg PO QID or dicloxacillin 250 mg PO QID for 7–14 days. Warm compresses, pain medications, and incision and drainage can be helpful. Marking location and looking for spread beyond the line of demarcation can be suggestive of antibiotic resistance. Consideration should be given to immediate treatment for MRSA, if appropriate.

Return to sport: Three days of antibiotic treatment have been completed without new lesions for 48 hours before competition, afebrile, cessation of pain, and healing of wound. It is not enough just to cover active infectious lesions to allow competition by the athlete.

Folliculitis (Occlusive Folliculitis, Steroid Folliculitis, Bikini Bottom)

Overview: Characterized by red-ringed papules, pustules, or crusts at hair follicles most commonly caused by *S. aureus*, *Candida*, or *Pseudomonas aeruginosa*, demodex (see Fig. 40.2). Steroids may also cause folliculitis. Infection may evolve to boils or carbuncles.

Presentation: Seen in areas of body that have been shaved or areas with friction from equipment or uniforms; spread is via skin to skin or fomites

Physical examination: Seen in areas of friction such as groin, thighs, buttocks, or gluteal folds

Diagnosis: History and characteristic rash, but Gram stain and bacterial culture are diagnostic

Treatment: Removal of irritant, topical antiseptics, antibiotic creams or ointment, and good hygiene; significant cases involving bacteria require cephalexin 250 mg PO QID or dicloxacillin 250 mg PO QID for 7–14 days.

Return to sport: No restriction with lesion coverage

Pseudomonas Folliculitis (Hot Tub Folliculitis)

Available online.

Furunculosis (Boil, Furuncle, Carbuncle)

Overview: Hair follicle infection by *S. aureus* or *Streptococcus* from trauma or direct contact with a furuncle on another athlete (see Fig. 40.2). Fomites can also spread infection.

Presentation: Begins as infection of hair follicle that often evolves to a loculated pustule

Physical examination: Usually on the upper extremities or trunk and present as erythematous nodules with or without purulence; often painful

Diagnosis: Lesion appearance; Gram stain and bacterial culture are diagnostic

Treatment: Purulent lesions should be incised and drained. Treatment is via topical or cephalexin 250 mg PO QID or dicloxacillin 250 mg PO QID for 7–14 days; if suspicious, presumptive treatment for MRSA should be considered before culture results are obtained. Infection can often be prevented by not sharing uniforms, towels, or equipment. Area of infection should be dried last and the towel immediately laundered.

Return to sport: Three days of antibiotic treatment have been completed without new lesions for 48 hours before competition and lesion coverage with a bio-occlusive dressing

Acne Mechanica (Sports Acne, Football Acne)

Overview: Acne breakout, including papules, pustules, comedones, nodules, and cysts, that is caused by bacterial infection in an area of tight-fitting clothing or ill-fitted equipment such as helmets or shoulder pads (see Fig. 40.2). Friction, heat, and occlusion lead to acne mechanica.

Presentation: The equipment causes erythema and friction at the site of contact with the skin. The site then often becomes infected.

Physical examination: Rash appears as erythematous papules and pustules on the back, shoulders, chin, or forehead.

Diagnosis: Characteristic rash in area of equipment/clothing; Gram stain and bacterial culture are definitive

Treatment: Topical antibiotics and astringents. More severe outbreaks can be treated with oral antibiotics. Good hygiene, wicking undergarments, and refitting of equipment can help prevent further breakout.

Return to sport: No restrictions

Pitted Keratolysis (Tennis Shoe Foot)

Overview: Bacterial infection caused by *Kytococcus sedentarius*, *Dermatophilus congolensis*, *Corynebacterium*, *Actinomyces*, or *Streptomyces*. These bacteria secrete proteinases that destroy the keratin of the stratum corneum of the skin, producing depressed lesions and pits on the sole of the foot but can be on hands as well (see Fig. 40.2).

Presentation: Infection in areas of macerated tissue from extended exposure to moist, warm conditions in nonbreathable shoes seen with cross-country runners or marathoners. Most cases exhibit no discomfort, but multifocal erosions can cause pain. Patients may have foul-smelling infectious lesions for months before presentation because of sulfur production from bacterial by-products.

Physical examination: The rash appears as scaly pits with associated foot odor.

Diagnosis: Characteristic rash or bacterial culture is definitive.

Treatment: Infection is treated with topical mupirocin, clindamycin, or erythromycin. Benzoyl peroxide may be helpful. Topical 20% aluminum chloride or botulinum toxin injection may decrease hyperhidrosis to create a less hospitable bacterial environment. The infection can be prevented with good hygiene, synthetic socks, and allowing ventilation of the feet.

Return to sport: No restrictions

Onychocryptosis (Ingrown Toenail)

Overview: Occurs when inappropriately cut nails or nails damaged from sport grow into the subcutaneous tissue causing infection by *Streptococcus* and *S. aureus* (see Fig. 40.2).

Presentation: Pain, inflammation, and erythema, followed by purulent drainage at the advancing nail edge

Physical examination: Seen on any toe

Diagnosis: Lesion appearance; bacterial culture is diagnostic

Treatment: Incision and drainage of the purulent pocket and trimming or cutting back of the nail; oral antibiotics, pain medications, and warm compresses also used; prevention by appropriate nail trimming and wearing of appropriately fitting footwear. Surgical destruction of part of the nail bed is often curative.

Return to sport: Passing of functional testing

FUNGAL INFECTIONS (FIG. 40.3)

Tinea Pedis/Cruris (Athlete's Foot/Jock Itch)

Overview: Caused by the fungus *Trichophyton rubrum*, *Trichophyton mentagrophytes*, *Epidermophyton floccusum*, or *Candida*. Scaly erythematous rash on plantar surface of the foot, between the toes, or in the groin, accompanied by a burning or itching sensation (see Fig. 40.3). In general, cases improve in 10–14 days and resolve in 4–6 weeks. Spread is by contact of skin with damp, warm conditions.

Presentation: Often seen in those with exposure to warm, damp conditions; in diabetics; and in immunocompromised

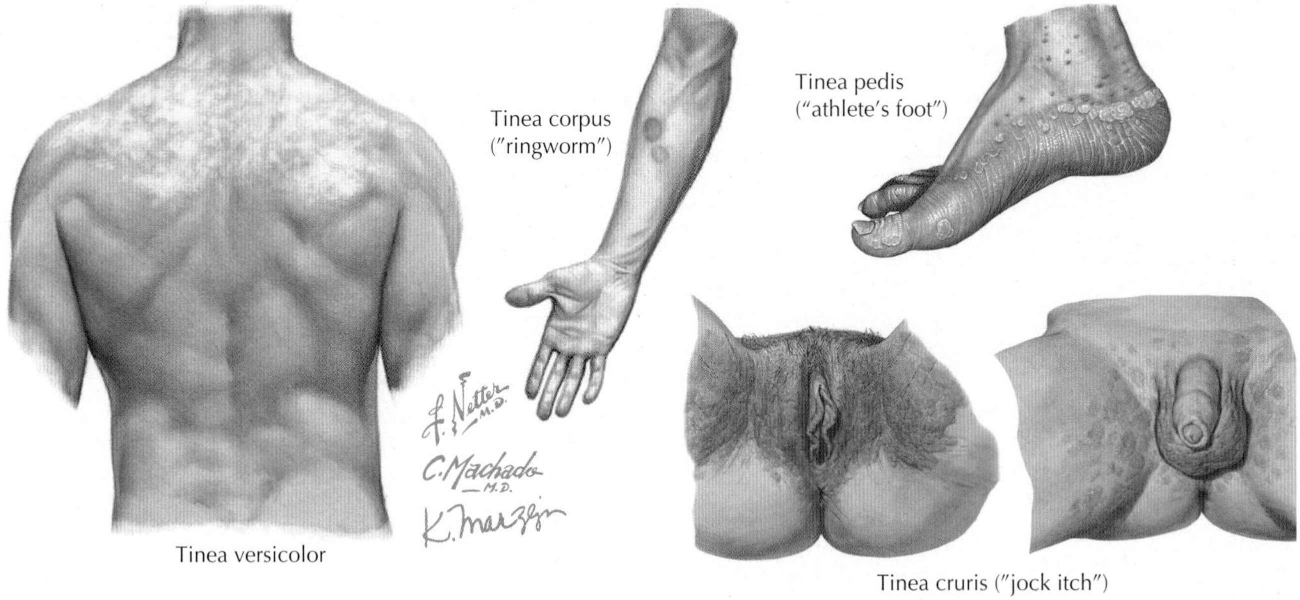
Tinea versicolor
Tinea corpus
("ringworm")
Tinea pedis
("athlete's foot")
Tinea cruris ("jock itch")

Figure 40.3 Common fungal infections.

individuals; athletes often present after trying over-the-counter medications; may spread from sharing of uniforms or towels

Physical examination: Infection is characterized by inflamed, flaky, red and white skin with tiny blisters and/or pimples. Skin may peel or crack, particularly between the toes in pedis. In cruris, it starts at crural folds and expands to thighs. Satellite lesions (i.e., erythematous bumps or blisters), may be seen at the leading edge of the rash or spreading out from the central rash.

Diagnosis: Characteristic rash, but examination of KOH skin scraping under microscope or fungal culture is definite

Treatment: Mild cases are treated with over-the-counter antifungals. Consider Tinactin or Desenex powders. Moderate cases are treated with prescription topical antifungals. Consider Lotrimin AF or Nizoral. Severe cases are treated with oral antifungals. Consider itraconazole (Sporanox) or terbinafine (Lamisil). Monitoring of liver functions is necessary with extended treatment. Antihistamine or low-potency steroid creams may be used for 1–2 days to decrease inflammation and itching. Keeping toes dry and separated promotes healing. Prevented by wearing footwear in the locker room and shower areas, changing socks often, and allowing breathable sneakers to dry. Socks in pedis should be put on before underwear.

Return to sport: No restrictions, as feet and groin are covered

Tinea Corporis (Ringworm)

Overview: Caused by *Microsporum*, *Trichophyton*, or *Epidermophyton*; called *ringworm* because of its characteristic circular appearance (see Fig. 40.3); spread is via fomites, skin to skin, or animals to humans

Presentation: The degree of rash is dependent on the host cellular-based immune response. Several athletes carry the spores but do not demonstrate the rash.

Physical examination: Most often seen on the torso, upper extremities, and head and neck. Rash begins as flat scaly spot in the shape of a small red or brown circle. It spreads as enlarging circle with a scaly border. There may be small papules, blisters, or scales on the leading edge. As it grows up to 5–8 cm, the center fades to a lighter brown or red color. The athlete may have several areas of infection in differing degrees of development, with leading edges being the most reactive. The rash may be pruritic.

Diagnosis: Characteristic rash, but examination of KOH skin scraping under microscope or fungal culture is definite

Treatment: Mild cases are treated with antifungal creams such as terbinafine, clotrimazole, miconazole, or ketoconazole applied BID to lesion and 2-cm border to lesion for 2–4 weeks. More severe cases usually require oral antifungal agents. Anecdotally, consider itraconazole (Sporanox) 200 mg PO daily for 1 week or terbinafine (Lamisil) 250 mg PO daily for 1 week. Monitoring of liver functions is necessary with extended treatment. Diffuse or refractory tinea corporis should be treated with terbinafine 250 mg PO daily or ketoconazole 200 mg PO daily for 2–4 weeks or itraconazole 200 mg for 3–4 weeks. Creams may be combined with oral treatment. It can take up to 3 months for this rash to completely resolve. Consider prophylaxis for those with recurrent infection. Prophylaxis can be via fluconazole 100 mg PO one time weekly, fluconazole 100 mg PO daily for 3 days at start of season and then again in 6 weeks, itraconazole 400 mg PO once every other week, or terbinafine 250 mg PO once a week. Coverage of the rash alone is not sufficient to prevent its spread. Cleaning of mats, equipment, and clothing can decrease transmission.

Return to sport: Conflicting literature, but most recommend 72 hours of drug treatment, either topical or oral, with coverage with gas-permeable dressing until flaking stops.

Tinea Capitis

Overview: Caused by the fungus *Trichophyton tonosurans*; spread is skin to skin or fomite and by contact with the fungus

Presentation: Lesions appear on the head and hair shafts.

Physical examination: Rash is characterized as a scaly, erythematous, pruritic plaques with raised, ring-shaped borders. Hair loss is often present.

Diagnosis: Characteristic rash, but examination of KOH skin scraping under microscope or fungal culture is definite

Treatment: Topical treatment alone is usually ineffective. Terbinafine 250 mg PO daily or ketoconazole 200 mg PO daily for 2–4 weeks or itraconazole 200 mg for 3–4 weeks plus ketoconazole 2% shampoo daily should be considered.

Return to sport: Most recommend oral treatment for at least 14 days and coverage with gas-permeable dressing until flaking stops.

Tinea Barbae

Overview: Caused by the fungus *Trichophyton mentagrophytes* and *T. verrucosum*; spread is skin to skin or fomite and by contact with the fungus
Presentation: Lesions appear on the bearded area and hair shafts.
Physical examination: Rash is characterized as a scaly, erythematous, pruritic plaques with raised, ring-shaped borders. Pimples or blisters may occur. Hair loss is often present, and hair is easy to remove.
Diagnosis: Characteristic rash, but examination of KOH skin scraping under microscope or fungal culture is definite
Treatment: Topical treatment alone is usually ineffective. Terbinafine 250 mg PO daily or ketoconazole 200 mg PO daily for 2–4 weeks or itraconazole 200 mg for 3–4 weeks plus ketoconazole 2% shampoo daily to beard should be considered.
Return to sport: Most recommend oral treatment for at least 14 days and coverage with gas-permeable dressing until flaking stops.

Tinea Versicolor

Overview: Fungal infection caused by *Pityrosporum orbiculare* or *P. ovale*; identified by hypopigmented or hyperpigmented areas on the skin (see Fig. 40.3). Spread is skin to skin or fomite and by contact with the fungus.
Presentation: Rash usually begins at nape of neck and extends to arms or trunk.
Physical examination: Characterized by hypopigmentation at the site of infection, which can last even after the infection has been treated. Rash is neither painful nor pruritic and often is found incidentally on physical examination.
Diagnosis: Observation of macular hypopigmented or hyperpigmented rash, but examination of KOH skin scraping under microscope or fungal culture is definite
Treatment: Topical or oral antifungals and selenium sulfide; good hygiene practices can often reduce the chances of infection
Return to sport: No restrictions

Tinea Unguium (Onychomycosis)

Overview: Fungal infection of nails caused most often by *Trichophyton rubrum*. Can involve matrix, bed, or plate. Identified by scaling, thickened, opaque, yellow-brown nails. Spread is skin to skin or fomite and by contact with fungus. Can be on fingers but mostly seen on toes.
Presentation: Initial complaints concern appearance of nail. Evolves to difficulty with ambulation. Can be associated with pain, paresthesia, and decreased motion in affected toe. Appearance can lead to social withdrawal and low self-esteem.
Physical examination: Exact examined appearance of the nail is determined by clinical subtype with distal lateral subungual onychomycosis most common.
Diagnosis: Characteristic-appearing nail is diagnostic, but examination of KOH scraping under microscope or fungal culture is definitive.
Treatment: Treatment options include topical ciclopirox solution (Penlac) for mild to moderate cases. For more severe cases, oral antifungals, including fluconazole, itraconazole, or terbinafine, can be considered. Use of less occlusive footwear in sport and use of footwear in locker room is preventive.
Return to sport: No restrictions

INFESTATIONS

Scabies

Overview: Parasitic infestation caused by *Sarcoptes scabiei* var. *hominis* mite; appear on the body as scattered groups of pruritic vesicles and pustules in runs or burrows (Fig. 40.4) Transmission from skin to skin or fomite to skin.
Presentation: Intense pruritus at the affected area; the pruritus is often worse at night
Physical examination: Burrows are seen most often on the sides of the fingers, palms, wrists, elbows, knees, axilla, waist, groin, and ankles. Breasts, penis, and scrotum may also be involved.
Diagnosis: Identification of rashes/burrows is usually diagnostic. Microscopic examination of skin scraping yields mites, ova, larvae, and/or feces.
Treatment: Permethrin cream 5% (Elimite) or crotamiton cream 10% (Eurax, Crotan). It is absolutely necessary to wash all uniforms, clothing, bathing items, and bedding with water greater than 122°F (50°C) according to the Centers for Disease Control and Prevention (CDC). Treatment of teammates with close contact with athlete and athlete's household members should be considered. Treatment may have to be repeated.
Return to sport: After all living mites have been eliminated by treatment. This is usually achieved in 24 hours, although itching may last for up to 1 week. Re-treatment is often necessary. A negative scraping should be obtained before return to play.

Pediculosis (Head, Body, or Pubic Lice)

Overview: Parasitic infestation of the skin of the scalp, trunk, or pubic area by *Pediculosis humanus* (see Fig. 40.4). Can be spread skin to skin or skin to fomites.
Presentation: Intense pruritus may lead to deep excoriations over the affected area.
Physical examination: Presence of nits or egg sacs usually on the hair of scalp, trunk, or pubic area.
Diagnosis: The presence of nits or egg sacs attached to the hair close to the skin is diagnostic. Visible nits are easiest to see on head or at the nape of the neck.
Treatment: Head lice shampoo with permethrin, phenothrin, or carbaryl. Treatment may have to be repeated in 3–7 days if lice remain. It is absolutely necessary wash all uniforms, clothing, bathing items, and bedding with water greater than 122°F (50°C) according to CDC.
Return to sport: After removal and elimination of all nits. This is usually 24 hours after treatment.

Cutaneous Larva Migrans

Available online.

ENVIRONMENTAL ENCOUNTERS

Seabather's Eruption, Swimmer's Itch

Available online.

Green Hair

Available online.

MECHANICAL FRICTION INJURIES (FIG. 40.5)

Blisters

Overview: Bullae that occur from repetitive friction combined with moisture in sports that lead to shearing and splitting of layers within the epidermis.
Presentation: Seen commonly on tips of toes, balls of the feet, and posterior calcaneus; formed from loose ill-fitting shoes or change in training pattern; most often seen early during a workout or early in a season
Physical examination: Bullae commonly found on posterior or plantar surfaces of foot but can occur anywhere friction occurs

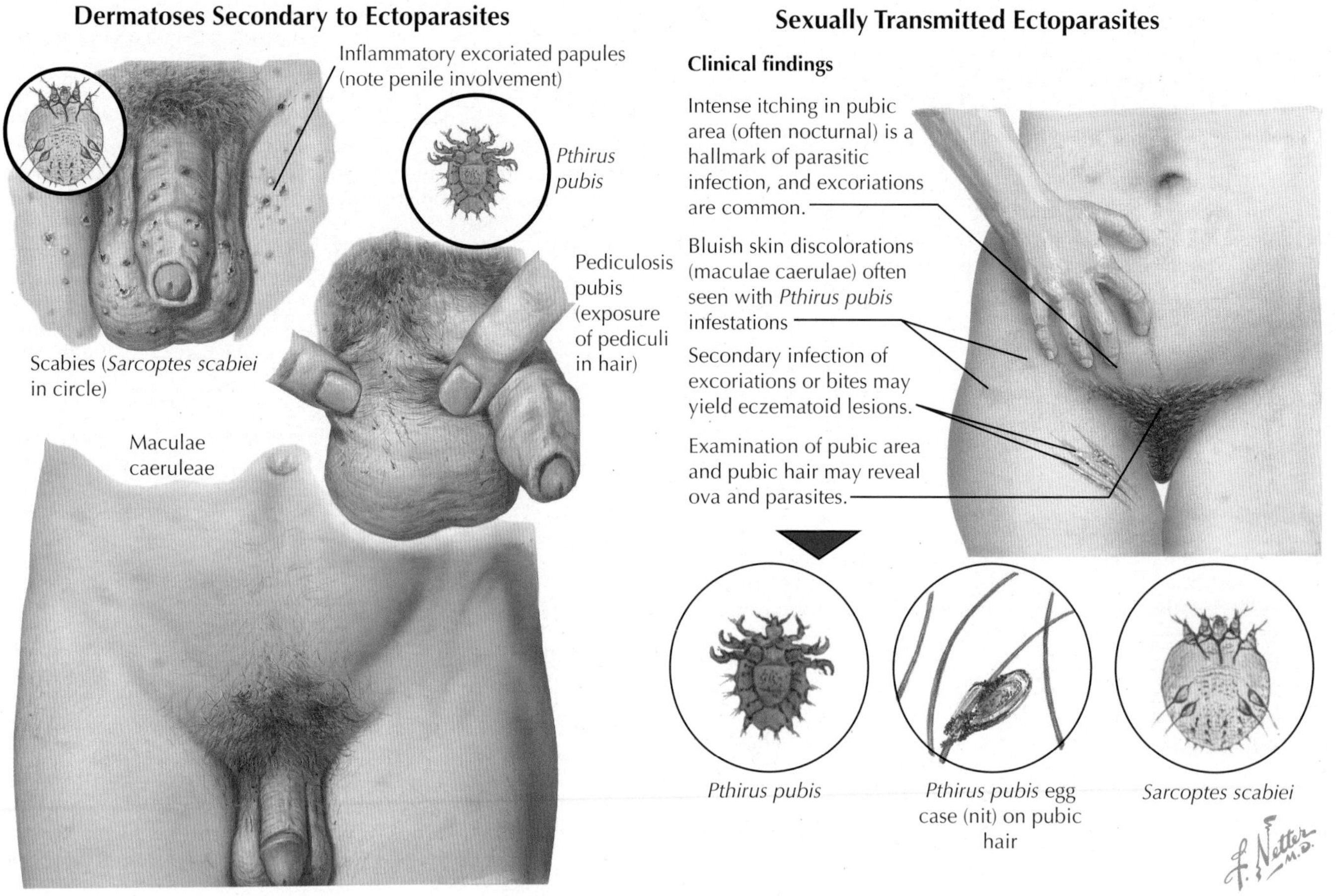

Dermatoses Secondary to Ectoparasites
Inflammatory excoriated papules (note penile involvement)
Pthirus pubis
Pediculosis pubis (exposure of pediculi in hair)
Scabies (Sarcoptes scabiei in circle)
Maculae caeruleae
Sexually Transmitted Ectoparasites
Clinical findings
Intense itching in pubic area (often nocturnal) is a hallmark of parasitic infection, and excoriations are common.
Bluish skin discolorations (maculae caerulae) often seen with Pthirus pubis infestations
Secondary infection of excoriations or bites may yield eczematoid lesions.
Examination of pubic area and pubic hair may reveal ova and parasites.
Pthirus pubis
Pthirus pubis egg case (nit) on pubic hair
Sarcoptes scabiei

Figure 40.4 Scabies and pediculosis.

Diagnosis: Characteristic bullae

Treatment: Blisters are best managed without breaking. They can be opened and drained if large or particularly painful. The goal of drainage is to allow adherence of separated tissue layers. The overlying tissue should be left intact. Use antibiotic creams if blister is open. Hydrocolloid dressings and Silvadene or antibacterial ointments ease pain. Use of moleskin around the blister is protective. Use of two sets of socks, synthetic socks, and hydrocolloidal antifriction products can prevent blisters, as can proper-fitting shoes.

Return to sport: No restrictions

Calluses (Tylomata)

Overview: Occur from repetitive trauma, which results in hyperkeratosis of the epidermis (see Fig. 40.5); can occur from change in equipment or surface

Presentation: They are the most common keratosis in sports and protect the skin; most often not painful

Physical examination: Occur most often on the palms and feet. Can be seen in clavicular region of weightlifting "clean and jerk."

Diagnosis: Characteristic lesion most often over pressure points

Treatment: If painful, calluses can be debrided by a scalpel or pumice stone, topical salicylic acid, or keratolytic emollients. Moleskin placed over a callus can decrease pressure and spread forces to other areas of the foot. Use of orthotics, synthetic socks, and change in footwear are often helpful. Gloves are helpful for calluses on hands.

Return to sport: No restriction

Corns

Overview: Accumulations of keratin that develop over bony prominences or pressure points (see Fig. 40.5)

Presentation: Most commonly seen on the toes

Physical examination: Keratin accumulation on bony areas of feet or toes

Diagnosis: Characteristic lesion

Treatment: Appropriately fitting footwear and padding may prevent development. Symptomatic corns can be treated with debridement, as described earlier.

Return to sport: No restrictions

Athlete's Nodules (Collogenomas, "Nike Nodules," "Knuckle Pad")

Available online.

Talon Noir and Tache Noir (Plantar or Palmar Petechiae, Black Heel or Palm, Black Dot Syndrome, Mogul's Palm)

Overview: Horizontal petechiae seen on the posterior or lateral heel or palms

Presentation: Occur in stopping and starting sports such as basketball on the feet and on the hands of gymnasts, golfers, and weightlifters; they are painless and resolve spontaneously.

Physical examination: Horizontal petechiae on feet or hands; no additional bleeding with paring, and skin lines are maintained

Diagnosis: Lesion itself is diagnostic; however, a skin scraping looking for occult blood is diagnostic.

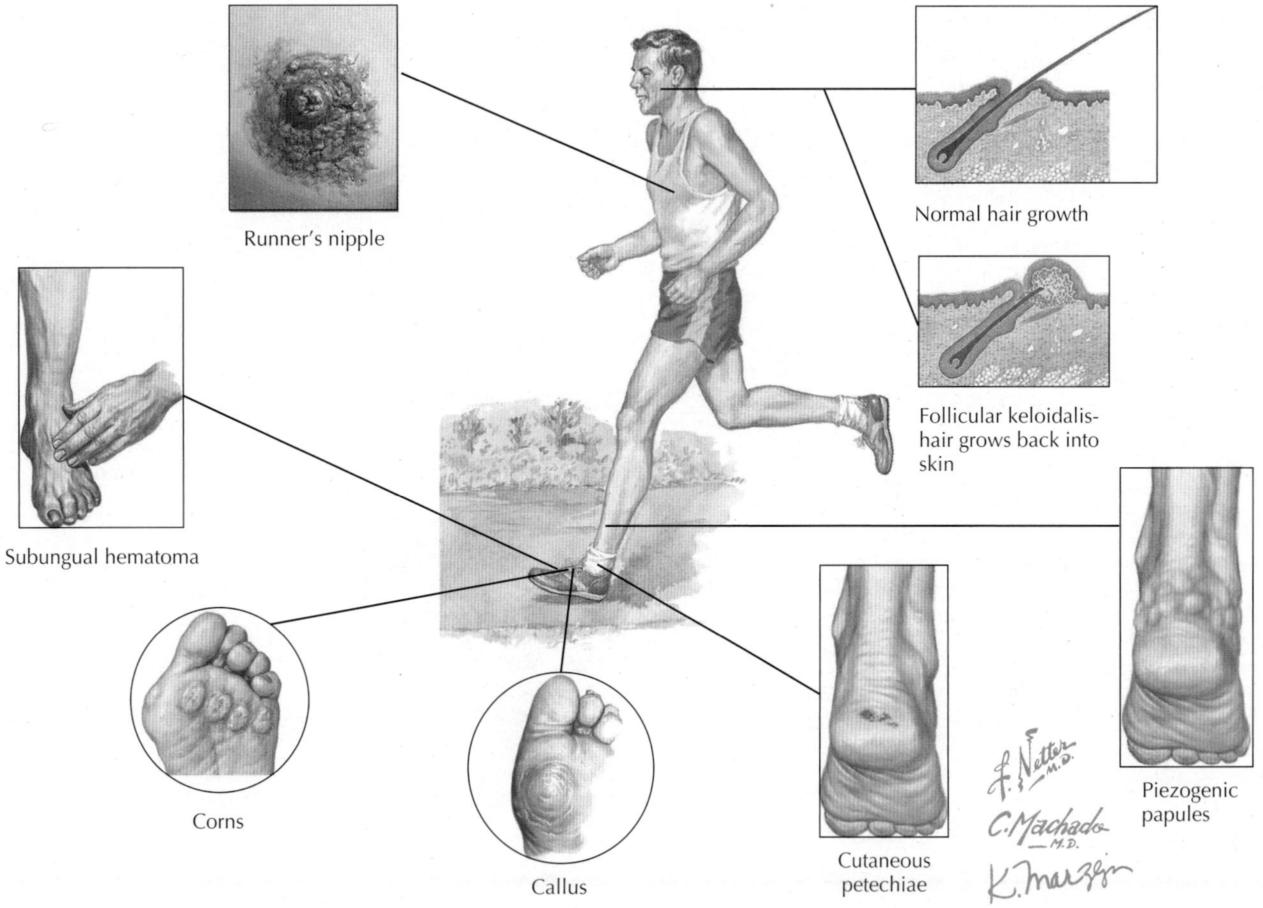

Runner's nipple
Normal hair growth
Subungual hematoma
Follicular keloidalis-hair grows back into skin
Corns
Callus
Cutaneous petechiae
Piezogenic papules

Figure 40.5 Common problems caused by friction and pressure.

Treatment: Use of appropriately fitting shoes and form-fitting socks
Return to sport: No restrictions

Piezogenic (Pedal) Papules

Overview: Small, often painful, fat papules on the outside aspect of the heels (see Fig. 40.5)
Presentation: Yellow or flesh-colored and found in long-distance runners as a result of fat herniation through the dermis; often painful
Physical examination: Fat collection seen on the medial, posterior, or lateral aspects of the heels when pressure is applied; often not painful when foot is not weight bearing
Diagnosis: Lesion is diagnostic
Treatment: Silicone gel heel cups or orthotics may reduce the symptoms. Compression stockings, electroacupuncture, injection of betamethasone with equal parts bupivacaine, deep punch biopsy, or small excision has also been used to treat.
Return to sport: No restrictions

Hematoma

Overview: Caused by separation of skin from underlying tissues by shear forces (see Fig. 40.5)
Presentation: Most common is auricular hematoma seen from contact of the ear with a wrestling mat
Physical examination: Blood-filled bullae from separation of the perichondrium and cartilage seen most commonly in the pinna of a wrestler's ear
Diagnosis: Lesion is diagnostic
Treatment: There is no consensus on treatment; however, when recognized, hematoma should be drained and splinted with a compression dressing to prevent development of a cauliflower ear, necrosis of the cartilage, or formation of fibroneocartilage of the ear.
Return to sport: After incision and drainage, allow with adhered compression dressing

Abrasions (Road Rash, Turf Burn, Raspberry)

Overview: Occur by contact of skin with artificial turf, mats, or ill-fitting equipment
Presentation: Loss of epidermis and/or dermis with bleeding and weeping secondary to skin contact with a surface; chronic abrasions can lead to skin changes, hair loss, and callus formation
Physical examination: Skin of an abrasion is erythematous and may ooze serous fluid. Debris may be present in the wound.
Diagnosis: Lesion is diagnostic
Treatment: Area should be cleaned with soap and water and protected with antifriction lubricants. Nonstick padding with petroleum jelly or antibiotic ointment is therapeutic. Monitor for missed debris or infection.
Return to sport: No restrictions upon covering of abrasion

Nail Dystrophies

Available online.

Subungual Hematoma (Black, Skier's, Hiker's, Climber's Toe)

Overview: Splinter hemorrhages often on the toes secondary to repetitive trauma (see Fig. 40.5)
Presentation: Can also be caused acutely by being stepped on or cleated or by pressure from tight shoes or rapid deceleration
Physical examination: Presence of blood underneath nails of fingers or toes
Diagnosis: Presence of blood under nails of hands or feet is diagnostic
Treatment: Drainage using a needle through the nail is therapeutic. Padding can then be applied for protection. Appropriately fitting shoes and change of running technique can prevent subungual hematomas.
Return to sport: No restrictions

Chafing

Overview: Denuding of epidermis because of mechanical contact between two opposing areas of the body
Presentation: Seen in areas of contact where skin meets skin or fabric meets skin; worsened by moisture and muscle bulk
Physical examination: Erythematous patch often at thighs, axilla, or neck
Diagnosis: Characteristic rash and location
Treatment: Removal of irritant, if possible; cold compresses, evaporation of moisture/sweat, lubricants, nonirritating clothing/equipment, and weight loss; antibiotic cream if infected
Return to play: No restrictions

Runner's Nipples (Jogger's, Weightlifter's Nipples)

Overview: Caused from friction between the nipple/areola complex and a tight-fitting cotton shirt during a run or lift (see Fig. 40.5)
Presentation: Nipples often present as raw and painful; bleeding and dryness may be present; most commonly seen in men, as women are often protected by sports bra
Physical examination: Erythematous, swollen, scaling, fissuring, or raw nipple/areola complex; bleeding may be present
Diagnosis: Rash is diagnostic
Treatment: Good hygiene followed by triple-antibiotic ointment, if infected; in men, these can be prevented by using Band-Aids, surgical tape, breast shields, or petroleum jelly before running or running shirtless, whereas prevention in women is the sports bra. Repeated cases can be treated with 0.1% tacrolimus.
Return to sport: As tolerated

COLD INJURIES (FIG. 40.6)

Frostnip

Overview: Superficial injury from the cold (see Fig. 40.6)
Presentation: Most common cold injury; it involves skin and subcutaneous tissues
Physical examination: Seen as flaking epidermis with possible vesicles associated with pain; most common area affected is the tip of the nose and ears; original presentation is white areas of skin with possible vessel formation
Diagnosis: Lesion is characteristic
Treatment: Gentle rewarming in 20-minute intervals, preventing the freeze–thaw cycle; covering of exposed skin with multiple layers is preventive
Return to sport: No restrictions

Frostbite

Overview: Deep tissue injury because of exposure to long periods of cold, particularly at subzero temperatures associated with wind and rain (see Fig. 40.6)
Presentation: Begins with numbness of the skin that progresses to blisters and then to tissue necrosis; exposed skin may harden as well
Physical examination: Seen most often on hands, feet, ears, and penis; athletes usually present with first- or second-degree frostbite
Diagnosis: Characteristic lesion
Treatment: Removal from cold environment; athletes should be placed in an area where there will not be a continuous freeze–thaw cycle; rewarming in water 102°F–111°F (39°C–44°C) for 20 minutes; affected area may become cold-sensitive. Wearing of multiple layers of clothing may be preventive.
Return to sport: As tolerated depending on the extent of injury

Pernio (Chilblains)

Overview: Development of painful nodules secondary to an area of vasoconstriction from nonfreezing temperatures

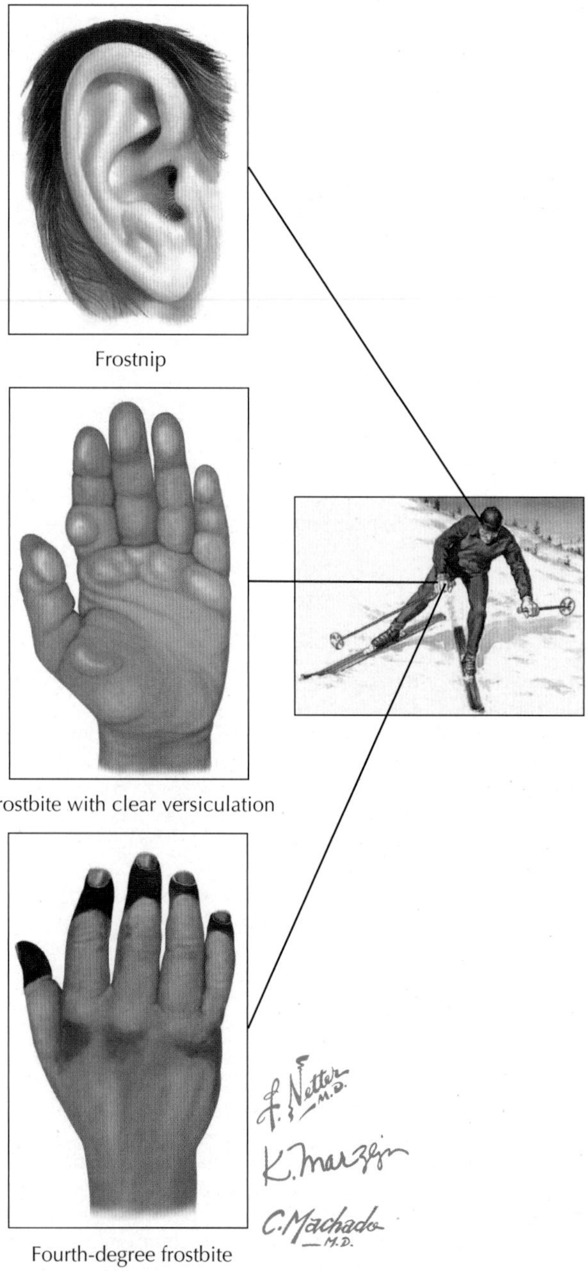
Frostnip
Frostbite with clear versiculation
Fourth-degree frostbite

Figure 40.6 Common cold-related injuries.

Presentation: Often associated with pruritis and/or paresthesias secondary to dermal damage
Physical examination: Painful nodules most often on exposed skin, particularly the extremities, are most often affected.
Diagnosis: Characteristic lesion
Treatment: Topical steroid ointment and/or vasodilators; coverage of exposed areas can prevent development; avoidance of cold is preventive; affected area may become cold-sensitive
Return to sport: As tolerated depending on the extent of injury

SUN AND HEAT INJURIES (FIG. 40.7)

Sunburn

Overview: Caused by skin exposure to ultraviolet (UV) rays; it is most common skin disorder (see Fig. 40.7)
Presentation: Usually occurs between 10 AM and 3 PM on exposed skin; water sports and ingestion of photosensitizing drugs put athletes at greater risk; athletes with fair skin are also at a higher risk
Physical examination: Erythema and pain to the most superficial layers of the skin; deeper burns can cause damage to the deeper skin layers, including nerves, causing blisters and bullae and resulting in significant discomfort. Repeated exposure can cause skin cancer, including melanoma.
Diagnosis: Characteristic rash
Treatment: Minor burns are treated with symptomatic treatment, including cold compresses, and possibly low-dose topical steroids, antihistamines, or anesthetics. Second-degree burns are treated with systemic corticosteroids and topical anesthetics. Avoid skin breakdown. Oral fluids may be necessary with severe burns. Prevention: exercising before 10 AM and after 3 PM. Sunscreens protecting against both UVA and UVB should be applied 30 minutes before exercise and repeated after excessive sweating and/or water exposure. Waterproof formulas allow for increased protection, covering exposed skin, protective clothing, and headgear.
Return to sport: No restrictions

Malignancies

Available online.

Photodermatitis

Overview: Immune reaction against the skin resulting from exposure to the sun's UV rays (see Fig. 40.7); can be caused secondary to medications, soaps, deodorants, or perfumes or by autoimmune conditions such as lupus or a vitamin deficiency
Presentation: May present similar to sunburn with erythema, pain, blisters, and some swelling. If athlete exhibits reactivity to a product, the athlete should be counseled to avoid products.
Physical examination: Can be seen on any part of body
Diagnosis: Characteristic rash and patient history
Treatment: Best achieved by avoidance of sun exposure; severe cases may be treated with corticosteroids or immunosuppressant therapy; alternative medication should be considered with those photosensitive to current prescription drugs
Return to sport: No restrictions

Atopic Dermatitis

Overview: Eczematous outbreaks that occur in response to heat, sweat, temperature changes, or exertion (see Fig. 40.7); mechanism unknown, but has polygenic inheritance pattern

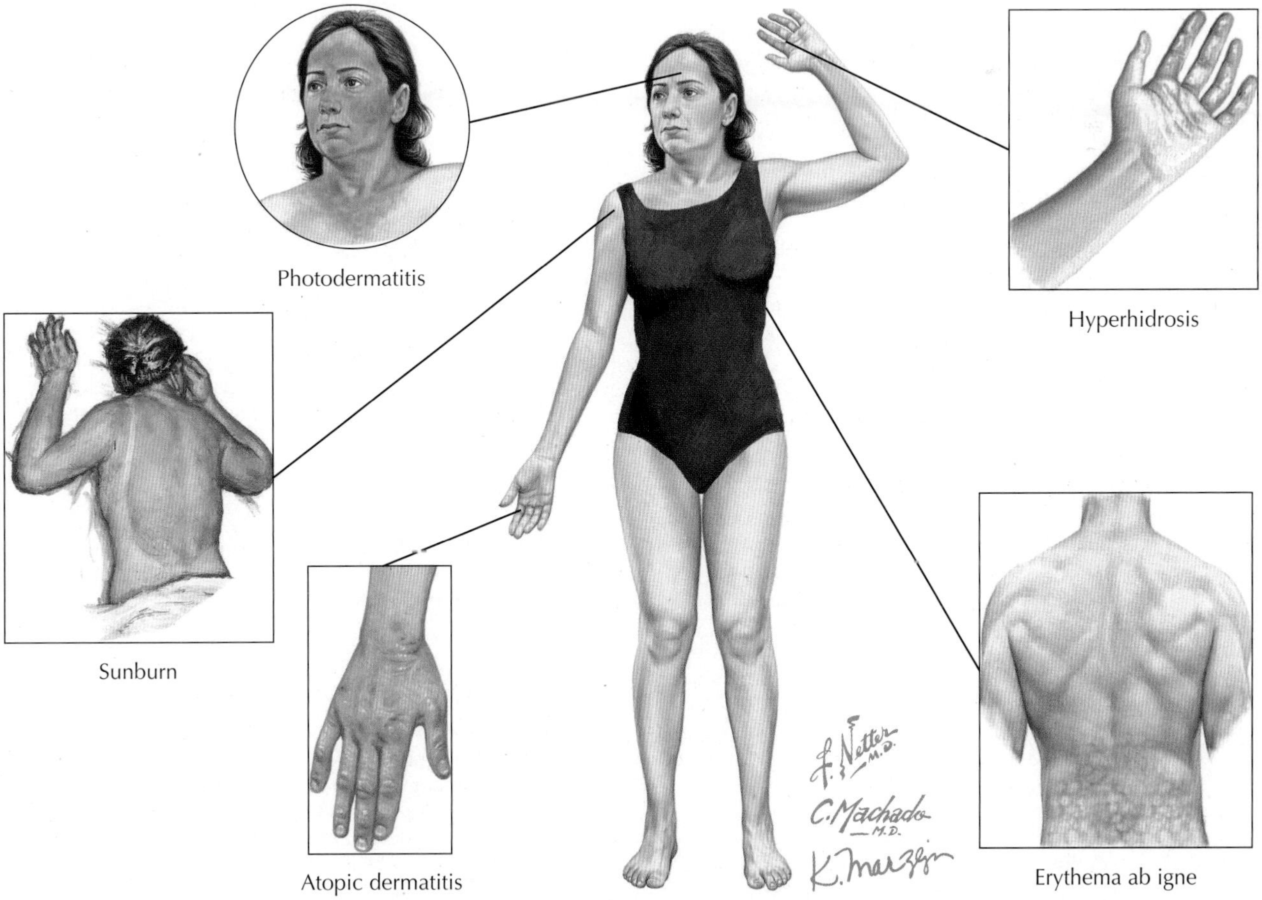
Photodermatitis
Hyperhidrosis
Sunburn
Atopic dermatitis
Erythema ab igne
F. Netter M.D.
C. Machado M.D.

Figure 40.7 Common sun- and heat-related problems.

Presentation: Often occur for the first time early in life and present as recurrent pruritic, dry, scaly patches; outbreaks wax and wane, often appearing early in life and resolving by the age of 30 years
Physical examination: Appear anywhere on body as pruritic, symmetric, and flexural eczematous lesions
Diagnosis: Diagnostic lesion and history of outbreaks
Treatment: Avoiding temperature changes and excessive sweating; sun exposure, emollients, and topical steroids are effective
Return to sport: No restrictions

Hyperhidrosis

Overview: Excessive sweating in the setting of sports usually because of stress but can be congenital (see Fig. 40.7)
Presentation: Benign but can interfere with vision or grip in sport
Physical examination: Findings of excessive sweat in the groin, axilla, palms, feet, forehead, and scalp
Diagnosis: History and presence of excessive sweating
Treatment: Aluminum chloride over time may decrease the excessive sweating
Return to sport: No restrictions

Miliaria Crystalline (Sudamina)

Overview: Characterized by "dew drop" vesicles on an erythematous base seen in hot and humid conditions; caused by retention of sweat in the superficial skin
Presentation: Produced by exercise in a hot environment
Physical examination: Found anywhere on the body
Diagnosis: Characteristic lesion
Treatment: Cold compresses
Return to sport: No restrictions

Miliaria Rubra (Prickly Heat)

Overview: Deeper, erythematous, and pruritic papules often lasting longer than those seen in miliaria crystallina; again, caused by retention of sweat, now in the living layers of epidermis or upper dermis
Presentation: Brought on by exercise in a hot environment; can evolve to miliaria pustulosa, when miliaria rubra papules become pustules
Physical examination: Can be found anywhere on the body
Diagnosis: Characteristic lesion
Treatment: Cold compresses; discontinuation of exercise and resumption in cooler temperatures
Return to sport: No restrictions

ALLERGIC REACTIONS AND DERMATITIS

Allergic/Irritant Contact Dermatitis

Overview: Caused by skin exposure to an allergen, urushiol, found in the sap of *Toxicodendron* plants—poison ivy is most common; other common allergens include nickel and elastic in sports equipment and tanning products in gloved sports; irritant contact dermatitis can be caused by calcium oxide seen in field-line markers when combined with water
Presentation: Poison ivy rash appears in linear rows approximating contact with the plant; other forms of contact dermatitis are seen at allergen contact site
Physical examination: Can occur anywhere on body as erythema and later scaling, exudative plaques with pain, and/or pruritus; vesicles may form
Diagnosis: Characteristic rash and history
Treatment: With poison ivy, exposed skin, nails, fomites, clothing, and shoes should be cleaned immediately to remove the resin. Upon removal, the exposed area is no longer contagious. Treatment is with topical or oral steroids, nonsedating antihistamines, and rash coverage. With other allergens, immediately remove allergen-containing equipment and follow previous treatment. With irritant contact dermatitis, the skin should be flushed with soap and water to eliminate the irritant, followed by the previous treatment.
Return to sport: After resin removal or removal of allergen/irritant and coverage of lesion

Urticaria (Hives)

Overview: Can occur because of several triggers, including exercise, often seen in runners; cholinergic, often seen in response to increased body temperature, emotional stress, or physical exertion; aquagenic, often seen in swimmers; and cold or solar urticaria, often seen in response to cold or hot temperatures (Fig. 40.8). Other sources in sports are pressure, dermatographic, and vibratory. Exercise-induced anaphylaxis can be related to foods, atopy, drugs, pollen, insect bites/stings, weather, humidity, and menses.
Presentation: Presents as raised, pruritic, edematous, and erythematous plaques; these can continue to evolve in seriousness depending on exposure. Bronchospasm can occur with cholinergic urticaria, but evolution to true anaphylaxis is rare.
Physical examination: Can occur anywhere on body—mostly on trunk and inner areas of the arms and legs
Diagnosis: Characteristic lesion and history
Treatment: Minor breakouts can be treated with antihistamines; systemic steroids are also used sometimes; evolving urticaria leading to anaphylaxis should be treated with epinephrine and airway and cardiovascular support; avoidance of triggers is preventive. Use of beta-agonist inhalers is of questionable benefit. Avoidance of exercise within 6 hours of exposure to triggers of exercise-induced anaphylaxis should be considered.
Return to sport: No return if athlete is in anaphylaxis; can consider return if athlete is protected and treated with minor symptoms

Stings

Overview: Insect stings should be planned for at sporting events
Presentation: Cause pain and pruritus at sting site along with swelling and erythema
Physical examination: Can be found anywhere on body
Diagnosis: Characteristic lesion
Treatment: Remove the stinger from the site without squeezing it to prevent more venom from penetrating the wound, decreasing the reactivity at the site and systemically; removal of the stinger can prevent secondary infection. After cleaning, topical anesthesia can provide pain relief from an immediate sting; more concerning is systemic reaction to the sting. Anaphylactic reactions to the sting, including swelling of the lips or tongue, shortness of breath, or sudden hypotension, should be immediately treated with epinephrine. EpiPens should be a part of any medical kit, and the athlete should carry EpiPen on person in the future.
Return to sport: No restrictions

TRAUMA

Lacerations

Overview: Break in the skin barrier; more problematic with bleeding. Athletes cannot compete with bleeding wounds or blood-soiled equipment or uniforms. With informed consent obtained in advance of the season, lacerations can be quickly and effectively closed and the athlete returned to play. Materials, including the use of a commercial blood removal agent, should be prepared in advance to allow for quick and effective cleaning and wound closure.

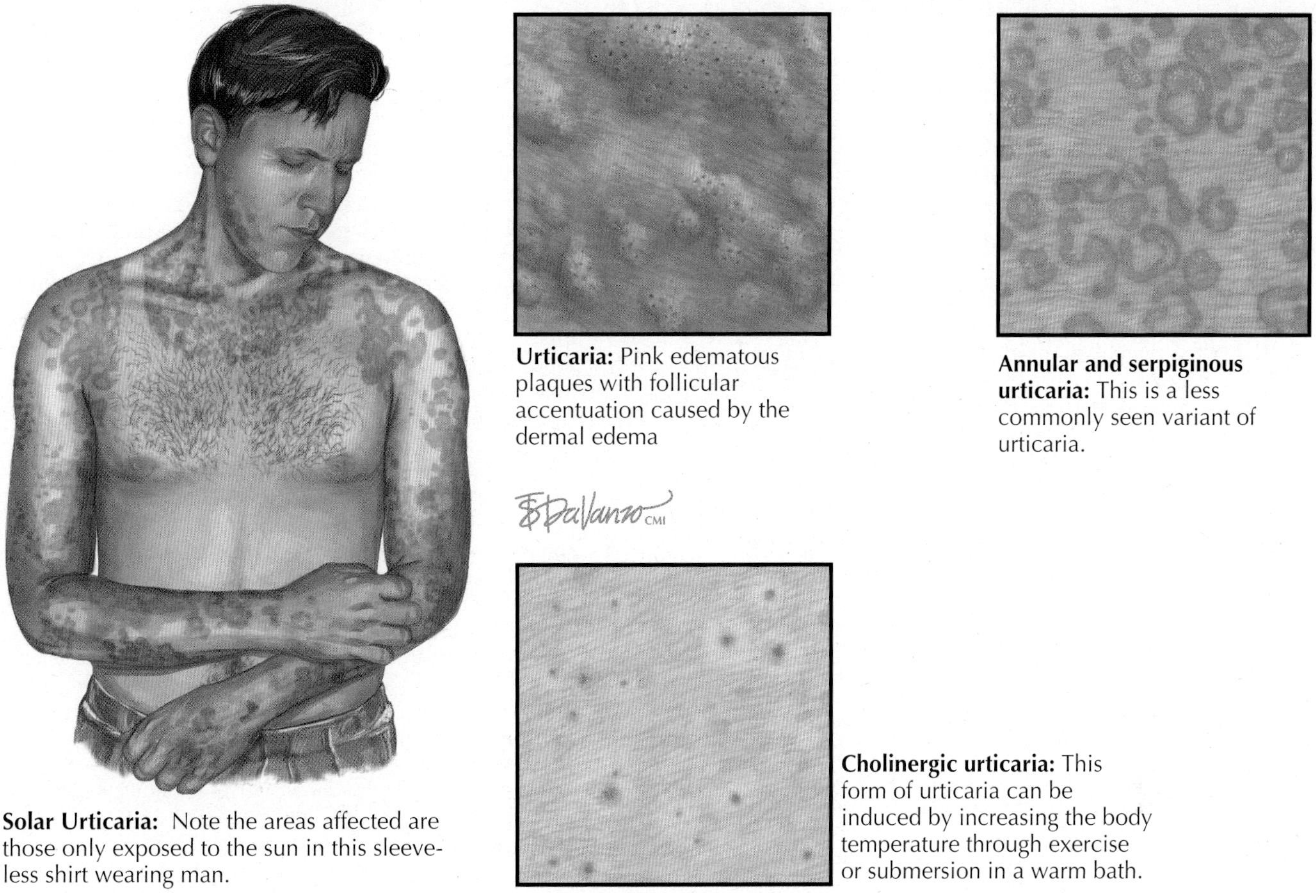

Solar Urticaria: Note the areas affected are those only exposed to the sun in this sleeveless shirt wearing man.

Urticaria: Pink edematous plaques with follicular accentuation caused by the dermal edema

Annular and serpiginous urticaria: This is a less commonly seen variant of urticaria.

Cholinergic urticaria: This form of urticaria can be induced by increasing the body temperature through exercise or submersion in a warm bath.

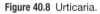

Figure 40.8 Urticaria.

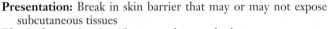

Presentation: Break in skin barrier that may or may not expose subcutaneous tissues

Physical examination: Seen anywhere on body

Diagnosis: Break in skin barrier, often with bleeding, and history of trauma is diagnostic.

Treatment: Universal precautions, including use of gloves and possibly a mask with shield, followed by anesthetizing the laceration. Cleaning and irrigation of wound with sterile saline to remove foreign debris. Do not damage the wound edges with irrigation. Betadine or other cleansing agents should be placed around the wound but not directly upon the wound itself because it can impede tissue healing. If time allows, sutures can be immediately placed during the competition. If not, and if adequate adherence of the wound edges can be obtained, the wound can be closed with Steri-Strips or glue and then sutured at halftime or after the competition, if necessary. Blood stain remover should be used to then remove blood from uniforms or equipment.

Return to sport: Closure of wound without active bleeding that is clean, dry, and covered and removal or cleaning of blood-stained uniforms or equipment.

RECOMMENDED READINGS

Available online.

41 CONNECTIVE TISSUE DISEASES AND RHEUMATOLOGIC PROBLEMS IN ATHLETES

Mark E. Lavallee • Ryan S. Stolakis

CONNECTIVE TISSUE DISORDERS

Marfan Syndrome

Overview: Inheritable autosomal-dominant genetic condition that affects the processing of fibrillin; it is caused by >1800 mutations in the gene encoding fibrillin-1 (FBN-1), located on chromosome 15 at the q21 loci. Approximately 10% of patients with Marfan phenotype have no identifiable mutation in the *FBN1* gene; mutations in TGF-beta receptor 2 and TGF-beta receptor 1 genes have been linked to these patients. Reported incidence is 1 in 3000–5000 individuals; an estimated 200,000 Americans have Marfan syndrome. Fibrillin, which is a major component of microfibrils, is found in large amounts in the aortic root > aorta > lens > joints > other connective tissues.

Presentation: Athletes with Marfan syndrome may have the following characteristics (Fig. 41.1):

- Tall (≥97th percentile) and thin
- Long thin arms, legs, hands, and feet
  - Arm span–to–height ratio is increased: (1:1.05)
- Aortic root disease, leading possibly to dilatation, regurgitation, and dissection
- Mitral valve prolapse (40%–54% in two series of Marfan syndrome patients)
- Joint laxity (including subluxations and dislocations)
- Reduced joint mobility, particularly in the elbows
- Joint pain
- Sixty percent have spinal curvature >20 degrees
- Pectus (chest wall) deformity (carinatum > excavatum)
- Visual problems (flat cornea/myopia)
- Dental crowding (high arched palate)
- Sports participation where tall, slender build is an advantage. An example would be Flo Hyman (United States Olympic Committee [USOC] volleyball)
- Arachnodactyly with (+) thumb and wrist signs
- Hindfoot valgus
- Vibration of the iris with eye movement—cardinal sign for ectopia lentis
- Increased risk for spontaneous pneumothorax
- Skin striae located in uncommon locations like upper arm, axillary region, or thigh

Physical examination: See Fig. 41.1

Diagnostics:

- American College of Cardiology (ACC), American Heart Association (AHA), and American Association for Thoracic Surgery (AATS) as of 2010 recommend echocardiogram to assess for aortic root dilation, aortic dissection, and valvular issues (e.g., mitral valve prolapse [MVP])
- Annual ophthalmologic evaluation is recommended
- Imaging of chest and abdomen: computed tomography (CT) scan with intravenous (IV) contrast, magnetic resonance imaging (MRI) with IV contrast, or ultrasound
- Genetic testing: Blood or tissue samples for *FBN1* mutation
  - First-degree relatives of patients with a gene mutation associated with aortic aneurysms/dissection should consider testing.
- Using diagnostic criteria (Table 41.1)
  - The Revised 2010 Ghent Nosology emphasizes cardinal clinical features of Marfan syndrome (aortic root dilatation/dissection and ectopia lentis) and on testing for mutations in the *FBN1* gene.
  - Application of diagnostic criteria to individuals aged <20 years requires special care because additional clinical features may present/develop later.

Treatment:

- **General:** Healthy lifestyle, including exercise and diet to control lipids and systemic blood pressure; Medic-alert bracelet/necklace stating the condition
- **Prevention:** Annual evaluation of eyes (ectopic lentis or lens dislocation), heart (valvular issues, aortic root dilatation, or dissection), and imaging of chest and abdomen (identifying/following aortic dissections, aneurysms, or dilatation)
- **Vascular:** Echocardiogram should be performed at the time of diagnosis and 6 months later to determine the rate of enlargement of the aortic root and ascending aorta. If stable over time, monitor annually for any changes in the aorta. Avoid strenuous activities that will increase intrathoracic pressure (e.g., powerlifting). If aortic pathology worsens, consider open surgical replacement of the aorta. Use of a beta-blocker has been correlated with increased survival. The dose should be adjusted to maintain the heart rate after submaximal exercise to <100 beats per minute (bpm) in adults and <110 bpm in children. The age at which beta-blockers should be initiated is still debated. Therapy targeting the renin–angiotensin system, such as losartan, may reduce aortic root dilatation rate in adults. Avoid calcium channel blockers. Valve replacement surgery is also an option, but it is not without severe risks for those with aortic valve insufficiency and ascending aorta dilation. The 2010 ACC/AHA/AATS guidelines recommend elective replacement of aortic valve at an external diameter ≥50 mm to avoid acute dissection or rupture. The 2015 Professional Advisory Statement from the Marfan Foundation stated that there is insufficient evidence for alternative approaches that reinforce rather than replace an aortic aneurysm.
- **Orthopedic:** Mild strength training to stabilize severe joint laxity; physical therapy (particularly joint and core strengthening, proprioceptive training modalities, and strengthening)
- **Psychology:** Provide empathy and psychological support as per the individual's and family's needs; genetic counseling is always strongly advised, as is putting the patient in contact with knowledgeable medical professionals and local/national support groups such as the National Marfan Foundation at www.marfan.org. It is not considered acceptable for children with Marfan syndrome to routinely observe exercise by their peers. This will promote stigmatization.
- **Pain control:** Encourage smoking cessation. Control pain with oral, injectable, transdermal, and topical medications, including acetaminophen, nonsteroidal anti-inflammatory drugs (NSAIDs), opioids, tramadol, transcutaneous electrical nerve stimulation (TENS) units, bracing, ring splints, and lastly, surgery. Nontraditional treatments like hypnosis, acupuncture, homeopathy, etc., may be effective.

Prognosis: In 1972, the mean age of death was 32 (range, 16–48) years. By 1995, the median cumulative probability of survival was 72 years.

Return to play:

- 46th Bethesda American College of Cardiology recommendations (2015):
  - May participate in low- and moderate-static/low-dynamic competitive sports if they *do not* have one of the following: aortic root dilation, moderate to severe mitral valve regurgitation, or family history of aortic dissection at an aortic diameter of <50 mm.
  - Athletes with aortic root dilation may only participate in low-intensity competitive sports.

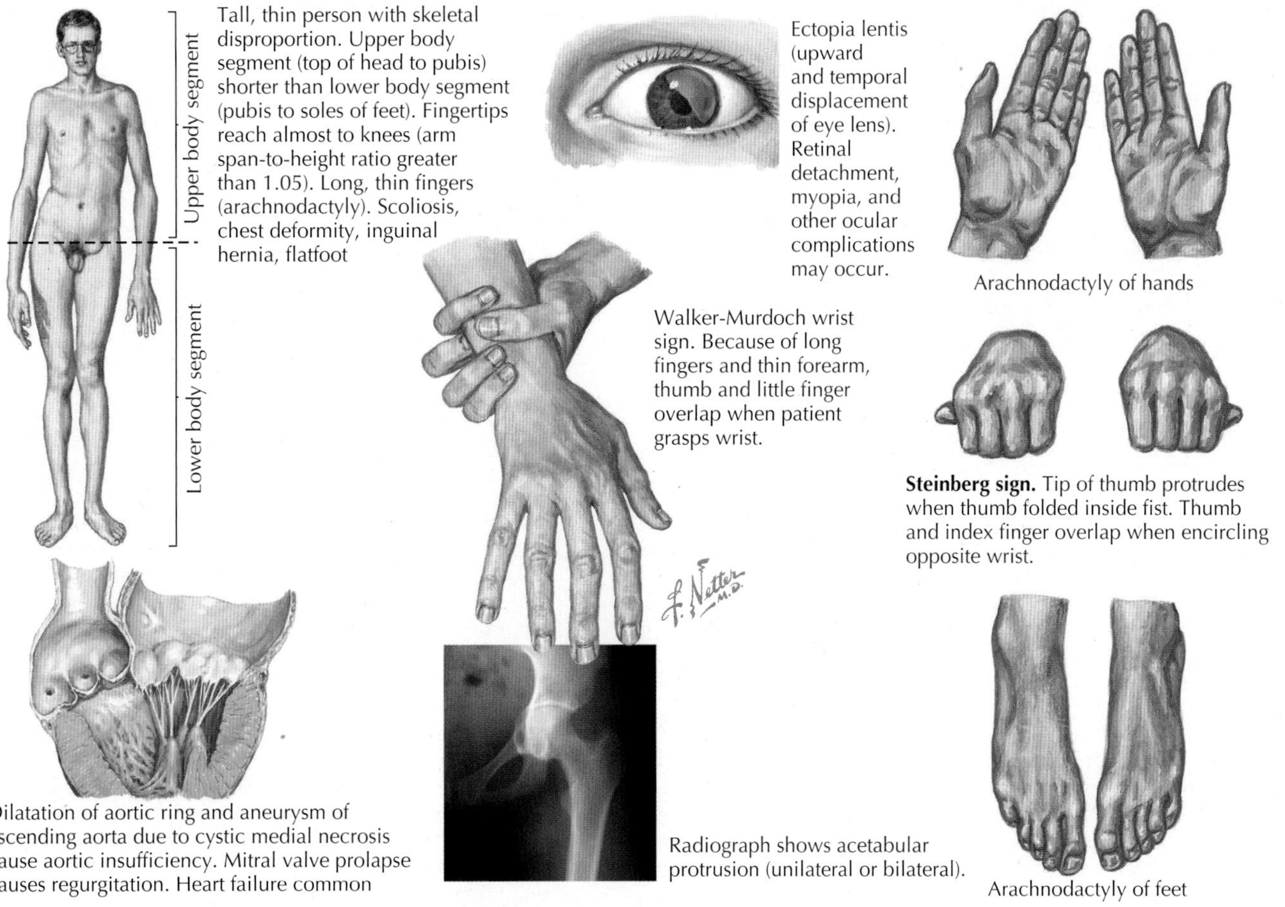
Upper body segment
Lower body segment
Tall, thin person with skeletal disproportion. Upper body segment (top of head to pubis) shorter than lower body segment (pubis to soles of feet). Fingertips reach almost to knees (arm span-to-height ratio greater than 1.05). Long, thin fingers (arachnodactyly). Scoliosis, chest deformity, inguinal hernia, flatfoot
Ectopia lentis (upward and temporal displacement of eye lens). Retinal detachment, myopia, and other ocular complications may occur.
Arachnodactyly of hands
Walker-Murdoch wrist sign. Because of long fingers and thin forearm, thumb and little finger overlap when patient grasps wrist.
Steinberg sign. Tip of thumb protrudes when thumb folded inside fist. Thumb and index finger overlap when encircling opposite wrist.
F. Netter M.D.
Dilatation of aortic ring and aneurysm of ascending aorta due to cystic medial necrosis cause aortic insufficiency. Mitral valve prolapse causes regurgitation. Heart failure common
Radiograph shows acetabular protrusion (unilateral or bilateral).
Arachnodactyly of feet

Figure 41.1 Characteristics of Marfan syndrome.

Table 41.1 GHENT NOSOLOGY

Family History?	Criteria	Systemic Symptoms
Yes (need at least 1 criterion for diagnosis)	Ectopia lentis Systemic score ≥7 points[a] Aortic criterion (aortic diameter Z ≥2 when age ≥20 years, Z ≥3 when age <20 years, or aortic root dissection)[a]	Wrist **AND** thumb sign: 3 points (wrist **OR** thumb sign: 1 point) Pectus carinatum deformity: 2 points (pectus excavatum or chest asymmetry: 1 point) Hindfoot valgus: 2 points (plain pes planus: 1 point) Pneumothorax: 2 points Dural ectasia: 2 points Protrusio acetabuli: 2 points Reduced upper segment/lower segment ratio **AND** increased arm span/height **AND** no severe scoliosis: 1 point Scoliosis or thoracolumbar kyphosis: 1 point Reduced elbow extension (≤170 with full extension): 1 point Facial features (at least 3 of the following 5 features: dolichocephaly [reduced cephalic index or head width/length ratio], enophthalmos, downslanting palpebral fissures, malar hypoplasia, retrognathia): 1 point Skin striae: 1 point Myopia >3 diopters: 1 point Mitral valve prolapsed (all types): 1 point
No (need at least 1 criterion for diagnosis)	Aortic criterion (aortic diameter Z ≥2 or aortic root dissection) **and** ectopia lentis[a] Aortic criterion (aortic diameter Z ≥2 or aortic root dissection) **and** a causal *FBN1* mutation Aortic criterion (aortic diameter Z ≥2 or aortic root dissection) **and** a systemic score ≥7 Ectopia lentis **and** a causal *FBN1* mutation that has been identified in an individual with aortic aneurysm	

[a]Diagnosis of Marfan syndrome can be made only in the absence of discriminating features of Shprintzen–Goldberg syndrome, Loeys–Dietz syndrome, or vascular Ehlers–Danlos syndrome and after TGFBR1/2, collagen biochemistry, or COL3A1 testing, if indicated.
Aortic root Z score determined by height, weight, age, and aortic root (in cm) at sinuses of Valsalva.

- Avoid sports with bodily collision.
- Avoid exercising to exhaustion.
- Same recommendation for aortic valve regurgitation.
- Prefer nonstrenuous, low-static, low-dynamic sports (e.g., golf, walking, billiards, riflery, and bowling).
- Encourage an active lifestyle.
  - Favor noncompetitive, isokinetic exercise performed at a nonstrenuous aerobic pace.
  - Avoid activities that involve high levels of isometric workloads and Valsalva maneuver (e.g., Olympic weightlifting, gymnastics, etc.).
  - Mild strength training (nonbreath-holding) if joint laxity is present; prefer multiple repetitions at lower resistance rather than maximal repetitions at higher resistance.
  - Be careful in environments with rapid atmospheric pressure changes (scuba diving or flying in an unpressurized cabin) or rapid decelerations (car racing or skydiving).
  - Control lipid levels, blood pressure, and blood sugar to decrease long-term injury to the vascular endothelium.
  - Educate the patient regarding the risks of participation.
  - Use protective eyewear whenever appropriate.
- Once orthopedic or ocular injury has healed and the injured area is adequately protected, the athlete may return to play. Support the patient with reasonable adaptive measures in order to participate.

Ehlers–Danlos Syndrome

Overview: Group of inheritable genetic conditions that affect connective tissue, particularly collagen in joints, vessels, skin, and internal organs; variable severity seen within each type and within the same family of pedigree; there are six types of Ehlers–Danlos syndrome (EDS), of which 95% seem to fall into the first three categories (hypermobility, classical, and vascular). Incidence is approximately 1 in 5000 live births. The term *generalized* or *benign joint hypermobility syndrome* (GJHS or BJHS) was first used by Kirk, Ansell, and Bywaters in 1967. The EDS hypermobility type was first described as a condition in 1946 and noted to be genetically based in 1970. The description of BJHS also uses the Beighton Scale and the same diagnostic criteria as EDS hypermobility type. Essentially, they are the same entity with only varying degrees of expressivity. A literature review seems to reveal no significant difference in the nosology between BJHS and aspects of EDS hypermobility type. BJHS seems to be a term preferred by those outside genetic circles (e.g., rheumatology, orthopedics, etc.), and EDS hypermobility type and Marfan syndrome are preferred by general medical and genetic groups. As of 2017, the Ehlers–Danlos Society published the new nosology, diagnostic criteria, treatment, and associated conditions in relation to EDS in the *American Journal of Medical Genetics*, March 17, 2017 edition. These can be accessed at Ehlers-Danlos.org.

Presentation:

- **Hypermobility:** Most common type in North America; autosomal dominant inheritance with unknown underlying genetic abnormality: mild to severe joint laxity, most often involving multiple joints subluxating or dislocating, mild skin involvement, chronic joint pain with often normal imaging studies, Beighton Scale score of ≥5/9, and 22% risk of developing aortic root dilatation in lifetime; 12% of pediatric patients with EDS show aortic root dilatation on their first echocardiogram. The incidence of hEDS is thought to be 1 in 5000 live births, and the frequency of MVP has been reported as 6%.
- **Classical:** Second most common type in North America with a prevalence estimated to be around 1 in 20,000; autosomal dominant inheritance; mutations found within the collagen genes *COL5A1* and *COL5A2*, interact with type 1 collagen molecules during fibrillogenesis. Skin hyperextensibility, wide atrophic scarring ("cigarette paper scar tissue"), and joint hypermobility are the major criteria. Minor criteria include easy bruising; soft, doughy skin; tissue friability; molluscoid pseudotumors; piezogenic papules; hernia; epicanthal folds around eyes, and first-degree family member with EDS. Diagnosis must have one major and two minor criteria or three minor criteria. There is a 33% lifetime risk of developing aortic root dilatation; 6% of pediatric patients with EDS show aortic root dilatation on their first echocardiogram; early osteoarthritis, particularly in smaller joints.
- **Vascular:** Third most common type in North America; autosomal dominant inheritance, mutations in the *COL3A1* gene; life-threatening (sudden death often from aortic/vascular or bowel rupture or can have spontaneous pneumothorax or uterine rupture in third trimester). Particular facial features include delicate nose; wide-set eyes; thin cheekbones; thin, translucent skin; very prominent veins on extremities and chest; skin friability; and mild to moderate joint laxity; a very significant risk (90% by the age of 40) of developing aortic pathology (e.g., root dilatation, aneurysm, and dissection). The incidence of vascular EDS is at least 1 in 100,000. This leads to a shortened lifespan with a median age of death of 48 years.
- **Kyphoscoliotic:** Very rare; autosomal recessive inheritance, mutations in the *PLOD1* gene: severe congenital hypotonia, progressive scoliosis, risk of ocular rupture, marfanoid body habitus, and diagnosis via urine test available. Incidence is estimated to be around 1 in 100,000.
- **Dermatosparaxis:** Very rare; autosomal recessive, mutations in the *ADAMTS2* gene: doughy, redundant skin; diagnosis via skin biopsy. Incidence is unknown.
- **Arthrochalasia:** Very rare; autosomal dominant inheritance, mutations in *COL1A1* or *COL1A2:* congenital hip dislocation, atrophic scars, joint hypermobility, and diagnosis via skin biopsy.
- **Other subtypes of EDS:** Be advised there are eight other recognized subtypes of EDS, but they are very rare. Visit Ehlers-Danlos.org for more information.

Physical examination: See Fig. 41.2

- Beighton Scale (score: ≥5/9)
- Excessive subtalar motion
- Pes planus
- Pinchable skin in the relaxed palmar aspect of hand
- Pectus deformity: excavatum more common than carinatum
- Touch tip of tongue to nose
- Skin hyperextensible to >3 cm at the mandibular angle or over olecranon
- Widened, atrophic scars (known as "cigarette paper scar tissue") (see Fig. 41.2)
- Piezogenic papules (often found near sole of feet)
- Subcutaneous spheroids (subcutaneous, firm, small, and mobile)
- Joint pain (acute or chronic, episodic)
- Joint laxity or hypermobility affecting multiple joints
- Joint subluxations and dislocations
- Family history
- Early osteoarthritis
- Postural orthostatic tachycardia syndrome (POTS) or dysautonomia
- Chiari malformation
- Mast cell activation
- Hernias (e.g., ventral, umbilical, and inguinal)
- MVP
- Dental malalignment/gingival issues
- Sudden death (from vascular or bowel rupture)

Diagnostics: Genetic testing, echocardiogram periodically, CT scan of chest and abdomen with IV contrast or ultrasound periodically, skin punch biopsy (4 mm) or blood serum put into a

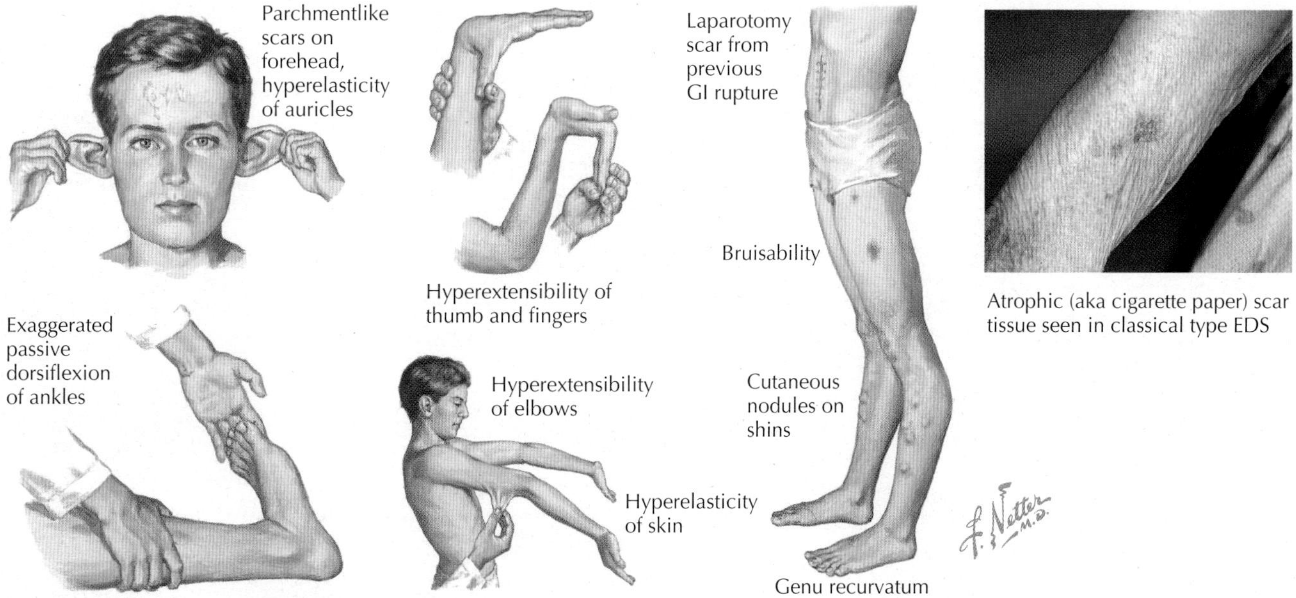
Parchmentlike scars on forehead, hyperelasticity of auricles
Hyperextensibility of thumb and fingers
Laparotomy scar from previous GI rupture
Bruisability
Atrophic (aka cigarette paper) scar tissue seen in classical type EDS
Exaggerated passive dorsiflexion of ankles
Hyperextensibility of elbows
Cutaneous nodules on shins
Hyperelasticity of skin
Genu recurvatum

Figure 41.2 Characteristics of Ehlers–Danlos syndrome. (Photograph from Goldman L, Ausiello D, Arend W, et al., eds. *Cecil Textbook of Medicine*. 23rd ed. Philadelphia: Elsevier; 2007.)

live medium for EDS and TGF-beta (e.g., *Chlamydia* culture), and radiographs and other imaging of affected joints

Treatment:

- **General:** Healthy lifestyle that includes exercise and diet to control lipids and systemic blood pressure; Medic-alert bracelet/necklace stating condition. The management strategies required in patients with EDS differ to some degree between EDS types and should be individualized depending on the severity of the disease.
- **Prevention:** Periodic evaluation of heart (e.g., valvular issues), chest/abdomen (e.g., identifying/following aortic dissections, aneurysms, or dilatation), and eyes (e.g., annual ophthalmologic evaluations in kyphoscoliotic type). Obtain baseline screening echocardiography in all patients, both children and adults. For classical and hypermobility types, follow-up examinations are performed every 2–5 years if initial screening studies are normal. No further testing is often needed beyond age 25 if the baseline and follow-up examination are normal. Regular ophthalmologic examinations should be performed in all patients with EDS.
- **Vascular:** Monitor any changes in the aorta and avoid strenuous activities that will increase intrathoracic pressure (e.g., powerlifting); if aortic pathology worsens, consider intraluminal prosthetic device versus elective open surgical replacement of aorta; encourage smoking cessation.
- **Orthopedic:** Mild strength training to stabilize severe joint laxity; physical therapy, particularly joint and core strengthening, proprioceptive training modalities, strengthening, and unweighted exercise (e.g., pool therapy, harnesses, and total gym).
- **Psychology:** Provide empathy and psychological support as per individual's and family's needs. Genetic counseling is always strongly advised, as is putting patient in contact with knowledgeable medical professionals and local/national support groups. Have the athlete visit the Ehlers–Danlos Society website at www.ehlers-danlos.org.
- **Pain control:** Oral, injectable, transdermal, and topical medications, including acetaminophen, NSAIDs, tramadol, TENS units, bracing, ring splints, ambulation-assist devices, and lastly surgery; use opioids only for acute trauma or as intermittent rescue medication because of the risk of dependence from chronic use.

Prognosis: Proportion of patients with EDS who will develop pathology within their aortic root or aorta: 90% vascular type, 33% classical type, and 22% hypermobility type. The lifespan for patients with classical and hypermobility types is not decreased. In vascular EDS, 80% of individuals experience a major event by age 40 years, and there is a shortened lifespan with a median age of death of 48 years.

Return to sport: Once orthopedic or integument injury has healed and the injured area is adequately protected, the athlete may return to play. Support the patient with reasonable adaptive measures in order to participate. According to the 46th Bethesda recommendations (2015):

- Individuals with vascular-type EDS may participate in low-static, low-dynamic sports if they do not have any of the following: aortic enlargement or dissection (or branch vessel enlargement), moderate to severe mitral regurgitation, or extracardiac organ system involvement that makes participation hazardous.
- Keep normal weight.
  - Underweight: Not enough muscle mass to stabilize loose joints
  - Overweight: Promotes early osteoarthritis
- Encourage an active lifestyle.
- Control lipids, blood pressure, and blood sugar to decrease long-term injury to vascular endothelium.
- Mild to moderate strength training is often helpful in joint stabilization.
- Encourage noncontact, nontraumatic sports, particularly for those with skin fragility (i.e., classical type) and severe joint laxity (i.e., hypermobility type).
- Do not recommend high-dynamic sports that could increase intraabdominal pressure and blood pressure because of the existing risk of aortic dilatation or colonic rupture.

Osteogenesis Imperfecta

Overview: Also known as *brittle bone syndrome*, osteogenesis imperfecta (OI) is an inheritable genetic disorder that affects collagen (type 1) (Fig. 41.3). OI is classified into a number of major subtypes based on genetic, radiographic, and clinical characteristics. The genetic defect (the *COL1A* gene) affects type 1 collagen, which is primarily found in the bone. A total of 16

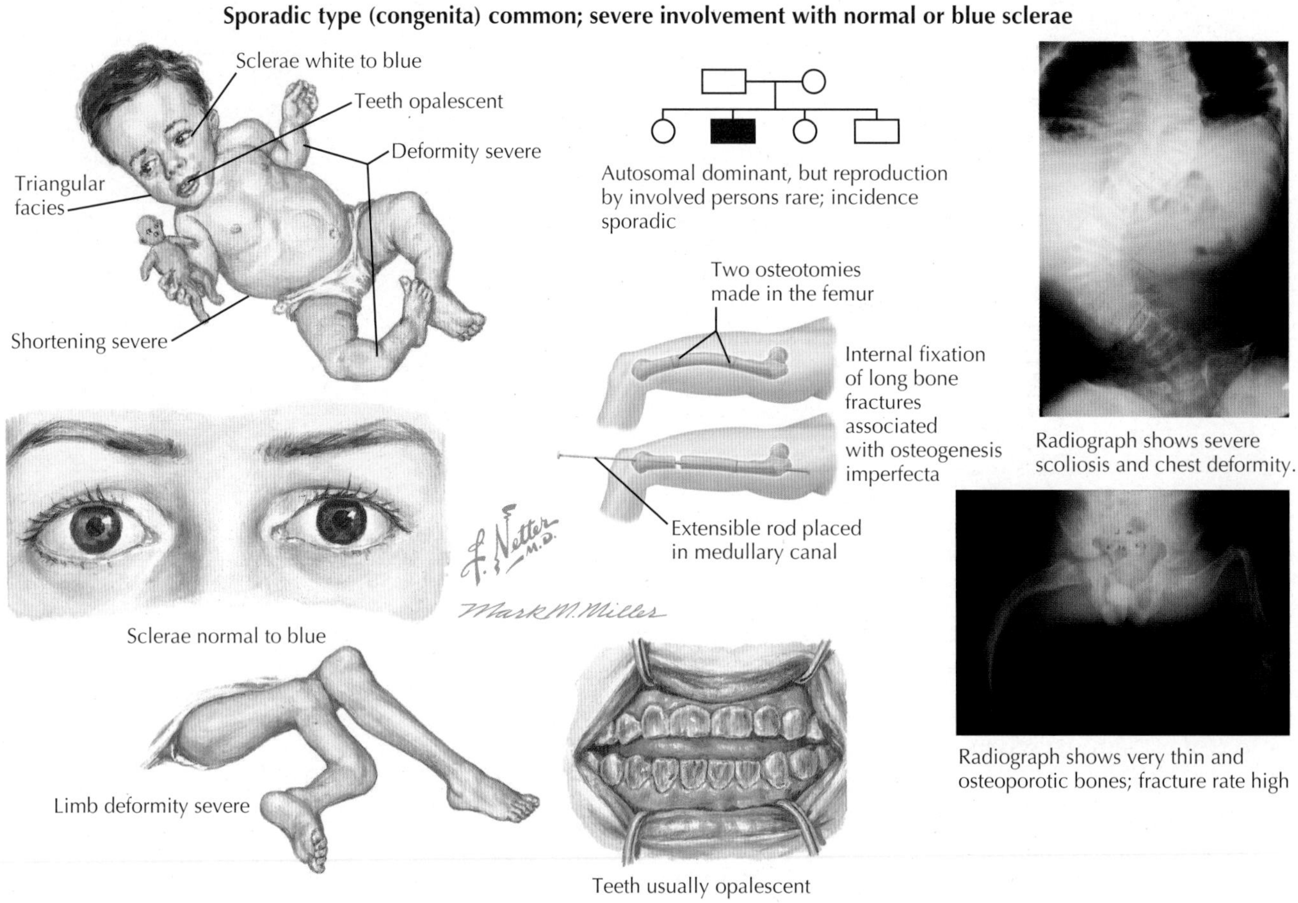
Sporadic type (congenita) common; severe involvement with normal or blue sclerae
Sclerae white to blue
Teeth opalescent
Deformity severe
Triangular facies
Shortening severe
Autosomal dominant, but reproduction by involved persons rare; incidence sporadic
Two osteotomies made in the femur
Internal fixation of long bone fractures associated with osteogenesis imperfecta
Extensible rod placed in medullary canal
Radiograph shows severe scoliosis and chest deformity.
Sclerae normal to blue
Radiograph shows very thin and osteoporotic bones; fracture rate high
Limb deformity severe
Teeth usually opalescent

Figure 41.3 Characteristics of osteogenesis imperfecta.

subtypes of OI have been documented. There are two major forms of OI: type I and type II. In the type I dominant (classical) form, the patient has extremely little or a poor quality of type 1 collagen. The type II dominant form has more severe manifestations, including long bone fractures and shortening and severe chest wall deformity.

Incidence: An estimated 20,000–50,000 individuals in the United States have OI.

Presentation:

- Long bones fracture easily. Most fractures occur before puberty. Often there may be "bowing" of long bone with or without fractures and excessive periosteal reaction.
- Normal or near-normal stature
- Loose joints and muscle weakness
- Sclera usually have blue, purple, or gray tint
- Triangular face
- Tendency toward spinal curvature
- Bone deformity absent or minimal
- Brittle teeth possible
- Hearing loss possible, often beginning in early 20s or 30s
- May die in utero (type II)
- Severe chest wall deformity (type II)
- Often nonambulatory in wheelchair (type II)

Physical examination (see Fig. 41.3):

- Dentinogenesis imperfecta (poorly formed teeth)
- Blue sclera
- Bone fragility
- Basilar skull deformity
- Pathogenic bowing of long bones and multiplicity of fractures
- Adult-onset hearing loss
- Osteoporosis
- Joint hyperextensibility
- Short stature/limb shortening or deformity in severe forms

Diagnostics: Laboratory findings may show elevated alkaline phosphatase and hypercalciuria. Radiographs may show bowing deformities and multiple fractures/callus formation. Bone scan may show multiple areas of increased uptake as a result of multiple areas of occult or stress fractures. Dual energy x-ray absorptiometry (DEXA) scan may show premature decrease in bone density consistent with osteopenia or osteoporosis. Of skin punch biopsy tests, both the collagen biopsy test and the DNA test are thought to detect almost 90% of all type I collagen (*COL1A1* or *COL1A2*) mutations. A negative type I collagen study does not rule out OI. When a type I collagen mutation is not found, other DNA tests to check for recessive forms are available.

Treatment:

- **General:** Healthy lifestyle, including exercise and diet. The goals of therapy for patients with OI are to reduce fracture rates, prevent long bone deformities and scoliosis, minimize chronic pain, and maximize mobility and other functional capabilities.
- **Prevention:** Protection or avoidance of contact or collision sports is paramount. Medic-alert bracelet/necklace stating condition and severity is recommended. Periodic evaluation of hearing, annual eye examination, bone mineral density

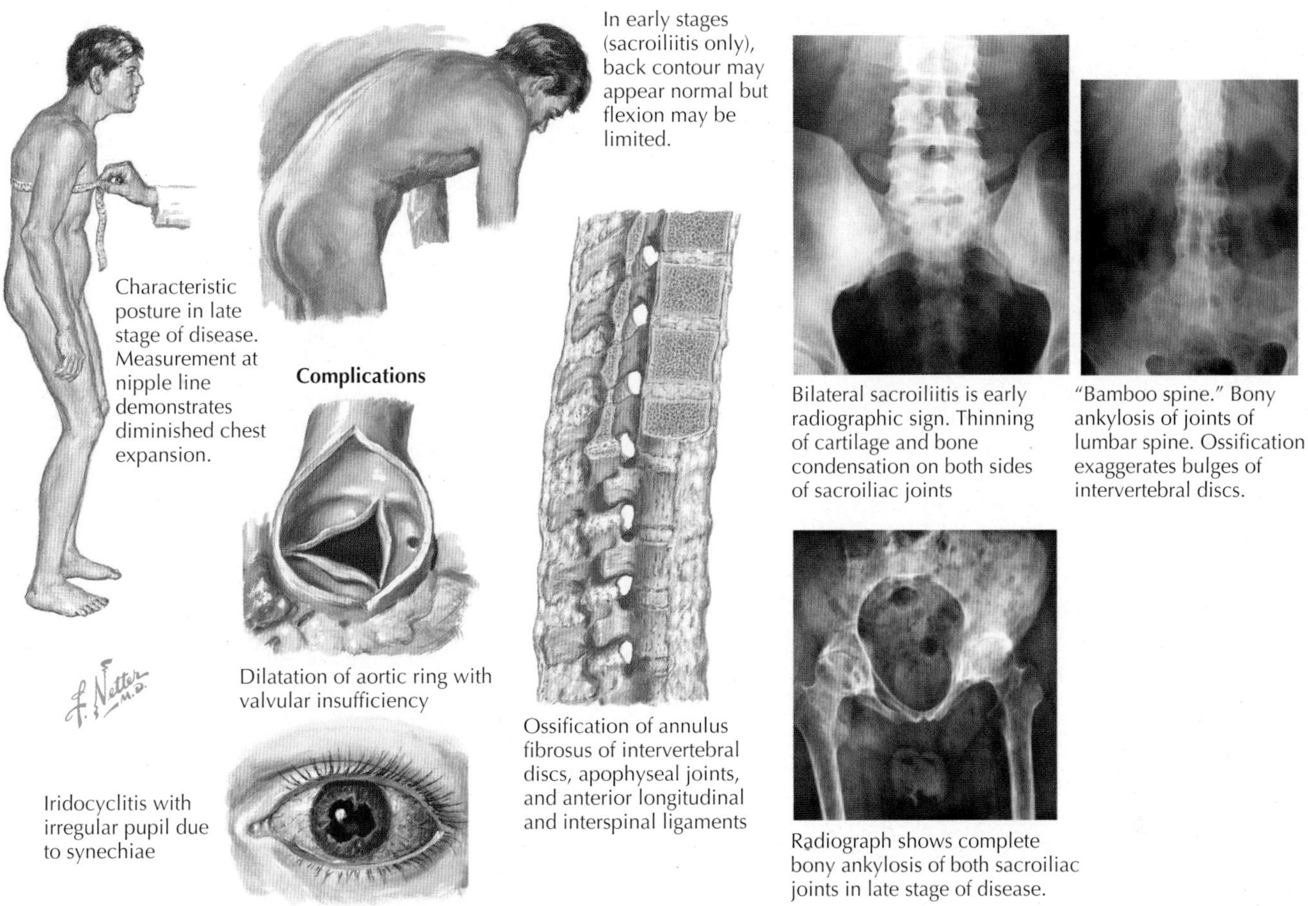
In early stages (sacroiliitis only), back contour may appear normal but flexion may be limited.
Characteristic posture in late stage of disease. Measurement at nipple line demonstrates diminished chest expansion.
Complications
Dilatation of aortic ring with valvular insufficiency
Iridocyclitis with irregular pupil due to synechiae
Ossification of annulus fibrosus of intervertebral discs, apophyseal joints, and anterior longitudinal and interspinal ligaments
Bilateral sacroiliitis is early radiographic sign. Thinning of cartilage and bone condensation on both sides of sacroiliac joints
"Bamboo spine." Bony ankylosis of joints of lumbar spine. Ossification exaggerates bulges of intervertebral discs.
Radiograph shows complete bony ankylosis of both sacroiliac joints in late stage of disease.

Figure 41.4 Characteristics of ankylosing spondylitis.

with DEXA scan, and spirometry to monitor for restrictive lung defects every 2 years (secondary to rib and vertebral fractures). Bisphosphonates are the mainstay of pharmacologic fracture-prevention therapy. However, women of reproductive age should abstain or prevent conception because of the teratogenicity of bisphosphonates.

- **Orthopedic:** Mild strength training to stabilize joint laxity; physical therapy may help (particularly after fractures) with pain control and improvement in function after prolonged immobilization. Often because of the nature of the fracture, open-reduction internal fixation is needed (see Fig. 41.3). Unweighted exercises may be beneficial (e.g., pool therapy, harnesses, and total gym). "Off-label" use of bisphosphonates has been advocated by some for between 2 and 5 years. A list of orthopedic clinics specializing in OI is available at www.oif.org.
- **Psychology:** Provide empathy and psychological support as per individual's and family's needs. Realize parents may have been suspected of child abuse in cases where the diagnosis is delayed, leading to feelings of guilt, frustration, and anxiety. Genetic counseling is always strongly advised, as is putting patient in contact with knowledgeable medical professionals and local/national support groups. Have athletes visit the Osteogenesis Imperfecta Foundation website at www.oif.org.
- **Pain control:** Oral, injectable, transdermal, and topical medications, including acetaminophen, NSAIDs, opioids, tramadol, TENS units, bracing, ring splints, ambulation-assist devices, and lastly surgery. Nontraditional treatments, including hypnosis, acupuncture, and homeopathy may help.

Prognosis: Depends on the type of OI. In general, patients have a full life expectancy, but morbidity seems to be directly correlated to the number of fractures. Type II has a significant higher morbidity, and patients are often wheelchair-bound if they survive the perinatal period.

Return to sport: Absolutely avoid contact/collision sports. Certain high-impact sports may be contraindicated, depending on severity of the condition. Joint and bone protection is crucial both in activities of daily life and in selection of athletic and recreational activities. No cardiovascular limitation noted by the 46th Bethesda Guidelines. Allowed once fracture(s) have both clinically and radiographically healed and matured.

SEROPOSITVE ARTHOPATHIES

Axial Spondyloarthritis

Overview: Formerly known as ankylosing spondylitis until 2009, axial spondyloarthritis (AS) is a chronic, inflammatory rheumatic disease that causes arthritis of the spine and sacroiliac joint (Fig. 41.4); the chronic inflammation and irritation of the spinal joints (vertebrae) can eventually cause the vertebrae to fuse together, a condition known as *ankylosis*. Can be classified as having either of two different subtypes: radiographic ankylosing spondylitis or nonradiographic ankylosing spondylitis.

Incidence: Approximately 350,000 Americans are estimated to have AS. Approximately 1.8% of the US population will develop it.

Presentation:

- Back pain: acute or chronic that improves with exercise and does not improve with rest.

- Usually presents in the third to fourth decade of life
- Probable male-to-female ratio is 2:1–3:1, although recent survey in the United States showed no significant difference in prevalence between men and women
- Sacroiliitis; will present as either bilateral or unilateral buttock pain
- Dactylitis ("sausage digits"): Present as diffuse swelling of the toes or fingers
- Occasional pain/inflammation in other joints (e.g., hips, shoulders, knees, and ankles)
- Morning stiffness
- Impairment in spinal mobility
- Postural abnormalities, especially hyperkyphosis
- Enthesitis; the region of attachment of tendons and ligaments to bone. Will have pain and tenderness at insertion sites.
- Be aware of coexisting diseases, especially acute anterior uveitis, psoriasis, and inflammatory bowel disease.

Physical examination: See Fig. 41.4
- Pain with back flexion (lumbar/sacral area)
- Decreased range of motion in spine (cervical to sacral)
- **Lateral spinal flexion examination:** Patient stands erect with heels and back against the wall. The first measurement is the distance from fingertips to floor. Then, the patient is asked to laterally flex the spine without rotating or bending the knees. Second measurement is the distance between fingertips and floor. Difference of >10 cm is normal.
- **Schober test:** Measure forward flexion of the lumber spine. Patient is erect, and a mark is placed 5 cm below the posterior superior iliac spine (PSIS), at midline at level of PSIS, and 10 cm above the PSIS over the spinous process. The patient is asked to bend forward without bending the knees. If the measurement between the two marks does not exceed 20 cm in length (start is 15 cm), the test is considered positive.
- Limited ability to fully expand chest with deep inhalation
- Ophthalmologic examination may show uveitis or iritis
- Limited internal and external rotation of the hips
- Enthesitis
- Sacroiliac tenderness and positive FABER test

Diagnostic:
- Refer to the 2013 Assessment of Spondyloarthritis International Society Modified Berlin Algorithm
- Blood work: HLA-B27 is positive in 90% of AS cases. Erythrocyte sedimentation rate (ESR) and C-reactive protein (CRP) are helpful for monitoring disease progression.
- Radiograph shows squaring of vertebral bodies, "bamboo spine," fusion of vertebrae
- Radiographic grading: modified Stokes Ankylosing Spine Score (SASS)
- MRI shows spondylitis (inflammation)/sacroiliitis.
- Indices for evaluating disease:
  - Bath Ankylosing Spondylitis Disease Activity Index (BASDAI)
  - Ankylosing Spondylitis Disease Activity Score (ASDAS)
  - Bath Ankylosing Spondylitis Functional Index (BASFI)
  - AS Quality of Life instrument (ASQoL)

Treatment:
- In most patients with symptomatic AS, we recommend an NSAID as initial therapy. Regardless of the NSAID used, the maximum dose is often required.
- Inadequate response to initial therapy with two different NSAIDs used consecutively in an adequate dose for at least 2–4 weeks each, we then recommend a tumor necrosis factor (TNF)-alpha inhibitor.
  - TNF-blockers: Adalimumab, etanercept, or infliximab
- Discontinue smoking because it can accelerate lung scarring and decrease pulmonary function.
- Drug-modifying antirheumatic drugs (DMARDs): Methotrexate or sulfasalazine.
- Oral glucocorticoids: Limited data suggest high doses may have some benefits for very short-term therapy.
- Injection (prednisone): Epidural versus facet
- Pain control: Aspirin, acetaminophen, NSAIDs, tramadol
- Physical therapy: Firm mattress, back extension exercises, stress core strength, maintain spine mobility and lung capacity, and improve posture

Prognosis: Variable

Most patients with limited disease do well, although a minority of patients develop severe skeletal symptoms or life-threatening complications. Approximately 1% will "burn out" or go into remission.

Return to sport: Continuous flexibility training and core strengthening and mild to moderate exercise within limits of disease activity; swimming is preferred because it avoids jarring impact of the spine. Patients can participate in carefully chosen aerobic sports when disease is inactive. Aerobic exercise is generally encouraged because it promotes full expansion of the breathing muscles and opens the airways.

Rheumatoid Arthritis

Overview: The most common chronic inflammatory arthritis, rheumatoid arthritis (RA) is thought to have a demographic, lifestyle, environmental, and genetic susceptibility and be caused by a complex interaction between T-cell and B-lymphocytes, macrophages, and fibroblast-like synoviocytes. Bimodal expressivity of this condition as juvenile-onset versus adult-onset RA.

Incidence: Approximately 1% of the population in Great Britain and the United States is affected by RA, or 40 per 100,000 persons. It is twice as common in women than men.

Presentation: Joint pain in multiple joints (usually symmetric), nontrauma-related, swollen joints, finger deformities or weakness (often episodic in nature), myositis/vasculitis, and drug-induced myopathy (e.g., glucocorticoids, statins, and antimalarials) (Fig. 41.5). Morning stiffness is common (>1 hour). It affects metacarpophalangeal and metatarsophalangeal joints early in the disease process.

Physical examination:
- Metacarpophalangeal joint inflammation, particularly early in the disease
- Heberden nodules (more common in osteoarthritis [OA])
- Bouchard nodules (see Fig. 41.5)
- Tender proximal interphalangeal (PIP) joints of the hand
- Fingernail: subungual hemorrhage or infarct (see Fig. 41.5)
- Synovitis of multiple joints
- Ulnar deviation of phalanges *(in long-term cases)*
- Symmetric joint pain and swelling; destruction of joint, synovium, and surrounding soft tissue
- Swan neck deformity
- Eye involvement: keratoconjunctivitis sicca and episcleritis (see Fig. 41.5)
- Lung involvement: pulmonary toxicity secondary to methotrexate or gold salts
- Cardiac involvement: pericarditis, myocarditis
- Foot deformities (see Fig. 41.5)
- Spine involvement

Diagnostic: History and physical examination and radiographic changes (joint space narrowing or destruction). Synovial fluid examination in affected joints usually reveals an inflammatory effusion, with a leukocyte count typically between 1500 and 25,000/mm^3 characterized by a predominance of polymorphonuclear (PMN) cells.
- Serum laboratory examination: rheumatoid factor, sedimentation rate, anti-CCP ab, CRP, antinuclear antibodies (ANA), and complete blood count (CBC) (anemia

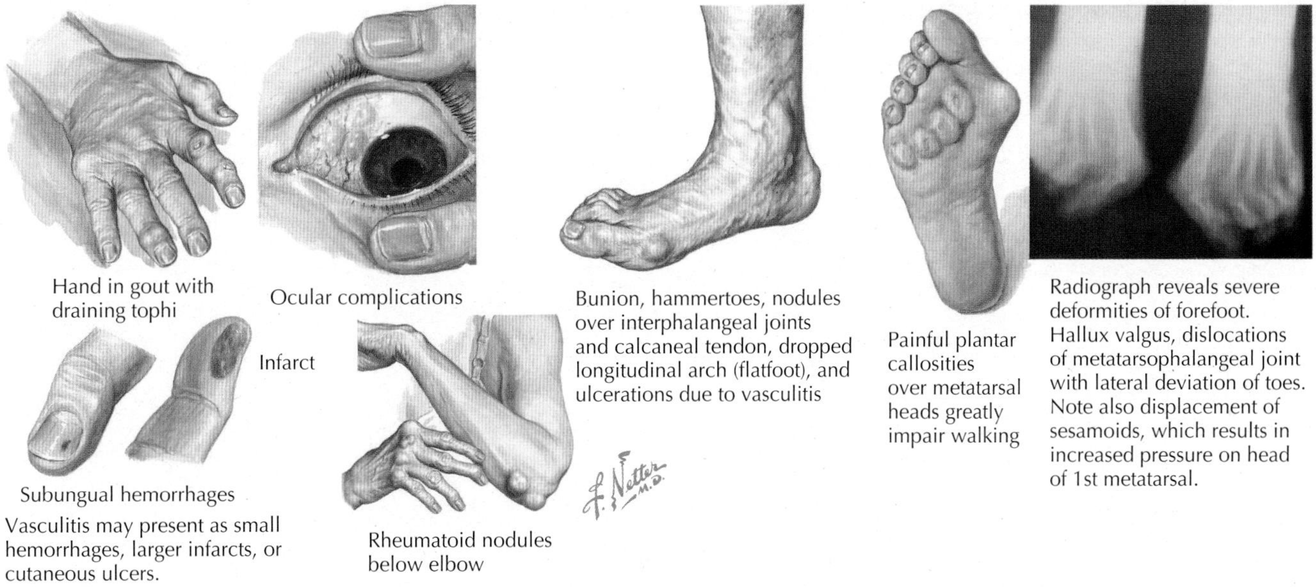
Hand in gout with draining tophi
Ocular complications
Infarct
Subungual hemorrhages
Vasculitis may present as small hemorrhages, larger infarcts, or cutaneous ulcers.
Rheumatoid nodules below elbow
Bunion, hammertoes, nodules over interphalangeal joints and calcaneal tendon, dropped longitudinal arch (flatfoot), and ulcerations due to vasculitis
Painful plantar callosities over metatarsal heads greatly impair walking
Radiograph reveals severe deformities of forefoot. Hallux valgus, dislocations of metatarsophalangeal joint with lateral deviation of toes. Note also displacement of sesamoids, which results in increased pressure on head of 1st metatarsal.
F. Netter M.D.

Figure 41.5 Characteristics of rheumatoid arthritis.

[normocytic hypochromic]) and neutropenia (consider Felty syndrome)

- About 75%–80% of patients with RA test (+) for RF, anti-CCP, or both.
- The 2010 American College of Rheumatology Classification Criteria includes the following clinical features for diagnosis: inflammatory arthritis of ≥3 joints for >6 weeks, positive RA and/or anti-CCP, elevated CRP or ESR, and exclusion of other diseases with similar clinical features.

Treatment:

- DMARDs: methotrexate, leflunomide, sulfasalazine, and minocycline
- Biologic DMARDs:
  - TNF-alpha inhibitors: infliximab, adalimumab, etanercept, golimumab, and certolizumab pegol
  - Other monoclonal antibodies: abatacept and rituximab
  - Targeted, synthetic DMARDs: tofacitinib
  - Interleukin-6 inhibitor: tocilizumab
- Prednisone oral burst then taper
- Intra-articular injections: steroids and hyaluronic acid
- Physical therapy
- Physical activity and healthy lifestyle
- Orthotics for foot deformities/pain
- Joint replacement surgery when conservative measures fail

Prognosis: Depends on severity, responsiveness to medications, and juvenile versus adult onset; in several cases, juvenile-onset RA may "burn out" and become quiescent in early adulthood. However, most patients have progressive disease, with either a slow or rapid course.

Return to sport: Avoid combative/collision/contact sports, particularly during the early phases of the condition as DMARDs are starting to work.

- Disease quiescent with complete functional recovery: moderate to vigorous activity (e.g., running)
- Disease quiescent with minimal to moderate crippling: mild to moderate activity (e.g., swimming and cycling)
- Asymptomatic with effusion and synovial changes in weight-bearing joints in active therapy: mild activity with participation at own tolerance
- Few evidence-based studies have shown that moderate athletic activity (e.g., swimming and cycling) had no negative impacts on deterioration of hand function and preserved hand function compared with nonactive controls.

Systemic Lupus Erythematosus

Overview: Systemic lupus erythematosus (SLE) is a chronic inflammatory immunologic disease that can affect multiple organ systems, including dermatologic, pulmonary, cardiac, renal, immune, musculoskeletal, and nervous systems, with the production of ANAs.

Presentation: SLE presents more often in young women than men. The organ systems that are involved early in the disease are the same organ systems that continue to be involved later in the disease process. Most patients present with fatigue, fever, myalgias, nonspecific abdominal pain and/or weight loss, and migratory asymmetric arthralgias; the small joints of hands, wrists, and knees are the most frequently involved.

- Cardiac disease is common and can involve most layers of the heart and conduction system. Pericarditis, with or without effusion, is the most common cardiac manifestation. Libman–Sacks endocarditis is usually clinically silent but can produce valvular insufficiency and can serve as a source of emboli.
- Renal involvement is clinically apparent in approximately 50% of SLE patients.
- Pulmonary manifestations include pleuritis, pneumonitis, interstitial lung disease, pulmonary hypertension, and alveolar hemorrhage.
- Hematologic abnormalities are common in SLE. Leukopenia is known to occur in about 50% of patients.

Physical examination and diagnostics: See Table 41.2. One can also refer to the 2019 European League Against Rheumatism (EULAR)/American College of Rheumatology classification criteria for SLE.

Treatment: The goals of therapy for patients with SLE are to ensure long-term survival, achieve the lowest possible disease activity, prevent organ damage, minimize drug toxicity, improve quality of life, and educate patients about their role in disease management.

- Fever usually responds to NSAIDs, acetaminophen, or low-dose corticosteroids.
- Limit exposure to sunlight.
- Difficult to differentiate between true SLE and drug-induced SLE. Review all recent medications/supplements.
- Infections may initiate or cause a relapse of SLE.
- Hydroxychloroquine or chloroquine

Table 41.2 SYSTEMIC LUPUS ERYTHEMATOSUS CLASSIFICATION CRITERIA

Criteria	Clinical Criteria	Immunologic Criteria
American College of Rheumatology (ACR): must satisfy at least 4 of 11 criteria	Malar rash Photosensitivity Discoid rash Oral ulcers Arthritis Serositis (pleuritis or pericarditis) Renal disorder (proteinuria >5 g/24 hr or cellular casts) Neurologic disorder (seizure or psychosis) Hematologic disorder (hemolytic anemia, leukopenia, lymphopenia, or thrombocytopenia)	Elevated ANA titer Antibodies (anti-DNA, anti-Sm, or antiphospholipid)
Systemic Lupus International Collaborating Clinics (SLICC): must satisfy 4 of 17 criteria, including at least 1 of 11 clinical criteria and 1 of 6 immunologic criteria, OR have a biopsy-proven nephritis compatible with SLE in the presence of ANA or anti-dsDNA antibodies	Acute cutaneous lupus (malar rash or subacute) Chronic cutaneous lupus (e.g., discoid rash, lupus panniculitis, chilblains lupus) Nonscarring alopecia Oral or nasal ulcers Joint disease (synovitis or tenderness of ≥2 joints) Serositis (typical pleurisy or pericardial pain for >1 day) Renal (proteinuria >5 g/24 hr or red blood cell casts) Neurologic (seizures, psychosis, mononeuritis multiplex, myelitis, peripheral or cranial neuropathy, or acute confusional state) Hemolytic anemia Leukopenia or lymphopenia Thrombocytopenia	Elevated ANA titer Anti-dsDNA antibody Anti-Sm antibody Antiphospholipid antibody Low complement (C3, C4, or CH50) Direct Coombs test (in absence of hemolytic anemia)

After excluding alternative diagnoses, SLE can be diagnosed using either ACR criteria or SLICC criteria.
From Petri M, Orbai AM, Alarcón GS. Derivation and validation of the Systemic Lupus International Collaborating Clinics classification criteria for systemic lupus erythematosus. *Arthritis Rheum*. 2012;64(8):2677–2686.

- NSAIDs and/or short-term use of low-dose glucocorticoids
- Other medications may include cyclophosphamide, methotrexate, azathioprine, mycophenolate, belimumab, and rituximab.

Prognosis: Variable, can be episodic with long periods of remission to rather progressive and debilitating; occasionally leads to significant morbidity and some mortality. The 5-year survival rate has dramatically increased to greater than 90% since the 1980s. Despite these improvements, patients with SLE still have mortality rates ranging from two to five times higher than that of the general population.

Return to sport: Protect from sun exposure because this can worsen or prolong dermatologic manifestations such as rashes. Assess the patient for signs of renal involvement by looking for proteinuria, calculating glomerular filtration rate via plasma creatinine levels, and rarely, by doing a renal biopsy on a scheduled basis if patient suffers a flare. Discourage patient from participating during a flare that includes fever because of increased risk of endocarditis, vasculitis, and worsening synovitis. Baseline echocardiogram and subsequent follow-up echocardiograms before clearing for endurance or competitive sports with moderate to severe intensity to look for any valvular insufficiency. Patients with a long history of SLE should be screened before starting a strenuous exercise regimen because they are at a higher risk of developing coronary artery disease. Stress, surgery, and pregnancy have been known to trigger relapses, so caution is warranted during such events.

SERONEGATIVE ARTHROPATHIES

Osteoarthritis

Overview: Most common joint disorder where approximately 240 million people are affected by OA, including over 30 million in the United States, which has increased from 21 million in 1990 to 27 million in 2005; approximately 5% of the population between ages 35 and 54 show signs of osteoarthritis in knee joint on radiographs; directly related to severity of occurrences of trauma, joint-related surgery, age, and activity wherein normal articular cartilage is damaged (Fig. 41.6). Currently, it is thought that metalloprotease enzymes (e.g., collagenase, stromelysin, and gelatinase) are active in the degradation of cartilage. Other mediators that seem to play a role in OA are cytokines, other proteases, nitric oxide, calcium crystals, sex hormones, aging, and familial genetics.

Presentation: Early morning stiffness and joint pain that generally improves with activity (see Fig. 41.6).

Physical examination:

- Heberden nodules: joint enlargement of the distal interphalangeal (DIP) joint
- Bouchard nodules: tendon nodules located around the PIP joint (see Fig. 41.6)
- Stiff, enlarged joint, often monoarticular or asymmetric
- Decreased range of motion
- Antalgic movement of that joint (seen often in weight-bearing joints)

Diagnostic: History and physical examination; radiographs (weight-bearing preferred in lower extremity); bone scan will show moderate to severe arthritic changes in all joints of the body.

Treatment:

- Pain control (acetaminophen, capsaicin, duloxetine, and NSAIDs)
- Physical therapy should address range of motion, core strength, mobility, modalities, mild strength training to stabilize joints, flexibility training, and home exercise program (HEP).
- Intra-articular injections: Steroids and hyaluronic acid. Platelet-rich plasma (PRP) and stem cell continue to show promise, but more research is needed.
- Weight loss if a patient is overweight
- Joint replacement surgery when conservative measures fail

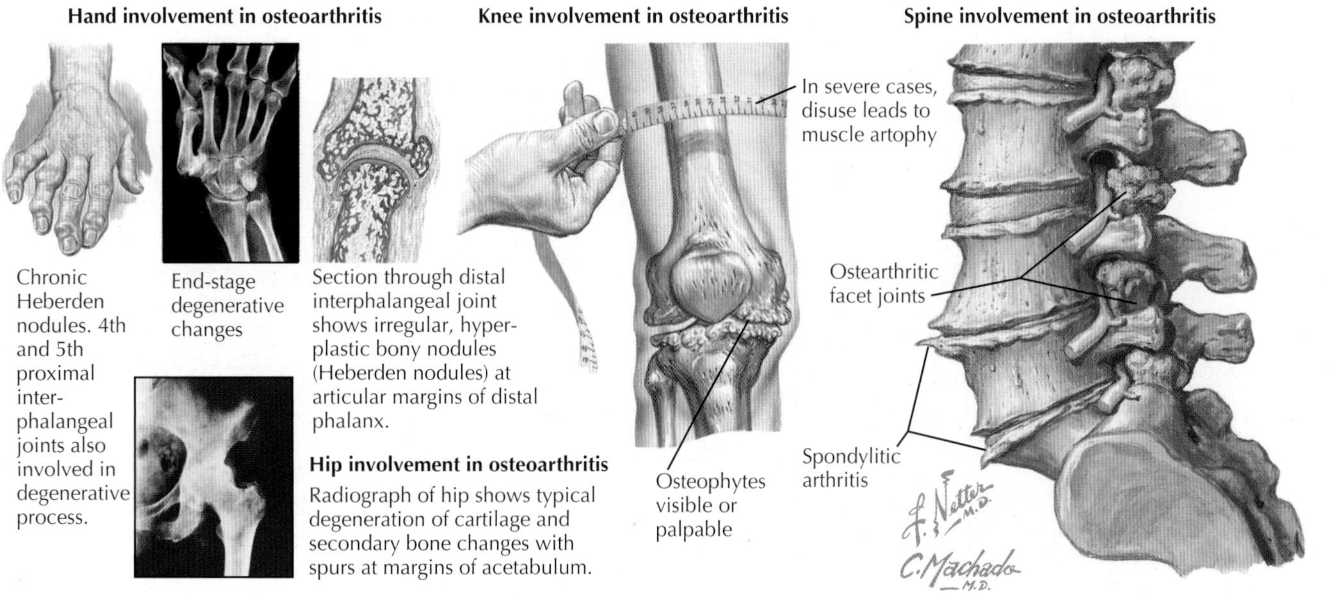
Hand involvement in osteoarthritis
Knee involvement in osteoarthritis
Spine involvement in osteoarthritis
Chronic Heberden nodules. 4th and 5th proximal inter-phalangeal joints also involved in degenerative process.
End-stage degenerative changes
Section through distal interphalangeal joint shows irregular, hyper-plastic bony nodules (Heberden nodules) at articular margins of distal phalanx.
Hip involvement in osteoarthritis
Radiograph of hip shows typical degeneration of cartilage and secondary bone changes with spurs at margins of acetabulum.
In severe cases, disuse leads to muscle artophy
Osteophytes visible or palpable
Ostearthritic facet joints
Spondylitic arthritis
F. Netter M.D.
C.Machado M.D.

Figure 41.6 Characteristics of osteoarthritis or degenerative arthropathy.

Prognosis: Varies among patients; depends on severity of the condition, number of joints involved, concomitant diseases, and activities (occupation/recreation)

Return to sport: As tolerated by pain and mechanical defects; long-term impact loading of affected joint(s) may advance the disease at a quicker pace

OTHER RHEUMATOLOGIC CONDITIONS

Buerger Syndrome (Thromboangiitis Obliterans [TAO])

Overview: Nontraumatic, nonatherosclerotic inflammatory occlusion of small to medium-sized arteries or vasculitis. It often presents with pain and claudication of lower extremities and is associated with heavy smokers and men younger than 50 years; also seen in users of smokeless tobacco.

Etiology: Unknown. The condition is distinguished from other forms of vasculitis by a highly cellular, inflammatory intraluminal thrombus with relative sparing of the vessel wall and, more specifically, sparing of the internal elastic lamina.

Incidence: The incidence of Buerger syndrome is approximately 12.6 per 100,000 persons in the United States. Incidence ranges from 1% to 5% in the population of Western Europe and approximately 80% among Ashkenazi Jews in Israel with peripheral arterial disease.

Presentation:

- Vascular involvement begins with the distal arteries and veins, followed by more proximal arterial occlusive disease.
- Male-to-female ratio: 3:1
- Coldness, numbness, and cyanosis of hands and feet
- Cold weather exacerbation: Raynaud phenomenon occurs in more than 40% of patients and may be asymmetric
- Multiple amputations and/or ischemic ulcers
- Arch pain (most common site of foot claudication)
- Pain at rest (at advanced stages)
- Three phases:
  - Acute phase: Inflammatory: Thrombi develop in the arteries and veins, typically of the distal extremities.
  - Intermediate phase: Progressive organization of thrombus
  - Chronic phase: Thrombus and fibrosis, no inflammation

Physical examination: See Fig. 41.7

- Mottled skin appearance
- Ulcers or gangrene on distal extremities
- Delayed capillary refill in extremities (2 seconds)
- Abnormal Allen test
- Tests for thoracic outlet syndrome (Wright, Addson, and Roos) may be positive
- Decreased or absent distal pulses
  - Ankle–brachial index (ABI) should be performed. Similarly, a wrist–brachial index (WBI) can be performed in the upper extremity.
- Twenty to fifty percent will also have migratory thrombophlebitis
- To differentiate atherosclerosis from Buerger syndrome:
  - Buerger syndrome usually affects both upper and lower extremities
  - Buerger syndrome does not affect proximal arteries
  - Associated with tobacco use; improves when tobacco use stops
  - History of thrombophlebitis
  - Age <45 years

Diagnostic:

- Serum laboratory examinations (normal): ESR, CRP, ANA, complement, rheumatoid factor (RF), anticentromere ab, Scl-70 ab, coagulopathy panel, serum cotinine (metabolite of nicotine) level, and toxicology panel (cocaine, amphetamine, cannabis)
  - These tests usually are normal or negative in patients. However, anticardiolipin antibodies may be present in some patients.
- Histopathologic examination of vessel identifies acute-phase lesions in a patient with an active tobacco history.
- Arterial angiography suggestive of TAO:
  - Early findings: Consistent with claudication
    - No evidence of atherosclerosis. No source of thromboembolism. Involvement of small and medium-sized vessels such as the plantar, tibial, peroneal, palmar, radial, and ulnar arteries.
  - Late findings: Show multiple fine "cork-screw"-shaped branches of distal arteries that end abruptly

Treatment:

- Eliminate contact with *all* tobacco products. Complete abstinence of tobacco and cannabis use will substantially lessen the likelihood of amputation.

- Echocardiogram to screen for intracardiac thrombus.
- Common methods to assist patient to quit smoking include hypnosis, nicotine replacement (via oral, inhaled, or transdermal), bupropion (Zyban), varenicline (Chantix), etc.
- Symptoms should improve if patient is compliant.
- Wear appropriate footwear and inspect feet daily.
- Avoid cold weather and vasoconstricting drugs.
- Iloprost decreases risk of amputation.

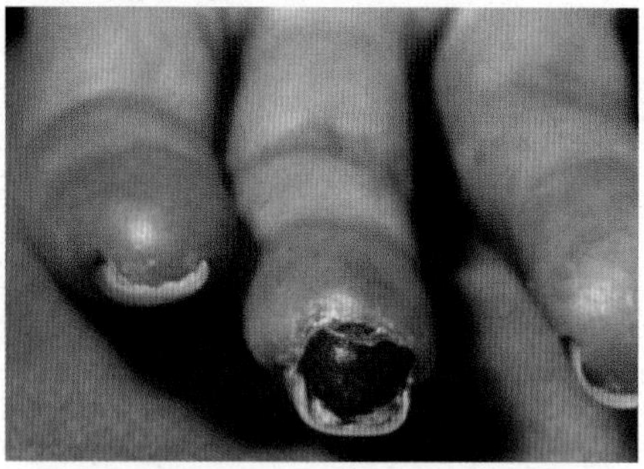

Ischemic finger of a young male patient with Buerger's syndrome

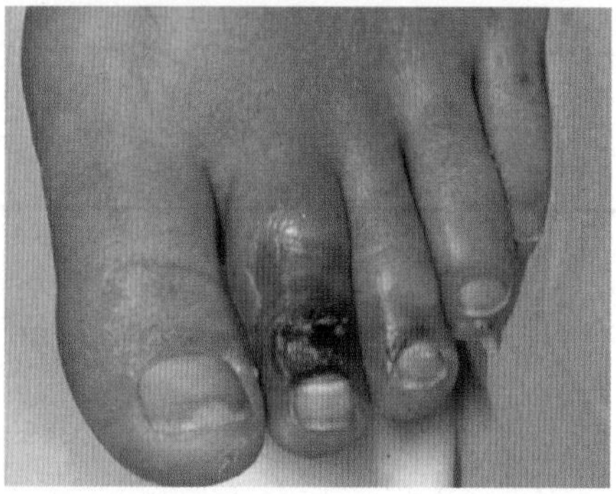

Ischemic toe of a 28-year-old woman with Buerger's syndrome

Figure 41.7 Characteristics of Buerger syndrome (thromboangiitis obliterans). (Photograph from Goldman L, Ausiello D, Arend W, et al. *Cecil Textbook of Medicine.* 23rd ed. Philadelphia: Elsevier; 2007.)

- Surgery for revascularization is rarely considered if patient is noncompliant with smoking cessation. Results are often less than optimal because the disease is so distal.
- Amputation if gangrene or osteomyelitis occurs.
- Clinical trials for phVEGF 165 (vascular endothelial growth factor) and cilostazol and PDE-3 inhibitors are underway and may show promise. PDE-5 inhibitors like tadalafil and sildenafil only show improvement with Raynaud phenomenon.

Prognosis: Good if patient stops smoking.

- In a study that followed 111 patients with proven TAO for a mean of 15.6 years, the incidence of major amputation was 11% at 5 years, 21% at 10 years, and 23% at 20 years. The risk of amputation in former smokers was eliminated by 8 years after smoking cessation.

Return to sport: Once symptoms have begun to abate, slow and progressive return to mild to moderate exercise is encouraged. Current literature review shows no evidence-based studies that recommend either sports participation or return to play.

Polymyalgia Rheumatica

Overview: A rheumatic condition that is associated with giant cell (temporal) arteritis (GCA), polymyalgia rheumatica (PMR) is characterized by chronic aching and morning stiffness in shoulders, hip girdles, neck, and torso in older persons.

Presentation: Prevalence is approximately 700 per 100,000 in persons older than 50 years. Of those with PMR, 10% also have GCA. In addition to the shoulder and hip stiffness and achiness, patient complains of malaise, fatigue, weight loss and anorexia, and mild fever.

Physical examination: See Fig. 41.8

- Decreased active range of motion at shoulder, neck, and hips
  - A classic finding is the inability to actively abduct the shoulder past 90 degrees
- Normal muscular strength, though weakness/atrophy has been noted because of disuse
- Often shoulder, neck, and hip musculature is not tender.
- Tenosynovitis around carpal tunnel has been noted.
- Soreness in affected joints seems to be related to a bursitis/synovitis.

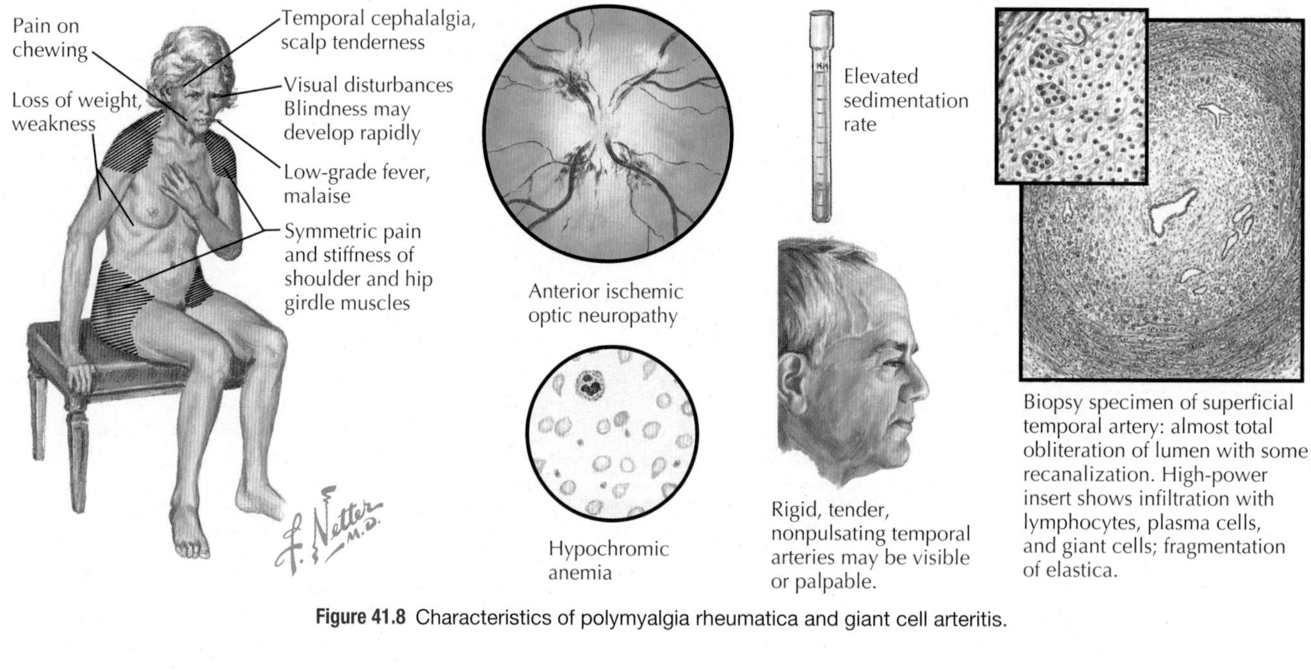
Pain on chewing
Loss of weight, weakness
Temporal cephalalgia, scalp tenderness
Visual disturbances Blindness may develop rapidly
Low-grade fever, malaise
Symmetric pain and stiffness of shoulder and hip girdle muscles
Anterior ischemic optic neuropathy
Hypochromic anemia
Elevated sedimentation rate
Rigid, tender, nonpulsating temporal arteries may be visible or palpable.
Biopsy specimen of superficial temporal artery: almost total obliteration of lumen with some recanalization. High-power insert shows infiltration with lymphocytes, plasma cells, and giant cells; fragmentation of elastica.

Figure 41.8 Characteristics of polymyalgia rheumatica and giant cell arteritis.

Diagnostic:

- Criteria, typical:
  - Older than 50 years
  - Bilateral, aching morning stiffness in neck, shoulders, or hips for at least 30 minutes and persisting for at least 2 weeks
  - A diagnostic cutoff value for elevations of CRP has not been established, but practically speaking, a normal CRP effectively excludes the diagnosis of PMR. The creatinine kinase (CK) level is always normal.
- *Differentiation from GCA:* PMR rarely expresses temporal tenderness, headache, jaw pain, visual loss, and noncranial ischemia (e.g., arm claudication)
- Hematologic: ESR is elevated, often >100 mm/hr, but up to 20% may have an ESR of ≤40 mm/hr.
- Rapid resolution of symptoms with low-dose glucocorticoids. Symptoms are generally 50%–70% better within 3 days in patients with PMR started on prednisone at a dose of 10–20 mg/day.
- Immunologic: PMR and GCA share the polymorphism on *HLA-DR4*. A secondary hypervariable region of the *HLA-DRB1* gene has been associated with PMR. Interleukin 6 (IL-6) may be elevated.
- Imaging:
  - Radiographs: Rarely reveal any changes of inflamed joints
  - MRI: May show inflammation of tenosynovial sheaths or bursae
  - Ultrasound: Effusions of shoulder bursa
  - Positron emission tomography (PET) scan: No proven clinical value in the care of patients with PMR

Treatment: Initial: moderate doses of corticosteroids (7.5–20 mg daily); **Chronic:** lower doses of corticosteroids are used (note: *ESR, CRP, and IL-6 levels may return to normal once corticosteroid treatment is started*); **Additional agents:** methotrexate, infliximab show no proven benefit.

- In most patients, an initial prednisone dose of 15 mg/day given orally is suggested. Majority of patients experience substantial improvement within days of starting treatment.

Prognosis: In most patients, PMR runs a self-limited course over months to years and corticosteroids can be discontinued. Ongoing surveillance for development of GCA symptoms should be assessed. There is no evidence of increased mortality associated with PMR. PMR is not erosive and does not cause structural damage.

Return to sport: Once a patient has been identified and appropriately treated, there are relatively few contraindications for participation outside of the issues associated with chronic steroid use (e.g., weight gain, glucose intolerance, osteoporosis, etc.).

RECOMMENDED READINGS

Available online.

SECTION VII

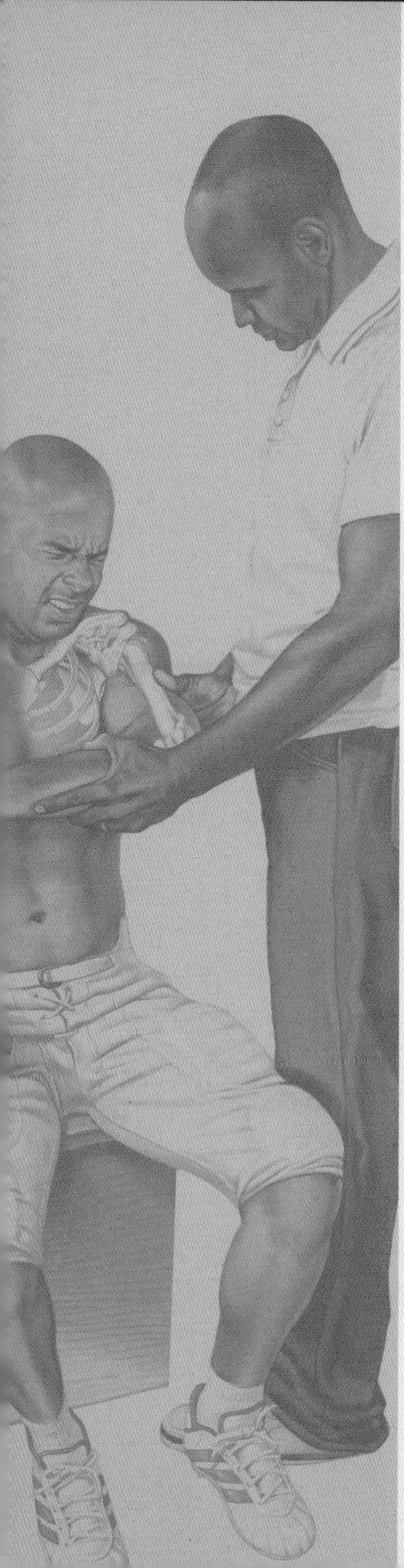

Injury Prevention, Diagnosis, and Treatment

MUSCULOSKELETAL INJURIES IN SPORTS 42

Eric C. McCarty • Torrance A. McCarty • Andrew G. Potyk

GENERAL CLASSIFICATION OF MUSCULOSKELETAL SPORTS INJURIES

Musculoskeletal sports injuries can be classified as **traumatic** or **overuse** injuries.

Traumatic Injuries

Description: Result from specific episode(s) of trauma, whether recent (acute) or in the more distant past (subacute or chronic)

Bone

Description: Traumatic injury to a bone most commonly results in a **fracture**, although rarely, another injury such as **subperiosteal hematoma can occur.**
Descriptive terms:

- **Closed fracture** is a fracture that does not produce an open wound in the skin.
- **Open fracture** is when an open wound in the skin communicates with the fracture site.
- Descriptive terms for direction of fracture line:
  - Fracture at right angles to the long axis of a bone is called **transverse.**
  - Fracture line at other angles to the long axis of a bone is called **oblique.**
  - Bone twisted apart creates **spiral** configuration of fracture.
- **Comminuted fracture** is when a bone is broken into three or more pieces.
- **Avulsion fracture** is a "pull-off" fracture; a piece of bone is pulled off by the ligament or by tendon attachment.
- **Greenstick fracture** is an incomplete fracture in children: one side of a bone is broken, whereas the other side appears bent.
- **Torus fracture** is localized buckling in the cortex of the bone, common in children.
- **Epiphyseal fracture** is a fracture that involves the growth center at the end of a long bone in children.

Joint

Description: Traumatic injury to a joint and supporting structures (capsule or ligaments) often results in an instability episode referred to as **dislocation** or **subluxation.** Rarely, other results such as joint contusion or hemarthrosis occur from a direct blow.
Classification:

- **Dislocation** is a complete displacement of joint surfaces so that they no longer make normal contact at all; important to distinguish **first-time** or **recurrent** dislocation
- **Subluxation** is a partial displacement of joint surfaces, usually transient in nature; important to distinguish **first-time** or **recurrent** subluxation
- Dislocation or subluxation implies damage to ligaments or other supporting structures of a joint; important to ascertain injury to those tissues; discussed in the following section

Ligament

Description: Traumatic injury to a ligament is referred to as **sprain** (Fig. 42.1)
Classification:

- **First-degree sprain:** Tear of only a few ligament fibers; mild swelling, pain, disability; no instability of joint created
- **Second-degree sprain:** Tear of a moderate number of ligament fibers, but ligament function is still intact; however, ligaments may be somewhat stretched. Moderate amount of swelling, pain, disability; slight to no instability of joint.
- **Third-degree sprain:** Complete rupture of a ligament; severe swelling and disability; definite joint instability; instability may be classified as:
  - **1+** joint surfaces normally stabilized by ligament(s) displaced 3–5 mm from their normal position
  - **2+** joint surfaces separated by 6–10 mm
  - **3+** joint surfaces separated by >10 mm

Muscle–Tendon Unit

STRAIN

Description: Traumatic injury to muscle or tendon caused by **indirect force** (i.e., contraction of muscle itself) is referred to as a **strain**
Classification:

- **First-degree strain:** Tear of only a few muscle or tendon fibers; mild swelling, pain, disability; can also be characterized by patient's ability to produce strong, but painful, muscle contraction
- **Second-degree strain:** Disruption of moderate number of muscle or tendon fibers, but muscle–tendon unit still intact; moderate amount of pain, swelling, disability; characterized by patient's weak and painful attempts at muscle contraction
- **Third-degree strain:** Complete rupture of muscle–tendon unit; may be at origin, muscular portion, musculotendinous junction, within tendon itself, or at tendon insertion; characterized by extremely weak attempts at muscle contraction

DEEP MUSCLE CONTUSION

Description: Traumatic injury to muscle caused by **direct force** may produce deep muscle contusion; typically affects quadriceps or brachialis muscles involved in contact or collision sports; may lead to **myositis ossificans** and therefore permanent loss of function

MYOSITIS OSSIFICANS

Description: Heterotopic bone formation caused by a deep muscle contusion or strain, particularly after marked hematoma formation
Common sites: Quadriceps; biceps, triceps, brachialis; hip girdle; groin; and lower leg
Risk factors: Severe contusion; continuing to play after injury; massaging injured area; early application of heat; passive, forceful stretching; overly rapid rehabilitation; premature return to sport; reinjury of same site; individual propensity to heterotopic bone formation
Calcification: Follows injury by 3–6 weeks

- May continue to develop for ≥6 weeks
- May remodel or reabsorb over 3–12 months, particularly if close to musculotendinous junction

Treatment:

- Treat strain or contusion with basic athletic first aid (see Chapter 43: "Comprehensive Rehabilitation of the Athlete") represented by the mnemonic **PRICES: P**rotection, **R**est, **I**ce, **C**ompression, **E**levation, and **S**upport; followed by progressive symptom-guided rehabilitation. Range of motion of the affected joint can be helpful, especially early on, to avoid stiffness. Nonsteroidal anti-inflammatories such as

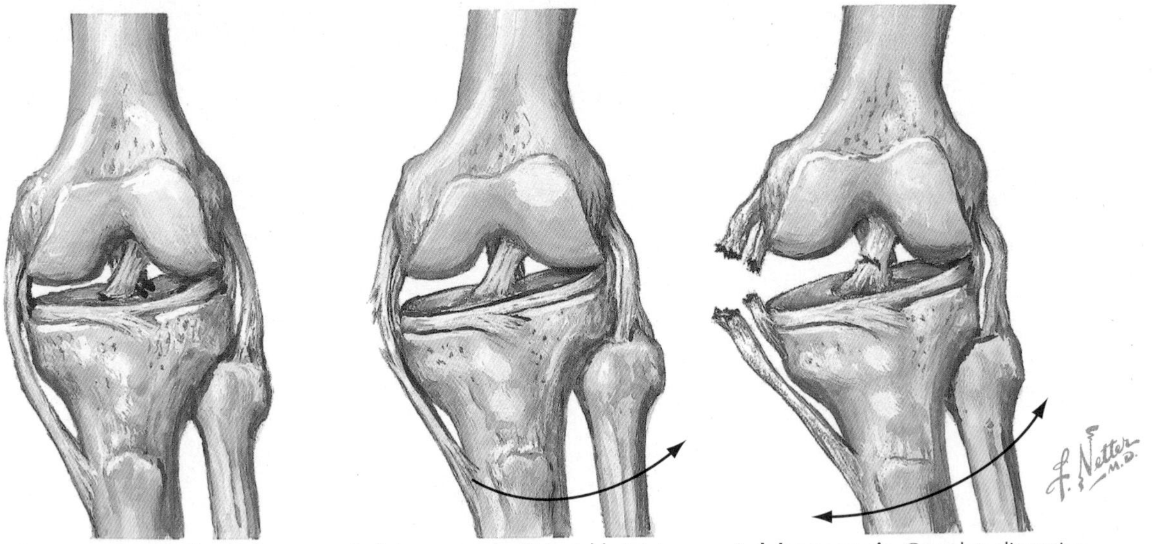

1st-degree sprain. Localized joint pain and tenderness but no joint laxity

2nd-degree sprain. Detectable joint laxity plus localized pain and tenderness

3rd-degree sprain. Complete disruption of ligaments and gross joint instability

Figure 42.1 Grading of ligament sprains.

indomethacin for 10 days can also be helpful in preventing calcifications from occurring.

- **Excision rarely necessary**
  - Warranted only in cases of persistent weakness or limited range of motion
  - Only after calcification matures (6–12 months)
  - High rate of recurrence if excised too early

EXERTIONAL RHABDOMYOLYSIS

Description: Breakdown of skeletal muscle cells with leakage of cellular contents, including myoglobin, creatine kinase (CK), and aldolase, through damaged sarcolemma into serum as a result of prolonged, heavy, or repetitious exercise

Presentation: Muscle pain and tenderness, muscle swelling, muscle cramps, and reddish-brown urine

Laboratory tests: Urinalysis (urine dipstick positive for hemoglobin; microscopic examination reveals few to no red blood cells); elevated CK (normal: 200 U/L; subclinical to mild rhabdomyolysis: 600 U/L; most clinical cases: 10,000 U/L; and severe cases: reports 200,000 U/L); and elevated serum myoglobin (normal, 5–70 g/L; elevated only up to 6 hours after injury if renal function is normal)

Etiology: Intense exercise causes local tissue hypoxia, resulting in elevation of adenosine triphosphate (ATP) and consequent failure of sodium–potassium pump with potassium efflux and calcium influx; anaerobic glycolysis with lactic acid overproduction and, in severe cases, metabolic acidosis; sarcolemma permeability; and, in severe cases, cell death

Common predisposing features: Heat, humidity, dehydration, poor physical conditioning (may also occur in well-conditioned athlete with very intense or repetitive exercise), high altitude, recent viral infection, sickle cell trait, and hereditary defects in ATP synthesis

Clinical course:

- Most cases are **subclinical** and never diagnosed or are **minimal** (visible myoglobinuria without muscle pain and spontaneous healing)
- **Mild to moderate cases** respond well to aggressive hydration; without nephrotoxic cofactors, dehydration, and acidosis, damage is usually not persistent; lasting systemic complications are rare; muscle has remarkable capacity for repair
- **Severe cases** are common in patients with dehydration or acidosis; they are characterized by **systemic complications:**
  - **Acute tubular necrosis and renal failure** caused by a combination of renal hypoperfusion, acidosis, and myoglobin sludging in renal tubules
  - **Acute compartment syndrome** (rhabdomyolysis causes muscle swelling, which increases intramuscular pressure, causing vicious cycle of damage; in athletes with chronic compartment syndrome, increased compartment pressure may reduce tissue perfusion and cause rhabdomyolysis)
  - Hyperkalemia
  - Hypocalcemia
  - Hyperphosphatemia
  - Diffuse intravascular coagulopathy (DIC)
  - Cardiac dysrhythmia

Treatment:

- **Aggressive early hydration** to maintain renal perfusion and clear myoglobin, thereby preventing acute tubular necrosis and renal failure
  - May require 4–12 L of normal saline during first 24 hours
  - Diuretic (furosemide) may be necessary to maintain kidney function
- **Alkalinization of urine with bicarbonate**
  - Myoglobin is less nephrotoxic and more soluble in alkaline urine
  - Uric acid is more soluble and less likely to crystallize in alkaline urine
  - **Caveat:** Alkalinization with bicarbonate may increase precipitation of calcium in injured muscles, causing heterotopic bone formation. Safer approach may be oral acetazolamide, 250 mg, three times daily, if plasma bicarbonate level is >13–15 mEq/L.
- Correct hyperkalemia, hyperphosphatemia, and hypocalcemia. Avoid intravenous (IV) calcium, except to treat tetany, because of the risk of heterotopic bone formation.
- **Fasciotomy,** if necessary for compartment syndrome
- Treat DIC if it does not resolve spontaneously
- Dialysis if necessary

Other Soft Tissues

Description: Traumatic injury to bursa with bursal swelling is referred to as **traumatic bursitis,** and it is usually caused by bleeding into bursa. Traumatic injuries to other soft tissues include various **contusions** and **hematomas.** Lacerations may involve musculoskeletal tissues.

Shearing injuries: Avulsions, abrasions, or blisters

MOREL–LAVALLÉE LESION

Description: A posttraumatic, closed, degloving soft tissue injury in which the skin and subcutaneous tissues are separated from fascia superficial to the underlying muscle plane, creating a space that fills with fluid and is susceptible to necrosis and infection.

Presentation: Diagnosis of Morel–Lavallée lesions is often missed or delayed. There may be a large swollen area where a hematoma develops, often in the pelvis area. There is soft tissue swelling with or without ecchymosis. Typically, there is asymmetry of the skin contour and hypermobility. Underlying soft fluctuance is also present with minimal or absent tenderness. Often, chronic lesions will have decreased sensation and cracked areas on the skin.

Imaging: Magnetic resonance imaging (MRI) is the preferred imaging modality of choice. In acute lesions, fluid collection will be a homogeneous collection that is hypointense on T1-weighted images and hyperintense on T2-weighted images. In chronic situations, the fluid will be hyperintense on both T1- and T2-weighted images (Fig. 42.2).

Etiology: A traumatic blow or sudden shearing force to any area with strong underlying fascia, most often around the pelvis or lower limb; the shearing force causes the thick layer of subcutaneous fat and skin to be ripped from its fascia underneath. As this occurs, the perforating vessels and lymphatics from the underlying muscle are torn, and blood and lymphatic fluid leak into a newly created cavity that has difficulty draining. The pressure of this area can cause skin and underlying necrosis. High-energy mechanisms are responsible for >50% of lesions.

Treatment:

- **Acute:** In isolated lesions, aspiration and compression may be acceptable. With any signs of infection, fracture, or skin necrosis, a percutaneous or open incision and drainage should be performed in the operating room.
- **Chronic:** Asymptomatic lesions can be observed and conservatively treated. Symptomatic lesions can be treated with percutaneous or open incision and drainage and may need sclerotherapy and possibly deadspace closure.

Overuse Injuries

Description: Account for >50% of injuries seen in sports medicine practices

General overuse concepts: If viewed as a function of Newton's third law of motion, athletic injury can be described as resulting from equal and opposite reactions, which, in turn, result in macrotrauma or microtrauma.

- Macrotrauma: Equal and opposite forces exceed strength of specific anatomic structure, and therefore the structure fails (see "Traumatic Injuries")
- Microtrauma: Microscopic subliminal injury from repeated activity; can be cumulative over time and result in inflammation; characterized by pain and dysfunction
- **Predisposition:** Equally important are intrinsic or extrinsic factors that predispose the athlete to overuse injury
  - **Intrinsic:** Malalignment of limbs, muscular imbalances, and other anatomic factors
  - **Extrinsic:** Training errors, faulty technique, incorrect surfaces and equipment, and poor environmental conditions
- **Degenerative processes:** May influence traumatic injuries as well, but more commonly have effect on overuse injuries; normal degenerative processes occur in many musculoskeletal tissues with aging; may add to likelihood of certain injuries such as rotator cuff and Achilles tendon problems
- **General classification:** Overuse injuries are classified according to four stages, depending on pain:
  - **Stage 1:** Pain after activity only
  - **Stage 2:** Pain during activity, does not restrict performance
  - **Stage 3:** Pain during activity, restricts performance
  - **Stage 4:** Chronic, unremitting pain, even at rest

Bones

Description: An overuse injury of bone may be a stress fracture or apophysitis.

Classification:

- **Stress fracture:** Most often found in lower extremity, but can also be found in spine and upper extremity when it is subjected to weight bearing (e.g., gymnastics, weight training)
- **Apophysitis:** In skeletally immature athletes, traction injuries can affect apophysis. Appear to result from repeated stress at tendinous insertion into bony growth center, followed by reactive bone formation; most common apophysitis is Osgood–Schlatter disease (see Chapter 55: "Knee Injuries")

Joints

Description: Overuse joint injuries almost invariably result from mechanical factors such as overload on the joint through repetitive high-impact stress or alignment issues. Although they may create a condition that could be called "arthritis," it may be

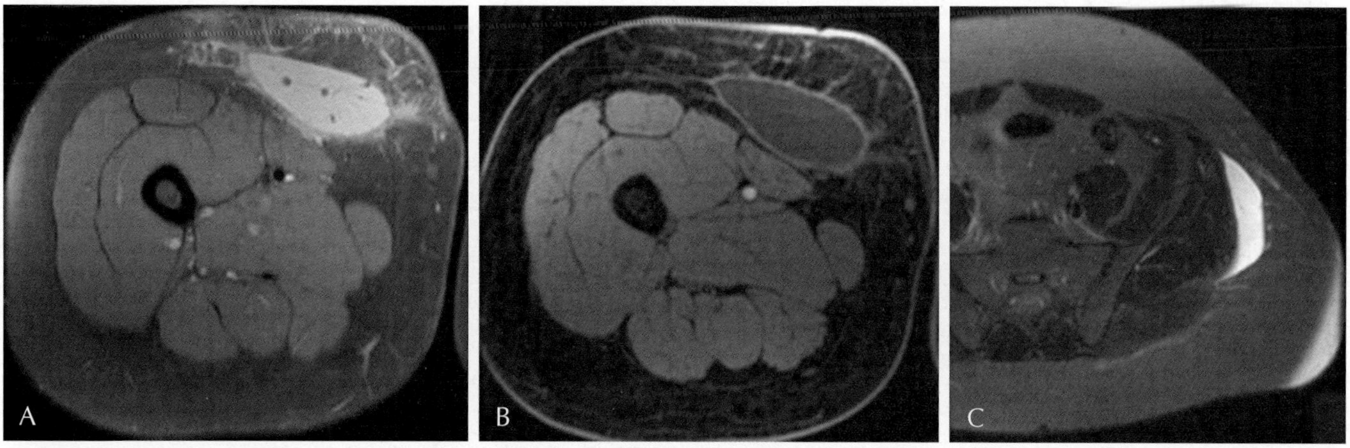
A
B
C

Figure 42.2 MRI demonstrating chronic subcutaneous fluid consistent Morel–Lavellée lesion on anterior lateral thigh. (From Greenhill D, Haydel C, Rehman S. Management of the Morel-Lavallée lesion. *Orthop Clin North Am*. 2016;47[1]:115-125.)

more valid when treating athletes to think of it as synovitis. **Synovitis** may be generalized with swelling, warmth, pain, and occasionally, redness.

Ligament

Description: There are a few examples of pure overuse injuries to ligaments. Theoretically, they may occur whenever a ligament is subjected to repeated stress. Examples include:
- **Medial elbow injuries:** Part of this spectrum may include overuse injury to medial collateral ligament of elbow, resulting from repetitive throwing with valgus loading.
- **Breaststroker's knee:** Probably most common example of pure ligament injury through overuse; typically involves medial collateral ligament of knee at femoral attachment, secondary to a breaststroke kick.
- **Plantar fasciitis:** Technically a ligament connecting bone to bone, the plantar fascia is commonly involved in overuse syndromes of the foot (see Chapter 60: "Foot Problems").

Description: Overuse injury of a muscle–tendon unit may be myositis, tendinitis, or tenosynovitis.

Classification:
- **Myositis** refers to overuse injuries of muscle tissues, which are rather nondescript; can involve practically any muscle in the body
- **Tendinitis** is an inflammatory reaction within the tendon tissue itself. Closely related to the concept of normal aging and degenerative changes within tendons (tendinosis), which may predispose to microtrauma. Common examples are bicipital tendinitis, lateral epicondylitis, and Achilles tendinitis.
- **Tenosynovitis** (peritendinitis) is an inflammatory change that involves tissue surrounding the tendon itself. Classic physical finding is crepitation, or "dry leather creaking" sensation, over the involved tendon as the tendon is moved through its sheath. Common locations include extensor tendons of forearm and tibialis anterior in lower leg.

Other Soft Tissues

Description: Most common overuse musculoskeletal injury involving other soft tissue is **bursitis**. Bursae lie between tissue planes and help reduce frictional stress between structures such as tendon and bone. Common sites for mechanical bursitis in athletes include subacromial bursa, greater trochanteric bursa of hip, and retrocalcaneal bursa in the ankle.

GENERAL TREATMENT OF MUSCULOSKELETAL INJURIES

- Basic athletic first aid: Use the PRICES mnemonic (discussed earlier).
- **Nonsteroidal anti-inflammatory drugs** (NSAIDs) are commonly used in treating musculoskeletal sports injuries. Several different types and brands exist. Choice should always be tempered by known side effects (e.g., renal damage).
- **Physical modalities:** Cold, heat, ultrasound, iontophoresis, and electrical muscle stimulation are commonly used.
- **Therapeutic exercises:** Most important, but the most commonly underused means of treating musculoskeletal sports injuries; important to correct not only deficits that may result from injury but also those that predispose to injury
- **Injection therapy:** Most commonly injected material is corticosteroid, with or without local anesthetic. **Studies have demonstrated a direct harmful effect of steroids on articular cartilage and a weakening effect on tendon** (see Chapter 62: "Injections in the Athlete").
  - **Never inject corticosteroid into major load-bearing tendons** (e.g., patellar tendon or Achilles tendon); **this would pose a significant risk factor for tendon rupture.**
  - **Acceptable** to inject corticosteroid into muscular trigger points, bursae, and small, nonweight-bearing joints (e.g., acromioclavicular joint) and large joints (e.g., knee, shoulder); however, numerous injections in a normal large joint is not recommended; also acceptable to inject corticosteroid into **muscular** attachments into bone, such as lateral epicondyle (**total number** of injections should be limited); ligament attachments to bone where subsequent rupture of ligament would not be disastrous (e.g., plantar fascia attachment to calcaneus); **tendon sheath,** but not the tendon itself (e.g., for de Quervain disease at wrist); and already degenerated joint in older athletes.
- **Braces, supports, and other devices:** Various products have been developed to aid in treatment of athletic injuries, ranging from simple compressive sleeves for various joints to expensive custom-made braces. They are discussed in chapters on anatomic parts and individual sports.
- Calcification excision: Rare

SELECTED MUSCULOSKELETAL EVALUATION TECHNIQUES

Flexibility Testing

Description: Flexibility is limited by length of muscle across joint. Lack of flexibility in two-joint muscles (muscles that cross two joints) is often indicated as cause of musculoskeletal problems. While assessing flexibility, consider whether the restriction seen is the result of muscular tightness or other sources, such as lack of joint range of motion or pain.

Heel cord flexibility: Athlete sits with knee extended and is asked to actively dorsiflex the ankle. Measurement is made goniometrically (Fig. 42.3). Normal value is at least 10 degrees beyond plantigrade. This may also be done with the knee flexed to assess tightness within soleus (normal value is at least 20 degrees beyond plantigrade).

Hamstrings flexibility: Athlete lies supine with hip maintained at a 90-degree flexion and is asked to actively extend knee without repositioning the hip (see Fig. 42.3). Measurement is made goniometrically. Normal value is less than 10 degrees short of full extension.

Quadriceps flexibility: Athlete lies prone and knee is passively flexed by examiner. Normal value is full knee flexion without tilting of pelvis (see Fig. 42.3).

Iliotibial band flexibility: Athlete lies on the opposite side, near edge of the examining table, facing away from the examiner (see Fig. 42.3). Hip on the side to be examined is slightly extended and passively adducted by gravity. Normal is when the knee drops level or below the table level; also called *modified Ober test.*

Strength Testing

Description: Although there are various ways to assess strength, the authors prefer the manual muscle "break" test technique. Athlete generates maximal contraction of muscle in shortened range, and examiner applies opposite force in attempt to move athlete from testing position. Common muscle testing rule is not to apply forces across adjacent joints, but athletes are generally able to adequately support adjacent joints, thus allowing examiner to apply more force to the area in question. Strength is usually graded on a 0–5 scale (0 = zero, 1 = trace, 2 = poor, 3 = fair, 4 = good, and 5 = normal). Most athletic applications are in the upper range of this scale and subjective in nature. Although more objective methods are available, the manual muscle test is the easiest to administer. Hip flexion, hip abduction, and supraspinatus strength tests are included because weakness may indicate a new or unrehabilitated condition more distal in the kinetic chain. Ankle dorsiflexion strength test is included because of a possible association with patellofemoral problems.

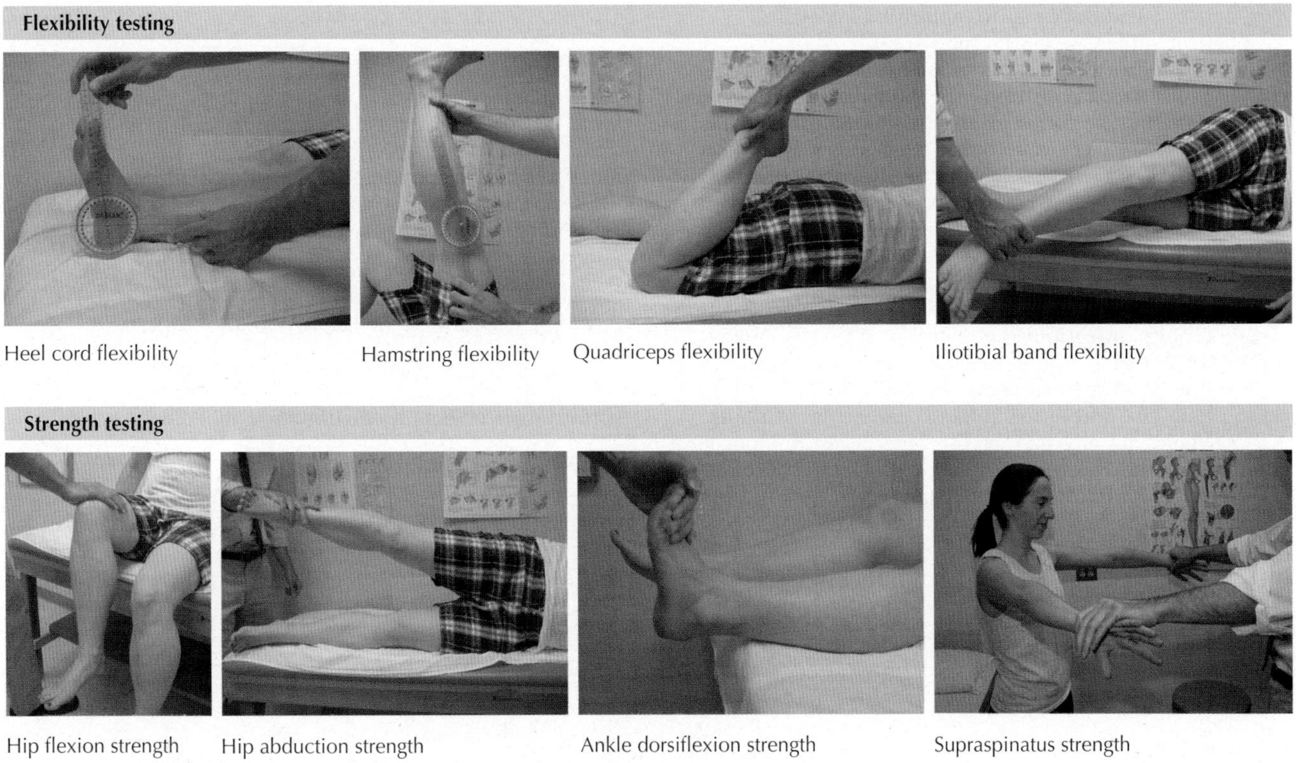
Flexibility testing
Heel cord flexibility
Hamstring flexibility
Quadriceps flexibility
Iliotibial band flexibility
Strength testing
Hip flexion strength
Hip abduction strength
Ankle dorsiflexion strength
Supraspinatus strength

Figure 42.3 Musculoskeletal evaluation techniques.

Hip flexion strength: Athlete sits at edge of the table with arms crossed. Athlete flexes hip and examiner performs a manual muscle "break" test (see Fig. 42.3). If a break occurs, observe whether the identified weakness is located in the hip or in the abdominal obliques.

Hip abduction strength: Athlete lies on the opposite side, facing away from the examiner. Athlete abducts hip and examiner performs a manual muscle "break" test (see Fig. 42.3). If a break occurs, observe whether the identified weakness is located in the hip or in the abdominal obliques.

Ankle dorsiflexion strength: Athlete sits with knee extended and is asked to dorsiflex the ankle. Examiner performs a manual muscle "break" test (see Fig. 42.3).

Supraspinatus strength: Athlete sits or stands with shoulders abducted to 90 degrees, horizontally adducted to 30 degrees, and in a "thumbs-down" position (fully internally rotated). Examiner performs a manual muscle "break" test, taking care to eliminate substitution from the trapezius (see Fig. 42.3).

MYOFASCIAL PAIN SYNDROME

Definitions

- **Myofascial trigger point:** Intensely irritable spot in muscle and/or adjacent fascia that stimulates and sends distress signals to the central nervous system.
  - Feels like an indurated nodule or a "ropey" taut band of muscle
  - Occurs only in characteristic anatomic sites (see later for typical sites in "Diagnosis")
  - Each site has specific "**reference zones**" of radiating/referred pain or paresthesia. Reference zone pain is often the presenting complaint.
  - **May trigger a spasm–pain–spasm cycle** (discussed in later section)
  - **Active trigger point**
    - Symptomatic reference zone pain
    - Palpation reproduces both trigger point tenderness and reference zone pain
  - **Latent trigger point**
    - Tender on examination
    - No reference zone pain
- **Myofascial pain syndrome** (myofascial syndrome): Presence of one or more active trigger points with characteristic reference zone pain
- **Scapulocostal syndrome:** Clustering of trigger point spasms in the trapezius, levator scapula, and posterior cervical muscles

Diagnosis

- **Knowledge of precise anatomic sites** of trigger points and reference zones; common trigger point sites:
  - Levator scapula, splenius capitis, trapezius, and sternocleidomastoid
  - Infraspinatus, supraspinatus, and rhomboids
  - Quadratus lumborum, gluteus medius, and tensor fascia lata
  - Biceps femoris, vastus lateralis, and adductor longus
  - Gastrocnemius/soleus
- **Initiating, precipitating, and perpetuating phenomena**
  - **Physical:**
    - Trauma (major/minor, old/recent)
    - Overuse (sports/exercise, work with repetitive motion, muscle cramps)
    - Inadequate warm-up
    - Cold exercise/work environment
    - Poor posture, poor body mechanics, anatomic abnormalities, and poorly designed or sized workstation (particularly computer worksite)
    - Disease (rheumatoid arthritis or multiple sclerosis)
  - **Mental:** fatigue, anxiety/stress, and depression
- **Palpation of trigger points:** "Rubbery" or "ropey," indurated, tight, and exquisitely tender

Pain–Spasm–Pain Cycle

- Trigger point activation
  - First pain

- Then local muscle activation and fatigue
- Thereafter, increase in pain spreads
- Then, additional trigger points recruited
- This causes more pain, which spreads farther
- "Key" or "matrix" trigger point recruits "satellite" trigger points

Treatment

- **Stretch and spray:** Passive stretching using vapocoolant (fluoromethane) for distraction
- **Massage:** Deep friction or pressure (acupressure); manual, elbow, and dowel
- **Trigger point injection**
  - 0.5% procaine
    - Other local anesthetics may be myotoxic.
    - Dilute 2% procaine with three parts of normal saline.
  - "Needling" by inserting an 18-gauge needle without local anesthetic may inactivate trigger points.
  - Typically, corticosteroids do not provide additional benefits because trigger points contain no inflammatory cells.
- **Therapeutic exercise** improves strength and flexibility.
- **Ice** (heat may exacerbate trigger points)
- Ultrasound
- Muscle energy manipulation techniques

Levator Scapula Syndrome

- Strain of levator scapula insertion with trigger point spasm of muscle body
- Treat trigger points as discussed earlier; may also need to treat muscle insertion with corticosteroid injection, iontophoresis, or phonophoresis

ACKNOWLEDGMENT

The authors would like to acknowledge the contributions of previous edition authors **W. Michael Walsh, MD; Ronnie D. Hald, PT, ATC; Laura E. Peter, MD; and Morris B. Mellion, MD**.

RECOMMENDED READINGS

Available online.

- Several recent studies have found that patients that add neuromuscular electrical stimulation (NMES) to postoperative exercises have stronger quadriceps and a more normal gait pattern than nonusers.
- Biofeedback can also be used to enhance voluntary control of injured musculature.
- Clinically, NMES is used after injury or surgery while the patient performs isometric and isotonic extremity exercises.
- NMES is typically used before biofeedback when the patient presents acutely with the inability to activate the musculature.
- Once independent muscle activation is present, NMES may still be used to recruit additional motor units, thus resulting in greater strength gains.
- NMES is typically used 4–8 weeks after ACL surgery or after selected shoulder surgeries.
- Biofeedback is used for patellofemoral patients when they are unable to actively recruit their vastus medialis; the biofeedback causes the patient to concentrate on neuromuscular control.
- The use of blood flow restriction training has been supported in the literature to increase muscle strength (nm) and muscle size (cross-sectional area).
- These changes are seen even with lower-intensity aerobic (<70 minutes of walking) and anaerobic (20% of 1 repetition maximum) exercise, which is especially beneficial within the rehabilitation setting.
- When the goal of rehabilitation is to retard muscle atrophy and increase muscle size, eccentrics should be emphasized.
- The dynamic lengthening that occurs during eccentric exercise places increased force demands on fewer active fibers, as compared with concentric exercise. This creates higher susceptibility of muscle tissue damage, thereby helping protect the muscle against future injury.
- In early phases of rehabilitation the clinician should be cautious with prescription of eccentric loading because of the higher intensity loads placed on tissue.

Restoration of Dynamic Stability

- Dynamic stability refers to the patient's ability to stabilize a joint during functional activities to avoid injury.
- Dynamic stability involves neuromuscular control and the efferent (motor) output to afferent (sensory) stimulation from the mechanoreceptors.
- Proximal stability should be established to allow for distal segmental mobility to occur within the kinetic chain.
- Dynamic stability of the glenohumeral joint is primarily achieved through interaction of rotator cuff muscles as they blend into the joint capsule.
- Contraction of the rotator cuff produces tension within the joint capsule, which centers the humeral head on the glenoid.
- Muscle weakness or strength imbalances of the posterior cuff muscles may have deleterious effects on shoulder mechanics.
- Emphasis should be placed on linking the upper extremity with the lower extremity. Exercises should link the scapula with the hip, hip with the knee, hip with patellofemoral joint, scapula with the glenohumeral joint, and the scapula with the elbow.
- Exercises to enhance dynamic stability are emphasized immediately after injury or surgery through the use of rhythmic stabilization drills.
- Alternating isometric contractions are performed to facilitate co-contractions of the anterior and posterior rotator cuff.
- Drills are progressed to include stabilization at end ROM and with the patient's eyes closed, particularly for overhead-throwing athletes, in whom dynamic stability is compromised during the throwing motion.

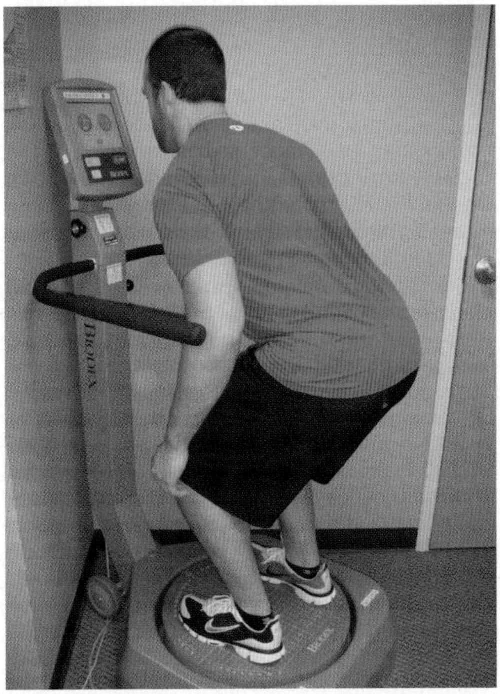

Mini-squats on a force platform that can provide objective feedback of the amount of weight distributed between lower extremities (Balance Trainer, Uni-Cam Inc., Ramsey, NJ).

Figure 43.3 Proprioceptive training.

Restoration of Proprioception and Neuromuscular Control

- Early proprioception and kinesthesia exercises are important for patients returning to sports because researchers have shown a decrease in these abilities after injury.
- Basic exercises designed to enhance the athlete's ability to detect the joint position and movement in space are performed to establish a baseline of motor learning for additional neuromuscular control exercises that will be integrated at a later time.

Proprioceptive Training

- Proprioceptive training initially begins with basic exercises such as joint positioning and closed kinetic-chain weight shifting.
  - Joint repositioning drills begin with an athlete's eyes closed; the rehabilitation specialist passively moves the extremity in various planes of motion and then returns to the starting position.
    - The patient is then instructed to actively reposition the extremity to the location.
    - A therapist may increase the challenge to the patient's proprioceptive system by altering external stimulus such as vision and hearing.
  - Weight shifting should be performed in the medial-lateral direction and in diagonal patterns.
    - Mini-squats on a force platform to ensure equal weight distribution are beneficial (Fig. 43.3).
    - Advancement to mini-squats on an unstable surface such as a tilt board may be used as the patient progresses.
- Several studies have shown that the wearing of an elastic bandage may have a positive effect on proprioception and joint position sense.
- As proprioception is advanced, drills to encourage preparatory agonist–antagonist co-activation during functional activities are incorporated.

Dynamic Stabilization Drills

- Dynamic stabilization drills begin with single-leg stance on flat ground and unstable surfaces, cone stepping, and lateral lunge drills.
- The patient may perform forward, backward, and lateral cone step-over drills to facilitate gait training, enhance dynamic stability, and train the hip to help control forces at the knee joint.
- Cone drills may be performed at various speeds to train the lower extremity to dynamically stabilize with different amounts of momentum.
- Lateral lunges are also performed, with the patient advancing from straight plane lateral lunges, to multiplanar/diagonal lunges, to lunges with rotation, and finally to lateral lunges onto foam (Fig. 43.4A).
- CLX TheraBand training can be used to target the musculature of the hip and core. Lateral slide drills with concomitant shoulder proprioceptive neuromuscular facilitation (PNF) D2 patterns not only link the upper extremities with the lower extremities but also place emphasis on the core and hips.
- Concentration may be challenged by adding a ball toss to any of these exercises, which challenges preparatory stabilization.
- Single-leg balance exercises are progressed by altering a patient's center of gravity and incorporating movement of the upper extremity and uninvolved lower extremity (see Fig. 43.4B).
- Perturbation training may also be incorporated into such exercises with single- or double-leg balance exercises on a tilt board (see Fig. 43.4C).
    - The patient performs an isometric hold of the tilt board with the knee flexed to 30 degrees while catching a light medicine ball.
    - The patient is instructed to stabilize the tilt board in reaction to the sudden outside force produced by the weighted ball.
    - The rehabilitation specialist can also challenge the athlete by providing manual perturbations by striking the tilt board with his or her foot to create a sudden disturbance in the static support of the lower extremity; this requires the patient to stabilize the board with dynamic muscular contractions.
- Exercises such as balance beam walking, lunges onto an unstable surface, and step-up exercises while standing on an unstable surface are also used to strengthen the knee musculature while requiring the muscles located proximally and distally within the kinetic chain to stabilize and allow coordinated functional movement patterns.
- Exercises that challenge dynamic stability are particularly important in the rehabilitation setting because research suggests that after injury participants demonstrate increased activity in brain regions that play a major role in working memory functions, memory processing, information processing, and attention in cognitive and sensorimotor tasks.
- Plyometric jumping drills are performed to facilitate dynamic stabilization and neuromuscular control (see Fig. 43.4D).
    - Plyometrics use the muscle's stretch-shortening properties to produce maximal contraction after a rapid eccentric loading of the muscle tissue.
    - Plyometric training is used to train the extremities to produce and dissipate forces to avoid injury.

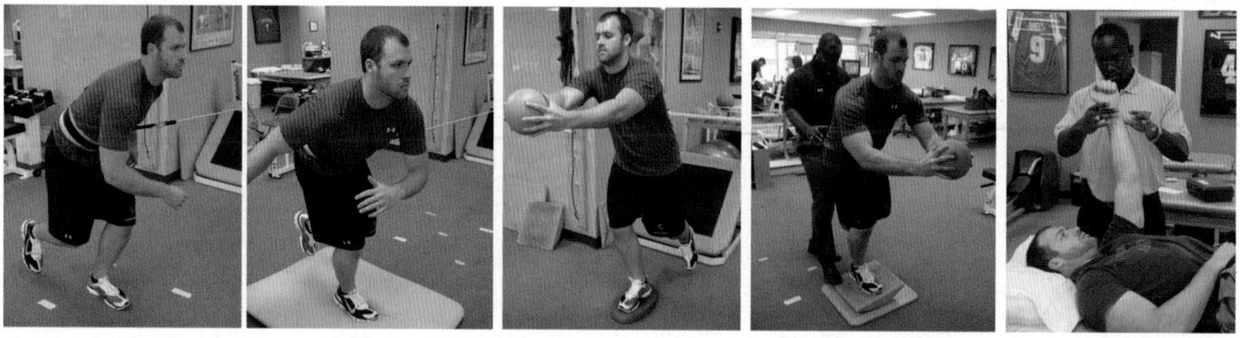

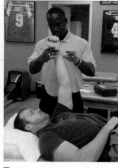

A. Lateral lunges using a sport-cord onto an unstable surface.

B. Single leg balance on an unstable surface while incorporating alternating upper extremities movements with a weighted ball to alter the patient's center of gravity.

C. Single leg balance on a tilt-board while the patient tosses a ball against a rebound device. The rehabilitation specialist may create a perturbation by striking the board.

D. Rhythmic stabilization to promote co-contraction of the rotator cuff. The patient is asked to hold the arm steady while the therapist gives alternating forces to the extremity.

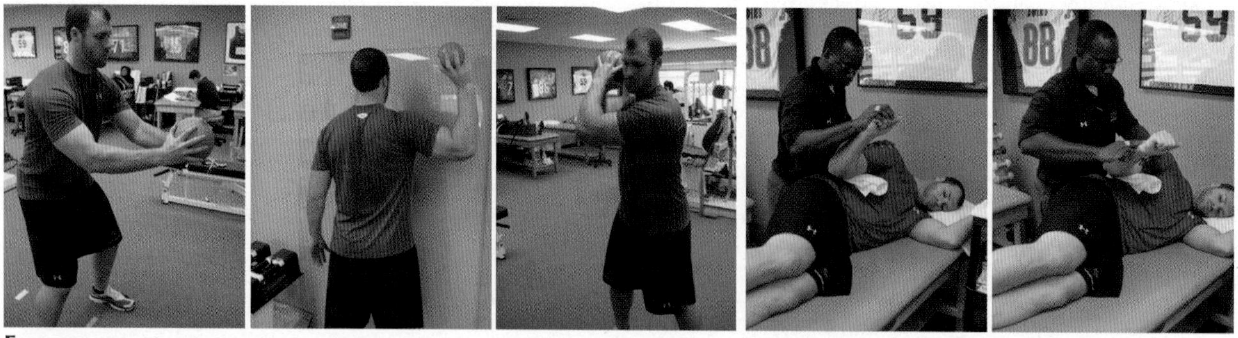

E. Upper extremity plyometrics. a. Chest pass using a trampoline and medicine ball. **b.** Single arm wall throws with the patient's arm at 90 degrees of abduction and 90 degrees of elbow flexion. **c.** Side to side throws using a medicine ball and trampoline.

F. Manual resistance during sidelying external resistance. The rehabilitation specialist resisted both external rotation and retraction of the scapula. Rhythmic stabilizations may also be performed at end range.

Figure 43.4 Dynamic stabilization drills.

Neuromuscular Control Drills

- The final aspect of rehabilitation regarding neuromuscular control involves enhancing muscular endurance.
  - Proprioceptive and neuromuscular control has been shown to diminish once muscular fatigue occurs.
  - Exercises such as bicycle, stair climbing, and elliptical machines are used to increase endurance.
  - High-repetition, low-weight resistance weight training can also increase muscular endurance.
- An additional strategy to protect the athlete from reinjury is to perform neuromuscular control drills at the end of treatment sessions after cardiovascular training.
  - This challenges the neuromuscular control of the knee joint after the dynamic stabilizers have been fatigued.
- Enhancement of neuromuscular control is equally important in the upper extremity.
  - Efficient dynamic stabilization and neuromuscular control of the glenohumeral joint are necessary for athletes to avoid injuries during competition.
  - Dynamic stabilization exercises for the upper extremity also begin with baseline proprioception and kinesthesia drills.
  - Rhythmic stabilization is also incorporated to facilitate co-contraction of the rotator cuff and dynamic stability of the glenohumeral joint (see Fig. 43.4E).
  - Exercise involves alternating isometric contractions designed to promote co-contraction and basic reactive neuromuscular control (see Fig. 43.4F).
- These dynamic stabilization techniques may be applied as the athlete progresses to provide advanced challenges to the neuromuscular control system.
- As an athlete progresses through the program, it is necessary to train the upper extremity to provide adequate dynamic stabilization in response to sudden forces, particularly at end ROM (referred to as *reactive neuromuscular control*).

Gradually Restore Muscular Strength and Endurance

- Gradually restore muscular strength after volitional muscle activity is achieved.
- Baseline levels of muscular strength are needed before the athlete can progress to the later stages of rehabilitation.
- Strengthening can be performed through various different methods of isotonic exercises.
  - Weight is gradually applied and increased as the athlete progressively improves strength.
- Isotonics can be used in the form of single- or multiple-joint exercises.
- Exercises can also be performed in either an open kinetic chain (OKC) or closed kinetic chain (CKC).
  - OKC exercise is defined as a movement wherein the distal extremity is not fixed, such as a leg extension.
  - CKC exercise is defined as an exercise wherein the distal extremity is fixed, such as a leg press.
  - These exercises both have a place in rehabilitation, although they have different effects on both muscular activity and biomechanics of the joint, as shown by multiple electromyographic activity studies.
- Muscular endurance is an important factor in rehabilitation programs.
  - Several activities related to athletics involve repetitive and microtraumatic events.
  - Training the musculature to endure these events is necessary to prevent injuries.
  - Fatigue has been shown to result in decreased proprioception and altered biomechanics of the joints, which may result in further pathology.

Normalization of Soft Tissue Mobility and Flexibility

- Rehabilitation of soft tissues to restore tissue balance applies to both soft tissue around the joints, such as retinacular tissue surrounding the patella, and muscular flexibility around each joint.
- Deviations in the balance of soft tissue forces will promote altered arthrokinematics and excessive forces to the joints.
- Muscular flexibility is vital to normal joint function because it allows the musculature to absorb force and align the joint in neutral position. For example:
  - Soft tissue tightness of the quadriceps muscle is common among people with patellar tendonitis and patellofemoral pain. In the upper extremity, patients commonly experience tightness of the anterior structures, which can lead to several pathologies such as impingement syndrome.
- It is critical for the clinician to identify the causes of loss of motion and treat involved structures based on assessment.

Emphasis on the Entire Kinetic Chain

- Rehabilitation must be focused not only on regaining strength and neuromuscular control of the affected joint but also on the surrounding areas. For example, neuromuscular control of the shoulder involves stability of not only the glenohumeral joint but also the scapulothoracic joint.
- Core stabilization drills are used to further enhance proximal stability with distal mobility of the extremities:
  - This is based on the kinetic chain concept, wherein imbalance at any point of the kinetic chain may result in pathology throughout.
  - Movement patterns, such as throwing, require a precise interaction of the entire body kinetic chain to be efficiently performed.
  - A multiphase approach is used, progressing from baseline core and trunk strengthening, to intermediate core strengthening with distal mobility, to advanced stabilization in sport-specific movement patterns.
- Imbalances of strength, flexibility, endurance, or stability may result in fatigue, abnormal arthrokinematics, and subsequent compensation.
- It is important to not neglect the uninjured extremity:
  - Numerous studies have indicated a crossover effect when the contralateral extremity is exercised, which may lead to improvements in proprioception and strength of the involved extremity.
  - The neuromuscular control system may have a certain amount of central mediating function receptive to bilateral training techniques.
  - When rehabilitating a patient with a joint injury, the rehabilitation specialist must consider having the patient perform either bilateral exercises or unilateral reciprocal exercises.

Gradual Return to Functional Activities

- After successful completion of the rehabilitation program, the athlete must begin a gradual return-to-sport program.
- Interval sport programs (ISPs) are designed to gradually return motion, function, and confidence to the athlete after injury or surgery by slowly progressing through graduated sport-specific activities.
  - Goal of this phase is to gradually and progressively increase functional demands on the athlete.
- Criteria before returning to sport-specific activities are:
  - Full-functional ROM
  - Adequate static and dynamic stability
  - Satisfactory muscular strength and endurance
  - Satisfactory clinical examination
- Once criteria are met, a gradual return-to-sport activity is initiated in a controlled manner.

- Healing constraints based on surgical technique and fixation, as well as the patient's tissue status, should be considered.
- ISP is set up to minimize chance of reinjury and emphasize precompetition warm-up and stretching.
- There should be no set timetable for completing the ISP because of individual differences.
  - Variability will exist based on skill level, goals, and injury of each athlete.
- The ISP is developed based on the specific sport and stresses observed during these athletic activities. For example, overhead-throwing athletes must perform an interval throwing program that includes a limited amount of throws using a flat-ground long toss.
- Other goals are to maintain a patient's muscular strength, dynamic stability, and functional motion established in the previous phase.
  - A stretching and strengthening program should be performed on an ongoing basis to maintain and improve these goals.
- Rate of progression with functional activities is dictated by the patient's unique tolerance for activities.
  - Exercise must be performed at a tolerable level without overstressing the healing tissue—referred to as the patient's *envelope of function*.
- The athlete's return to sport-specific drills progresses through a series of transitional drills designed to progressively challenge the neuromuscular control system. Examples include:
  - Pool running before flat-ground running
  - Backward and lateral running before forward running
  - Plyometrics before running-and-cutting drills and, finally, sport-specific drills
- Integration of functional activities is necessary to train the injured patient to perform specific movement patterns necessary for daily activities.
- The intention of sport-specific training is to stimulate the functional activities associated with sports while incorporating peripheral afferent stimulation with reflexive and preprogrammed muscle control and co-activation.
  - Drills may be modified based on specific functional movement patterns that are unique to the patient's sport.
- Sport-specific training can include side-to-side shuffle, cariocas, sudden starts and stops, 45-degree cutting, 90-degree cutting, and various combination movements.
- Sport-specific patterns learned throughout the rehabilitation program are integrated to provide challenges in a controlled setting.
- Drills are performed to train the neuromuscular control system to perform during competition in a reflexive pattern.

Lower Extremity Return to Play

- Many components go into determining whether an individual is ready to return to play or not. Although subjective examination is critical, clinicians should aim to obtain as much objective data as they can to justify their decision to allow an individual to return to activity.
- The subjective scales used to determine an individual's perception of their own readiness for activity include the clinical knee rating score (Barber and Noyes, 1999), the international knee documentation scale (Irrgang, 2006), and the Tampa scale for kinesiophobia (Woby et al., 2005).
- Objectively, many measures can be used to determine an individual's preparedness for activity.
- Isokinetic testing utilizing a Biodex (if available) is a great clinical tool to objectively measure a participant's strength. After performing a standardized warm-up, the individual will perform 10 to 15 repetitions of leg extension and curl from 100 to 0 degrees against a distal pad set to 180 degrees per second and 300 degrees per second.
  - Overall, the individual should score within 85%–90% during bilateral strength comparison at both speeds. Additionally when set to 300 degrees per second, the individual should demonstrate bilateral extension strength within 12% and flexion within 9%.
  - When analyzing the measurements during participation at 180 degrees per individual should have:
    - Peak torque time body weight for quadriceps: males: 60%–65% and females: 50%–55%
    - Quadriceps to hamstrings ratio: males: 66%–70% and females: 69%–75%
    - Bilateral quadriceps comparison: 85%–90%
    - Time to peak torque at 0.2 of a second: 90%>
- **Sport-specific tests are important to perform in addition to:**
  - Front step-down
  - Hop tests (single leg, crossover, triple)
  - Agility and shuttle runs
  - Y balance test
  - Functional movement screen
  - A score <14 (+ asymmetry) was predictive of injury risk with a specificity of 91 and sensitivity of 54 (Keisel et al., 2007)

SPECIFIC REHABILITATION PROGRAMS

Anterior Cruciate Ligament

- Over a 20-year period, ACL surgery procedures have increased by 58% with 148,714 ACL surgeries performed in 2013 (PearlDiver Technologies. PearlDiver supercomputer database.
- ACL rehabilitation programs have dramatically changed over the past 20 years.
- Currently, a scientifically based program that takes into account the patient's functional demands is critical to maximize outcomes.
- Emphasis is now on immediate ROM, full passive knee extension, immediate weight-bearing, and activation of the quadriceps musculature through NMES.
- The rehabilitation program begins preoperatively through education of the patient and family on both the surgical procedure and rehabilitation progression.
- Preoperative goals include reduction of pain and swelling, restoration of ROM, gait normalization, and prevention of muscular atrophy.
- Postoperative rehabilitation begins 1–2 days after surgery.
- Initial sessions include the initiation of ROM activities and to assure patient that weight-bearing with the use of crutches is encouraged.
  - Primary goals at this point are to reduce swelling, restore full extension, and activate quads. Expectations are that the patient should be able to bear full weight in a hinged brace without the use of crutches at 10–14 days after surgery.
  - Expectations are that the patient should be able to bear full weight in a hinged brace without the use of crutches at 10–14 days after surgery.
- Full passive knee extension is attained as quickly as possible with gradual restoration of flexion ROM and patella mobility.
- OKC exercises with the use of NMES, followed by incorporation of CKC exercises, can be introduced 2 weeks after surgery.
- Machine weights may be introduced approximately 3–4 weeks after surgery, including leg press and multi-hip (abduction, extension, and adduction).
- Hip- and core-strengthening exercises are essential from a functional standpoint to prevent faulty biomechanical stresses on the knee. Activities should aim to control femur internal rotation, lateral trunk displacement, valgus knee collapse, and pelvic drop.
- CKC exercises and neuromuscular control drills may be progressed as tolerated to include perturbation training on unstable surfaces.
- Light plyometric jumping may be initiated 8–10 weeks after surgery.
- Functional activities such as jogging may begin shortly after plyometrics with progression to running and jumping at 10–14 weeks.

- Careful attention should be paid to avoid overstressing the athlete during this phase; the development of patella tendonitis is possible, particularly if adequate quadriceps strength has not yet returned.
- Educating the female athlete on appropriate jumping and landing techniques should be included; this has been shown to reduce the incidence of future ACL injuries in the athletic population.
- Finally, the athlete can gradually return to cutting sports such as baseball, football, and tennis approximately 4–6 months after surgery, but a return to jumping sports (e.g., basketball and volleyball) should be delayed until 6–8 months after surgery.

Superior Labral Anterior to Posterior Repairs

- Nonoperative rehabilitation is often successful in type I and II SLAP lesions with a sequential, multiphased program.
- Better understanding of the normal labral anatomy and healing constraints after a repair procedure will make a successful return to unrestricted function very likely.
- Successful return to the patient's prior level of function can be attained through communication by the surgeon with the rehabilitation team and patient; activity should be restricted until adequate healing response is obtained.
- Before initiating rehabilitation, a thorough subjective and clinical examination should be performed to identify the nature of the labral pathology and mechanism of injury.
  - This will aid the rehabilitation specialist after surgery while advancing the patient through the protocol.
- There are certain restrictions to a patient's rehabilitation process that can be unique based on the method of injury. For example:
  - Patients who have sustained labral injury after falling onto an outstretched hand would be encouraged to avoid closed-chain and weight-bearing activities.
  - Patients with traction injuries should avoid heavy biceps resistance activities, particularly those involving the eccentric phase of muscle contraction.
  - Overhead-throwing athletes with superior labral injuries should avoid excessive external rotation until an adequate healing time (at least 8 weeks) has passed.
- Mechanism of injury is a crucial factor to consider as the patient progresses through the rehabilitation program.
- Rehabilitation after a SLAP type II repair presents a significant challenge but should render the patient with good to excellent outcomes.
  - This type of labral lesion is commonly seen in overhead-throwing athletes with the biceps tendon detached from its glenoid rim attachment.
- Initially, the goal of rehabilitation is to control the forces placed on the healing tissue.
- Gradual passive and active-assisted ROM activities are performed below 90 degrees of flexion for the first 4 weeks (see Fig. 43.1).
  - Passive external rotation is allowed only to approximately 15 degrees in the scapular plane.
  - The patient is instructed to sleep in an immobilizer for 4 weeks.
- ROM activities are progressed beyond 90 degrees of flexion, with full flexion at 6–8 weeks after surgery.
- External rotation ROM is progressed to 90 degrees of abduction at 4 weeks after surgery, and motion is gradually increased until completely restored (115–125 degrees) by approximately 8 weeks after surgery.
- Isometric strengthening activities are immediately performed to prevent muscle atrophy as a result of the immobilization.
- Rhythmic stabilization drills are also initiated with the patient in the supine position and the shoulder in the scapula plane and neutral rotation.
- These activities promote dynamic stability and neuromuscular control of the humeral head within the glenoid while the scapula is stabilized by the table.
- Active joint-repositioning exercises after passive displacement are also used to enhance proprioception.
- External rotation/internal rotation tubing exercises are initiated during week 3–4 with the arm at 0 degrees abduction along with lateral raises, full can (scaption), and scapula stabilization drills.
- At approximately week 6–7, the Thrower's Ten program is initiated; this program places emphasis on external rotator and scapula strengthening.
- No isolated biceps strengthening should be performed for the first 8 weeks to protect the healing biceps attachment into the labrum.
- Isotonic strengthening can be progressed by 1 pound per 7–10 days as long as there is no increase in pain or soreness.
- More aggressive strengthening such as manual resistance exercises, PNF, and two-handed plyometrics may be added at 10–12 weeks after surgery.
- Functional activities such as one-handed plyometrics in the 90/90 position into a trampoline may be initiated approximately 2–3 weeks after initiation of two-handed plyometric drills.
- At week 12, machine weights such as lat pull-downs and seated presses may be incorporated.
- The interval hitting program may also be initiated at week 12; this comprises a gradual progression beginning with hitting of a tee, progressing to soft toss, and finally taking batting practice off a live pitcher.
- At week 16, the athlete may begin the interval throwing program.
  - Athlete begins at 45 feet and progresses to 60, 90, and 120 feet.
  - After the 120-foot phase, the athlete may begin flat-ground throwing using pitching mechanics.
  - After completion of the flat-ground throwing step is when the athlete can begin throwing fastballs off the mound at 50% of the athlete's normal velocity.
  - Velocity and number of pitches are gradually increased.
  - The throwing program takes approximately 4–6 months depending on timing of the upcoming season, position played, or any concomitant procedures performed during surgery that may delay onset or progression of the program.
- Typically, return to play after a type II SLAP repair occurs at approximately 9–12 months after surgery.
- Rehabilitation should be based on the specific injury (mechanism or location), the surgery performed, and the ultimate functional goals of the patient.
- Gradual restoration of ROM, strength, endurance, and dynamic stability is critical, but it must be applied in a controlled manner to minimize stress on the healing tissue.
- The ultimate goal is to return the patient to prior level of function as safely and as quickly as possible without deleterious consequences.

Ulnar Collateral Ligament Reconstruction

- Overhead-throwing athletes are susceptible to numerous elbow injuries because of the strong forces that act on the elbow during the throwing motion.
- The ulnar collateral ligament (UCL) is the primary medial stabilizer of the elbow and is subject to high valgus stresses, particularly during the late cocking phase of the throwing motion.
- Injuries are caused by chronic stresses or repetitive microtrauma to the medial soft tissue structures that result from the athlete's attempts to stabilize the elbow joint.
- There exists a medial shear force of 300 N and a compressive force of 900 N.

- The valgus stress that is applied to the medial elbow during the late cocking and acceleration phase of throwing is 64 N, which exceeds the strength of the UCL.
- Surgical reconstruction is employed to regain normal stabilizing function of the UCL, particularly the anterior bundle.
  - Autologous graft sources are typically either the palmaris longus tendon or the gracilis tendon.
  - Ulnar nerve transposition is often concomitantly performed at the time of reconstruction as well.
- Rehabilitation after UCL reconstruction is vital to fully restore normal function and return the athlete to competition as quickly and safely as possible.
  - Rehabilitation must be progressed to restore full ROM, strength, dynamic stability, and neuromuscular control while protecting the healing tissues.
- Rehabilitation generally commences before surgery through an educational component with the athlete and the family; this should include progression, brace use, and prognosis.
- Preoperative ROM measurements are generally obtained to gauge how much motion recovery after surgery should be expected.
- A general strength assessment is also performed of both the elbow joint and the shoulder joint musculature.
- Immediately after surgery, the elbow is placed in a 90-degree splint for the first 5 days; this allows for adequate healing of the UCL graft and soft tissue sling of the transposed ulnar nerve.
- The patient performs wrist ROM and gripping exercises to improve overall circulation of the distal upper extremity.
- After approximately 5 days, the athlete is placed in a hinged elbow brace, which is adjusted to allow 30–100 degrees of ROM.
  - Motion is increased 10 degrees in each direction per week until full ROM is obtained at approximately 4–5 weeks after surgery.
- Strengthening exercises progress from isometric contractions to isotonic exercises by week 4.
- The full Thrower's Ten program may be performed using light weights by week 6.
- Progressive resistance exercises for the elbow and shoulder dynamic stabilizers are emphasized through postoperative weeks 8–10.
- Wrist flexor and extensor stretches to increase flexibility are also incorporated at this time.
- Aggressive exercises involving eccentric and plyometric contractions are included, starting at weeks 9–12.
- Two-handed plyometrics are added at week 10, and one-handed plyometrics are added approximately 2–3 weeks later.
- Interval throwing begins at approximately week 16.
- Return to competitive throwing usually occurs at approximately 8–10 months after surgery.

RECOMMENDED READINGS

Available online.

PHYSICAL MODALITIES IN SPORTS MEDICINE 44

Sophia Gonzalez • Catherine Miller

GENERAL PRINCIPLES

A modality is the application of a therapeutic treatment in order to elicit an adaptive response within the body. The aim of modalities is to create an optimal healing environment. They are external treatments best thought of as an adjunct to the body's own recovery process. Although they should not be the only treatment, they show value in the sports medicine realm by speeding up the return-to-play process. Some experts may claim that certain modalities are an integral part of healing and recovery from injury, although minimal evidence exists to support many claims.

THERMOTHERAPY

Thermotherapy uses devices to conduct thermal energy via direct contact with skin to increase tissue temperature. The depth of thermal energy conduction is dependent on the method and duration of treatment application.

An increase in tissue temperature has the following therapeutic effects:

- Vasodilation
- Increased blood flow
- Increased cell metabolism
- Increased elasticity of collagen tissues
- Decreased pain
- Decreased muscle spasm
- Decreased joint stiffness

Methods of Thermotherapy

- Moist heat pack
  - Canvas covers filled with silica gel that come in varying sizes
  - Heated in hot water tanks (approximately 160°F [71°C])
  - Placed in insulating layers of clean towels or cloth covers
  - Heat dissipates quickly
  - Easier to get the patient in a comfortable position
  - Treatment duration: 10–20 minutes
- Dry heat pad
  - Plug-in electrical or microwaveable varieties
  - Do not heat tissue as rapidly and comfortably as moist heat packs
  - Skin can be burned by prolonged or overly intense heat exposure
  - Treatment duration: 10–20 minutes
- Whirlpool
  - The body part is immersed in a tub of water that has a motor for circulation
  - Water temperature usually ranges between 92°F and 110°F [33°C and 43°C], lower temperatures used with larger treatment areas
  - Water circulation keeps the temperature next to the skin constant and has a massaging effect
  - Care must be taken to keep open wounds and tank clean to prevent transmission of bacteria and infection
  - Treatment duration: 10–20 minutes
- Paraffin bath
  - Mixture of wax and mineral oil melted to a liquid state (126°F–130°F [52°C–54°C])
  - Low specific heat of wax allows for comfort at higher temperatures
  - Apply multiple coats to a body part by dipping or brushing on, then allow to cool, which transfers heat into body tissues
  - Effective with irregularly shaped body parts such as hands and feet
  - Treatment duration: 10–15 minutes

Active Warm-Up

Exercise is the most effective at deep heating, as heat is a by-product of muscular work. Heat is transmitted from muscle into other body tissues and is carried away by the bloodstream. The more intense the exercise, the greater and quicker the heating. The benefits of using active exercise for tissue heating go beyond the thermal effects. Active warm-up increases vasodilation for increased speed of oxygen flow, heart rate elevation, achievement of metabolic steady state faster than with passive heating, and possibly lower lactate accumulation.

Thermotherapy Indications

- Subacute conditions
- Chronic inflammatory conditions
- Pain modulation
- General relaxation
- Decreased range of motion
- Hematoma
- In preparation for therapeutic exercise
- Injuries wherein the goal of treatment is to increase circulation

Thermotherapy Contraindications

- Acute injuries (risk of increased swelling)
- Circulatory insufficiency
- Poor thermal regulation
- Anesthetic areas
- Fever
- Skin conditions
- Uncovered open wounds
- Tumors
- Thrombophlebitis
- Nerve sensitivities

Thermotherapy Precautions

- Fair skin that burns easily
- Areas of decreased sensation
- Dermatologic problems and disease transmittal
- Vasovagal response

CRYOTHERAPY

Cryotherapy involves the loss of thermal energy via skin with the application of a cold modality. As with thermotherapy, the depth of thermal energy conduction is dependent on the method and duration of treatment application. A decrease in tissue temperature has the following therapeutic effects:

- Vasoconstriction
- Decreased blood flow
- Decreased swelling
- Reduction in inflammatory mediators
- Reduction in pain-producing substances
- Decreased cell metabolism
- Reduced elasticity in collagen tissues
- Analgesia

- Decreased muscle spasm
- Increased joint stiffness

Methods of Cryotherapy

- Ice bag
  - More conforming to the body part, which also results in greater cold effects
  - Treatment duration: 15–20 minutes
- Reusable ice pack
  - Silica gel pack kept in a freezer that allows for multiple uses
  - To avoid potential skin irritation because of lower temperatures specific to reusable ice packs, apply insulating layer between the pack and skin
  - Treatment duration: 15–20 minutes
- Chemical cold pack
  - Water and ammonium nitrate separated within a pack until ready to use
  - Chemicals mix when barrier is broken by squeezing
  - More expensive than ice bag or reusable ice pack
  - Chemicals can irritate skin if bag leaks
  - Treatment duration: 10–15 minutes
- Ice cup massage
  - Water frozen in paper or plastic cups applied directly to skin in circular massaging motions
  - Limited to small treatment areas and requires active participation
  - Treatment duration: 5–10 minutes (or until analgesia is achieved)
- Cold-water immersion
  - The body part is immersed in a tub of water and ice
  - Whirlpool uses a motor for circulation that keeps the temperature next to the skin constant and has a massaging effect
  - Water temperature usually ranges between 50°F and 65°F (10°C and 18°C), higher temperatures used with larger treatment areas
  - Care must be taken to keep open wounds and tank clean to prevent transmission of bacteria and infection
  - Treatment duration: 10–20 minutes
- Whole-body cryotherapy (cryosauna)
  - A device (chamber- or barrel-like) that exposes the minimally dressed patient to extreme cold (<–212°F [–100°C]) via liquid nitrogen and refrigerated air
  - Currently, research on the effectiveness of whole-body cryotherapy is inconclusive, with the majority supporting effectiveness for relieving inflammatory conditions and symptoms and improving postexercise recovery
  - Treatment duration: no longer than 3 minutes
- Vapocooling sprays
  - Chemical spray (ethyl chloride) topically applied on skin that cools immediately and evaporates quickly
  - Used whenever quick numbing is desired; trigger point treatment
- Cryokinetics
  - Combination of cryotherapy with exercise in order to achieve normal range of motion using analgesia of the injured area
  - Exercise is done progressively and in pain-free ranges and can have multiple applications of cryotherapy

Cryotherapy Indications

- Pain modulation
- Swelling control
- Desired analgesia effect
- Muscle recovery
- Muscle spasm
- Heat-related illness
- Inconclusive evidence for improvement of delayed-onset muscle soreness

Cryotherapy Contraindications

- Uncovered open wounds
- Circulatory insufficiency
- Cold allergy/urticaria
- Anesthetic area
- Advanced diabetes
- Peripheral vascular disease
- Raynaud phenomenon
- Rheumatoid arthritis
- Lupus
- Hypertension
- History of vascular impairment (i.e., frostbite or arteriosclerosis)
- Paroxysmal cold hemoglobinuria
- Hypothyroidism (cryosauna)
- Acute respiratory disorders (cryosauna)

Cryotherapy Precautions

- Hypertension requires careful monitoring, and treatment should be discontinued if increases are shown
- Elderly patients
- Extended treatment could cause injury to superficial peripheral nerves
- Claustrophobia (cryosauna)

THERMOTHERAPY VERSUS CRYOTHERAPY

- In general, thermotherapy is used for stiffness and cryotherapy is used for pain
- Only cryotherapy should be used with injuries in the acute inflammatory phase (~24–72 hours postinjury)
- Thermotherapy can be safely applied when out of the acute inflammatory phase
- Only thermotherapy should be used before activity, exercise is the most optimal modality to achieve deep heating effects

CONTRAST THERAPY

- Alternating thermotherapy and cryotherapy applications to achieve neurogenic and cardiovascular effects for pain control, reducing fatigue, reducing delayed-onset muscle soreness, and swelling control
- Most common method involves whirlpool; however, other methods may be used
- Evidence suggests contrast therapy is superior to passive recovery but shows little difference compared with other recovery interventions
- Treatment duration: warm:cold 1–3:1 for 10–20 minutes; no data for optimal dosage

THERAPEUTIC ULTRASOUND

Therapeutic ultrasound (US) uses acoustic energy inaudible to the human ear to create metabolic changes at the cellular level via a coupling agent. Continuous US delivers a constant stream of energy, whereas pulsed US delivers energy in time-specific bursts. Treatment frequency is generally between 0.7 and 3.3 megahertz (MHz). Frequency and depth of penetration have an inverse relationship; 1 MHz penetrates 2–5 cm into the skin and 3MHz penetrates 1–2 cm into the skin. US can have the following therapeutic effects depending on the parameters chosen:

- Thermal effects (continuous US):
  - Increased tissue temperature 1–5 cm below skin surface
  - Increased circulation, which may increase metabolic rate
  - Increased soft tissue extensibility
  - Reduced muscle spasm
  - Pain modulation

- Nonthermal effects (pulsed and continuous US):
  - Acoustic streaming movement of fluids along cell membranes
  - Cavitation formation of gas-filled bubbles that can change cellular diffusion gradients
  - Micromassage-microscopic movement of fluids that is theorized to stimulate mechanoreceptors
- The treatment area is two to three times the size of the device's sound head, called the *effective radiating area (ERA)*. If a larger area is desired, multiple treatments will be needed or another modality should be considered.
- Sound head must be kept moving (~2 inches/second) during the treatment to mitigate adverse effects and discomfort
- Treatment duration: 1–10 minutes dependent on desired treatment effects

US Indications

- Pain modulation
- Muscle spasm reduction
- Increase soft tissue extensibility
- Bone and wound healing
- Plantar wart management

US Contraindications

- Bleeding or active infection
- Deep vein thrombosis or thrombophlebitis
- Cancer
- External fixation devices
- Around eyes, heart, skull, genitals, or central nervous system tissue
- Over the trunk during pregnancy

US Precautions

- Epiphyseal plates
- Fracture or bone pathology
- Injury in the acute inflammatory phase

Phonophoresis

Phonophoresis involves the use of therapeutic US to assist the diffusion of topical medications through the skin and into the target tissues. Improving cellular permeability is the main proposed mechanism, and both thermal and nonthermal parameters may be used depending on the treatment goal. Common medications used are topical analgesics and anti-inflammatories. Medication absorption is influenced by the following:

- Water content of skin
- Patient age
- Thickness of skin
- Vascularity

Ultrasonic Osteogenesis Stimulator

Ultrasonic osteogenesis stimulators use low-intensity pulsed US to facilitate fracture healing. These devices are separate machines from traditional therapeutic US machines with different settings. Treatment duration is 20 minutes/day.

ELECTRICAL STIMULATION

Electrical stimulation uses electrical current delivered via wired electrodes to create cellular changes in the target tissue. Different therapeutic effects are achieved by manipulating the following parameters: waveform, modulation, intensity, duration, frequency, polarity, and electrode placement (Table 44.1). Equipment used includes therapeutic electrical generators, both portable and nonportable, and electrodes. Modern devices have preprogrammed parameters to ensure patient safety and ease of use. Electrical stimulation has the following therapeutic effects:

- Increased cellular metabolism via mitochondrial stimulation
- Pain modulation
- Elicit muscle contraction to increase blood flow locally
- Stimulation of sensory, motor, and/or nerve fibers

Types of Current

- Direct/monophasic
  - Continuous, unidirectional flow of charged particles
  - Electrodes represent positive and negative poles to facilitate current flow in one direction
- Alternating/biphasic
  - Continuous bidirectional flow of charged particles
  - Current flow moves toward one pole of the circuit then changes direction to the opposite pole; no polar effects
- Pulsatile
  - Discontinuous delivery of electrical current
  - Can be direct or alternating
  - Has an on period and an off period, stimulating electrical current delivery in "pulses"

Electrode Placement

- Monopolar
  - Large dispersive pad placed away from treatment area and a small active pad placed over the treatment area
  - Used for polar effects such as wound healing, edema reduction, and medication delivery
- Bipolar
  - Two pads of the same size
  - Treatment area between the electrodes
- Quadripolar
  - Two pairs of electrodes with alternating currents that bisect each other
  - Treatment area between the electrodes where the current intersects

Methods of Electrical Stimulation

- **Transcutaneous electrical nerve stimulation (TENS).** The main goal of TENS is pain modulation:
  - High-rate (sensory) TENS achieves fast-acting, short-duration pain management through stimulation of large-diameter (A-beta) nerve fibers
  - Low-rate (motor) TENS achieves slow-acting, long-duration pain management through stimulation of smaller-diameter (A-delta) nerve fibers
  - Noxious (hyperstimulation) TENS achieves pain management through stimulation of the smallest (C) nerve fibers
- **Interferential current (IFC).** The main goal of IFC is pain modulation.
- **High-voltage** The main goal of high-voltage is to use the polar effects for wound healing and edema reduction.
  - High rate (sensory) used for wound healing.
  - Low rate (motor) used for edema reduction.
- **Neuromuscular electrical stimulation (NMES).** The main goal of NMES is muscular strengthening via increased alpha motor neuron recruitment. Larger fast-twitch fibers are recruited first and are more easily fatigued, resulting in muscular strengthening. The muscle strengthening is amplified if voluntary muscle contraction is combined with electrical stimulation. This is also used for stimulation of denervated muscle via regeneration of alpha motor neurons.

Table 44.1 ELECTRICAL STIMULATION TREATMENT PARAMETERS

Goal	*Pain Management*					*Wound Healing*	*Edema Reduction*	*Muscle Strengthening*	
	TENS			*IFC*		*High-Voltage*		*NMES*	
Method	**Sensory**	**Motor**	**Hyperstimulation**	**Sensory**	**Motor**	**Sensory**	**Motor**	**Low Rate**	**Medium Frequency (Russian)**
Current type	Alternating	Alternating	Alternating	Alternating	Alternating	Pulsed direct	Pulsed direct	Direct	Direct
Pulse frequency (Hz)	50–110	1–5	1–4	50–100	1–5	80–105	4–10	35–80	2500
Phase duration (μsec)	50–125	200–500	250–10 msec	Machine default	Machine default	Fixed	250	200–300	Machine default
Intensity	Comfortable paresthesia, no muscle contraction	Visible muscle contraction	Highest tolerable noxious sensation	Highest tolerable paresthesia, no muscle contraction	Highest comfortable muscle contraction	Below motor threshold	Visible muscle contraction	Maximum tolerable muscle contraction	Maximum tolerable muscle contraction
Electrode placement	Bipolar	Bipolar	Monopolar with point probe	Quadripolar or bipolar with premodulated current	Quadripolar or bipolar with premodulated current	Monopolar	Monopolar	Bipolar	Bipolar
Duty cycle (on:off)	100%	100%	100%	100%	100%	100%	1:1 with low on ramp	10s:50s with 1–2s on ramp	10–15s: 50–120s with 0.5–2s on ramp
Treatment duration	30–60 minutes, continuous	40–60 minutes	2 × 30 seconds for each point; 10–20 points max	20–30 minutes	20–30 minutes	60 minutes/ day 5 days/ week	30 minutes	8–10 repetitions	8–10 repetitions

Electrical Stimulation Indications

- Pain modulation
- Inflammation
- Swelling
- Muscle spasms
- Muscle atrophy
- Muscle weakness

Electrical Stimulation Contraindications

- Heart/respiratory conditions (current through chest/neck)
- Over anterior neck, eyes, transthoracically
- Pacemakers
- Over abdomen, pelvis, or lumbar areas during pregnancy
- Tumors
- Active infections
- Thrombophlebitis
- Unstable fracture
- Exposed or superficial metal implants
- Electronic monitoring equipment

Electrical Stimulation Precautions

- Obesity
- Osteoporosis
- Epilepsy
- Impaired sensation
- Skin irritation or sensitivity
- Impaired cognition or communication

IONTOPHORESIS

Iontophoresis involves the use of direct current electrical stimulation to assist the diffusion of medications through the skin and into the target tissues. Common medications used are topical analgesics and anti-inflammatories.

- Intensity: 1–4 mA (based on machine, electrode size used, and patient comfort)
- Electrode placement: monopolar
- Polarity: choose opposite of polarity of medication.
  - Common medications and associated polarities:
    - Salicylate (–),
    - Hydrocortisone (+)
    - Lidocaine (–)
    - Dexamethasone (–)
- Current dosage: 40–80 mA with 70–80 mA optimal
- Treatment duration: 20–40 minutes dependent on dosage and tolerable current

COMBINED THERAPY (COMBO)

Combo uses parameters of therapeutic US and electrical stimulation combined via a multiuse machine. This allows for increased therapeutic effects of localized analgesia, pain management, and reduced muscle spasm compared with either modality alone. The US head is used as the active electrode, and a dispersive pad is placed away from the treatment site.

BIOFEEDBACK

Biofeedback is a training technique that uses various devices to provide visual or auditory input via a physiologic stimulus. It is used to optimize muscle activity patterns to improve functional outcomes. This feedback could assist an individual in increasing the activity in weakened muscles or decreasing the activity in overactive muscles. It is important to note that biofeedback is an assessment of muscular activity, not muscular strength.

Examples of Biofeedback

- Mirror
- Surface electromyography (sEMG)
- Games that provide real-time input; Wii Fit or virtual reality
- Force platform for proprioceptive training

Biofeedback Indications

- Improve neuromuscular activation
- Inhibit neuromuscular activation
- Pain modulation via motor recruitment or inhibition
- Increase awareness of physiologic states such as heart rate, blood pressure, temperature control, brainwave activity

Biofeedback Contraindications

- Dermatologic sensitivity or irritation
- Diminished patient engagement in therapy
- Impaired visual or auditory senses
- Lack of detectable neuromuscular activity

LOW-LEVEL LASER THERAPY

Low-level laser therapy (LLLT), also known as *cold lasers*, uses light energy delivered to a small target area of the body. Treatment dosage is determined by the wavelength of the light (longer wavelengths penetrate deeper into tissue up to 15 mm), the fixed power output of the machine, duty cycle, treatment time (set by the machine), and energy density. The energy density is the actual amount of energy delivered per square centimeter of the probe. Parameters vary across studies ranging from 2 to 500 J/cm^2 depending on diagnosis. LLLT has the following therapeutic effects:

- Increased adenosine triphosphate (ATP) production
- Increased DNA/RNA synthesis leading to cell proliferation and repair
- Increased cell permeability
- Increase in vascularization
- Increase in collagen and connective tissue synthesis
- Increase in endorphin production
- Reduction of pain
- Reduction of inflammation by inhibiting prostaglandin production
- Minimal raise in tissue temperature (no greater than 97.7°F [36.5°C])

LLLT Indications

- Pain modulation
- Inflammation
- Wound care and tissue repair

LLLT Contraindications

- Cancerous tissue
- Directly into eyes
- During first trimester of pregnancy
- Unfused epiphyseal plates
- Hemorrhaging regions
- Local irradiation to endocrine glands
- Within 6 months of radiation therapy

LLLT Precautions

- Hazard if directly viewed
- Occasionally pain is experienced the following day after treatment

- Continued occurrence of patient dizziness and syncope with treatment
- Fever or infection
- Photophobia, sensitivity to light, or epileptics
- Confused or disoriented patients
- Areas of decreased sensation

DRY NEEDLING

Dry needling uses thin filiform needles through the skin to penetrate neuromuscular tissue. The needle is the same as used in acupuncture, but the target tissue and treatment philosophy differ. Dry needling should only be attempted by clinicians who have undergone specialized training, have practical experience, and understand the state regulations regarding dry needling. Dry needling has the following therapeutic effects:

- Initiation of the healing process at needled area
- Vasodilation to needled area
- Release of nerve growth factor
- Decrease trigger point sensitivity
- Pain modulation
- Improve range of motion
- Reduce overall pain sensitivity response

Dry Needling Indications

- Musculoskeletal pain
- Muscle spasm or tension
- Trigger points
- Headaches

Dry Needling Contraindications

- Local skin lesions or rashes
- Local or systemic infections
- Severe hyperalgesia
- Metal (nickel and chromium) allergies
- Blood and systemic diseases (i.e., leukemia)
- Clotting disorders
- Cancerous tissue
- Vascular disease
- Varicose veins
- First trimester of pregnancy
- Needle phobia
- Lymphedema
- Spray tans
- Inability of patient to communicate
- Implants or prosthetic tissue
- HIV, AIDS, or hepatitis

Dry Needling Precautions

- If too deep of penetration, underlying structures can be punctured, leading to pneumothorax

MYOFASCIAL DECOMPRESSION

Myofascial decompression is also known as *cupping therapy*. It uses plastic or glass cups to lift the skin and subdermal tissue via heat or suction forces. This creates a vacuum of negative pressure to elicit hyperemia and incite an acute inflammatory process. Each cup is placed on palpable myofascial trigger points or acupoints. Treatment duration is typically 3–10 minutes and can be coupled with light active exercise. Cupping therapy has primarily short-term benefits for the treatment of musculoskeletal pain with side effects including petechiae, erythema, and possible soreness. Although rare, potential adverse events include headaches, nausea, dizziness, vasovagal response, and hyperpigmentation. Myofascial decompression can serve as a safe, noninvasive alternative to dry needling. Myofascial decompression has the following therapeutic effects:

- Pain modulation
- Increased superficial blood flow

Myofascial Decompression Indications

- Myofascial adhesions
- Areas of decreased blood flow
- Improve local circulation
- Pain modulation
- Stimulate acute inflammatory cycle

Myofascial Decompression Contraindications

- Open wounds, sunburn, rash
- Hemophilia
- Pacemaker
- Contusion
- Patients using anticoagulants
- Cancer
- Organ failure

Myofascial Decompression Precautions

- Acute injuries or inflammation
- Skin sensitivity
- Pregnancy
- Anemia

INSTRUMENT-ASSISTED SOFT TISSUE MOBILIZATION

Instrument-assisted soft tissue mobilization (IASTM) uses instruments to apply force across the skin to detect and treat soft tissue restrictions. Common techniques include gua sha, Graston technique, and fascial abrasion technique (FAT). These often require proprietary training and specific equipment. The instruments used come in different materials, often plastic, metal or ceramic, and different shapes with contours designed for various treatment sites. To date, the evidence on effectiveness is confined to case series and case studies. Some higher levels of evidence exist but have contradictory findings on effectiveness. IASTM has the following therapeutic effects:

- Increased local blood flow
- Attempt to free restrictions from myofascial adhesions
- Stimulate acute inflammatory cycle
- Release of growth factors
- Stimulate macrophage-mediated phagocytosis
- Remodel degenerated tissue

IASTM Indications

- Musculoskeletal pain
- Myofascial adhesions
- Neural restrictions

IASTM Contraindications

- Open wounds
- Infection
- Diabetic ulcers
- Compromised skin integrity
- Primary tumor
- Over abdomen during pregnancy
- Over pacemaker
- Acute deep vein thrombosis
- Lymphedema greater than stage 1

IASTM Precautions

- Temporary bruising and/or soreness may occur
- Hemophilia or clotting disorders
- Autoimmune disease
- Fibromyalgia
- Cancer
- Vascular disease
- Obesity
- Surgical hardware
- Growth plates
- Reflex sympathetic dystrophy
- Stage 1 lymphedema
- Medications: nonsteroidal anti-inflammatories, steroids, Botox

VIBRATION THERAPY

Whole-Body Vibration

Whole-body vibration (WBV) therapy uses a platform that patients stand or do exercises on while the machine vibrates at varying intensities. The theory behind this modality is that chronic vibration will produce enhanced neuromuscular effects when combined with strength training. It is used as an adjunct to rehabilitation exercises and is not often a singular treatment. Although many studies support the use of WBV, the evidence is inconclusive because of differing vibration intensities, populations, and treatment parameters used throughout the literature.

WBV Indications

- Proprioceptive training
- To be used in combination with strength training
- Enhanced neuromuscular input
- Gradually increase loading to bone and tissue returning from injury

WBV Contraindications

- Unstable fracture
- Vestibular pathology

Deep Oscillation Therapy

Deep oscillation therapy involves a machine that provides an oscillation frequency from 5 to 250 Hz aimed at improving pain and swelling outcomes after acute injury. It is also known as *electrostatic massage*, where the clinician attaches electrodes to the patient and themselves in order to complete an electrical current to send the oscillations to the body part being treated. There is weak evidence to support this modality; however, it may be a beneficial concurrent treatment when using manual therapy for pain control and relaxation effects.

Massage Therapy Gun

Massage therapy guns are devices with powerful motors used to provide massaging effects at variable frequencies for a set duration. They mimic some manual therapies; however, they are not able to adjust pressure based upon tissue tension as a massage therapist would. Treatment duration may last from 3 to 20 minutes depending on the depth of the tissue being treated.

Massage Therapy Gun Indications

- Muscular stiffness
- Muscular soreness
- Recovery benefits
- Pain modulation

Massage Therapy Gun Contraindications

- Fracture
- Acute injury
- Wound
- Swelling

BLOOD FLOW RESTRICTION

Blood flow restriction training (BFR) uses measured (50%–80%) arterial occlusion on the proximal aspect of the limb with exercise. There are many different types of equipment available with different occlusion capabilities. BFR has the following therapeutic effects:

- Increases in blood lactate
- Increase myocyte hydration, which triggers pathways for cell growth
- Increases in growth hormone production and insulin-like growth factor (IGF-1)
- Inhibits myostatin and TGF-beta
- Promotes angiogenesis and osteogenesis
- Decrease fibrosis of muscle tissues
- Muscle hypertrophy and increased strength distal and proximal to the occlusion
- Decrease rate of atrophy with increase in muscle fiber recruitment
- Cellular swelling and increased capillary permeability
- Increase in $\dot{V}O_2$ max

BFR Exercise Prescription

- Methods of exercise:
  - Simple, not complex, movements
    - Open chain
    - Closed chain
    - Low-level aerobic
- Treatment dosage: 3–4 exercises of 75 reps: 1 × 30, 3 × 15
- Rest: 30 seconds rest with occlusion between sets; 1-minute rest from occlusion between exercises
- External load: 15%–30% 1RM
- Goal: fatigue in fourth set; if not achieved, increase load—do not increase sets or reps
- Treatment duration: 15–30 minutes with on:off times of occlusion

Side Effects of BFR

- Increase in acute (<24 hours) delayed-onset muscle soreness
- Acute increase in heart rate to maintain cardiac output
- Potential bruising
- Acute numbness from occlusion pressure
- Acute residual swelling in the limb
- Abnormal responses would include total numbness, excessive tingling, technique breakdown, and vasovagal response

BFR Indications

- For patients unable to increase the mechanical load stress, BFR can be used to increase the metabolic stress
- Presurgical and postsurgical cases
- Stress injuries
- Joint injuries
- In-season maintenance
- Muscle disuse or atrophy

BFR Contraindications

- History of blood disorders
  - Deep vein thrombosis
  - Coagulation conditions
  - Hemophilia
  - Sickle cell disease

- Medications known to increase clotting risk
- Impaired circulation
- Varicose veins
- Fever
- Active infection
- Pregnancy
- Cardiopulmonary conditions
- Unstable or severe hypertension
- Lymphedema
- Limb with port or vascular access or indwelling catheter
- Tumor/cancer distal to tourniquet
- Open fracture
- Open wound
- Increased intracranial pressure

BFR Precautions

- Ischemic heart disease
- Severe aortic stenosis
- Hypertrophic obstructive cardiomyopathy
- Peripheral artery disease
- Sickle cell trait
- Increased injury risk if done with or directly before:
  - Olympic lifts
  - Plyometrics
  - Agility work

INTERMITTENT SEQUENTIAL PNEUMATIC COMPRESSION

Intermittent sequential pneumatic compression (ISPC) uses garments wrapped around a body part to apply pressure in a graded pattern via a motor pump. The garments have multiple compartments that subsequently fill with air and then release the pressure to simulate a massaging effect. Treatment duration ranges from 5 to 30 minutes depending on the pressure selected and indication of treatment. It is often used in the lower extremities for patients postoperatively to prevent deep vein thrombosis, improve venous return, and treat venous thromboembolism. In sports medicine ISPC has been used as a recovery modality postexercise with proposed benefits including swelling reduction, decreased soreness, improving blood flow, and eliminating metabolic waste. To date there has been little literature to support objective measures; however, many athletes report subjective improvements after treatments compared with passive recovery methods. ISPC has the following therapeutic effects:

- Decreased delayed-onset muscle soreness
- Pain modulation
- Increased blood flow
- Potentially decreased recovery time
- Placebo effect

ISPC Indications

- Postexercise
- Improve venous return and mitigate swelling
- Lymphedema
- Postoperatively to prevent deep vein thrombosis

ISPC Contraindications

- Poor circulation
- Paresthesia
- Acute fracture sites
- Acute surgical fixations
- Uncovered wounds
- Open wounds

ISPC Precautions

- Patient intolerance of amount of pressure

TRACTION

Traction is the application of an external force by gently drawing or pulling to the cervical or lumbar spine. Dosage is determined by manipulating the mode, intensity, treatment duration, and frequency (Table 44.2). Traction has the following therapeutic effects:

- Separation of joint surfaces
- Elongation of soft tissue surrounding the joint
- Decreased central or peripheral pain
- Increased muscle relaxation
- Stimulation of mechanoreceptors (intermittent load)
- Improved metabolic activity (intermittent load)
- Increased joint mobility

Methods of Traction

- **Continuous bed:** continuous low loads for several hours per day, up to 10–14 days, not often used because the lack of improvement in back pain with prolonged bed rest
- **Mechanical:** machine applies the static or intermittent traction force to patient on the table
- **Active:** traction that occurs during an activity, such as exercise, typically done via tilted table.

Table 44.2 TRACTION TREATMENT PARAMETERS

	Initial Session		Subsequent Sessions	
Mode	**Static:** 100% hold: 0% relax **Intermittent:** Disc protrusion: 60 sec hold: 20 sec relax Joint distraction: 20–60 sec hold: 15 sec relax Muscle spasm: 1–5 sec hold: 5 sec relax			
Intensity	**Cervical**	**Lumbar**	**Cervical**	**Lumbar**
	Joint distraction:10–25 pounds Muscle spasm, disc protrusion, soft tissue stretch: 12–15 pounds	Joint distraction: at least 50% body weight Muscle spasm, disc protrusion, soft tissue stretch: 25% body weight	3- to 5-pound increase per session Over the door: maximum of 20 pounds	5- to 15-pound increase per session
Duration	5–10 minutes	Static: 5–10 minutes Intermittent: 10–15 minutes	20–30 minutes	
Frequency	Clinic: 2–3/day Home: no >2×/day			

- **Manual:** clinician provides the traction force
- **Positional:** uses devices such as towel rolls, wedges, arm rests, and cushions to create traction force
- **Portable:** moveable devices that can be used in various positions and can vary the amount of force applied
- **Inversion:** uses gravity and can be done with different devices that cause the patient to be inverted; care should be taken for elevation in blood pressure and eye pressure
- **Aquatic:** traction force created in deep water with a flotation belt and ankle or hip weights; this can also be used with exercise for active traction
- **Self:** traction force is applied by the patient

Traction Indications

- Disc herniation
- Muscle spasm
- Lumbar or cervical pain
- Lumbar or cervical radiculopathy
- Nerve root impingement
- Joint inflammation
- Generalized hypomobility

Traction Contraindications

- Fracture
- Cord compression
- Status post–spinal surgery
- Spinal tumor
- Acute injury or inflammation
- Inflammatory diseases
- Spinal infections
- Osteoporosis
- Pregnancy
- Down syndrome because of hypermobility
- Peripheralization of symptom with application

Traction Precautions

- Injury at the site of the belts
- Displacement of disc fragment
- Medial disc protrusion
- Claustrophobia or anxiety
- Patient unable to tolerate the position for application
- Vertebral artery compromise
- Temporomandibular joint dysfunction
- Dentures

RECOMMENDED READINGS

Available online.

45 HEAD INJURIES

Torb Morkeberg • Siatta B. Dunbar • Margot Putukian

GENERAL PRINCIPLES

- Head injuries in sports are comparatively mild compared with those in high-velocity motor vehicle accidents (MVAs), yet they remain significant and important injuries for team physicians to evaluate and manage.
- **Concussion** is the most common head injury in sports. Information is evolving regarding pathophysiology, diagnosis, natural history, and treatment of concussion in sports.
- Consider focal, vascular, and associated injuries (e.g., cervical spine, skull fractures, intracranial hemorrhage) when evaluating head-injured athletes.
- Cumulative injury, persisting symptoms after concussion, and other sequelae of head injury may contribute to significant morbidity.

TYPES OF HEAD INJURY

Head injuries occur across a large spectrum, from minor to catastrophic. Classifications such as diffuse versus focal or nonstructural versus structural are not absolute, but they permit the organized discussion of specific pathologies.

Diffuse Brain Injury

Diffuse Axonal Injury (DAI)

- Involves diffuse axonal disruption in the white matter of the brain and brainstem
- Severity of injury determined by clinical course
  - Mild DAI: comatose for 6–24 hours; mortality rate is approximately 15%
  - Moderate DAI: comatose for more than 24 hours; often associated with basilar fracture; mortality rate is approximately 25%
  - Severe DAI: prolonged coma, severe disability, or persistent vegetative state common if patient survives; high mortality rate.
- Caused by **shear or tensile forces;** often results from falls or MVAs
- **Presentation:** All patients present in coma, may exhibit decorticate or decerebrate posturing, severe posttraumatic amnesia, and cognitive deficits after awakening (moderate DAI). Can include hypertension and hyperpyrexia, increased intracranial pressure (ICP), and herniation syndromes.
- **Treatment:** Supportive during coma; medical or surgical measures as needed for increased ICP and associated injuries.

Sport-Related Concussion

- The Fifth International Conference on Concussion in Sport (CIS) defined sports-related concussion (SRC) as a "subset of traumatic brain injury."
  - It is a "complex pathophysiologic process affecting the brain, induced by traumatic biochemical forces."
- Several common features that incorporate clinical, pathologic, and biomechanical injury constructs that may be used in defining the nature of a concussive head injury include:
  - May be caused by direct impact to head or elsewhere on body with "impulsive" force transmitted to head.
  - Results in the rapid onset of short-lived impairment of neurologic function that usually resolves spontaneously, though symptoms may arise over minutes to hours.
  - May result in neuropathologic changes, but acute clinical symptoms reflect functional rather than structural disturbance.
  - Results in a graded set of clinical syndromes that may or may not involve loss of consciousness. The resolution of symptoms typically follows a sequential course, but in some cases may be prolonged.
  - The clinical signs and symptoms cannot be explained by drug, alcohol, or medication use; other injuries (such as cervical injuries, peripheral vestibular dysfunction); or other comorbidities (e.g., psychological factors or coexisting medical conditions).
  - Typically associated with grossly normal structural neuroimaging studies
    - Advanced neuroimaging (e.g., diffuse tensor imaging, functional magnetic resonance imaging (MRI), magnetic resonance spectroscopy) may demonstrate abnormalities; **however, imaging will remain normal in many clinical cases.**
    - **Advanced imaging currently remains a research tool.**
- SRC is the **most common head injury in athletes;** in the majority of cases resolves completely (within 2 weeks in adults and 4 weeks in adolescents and children).
- In the sports tracked by the National Collegiate Athletics Association, the incidence of SRC is shown in Table 45.1.
- Caused by **acceleration/deceleration** (tensile), **rotational** (shearing), and/or **impact** (compressive) forces. Coup injuries often result from direct impact, whereas contrecoup injuries occur from acceleration/deceleration forces (e.g., athlete falls and strikes ground with head).
- **Presentation:** The hallmark of concussion is confusion; other signs and symptoms may occur immediately or several minutes later. In some situations, they may be delayed (Table 45.2).
- **Treatment:** initial period of rest (physical and cognitive), education, protection from further injury, and serial follow-up evaluations (see detailed discussion later)

PATHOPHYSIOLOGY OF SRC

- SRC is associated with neurochemical and metabolic changes with changes in glutamate, potassium, lactate, and glucose, in addition to changes in cerebral blood flow.
- Force on the brain may cause stretching of neuronal cell membranes and axons, resulting in a complex cascade of ionic, metabolic, and pathophysiologic events.
- There are no current objective biomarkers, neuroanatomic or neurophysiologic, that can be used practically and reliably to determine if an athlete has a concussion, though several options are actively being researched. See the "Additional Diagnostic Testing" section. After concussion, the brain cells may be in state of **injury-induced vulnerability;** a second injury during this time of heightened vulnerability may produce additional deficits.
  - Injury-induced vulnerability is characterized by a **fuel need–fuel delivery mismatch.** The brain's need for glucose increases acutely (hyperglycolysis), and cerebral blood flow and oxidative metabolism are relatively reduced.
  - Increased levels of extracellular potassium probably activate adenosine triphosphate (ATP)–dependent sodium–potassium pumps, which increases energy consumption and adds to metabolic stress (e.g., need for glucose).

Table 45.1 NCAA INJURY SURVEILLANCE SYSTEM DATA FOR 1988–1989 THROUGH 2003–2004

Head Protection Required	% of All Game Injuries	No Head Protection	% of All Game Injuries
Men's ice hockey[a]	7.9	Women's lacrosse[a]	6.3
Women's ice hockey	18.3	Wrestling	3.3
Men's lacrosse[a]	5.6	Women's soccer	5.3
Football[a]	6.0	Men's soccer	3.9
Spring football[a] (practice)	5.6	Field hockey	3.9
Softball	4.3	Women's basketball	4.7
Baseball	2.5	Men's basketball	3.2
Concussion Injuries in Games and Practices Per 1000 Athlete Exposures			
Head Protection Required		**No Head Protection**	
Football[a]	0.37	Wrestling	0.25
Men's ice hockey[a]	0.41	Men's soccer	0.28
Women's ice hockey	0.91	Women's soccer	0.41
Men's lacrosse[a]	0.26	Women's lacrosse[a]	0.25
Spring football[a]	0.54	Field hockey	0.18
Softball	0.14	Women's basketball	0.22
Baseball	0.07	Men's basketball	0.16

[a]Mouth guard required.
Data from Hootman J, Agel J, Dick R. Epidemiology of collegiate injuries for 15 sports: summary and recommendations for injury prevention initiatives. *J Athl Train*. 2007;42(2):311–319.

Table 45.2 SIGNS AND SYMPTOMS OF CONCUSSION

Early (Minutes to Hours)	Late (Days to Weeks)
Cognitive	Persistent low-grade headache
Confusion	Lightheadedness
Vacant stare	Poor attention and concentration
Slow to answer questions or follow instructions	Memory dysfunction
Easily distracted	Anomia (cannot think of word one wants to say)
Inability to focus	Easy fatigability
Feeling "in a fog"	Irritability and frustration
Disoriented: unaware of time/date/place	Difficulty with focusing vision
Slurred or incoherent speech	Photophobia
Memory deficits	Phonophobia
Repeatedly asks same question (e.g., what happened?)	Anxiety and/or depression
Retrograde amnesia (RGA): cannot remember events before injury	Sleep disturbance
Posttraumatic amnesia (PTA): cannot remember events after injury	Persistent cognitive deficits
Loss of consciousness	Postconcussive syndrome
Somatic	
Gross incoordination: cannot walk straight line	
Headache	
Dizziness, disequilibrium or vertigo	
Visual disturbances (blurry vision, photophobia)	
Phonophobia	
Fatigue	
Nausea and/or vomiting	
Seizure	
Affective	
Emotional lability: may cry for no apparent reason	
Irritability	
Nausea and/or vomiting	
Seizure	

- Glutamate (excitatory amino acid) levels increase extracellularly and may contribute to an increased flux of potassium.
- Increased intracellular calcium may be related to regional reduction of cerebral blood flow.

Focal Brain Injury

Subdural Hematoma

- Low-pressure venous bleed into potential space (subdural) between the arachnoid and dura mater; classified by time to clinical presentation (Fig. 45.1).
  - **Acute:** within 24 hours; often associated with other intracranial pathology (e.g., contusion, axonal injury)
  - **Subacute:** 24 hours to 2 weeks
  - **Chronic:** 2 weeks or more
- Leading cause of death related to head injury; overall mortality rate of 35%–50%; loss of consciousness implies poor prognosis.
- Elderly and alcoholics at greatest risk because of increased space between brain (atrophy) and dura.
- Caused by brain movement within the skull: acceleration–deceleration, rotational, shearing injuries.
- **Presentation:** Decreased/altered level of consciousness, lucid interval followed by declining mental status and headache; patients may have pupil inequality, motor deficit (e.g., unilateral weakness or paralysis), or other indicators of brain swelling.
- **Treatment:** Usually prompt surgical evacuation (see Fig. 45.1).
  - Surgery within 2–4 hours after onset of neurologic deterioration is associated with a lower mortality.
  - Craniotomy may be associated with better outcomes than burr hole evacuation.
  - Nonoperative management may be an option for patients with small hematoma (<10 mm and <5 mm of midline shift on head computed tomography [CT]).
  - Patient may be observed if prognosis is poor (e.g., prolonged loss of consciousness) or if elderly and asymptomatic.

Epidural Hematoma

- High-pressure arterial bleed between inner table of skull and dura mater (epidural space); middle or other meningeal arteries often disrupted; 80% associated with a skull fracture in the temporoparietal region; occasionally caused by tear of underlying dural sinus (most common in posterior fossa) (Fig. 45.2). Mortality rate is low if diagnosed acutely; comatose state is associated with the highest mortality rate (<20%); mortality rate higher with associated injuries.
- **Presentation:** Decreased level of consciousness followed by lucid interval, deteriorating mental status with eventual loss of consciousness, headache, confusion, sleepiness, nausea, vomiting.
- **Late signs:** Ipsilateral dilated pupil, contralateral muscle weakness, coma
- **Lucid interval may last for several hours and lead to false reassurance and a missed diagnosis.**
- **Treatment:** Surgical evacuation of hematoma.
  - Craniotomy may be preferred over burr hole, as it allows for more complete evacuation.

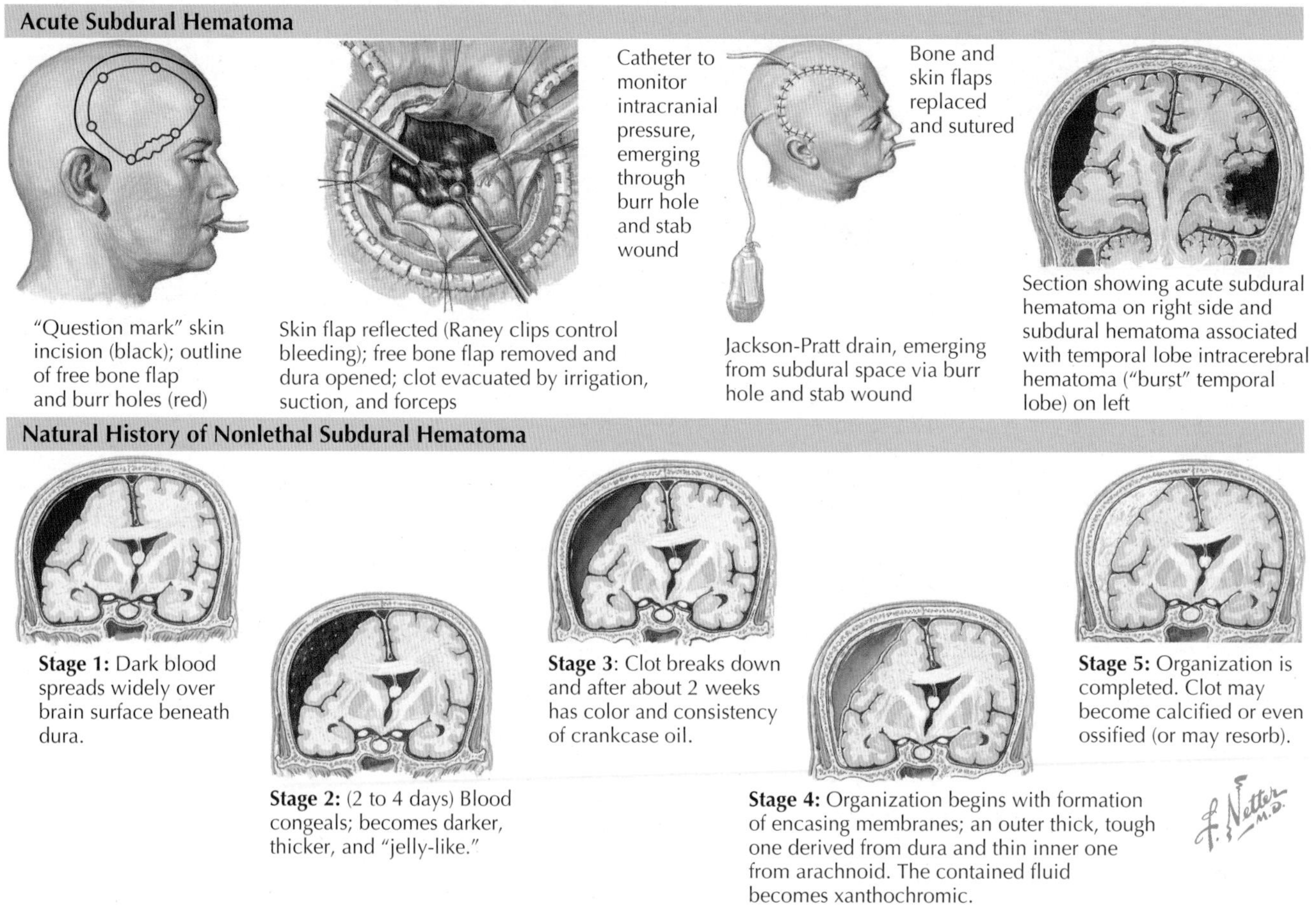
Acute Subdural Hematoma
"Question mark" skin incision (black); outline of free bone flap and burr holes (red)
Skin flap reflected (Raney clips control bleeding); free bone flap removed and dura opened; clot evacuated by irrigation, suction, and forceps
Catheter to monitor intracranial pressure, emerging through burr hole and stab wound
Bone and skin flaps replaced and sutured
Jackson-Pratt drain, emerging from subdural space via burr hole and stab wound
Section showing acute subdural hematoma on right side and subdural hematoma associated with temporal lobe intracerebral hematoma ("burst" temporal lobe) on left
Natural History of Nonlethal Subdural Hematoma
Stage 1: Dark blood spreads widely over brain surface beneath dura.
Stage 2: (2 to 4 days) Blood congeals; becomes darker, thicker, and "jelly-like."
Stage 3: Clot breaks down and after about 2 weeks has color and consistency of crankcase oil.
Stage 4: Organization begins with formation of encasing membranes; an outer thick, tough one derived from dura and thin inner one from arachnoid. The contained fluid becomes xanthochromic.
Stage 5: Organization is completed. Clot may become calcified or even ossified (or may resorb).
F. Netter M.D.

Figure 45.1 Subdural hematoma.

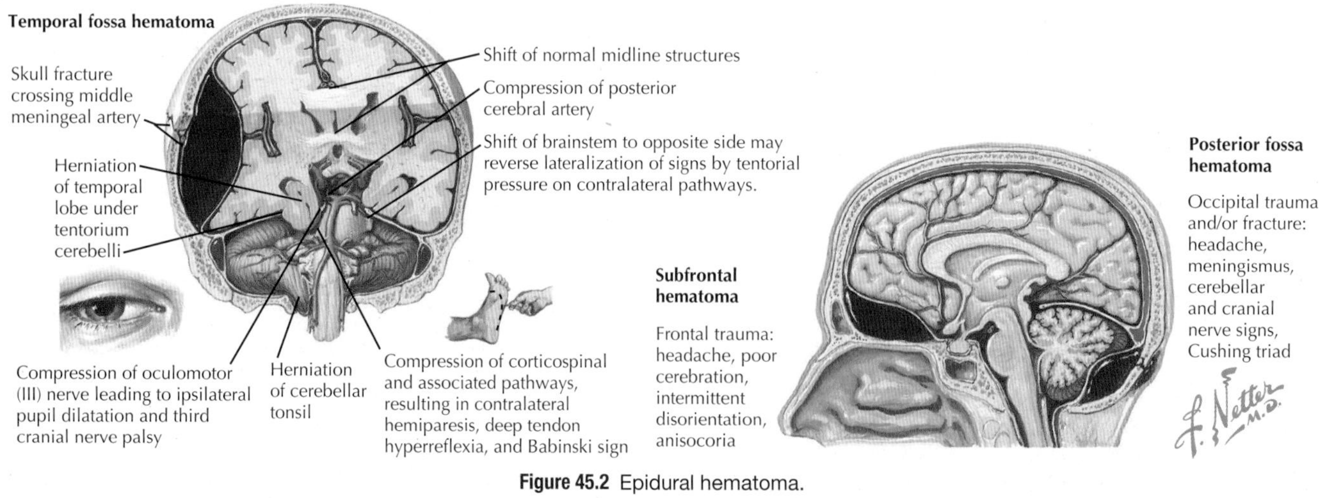
Temporal fossa hematoma
Skull fracture crossing middle meningeal artery
Herniation of temporal lobe under tentorium cerebelli
Shift of normal midline structures
Compression of posterior cerebral artery
Shift of brainstem to opposite side may reverse lateralization of signs by tentorial pressure on contralateral pathways.
Compression of oculomotor (III) nerve leading to ipsilateral pupil dilatation and third cranial nerve palsy
Herniation of cerebellar tonsil
Compression of corticospinal and associated pathways, resulting in contralateral hemiparesis, deep tendon hyperreflexia, and Babinski sign
Subfrontal hematoma
Frontal trauma: headache, poor cerebration, intermittent disorientation, anisocoria
Posterior fossa hematoma
Occipital trauma and/or fracture: headache, meningismus, cerebellar and cranial nerve signs, Cushing triad
F. Netter M.D.

Figure 45.2 Epidural hematoma.

Intracerebral Hemorrhage/Hematoma

- Bleeding from small-caliber arterioles within the brain parenchyma; frontal and temporal lobes are affected most often; may be accompanied by **brain laceration** (Fig. 45.3). Caused by tensile or shearing forces that stretch the brain (coup or contrecoup mechanism of injury).
- **Presentation** varies with the size and location of lesions, as well as any associated pathology (e.g., contusion, postinjury edema); loss of consciousness (<50%), headache, confusion, nausea, vomiting, focal deficits (affected areas) (see Fig. 45.3). Symptoms may develop over hours or days.
- **Treatment:** Many require emergent intervention to lower ICP and/or stop bleeding; depends on severity of clinical presentation, bleed, and associated pathology

Subarachnoid Hemorrhage (SAH)

- Bleeding between the arachnoid and pia mater (subarachnoid space) into the cerebrospinal fluid (CSF); may be **traumatic** or **spontaneous.**
- Traumatic SAH results in small tears of subarachnoid vessels; spontaneous SAH (and sometimes traumatic SAH) is often associated with intracranial aneurysms and arteriovenous

Pathology	CT scan	Pupils	Eye movements	Motor and sensory deficits	Other
Caudate nucleus (blood in ventricle) 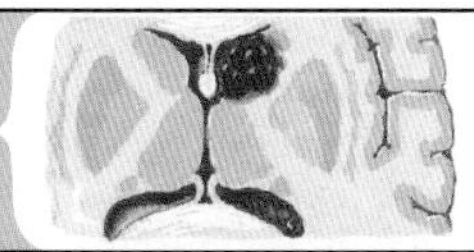	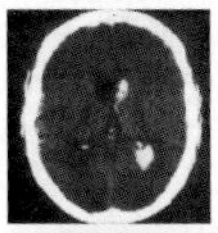	Sometimes ipsilaterally constricted	Conjugate deviation to side of lesion; slight ptosis	Contralateral hemiparesis, often transient	Headache, confusion
Putamen (small hemorrhage) 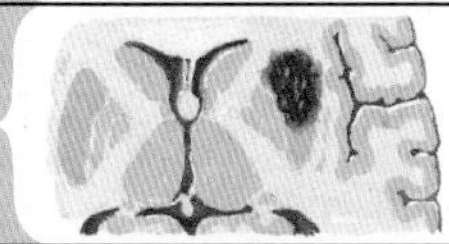	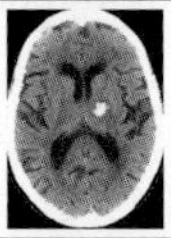	Normal	Conjugate deviation to side of lesion	Contralateral hemiparesis and hemisensory loss	Aphasia (if lesion on left side)
Putamen (large hemorrhage) 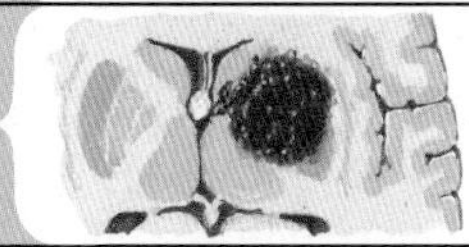	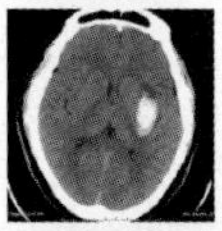	In presence of herniation, pupil dilated on side of lesion	Conjugate deviation to side of lesion	Contralateral hemiparesis and hemisensory loss	Decreased consciousness
Thalamus 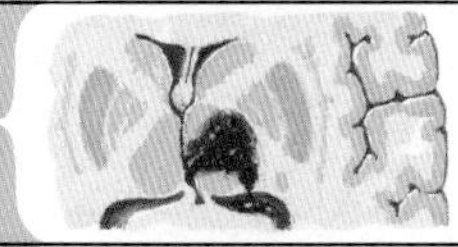	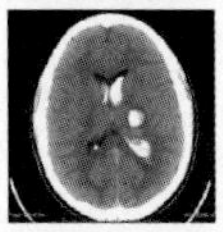	Constricted, poorly reactive to light bilaterally	Both lids retracted; eyes positioned downward and medially; cannot look upward	Slight contralateral hemiparesis, but greater hemi-sensory loss	Aphasia (if lesion on left side)
Occipital lobar white matter 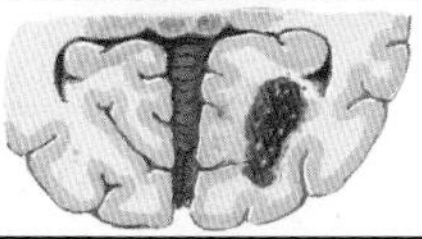	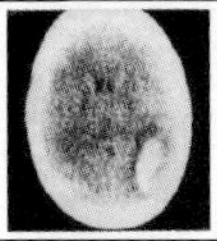	Normal	Normal	Mild, transient hemiparesis	Contralateral hemianopsia
Pons 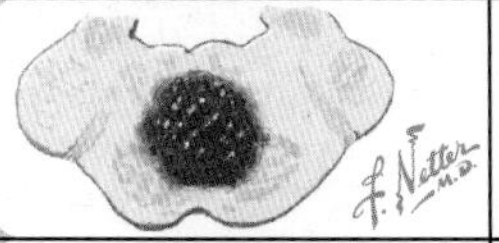	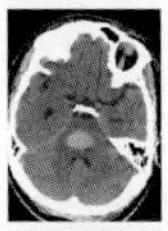	Constricted, reactive to light	No horizontal movements; vertical movements preserved	Quadriplegia	Coma
Cerebellum 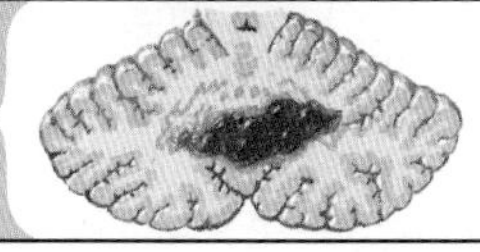	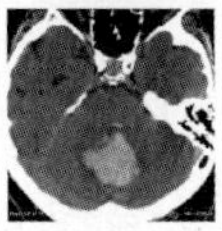	Slight constriction on side of lesion	Slight deviation to opposite side; movements toward side of lesion impaired, or sixth cranial nerve palsy	Ipsilateral limb ataxia; no hemiparesis	Gait ataxia, vomiting

Figure 45.3 Intracerebral hemorrhage: Clinical manifestations related to site.

malformations, and sometimes with hypertension and arteriosclerosis (Fig. 45.4).

- Presentation depends on associated pathology and whether SAH is traumatic or spontaneous. Symptoms include headache (often described as the "worst ever"), photophobia, nausea, vomiting, dizziness, confusion, neck stiffness, and focal deficits (affected areas).
- Must be differentiated from a "bad" migraine or meningitis. Lumbar puncture done only after funduscopic examination (to rule out papilledema) and CT scan. Xanthochromia of the CSF may be the most specific finding with SAH.
- Treatment varies with individual case and pathology; may involve surgical intervention (e.g., clipping of aneurysm), medical management (e.g., calcium channel blocker for vasospasm), and conservative measures.

Other Injuries

Scalp Laceration

- The scalp has many layers and a generous blood supply. Large lacerations or avulsions may be a significant source of bleeding.
- All scalp lacerations should be examined for "step-off" deformities that indicate an underlying depressed skull fracture.
- Hemostasis may be obtained with direct pressure (if no skull fracture is present) followed by quick, careful closure of the wound.

Skull Fracture

- Less common in sport, but must always be considered.
- Classified as linear or depressed (open or closed).
- Caused by direct impact; usually the force of impact is large enough to cause underlying brain injury.
- Presentation varies with the type of fracture and associated brain injury.
- **Nondepressed linear fractures** may cause only localized pain and swelling; basilar fractures (linear) often occur in petrous portion of temporal bone and may present with hemotympanum, otorrhea, or rhinorrhea (CSF leak); periorbital ecchymosis (raccoon eye); or retroauricular ecchymosis (Battle sign) (Fig. 45.5).
- **Depressed fractures** are noted by palpating "step-off" beneath skull laceration (considered open if scalp is disrupted) (see Fig. 45.5). Neurosurgical consultation is advised with all depressed skull fractures. Treatment is individualized.

EVALUATION

Evaluation and management of head-injured athletes must be complete, rigorous, and performed by trained personnel. Standardized approach with careful attention to evaluate for "red flags" should be used.

On-Field Evaluation of Head Injuries

- The use of the most recent version of the Sport Concussion Assessment Tool (SCAT) or child SCAT (for ages 5–12) developed by the CIS group, provides a standardized on-field and off-field assessment for medical professionals to use to evaluate head injuries and includes useful educational information for management (see https://bjsm.bmj.com/content/bjsports/early/2017/04/26/bjsports-2017-097506SCAT5.full.pdf).

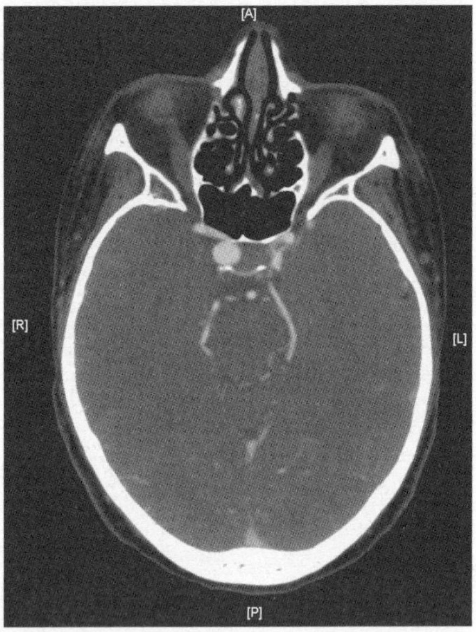
[A]
[R]
[L]
[P]

CT Angio source image showing an aneurysm.

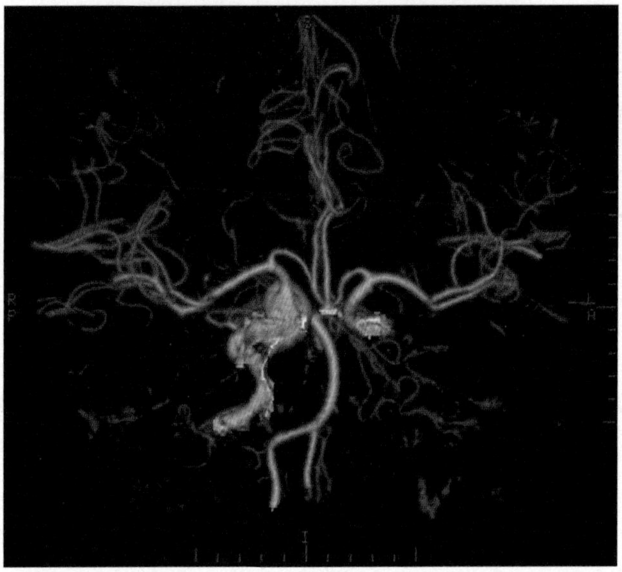

CTA 3-D reconstruction showing detailed anatomy of the aneurysm.

Figure 45.4 Subarachnoid hemorrhage.

- Airway, **B**reathing, **C**irculation, **D**isability, Exposure **(ABCDE)**
- Evaluation for "red flags," including neck pain or tenderness; double vision; weakness or tingling/burning in arms or legs; severe or increasing headache; seizure or convulsion; loss of consciousness; deteriorating conscious state; vomiting; increasingly restless, agitated, or combative. Athletes with any "red flags" after a direct or indirect blow to the head should be removed from play and evaluated by a physician or licensed healthcare provider. In these situations or those that may present additional risk (e.g., athlete with hemophilia, on anticoagulants), transport to a trauma center may be indicated.
- **Glasgow Coma Scale: best evaluates eye, verbal, and motor response. Useful for predicting prognosis in severe head injury.**
- **If athlete is unconscious** or confused; has a neurologic deficit, bony cervical spine tenderness, or restricted range of motion; or there is suspicion for cervical or skull fracture, protect the airway, immobilize the cervical spine, and transport to a trauma center for further evaluation.
- **If athlete is conscious** and has no neck pain and a normal brief neurologic evaluation, he or she can be brought to the sideline for further assessment and observation.
- **Evaluation of associated injuries**
  - Unstable cervical spine injury should be assumed until proven otherwise; ask about neck pain and palpate for tenderness.
  - Maintain a high suspicion for vascular or focal injuries (change in level of consciousness, focal deficits, and other signs or symptoms [red flags]).
  - Assess for skull fracture (see the "Skull Fracture" section).
- **Observable signs:** Several observable signs have been shown to predict the likelihood of diagnosed concussion after a direct or indirect blow to the head. These include:
  - **Lying motionless:** The athlete does not appear to move or react purposefully, respond, or reply appropriately to the game situation (including teammates, opponents, referees, or medical staff).
  - **Motor incoordination:** The athlete appears unsteady (e.g., loses balance, staggers/stumbles, struggles to get up, falling) or in the upper limbs (including fumbling).
  - **Impact seizure:** The athlete exhibits involuntary clonic movements that comprise periods of asymmetric and irregular rhythmic jerking of axial or limb muscles.
  - **Tonic posturing:** The athlete exhibits involuntary sustained contraction of one or more limbs (typically upper limbs), so that the limb is held stiff despite the influence of gravity or the position of the athlete. The tonic posturing could involve other muscles such as the cervical, axial, and lower limb muscles. Tonic posturing may be observed while the athlete is on the playing surface or while falling, where the player may also demonstrate no protective action.
  - **No protective action—floppy:** The athlete falls to the playing surface in an unprotected manner (i.e., without stretching out hands or arms to lessen or minimize the fall). There may be loss of motor tone (which may be observed in the limbs and/or neck) before landing on the playing surface.
  - **Blank/vacant look:** The athlete exhibits no or blunted facial expression or apparent emotion in response to the environment (may include a lack of focus/attention of vision). This is best appreciated in comparison to the athlete's normal or expected facial expression.

Off-Field Assessment

- **Thorough history at time of injury and focused neurologic examination with attention to symptoms, mental status, cognitive functioning, and postural stability.**
- Determine if any loss of consciousness occurred (based on others' report), as well as whether any loss of memory of the event before (retrograde amnesia) and/or after (posttraumatic amnesia) the injury.
- Ask athlete to recount the specifics of events (e.g., game score, special plays, teammates), events before game, previous game score. Teammates and coaching staff may be useful in validating information. Maddock's questions in the SCAT are more useful than asking standard orientation questions in athletes: What venue are we at today? Which half is it now? Who scored last in this match? What team did you play last week/game? Did your team win the last game?
- Neurologic assessment: oculomotor examination; cranial nerve function; early cognitive, somatic, and affective signs and symptoms (see Table 45.2)
- Short-term memory, delayed-term memory, and concentration assessment
- Examples include asking the athlete about teammates, coach, specific plays, home phone numbers, etc.
- Perform the Sideline Assessment of Concussion (SAC), which has been validated to assess for SRC acutely and is a component of the SCAT. This includes standard orientation questions and both immediate and delayed memory and concentration.

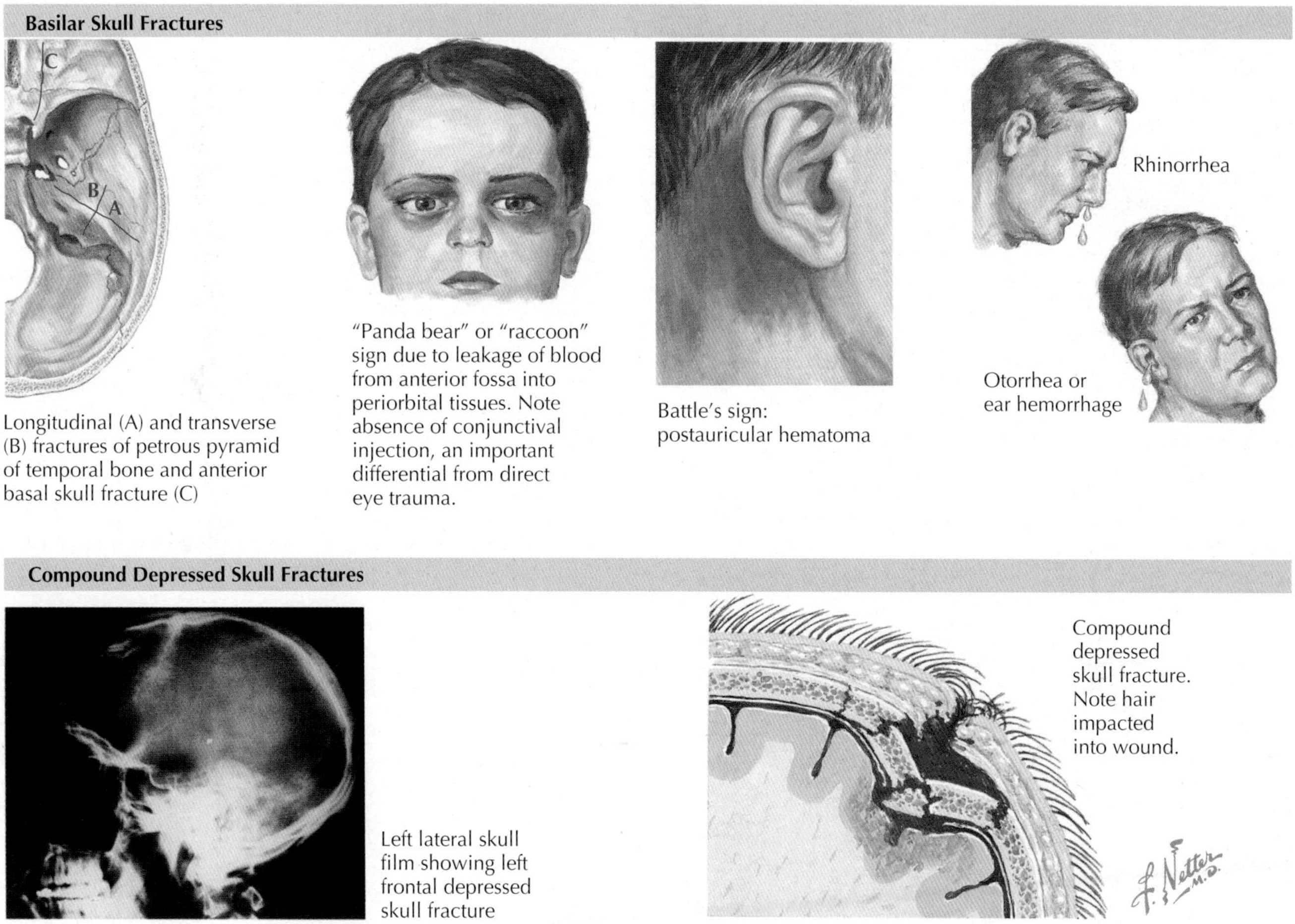
Basilar Skull Fractures
C
B
A
Longitudinal (A) and transverse (B) fractures of petrous pyramid of temporal bone and anterior basal skull fracture (C)
"Panda bear" or "raccoon" sign due to leakage of blood from anterior fossa into periorbital tissues. Note absence of conjunctival injection, an important differential from direct eye trauma.
Battle's sign: postauricular hematoma
Rhinorrhea
Otorrhea or ear hemorrhage
Compound Depressed Skull Fractures
Left lateral skull film showing left frontal depressed skull fracture
Compound depressed skull fracture. Note hair impacted into wound.
F. Netter M.D.

Figure 45.5 Skull fracture.

- Orientation (month, date, day, year, and approximate time)
- Immediate memory (standardized list of 5 or 10 words—significant improvement in performance if use a 10-word list instead of a 5-word list, which has a significant ceiling effect).
- Concentration (digit span backward—start with three digits then increase, e.g., 1-4-2, 6-9-3-1, 5-8-3-4-6…)

- Delayed memory (remember the 10 words provided previously). This should be done 5 minutes after the immediate recall of the words has been performed, and this time is typically after the off-field evaluation is completed. Perform a neurologic screen, which can include having the athlete read aloud and follow instructions, confirming full range of pain-free passive cervical spine movement, having the athlete look side to side and up and down without double vision, perform finger to nose and tandem gait.
- Assess balance; may use computerized platform or clinical assessment. The modified Balance Error Scoring System (mBESS) can be utilized. It includes three different stances for 20 seconds each with eyes closed, with the provider counting errors during all three stances. The mBESS has been validated as a tool to assess balance in the setting of SRC and is a component of the SCAT.
- Assess horizontal and vertical gaze in addition to near point convergence (NPC). Emerging data suggest that abnormalities in NPC may be associated with prolonged symptoms after SRC.
- Assess upper and lower extremity motor and sensory function
- **History of prior concussions and risk factors**
  - Details of previous injuries, including alterations in level of consciousness, associated injuries, time lost from participation, and date of most recent concussion.
  - Pay particular attention to repeat concussions with lesser impact forces and/or increasing duration of symptoms.
  - Those with a history of at least three concussions had a threefold greater chance of sustaining another concussion.
  - Assessment of other possible risk factors: history of depression, attention-deficit disorder (ADD) attention-deficit/hyperactivity disorder (ADHD), or migraines; age (<18 years of age); intoxication; use of anticoagulants; hemophilia; inadequate postinjury supervision.
  - **Close observation and serial assessments are important.**
- Athlete's equipment (e.g., helmet, stick, and glove), as applicable, should be held to prevent re-entry into game, and the coach should be made aware that the athlete is not available to participate. Athletes should be serially evaluated after an injury, and a disposition plan should be arranged with the athlete, parent, and/or other teammates/roommates such that the athlete can be watched for signs of deterioration and transported to an appropriate facility if need be.
- The disposition plan should also include when the athlete will be seen in follow-up and instructions on what to do activity-wise in the interim.
- If neuropsychological testing (NPT) is available, consider performing postinjury NPT at least 24–48 hours after injury.

Standardized Assessment Tools

- Developed to establish valid standardized, systematic sideline evaluation for the immediate assessment of concussion in athletes. The SAC and SCAT are both examples. The SAC has been validated when used acutely to differentiate concussed vs.

nonconcussed athletes. The SCAT was developed by the CIS group and has been updated and revised regularly. Computerized neurocognitive tests also are standardized assessment tools that assess neurocognitive function, and some platforms also include symptom scores.

- **Not meant to replace individual assessments, clinical judgement,** or more comprehensive formal clinical NPT; **do not diagnose concussion.**
- The SCAT 3 was updated to SCAT 5 in 2017, and the SCAT6 will be published after the CIS Conference in October 2021.
- The SCAT 5 includes a SAC with 10-word lists (as opposed to the 5-word lists of SCAT 3) for immediate and delayed memory and longer digit backwards sequencing. This increases SCAT 5's clinical utility by decreasing the ceiling effect, which was a weakness of the SCAT 3. There is a child SCAT 5 for ages 5–12 years old.
- Previous data on older versions of the SCAT show:
  - When baseline assessments were used and could be available for postinjury assessments, a drop in score of 3.5 points on the SCAT 2 was demonstrated to have a sensitivity of 96% and a specificity of 81%.
  - Studies on the SCAT 3 show that its sensitivity and specificity are highest within 3–5 days of injury.

Other Testing to Consider in Evaluating Head Injury

- Vestibular/Ocular Motor Screening (VOMS) tool. NPC appears to be the most useful. Some components of the VOMS may be difficult to perform for the athlete who is symptomatic and/or has a history of motion sickness.
- King–Devick (KD) test (saccadic eye movements).

Delayed Evaluation

- Serial sideline, postgame, training room, or office.
- One goal is to uncover persisting symptoms.
  - The Berlin 5th International Conference defines persisting symptoms as lasting over 10–14 days in adults and over 4 weeks in children.
- All athletes with head injury should be reassessed serially as needed. Graded symptom checklist can be useful in following serially over time, as well as how the athlete is doing in school and with limited activity.
- Additionally, if abnormalities are initially noted on the sideline assessment, they may be useful to repeat (e.g., mBESS, SAC component of SCAT, or NPC)
- Consideration of repeat or additional formal neuropsychological testing (e.g., computerized and/or standard paper/pencil testing).

INJURY SEVERITY AND MANAGEMENT OF CONCUSSION

- Numerous concussion grading systems and return-to-play (RTP) guidelines are available. **Many are empirical and lack outcome or evidence-based research.**
- Early guidelines used loss of consciousness as an indicator of injury severity, which has subsequently been shown not to be true unless prolonged.
- Newer guidelines, such as those published by the National Athletic Trainers Association, the American Medical Society for Sports Medicine, the Berlin 5th International Conference on Concussion in Sport, the American Academy of Neurology, and the Team Physician Concussion Consensus (TPCC) Statement, likely represent the most comprehensive guidelines available.
- Diagnosis is a clinical one, based on a combination of different domains, including clinical symptoms (e.g., headache), signs (e.g., loss of consciousness, amnesia), behavior (e.g., irritability), and/or balance changes and cognition (e.g., slowed reaction times).
- The TPCC guidelines encourage determining the severity of a concussion only after all symptoms resolve and cognitive and neurologic examinations normalize.
  - Severity of injury is based on nature, burden, and duration of symptoms.
- Berlin 5th International Consensus Statement recommends an individualized RTP with a graduated return-to-sport and a graduated return-to-school strategy.
- Both the return-to-sport and return-to-school strategies incorporate incremental increases in physical and cognitive load over time.
- After an initial acute period of rest, there is strong evidence to suggest light activity is appropriate as early as 24–48 hours postinjury and may also be associated with earlier recovery. This low-level activity can be going for a brisk walk or low-level bicycling/treadmill use and can be initiated even if the athlete has a low level of symptoms.
- Avoiding vigorous exertion too early is important.
- Exercise can be gradually increased in both intensity and duration and should be monitored, stopping if symptoms worsen or develop.
  - The Buffalo Concussion Exercise Treatment Protocol is a standardized exercise protocol that has been well studied. It is a treadmill protocol/program that establishes a clear symptom threshold, stays below that threshold, and progressively increases the threshold as tolerated.

Return-to-Play Guidelines

- For RTP, the emphasis is placed on individualized assessment, not on a rigid timeline.
- Newer guidelines are all consistent; no same-day RTP for an athlete diagnosed with or suspected to have concussion.
- An initial period of rest is important.
  - Likely leads to less discomfort and promotes recovery by minimizing brain energy demands.
  - Often 24–48 hours indicated (though exact duration will vary).
- All agree that **symptomatic athletes should not be allowed to return to contact or full play.**
- Conservative considerations with emphasis on a period of prolonged avoidance of contact activities should be considered in athletes with a history of repeat concussions, young athletes, and athletes with a history of prolonged signs or symptoms, among others.
- The **timing** and **speed** of progression are controversial.
  - Physiologic recovery may take more time than clinical recovery.
  - Having a low symptom burden early (first day postinjury) is a favorable prognostic indicator.
  - The strongest and most consistent predictor of slow recovery is symptom burden and severity acutely postinjury.
  - If problems like migraine headache or depression arise, more likely to have symptoms lasting 1 month.
  - Some evidence to suggest that teenagers particularly might be at highest risk for persisting symptoms.
    - Recovery is often slower in younger athletes.
  - It can be a challenge to determine whether persisting symptoms after concussion are preexisting, coexisting, or a result of other psychosocial factors.
- If there are persisting symptoms after concussion, treatment should be targeted towards the specific symptoms, and a multidisciplinary team may be beneficial. Additional testing, including formal NPT, balance testing, mental health screening, and follow-up imaging, should be considered as indicated by the specific symptom(s).

- A collaborative approach needs to consider cognitive stress, school accommodations, etc.
- Cognitive work should be modified such that it should not exacerbate symptoms.
- Athletes with persisting symptoms should be assessed for headache, sleep disorder, mood disturbance, cognitive deficits, and vestibular/ocular symptoms.
- For these types of persisting symptoms, cognitive behavioral therapy and pharmacotherapy may be considered.
- Targeted physical therapy is specifically indicated for cervical/vestibular/ocular symptoms. This should be performed by a clinician with experience in the following forms of rehabilitation. Several common impairments (with their associated forms of rehab include):
  - Benign paroxysmal positional vertigo: canalith repositioning maneuvers.
  - Vestibulo-ocular reflex impairment: gaze stability testing.
  - Visual motion sensitivity: graded exposure to visually stimulating environments (possibly using virtual reality).
  - Impaired postural control: sensory organization, divided attention, and dynamic balance training.
  - Cervicogenic dizziness: manual therapy and balance/oculomotor training.
  - Exercise-induced dizziness: progressive dynamic exertion.

PREVENTION

- Before making rule or equipment changes, consider incidence of injury and how changes may affect the sport.
- Mixed evidence for mouthguard use.
  - Meta-analysis suggests nonsignificant trend toward a protective effect in collision sports (needs to be further evaluated).
  - Mouthguards can decrease tooth injury.
- Strong evidence for prohibiting body checking in youth (under age 13) ice hockey.
- Some evidence for vision training in collegiate football players reducing concussion.
- Limiting contact in youth football practices leads to less frequent head contact.
  - Unclear if this includes fewer concussions.
- Stricter rule enforcement of red cards for high elbows in heading in professional soccer may lead to reduction in risk of head contact and concussion.
- Mixed evidence on helmets.
  - The proper enforcement of existing rules (avoiding head-to-head hits) is essential.
  - Helmets can at least decrease the incidence of skull fractures because of their protective plastic shell.
  - Use of helmets significantly decreases the risk of head injury in bicycling, baseball, skiing, snowboarding, and softball, without negatively affecting the sport.
  - One study on ice hockey reported that 75% of 246 head injuries involve violence unrelated to on-ice activities (high sticking, deliberate pushing, or fistfights).
- These measures do not appear to lead to significant reduction in concussion risk:
  - Fair play rules in youth ice hockey.
  - Tackle training without helmets and shoulder pads in youth American football.
  - Tackle technique training in professional rugby.

Additional Diagnostic Testing

- A CT scan should be the first tool used if there is a concern about intracranial bleeding or fracture; better at detecting blood, fracture; as good as MRI at identifying surgical lesions.
- Electroencephalogram (EEG), MRI, and CT scan may present normally despite significant clinical symptoms and abnormalities in cognitive function.
- Positron emission tomography (PET), diffusion tensor imaging (DTI), and functional MRI scans may play roles; correlate with pathophysiologic data. Clinical applicability is not practical in most settings at this time; mainly research tools.
- Neuropsychological testing (see later discussion).
- Laboratory evaluation of athletes with significant head injuries should be individualized. Consider complete blood count, electrolytes, serum glucose, urinalysis, coagulation studies, toxicologic and ethanol screens, and blood type and crossmatch.
- Cervical spine x-rays should be considered in all athletes with significant head injuries. Skull films may help localize and determine severity of depression of underlying skull fractures.
- MRI should be considered for athletes with persisting symptoms, but are not typically useful acutely (where CT scans may be indicated)
- Proteomic markers of injury and recovery in severe forms of neurotrauma/traumatic brain injury (TBI) are showing promise.
  - However, low level of evidence for diagnosing concussion.
- Fifty fluid biomarkers have potential for research, especially regarding pathophysiology of concussion and neurobiological recovery
  - There is a low level of evidence to use these clinically for SRC.
  - If these become practical clinically, there is hope they can decrease use of head CT in the emergency department setting.

NEUROPSYCHOLOGICAL TESTING

- **NPT provides assessment and quantification of brain function** by examining brain–behavior relationships. Neuropsychologists are likely best trained to interpret NPT results.
- Tests measure a broad range of cognitive functions: speed of information processing, memory, attention and concentration, reaction time, scanning and visual tracking ability, and problem-solving abilities.
- Preliminary studies used in athletics utilizing paper and pencil testing demonstrate NPT as a useful tool in the assessment of concussion.
- Newer and more portable computerized neurocognitive test batteries are available, including Immediate Post-Concussion Assessment and Cognitive testing (ImPACT), CogState/CogSport, Automated Neuropsychological Assessment Metrics (ANAM), and Headminder, Central Nervous System Vital Signs.
  - These computerized tests are shorter and easier to perform than the standard paper and pencil tests. Controversy surrounds the optimal protocol of tests and most appropriate time for usage.
- Several studies using computerized NPT have shown the "value added" of NPT in addition to symptoms in demonstrating cognitive deficits in athletes after concussion.
- May be useful in assessment and recovery phases of head injury. Most clinicians advocate usage after acute injury and symptoms have resolved, compared with preinjury baseline assessment.
- NPT is currently used by several sport leagues, including the National Football League, the National Hockey League, Major League Soccer, US Soccer, and US Lacrosse, as well as at various college and high school programs, as one component in the management of concussion.
- NPT may detect acute and chronic head injury; it is more sensitive in assessing cognitive function than classic medical testing (neurologic examinations using MRI, CT, and/or EEG).
- NPT provides additional useful information in the assessment of concussion and may supplement, but not replace,

comprehensive individualized assessments. NPT is "only one tool in the toolbox."
- NPT may become more widely available for sideline use in the future, especially with the development of more sophisticated programs for laptop and handheld computers.
  - Essential for consideration is how NPT is conducted and who is interpreting the results.

Take-Home Messages for Concussion

- Important to individualize treatment.
- Any athlete suspected of having a concussion or other head injury should be removed from play and evaluated by a licensed healthcare provider. No athlete should be allowed to participate with acute symptoms.
- **No athlete should be returned to play the same day of a diagnosed or suspected concussion.**
- Any athlete with worsening symptoms, altered mental status, other symptoms of intracranial bleeding, or other "red flags" should be transferred immediately to a trauma facility with 24/7 imaging capabilities.
- Athletes with suspected cervical spine injury should be immobilized and transported immediately to a trauma facility.
- Severity of injury is more closely related to the burden, severity, and duration of symptoms.
- Children and adolescents often take longer to recover.
- It is important to differentiate the role of exercise in the treatment of SRC from initiating the RTP progression.
  - After an acute period (24–48 hours) of cognitive and physical rest, exercise is useful in speeding recovery. Strict rest after SRC slows recovery and increases the probability of persisting symptoms.
  - Exercise that does not exacerbate symptoms or create new symptoms can be initiated after 24–48 hours.
  - Athletes should be at their baseline level of symptoms, cognitive function, and balance before returning to contact or competitive sport. This RTP progression is individualized, gradual, and incremental in load and should be monitored by the medical staff.

HEAD INJURY COMPLICATIONS

Second-Impact Syndrome (SIS)

- First described in 1973 and nearly all cases in adolescent males. Some cases in adult male boxers. Cases in college-aged athletes described the condition as "second impact dysautoregulation."
- **Controversy regarding whether SIS exists**
- Rapid brain swelling and herniation after second head injury in athlete still recovering from initial head injury (during period of injury-induced vulnerability)
- Vascular congestion, increased ICP, and brain (uncal) and brainstem herniation probably result from loss of autoregulation of cerebral vasculature
- Second impact may be mild (e.g., a blow to chest or back that "snaps" the head). Athlete may initially appear dazed. Precipitous collapse, rapidly dilating pupils, coma, and respiratory failure ensue in seconds to minutes; end result is often death.
- Underscores the importance of:
  - Educating athletes on reporting symptoms right away
  - Immediately removing athletes with SRC or suspected SRC from play until evaluated by a healthcare provider
  - Complete clinical recovery before initiating RTP

Posttraumatic Seizure

- Three types of seizures may follow head injury: immediate, early, and late.
- **Immediate posttraumatic seizures (concussive convulsions)** are associated with no underlying structural or permanent brain injury, occur seconds after impact, and involve a brief tonic phase followed by bilateral myoclonic jerking.
- Seizures cease spontaneously and are followed by concussive symptoms.
- Are often associated with brief loss of consciousness.
- Do not require anticonvulsant therapy. Recurrence uncommon.
- **Early** (<1 week) or **late** (>1 week) **posttraumatic seizures** may be partial or generalized. Many involve the temporal lobe, and most are associated with underlying brain pathology (e.g., contusion, hemorrhage, skull fracture) and require long-term anticonvulsant therapy. Seizures may recur in 20%–25% of early and in up to 70% of late cases of posttraumatic epilepsy.
- **Differential diagnosis** for posttraumatic seizures includes idiopathic generalized epilepsy (poorly controlled or new onset), focal (partial) epilepsy associated with preexisting brain lesion or seizure focus, secondary epilepsy (e.g., drug-induced), convulsive syncope, and posttraumatic seizures.
- **Risk factors** for chronic posttraumatic seizures include depressed skull fracture, dural penetration, prolonged posttraumatic amnesia, acute intracranial hemorrhage, and early or late posttraumatic epilepsy.

Chronic Traumatic Brain Injury (CTBI)

- CTBI (also called *chronic traumatic encephalopathy [CTE]* and dementia pugilistica) represents chronic and cumulative neurologic dysfunction after repetitive head trauma. Observed most often in boxers, with more recent reports in professional wrestlers and American football players.
- Area of significant ongoing research.
- Characterized by central nervous system dysfunction that may include cognitive impairment, ataxia, behavioral changes, parkinsonism, and pyramidal tract dysfunction.
- Apolipoprotein E4 allele mutation has been noted to be a risk factor for CTBI in boxers.
- Tau deposition is noted, though it is unclear if this is a/the cause or simply a by-product/marker of disease. Varying degree and durations of neuropsychological dysfunction have been observed after head injuries (both in sports-related and nonsports-related trauma).
- A cause-and-effect relationship has not yet been demonstrated between CTBI or concussions/exposure to contact sports. As such, the notion that repeated concussion or subconcussive impacts cause CTE remains unknown.
- Some retrospective studies have reported increased risk of neurodegenerative disease in former professional football players. At the same time, former high school football players do not show a higher prevalence of neurodegenerative disease when compared with nonfootball peers.
- Most widely described risk factor to date is extensive exposure to both multiple concussions and repetitive head impacts.
  - Degree of necessary exposure is likely specific to the individual and subject to multiple modifying risk factors.
- Other risk factors for reduced cognitive performance may include cognitive dysfunction and learning disability.
- Potential links to Alzheimer disease, depression, and suicide have been reported.
- Athletes and former athletes who present with neuropsychiatric symptoms and signs that have been ascribed to CTE should be evaluated for potentially treatable comorbid conditions that share symptoms and not be assumed to have CTE.

RECOMMENDED READINGS

Available online.

NECK INJURIES 46

R. Lance Snyder

GENERAL PRINCIPLES

Cervical spine injuries are most often seen in football and hockey but have occurred in wrestling, rugby, baseball, lacrosse, skiing, snowboarding, equestrian sports, and mountain biking.

Anatomy

- There are seven cervical vertebrae and eight cervical nerves.
- Spinal nerves exit above the vertebral body for which they are named; for example, the sixth cervical nerve exits at the C5–C6 disc space.
- The cervical spine is divided into upper and lower segments. The upper segment includes C1 (the atlas) and C2 (the axis). The spinal cord occupies a little space because the canal is funnel shaped in the sagittal plane. The atlas (C1) and the occiput account for 40% of cervical flexion. Together they account for 5–10 degrees of lateral bending. The axis (C2) has a finger-like projection, the dens, about which the atlas rotates; this accounts for 60% of cervical rotation. The key for C1 and C2 stability is the transverse atlantal ligament, which lies posterior to the body of C2 and connects C1 to C2. Distraction of this ligament can cause atlantoaxial instability (Fig. 46.1).
- The lower segment of the cervical spine includes C3–T1. The bony structure is relatively constant, with anterior column support provided by the anterior longitudinal ligament, the vertebral bodies, and the discs. Posterior column support is provided by the posterior longitudinal ligament, facet articulation, facet capsule, interspinous ligament, and supraspinous ligament. The spinal cord occupies 75% of the canal at this level. Clinically, the space available for the spinal cord (SAC) ranges between 13 and 23 mm. The cord is stenotic when the available space is <13 mm. Cord compression may occur when the space is less than 10 mm. The Torg ratio is calculated by taking the space available for the cord and dividing it by the anterior-to-posterior dimension of the vertebral body. Stenosis is indicated by a ratio less than 0.8 and increased risk for neurologic injury.

HISTORY AND PHYSICAL EXAMINATION

History

- First, the physician should enquire if and where the athlete has symptoms. Does the athlete have full movement and sensation of the extremities? The physician should enquire about neck pain and does the athlete remember the injury.
- The physician should then ask about the injury, including the direction of the athlete's helmet at the time of injury and the radiation of symptoms and their resolution.

Physical Examination

- The athlete must be removed from the field in a safe and protected manner. Six people who have practiced the maneuver before injury must logroll the athlete onto a spine board and safely transport the athlete to the sidelines. The helmet should not be removed, but the airway must be protected and maintained. The physician and trainers should be familiar with the removal of all types of face masks. A power screwdriver is essential to accelerate face mask removal. This is appropriate for football and hockey.
- A patient with pain must be examined with palpation. A step-off may indicate instability.
- A fracture of the cervical spine may present with minimal pain, and the physician and the medical staff should be aware of this fact. Unstable fractures may present as radicular pain.
- Athletes who are suspected to have cervical spine injuries should be immobilized.
- If only radicular symptoms are present, the athlete should be examined for range of motion of the cervical spine, followed by a neurologic evaluation.
- Although this examination is not a complete and thorough workup, it should be performed at a later date.
- Strength is tested by comparing both sides at a scale of 0–5 (5/5 indicates full strength). The deltoids are checked with the corresponding C5 nerve root. The biceps correspond to C6 and the triceps correspond to C7.
- Sensation is checked with the thumb dorsally placed corresponding to C6, the long finger corresponding to C7, and the little finger corresponding to C8.
- Reflexes are then checked with the biceps reflex corresponding at the elbow to C6 and the triceps to C7.
- Spurling test may be performed if fractures have been ruled out, with the athlete's head being rotated and extended toward the affected extremity (Fig. 46.2).
- A positive Spurling sign is elicited when pain is exacerbated with this maneuver and is often caused by impingement of a nerve root with a disc herniation or osteophyte.

CERVICAL SPINE INJURIES

Stingers or Burners

Description: This is a stretch injury of the nerve root.

Mechanism: Typically, hyperextension of the neck with lateral deviation of the head causing traction of the upper trunk of the brachial plexus or pinching the cervical nerve root at the level of the foramen.

Presentation: Typically, there is a stinging or burning pain into the shoulder, arm, or hand, which may be accompanied by weakness of the affected upper extremity. There may be numbness or tingling. Symptoms typically last from seconds to minutes but can last from days to weeks. The incidence of such injuries is 65% in college football athletes, with an 87% risk of recurrence.

Differential diagnoses: Cervical fracture or cervical herniation.

Diagnostics: Cervical radiographs should be recorded in flexion and extension to rule out instability. Ideally, the T1 vertebral body must be included in the radiographs. Magnetic resonance imaging (MRI) or electromyography (EMG) may be required if symptoms persist. An EMG is typically not ordered until 6 weeks after the injury, but can help distinguish a nerve root from a brachial plexus problem.

Treatment: The athlete is rested until full strength has returned and sensation has returned to normal. Pad modification to prevent lateral deviation of the cervical spine may be beneficial. In addition, positional change may be beneficial (e.g., change from right to left guard).

Prognosis: The athlete is allowed to return to play when full range of motion, strength, and sensation have returned. The return-to-play prognosis for such injuries is typically extremely good.

Transient Quadriparesis

Description: Pathologic insult to the spinal cord, which may or may not be accompanied by transient hypoxemia to the spinal cord.

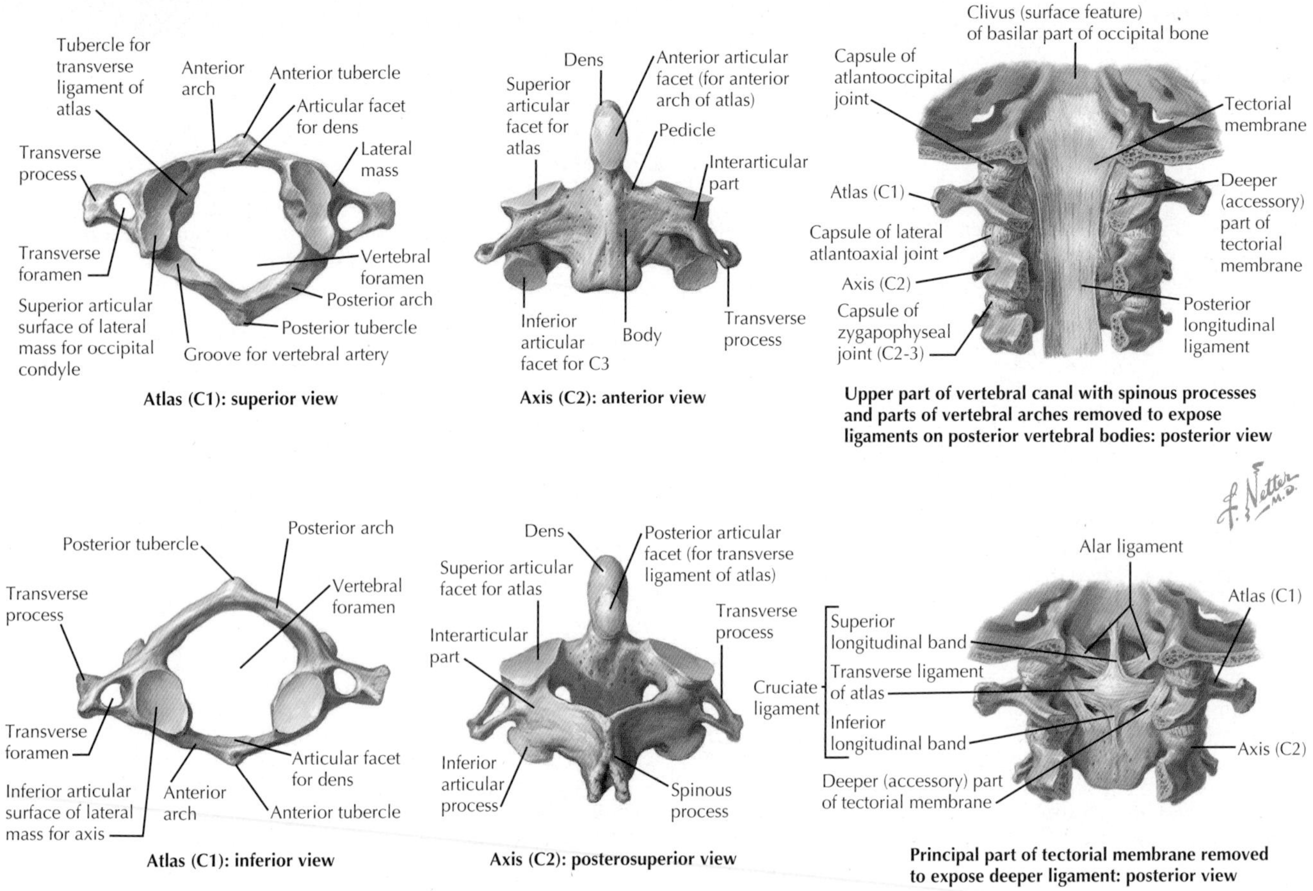
Tubercle for transverse ligament of atlas
Anterior arch
Anterior tubercle
Articular facet for dens
Lateral mass
Transverse process
Transverse foramen
Vertebral foramen
Posterior arch
Superior articular surface of lateral mass for occipital condyle
Posterior tubercle
Groove for vertebral artery
Atlas (C1): superior view
Dens
Superior articular facet for atlas
Anterior articular facet (for anterior arch of atlas)
Pedicle
Interarticular part
Inferior articular facet for C3
Body
Transverse process
Axis (C2): anterior view
Clivus (surface feature) of basilar part of occipital bone
Capsule of atlantooccipital joint
Tectorial membrane
Atlas (C1)
Deeper (accessory) part of tectorial membrane
Capsule of lateral atlantoaxial joint
Axis (C2)
Capsule of zygapophyseal joint (C2-3)
Posterior longitudinal ligament
Upper part of vertebral canal with spinous processes and parts of vertebral arches removed to expose ligaments on posterior vertebral bodies: posterior view
Posterior tubercle
Posterior arch
Transverse process
Vertebral foramen
Transverse foramen
Articular facet for dens
Inferior articular surface of lateral mass for axis
Anterior arch
Anterior tubercle
Atlas (C1): inferior view
Dens
Posterior articular facet (for transverse ligament of atlas)
Superior articular facet for atlas
Transverse process
Interarticular part
Inferior articular process
Spinous process
Axis (C2): posterosuperior view
Alar ligament
Atlas (C1)
Superior longitudinal band
Cruciate ligament
Transverse ligament of atlas
Inferior longitudinal band
Axis (C2)
Deeper (accessory) part of tectorial membrane
Principal part of tectorial membrane removed to expose deeper ligament: posterior view

Figure 46.1 Anatomy of a vertebra.

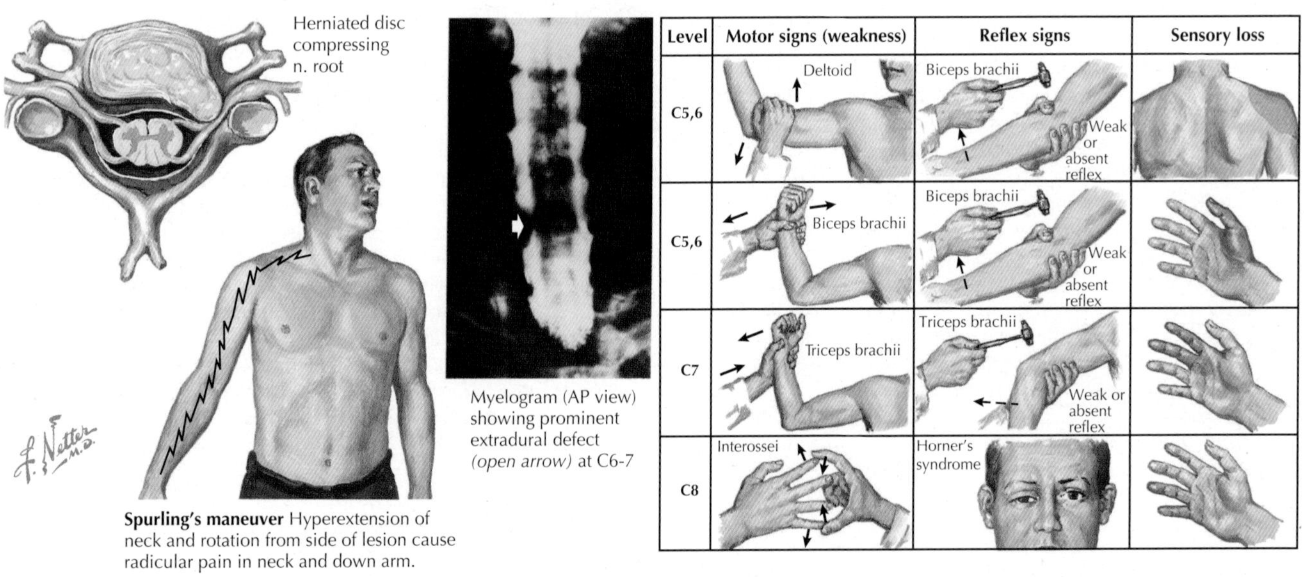
Herniated disc compressing n. root
Myelogram (AP view) showing prominent extradural defect (open arrow) at C6-7
Spurling's maneuver Hyperextension of neck and rotation from side of lesion cause radicular pain in neck and down arm.
Level
Motor signs (weakness)
Reflex signs
Sensory loss
C5,6
Deltoid
Biceps brachii
Weak or absent reflex
C5,6
Biceps brachii
Biceps brachii
Weak or absent reflex
C7
Triceps brachii
Triceps brachii
Weak or absent reflex
C8
Interossei
Horner's syndrome

Figure 46.2 Cervical disc herniation: Clinical manifestations.

Mechanism: With flexion of the cervical spine, the cord is pinched between the superior spinolaminar line and the superior aspect of the posterior lower vertebral body.

Presentation: An athlete will typically experience sudden paralysis after a tackle or being struck. The paralysis may occur in all four limbs or be limited to the upper body. Weakness is typically short-lived, lasting only minutes, but can last from hours to days. Sensory changes may be present as well.

Physical examination: The airway must be cleared and maintained if there is loss of consciousness. A gross neurologic examination must be performed. The physician must check for upper motor neuron signs such as hyperreflexia. Reflexes of the upper and lower extremity must be tested. Strength and sensation of the upper and lower body must be assessed as well.

Differential diagnoses: Cervical herniation, cervical fracture, and cervical fracture with dislocation.

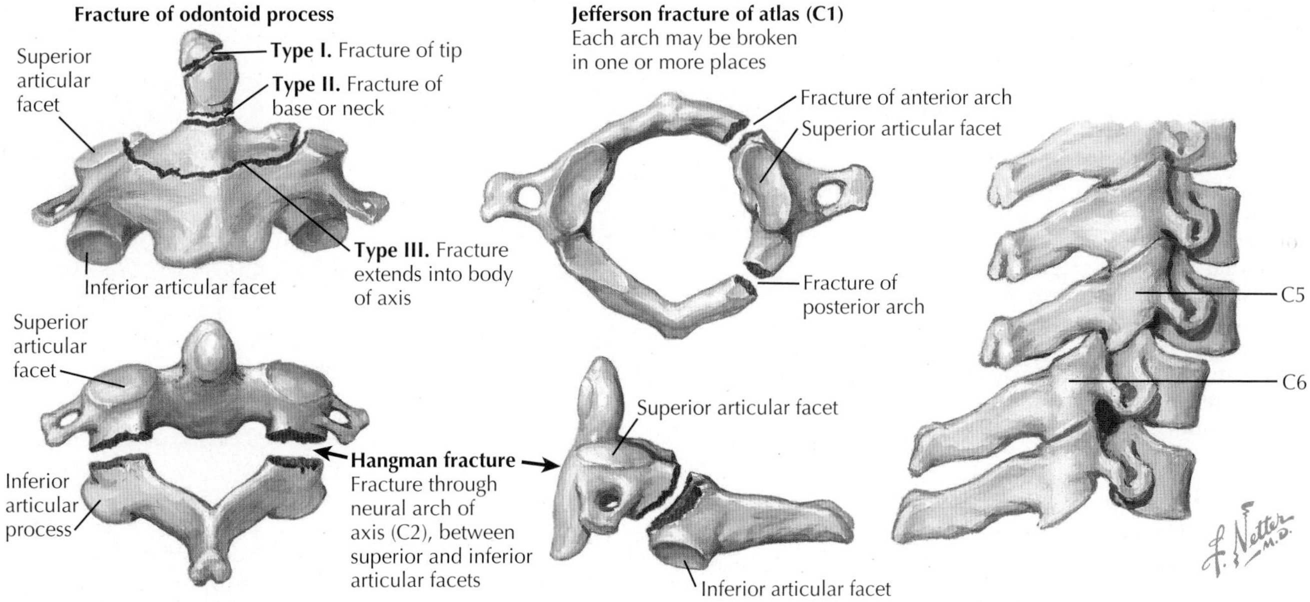
Fracture of odontoid process
Superior articular facet
Type I. Fracture of tip
Type II. Fracture of base or neck
Type III. Fracture extends into body of axis
Inferior articular facet
Jefferson fracture of atlas (C1)
Each arch may be broken in one or more places
Fracture of anterior arch
Superior articular facet
Fracture of posterior arch
C5
C6
Superior articular facet
Inferior articular process
Hangman fracture
Fracture through neural arch of axis (C2), between superior and inferior articular facets
Superior articular facet
Inferior articular facet

Figure 46.3 Fracture and dislocation of cervical vertebrae.

Diagnostics: Radiography.

The Torg ratio is determined by comparing the space from the back of the vertebral body to the spinolaminar line with the width of the vertebral body. The port ratio should be >0.8; a value less than this indicates spinal stenosis and the risk of recurrence. Anteroposterior (AP) and lateral radiographs should be obtained. A computed tomography (CT) scan can help to delineate any fractures in the bony structures. An MRI will help delineate any pathologic damage to soft tissue structures. An MRI has also been used to outline cerebrospinal fluid around the cord and thus *functional reserve*.

Treatment: Careful observation of the athlete; serial observation and neurologic examinations should be performed. Diagnostic studies must be performed as well. There is not clear evidence regarding the use of steroids in such cases. Administration of a steroid regimen within 8 hours of neurologic damage has shown some improvement in certain cases. Typically, the dosage of methylprednisolone is 30 mg/kg bolus over 15 minutes and then 15 mL/kg over 23 hours.

Prognosis: Return to play is highly controversial. Several doctors believe that if there is no stenosis and no evidence of structural damage, athletes should be allowed to return to play; however, athletes must have regained full strength and sensation before returning to play.

Cervical Disc Herniations

Description: Herniated disc material protrudes through a tear in the annulus causing compression on a root and, rarely, the spinal cord (see Fig. 46.2)

Mechanism of injury: Compression and rotation of the disc cause the annulus to tear. Pressure on the nucleus causes retropulsion through the tear.

Presentation: A nerve root exits in the neuroforamen at the level above its vertebral body; therefore, a herniation at C5–C6 will cause compression of the sixth cervical nerve root. Athletes will likely experience corresponding radicular pain, which often radiates, along with weakness of the corresponding muscles.

Physical examination: A Spurling sign may be present, which is pain radiating into the upper extremity when an athlete's head is extended and rotated toward the affected side. The athlete must be examined for sensory loss in a dermatomal pattern and checked for muscular weakness correlating to the corresponding nerve root.

Diagnosis: MRI is typically diagnostic and will indicate presence of a hard or soft disc between the affected vertebral bodies.

Treatment: Oral steroids or epidural injections are often beneficial. Anterior cervical discectomy and fusion or a foraminotomy of the cervical lamina may be needed to decompress the nerve root.

Prognosis and return to play: Athletes may be allowed to return to play when they have regained full function without any neurologic damage.

Spear Tackler Spine

Description: Athletes who experience multiple episodes of cervical neuropraxia; often seen in football players with the propensity to hit or tackle using the crown of the head. The National Football League (NFL) and the National Collegiate Athletic Association (NCAA) have banned the use of this technique; thereafter, the incidence of such catastrophic cervical spine injuries has correspondingly decreased.

Diagnostic: Radiographs may show cervical stenosis with a positive Torg ratio (<0.8). Moreover, degenerative abnormalities may also be observed on radiographs. Video analysis of athletes with the crown of the head and helmet intact is a common recent practice.

Prognosis: Athletes should not be allowed to return to athletic activity.

FRACTURES

C1 Fractures (Jefferson Fracture)

Description: Traumatic burst fracture of C1 (Fig. 46.3)

Mechanism of injury: Axial load

Presentation: Athletes often present with neck pain. Such an injury is unlikely to cause a neurologic injury because of the wide amount of space available for the spinal cord in this area.

Physical examination: Palpate for any tenderness. Check for lack of range of motion.

Differential diagnosis: Cervical strain

Diagnostics: Plain radiographs and CT scan are diagnostic.

Treatment: This is an unstable injury, and the athlete must be referred to an orthopedic spine surgeon or neurosurgeon.

Prognosis and return to play: The athlete will likely never return to play.

C2 Fracture (Hangman's Fracture)

Description: Traumatic spondylolisthesis of C2 (see Fig. 46.3)
Mechanism of injury: Axial load and extension
Presentation: Athletes will experience pain and may experience a sense of instability.
Physical examination: Palpation of the neck is performed, and range of motion is assessed. Such an injury typically does not result in paralysis or death because it actually widens the amount of area available to the spinal cord.
Differential diagnoses: Cervical strain
Diagnostics: Lateral radiographs can be diagnostic if there is displacement of the fracture. CT scans can further define the injury.
Treatment: The head should be immobilized, and the athlete must be referred to a spine specialist.
Prognosis and return to play: Poor

Burst Fractures

Description: This injury involves a fracture of the vertebral body in the coronal and sagittal plane. There can be retropulsion of fragments, which often results in spinal cord damage (Fig. 46.4).
Mechanism of injury: When a pure axial load is applied to straighten the cervical spine, failure can result because of bone and soft tissue inability to dissipate the force.
Presentation: Athletes commonly complain of neck pain, which may be the only symptom. There may be a root lesion accompanied by incomplete or complete paralysis.
Physical examination: Pain in the neck region. Often there is loss of motion in the cervical spine. There may be a sensory or muscular strength loss.
Differential diagnoses: Cervical strain
Diagnostics: Radiographs, CT scans, and MRI should be performed. A flexion and extension series should not be performed when there is an obvious fracture. The physician must be aware of the seemingly mild anterior teardrop fracture, which may indicate an unstable sagittal split in the anterior and posterior columns of the spine. Radiographs must include C1–T1 on the lateral films. An indication of fracture is loss of height (≥3 mm) of a vertebral body when compared with another vertebral body. An angulation of >11 degrees between the adjacent vertebral bodies is also a mark of instability. Measurements must be recorded between the vertebral bodies, not just between the vertebral body and the inferior vertebral body line (Fig. 46.5).
Treatment: The ABCs of trauma management must be applied. Sports medicine team members mostly practice turning the patient from the prone to the supine position and transport the patient onto a spine board. This often requires at least six individuals because of the relatively large size of an athlete. Helmets should not be removed on the field, but face masks can be removed to gain airway access while the cervical spine is stabilized. The medical professional must be familiar with the head gear the athlete is wearing and have all the necessary tools, nonelectric and electric, to remove the face mask. Equipment differs from sport to sport, and this should be recognized. Anatomic differences between pediatric and adult athletes must be also taken into account. Once the athlete is stabilized, transport him or her to the emergency department for further treatment.

DISLOCATIONS

Description: An injury wherein one or both facets are dislocated; an associated facet fracture may be present as well (Fig. 46.6)
Mechanism of injury: A flexion distraction injury

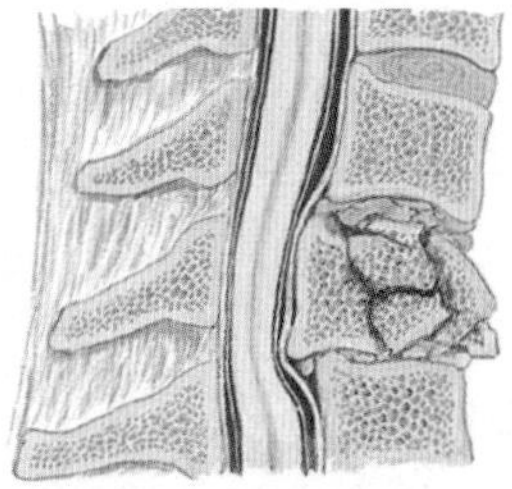

Type III. Fracture through entire vertebral body with fragmentation of its anterior portion. Posterior cortex intact but projects into spinal canal causing damage to cord and/or nerve roots.

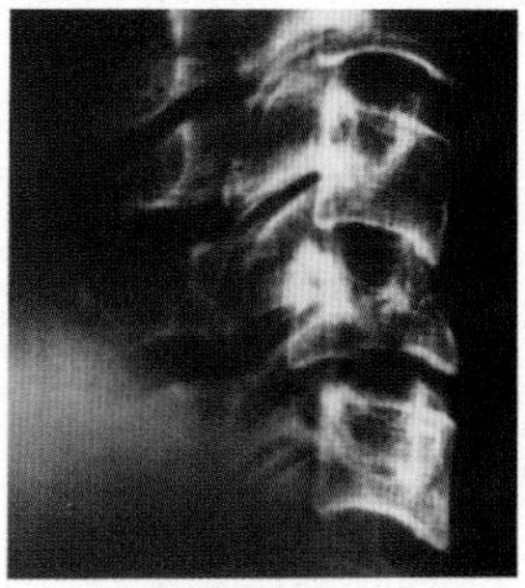

X-ray film: Type III fracture of C5

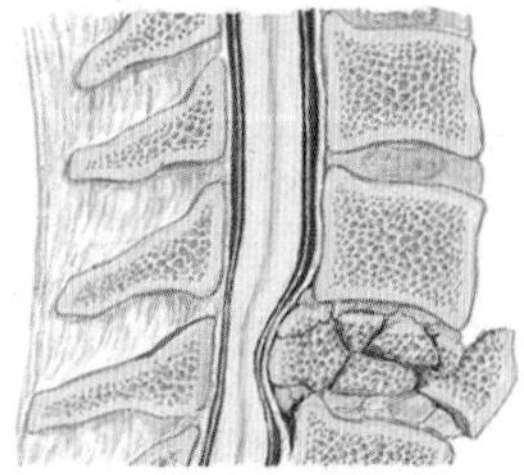

Type IV. "Burst" fracture. Entire vertebral body crushed, with intraspinal bone fragments.

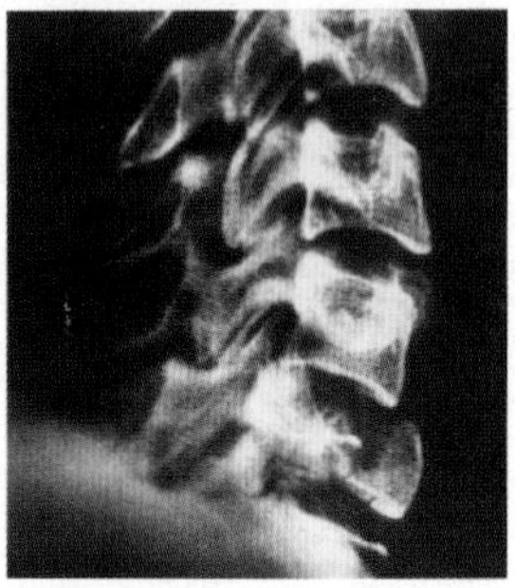

X-ray film: Type IV fracture of C6

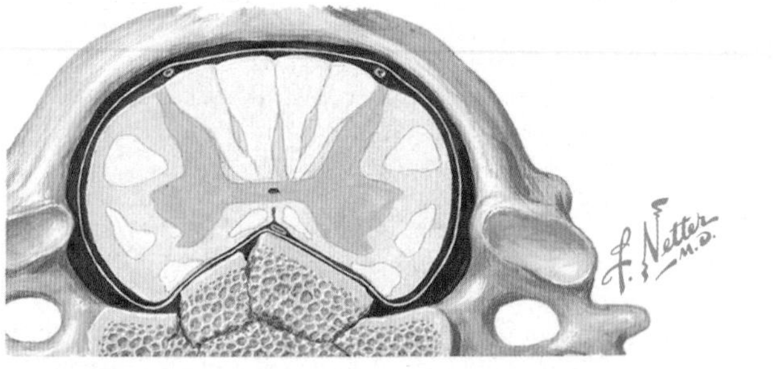

Dislocated bone fragments compressing spinal cord and anterior spinal artery. Blood supply to anterior two thirds of spinal cord is impaired.

Figure 46.4 Compression fractures of cervical spine.

Presentation: Pain or tenderness in the cervical spine; pain with range of motion; muscular strength or sensation loss. There may be associated neurologic injury, which can include nerve root injury or a complete lesion.
Differential diagnoses: Cervical strain and cervical disc herniation
Diagnostics: Radiographs will usually show >25% displacement on the posterior vertebral body line from the adjacent posterior vertebral body line for unilateral facet dislocation. There may be >50% displacement for a bilateral facet dislocation. A >3.5-mm displacement of the posterior vertebral line of one vertebral body compared with the other indicates instability. CT scans should be performed as well, which will delineate fractures of facets and provide an overall indication of the force and treatment pattern. MRI will indicate the presence of myelomalacia or cord damage in addition to the presence of a herniated disc. A herniated disc is observed in up to 55% of cases with bilateral facet dislocation.

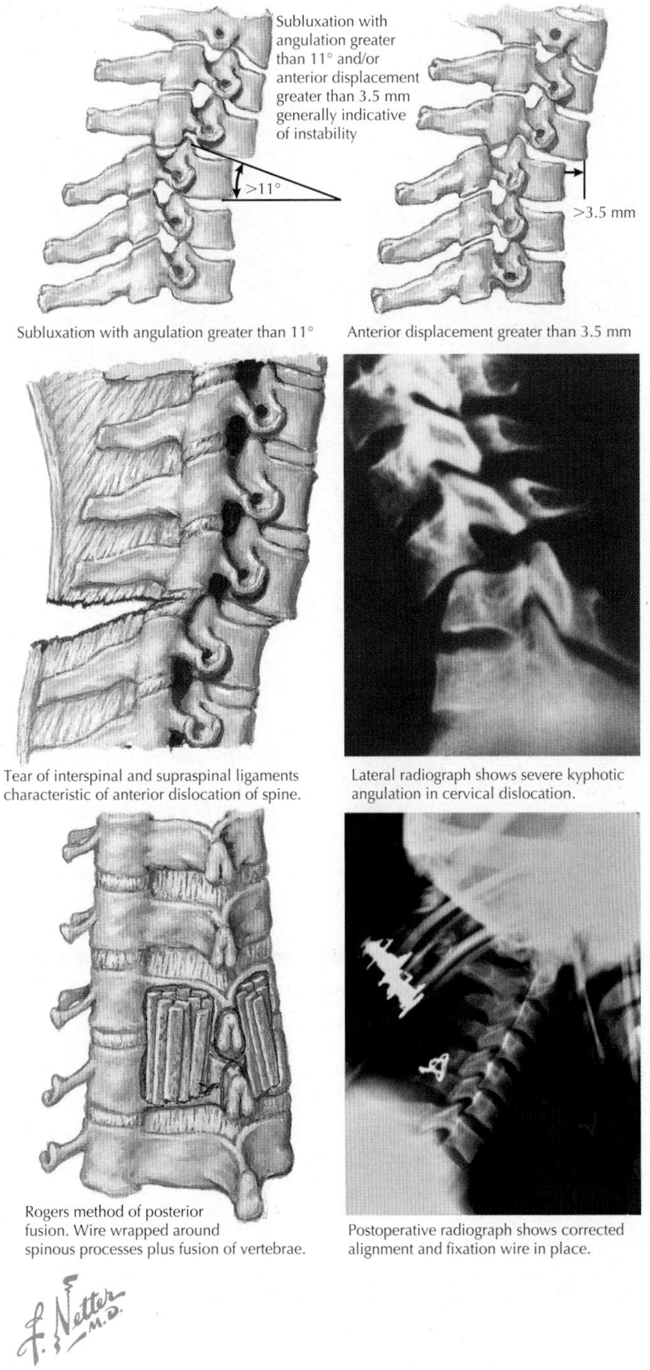
Subluxation with angulation greater than 11° and/or anterior displacement greater than 3.5 mm generally indicative of instability
>11°
>3.5 mm
Subluxation with angulation greater than 11°
Anterior displacement greater than 3.5 mm
Tear of interspinal and supraspinal ligaments characteristic of anterior dislocation of spine.
Lateral radiograph shows severe kyphotic angulation in cervical dislocation.
Rogers method of posterior fusion. Wire wrapped around spinous processes plus fusion of vertebrae.
Postoperative radiograph shows corrected alignment and fixation wire in place.
F. Netter M.D.

Figure 46.5 Subluxation and ligamentous instability of cervical spine.

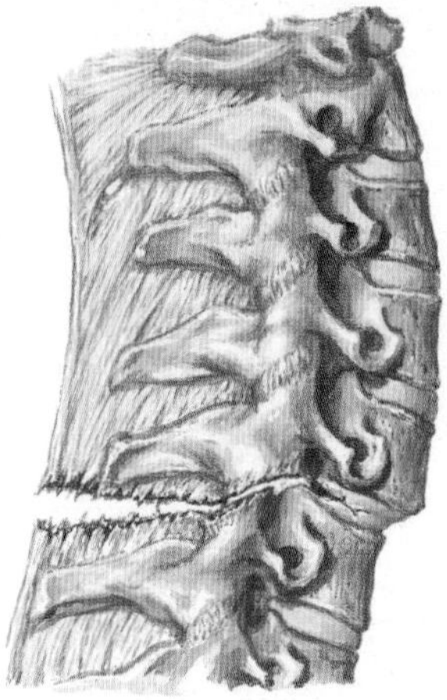

Anterior dislocation of C5 on C6 with tear of interspinous ligament, facet capsules, and posterior fibers of intervertebral disc

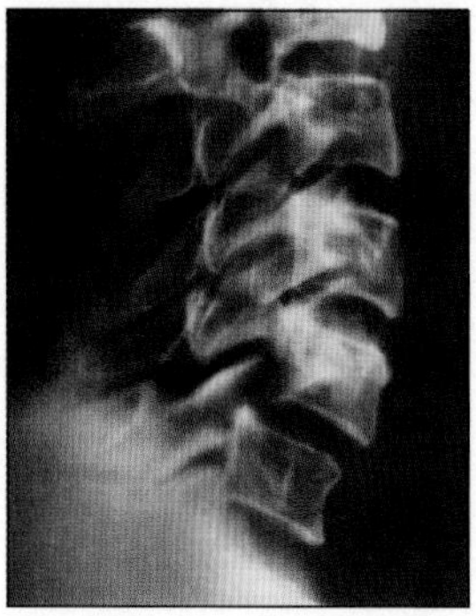

X-ray film showing moderate (1st-degree) dislocation of C5. If there is no evidence of spinal cord injury, spontaneous healing may occur following reduction by traction and prolonged bracing.

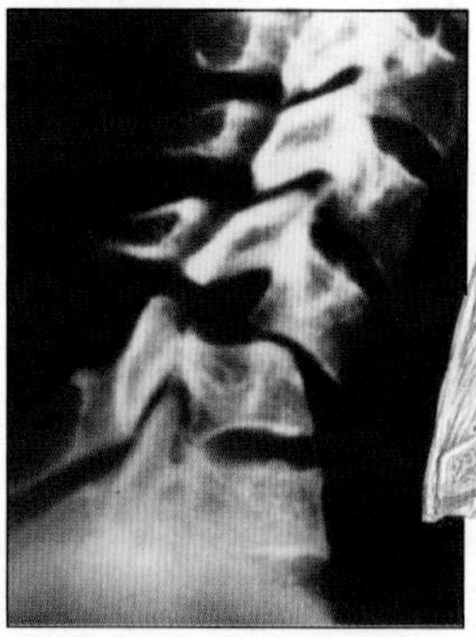

X-ray film: 3rd-degree dislocation of C5

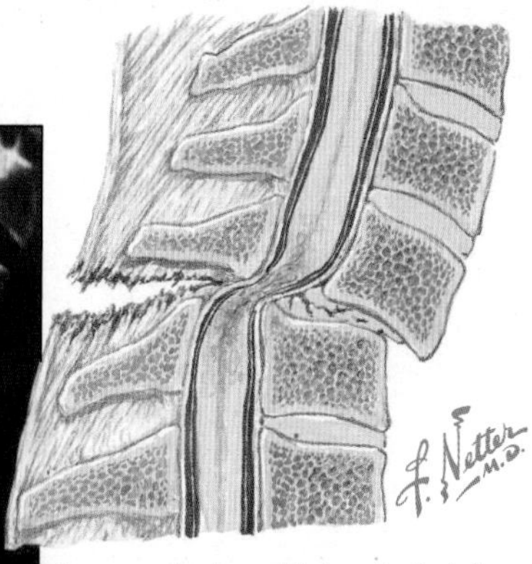
F. Netter M.D.

Severe spinal cord injury in 3rd-degree cervical dislocation. Any evidence of cord or nerve root damage is indication for prompt:
· **Reduction** by traction
· **Decompression** by disc removal
· **Fixation** by interbody fusion

Figure 46.6 Dislocation of cervical spine.

Treatment: On the field, the head and neck are mobilized until the athlete is safely transported to the hospital. The helmet should not be removed. An orthopedic spine surgeon or neurosurgeon should then be consulted. Reduction is typically performed with weight applied to Gardner–Wells tongs; this procedure is usually performed with the patient awake to ensure no worsening of any neurologic injury. The herniated fragment can retropulse into the spinal cord canal. Certain physicians use prereduction MRI to identify any herniated discs and reduce the likelihood of retropulsion.

RECOMMENDED READINGS

Available online.

EYE INJURIES

47

David E. Olson • Jaimi Weber • Brian F. Allen

GENERAL PRINCIPLES

- A 2013 study estimated over 30,000 emergency department visits annually for sports- and recreation-related eye injuries. The majority of these injuries occurred in individuals younger than 25 years, with a peak during adolescence, and 80% occurred in males.
- Approximately 1.5% of all sports-related injuries involve the eye or ocular adnexa. These injuries have a high morbidity rate, and long-term visual impairment can lead to additional medical and socioeconomic sequelae. The highest rate of visual impairment occurs with projectile-firing devices, such as paintball, air, or pellet guns.
- In the United States, basketball is the leading sports-related cause of eye injuries, followed by baseball/softball and cycling. In Europe and South America, soccer is the leading cause.
- Although eye protectors cannot completely eliminate the risk of injury, appropriate and well-fitted eye protection can reduce the risk of significant eye injury by as much as 90%.
- The American Association of Pediatrics and the American Academy of Ophthalmology 2004 position statement on protective eyewear in young athletes categorizes sports by the risk of eye injury to the unprotected eye (Table 47.1). Although there is no ideal collecting system for data, there are national reporting systems at the high school (High School Reporting Information Online [HS RIO]) and collegiate levels (National Collegiate Athletic Association Injury Surveillance Program [NCAA ISP]) (Table 47.2).

Mechanisms of Eye Injuries in Sports

- Eye injury severity is correlated with total impact force, rate of force onset, and kinetic energy of impacting object.
- Ocular injuries fall into several broad categories (Table 47.3).
- Open globe injuries are full-thickness wounds to the eye wall (cornea or sclera) and may result from a blunt or penetrating trauma. Activities that cause ruptured globes typically have a stick or projectile that fits into the orbit. An underlying history of eye surgery or eye disease may increase the risk of open globe injury.
- Lacerations may be caused by objects that "slice" or penetrate the eye, which may lead to open globe injuries.
- Closed globe injuries are those that do not completely penetrate the cornea or sclera. These include lamellar lacerations, corneal abrasions, contusions, hyphema, or injury to the choroid, macula, retina, or optic nerve.
- Blunt injuries, typically causing contusions, globe rupture, or adnexal injury, account for most sports-related eye injuries. Contusions are usually caused by blunt objects smaller than the orbit (e.g., golf ball or finger). In addition, several objects will deform significantly on impact (e.g., soccer ball), producing a "knuckle" that will impact the eye (Fig. 47.1). With objects smaller than the orbit, there is generally a greater force transmitted to the internal structures of the eye, whereas with larger objects, there is an increased risk of orbital wall fracture and occult internal ocular injuries.
- Radiant energy or ultraviolet (UV) burn injuries are less common but may occur in activities that take place at a high altitude or on snow.

Principles of Protection From Eye Injuries in Sports

- Protective devices work by deflecting the impact energy away from the eye and dissipating the energy over time and area. This is typically accomplished with either a lens or a mechanical grid (e.g., wire-framed face guard or mesh-fencing helmet).
- Inappropriate fit of protective gear can decrease the protection offered, placing the eye at an increased risk.
- Gear must be comfortable and not interfere with athletic performance.
- Contact lenses offer no protection. Athletes who wear corrective lenses should wear one of these three options:
  - Contact lenses plus the appropriate protective eyewear
  - Polycarbonate lenses in sports frames that pass the appropriate American Society for Testing and Materials (ASTM) standard
  - Over-the-glasses protector that conforms to the appropriate ASTM standard

Certification and Selection of Eyewear

- Organizations that certify sports protective eyewear include the Protective Eyewear Certification Council (PECC), Canadian Standards Association (CSA), Hockey Equipment Certification Council (HECC), and National Operating Committee on Standards in Athletic Equipment (NOCSAE). The equipment approved by these organizations commonly bears their seal and should be selected when available (Table 47.4).
- ASTM International has written performance standards based on design and strength, upon which many of these organizations base their certification (see Table 47.4).
- For sports with no appropriate ASTM standards or certified equipment, the American National Standards Institute (ANSI) should be considered.

Preparticipation Eye Examination

- Preparticipation eye examinations should include the assessment of visual acuity, visual fields, pupillary size and responsiveness, eye movements, and ophthalmoscopy.
- Documentation of anisocoria is imperative in order to determine if it is preexisting or caused by an acute injury. Up to 20% of the population may have physiologic anisocoria of >0.4 mm. In physiologic cases, there will be no associated visual field defects or diplopia. The afferent and efferent pupillary light reaction will also be normal.
- Assess athlete's history for high degree of myopia, surgical aphakia, retinal detachment, eye surgery, infection, or injury and family history for retinal detachment, retinal tears, or diabetic retinopathy. All these conditions increase risk of serious eye injury and thus require ophthalmologic consultation before participation in high-risk or very high-risk sports.

Visual Risk Factors

- Best-corrected visual acuity worse than 20/40 in either eye or spectacle correction for myopia or hyperopia >6 diopters; disease, degeneration, or structural weakness of the eye itself; thin sclera; history of retinal degenerative disease; and history of eye surgery that weakens the outer wall of the eye, particularly cataract or refractive surgery. Athletes with such risk factors should be evaluated by an ophthalmologist before engaging in high-risk or very high-risk sports.
- Disability from high corrective spectacle lenses can sometimes be mitigated by contact lenses; however, contact lenses themselves can be a risk factor.

Table 47.1 RISK CATEGORIES FOR SPORTS

High Risk	**Small, Fast Projectiles** • Air rifle/BB gun • Paintball • Hard projectiles, fingers, "sticks," close contact • Baseball/softball/cricket • Basketball • Fencing • Field hockey • Ice hockey • Lacrosse (in men and women) • Squash/racquetball • Street hockey **Intentional Injury** • Boxing • Full-contact martial arts
Moderate Risk	• Fishing • Football • Soccer/volleyball
Low Risk	• Bicycling • Noncontact martial arts • Skiing
Eye Safe	• Gymnastics • Track and field

Modified from Vinger PF. A practical guide for sports eye protection. *Phys Sports Med.* 2000;28(6):49–69; Committee on Sports Medicine and Fitness. Protective eyewear for young athletes. *Pediatrics.* 2004;113(3):619–622.

Table 47.2 RATE OF EYE INJURIES AS REPORTED IN NCAA ISP

	Rate of Eye Injury Per 100,000 Athlete-Exposures	
	Men	**Women**
Wrestling	10.06	
Field hockey		5.61
Basketball	5.13	7.24
Softball		2.39
Baseball	1.64	
Soccer	2.09	2.55
Volleyball		1.32
Football	0.83	
Lacrosse	0.70	

Data from Boden BP, Pierpoint LA, Boden RG, Comstock RD, Kerr ZY. Eye injuries in high school and collegiate athletes. *Sports Health*. 2017;9(5):444–449.

- Functionally one-eyed athletes face additional risk. A person is functionally one-eyed when loss of the better eye would result in significant changes in lifestyle because of poor vision in the remaining eye.
  - A child with vision worse than 20/40 should be considered functionally one-eyed. Assessment of adults is more difficult because their judgment and values determine the visual impairment they are willing to accept. Special considerations are necessary for such athletes.
  - The only sports absolutely contraindicated for functionally one-eyed athletes are boxing and full-contact martial arts because the risks of serious injury are high and there is no effective eye protection. Wrestling and noncontact martial arts have a lower incidence of eye injury, but also do not have effective eye protection. They should be discouraged for functionally one-eyed athletes and banned for monocular athletes.

Table 47.3 RELATIVE FREQUENCY OF EYE INJURIES

Most Common	**Relatively Infrequent**	**Eye Emergencies**
Corneal abrasion	Chemical burns	Globe disruption
Corneal foreign body	Vitreous hemorrhage	Retinal detachment
Conjunctival foreign body	Retinal edema or hemorrhage	Lens dislocation
Subconjunctival hemorrhage	Hyphema	Blowout fracture of the orbit
Eyelid laceration	Injury to the lacrimal system	Optic nerve injury

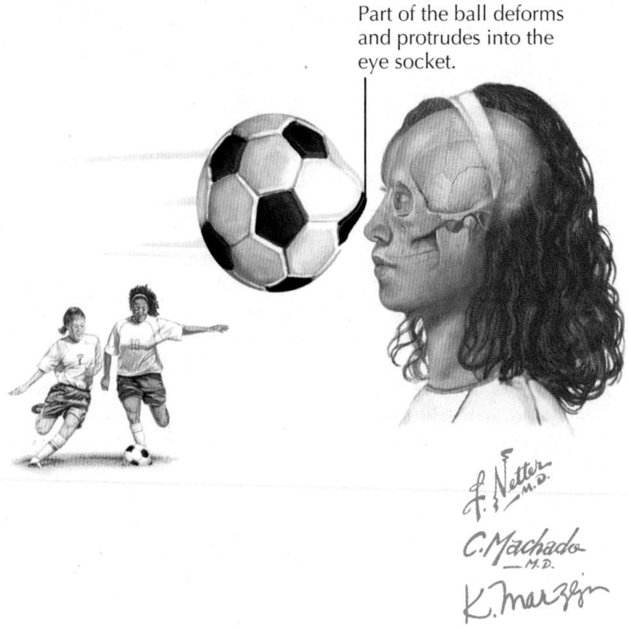
Part of the ball deforms and protrudes into the eye socket.
F. Netter M.D.
C. Machado M.D.

Figure 47.1 Large object causing injury to the globe.

Examination and Functional Testing After Injury

History

- Mechanism of injury is important. Historical features such as type of trauma (blunt vs. penetrating), direction of force, object size, and whether eye protection was worn influence the type of injury.
- Relevant signs and symptoms include pain, decreased visual acuity, diplopia, flashers, floaters, and halos around lights.
- Intraocular injuries or foreign bodies may be painless because the lens, retina, and vitreous have no pain sensation.

Physical Examination

Inspection: Look for signs of external trauma, bruising, fullness, or subcutaneous emphysema. Mild external trauma can be a sign of more severe internal ocular injury. Do not manipulate or forcibly open an eye if mechanism and examination cannot rule out a ruptured globe.

Visual acuity: This is the single most important physical examination feature in evaluation of the eye. Visual acuity can be determined with a Snellen eye chart if one is available. Alternatively, have the patient read printed material from different distances. Changes in visual acuity are more important than absolute values. Any acute decrease in acuity necessitates immediate further evaluation and referral (Box 47.1).

Table 47.4 STANDARDS AND CERTIFYING ORGANIZATIONS FOR SELECTED SPORTS

Sport	Eye Protection	Standards	Certifying Organizations
Baseball	Polycarbonate or wire face guard attached to a helmet while batting; sports goggles with polycarbonate or TriVex lenses while on the field	ASTM F910	PECC
Basketball	Sports goggles with polycarbonate or TriVex lenses	ASTM F803	PECC
Field hockey	Full face mask for the goalie; sports goggles with polycarbonate lenses or wire mesh goggles while on the field	ASTM F803	PECC
Football	Wire face mask and polycarbonate eye shield attached to the helmet		NOCSAE
Ice hockey	Helmet with full face protection	ASTM F1587 ASTM F513	CSA/HECC
Men's lacrosse	Helmet with full face protection		NOCSAE
Women's lacrosse	Full face protection or sports goggles with either polycarbonate lenses or wire mesh goggles	ASTM F803	PECC
Paintball	Full face protection	ASTM F1776	PECC
Racket sports	Sports goggles with polycarbonate or TriVex lenses	ASTM F803	CSA/PECC
Skiing	High impact–resistant eye protector	ASTM F659	PECC

From the American Academy of Ophthalmology (AAO). www.aao.org.

Confrontational visual field testing: Examiner tests visual fields in all four quadrants of each eye using his or her own eye as a control.

Ocular motor testing: Check the cardinal eye movements. Deficiencies in upward gaze may suggest entrapment with orbital blowout fracture or neuro-ophthalmologic pathology. There will often be associated diplopia. Do not perform this evaluation if globe laceration is suspected.

Pupillary examination: Initially, evaluate the pupils for uniform roundness and symmetry. Anisocoria may denote an injury along the pupillary pathways. Check direct and consensual responses. If a defect is found, a swinging flashlight examination may be performed to help localize the injury by quickly moving the light back and forth between the eyes.

- Afferent pupillary defect, or injury to the retina or optic nerve (cranial nerve [CN] II), results in paradoxical dilation when the light hits the ipsilateral eye. In this case, the consensual response would be intact because the efferent pathway (CN III) from the contralateral eye would be maintained. This is known as a *Marcus Gunn pupil.*
- An efferent lesion would limit direct and consensual response in a lesion ipsilateral to the affected eye.

Anterior chamber assessment: Can be accomplished by shining a light from the temporal side of the eye toward the medial aspect. Inspect the iris for a symmetric round opening and presence of hyphema.

- Assess depth of anterior angle. Increased medial shadowing can suggest a narrow angle, though a special slit lamp examination is needed to visualize and fully assess the anterior angle.
- Assess for a layer of blood that accumulates at the 6 o'clock position. Look at the iris for uniformity. The iris may prolapse into the wound, producing an irregular pupil.

Ophthalmoscopy: Often impractical on the sideline, but can add useful information for a more complete ophthalmologic examination; very useful in evaluation of acute visual loss

Red reflex: Normally is evenly colored and without shadows.

- Hyphema, acute swelling of the lens, and vitreous hemorrhage may lead to loss of this reflex.
- Retinal edema occurs in contusion injuries to the globe in addition to retinal detachments. This leads to interruption of circulation and may alter the intensity of the red reflex.

Fundoscopic examination: Assess optic disk margins, cup-to-disk ratio, blood vessels, and retina. This is ideally performed after pupillary dilation.

- Contraindications to pupillary dilation include (1) need for neurologic monitoring, including pupillary response, with significant head trauma; (2) suspected acute angle glaucoma or narrow anterior chambers; and (3) iris-supported ocular lens implants.

Neurologic: Decreased sensation or numbness in the V2 distribution may accompany orbital floor fractures.

Special tests:

- **Fluorescein staining:** Instill anesthetic drops such as proparacaine hydrochloride 0.5% and have the patient blink. Fluorescein strips can then be moistened with sterile water and touched to the inferior cul-de-sac, with care taken to not brush the cornea. Use a cobalt light or Wood's light to examine for defects, which fluoresce yellow-green.
- **Applanation tonometry:** Hand-held electronic tonometers are convenient for measuring intraocular pressure (IOP). Topical anesthetic drops should be instilled before use. Normal IOPs range from 10 to 21 mmHg.
- Pressure can be estimated by palpating the globe and using palpated tension in the fellow eye for a rough comparison.
  - Care should be taken to avoid compression of a ruptured or perforated globe by this test.
  - IOP may be elevated with hemorrhage or swelling of orbital contents and may be decreased in certain cases of blunt injury to the globe.

BOX 47.1 INDICATIONS FOR REFERRAL

- Any loss of visual acuity
- Visual field cuts
- Pupil asymmetry or abnormal pupillary reaction
- Perception of flashing lights
- Orbit asymmetry
- Hyphema
- Laceration of eye or complex laceration of lids
- Orbital pain with movement of the eye
- Halos around lights
- Abnormal EOM
- Abnormal mass on inspection
- Diplopia

EOM, Extraocular movements.

COMMON SPORTS INJURIES

Corneal Abrasion

Description: Results from cutting, scratching, or abrading the thin protective surface of the anterior ocular epithelium. Corneal disruption near the central visual axis interferes with visual acuity.

Patients often report a history of ocular trauma or foreign body sensation and subsequent acute pain. Aggressive eye rubbing can also cause injury. Predisposing factors include foreign body, contact lens, and previous history of corneal abrasion.

Signs and symptoms: Red eye, pain, photophobia, conjunctival injection, tearing, foreign body sensation, gritty feeling, and decreased visual acuity if central corneal area is involved; symptoms are worsened by blinking, rubbing, and light exposure.

Examination: After fluorescein staining, corneal abrasions and foreign bodies will appear yellow-green against a blue background illumination. Topical anesthetic may be necessary to allow examination. Additional ocular injury must be ruled out, and any foreign bodies should be removed. Small conjunctival lacerations heal quickly and may mask penetrating globe injuries.

Treatment:

- Healing is best facilitated by pain management and controlling lid movement.
- Postinjury infection is uncommon; however, topical antibiotics may be useful in cases where contamination with debris has occurred, as well as in immune-compromised patients. Bacitracin, erythromycin, or gentamicin ointment has better lubricating properties than drops and is considered first-line treatment.
- In contact lens wearers, a gram negative/antipseudomonal antibiotic such as ciprofloxacin should be administered. Contact lens use should be discontinued until abrasion is completely healed and antibiotic course completed. **An ophthalmologist should follow these patients within 24 hours.**
- Patching is no longer recommended. A 2016 Cochrane review failed to show an increase in healing rate or pain relief with patching. Patching may cause increased pain, decreased oxygen delivery, and increased moisture, resulting in increased risk of infection.
- For large abrasions with significant pain and photophobia, topical nonsteroidal anti-inflammatory drugs (NSAIDs) such as Voltaren or Acular are useful in reducing pain.
  - **Topical mydriatics have not been proven to be beneficial.** Mydriatics were previously thought to relieve ciliary muscle spasm. However, one randomized controlled trial (RCT) showed that pain was similar in patients using eye lubricant alone or combined with topical NSAID.
  - Topical anesthesia can be effective in relieving discomfort and allowing for an appropriate examination. These medications traditionally were avoided because they were thought to increase the risk of corneal ulceration. However, a recent study showed that topical tetracaine can be safely used with a frequency up to every 30 minutes for a 24-hour period. In this study, 116 total patients were studied, and the effectiveness of topical tetracaine versus topical saline was compared. There was no increase in healing time with topical anesthesia use as determined by repeat fluorescein examination at 48 hours. Moreover, this group reported significantly greater drug effectiveness compared with the saline drop group. Based on this study, topical tetracaine can be considered on a case-by-case basis for a 24-hour period to allow an athlete to return to play the same day.
  - In general, avoid topical corticosteroid preparations except in complicated cases because they can encourage fungal and viral infections; consider an ophthalmology consult if they are being considered.

Prognosis: Uncomplicated corneal epithelial injuries heal completely within 24–72 hours without scarring. Although frequently contaminated, they rarely become infected. **Recurrent epithelial erosion** is infrequent, but patients must be warned that this may occur.

Foreign Bodies on Eye and Eyelid Surfaces

Description: May result from penetrating ocular trauma, which is the most common cause of blindness in teenage and young males. The size, shape, and momentum of the object at impact affect the depth of ocular penetration. Superficial corneal foreign bodies are much more common than deeper penetrating objects, which can lodge within the orbit and cause retinal injury. Corneal scarring or infection may occur.

Signs and symptoms: Same as for abrasions

Examination:

- Minute foreign bodies may require magnification to be appropriately visualized and removed.
- If a metallic foreign body has been embedded for hours to days, a rust ring may be present.
- Localization can be enhanced by fluorescein stain; topical anesthetic may be necessary to facilitate examination. Fluorescein stain will appear yellow-green against blue background.
- Upper and lower conjunctival fornices should be carefully examined for foreign bodies.
- Upper eyelid should be everted and conjunctival surface inspected for foreign bodies.
- A Seidel test will help detect leaking aqueous or exposed vitreous. In this test, fluorescein ophthalmic strips are wetted with normal saline and applied to the superior conjunctiva, allowing dye to flow over the cornea. The concentrated fluorescein is dark orange, but if it becomes diluted with aqueous, it turns bright green under blue light. The presence of an intraocular foreign body (IOFB) suggests globe penetration. The patient may be asymptomatic if foreign bodies are below the epithelial or conjunctival surface. Over a few days, the epithelium may grow over small corneal foreign bodies, with pain reduction. If a corneal infiltrate is noted, an infectious cause should be considered. Foreign bodies can cause small sterile inflammatory reactions around the object. However, if a large infiltrate, ulceration, significant anterior chamber reaction, or significant pain is present, it should be managed as an infection.
- If there is concern for IOFB, helical computed tomography (CT) scan with 1-mm axial and coronal cuts or biomicroscope ultrasound can be considered. Referral should be made to an ophthalmologist for a dilated examination and management.

Treatment: For corneal foreign bodies, apply short-acting topical anesthetics. If there is a likelihood of penetration through >25% of the globe wall, immediate referral should be made to an ophthalmologist for surgical removal. Otherwise, foreign body removal should be performed using irrigation, sterile needle, or foreign body removal instrument. Cotton-tip applicators are not appropriate because the large surface area may cause an epithelial defect.

- Always approach foreign bodies tangentially and aim just beneath them to avoid accidental corneal perforation.
- Often, vigorous flushing with a forceful stream of irrigation solution (e.g., normal saline from a squeeze bottle) is enough to dislodge foreign bodies.
- For metallic foreign bodies, a magnetic spud may be helpful.
- Topical antibiotic ointments such as bacitracin or Ciloxan should be prescribed to prevent infection.
- Rust rings may be removed by a well-trained physician with an Alger brush or automated burr. Rust rings should be visualized using a slit lamp.

Eyelid Lacerations

Description: May occur in association with blunt trauma and from sharp objects and can result from the propulsion and shattering of eye protection equipment (Fig. 47.2).

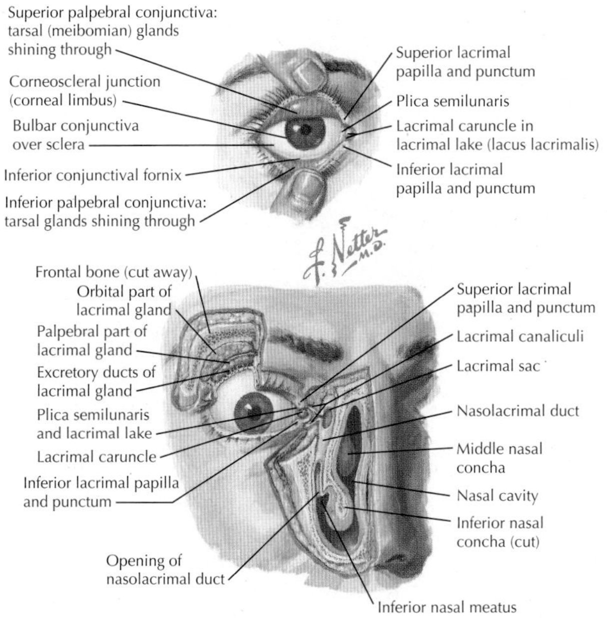
Superior palpebral conjunctiva: tarsal (meibomian) glands shining through
Corneoscleral junction (corneal limbus)
Bulbar conjunctiva over sclera
Inferior conjunctival fornix
Inferior palpebral conjunctiva: tarsal glands shining through
Superior lacrimal papilla and punctum
Plica semilunaris
Lacrimal caruncle in lacrimal lake (lacus lacrimalis)
Inferior lacrimal papilla and punctum
Frontal bone (cut away)
Orbital part of lacrimal gland
Palpebral part of lacrimal gland
Excretory ducts of lacrimal gland
Plica semilunaris and lacrimal lake
Lacrimal caruncle
Inferior lacrimal papilla and punctum
Opening of nasolacrimal duct
Superior lacrimal papilla and punctum
Lacrimal canaliculi
Lacrimal sac
Nasolacrimal duct
Middle nasal concha
Nasal cavity
Inferior nasal concha (cut)
Inferior nasal meatus

Figure 47.2 Orbit eyelids and lacrimal apparatus.

Signs and symptoms: Swelling, hemorrhage, and anatomic disruption of lids. Damage may be subtle, and appearance may be normal.

Examination: Evaluation of normal anatomic relationship of lid margins and front surface of the globe, as well as symmetry with uninjured side; opening and closing functions are specifically assessed, particularly to verify that lids can be spontaneously closed. Rule out the possibility of upper eyelid ptosis or lacerations in lacrimal drainage (canalicular) system. The globe must be thoroughly inspected for signs of damage.

Treatment: Lacerations require individual suturing of lid tissue layers and additional repairs specific to any injuries involving integrity of the lacrimal drainage apparatus. **Particular injuries requiring ophthalmology referral include:**
- Lacerations involving the upper or lower lid margin
- Lacerations suspected to involve the lacrimal sac or duct
- Lacerations with exposure of orbital fat
- Horizontal lacerations with ptosis and possible disruption of the tarsal plate
- Any laceration with avulsion of eyelid tissue

Prognosis: Because of the rich vascular supply to eyelids, healing is rapid and deformities are minimal in cases of minimal tissue loss and good anatomic approximation.

Blunt Trauma to Orbit

Blunt injuries to the globe are the most common sports-related eye injury and may be associated with ruptured globe or hyphema. They result from facial blows directed toward orbital contents or from sudden pressure increases transmitted to the eye from surrounding orbital tissue.

Ruptured Globe

Description: Occurs when the full thickness of the cornea or sclera is breached and has the potential for serious eye morbidity.

Epidemiology: Sports-related open globe injuries occurrence from most to least common: fishing, hunting/shooting, baseball/softball, golf, basketball, and racket sports.

Mechanism of injury: Rupture occurs when hard objects increase IOP, causing rupture at weak point. Globe lacerations occur when sharp (e.g., sticks) or small hard objects (e.g., shrapnel, BBs, shattered eye protection) enter globe at high velocity.

Physical examination:
- Evaluate anterior segment of globe for signs of subconjunctival hemorrhage.
- Pupil should be round, central, and symmetric with fellow eye.
  - Corneal lacerations frequently incarcerate iris tissue, causing distortion and displacement of the pupil.
  - Scleral lacerations also may displace the pupil because of herniations of the uveal tract through the defect.
  - Prolapsed uveal tissue presents as a dark brown or black mass, even in those with fair complexion and blue eyes.
  - Globe lacerations may result in subluxation of crystalline lens.
  - Intraocular bleeding is a frequent complication, causing obscuration of ocular media and loss of red reflex.
  - IOP may be decreased.

Treatment: Emergent ophthalmology referral:
- Manage other trauma, including other head or neck trauma.
- Patients should not be given anything orally.
- **Rigid** shield over affected eye at all times. Patches are not sufficient.
- Avoid ointments and other topical medications.
- Tetanus status should be updated.
- Other considerations to discuss with ophthalmologist include narcotics, prophylactic antibiotics, and imaging. Imaging is often necessary to rule out associated foreign body.
- Penetrating objects that remain in place should be secured in place without removal and covered for protection. A Styrofoam cup may be a useful adjunct for this.

Prognosis: In patients with penetrating eye trauma, predictors of excellent final visual acuity (defined as 20/60 or better) are initial postinjury visual acuity of 20/200 or better, wound location anterior to the plane of insertion of the four rectus muscles, wound length ≤10 mm, and sharp mechanism of injury. Predictors of poor outcomes include initial visual acuity of light perception or no light perception, wounds extending posterior to rectus muscle insertion plane, wound length >10 mm, blunt or missile injury, associated hyphema, lid involvement, vitreous loss, and retinal detachment. Only 50% of children with ruptured globe injuries recover good visual acuity.

Return to play: After a ruptured globe injury, return-to-play decisions should include ophthalmology consultation and discussion of risks of future participation.

Orbital Fracture

Description: An orbital blowout fracture occurs when blunt trauma to the eye or orbit is transmitted to the bony walls of the orbit, causing fracture. This may result in entrapment of contents of the orbit, including the eye muscles, leading to restricted gaze and diplopia (Fig. 47.3).

Signs and symptoms: A high index of suspicion for this injury should be present when an object larger than the ocular orbit strikes the eye. History should elicit the mechanism, change in visual acuity, pain, previous visual impairment, and use of eye protection. Additional symptoms suggestive of injury are diplopia, particularly with upward gaze, and ipsilateral nosebleed.

Examination:
- Rule out ruptured globe.
- Findings include:
  - Enophthalmos (posterior displacement of eye), which may have the appearance of relative ptosis
  - Periorbital ecchymoses/abrasions suggest mechanism sufficient to cause injury.
- Restricted vertical gaze occurs with orbital floor fractures that result in inferior rectus muscle entrapment tethering the eye.
- Decreased sensation or numbness in V2 distribution can occur as a result of neurapraxia because V2 runs through the orbital floor/maxillary sinus roof.

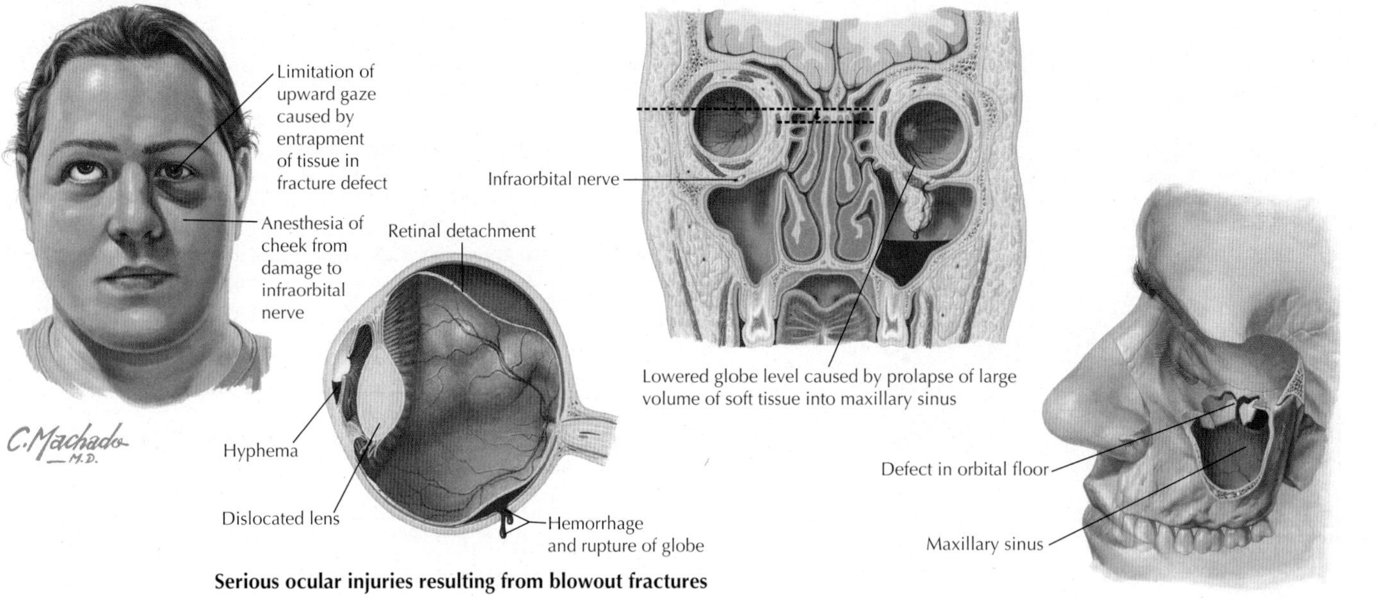
Limitation of upward gaze caused by entrapment of tissue in fracture defect
Anesthesia of cheek from damage to infraorbital nerve
Retinal detachment
Infraorbital nerve
Lowered globe level caused by prolapse of large volume of soft tissue into maxillary sinus
Hyphema
Dislocated lens
Hemorrhage and rupture of globe
Defect in orbital floor
Maxillary sinus
C. Machado M.D.
Serious ocular injuries resulting from blowout fractures

Figure 47.3 Orbital blowout fractures.

- Coronal CT with 2-mm slices enables visualization of soft tissue densities, such as prolapsed orbital fat, extraocular muscle, and hematoma.
- Plain radiographs can have a false-negative rate of up to 50%.
- Magnetic resonance imaging (MRI) does not visualize bone well.

Treatment: Surgical treatment is usually necessary only when there is interruption or herniation of orbital tissue. Diplopia may be transient; thus, surgery should be deferred until a significant portion of the contusion injury has resolved. Conversely, in cases with little contusion injury and obvious interruption or herniation of orbital tissue, there is no need to delay definitive repair.

Prognosis: Varies depending on degree of injury; prognosis is best when orbital tissue damage is minimal. Prolonged tissue entrapment and inflammation can result in fibrosis and contractures, which can lead to permanent functional disabilities.

Hyphema

Description: Presence of blood in the anterior chamber. Projectiles that strike exposed portion of the eye are a common cause of hyphema. Anteroposterior globe compression leads to expansion of the globe with tearing of the blood vessels of the iris or ciliary body. There is a high frequency of concomitant injury, including blunt or penetrating trauma. Baseball and softball players are commonly affected. Hyphema frequently occurs in microscopic quantities and, consequently, can be easily overlooked.

Signs and symptoms: Because many hyphemas are small, visual acuity may be unaffected. There may be a mild injection of the globe with moderate transient discomfort and photophobia. In addition to hyphema, other injuries associated with contusion injuries may be found, including papillary paralysis, pupillary contour irregularities, and tearing of the uveal tract.

Examination: Slit lamp examination is necessary to identify any turbid microscopic hyphema before it has had time to settle out in the anterior chamber; however, careful penlight examination can identify hyphema in acute settings. IOP should be measured. Of hyphema patients, 25% have other ocular injuries, including vitreous or retinal hemorrhage or dislocated lens.

Treatment:
- Immediate referral to an ophthalmologist.
- Manage as if a ruptured globe were present.
- Shielding of the eye should be accomplished with a protective metal shield for 2 weeks.
- Activity should be severely restricted with bed rest for 4 days followed by light activity for 2 weeks. Topical cycloplegics (e.g., atropine sulfate twice daily for 2 weeks) and topical corticosteroids should be given. Salicylates and NSAIDs should be restricted. Acetaminophen can be given for pain relief. Topical beta-blockers, (e.g., timolol) are often used if there is associated increased IOP. In nontraumatic cases, assess for coagulopathy and treat accordingly.
- Examine 3 consecutive days to monitor for re-bleeding or IOP elevation. Recurrent bleeding is most frequent during initial 5 days after injury and occurs in 4%–6% of cases. Increased IOP may lead to glaucoma. Patients with sickle cell trait or disease are more susceptible to this complication. **Increased IOPs may accompany hyphemas of any size.**
- Corneal blood staining is possible.
- Sickle cell status should be established in all African-American patients or Hispanic patients who have an IOP >21 mmHg.
- Patients should be re-evaluated 2 weeks after the injury even if there are no other problems.

Prognosis: Excellent, particularly if blood clears rapidly, no recurrent bleeding, or other injuries. Usual duration of an uncomplicated hyphema is 5–6 days.
- **Recurrent bleeding may lead to permanent loss of visual acuity.**
- Most microhyphemas can be treated on an outpatient basis, unless re-bleeding or IOP is uncontrolled. If hyphema occupies greater than one-third of anterior chamber or IOP is over 30 mmHg, hospitalization is recommended.

Vitreous Hemorrhage

Description: When vitreous hemorrhage is caused by trauma, significant force is involved and additional eye injury is generally present. It can result from blunt trauma, shaking, or proliferative retinopathy. Blood obscures light path through the vitreous cavity and reduces visual acuity.

Signs and symptoms: Assessing and documenting the patient's vision before symptoms of hemorrhage are crucial. Patients may report seeing "floaters, visual haze, smoke, shadows, or cobwebs." More severe hemorrhages may result in sensation of dark streaks that break up into numerous, minute black spots, or vision reduction to only light perception. Isolated vitreous bleeding is not associated with symptoms such as pain or discomfort.

Examination: Measure visual acuity and pupillary response; on fundoscopic examination, fundus detail is often blurred or disappears entirely and may be seen as a "black reflex." On slit lamp examination, fresh blood is identified readily by adjusting the slit beam to a tangential position and viewing the anterior vitreous directly behind the lens.

Treatment: Generally nonoperative; severe cases may require surgical removal of blood and vitreous, which is often performed at the time of repair of associated ocular injuries.

Prognosis: Guarded

Retinal Hemorrhages and Detachment

Description: Can result from direct trauma to eye by transmission of force to the retinal surface; this produces immediate loss of visual function within the detached segment. In the absence of treatment, the entire retina eventually becomes involved, and total retinal detachment develops. Can be caused by retinal instability seen with violent exercise performed in conditions of decreased oxygen saturation or elevated venous pressure from Valsalva maneuvers; such findings have been documented in activities such as mountain climbing and weightlifting. **Retinal detachment** produces immediate loss of visual function within the detached segment. Any form of blunt or perforating trauma can produce retinal detachment. Indirect trauma, such as severe head injury, myopia, and vitreous traction, are risk factors.

Signs and symptoms: Assessing and documenting the patient's vision before hemorrhagic symptoms develop is crucial. Multiple asymptomatic areas of retinal hemorrhage and edema are not uncommon, particularly if affected areas are confined to the peripheral retina. Macular involvement results in decreased visual acuity or distortion of visual perception. Patients often report positive scotoma at the edge of the visual field or seeing "floaters, visual haze, smoke, shadows, or cobwebs." As detachment progresses, the patient may describe visualization of "lightning flashes" or "flying sparks." An enlarging scotoma may be seen as a waving black curtain encroaching on central vision. Severe hemorrhages may result in the sensation of dark streaks that break up into numerous, minute black spots, or vision reduction to only light perception.

Examination: Visual field and acuity measurement; fundoscopic examination reveals both flame-shaped hemorrhages and round-blot hemorrhages or may show a "black reflex." On slit lamp examination, fresh blood is readily identified by adjusting the slit beam to a tangential position and viewing the anterior vitreous directly behind the lens. As the retina becomes more elevated, it is necessary to add additional convex or plus lenses to the fundoscopic viewing port to maintain sharp focus on the internal retinal surface. It is necessary to dilate the pupil widely to visualize a detachment during its early stages because detachments begin in the far periphery.

Treatment: Symptomatic; surgical intervention is almost invariably necessary after actual retinal separation has occurred. If surgery is not indicated, close observation for 1–2 weeks allows time for spontaneous clearing of mild hemorrhage, but it may take several months for complete vision to return. Upright positioning for sleep may enhance settling of the hemorrhage. Emergent consultation is required if hemorrhage results from trauma.

Prognosis: Varies depending on location, extent, and severity; poor chance for recovery of good central vision if macula is involved.

Dislocated Lens

Description: Results from tearing of lens zonules and loss of support in its normal position; may result in subluxation or movement of the lens away from the site of injury, causing it to decenter slightly but remain in a relatively normal position. More extensive damage may entirely displace the lens, causing it to fall either into the anterior or posterior chamber.

Signs and symptoms: Visual acuity is affected by even the slightest shift in position of the crystalline lens:
- Lens decentering causes irregular astigmatism with poor near vision secondary to loss of accommodation power and decreased distance visual acuity.
- Complete dislocation results in aphakia.
- Shifts of lens position, although slight, can also cause loss of iris stability and resulting tremulousness with slight ocular movements or vibrations (iridodonesis).
- Monocular diplopia

Examination:
- Visual acuity may be initially reduced but can frequently be corrected by change in refraction.
- Slit lamp examination may reveal iris undulations (iridodonesis) at the pupillary margin after rapid eye movements.
- Strabismus is not uncommon secondary to amblyopia.
- Pupillary dilatation can aid in assessment of lens position and evaluation of the retina.
- Enophthalmos with facial myopathic appearance may be seen in patients with Marfan syndrome.
- IOP should be assessed because lens dislocation can result in secondary glaucoma.
- If Marfan syndrome, homocystinuria, or other collagen vascular diseases are suspected, cardiac workup should be performed, including a cardiac echocardiogram. Check serum and urine levels of homocysteine or methionine for homocystinuria. Genetic-associated lens dislocation is usually bilateral.

Treatment: Variable and may necessitate surgical removal of the lens; immediate referral should be made to an ophthalmologist if this injury is suspected

Prognosis: Varies with extent of injury

Chamber Angle Recession

Description: Generally results from blunt trauma to globe, causing a sudden increase in anterior chamber pressure, which is transmitted to lens–iris diaphragm, propelling it backward. Dynamics are similar to that of lens dislocation; however, in angle recession, lens position is usually normal. In a few cases, force of injury is sufficient to produce associated injury to trabecular meshwork, which may eventually lead to glaucoma.

Signs and symptoms: In cases wherein glaucoma develops, onset is almost invariably delayed from the time of the injury and progresses slowly. As with other forms of chronic glaucoma, visual loss is insidious, beginning with the peripheral areas of the visual field. Angle recession glaucoma should always be suspected in cases of unilateral chronic glaucoma.

Examination: Usual methods for evaluating chronic glaucoma, including evaluation of IOP and visual field examination, with special attention to classic field defects commonly seen in chronic glaucoma.

Treatment: Angle recession glaucoma is frequently not responsive to medical therapy and may require surgical treatment.

Prognosis: Varies with extent of pressure elevation, length of time it has been present, and responsiveness to treatment.

Red Eye

Description: Aim of management should be differentiation of the symptom of red eye and assessment of underlying disease. Redness can be caused by hyperemia with dilation of conjunctival, episcleral, or scleral vessels (caused by trauma, chemical burns, or immunologic reactions); inflammatory reactions from infections (bacterial, viral, or fungal); or chronic reactions of external eye from systemic causes (Box 47.2).

BOX 47.2 MOST COMMON CAUSES OF RED EYE

- Conjunctivitis
- Episcleritis and scleritis
- Keratitis and corneal ulcer
- Iritis and intraocular infections (endophthalmitis)
- Glaucoma (acute and chronic)
- Dry eye
- Subconjunctival hematoma (hyposphagma)
- Corneal and conjunctival foreign body
- Corneal abrasion
- Corneal flash burn
- Chemical burns
- Blunt or penetrating trauma to the eye
- Allergic reaction
- Blepharitis

Signs and symptoms: Important aspects of history:
- Association with pain
- Pain, itching, and visual decrease or loss
- Mucopurulent discharge, watering, blepharospasm (lagophthalmos), or systemic (e.g., fever, nausea) findings
- Foreign body sensation
- Decreased visual acuity

Examination: Should include anatomic location of redness (eyelids, conjunctiva, cornea, sclera and episclera, or intraocular); measurement of IOP (to rule out acute closed angle glaucoma) and visual acuity (evaluation if decreased, needs urgent referral to ophthalmologist). Measure pupil size and response to light. Fluorescein testing may be necessary.

Treatment and prognosis: Depends on the cause of symptoms; athletes should not return to play until cause is ascertained

INJURY PREVENTION

Risk Factors to Be Considered

- Physical development and skill level
  - Beginners may have increased risk because of lack of necessary refinement of skill of sport.
  - Advanced players, particularly in certain high-risk sports, may play more aggressively and be at a higher risk.
- **Existing visual impairment** increases the risk of injury.
- **Preexisting eye disease** may present an increased risk to athletes in all risk groups.
  - Conditions that may lead to serious eye disorders or get worse after even minor trauma to the eye include retinal detachment, retinal degeneration, severe myopia, thin sclera, and prior ocular surgery.
  - Systemic disease with eye involvement and previous serious ocular injuries may be risk factors as well.

Types of Eye Protectors

Total head protector: Combination of helmet and face shield designed to protect eyes, teeth, jaw, and larynx and transfer forces to skull; designed for use in high-risk sports that require total head protection: football, hockey, and lacrosse

Full face protector: Designed for use in conjunction with eye protectors for high-risk sports that do not require protection for brain: fencing and certain positions in baseball and softball

Helmet with separate eye protectors: For use in sports with low risk of injuries to lower face and neck: cycling, snowmobiling, skiing, automobile racing, and bobsled racing

Helmet only: Designed to protect brain only; afford little protection to face or eyes; used in boxing and cycling

Sports eye protectors: Used only to protect eyes and are recommended in all high-risk sports for which additional head and face protection is impractical: all racquet sports, baseball, soccer, basketball, and softball (see Table 47.4)

"Sports" sunglasses: Most are inadequate for both impact resistance and UV radiation blockage. Adequate eyewear of this type should:
- Contain manufacturer's statement on intended sport use
- Block light from sides and below
- Protect from glare (transmit 30% of light)
- Be lightweight, cosmetically acceptable, and aerodynamically designed to prevent drying in wind

RECOMMENDED READINGS

Available online.

MAXILLOFACIAL INJURIES 48

Mark J. Erickson • Paul Escher • Michael K. Case • Scott A. Escher

GENERAL PRINCIPLES

Epidemiology

- Three to twenty-nine percent of facial injuries are a result of sporting activities.
- Sixty to ninety percent of facial injuries in sports occur in males aged 10–29 years.
- Approximately 75% of facial fractures involve the zygoma, mandible, or nose.
- Most commonly injured teeth are maxillary central incisors, followed by lateral incisors and mandibular incisors.

Initiation of Care of the Head-Injured Athlete

Airway Injury or Compromise

- Perform primary survey, following the ABCDEs (airway, breathing, circulation, disability/neurologic assessment, exposure) of basic life support.
- May need to secure airway before making any other assessment.
- If neck is injured, use jaw thrust maneuver and maintain cervical spine precautions.
- May be difficult to maintain airway with unstable mandibular fracture and some soft tissue injuries.
- Can use oral airway or endotracheal tube as indicated in unconscious patients. A nasal trumpet works well in an awake patient without a midface fracture.
- Cricothyrotomy may be the only option in emergency.

Cervical Spine Injury and Concussion (See Chapter 45: "Head Injuries" and Chapter 46: "Neck Injuries")

- The spine must be stabilized if there is any doubt regarding injury or if the athlete shows altered mental status.
- With facial injuries, providers must check for associated cervical spine injuries or concussion. Approximately 1 in 20 mandibular fractures will have an associated cervical spine injury.

History

- Check for history of abnormalities such as crooked nose, missing teeth, malocclusion, or anisocoria to look for preexisting condition.

Physical Examination

INSPECTION

- Observe for facial asymmetry, facial nerve function, midface widening (intercanthal distance), ocular asymmetry, and malocclusion from multiple angles.
- Early examination before swelling causes any asymmetry is optimal.
- Bleeding or bruising may be indicative of other possible injuries.

PALPATION

- Systematically palpate bony structures, including maxilla and mandible, bimanually with gloved fingers in the oral cavity.
- Conduct sensory examination for possible nerve injuries, including all three branches of the trigeminal nerve (Fig. 48.1).

RANGE OF MOTION

- Assess mandibular motion. Pain with opening or closing can indicate mandible fracture, hemarthrosis, or zygomatic arch fracture.
- Ocular motions can be altered in certain facial fractures, indicating ocular muscle entrapment or nerve injury, which may require more immediate treatment.

Imaging Studies

CONVENTIONAL RADIOGRAPHY

- Conventional radiography is rarely used for facial bone evaluation and adds little to the clinical examination.
- Panoramic radiographs are often used for dental root injuries.

CROSS-SECTIONAL IMAGING

- Computed tomography (CT) and magnetic resonance imaging (MRI) are much superior to conventional radiographs in identifying both normal and abnormal anatomy, particularly in the pediatric population.
- Facial bone CT offers better anatomic details, particularly bony anatomy, and is the study of choice over plain radiographs in trauma. Three-dimensional CT reconstructions can be a valuable diagnostic tool and aid in surgical planning. The speed of CT makes it preferred over MRI for initial workup, particularly in unstable patients.
- MRI is superior in soft tissue imaging, does not use ionizing radiation, and displays vascular anatomy without using contrast, but is rarely used in trauma.

COMMON SOFT TISSUE INJURIES

Lacerations

Examination: Assess for both sensory and motor nerve injuries in addition to underlying bone damage. With the ears or nose also assess for cartilage exposure and tissue avulsion, as these injuries may require care by a facial trauma specialist.

Treatment: Cleanse with sterile water or irrigating solution. Administer local anesthesia with lidocaine and epinephrine to help with hemostasis. Certain experts advocate not using epinephrine on ear or nose, sometimes preferring regional anesthetic approaches. Deep wounds may require layered closure with a dissolving suture to re-approximate subcuticular tissues. Skin closure can be with 5-0 or 6-0 suture or tissue adhesive if skin edges are closely aligned; appropriate alignment of certain anatomic structures (e.g., eyebrows and vermilion border of lip) is important for cosmesis. If laceration is minor, bleeding can be controlled, and wound can be covered with occlusive dressing, the athlete may return to competition.

COMMON EAR INJURIES

Auricular Hematoma ("Cauliflower Ear")

Mechanism of injury: Caused by shear forces (e.g., in wrestlers without head protection) that results in blood and/or serum accumulation between the ear cartilage and the perichondrium or between sheared layers of perichondrium.

Examination: Swelling or fluctuance in the cartilaginous area, usually in outer or lateral regions (Fig. 48.2)

Treatment: May usually continue participation in the event where the injury occurs; initially treated by aspiration of hematoma or incision and drainage after anesthetizing:

- Permanent disfigurement can occur if not appropriately treated.
- Field-block anesthesia by infiltrating the posterior sulcus, as well as the skin anterior to the helix and tragus, with 1% or 2% lidocaine without epinephrine; care should be taken to avoid injecting near the facial nerve.
- Hematoma will recur if not bolstered to hold the packing onto the area with slight pressure. Bolster can be a dental roll on both sides of the pinna held in place by a 3-0 or 4-0

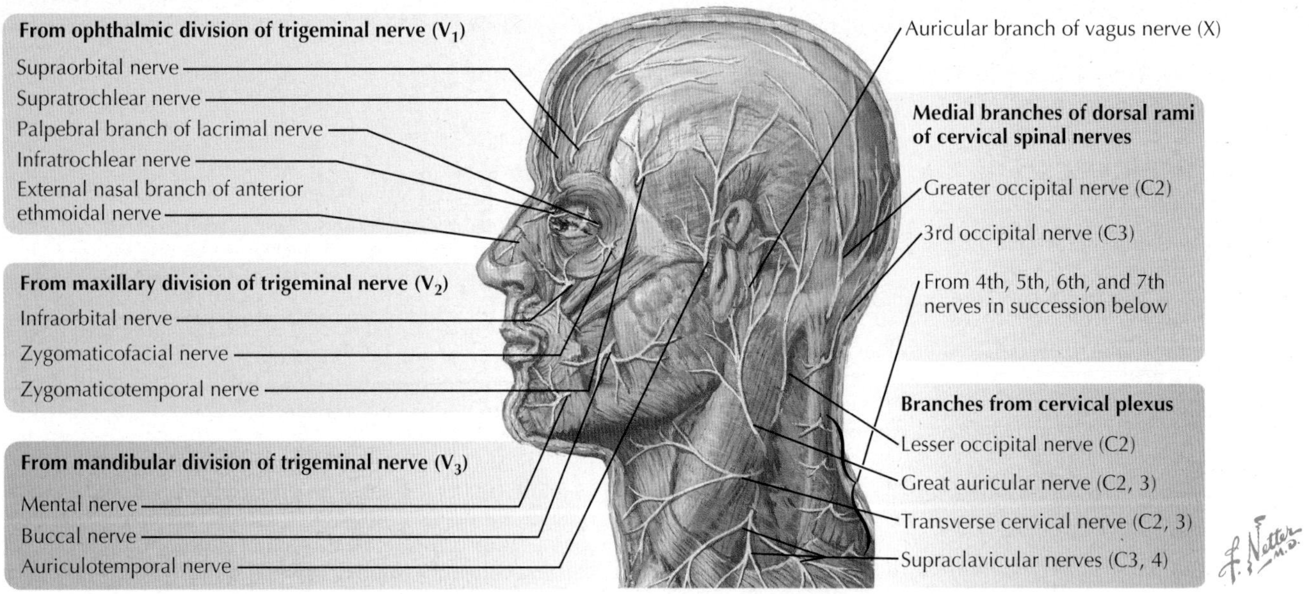
From ophthalmic division of trigeminal nerve (V_1)
Supraorbital nerve
Supratrochlear nerve
Palpebral branch of lacrimal nerve
Infratrochlear nerve
External nasal branch of anterior ethmoidal nerve
From maxillary division of trigeminal nerve (V_2)
Infraorbital nerve
Zygomaticofacial nerve
Zygomaticotemporal nerve
From mandibular division of trigeminal nerve (V_3)
Mental nerve
Buccal nerve
Auriculotemporal nerve
Auricular branch of vagus nerve (X)
Medial branches of dorsal rami of cervical spinal nerves
Greater occipital nerve (C2)
3rd occipital nerve (C3)
From 4th, 5th, 6th, and 7th nerves in succession below
Branches from cervical plexus
Lesser occipital nerve (C2)
Great auricular nerve (C2, 3)
Transverse cervical nerve (C2, 3)
Supraclavicular nerves (C3, 4)
F. Netter M.D.

Figure 48.1 Cutaneous nerves of head and neck.

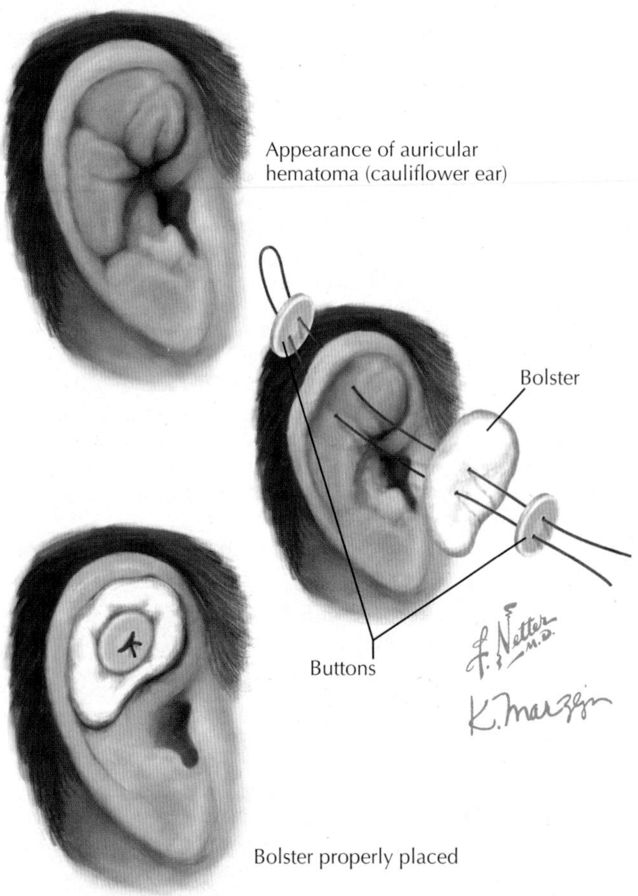
Appearance of auricular hematoma (cauliflower ear)
Bolster
Buttons
Bolster properly placed
F. Netter M.D.
K. Marzen

Figure 48.2 Cauliflower ear.

monofilament nonabsorbable suture. Alternatively, a button or silicone splint can be placed on either side of the ear. To prevent further trauma, the wrestler must use headgear and leave the bolster in place for 7 days (see Fig. 48.2).

- Always use antibiotics with *Staphylococcus* coverage with a bolster in place.
- If infection occurs, bolster must be removed and the area must be incised, drained, and treated with an antibiotic that covers *Staphylococcus* and *Pseudomonas.*

Prevention: Appropriately fitted headgear

Ear Laceration (Including Aforementioned Lacerations)

- Sew the ear in layers with cartilage, perichondrium, and finally skin. On the lateral portion of the ear, all three layers may have to be sutured together.
- Attempt to minimize sutures in cartilage.
- Use an undyed absorbable 6-0 suture for cartilage and perichondrium.

Otitis Externa ("Swimmer's Ear")

Mechanism of injury: Disruption of the thin ear canal skin. Water-sport athletes are at particularly high risk; usually caused by *Pseudomonas aeruginosa* or *Staphylococcus aureus*

Examination:

- Pain and discomfort with motion of pinna
- Swollen, inflamed, and erythematous external auditory canal
- Purulent discharge

Treatment:

- Suction ear to remove debris.
- Antibiotics/corticosteroid combination drops; quinolones are the best choice.
- May need a wick to allow antibiotics to penetrate to innermost portion of the ear canal if marked swelling is present; leave in place for 3–5 days.
- Consider treating significant infections with an oral antibiotic that has *Pseudomonas* coverage.
- Stay out of water until asymptomatic.

Prevention: Dry ears after swimming; use of hair dryer to ear can help reduce moisture. A combination of alcohol and vinegar or commercially available alcohol-based products such as Swim Ear® can help lessen moisture and may reduce incidence of otitis externa.

Tympanic Membrane Perforation

Mechanism of injury: Can occur while skydiving or scuba diving because of pressure changes; from a blow to the ear or a fall onto the ear while water skiing

Examination:
- Conductive hearing loss and serous or bloody drainage from ear
- Visible perforation in tympanic membrane
- Associated vertigo can signify ossicular disruption

Treatment: Eighty-five to ninety percent will heal without treatment; if not healed within 2–3 weeks, refer to an otolaryngologist. For water sports, use earplugs to keep water out of ear canals until perforation heals. Avoid sports with large changes in pressure, such as platform diving, until perforation heals. If injury occurred in river or lake, consider antibiotic eardrops. For suspected ossicular disruption, the athlete must be immediately referred to an otolaryngologist.

COMMON DENTAL INJURIES

Mechanism of injury: Traumatic event causing direct or indirect trauma to teeth resulting in displacement of affected teeth, alveolar ridge fracture, or tooth nerve damage.

History:
- Spontaneous pain may indicate pulp exposure.
- Tender teeth with chewing may indicate injury to the periodontal ligament or a cracked tooth.
- Teeth sensitivity to extremes of temperature may indicate pulp exposure or inflammation.
- Changes in bite patterns (e.g., malocclusion) suggest facial fracture or dental subluxation.

Examination: Examine teeth for fractures and laxity, bite for occlusal discrepancies, and soft tissues for associated lacerations and bruising. Panoramic radiographs or CT should be performed with dental fractures or loosening. Assess for root or bony fractures or, in case of younger athletes, for permanent tooth bud displacement.

Treatment:
- ***Primary teeth:*** Primary goal is to prevent injury to permanent teeth.
  - Injuries needing urgent dental evaluation:
    - Displaced or significantly loose primary teeth
    - Do not replace avulsed or extruded (completely dislocated) teeth because this may injure the underlying permanent teeth.
    - Crown fractures involving the pulp need prompt referral to prevent infection.
  - Injuries needing dental evaluation within a few days:
    - Mildly subluxed teeth, which appear in normal position but have pain with chewing, should be treated with a soft diet
    - Crown fractures not involving the pulp
    - Root fractures
- ***Permanent teeth:*** Permanent teeth that are subluxed (loosened) or luxated (loosened with displacement) should be examined by a dentist as soon as possible, but no on-field reduction is needed. Fractures involving pulp can be painful. Fractures of teeth can be treated hours after injury.
- Avulsed or displaced teeth: Preservation of the delicate periodontal ligament cells on the root is necessary for tooth survival. Little chance for dental survival after 1 hour out of socket, especially if left dry. Needs immediate dental referral for emergent reimplantation. Field care:
  - Handle only by crown
  - May rinse with saline or tap water, but do not rub or clean root
  - Reimplantation of the tooth, if possible, is best option. Athlete can keep tooth in place with finger pressure or by biting on a gauze pad.
  - If tooth cannot be reimplanted immediately, a transport medium can be used until arrival at appropriate facility. The tooth can be held in the mouth (under the tongue or buccal vestibule) if compliance and age allow, or it can be placed in Hank balanced salt solution, (e.g., Save-A-Tooth®). This will maintain viability of periodontal ligament cells longer, increasing the likelihood of successful reimplantation. Other alternatives are cold milk and saline solution. Water should not be used because of its hypotonicity.
  - Tetanus prophylaxis should be given if tooth is contaminated with dirt and last tetanus shot was more than 5 years ago.

Prevention: Mouth guards can prevent dental injury. Basketball players are seven times more likely to have an orofacial injury when not wearing a mouth guard.

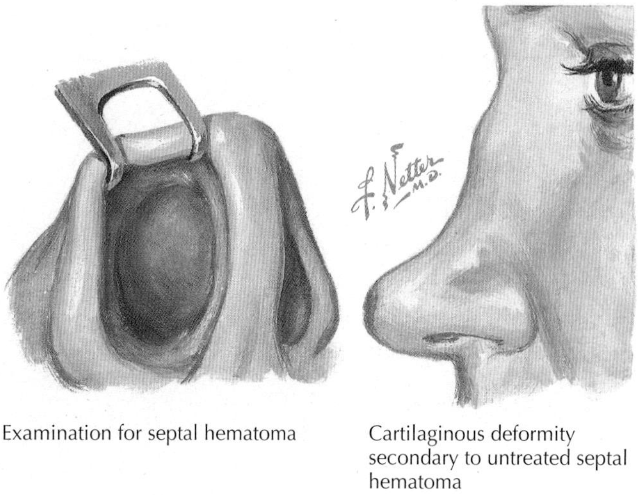
Examination for septal hematoma
Cartilaginous deformity secondary to untreated septal hematoma
F. Netter M.D.

Figure 48.3 Nasal fracture.

NASAL FRACTURE

Mechanism of injury: Trauma to nose. Nasal fractures constitute 50% of facial fractures in adults. Injury to bone–cartilage interface can be similar to nasal bone fracture, and diagnosis is made clinically.

Examination: Signs and symptoms include epistaxis, nasal asymmetry, crepitus on palpation, swelling, and nasal airway obstruction. Assess for septal hematoma (Fig. 48.3), submucosal swelling on one or both sides of septum. Septal hematoma causes injury to nasal cartilage blood supply.

Imaging: Although radiographs may show fracture, they are not necessary. Radiographs may be normal if injury is at the bone–cartilage interface. Some experts advocate prereduction photograph for medicolegal purposes.

Treatment:
- Control hemorrhage with compression or nasal packing; most bleeding will stop with time. Topical vasoconstriction or clotting agents, such as Arista® may be used.
- It is imperative to treat septal hematoma within 24–48 hours to prevent permanent damage to underlying nasal cartilage (i.e., saddle nose deformity) (see Fig. 48.3). Use antibiotic with *Staphylococcus* coverage if packing or hematoma is present.
- Reduce displaced fractures immediately or wait 5–7 days for swelling to diminish; waiting longer can make reduction more difficult.
- Control fracture with splinting; complex fractures may require operative reduction.

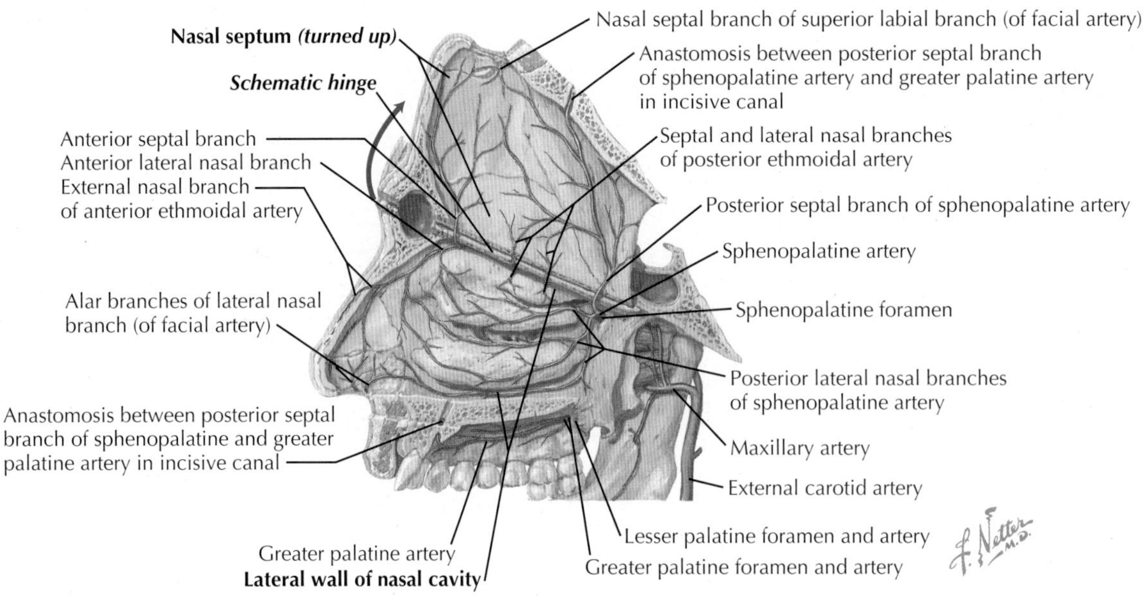
Nasal septum (turned up)
Schematic hinge
Anterior septal branch
Anterior lateral nasal branch
External nasal branch
of anterior ethmoidal artery
Alar branches of lateral nasal
branch (of facial artery)
Anastomosis between posterior septal
branch of sphenopalatine and greater
palatine artery in incisive canal
Greater palatine artery
Lateral wall of nasal cavity
Nasal septal branch of superior labial branch (of facial artery)
Anastomosis between posterior septal branch
of sphenopalatine artery and greater palatine artery
in incisive canal
Septal and lateral nasal branches
of posterior ethmoidal artery
Posterior septal branch of sphenopalatine artery
Sphenopalatine artery
Sphenopalatine foramen
Posterior lateral nasal branches
of sphenopalatine artery
Maxillary artery
External carotid artery
Lesser palatine foramen and artery
Greater palatine foramen and artery
F. Netter M.D.

Figure 48.4 Arteries of nasal cavity: Nasal septum turned up.

Return to play:

- Restrict aerobic activity for a few days
- Facial protection can be off-the-shelf or individually fabricated. Athletes can return to contact/collision sports with face mask in approximately 4 weeks. Many athletes return earlier than 4 weeks with the understanding that they may refracture and require further treatment.

EPISTAXIS

Mechanism of injury: Usually occurs spontaneously at Kiesselbach plexus on nasal septum in the area of thin nasal mucosa overlying blood vessels. The second most common cause is trauma. Posterior bleeding is less common and can be difficult to control.

Examination: Anterior rhinoscopy if initial treatment does not resolve epistaxis and bleeding site is not readily identified. If bleeding site is difficult to find, a nasal endoscope can be used, particularly if posterior bleed is suspected.

Treatment: Most nosebleeds resolve spontaneously in a few minutes; apply pressure to upper lip over the superior labial artery. Pinch nostrils against nasal septum, which helps constrict blood flow from anterior ethmoidal and sphenopalatine arteries (Fig. 48.4). If the bleeding site is at Kiesselbach plexus, a folded dental roll temporarily inserted into the naris will apply pressure over the bleeding site and may allow the athlete to finish the contest. If time allows, consider vasoconstriction of the area with topical oxymetazoline, cocaine, epinephrine 1:100,000, or a combination of lidocaine, epinephrine, and tetracaine. Subsequently, chemically cauterize the area with a silver nitrate stick or use electrocautery. Electrocautery should be restricted to one side, as bilateral use can result in septal perforation. Anterior nasal bleeding that does not stop with these maneuvers can be treated with nasal packing. Posterior bleeds and those anterior bleeds not controlled with nasal packing need an urgent visit with an otolaryngologist. Petrolatum jelly applied nightly to the nasal septum can prevent drying and cracking of the mucosa and may help prevent epistaxis.

MANDIBULAR FRACTURES

Mechanism of injury: Usually direct trauma to jaw

Examination: Signs and symptoms include pain with palpation, laceration of overlying oral mucosa, sublingual ecchymosis, loose teeth, malocclusion, loose segments of jaw, inability to open or close jaw, and numbness if injury involves mandibular nerve (Fig. 48.5).

Imaging: There are multiple radiographic modalities to evaluate for fractures. Panoramic radiographs are superior to other plain films for the evaluation of mandibular trauma. Advances in CT make it a readily available, easily obtained, and fast modality. Although CT shows bone anatomy well, a panoramic radiograph shows dental root injury better.

Treatment: If the athlete can breathe through the nose, initially immobilize with an Ace wrap until followed up with imaging. Eventual surgical treatment consists of reduction followed by bony immobilization with maxillomandibular fixation (wiring of teeth) or internal fixation (bone plating) (Fig. 48.6).

Rehabilitation: Physical therapy after jaw wiring may be needed to improve jaw opening. Early mobilization is key to preventing ankylosis of mandibular condylar fractures.

Return to play: Return to noncontact sports in 4 weeks; contact sports in 2–3 months.

Maxillary Fractures

Mechanism of injury: Usually from direct trauma to midface; classified by Le Fort schema (Fig. 48.7). Le Fort II and III fracture patterns may be more likely to have associated brain, cervical, vascular, or ocular injuries.

Examination: Signs and symptoms include asymmetry or altered contour of face; flattening of the midface; midface mobility when applying a force directed anteriorly to the anterior maxillary alveolus; epistaxis; malocclusion and loose dentition; and diplopia or globe malposition. Document function of all cranial nerves. Injury to the infraorbital nerve is common in midface fractures, resulting in altered sensation of cheek and upper lip.

Radiology: Facial bone CT scan to evaluate for maxillary fractures. Waters view plain film can be helpful if no CT scan is available.

Treatment: Secure airway. If athlete is able, a forward sitting position will allow blood to drain outside the body and may facilitate mouth breathing. Nasotracheal airway is contraindicated without fiber-optic placement in these injuries because of concern for intracranial involvement. Most surgeons advocate open reduction with internal fixation with titanium miniplates and microplates as soon as medically prudent based on other injuries. Le Fort I fractures can be treated with intermaxillary fixation (wiring). Pediatric fractures can develop further deformity with growth, and parents should be made aware of

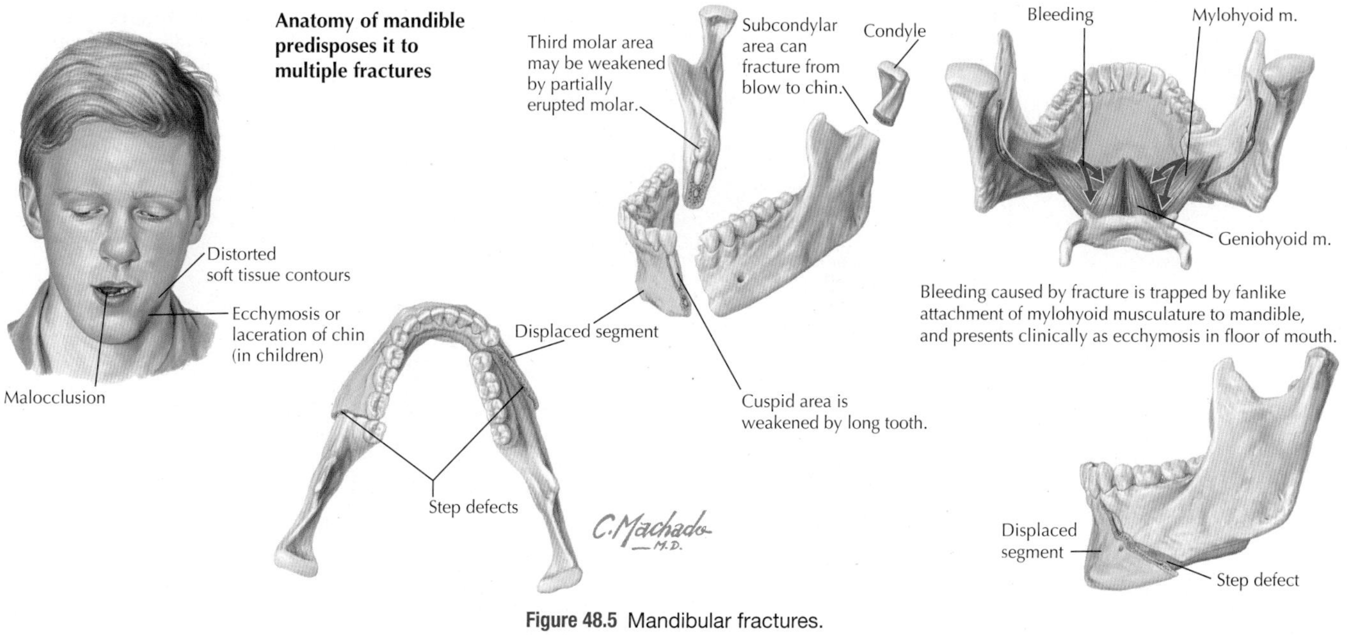
Anatomy of mandible predisposes it to multiple fractures
Distorted soft tissue contours
Ecchymosis or laceration of chin (in children)
Malocclusion
Third molar area may be weakened by partially erupted molar.
Subcondylar area can fracture from blow to chin.
Condyle
Displaced segment
Step defects
Cuspid area is weakened by long tooth.
C.Machado M.D.
Bleeding
Mylohyoid m.
Geniohyoid m.
Bleeding caused by fracture is trapped by fanlike attachment of mylohyoid musculature to mandible, and presents clinically as ecchymosis in floor of mouth.
Displaced segment
Step defect

Figure 48.5 Mandibular fractures.

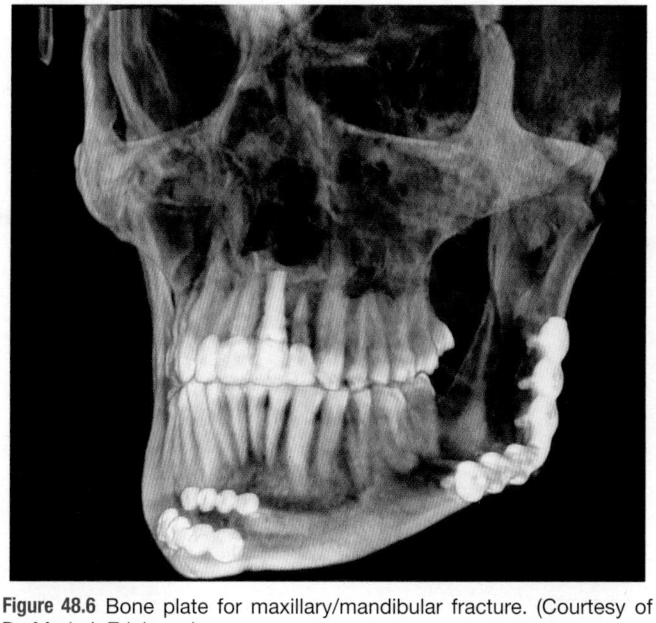

Figure 48.6 Bone plate for maxillary/mandibular fracture. (Courtesy of Dr. Mark J. Erickson.)

this possibility. Resorbable plates can be used in certain cases in children.

ZYGOMA FRACTURES

Mechanism of injury: Usually from direct force to cheek. A zygomatic arch fracture can occur in isolation or in association with a zygomatic complex fracture that includes the zygoma, zygomatic buttress of the maxilla, lateral orbital wall, orbital rim, and possibly the orbital floor.

Examination: Signs and symptoms include:

- Facial asymmetry
  - Flattening of malar eminence of the involved side because of displacement of the complex and/or the masseter muscle pulling the malar eminence inferiorly. This may not be apparent until swelling resolves.
  - Enophthalmos (sinking of the eyeball into the orbital cavity) if orbital floor is sufficiently damaged.
- Restriction of ocular range of motion and/or diplopia may be seen if inferior rectus or inferior oblique muscles are entrapped indicating orbital floor fracture.
- Pain with mastication because of zygomatic arch depression and the action of the temporalis muscle
- Numbness of affected cheek
- See Fig. 48.8 for hallmarks of zygomatic fractures.

Imaging: CT scan is preferred with axial, sagittal, and coronal imaging usually sufficient for surgeon to plan treatment. Plain films such as the Caldwell, Waters, and submentovertex views have historically been used, but are now rarely employed as a primary imaging modality.

Treatment: Nonsurgically if <2 mm of displacement; however, cosmetic deformity can become apparent when facial swelling diminishes. Surgical fixation after reduction is often performed 3–7 days after injury. Athletes with nonsurgically treated fractures should use a soft diet for 1–2 weeks to minimize tension on fracture from masseter muscle; those with surgically treated fractures can use soft diet for 1 week.

Return to play: Return to noncontact sports in 3–4 weeks and contact sports in 6–8 weeks

Frontal Sinus Fracture

Mechanism of injury: Direct trauma to sinus; an uncommon fracture, especially in the pediatric population because of lack of developed sinuses; anterior wall of sinus is strongest portion of sinus.

Examination: Signs and symptoms include frontal headache, epistaxis, forehead numbness from supraorbital nerve injury, anosmia if associated fracture of anterior cranial fossa floor, cerebrospinal fluid leakage if posterior wall of frontal sinus fractured, and depression of frontal area of skull.

Imaging: CT imaging of face and head.

Treatment: Referral to a maxillofacial surgeon is indicated. Nondisplaced fractures limited to the anterior wall of the frontal sinus may be treated nonsurgically. Certain frontal sinus fractures must be surgically explored to prevent complications such as deformity, damage to the frontonasal duct, and subsequent mucocele formation. Posterior wall fractures may result in damage to the dura and possible infection of the meninges and brain, and in such cases referral to a neurosurgeon is indicated.

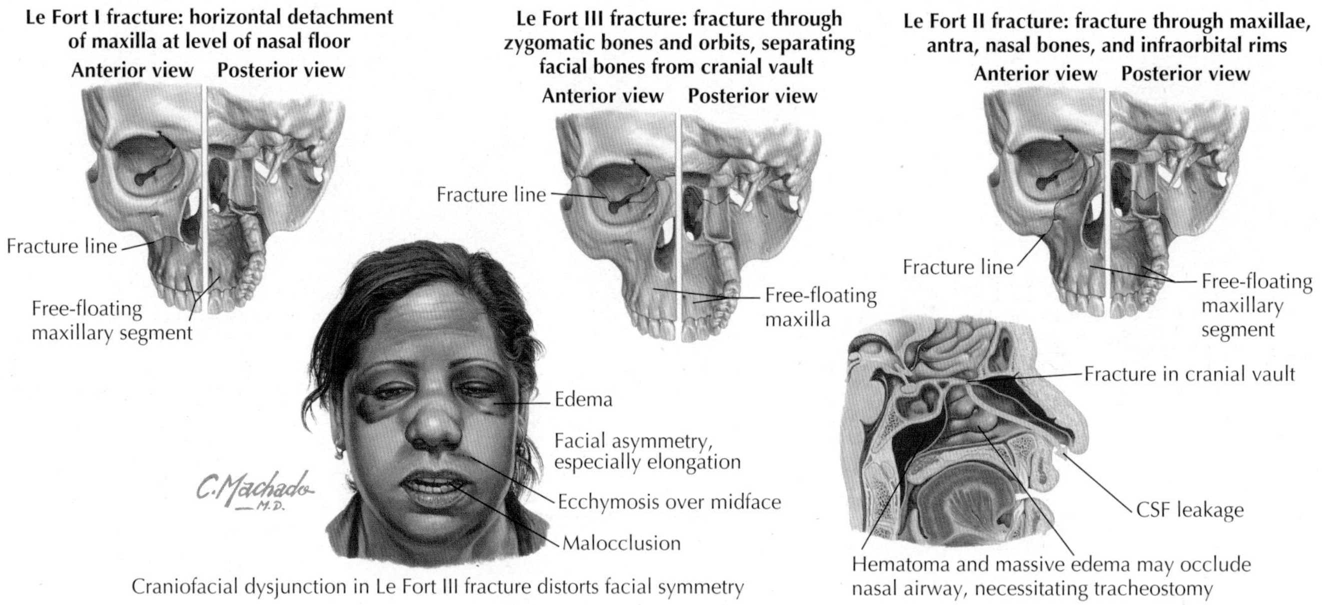
Le Fort I fracture: horizontal detachment of maxilla at level of nasal floor
Anterior view
Posterior view
Fracture line
Free-floating maxillary segment
Le Fort III fracture: fracture through zygomatic bones and orbits, separating facial bones from cranial vault
Anterior view
Posterior view
Fracture line
Free-floating maxilla
Le Fort II fracture: fracture through maxillae, antra, nasal bones, and infraorbital rims
Anterior view
Posterior view
Fracture line
Free-floating maxillary segment
Edema
Facial asymmetry, especially elongation
Ecchymosis over midface
Malocclusion
C. Machado M.D.
Craniofacial dysjunction in Le Fort III fracture distorts facial symmetry
Fracture in cranial vault
CSF leakage
Hematoma and massive edema may occlude nasal airway, necessitating tracheostomy

Figure 48.7 Midface fractures: Le Fort.

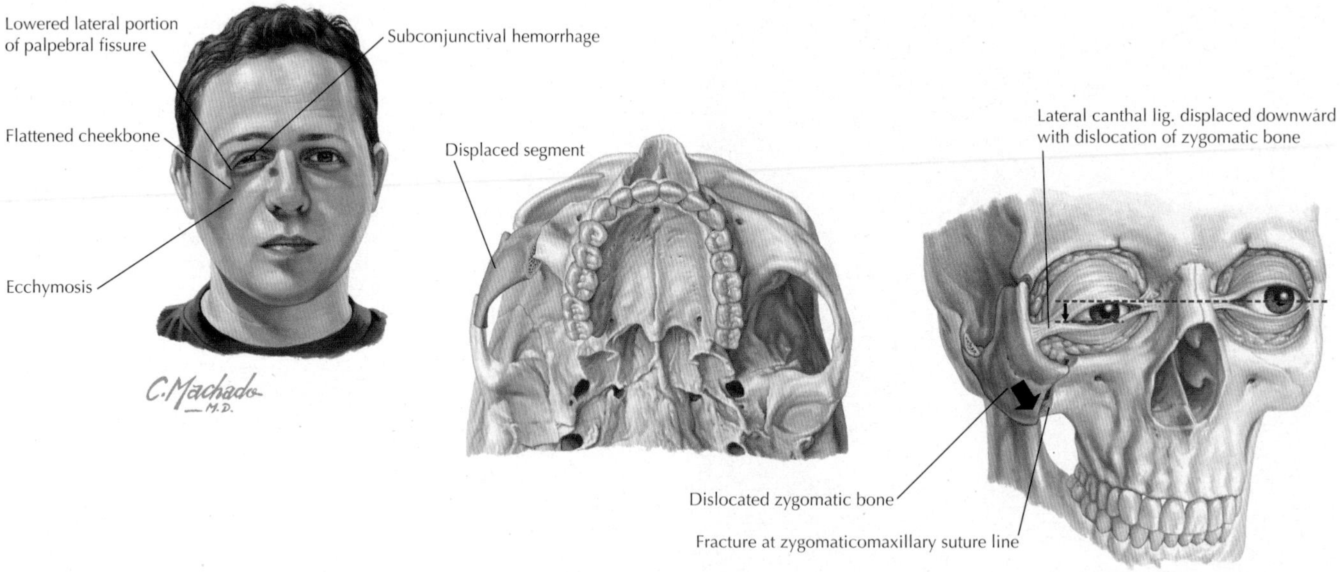
Lowered lateral portion of palpebral fissure
Subconjunctival hemorrhage
Flattened cheekbone
Ecchymosis
C. Machado M.D.
Displaced segment
Lateral canthal lig. displaced downward with dislocation of zygomatic bone
Dislocated zygomatic bone
Fracture at zygomaticomaxillary suture line

Figure 48.8 Zygomatic fractures.

ORBITAL AND OPHTHALMIC INJURIES

See Chapter 47: "Eye Injuries."

RECOMMENDED READINGS

Available online.

SHOULDER INJURIES 49

Eric C. McCarty • John Wilson Belk • Jonathan T. Bravman

HISTORY

- A careful history will help establish the diagnosis and formulate a treatment plan.
- Important factors include the chief complaint, mechanism of injury, hand dominance, what sport the athlete plays, and prior treatments.
- Common complaints are "pain with overhead activities," "loss of range of motion," "pain at night when I lie on that side," and "a feeling of the shoulder coming out of the joint."

PHYSICAL EXAMINATION

Evaluation of shoulder pathology should include an examination of the cervical spine to rule out referred pain.

Inspection

- It is important to visualize the entire shoulder during an examination and compare it with the unaffected side (including the scapula).
- Check for muscle atrophy, which can indicate neurologic dysfunction or chronic injury.
- Examine for scapular dyskinesia or winging.
- Note bony prominence that could represent acromioclavicular (AC) separation, clavicle fracture, sternoclavicular (SC) subluxation, or degenerative disease.

Palpation

- Palpate bony landmarks for tenderness or crepitus—AC joint, clavicle, SC joint, greater tuberosity, and coracoid.
- Extension and internal rotation of the arm deliver a greater tuberosity from under the acromion.

Motion

- It is important to compare active and passive range of motion with the unaffected side. Forward flexion, abduction, and external rotation are measured in degrees from neutral rotation. Internal rotation is measured in relation to the spinal level that can be reached posteriorly (Fig. 49.1A).
- Does motion cause pain or produce a feeling of instability?
- The normal ratio of glenohumeral (GH) to scapulothoracic motion is 2:1 (see Fig. 49.1B).

Manual Muscle Testing

Supraspinatus: (Jobe test) Resistance is applied with the patient's arm abducted 90 degrees, forward flexed 30 degrees, and internally rotated (thumb pointing down).

Infraspinatus/teres minor: Resistance to external rotation with the arm adducted and the elbow preferentially flexed 90 degrees assesses the infraspinatus. Resistance to external rotation with the arm abducted and the elbow flexed 90 degrees assesses both the infraspinatus and teres minor (see Fig. 49.1).

Subscapularis: Resistance to internal rotation with the arm adducted and the elbow flexed 90 degrees (see Fig. 49.1F)

SPECIFIC TESTS

Impingement

Positive tests produce pain at the anterior or lateral aspect of the shoulder.

Hawkins test: The arm is passively forward flexed to 90 degrees and then forcibly internally rotated (Fig. 49.2A).

Neer sign: The patient's arm, with the forearm pronated, is passively forward flexed while the scapula is stabilized (see Fig. 49.2B).

Painful arc: The patient actively elevates the arm in the scapular plane and then lowers it in the same plane. Pain during range of motion between 60 and 120 degrees is positive.

Coracoid impingement sign: The patient's arm is passively placed in a position of forward flexion, adduction, and internal rotation with pain produced directly over the coracoid.

Rotator Cuff Tear

Jobe test: Isolates the **supraspinatus** (see earlier discussion); pain can also be indicative of subacromial impingement

Champagne toast: The arm is abducted against resistance at 30 degrees of abduction, 30 degrees of forward flexion, and mild external rotation; this test isolates the **supraspinatus.**

Drop arm sign: The patient fully elevates the arm in the plane of the scapula and then tries to lower it slowly. Sudden dropping of the arm or pain while doing so suggests a supraspinatus tear.

External rotation lag sign: With the arm adducted and the elbow flexed 90 degrees, the arm is passively brought to maximal external rotation. Inability of the patient to actively maintain the arm in the externally rotated position indicates a **massive tear** involving the **infraspinatus** (see Fig. 49.2C).

Lift-off test: The dorsum of the patient's hand is placed against the lumbar spine (see Fig. 49.2D). The patient then lifts the hand away from the back, maintaining the elbow in the coronal plane. Inability to do so indicates a lower **subscapularis** tear.

Belly-press test: The patient places both hands on the abdomen, internally rotates to bring the elbows forward beyond the coronal plane, and then presses the hands into the abdomen. Inability to move the elbow beyond the coronal plane indicates an upper **subscapularis** tear (see Fig. 49.2D).

Hornblower sign: The patient is asked to hold the arm in a 90-degree abduction and a 90-degree external rotation. A positive sign, wherein the arm falls into internal rotation, represents a **teres minor** pathology.

Biceps Tendon Pathology

Speed test: With the forearm supinated and the elbow extended, the patient forward flexes the arm against resistance. A positive test produces anterior shoulder pain.

Yergason test: With the elbow in 90 degrees of flexion, the patient supinates the forearm against a resistive force. A positive test produces pain in the biceps region.

Upper cut test: With the elbow in 90 degrees of flexion and the forearm supinated, an upward and cross-body motion is performed against resistance. A positive test will induce pain.

Instability

It is important to perform these tests on the contralateral extremity for comparison and assessment of the patient's normal laxity.

Anterior

Apprehension test: Best performed supine (table stabilizes the scapula); the arm is passively abducted to 90 degrees and then progressively externally rotated while the patient's response is

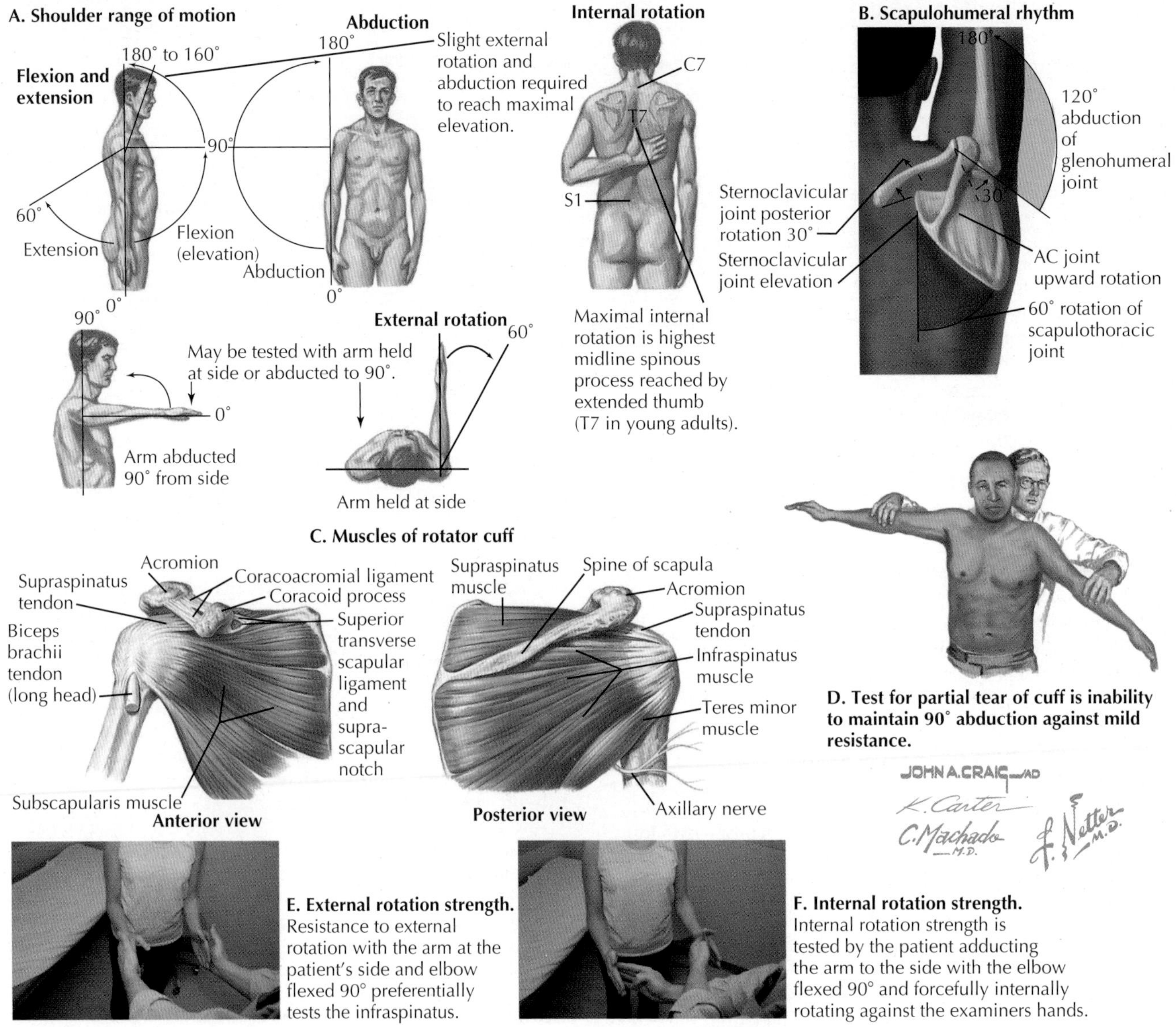
A. Shoulder range of motion
Flexion and extension
180° to 160°
90°
60°
Extension
Flexion (elevation)
0°
Abduction
180°
Slight external rotation and abduction required to reach maximal elevation.
Abduction
0°
90°
0°
Arm abducted 90° from side
External rotation
60°
May be tested with arm held at side or abducted to 90°.
0°
Arm held at side
Internal rotation
C7
T7
S1
Maximal internal rotation is highest midline spinous process reached by extended thumb (T7 in young adults).
B. Scapulohumeral rhythm
180°
120° abduction of glenohumeral joint
30°
Sternoclavicular joint posterior rotation 30°
Sternoclavicular joint elevation
AC joint upward rotation
60° rotation of scapulothoracic joint
C. Muscles of rotator cuff
Acromion
Coracoacromial ligament
Supraspinatus tendon
Coracoid process
Biceps brachii tendon (long head)
Superior transverse scapular ligament and supra-scapular notch
Subscapularis muscle
Anterior view
Supraspinatus muscle
Spine of scapula
Acromion
Supraspinatus tendon
Infraspinatus muscle
Teres minor muscle
Axillary nerve
Posterior view
D. Test for partial tear of cuff is inability to maintain 90° abduction against mild resistance.
JOHN A.CRAIG_AD
K. Carter
C.Machado M.D.
F. Netter M.D.
E. External rotation strength. Resistance to external rotation with the arm at the patient's side and elbow flexed 90° preferentially tests the infraspinatus.
F. Internal rotation strength. Internal rotation strength is tested by the patient adducting the arm to the side with the elbow flexed 90° and forcefully internally rotating against the examiners hands.

Figure 49.1 Physical examination of shoulder.

noted. A positive test produces a patient response of "apprehension" by reproducing the patient's symptoms of anterior instability.

Relocation test: A posteriorly directed force is applied to the proximal humerus while performing the **apprehension test.** The test is positive when the patient's "apprehension" is relieved and greater external rotation can be achieved. **Note:** If the **apprehension test** produces pain (as opposed to a feeling of instability) that is relieved by the **relocation test**, it is suggestive of **internal impingement (Jobe relocation test).**

Load and shift test: The humeral head is loaded to center it within the glenoid. It is then translated anteriorly and posteriorly. The amount of translation is graded as follows: grade 0, minimal; grade I, up to the rim of the glenoid; grade II, over the glenoid rim but spontaneously reduces; or grade III, over the glenoid rim and does not spontaneously reduce.

Posterior

Load and shift test: See previous discussion.

Posterior stress test: Performed supine; the arm is flexed to 90 degrees and internally rotated. A posteriorly directed force is then applied to the humerus. A positive test causes subluxation.

Jerk test: Performed upright; the arm and the elbow are flexed 90 degrees. The arm is internally rotated and the humerus is loaded posteriorly. A positive test can cause posterior subluxation of the humeral head that is then reduced with a "jerk" when extending the arm.

Multidirectional

Sulcus sign: Traction is applied to the arm in an inferior direction while observing the area lateral to the acromion for a "sulcus." Presence of a sulcus >1 cm indicates **inferior** laxity.

Labrum

Clunk test: Performed supine; the arm is fully abducted, and the examiner's hand is placed on the posterior aspect of the humeral head. An anterior force is applied to the humerus, while the other hand rotates the humerus. Positive findings include a "clunk," pain, and grinding.

O'Brien test (active compression test): The arm is positioned in 90 degrees of flexion and 10–15 degrees of adduction. A downward force is applied by the examiner as the patient resists, first with the arm internally rotated (thumb down) and then with the arm externally rotated (thumb up). A positive test

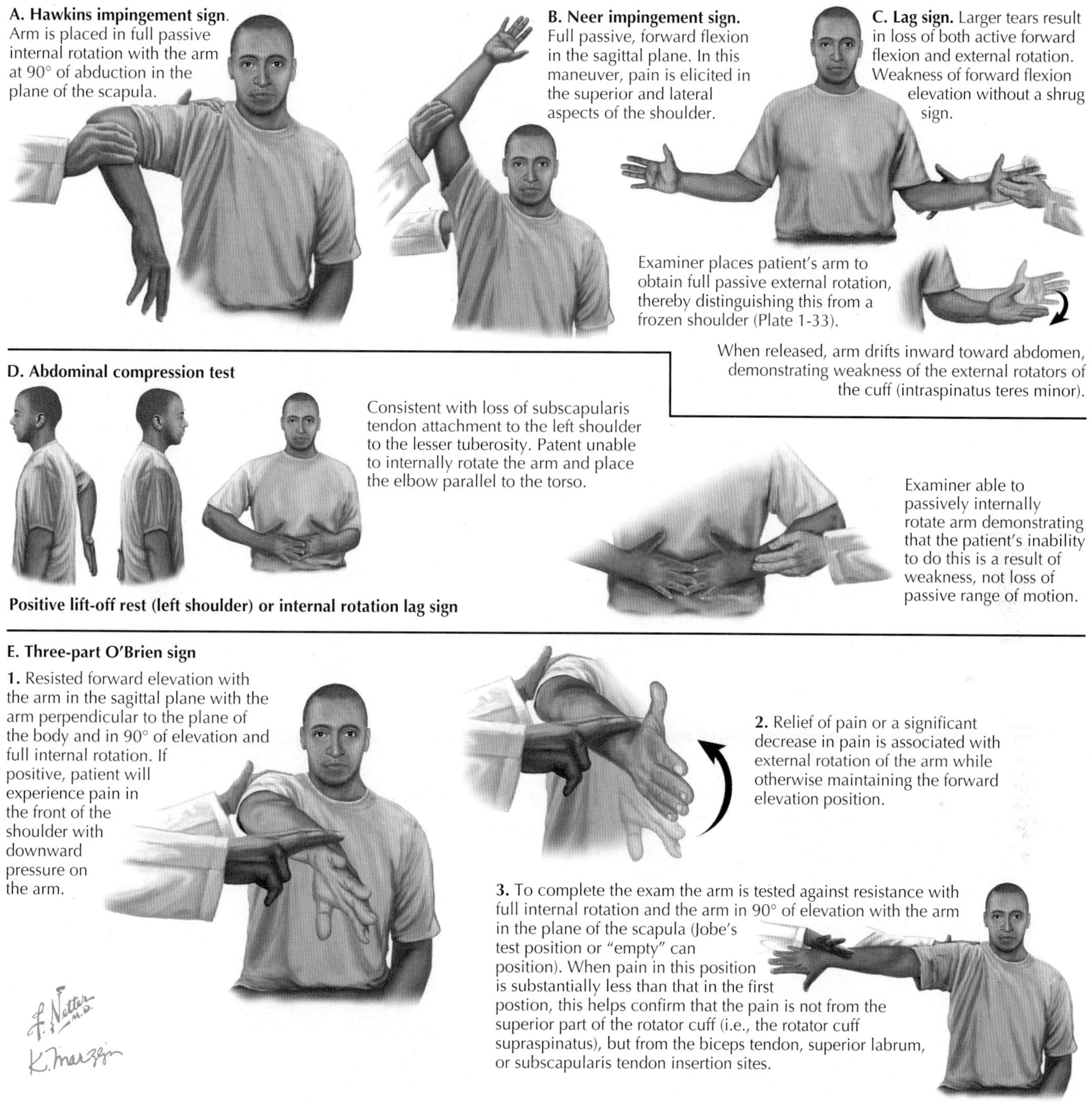
A. Hawkins impingement sign.
Arm is placed in full passive internal rotation with the arm at 90° of abduction in the plane of the scapula.
B. Neer impingement sign.
Full passive, forward flexion in the sagittal plane. In this maneuver, pain is elicited in the superior and lateral aspects of the shoulder.
C. Lag sign. Larger tears result in loss of both active forward flexion and external rotation. Weakness of forward flexion elevation without a shrug sign.
Examiner places patient's arm to obtain full passive external rotation, thereby distinguishing this from a frozen shoulder (Plate 1-33).
When released, arm drifts inward toward abdomen, demonstrating weakness of the external rotators of the cuff (intraspinatus teres minor).
D. Abdominal compression test
Consistent with loss of subscapularis tendon attachment to the left shoulder to the lesser tuberosity. Patent unable to internally rotate the arm and place the elbow parallel to the torso.
Examiner able to passively internally rotate arm demonstrating that the patient's inability to do this is a result of weakness, not loss of passive range of motion.
Positive lift-off rest (left shoulder) or internal rotation lag sign
E. Three-part O'Brien sign
1. Resisted forward elevation with the arm in the sagittal plane with the arm perpendicular to the plane of the body and in 90° of elevation and full internal rotation. If positive, patient will experience pain in the front of the shoulder with downward pressure on the arm.
2. Relief of pain or a significant decrease in pain is associated with external rotation of the arm while otherwise maintaining the forward elevation position.
3. To complete the exam the arm is tested against resistance with full internal rotation and the arm in 90° of elevation with the arm in the plane of the scapula (Jobe's test position or "empty" can position). When pain in this position is substantially less than that in the first postion, this helps confirm that the pain is not from the superior part of the rotator cuff (i.e., the rotator cuff supraspinatus), but from the biceps tendon, superior labrum, or subscapularis tendon insertion sites.
F. Netter M.D.
K. Marzen

Figure 49.2 Special tests.

causes pain felt deep within the joint that is reduced or relieved with the arm externally rotated, which indicates superior/posterior labral pathology (see Fig. 49.2D).

Kim test: Performed upright; with the arm in a 90-degree abduction, a strong axial load is applied. While the arm is elevated to 45 degrees upward and diagonally, a downward and backward force is applied. A positive test is sudden onset of posterior shoulder pain, which indicates a posteroinferior labral lesion.

Biceps load test: Performed supine; the arm is abducted 120 degrees, maximally externally rotated, the forearm supinated, and the elbow flexed 90 degrees. Active elbow flexion is then performed against resistance. A positive test produces pain suggestive of a superior labrum anterior and posterior (SLAP) tear.

Anterior slide test: The patient's hands are placed on the hips with the thumbs pointing posteriorly. An axial load is applied at the elbow toward the GH joint against patient resistance. A positive test produces pain suggestive of a SLAP tear.

Modified dynamic labral shear: The arm is flexed 90 degrees at the elbow, abducted in the scapular plane to above 120 degrees, and externally rotated to tightness. The arm is then lowered from a 120- to a 60-degree abduction, keeping the arm maximally externally rotated. A positive test produces pain or a painful click and indicates superior labral pathology.

Acromioclavicular Joint

Direct palpation over the AC joint causes pain.

Cross-arm adduction test: The arm is flexed 90 degrees and then adducted across the chest. A positive test causes pain at the AC joint.

O'Brien test: Can cause pain localized to the AC joint and should be distinguished from pain deep within the shoulder

IMAGING OF THE SHOULDER

Radiographs

Anteroposterior (AP): Taken in the plane of the thorax; provides an oblique view of the GH joint because of the anteverted position of the scapula on the posterolateral aspect of the thoracic cage (Fig. 49.3A).

True AP (Grashey view): Taken in the plane of the scapula; provides a true AP view of the GH joint by angling the beam approximately 45 degrees in the medial-to-lateral direction or by rotating the patient and placing the scapula flat on a radiograph cassette

Axillary view: Important for evaluating dislocations; useful for evaluating fractures of the coracoid and the anterior or posterior glenoid rim; will additionally reveal an os acromiale

West Point axillary lateral: Provides a tangential view to the anteroinferior glenoid rim, useful for evaluating instability cases

Scapular Y-view: Lateral radiographs recorded in the scapular plane; helpful in evaluating the relationship of the humerus to the glenoid fossa; tilting the beam caudally by 10 degrees produces a supraspinatus **outlet view,** which allows assessment of acromion morphology

Stryker notch view: The patient is placed supine with the hand on the superior aspect of the head with the finger directed posteriorly. The beam is aimed 10 degrees cephalad at the coracoid; evaluates compression fractures or defects in the posterolateral aspect of the humeral head (Hill–Sachs lesion) (see Fig. 49.3B)

Serendipity view: A 40-degree cephalic tilt view for visualization of the SC joint

Zanca view: Provides clear view of the AC joint by directing the x-ray beam 10–15 degrees cephalad; allows assessment of AC separations, distal clavicular osteolysis, and distal clavicle fractures

Magnetic Resonance Imaging

Magnetic resonance imaging (MRI) is the gold standard for evaluating soft tissue structures and cartilage; magnetic resonance arthrogram (MRA) preferred for labral pathology

SPECIFIC SHOULDER INJURIES

Instability

Description: Defined as symptomatic, abnormal translation of the humeral head on the glenoid; instability can be classified in several ways—*direction of instability* **(anterior, posterior, multidirectional)**, *traumatic versus atraumatic*, and *degree of instability*

Anterior Glenohumeral Instability

Description: Most common direction of instability

Mechanism of injury: Direct or indirect trauma leading to tearing and attenuation of the anterior capsulolabral complex; direct trauma involves a blow to the posterior shoulder; indirect trauma involves injury to the arm in a position of abduction, extension, and external rotation

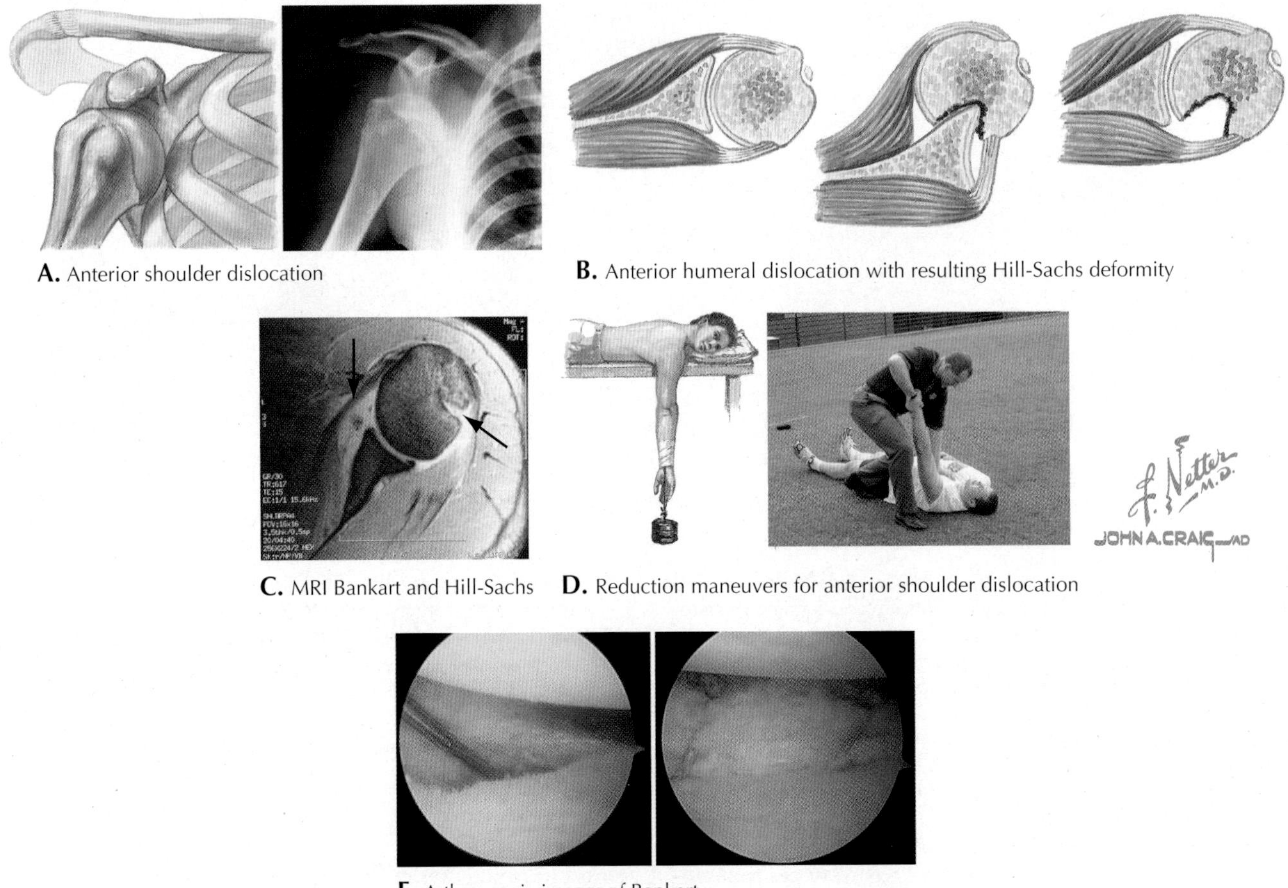

A. Anterior shoulder dislocation

B. Anterior humeral dislocation with resulting Hill-Sachs deformity

C. MRI Bankart and Hill-Sachs

D. Reduction maneuvers for anterior shoulder dislocation

E. Arthroscopic images of Bankart

Figure 49.3 Anterior glenohumeral instability.

Presentation: Can present with pain, feeling of weakness, instability, or recurrent dislocations; dislocations in younger patients are associated with *Bankart lesions*, whereas patients aged over 40 years typically have associated rotator cuff tears. A Bankart lesion is an avulsion of the anteroinferior glenoid labrum.

Physical examination: In acute dislocations, the lateral shoulder will lose its normal contour with fullness present anteriorly. The arm is held in slight abduction and in external rotation. A careful neurovascular examination is important. The nerve most commonly injured is the axillary nerve. The following examination maneuvers will be positive in patients with recurrent anterior instability: **apprehension test, relocation test,** and **load and shift test.**

Differential diagnosis: Multidirectional instability (MDI), rotator cuff tear, SLAP lesion, and proximal humerus fracture

Diagnostics:

- **Radiographs:** A standard shoulder series (AP, axillary, and scapular-Y) to ensure the humeral head is reduced. The **Stryker notch** view can detect a Hill–Sachs lesion. The **West Point axillary view** will provide better evaluation of the anterior glenoid rim for possible *bony Bankart lesions.*
- **3D computed tomography (CT):** Gold standard to evaluate bony pathology (particularly in recurrent instability to evaluate critical glenoid bone loss)
- **MRI or MRA:** Will demonstrate *Bankart lesions*, anterior capsule pathology, and presence of Hill–Sachs lesion (with associated T2 edema in acute injuries) (see Fig. 49.3C)

Treatment:

- Acute anterior dislocations require urgent reduction. Several reduction methods have been described. The Stimson technique is a relatively atraumatic technique. The patient is placed prone, and weights are placed on the affected wrist (see Fig. 49.3D). A variation of this technique can be performed on the field by placing the athlete in the supine position and applying traction on the wrist in forward flexion and counter traction on the chest (see Fig. 49.3D). Another technique is the Milch technique; this is performed with the physician placing a hand on the superior aspect of the dislocated shoulder while using a thumb to stabilize the humeral head in a fixed position. The arm is then abducted with application of a gentle longitudinal traction while the humeral head is manipulated with the thumb over the glenoid rim. Slight external rotation can help facilitate the manipulation of the humeral head over the glenoid rim. Intra-articular injection of a local anesthetic has been shown to be effective in aiding reduction, although relaxation with an intravenous (IV) sedative may be necessary.
- The value of postreduction treatment with sling immobilization (particularly in external rotation) is controversial. There is no consensus in the literature on the utility of sling use, period of immobilization, or degree of rotation. It is currently recommended for 4–6 weeks of immobilization in neutral rotation.
- Initial treatment is physical therapy focusing on strengthening dynamic stabilizers of the GH joint (rotator cuff muscles, deltoid and scapula stabilizers) and maintaining GH motion.
- Recurrent instability should be surgically treated with anterior stabilization. Current arthroscopic techniques have results equivalent to those with open techniques (see Fig. 49.3E). Bony deficiencies of the anterior glenoid or large, engaging Hill–Sachs lesions may have to be addressed for successful outcomes.

Prognosis and return to play: The re-dislocation rate is approximately 90% in patients aged <20 years and decreases with increasing age. The decision to treat initially with surgical stabilization versus nonoperative therapy must take into account several factors such as patient age, activity level, and the specific sport. Return to play after nonoperative therapy requires near-normal range of motion, strength, and functional ability. Return to play after surgical stabilization is typically after 4–6 months.

Posterior Glenohumeral Instability

Description: Tear or stretching of posterior capsulolabral structures leading to dislocation or subluxation

Mechanism of injury: Posterior subluxation or dislocation can result from a traumatic event with the arm in a position of flexion, adduction, and internal rotation causing a *reverse Bankart lesion* (see Fig. 49.3E); more commonly, it can result from repetitive microtrauma causing a labral tear or capsular attenuation. This mechanism is commonly associated with an offensive lineman in football jamming his opponents while blocking.

Presentation: Posterior dislocation is rare compared with an anterior dislocation and is easily missed upon initial evaluation. Patients presenting after a seizure or electrical shock should raise suspicion of a posterior dislocation. More commonly, posterior instability presents as pain or a feeling of instability posteriorly with a load to the arm in a position of forward flexion, adduction, and internal rotation.

Physical examination: In acute posterior dislocations, the arm is held in adduction and internal rotation. A prominent coracoid anteriorly and posterior fullness are present. The following maneuvers will be positive in patients with recurrent posterior instability: **load and shift test, posterior stress test,** and **jerk test.**

Differential diagnosis: MDI, rotator cuff tear, SLAP tear, and proximal humerus fracture

Diagnostics:

- **Radiographs:** A standard shoulder series (AP, scapular-Y, and axillary view) to ensure the humeral head is reduced. AP view may reveal "lightbulb sign." Plain radiograph films will also reveal reverse Hill–Sachs lesions indicative of a posterior dislocation and allow for evaluation of bony contributions to posterior instability, such as glenoid fractures, hypoplasia, or excessive retroversion (Fig. 49.4 A, B, and C).
- **CT:** Improved assessment of glenoid deformities contributing to instability (i.e., retroversion)
- **MRI or MRA:** Will demonstrate *reverse Bankart lesions* (posterior labral tear) or a redundant, attenuated posterior capsule (see Fig. 49.4D)

Treatment:

- Acute posterior dislocations require reduction. This is often more difficult than reduction of an anterior dislocation. With the patient supine, traction is applied in line with the deformity while the humeral head is guided into the joint. Avoid external rotation to prevent proximal humerus fracture.
- For recurrent posterior instability, a majority will improve with physical therapy focusing on dynamic stabilizers of the shoulder, particularly the posterior deltoid and external rotators. Surgery is indicated for patients who fail nonoperative treatment. Surgery is directed at the pathology with capsular plication for attenuated capsule and repair of *reverse Bankart lesions.* Bony abnormalities of the glenoid must be identified and addressed if present.

Prognosis and return to play: Criteria are similar to those for anterior instability.

Multidirectional Instability

Description: Symptomatic instability in more than one direction—inferior plus anterior or posterior

Mechanism of injury: Often atraumatic in the setting of generalized laxity or from repetitive microtrauma, most common in overhead athletes such as swimmers and volleyball players; the

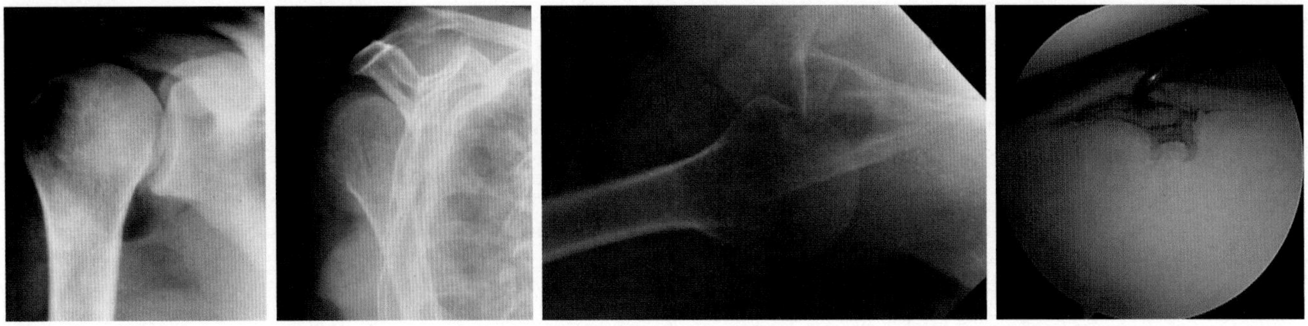

A. Anteroposterior radiograph. Difficult to determine if humeral head within, anterior, or posterior to glenoid cavity.

B. Lateral radiograph (parallel to plane of body of scapula). Humeral head clearly seen to be posterior to glenoid cavity.

C. True axillary view. Also shows humeral head posterior to glenoid cavity.

D. Posterior labral tear.

Figure 49.4 Posterior glenohumeral instability.

primary pathology is an attenuated inferior capsule with associated globally increased capsular volume

Presentation: A majority are young adults and often bilateral. Patients present with pain, instability, and occasionally transient neurologic symptoms. Symptoms when carrying heavy objects at one's side are indicative of inferior instability.

Physical examination: Examine for signs of generalized laxity, such as hyperextension of the elbows or ability to bring the thumb to the forearm (Beighton score). A positive **sulcus** and/or **Gagey sign** indicates inferior instability. Apply the tests described earlier to evaluate for anterior and posterior instability.

Differential diagnosis: Unidirectional instability, rotator cuff tear, and SLAP lesions

Diagnostics:

- **Radiographs:** Usually normal but may reveal a Hill–Sachs or bony Bankart lesion
- **MRA:** Can demonstrate excessive capsular volume and if have superimposed unidirectional instability, will demonstrate a Bankart lesion

Treatment: A majority of patients respond to physical therapy to strengthen the dynamic stabilizers of the shoulder. Those who fail nonoperative treatment are candidates for surgical stabilization via capsular shift/plication.

Prognosis and return to play: Even with surgical stabilization, a majority of patients return to a competitive level. The time frame for return to play after surgery is similar to unidirectional instability.

Biceps Tendon Pathology

Tendonitis

Description: *Primary* tendonitis is an isolated inflammatory condition of the long head of the biceps (LHB) brachii tendon in the intertubercular (bicipital) groove. More commonly, it occurs as a *secondary* process in conjunction with pathologic changes to surrounding structures in the shoulder such as rotator cuff pathology, impingement syndrome, bursitis, and AC joint disorders. This results in fraying or degeneration of the proximal LHB tendon.

Mechanism of injury: Overuse injury causing repetitive trauma to the LHB tendon. Chronic inflammation can lead to the tendon sheath becoming thickened and the tendon developing degenerative changes. These changes lead to scar tissue formation and the LHB becomes fixed within the bicipital groove.

Presentation: Pain in the anterior aspect of the shoulder that may radiate down the biceps; usually, a history of overuse and no history of trauma

Physical examination:

- Tenderness anteriorly over the bicipital groove
- Speed, Yergason, and upper cut tests are positive
- Because of its association with impingement, Hawkins and Neer tests are often positive.

Differential diagnosis: Rotator cuff pathology and labral tear

Diagnostics:

- Radiographs are normal in primary bicipital tendonitis; they may show an acromial spur suggestive of impingement associated with secondary bicipital tendonitis.
- Ultrasound will show thickened tendon within the bicipital groove, but this test is heavily reliant on operator technique.
- MRI is the gold standard and may show edema in or around the tendon or a thickened or split tendon. MRI is additionally helpful at showing associated pathology.

Treatment: Begins with nonoperative therapy consisting of rest and nonsteroidal anti-inflammatory drugs (NSAIDs), followed by range-of-motion exercises. Corticosteroid injections have utility in the bicipital sheath (via ultrasound guidance) or in the intra-articular space or subacromial space (particularly for secondary tendonitis). Surgery is indicated for those who fail conservative therapy. Surgical options include tenotomy or tenodesis with concomitant management of associated pathology.

Prognosis and return to play: Once pain has resolved enough to allow near-normal range of motion and strength. For isolated biceps tenodesis, a sling is typically used for 3–4 weeks with light work allowed at 4 weeks and completely unrestricted activity at 3–4 months.

Instability/Subluxation

Description: The LHB tendon subluxates out of the bicipital groove.

Mechanism of injury: Invariably associated with complete or partial tear of the subscapularis and structures of the rotator interval that comprise the bicep pulley system

Presentation: Similar to bicipital tendonitis; patients may also report popping during shoulder motion

Physical examination: Similar to bicipital tendinitis

Differential diagnosis: Bicipital tendonitis and rotator cuff pathology

Diagnostics: Radiographs will be normal. MRI will reveal injury to the subscapularis and dislocation of the proximal biceps tendon from the bicipital groove, if present. Ultrasound is both sensitive and specific for diagnosing subluxation.

Treatment: Conservative therapy is similar to that for bicipital tendonitis. Surgical intervention (tenotomy or tenodesis) is more appropriate as primary treatment in young active patients

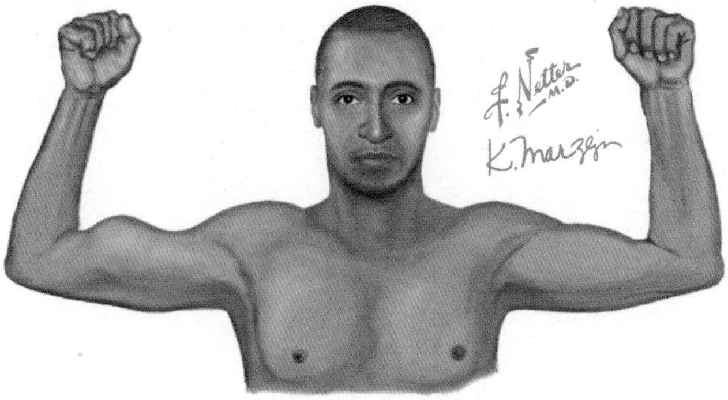

Rupture of tendon of long head of right biceps brachii muscle indicated by active flexion of elbow

Figure 49.5 Rupture of long head biceps brachii muscle.

or in those who fail conservative therapy. It is important to address associated cuff pathology as well.

Prognosis and return to play: Those undergoing tenotomy can return to play when near-normal strength and range of motion have returned. Tenodesis procedures will require 4–6 months to allow adequate healing and rehabilitation.

Rupture

Description: Disruption of the LHB tendon

Mechanism of injury: Most commonly caused by forceful elbow flexion against resistance

Presentation: In acute traumatic ruptures, patients present with pain and ecchymosis anteriorly. Ruptures in older patients are often the result of attritional degeneration or chronic tendonitis. Such patients are often unaware that they have sustained a rupture.

Physical examination: Acutely, patients will experience tenderness over the anterior shoulder and the upper arm. Swelling and ecchymosis will be present. The classic "Popeye" deformity will be present because the biceps will be more prominent in the middle of the arm (Fig. 49.5). Patients may experience a slight decrease in the strength of elbow flexion and forearm supination.

Differential diagnosis: Proximal humerus fracture, bicipital tendonitis/instability/subluxation, rotator cuff tear, and pectoralis tear

Diagnostics: Radiographs are unremarkable. MRI will confirm the diagnosis.

Treatment: Pain control and therapy to maintain motion in the elderly. Surgical tenodesis may be more appropriate for young active patients or those concerned with the cosmesis of the "Popeye" deformity.

Prognosis and return to play: Same as discussed earlier for tenotomy and tenodesis

SLAP Lesion

Description: The SLAP lesion describes any injury to the superior glenoid labrum.

Mechanism of injury: Several are atraumatic with an insidious onset of pain. Traumatic mechanisms include traction, compression, and direct blow injuries. Traction injuries occur in overhead-throwing athletes or in a sudden pull in an inferior or superior direction, such as catching oneself from falling. Compression injury occurs when falling onto an outstretched, slightly abducted arm.

Classification: The original classification described four types of lesions, as described here (Fig. 49.6). Several additional types have since been added.

- **Type I:** Fraying of the superior labrum but the biceps anchor and labrum are still attached.

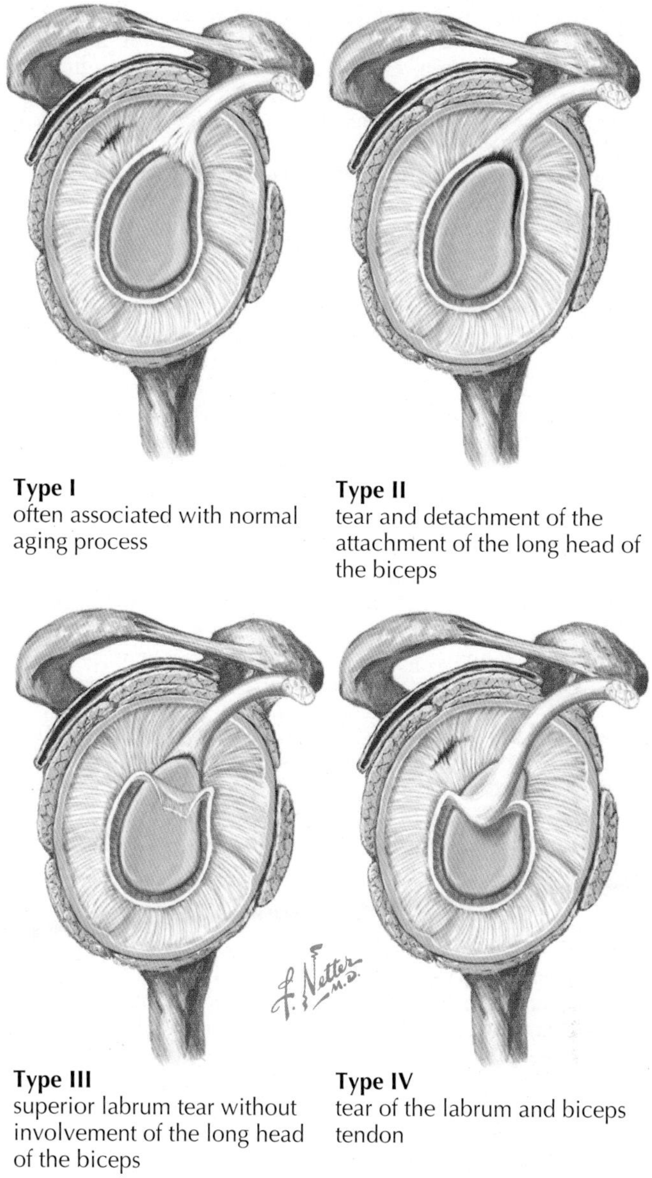
Type I
often associated with normal aging process
Type II
tear and detachment of the attachment of the long head of the biceps
Type III
superior labrum tear without involvement of the long head of the biceps
Type IV
tear of the labrum and biceps tendon

Figure 49.6 Superior labrum anterior and posterior (SLAP) injury.

- **Type II:** Most common clinically significant lesion; the superior labrum and biceps anchor are detached from the superior glenoid; further classified as anterior, posterior, or combined; posterior and combined type II SLAPs are often associated with throwing athletes because of the *"peel-back" phenomenon* as the arm is abducted while in an externally rotated position.
- **Type III:** A bucket handle tear of the superior labrum, but the biceps anchor is still attached to the glenoid
- **Type IV:** The bucket handle tear of the superior labrum extends into the biceps tendon

Presentation: Patients frequently complain of pain, particularly during overhead activities, and decreased function. Patients also report mechanical symptoms of popping, clicking, or catching with motion. Symptoms are usually difficult to distinguish from those associated with impingement or rotator cuff tears.

Physical examination: Several examination maneuvers have been described, but no one test has proven to be consistently successful in diagnosing a SLAP tear. SLAP lesions are often associated with rotator cuff tears or instability, complicating the diagnosis. The following examination maneuvers are considered positive for SLAP lesions if the patient describes pain as deep within the joint: **O'Brien test, biceps load test, anterior slide test modified dynamic labral shear, positive apprehension test,** and **positive relocation test.**

Differential diagnosis: Instability, impingement, rotator cuff tear, and GH arthritis

Diagnostics: MRI and MRA are the best imaging studies to evaluate for a SLAP lesion. Great variability in the normal appearance of the superior labrum exists, making interpretation difficult, but presence of a superior paralabral cyst has a high correlation with a SLAP lesion.

Treatment: Nonoperative treatment begins with rest, NSAIDs, and physical therapy to focus on strengthening and stretching because several overhead athletes will have an associated tight posterior capsule and loss of internal rotation. Patients who fail conservative therapy are indicated for surgery. Surgical treatment is dictated by the type of SLAP lesion. In general, types I and III lesions require debridement, type II lesions require repair, and type IV lesions require repair or tenodesis depending on the extent of involvement of the biceps tendon.

Prognosis and return to play: Throwing athletes require 6–7 months to fully rehabilitate; nonthrowing athletes typically return to sport at 4–6 months.

Rotator Cuff Pathology

Impingement Syndrome

Description: Impingement syndrome encompasses a spectrum of pathologies, including subacromial bursitis, rotator cuff tendinopathy, and partial-thickness rotator cuff tears. Three types of impingement entities have been described: **subacromial impingement**, **internal impingement,** and **subcoracoid impingement.**

Mechanism of injury:

- **Subacromial impingement:** Impingement of the rotator cuff on the undersurface of the acromion and coracoclavicular ligament (Fig. 49.7); this can be the result of acromion morphology, rotator cuff muscle fatigue, degenerative tendinopathy, or AC joint spurring/hypertrophy.
- **Internal impingement:** Particularly in throwers, the articular surface of the rotator cuff comes into contact with the superior glenoid labrum. Although considered anatomically normal, overuse combined with instability or loss of internal rotation leads to combined articular-sided rotator cuff and SLAP tears.
- **Subcoracoid impingement:** Contact between the rotator cuff and a prominent coracoid; the prominence can be idiopathic or iatrogenic (after osteotomy).

Presentation:

- **Subacromial impingement:** Presents with symptoms typical for rotator cuff pathology; this includes anterolateral shoulder pain that radiates to the lateral arm. Pain is exacerbated by overhead activities. Pain at night and when lying on the affected shoulder is extremely common.
- **Internal impingement:** Posterior-superior shoulder pain or pain described as deep in the joint; exacerbated by activities that place the arm in an abducted, externally rotated position
- **Subcoracoid impingement:** Anterior shoulder pain exacerbated by activities that involve forward flexion and internal rotation

Physical examination (see the earlier "special test" section for description of tests): Neer impingement sign, Hawkins test, painful arc, coracoid impingement sign, and Jobe relocation test

Differential diagnosis: Instability, GH arthritis, adhesive capsulitis, cervical radiculopathy, calcific tendonitis, AC joint arthritis, and thoracic outlet syndrome

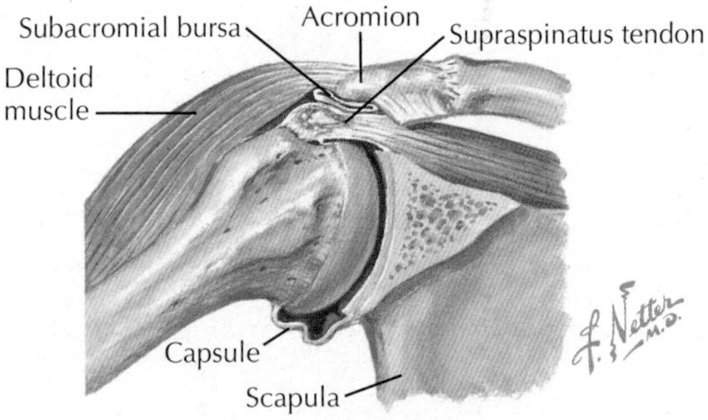
Subacromial bursa
Acromion
Supraspinatus tendon
Deltoid muscle
Capsule
Scapula
F. Netter M.D.

Rotator cuff disease

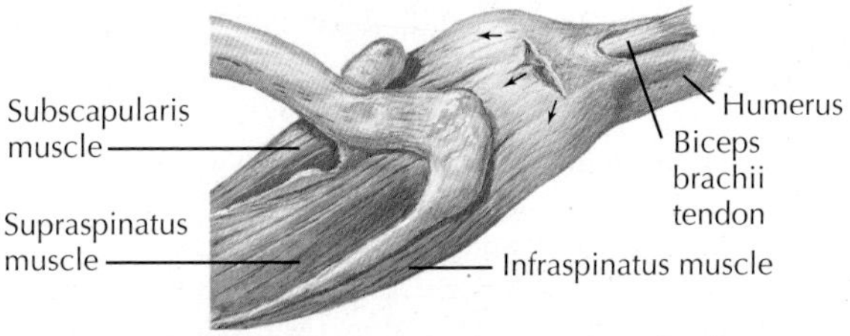
Subscapularis muscle
Supraspinatus muscle
Humerus
Biceps brachii tendon
Infraspinatus muscle

Acute rupture (superior view). Often associated with splitting tear parallel to tendon fibers. Further retraction results in crescentic defect as shown at right.

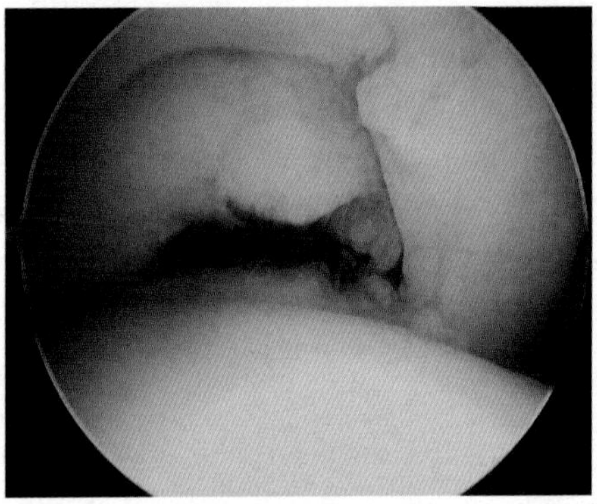

Arthroscopic image of small rotator cuff tear as viewed from the joint

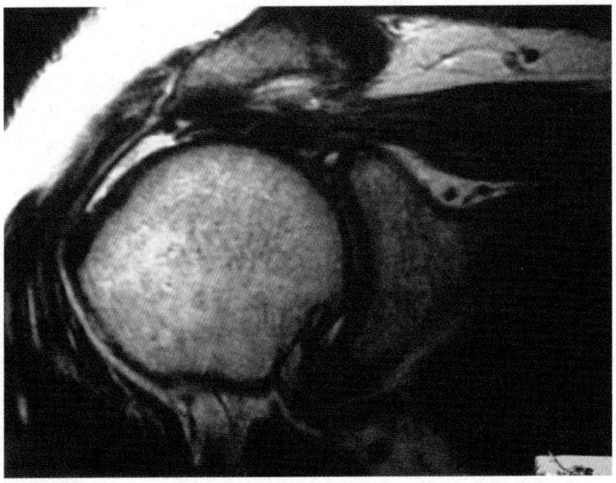

MRI large cuff tear

Figure 49.7 Rotator cuff injury.

Diagnostics:

- **Neer test:** A subacromial lidocaine injection is given. Resolution of pain when performing Neer impingement sign maneuver is a positive test.
- **Coracoid impingement test:** Lidocaine injection just lateral to the coracoid; resolution of symptoms when performing the coracoid impingement sign maneuver indicates a positive test.
- **Radiographs:**
  - AP of the shoulder to rule out GH arthritis
  - Outlet view allows evaluation of acromion morphology (type I—flat, type II—curved, type III—hooked). Type III acromions are associated with a greater incidence of rotator cuff pathology.
  - Axillary view allows evaluation of the coracoid.
- **MRI:** Will demonstrate rotator cuff tendinopathy, partial- or full-thickness rotator cuff tears, and subacromial bursitis
- **Coracohumeral index:** Distance between the coracoid and humerus can be measured on a CT or MRI. Normal is 8.6 mm with the arm in maximal internal rotation; symptomatic patients display a mean distance of 5.5 mm.

Treatment:

- NSAIDs and physical therapy to strengthen the rotator cuff and scapular stabilizers; subacromial corticosteroid injections are used in subacromial impingement.
- A majority of patients improve with conservative therapy, but those who fail may be indicated for surgical decompression. *Subcoracoid decompression* involves a partial resection of the coracoid; it involves bursectomy and acromioplasty. Surgical treatment for *internal impingement* is directed at the SLAP lesion and rotator cuff tear as necessary.

Prognosis and return to play: Athletes involved in overhead activities can return to sports once pain has resolved enough to allow for normal range of motion and near-normal strength.

Rotator Cuff Tear

Description: Disruption of the tendon or tendons of the rotator cuff muscles; the supraspinatus tendon is most commonly involved (see Fig. 49.7)

Mechanism of injury: Tears can occur acutely from direct or indirect trauma. Alternatively, chronic tears can be the result of long-standing tendinopathy that eventually progresses to a tear.

Presentation: Similar to subacromial impingement, patients present with anterolateral shoulder pain exacerbated by overhead activities. Night pain and pain while sleeping on the affected side are common. Weakness may be present depending on the acuity or size of the tear.

Physical examination: Inspection for atrophy of the supra or infraspinatus, which if present, indicates a chronic condition. Evaluate active and passive range of motion. Positive findings during the following examination maneuvers are suggestive of a rotator cuff tear:

- Supraspinatus testing
  - Strength testing
  - Champagne toast
  - Jobe test
  - Drop-arm sign
  - Impingement tests
- Infraspinatus
  - External rotation strength at 0 and 90 degrees; also tests teres minor
  - External rotation lag sign
- Teres minor
  - Hornblower's (indicative of massive tear)
- Subscapularis
  - Internal rotation strength
  - Lift-off test
  - Belly-press test

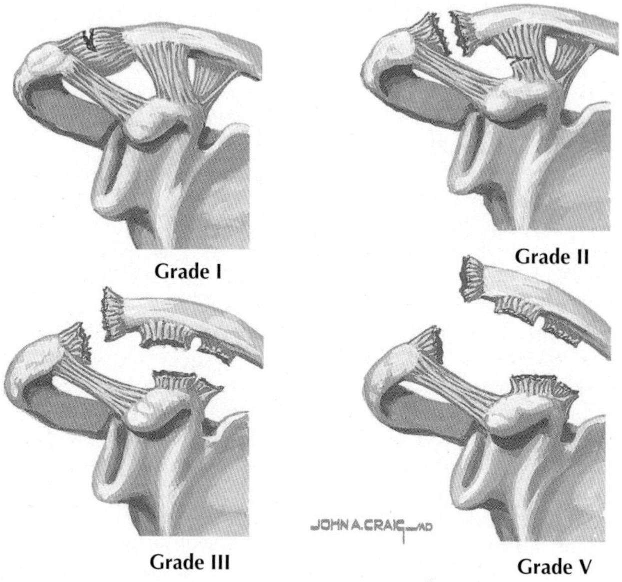
Grade I
Grade II
Grade III
Grade V
JOHN A.CRAIG_MD

Figure 49.8 Acromioclavicular dislocation.

Differential diagnosis: Impingement, AC joint arthritis, biceps pathology, GH instability, adhesive capsulitis, and cervical radiculopathy

Diagnostics:

- **Radiographs:** AP view to identify proximal migration of the humeral head, which would indicate a massive/chronic and typically irreparable tear (acromiohumeral distance <7 mm)
- **MRI:** Extremely sensitive and specific for rotator cuff disease; can distinguish partial- and full-thickness tears. Other notable findings that can influence treatment plan and prognosis are fatty infiltration and atrophy of the rotator cuff muscles and degree of tear retraction (see Fig. 49.7).
- **Ultrasound:** Extremely sensitive and specific for rotator cuff tears; cheaper than MRI, but is highly operator dependent

Treatment: Decision-making should be individualized and take into account the patient's age and activity level. Nonoperative treatment tends to be less successful in patients who present with a symptom duration of >1 year and significant weakness. Nonoperative treatment is similar to that for impingement. Patients who fail nonoperative treatment are indicated for surgical repair. Acute traumatic tears are best treated with prompt surgical repair.

Prognosis and return to play: Overhead athletes undergoing surgical repair may require 6 months to 1 year before being able to fully return to sports. Only 50% of professional athletes return to same level of play as before the injury, but most recreational athletes are able to return to prior level of play.

Acromioclavicular Joint Injuries

Sprains/Separations

Description: Involves sequential injury to the AC and coracoclavicular (CC) ligaments; includes involvement of the deltoid and trapezius muscle and fascia in higher-degree injuries

Classification:

- **Type I:** Sprain of the AC ligament; AC and CC ligaments are intact; normal radiographs (Fig. 49.8)
- **Type II:** Rupture of the AC ligament; CC ligaments are intact; radiographs will show slight elevation of the clavicle. The AC joint is unstable to examination, but a stress radiograph will *not* produce 100% separation.
- **Type III:** Complete rupture of the AC and CC ligaments with 100% superior displacement of the clavicle

- **Type IV:** Complete separation of the AC joint with the clavicle displaced posteriorly through the trapezial fascia
- **Type V:** More severe type III with complete rupture of the AC and CC ligaments; also involves disruption of the trapezial and deltoid fascia off of the acromion and clavicle. The clavicle is superiorly displaced by 100%–300%.
- **Type VI:** A rare inferior dislocation of the clavicle into a subcoracoid (lodged behind the conjoined tendon) or subacromial position

Mechanism of injury: A vast majority of such injuries are the result of direct trauma by a fall or blow onto the shoulder with the arm adducted. An indirect mechanism involves falling onto an outstretched hand, which drives the humerus proximally into the acromion.

Presentation: The patient will usually report the aforementioned mechanism and complain of pain at the anterior/superior aspect of the shoulder. Common examples include hockey players being checked into the boards, football players taking a blow to the shoulder pads, or a cyclist falling off of a bike.

Physical examination: Tenderness will be present over the AC joint. Prominence of the distal clavicle will be evident in types II, III, and V. Stability of the distal clavicle can be assessed, although it may be difficult in the acute setting. The **cross-arm adduction test** will be positive. The **O'Brien test** has been shown to have a high specificity for AC sprains if the pain localizes to that region.

Differential diagnosis: Clavicle fracture, distal clavicular osteolysis, and shoulder contusion

Diagnostics: In standard radiographs of the shoulder, the AC joint is overpenetrated and poorly visualized.

- **Bilateral AP:** Used to compare displacement of AC and CC with uninjured side
- **Zanca view:** See earlier discussion under "Imaging of the Shoulder"
- **Axillary view:** Allows evaluation for anterior or posterior displacement of the clavicle
- **MRI:** Can directly visualize the CC ligaments, allowing for more definitive classification of injury

Treatment:

- Types I and II are nonoperatively treated with a brief period of immobilization in a sling, ice, and analgesics followed by physical therapy. A local anesthetic injection can be used for in-game situations to allow the athlete to resume play. Chronic type II injuries that are symptomatic can be surgically treated with distal clavicle excision and anatomic reconstruction.
- Type III: Treatment is controversial, but most lean toward nonoperative treatment. If the patient has persistent pain or is unable to return to the desired level of activity, distal clavicle excision and anatomic reconstruction can be performed. Certain experts favor early operative management for high-level throwing athletes.
- Typically, types IV, V, and VI are surgically treated.

Prognosis and return to play: Those nonoperatively treated will be able to return to sports in 1–6 weeks depending on the severity of the injury and sport played. Those surgically treated will require 4–6 months before returning to sports.

Distal Clavicle Osteolysis

Description: A painful condition of the AC joint caused by lysis and resorption of the distal clavicle

Mechanism of injury: Overuse injury producing repetitive microtrauma to the distal clavicle that leads to bone resorption

Presentation: Most common in young males and often bilateral; frequently associated with weightlifting. Patients present with pain over the anterior/superior aspect of the shoulder. Pain is exacerbated with more demanding activities. Weightlifters are more symptomatic with specific exercises such as bench pressing, dips, and push-ups.

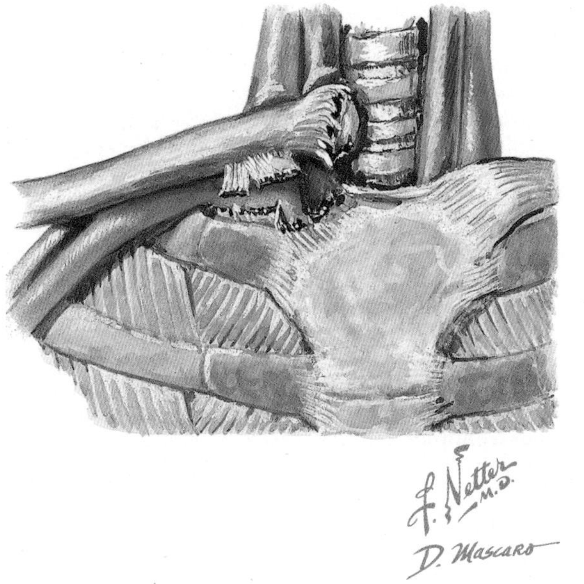
F. Netter M.D.
D. Mascaro

Figure 49.9 Dislocation of acromioclavicular or sternoclavicular joint.

Physical examination: Tenderness over the AC joint; there may be a prominence of the distal clavicle and crepitus with motion. The **cross-arm adduction test** will elicit pain. Stability of the distal clavicle should be assessed because this may affect surgical planning.

Differential diagnosis: Rotator cuff disease, infection, hyperparathyroidism, clavicle fracture, and AC separation

Diagnostics:

- Zanca view reveals osteopenia and expansion of the distal clavicle. Joint space widening and cysts may be present as well.
- MRI will reveal T2 edema in the distal clavicle and periarticularly throughout the AC joint.
- Bone scan is sensitive and is useful in cases wherein radiographic findings are not obvious.
- A diagnostic injection of local anesthetic into the AC joint is useful in cases wherein the diagnosis is unclear.

Treatment: Initial treatment should be nonoperative and comprises modification of activities and weightlifting technique, NSAIDs, and corticosteroid injections. Distal clavicle resection is indicated in patients who fail nonoperative treatment or cannot tolerate the extended course usually required for complete resolution of symptoms.

Prognosis and return to play: Those nonoperatively treated with a local injection or symptomatic treatment can return to sports as tolerated; those surgically treated will require at least 4–6 weeks before returning to sports.

Sternoclavicular Joint Injuries

Sprains, Subluxations, and Dislocations

Description: Involves injury (ranging from stretching to partial tearing to complete rupture) of the ligaments of the SC joint; these ligaments (intra-articular disc ligament, extra-articular costoclavicular ligament, capsular ligament, and interclavicular ligament) provide most of the stability to this extremely incongruent joint. Acute sprains are classified as mild (stable joint), moderate (joint subluxation), and severe (joint dislocation). Dislocations are further classified according to the direction of dislocation: anterior (more common) or posterior (Fig. 49.9). In the skeletally immature, the injury may be through the medial clavicular physis, which is the last of the long bones in the body to close. Can also present as spontaneous, atraumatic anterior subluxation.

Mechanism of injury: These injuries are the result of direct or indirect forces.

- Indirect forces are more common and are applied to the SC joint from the anterolateral or posterolateral aspects of the shoulder. Compression and rolling forward of the shoulder cause a posterior dislocation, whereas compression and rolling backward of the shoulder cause an anterior dislocation. Such mechanisms can be seen in football pile-ons.
- Direct force applied over the anteromedial aspect of the clavicle will result in a posterior dislocation.

Presentation:

- Acute traumatic dislocations or physeal fractures present with significant pain and will often be supporting the arm with the uninjured side. Pain is exacerbated by shoulder motion. Dislocations will give an appearance of shortening of the shoulder. Patient will often tilt head toward injured side to minimize traction of sternocleidomastoid.
- A majority of spontaneous, atraumatic subluxations are not painful and occur with overhead elevation of the arm. The subluxation reduces when the arm is brought back down. These patients are usually in their teens to 20s, and numerous patients have generalized ligamentous laxity.

Physical examination:

- Anterior dislocations: Tenderness and swelling exist over a prominent medial end of the clavicle.
- Posterior dislocations: The medial end of the clavicle may not be palpable because it sits posterior to the sternum. Significant swelling anteriorly over the SC joint has been known to mask a posterior dislocation. Patients may have difficulty breathing or swallowing. Venous congestion can be present in the neck or extremity. Compression on the trachea or great vessels can make these injuries a medical emergency.

Differential diagnosis: Sternum fracture, rib fracture, and contusion

Diagnostics:

- **Radiographs:** Because of its location and the surrounding anatomy, the SC joint is difficult to image by using plain radiography. Several special views have been developed over time to maximize visualization.
- **Serendipity view (see earlier description under "Imaging of the Shoulder"):** Anterior dislocations will appear displaced superiorly to a horizontal line off of the normal clavicle. Posterior dislocations will appear displaced inferiorly.
- **Heinig view:** A lateral view centered at the manubrium and shot tangential to the SC joint and parallel to the opposite clavicle
- **CT scan:** The best imaging modality to evaluate the SC joint

Treatment:

- Mild sprain: Ice in the initial 12–24 hours; sling immobilization for comfort for initial 3–4 days, followed by a progressive range of motion and return to activities
- Moderate sprain/subluxation: Ice in the initial 12–24 hours; figure-of-eight strap to hold shoulders back and reduce SC subluxation; sling to support upper extremity
- Dislocation:
  - Anterior: Gentle reduction followed by figure-of-eight strap for 6 weeks and a sling; anterior dislocations are often unstable after reduction and may re-dislocate after figure-of-eight strap is discontinued. Conservative versus surgical treatment is then based on patient's symptoms and whether activities are limited.
  - Posterior: Closed reduction is the treatment of choice for acute injuries. It usually requires general anesthesia and results in a stable SC joint. Appropriate consultants should be available, given the associated vascular injuries that have been known to occur. Again, postreduction care includes a figure-of-eight strap and a sling.
- Atraumatic spontaneous subluxation: Symptoms resolve spontaneously. Surgery is not indicated.
- Physeal fracture: Reduction and immobilization similar to dislocations; however, period of immobilization is shorter (3–4 weeks) because of fracture healing.

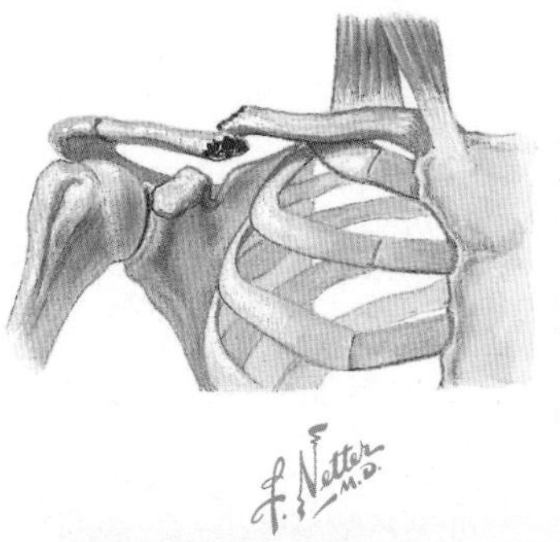
F. Netter M.D.

Fracture of middle third of clavicle (most common). Medial fragment displaced upward by pull of sternocleidomastoid muscle; lateral fragment displaced downward by weight of shoulder. Fractures occur most often in children.

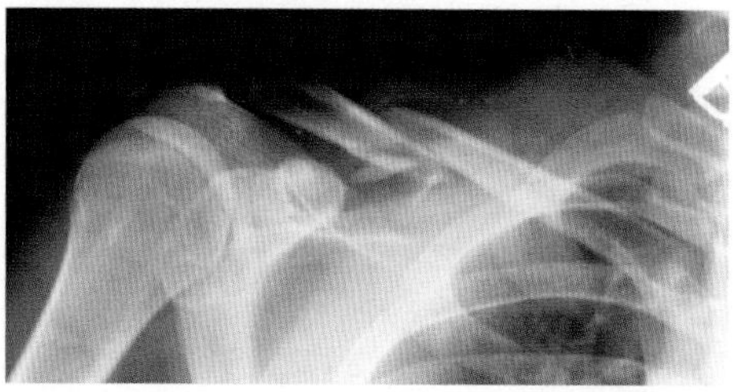

Anteroposterior radiograph. Fracture of middle third of clavicle.

Figure 49.10 Fracture of the clavicle.

Prognosis and return to play: Patients report good to excellent outcomes with both operative and nonoperative management. Patients with mild and moderate sprains can return to sports in 2–4 weeks once the pain has resolved and motion has returned. Those with anterior dislocations should be withheld from sports for 6–8 weeks. Those with posterior dislocations should be withheld for a longer duration to allow for complete ligament healing, given the potential complications associated with a recurrent posterior dislocation.

Clavicle Fracture

Description: Accounts for about 2.5% of all fractures; 80% occur in the middle third of the clavicle

Mechanism of injury: Similar mechanism as AC joint separations or direct blows to the clavicle

Presentation: The patient is usually splinting the injured extremity and can give a clear history of the injury-causing event (Fig. 49.10). A visible deformity with marked swelling and ecchymosis may be present in displaced fractures.

Physical examination:

- Important to check the neurovascular status of the involved extremity
- Evaluate the overlying skin at the fracture site to determine if it is at a risk of breakdown, converting a closed fracture into an open fracture.
- Rule out any associated musculoskeletal injuries to the cervical spine or ipsilateral upper extremity and any visceral injuries such as a pneumothorax.

Differential diagnosis: AC separation, SC dislocation, scapula fracture, contusion, and congenital pseudoarthrosis

Diagnostics: Standard radiograph series of the shoulder to evaluate for associated shoulder girdle injuries (see Fig. 49.10);

a standard AP radiograph will not adequately demonstrate true displacement of the fracture. Therefore, an additional 45-degree cephalic tilt or axillary view with slight cephalic tilt is recommended.

Treatment: Historically, middle clavicle fractures have been nonoperatively treated with immobilization in a sling with good results in terms of union and function despite the deformity associated with healing of displaced fractures. More recently, the literature suggests higher nonunion rates and lesser outcomes associated with shortening of the clavicle (>2 cm). Surgical treatment has been shown to have fewer nonunions, faster time to union, and greater functional outcomes. Surgery also has implant-related complications resulting in multiple surgeries. With no proven advantage to surgical versus conservative management, the decision should be individualized based on the patient's goals and wishes. Surgical treatment is indicated in fractures that are open, tenting the skin, or associated with a neurovascular injury.

Prognosis and return to play: Noncontact athletes can return to sports once evidence of radiographic healing is present and full, painless, active range of motion with near-normal strength has returned. Contact athletes should be withheld for 2–3 months to allow for adequate healing.

Proximal Humeral Epiphysitis (Little Leaguer's Shoulder)

Description: Growth plate injury (epiphysiolysis) of the proximal humerus

Mechanism of injury: Caused by overuse and repetitive microtrauma in overhead, skeletally immature athlete; poor throwing technique can contribute to the cause of injury

Presentation: Diffuse shoulder pain, worse with throwing or extremes of motion; usually gradual in onset and may present after a recent increase in throwing activity

Physical examination: Pain with palpation about the proximal humeral physis and possibly at extremes of shoulder range of motion; patients may present with external rotation contractures and decreased internal rotation

Differential diagnosis: Osteochondrosis of the proximal humerus, instability, and impingement

Diagnostics: Radiographs of the shoulder, including an AP with the arm externally rotated, allows evaluation of the physis; usually reveals physeal widening but may demonstrate metaphyseal fragmentation and periosteal reaction depending on severity. MRI will reveal the injury in occult cases not detected on radiographs.

Treatment: Most of these injuries are subtle with minimal displacement. Treatment for these cases begins with cessation of throwing for approximately 3 months. Then, a progressive throwing program should be initiated. Attention should be given to the athlete's throwing mechanics. In cases of significant displacement and/or angulation, treatment is based on the age and growth remaining of the patient.

Prognosis and return to play: Adherence to the treatment protocol of rest, followed by a throwing program with appropriate mechanics, will return a vast majority to play without return of symptoms.

Glenohumeral Internal Rotation Deficit (GIRD)

Description: Loss of GH internal rotation of >25 degrees; overhead athletes will often gain external rotation adaptively to increase velocity. The gain in external rotation usually leads to a loss of internal rotation. If the loss of internal rotation exceeds the gain in external rotation, it is considered pathologic.

Mechanism of injury: Posterior-inferior capsular contracture; the posterior capsular contracture alters the kinematics of the shoulder, leading to SLAP lesions (most commonly type II) or impingement.

Presentation: Patients complain of shoulder pain and decreased performance. They may report difficulty reaching across their body or up their back.

Physical examination: External and internal rotation are documented with the patient supine and the scapula stabilized. Impingement tests and O'Brien test will be positive if impingement or a SLAP tear has developed.

Differential diagnosis: Adhesive capsulitis and physiologic loss of internal rotation (internal rotation loss is *not* greater than external rotation gain)

Diagnostics: Diagnosis is clinical. MRI will demonstrate associated SLAP lesions or cuff pathology indicative of impingement. Bennet lesion (posterior capsular calcification) may be present.

Treatment: Physical therapy to focus on posterior capsular stretching. Patients who do not regain internal rotation with a therapy program are candidates for arthroscopic release of the posterior-inferior capsule. Patients with recalcitrant pain despite improvement in internal rotation may have a SLAP lesion that needs to be surgically addressed.

Prognosis and return to play: Ninety percent of patients respond to a stretching program in 2 weeks. A prophylactic stretching program will protect against GIRD and the potential development of an associated SLAP lesion.

Adhesive Capsulitis (Frozen Shoulder)

Description: Characterized by pain and gradual loss of both active and passive motion of the GH joint caused by soft tissue contracture; risk factors include female gender, middle age, smoking, immobilization, and endocrine disorders such as diabetes and thyroid disease.

Mechanism of injury: Capsulitis can be idiopathic, which is termed "primary adhesive capsulitis." Etiology is unknown. When the condition is caused by a known intrinsic or extrinsic cause, such as postsurgical or posttraumatic, it is termed "secondary adhesive capsulitis."

Presentation: Depends on stage of the disease, but the hallmarks are pain and limited active and passive motion; four stages have been described.

- Stage 1 ("painful stage"): Pain with active and passive range of motion; positive rest and night pain; symptoms present <3 months
- Stage 2 ("freezing stage"): Chronic pain and progressive loss of range of motion; positive rest and night pain; symptoms present 3–9 months
- Stage 3 ("frozen stage"): Significant shoulder stiffness; minimal rest and night pain; symptoms present 9–15 months
- Stage 4 ("thawing stage"): Minimal pain and progressive improvement in range of motion

Physical examination: Tenderness to palpation over deltoid insertion and on deep palpation over anterior and posterior capsule; careful examination of passive and active range of motion of the GH joint; make sure to stabilize the scapula so as not to be fooled by scapulothoracic motion, which can be increased to compensate for a lack of GH joint motion.

Differential diagnosis: GH arthritis, rotator cuff disease, and polymyalgia rheumatica

Diagnostics: Clinical diagnosis is adhesive capsulitis. Radiographs are unremarkable but are useful to rule out other pathologies. MRI findings include thickening of the coracohumeral ligament and joint capsule, including the rotator interval.

Treatment:

- Options include benign neglect, physical therapy, NSAIDs, intra-articular corticosteroid injections, manipulation under anesthesia, hydrodilatation, and surgical capsular release.

- Treatment should be individualized depending on the stage of disease at presentation. NSAIDs and corticosteroid injections are beneficial for the inflammatory process associated with stages 1 and 2. Physical therapy during these stages focuses on gentle range-of-motion exercises and modalities for pain and inflammation. Range-of-motion exercises should be more aggressive during stages 3 and 4.
- Surgery is indicated for those who fail nonoperative treatment.
- Secondary adhesive capsulitis may be treated more aggressively.

Prognosis and return to play: A majority of patients will improve with conservative therapy but it is a protracted course. Up to 35% of patients can have minimal pain and minor residual deficits in motion, although functional limitations may exist in the long term.

Pectoralis Major Tear

Description: Tear of the pectoralis major tendon; more commonly isolated to the sternal head; usually a distal injury occurring as a tendon avulsion or rupture at the myotendinous junction; can occur as a proximal injury to the muscle belly

Mechanism of injury: Distal injuries are associated with strenuous activity such as football, wrestling, and weightlifting (during eccentric phase of bench press exercise). Proximal injuries to the muscle belly usually are the result of direct trauma.

Presentation: Patients may remember a specific incident and report feeling a tearing sensation and a "pop"; complaints of pain around the chest, axilla, and upper arm, associated with weakness and painful limited motion

Physical examination: Acutely, swelling and ecchymosis will be present over the anterior chest wall and the upper arm (if distal injury). Weakness will be evident with resisted adduction and internal rotation. Distal injuries will often have a palpable defect in the axilla and noticeable asymmetry compared with contralateral side in complete tears.

Differential diagnosis: Biceps tendon rupture, anterior dislocation that spontaneously reduced, rotator cuff tear, and contusion

Diagnostics: Although radiographs are usually normal, avulsion injuries and loss of the normal pectoralis major shadow may be detected. MRI is the modality of choice. It can distinguish between partial and complete tears and acute and chronic tears.

Treatment: Nonsurgical management applies only to proximal injuries or partial tears distally. Treatment consists of rest, ice, and physical therapy to maintain shoulder motion. Resisted strengthening should be incorporated after 6 weeks. Surgical management is indicated for complete distal tears.

Prognosis and return to play: Athletes undergoing surgical repair can expect a return to full or near-full strength.

Proximal Humerus Fracture

Description: Commonly described by the Neer classification, which divides the proximal humerus into four parts: humeral head, greater tuberosity, lesser tuberosity, and humeral shaft; a fracture fragment is considered a part if it is displaced >1 cm (0.5 cm if the greater tuberosity) or angulated >45 degrees (Fig. 49.11).

Mechanism of injury: Sports-related fractures are usually caused by a high-energy impact or are avulsion fractures of the greater or lesser tuberosity associated with a dislocation. Fractures in the older population result from a fall onto the shoulder or an outstretched arm.

Presentation: Pain, swelling, ecchymosis, and inability to move the shoulder; patients often splint their arm against their body and support it with the uninjured arm

Physical examination: Tenderness and swelling about the shoulder will be present. Pain and crepitus with range of motion; a good neurovascular examination is important

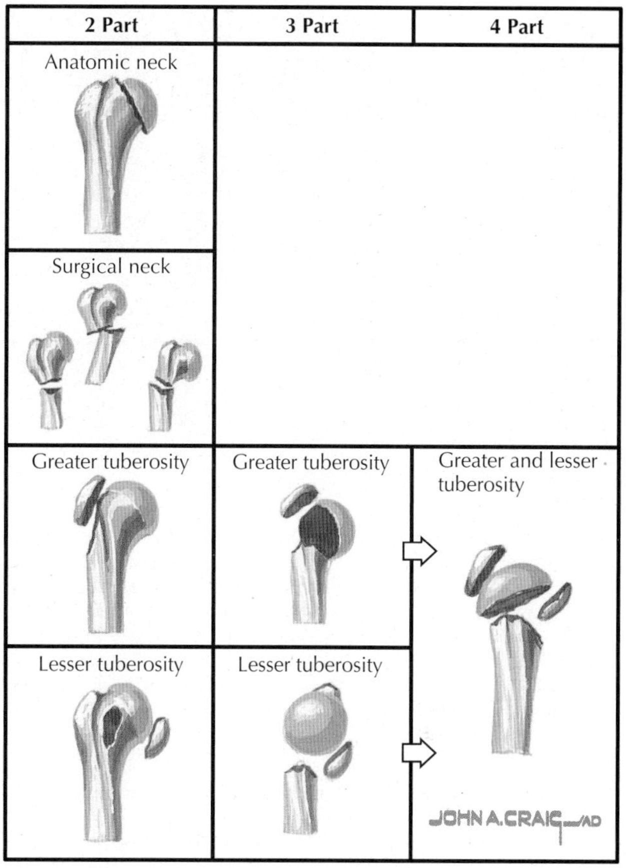
2 Part
3 Part
4 Part
Anatomic neck
Surgical neck
Greater tuberosity
Greater tuberosity
Greater and lesser tuberosity
Lesser tuberosity
Lesser tuberosity
JOHN A.CRAIG_AD

Figure 49.11 Neer classification of proximal humerus fractures.

Differential diagnosis: Dislocation, rotator cuff tear, contusion, clavicle fracture, and scapula fracture

Diagnostics: Plain radiographs are diagnostic.

- Standard trauma series of the shoulder (AP, axillary, and scapular-Y views.) The axillary view is critical to rule out a concomitant dislocation. If the patient is not able to tolerate a traditional axillary view, a *Velpeau axillary* can be taken without moving the arm (Fig. 49.12).
- CT is essential to evaluate the amount of displacement of the greater tuberosity and articular involvement.

Treatment: Most fractures are minimally displaced and can be treated in a sling with early passive range of motion. Displaced fractures (>1 cm) require open reduction and internal fixation. Recent data support arthroplasty solutions (reverse total shoulder) in the setting of displaced four-part fractures in elderly patients.

Prognosis and return to play: Noncontact, nonoverhead athletes can return in 2–3 months, once adequate fracture healing has occurred. Overhead athletes will require a longer recovery time to allow for return of full range of motion and strength.

Neurologic Syndromes Affecting the Shoulder

Parsonage–Turner Syndrome (or Brachial Neuritis)

Description: Inflammation of nerves of the brachial plexus

Mechanism of injury: Unknown etiology; often associated with preceding upper respiratory tract infection or unusually heavy exercise

Presentation: Initial complaint is spontaneous pain in the shoulder or the arm. As the pain resolves, weakness ensues.

Physical examination: Affected nerve distribution is variable, but those most commonly affected are the axillary,

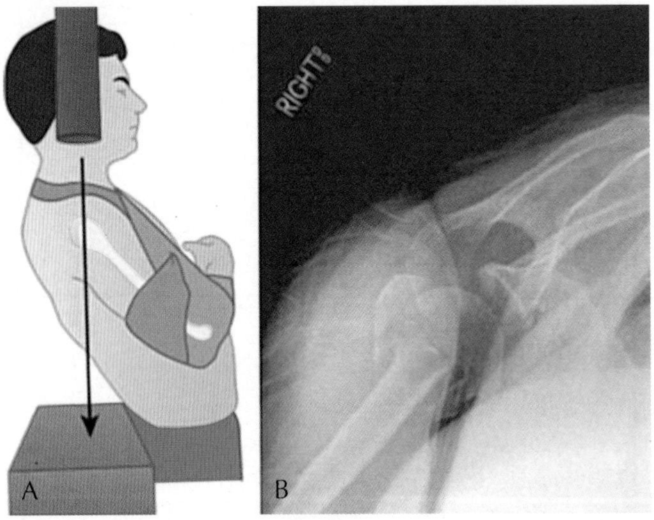
A
RIGHT
B

Figure 49.12 A, Velpeau axillary view may be taken; this allows the patient to keep the arm immobilized in the sling. The patient leans back and over the plate while the beam is directed from superior to inferior. **B,** Velpeau axillary radiograph showing proximal humerus fracture. Note that the head is located and the greater tuberosity is displaced posteriorly. (From Cuomo F, Zuckerman JD. Proximal humerus fracture. In: Browner BD, ed. *Techniques in Orthopaedics*. vol 9. New York: Raven Press; 1994:143.)

musculocutaneous, suprascapular, and long thoracic nerves. Weakness in the corresponding muscle groups would be noted. Muscle atrophy may be apparent. Sensation is usually intact.

Differential diagnosis: Rotator cuff tear, adhesive capsulitis, suprascapular nerve entrapment, cervical spine pathology, and Pancoast tumor

Diagnostics: Imaging is not generally useful for diagnosis of brachial neuritis but is recommended to rule out intrinsic pathology. MRI is the imaging modality of choice. Electromyography (EMG) can be useful in diagnosing and in localizing the nerves involved.

Treatment: Pain control during the painful phase; physical therapy to maintain range of motion and progression to strengthening exercises as weakness resolves; certain studies have recommended early use of corticosteroids, but this is yet to be proven.

Prognosis and return to play: Self-limiting condition with overall good prognosis; time frame for complete recovery is variable: 36% recover by 1 year, 75% by 2 years, and 89% by 3 years.

Suprascapular Neuropathy

Description: The suprascapular nerve provides motor function to the supraspinatus and infraspinatus muscles. Injury to the nerve can cause paralysis of these muscles.

Mechanism of injury: Can occur from a compressive lesion or from positional traction on the nerve caused by overuse (e.g., volleyball players or baseball pitchers); injury usually occurs at one of two locations: suprascapular notch or spinoglenoid notch. Compression at these locations can result from a ganglion or paralabral cyst (in the setting of labral tear), hypertrophied/calcified transverse scapular ligament, narrow suprascapular notch, or lipoma (Fig. 49.13).

Presentation: Vague deep pain in posterolateral shoulder with possible radiating down the arm or into the neck; difficulty elevating the arm past horizontal

Physical examination: Should focus on strength testing of the rotator cuff and shoulder girdle muscles; important to inspect for atrophy of the supraspinatus and/or infraspinatus muscles, which would be present in later stages. Distinguishing the involvement of both the supraspinatus and infraspinatus versus the infraspinatus alone indicates the location of injury. Injury at the suprascapular notch will involve both muscles, whereas injury at the spinoglenoid notch will be isolated to the infraspinatus.

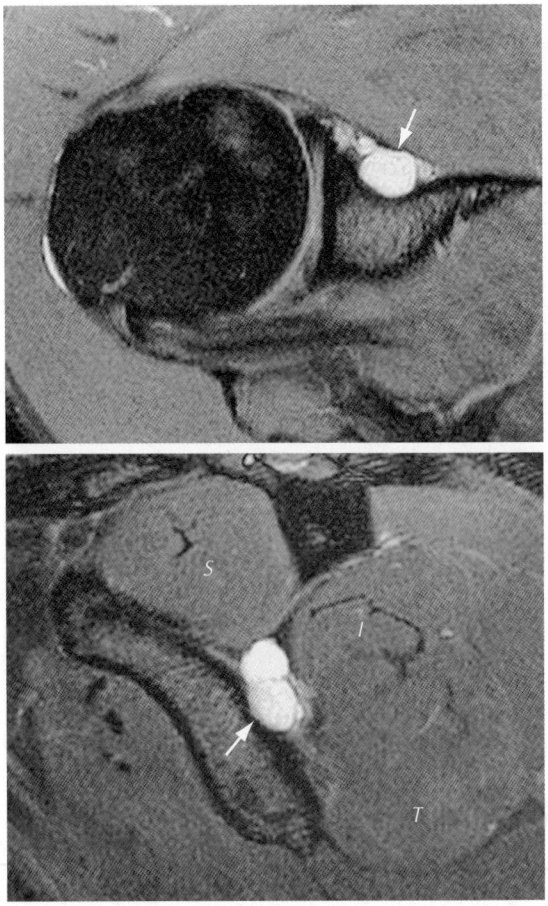
S
I
T

Figure 49.13 Spinoglenoid cyst. (From DeLee J, Drez D, Miller M. *DeLee & Drez's Orthopaedic Sports Medicine: Principles and Practice*. 2nd ed. Philadelphia: Saunders, Elsevier; 2002.)

Differential diagnosis: Cervical spine pathology, rotator cuff tear, and Parsonage–Turner syndrome

Diagnostics: Plain radiographs are usually normal. EMG can be helpful for diagnosis and to localize site of compression. MRI will demonstrate discrete compressive lesions and muscle atrophy.

Treatment: A majority of patients respond to conservative therapy consisting of activity modification, NSAIDs, analgesics, and physical therapy to strengthen the rotator cuff and scapular stabilizers. Surgical intervention is indicated in patients who fail conservative therapy, show signs of atrophy, or have structural compression. Ganglion cysts in the spinoglenoid notch are often the result of superior labral pathology. Treatment to address this intra-articular pathology also successfully decompresses the cyst.

Prognosis and return to play: A majority of nonoperative patients have good to excellent results at 6 months. Patients can return to play once near-normal strength and motion have returned.

Scapular Dyskinesia

Description: Abnormal motion of the scapula in relation to the thoracic cage and a visible altered position of the scapula; dyskinesia of the scapula leads to altered kinematics of the GH and

AC joints. SICK scapular syndrome is a severe form of scapular dyskinesia, in that the scapula is in malposition at rest and in motion. Findings can be remembered by the acronym **SICK** (**S**capular malposition, **I**nferior medial border prominence, **C**oracoid pain and malposition, and dys**K**inesia of the scapula).

Mechanism of injury: Most commonly the result of abnormal muscle activation and coordination; contracture of shoulder muscles, ligaments, and capsular structures (e.g., GIRD) can contribute to dyskinesia. Bony abnormalities that affect shoulder girdle motion, such as malunited clavicle fractures or AC joint injuries, can play a role.

Classification:

- **Type I:** Prominence of the inferior-medial scapular border
- **Type II:** Prominence of the medial scapular border
- **Type III:** Prominence of the superomedial scapular border; types I and II are associated with labral pathology, whereas type III is associated with impingement and rotator cuff pathology

Presentation: Among throwing athletes, patients often complain of pain anteriorly and decreased performance level. Onset is usually insidious.

Physical examination:

- Examine for any abnormal static scapular position such as winging, elevation, depression, or rotation; also during shoulder motion to evaluate dynamic asymmetry
- Patients with SICK syndrome will have pain anteriorly over the coracoid caused by tightness of the pectoralis minor.
- Scapular pinch test: Isometric retraction of the scapulas will elicit a burning sensation in <20 seconds in those with scapular muscle weakness.
- Scapular assistance test: Determines if scapular dyskinesia is contributing to impingement signs; the scapula is stabilized by the examiner with forward flexion of the extremity; if impingement pain resolves or improves, the test is positive.
- Scapular retraction test: Scapula is stabilized in a retracted position. The test is positive if either the rotator cuff strength is improved or pain and impingement with the Jobe relocation test is improved.

Differential diagnosis: Serratus anterior injury, long thoracic nerve injury, trapezius injury, and spinal accessory nerve injury

Diagnostics: Radiographs will be normal. MRI will reveal associated pathology to the rotator cuff or labrum.

Treatment: The mainstay of treatment is physical therapy. This focuses on the periscapular muscles and their coordination in repositioning the scapula. Stretching of tight structures such as the posterior capsule and pectoralis minor is important. Therapy should include the trunk and lower extremities because of their involvement in the kinetic chain of throwing. Surgical treatment may be necessary to address associated rotator cuff or labral pathology.

Prognosis and return to play: Once the scapula is symmetric with the contralateral side, the throwing athlete can return to play, approximately 3 months.

ACKNOWLEDGMENT

The authors would like to acknowledge the work of **Charles T. Crellin, MD,** and **Kevin M. Honig, MD,** for their contribution to the previous edition.

RECOMMENDED READINGS

Available online.

50 ELBOW INJURIES

Eric N. Bowman • Matthew V. Smith • Rick W. Wright • Joseph D. Lamplot

GENERAL PRINCIPLES

History and Physical Examination

History

- Hand dominance
- Location: medial, lateral, anterior, or posterior
- Type of pain: radiating, numbness/tingling, stiffness, mechanical symptoms (locking/catching)
- Duration of symptoms
- Mechanism of injury
- Pain modifiers
- Activity related: gripping, lifting, pushing, throwing, punching
- History of previous injuries
- Recent changes in technique or training regimen
- Treatments rendered and response

Physical Examination

- Inspection
    - Compare with uninjured side
    - Skin changes
    - Swelling
    - Ecchymosis
    - Muscle atrophy/hypertrophy
    - Carrying angle (cubitus valgus/varus)
        - Normal 10–20 degrees valgus, often greater in females
- Neurovascular examination
    - Sensation
        - Median, ulnar, radial, medial, and lateral antebrachial cutaneous (LABC) nerves
        - Two-point discrimination at fingertips (≤5 mm is normal)
    - Motor
        - Median, ulnar, and radial nerves
    - Ulnar nerve subluxation, irritability
- Range of motion (ROM) (Fig. 50.1)
    - Elbow flexion/extension
    - Forearm pronation/supination
- Palpation:
    - Tenderness of key anatomic structures
- Manual strength testing
- Stability
    - Valgus–varus laxity
    - Posterolateral rotary laxity
    - Ulnar collateral ligament laxity
- Provocative maneuvers

Ancillary Tests

- **Radiographs:** Anteroposterior (AP) and lateral
    - Special views:
        - Forty-five-degree flexion (capitellum)
        - Oblique (radial head)
        - Axial projections (olecranon fossa or gun-sight, Jones)
        - Gravity/manual stress
- **Computed tomography (CT) scan:** Articular congruity, loose bodies, fracture dislocation, osteophytes/exostosis, tendon calcification, heterotopic ossification
- **Magnetic resonance imaging (MRI) ± magnetic resonance arthrogram (MRA):** Soft tissue mass, ligament attenuation/rupture, chondral defect, loose bodies
- **Arthroscopy (diagnostic):** Loose bodies, chondral lesions, synovitis
- **Electromyogram (EMG)/nerve conduction study (NCS):** Nerve compression
- **Ultrasound:** Dynamic evaluation for ligament laxity or ulnar nerve instability

ANTERIOR ELBOW INJURIES

Distal Biceps Rupture

Description: Traumatic avulsion of the distal bicep tendon from the bicipital tuberosity of the proximal radius

Mechanism of injury: Eccentric muscle contraction against an extension load on a flexed elbow

Presentation: Less than 10% of biceps ruptures occur at the elbow. Most often occur in males (90%), dominant extremity (80%), in ages 30–50. Risk factors: smoking, anabolic steroids, and mechanical attrition. Often an acute pop or tearing sensation in the proximal forearm or antecubital fossa with an eccentric contraction, with subsequent pain and weakness. Tears may be complete or partial (radial sided).

Physical examination: Tenderness to palpation in the antecubital fossa, acute swelling, and ecchymosis are common. Palpable tendon defect in complete tears indicates tendon retraction ("Popeye sign"), though may not occur because of adhesion to the lacertus fibrosus. Pain and weakness with supination (40%–50% loss) and flexion.

- Hook test: Flex the elbow to 90 degrees in full supination, and insert a finger from the lateral side into the antecubital fossa to palpate for a cordlike structure
- Biceps squeeze test: Rest the elbow on patient's lap in slight pronation and midflexion, firmly squeeze the biceps muscle belly and observe for supination

Differential diagnosis: Biceps tendonitis, bicipital-radial bursitis, LABC nerve entrapment

Diagnostics: Primarily a clinical diagnosis

- **Radiographs:** Rule out associated elbow injuries and evaluate for irregularities around the radial tuberosity
- **Ultrasound:** Demonstrates extent of injury; cost-effective but user dependent
- **MRI:** Should be performed with the patient prone, shoulder abducted overhead, elbow flexed to 90 degrees, and forearm fully supinated; identify complete vs. partial tear and amount of retraction

Treatment:

- Nonsurgical: Activity modification, rest for low-grade partial tears
- Surgical: Complete or high-grade partial tears; acute repair superior to nonsurgical treatment; grafting may be required in chronic cases; one- and two-incision repair techniques described; concern for heterotopic bone formation/radioulnar synostosis with the two-incision technique; most common complication with either approach is LABC nerve palsy (15%–40%), higher with the one-incision technique (most resolve within 6 months)

Prognosis and return to sport: A season-ending injury; patients surgically treated early can be expected to have near-full return of power and function; return to sport 4–6 months; re-rupture rate of 5%.

Pronator Syndrome (Median Nerve Entrapment)

Description: Compression of the median nerve at the elbow with resultant nerve irritation (Fig. 50.2)

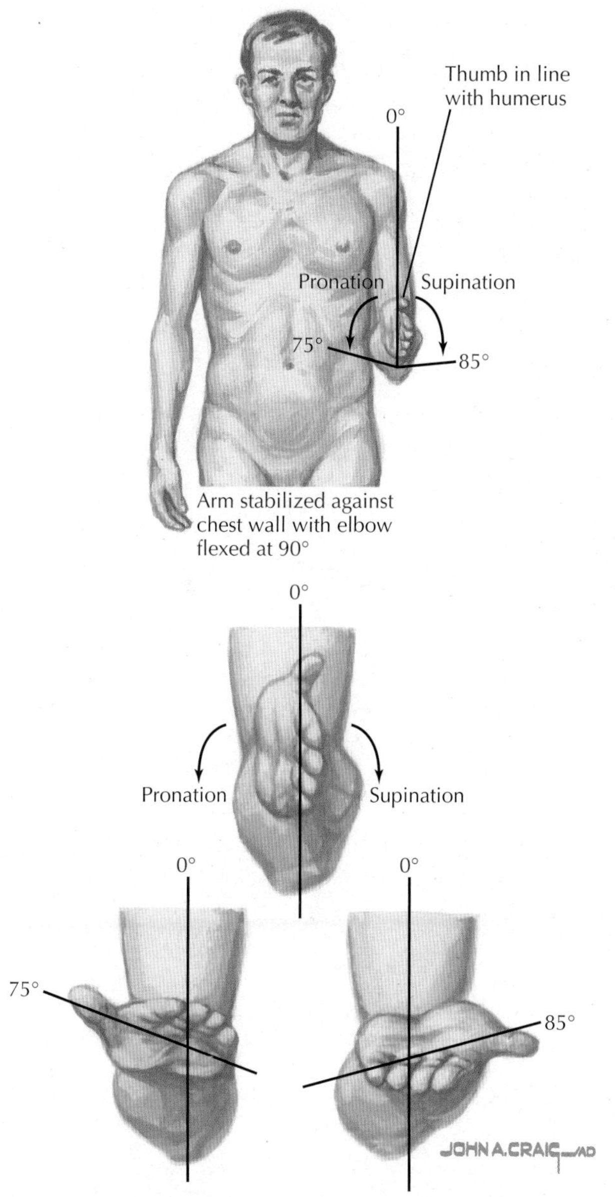
Thumb in line
with humerus
0°
Pronation
Supination
75°
85°
Arm stabilized against
chest wall with elbow
flexed at 90°
0°
Pronation
Supination
0°
0°
75°
85°
JOHN A.CRAIG_MD

Figure 50.1 Measurement of pronation/supination.

Mechanism of injury: No specific mechanism of injury has been associated; four possible sites of compression have been identified: beneath the ligament of Struthers in patients with a supracondylar process; an accessory head of the flexor pollicis longus (Gantzer muscle); lacertus fibrosus; tendinous arch of the flexor digitorum superficialis (FDS) ("sublimis bridge")

Presentation: Similar to carpal tunnel syndrome with paresthesias in the volar radial three and a half digits and volar forearm/wrist pain; distinguished from carpal tunnel syndrome by decreased sensation over the thenar eminence in the distribution of the palmar cutaneous branch of the median nerve. Symptom severity may increase with activity such as weightlifting, competitive driving, and underarm pitching. Nighttime symptoms are less common than those in carpal tunnel syndrome.

Physical examination: Symptoms recreated with resisted pronation/supination or resisted middle finger proximal interphalangeal (PIP) flexion, caused by compression of FDS heads; may have a positive Tinel sign over volar forearm

- Pronator compression test: Apply pressure for 30 seconds to the proximal edge of pronator muscle belly, which reproduces pain and paresthesias

Differential diagnosis: Carpal tunnel syndrome, cervical spine or brachial plexus nerve compression, flexor–pronator tendonitis, biceps tendonitis

Diagnostics:

- **Radiographs:** Often normal but can reveal a supracondylar process (5 cm proximal to the medial epicondyle; 1% of population)
- **EMG/NCS:** Help rule out other sites of compression; however, are often nondiagnostic

Treatment:

- Nonsurgical: Activity modification, forearm flexor stretching, and nonsteroidal anti-inflammatory drugs (NSAIDs)
- Surgical: Complete decompression of the median nerve throughout its course in the proximal forearm after failed conservative treatment: release of the ligament of Struthers, lacertus fibrosus, deep head of the pronator teres, and the FDS arch

Prognosis and return to sport: Early active range of motion (ROM), full return to activity by 6–8 weeks, and return to sport dependent upon restoration of strength and ROM.

POSTERIOR ELBOW INJURIES

Triceps Rupture

Description: Traumatic avulsion of the triceps tendon from its insertion on the olecranon process of the ulna, occasionally with a bony fragment attached

Mechanism of injury: Most commonly occurs from forceful eccentric contraction of triceps such as fall onto outstretched hand or weightlifting

Presentation: Twice as common in males, most often 30–50 years; Risk factors include anabolic steroids, systemic corticosteroids, and certain metabolic/systemic (endocrine or rheumatologic) disorders. Patients report a painful pop or a tearing in the posterior elbow during an eccentric load, with subsequent loss of elbow extension strength.

Physical examination: Tenderness to palpation along olecranon and distal triceps, ecchymosis, and edema; palpable defect of triceps tendon or step-off at olecranon; weak elbow extension/inability to hold elbow extended against gravity

- **Modified Thompson squeeze test:** Compressing the triceps muscle belly fails to cause elbow extension

Differential diagnosis: Triceps tendonitis, olecranon bursitis, olecranon stress fracture, posterior elbow impingement

Diagnostics:

- **Radiographs:** "Flake sign" (small bony avulsion fragment from olecranon process) observed in 80% of cases and pathognomonic for triceps rupture
- **MRI or ultrasound:** Can help distinguish partial from complete tendon rupture

Treatment:

- Nonsurgical: Mainly for elderly, sedentary patients or low-grade partial tears; immobilization with the elbow in 30 degrees of flexion for approximately 3–4 weeks, followed by progressive flexion
- Surgical: Most complete ruptures or high-grade partial ruptures are managed with early, primary surgical repair

Prognosis and return to sport: A season-ending injury for complete tears with at least 4–6 months of recovery/rehabilitation. Most athletes are able to return to preinjury level of sport, with slight loss of extension and strength. Re-rupture rate up to 20%.

Valgus Extension Overload

Description: Repetitive forceful shearing of the olecranon within its fossa causing chondromalacia and olecranon osteophyte formation

Mechanism of injury: Overuse injury frequently seen in throwing athletes. Bony constraints provide secondary stability to valgus stress to the elbow, which increases with extension; the

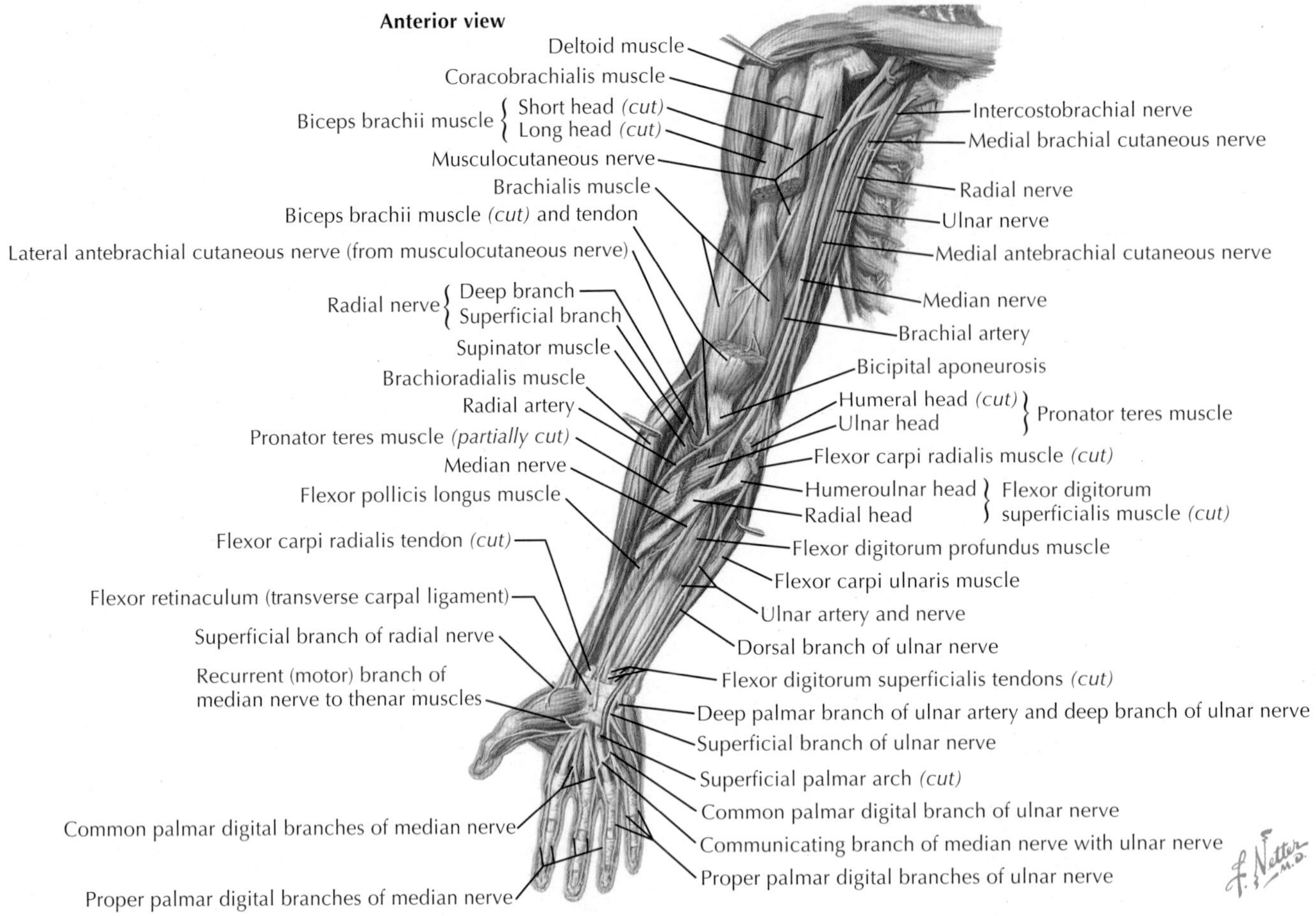
Anterior view
Deltoid muscle
Coracobrachialis muscle
Biceps brachii muscle
Short head (cut)
Long head (cut)
Musculocutaneous nerve
Brachialis muscle
Biceps brachii muscle (cut) and tendon
Lateral antebrachial cutaneous nerve (from musculocutaneous nerve)
Radial nerve
Deep branch
Superficial branch
Supinator muscle
Brachioradialis muscle
Radial artery
Pronator teres muscle (partially cut)
Median nerve
Flexor pollicis longus muscle
Flexor carpi radialis tendon (cut)
Flexor retinaculum (transverse carpal ligament)
Superficial branch of radial nerve
Recurrent (motor) branch of median nerve to thenar muscles
Common palmar digital branches of median nerve
Proper palmar digital branches of median nerve
Intercostobrachial nerve
Medial brachial cutaneous nerve
Radial nerve
Ulnar nerve
Medial antebrachial cutaneous nerve
Median nerve
Brachial artery
Bicipital aponeurosis
Humeral head (cut)
Ulnar head
Pronator teres muscle
Flexor carpi radialis muscle (cut)
Humeroulnar head
Radial head
Flexor digitorum superficialis muscle (cut)
Flexor digitorum profundus muscle
Flexor carpi ulnaris muscle
Ulnar artery and nerve
Dorsal branch of ulnar nerve
Flexor digitorum superficialis tendons (cut)
Deep palmar branch of ulnar artery and deep branch of ulnar nerve
Superficial branch of ulnar nerve
Superficial palmar arch (cut)
Common palmar digital branch of ulnar nerve
Communicating branch of median nerve with ulnar nerve
Proper palmar digital branches of ulnar nerve

Figure 50.2 Nerves of the upper extremity.

olecranon traumatically abuts the posteromedial olecranon fossa near full extension, often secondary to incompetent medial structures (medial ulnar collateral ligament [UCL] attenuation or tear).

Presentation: Pain localized to the medial aspect of olecranon in acceleration/deceleration phases of throwing; limited extension because of impinging osteophytes; mechanical symptoms from loose bodies; exacerbated by UCL laxity; throwing athletes may complain of premature fatigue, loss of velocity or control.

Physical examination: May demonstrate loss of terminal extension; posterior pain with pronation, valgus, and extension; possible pain or laxity of the UCL with valgus stress; possible ulnar nerve irritation; occasional loose bodies/crepitus

Differential diagnosis: Olecranon bursitis, olecranon stress fracture, triceps tendonitis

Diagnostics:

- **Radiographs:** May reveal posteromedial osteophytes, loose bodies, hypertrophic bone formation, calcification of the UCL, or medial epicondyle avulsion fractures; a 110-degree flexion oblique view can profile the posteromedial ulnar-humeral joint
- **MRI:** Define status of the articular cartilage and identify loose bodies

Treatment:

- Nonsurgical: Activity modification, NSAIDs, therapy with focus on eccentric strengthening of wrist flexors, shoulder flexibility, and core strengthening; progression to a supervised throwing program with correction of form/mechanics
- Surgical: Arthroscopic debridement; recommend <3 mm of bone resection because of subsequent increased force on the UCL

Prognosis and return to sport: A progressive throwing program should begin approximately 6 weeks after surgery. Most throwing athletes return to preinjury level within 3–4 months after surgery; patients with loose bodies or posterior impingement have better prognosis than those with degenerative changes.

Olecranon Stress Fracture

Description: Stress across the proximal portion of the ulna results in a fracture, usually through the epiphyseal plate

Mechanism of injury: Similar to valgus extension overload; repetitive abutment of the medial olecranon into the olecranon fossa during the deceleration phase of throwing. May indicate UCL insufficiency.

Presentation: Typically adolescent throwers; usually presents with insidious onset of pain in the posteromedial elbow

Physical examination: Tenderness to palpation over the posteromedial olecranon; pain with forced passive elbow extension and resisted extension; patients may demonstrate limited terminal extension.

Differential diagnosis: Triceps tendonitis, olecranon bursitis, valgus extension overload

Diagnostics:

- **Radiographs:** May show a transverse or oblique fracture line and/or sclerosis, typically through the epiphyseal plate; may present as delayed physeal fusion or widening; contralateral radiographs useful in skeletally immature patients because of variability in location of the olecranon physis
- **MRI:** May better characterize if radiographs are nondiagnostic

Treatment:
- Nonsurgical: Throwing cessation; may temporarily immobilize; return to sport after radiographic evidence of fracture healing and resolution of symptoms (may take 3–6 months)
- Surgical: Failure to respond to conservative therapy (delayed or nonunion); compression screw (oblique fractures) or tension band fixation (transverse fractures)

Prognosis and return to sport: Fractures typically heal with nonsurgical management or surgical fixation if required; athletes generally return to sport within 3–6 months.

Olecranon Bursitis

Description: Inflammation of the bursa overlying the triceps tendon and olecranon of the ulna; can be acute or chronic, septic or aseptic (Fig. 50.3)

Mechanism of injury: Typically from direct trauma to the posterior elbow; may be secondary to a single direct blow or repetitive trauma. Infection may lead to septic bursitis. Also associated with systemic conditions, including immunosuppression, crystalline diseases, diabetes, and alcoholism.

Presentation: Acute or gradual onset of bursal edema, erythema, and tenderness. Septic cases may be more painful with motion and may demonstrate associated cellulitis or systemic symptoms.

Physical examination: Focal posterior elbow swelling; mobile, fluctuant mass that changes in size; may have associated laceration/abrasion; typically normal ROM

Differential diagnosis: Gouty tophus, calcium pyrophosphate deposition, cellulitis

Diagnostics:
- **Radiographs:** May demonstrate bursal calcification or olecranon spurring
- **MRI:** If concern for additional abscess
- Aspiration should be performed under sterile conditions if concern for septic bursitis: fluid analysis for cell count and differential, Gram stain, culture, and crystal analysis; *Staphylococcus aureus* most common cause of septic bursitis

Treatment:
- Nonsurgical: Acute aseptic cases effectively treated with rest, short-term immobilization (3–5 days), compressive dressing, ice, NSAIDs, and avoidance of direct pressure; chronic aseptic cases can be treated with cautious aspiration and injection of corticosteroids, with a compressive dressing; corticosteroid injections are controversial and may increase the risk of septic bursitis or cause skin/fat atrophy
- Surgical: Excision of bursa/olecranon osteophyte for recalcitrant cases; wound complications common, especially with gouty tophi; septic bursitis should be aspirated, with possible surgical excision, followed by culture-directed intravenous antibiotics (1–3 weeks) followed by oral (2–3 weeks)

Prognosis and return to sport: Aseptic bursitis should be initially managed conservatively, though there is a high risk of recurrence. Surgical resection only for recalcitrant cases or septic cases not responding to antibiotics. High risk of wound complications or recurrence. Appropriate protective padding should be used during sports.

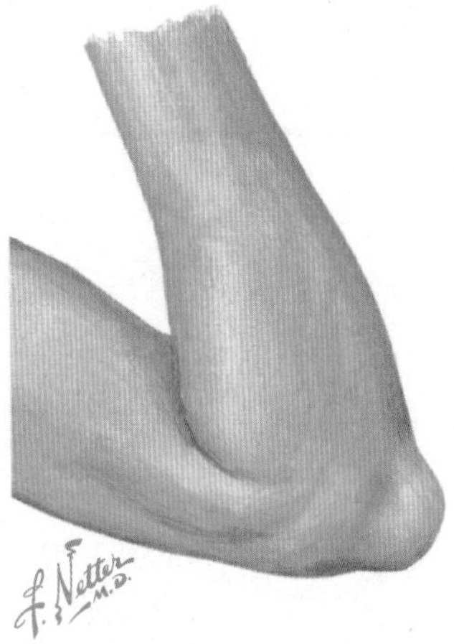
F. Netter M.D.

Figure 50.3 Olecranon bursitis (student's elbow).

MEDIAL ELBOW INJURIES

Medial Epicondylitis

Description: Also known as "golfer's elbow"; chronic symptomatic degeneration of the forearm common flexor tendons near the medial epicondyle from repetitive activities involving wrist flexion and pronation

Mechanism of injury: Repetitive eccentric loading of wrist flexors and forearm pronators. Potentially coexistent with valgus overload in overhead athletes; the common flexor tendon acts as a dynamic stabilizer of the elbow and eccentrically contracts during ball release. Peritendinous inflammation subsequently leads to angiofibroblastic hyperplasia, followed by tendon fibrosis, with potential tendon rupture and/or calcification within tendon.

Presentation: Insidious onset of medial elbow pain localized to medial epicondyle; may radiate to proximal forearm. Ten percent of tendinopathies about the elbow; pain with flexion of the wrist, including grip; dominant arm (75%), age 30–50 years, common in sports requiring repetitive wrist flexion (golf, weightlifting, baseball, racquet sports); exacerbated during swinging or late cocking/early acceleration phase of throwing. Twenty percent with concurrent ulnar neuropathy.

Physical examination: Usually normal ROM; pain approximately 5–10 mm distal and volar to medial epicondyle with occasional soft tissue swelling; symptoms exacerbated with resisted wrist flexion and forearm pronation in elbow extension; grip strength may be decreased compared with the contralateral side. Examine for concurrent pathology (i.e., ulnar neuritis, valgus instability).

Differential diagnosis: UCL injury, flexor–pronator strain/tear, ulnar neuritis, cubital tunnel syndrome, pronator teres rupture, cervical radiculopathy

Diagnostics: Primarily a clinical diagnosis. MRI and ultrasound do not necessarily correlate with symptoms.
- **Radiographs:** Typically normal but may demonstrate calcification of common flexor tendon
- **MRI:** Identify pathologic changes in common flexor tendon, pronator teres, or UCL
- **Ultrasound:** Demonstrates tendinopathy

Treatment:
- Nonsurgical: Activity modification, NSAIDs, physical therapy with focus on eccentric stretching and strengthening, bracing to off-load tendon; corticosteroid or platelet-rich plasma injection if symptoms persist (with caution, as multiple injections may weaken tendon); address athletic form/mechanics
- Surgery: Rare and only in refractory cases: open tendon debridement and repair; address concurrent pathology

Prognosis and return to sport: Nonsurgical treatment is successful in approximately 90% of cases (6- to 12-week course). Among surgical cases using various approaches, 80% of patients return to full activity by 6 months.

Ulnar Collateral Ligament Injury

Description: Partial or complete tears of the UCL (Fig. 50.4)

Mechanism of injury: Repetitive valgus stress (pitching, throwing, or racket sports) causes tensile loading of the UCL, resulting in ligament attenuation or tears. The anterior band of the anterior ligament is the strongest, most important stabilizer.

Presentation: Typically, insidious medial elbow pain in late cocking/early acceleration phases of throwing; occasionally acute/traumatic. Often asymptomatic at rest; throwing athletes often report decrease in velocity and accuracy. Pain returns when throwing exceeds approximately 75% of normal velocity. Patients with acute ruptures may describe acute pop. May have associated ulnar neuritis symptoms, flexor-pronator muscle/tendon strain, and valgus extension overload symptoms.

Physical examination:

- Tenderness along the ligament from the medial epicondyle (posterior to the common flexor tendon origin) to the sublime tubercle of the ulna

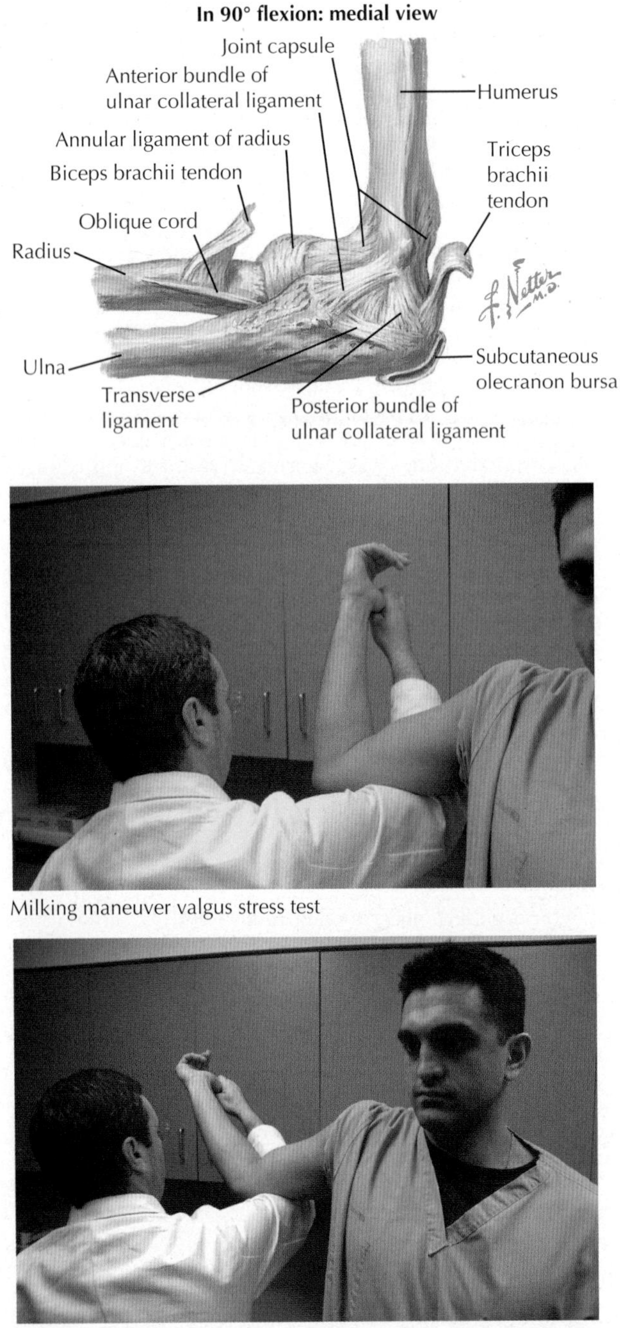
In 90° flexion: medial view
Joint capsule
Anterior bundle of ulnar collateral ligament
Humerus
Annular ligament of radius
Biceps brachii tendon
Triceps brachii tendon
Oblique cord
Radius
Ulna
Subcutaneous olecranon bursa
Transverse ligament
Posterior bundle of ulnar collateral ligament

Milking maneuver valgus stress test

Moving valgus stress test

Figure 50.4 Ulnar collateral ligament sprain.

- Moving valgus stress test from 30 degrees of flexion (testing the anterior band) to 90 degrees of flexion (entire UCL): Abduct shoulder to 90 degrees in maximal external rotation with full flexion and valgus stress applied to the elbow, then quickly extending the elbow to 30 degrees
- Milking maneuver: Abduct shoulder to 90 degrees, flex elbow to 90 degrees, and supinate forearm while pulling the patient's thumb posteriorly to apply valgus load
- Valgus extension overload test: Passive snapping of elbow into extension while maintaining valgus stress, indicates symptomatic posteromedial olecranon osteophyte (see Fig. 50.4)
- Note presence or absence (15% of population) of palmaris longus for possible reconstruction

Differential diagnosis: Ulnar neuritis, medial epicondylitis, flexor–pronator tendon rupture/strain, valgus extension overload

Diagnostics:

- **Radiographs:** May demonstrate acute, bony, proximal UCL avulsions or chronic traction spurs/calcifications in UCL or posteromedial olecranon osteophytes; comparative bilateral valgus stress radiographs may demonstrate medial gapping
- **Ultrasound:** Dynamic, may delineate UCL integrity and joint laxity
- **MRA:** Modality of choice to assess the extent of UCL damage and to identify concurrent elbow pathology; evaluate for attenuation of ligament, avulsion, rupture, or distal "T-sign"

Treatment:

- Nonsurgical: Partial or proximal tears; throwing cessation and physical therapy focused on appropriate throwing mechanics, shoulder ROM, and core strengthening, followed by a graduated, supervised throwing program
- Surgical: UCL reconstruction for complete ruptures in throwing athletes or partial ruptures in high-level athletes; typically use palmaris or gracilis autograft; concurrent treatment of additional elbow pathology; potential role for ligament repair in certain tear patterns

Prognosis and return to sport: Variable outcomes with nonsurgical management; proximal and partial tears have better nonoperative prognosis than distal tears. Typically, a season-ending injury; nonoperative treatment typically 3 months or longer. Return to competitive throwing after reconstruction usually 12–16 months after surgery with approximately 80%–90% returning to preinjury level of competition.

Medial Epicondyle Stress Lesions

Description: Also known as "little leaguer's elbow"; medial epicondyle apophyseal edema, fragmentation, separation, or avulsion

Mechanism of injury: Skeletally immature throwing athletes experience repetitive high-tensile stress on the medial epicondyle apophysis from flexor–pronator and UCL strain. Occurs at the physis because it is the weakest link in skeletally immature patients; UCL tears less likely. Correlated with excessive number of pitches; acute trauma is less common.

Presentation: Medial elbow pain with throwing, loss of throwing velocity and accuracy

Physical examination: Tenderness at medial epicondyle; pain with valgus stress test without instability

Differential diagnosis: UCL injury, ulnar neuritis, medial epicondyle fracture, flexor–pronator strain

Diagnostics:

- **Radiographs:** Bilateral, the injured side may demonstrate apophyseal widening, fragmentation, or avulsion with displacement
- **MRI:** May show edema at the apophysis

Treatment:

- Nonsurgical: Physeal widening and minimally displaced fractures (<0.5 cm) are managed with brief immobilization (1–3 weeks), followed by ROM protecting against valgus force and resisted flexion/pronation until symptoms resolve; avoid throwing for 3 months followed by progressive throwing program with focus on appropriate mechanics
- Surgical: Fixation of significantly displaced fractures (>0.5–1 cm) and fragments incarcerated in the joint

Prognosis and return to sport: Full recovery generally achieved at 4–6 months; recurrence is possible, particularly with poor throwing mechanics.

Ulnar Nerve Compression (Cubital Tunnel) Syndrome

Description: Symptomatic dysfunction of the ulnar nerve at the level of the elbow because of compression, traction, and friction

Mechanism of injury: May be incited by trauma, repetitive elbow flexion (traction), cubitus valgus deformity, or subluxation of the ulnar nerve at the medial epicondyle; nerve most commonly compressed at flexor carpi ulnaris (FCU) aponeurosis (also arcade of Struthers, Osborne ligament/medial collateral ligament [MCL]); associated with medial epicondylitis; also seen in weightlifters concentrating on triceps strengthening.

Presentation: Insidious onset of medial elbow and forearm pain with paresthesias of the ring and small fingers, possible grip weakness; ROM normal; often awakens patient at night, as elbow is frequently flexed while sleeping, thereby increasing traction on the nerve.

Physical examination: Two-point discrimination diminished in small finger and ulnar aspect of ring finger: positive Tinel sign over cubital tunnel; positive ulnar nerve compression test; subluxation of the ulnar nerve with elbow flexion. Weakness of grip, small finger flexor digitorum profundus (FDP) flexion, interossei (Wartenberg sign: abducted small finger), and adductor pollicis (Froment sign: weak pinch); chronic claw-hand deformity may develop.

Differential diagnosis: Cervical radiculopathy, thoracic outlet syndrome, ulnar nerve compression at the wrist (Guyon canal: sensory disturbance on dorsal ulnar hand in distribution of dorsal cutaneous branch), UCL injury, medial epicondylitis (often comorbid)

Diagnostics: Primarily a clinical diagnosis.

- **EMG–NCS:** May show slowing of conduction velocity across the elbow
- **Radiographs:** Usually normal but may have osteophyte or cubitus valgus deformity

Treatment:

- Nonsurgical: NSAIDs, modification of training (avoid triceps strengthening exercises), nighttime extension splinting, elbow pads, and avoidance of direct medial elbow pressure; 50% effective
- Surgical: Decompression of the cubital tunnel with or without nerve transposition (subcutaneous, submuscular, or intramuscular); in situ decompression equivalent outcomes to transposition, has lower complication rate but higher revision rate

Prognosis and return to sport: Dependent on severity and chronicity of neuropathy; if nonsurgically treated, may return to sport based on symptoms; if surgically treated, may return to full activity at approximately 4–6 weeks.

LATERAL ELBOW INJURIES

Lateral Epicondylitis

Description: Also known as "tennis elbow"; chronic symptomatic degeneration of the forearm common extensor tendons near the lateral epicondyle; most commonly affecting the extensor carpi radialis brevis (ECRB) tendon (Fig. 50.5)

Mechanism of injury: Excessive stress or repetitive contraction of wrist extensors leads to extensor tendon degeneration followed by angiofibroblastic hyperplasia; late-stage disease may lead to partial or complete rupture and/or calcification within the tendon

Presentation: Pain with repetitive movements requiring resisted wrist extension or gripping; increased risk with racket sports, dominant arm, age 35–55 years

Physical examination: Tenderness to palpation over the lateral epicondyle and extensor tendons; pain with resisted wrist and long-finger extension with the forearm in pronation; pain with resisted supination; diminished grip strength; chair test: pain with lifting chair with forearm pronated (see Fig. 50.5)

Differential diagnosis: Posterior interosseous branch of the radial nerve (posterior interosseous nerve [PIN]) entrapment (radial tunnel syndrome, concurrent in 5%–10%), radiocapitellar arthrosis, osteochondritis dissecans, cervical radiculopathy

Diagnostics: Primarily a clinical diagnosis. MRI and ultrasound do not necessarily correlate with symptoms.

- **Radiographs:** Usually normal (may demonstrate calcific changes within the tendon), rule out radiocapitellar arthrosis
- **MRI:** May show inflammation of the ECRB or define the extent of tendon tearing
- **Ultrasound:** May identify structural changes in affected tendons

Treatment:

- Nonsurgical: Activity modification, NSAIDs, physical therapy with focus on eccentric stretching and strengthening; address athletic form/mechanics; counterforce bracing or wrist brace (limiting wrist extension) to off-load tendon; corticosteroid or platelet-rich plasma injection if symptoms persist (with caution, as multiple injections may weaken the tendon); ultrasound-guided percutaneous debridement appears to be effective
- Surgical: Only for refractory cases, typically with extensive (>50%) tendon rupture: open or arthroscopic release of the common extensor origin followed by debridement and repair

Prognosis and return to sport: Nonsurgical treatment is successful in approximately 90% of cases (6- to 12-week course). In surgical cases, 85%–90% patients return to full activity by 6 months.

Osteochondritis Dissecans (OCD) of the Capitellum

Description: Localized capitellar lesion involving the articular cartilage and subchondral bone (Fig. 50.6)

Mechanism of injury: Repetitive microtrauma to capitellum from high valgus stresses leads to osteochondral injury; if the overlying cartilage is stable, the underlying subchondral defect may heal; unstable lesions may lead to separation, fragmentation, and loose body formation

Presentation: Insidious onset of activity-related lateral elbow pain in adolescents/young adults (age 11–21 years); consider Panner disease in patients aged ≤10 years; more common in throwing sports (dominant arm) and gymnastics (possibly bilateral). Pain resolves with rest during the earlier stages of disease. Pain with activities of daily living, mechanical symptoms, and stiffness occur in later stages.

Physical examination: Swelling and tenderness over radiocapitellar joint; occasional loss of terminal extension; positive radiocapitellar compression test with pronation and supination and axial load with elbow in extension; crepitus and mechanical symptoms with ROM suggest loose body

Differential diagnosis: Panner osteochondrosis, radiocapitellar chondrosis, lateral epicondylitis

Diagnostics:

- **Radiographs:** Radiolucency of the capitellum, with flattening of the articular surface, possible sclerotic rim; possible fragmentation or loose body; obtain contralateral comparison, 45-degree flexion, and oblique views

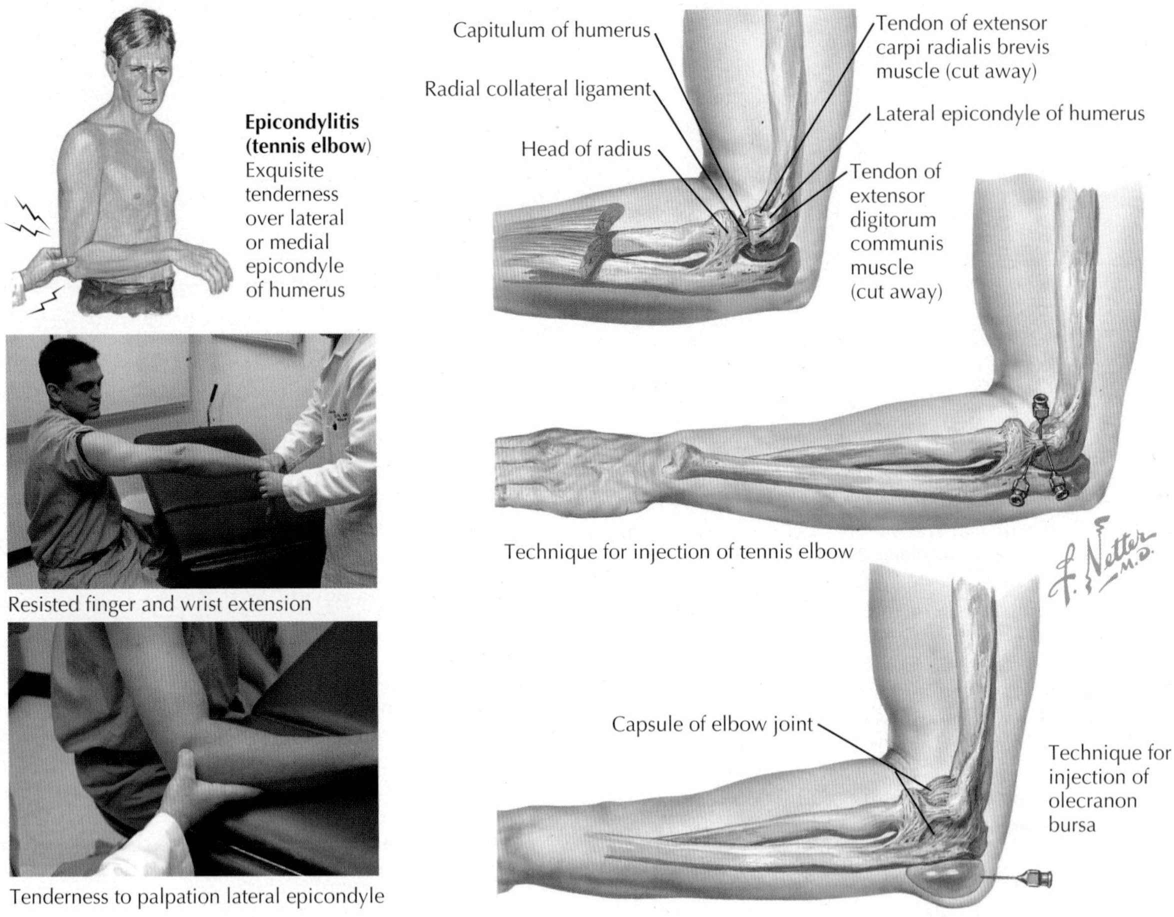
Epicondylitis (tennis elbow) Exquisite tenderness over lateral or medial epicondyle of humerus
Resisted finger and wrist extension
Tenderness to palpation lateral epicondyle
Capitulum of humerus
Radial collateral ligament
Head of radius
Tendon of extensor carpi radialis brevis muscle (cut away)
Lateral epicondyle of humerus
Tendon of extensor digitorum communis muscle (cut away)
Technique for injection of tennis elbow
Capsule of elbow joint
Technique for injection of olecranon bursa

Figure 50.5 Tennis elbow.

- **MRI:** Best for assessing extent of chondral damage; early low-signal changes on T1 images; T2 images helpful in visualizing intervening fluid in lesion consistent with fragment separation

Treatment:

- Nonsurgical: Stable lesions: intact articular cartilage; rest with activity restriction, physical therapy, and gradual return to activities in 3–6 months; follow with serial radiographs
- Surgical: Failed conservative treatment or unstable lesion; stable lesions: drilling (antegrade or retrograde); unstable lesions: fragment fixation if possible; arthroscopic loose body removal, debridement, microfracture if fragment cannot be salvaged; possible open osteochondral autograft/allograft for large lesions (>1 cm^2) or lesions violating the lateral column of the capitellum

Prognosis and return to sport: Early diagnosis and treatment are essential. For early lesions, athletes will miss remainder of the season, but long-term results are consistently good; for high-grade, unstable lesions, disability widely varies, with return to preinjury level less likely, though long-term functional results are generally good. Occasional loss of terminal extension and mild pain with activities of daily living; up to 50% may develop arthritic changes.

Posterior Interosseous Nerve Compression Syndrome

Description: Also known as "radial tunnel syndrome"; compressive neuropathy of the PIN causing pain without motor or sensory dysfunction

Mechanism of injury: Compression of the PIN within one or multiple of the following locations: fibrous bands volar to radiocapitellar joint, radial recurrent vessels, medial edge of ECRB, arcade of Frohse (most common), or distal aspect of the supinator

Presentation: Aching lateral elbow pain radiating from the lateral epicondyle into dorsoradial forearm; aggravated by pronation–supination activities and lifting objects; extensor weakness of the wrist and fingers secondary to pain

Physical examination: Tenderness to palpation over supinator arch (approximately 4 cm distal to lateral epicondyle); may have positive Tinel sign along course of PIN; pain with resisted long-finger extension, with resisted wrist extension and supination, and with passive pronation in wrist flexion (passive stretch of supinator).

Differential diagnosis: Lateral epicondylitis, cervical radiculopathy, extensor tendon rupture, distal PIN syndrome (wrist)

Diagnostics: Primarily a clinical diagnosis.

- **Radiographs:** Osteophyte at radiocapitellar joint (rare)
- **MRI:** May demonstrate atrophy of supinator/extensors (prolonged denervation), may help identify sites of compression or rule out other pathology
- Diagnostic injection of local anesthetic into radial tunnel

Treatment:

- Nonsurgical: Activity modification avoiding prolonged elbow extension with forearm pronation and wrist flexion, temporary dorsiflexion wrist splint, physical therapy for stretching, strengthening and nerve glides; corticosteroid injection in radial tunnel
- Surgery: Radial tunnel decompression in recalcitrant cases

Prognosis and return to sport: Nonsurgical management usually successful (80%); full return to sports usually by 4–8 weeks; surgical release also highly effective (80%); return to sport 6–8 weeks.

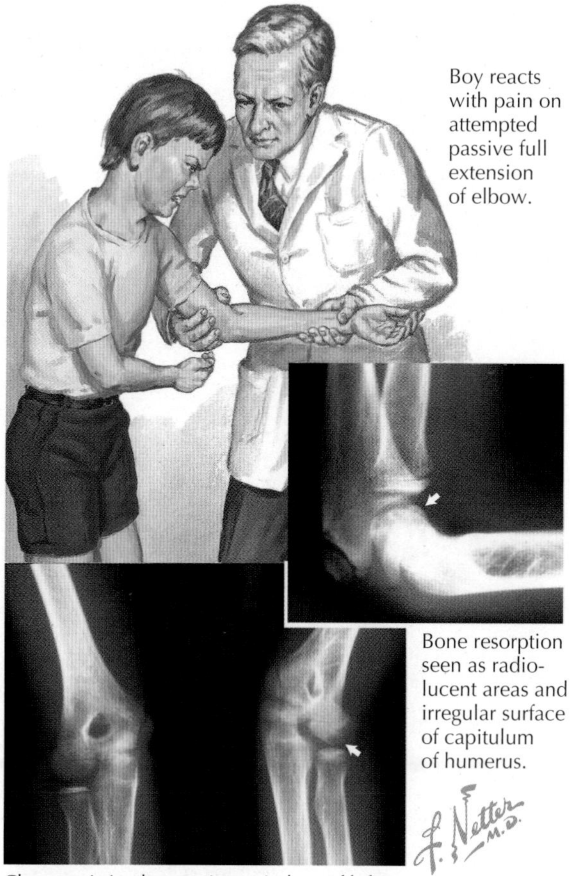
Boy reacts with pain on attempted passive full extension of elbow.
Bone resorption seen as radiolucent areas and irregular surface of capitulum of humerus.
Characteristic changes in capitulum of left humerus *(arrow)* compared with normal right elbow.

Figure 50.6 Osteochondritis dissecans capitellum.

Fractures and Dislocations

Description: Fracture of the radius, ulna, or humerus, with or without dislocation or subluxation of the elbow joint (Fig. 50.7)
Mechanism: Usually a fall onto outstretched arm or onto the olecranon; may be associated with high-energy trauma
Presentation: History of acute trauma; severe pain, exacerbated by subtle movement; possible instability
Physical examination: Tenderness, deformity, swelling, and ecchymosis; limited and severely painful motion and crepitus; possible neurologic or vascular compromise; and varus/valgus instability
Differential diagnosis: Associated ligamentous injury
Diagnostics:

- **Radiographs:** Fractures of radial head or neck, olecranon or coronoid, and distal humerus; dislocation with or without fracture; *Monteggia fracture:* proximal ulnar fracture with associated radial head dislocation, traction-view radiograph of elbow to delineate fracture pattern; *supracondylar humerus fracture:* intra-articular swelling ("sail sign") may indicate an occult fracture, particularly in children
- **CT:** Assess fracture pattern and degree of comminution
- **MRI:** Assess ligamentous or chondral damage after acute fracture care

Treatment: Document neurovascular examination; if compromised, then prompt reduction is indicated; temporarily immobilize with a splint; refer urgently for evaluation and further treatment as indicated (closed reduction, open reduction and internal fixation, and staged ligamentous repair)
Prognosis and return to sport: Usually a season-ending injury; simple dislocations usually have good outcomes with early ROM; return to preinjury level of sports less likely after complex fractures/dislocations; stiffness is common after elbow injuries; therefore, early ROM is important if stable (nondisplaced radial head/neck fractures)

Posterolateral Rotatory Instability (PLRI)

Description: Disruption of the lateral ligamentous complex leading to instability of the radiocapitellar and ulnohumeral joint
Mechanism: Injury often from a fall onto an outstretched arm with axial load and forearm supination resulting in posterolateral dislocation or subluxation; injury to the lateral ligament complex results; may also be iatrogenic from lateral elbow surgery

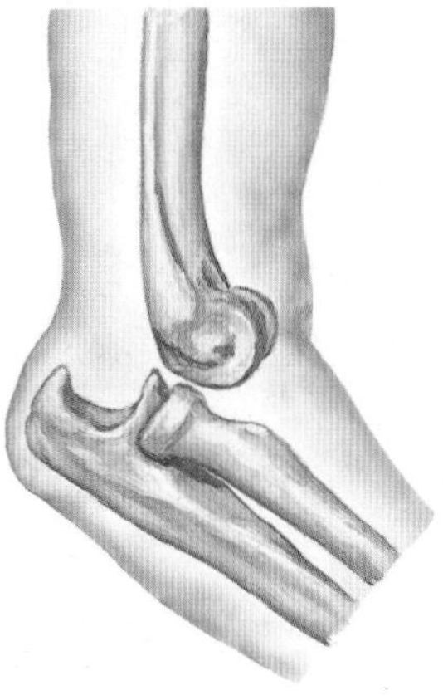
Posterior dislocation. Note prominence of olecranon posteriorly and distal humerus anteriorly.

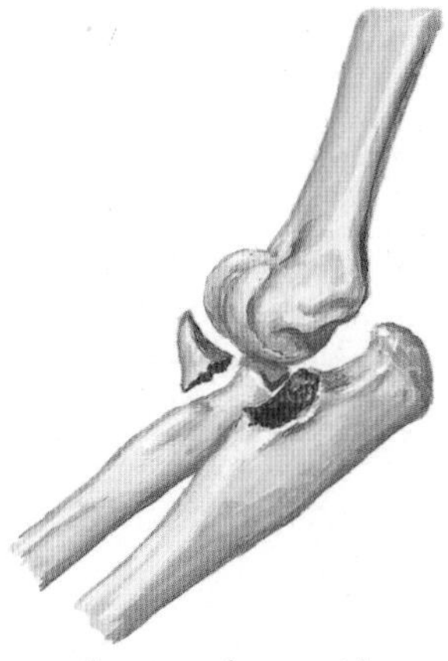
Fracture of coronoid process of ulna with posterior dislocation of elbow. Coronoid fracture may occur occasionally without dislocation.

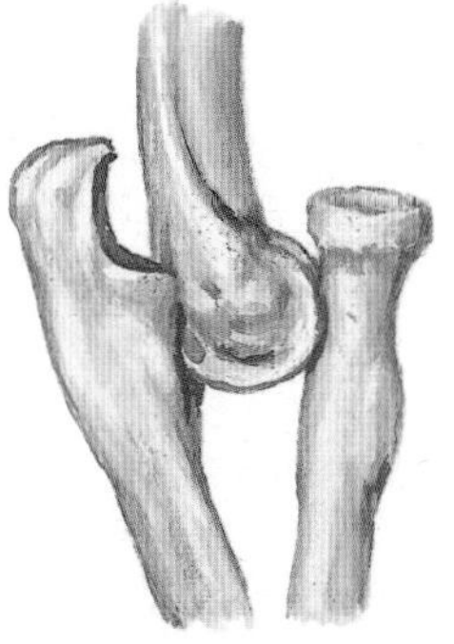
Divergent dislocation, anterior-posterior type (rare). Medial-lateral type may also occur (extremely rare).

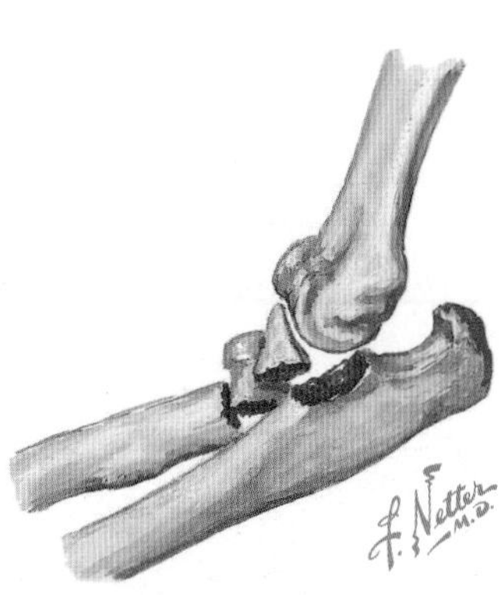
Posterior dislocation with fracture of both coronoid process and radial head. Rare but serious; poor outcome even with good treatment. May require total elbow replacement.

Figure 50.7 Dislocations of the elbow.

Presentation: Lateral elbow pain; feeling of instability with axial load and forearm supination (pushing out of a chair); instability may manifest as a mechanical catch or pop with elbow extension

Physical examination: Tenderness, deformity, swelling, and ecchymosis acutely; may have varus laxity

- Apprehension/lateral pivot shift test: Apprehension or visible shifting of the elbow with valgus stress while moving the elbow from flexion to extension
- Chair-rise test: Pain or instability reproduced as patient tries to push themselves out of a chair with their hands.

Differential diagnosis: Loose body, fracture, lateral epicondylitis, synovial plica

Diagnostics:

- **Radiographs:** Rule out fracture; lateral radiograph is critical to evaluate for posterior radial head subluxation with the elbow extended and the forearm in supination; AP radiograph to evaluate for lateral ulnohumeral gapping
- **MRI:** After acute injury if the elbow is grossly unstable or if there is concern for osteochondral injury

Treatment:

- Nonsurgical: Acutely, if radiographs stable, splint in pronation for 2 weeks at 90 degrees; start early motion with the forearm in pronation; allow supination with elbow flexion above 90 degrees; after 6 weeks, allow supination in extension if the radiocapitellar articulation remains concentric.
- Surgical: Early repair indicated for an acute, unstable injury; lateral ligament reconstruction for chronic PLRI or failure of nonsurgical treatment.

Prognosis and return to sport: Usually a season-ending injury; 4–6 months for return depending on the sport

RECOMMENDED READINGS

Available online.

HAND AND WRIST INJURIES 51

Jeffry T. Watson

GENERAL PRINCIPLES

Overview

- Fortunately, most sports-related hand and wrist injuries, when addressed in a timely manner, do not represent a significant threat to limb viability, long-term function, or eventual return to sports.
- Perhaps the greatest morbidity from these injuries results from delayed presentations or missed injuries, a common feature in athletes motivated to compete.
- Hand function is closely linked to full flexion of the ulnar three digits (for power grip), prehension grip in the radial three digits (fine manipulation), and a stable, mobile wrist.
- Do not minimize or underestimate subtle losses of finger flexion after open or closed potential injuries to the flexor mechanism. Delayed diagnosis and treatment of jersey fingers or flexor tendon disruption invites significant morbidity and limits treatment options.
- Return to play (RTP) for hand injuries, as with other musculoskeletal conditions, will be influenced by level of participation (amateur vs. professional), sport/position, and tissue-specific healing requirements. As a general trend, we are apprehensive about power grip/contact sports (i.e., football/rugby) with K-wires in place, especially those crossing a joint.

Physical Examination

- Dictated by the context of the injury. No single, comprehensive evaluation applies to all maladies.
- Attention is directed toward the individual part and system (bone, joint, tendon, nerve, etc.) in question.

Observation/Inspection

- Focal swelling, digital perfusion, digital malrotation, digital cascade, and any penetrating injury must be noted.
- Any difference in posture of one digit relative to the others should not be dismissed or minimized, as this often signifies a displaced fracture, tendon disruption, or joint subluxation.
- In the absence of a penetrating injury, isolated pallor of a digit usually represents spasm of the digital vessels. Although this often resolves with digital warming or reduction of associated displaced fractures or dislocations, digital viability remains in question until perfusion is actually observed.
- Even in closed fractures, the digital vessels can tear or thrombose, representing a surgical emergency.
- Dorsal swelling of the hand is a nonspecific finding and may not represent a significant injury.

Palpation

- Careful palpation of specific bones or ligaments in question is FUNDAMENTAL to hand/wrist assessment. There are not many "referred-pain" injuries in the hand or wrist—tenderness to palpation does not lie.
- Focused palpation will usually localize the injured structure within an area of generalized edema demonstrating diffuse swelling; for example, a swollen wrist after distal radius fracture or perilunate injury.
- Focal tenderness over the scaphoid or scapholunate ligament, even in the setting of normal radiographs, suggests an underlying ligament tear or fracture with poor prognosis if not recognized and treated.

SPECIFIC INJURIES AND CONDITIONS

Nail Bed Injury

Description: Any tear or disruption of the sterile or germinal matrix of the nail bed; may or may not be associated with an underlying distal phalanx fracture or actual disruption of the nail plate (Fig. 51.1). Associated distal phalangeal fractures, particularly of the midshaft, may be open and require aggressive debridement/washout.

Mechanism of injury: Usually caused by dorsal crush of the fingertip (such as when the fingertip is crushed by another player's cleated shoe); however, may also occur with axial load to the fingertip that results in flexion fracture of the distal phalangeal shaft and tear of the overlying nail bed.

Presentation: If the nail bed is disrupted, subungual hematoma results. The tear may extend peripherally beyond the borders of the nail fold into the surrounding skin (see Fig. 51.1).

Physical examination: Gross instability of the fingertip with nail bed injury is suggestive of a concomitant distal phalangeal shaft fracture.

Differential diagnosis: If the base of the nail plate is flipped out dorsally over the nail fold, consider an open fracture of the proximal portion of the phalanx. In skeletally immature patients, the presence of the physis at this location may result in failure to recognize what is, in fact, a Seymour (open Salter–Harris I distal phalangeal) fracture.

Diagnostics: Physical examination is usually sufficient. Anteroposterior (AP) and lateral radiographs reveal an underlying distal phalanx fracture.

Treatment: For a small subungual hematoma encompassing a portion of the nail plate, no intervention is necessary. Decompression of the hematoma through needle fenestration of the nail plate can offer pain relief; however, this may increase the likelihood of wound sepsis if performed on a playing field (see Fig. 51.1). For **larger hematomas** (50% of the nail plate) with tearing beyond the nail fold borders, formal repair is recommended. Under a digital block anesthetic and digital tourniquet the nail plate should be removed, the wound irrigated, and the nail matrix repaired with either a topical skin adhesive or a 7-0 resorbable suture. The adjacent skin rip is repaired with a 5-0 nylon suture. An underlying phalangeal tuft fracture is nonsurgically managed. However, an associated unstable distal phalangeal shaft fracture requires washout and pin stabilization, usually crossing the distal interphalangeal (DIP) joint.

Prognosis and RTP: If no nail bed repair is required, immediate RTP is alright. After nail bed repair, the fingertip (including DIP joint) should be dressed and splinted to protect from impact. If there is an associated unstable phalangeal shaft fracture requiring pin fixation, RTP should be delayed until pin removal in gripping sports. Prognosis for nail plate growth is directly related to anatomic restoration of the nail bed. If there is a wide scar in the matrix, a ridge or split in the nail plate will occur. Open fractures through the nail bed require urgent surgical debridement in the operating room. Displaced distal phalangeal shaft fractures are often unstable and require pinning.

Mallet Finger

Description: Loss of terminal extensor mechanism attachment to the distal phalanx with resultant flexion deformity of the DIP joint

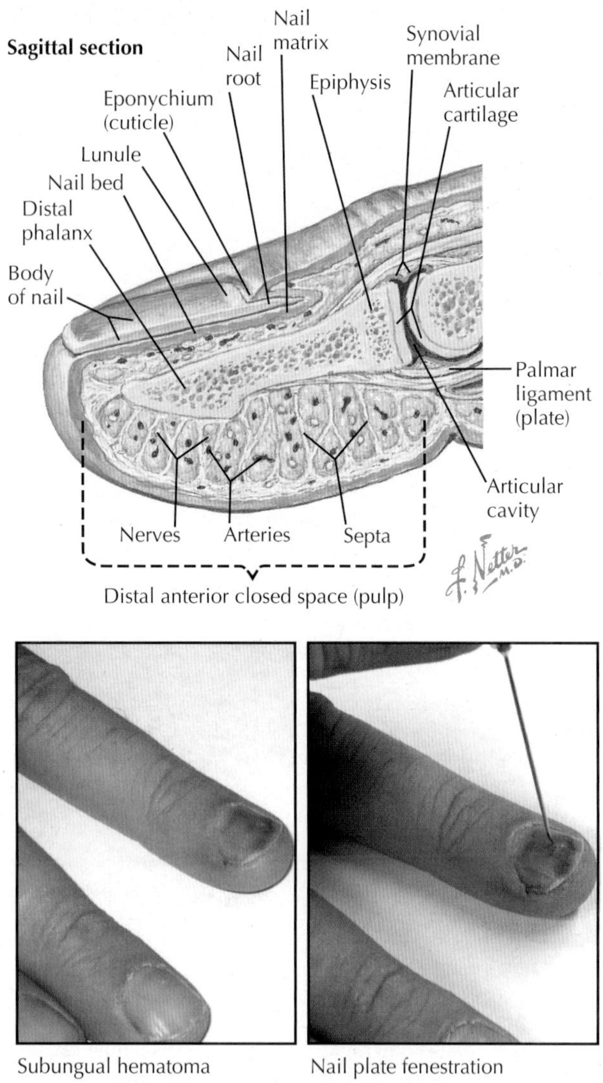
Sagittal section
Nail matrix
Nail root
Synovial membrane
Epiphysis
Articular cartilage
Eponychium (cuticle)
Lunule
Nail bed
Distal phalanx
Body of nail
Palmar ligament (plate)
Articular cavity
Nerves
Arteries
Septa
Distal anterior closed space (pulp)
Subungual hematoma
Nail plate fenestration

Figure 51.1 Nail bed injury.

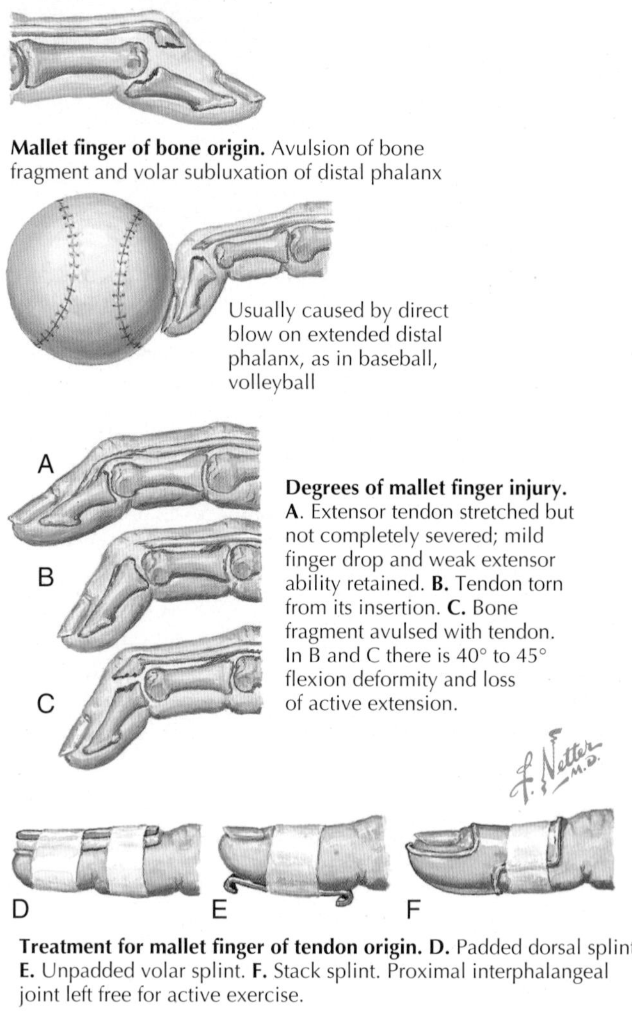
Mallet finger of bone origin. Avulsion of bone fragment and volar subluxation of distal phalanx
Usually caused by direct blow on extended distal phalanx, as in baseball, volleyball
A
B
C
Degrees of mallet finger injury. **A.** Extensor tendon stretched but not completely severed; mild finger drop and weak extensor ability retained. **B.** Tendon torn from its insertion. **C.** Bone fragment avulsed with tendon. In B and C there is 40° to 45° flexion deformity and loss of active extension.
D
E
F
Treatment for mallet finger of tendon origin. D. Padded dorsal splint. **E.** Unpadded volar splint. **F.** Stack splint. Proximal interphalangeal joint left free for active exercise.

Figure 51.2 Mallet finger.

Mechanism of injury: Sudden forced flexion of the DIP joint during active extension through the terminal tendon, often as a result of a ball jamming the fingertip (Fig. 51.2)

Presentation: The DIP joint is maintained in flexion with an inability to actively bring the joint into full extension. Varying degrees of pain, often with minimal or no pain; swelling or ecchymosis may be noted over the dorsal aspect of the joint.

Differential diagnosis: Distal phalanx fracture or DIP dislocation

Diagnostics: Posteroanterior (PA) and lateral radiographs of a digit to assess if injury is limited to the soft tissue (tendon only) or has associated bony avulsion (see Fig. 51.2). Lateral radiographs determine stability based on the size of the bony component and whether palmar subluxation is present.

Treatment: Acute mallet injuries with no subluxation on the lateral radiographs require *full-time* splinting of the DIP joint in extension for 6–8 weeks (see Fig. 51.2). Displaced bony components with joint involvement of >30% and/or palmar subluxation often require surgery to restore joint congruity. The DIP joint will usually require transarticular pinning in full extension with surgery. Primary surgical repair of acute, closed, soft tissue mallet injuries has not proven to be superior and may have more significant complications.

Prognosis and RTP: Noncompliance with splint wear will negatively affect the outcome and usually results in mild-to-moderate degrees of extension lag. The functional effect of this is variable. Most athletes nonsurgically treated will RTP within a week (while splinted). With surgical treatment, RTP will depend on the athlete's ability to protect a transarticular pin. Any activity requiring grip is likely to result in bending or breakage of the pin.

Most patients will have some degree of extensor lag, even with full compliance, and should be advised of this. If lag is excessive and interferes with function, revision surgical options may be considered.

Jersey Finger

Description: Traumatic avulsion of the flexor digitorum profundus (FDP) from the distal phalanx (Fig. 51.3); the tendon may detach alone or avulse a palmar fragment of the distal phalanx; ring finger is most commonly affected

Mechanism of injury: Forced passive extension of DIP joint during active flexion of DIP joint

Presentation: Typically seen in football and rugby players attempting to grab a jersey; variable degree of pain, although the player may complain of pain proximally in the finger or palm at the level of the retracted tendon. Usual concern is inability to flex the involved DIP joint. Unfortunately, many are delayed presentations.

Physical examination: Ecchymosis may be present at DIP joint, depending on timing of presentation. The flexor tendon stump may be tender or palpable in the palm or along the digit,

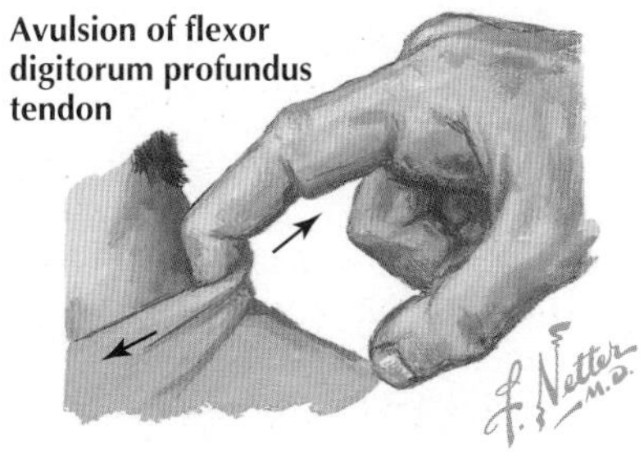
Avulsion of flexor
digitorum profundus
tendon

Caused by violent traction on flexed distal phalanx, as in catching on jersey of running football player

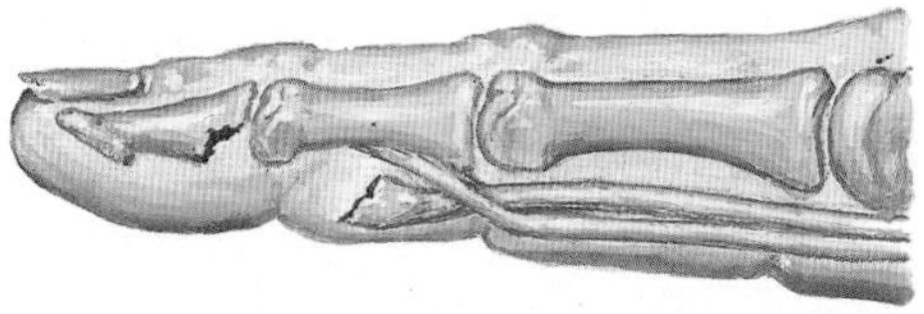

Flexor digitorum profundus tendon may be torn directly from distal phalanx or may avulse small or large bone fragment. Tendon usually retracts to about level of proximal interphalangeal joint, where it is stopped at its passage through flexor digitorum superficialis tendon; occasionally, it retracts into palm. Early open repair of tendon and its torn fibrous sheath indicated.

Figure 51.3 Jersey finger.

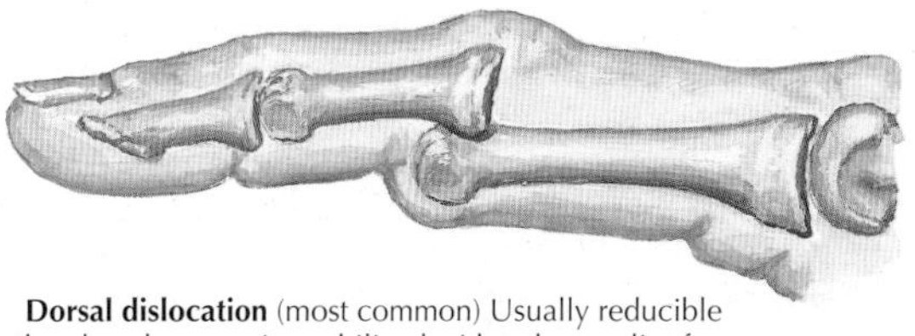

Dorsal dislocation (most common) Usually reducible by closed means, immobilized with palmar splint for 3 weeks, then active range-of-motion exercises begun

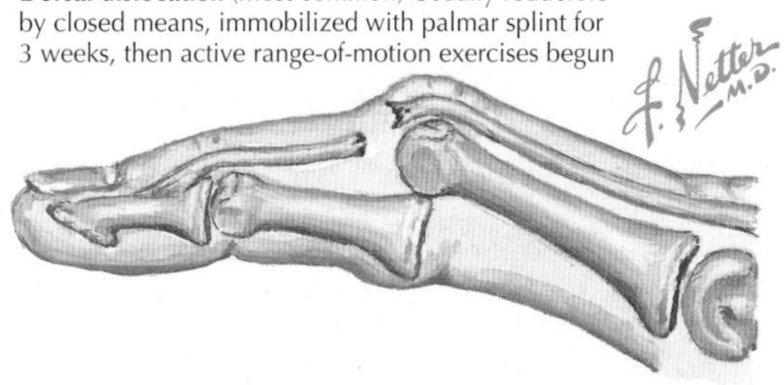

Palmar dislocation (uncommon) Causes boutonniere deformity. Central slip of extensor tendon often torn, requiring open fixation, followed by dorsal splinting to allow passive and active exercises of distal interphalangeal joint

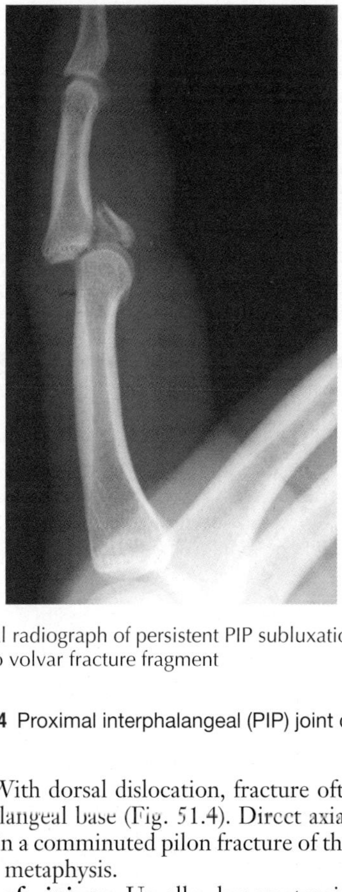

Lateral radiograph of persistent PIP subluxation due to volvar fracture fragment

Figure 51.4 Proximal interphalangeal (PIP) joint dislocation.

depending on the level of proximal retraction. Bony avulsions tend to become incarcerated along the flexor sheath (often at the A4 pulley over the middle phalanx). *Loss of active DIP joint flexion* is the most specific finding.

Differential diagnosis: Distal phalanx fracture and DIP joint dislocation

Diagnostics: PA and lateral radiographs of injured digit to check for bone avulsion fragment; ultrasound or magnetic resonance imaging (MRI) may identify a retracted tendon rupture.

Treatment: Surgical reattachment of the flexor tendon within 7–10 days if the tendon has retracted into the palm; if tendon has retracted only to the middle phalanx or proximal interphalangeal (PIP) level, reattachment may be successful with a delay of up to a few weeks. For flexor tendon avulsions with a bony component, internal fixation is necessary to restore continuity of the flexor tendon. DELAYED presentations outside of these time windows should be approached with caution. An excessively tight attempted primary repair will hinder function of the involved and surrounding digits with far greater morbidity than loss of active DIP flexion from the initial injury. Also, single- or two-staged grafting procedures in the setting of intact FDS function risks prolonged convalescence and scarring with potential loss of BOTH DIP and PIP function.

Prognosis and RTP: Soft tissue FDP avulsions require 12 weeks of protected activity before return to full gripping and grasping activities. Bony avulsions amenable to open reduction and internal fixation (ORIF) require at least 6 weeks of protected activity. Both types of FDP avulsions also require extensive hand therapy after surgery.

Proximal Interphalangeal Joint Dislocation and Fracture-Dislocation

Description: Usually, the middle phalanx displaces dorsally to the proximal phalanx. However, rotatory (with the proximal phalanx condyle protruding between the lateral band and central slip), volar, and lateral dislocations, though less frequent, do occur. With dorsal dislocation, fracture often occurs at the middle phalangeal base (Fig. 51.4). Direct axial load, however, may result in a comminuted pilon fracture of the entire articular surface and metaphysis.

Mechanism of injury: Usually, hyperextension of PIP joint with varying degrees of axial loading; often occurs from a ball, another participant, or ground jamming into the finger.

Presentation: Usually with pain and swelling around the PIP joint with or without angular deformity; patient will be apprehensive to active or passive motion

Physical examination: Pain localized to PIP joint with swelling; collateral ligaments will be tender because they are disrupted; occasionally will have skin laceration or a palmar skin tear

Differential diagnosis: Volar plate injury without dislocation; phalangeal, articular, or periarticular fracture

Diagnostics: PA and lateral radiographs of the injured digit *must* be performed to verify congruent reduction and rule out fracture or subluxation but can be delayed for a few days if "on the field"

reduction is clinically stable. If the initial reduction attempts seem unsuccessful, radiographs should be obtained before repeated efforts. Reduction may be impeded from a fracture component or different orientation of dislocation (see Fig. 51.4).

Treatment: Digital blocks with 1% lidocaine without epinephrine may be helpful. Closed reduction employing longitudinal traction, slight extension, and dorsal pressure over the middle phalanx for dorsal dislocations. After reduction, range of motion (ROM) and joint stability must be evaluated. **Radiographic or fluoroscopic confirmation of reduction is required within a few days.** Without a significant periarticular fracture, instability requiring surgery is unlikely. For **rotatory dislocation,** manipulation with the metacarpophalangeal (MCP) and PIP in flexed position facilitates reduction. **Volar dislocation** is reduced with slight PIP flexion and dorsal translation of the middle phalangeal base. After reduction of volar dislocation, it is *crucial* to protect the central extensor slip insertion (which generally is always disrupted in a volar dislocation; Fig. 51.5) with immobilization of PIP in full extension in order to avoid inevitable progression to boutonniere deformity. For **fracture-dislocations,** closed reduction with longitudinal traction and a subsequent dorsal blocking splint to hold the flexed PIP joint may be adequate, depending on the size of the fractured palmar joint margin. In general, if the fracture involves <40% of the articular surface, this technique is useful. The joint is gradually moved into greater degrees of extension with weekly radiographic verification of maintained reduction over the ensuing 4–6 weeks. Fractures with persistent dorsal subluxation after closed reduction require surgical stabilization.

Prognosis and RTP: RTP is usually minutes after closed reduction of dorsal dislocations. Buddy taping to adjacent digits or aluminum extension block splinting should suffice; **early follow-up radiographs are mandatory.** Athletes with stable reduction of dorsal dislocation without associated fracture can continue playing most sports, avoiding forced passive hyperextension for the initial 3 weeks. Volar dislocations need to be splinted in full extension for approximately 6 weeks to protect the central slip. During this time, active DIP motion is employed to promote gliding of lateral bands. Swelling and stiffness may persist for several months. Open surgical treatment of fracture-dislocations requires no forceful grip or impact for 4–6 weeks and usually results in some loss of PIP motion.

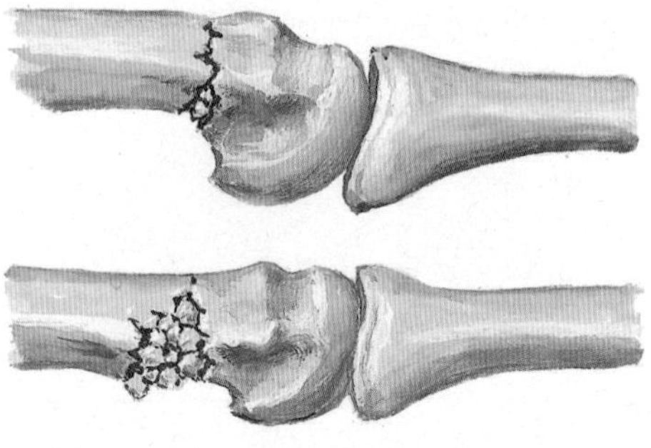

In fractures of metacarpal neck, volar cortex often comminuted, resulting in marked instability after reduction, which often necessitates pinning

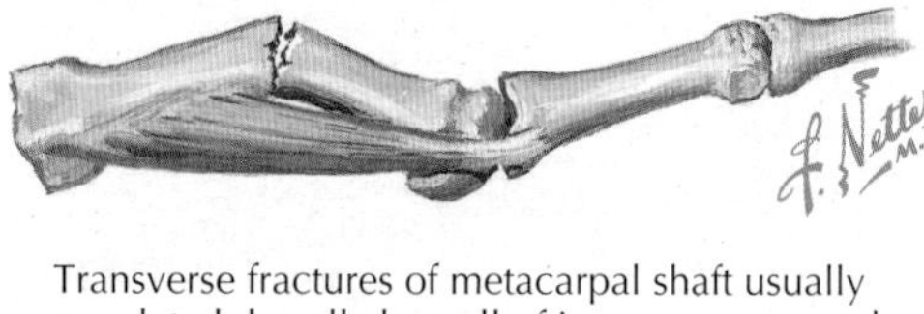

Transverse fractures of metacarpal shaft usually angulated dorsally by pull of interosseous muscles.

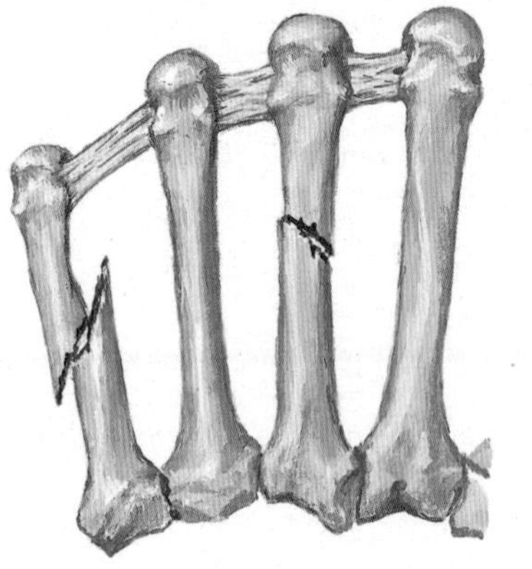

Oblique fractures tend to shorten and rotate metacarpal, particularly in index and little fingers because metacarpals of middle and ring fingers are stabilized by deep transverse metacarpal ligaments.

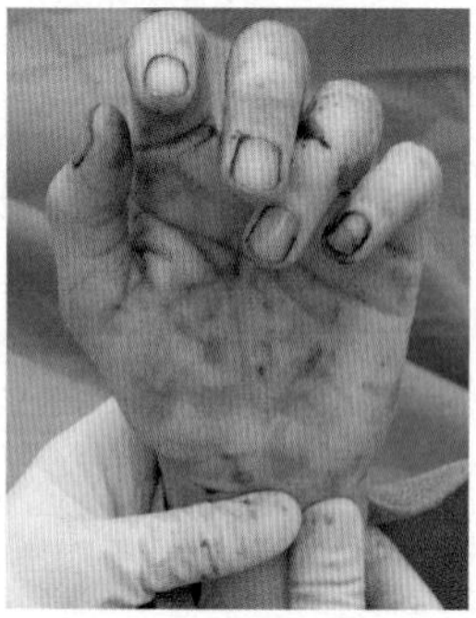

Clinical scissoring due to malrotation of 4th and 5th metacarpal fractures

Figure 51.5 Metacarpal fracture.

Metacarpal Fracture

Description: Fracture of metacarpal neck, shaft, or base. Perhaps the most common fracture in contact sports.

Mechanism of injury: Axial load or clenched fist impact are common mechanisms for distal or proximal metaphyseal fractures. Direct dorsal impact (such as a baseball striking a batter's hand or another participant stepping on the hand) often results in shaft fractures (see Fig. 51.5).

Presentation: Localized swelling, with or without angular deformity of digits

Physical examination: Point tender over metacarpal fracture with swelling; angular and sometimes rotational deformity (scissoring) of digits (see Fig. 51.5). Scissoring is more easily detected if patient is able to offer some degree of digital flexion.

Differential diagnosis: Contusion or MCP joint dislocation

Diagnostics: PA, lateral, and oblique radiographs of the hand

Treatment: Most can be treated nonoperatively, but fracture characteristics and level of athlete and position determine strategy. Generally, displaced intra-articular head or base fractures merit surgical treatment. For neck and shaft fractures, we can accept more angular deformity in the fourth and fifth metacarpals. Isolated second and fifth or multiple metacarpal shaft fractures lack surrounding ligamentous stabilizers and are prone to objectionable rotation deformity ("scissoring") when treated nonoperatively. If athlete can participate in sport with a rigid cast or splint for appropriate patterns or can sit out long enough to heal, nonoperative management may suffice using spanning wrist/hand splint for 3–4 weeks. Any reduction of metacarpal neck fractures is practically difficult to maintain using a splint or cast. Pinning often leads to joint stiffness; hence, most metacarpal neck fractures are allowed to heal with some flexion deformity as long as there is no clinically significant rotational component or associated loss of PIP flexion.

Intramedullary screw fixation has become useful for problematic transverse or very short oblique neck or shaft fractures in skeletally mature (closed physes) athletes. This technique requires less dissection, smaller exposure, and less potential need for hardware removal than plating. Also, unlike pins, does not bind the surrounding soft tissues. The metacarpal head entry hole is dorsal to the contact area with the proximal phalanx and thus far has not created problems with MCP arthritis. Plate and screw fixation is better for long oblique patterns, comminution, or intra-articular involvement.

Prognosis and RTP: Stable fractures not requiring surgery usually require 3–4 weeks of splinting while swelling and soreness subside. RTP depends on whether sport and position allow for immobilization device. Transition to hand-based splints may allow skilled position players to return within 1–2 weeks depending on level of discomfort. Surgically treated fractures often require 2–4 weeks before ROM and pain allow return to sports. Playing with sutures in place is controversial and invites potential wound problems. Playing with indwelling pins/K-wires can also result in displacement, pin migration, or pin failure.

Injuries to the PIP Joint: Central Extensor Slip Insertion/Boutonniere Deformity

Description: Central slip of the extensor tendon inserts on the dorsal base of the middle phalanx. Disruption of this insertion results in loss of full active PIP joint extension. Over time, adjacent lateral band tendons migrate and become fixed palmar to the axis of rotation of the PIP joint, resulting in a boutonniere deformity characterized by PIP flexion and DIP hyperextension (Fig. 51.6).

Mechanism of injury: May occur with forced passive PIP flexion against active extension through the central slip tendon, resulting in avulsion; volar PIP dislocations often result in avulsion of the central slip insertion; dorsal PIP laceration through the central slip (hockey skate) will result in boutonniere deformity if left untreated.

Presentation: Often has a subtle presentation, and a high index of suspicion is required. Nonspecific presence of swelling is usually present about the PIP joint, and the joint may be maintained in slight flexion (see Fig. 51.6). However, in the immediate phase, the patient may be able to maintain PIP extension through the lateral bands, which have not yet palmarly migrated.

Physical examination: Palpate for tenderness directly over the central slip insertion on the dorsal middle phalangeal base. Collateral ligament tenderness may also be present, but tenderness at the central slip insertion should raise concern. A sensitive method to assess disruption of the central slip is the Elson test (see Fig. 51.6). A digit is placed on a table with the PIP joint flexed over the edge. While the proximal phalanx is held firmly flat on the table by the examiner, the patient attempts active extension of the PIP joint. Any pressure felt by the examiner on the dorsum of the middle phalanx suggests some continuity of the central slip insertion. If the central slip has torn and retracted proximally, there will be loss of active PIP extension and reduced passive DIP flexion (normally floppy and supple) during the attempt.

Differential diagnosis: Nonspecific swelling around the PIP joint could represent anything from mild collateral ligament injuries to periarticular fractures.

Diagnostics: PA and lateral plain radiographs are needed to rule out periarticular fractures or avulsion of the dorsal margin of middle phalangeal base.

Treatment: For closed injuries noted early (within 2–3 weeks), the lateral bands may not have yet become fixed in a position palmar to the axis of rotation. Closed treatment with *full-time* PIP splinting in full extension and active DIP flexion/extension exercises often results in healing of the central slip to its insertion bed while preserving lateral band mobility; should be continued for 6–8 weeks. Open lacerations require primary surgical repair of the tendon followed by protection of the repair with full PIP extension splinting and active DIP motion, as discussed earlier. Delayed presentations with fixed boutonniere postures are exceedingly difficult to treat. Salvage procedures in the form of terminal extensor tendon releases and even PIP fusion may be required depending on the degree and rigidity of the contracture.

Prognosis and RTP: Primary prognostic factors are prompt diagnosis and initiation of closed treatment. The digit must be protected from PIP flexion for at least 6 weeks. Fixed boutonniere deformities have a poor prognosis in terms of regaining full active motion.

Flexor Pulley Injuries

Description: The annular and cruciate pulleys of the flexor sheath (Fig. 51.7) form a fibro-osseous channel of "straps" that maintain the flexor tendons in close proximity to the phalanges. Annular pulley disruption, particularly multiple ruptures involving A2, A3, or A4, can result in clinically significant bowstringing of flexor tendons with resultant diminution of active digital flexion or slight PIP joint flexion contracture. Mainly seen in rock climbers, usually involving the middle and ring fingers. Also a common injury in higher-level baseball pitchers.

Mechanism of injury: Generally abrupt extension force to flexed digit (note same mechanism as jersey fingers). Often occurs with hand in "crimp" position (PIP flexed with MCP, DIP

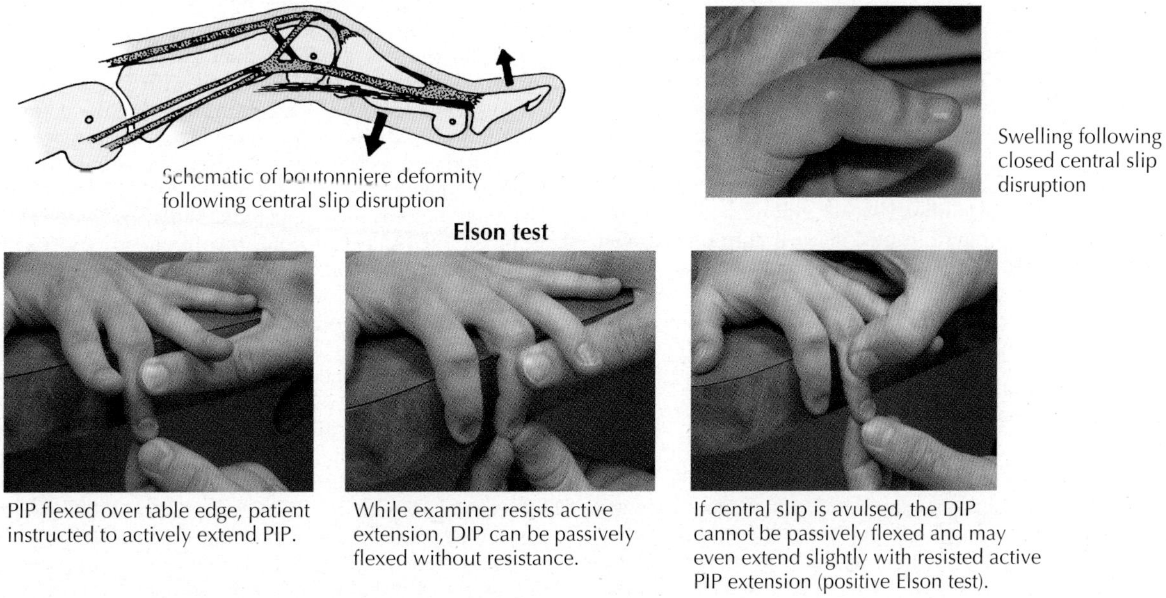
Schematic of boutonniere deformity following central slip disruption
Swelling following closed central slip disruption
Elson test
PIP flexed over table edge, patient instructed to actively extend PIP.
While examiner resists active extension, DIP can be passively flexed without resistance.
If central slip is avulsed, the DIP cannot be passively flexed and may even extend slightly with resisted active PIP extension (positive Elson test).

Figure 51.6 Injuries to the PIP joint central extensor slip insertion/boutonniere deformity. (From Green D, Hotchkiss R, Pederson W, eds. *Green's Operative Hand Surgery*. 5th ed. Philadelphia: Churchill Livingstone, Elsevier; 2005.)

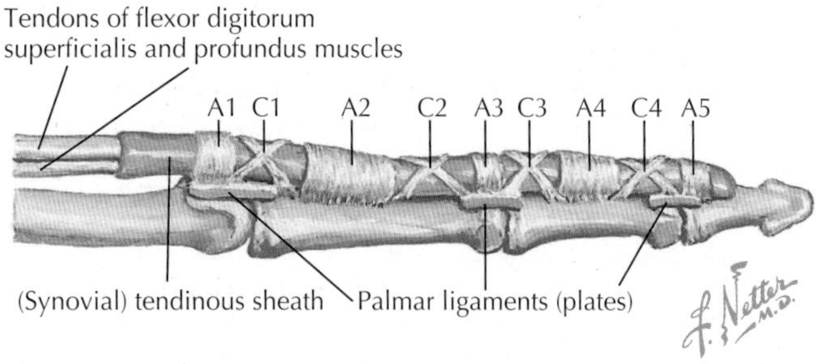
Tendons of flexor digitorum superficialis and profundus muscles
A1 C1 A2 C2 A3 C3 A4 C4 A5
(Synovial) tendinous sheath
Palmar ligaments (plates)
F. Netter M.D.

Figure 51.7 Flexor tendon sheath pulley system.

joints extended), which subjects the A2, A3, and A4 pulleys to maximal tearing force, perhaps when a climber loses footing and abruptly loads the supporting hand.

Presentation: Usually acute palmar digital pain accompanied by palpable or audible pop that precludes further loading of flexors.

Physical examination: May hold digit in slight flexed position because of pain or bowstringing associated with multiple pulley ruptures. Slight swelling or bruising can present with subacute presentations. Usually tender to palpation either palmar or lateral to injured pulley.

Differential diagnosis: Fracture, flexor tendon (flexor digitorum superficialis [FDS], FDP) rupture.

Diagnostics: PA and lateral digital x-rays to check for fracture. Ultrasound is an inexpensive, effective way to evaluate for bowstringing, but is clearly dependent on having a skilled operator. MRI is the gold standard and also allows for easier evaluation of a potential tendon injury. A tendon–bone distance (TBD) of >2 mm suggests at least a single tendon rupture (Fig. 51.8).

Treatment: Depends on actual grade of pulley injury (Schoffll classification, see later) and participation requirements:

- Grade 1: Pulley strain, <2 mm TBD: functional therapy, protective tape. Gradual RTP 4–6 weeks, taping through 3 months.
- Grade 2: Complete A4 or partial A2 or A3 rupture: 2 weeks immobilization, 2–4 weeks functional therapy, progressive RTP 4–8 weeks, tape pulley protection months.
- Grade 3: Complete A2 or A3 rupture: immobilization 2 weeks, functional therapy 4 weeks, progressive RTP 6–12 weeks, tape or thermoplastic rigid ring (Fig. 51.9) through 3 months.
- Grade 4: Single A2, A3, or multiple ruptures with associated lumbrical or collateral ligament injury: Surgical repair (various described techniques using free tendon graft or slip of FDS to recreate pulley).

Prognosis and RTP: Fortunately, many of these are grade 1–2 injuries without significant bowstringing and can be managed nonoperatively with taping/splinting support and gradual return to participation as outlined earlier. Surgical reconstruction, using a tendon autograft, can be delayed until off-season, and the athlete can be allowed to participate with taping until then, if able. Postoperative rehabilitation entails early protected ROM to avoid adhesions, with full participation delayed until 6 months.

Phalangeal Fractures

Description: May occur as simple transverse patterns with minimal displacement or as more complicated, comminuted patterns with marked displacement and associated soft tissue injury; in the distal phalanx, tuft fractures occur in the very tip of the bone, usually resulting from some form of crush to the fingertip, and often have a stellate pattern; distal phalangeal shaft and base fractures may result from a crush or bending force and can be more unstable than tuft fractures (Fig. 51.10).

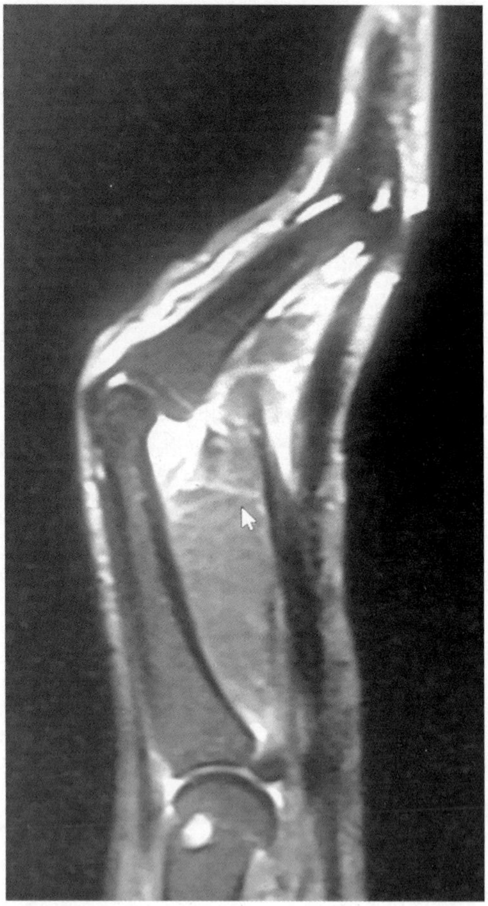

Figure 51.8 Sagittal MRI with flexor bowstringing from multiple annular pulley (A2, A3, A4) ruptures.

Mechanism of injury: Excessive axial, torsional, or bending forces; rate and direction of loading will determine the fracture pattern; sudden axial load from a ball to crush from another competitor's foot can result in various types of fractures, such as periarticular fractures or fracture-dislocations

Presentation: Nondisplaced fracture—pain, swelling, and associated apprehension to movement; fractures from crush injuries will often have a concomitant soft tissue injury component. Tuft fractures or displaced shaft fractures usually present with a subungual hematoma. Fractures with more comminution or displacement will likely result in some angular deformity of the digit. Be aware of any open wound around a displaced phalangeal shaft fracture, as this may communicate with the fracture site.

Physical examination: Inspect soft tissues, checking for open wounds or subungual hematoma. If the base of the nail plate has flipped out of the nail fold, this frequently represents a distal phalangeal shaft or metaphyseal open fracture through the nail bed. Point tenderness to palpation over the phalanx should raise suspicion. Angulation likely represents a fracture or fracture-dislocation, more easily detected if the patient can flex the digits (see Fig. 51.10). Open wound over the radial or ulnar neurovascular bundle mandates two-point discrimination sensory testing along that side of the fingertip. Perfusion of the digit should also be verified in settings of injuries with more energy imparted or displacement (crush injuries).

Differential diagnosis: Dislocations of the MCP or interphalangeal (IP) joints may be mistaken for phalangeal fractures; clarified using plain radiographs.

Diagnostics: PA and lateral plain radiographs of the digit should suffice for determination of fracture pattern and differentiation from joint involvement.

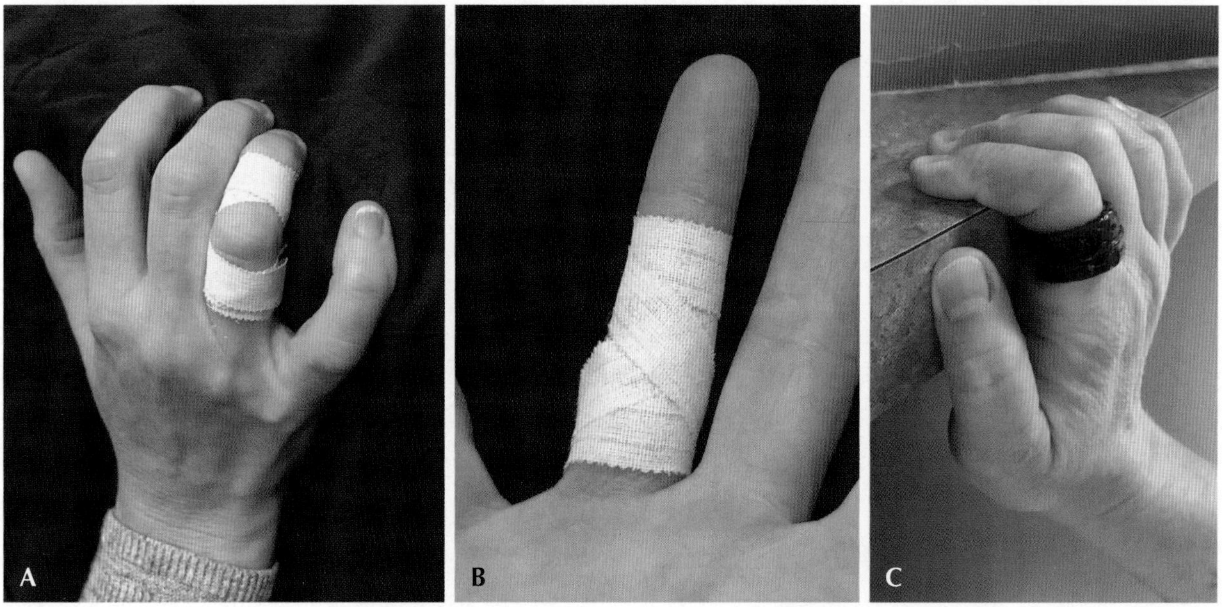
A
B
C

Figure 51.9 Taping and rigid splinting for pulley injuries.

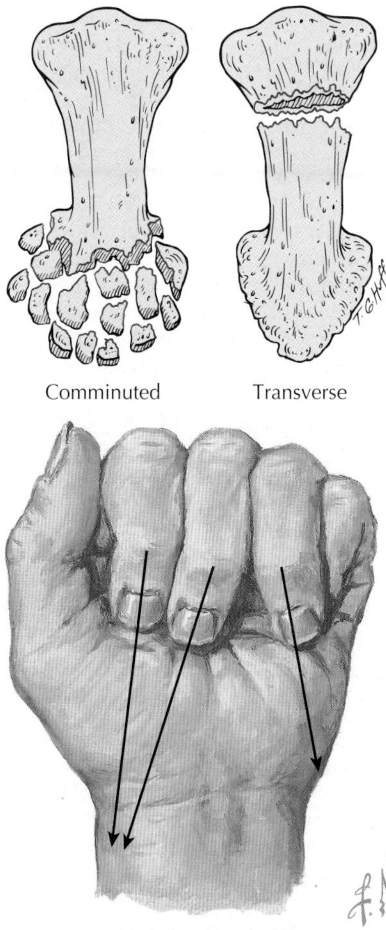
Comminuted
Transverse
Results of healing ring finger in rotational malalignment

Figure 51.10 Phalangeal fractures. (From Browner B, Jupiter J, Levine A, Trafton P. Skeletal trauma. In: *Basic Science, Management, and Reconstruction*. 3rd ed. Philadelphia: Saunders, Elsevier; 2002.)

Treatment: Potentially open fracture or nonperfused digit requires emergent surgical treatment and withdrawal from competition. Otherwise, the injured digit may be bandaged in a bulky dressing together with the other digits to allow RTP. Formal radiographic and clinical evaluation of closed perfused injuries should be performed within 48 hours. **Nondisplaced stable fractures** can usually be treated with custom splinting and gentle active-assist ROM exercises over 2–3 weeks. **Displaced fractures** must be reduced; digital block anesthetic is usually sufficient. Anything other than complete anatomic reduction of a transverse fracture is unstable and will require pin or plate and screw fixation. Tuft fractures can be managed without splinting, which allows load bearing as tenderness subsides. Unlike tuft fractures, displaced distal phalangeal shaft fractures are unstable and often require pin fixation.

Prognosis and RTP: Primary complications usually include stiffness and angular deformity. RTP is dictated by fracture stability (or fixation rigidity), union, and participation requirements. If fixation requires pin placement across a joint, the athlete should not be allowed to participate in any sport requiring forceful grip or ball handling until the pin has been removed. Similarly, even the most stable plate and screw constructs are prone to failure under such loads, and return to activity before at least early callus formation after the third week risks fixation failure and deformity.

Thumb Metacarpophalangeal Joint Ligament Injuries

Description: Often referred to as "skier's" or "gamekeeper's" thumb (for ulnar collateral ligament [UCL] failure) and "reverse gamekeeper's" thumb (for radial collateral ligament [RCL] failure), these injuries can result in chronically impaired and painful grip when left untreated. UCL failure can occur anywhere along the length of the ligament; detachment usually occurs with or without an avulsion fracture at the site of insertion into the base of the proximal phalanx (Fig. 51.11). The tendon or aponeurosis of the adductor pollicis can become interposed between the torn ligament and its insertion on the phalanx, thus preventing healing; this is called a *Stener lesion* (see Fig. 51.11).

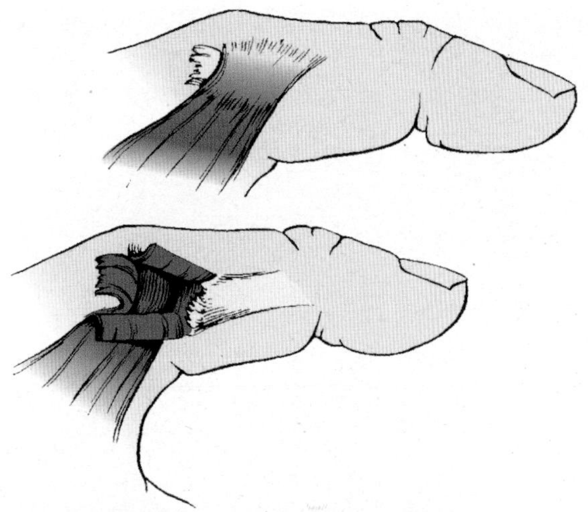

Schematic of Stener lesion

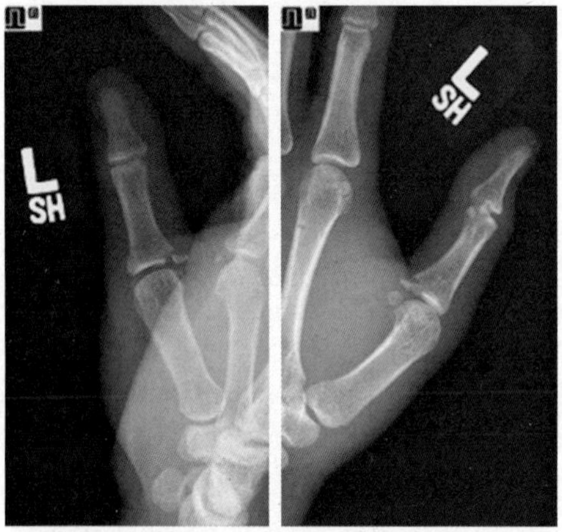
L
SH
L
SH

Radiograph showing UCL avulsion fracture

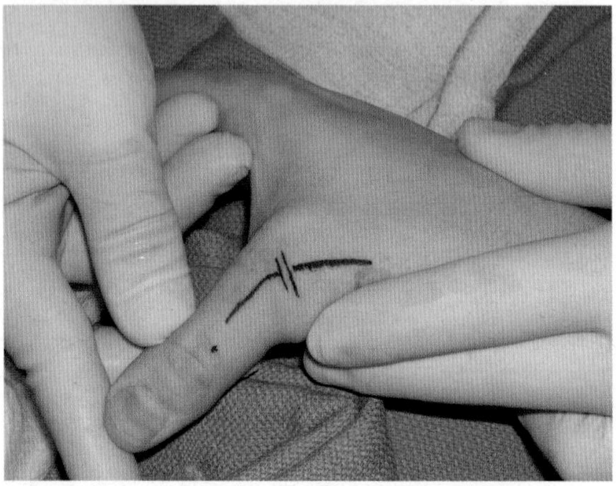

Valgus MCP stress test demonstrating UCL instability

Figure 51.11 Thumb metacarpophalangeal (MCP) joint ligament injuries. (From DeLee J, Drez D, Miller M. *DeLee & Drez's Orthopaedic Sports Medicine: Principles and Practice*. 2nd ed. Philadelphia: Saunders, Elsevier; 2002.)

Mechanism of injury: UCL injuries (10 times more frequent than RCL injuries) result from sudden valgus force to the thumb, often after a fall onto the thumb or impact from a ball. RCL injuries result from sudden varus force to the thumb and are often underappreciated and underdiagnosed.

Presentation: Painful, impaired grip; usually, the MCP joint is diffusely swollen in the subacute phase; resting angular deformity may or may not be visible at the MCP joint. In RCL injuries, as swelling subsides, the metacarpal head may appear prominent because of "sagging" of the radial aspect of the joint from capsuloligamentous incompetence.

Physical examination: In acute and subacute phases, tenderness to direct palpation over the injured ligament is present. Assess UCL stability with passive valgus stress of the extended proximal phalanx while stabilizing the metacarpal with the other hand (see Fig. 51.11). Although it has been suggested that pain and deviation of >30 degrees are indicative of a UCL tear, this laxity should be compared with the contralateral uninjured thumb. Several patients with inherent ligamentous laxity will have that degree of mobility in that joint; repeating the maneuver with the phalanx in 30 degrees of flexion will isolate the UCL and eliminate the stabilizing effect from an intact volar plate. RCL is evaluated in a similar manner, except the phalanx is passively deviated in the ulnar direction while the metacarpal is stabilized.

Differential diagnosis: Metacarpal head or phalangeal base fractures

Diagnostics: PA and lateral plain radiographs required to evaluate for fractures. In RCL injuries, the lateral view may reveal sagging of the proximal phalanx relative to the metacarpal. MRI may be helpful in clarifying both UCL and RCL injuries. Stener lesion, an important feature in determining treatment, *may* be evident on MRI, but is not always that clear.

Treatment: For UCL injuries, the degree of tear, avulsion fracture displacement, and presence or absence of a Stener lesion is considered. Partial tears with minimal relative laxity can usually be managed by thumb spica cast (including the IP joints) immobilization for 4–6 weeks, followed by a 2-week period of splinting and ROM exercises. A Stener lesion requires surgery to remove the interposed tendon and repair the ligament to its insertion bed. Use of an "internal brace" of suture tape has become popular, as it has higher load to failure than isolated direct repair and may allow earlier RTP and less use of temporary transarticular pins. Controversy surrounds complete tears wherein a Stener lesion is not apparent. Several experts advocate direct primary repair, whereas others may recommend casting. There is no consensus regarding management of acute RCL injuries. However, if sagging of the radial side of the joint is present clinically or on radiographs, surgical repair of the radial collateral complex (including associated capsular hood tear) over immobilization alone is preferred.

Prognosis and RTP: If the ligament complex heals, return to full activity in a 2- to 3-month window; however, may participate in cast if sport/position allows. After surgical repair, may RTP within 2 weeks (when wound is stable) in cast, play unprotected at 3 months. A small proportion of patients may continue to have pain with forceful grip, even with a clinically stable repair, thus requiring more prolonged splinting. If untreated, symptomatic instability persists and eventual osteoarthritis may develop.

Metacarpophalangeal Dislocation (Thumb or Finger)

Description: Complete dislocation of thumb or finger proximal phalanx (usually dorsal) in relation to the corresponding metacarpal joint, classified as either *simple* or *complex*; simple dislocation can be manually reduced; complex dislocation requires open reduction to remove the interposed tissue. In both simple and complex dislocations, the volar plate usually detaches from its metacarpal attachment and retains its attachment on the proximal phalanx. However, in a complex dislocation, the entire volar plate is interposed in the MCP joint, preventing manual reduction (Fig. 51.12). Apart from the interposed volar plate, the flexor tendons and tendons from intrinsic musculature can pass around opposite sides of the metacarpal head, creating a "noose effect" that blocks reduction when traction is applied.

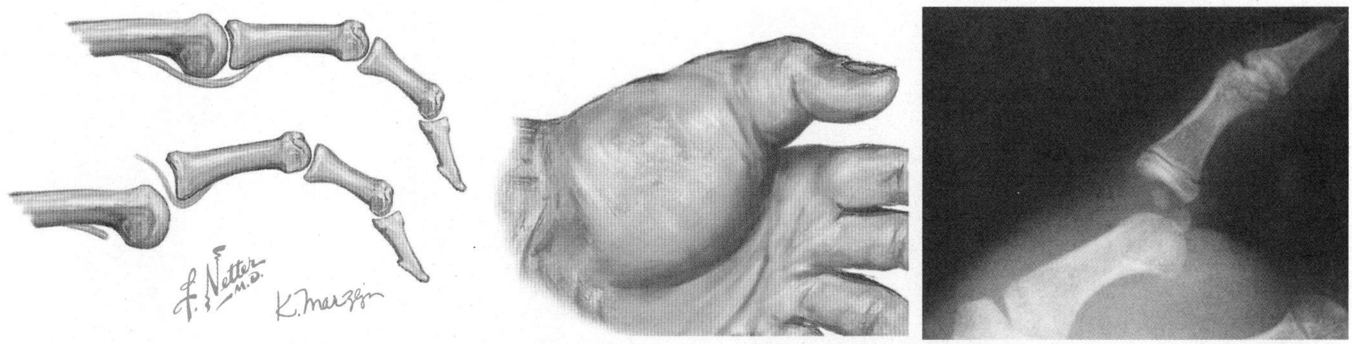

Metacarpophalangeal (MCP) joint dislocation is typically dorsal, and frequently the volar plate becomes incarcerated dorsally.

Thumb MCP dislocation is clinically apparent with shortened thumb and fullness in thenar eminence.

Complex thumb MCP dislocation, showing joint space widening and entrapped sesamoids within joint

Figure 51.12 Metacarpophalangeal (MCP) dislocation.

Mechanism of injury: Hyperextension injury to a digit at the level of the MCP joint

Presentation: Acute pain, swelling, and hyperextension of the MCP joint; border digits are most commonly affected

Physical examination: Differentiate between a simple and complex dislocation. Affected joint is typically hyperextended to approximately 70–90 degrees in a simple dislocation, whereas less hyperextension is seen in a complex dislocation. A volar skin "dimple" near the region of the A1 pulley is a pathognomonic finding of a complex dislocation. If a dimple is present, one must take care to evaluate the overlying skin for threatened skin or pressure necrosis. A careful neurovascular examination of the digit should be performed.

Differential diagnosis: A fracture at the level of the MCP joint may occur in conjunction with a dislocation.

Diagnostics: Physical examination is the mainstay in initial diagnosis. Although reduction may be attempted on the field, *eventual* PA, lateral, and oblique radiographs are required because up to 50% of such injuries have an associated fracture. Before reduction or after failed attempted reduction, simple dislocations will demonstrate the proximal phalanx hyperextended 70–90 degrees; complex dislocation may demonstrate excessive joint widening or entrapped sesamoids (see Fig. 51.12).

Treatment: Closed reduction is the initial treatment strategy, taking care to avoid converting a simple dislocation to a complex one. Technique includes wrist flexion (to relax flexor tendons), gentle traction, and volar translation of the base of the proximal phalanx relative to the metacarpal head to slide the phalanx into position. Excessive hyperextension and axial traction should be avoided because it may convert a simple to a complex dislocation by flipping the volar plate, lumbrical tendon, thenar tendon (in the thumb), or flexor tendon dorsal to the metacarpal head. For an irreducible dislocation, an open reduction must be performed, using either a dorsal or volar approach. After reduction of thumb MCP dislocations, grade III UCL tears with associated gross instability may be better managed with direct ligament repair, similar to skier's thumb (see earlier).

Prognosis and RTP: Simple dislocations in the fingers should be protected from hyperextension with a splint for at least 2 weeks while allowing early active flexion. Depending on the specific sport, consider prolonged protection against hyperextension with splint during participation. Consider slightly prolonging the protection of complex repairs. Thumb MCP dislocations mandate a more guarded approach to mobilization and RTP. Stability is a greater priority than mobility here. Rigid immobilization for 4 weeks is recommended with protection against forced hyperextension/hyperabduction for another 2 weeks. After surgical ligament repair, such protection against impact should be considered for 2–3 months.

Second to Fifth Carpometacarpal Dislocation

Description: Complete dislocation of the metacarpal in relation to the adjacent carpus; metacarpals dislocate dorsally relative to the carpus; often associated with fractures along the carpal joint margin, which significantly increases instability after reduction.

Mechanism of injury: High-energy axial load on the metacarpals; fifth and fourth rays may dislocate in isolation because of a more mobile articulation with the hamate. Index and long carpometacarpal (CMC) joints typically dislocate only in high-energy injuries wherein all four CMC joints are dislocated.

Presentation: Significant dorsal swelling and apprehension to grip

Physical examination: Inspection for an open injury; careful palpation of each digit is required to look for associated fractures. A neurovascular examination is imperative. Tense swelling in setting of high-energy injuries should raise concern for hand compartment syndrome.

Differential diagnosis: Metacarpal fractures, severe contusion, and carpal dislocations

Diagnostics: AP, lateral, and oblique radiographs are the mainstay. Radiographic evidence of dislocation is rather obvious when all four CMC joints are involved; however, radiographic findings are more subtle when dislocations occur in isolation. A "true lateral" radiograph of the involved digit must be obtained. Lateral views of small and ring fingers require approximately 30 degrees of pronation at the wrist; lateral views of the index and long finger may require more supination. Distraction or traction views may be useful. Computed tomography (CT) scans can be particularly helpful in cases of fracture-dislocations.

Treatment: These injuries are inherently unstable, although isolated dislocations may be stable after a closed reduction maneuver is performed. Reduction maneuver entails axial traction in conjunction with a palmar-directed force on the dorsal base of the affected metacarpal. Most injuries require closed or open reduction combined with internal fixation (usually temporary pins).

Prognosis and RTP: Because of the unstable nature of these injuries, RTP involving gripping or hand contact occurs after 6–8 weeks to allow for sufficient healing. In an isolated CMC dislocation that is stable upon closed reduction, return may be earlier with protective bracing or casting.

Scaphoid Fracture

Description: A common injury in sports; a precarious retrograde vascular supply renders the scaphoid prone to slow healing and nonunion, particularly in fractures of the waist or proximal pole. Left untreated, scaphoid fractures in adolescents or young adults will invariably progress to symptomatic nonunion

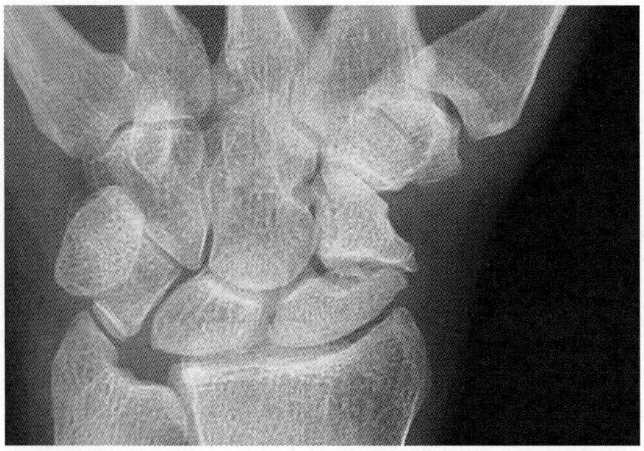

Radiograph of scaphoid nonunion with collapse and secondary osteophyte formation

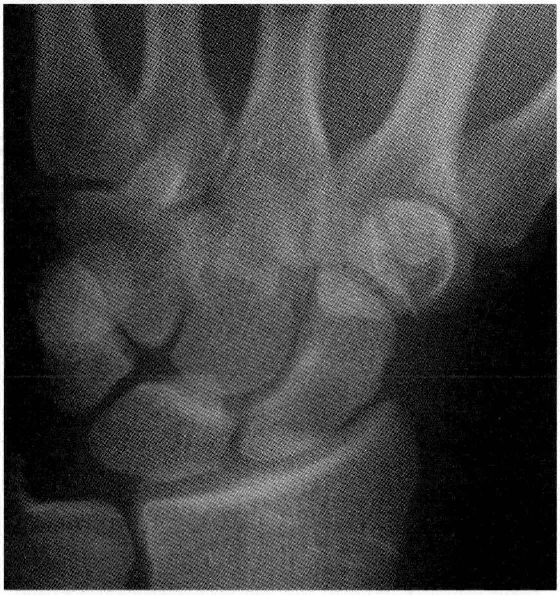

Normal x-ray of acute fracture

Figure 51.13 Scaphoid fractures.

and secondary arthritic collapse (Fig. 51.13). In isolation, this fracture results in no visible deformity and often no more pain than a minor joint sprain. As such, the diagnosis is frequently missed or the athlete often does not complain of wrist pain until weeks or months later.

Mechanism of injury: Frequently results from a fall on the outstretched hand with an extension load across the distal radius and carpus. The proximal pole is locked in the scaphoid fossa of the radial articular surface, resulting in failure of the waist or proximal pole of the scaphoid. A less frequent mechanism is an axial load through the carpus.

Presentation: Radial-sided wrist pain, usually after a fall or sudden axial load through the wrist. Usually no visible deformity, including lack of swelling. Patient will often still be able to move the wrist in the mid-ROM, particularly in more delayed presentations.

Physical examination: Tenderness to palpation directly over the fracture; in waist fractures, this is in the anatomic snuffbox. However, the proximal pole should be assessed by palpation at the scapholunate joint just distal to the dorsal radial tubercle. The distal scaphoid pole can be palpated at the scaphotrapezial joint, deep to the intersection of the flexor carpi radialis tendon and wrist flexion crease. Forced passive wrist extension also usually produces pain at the fracture site.

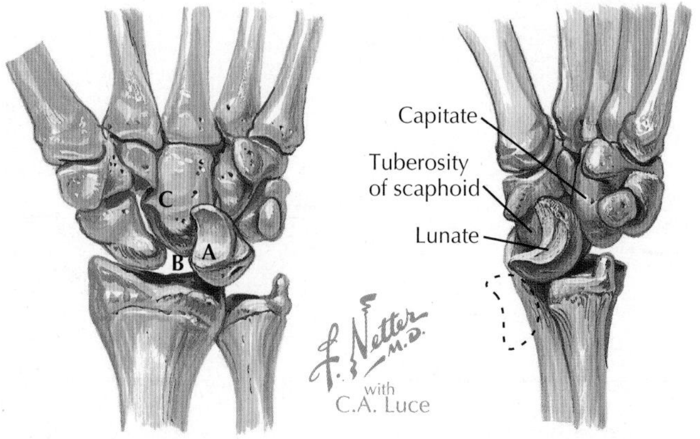
C
B
A
Capitate
Tuberosity of scaphoid
Lunate
F. Netter M.D.
with
C.A. Luce

Palmar view shows (A) lunate rotated and displaced volarly, (B) scapholunate space widened, (C) capitate displaced proximally and dorsally.

Lateral view shows lunate displaced volarly and rotated. Broken line indicates further dislocation to volar aspect of distal radius.

Figure 51.14 Volar lunate dislocation. Note that in *perilunate* dislocation, the lunate remains in place relative to the radius while the capitate dislocates relative to the lunate (see Fig. 51.15).

Differential diagnosis: Distal radius fractures, injuries to the scapholunate ligament, and perilunate or lunate dislocations (markedly more painful with visible deformity)

Diagnostics: PA, oblique, lateral, and clenched-fist/ulnar deviation radiographs are essential. If plain radiographs are negative, bone scan or MRI may demonstrate the presence of a nondisplaced fracture, although MRI may offer more specificity (see Fig. 51.13). However, simple repeat radiographs 2–3 weeks later after cast immobilization may reveal bone changes around a previously unrecognizable fracture. To determine displacement and potential surgical planning, CT scan offers the best bony detail.

Treatment: Displaced fractures are managed with arthroscopic or ORIF, as are fractures associated with other carpal fractures or ligament injuries. With displacement, the union rate precipitously decreases with immobilization alone. Controversy surrounds management of a truly nondisplaced scaphoid waist fracture because similar union rates and functional results have been demonstrated with immediate cast immobilization compared with immediate percutaneous screw fixation. Immediate fixation may allow players to return to competition sooner while casted than without internal fixation. Proximal pole fractures, even when nondisplaced, are often primarily managed with screw fixation because of the poor vascularity of that portion of the bone and high nonunion rate.

Prognosis and RTP: Union rate with immobilization of nondisplaced or impacted distal pole fractures is >90%. Union rate of nondisplaced waist fractures with immobilization ranges from 85% to 95%. Proximal pole fracture union rates drop significantly. RTP is dictated by the fixation stability and the degree of fracture union. With anatomic reduction and screw fixation, a player may be able to RTP *in a cast* within a few weeks or once the wounds have adequately healed. Until union occurs, the wrist must be protected against forced flexion or extension. Fifty percent trabecular bridging across the fracture demonstrated by CT scan should allow unprotected RTP.

Perilunate Injuries

Description ***(scapholunate tears, perilunate, and lunate dislocations)*****:** Injuries involving combinations of ligaments and bones surrounding the lunate (Fig. 51.14). Consider as a sequence of failure, with carpus supinating around the lunate. The scapholunate

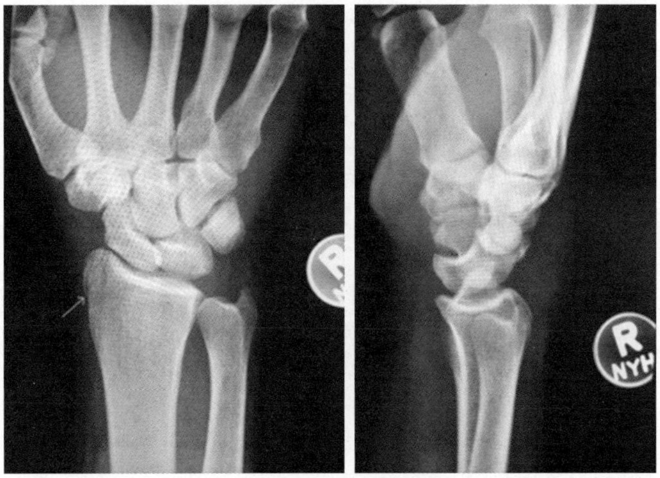

Figure 51.15 Radiographs of *perilunate* dislocation.

ligament fails before force progresses through the midcarpal joint and ruptures the lunotriquetral ligament. Volar dislocation of the lunate into the carpal canal represents the final stage.

Mechanism of injury: Wrist hyperextension and ulnar deviation during axial loading

Physical examination: Localized wrist pain, point tenderness over dorsal carpus, limited motion. Bleeding or lunate displacement into the carpal canal can create median sensory deficits and often painful dysesthesias. With lunate dislocation, bone may be palpable at the wrist flexion crease.

Differential diagnosis: Scaphoid fracture and distal radius fracture

Diagnostics: PA, lateral, and scaphoid radiograph of wrist; any malalignment of the lunate relative to the radius or capitate on the lateral view is evidence of perilunate injury (Fig. 51.15). For an isolated complete scapholunate tear, may see widening >3 mm on PA view, increased scaphoid flexion, and lunate extension on lateral view. With normal radiographs and profound carpal tenderness or swelling, MRI is indicated.

Treatment: All acute perilunate fractures and dislocations require surgical repair of the ligaments and/or bony elements. Combinations of K-wires, suture anchors, and screws are used.

Prognosis and RTP: K-wires are removed at 8 weeks, and cast immobilization is usually required for 12 weeks. Most injuries take at least 5–6 months before ROM and strength stabilize, but the construct may be stable enough for loading at 12 weeks.

Distal Radius Fractures

Description: One of the most common upper limb injuries seen in orthopedics; in an athlete with open physes, fractures through the growth plate are particularly common after falls onto the outstretched hand. Fracture patterns may be limited to the metaphysis or also involve radiocarpal or ulnocarpal articulations. Degree of comminution is determined by the quality of the bone and injury load.

Mechanism of injury: Fall onto the outstretched hand is the most common mechanism.

Presentation: Nondisplaced fractures may have no visible deformity other than mild swelling with complaints of wrist pain after a fall. The more common dorsally displaced patterns may demonstrate a "dinner fork" deformity just proximal to the carpus. Patients will be apprehensive regarding any motion of the wrist. These injuries are typically more painful than scaphoid fractures; hence, most patients will be forced to withdraw from play.

Physical examination: Assessment of skin integrity and neurovascular status; open fractures, seen with higher-energy injuries with greater degrees of displacement at the fracture site, fortunately are uncommon in athletic competition. With greater dorsal displacement at the fracture site, there is a higher risk of traction injuries to the median nerve. Sensation of the radial three and a half digits should be assessed before any manipulation. In nondisplaced fractures, the patient will reliably be tender to palpation directly over the fracture site.

Differential diagnosis: Carpal fractures and ligament injuries should always be considered; usually differentiated by direct palpation because the patient will usually be tender over the fractured radial metaphysis as opposed to the carpus. Nevertheless, these injuries can occur in combination, and tenderness over the scaphoid and the radius should lead to assessment with appropriate plain radiographs.

Diagnostics: PA and lateral plain radiographs usually sufficient; CT may be useful for surgical planning for fractures with intra-articular displacement or comminution

Treatment: Nondisplaced fractures can be splinted in the neutral position and transitioned to a cast as swelling subsides. Usually 4–6 weeks to heal for preadolescent or adolescent. For fractures with obvious clinical displacement, there is little to be gained from immediate manipulation or attempted reduction before obtaining plain radiographs or having adequate analgesia. Supportive splinting of the wrist should be applied until then. Common guidelines for accepted displacement of extra-articular fractures in skeletally mature individuals of ≤10 degrees of dorsal tilt of the articular surface. For intra-articular patterns, most practitioners accept ≤2 mm of gap or a 1-mm step-off of the joint surface. If the reduction cannot be maintained with closed manipulation and splinting, ORIF is recommended. For nondisplaced or minimally displaced fractures, ORIF may allow earlier ROM and use of a removable splint.

Prognosis and RTP: Participation in contact sports or load-bearing of the fractured radius is usually precluded until stable union is evident, minimum of 4–6 weeks, depending on patient age and fracture pattern. Restoration of normal anatomy ensures optimal prognosis in skeletally mature individuals, whereas younger patients with open physes may still exhibit some remodeling, mainly in the sagittal plane.

Bennett and Rolando (First Metacarpal Base) Fractures

Description: Intra-articular fractures of the base of the thumb metacarpal. A Bennett fracture pattern includes a constant piece on the volar–ulnar aspect of the thumb metacarpal base that is held in a normal anatomic position to the adjacent trapezium by the strong *deep anterior oblique (beak) ligament*, whereas the remainder of the metacarpal base subluxates or dislocates dorsally. A Rolando fracture pattern has the same volar–ulnar fragment and an associated dorsal fragment as well; thus, it is often described as a T- or Y-shaped thumb metacarpal base fracture (Fig. 51.16).

Mechanism of injury: Results due to an axially directed force through the shaft of the flexed thumb metacarpal

Presentation: Acute pain and swelling localized to the base of the thumb metacarpal after a contact or impact injury; pain is associated with any attempt to move the thumb.

Physical examination: Pain and swelling localized to the base of the thumb metacarpal

Differential diagnosis: Thumb metacarpal shaft fracture and thumb trapeziometacarpal dislocation must be considered.

Diagnostics: Accurate injury classification requires quality radiographs. True AP views of the thumb CMC joint, with the wrist pronated and dorsum of the first metacarpal placed flat against

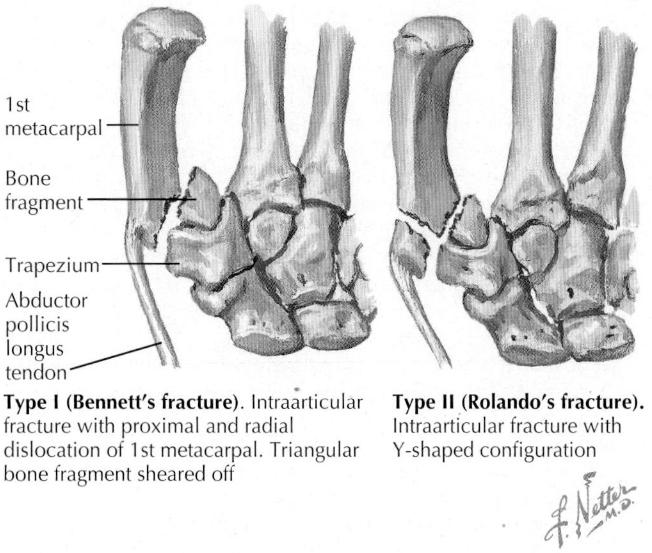
1st metacarpal
Bone fragment
Trapezium
Abductor pollicis longus tendon
Type I (Bennett's fracture). Intraarticular fracture with proximal and radial dislocation of 1st metacarpal. Triangular bone fragment sheared off
Type II (Rolando's fracture). Intraarticular fracture with Y-shaped configuration
F. Netter M.D.

Figure 51.16 Bennett and Rolando (first metacarpal base) fractures.

the plate combined with lateral view, should suffice. Traction views may also be helpful.

Treatment: These fractures are unstable, and surgical management is recommended to maintain CMC joint congruity. Bennett fractures are often successfully managed with closed reduction and percutaneous pin fixation, whereas Rolando fractures typically require ORIF techniques.

Prognosis and RTP: Overall prognosis is good if articular congruity and length of the metacarpal is restored. A typical course of 6 weeks of immobilization is required before gradual RTP, with protective bracing depending on sport-specific demands.

Hook of Hamate Fracture

Available online.

Injuries to the Triangular Fibrocartilage Complex

Available online.

Flexor Tendon Laceration

Available online.

RECOMMENDED READINGS

Available online.

THORAX AND ABDOMINAL INJURIES 52

Ginger L. Cupit • Sameer Dixit • Cindy J. Chang

GENERAL PRINCIPLES

Overview

- Injuries to the thorax and abdomen are more often seen in sports involving sudden deceleration and impact (e.g., football, ice hockey, skiing, and snowboarding).
- Early recognition and management of these potentially life-threatening injuries are imperative. Serial assessments and a high index of suspicion are essential for accurate evaluation. Once severe injury is recognized, emergency medicine fundamentals and stabilization should be initiated until transfer to a hospital occurs.
- Torso injuries overlap with injuries to the skeletal system (e.g., traction apophysitis of iliac crest presenting as lower abdominal pain; shoulder conditions can radiate to the thorax; similarly, thoracic and abdominal conditions can radiate to the extremities, confusing the source of symptoms).

Anatomic and Physiologic Issues

- Combination of upper abdomen injuries can be divided into three regions:
  - Midline region: Left lobe of liver, pancreas, duodenum, transverse colon, small bowel and mesentery, aorta, inferior vena cava, sternum, lower ribs, and heart.
  - Right region: Liver, kidney, adrenal gland, hemidiaphragm, lung, pneumothorax or hemothorax, and ribs.
  - Left region: Other paired organs, but spleen instead of liver.
- In sports, organs can suffer damage usually resulting from compressive forces (e.g., tackle or bicycle handlebar) that push solid or viscus organ against the spine.
- Deceleration forces and penetrating injuries are uncommon in athletics, although "almost penetrating" injuries are possible (e.g., hockey stick or ski pole) without causing a wound.
- Abdominal organs in children are more susceptible to injury from trauma because of their relative position (more anterior and lower because of the more horizontal nature of the diaphragm), still developing abdominal musculature, and pliable nature of cartilaginous ribs.
- **"Getting the wind knocked out"** is more common than significant trauma to visceral organs. An unguarded blow to the epigastric region causes temporary reflex spasm of the diaphragm. Loosening of restricting garments and flexion at the knees and hips usually restores normal respiration. Because of the risk of intra-abdominal injury, serial observation and follow-up are necessary.

Epidemiology, Injury Statistics, and Sports-Specific Issues

Sport-specific data are limited.

Myocardial injury: Up to 76% of patients may sustain blunt chest trauma with direct compression of the heart between the anterior chest wall and vertebral column. Most common cardiac injury is cardiac contusion (60%) among pediatric patients. Most common causes are motor vehicle accident (MVA) (50%), sports injuries, and falls. Sudden cardiac death (36%) was the most common catastrophic injury in high school and intercollegiate athletes in 2019.

Abdominal injury: Second most common sport-related internal organ injury is the spleen, which can occur in 5.6 per 1,000,000 children, and in college it can occur in up to 57%. Most of these injuries were sustained during football, ice hockey, soccer, or horseback riding.

Thoracic and pulmonary injuries: Study assessing chest wall injuries in high school athletes demonstrated that only 2% required surgical intervention, with two-thirds of surgeries being from football or wrestling. Despite potential for catastrophic outcomes of chest wall injuries, most injuries were contusions/strains (63%), and nearly 60% of athletes were able to return to play in <1 week.

History and Physical Examination

History

- Accurate account of events leading to injury is important in establishing diagnosis.
- History and physical examination (PE) are sometimes unreliable, particularly in children and if there is an altered level of consciousness.
- Seemingly minor trauma can cause delayed splenic rupture or other injuries; careful history-taking, including past injuries, surgeries, and illnesses, is paramount.
- Previously undiagnosed preexisting condition such as inflammatory bowel disease, liver hemangioma, and infectious mononucleosis can cause major clinical symptoms after trauma to affected organ.
- Detailed history of patient's pain and use of pain scale upon initial presentation and during serial evaluations are useful.

Physical Examination

- See Chapter 4: "Sideline Preparedness and Emergencies," for discussion of initial evaluation of injuries to thorax and abdomen.

General Appearance and Vital Signs

- If thoracic and abdominal injuries are both present, thoracic injuries are usually more symptomatic and will distract attention from abdominal pain, which is usually less localized and specific.
- Abdominal pain can be vague and diffuse or localized to a quadrant. Abdominal pain is sensitive but not specific to the presence of injury; 50% of individuals with pain have no significant injury. Always examine the chest and spine when evaluating an abdominal complaint; consider examining inguinal and pelvic regions.
- Frequent monitoring of vital signs, including orthostatics, is important to gauge cardiovascular status; in addition, respiratory rate, rhythm, and use of accessory respiratory muscles should be observed. If difficult to obtain blood pressure by auscultation, deflate the cuff until palpable return of brachial or radial pulse; the systolic pressure obtained by auscultation is approximately 10 mmHg higher.

Inspection

- Observe effort of breathing; listen for abnormal breathing sounds.
- Look for asymmetry, deformity, swelling, bruising, lacerations, and scars.
- Confirm that trachea is in midline and chest has normal anteroposterior (AP) diameter.
- Evaluate abdominal contour and signs of increasing abdominal girth; observe for peristaltic or pulsating movements.
- Observe for splinting or guarding of torso and upper extremities (UEs) or any change in neck position.

Auscultation, Percussion, and Palpation

- Auscultate anteriorly and posteriorly, comparing for asymmetry. If breath sounds are decreased, normal lung has been displaced by air (suspect pneumothorax) or fluid (hemopneumothorax or pleural effusion).
- Percuss anterior and posterior chest, comparing both sides, and for normal diaphragmatic excursion with inspiration (symmetrical 3–5 cm). If hyperresonant, suspect pneumothorax; if dull, suspect fluid. Percuss all four quadrants; percuss liver span (range 6–12 cm), check for splenic enlargement.
- Auscultate before palpating, as bowel sounds can change with manipulation. Listen for bruits over aorta and renal and iliac arteries. Gently palpate to check for areas of tenderness, noting facial expression and guarding. Follow with deep palpation to further delineate areas of pain or presence of abdominal masses. Include a complete evaluation of the genitourinary system.
- For bony and soft tissue injuries of the thorax, perform neck, thoracic spine, and shoulder range-of-motion (ROM) and strength tests and palpate for crepitus, deformities, or tenderness.

SPECIFIC INJURIES AND PROBLEMS

Chest Wall Injuries

Sternal Fracture

Description: Incidence of associated intrathoracic trauma is high in acute injury, particularly rib fractures and soft tissue contusions. Incidence may be increasing: in a recent case series of 22 patients, 11 injuries were related to sports.

Mechanism of injury (MOI): High-impact injuries and acute hyperflexion of cervicothoracic spine

Presentation: Chest pain (CP), localized tenderness over sternum, and shortness of breath (SOB)

PE: Bruising, swelling, localized pleuritic pain, palpable pain, visible defect suggesting displacement

Differential diagnosis/associated injuries: Stress fracture of sternum (develops when great stress placed on upper body during wrestling or golf), manubriosternal joint dislocation, sternoclavicular or costochondral injury, or sternal contusion; associated with myocardial contusion, injury of internal mammary vessels, retrosternal and mediastinal hematoma, pulmonary laceration or contusion, and rib and thoracic vertebrae fractures

Diagnostics: Lateral chest film is best to evaluate fractures (upper fragment usually displaced anteriorly over lower fragment) but often misses them; posteroanterior (PA) radiograph to evaluate possible pneumothorax or widened mediastinum; cervical, thoracic, and lumbar spine radiographs if flexion/compression mechanism; computed tomography (CT) scan gold standard (axial cuts alone can miss transverse fractures; sagittal and coronal reconstruction views needed); ultrasound (US) has higher sensitivity and specificity than conventional radiographs in diagnosing abrupt discontinuity of bone; in experienced hands, US can rule out associated conditions such as pleural effusions. If intrathoracic trauma suspected based on history and PE, perform electrocardiogram (ECG) and chest x-ray (CXR) and consider chest CT to evaluate for cardiac and aortic injuries; incidence of myocardial damage is <2.5%. Important to reassess for myocardial contusion and arrhythmia with repeat ECG 6 hours later.

Treatment: If displaced, reduction possible by lying supine and then lifting both arms above the head while hyperextending thoracic spine at a level just below the scapular spines; **because of possible associated intrathoracic trauma, observation in hospital with cardiac monitor is advisable during reduction.** Displaced fractures may require open reduction and internal fixation (ORIF), particularly if respiration is compromised. If sternal fracture is isolated without associated injury (normal vital signs, CXR, ECG, no dysrhythmias), patient can be safely managed as outpatient, although in one prospective study 12.5% had clinically insignificant delayed hemothorax.

Prognosis and return to play (RTP): Nonunion of sternal fractures rare, but suspect when pain persists over sternum; if an isolated fracture with no underlying thoracic injuries, progressive RTP limited by pain; avoid contact sports until fracture healed and pain resolved (range 6–12 weeks); if risk of reinjury is high, consider chest protector during sport.

Dislocation of Sternoclavicular Joint (SCJ)

Description: Relatively infrequent, constituting ≤1% of somatic dislocations and 3% of shoulder-girdle lesions; only 50% of the clavicular joint surface contacts the sternal articular surface; posterior sternoclavicular ligament is stronger than anterior ligament; anterior disruption more common than posterior disruption (ratio ranges from 9:1 to 20:1); superior dislocation rare

Allman classification:

- **Grade I:** Sprain with no ligamentous disruption or instability; normal alignment
- **Grade II:** Rupture of sternoclavicular ligament; joint is partially displaced/widened
- **Grade III:** Dislocation with gross disruption of capsule and both sternoclavicular and costoclavicular ligaments

MOI: Caused by falls and direct or indirect trauma to shoulder girdle; injury most often seen in contact sports (e.g., martial arts, football, and rugby); indirect trauma can be seen in gymnastics; for anterior dislocation, force applied at anterolateral aspect of shoulder or along abducted arm is transmitted along clavicle to SCJ, compressing and rolling the shoulder back and displacing the clavicle. For posterior dislocation, force applied to posterolateral aspect of shoulder when arm is adducted and flexed is transmitted to SCJ, compressing and rolling the shoulder forward and displacing the clavicle (Fig. 52.1). Posterior

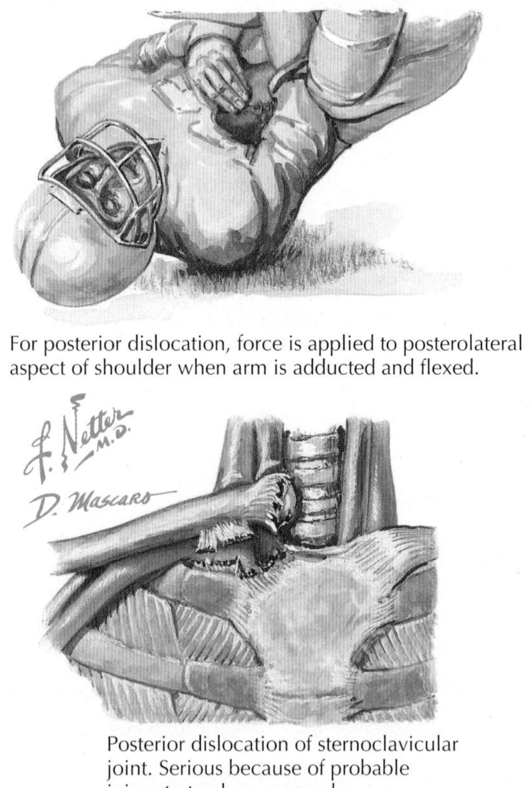
For posterior dislocation, force is applied to posterolateral aspect of shoulder when arm is adducted and flexed.
F. Netter M.D.
D. Mascaro
Posterior dislocation of sternoclavicular joint. Serious because of probable injury to trachea or vessels

Figure 52.1 Posterior dislocation of sternoclavicular joint.

dislocation can also result from direct blow on anterior aspect of medial end of clavicle.

Presentation: Severe pain, particularly with arm movement especially raised >90 degrees; pain exacerbated by coughing, sneezing, or deep breathing; because neck muscles spasm, head is tilted toward injured side. Increased discomfort in supine position. Other symptoms include hoarseness, dysphagia, dyspnea, numbness, and weakness or venous engorgement of ipsilateral arm.

PE: Bruising, pain, and significant swelling at joint; noticeable prominence of medial end of clavicle in anterior dislocation; in posterior dislocation, loss of normal prominence but often missed because of swelling; obtain vital signs; observe ease of respiration, dyspnea or dysphagia, and neurologic/vascular status of affected UE to rule out pressure on adjacent vital structures.

Differential diagnosis/associated injuries: SCJ sprain or subluxation; fracture of medial clavicle; fracture of medial physeal growth plate of clavicle (ossification begins at age 16–19; fusion occurs at age 22–25). SCJ pseudo-dislocations in patients <25 classified as Salter–Harris I or II fractures; important to recognize, as displaced epiphysis can block reduction of SCJ. **More serious injuries associated with posterior SCJ dislocations; a 25%–30% incidence of injury to vital structures traversing the thoracic outlet, including major vessels of the neck, brachial plexus, dome of pleurae, trachea, esophagus, and larynx; 12.5% mortality rate in this group of injuries.**

Diagnostics: Plain radiographs (Rockwood "serendipity" view) with 40-degree cephalic tilt centered at sternum (45 inches tube distance for children and 60 inches for adults; anterior dislocation = superior appearance and posterior = inferior); CXR to rule out pneumothorax; axial CT images (3-mm cuts) have greater sensitivity and specificity and are imaging modality of choice; use coronal plane paraxial CT reconstruction if superior component of dislocation is suspected; CT angiography allows assessment of adjacent mediastinal structures; magnetic resonance imaging (MRI) if more detailed information needed regarding soft tissue and possible physeal injuries); US has been used for successful diagnosis but lacks anatomic detail of CT; occasionally, arteriography/venography may be needed.

Treatment:

- **Grade I and II injuries:** Sling as needed initially for pain; avoid stress to joint for 2–4 weeks for adequate healing, with goal to avoid increased symptomatic mobility at the joint; early functional therapy
- **Grade III injuries:** Immediate closed reduction for posterior dislocations with impending airway or bleeding complications; otherwise, reduce in operating room under anesthesia in presence of a cardiothoracic or trauma surgeon. Closed reduction of posterior dislocations have reported 30%–50% success rate and higher if done <10 days of initial injury. Anterior dislocations can be reduced in outpatient settings by applying gentle pressure over displaced medial aspect of clavicle. If closed reduction fails, open reduction can be considered in severe cases; however, anteriorly displaced medial clavicle often becomes relatively asymptomatic with activities of daily living (ADLs). Chronic joint instability may cause pain and persistent functional limitation in active patients; this is an indication for surgical intervention.
- **For chronic SCJ dislocation:** Check for hypermobility of surrounding structures (including acromioclavicular and glenohumeral joints). Consider a limited course of corticosteroid and prolotherapy injections for symptomatic patients. Soft tissue reconstruction can be performed.

Prognosis and RTP: Up to 6–8 weeks of immobilization after successful reduction; healing can be inadequate and mild SCJ instability may persist, with a propensity for recurrent subluxation. Usually after surgery, 3 months before RTP. Osteomyelitis of clavicle can be a late complication. Operative stabilization can be difficult, with unpredictable results. In cases of recurrent stabilization failure or painful arthroses, resection of medial clavicle as salvage procedure.

Rib Fractures

Description: Common; can be complete, incomplete, or stress fractures (Fig. 52.2); often associated with other injuries, including other fractures and organ trauma; nondisplaced fractures more common; if displaced, other injuries include laceration of intercostal artery and pneumothorax; uncommon in children because thorax is more pliable.

MOI:

- Blunt trauma: Force usually applied in AP plane; fractures located at posterior angles of fifth to ninth ribs
- Direct force over small area of chest wall leads to fracture beneath point of impact
- Violent muscle contraction: **Floating rib** or **avulsion fractures** of attachments of external oblique muscle to lower three ribs; reported in baseball pitchers and batters. Forceful contraction against significant resistance of other muscles that attach to ribs can also result in fractures.
- **Fracture of first rib:** Direct external trauma is rare cause because of protection of shoulder girdle. Other causes are indirect trauma from falling on outstretched arm, violent muscular pull (e.g., hyperabduction of arm), or repetitive stresses.
- **Stress fractures of ribs:** Caused by excessive forceful muscular traction at attachments to ribs. Chronic opposing pulls of scalene muscles and upper digitations of serratus anterior may fracture **first rib** at its thinnest and most anatomically weak segment, where the subclavian artery crosses (subclavian sulcus), as with **weightlifting, pitching, and other throwers.** Anterolateral stress fractures of **fourth** and **fifth ribs,** and other ribs have been reported in **rowers** because of excessive action of serratus anterior muscle (see Chapter 85: "Rowing").

Presentation: History of traumatic event with intense localized pain over involved rib. **If first rib injured, may complain of shoulder, scapular, or neck pain; may complain of abdominal pain if lower ribs (11th and 12th) involved.** With stress fractures, insidious onset of pain associated with specific activities and possible radiation of pain. If fracture is unstable, pain is acute and knifelike. Pain aggravated by deep inspiration, coughing, or sneezing and with twisting or side flexion (causing tension on fractured rib); may report dyspnea.

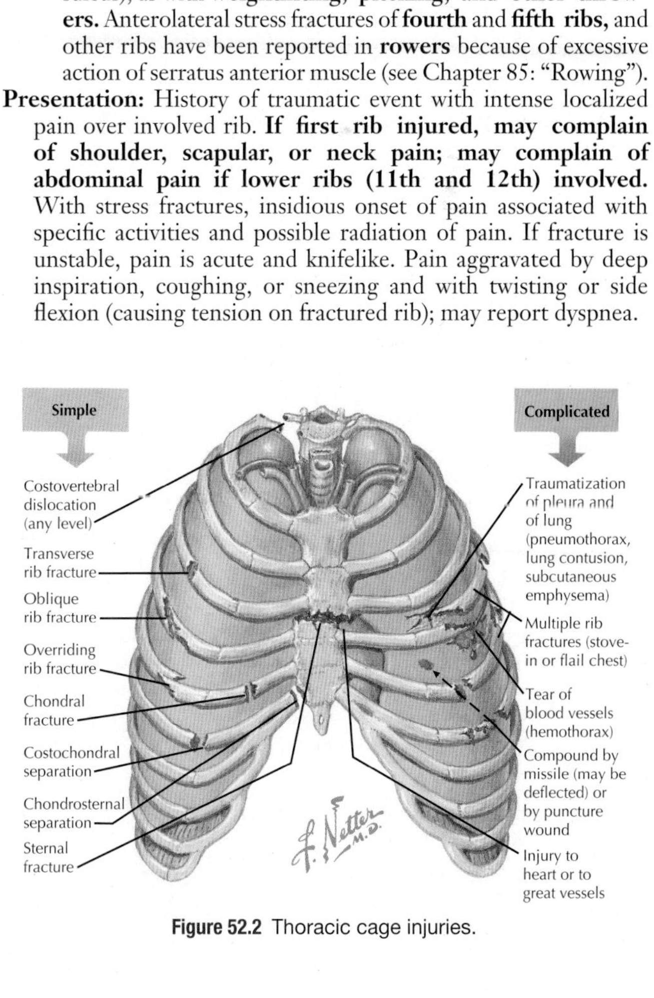
Simple
Complicated
Costovertebral dislocation (any level)
Transverse rib fracture
Oblique rib fracture
Overriding rib fracture
Chondral fracture
Costochondral separation
Chondrosternal separation
Sternal fracture
Traumatization of pleura and of lung (pneumothorax, lung contusion, subcutaneous emphysema)
Multiple rib fractures (stove-in or flail chest)
Tear of blood vessels (hemothorax)
Compound by missile (may be deflected) or by puncture wound
Injury to heart or to great vessels
F. Netter M.D.

Figure 52.2 Thoracic cage injuries.

PE: Localized tenderness, ecchymosis, and edema; crepitus over fracture site; palpable deformity of rib if fracture displaced; shallow and rapid breathing; with AP and transverse compression of rib cage, pain at site of suspected injury; subcutaneous emphysema with pleural injury.

Differential diagnosis/associated injuries:

- Severe rib contusion, costochondral separation, muscle strain (e.g., forceful contraction of thoracic muscles during tennis serve), and other medical causes of CP (e.g., pneumothorax, pleurisy, and herpes zoster).
- Incidence of intrathoracic injuries increases as more ribs are fractured.
- **If first rib fracture displaces posteriorly, check for vascular injury** (e.g., subclavian artery and aorta).
- **Fracture of lower two ribs may damage kidneys, liver, or spleen**; splenic trauma reported in up to 20% of left lower rib fractures; liver trauma in up to 10% of right lower rib fractures.
- **Flail chest:** Fracture of at least three consecutive ribs, each in two locations, causing free-floating segment of chest wall; high risk of internal injury, particularly lung and thoracic aorta. Paradoxical chest wall movement results in impaired ventilation and respiratory failure.

Diagnostics: CXR establishes diagnosis in 90% of cases if acute fracture; can also exclude complications, such as pneumothorax. Oblique views may detect anterior and lateral fractures. Bone scan if stress fracture suspected; US more sensitive than conventional radiography; CT scan most appropriate imaging modality if suspect posterior displacement of first rib; reformatting CT images to a single-in-plane image improves detection of rib fractures; if cardiac complications are possible, follow-up with ECG and echocardiogram. If upper thoracic ribs are fractured, consider angiography. If renal injury suspected, perform intravenous (IV) pyelogram or other imaging modalities.

Treatment: Pain relief using ice, nonsteroidal anti-inflammatory drugs (NSAIDs), and analgesics; bone stimulators have been approved by Food and Drug Administration (FDA) for nonunion of a stress fracture if ≥3 months from diagnosis and imaging at least 90 days after diagnosis demonstrates fracture line that has not healed after conventional nonsurgical management. Intercostal nerve block for relief of severe pain: after aspirating, infiltrate with 3–5 mL of lidocaine or bupivacaine just below lower border of the fractured rib, in close approximation to intercostals vessels and nerve (can also block two ribs above and below); risk of causing pneumothorax; multiple fractures may require ORIF. Encourage deep breathing to prevent atelectasis and pneumonia, although incidence of latter in general population is 1.6% in isolated minor rib fractures, with risk rising if ≥2 fractures; avoid/minimize rib belt or taping. Activity modification until symptoms resolve, then gradual resumption of training; changes in technique (if thought to contribute to cause of fracture); nutritional evaluation and pertinent laboratory tests if bone insufficiency suspected.

Prognosis and RTP: RTP when no pain on palpation, no use of analgesics, full ROM of thoracic cage, and ability to sprint/twist without significant discomfort; typically minimum 3 weeks and 6–8 weeks before return to contact sports; ability to protect fracture site should be considered; early return inadvisable because of danger of pneumothorax; close follow-up essential to avoid delayed complications (e.g., excessive callus formation of first rib can cause thoracic outlet syndrome [TOS] or Horner syndrome).

Costochondral Sprain and Separation ("Rib-Tip" or "Slipping Rib Syndrome")

Description: Frequently occurs in contact sports (football, ice hockey, wrestling, lacrosse, rugby) and running, field hockey, rowing, swimming, softball, soccer; weakness or separation of costal cartilage as it attaches to sternum (sternocostal ligament) or separation of anterior margin of rib from anterior end of costal cartilage (costochondral ligament); separation can be congenital or acquired; its hypermobility leads to possible subluxation of cartilaginous rib tip under rib above and impingement of intercostal nerve lying between them; more frequently involves 10th rib, followed by 9th or 8th. More common in females (4:1); often overlooked or misdiagnosed; most >1 year before correct diagnosis is made.

MOI: Forced compression of rib cage, twisting injury, or stretching injury to joint when arm is forcefully pulled to the side; onset sometimes insidious, occurring long after initial trauma because loose ribs can cause further stretching of supporting ligaments

Presentation: Often severe upper abdominal pain or lower CP; usually one dominant symptomatic side; history of feeling a pop; initial sharp discomfort, with severe pain lasting for several days before slowly decreasing in intensity. Pain patterns can include constant dull, achy, or burning sensation; intermittent unilateral pain in anterior ends of lower costal cartilages; or severe sharp pain triggered by respiratory movements, sneezing, and coughing or during bending, twisting, or lifting maneuvers, with painful click as cartilage and bone override one another. Pain can radiate toward epigastrium or spine. Because of crossover in innervation of intercostal nerves and visceral sympathetic nerves at spinal cord, abdominal pain can be associated with nausea and vomiting if severe.

PE: Localized swelling and tenderness at involved joint; possible deformity because of cartilage displacement. Reproducible pain and sometimes clicking when curling fingers under costochondral junction in question and lifting region superiorly and anteriorly to palpate subluxing rib ("hooking maneuver"). Can reproduce pain by pushing posteriorly and superiorly on affected rib to move it under rib above ("rib push maneuver"). Almost 20% are hypermobile.

Differential diagnosis/associated injuries:

- **Costochondritis or costosternal syndrome:** Both traumatic and nontraumatic; self-limiting; multiple sites of tenderness (usually second to sixth costal cartilages) but without swelling
- **Tietze syndrome:** Traumatic and nontraumatic; self-limiting; usually only second or third costochondral junction involved with localized swelling
- **Other causes of upper abdominal and lower CP:** Gastric ulcer, cholecystitis, pancreatitis, pleuritic CP, renal colic, rib fracture, oblique or intercostal strain

Diagnostics: CXR if chronic to rule out tumors, Paget disease, or rheumatoid arthritis; imaging with CT or MRI of unknown benefit; dynamic US during rib push and crunch maneuvers best modality to demonstrate abnormal mobility of ribs

Treatment: Ice and NSAIDs; injection of lidocaine or bupivacaine with or without corticosteroid at costochondral junction or for intercostal nerve block; physical therapy for correction of possible posterior dysfunction at corresponding costovertebral joint; surgical resection of affected rib and costal cartilage or resorbable plating of ribs and cartilage for intractable pain

Prognosis and RTP: May take 9–12 weeks to resolve (slow healing); subject to incomplete resolution or recurrence of pain (25%–30%)

Rupture of Pectoralis Major

Description: Most important adductor and internal rotator of shoulder and cosmetically forms anterior wall of axilla. Ruptures can be partial (grades I and II) or complete (grade III). Excessive tension on muscle causes tear of muscle belly, musculotendinous junction, or tendinous insertion on humerus lateral to bicipital groove; latter most common. Tears of proximal sternal origin are rare; may be associated with anabolic steroid use (muscle hypertrophy not accompanied by tendon adaptation); increased incidence over past several years

MOI: Excessive tension on maximally and eccentrically contracted muscles while affected UE is externally rotated, extended, or abducted. Commonly seen with bench pressing, waterskiing, wrestling, boxing, football, and other sudden violent deceleration maneuvers with sudden stretching and co-contraction of muscle (grasping at objects to prevent fall, punching, or blocking with outstretched arm).

Presentation: Sudden stress or direct blow to shoulder while arm abducted and extended; sudden onset of extreme pain on medial aspect of UEs or in chest wall; tearing, snapping, or popping sensation; significant swelling and ecchymosis; painful limitation of motion; weakness of involved UE; after resolution of swelling and ecchymosis, complaints of asymmetry and persistent weakness.

PE: Swelling and hemorrhage into arm and across anterior chest wall; weakness and pain during resisted internal rotation, flexion, and adduction of arm; deformity of chest wall and palpable muscle bulge with resisted adduction; with abduction, defect in anterior axillary fold if tendon is avulsed at insertion; shoulder ROM limited by pain

Differential diagnosis/associated injuries: Pectoralis muscle tendonitis/tendinosis and congenital absence of pectoralis major muscle

Diagnostics: CXR reveals soft tissue swelling and absent pectoralis major muscle shadow but limited in diagnosis and characterization of ruptures; shoulder radiographs to rule out bony avulsions/fractures. US shows uneven echogenicity and muscle thinning; useful when clinical examination is in question and prompt MRI unavailable; MRI with appropriate sequences accurately defines extent of injury (grade), location, and amount of retraction; guides treatment plan

Treatment: Extent of tear may be difficult to diagnose because of ecchymosis, swelling, and extreme pain; serial examinations important; partial tear treated conservatively with initial ice, analgesia, sling for comfort, and activity restriction. Start passive and active ROM early; by 6–8 weeks resisted strengthening exercises. Activities resumed slowly as allowed by pain and function; complete tear surgically repaired in competitive athletes, particularly those who depend on chest and shoulder strength; without surgical repair, weakness can result, particularly adduction and flexion; repair recommended in bodybuilders for improved cosmesis. Several cases present with delayed diagnosis and thus adhesions, muscle retraction, and atrophy, but late repair compatible with significant strength improvement. After surgery, immobilization for 4–6 weeks to protect repair; passive pendulum exercises and passive forward flexion with arm adducted to 130 degrees can begin immediately. Within 6–12 weeks, progress to full passive ROM and add periscapular and isometric strengthening program (avoiding shoulder adduction, internal rotation, and horizontal adduction); by 12 weeks, resistive strengthening exercises begin; by 6 months, light free weights and push-ups

Prognosis and RTP: Surgical repair of distal pectoralis major tears results in almost full recovery of peak torque and work performed (95%). Full recovery of those managed nonsurgically in 56%, but normal ADLs are not affected; nonsurgical management recommended for tears at sternoclavicular origin, although delayed repairs for persistent pain are successful; RTP after surgery averages 5.5 months.

Breast Injuries

Description: Contusions, hematomas, runner's/cyclist's nipple, and breast pain

MOI and presentation: Direct trauma with resultant bleeding and swelling; common in softball and basketball; nipple chafing, pain, eczema, and occasional bleeding from friction and abrasion by clothing during prolonged activity or evaporation of perspiration over chest (see Chapter 40: "Skin Problems in the Athlete"); breast pain often experienced during athletic activity, particularly during running, because of strain on Cooper ligaments (connective tissue that holds and supports breast on chest wall); query if pain is cyclical, and if so, its duration

PE: Examine for additional signs suggestive of other breast conditions, such as a mass, skin changes, or bloody nipple discharge. In runner's nipple, usually bilateral involvement with erythema, edema, oozing, crusting, and occasionally lichenification; systematically examine four breast quadrants in both lying and sitting positions with hands on hips and then above head. Examine axillary, supraclavicular, and infraclavicular lymph nodes.

Differential diagnosis/associated injuries: Pectoralis major strain, costochondritis, rib fractures if significant trauma, fibrocystic breast disease, cyclic mastalgia, contact dermatitis, bacterial or yeast infection of nipple, Paget disease, and breast cancer

Up to 3.3% of women with breast cancer present with breast pain. Individuals with concomitant atopy are predisposed to develop jogger's nipples. For those with breast augmentation and blunt chest trauma, implant rupture can lead to spherical capsular contracture.

Diagnostics: Generally, diagnostic studies not required if no breast masses palpated and no nipple discharge; if pain is focal, US can be considered in women <30 and with or without mammography in women between 30 and 39, and both for women >40

Treatment, prognosis, and RTP:

- See Chapter 40: "Skin Problems in the Athlete" for information on runner's nipple
- **For contusions:** Ice, NSAIDs, and appropriate support; added protective padding. Hematomas rarely require aspiration.
- Can lead to posttraumatic scarring and retraction or thrombophlebitis of superficial veins (Mondor disease); follow up closely to differentiate from breast carcinoma
- Premenarchal athletic injuries to breast bud (Tanner stages I–II; ages 10–11 years) can cause appreciable breast asymmetry (as much as one cup size or more)
- Hormonal therapy may help diminish breast tenderness during phases of menstrual cycle.
- Nicotine may increase breast pain; it increases epinephrine levels, which stimulates cyclic adenosine monophosphate (AMP), a regulator of mammary tissue metabolism.
- During pregnancy, specialized breast support is imperative, as breasts can enlarge by 800 mL.

Lung Injuries

Pulmonary Contusion

Description: Blood and protein leak into alveoli and interstitial spaces, leading to atelectasis and consolidation (Fig. 52.3).

MOI: Blunt trauma

Presentation: CP, SOB, cough, and hemoptysis (see Fig. 52.3)

PE: Hypoxemia (hallmark clinical sign), tachypnea, rales, wheezing, and diminished breath sounds; PE may be normal

Differential diagnosis/associated injuries: Other causes of CP and hemoptysis (pulmonary embolism and pneumonia); with history of chest trauma, injury to pulmonary parenchyma most likely; flail chest greatly associated with pneumothorax or hemothorax; aortic rupture

Diagnostics: Initial CXR may not show severity of injury; nonsegmental patchy infiltrates or consolidation evident between 4 and 48 hours after injury (see Fig. 52.3). CT scans highly sensitive; pulmonary contusions are detected twice as frequently with CT compared with CXR. However, CXR provides clinically valuable information at minimal cost and should be considered a primary imaging tool. US is also highly sensitive and specific. Pulse oximeter or blood gas analysis is helpful.

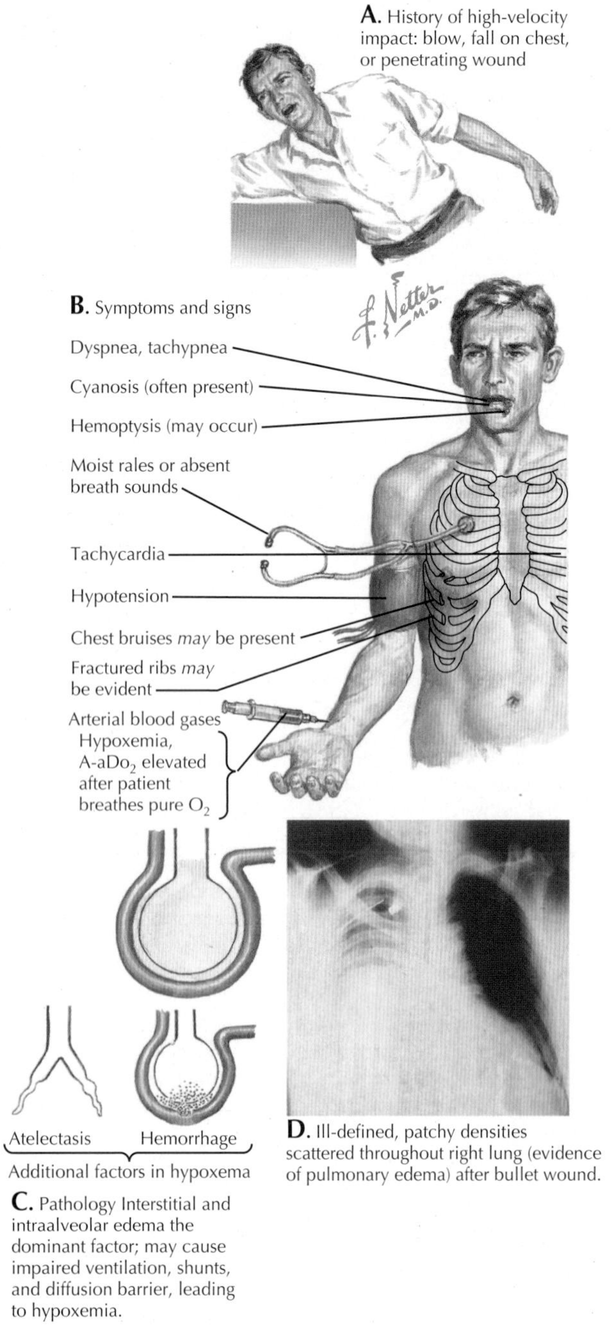
A. History of high-velocity impact: blow, fall on chest, or penetrating wound
B. Symptoms and signs
Dyspnea, tachypnea
Cyanosis (often present)
Hemoptysis (may occur)
Moist rales or absent breath sounds
Tachycardia
Hypotension
Chest bruises *may* be present
Fractured ribs *may* be evident
Arterial blood gases
Hypoxemia, A-aDo$_2$ elevated after patient breathes pure O$_2$
Atelectasis
Hemorrhage
Additional factors in hypoxema
C. Pathology Interstitial and intraalveolar edema the dominant factor; may cause impaired ventilation, shunts, and diffusion barrier, leading to hypoxemia.
D. Ill-defined, patchy densities scattered throughout right lung (evidence of pulmonary edema) after bullet wound.

Figure 52.3 Pulmonary contusion.

Treatment: Supportive therapy; frequent vital sign checks, oxygen support, pain control, and early mobilization. Watch for onset of pneumonia and acute respiratory distress syndrome (ARDS), which may require mechanical ventilation.

Prognosis and RTP: No sport-specific guidelines exist. With mild pulmonary contusion and no CXR findings, gradual RTP after symptoms resolve (within 2–10 days). Traumatic pseudocysts can develop; follow-up imaging to avoid an infection and possible surgical excision. Consider flak jacket for contact sports. Those who recover even from severe pulmonary contusions do not suffer any significant late respiratory problems.

Pneumothorax

Description: Refers to air within chest cavity in pleural space (separation of visceral and parietal pleura), which leads to collapse of lung; classified as **spontaneous** or **traumatic**; described by approximate percentage of hemithorax occupied by free air (e.g., 10%, 50%)

MOI: Typically blunt trauma; spontaneous pneumothorax occasionally precipitated by strenuous physical activities, particularly in tall, thin, young males who smoke; risk increases by defects in lung periphery; these bullae are usually located in lung apex.

Presentation: Gradual or sudden pleuritic CP and dyspnea (depending on size and rate of collapse of lung); pain referred to shoulder

PE: Shallow, rapid respirations; cyanosis; tachycardia; hyperresonance to percussion and decreased or absent breath sounds over affected lung; tracheal shift to contralateral side; possible subcutaneous emphysema

Differential diagnosis/associated injuries: Traumatic rupture of left hemidiaphragm with herniated stomach bubble mistaken for loculated pneumothorax; skin folds act as "Mach bands" and are presumed to be visceral pleural lines; associated with rib fracture(s)

Hemothorax: Blood accumulates in pleural space as a result of bleeding of intercostal or mammary blood vessels and lung parenchyma injury; massive bleeding with aortic or myocardial rupture and injuries to hilar structures; usually associated with pneumothorax. Symptoms include dullness to percussion, decreased breath sounds, and hypotension.

Pneumomediastinum: Excessive intra-alveolar pressures (from exacerbation of asthma, coughing, vomiting, seizures, Valsalva maneuver) lead to rupture of perivascular alveoli; air escapes into surrounding connective tissue, with dissection into mediastinum. Symptoms include CP, persistent cough, sore throat, and substernal CP radiating to back, neck, or shoulders. Subcutaneous emphysema is most consistent physical finding.

Diagnostics: Upright PA CXR shows absence of lung markings in periphery and increased density of collapsed part of lung. White visceral pleural line is evident. Lateral width of 1 cm corresponds to 10% pneumothorax. Small pneumothorax on nondependent side more easily detected in lateral decubitus view; mediastinal shift seen with large pneumothorax. US is popular in acute settings showing absent lung sliding and B-lines; B-lines represent adherence of visceral pleura to parietal pleura.

Treatment: If minimal (15%–30%), stable, and asymptomatic, observation with serial examinations and CXR; avoid unnecessary physical exertion; if large enough to cause SOB and discomfort, transport to hospital for possible tube thoracostomy. In **open pneumothorax** with chest wall defect, ambient air enters the injured hemithorax during inspiration, and the mediastinum shifts to the uninjured side. In expiration, the mediastinum swings back to the injured side, and expiratory air from the normal lung enters the collapsed lung. Place foil, cloth, or other item over wound, securing it only on three sides to avoid development of tension pneumothorax.

Prognosis and RTP: No vigorous activities and air travel for 2–3 weeks after chest tube removal; gradual and monitored RTP. Educate regarding risk of further episodes (reported up to 50% of cases of primary spontaneous pneumothorax).

Tension Pneumothorax

Description: Progressive enlargement of a pneumothorax because of communication between the airways or exterior and interpleural space (Fig. 52.4); **flap valve effect** created; with inspiration, air is drawn into the pleural cavity, whereas with expiration, air stays trapped. Positive intrapleural pressure develops, shifting the mediastinum, and further impairs ventilation of compressed noninjured lung. **Absolute medical emergency**; progressive hypoxia and hypotension lead to death.

MOI: Similar to pneumothorax

Presentation: Rapidly increasing SOB, asymmetry of respiration (see Fig. 52.4)

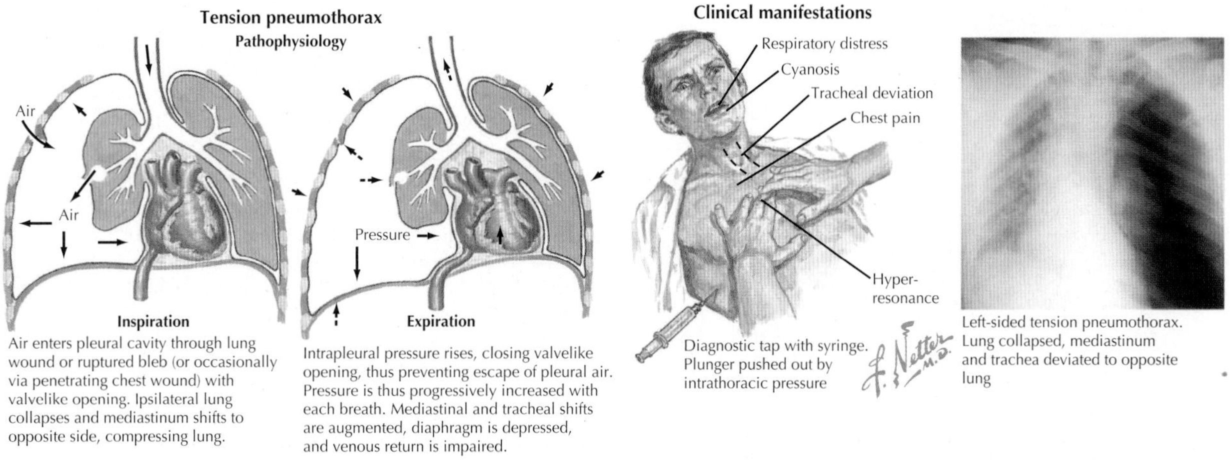
Tension pneumothorax
Pathophysiology
Air
Air
Pressure
Inspiration
Air enters pleural cavity through lung wound or ruptured bleb (or occasionally via penetrating chest wound) with valvelike opening. Ipsilateral lung collapses and mediastinum shifts to opposite side, compressing lung.
Expiration
Intrapleural pressure rises, closing valvelike opening, thus preventing escape of pleural air. Pressure is thus progressively increased with each breath. Mediastinal and tracheal shifts are augmented, diaphragm is depressed, and venous return is impaired.
Clinical manifestations
Respiratory distress
Cyanosis
Tracheal deviation
Chest pain
Hyper-resonance
Diagnostic tap with syringe. Plunger pushed out by intrathoracic pressure
Left-sided tension pneumothorax. Lung collapsed, mediastinum and trachea deviated to opposite lung

Figure 52.4 Tension pneumothorax.

PE: Distended neck veins, cyanosis, hypotension and tachycardia, dyspnea and tachypnea, shift of trachea away from injured side, and absent breath sounds on involved side; hyperresonance on percussion of involved side

Diagnostics: CXR (only if immediately available) shows a distinct shift of mediastinum to contralateral side and flattening of ipsilateral hemidiaphragm.

Treatment: Usually emergently treated before confirmatory CXR with needle decompression; large-bore needle (14–16 gauge) inserted into second intercostal space in midclavicular line on affected side, just over superior aspect of the rib to avoid intercostal vessels; transport to hospital and chest tube placement for definitive treatment. If breathing is spontaneous, hemodynamically stable, and no evidence of respiratory compromise, obtain portable CXR, then place chest tube once diagnosis confirmed.

Prognosis and RTP: No specific RTP guidelines; treated as discussed previously with gradual RTP

Cardiac and Great Vessel Injuries

Myocardial Contusion

Description: Most common blunt cardiac injury; can lead to impaired circulation, arrhythmia, or bleed into pericardium, resulting in cardiac tamponade at time of injury or as late complication several weeks after injury; generally, myocardial contusion refers to structural damage of heart as described in this section; commotio cordis refers to sudden disturbance in heart rhythm via mechanical impact in the absence of structural damage (see Chapter 35: "Cardiac Disease in Athletes")

MOI: Compression of heart between spine and sternum; most commonly from baseball or hockey puck

Presentation: Crushing and sudden deceleration injuries; impact to anterior chest wall; difficult to diagnose because signs typically transient and vary with degree of myocardial damage; athletes may experience CP or sudden cardiac arrest. CP is nonpleuritic; relieved by oxygen but not nitroglycerin

PE: Tachycardia, arrhythmias, chest wall bruising, and signs of decreased cardiac output; cardiac examination usually normal but may show friction rub or murmur

Differential diagnosis/associated injuries: Acute coronary occlusion; sternal or rib fractures, commotio cordis, pneumothorax

Diagnostics:

- **ECG:** Nonspecific, but 70%–85% show abnormalities of ST-segment and T-wave changes, sinus tachycardia, and intraventricular conduction disturbances; seen on initial evaluation and subsequent 3 days after injury; usually transient
- **Biomarkers:** Negative troponin I assay in addition to normal ECG is required to exclude myocardial injury; creatine kinase-MB (CK-MB) is neither sensitive nor specific; not recommended
- **Holter monitor:** If arrhythmias present, most are premature ventricular contractions; atrial fibrillation and other supraventricular arrhythmias also noted
- **Echocardiography:** Transthoracic echocardiogram (TEE) can narrow differential diagnosis of blunt chest trauma and assess cardiac function in the setting of rising cardiac markers. TEE may be a more effective tool to follow suspected contusion and manage myocardial decompensation.
- **Cardiac MRI:** Evolving literature for use of cardiac MRI to identify.

Treatment: For mild contusion, admit for observation and watch for dysrhythmias (more likely to occur in initial 24 hours after injury); more severe contusion associated with other injuries may require invasive monitoring and inotropic medications

Prognosis and RTP: Gradual RTP when stable and showing signs of fully healing from a diagnostic and clinical standpoint. Manufacturers have developed softer baseballs in an attempt to decrease the incidence of morbidity and mortality. Use of chest protector, particularly during batting, is advocated.

Cardiac Tamponade

Description: Accumulation of blood or edematous exudate into pericardial sac; volume and rate of accumulation of fluid determine symptoms; tension created within pericardial sac limits venous inflow and diastolic filling, and cardiac output is diminished (Fig. 52.5); shock and death can rapidly evolve without early recognition and treatment

MOI: Blunt trauma commonly from high-energy collisions

Presentation: Symptoms are variable, but in acute cases, will present with dyspnea, tachycardia, and tachypnea; cold and clammy extremities caused by hypoperfusion

PE: "Beck triad"—hypotension, jugular venous distention, and distant heart sounds; pulsus paradoxus (fall in blood pressure of >10 mmHg on inspiration)—tachycardia and weak pulse

Diagnostics:

- **CXR:** Cardiomegaly, water bottle–shaped heart, pericardial calcifications, or evidence of chest wall trauma
- **ECG:** Low voltage most common; also sinus tachycardia, electrical alternans, and PR-segment depression
- **Echocardiography:** Can dynamically access pericardial effusion and collapse of right ventricle

Treatment: IV fluids and **urgent transport to a hospital**; pericardiocentesis guided by echocardiography and emergent thoracotomy (see Fig. 52.5)

Prognosis and RTP: No evidence-based guidelines; decisions should involve cardiologist and/or cardiothoracic surgeon

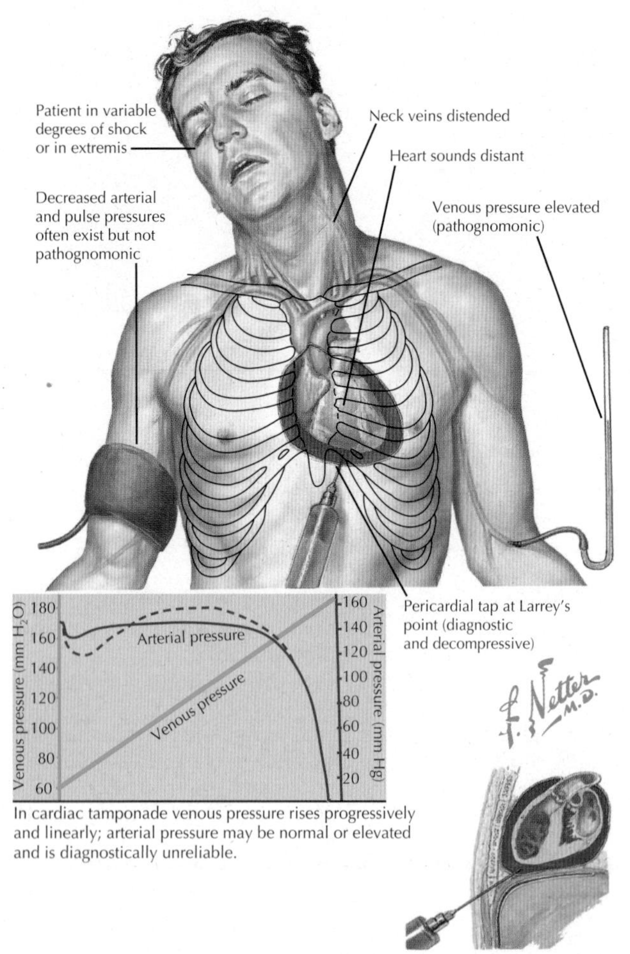

Patient in variable degrees of shock or in extremis
Neck veins distended
Heart sounds distant
Decreased arterial and pulse pressures often exist but not pathognomonic
Venous pressure elevated (pathognomonic)
Pericardial tap at Larrey's point (diagnostic and decompressive)
Venous pressure (mm H_2O)
Arterial pressure (mm Hg)
Arterial pressure
Venous pressure
180
160
140
120
100
80
60
160
140
120
100
80
60
40
20
In cardiac tamponade venous pressure rises progressively and linearly; arterial pressure may be normal or elevated and is diagnostically unreliable.

Figure 52.5 Cardiac tamponade.

Coronary Artery Dissection and Occlusion

Description and MOI: Rare, usually resulting from rapid deceleration of body (e.g., high-speed vehicular collisions); creates enormous shearing forces that may result in intimal dissection or disruption of coronary artery near its origin; intraluminal thrombus can form adjacent to injured arterial wall; can be asymptomatic; may cause angina, myocardial infarction, or death

Presentation: Dyspnea, diaphoresis, severe CP with or without radiation of pain, nausea

PE: Sinus tachycardia, hypotensive or hypertensive, may hear murmur particularly if injury affects valvular function or wall motion

Diagnostics:

- **ECG:** May show ST elevation
- **Biomarkers:** Cardiac troponin may be elevated
- **Echocardiography:** Evaluate wall motion abnormality
- **Coronary angiogram:** Evaluate coronary vasculature

Treatment: Conservative, because lesion may heal with medical management: IV morphine, nitroglycerin; anticoagulation with heparin and acetylsalicylic acid; beta-blocker, statin, or later angiotensin-converting enzyme (ACE) inhibitor. Watch for postinfarction complications, including complete heart block, ventricular arrhythmias, left ventricular failure, ventricular aneurysm, and pulmonary emboli. With ongoing ischemia, coronary angiography can confirm diagnosis and assess extent of injury.

Prognosis and RTP: Dependent on extent of injury and treatment used; decisions should be made in conjunction with cardiologist

Traumatic Aortic Rupture

Description: Only 0.3% of blunt trauma admissions had aortic injury and isolated aortic injury is rare (0.03%); approximately 80%–90% fatality rate at accident scene; disruption extends through full thickness of aortic wall, with rapid exsanguination into mediastinum and pleural spaces; rupture sufficiently contained by adventitia to allow long enough survival to reach medical attention in only 20%; potentially higher risk with **Marfan syndrome** (cystic medial necrosis causes aortic dilatation), and these athletes are restricted from contact and high-exertion sports

MOI: High-speed, deceleration-type injuries (e.g., motor sports, bicycling, skiing, snowboarding); tremendous torques that result from sudden deceleration affect junction of fixed and mobile parts of great vessels, as between aortic arch and fixed descending aorta

Presentation: Sudden anterior chest or interscapular pain that can migrate, dyspnea, hoarseness, occasionally neurologic deficits seen; can be difficult to detect initially

PE: One-third to one-half of patients have minimal to no external signs of chest trauma; using only systolic blood pressure ≤90 mmHg to determine hemodynamic instability can miss 50% of patients; can have hypertension in UEs with pulse pressure widening; with **ascending aortic injury,** aortic diastolic murmur radiating to back because of incompetence of aortic valve; acute coarctation syndrome in up to 25% of **descending aortic injuries:** caused by partial obstruction of aortic lumen, UE hypertension, diminution of femoral pulses and leg blood pressure, and systolic murmur

Diagnostics:

- **CXR:** Most consistent findings are obscuring of aortic knob shadow and widening of superior mediastinum, but the latter has low sensitivity for aortic injury (33%). Other findings: deviation of trachea to the right, depression of left mainstem bronchus, left apical extrapleural density, and left pleural effusion. Seven-point NEXUS Chest CT decision instrument (DI) screening tool has 100% sensitivity for aortic injury.
- **ECG:** May show left ventricular hypertrophy or myocardial ischemia or infarction
- **TEE:** Highly sensitive and specific; valuable in hemodynamically unstable patients
- **CT angiogram:** Highly sensitive and specific; can help identify grade of injury to determine treatment plan
- **Cardiac MRI:** Evolving literature for use of cardiac MRI to identify.

Treatment: Medical therapy to avoid sudden rupture, including antihypertensive agents and beta-blockers; emergent operative repair results in 75%–90% survival

Prognosis and RTP: Mortality and morbidity rates for repair of this condition are among the highest in cardiovascular surgery; RTP decisions should be made with consultation of a cardiologist and/or cardiothoracic surgeon.

Thoracic Outlet Syndrome

Description: Spectrum of signs and symptoms resulting from compression of neurovascular bundle (brachial plexus [nTOS], subclavian and axillary arteries [aTOS], and veins [vTOS]) in interval between intervertebral foramina and axilla (Fig. 52.6); clinical presentations differ according to different degrees of compression. Greater incidence in women with nTOS, whereas vascular TOS is more common in athletic men.

MOI: Related to areas of compression:

- **Supraclavicular region:** Interscalene triangle bordered by anterior and middle scalene muscles that attach to first rib. Contributing factors: hypertrophy of scalene muscles; long transverse process of C7, cervical ribs, or other rib anomalies; and fibrous band changes in alignment and angulation of first rib, as may occur with age and postural changes.

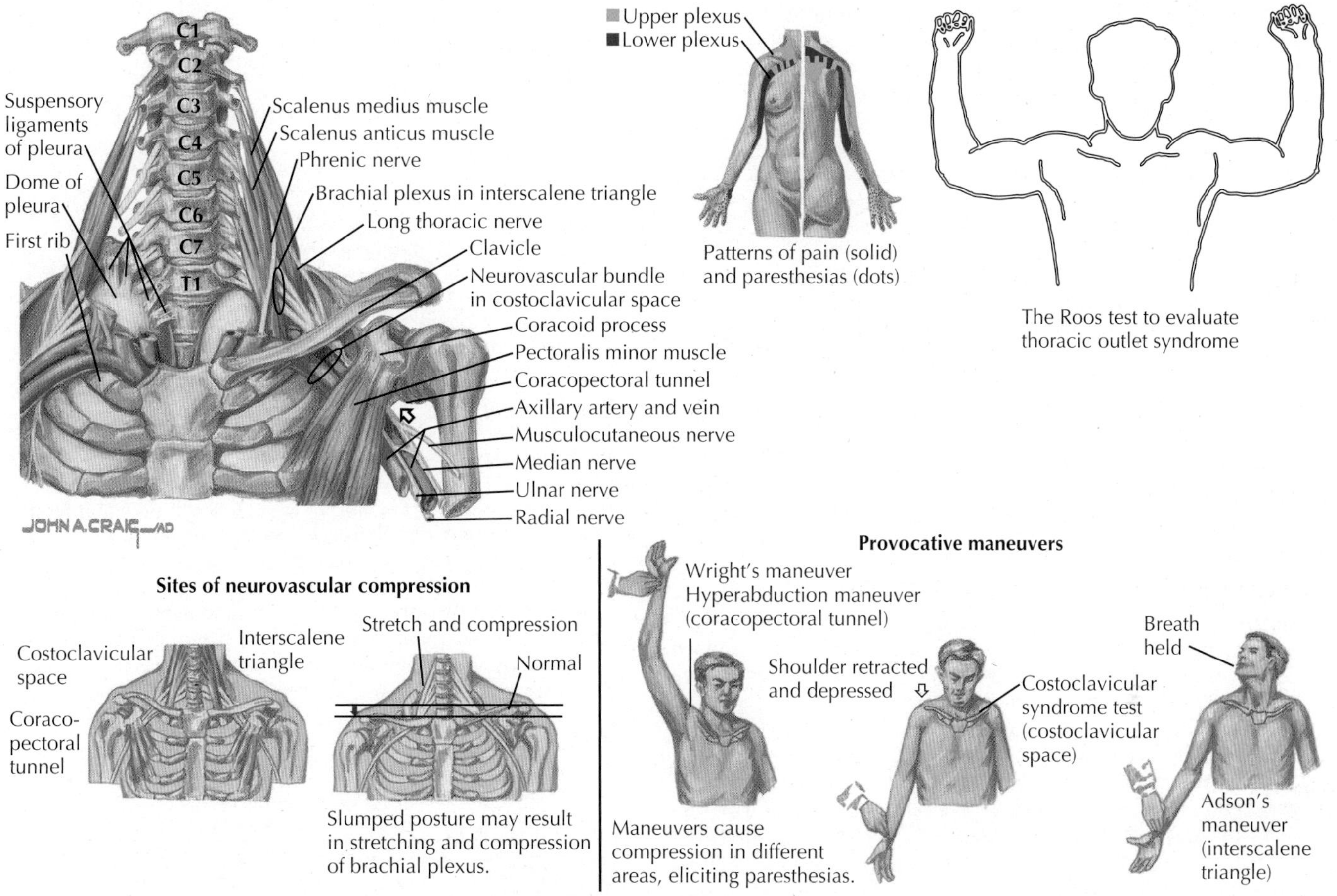
C1
C2
C3
C4
C5
C6
C7
T1
Suspensory ligaments of pleura
Dome of pleura
First rib
Scalenus medius muscle
Scalenus anticus muscle
Phrenic nerve
Brachial plexus in interscalene triangle
Long thoracic nerve
Clavicle
Neurovascular bundle in costoclavicular space
Coracoid process
Pectoralis minor muscle
Coracopectoral tunnel
Axillary artery and vein
Musculocutaneous nerve
Median nerve
Ulnar nerve
Radial nerve
JOHN A.CRAIG_AD
Upper plexus
Lower plexus
Patterns of pain (solid) and paresthesias (dots)
The Roos test to evaluate thoracic outlet syndrome
Sites of neurovascular compression
Costoclavicular space
Interscalene triangle
Coraco-pectoral tunnel
Stretch and compression
Normal
Slumped posture may result in stretching and compression of brachial plexus.
Provocative maneuvers
Wright's maneuver
Hyperabduction maneuver (coracopectoral tunnel)
Shoulder retracted and depressed
Costoclavicular syndrome test (costoclavicular space)
Breath held
Adson's maneuver (interscalene triangle)
Maneuvers cause compression in different areas, eliciting paresthesias.

Figure 52.6 Thoracic outlet syndrome.

- **Subclavicular or costoclavicular region:** Between "mobile" clavicle and "fixed" first rib; changes in shape and mobility of clavicle, such as callus from fracture or alteration in shoulder motion, can narrow interval; subclavius muscle lies behind clavicle and just anterior to subclavian vein
- **Infraclavicular region:** At coracoid process of scapula; compression by pectoralis minor, which inserts at coracoid, during full abduction; subcoracoid area thickens the costocoracoid membrane; another contributing factor is any lesion involving the pleura, such as a neoplasm

Presentation:

- **Neural compression symptoms:** Pain from root of neck to shoulder and diffusely down arm; if lower trunk of brachial plexus compressed (most common), paresthesias involving medial aspect of elbow, forearm, and hand, particularly little and ring fingers; weakness and occasionally atrophy of affected hand; sometimes just a vague ache and heaviness in shoulder, upper arm, and upper anterior and posterior chest, including trapezius and suboccipital region; if patient sleeps with arms above head, may awaken with symptoms at night
- **Arterial compression symptoms:** Hand feels cold and arm becomes numb and fatigued with rapid overhead movement
- **Venous compression symptoms:** Swelling and discoloration of arm after exercise and prominent superficial venous pattern over ipsilateral shoulder and chest

PE: Neck, cervical spine, shoulder, elbow, and hand; check supraclavicular fossa for masses or bruits; careful neurologic examination

- **Adson maneuver:** Arm abducted and externally rotated while head extended and turned to side of lesion; radial pulse monitored while deep breath is taken and held; positive test equals diminution or total loss of pulse; positive in up to 30% of asymptomatic population
- **Wright maneuver:** Similar to Adson except arm is hyperabducted, with hand brought over head with elbow and arm in coronal plane; 70%–90% sensitivity and 29%–53% specificity
- **Military brace position or costoclavicular syndrome test:** Shoulders are retracted and pulled down to narrow the interval between the clavicle and first rib and reproduce symptoms, including absence of radial pulse; effective test in those with symptoms when wearing backpack
- **Overhead exercise test (Roos test):** Arms are abducted to 90 degrees, shoulders externally rotated, and elbows flexed to 90 degrees (see Fig. 52.6); hands opened and closed slowly for 3 minutes to reproduce symptoms of fatigue, cramping, numbness and tingling, or coolness or paleness of extremity; false-positive rate as high as 47% in normal individuals

Differential diagnosis/associated injuries: Shoulder instability and "dead arm syndrome"; cervical spine pathology; peripheral neuropathies; Raynaud phenomenon (can be present with both TOS and collagen vascular diseases); complex regional pain syndrome; Pancoast tumor or other space-occupying lesion in thoracic outlet; **myofascial syndrome** (periscapular region, base of neck, and chest wall are common areas of pain and fatigue; trigger points found in supraspinous fossa near rhomboids, levator scapula, and infraspinatus can cause pain to radiate down arm)

Diagnostics: Cervical spine radiographs to assess for cervical ribs; CXR to evaluate lung apex; electrodiagnostic studies when suspecting nTOS; injection of local anesthetic into anterior scalene can help diagnose nTOS; CT angiography and venography have supplanted conventional venography or arteriography to evaluate vascular structures. US can be useful to evaluate for vascular TOS, but is operator dependent; MRI is optimal for brachial plexus nerve compression and can be combined with MR angiography to evaluate vascular findings or anatomic detail for surgical planning.

Treatment: Conservative management results in 50%–90% recovery. Strengthen shoulder girdle suspensory muscles; NSAIDs; steroid or anesthetic injection into anterior scalene; stretch scalenes, lateral neck flexors, and pectoral muscles. Other measures include weight reduction, posture training, and appropriate brassiere support. Avoid hyperabduction of shoulder and carrying heavy packages in affected hand. Surgery considered only if diagnosis is firm and conservative treatment has failed (4–6 months), with symptoms of intractable pain or major neurologic or vascular complications. First rib resection is most dependable, but surgical procedure varies depending on anatomic basis for symptoms.

Prognosis and RTP: Conservative treatment generally results in recovery from injury; RTP guided by patient's clinical symptoms

Vascular Injuries of Subclavian and Axillary Veins

Description: "Effort thrombosis" (Paget–Schroetter syndrome), or primary thrombosis, describes traumatic thrombosis of subclavian or axillary vein; rare phenomenon; associated most often with baseball (27%) and weightlifting (20%)

MOI: May occur after single traumatic event around the shoulder or clavicle (clavicular fracture, axillary hematoma, injury to axillary or subclavian vein); **more commonly associated with repetitive overhand motions causing trauma to a vessel** (e.g., hyperabduction, external rotation); primary thrombosis is related to inherent anatomic structure of thoracic outlet and axillary region, with compression at various points causing damage to vein walls.

Presentation: Pain and diffuse swelling in arm; numbness, heaviness, and easy fatigability; distention of superficial arm veins with cyanosis (bluish discoloration) of skin; onset of symptoms commonly within 24–72 hours of activity

PE: Increased girth of affected UE, and perhaps weakness of UE, particularly if venous occlusion long-standing; symptoms often reproduced with exercise test of affected UE or by putting arms into extreme hyperabduction

Differential diagnosis/associated injuries: Rule out secondary causes of thrombosis (sarcoidosis, infection, drug use, hypercoagulable states, and metastatic tumor) and poor circulation; lymphedema; arterial occlusion, including **aneurysms of subclavian or axillary arteries**, also reported in athletes; classic symptom is early fatigue during act of throwing; other symptoms: absent pulses, cyanosis, decreased skin temperature, and finger ischemia secondary to digital embolization. If UE thrombosis is confirmed, watch for signs of pulmonary embolus (incidence approximately 12%).

Diagnostics: D-dimer to exclude thrombosis etiology; initial imaging with duplex Doppler studies; if US is equivocal, can use venography; CXR and cervical spine radiography (AP view); given frequent bilateral presentation, consider evaluation of both UEs

Treatment: NSAIDs and arm elevation for pain relief. For mild, intermittent symptoms and if present >2 weeks from onset can be treated with anticoagulation (e.g., apixaban, rivaroxaban, warfarin) for a minimum of 3 months; for patients who present acutely with moderate-to-severe symptoms <2 weeks thrombolysis with fibrinolytic agents such as streptokinase or urokinase and afterwards bridge to oral anticoagulation; thrombectomy and surgical correction of involved thoracic outlet and axillary structures if documented external compression

Prognosis and RTP: No participation in contact sports while on oral anticoagulants; most athletes RTP in 1 year

Abdominal Injuries

Rectus Sheath Hematoma

Description: Major muscle groups of abdominal wall are rectus abdominis muscles, external and internal obliques, and transversus

MOI: Direct blow to abdominal wall, causing hemorrhage into muscle; may damage either epigastric artery or intramuscular vessels, causing hematoma within sheath, which usually self-tamponades; with violent stretching movements, inferior epigastric artery can rupture and hemorrhage without associated indirect injury to muscle tissue

Presentation: Sudden abdominal pain, particularly with trunk flexion or rotation; local tenderness, rapid swelling, greatest comfort in supported flexed position; may have nausea and vomiting. Rectus sheath hematoma can mimic an acute abdomen.

PE: Abdomen may be somewhat rigid with guarding, increased tenderness over rectus; fixed (within rectus sheath) palpable mass most often below the umbilicus in sitting or lying position; other signs: bluish discoloration around periumbilical region 72 hours after injury (Cullen sign) and pain with resisted trunk or hip flexion; hyperextension of spine causes pain in anterior abdominal wall.

Diagnostics: Laboratory studies: Complete blood count (CBC), international normalized ratio (INR), protime (PR), and partial thromboplastin time (PTT). Based on emergency medicine literature, US can be a useful diagnostic tool. MRI or CT scan may be used to assist in differentiation between intra-abdominal injury and hematoma (Fig. 52.7).

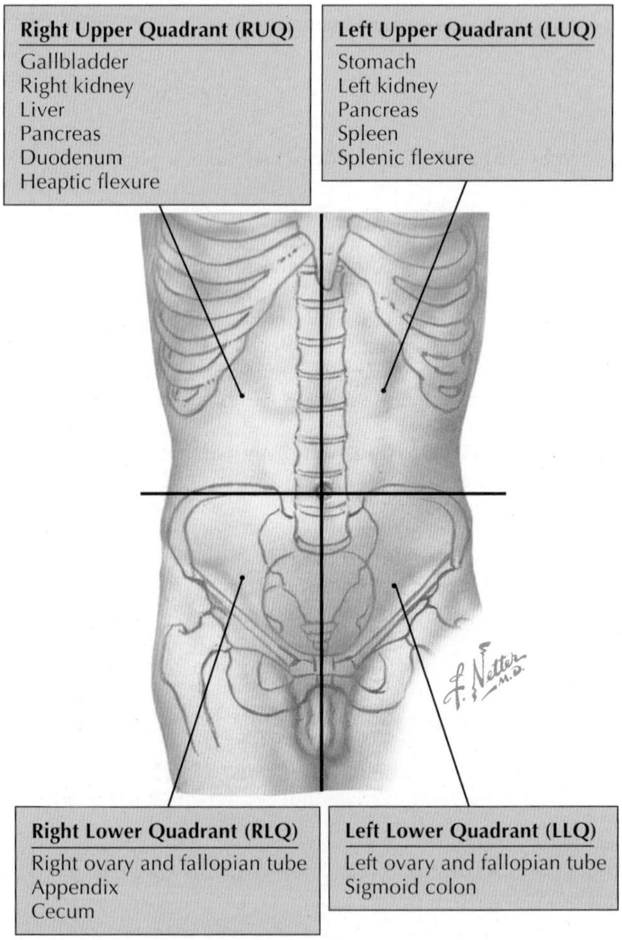
Right Upper Quadrant (RUQ)
Gallbladder
Right kidney
Liver
Pancreas
Duodenum
Heaptic flexure
Left Upper Quadrant (LUQ)
Stomach
Left kidney
Pancreas
Spleen
Splenic flexure
Right Lower Quadrant (RLQ)
Right ovary and fallopian tube
Appendix
Cecum
Left Lower Quadrant (LLQ)
Left ovary and fallopian tube
Sigmoid colon
F. Netter M.D.

Figure 52.7 Quadrants of abdomen.

Treatment: Ice, activity modification, and NSAIDs; local heat after 48–72 hours. Avoid activities requiring rotation, stretching, or flexion of trunk or lower extremities. Rehabilitation concentrates on restoring flexibility, strength, and endurance of all abdominal muscles. If hemorrhage extensive and superficial epigastric artery is torn, may require operative evacuation of hematoma and ligation of artery

Rupture of Diaphragm

Description: Herniation of abdominal contents into chest (Fig. 52.8); twice more common on left side with blunt trauma (there is some degree of protection from the liver on the right); easily overlooked because of delayed onset of symptoms

MOI: Blunt chest or abdominal trauma from high-energy injuries

Presentation: CP, epigastric pain, referred shoulder pain, SOB, vomiting, dysphagia, and intestinal obstruction

PE: Decreased breath sounds, excessive percussion of tympany in chest; bowel sounds in chest and scaphoid abdomen

Differential diagnosis/associated injuries: Hemothorax, pneumothorax, pulmonary contusion, blunt thoracic aortic tear, and elevated hemidiaphragm because of other reasons; associated with splenic rupture in 26% of patients, liver lacerations in 37%, hollow viscus injuries in 26%, pelvic fracture in 40%, rib fracture in 52%, and thoracic aortic tears in 5%

Diagnostics: CXR and abdominal films show dilated stomach in lower chest. Presence of nasogastric tube terminating in air space is confirmatory. Abdominal CT with reformatted images: for left-sided hernias, 87% sensitivity and 100% specificity; for right-sided hernias, 50% sensitivity and 100% specificity; MRI with clinical suspicion and indeterminate CXR and CT findings.

Treatment: Immediate surgical repair with laparotomy; thoracotomy may be necessary for patients with chronic injury; watch for complications of pneumonia and abscess

Prognosis and RTP: Mortality rate 1%–28% due to associated injuries. Complications include missed diaphragmatic injuries; delayed diagnosis may result in intestinal herniation, ischemia, and necrosis; no RTP literature

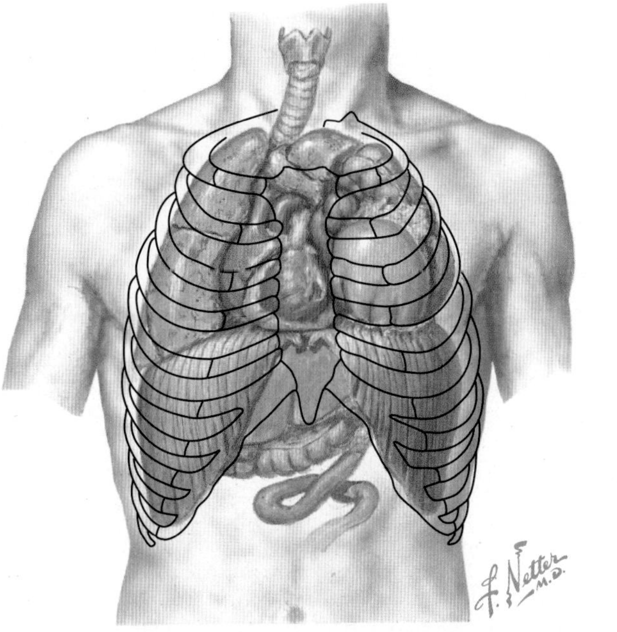

May result from blunt impact or compression or from penetrating wound. Stomach and other abdominal viscera herniated into left thorax; left lung collapsed, right lung compressed; mediastinum shifted and trachea deviated to right.

Figure 52.8 Rupture of diaphragm.

Splenic Rupture

Description: Spleen most commonly injured organ in sport and **most frequent cause of death related to abdominal injury.** Although rib cage offers a certain amount of protection, rib fractures can leave the spleen more vulnerable to injury. Spleen's capacity for encapsulating bleeding delays overt signs and symptoms of rupture; may be days before clinical deterioration. Spleen can enlarge and weaken during certain illnesses (infectious mononucleosis and sarcoidosis), making it more susceptible to rupture.

MOI: Direct trauma to left lower chest from falls, sporting injuries, or MVAs

Presentation: Initial sharp pain in left upper abdomen, then continuation of dull, left-sided flank pain; abdominal distention; referred pain to either right or, more commonly, left shoulder **(Kehr sign)** from free intraperitoneal blood irritating the diaphragm. Neck pain may be referred from phrenic nerve pressure **(Saegesser sign).**

PE: Generalized abdominal tenderness; may have rebound tenderness and rigid abdomen; tenderness over 10th, 11th, or 12th ribs; tachycardia, hypotension, diaphoresis, and rapid respirations suggest internal bleeding; fixed dullness in left flank **(Ballance sign)**

Differential diagnosis/associated injuries: Left-sided 11th and 12th rib fractures and abdominal contusions

Diagnostics: Imaging studies: Flat-plate abdominal radiographs may show fading splenic outline and growing splenic shadow. CT scan with contrast (greater sensitivity and specificity and greater anatomic detailing of spleen and surrounding structures than radionuclide scan) is current diagnostic imaging standard; US; arteriogram; peritoneal lavage (useful but can miss subcapsular tear)

Laboratory studies:

- Decreased hemoglobin and hematocrit levels
- Markedly elevated white blood count if subcapsular hematoma has developed
- Diagnostic peritoneal lavage is positive unless bleeding is encapsulated (10 mL of free blood, >100,000 red blood cells/mm^3, or >500 white blood cells/mm^3)

Treatment:

- If splenic injury suspected, immediate transport to hospital; if hypotensive, give bolus of IV fluids; keep flat or in modified Trendelenburg position to direct blood flow to heart
- Various grading systems, based on anatomic location of splenic injury on CT scan, help guide treatment and predict outcomes. If hemodynamically stable and splenic injury is minimal or subcapsular, nonsurgical management with observation in critical care setting is preferred treatment; splenic preservation is preferred over splenectomy, particularly in pediatric population.
- Exploratory laparoscopy/laparotomy indicated if continued hemodynamic instability or if require >4 units of blood during a 48-hour period; first choice: repair of capsular lacerations (splenorrhaphy); splenectomy only for extensive injury and uncontrolled hemorrhage; after splenectomy, vaccinate for encapsulated organisms (*Streptococcus pneumoniae*, *Haemophilus influenzae*, and *Neisseria meningitides*).
- Beware of **"delayed rupture"** of spleen; occurs >7 days after initial negative CT scan; need high index of suspicion and liberal utilization of other imaging techniques.

Prognosis and RTP: After 3 months in nonsurgical patients (may be longer depending on results of follow-up studies; interval studies useful in predicting RTP); after 3–6 months in postsplenectomy patients; postsplenectomy patients often return before those treated conservatively; may RTP when surgical scars are healed and able to tolerate activity

Liver Laceration

Description: Relatively rare; usually results from high-speed accidents during motor racing and skiing; capsular hematoma most common liver injury in athletes

MOI: Blows to right upper quadrant (RUQ)

Diagnosis: Pain in RUQ, right shoulder, or neck pain

PE: Pain and tenderness to palpation over RUQ; tachycardia and hypotension; may be associated with right lower rib fractures

Differential diagnosis/associated injuries: Pancreatic injury; obtain serum amylase levels

Diagnostics: CT scan with contrast, US, arteriogram, liver enzymes (aspartate aminotransferase [AST] or alanine aminotransferase [ALT] 130 IU/L indicates liver injury), and peritoneal lavage

Treatment: Grading systems based on anatomic location of lesions on CT scan help determine treatment and prognosis; 50%–80% of liver injuries stop bleeding spontaneously. Rest, observation, and IV fluids for hemodynamically stable patients with no signs of peritoneal irritation and no other intra-abdominal injuries that may require surgical repair; laparotomy may be necessary to control bleeding.

Prognosis and RTP: Length of time varies; interval radiographic studies help predict; RTP guidelines not established; athletes must show anatomic and functional healing before participation.

Rupture of Stomach and Intestines

Description: Injuries are rare

MOI: Forceful kick or blow to abdomen; falls off horse or against equipment, as in gymnastics; pile-ons and spearing in football; handlebar accidents in cycling; diving decompression accidents

Presentation: Persistent abdominal pain with signs of chemical or bacterial peritonitis, including fever, nausea, and vomiting; referred shoulder pain from irritation of diaphragm; may have blood in stool if intramucosal hemorrhage present

PE: Localized pain, guarding, rebound tenderness, absence of normal bowel sounds, rigid abdomen; clammy, sweaty skin; hypotension and tachycardia; absence of normal respiratory motion of abdomen; gross or occult blood on rectal examination

Associated injuries: Intramural hematoma of duodenum may manifest as gastric outlet or high small bowel obstruction

Diagnostics: Plain radiograph with upright and decubitus abdominal views shows free air under diaphragm or along abdominal wall; keep athlete in appropriate positions for 3 minutes before views are taken; peritoneal lavage not helpful for duodenal or large intestine injuries because of retroperitoneal position; nasogastric tube placement to check for blood if damage to stomach suspected; meglumine diatrizoate (Gastrografin) swallow; CT abdomen

Treatment: Urgent transport to hospital if increasing pain, signs of peritonitis, or circulatory collapse develops; infuse IV fluid until transport arrives; serial examinations, nasogastric tube, and IV fluids; abdominal exploration and repair

Prognosis and RTP: Length of time may vary; RTP guidelines not established; decisions should be made with a general surgeon

Pancreatic Injury

Description: Injuries rare; pancreas is relatively immobile and in protected retroperitoneum; injuries to pancreas most often occur with direct contact; reported injuries include lacerations and contusions to body and duct of pancreas

MOI: Similar to injuries to stomach and intestine

Presentation: Abdominal pain; can diminish within initial 2 hours after injury then subsequently increase in following 6–8 hours

PE: Abdominal or epigastric pain, abdominal wall ecchymosis; rebound tenderness is rare

Diagnostics: Often, normal amylase immediately after trauma; amylase neither sensitive nor specific for pancreatic injuries, but serial monitoring found to be more specific; lipase more sensitive; hemoglobin (Hgb) and hematocrit (Hct) generally normal because blood loss usually minimal

- **Peritoneal lavage:** Not helpful because of retroperitoneal position of pancreas
- **CT contrast-enhanced:** Efficient screening modality for pancreatic trauma
- **Focused sonography for abdominal trauma (FAST):** Often used in trauma centers as screening in blunt abdominal trauma while checking for intraperitoneal fluid
- **Endoscopic retrograde cholangiopancreatography (ERCP):** Evaluates pancreatic duct; highly sensitive; risk of pancreatitis, hemorrhage, and gastrointestinal tract perforations
- **Magnetic resonance cholangiopancreatography (MRCP):** Noninvasive and accurate method of imaging pancreatic duct

Treatment: Principally supportive, IV fluid hydration, management of metabolic complications, fasting to avoid pancreatic stimulation, parental or enteral jejunal feedings

Prognosis and RTP: Higher morbidity and mortality when pancreatic injuries not recognized in initial 24 hours; no RTP guidelines; progressive RTP after anatomic and functional healing

Hernias

Description: Three most common hernias in adults are indirect inguinal (50%–70%), direct inguinal (men >40 years), and femoral (women). Hernias involving anterior abdominal wall include incisional, periumbilical, and linea alba defects (spigelian hernias); potential for **incarceration** (irreducible hernia) and **strangulation** (twisting of hernia) causing bowel obstruction and toxicity

MOI: Repetitive heavy lifting activities cause increased intra-abdominal pressure, which can contribute to development of hernias, particularly with predisposing weakness of abdominal muscle and fascia; hernias also reported secondary to trauma, such as impact from bicycle handlebar on abdominal wall

Presentation: Aching sensation and occasionally tender swelling in area of hernia; may be scrotal swelling with indirect hernia, as sac extends into inguinal canal

PE: Indirect and direct inguinal hernias are palpated by invaginating scrotum with a finger to palpate external inguinal rings and inguinal canals. Athletes asked to do Valsalva maneuver; elliptical mass descending along spermatic cord and bulging against tip of finger is indirect hernia (Fig. 52.9); globular mass close to pubis that bulges against bottom of finger is direct hernia; **femoral hernias** occur below the inguinal ligament, two fingerbreadths medial to femoral artery (see Fig. 52.9); hernias more prominent when athlete stands or increases intra-abdominal pressure.

Diagnostics:

- **Herniography:** Intraperitoneal injection of contrast material to diagnose occult hernia sacs; 84% incidence of inguinal hernia by herniography in soccer players with groin pain; only 8% had hernias detectable by PE
- Bone scan: Increased uptake in musculature in initial phase
- MRI: Examine soft tissues in groin region
- CT scan: Contrastographic medium combined with CT scan
- US: Helpful in hands of experienced clinician

Differential diagnosis/associated injuries:

- **Defined clinical entities for groin pain: adductor related, iliopsoas-related, inguinal-related, and pubic related in addition to hip pathology.**
- **Adductor related:** Adductor tenderness and pain with resisted adduction.

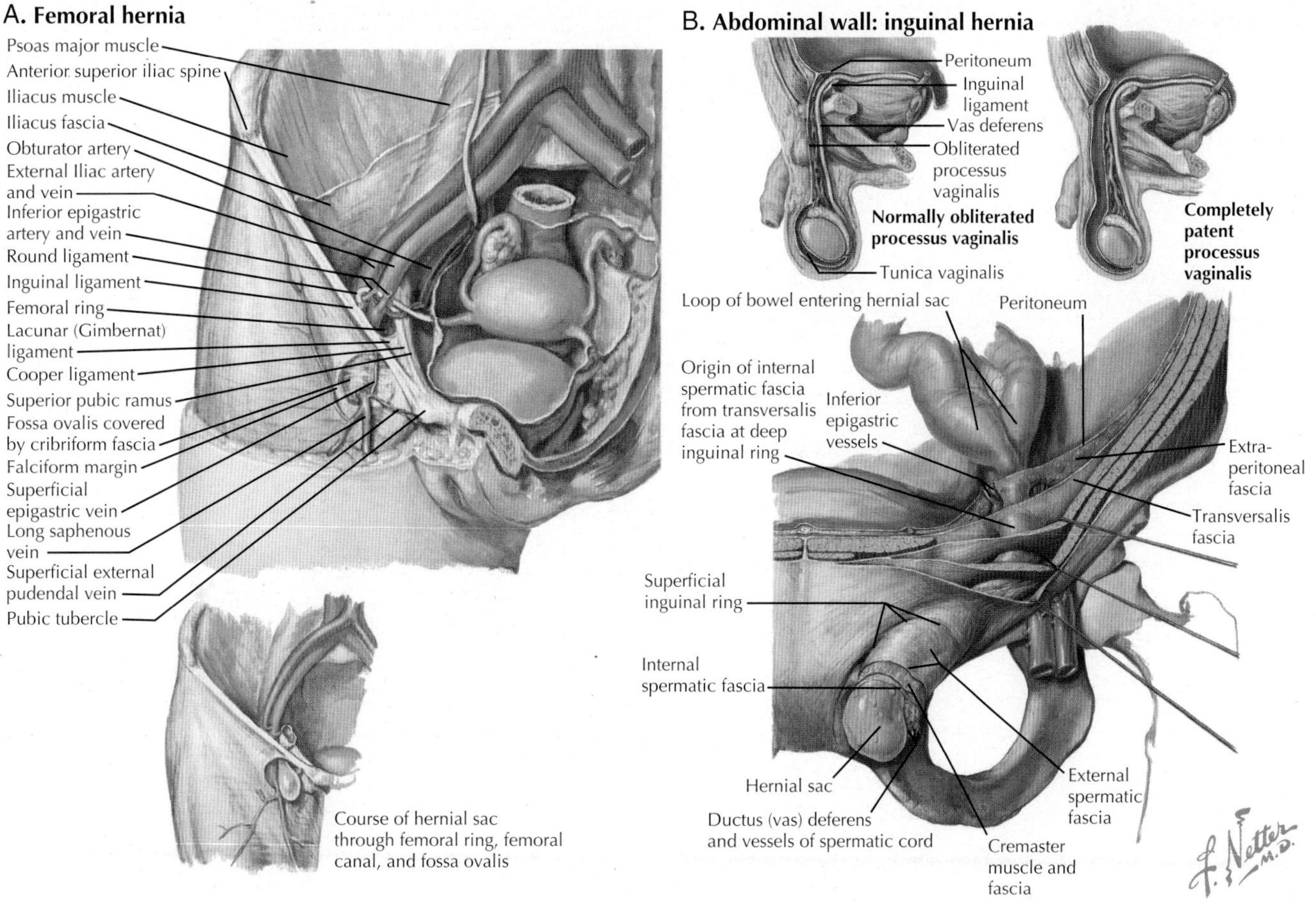
A. Femoral hernia
Psoas major muscle
Anterior superior iliac spine
Iliacus muscle
Iliacus fascia
Obturator artery
External Iliac artery and vein
Inferior epigastric artery and vein
Round ligament
Inguinal ligament
Femoral ring
Lacunar (Gimbernat) ligament
Cooper ligament
Superior pubic ramus
Fossa ovalis covered by cribriform fascia
Falciform margin
Superficial epigastric vein
Long saphenous vein
Superficial external pudendal vein
Pubic tubercle
Course of hernial sac through femoral ring, femoral canal, and fossa ovalis
B. Abdominal wall: inguinal hernia
Peritoneum
Inguinal ligament
Vas deferens
Obliterated processus vaginalis
Normally obliterated processus vaginalis
Tunica vaginalis
Completely patent processus vaginalis
Loop of bowel entering hernial sac
Peritoneum
Origin of internal spermatic fascia from transversalis fascia at deep inguinal ring
Inferior epigastric vessels
Extra-peritoneal fascia
Transversalis fascia
Superficial inguinal ring
Internal spermatic fascia
Hernial sac
Ductus (vas) deferens and vessels of spermatic cord
Cremaster muscle and fascia
External spermatic fascia
F. Netter M.D.

Figure 52.9 Hernias.

- **Iliopsoas-related groin pain:** Groin pain reproduced by passive hip flexion caused by inflammation of bursa between pectineus and psoas muscle; pain on resisted hip flexion and/or pain on stretching the hip flexors.
- **Pubic-related groin pain:** Local tenderness of pubic symphysis and adjacent bone.
- **Inguinal related:** Pain aggravated with resistance testing of abdominal muscles OR on Valsalva/cough/sneeze. Often presents as gradually worsening, poorly localized groin pain aggravated with activity. Herniography shows bulging or areas of weakness of wall. Dynamic US can demonstrate weakening of pelvic floor musculature with Valsalva. Surgical exploration reveals tears in floor of inguinal ring (transversalis fascia). Ilioinguinal nerve is occasionally trapped in scar tissue within torn aponeurosis.
- Other: Muscular strain, hydrocele, or varicocele

Treatment: Treatment for inguinal-related groin pain ("athletic pubalgia"/"sports hernia") is discussed in Chapter 66: "Football" and Chapter 80: "Ice Hockey." Prompt surgical repair for large or symptomatic hernias; avoid activities that stretch or pull the abdominal muscles for 2–4 weeks after repair; then gradually resume progressive exercise and conditioning; by 4 weeks, begin abdominal, back, and pelvic strengthening

RTP: Return to noncontact sports after 6–8 weeks for indirect hernia repairs: RTP at 8–10 weeks; more extensive repairs of direct inguinal, femoral, and anterior abdominal wall hernias require longer recovery: contact sports at 12 weeks.

RECOMMENDED READINGS

Available online.

53 THORACIC AND LUMBOSACRAL SPINE INJURIES

Brock E. Schnebel

GENERAL PRINCIPLES

- With an increased number of adults and adolescents participating in fitness programs and competitive sports, there has been an increase in thoracic and lumbar spinal problems.
- Most injuries are soft tissue injuries, and appropriate training and avoidance of aggravating activities may allow participation while the pain resolves.
- Treatment of an athlete can be complicated by his or her competitiveness and the fact that the athlete will be returning to the activity that precipitated the injury.
- The primary treatment objective is the protection and preservation of the nervous system.
- Spine injuries occur with a reported incidence of 7%–27% among sports-related injuries.
- The use of biologic injections (platelet-rich plasma [PRP], stem cells) for treatment of spinal issues is controversial at this time.

Anatomy

- The spine is a mechanical structure consisting of bones, joints, ligaments, and muscles surrounding and distributing neural elements.
- The thoracic spine is more stable than the lumbar and cervical spine and is less mobile because of the thoracic cage.
- The spinal column is composed of 33 vertebrae divided into five sections: cervical (7), thoracic (12), lumbar (5), sacral (5), and coccygeal (4) (Fig. 53.1).

Osseous

Vertebral body: Large, strong, anterior weight-bearing structure (see Fig. 53.1)

Posterior vertebral arch: Semicircular-shaped structure surrounding the central canal, above and below the **vertebral foramen** through which the roots pass; composed of **pedicles,** which project dorsally off the body, one on each side, and the **lamina,** which connects the pedicles; from the pedicles and lamina, project the **transverse process**; from the lamina, project the **spinous process**; these are locations for muscular attachments. Each lamina articulates with the lamina above and the lamina below through **facet joints.** These **synovial-lined** facet joints are formed by a **superior articular process** from the lamina below and an **inferior articular process** from the lamina above and are surrounded by a facet capsule or ligament (see Fig. 53.1).

Pars interarticularis: Literally, the "part between the joints," or the area between these facet joints; relevant because it is the weak link anatomically and is susceptible to injury and stress fracture

Sacrum: Coalesced lower segments of the spine that articulate with the pelvis

Costovertebral joints: Area of articulation of the thoracic vertebrae with its rib

Disc: Major ligament connecting each vertebral body; composed of two types of tissue: annulus fibrosus (outer layer of fibers that functions to hold the nucleus pulposus and restrains the vertebral bodies) and nucleus pulposus (gelatinous structure located in the annulus)—both are responsible for load-bearing

Ligaments

Anterior longitudinal ligament: Strong bond of fibrous tissue that runs the entire length of the spine along the anterior vertebral bodies (see Fig. 53.1)

Posterior longitudinal ligament: Weaker than the anterior ligament; runs along the posterior surface of the vertebral bodies

Ligamentum flavum: Very strong ligament attaching the lamina above to the lamina below

Facet capsule: Connects each superior articulating process with its corresponding inferior articulating process

Interspinous ligament: Connects each spinous process to the one below

Supraspinous ligament: Runs along the dorsal surface of the tips of the spinous processes

Costotransverse ligaments: Thoracic area

Muscles and Fascia

Thoracolumbar fascia: Investing tissue that separates the muscular compartments and fuses with the aponeuroses of several muscles (see Fig. 53.1)

Anterior groups of muscles: Anterior to the transverse processes; include psoas, intertransversalis, quadratus, and levator costae

Posterior groups of muscles: Posterior to the transverse process; include superficial muscles, erector spinae (semispinalis, longissimus, and iliocostalis), deep muscles, multifidus, rotares, and interspinalis

Accessory group of muscles: Includes abdominal muscles, latissimus dorsi, rhomboids, and gluteus maximus

Neural Elements

- Neural elements of the spine include the spinal cord from the occiput to about L1, the conus medullaris or lower portion of the cord thickened by the mass required to innervate the lower extremities located from T11 to L1, and the cauda equina from L1 to the sacrum; the nerve roots exit at each level on both sides of the canal via the vertebral foramina (see Fig. 53.1).

Vascular Elements

- Vascular elements of the spine include a complex system of intradural and extradural arteries and veins that supply the neural elements.

Biomechanics

- The spinal column has five principal functions:
  - Support of the head
  - Support of the abdominal contents and pelvic girdle
  - Point of attachment for the thoracic cage and muscles
  - Protection of the spinal cord and the neural elements within while allowing motion
  - The biomechanical transfer of the weight and bending movements of the head and trunk to the pelvis
- Understanding several basic concepts of biomechanics helps us understand how specific activities can exacerbate symptoms in certain syndromes:
  - In the spine, flexion of the lumbar spine increases the size of the intervertebral canal and the intervertebral foramina.
  - Extension decreases the size of the intervertebral canal and the intervertebral foramina.
  - Flexion increases dural sac and nerve root tension.
  - Extension decreases dural sac and nerve root tension.
  - Front flexion, axial loading, and an upright posture increase intradiscal pressure: pressure is greater while sitting, less while standing, and least while lying down.

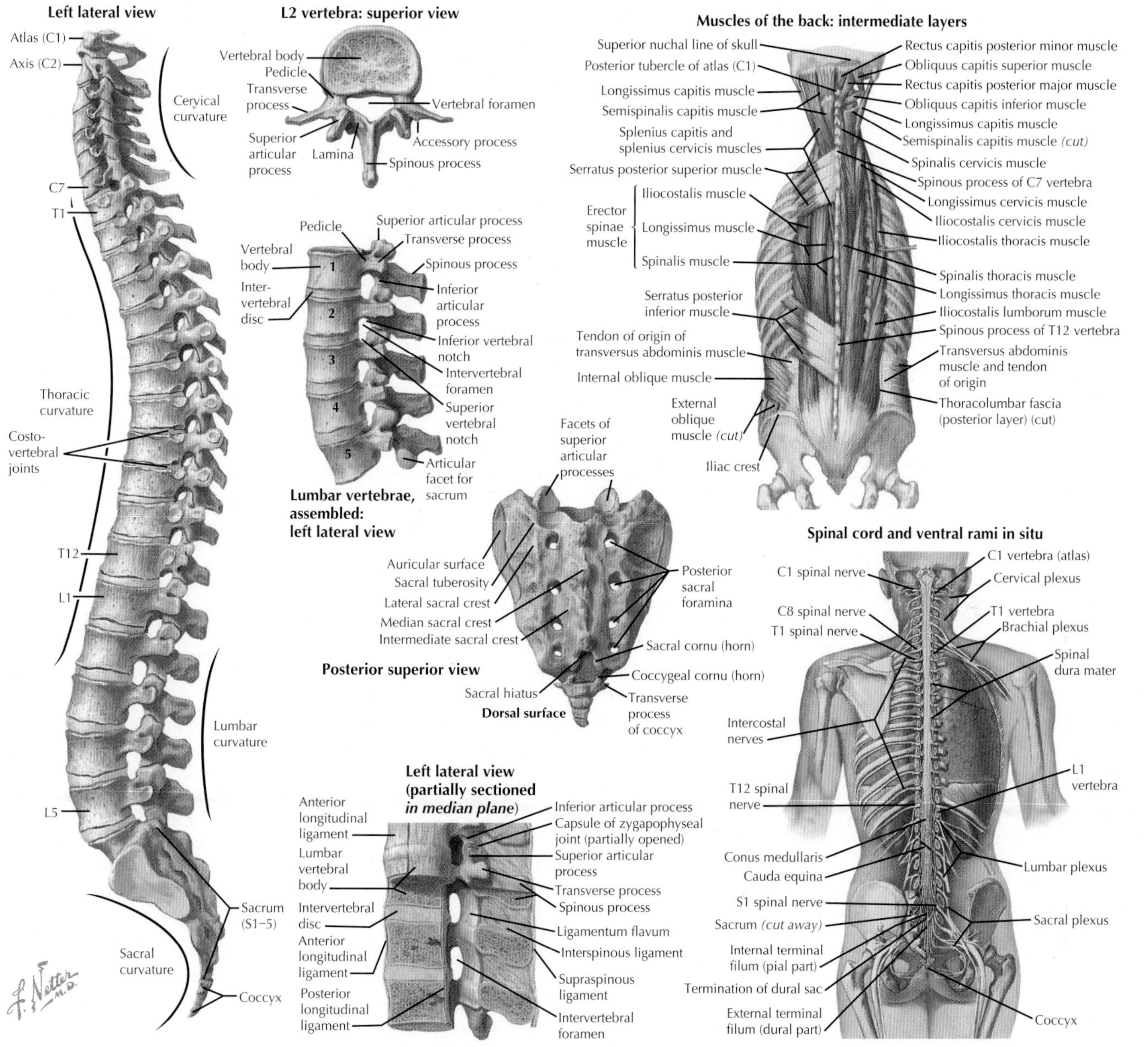
Left lateral view
Atlas (C1)
Axis (C2)
Cervical curvature
C7
T1
Thoracic curvature
Costo-vertebral joints
T12
L1
Lumbar curvature
L5
Sacrum (S1–5)
Sacral curvature
Coccyx
L2 vertebra: superior view
Vertebral body
Pedicle
Transverse process
Vertebral foramen
Superior articular process
Lamina
Accessory process
Spinous process
Pedicle
Superior articular process
Transverse process
Vertebral body
Spinous process
Inter-vertebral disc
Inferior articular process
Inferior vertebral notch
Intervertebral foramen
Superior vertebral notch
Articular facet for sacrum
Lumbar vertebrae, assembled: left lateral view
Muscles of the back: intermediate layers
Superior nuchal line of skull
Posterior tubercle of atlas (C1)
Longissimus capitis muscle
Semispinalis capitis muscle
Splenius capitis and splenius cervicis muscles
Serratus posterior superior muscle
Erector spinae muscle
Iliocostalis muscle
Longissimus muscle
Spinalis muscle
Serratus posterior inferior muscle
Tendon of origin of transversus abdominis muscle
Internal oblique muscle
External oblique muscle (cut)
Iliac crest
Rectus capitis posterior minor muscle
Obliquus capitis superior muscle
Rectus capitis posterior major muscle
Obliquus capitis inferior muscle
Longissimus capitis muscle
Semispinalis capitis muscle (cut)
Spinalis cervicis muscle
Spinous process of C7 vertebra
Longissimus cervicis muscle
Iliocostalis cervicis muscle
Iliocostalis thoracis muscle
Spinalis thoracis muscle
Longissimus thoracis muscle
Iliocostalis lumborum muscle
Spinous process of T12 vertebra
Transversus abdominis muscle and tendon of origin
Thoracolumbar fascia (posterior layer) (cut)
Facets of superior articular processes
Auricular surface
Sacral tuberosity
Lateral sacral crest
Median sacral crest
Intermediate sacral crest
Posterior sacral foramina
Sacral cornu (horn)
Coccygeal cornu (horn)
Transverse process of coccyx
Posterior superior view
Sacral hiatus
Dorsal surface
Left lateral view (partially sectioned in median plane)
Anterior longitudinal ligament
Lumbar vertebral body
Intervertebral disc
Anterior longitudinal ligament
Posterior longitudinal ligament
Inferior articular process
Capsule of zygapophyseal joint (partially opened)
Superior articular process
Transverse process
Spinous process
Ligamentum flavum
Interspinous ligament
Supraspinous ligament
Intervertebral foramen
Spinal cord and ventral rami in situ
C1 spinal nerve
C1 vertebra (atlas)
Cervical plexus
C8 spinal nerve
T1 spinal nerve
T1 vertebra
Brachial plexus
Spinal dura mater
Intercostal nerves
T12 spinal nerve
L1 vertebra
Conus medullaris
Cauda equina
Lumbar plexus
S1 spinal nerve
Sacrum (cut away)
Sacral plexus
Internal terminal filum (pial part)
Termination of dural sac
External terminal filum (dural part)
Coccyx

Figure 53.1 Anatomy of the spine.

- With flexion, the annulus bulges anteriorly.
- With extension, the annulus bulges posteriorly.
- Nuclear shift in an injured disc is poorly documented, but the disc probably shifts in the direction of the annular bulge.
- Rotation and torsion produce annular tears and disc herniations.

History and Physical Examination

History

- Information obtained during history taking and physical examination is critical. The following questions are particularly relevant.
  - **When and how did your symptoms start?** Mechanism of injury can help locate the damage. Onset can be telling because a gradual onset can be more related to a stress injury, and a rapid severe onset may indicate a more acute injury.
  - **What is the location of the pain?** Neurologic involvement is likely when a patient perceives more pain in the leg than in the back. The percentage of back to leg pain is relevant. Associated neurologic symptoms such as numbness, dysesthesia, weakness, or spasticity are important to note. There are multiple nociceptive sources in the spine.
  - **When does it hurt?** Night pain may be more ominous and associated with tumors. Pain with motion and relieved by rest implies mechanical pain. Constant pain unaffected by rest may indicate an inflammatory component.
  - **What makes it worse?** Discogenic pain is usually worse with flexion or prolonged sitting and increases with a Valsalva maneuver (cough or strain with defecation). Pain from a spondylolysis is worse than that with hyperextension. Pain from spinal stenosis (pseudoclaudication) is worse with ambulation or prolonged standing. Sacroiliac (SI) joint dysfunction can be worse with hyperextension.

Table 53.1 COMMON NERVE ROOT FINDING

Root	Strength	Sensation, Dermatomal Distribution	Reflex
L1–L2	Iliopsoas	Inguinal area and upper two-thirds of anterior thigh	
L3	Quadriceps	Oblique band of distal third of anterior thigh immediately above patella	
L4	Tibialis anterior and quadriceps	Medial side of lower leg and foot	Patellar tendon
L5	Extensor hallucis longus and tibialis anterior	Anterior aspect of lower leg and dorsum of foot	Not reliable (posterior tibialis reflex present in only 40%–50% of population)
S1	Peroneus longus and brevis gastrocnemius	Lateral aspect of lower leg and lateral foot	Achilles tendon reflex

- **What makes it better?** Discogenic pain can be improved by lying down with knees and hips flexed (opens foramina and unloads disc). Spinal stenosis symptoms can improve by bending forward (as in walking over a grocery cart) or by sitting.
- **How do you train?** This may reveal a voluntary restriction that helps with a diagnosis or reveals a training error compatible with a specific syndrome.
- **Do you have any of these factors?** Bowel, bladder, or sexual dysfunction may indicate significant neurologic involvement of the cord, conus, or cauda equina. Weight loss, anorexia, night pain, and pain at rest may suggest neoplasia. Fever may indicate infection. A visceral type of pain with referral may indicate kidney, prostate, bowel, or vascular pathology.

Physical Examination

- Should address inspection, palpation, and percussion and identify:
  - Exact location of tenderness, dysesthesias, or numbness
  - Maneuvers that reproduce the pain
  - Presence of neural tension signs
  - Deficits in range of motion (ROM)
  - Any neurologic deficit

Inspection of posture and stance: Patients in a sitting position may tend to tripod or lean back to unload the spine. When standing, a list to one side may suggest nerve root compression. The appearance of a flat back with a vertical sacrum may be seen in advanced spondylolisthesis. Scoliosis may be detected in a standing position.

Inspection of gait: Myelopathic patients may walk with spasticity. A forward flexed posture can be seen in stenosis. Patients with discitis may have a rigid short-stride gait.

Inspection of ROM: May be limited by painful conditions; extension may be limited in stress fractures and facet syndromes. Discogenic pain may limit flexion.

Palpation: May detect muscle spasm, deformity with a palpable mass, scoliosis, spondylolisthesis, or a gibbus deformity; tenderness may be present at the sciatic notch.

Percussion: May elicit tenderness in trauma or infection, and costovertebral angle tenderness may imply a kidney problem

Neurologic: Most critical portion of the examination (Table 53.1 and Fig. 53.2); **upper motor neuron findings** of spasticity, weakness, numbness, hyperreflexia, and clonus may indicate spinal cord pathology; **lower motor neuron findings** of flaccid muscles, weakness, numbness, and hyporeflexia may indicate cauda equina or root injury. Sensory levels on the trunk will help determine the level of spinal cord injury, if present. A rectal and cremasteric reflex examination is recommended with any spinal cord injury.

Special Tests

Pain From Neural Source

Straight leg raise (SLR) test: Tension test that indicates nerve irritation in the sciatic nerve if positive with radicular pain at <60–70 degrees of leg elevation (Fig. 53.3)

SLR test with foot dorsiflexion (Lasègue test): Tension test suggesting sciatic nerve irritation if painful

SLR test while sitting: Positive when extending the knee while patient is sitting causes radicular pain; patient may lean back to gain relief. A positive and a negative SLR test while sitting can be inconsistent and suggest other etiologies.

Crossed SLR test: Positive test may be pathognomonic for a herniated disc. With the patient sitting, the examiner lifts the unaffected leg; in the presence of a herniated disc, this may produce pain in the affected leg.

Femoral stretch test: In a side-lying position with knee flexed 90 degrees, the hip is extended, stretching the femoral nerve. Pain on the anterior thigh suggests femoral nerve or upper lumbar root irritation.

Pain From Structural Source

Jackson one-legged standing hyperextension test: If painful, it suggests a stress fracture (spondylolysis), a facet syndrome, or SI joint dysfunction.

Flexion, abduction, and external rotation of hip (FABER) or Patrick test: Can suggest hip joint or SI joint dysfunction

Supine-to-long sitting test: Examiner tests leg length at the medial malleoli with the patient first supine and then sitting with both legs extended at the knees. A change in relative leg length may indicate SI joint dysfunction.

Radiographic and Ancillary Testing

Plain radiographs: May be unnecessary in the acute phase in a nonathletic clinic setting, but in high-velocity and collision sports, early radiographic evaluation may be needed. Plain radiographs may reveal an acute fracture or spondylolysis that may alter treatment. Plain radiographs may also reveal spondylolisthesis, degenerative changes, signs of infection in discitis (endplate irregularities), or congenital anomalies. Anteroposterior (AP) and lateral radiographs of the lumbar spine may be augmented by right and left obliques if a spondylolysis is suspected.

Bone scan: May be used to reveal lesions that are not yet visible on plain radiographs (e.g., stress fractures in the pars interarticularis); because a positive bone scan indicates increased metabolic activity, this scan may reveal bone tumors or infection in addition to occult fractures. It may take up to 5 days after the onset of symptoms for a bone scan to be positive.

Computed tomography (CT) scan: To evaluate osseous lesions and to help stage stress reactions

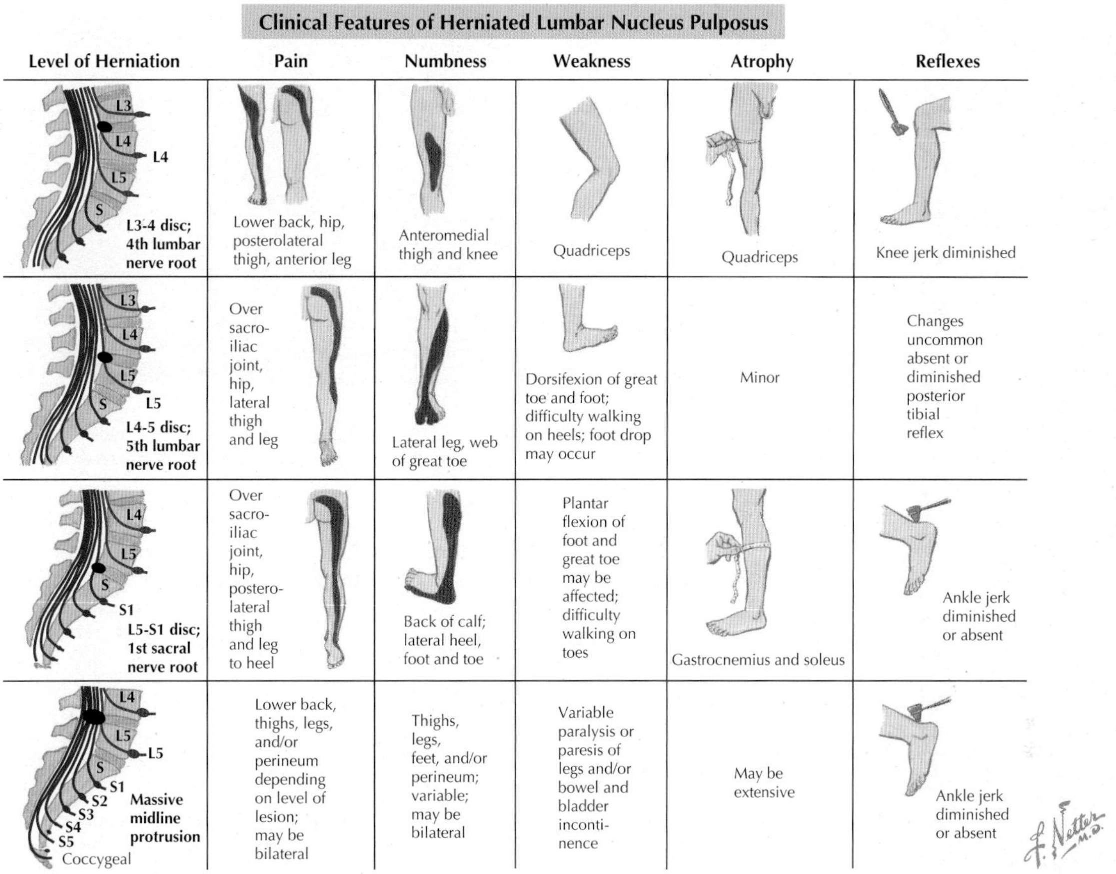
Clinical Features of Herniated Lumbar Nucleus Pulposus
Level of Herniation
Pain
Numbness
Weakness
Atrophy
Reflexes
L3
L4
L4
L5
S
L3-4 disc; 4th lumbar nerve root
Lower back, hip, posterolateral thigh, anterior leg
Anteromedial thigh and knee
Quadriceps
Quadriceps
Knee jerk diminished
L3
L4
L5
S
L5
L4-5 disc; 5th lumbar nerve root
Over sacro-iliac joint, hip, lateral thigh and leg
Lateral leg, web of great toe
Dorsifexion of great toe and foot; difficulty walking on heels; foot drop may occur
Minor
Changes uncommon absent or diminished posterior tibial reflex
L4
L5
S
S1
L5-S1 disc; 1st sacral nerve root
Over sacro-iliac joint, hip, postero-lateral thigh and leg to heel
Back of calf; lateral heel, foot and toe
Plantar flexion of foot and great toe may be affected; difficulty walking on toes
Gastrocnemius and soleus
Ankle jerk diminished or absent
L4
L5
L5
S
S1
S2
S3
S4
S5
Massive midline protrusion
Coccygeal
Lower back, thighs, legs, and/or perineum depending on level of lesion; may be bilateral
Thighs, legs, feet, and/or perineum; variable; may be bilateral
Variable paralysis or paresis of legs and/or bowel and bladder inconti-nence
May be extensive
Ankle jerk diminished or absent

Figure 53.2 Dermatomal distribution of nerves.

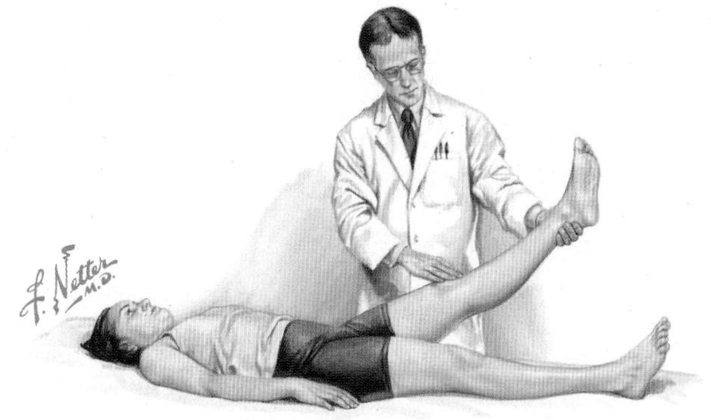

Straight leg raising test
Perform with the knee extended. Flex hip until resistance and/or pain is noted. Test places sciatic nerve, as well as hamstrings on stretch. Patients with herniated disc causing compression of sacral nerve roots often experience back pain radiating to lower extremity.

A *crossed straight leg raising test* is pain in the affected extremity when the contralateral leg is raised and is highly specific for nerve root entrapment.

Figure 53.3 Straight leg raise test.

Magnetic resonance imaging (MRI): To help detect discogenic lesions such as degenerative disease with desiccation, disc herniations, spinal cord lesions, fractures, stress reactions, and compressive lesions

Myelography and CT myelography: May also be used to show compressive lesions

Electromyography (EMG) and nerve conduction velocity (NCV): May help in localizing the location of a nerve compression lesion; it may take up to 3 weeks before denervation changes occur such that they are revealed on an EMG

Laboratory studies: Can be useful in diagnosing discitis, inflammatory spondylitis, or neoplasia, but these studies are rarely needed

SPECIAL INJURIES AND PROBLEMS

Traumatic Injuries to the Thoracic or Lumbar Spine

Description: Motor sports, high-velocity sports, and collision sports are capable of producing significant forces to the thoracic and lumbar spine. Fractures, fracture dislocations, and dislocations can occur with and without neurologic injury (Fig. 53.4). Blunt trauma may produce rib fractures and transverse process fractures. Any of the ligamentous structures may be injured, requiring very specific treatments.

Mechanism of injury: Trauma

Presentation: Pain, limited motion, and possible neurologic findings with neurologic distribution of pain

Physical examination: Local tenderness, possible deformity, neurologic findings with lower motor neuron findings with a lumbar injury (cauda equina) or upper motor neuron findings with a cord injury

Differential diagnosis: Be aware of injuries at multiple levels.

Diagnostics: Imaging techniques, CT, MRI

Treatment: After on-field management and transfer to a care facility, further treatment plans can be made depending on examination and imaging. Certain traumatic injuries can be managed nonsurgically, but surgical intervention may be required in others.

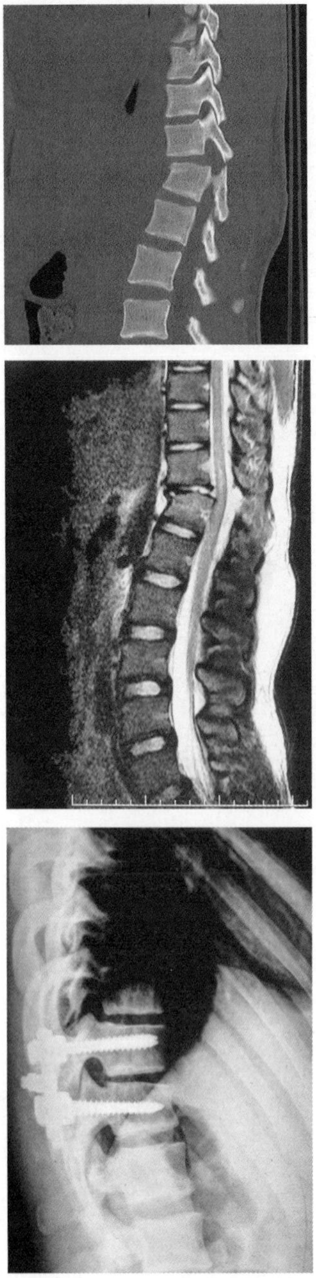

A. CT shows facet dislocation.

B. MRI shows edema in cord, kyphotic deformity, and rupture of the ligamentum flavum.

C. Plain film shows internal fixation postoperative.

Figure 53.4 A National Collegiate Athletic Association (NCAA) football player sustained an accidental injury in the weight room, resulting in a fracture dislocation of T11 on T12, with a conus medullaris spinal cord injury.

Prognosis and return to sport: Dependent on specific injury and neurologic involvement

Thoracic Disc Herniation

Description: The extrusion of nucleus pulposus out of its contained position in the annulus fibrosus; nuclear material may cause a protrusion in the annulus (contained) or escape from the annulus, termed an *extrusion* or *free fragment*

Mechanism of injury: Annular tears occur with torsional loads under pressure; through these tears, the nucleus can extrude gradually or suddenly. Most herniations occur at the posterolateral portion of the annulus, where the annulus fibrosus merges with the posterior longitudinal ligament.

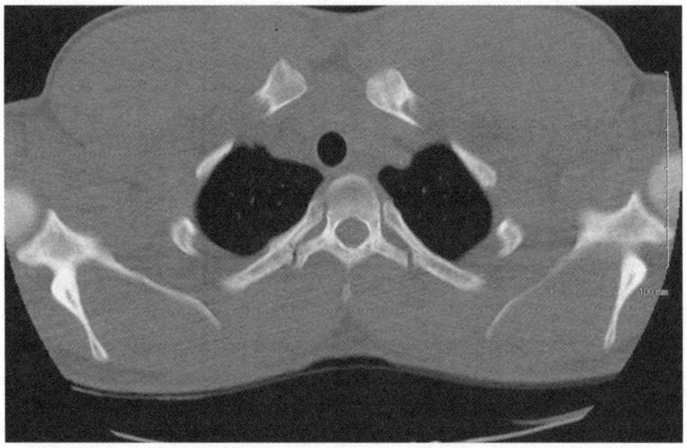

Figure 53.5 CT scan performed after a bone scan of a NCAA football player shows a posterior rib fracture that enters the costotransverse joint; this may manifest as a thoracic disc herniation.

Presentation: Thoracic herniations may present as chest wall pain, thoracic back pain, exiting root pain along a rib, or myelopathy if the cord is involved. Upper thoracic herniations may present as a cervical problem with pain radiating to the medial brachium. Lower thoracic herniations may present as lumbar disease.

Physical examination: If the patient is myelopathic, he or she will have upper motor findings of spasticity, weakness, clonus, and positive Babinski. Exiting nerve root distribution of numbness or hyperesthesia may be present.

Differential diagnosis: Cervical and lumbar herniated discs, tumors (benign, primary, metastatic, neural, bone, or malignant), and fractures (both stress and traumatic) of the spine or rib (Fig. 53.5)

Diagnostics: Diagnosis is confirmed with MRI or myelogram with CT

Treatment: Nonoperative treatment is with medications and physical therapy with a stabilization program; surgical interventions indicated for significant progressive myelopathy and unrelenting radiculopathy

Prognosis and return to sport: Variable; return should be slow and cautious with intense rehabilitation

Apophysitis

Description: Injury or inflammation of the ring apophysis of the spine

Mechanism of injury: Caused by repetitive traction on the anterior longitudinal ligament or repetitive compressions with endplate microfractures

Presentation: Presents as back pain that increases with activity and is relieved by rest

Physical examination: Normal; unlike Scheuermann disease, there will not be a kyphosis

Differential diagnosis: Stress fractures, traumatic fractures, and spondyloarthropathy

Diagnostics: Plain radiographs will reveal irregularities of the ventral apophysis; bone scan may have increased activity.

Treatment: Rest

Prognosis and return to sport: Excellent; return is variable depending on length of symptoms

Slipped Apophyseal Ring

Description: Posterior fracture of the ring apophysis with protrusion of the bone rim and disc into the canal (Fig. 53.6)

Mechanism of injury: Same as a herniated disc but in the skeletally immature

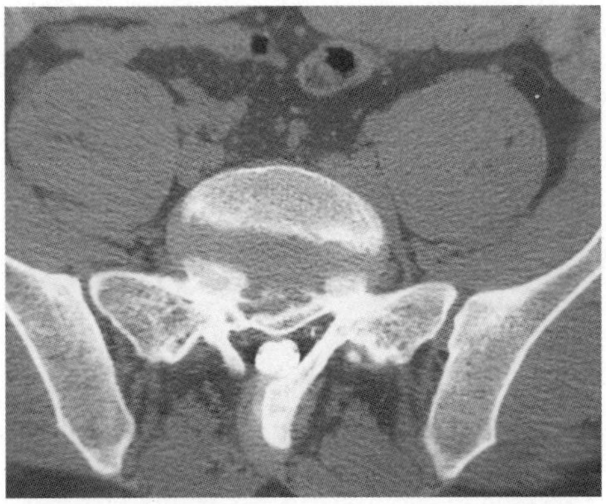

A. Axial CT with bone remodeling

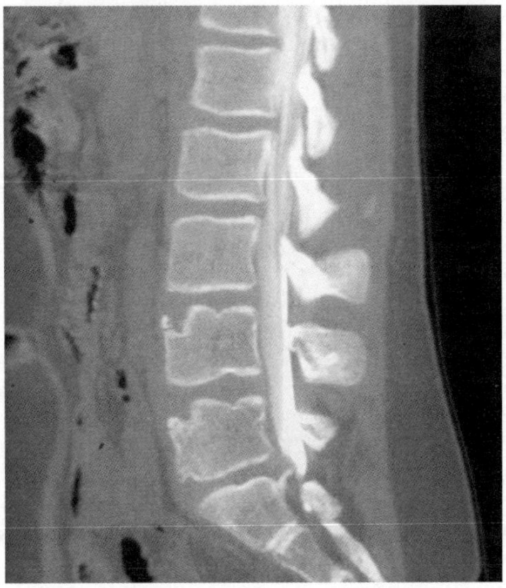

B. Sagittal cut showing protrusion of disc and calcified slipped apophysis at superior S1 and Schmorl's nodes at anterior L4 and L5

Figure 53.6 Slipped apophyseal ring: CT scan of a junior high basketball player with back and leg pain shows a slipped apophyseal ring at superior aspect of S1 and anterior Schmorl nodes at L4 and L5.

Presentation: Can produce back pain only, particularly if the disc herniates anteriorly or into the vertebral body producing a Schmorl node, which is common (see Fig. 53.6); can present with leg pain if the protrusion enters the canal and will behave like a herniated disc
Physical examination: May have same findings as a herniated disc: list, weakness/numbness, tension findings, and reflex deficit
Differential diagnosis: Herniated disc, stress fracture, and SI joint pain
Diagnostics: MRI, myelogram with CT, EMG, and NCV
Treatment: Similar to herniated nucleus pulposus (see later section)
Prognosis: Same as herniated nucleus pulposus (see later section)

Acute Lumbar Strain

Description: Muscle or muscle–tendon unit strain
Mechanism of injury: Fatigue failure or overstretch injury to a muscle–tendon unit about the lumbar spine; usually with bending, rotation, and/or inappropriate lifting
Presentation: Acute onset, back pain, no neurologic complaints
Physical examination: Localized tenderness, with or without spasm

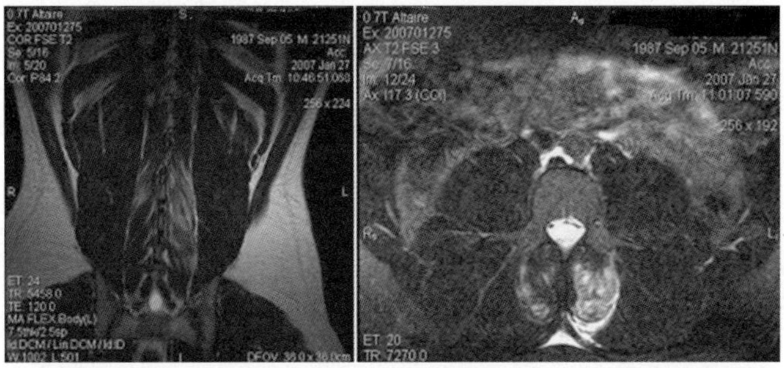

Figure 53.7 Lumbar myonecrosis with potential paravertebral compartment syndrome: MRI shows edema in paravertebral muscles.

Differential diagnosis: Stress reaction or fracture and SI joint pain
Diagnostics: Radiographs may not be required by history or examination but will be normal or show a straight spine related to the spasm
Treatment: Conservative care with rest, modalities, and occasional use of medications; to prevent recurrences, a rehabilitation program with spine stabilization exercises will be helpful; this is based on core strength and teaches the principle of muscle fusion; use of core muscles to brace the spine. The goal is to find the neutral position or position of least pain and use it protectively. Overall, flexibility and strength are stressed through a well-defined program. Progressive aerobic training and sport-specific training are added as skills improve.
Prognosis: Excellent

Lumbar Myonecrosis and Potential Compartment Syndrome

Description: Rare reports of compartment syndrome of the lumbar paraspinal muscles; more recently, events of lumbar myonecrosis with rhabdomyolysis have been reported; associated with sickle cell trait in athletes and can be significant
Mechanism of injury: Overuse, possibly associated with sickle cell trait
Presentation: After aggressive exercise, back pain, muscular spasm, cramping sensation, dark urine occur if rhabdomyolysis significant; back pain more severe and not motion-related compared with lumbar strain
Physical examination: Posturing, spasm, and neurologically intact
Differential diagnosis: Lumbar strain, acute fracture, and acute stress fracture
Diagnostics: MRI will show edema in paraspinous muscles and possible enlargement (Fig. 53.7); laboratory studies (creatine kinase); sickle cell testing
Treatment: Rest when it occurs, observe to check for progression of rhabdomyolysis; treatment of potential causes of rhabdomyolysis, hospitalization if needed; long-term management with appropriate guidance
Prognosis: Excellent if detected early and protective measures taken

Discogenic Syndromes

Annular Tears

Description: A tear of the annulus fibrosus; nucleus material may or may not be extruded or displaced. As the tear occurs at the periphery, it is more likely to be painful and may be associated with referred radicular pain or a chemical neuritis.
Mechanism of injury: Rotational stress or rotation with compression

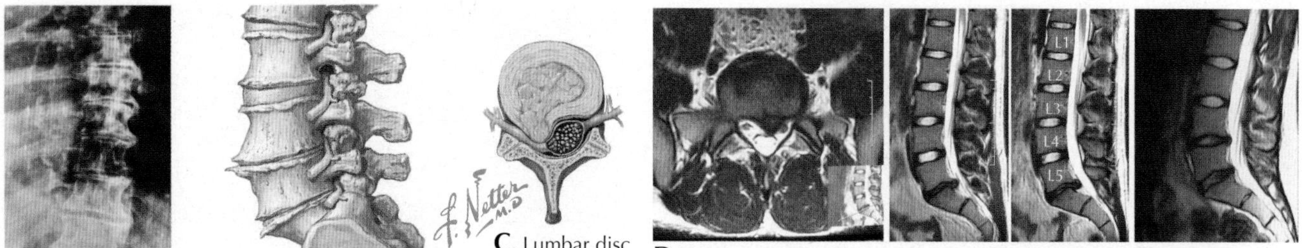
L1
L2
L3
L4
L5

A. Radiograph of thoracic spine shows narrowing of intervertebral spaces and spur formation.

B. Degeneration of lumbar intervertebral discs and hypertrophic changes at vertebral margins with spur formation. Osteophytic encroachment on intervertebral foramina compresses spinal nerves.

C. Lumbar disc herniation. Schematic cross section showing compression of nerve root.

D. Axial and sagittal MRI of NCAA baseball player shows a herniated disc at L5–S1compressing the S1 nerve root.

E. MRI shows disc degeneration at two levels in a NCAA softball player.

Figure 53.8 Discogenic syndromes.

Presentation: Pain, local back and possible dermatomal distribution of referred pain, often with spasm and postural changes; limited motion

Physical examination: Neurologically normal examination, but may be posturing, with spasm

Differential diagnosis: Early herniated nucleus pulposus (HNP), stress fracture, acute lumbar strain, fracture, and SI joint pain

Diagnostics: Plain radiographs may be normal or show degenerative changes; straight spine if spasm significant; MRI may be normal but may show an area of increased signal intensity in the annulus, particularly at the outer annulus on T2-weighted images.

Treatment: Modalities: possible nonsteroidal anti-inflammatory drugs (NSAIDs) or Medrol dose pack and physical therapy with a spine stabilization program

Prognosis: Excellent, but may cause prolonged and often recurrent symptoms

Herniated Nucleus Pulposus

Description: The nucleus pulposus partially or completely extrudes through the annulus fibrosus, protruding into the neural elements or extruding into the canal, and possibly sequestered away from the annulus (Fig. 53.8). Herniation usually occurs to one side or the other of the posterior longitudinal ligament, which is a restraint, but it may exit centrally through the posterior ligament. It can also exit far laterally to involve the root in the foramen. It is most common at the lower segments and during the third or fourth decade of life.

Mechanism of injury: Repetitive flexion and rotation increases the load on the disc; Nachemson has measured the intradisc pressures in various positions, and this pressure is increased with flexion.

Presentation: May present as back pain as the annulus tears in the process of the disk extruding; as it extrudes and as the nerve becomes involved, the back pain will become associated with buttock pain or extremity pain. The back pain may lessen as the radicular pain, numbness, and dysesthesias progress along a dermatomal distribution. Weakness is possible. Pain is usually worse with prolonged sitting, flexion, or Valsalva maneuvers. If severe compression occurs, part or all of the cauda equina may be involved, leading to weakness, bowel, bladder, and sexual dysfunction (cauda equina syndrome).

Physical examination: Patient may have a list, may tripod, may have limited ROM, and may have spasms. Tension tests are positive, and a neurologic examination may reveal numbness and weakness.

Differential diagnosis: Stress fracture to lumbar spine, sacrum, or pelvis; annular tear with referred pain; plexopathy; peripheral neuropathy or nerve injury; SI joint pain; and fracture (see Figs. 53.6 and 53.7)

Diagnostics: Plain radiographs may be normal or show a narrow disc space. MRI will show the lesion (see Fig. 53.8). Myelogram and myelo-CT will also reveal the lesion but are more invasive. An MRI with gadolinium may be required to distinguish postsurgical scarring from a recurrent herniated disc. EMG and NCV studies may be helpful to rule out a peripheral neuropathy that can masquerade as a radiculopathy. This may be needed because 32% of imaging techniques may be positive in asymptomatic subjects. A positive study is not diagnostic unless it confirms the clinical picture.

Treatment: Conservative with medications, possible Medrol dose pack, followed by NSAIDs; epidural steroid treatment may be used. Surgery may be required for intractable pain, progressive neurologic deficit, or lack of improvement after 8–12 weeks. Cauda equina syndrome requires urgent surgical care.

Prognosis and return to sport: Several patients completely recover with nonsurgical care; this, followed by aggressive rehabilitation and a prolonged care program, can lead to return to sport. In certain studies, 70%–90% of athletes treated surgically were able to return to an elite level. Strength programs and lifting as a part of training should be appropriately adjusted.

Spinal Stenosis

Description: Narrowing of the space available for the nerves; may be congenital with short pedicles or a narrow interpedicular distance or acquired related to trauma or degeneration. It may be central (spinal canal) or foraminal.

Mechanism of injury: Congenital, traumatic, or degenerative; may be caused by a synovial cyst or herniated disc

Presentation: Neurologic symptoms, radicular pain, neurogenic claudication, and postural radicular pain

Physical examination: May be normal; if severe, may have neurologic findings

Differential diagnosis: Herniated disc, stress fracture, fracture, SI joint pain, and peripheral neuropathy

Diagnostics: Imaging by MRI or myelo-CT; EMGs and NCV may be useful (Fig. 53.9)

Treatment: Specific to cause; if symptoms are related to a synovial cyst, then aspiration or injection may be useful. If congenital, then surgical decompression may be required; if acquired

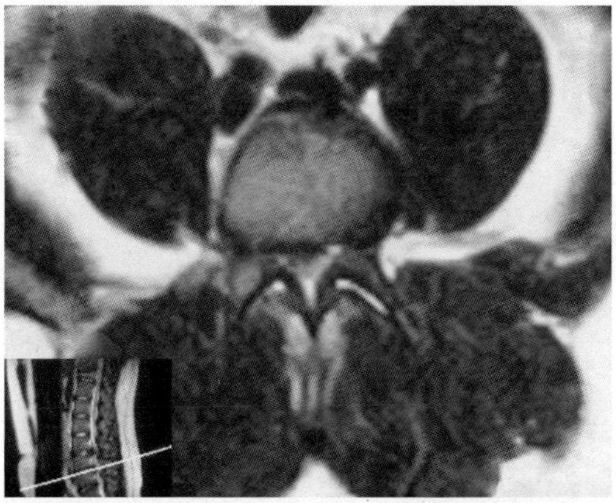

A. Axial image shows congenitally short pedicles and triangular narrowed canal.

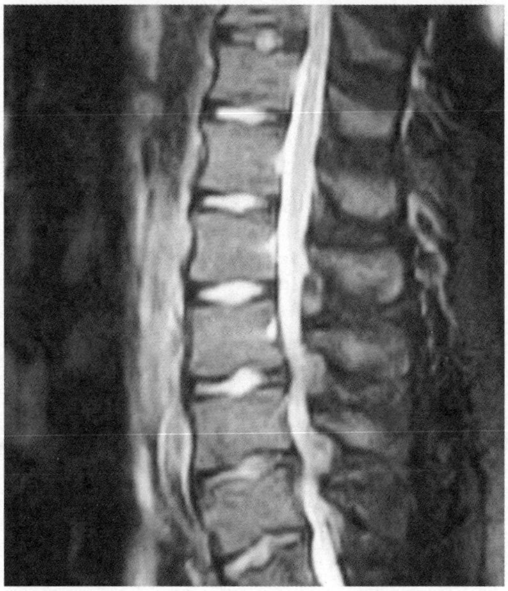

B. Sagittal image shows degeneration with acquired changes exacerbating a congenital stenosis.

Figure 53.9 Spinal stenosis: MRI of NCAA football player shows spinal stenosis.

degenerative, then conservative measures such as medication and epidural steroids may help prolong an athletic career.

Prognosis and return to sport: Variable

Stress Reaction, Stress Fracture, Spondylolysis

Description: A spectrum of overuse injuries to the pars interarticularis or pedicle area of the bone; very common in athletes

Mechanism of injury: Repetitive shear forces, worse with repeated extension and hyperextension maneuvers that load this portion of the bone

Presentation: Back pain, occasionally with some radicular pain; worse with extension; present as a bone stress reaction without a fracture on one or both sides, or as a nonunion of a stress fracture, known as *spondylolysis* (spondylo = spine, lysis = defect), on one or both sides (Fig. 53.10). Pain can be present on one or both sides, worse with motion or running; often has onset in strength and conditioning workouts

Physical examination: Extension and one-legged extension tests are positive; neurologic examination is negative; tension tests are negative. Pain may occur with rotation or side bending.

Differential diagnosis: Annular tear, HNP, SI joint pain, and stress fractures; in the sacrum or pelvis, facet syndrome, osteoid osteoma, or lesions of the posterior elements

Diagnostics: Plain radiographs include AP, lateral, and oblique views. They may be normal early in a reaction, and certain defects are not clearly seen. Oblique radiographs can show a defect as "the neck of the Scotty dog" (see Fig. 53.10). Sometimes, the defect can be seen on a lateral radiograph. If plain radiographs are negative, nuclear imaging will be helpful. A whole-body conventional biplanar bone scan can not only visualize the pars area but also rule out a sacral or pelvic stress fracture that mimics a lumbar injury. A bone scan combined with single photon emission computerized tomography (SPECT) will improve sensitivity and localization of small abnormalities by screening out other tissues. A positive scan indicates an acute lesion and suggests bone healing potential.

Treatment: Guided by symptoms and images; restrictions are controversial, particularly bracing. Younger age—preteen and early teen—may indicate more healing potential and more of a tendency to brace.

- Normal plain radiograph, positive scan indicates an acute lesion; a positive scan indicates metabolic activity and some potential for healing. A modified Boston orthosis may be indicated. Limit activities for 4–8 weeks; rehabilitation exercises to begin as symptoms abate. Strength and neutral position are stressed. Occasionally with a positive scan, a thin-slice CT may help evaluate the lesion and help with treatment. If CT scan normal, no brace; if CT scan shows acute fracture line, brace; if CT scan shows fracture with sclerotic margins (chronic lesion), no brace required
- Positive plain radiograph and positive scan indicate a semi-acute lesion. A 0-degree antilordotic modified Boston orthosis may be indicated; Micheli reported success with use of this orthosis for 23 hours/day for 12 weeks, but the use is variable. The goal is to be pain free before beginning rehabilitation exercises. The lesion may not heal with bone, so progression is based on symptoms.
- Positive plain radiographs with a negative bone scan indicate a chronic lesion or nonunion. A negative scan suggests minimal metabolic activity and poor healing potential. Start rehabilitation when symptoms abate. Occasionally, surgery is required if pain is intractable.

Prognosis and return to sport: Excellent

Spondylolisthesis

Description: One vertebral body is slipping relative to another (spondylo = spine, listhesis = slippage) (see Fig. 53.10); usually, the upper body is slipping forward on the body below, resulting in a kyphotic deformity at the slip and a reactive lordosis above.

- There are five types of spondylolisthesis:
  - Dysplastic (abnormal anatomy)
  - Isthmic (caused by a defect in the pars); this is most common in young athletes
  - Degenerative (caused by lax facet joints and a degenerative disc that allows the slippage)—more common with age
  - Traumatic (high-velocity injuries)
  - Pathologic (tumors or osteopenic bone)
- Isthmic (the most common type in young athletes) is most common from L5 to S1 and can be graded on a scale of I–V based on the amount of forward displacement of the higher vertebra on the vertebra below.
  - 0%–25% is grade I
  - 25%–50% is grade II
  - 50%–75% is grade III
  - 75%–100% is grade IV
  - Complete displacement or spondylolisthesis is grade V

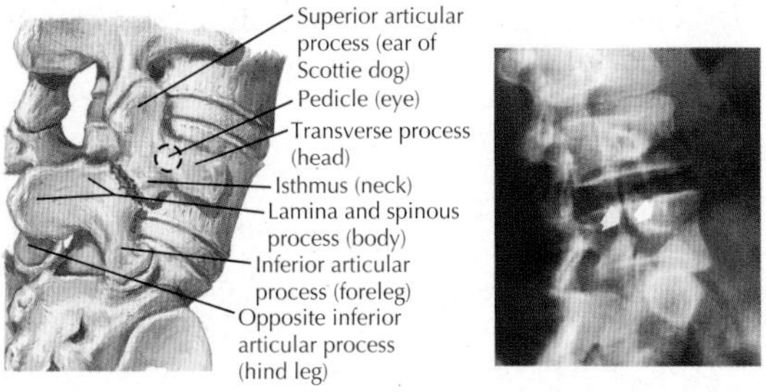
Superior articular process (ear of Scottie dog)
Pedicle (eye)
Transverse process (head)
Isthmus (neck)
Lamina and spinous process (body)
Inferior articular process (foreleg)
Opposite inferior articular process (hind leg)

Spondylolysis without spondylolisthesis. Oblique view demonstrates formation of radiographic Scottie dog. On oblique radiograph, dog appears to be wearing a collar.

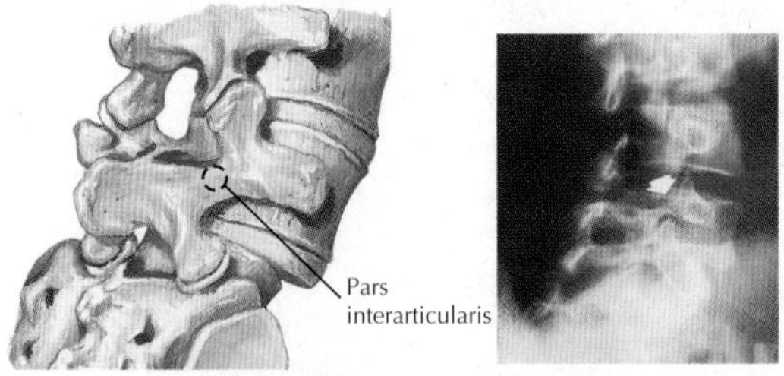
Pars interarticularis

Dysplastic (congenital) spondylolisthesis. Luxation of L5 on sacrum. Dog's neck (isthmus) appears elongated. Dysplastic facets may lead to lystesis.

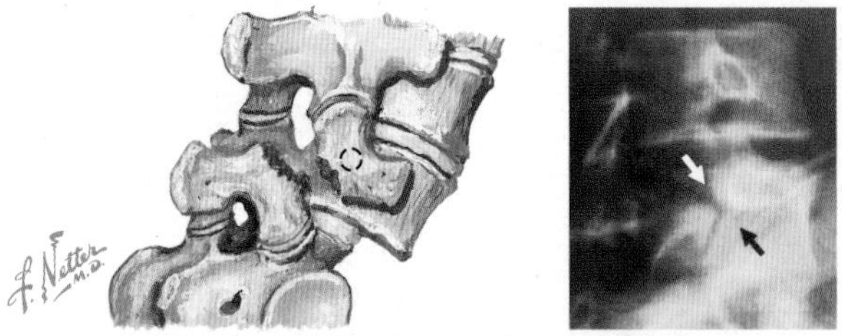

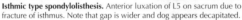

Isthmic type spondylolisthesis. Anterior luxation of L5 on sacrum due to fracture of isthmus. Note that gap is wider and dog appears decapitated.

Figure 53.10 Spondylolysis and spondylolisthesis.

Mechanism of injury: Isthmic spondylolisthesis occurs as a result of repetitive overuse at a young age, probably related to extension activities. Progression of slips is most likely to occur between ages 9 and 12 years in girls and 10 and 14 years in boys.

Presentation: Patients with grade I and II slips may be asymptomatic and may be participating in sport not knowing about the defect. They may have back pain and occasional radicular pain; pain is worse with extension activities. Patients with higher-grade lesions may have been limited by their pain and face more difficulty with sports because of back pain, stiffness, and hamstring tightness. Localized back pain is common, and radicular pain may develop as a result of nerve root compression by hypertrophic callus or the deformity or instability.

Physical examination: With high-grade slips, there will be vertical sacrum, flat buttocks, and compensating tight hamstrings. There may be a palpable step-off at the deformity and a short waist. Neurologic examination is usually normal.

Differential diagnosis: Just because a patient has a spondylolisthesis does not mean that it is the origin of the pain. Other possibilities include SI joint pain, degeneration of other levels, and stress fracture at other levels.

Diagnostics: Standing plain radiographs usually reveal the abnormality, and a lateral projection allows grading. Repeat radiographs should be obtained yearly if the diagnosis is made before the age of 10 years because progression can occur. CT and MRI are useful if other sources are suspected.

Treatment: Conservative in most cases and involves trunk stabilization exercises; occasional limits may be required for symptomatic events. Surgical fusion may be required with high-grade slips or with slips associated with neurologic symptoms related to nerve root compression or stenosis.

Prognosis and return to sport: For low-grade slips, excellent to good; but high-grade slips can be more problematic and limiting

Inflammatory Causes of Pain

Facet Syndrome

Description: Pain syndrome emanating from an irritated facet joint

Mechanism of injury: This synovial fluid–lined joint can become inflamed with injury and have associated hyaline cartilage damage. Synovitis may occur. Facet trophism (asymmetry) may lead to injury.

Presentation: Painful with extension and bending to the involved side

Physical examination: Pain reproduced with maneuvers noted earlier; neurologically intact

Differential diagnosis: Stress fracture, fracture, discogenic disease, and SI joint pain

Diagnostics: Plain radiographs may show joint changes. Bone scan may reveal increased activity in the joint, and a CT scan may show arthritic changes.

Treatment: NSAIDs may be helpful. A facet injection may be diagnostic and therapeutic.

Prognosis and return to sport: Participation limited by pain

Sacroiliac Joint Dysfunction

Description: Pain syndrome emanating from an irritated SI joint; commonly confused with low back pain. These joints are very strong and allow limited motion while being constrained with strong anterior and posterior ligaments; possess a synovial membrane

Mechanism of injury: Injury, contracture, or inflammation of the SI joint

Presentation: Patients may present with a traumatic history, or they may be involved in jumping sports that require repetitive single-leg landing. Pain is usually over the SI joint but may also be referred into the leg, suggesting radiculopathy.

Physical examination: Local tenderness, a positive supine-to-long sitting test, a painful extension test, a painful FABER test, and pain when stresses are applied to the SI joint

Differential diagnosis: Discogenic pain, stress fracture, facet joint pain, and muscle injury

Diagnostics: Radiographs normal unless late in the course of severe spondyloarthropathy

Treatment: Mobilization exercises, NSAIDs, modalities, and occasionally, corticosteroid injections into the SI joint

Prognosis and return to sport: Limited only by pain

RETURN-TO-PLAY DECISIONS

- Each condition has its own criteria and may allow return to sport at certain, but not all, levels.
- Consultation with a spine specialist is recommended to help make the decisions and to discuss the risks and benefits of participation with the patient and family.

- The following findings may prohibit participation in contact sports:
  - Intersegmental instability on flexion–extension radiographs (e.g., instability that could potentially lead to neurologic impairment)
  - Spinal cord impingement with myelopathy
  - Significant neurologic impairment or risk of impairment with a herniated disc or obstructing lesion
  - Limiting pain
  - A previous spinal fusion
- After treatment, certain athletes can be placed into the following risk categories and allowed to return to sport with the understanding that there is a level of risk involved:
  - Minimal risk: The increase in risk is small compared with play before the injury.
  - Moderate risk: There is a reasonable chance that symptoms will recur, and the patient is at a risk of permanent injury.
  - Extreme risk: The risk that symptoms will recur and cause permanent damage is high.

LESS COMMON THORACIC AND LUMBOSACRAL SPINE ISSUES

Available online:
- Degenerative disc disease
- Postural roundback (flexible)
- Scheuermann disease
- Atypical Scheuermann disease
- Scoliosis
- Ankylosing spondylitis
- Infections

RECOMMENDED READINGS

Available online.

54 PELVIS, HIP, AND THIGH INJURIES

Matthew J. Kraeutler • Jorge Chahla • Cecilia Pascual-Garrido

GENERAL PRINCIPLES

Overview

The understanding of hip pathology has substantially improved recently because of more specific clinical tests, better imaging diagnosis, and discovery of new entities. Hip pathologies include femoroacetabular impingement (FAI), borderline dysplasia, femoral anteversion, hip instability, and femoral head deformities such as slipped capital femoral epiphysis (SCFE) and Perthes disease. Understanding of the hip anatomy, physiology, biomechanics, different pathologies, and treatment options is key to offering high-quality care to patients.

This chapter will discuss hip and pelvis anatomy; various hip pathologies; and treatment options that the orthopedic surgeon, physical therapist, or athletic trainer will encounter through their regular practice.

HIP AND PELVIS ANATOMY

Bony Anatomy

Acetabulum

- The acetabular fossa constitutes the inferior portion of the acetabulum and is surrounded by the lunate surface in its superior and lateral aspects (Fig. 54.1).
- When performing a hip arthroscopy, it is critical to understand the location of the pathology. To more easily locate chondrolabral hip lesions, the socket is considered a clock in which 12 o'clock represents the most superior aspect of the acetabulum and continuing anteriorly with successive hours. Unlike the knee, the 3 o'clock position is always anterior for both right and left hips.
- Different bony landmarks have been described to help the surgeon with an accurate location during arthroscopy:
  - The superior extent of the anterior labral sulcus (psoas-u) indicates the 3 o'clock position on the acetabular rim. It corresponds to the location of the iliopsoas tendon anteriorly.
  - The stellate crease is located superior to the apex of the acetabular fossa and corresponds to the 12:30 position (Fig. 54.2).
- The abduction angle of the acetabulum relative to the horizontal plane averages 45 degrees with 20 degrees of anteversion.

Femoral Head

- The femoral head forms roughly two-thirds of a sphere whose surface is completely articular except for the fovea capitis femoris, where the ligamentum teres is attached (Figs. 54.3 and 54.4).
- The neck-shaft angle averages 130 degrees, and the femoral neck is anteverted 14 degrees on average relative to the bicondylar axis at the knee.

Soft Tissue Anatomy

Labrum

- The labrum is a fibrocartilaginous structure attached to the acetabular rim.
- It is responsible for guaranteeing the suction seal, a key function in fluid dynamics, ensuring wider coverage of the femoral head and providing negative intra-articular pressure that provides stability to the hip joint.
- Labral pathology is normally observed in the anterosuperior area of the socket (12 to 2 o'clock position). This area correlates to the location where impingement normally occurs.

Capsule

- The hip capsule is formed by the iliofemoral ligament anteriorly, the ischiofemoral ligament posteriorly, and the pubofemoral ligament inferiorly (Fig. 54.5).
- Near the acetabular origin, the superior and superolateral aspect of the capsule is the thickest portion (3.7–4.0 mm).
- The capsule is inserted at a mean of 26.2 mm distal to the chondral head–neck junction of the proximal femur. The capsule has a spiral configuration that tightens in terminal extension and external rotation.

Muscles

Hip Abductors

- Gluteal group: The gluteal muscles include the gluteus maximus, gluteus medius, gluteus minimus, and tensor fasciae latae.
- The gluteus medius muscle stabilizes the hip and controls hip motion, particularly in weight-bearing. Weakness or insufficiency of this muscle leads to a Trendelenburg gait.

Hip Adductors

- Adductor group: Adductor brevis, adductor longus, adductor magnus, pectineus, and gracilis muscles. The adductors originate on the pubis and insert on the medial, posterior surface of the femur, with the exception of the gracilis, which inserts distally on the pes anserine on the tibia. There is a pubic aponeurosis, which is a confluence of the adductor and gracilis origins. It is also referred to as the rectus abdominus/adductor aponeurosis. There is a clinical association between FAI and sports hernia/core muscle injury/athletic pubalgia.

Hip Flexors

- Iliopsoas group: Composed of the iliacus and psoas major muscles. The iliacus originates on the iliac fossa of the ilium and joins the psoas major muscle that runs from the lumbar bodies (2, 3, 4) and inserts distally into the lesser trochanter.
- The rectus femoris is a weaker flexor with the knee in extension. However, because of its proximity to the capsule and its complex anatomy, it serves as an important differential diagnosis for hip pain.
- The direct head of the rectus femoris attachment has a shape of a "tear drop" occupying the entire footprint of the superior facet of the anterior inferior iliac spine (AIIS). The indirect head has a broad insertion over the acetabular rim (Fig. 54.6).

Hip Short External Rotators

- This group consists of the obturator externus and internus, the piriformis, the superior and inferior gemelli, and the quadratus femoris (Fig. 54.7). The piriformis muscle originates in the anterior surface of the sacrum and inserts into the superior boundary of the greater trochanter; the superior gemellus originates at the ischial spine and joins the piriformis tendon in its insertion at the greater trochanter. The obturators (internus and externus) insert on the medial and lateral surface of the obturator membrane and then travel to the medial surface of the greater trochanter and the trochanteric fossa, respectively. The inferior gemellus muscle originates on the superior aspect of the ischial tuberosity and inserts distally into the piriformis tendon (indirectly to the greater trochanter). Lastly, the quadratus femoris muscle originates at the lateral edge of the ischial tuberosity and inserts on the intertrochanteric crest.

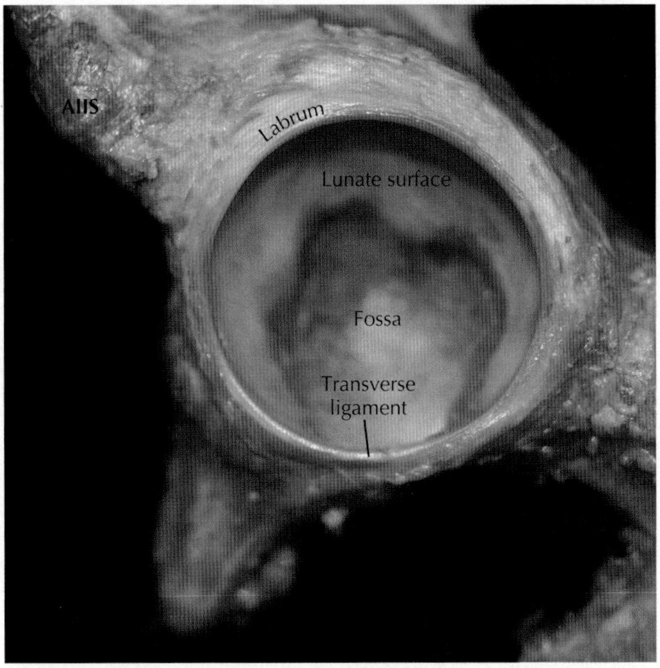
AIIS
Labrum
Lunate surface
Fossa
Transverse ligament

Figure 54.1 Cadaveric image of a left hip demonstrating osseous and soft tissue (including the labrum and the transverse ligament) components of the acetabulum. *AIIS,* Anterior inferior iliac spine.

Neurovascular Structures

- The extracapsular arterial ring at the base of the femoral neck is formed posteriorly by a large branch of the medial femoral circumflex artery (MFCA) and anteriorly by smaller branches of the lateral femoral circumflex artery (LFCA). The superior and inferior gluteal arteries have minor contributions to the blood supply. Retinacular arteries and the internal ring arise from the ascending cervical branches. Finally, the artery of the ligamentum teres is derived from the obturator artery or the MFCA (Fig. 54.8).
- The blood supply to the femoral head is mainly from the deep branch (posterior) of the MFCA. During anterior controlled hip dislocation, this vessel is protected by the obturator externus muscle. The ligamentum teres branch, which is important during developmental phases of the femoral head, does not play an important role in the adult hip.
- The lower extremity receives its innervation from the lumbosacral plexus, which forms the sciatic, femoral, and obturator nerves, in addition to various smaller branches.
- The hip receives innervation from the L2 to S1 nerve roots, but principally from L3. This explains the presence of medial thigh pain often accompanying hip pathology because symptoms may be referred to the L3 dermatome.
- The lateral femoral cutaneous nerve, providing sensation to the lateral thigh, exits the pelvis under the inguinal ligament, close to the anterior superior iliac spine (ASIS).

HISTORY AND PHYSICAL EXAMINATION

History

- Acute onset of hip pain is more likely to be the result of a specific pathology, which may be diagnosed through physical examination and imaging.
  - These injuries are typically easier to treat and carry a more favorable prognosis.
- Gradual onset of hip pain is likely to be the result of (1) chronic disease or (2) pain syndromes, which may be difficult to diagnose.
  - These injuries typically carry a worse prognosis and require more complex methods of treatment.

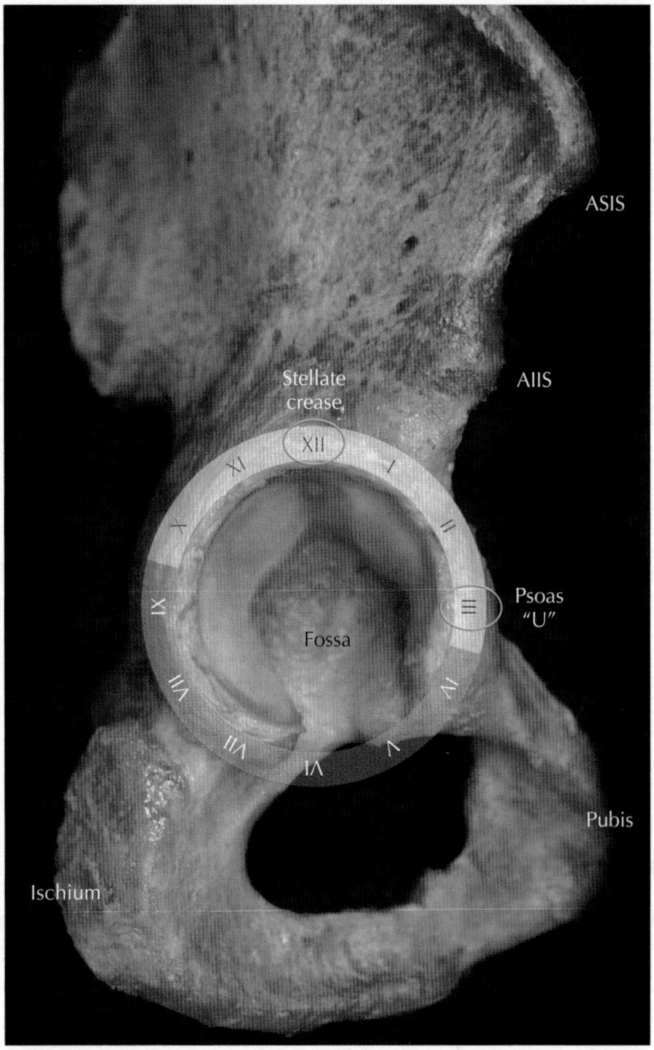
ASIS
Stellate crease
AIIS
XII
I
II
III
IIII
V
VI
VII
VIII
IX
X
XI
Psoas "U"
Fossa
Pubis
Ischium

Figure 54.2 Cadaveric image of a right hip showing the most relevant osseous landmarks in hip arthroscopy and their position using a superimposed clock. *AIIS,* Anterior inferior iliac spine; *ASIS,* anterior superior iliac spine.

Inspection

- Examine patient's gait and stance.
- Examine patient's posture in supine and seated positions, looking for internal or external rotation of the injured limb at rest or a flexion contracture of the hip joint.
- Look for asymmetry in leg length, muscle atrophy, or pelvic obliquity.

Range of Motion

- When performing these measurements, it is important to assess if the range of motion (ROM) is limited or excessive. This will help differentiate between two different pathologies (impingement vs. dysplasia).
- Clinically, leg length can be measured from the ASIS to the medial malleolus.
- ROM should be measured bilaterally to compare the injured and noninjured sides. Hip flexion, extension, abduction, adduction, and internal and external rotation should be measured. Internal and external rotation should be assessed both with the patient supine, at 90 degrees of hip flexion, and prone with the hip at neutral. This last position will help define the patient's femoral

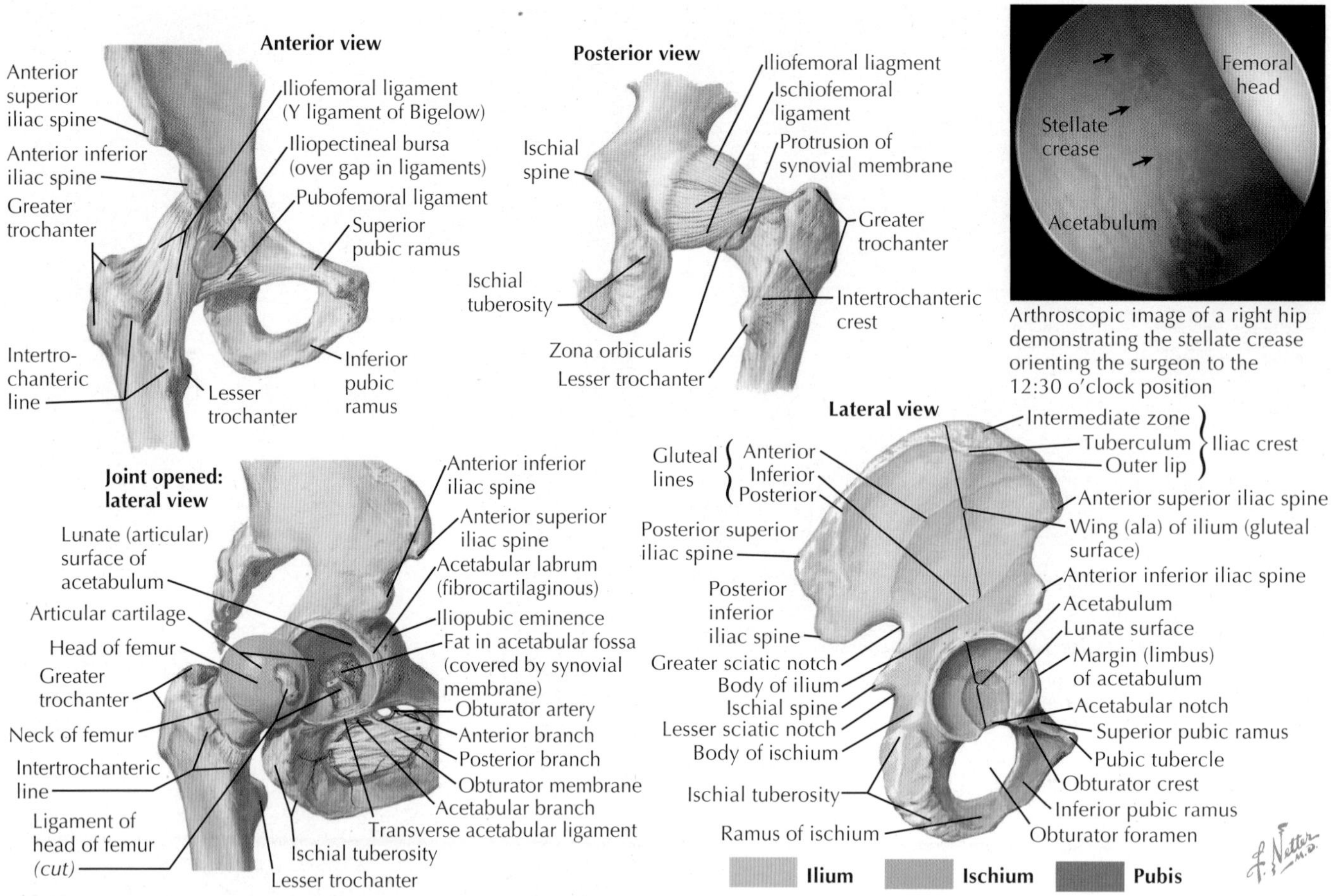
Anterior view
Anterior superior iliac spine
Anterior inferior iliac spine
Greater trochanter
Intertro-chanteric line
Iliofemoral ligament (Y ligament of Bigelow)
Iliopectineal bursa (over gap in ligaments)
Pubofemoral ligament
Superior pubic ramus
Lesser trochanter
Inferior pubic ramus
Posterior view
Ischial spine
Ischial tuberosity
Iliofemoral liagment
Ischiofemoral ligament
Protrusion of synovial membrane
Greater trochanter
Intertrochanteric crest
Zona orbicularis
Lesser trochanter
Femoral head
Stellate crease
Acetabulum
Joint opened: lateral view
Lunate (articular) surface of acetabulum
Articular cartilage
Head of femur
Greater trochanter
Neck of femur
Intertrochanteric line
Ligament of head of femur (cut)
Anterior inferior iliac spine
Anterior superior iliac spine
Acetabular labrum (fibrocartilaginous)
Iliopubic eminence
Fat in acetabular fossa (covered by synovial membrane)
Obturator artery
Anterior branch
Posterior branch
Obturator membrane
Acetabular branch
Transverse acetabular ligament
Ischial tuberosity
Lesser trochanter
Lateral view
Gluteal lines
Anterior
Inferior
Posterior
Posterior superior iliac spine
Posterior inferior iliac spine
Greater sciatic notch
Body of ilium
Ischial spine
Lesser sciatic notch
Body of ischium
Ischial tuberosity
Ramus of ischium
Intermediate zone
Tuberculum
Outer lip
Iliac crest
Anterior superior iliac spine
Wing (ala) of ilium (gluteal surface)
Anterior inferior iliac spine
Acetabulum
Lunate surface
Margin (limbus) of acetabulum
Acetabular notch
Superior pubic ramus
Pubic tubercle
Obturator crest
Inferior pubic ramus
Obturator foramen
Ilium
Ischium
Pubis
F. Netter M.D.

Arthroscopic image of a right hip demonstrating the stellate crease orienting the surgeon to the 12:30 o'clock position

Figure 54.3 Bony anatomy of the hip.

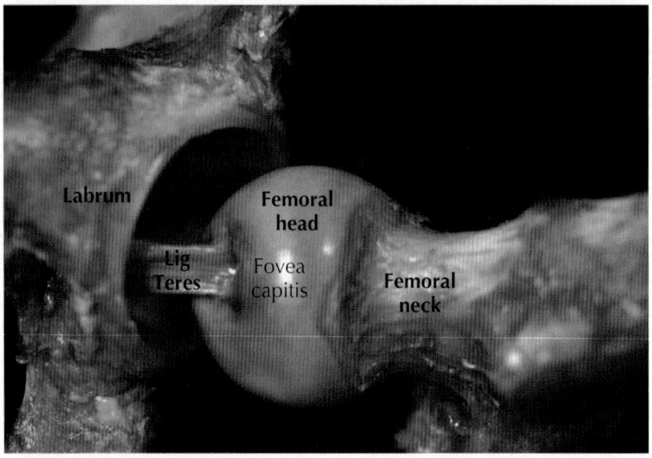
Labrum
Femoral head
Lig Teres
Fovea capitis
Femoral neck

Figure 54.4 Cadaveric image of a left hip under distraction demonstrating its anatomic relationship with the acetabulum. The ligamentum teres is in tension.

version. Patients with excessive anteversion of the femur will have excessive internal rotation when they are prone with the hip neutral.

Palpation

- The patient should be asked to point to the single most painful location. This will provide helpful clues as to the potential diagnoses.
  - Patients with hip pain will normally do the "C sign," grabbing their hip in a C-shape with their hand.
  - Patients with posterior pelvic pain may also have associated groin pain, lateral thigh pain, or anterior thigh pain.
  - Posterior pelvic pain may be associated with labral tear, developmental dysplasia of the hip, and/or femoroacetabular impingement.
- Palpation should begin away from the source of the patient's pain and progressively move closer to the painful location.
- The following anatomic sites should be palpated to assess for significant pain: lumbar vertebrae, sacroiliac (SI) joint, ischium, iliac crest, greater trochanter, trochanteric bursa, muscle bellies of the thigh and hamstrings, and pubic symphysis.

SPECIFIC TESTS

- Before performing these tests, it is important to ask the patient to score the test. Tests are normally scored as follows:
  - + Patient feels pain but he or she has never felt this pain before
  - ++ Patient has felt this pain before but it is not the pain that brings him or her to the office on the day of the visit
  - +++ Patient states that the pain that was reproduced during the test is the pain that brings him or her to the office today

Impingement:

- **FABER:** Stands for **F**lexion, **AB**duction, and **E**xternal **R**otation of the hip (Fig. 54.9A). Pain during these movements represents a positive test indicating SI joint (if pain is located posteriorly) or hip (if pain is reproduced anteriorly in the groin) pathology.
- **FADIR:** Stands for **F**lexion, **AD**duction, and **I**nternal **R**otation of the hip (see Fig. 54.9B). Pain during these movements represents a positive test indicating either femoroacetabular impingement or anterior labral tear.

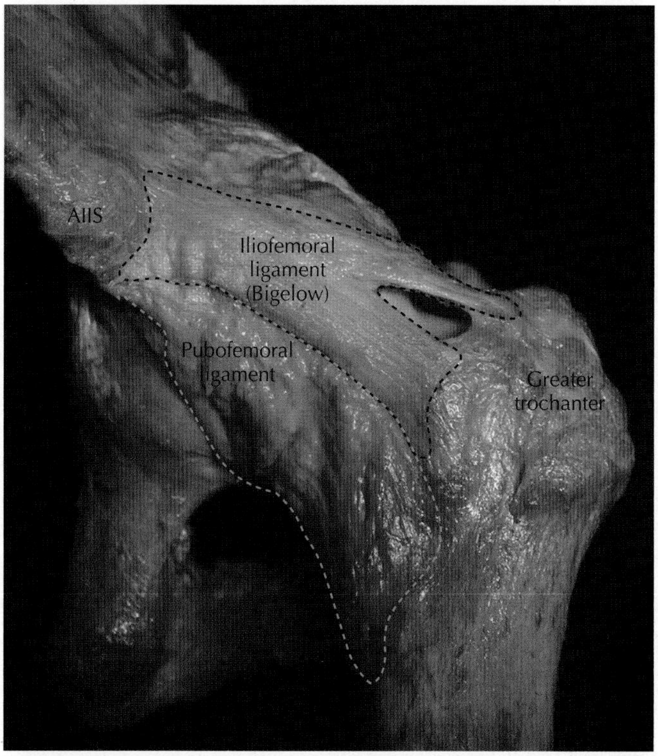
AIIS
Iliofemoral
ligament
(Bigelow)
Pubofemoral
ligament
Greater
trochanter

Figure 54.5 Cadaveric image of a left hip showing the different parts of the hip capsule. The iliofemoral ligament is demarcated in black and the pubofemoral ligament in green. The iliofemoral ligament is normally incised during arthroscopy in an interportal or T-shaped fashion.

Iliopsoas: The Thomas test is used to test for a hip flexion contracture. The patient lies supine on the examination table and flexes the uninjured hip so that the knee is brought to the chest. If the contralateral leg remains on the table, there is no hip flexion contracture, whereas the leg will raise off of the table if a contracture is present. The bicycle test is also used to assess for the presence of pain and snapping corresponding with iliopsoas tendinitis (see Fig. 54.9C).

Posterior impingement: The patient lies supine with the unaffected hip flexed as in the Thomas test. The examiner places the affected limb in extension, external rotation, and slight abduction while applying an overpressure into hip extension (see Fig. 54.9D). Pain at the posterior hip indicates posterior impingement of the labrum. Posterior impingement could be observed in patients with anteverted femurs or patients with large femoral head deformities such as SCFE or Perthes disease with posterior impingement.

Adductor squeeze test: Used to test the strength of the adductors. The patient lies supine on the examination table with both hips flexed to 45 degrees. The examiner places both fists between the knees and asks the patient to squeeze (adduct) both knees simultaneously (see Fig. 54.9E). A noticeably lower force exerted by one of the knees indicates adductor muscle weakness. Pain can also be quantified. Adductor tendinosis is frequently seen in patients with hip FAI.

Piriformis test: Used to test for piriformis syndrome. The patient lies on the side of the unaffected hip with both knees flexed. The patient then attempts to abduct the top knee against resistance from the examiner and holds it for 30 seconds (see Fig. 54.9F). A positive test is indicated by pain in the buttock or shooting pain/numbness radiating to the posterior thigh or lower leg.

Cross-body sit-up test: Patient is lying supine and is asked to bring the contralateral shoulder to the knee on the affected side against resistance. Pubic/groin pain indicates a positive test with a high sensitivity for core muscle injury.

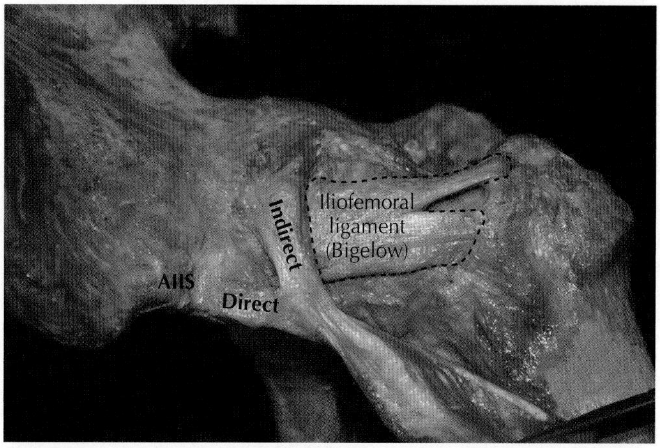
Iliofemoral
ligament
(Bigelow)
Indirect
AIIS
Direct

Figure 54.6 Anterior view of a cadaveric dissection showing the proximal insertions of the rectus femoris (direct to the AIIS and indirect above the capsule) and their relationship to the hip capsule.

SPECIFIC INJURIES

Proximal Hamstring Injuries

Description: Hamstring strain is the most common injury. This typically occurs during sprinting when there is a sudden stretch on the musculotendinous junction. In severe cases, complete avulsion may occur at the ischium. This is a common injury seen in water skiers. Chronic tendinopathy is frequently seen in older patients as a degenerative process.

Symptoms: Sudden pain during exercising, especially sprinting. Pain may be along the posterior thigh up to the ischium. A bruise is normally evident in the buttock area. Some patients may also report some numbness and tingling in the area corresponding to the sciatic nerve. This has been related to the presence of a hematoma that compresses the sciatic nerve.

Diagnosis: History usually provides clues to the diagnosis. Magnetic resonance imaging (MRI) is necessary to confirm the diagnosis and define treatment (Fig. 54.10).

Treatment: For hamstring strains, supportive treatment (rest, ice, compression, and elevation [RICE]) is sufficient. Once the pain subsides, stretching and strengthening exercises should be done. For complete avulsion injuries, it is important to define the degree of retraction. If the hamstring is retracted more than 3 cm, early surgical intervention (within 6 weeks) is associated with quicker return to sports and less morbidity. This surgery is normally performed open, though some advanced hip arthroscopists may perform the procedure in a closed arthroscopic fashion. For those patients with less than 3 cm of retraction, nonoperative treatment with platelet-rich plasma (PRP) can be offered initially.

Prognosis: Depends on extent of initial injury and patient's activity level. For hamstring strains, patients should be pain-free with full ROM before return to play. For complete avulsion injuries, return to sports varies based on timing of surgical intervention and typically ranges from 16 to 29 weeks after surgery.

Rectus Femoris Injuries

Description: Similar to proximal hamstring injuries, strains of the rectus femoris ("hip flexor strain") are more common than complete avulsions. The rectus femoris is the most commonly strained muscle in the quadriceps group. These injuries typically occur when attempting to kick a ball, as in soccer or football, especially when the patient's foot hits another player in the middle of the kicking motion.

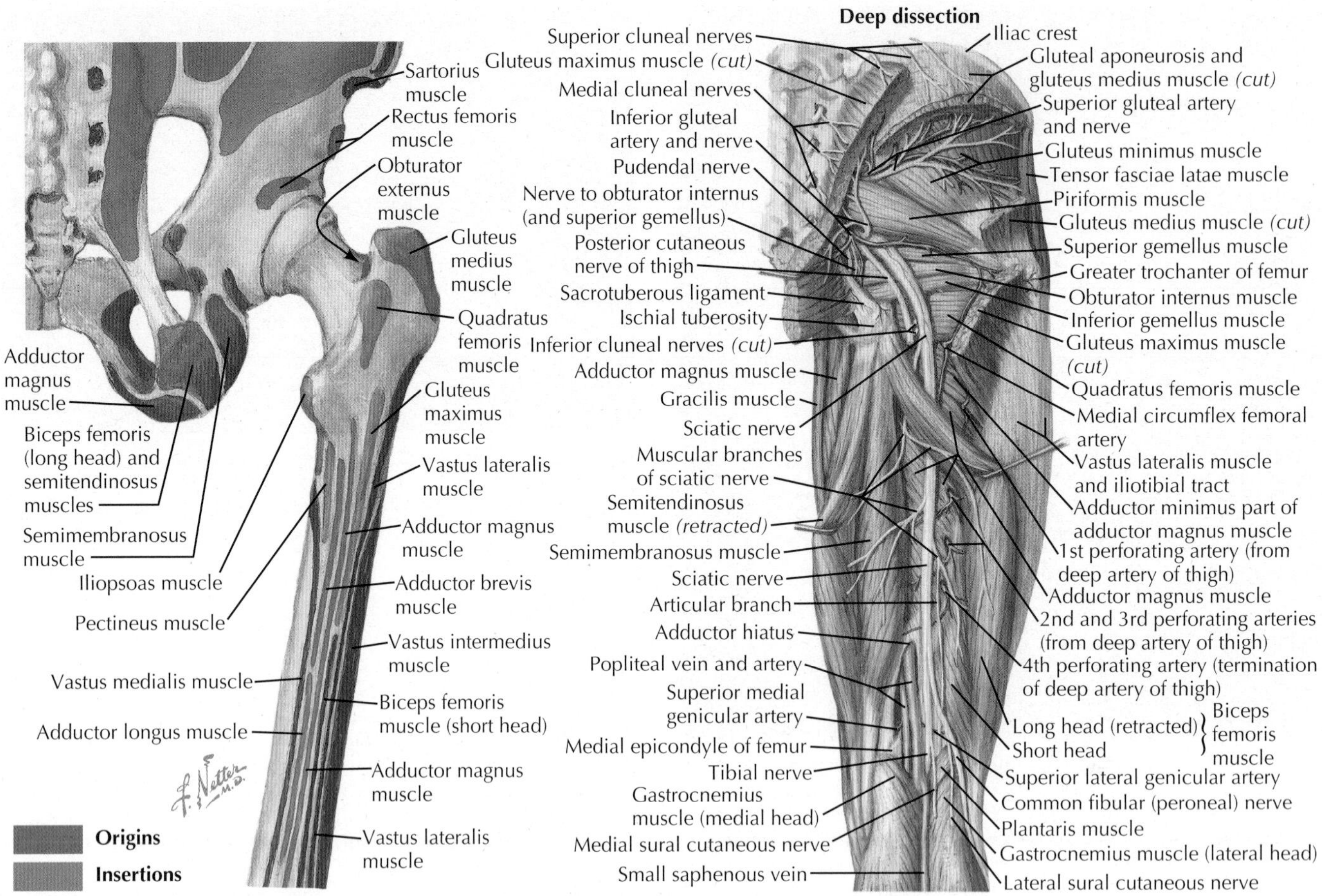
Sartorius muscle
Rectus femoris muscle
Obturator externus muscle
Gluteus medius muscle
Quadratus femoris muscle
Adductor magnus muscle
Gluteus maximus muscle
Biceps femoris (long head) and semitendinosus muscles
Vastus lateralis muscle
Semimembranosus muscle
Adductor magnus muscle
Iliopsoas muscle
Adductor brevis muscle
Pectineus muscle
Vastus intermedius muscle
Vastus medialis muscle
Biceps femoris muscle (short head)
Adductor longus muscle
Adductor magnus muscle
Vastus lateralis muscle
Origins
Insertions
Deep dissection
Superior cluneal nerves
Gluteus maximus muscle (cut)
Medial cluneal nerves
Inferior gluteal artery and nerve
Pudendal nerve
Nerve to obturator internus (and superior gemellus)
Posterior cutaneous nerve of thigh
Sacrotuberous ligament
Ischial tuberosity
Inferior cluneal nerves (cut)
Adductor magnus muscle
Gracilis muscle
Sciatic nerve
Muscular branches of sciatic nerve
Semitendinosus (retracted)
Semimembranosus muscle
Sciatic nerve
Articular branch
Adductor hiatus
Popliteal vein and artery
Superior medial genicular artery
Medial epicondyle of femur
Tibial nerve
Gastrocnemius muscle (medial head)
Medial sural cutaneous nerve
Small saphenous vein
Iliac crest
Gluteal aponeurosis and gluteus medius muscle (cut)
Superior gluteal artery and nerve
Gluteus minimus muscle
Tensor fasciae latae muscle
Piriformis muscle
Gluteus medius muscle (cut)
Superior gemellus muscle
Greater trochanter of femur
Obturator internus muscle
Inferior gemellus muscle
Gluteus maximus muscle (cut)
Quadratus femoris muscle
Medial circumflex femoral artery
Vastus lateralis muscle and iliotibial tract
Adductor minimus part of adductor magnus muscle
1st perforating artery (from deep artery of thigh)
Adductor magnus muscle
2nd and 3rd perforating arteries (from deep artery of thigh)
4th perforating artery (termination of deep artery of thigh)
Long head (retracted)
Short head
Biceps femoris muscle
Superior lateral genicular artery
Common fibular (peroneal) nerve
Plantaris muscle
Gastrocnemius muscle (lateral head)
Lateral sural cutaneous nerve

Figure 54.7 Muscles and insertions of pelvis, hip, and thigh.

Symptoms: Acute pain at the midline of the anterior thigh is most common. Pain or weakness may also be noted with resisted hip flexion or knee extension. A visible defect may be seen with complete avulsion of the rectus femoris tendon, though these injuries are rare.

Diagnosis: Similar to hamstring strains, history and physical examination are usually sufficient for diagnosis, though MRI (Fig. 54.11) may be used to determine severity and confirm a complete avulsion of the rectus femoris from its origin on the AIIS.

Treatment: In cases of muscle strain, RICE and strengthening exercises are useful. With proximal rupture of the rectus femoris, nonoperative management is an option, though surgical treatment with bone anchoring sutures should be indicated in patients with loss of hip flexion strength and high-level athletes who wish to return to normal activity.

Prognosis: With conservative treatment, patients with rectus femoris strains do very well. Prognosis is also very good in patients who undergo surgical treatment for complete avulsion injuries, with return to sports at an average of 4 months after surgery.

Gluteus Avulsion

Description: Avulsion of the gluteus could compromise the gluteus maximus, medius, or minimus. These injuries are more common in older patients. However, it can be seen after an abrupt trauma in young, active patients. Gluteus medius avulsions may be chronic ("rotator cuff tear of the hip") or may occur iatrogenically during total hip arthroplasty (THA) through an anterolateral or transgluteus approach.

Symptoms: Lateral hip pain and weakness of hip abduction. Patients who suffer gluteal avulsions during THA will typically also present with a limp.

Diagnosis: An MRI should always be indicated in those patients with chronic lateral hip pain. Many patients are mistakenly diagnosed with chronic bursitis. The MRI confirms the presence of gluteal tears from the greater trochanter or within the tendon.

Treatment: Operative treatment with transosseus sutures or suture anchors is necessary in cases of gluteal tears with retraction. The repair is done in a SpeedBridge fashion (double row). Use of an Achilles tendon allograft has been described for patients with large chronic abductor tears. Early operative management is preferred before the onset of muscle atrophy.

Prognosis: Surgical management is highly successful in relieving pain and weakness in patients with chronic tears. Patients with iatrogenic avulsions have less predictable improvement in strength after surgery.

Femoroacetabular Impingement

Description: Results from abnormal contact between the femoral head and the acetabulum. There are three subtypes of FAI: cam, pincer, and mixed.

- Cam: The femoral head is not round and therefore cannot rotate smoothly inside the acetabulum. The uneven surface of the femoral head results in an increased load on certain aspects of the acetabular cartilage during hip motion (zone of collision) (Fig. 54.12).
- Pincer: An acetabular abnormality whereby extra bone extends beyond the normal rim of the acetabulum, thereby impinging upon the femoral head and the labrum.
- Mixed: Patients may also have a combination of both cam and pincer types of impingement (Fig. 54.13).

Symptoms: Limited ROM, especially in flexion and internal rotation, with concomitant groin/hip pain.

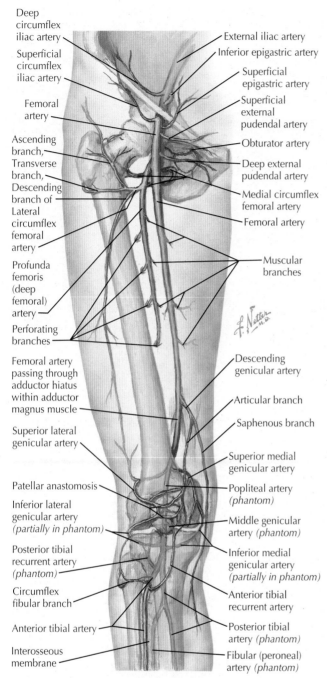

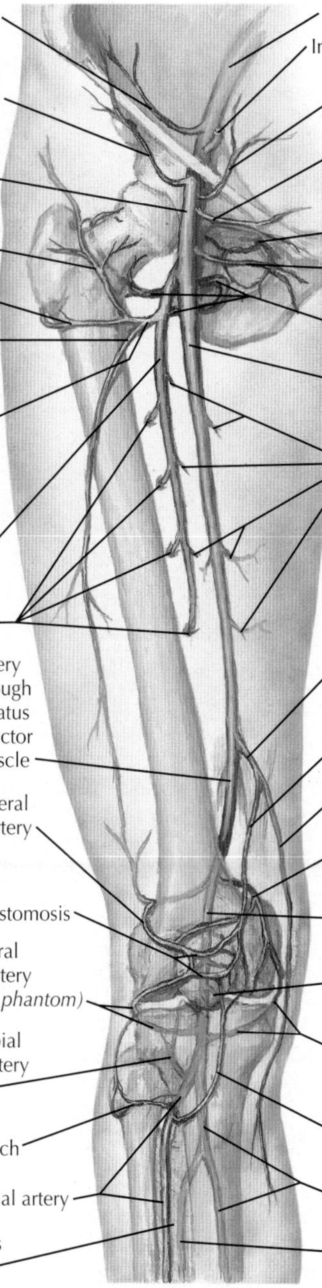
Deep circumflex iliac artery
Superficial circumflex iliac artery
Femoral artery
Ascending branch,
Transverse branch,
Descending branch of
Lateral circumflex femoral artery
Profunda femoris (deep femoral) artery
Perforating branches
Femoral artery passing through adductor hiatus within adductor magnus muscle
Superior lateral genicular artery
Patellar anastomosis
Inferior lateral genicular artery (partially in phantom)
Posterior tibial recurrent artery (phantom)
Circumflex fibular branch
Anterior tibial artery
Interosseous membrane
External iliac artery
Inferior epigastric artery
Superficial epigastric artery
Superficial external pudendal artery
Obturator artery
Deep external pudendal artery
Medial circumflex femoral artery
Femoral artery
Muscular branches
Descending genicular artery
Articular branch
Saphenous branch
Superior medial genicular artery
Popliteal artery (phantom)
Middle genicular artery (phantom)
Inferior medial genicular artery (partially in phantom)
Anterior tibial recurrent artery
Posterior tibial artery (phantom)
Fibular (peroneal) artery (phantom)

Figure 54.8 Arteries of the hip, pelvis, and thigh.

Diagnosis: Physical examination, such as the FADIR test, may provide clues to the diagnosis, although imaging is necessary to confirm FAI. Anteroposterior (AP) and true lateral views of the pelvis should be obtained. MRI or computed tomography (CT) may provide more information on the femoroacetabular incompatibility.

Treatment:

- Acetabular rim trimming: For patients with pincer or mixed-type deformities, arthroscopic removal of extra acetabular bone (acetabuloplasty) may be helpful. The labrum is normally hypoplastic in these patients and red secondary to inflammation. No more than 4–6 mm of the acetabular rim should be removed, as more than this results in increased loads in the hip joint. It is crucial to use CT preoperatively to determine the amount of rim that should be trimmed. Excessive rim trimming can lead to a dysplastic hip.
- Labral repair: The femoroacetabular mismatch in FAI results in frequent bone–bone contact, which can damage the labrum. Thus, labral repair should be performed at the same time as other procedures for FAI.
- Labral reconstruction: For irreparable labral tears, labral reconstruction may be necessary. This can be performed arthroscopically with autograft or allograft tissue to replace the labrum.
- Femoral osteochondroplasty: In patients with cam-type lesions, the femoral head–neck junction may be flat or convex, whereas normally it is concave. To alleviate the resulting abnormal contact between the femoral head–neck junction and the acetabular cartilage, an open or arthroscopic procedure may be performed to resect some of the bone overgrowth (Fig. 54.14).

Prognosis: A high percentage of patients are able to return to sport after surgery for FAI, with the majority of these returning to the same level of activity as before symptoms began.

Hip Instability: Borderline Dysplasia and Developmental Dysplasia of the Hip (DDH)

Description:

- Typical anatomic changes in DDH include a misshapen femoral head, a shallow acetabulum with loss of anterolateral coverage, decreased acetabular lateral tilt, and excessive anteversion of the acetabulum and proximal femur.
- The combination of these bony abnormalities can result in anterior hip instability and early degenerative changes because of these abnormal hip joint forces.
- The center-edge angle (CEA) of Wiberg is the angle formed by a vertical line drawn from the center of the femoral head and a line from the center of the femoral head to the most lateral edge of the acetabulum. Values less than 20 degrees are considered abnormal (dysplastic). Values between 20 and 25 degrees are considered borderline dysplasia.
- The anterior center-edge angle (ACE), or Lequesne angle, is measured on the false-profile view. Designed to assess anterior coverage of the femoral head, it can be calculated by measuring the angle between a vertical line through the center of the femoral head and a line connecting the center of the femoral head and the most anterior point of the acetabular sourcil.
- The measurement of the Tönnis angle can be determined by drawing three lines on the AP pelvic radiograph: (1) a horizontal line connecting the base of the acetabular teardrops (reference line); (2) a horizontal line parallel to line 1, running through the most inferior point of the sclerotic acetabular sourcil (point I); and (3) a line extending from point I to a point L at the lateral margin of the acetabular sourcil (the sclerotic weight-bearing portion of the acetabulum). The Tönnis angle is formed by the intersection of lines 2 and 3. Acetabula with a Tönnis angle of 0–10 degrees are considered normal, whereas those with an angle of >10 degrees or <0° degrees are considered to have increased and decreased inclination, respectively. Acetabula with increased Tönnis angles are subject to structural instability, whereas those with decreased Tönnis angles are at risk for pincer-type FAI.

Symptoms:

- Dysplasia is more frequent in females. Patients normally present in the office complaining of hip pain. They are normally flexible and have preserved or excessive ROM, especially internal rotation (IR).
- Patients may also describe popping secondary to iliopsoas irritation.
- Patients typically have pain while standing up, which differs from patients with FAI, who will report pain during sitting.

Diagnosis:

- Physical examination, together with x-ray, MRI, and CT, are necessary to make an accurate diagnosis of dysplasia.

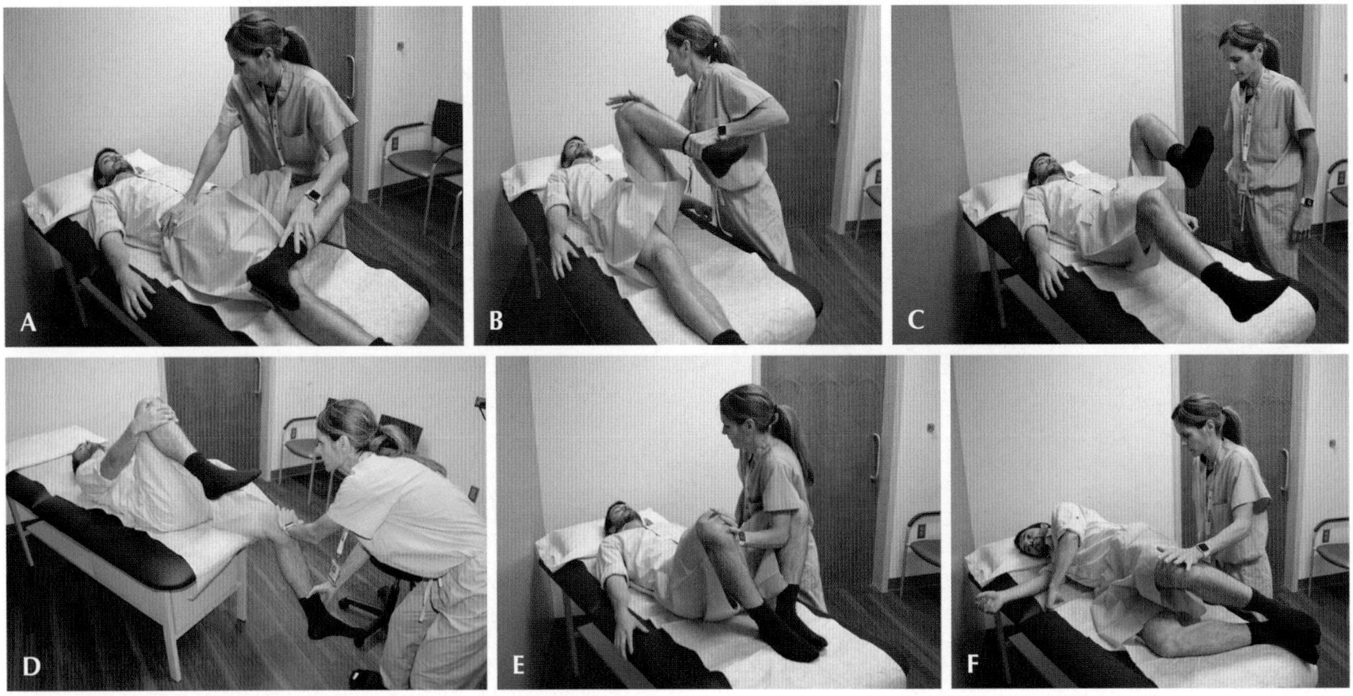

Figure 54.9 Physical examination. **A,** FABER (Flexion, ABduction, External Rotation). **B,** FADIR (Flexion, ADduction, Internal Rotation). **C,** Bicycle test. **D,** Posterior impingement test. **E,** Adductor squeeze test. **F,** Piriformis test.

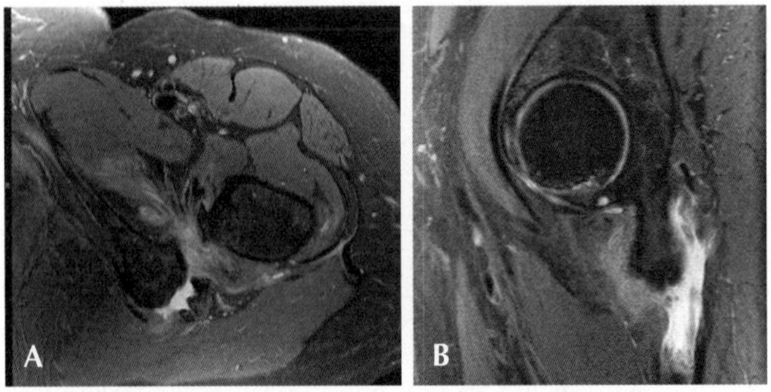

Figure 54.10 **(A)** Axial and **(B)** coronal MRI of the left hip showing complete avulsion of the proximal hamstring tendons.

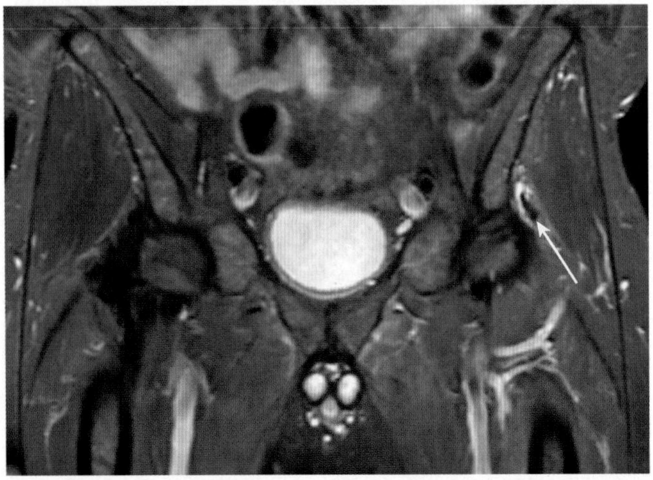

Figure 54.11 Hip coronal MRI showing a left rectus femoris avulsion *(white arrow)* from its origin on the anterior inferior iliac spine.

- X-ray: AP pelvis, Dunn view, and false profile should be evaluated. The AP pelvis should be a true AP pelvis for accurate measurements of the CEA and Tönnis angle. Dunn view will determine the presence of a concomitant FAI cam lesion, and the false profile is used to measure the ACE angle.
- CT: This is critical to evaluate the version of the socket, femoral version, and presence of a concomitant cam lesion. Most of these patients will present with an anteverted socket (>20 degrees) and an excessively anteverted femur (>20 degrees). It is important to determine the presence of dysplasia in a tridimensional way. Dysplasia could be lateral or anterior. Lateral dysplasia includes those that undercover the femoral head laterally (CEA <20 degrees). Others may present with a normal CEA but with an excessively anteverted (excessive ACE) socket, which undercovers the femoral head anteriorly.

Treatment: Will depend on the age of the patient, status of the cartilage, and presence of concomitant cam lesions. In patients with degenerative cartilage, surgery to preserve the hip joint is contraindicated. For young and active patients with healthy cartilage, surgery is indicated. Normally a hip arthroscopy is indicated, followed by a periacetabular osteotomy (PAO). Hip arthroscopy should be performed before PAO to treat intra-articular pathology, including labral tears, ligamentum teres tears, and cartilage damage. In these cases, a PAO is indicated to correct the dysplastic socket. Normally, surgery is performed to correct the anterior and lateral coverage. However, in some situations a reverse PAO is indicated. This is indicated for patients with an excessively retroverted socket and posterior instability.

PERITROCHANTERIC SPACE DISORDERS

Gluteal Bursitis

Ischial Bursitis

Description: Also known as *ischiogluteal bursitis* and results from inflammation of the ischiogluteal bursa found between the gluteus maximus and the ischial tuberosity.

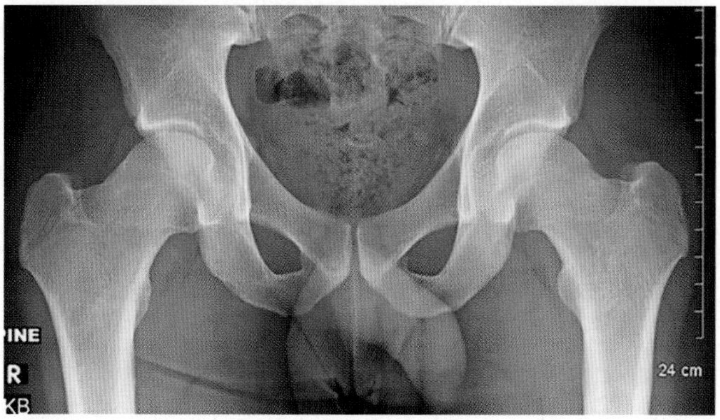
INE
R
KB
24 cm

Figure 54.12 Plain AP hip radiograph demonstrating bilateral cam impingement in a male patient.

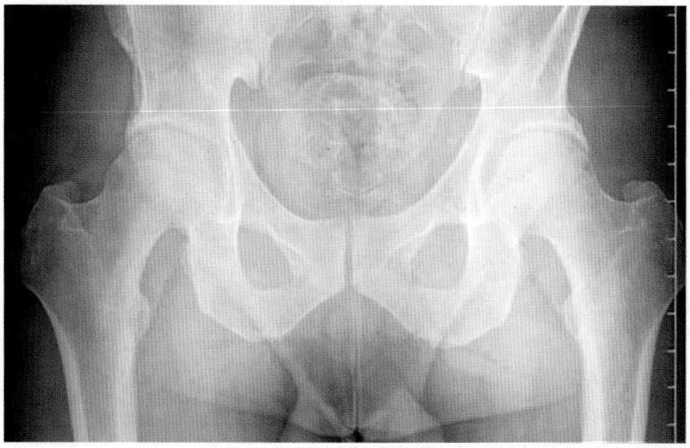

Figure 54.13 Plain AP hip radiograph with bilateral mixed-type FAI (pincer and cam deformities).

Symptoms: Pain at the medial buttock. May be difficult to distinguish from hamstring strain.

Diagnosis: Pain elicited by pressure over the ischial tuberosity with the patient in the lateral decubitus position. Absence of pain with stretching distinguishes ischial bursitis from a hamstring injury.

Treatment: Conservative treatment with anti-inflammatory medications and modification of training regimen. The use of corticosteroid injections into the ischiogluteal bursa and ischiogluteal bursectomy is poorly studied.

Prognosis: Return to sports may be allowed based on relief of symptoms. In refractory cases, more extensive diagnostic tests such as MRI may be necessary to rule out other pathologies such as hamstring tendon avulsions.

Trochanteric Bursitis

Description: Inflammation of the trochanteric bursa found just superficial to the greater trochanter.

Symptoms: Pain in the buttock or lateral hip, exacerbated by lying on the affected side, going from a seated to a standing position, or running on banked surfaces such as roadsides.

Diagnosis: Pain elicited by pressure at the lateral edge of the greater trochanter. An MRI is sometimes necessary to confirm the diagnosis and exclude the presence of a tear or tendinopathy of the glut.

Treatment: Conservative treatment with anti-inflammatory medications, modification of training regimen, and corticosteroid injections into the trochanteric bursa. In refractory cases, arthroscopic bursectomy, iliotibial band release, or trochanteric reduction osteotomy are options.

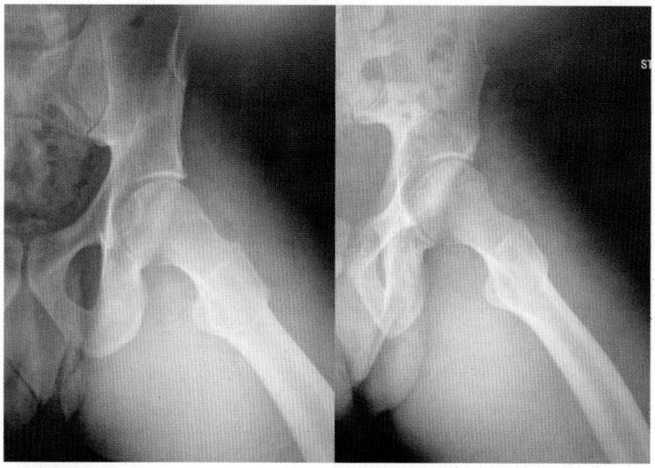

Figure 54.14 Dunn view of a left hip before *(left)* and after *(right)* cam resection.

Prognosis: Return to sports may be allowed based on relief of symptoms. Improvement in symptoms has been shown in the majority of patients undergoing various surgical treatments for trochanteric bursitis, though return to sport has not been well-defined in these patients.

Piriformis Syndrome

Description: Results from entrapment of the sciatic nerve under the piriformis muscle at the sciatic notch.

Symptoms: Pain and symptoms of sciatica with sitting, as this compresses the piriformis muscle against the sciatic nerve.

Diagnosis: Typically a diagnosis of exclusion. Sacroiliac dysfunction and lumbar disc herniation should be ruled out through pelvic radiographs and MRI of the lumbar spine, respectively.

Treatment: Massage of the piriformis muscle in addition to physical therapy with piriformis stretching exercises may improve symptoms in mild cases. Use of nonsteroidal anti-inflammatory medications may reduce inflammation at the site of nerve compression. Corticosteroid injections directly into the piriformis muscle may reduce muscle spasms and pain. For more severe cases, Botox injections in the piriformis muscle may be more effective in relaxing the muscle. For patients who do not respond to conservative treatment for 6 months or more, release of the distal tendon of the piriformis muscle may be performed.

Prognosis: Return to sports may be allowed based on relief of symptoms. Good outcomes have been shown in the majority of patients undergoing surgical release.

SUMMARY

History, physical examination, and imaging are the keys to accurate diagnosis of hip pathology. There have been significant advancements in arthroscopic techniques for surgical repair of hip pathology in recent years, which have resulted in an increase in the number of less invasive hip procedures.

RECOMMENDED READINGS

Available online.

55 KNEE INJURIES

Eric C. McCarty • John Wilson Belk • Christopher C. Madden

PHYSICAL EXAMINATION

Anatomy of the Knee

See Fig. 55.1.

Observation and Measurement

Standing

Alignment of lower extremities: View the patient from the front, side, and back.

Angular and rotational deformities: Excessive valgus, varus, recurvatum, flexion contracture, and femoral or tibial torsion

Foot alignment and mechanics: Excessive cavus or pes planus; heels should invert and arches increase on toe rising

Leg length inequality: Best judged by pelvic levelness on standing

Difference in size of legs: Atrophy of one limb versus hypertrophy of opposite limb

Popliteal masses: May be seen better in the prone position

Sitting

Patellar position: With patient's knees flexed 90 degrees, check from the side to judge a high or low position. The anterior patellar surface normally faces the wall in front of the patient sitting with legs over the side of the examination table. View from the front to judge lateral posture. The patella should appear centered in the soft tissue outline of the knee.

Osgood–Schlatter changes: Enlarged and/or tender tibial tuberosity

Vastus medialis obliquus/vastus lateralis (VMO/VL) relationship: With the patient's knees held actively at 45 degrees of flexion (Fig. 55.2), the distal one-third of the vastus medialis should normally present as a substantial muscle from the adductor tubercle, inserting into the upper one-third to one-half of the medial patella. Dysplastic VMO appears hollow in this normal muscular location (see Fig. 55.2); also observe for apparent hypertrophy of VL.

Patellar tracking: Observe on active flexion and extension; watch for excessive displacement of the patella.

Lying

SUPINE

Range of motion: Both active and passive; compare the injured with the uninjured side

Muscle bulk: Thigh and calf; can measure circumferences

Quadriceps (Q) angle: With quadriceps contracted, measure the angle between the line from the anterior superior iliac spine to the midpoint of the patella and the line from the midpoint of the patella to the tibial tuberosity (see Fig. 55.2); normal in males is ≤10 degrees and in females is ≤15 degrees.

Hamstring and heel cord tightness: See Chapter 42: "Musculoskeletal Injuries in Sports."

PRONE

Range of motion: Lack of full knee flexion may show quadriceps tightness

Popliteal masses: Compare contours with those of the opposite knee

Walking/Running

Mechanics of gait: Stance and swing phase from side to side is even; look for limp, other asymmetry, excessive limb rotation, or limb malalignment.

Patellofemoral tracking: Observe the patella closely from the front view.

Palpation

Joint effusion: With the patient's knee extended, milk fluid from the suprapatellar pouch, and palpate along medial and lateral sides of the patella (see Fig. 55.2). Try to distinguish intra-articular effusion that can be moved about from extra-articular swelling that feels more like thick soft tissue, which is not movable.

Significant areas of tenderness:

- Menisci: medial and lateral joint lines
- Ligament attachments: medial femoral epicondyle, adductor tubercle, lateral femoral epicondyle, proximal medial tibia
- Tendons: patellar tendon, quadriceps tendon, popliteus tendon, hamstrings
- Bursae: prepatellar, pes anserinus, tibial collateral ligament, deep infrapatellar
- Other: patellar facets, extensor retinaculum

Crepitation: During range of motion—from any rough joint surface (particularly patellofemoral joint), fractures, or soft tissue thickness; **patellofemoral compression**—longitudinal and/or transverse compression of the patella against the femur. Examine for crepitation or ask regarding any elicited pain.

Muscle tone: Overall turgor of muscle tissue; may be decreased early after injury, even if the bulk still measures normal

Specific Tests

Perform all tests on an uninjured knee first to establish "normal" baseline for that patient (Table 55.1).

Ligaments

MEDIAL

Valgus stress test at 30 and 0 degrees: The patient is supine and relaxed, with the thigh supported on the table. The examiner applies valgus force at the foot while using other hand as a fulcrum along the lateral side of the joint. Watch and feel for medial joint line opening. Perform first with the knee flexed to 30 degrees, then with maximum possible extension or hyperextension (Fig. 55.3).

Anterior drawer test with external rotation of tibia: The patient is supine and relaxed, with the hip flexed to 45 degrees and knee to 90 degrees. Externally rotate the foot 30 degrees; then, pin the foot to the table with the examiner's thigh. Grasp the proximal tibia with both hands and pull toward the examiner. A positive test is excessive anterior rotation of the medial tibial condyle (see Fig. 55.3).

LATERAL

Varus stress test at 30 and 0 degrees: The patient is in the same position as for the abduction stress test. Reverse the hand position so that one hand applies varus stress while the other acts as a fulcrum along the medial side of the joint. Watch and feel for lateral joint line opening. Perform the test at 30 degrees of flexion and then at full possible extension or hyperextension (see Fig. 55.3).

External rotation recurvatum test: The patient is supine and relaxed. Lift the entire lower extremity by the first toe. Observe for excessive recurvatum and external rotation of the proximal tibia (tibial tuberosity) and apparent varus deformity of the knee; indicates posterolateral corner injury

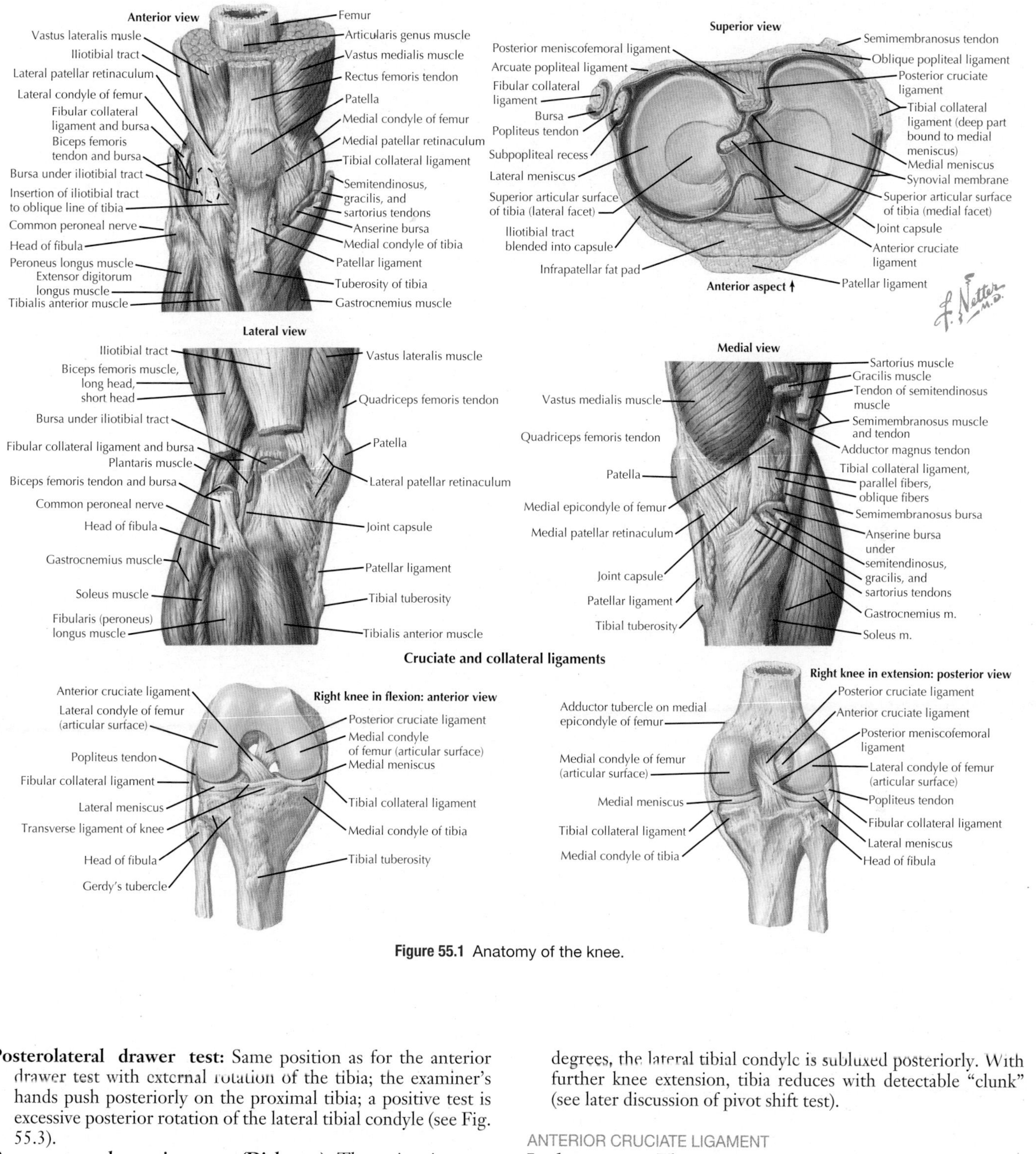
Anterior view
Femur
Vastus lateralis musle
Articularis genus muscle
Iliotibial tract
Vastus medialis muscle
Lateral patellar retinaculum
Rectus femoris tendon
Lateral condyle of femur
Patella
Fibular collateral ligament and bursa
Medial condyle of femur
Biceps femoris tendon and bursa
Medial patellar retinaculum
Tibial collateral ligament
Bursa under iliotibial tract
Semitendinosus, gracilis, and sartorius tendons
Insertion of iliotibial tract to oblique line of tibia
Common peroneal nerve
Anserine bursa
Head of fibula
Medial condyle of tibia
Peroneus longus muscle
Patellar ligament
Extensor digitorum longus muscle
Tuberosity of tibia
Tibialis anterior muscle
Gastrocnemius muscle
Superior view
Posterior meniscofemoral ligament
Semimembranosus tendon
Arcuate popliteal ligament
Oblique popliteal ligament
Fibular collateral ligament
Posterior cruciate ligament
Bursa
Popliteus tendon
Tibial collateral ligament (deep part bound to medial meniscus)
Subpopliteal recess
Medial meniscus
Lateral meniscus
Synovial membrane
Superior articular surface of tibia (lateral facet)
Superior articular surface of tibia (medial facet)
Iliotibial tract blended into capsule
Joint capsule
Anterior cruciate ligament
Infrapatellar fat pad
Anterior aspect
Patellar ligament
F. Netter M.D.
Lateral view
Iliotibial tract
Vastus lateralis muscle
Biceps femoris muscle, long head, short head
Quadriceps femoris tendon
Bursa under iliotibial tract
Patella
Fibular collateral ligament and bursa
Plantaris muscle
Lateral patellar retinaculum
Biceps femoris tendon and bursa
Common peroneal nerve
Head of fibula
Joint capsule
Gastrocnemius muscle
Patellar ligament
Soleus muscle
Tibial tuberosity
Fibularis (peroneus) longus muscle
Tibialis anterior muscle
Medial view
Sartorius muscle
Gracilis muscle
Tendon of semitendinosus muscle
Vastus medialis muscle
Semimembranosus muscle and tendon
Quadriceps femoris tendon
Adductor magnus tendon
Tibial collateral ligament, parallel fibers, oblique fibers
Patella
Medial epicondyle of femur
Semimembranosus bursa
Medial patellar retinaculum
Anserine bursa under semitendinosus, gracilis, and sartorius tendons
Joint capsule
Patellar ligament
Gastrocnemius m.
Tibial tuberosity
Soleus m.
Cruciate and collateral ligaments
Right knee in flexion: anterior view
Anterior cruciate ligament
Lateral condyle of femur (articular surface)
Posterior cruciate ligament
Medial condyle of femur (articular surface)
Popliteus tendon
Medial meniscus
Fibular collateral ligament
Lateral meniscus
Tibial collateral ligament
Transverse ligament of knee
Medial condyle of tibia
Head of fibula
Tibial tuberosity
Gerdy's tubercle
Right knee in extension: posterior view
Posterior cruciate ligament
Adductor tubercle on medial epicondyle of femur
Anterior cruciate ligament
Posterior meniscofemoral ligament
Medial condyle of femur (articular surface)
Lateral condyle of femur (articular surface)
Medial meniscus
Popliteus tendon
Tibial collateral ligament
Fibular collateral ligament
Medial condyle of tibia
Lateral meniscus
Head of fibula

Figure 55.1 Anatomy of the knee.

Posterolateral drawer test: Same position as for the anterior drawer test with external rotation of the tibia; the examiner's hands push posteriorly on the proximal tibia; a positive test is excessive posterior rotation of the lateral tibial condyle (see Fig. 55.3).

Prone external rotation test (Dial test): The patient is prone with the knees together, and the feet are externally rotated at 30 degrees of knee flexion and then at 90 degrees. The external rotation of the foot relative to the thigh is compared with the contralateral side. The test is positive if there is >10 degrees of rotation of the affected side compared with that of the normal side. If asymmetry is present only at 30 degrees, then isolated posterolateral corner injury is likely. If asymmetry is present at both 30 and 90 degrees, combined injury to the posterior cruciate ligament (PCL) and posterolateral corner is present (see Fig. 55.3).

Reverse pivot shift test: Performed with the tibia in external rotation rather than internal rotation; with knee flexed 90 degrees, the lateral tibial condyle is subluxed posteriorly. With further knee extension, tibia reduces with detectable "clunk" (see later discussion of pivot shift test).

ANTERIOR CRUCIATE LIGAMENT

Lachman test: The patient is supine and relaxed; the examiner grasps the distal femur with one hand, while other hand grasps the proximal tibia; knee flexed to approximately 15–20 degrees; apply anterior force to proximal tibia while holding distal femur in place. Positive test is excessive anterior translation of the tibia beneath the femur and lack of a firm endpoint (see Fig. 55.3).

Anterior drawer test in neutral rotation: Same position as for anterior drawer with external rotation of the tibia except that foot and tibia are in neutral rotation; anterior pull is applied to the proximal tibia. Positive test is anterior translation of both tibial condyles from beneath the femur (see Fig. 55.3). *Note:* This test is influenced by structures other than anterior cruciate

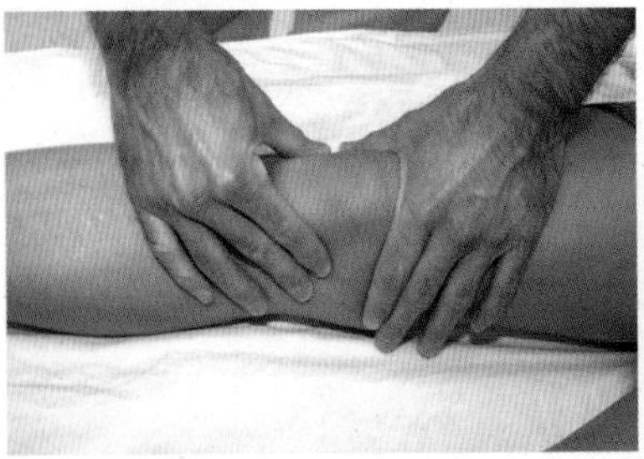

Effusion. Fluid is milked from suprapatellar pouch with one hand and with other and the fluid is palpated on the sides of the patella.

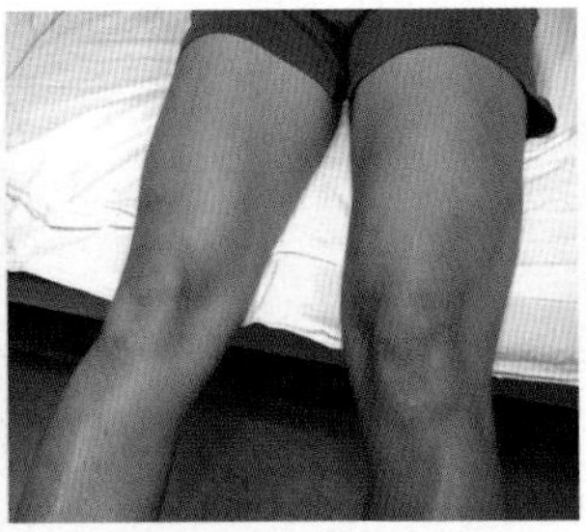

Vastus medialis obliquus (VMO). Patient with marked VMO dysplasia. This is probably the most important predisposition to all extensor mechanism syndromes.

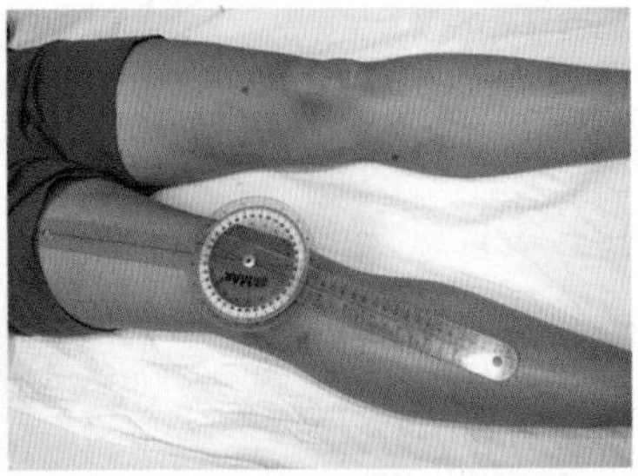

Quadriceps (Q) angle measurement. With quadriceps contracted, proximal arm of goniometer is directed toward anterior superior spone, pivot point of goniometer is directed toward anterior superior spone, pivot point of goniometer is placed over the center of patella, and distal arm of goniometer is placed on tibial tuberosity. Normal in males, up to 10 degrees; females, 15 degrees.

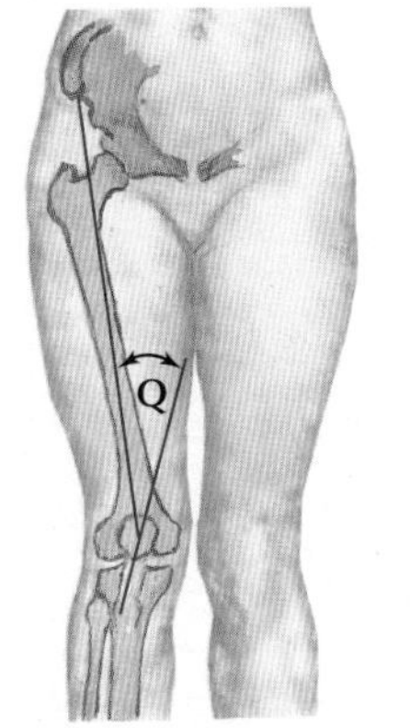
Q

Q angle formed by intersection of lines from anterior superior iliac spine and from tibial tuberosity through midpoint of patella. Large Q angle predisposes to patellar subluxation.

Figure 55.2 Observations and measurement of the knee.

Table 55.1 KEY PHYSICAL EXAMINATION TESTS AND INJURED STRUCTURES

Test	Injured Structure
Valgus stress test at 30 degrees and 0 degrees	30 degrees: Medial collateral ligament 0 degrees: Posteromedial corner, medial collateral ligament, posterior cruciate ligament, possibly anterior cruciate ligament
Varus stress test at 30 degrees and 0 degrees	30 degrees: Lateral collateral ligament 0 degrees: Posterolateral corner, lateral collateral ligament, posterior cruciate ligament
Lachman test	Anterior cruciate ligament
Anterior drawer test	Anterior cruciate ligament, but affected by other structures such as collaterals
Pivot shift test/jerk test	Anterior cruciate ligament
Posterior drawer test	Posterior cruciate ligament
Gravity or sag test	Posterior cruciate ligament
Posterolateral drawer test	Posterolateral corner structures
External rotation recurvatum test	Posterolateral corner structures
McMurray test	Menisci
Apley compression test	Menisci
Apprehension test	Medial patellofemoral ligament and retinaculum
Prone external rotation test (dial test)	Posterolateral corner structures

ligament (ACL). Do not rely on this test for diagnosis of ACL tear.

Pivot shift test and jerk test: The patient is supine and relaxed. Begin with knee fully extended (pivot shift test) or flexed to 90 degrees (jerk test); foot and tibia internally rotated; valgus applied at knee; knee progressively flexed (pivot shift test) or extended (jerk test). At approximately 30 degrees, watch and feel for anterior subluxation of lateral tibial condyle: tibia suddenly reduces with further flexion (pivot shift test) or extension (jerk test) (see Fig. 55.3).

POSTERIOR CRUCIATE LIGAMENT

Posterior drawer test: Same position as for anterior drawer test in neutral rotation; posterior force is applied to proximal tibia. Positive test is straight posterior displacement of both tibial condyles (see Fig. 55.3). *Caution:* Ensure a neutral position as the starting point. Compare position of the tibia relative to the femur with normal knee. It is easy to start from a posteriorly displaced position and interpret reduction to neutral as a positive anterior drawer sign rather than starting at neutral and interpreting as a positive posterior drawer sign.

Gravity or sag test: The patient is supine and relaxed. Flex hips to 45 degrees and knees to 90 degrees with feet flat on table. With quadriceps relaxed, observe from the lateral side for posterior displacement of one tibial tuberosity compared with the other; then flex the hips to 90 degrees, support both legs by the ankles and feet, and observe again (see Fig. 55.3).

Valgus or varus stress test at 0 degrees: As described for abduction and adduction stress tests at 30 and 0 degrees; positive test in full extension in acute case is often the result of PCL rupture in addition to injury to associated collateral ligaments (see Fig. 55.3).

Menisci

Joint line tenderness: Tenderness along the medial or lateral joint lines is among the most sensitive findings for a meniscal tear (see Fig. 55.3).

McMurray test: The patient is supine and relaxed. Have patient flex knee maximally with external tibial rotation (medial meniscus) or internal tibial rotation (lateral meniscus). While maintaining rotation, patient brings the knee into full extension. Positive test is a painful pop occurring over the medial (medial meniscus) or lateral (lateral meniscus) joint line (see Fig. 55.3).

Apley compression test: The patient is in joint line prone position. Knee is flexed to 90 degrees with external tibial rotation (medial meniscus) or internal tibial rotation (lateral meniscus). Apply axial compression to joint line tibia while joint line patient flexes and extends joint line knee. Positive test is a painful pop over joint line medial (medial meniscus) or lateral (lateral meniscus) joint line (see Fig. 55.3).

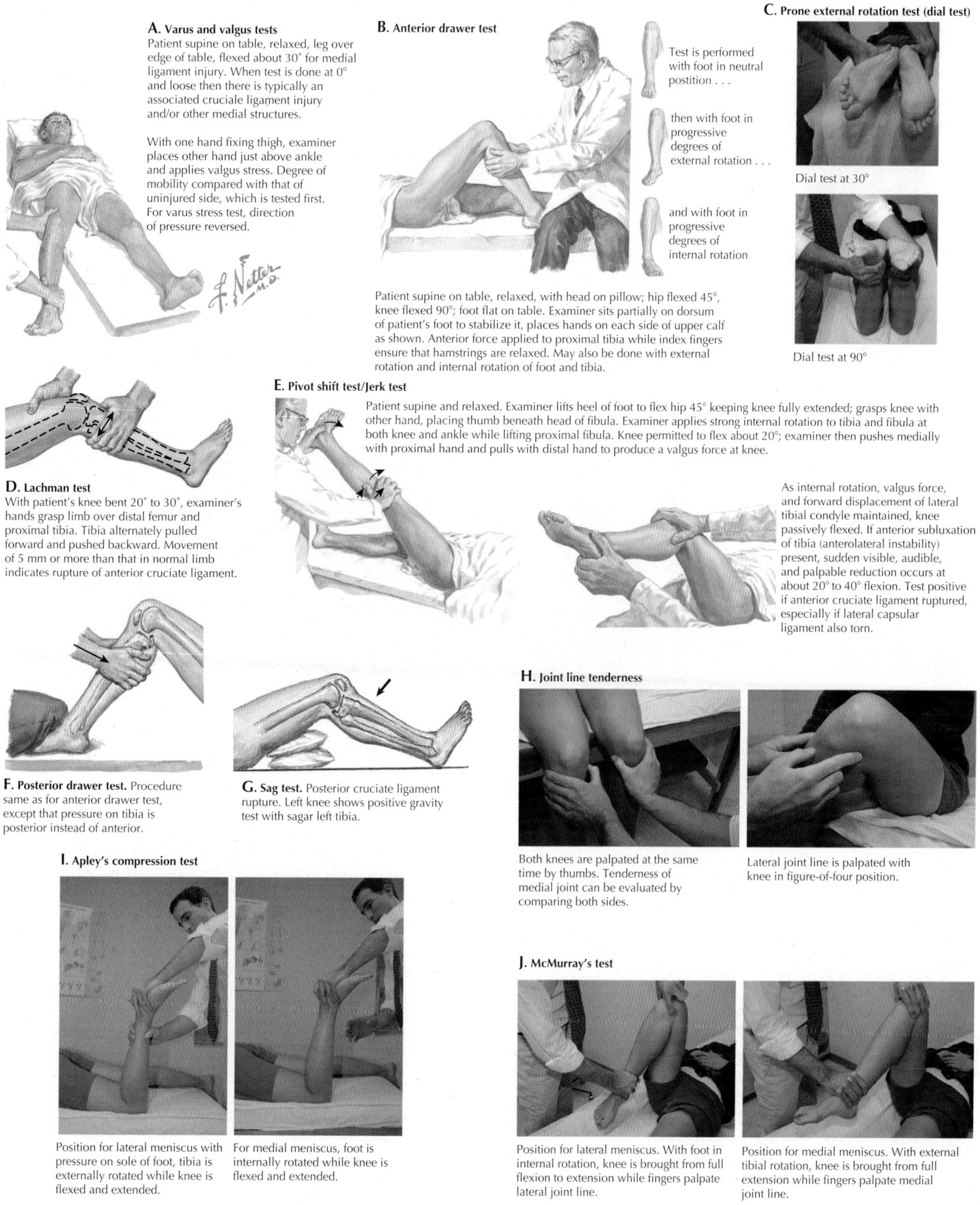
A. Varus and valgus tests
Patient supine on table, relaxed, leg over edge of table, flexed about 30° for medial ligament injury. When test is done at 0° and loose then there is typically an associated cruciale ligament injury and/or other medial structures.
With one hand fixing thigh, examiner places other hand just above ankle and applies valgus stress. Degree of mobility compared with that of uninjured side, which is tested first. For varus stress test, direction of pressure reversed.
B. Anterior drawer test
Test is performed with foot in neutral postition . . .
then with foot in progressive degrees of external rotation . . .
and with foot in progressive degrees of internal rotation
Patient supine on table, relaxed, with head on pillow; hip flexed 45°, knee flexed 90°; foot flat on table. Examiner sits partially on dorsum of patient's foot to stabilize it, places hands on each side of upper calf as shown. Anterior force applied to proximal tibia while index fingers ensure that hamstrings are relaxed. May also be done with external rotation and internal rotation of foot and tibia.
C. Prone external rotation test (dial test)
Dial test at 30°
Dial test at 90°
D. Lachman test
With patient's knee bent 20° to 30°, examiner's hands grasp limb over distal femur and proximal tibia. Tibia alternately pulled forward and pushed backward. Movement of 5 mm or more than that in normal limb indicates rupture of anterior cruciate ligament.
E. Pivot shift test/Jerk test
Patient supine and relaxed. Examiner lifts heel of foot to flex hip 45° keeping knee fully extended; grasps knee with other hand, placing thumb beneath head of fibula. Examiner applies strong internal rotation to tibia and fibula at both knee and ankle while lifting proximal fibula. Knee permitted to flex about 20°; examiner then pushes medially with proximal hand and pulls with distal hand to produce a valgus force at knee.
As internal rotation, valgus force, and forward displacement of lateral tibial condyle maintained, knee passively flexed. If anterior subluxation of tibia (anterolateral instability) present, sudden visible, audible, and palpable reduction occurs at about 20° to 40° flexion. Test positive if anterior cruciate ligament ruptured, especially if lateral capsular ligament also torn.
F. Posterior drawer test. Procedure same as for anterior drawer test, except that pressure on tibia is posterior instead of anterior.
G. Sag test. Posterior cruciate ligament rupture. Left knee shows positive gravity test with sagar left tibia.
H. Joint line tenderness
Both knees are palpated at the same time by thumbs. Tenderness of medial joint can be evaluated by comparing both sides.
Lateral joint line is palpated with knee in figure-of-four position.
I. Apley's compression test
Position for lateral meniscus with pressure on sole of foot, tibia is externally rotated while knee is flexed and extended.
For medial meniscus, foot is internally rotated while knee is flexed and extended.
J. McMurray's test
Position for lateral meniscus. With foot in internal rotation, knee is brought from full flexion to extension while fingers palpate lateral joint line.
Position for medial meniscus. With external tibial rotation, knee is brought from full extension while fingers palpate medial joint line.

Figure 55.3 Special tests.

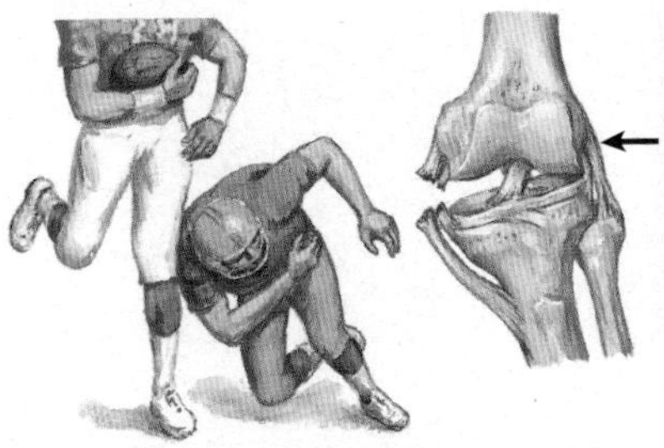

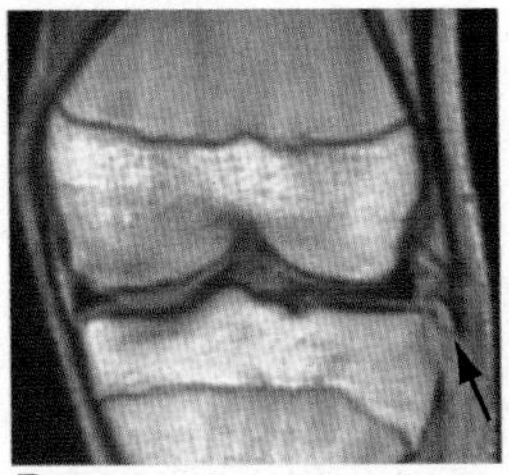

C. Anterior cruciate ligament rupture

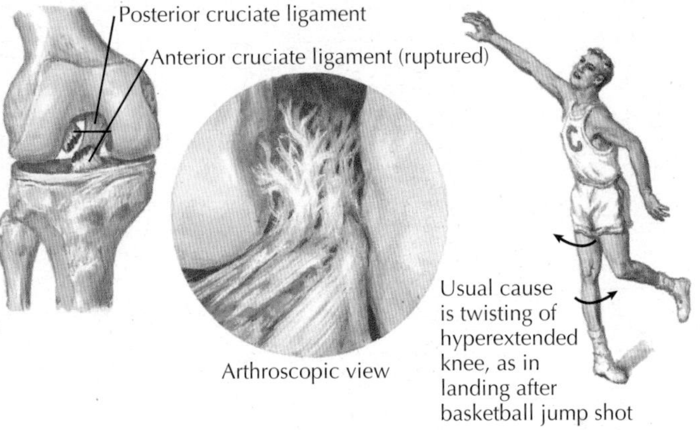
Posterior cruciate ligament
Anterior cruciate ligament (ruptured)
Arthroscopic view
Usual cause is twisting of hyperextended knee, as in landing after basketball jump shot

A. Medial collateral ligament injury. Usual cause is forceful impact on posterolateral aspect of knee with foot anchored, producing valgus stress on knee joint. Valgus stress may rupture tibial collateral and capsular ligaments.

B. Lateral ligament injury. Segond fracture of the knee. Coronal proton density-weighted MRI demonstrates avulsion of the bony insertion of the iliotibial band *(arrow)*. Avulsions of the lateral collateral ligament complex have a close association with ACL injury. (From Adam A, Dixon A, Grainger R, Allison D. *Grainger & Allison's Diagnostic Radiology,* 5th ed. Philadelphia: Elsevier; 2008.)

D. Posterior cruciate ligament injury. Usual causes include hyperextension injury, as occurs from stepping into hole, and direct blow to flexed knee.

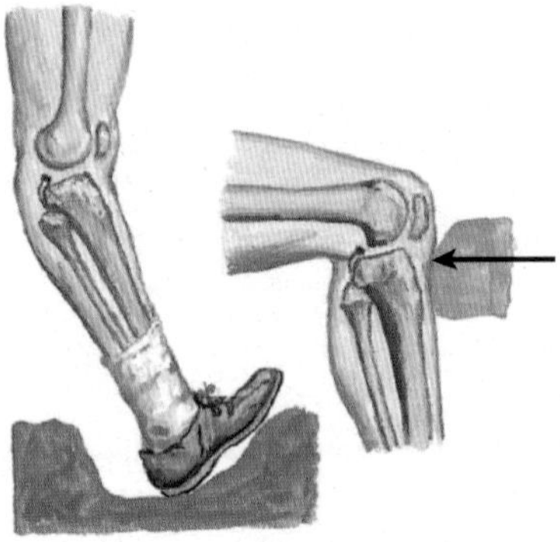

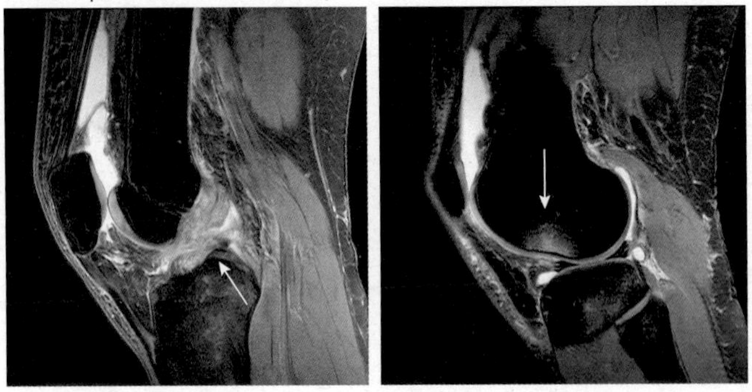

Acute anterior cruciate ligament tear. Fat-suppressed proton density–weighted image *(left)* shows irregular distorted fibers of torn ACL *(arrow)*. Hyperintense bone marrow edema *(right)* in lateral femoral condyle (*arrow*) is a secondary sign often seen with acute ACL injury. (Reused with permission from Witte D. Magnetic Resonance Imaging in Orthopaedics in *Campbells Orthopedics.* Elsevier; 2013).

Figure 55.4 Knee ligament injuries.

Thessaly test: The patient is standing with 20 degrees of knee flexion on the affected limb. Apply recurrent external and internal rotation of the knee. Positive test is pain, discomfort, or clicking.

Patella

Hypermobility/apprehension test: The patient is supine and relaxed. The examiner sits on edge of the table with the patient's knee flexed approximately 30–45 degrees across the examiner's thigh. With the patient's quadriceps relaxed, the examiner uses both thumbs to forcefully displace the patella over the lateral femoral condyle. Positive test is increased lateral mobility of the patella compared with the opposite knee or other patients; more important is discomfort or extreme apprehension that the patella is going to dislocate because of lateral displacement.

Plica tests: The patient is supine and relaxed. With the tibia internally rotated, the examiner passively flexes and extends knee from 30 to 100 degrees of flexion. Examining the fingers placed along the medial patellofemoral joint may feel a click, possibly some tenderness, or even a pop of a pathologic plica.

KNEE LIGAMENT INJURIES

Medial Ligaments

Description: Injury to medial (tibial) collateral ligament and/or medial capsular ligament (Fig. 55.4)

Mechanism of injury: Valgus force applied to the knee with external tibial rotation; may be noncontact twist or a blow to lateral side of joint

Presentation: Initial pain on medial side of the knee; with complete tear, complaints of the knee giving way into valgus

Examination: Positive valgus stress test at a 30-degree flexion; compare with opposite knee. An injured medial collateral ligament (MCL) along with disrupted ACL or PCL will result in more gap occurring with a valgus stress test, particularly noticeable when the knee is tested in extension. Frequently, but not always, positive anterior drawer sign results with the tibia in external rotation. The medial tibial condyle rotates anteriorly.

Imaging: Abduction stress radiographs may be used to distinguish ligament injury from epiphyseal fracture in skeletally immature athletes. Fracture opens at the growth plate; ligament tear opens at the joint line; perform in 20–30 degrees of flexion.

Differential diagnosis: In young patients, epiphyseal fracture of the distal femur or proximal tibia; patellar dislocation (may be associated with MCL tear); medial meniscus tear (may be associated with MCL tear)

Treatment:

- **Grades I and II sprains:** Rest, ice, compression, and elevation (RICE); crutches; rehabilitation
- **Grade III sprain (complete ligament tear):** With other associated injuries, surgery may be considered (currently rare); if no surgery indicated, immobilization should be used for short period after acute injury; begin rehabilitation program as soon as possible; with only mild instability, rigid immobilization may not be necessary. RICE and functional rehabilitation may be adequate treatment.

Lateral Ligaments

Description: Sprain or tear of lateral (fibular) collateral ligament and/or lateral capsular ligament; may be associated injuries to popliteus tendon, iliotibial band, popliteofemoral ligament, and peroneal nerve

Mechanism of injury: Varus or twisting injury; may be contact or noncontact. Posterolateral ligaments often injured by a hyperextension mechanism, frequently with a blow to the anteromedial tibia

Presentation: Pain is present over the lateral ligament complex. Knee may give way on twisting, cutting, or pivoting. In chronic cases, posterolateral corner injury gives a feeling of giving way into hyperextension when standing, walking, or running backward.

Examination: Compare with opposite knee; in acute case, may be increased varus stress test at 30 degrees of flexion and positive posterolateral drawer sign; chronic cases show a positive reverse pivot shift test and external rotation recurvatum test. External rotation recurvatum may also be apparent on standing, giving increased varus appearance to the knee.

Imaging: Lateral capsular sign shows avulsion of the midportion of the lateral capsular ligament with a small fragment of proximal lateral tibia. Associated with a high incidence of anterior cruciate tear and indicates anterolateral instability (see Fig. 55.4). Arcuate sign shows avulsion of proximal fibula with the posterolateral ligament complex; indicates posterolateral instability.

Differential diagnosis: Chronic posterolateral injury may be confused with medial compartment arthritis because of progressive varus appearance; difficult to differentiate from posterior cruciate injury. Acute lateral ligament injury may be confused with lateral meniscus tear. Injury to the middle third of the lateral capsular ligament, as shown by lateral capsular sign on radiograph, usually associated with ACL injury.

Treatment:

- **Grade I and II sprains:** RICE, crutches, rehabilitation
- **Grade III sprain (complete ligament tear):** Surgical repair is usually preferable if injury involves more than just lateral (fibular) collateral ligament. Immobilization is not really useful by itself. Mild instability may be treated by RICE and functional rehabilitation.

Anterior Cruciate Ligament

Description: Tear of part or all of two major bundles (posterolateral and anteromedial) of ACL; may be associated with tears of middle one-third of lateral capsular ligament. ACL is torn from femur or tibia, or torn in its midportion; may avulse tibial spine in young patients (see Fig. 55.4).

Mechanism of injury: Hyperextension, varus/internal rotation, and extremes of valgus and external rotation are possible causes.

Presentation: Usually a loud pop occurs; may be followed by autonomic symptoms of dizziness, sweating, faintness, and slight nausea. A large swelling usually occurs within first 2 hours after an acute injury (hemarthrosis). Conversely, most acute hemarthroses (85%) are anterior cruciate tears; in chronic cases, complaints of giving way on twisting, pivoting, and cutting.

Examination: Acute, large hemarthrosis; positive Lachman test; chronic, positive Lachman test, positive pivot shift test or jerk test; perhaps a positive anterior drawer sign, but not reliable; do not rely on the anterior drawer sign

Imaging: Lateral capsular sign; avulsion of the tibial spine may be seen in young patients; magnetic resonance imaging (MRI) useful in acute injury to confirm diagnosis and evaluate for injuries to other structures; reported accuracy rates as high as 95% in detecting ACL tears (see Fig. 55.4). Subchondral bruising of the middle one-third of the lateral femoral condyle and posterior one-third of the lateral tibial plateau (kissing lesion) is present on MRI in over half of acute ACL tears.

Differential diagnosis: Acute, differentiate from other causes of hemarthrosis (e.g., osteochondral fracture, peripheral meniscus tear, and patellar dislocation); chronic, differentiate from other types of ligamentous laxity and/or meniscal tears

Treatment:

- Acute
  - Various methods delineate degree of damage and associated injuries
  - Knee may be treated symptomatically, followed by repeated evaluations over initial 2–3 weeks after injury.
  - Most active patients engaged in agility sports require surgical reconstruction.
  - Graft recommendations vary on patient sex, age, and activity level
  - Reconstruction is now usually delayed at least 3 weeks after injury to allow decrease in swelling and increase in range of motion.
  - For mild laxity with a firm endpoint (partial ACL injury) and no other associated injury, may treat with PRICES (protect, rest, ice, compression, elevation), functional rehabilitation, and protective bracing
  - Apparent partial injuries often progress to more obvious complete tears.
- Chronic
  - May attempt functional stabilization through rehabilitation, bracing, lifestyle modification; often requires surgical reconstruction
- Re-rupture
  - Revision ACL reconstruction often indicated, may require additional stabilization procedure (lateral extra-articular tenodesis, anterolateral ligament reconstruction).
  - Consider further investigation into patient's native patellofemoral kinematics to evaluate risk for excessive anterior tibial translation.

Posterior Cruciate Ligament

Description: Tear of part or all of two major bundles of the PCL (posteromedial and anterolateral)

Mechanism of injury: Valgus/varus in full extension; in rare cases, severe twist; direct blow to the anterior proximal tibia, as in fall on artificial turf or other hard playing surface

Presentation: Usually less swelling than with ACL; otherwise, in acute stage, nothing particularly distinguishing; chronically, feeling of femur sliding anteriorly off tibia, particularly when rapidly decelerating or descending slopes or stairs

Examination: Acute, if produced by varus or valgus mechanism, may find abduction or adduction stress test positive in full extension; if produced by blow to anterior tibia, posterior drawer sign may be positive; chronic, rely on posterior drawer sign and gravity test (see Fig. 55.4)

Imaging: Cross-table lateral view radiographs may show sag of tibia compared with opposite side; may accentuate by doing posterior drawer sign while taking cross-table lateral view; may see bony avulsion with tibial attachment of the PCL; MRI shows posterior cruciate well and may help confirm diagnosis and evaluate for other injuries (see Fig. 55.4).

Differential diagnosis: Most difficult is distinguishing posterior cruciate injury from posterolateral corner injury; posterior drawer sign and posterolateral drawer sign may appear the same. Both injuries may exist in the same knee.

Treatment: Acute, most important to delineate degree of injury; may require examination under anesthesia and arthroscopy; for mild laxity (isolated PCL tear), may treat with PRICES, functional rehabilitation, protective bracing; for moderate or severe laxity, surgical repair/reconstruction is usually required

Chronic, may attempt functional stabilization through rehabilitation and bracing; often requires surgical reconstruction if instability is more than mild

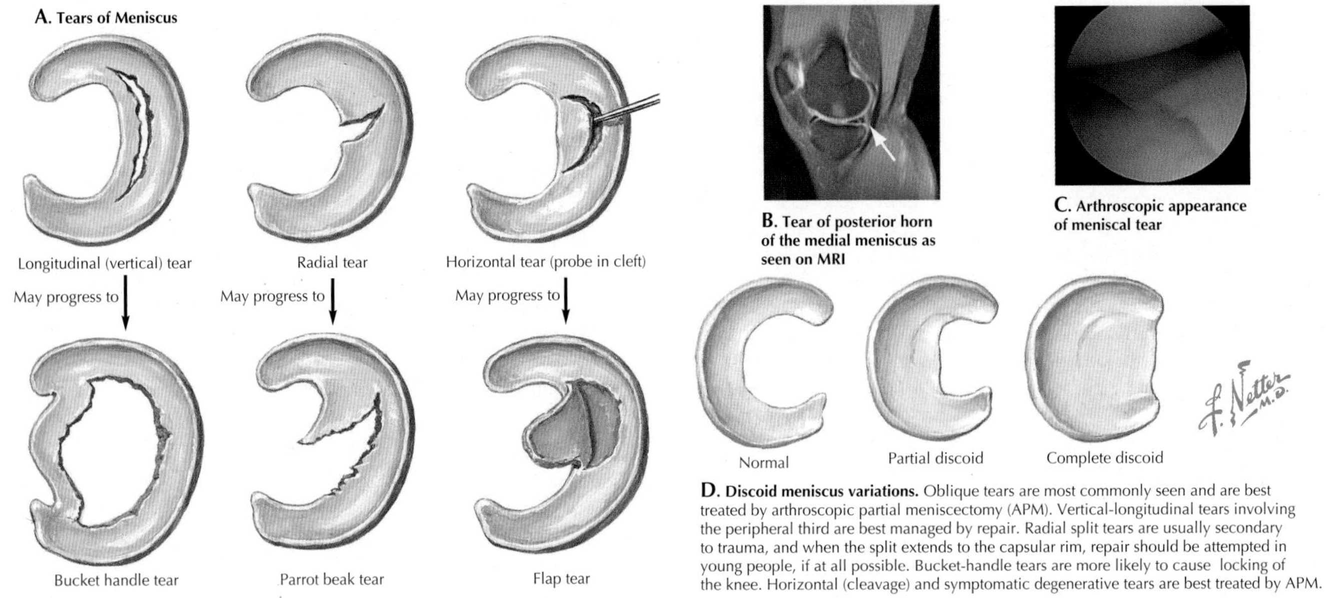
A. Tears of Meniscus
Longitudinal (vertical) tear
Radial tear
Horizontal tear (probe in cleft)
May progress to
May progress to
May progress to
Bucket handle tear
Parrot beak tear
Flap tear
B. Tear of posterior horn of the medial meniscus as seen on MRI
C. Arthroscopic appearance of meniscal tear
Normal
Partial discoid
Complete discoid
D. Discoid meniscus variations. Oblique tears are most commonly seen and are best treated by arthroscopic partial meniscectomy (APM). Vertical-longitudinal tears involving the peripheral third are best managed by repair. Radial split tears are usually secondary to trauma, and when the split extends to the capsular rim, repair should be attempted in young people, if at all possible. Bucket-handle tears are more likely to cause locking of the knee. Horizontal (cleavage) and symptomatic degenerative tears are best treated by APM.
F. Netter M.D.

Figure 55.5 Meniscal injuries. (MRI and arthroscopy images from Hart J, Miller M. *Netter's Musculoskeletal Flash Cards*. Philadelphia: Elsevier; 2007.)

MENISCAL INJURIES

Medial Meniscus

Description: Disruption of medial semilunar cartilage of the knee; may be from single traumatic episode, degenerative processes, or a combination; tears take different forms, such as radial, longitudinal, or horizontal. Most important surgical factor is whether the tear is peripheral in the vascular zone or more central in the nonvascular zone; more common than lateral meniscus tears because medial meniscus is less mobile.

Mechanism of injury: Twisting or squatting; may be in association with ligament injuries as a result of any of their precipitating mechanisms

Presentation: Usually mild swelling and joint line pain; in an acute setting, important to know whether knee lacked full extension from time of injury (locked knee from displaced fragment) or knee lacked full extension next day (pseudolocking from hamstring spasm). In a chronic setting, recurrent locking is typical. Otherwise, symptoms may include slipping or catching over the joint line.

Examination: Positive McMurray, Thessaly, and Apley tests; results may vary considerably from one examination session to the next. Joint line tenderness and mild effusion may be present. Chronically, quadriceps atrophy is common. With peripheral meniscus detachment and positive anterior drawer test, loud "clunk" may be elicited as the meniscus displaces during the anterior drawer test.

Imaging: Plain radiographs are usually normal, unless meniscal tear has been present for a significant amount of time. Thereafter, they may show joint line spurring and/or narrowing. MRIs have now supplanted arthrograms for diagnosis of meniscal injury. For medial meniscus, MRI has a sensitivity as high as 94% (Fig. 55.5).

Differential diagnosis: Ligamentous injury (causing pain in the same area), patellar problems (anteromedial joint pain that is confused with pain from medial meniscus injury), pathologic synovial plica (similar pain, swelling, catching, and popping), loose bodies may cause locking, medial compartment arthritis (medial joint pain similar to that from torn meniscus)

Treatment: Suspected meniscus tear with no ligamentous instability may be managed initially through symptomatic treatment and functional rehabilitation. If no improvement, or if time constraints do not allow initial conservative treatment, diagnostic arthroscopy is pathologically the most certain way of diagnosing and treating meniscal injury. MRI may help decide whether to proceed with surgical treatment or continue with nonsurgical care. Most meniscal tears still require arthroscopic partial meniscectomy. Meniscectomy increases the risk of development of future arthritic changes in the knee. Vertical tears in the peripheral vascular zone are now routinely treated by meniscal repair rather than removal of the meniscus.

Lateral Meniscus

Description: Disruption of lateral semilunar cartilage of the knee; may be from single traumatic episode, degenerative processes, or combination; with lateral meniscus injury, may also encounter injuries of congenital discoid meniscus (see Fig. 55.5). Tears take different forms, such as radial, longitudinal, or horizontal (see Fig. 55.5). Most important surgical factor is whether the tear is peripheral in the vascular zone or more central in the nonvascular zone. Lateral meniscus tears are less common than medial meniscus tears because the lateral meniscus is more mobile (see Fig. 55.5).

Mechanism of injury: Same as for medial meniscus injury

Presentation: Same as for medial meniscus injury, although often more pain and fewer mechanical symptoms than with medial meniscus tears; patients may give history of a cystic lesion directly over the lateral joint line.

Examination: Much the same as for medial meniscus injury; may palpate localized puffiness or distinct cystic lesion over lateral joint line

Imaging: Same findings as for medial meniscus injury; in children with congenital discoid lateral meniscus, widening of the lateral joint space may be seen. In contrast to medial meniscus, MRI has somewhat less sensitivity (approximately 78%) in detecting lateral meniscus tears.

Differential diagnosis: Lateral ligamentous injury, loose bodies, degenerative arthritis of lateral compartment; popliteus tendinitis; iliotibial band friction syndrome

Treatment: Same as for medial meniscus injury; special considerations in youngsters with lateral discoid meniscus include whether to remove or repair and how much meniscus to remove

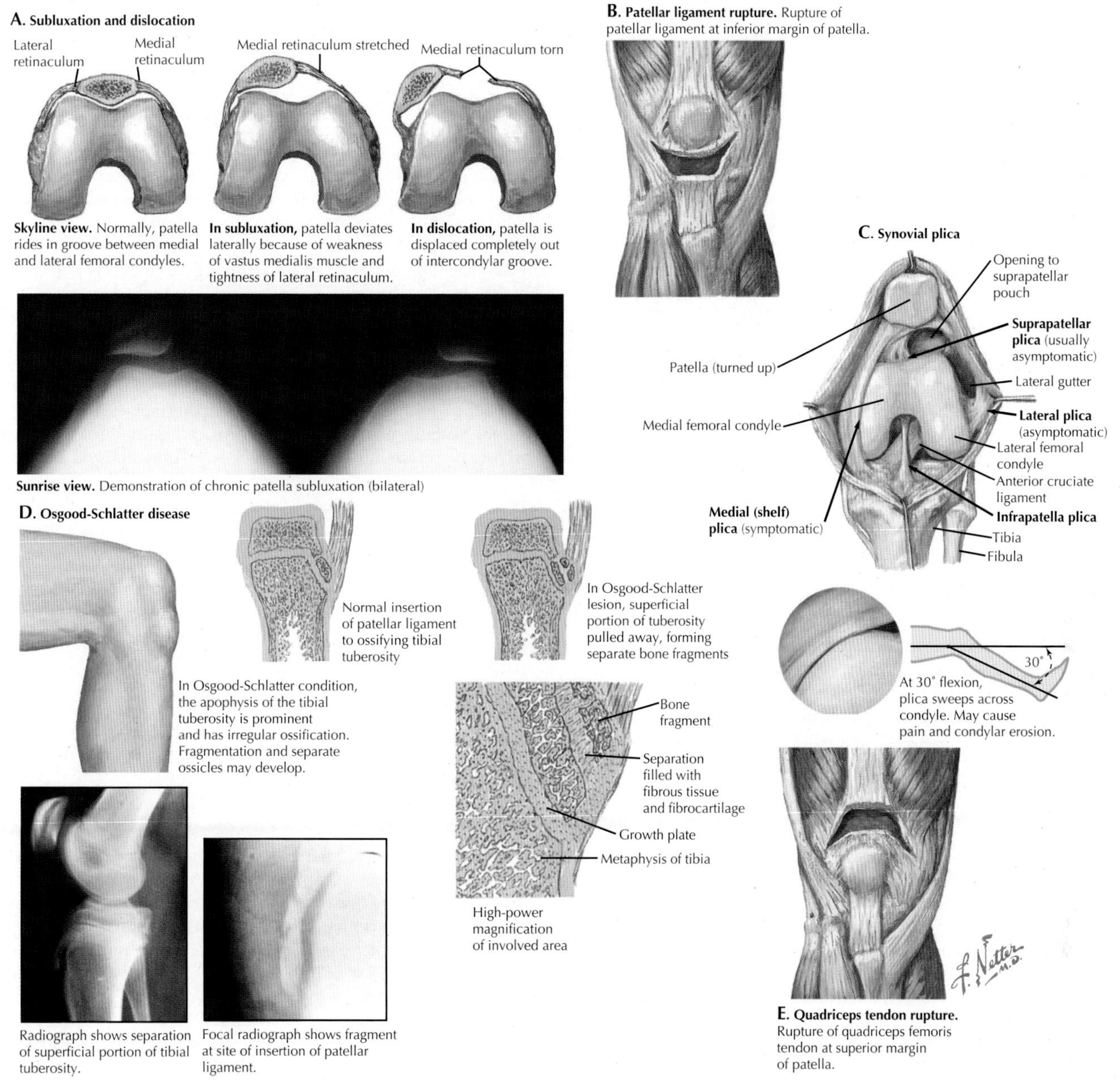
A. Subluxation and dislocation
Lateral retinaculum
Medial retinaculum
Medial retinaculum stretched
Medial retinaculum torn
Skyline view. Normally, patella rides in groove between medial and lateral femoral condyles.
In subluxation, patella deviates laterally because of weakness of vastus medialis muscle and tightness of lateral retinaculum.
In dislocation, patella is displaced completely out of intercondylar groove.
Sunrise view. Demonstration of chronic patella subluxation (bilateral)
B. Patellar ligament rupture. Rupture of patellar ligament at inferior margin of patella.
C. Synovial plica
Opening to suprapatellar pouch
Suprapatellar plica (usually asymptomatic)
Patella (turned up)
Lateral gutter
Medial femoral condyle
Lateral plica (asymptomatic)
Lateral femoral condyle
Anterior cruciate ligament
Medial (shelf) plica (symptomatic)
Infrapatella plica
Tibia
Fibula
D. Osgood-Schlatter disease
Normal insertion of patellar ligament to ossifying tibial tuberosity
In Osgood-Schlatter lesion, superficial portion of tuberosity pulled away, forming separate bone fragments
In Osgood-Schlatter condition, the apophysis of the tibial tuberosity is prominent and has irregular ossification. Fragmentation and separate ossicles may develop.
Bone fragment
Separation filled with fibrous tissue and fibrocartilage
Growth plate
Metaphysis of tibia
High-power magnification of involved area
30°
At 30° flexion, plica sweeps across condyle. May cause pain and condylar erosion.
Radiograph shows separation of superficial portion of tibial tuberosity.
Focal radiograph shows fragment at site of insertion of patellar ligament.
E. Quadriceps tendon rupture. Rupture of quadriceps femoris tendon at superior margin of patella.

Figure 55.6 Extensor mechanism problems. (Sunrise view from Miller M, Cole B. *Textbook of Arthroscopy*. Philadelphia: Elsevier; 2004.)

EXTENSOR MECHANISM PROBLEMS

Instability Syndromes

Dislocation

Description: Complete, usually lateral displacement of the patella from femoral trochlea that persists until reduced, usually by extending knee

Mechanism of injury: Valgus and/or twisting with strong quadriceps contraction

Predisposing factors: All the stigmata indicating congenital extensor mechanism malalignment, such as VMO dysplasia, VL hypertrophy, high and lateral patellar posture, increased Q-angle, and bony deformity; usually more easily seen in acute cases on the opposite uninjured side

Presentation: May or may not be previous symptoms of instability or patellofemoral pain; feeling of patellar dislocation when injury occurred; report of lying on ground with knee flexed; report of "something coming out" medially, which usually represents uncovered medial femoral condyle rather than the patella going medially; report of "something going back into place" when the knee is extended. Swelling occurs within the initial 2 hours.

Examination: Depends on whether the patella is still dislocated or has been reduced; predisposing physical findings seen on the opposite knee; if the patella is still dislocated, will be located over lateral femoral condyle with prominence of uncovered medial femoral condyle (Fig. 55.6); if the patella has been reduced, there may be large hemarthrosis with hypermobility and marked apprehension on hypermobility testing; may also find associated medial ligamentous instability

Imaging: Unusual to find the patella still dislocated on radiograph because positioning on the radiograph table usually reduces dislocation; infrapatellar view may show an avulsion of the medial edge of the patella. Large osteochondral fracture may be visible; important to take infrapatellar view with knee flexed only 30–45 degrees, rather than a traditional "sunrise" or "skyline" view with the knee flexed beyond 90 degrees. Patella alta can be objectively measured on lateral view. Lesions of medial supporting structures often visualized on MRI.

Differential diagnosis: In acute cases, differentiate from ligamentous tears; in chronic recurrent cases, distinguish from meniscus disorders

Treatment: If patella dislocated, knee extension and gentle pressure along the lateral patellar edge usually reduces it easily and without anesthesia. Aspiration may be indicated for comfort or to search for fat in blood secondary to osteochondral fracture. Perceptions about rigid immobilization are changing, even with first-time dislocation, because of harmful effects of immobilization on the knee joint. Immobilize first-time dislocation only as needed for symptoms, followed by an extensive rehabilitation program and functional patellar bracing. Obvious disruption of VMO insertion into the medial patellar edge or rupture of the medial patellofemoral ligament from the adductor tubercle provides best outcomes with early surgical repair. Treat recurrent dislocation symptomatically with crutches, followed by functional rehabilitation and bracing. Consider surgical realignment of extensor mechanism if there is residual functional disability despite extensive conservative treatment. Surgical realignment is not always successful and should be the last resort.

Subluxation

Description: Transient partial displacement of the patella from the femoral trochlea; may occur acutely, as in patellar dislocation, or may be intermittent. There is spontaneous reduction of displacement.

Mechanism of injury: Same as for patellar dislocation; may occur with less severe force or in normal everyday activity

Predisposing factors: Same as for patellar dislocation

Presentation: Patient may or may not have a history of complete dislocation or patellofemoral pain. Feeling of slipping when cutting, twisting, or pivoting; mild recurrent swelling.

Examination: Predisposing physical findings seen in both knees but may be more obvious on asymptomatic side, particularly if there has been an acute injury on the symptomatic side; mild effusion; positive hypermobility and apprehension test

Imaging: Infrapatellar radiograph view must be performed with appropriate technique and knee flexed only 30–45 degrees; may show lateral tilt and/or lateral subluxation or be normal in appearance. Patellofemoral indices (Merchant, Laurin, and Brattstrom) show a tendency toward patellofemoral problems but do not give specific diagnosis (see Fig. 55.6).

Differential diagnosis: Chronic knee ligament instability, causing giving way of the knee

Treatment: For acute subluxation, use temporary symptomatic immobilization, followed by functional rehabilitation and bracing of the patella; if no acute episode, treat with functional rehabilitation, bracing, and nonsteroidal anti-inflammatory drugs (NSAIDs). Patients disabled by subluxation may require arthroscopic lateral release or open extensor mechanism reconstruction. Surgical treatment has less-than-perfect results and should be considered as the last resort (see Fig. 55.6).

Painful Syndromes

Patellofemoral Pain Syndrome

Description: Various syndromes characterized by anterior knee pain as major symptom; an imprecise term wherein pain is not explained by a more readily definable cause; often called "chondromalacia patella," a term that should be reserved for articular cartilage damage actually observed

Mechanism of injury: May result from extensor mechanism malalignment, with or without an instability syndrome; may occur as overuse injury with extreme and/or repetitive loading of patellofemoral joint (e.g., knee flexion, running, and jumping)

Predisposing factors: Same as for instability syndromes

Presentation: Anterior knee pain, often worse with sitting in tight space with knee flexed and on descending stairs or slopes; mild swelling (may be bilateral); may be snapping and popping around patella

Examination: Findings predisposing to extensor mechanism problems in both legs; pain on patellofemoral compression test; crepitation about patella on range of motion; tenderness to palpation around patella. Mild effusion may be present. Foot malalignment or leg length inequality may aggravate the symptoms.

Imaging: Same as for subluxation; may be normal

Differential diagnosis: In preadolescents and young adolescents, consider referred pain from hip disorder (e.g., Legg–Calvé–Perthes disease and slipped capital femoral epiphysis), osteochondritis dissecans of femur or patella, bone tumor—particularly in case of unilateral symptoms. In older patients, osteoarthritis or some other inflammatory joint disease.

Treatment: Functional rehabilitation program, NSAIDs, functional bracing of the patella, orthotics for foot malalignment; if other treatments are unsuccessful, surgical treatment may be considered—either lateral release or extensor mechanism reconstruction. Because results are unpredictable, surgery should be considered as the last resort. Always look for other more specific causes of anterior knee pain.

Patellar Tendinitis ("Jumper's Knee")

Description: Inflammation of the patellar tendon, usually at its attachment to the inferior pole of the patella. Rupture of the patellar tendon may occur with or without a history of tendinopathy (see Fig. 55.6).

Mechanism of injury: Usually excessive jumping or bounding activity or other high patellofemoral stress activity; less commonly from running

Predisposing factors: Same as for other extensor mechanism disorders; possibly ankle dorsiflexor muscle weakness, perhaps secondary to ankle injury

Presentation: Activity, such as jumping sport, typically associated with this problem; complaint of infrapatellar pain, originally after exercise, later during exercise and while at rest; rupture occurs with forceful knee flexion against resistance

Examination: Tenderness at inferior pole of the patella; less commonly, tenderness over body of the patellar tendon. Other findings of extensor mechanism malalignment; weakness of ankle dorsiflexors; hamstring, heel cord, and/or quadriceps muscle tightness; patellar tendon incongruity and significant knee extension weakness noted

Imaging: Radiographs occasionally show irregularity at inferior pole of the patella; may show extensor mechanism malalignment, including patella alta (particularly with rupture). MRI may demonstrate degenerative changes in tendon, which are often read as a partial tear of the patellar tendon by the radiologist but are, in fact, representative of changes in the tendon consistent with patellar tendinosis (see Fig. 55.6).

Differential diagnosis: Usually firm diagnosis not difficult with this entity; may consider some other soft tissue lesion of the patellar tendon or fat pad, such as tumor; otherwise, could be any of other causes of patellofemoral pain

Treatment: Rehabilitative exercise program, concentrating on hamstring, heel cord, and quadriceps flexibility and strength; eccentric strengthening exercises for ankle dorsiflexors are important; anti-inflammatory medication; ultrasound, using hydrocortisone phonophoresis; questionable benefit from infrapatellar strap; more invasive but relatively safe measures used to treat recalcitrant patellar tendinosis include prolotherapy (injection at multiple points in the tendon with "sugar water") and injection of platelet-rich plasma gel. Surgical treatment should be the last resort because of unpredictable results. Immediate surgical repair is indicated with rupture.

Synovial Plica

Description: Structurally, remnant of embryologic walls that divide knee into medial, lateral, and suprapatellar pouches; appears as a fold of synovium attached to the joint periphery and to the underside of the quadriceps tendon (suprapatellar plica); may also present as a free edge along medial patellofemoral joint (medial plica) or may be in both locations; rarely seen in other configurations; edge protruding into joint may be of various sizes (see Fig. 55.6)

Mechanism of injury: Overuse with repetitive flexion and extension (e.g., running); direct blow to medial patellofemoral joint (e.g., falling on turf or dashboard injury)

Predisposing factors: Congenital presence of plica; other extensor mechanism malalignment predispositions may increase the likelihood of symptoms because of plica

Presentation: Complaints of anterior knee pain, pain over suprapatellar or medial peripatellar regions with long periods of knee flexion (particularly when accompanied by distinct snap or pop when knee is extended) and painful catching episodes over the medial patellofemoral joint

Examination: Often difficult to palpate plica; best performed with passive flexion and extension with tibia held internally rotated. Fingers should lie over the medial patellofemoral joint; may see other extensor mechanism malalignment stigmata; heel cord tightness and hamstring tightness aggravate significantly.

Imaging: Not helpful

Differential diagnosis: Other painful patellofemoral conditions; possibly medial meniscus injury or loose body; patients often dismissed as "neurotic" because of lack of findings in the face of significant symptoms.

Treatment: If inflammatory process is not reversible and plica is fibrotic, persistent symptoms require arthroscopic removal of plica; promises good relief of symptoms and good future functioning. If the inflammatory process in the synovium is still reversible:

- The condition may improve with hamstring stretching, heel cord stretching, or VMO exercises (if VMO is dysplastic)
- NSAIDs, ice, activity modification
- Simple external patellar support may help
- Phonophoresis and/or a corticosteroid injection to plica area may also be beneficial.

Osgood–Schlatter Disease

Description: Painful enlargement of the tibial tuberosity at the patellar tendon insertion. Rather than being a disease, the condition is caused by mechanical stress and excessive tension on growing tibial tuberosity apophysis; occurs in preadolescence and early adolescence, usually during a rapid growth period (see Fig. 55.6).

Mechanism of injury: Overuse in normal childhood activities, including sports; rarely, acute onset of popping and pain over tibial tuberosity

Predisposing factors: Patella alta, other evidence of extensor mechanism malalignment and altered extensor mechanics; tight hamstrings, heel cords, and quadriceps muscles predispose to symptoms

Presentation: Complaints of painful enlargement of tibial tuberosity

Examination: Enlarged, tender tibial tuberosity; stigmata of extensor mechanism malalignment, particularly patella alta; tight hamstrings, heel cords, and quadriceps muscles

Imaging: Enlarged tibial tuberosity, irregularity of tibial tuberosity, loose ossicle separated from the tuberosity, and patella alta shown in radiographs

Differential diagnosis: Other forms of patellar tendinitis; in acute episodes, avulsion fracture of tibial tuberosity; tumorous processes of tibial tuberosity

Treatment: Hamstring stretching, heel cord stretching, and quadriceps stretching exercises; VMO-strengthening exercises; activity modification as necessitated by symptoms; simple modalities; local padding

Quadriceps Tendinitis (Including VL Tendinitis and VMO Tendinitis) and Rupture

Description: Inflammation of the quadriceps tendon at its insertion into superior edge of the patella; may involve only VL insertion into superolateral pole of the patella or VMO insertion into superomedial pole of the patella. Rupture of the quadriceps mechanism may occur with or without a history of tendonitis after forceful knee flexion against resistance (see Fig. 55.6).

Mechanism of injury: Same as for patellar tendinitis

Predisposing factors: Extensor mechanism malalignment

Presentation: Complaints of suprapatellar pain

Examination: Tenderness at superior pole of the patella; may be over central rectus femoris insertion, superolateral VL insertion, or superomedial VMO insertion. Other findings of extensor mechanism malalignment; hamstring, heel cord, and quadriceps muscle tightness; quadriceps tendon defect and inability to extend knee present with rupture

Imaging: Usually there are no radiographic findings with tendonitis but may observe patella baja with rupture

Differential diagnosis: Suprapatellar pain from synovial plica, bone tumor of distal femur

Treatment: Same as for patellar tendonitis; immediate surgical repair for rupture

MISCELLANEOUS KNEE CONDITIONS

Bursitis

Description: Inflammation of any of various bursae around knee, evidenced by swelling and/or pain; typically prepatellar bursa, pes anserinus bursa, tibial collateral ligament bursa, and deep infrapatellar bursa (Fig. 55.7)

Mechanism of injury: Usually overuse; may be the result of direct blow with bleeding into bursa

Predisposing factors: For pes anserinus bursitis, tight hamstrings seem to predispose

Presentation: Complaints of swelling (if prepatellar bursa), pain in the prepatellar region (for prepatellar bursitis), pain in the distal patellar tendon region (for deep infrapatellar bursitis), pain in the proximal medial tibia (for pes anserinus bursitis), or pain over the medial joint line (for tibial collateral ligament bursitis)

Examination: For prepatellar bursa, check for localized swelling and tenderness; for others, tenderness over described areas

Imaging: Not helpful for diagnosis

Differential diagnosis: For deep infrapatellar bursitis, other causes of patellar tendon pain; for tibial collateral ligament bursitis, medial meniscus tear; for prepatellar bursitis, usually no differential; for pes anserinus bursitis, pain from pes anserinus tendons, tumors, other causes of proximal medial tibial pain

Treatment:

- Acute prepatellar bursitis: ice, compression, possible aspiration, and padding
- Chronic prepatellar bursitis: NSAIDs, compression, hamstring stretching, ultrasound, possible aspiration, and corticosteroid injections
- Pes anserinus bursitis: hamstring stretching, ultrasound, NSAIDs, and corticosteroid injections
- Tibial collateral ligament bursitis: injection, both as diagnostic test and as treatment
- Deep infrapatellar bursitis: hamstring stretching, possible injection behind the patellar tendon

Other Tendonitis

Description: Inflammation of any other tendinous structures about knee, typically semimembranosus, popliteus, or biceps femoris tendons; inflammation of the gastrocnemius tendon is rare.

Mechanism of injury: Usually overuse; much less commonly, single episode of strain. Popliteus tendinitis is usually a running injury

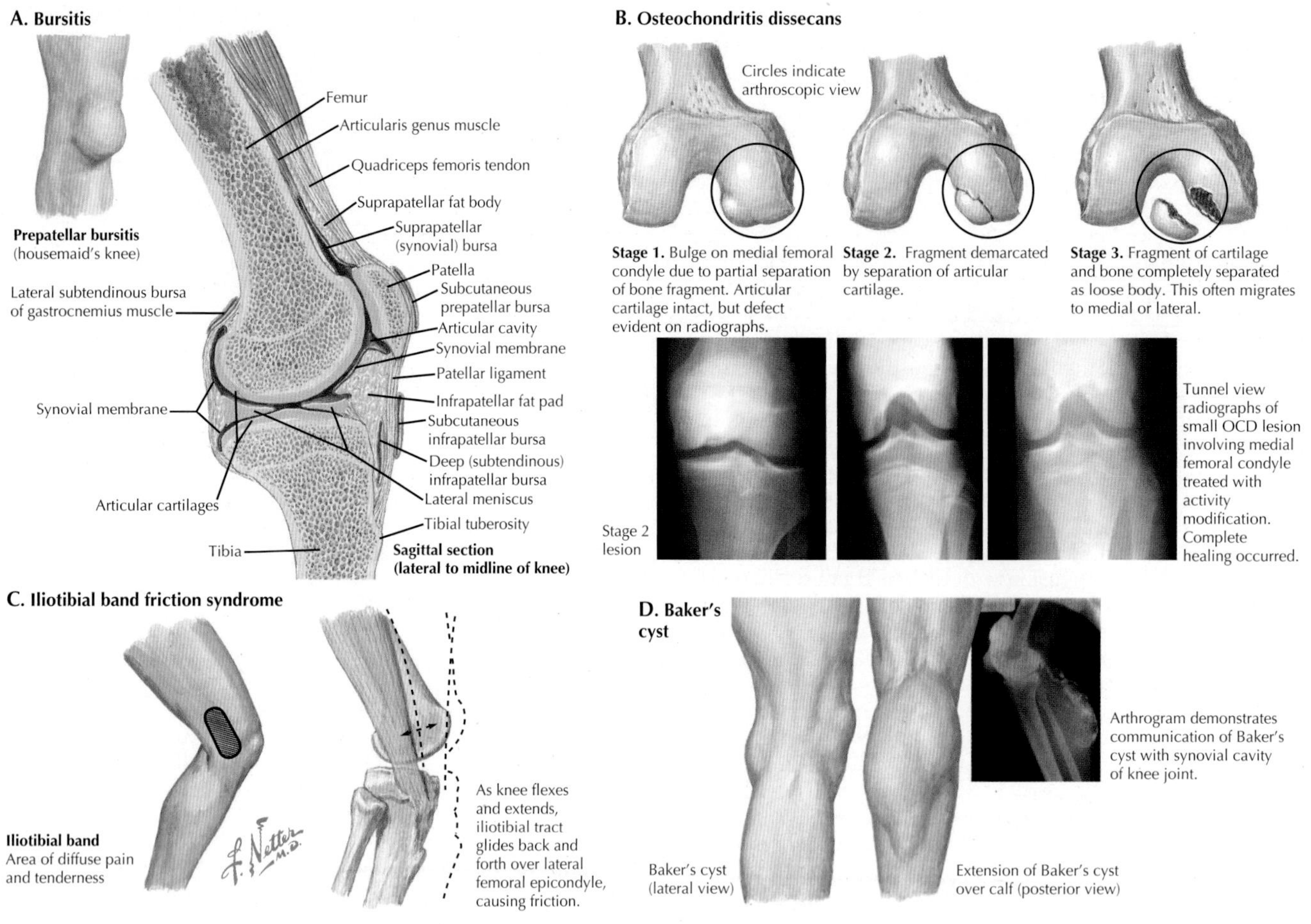
A. Bursitis
Femur
Articularis genus muscle
Quadriceps femoris tendon
Suprapatellar fat body
Suprapatellar (synovial) bursa
Patella
Subcutaneous prepatellar bursa
Articular cavity
Synovial membrane
Patellar ligament
Infrapatellar fat pad
Subcutaneous infrapatellar bursa
Deep (subtendinous) infrapatellar bursa
Lateral meniscus
Tibial tuberosity
Prepatellar bursitis (housemaid's knee)
Lateral subtendinous bursa of gastrocnemius muscle
Synovial membrane
Articular cartilages
Tibia
Sagittal section (lateral to midline of knee)
B. Osteochondritis dissecans
Circles indicate arthroscopic view
Stage 1. Bulge on medial femoral condyle due to partial separation of bone fragment. Articular cartilage intact, but defect evident on radiographs.
Stage 2. Fragment demarcated by separation of articular cartilage.
Stage 3. Fragment of cartilage and bone completely separated as loose body. This often migrates to medial or lateral.
Stage 2 lesion
Tunnel view radiographs of small OCD lesion involving medial femoral condyle treated with activity modification. Complete healing occurred.
C. Iliotibial band friction syndrome
Iliotibial band
Area of diffuse pain and tenderness
As knee flexes and extends, iliotibial tract glides back and forth over lateral femoral epicondyle, causing friction.
D. Baker's cyst
Arthrogram demonstrates communication of Baker's cyst with synovial cavity of knee joint.
Baker's cyst (lateral view)
Extension of Baker's cyst over calf (posterior view)

Figure 55.7 Miscellaneous knee conditions.

Predisposing factors: For semimembranosus, pes anserinus or biceps femoris tendinitis, and hamstring tightness predisposes
Presentation: Complaints of pain over appropriate tendon area; for popliteus tendinitis, lateral knee pain, particularly while running downhill
Examination: Tenderness over appropriate tendon; tight hamstrings; for popliteus tendinitis, painful resisted internal rotation of tibia with knee flexed; for all, initially pain on stretching tendon, later pain on active contraction of tendon
Imaging: Usually not helpful
Differential diagnosis: Hamstring tendinitis occasionally to be differentiated from sciatica; semimembranosus tendinitis may be confused with medial meniscus disorders; for popliteus tendinitis, lateral meniscus injury, and iliotibial band friction syndrome
Treatment: Usual anti-inflammatory methods; hamstring stretching exercises; patient may require corticosteroid injections. Immobilization is inappropriate except in the acute phase because of adverse effects on collagen tissue and muscle atrophy.

Neuromas

Description: Nonneoplastic enlargement of nerve, usually from direct trauma; typically involves various portions of saphenous nerve around knee
Mechanism of injury: Direct blow, previous surgery
Predisposing factors: Previous surgical incisions
Presentation: Pain, particularly nervelike quality (i.e., paresthesias, burning, and other alterations of sensation)
Examination: Tenderness over neuroma, positive Tinel sign, objective changes in sensation in appropriate distribution
Imaging: Not helpful
Differential diagnosis: More central sources of nerve compression
Treatment: Injection, surgical excision

Loose Bodies ("Joint Mouse," Chondral Fracture, Osteochondral Fracture, Osteochondritis Dissecans)

Description: Cartilaginous or osteocartilaginous fragments usually free-floating within knee joint (though may be attached to synovium more or less firmly) (see Fig. 55.7)
Mechanism of injury: Dislocation of the patella (see "Instability Syndromes"), other trauma to joint surface; may be result of preexisting osteochondritis dissecans; rarely the result of synovial osteochondromatosis
Predisposing factors: Predisposition to patellar dislocation, preexisting osteochondritis dissecans
Presentation: Consistent with previous patellar instability, twisting or direct blow injury, locking episodes, subcutaneous mass that comes and goes and may be felt in various locations around the knee
Examination: Patellar findings; may feel movable mass, usually around patellofemoral joint, although it may be at the anteromedial or anterolateral joint line
Imaging: In radiographs, purely cartilaginous fragments are not visible; tunnel view may reveal small osteochondritis dessicans (OCD) lesion on lateral aspect of medical femoral condyle; very small bony loose bodies may be obscured; most loose bodies of significance containing bone are visible; source (e.g., osteochondritis dissecans) may be seen. MRI, tomogram, computed tomography (CT), or arthrogram may help in delineation (see Fig. 55.7).

Differential diagnosis: Meniscal tears as source of locking

Treatment: Symptomatic loose bodies require surgical removal, usually arthroscopically; a few loose bodies may require replacement and internal fixation. Patellofemoral instability may require treatment. OCD may require other treatment. Large chondral or osteochondral fractures may require surgical debridement of joint surface in addition to prolonged and protected weight bearing.

Cysts (Popliteal Cyst, Popliteal Ganglion, Baker's Cyst, Meniscus Cyst)

Description: Fluid-filled lesion about the knee arising usually as extension of synovial space, either into normal bursal structure or into soft tissue surrounding knee (see Fig. 55.7)

Mechanism of injury: Normally, no specific injury is involved

Predisposing factors: None

Presentation: Localized swelling in popliteal space or over meniscus

Examination: Cystic swelling in medial popliteal space or over mid–joint line, usually lateral joint line

Imaging: Plain films are no help; MRI is very helpful in delineating cysts (see Fig. 55.7)

Differential diagnosis: Other tumorous lesions about knee

Treatment: Aspiration and injection with corticosteroids not very likely to give permanent cure; surgical excision is usually curative. Presence of cyst is usually secondary to another process in knee that leads to excessive synovial fluid, thus causing a cyst; most likely meniscal tear causing popliteal cyst, or lateral meniscus tear causing lateral meniscus cyst. Underlying disorders must be treated.

Iliotibial Band Friction Syndrome

Description: Chronic inflammatory process involving soft tissues adjacent to lateral femoral epicondyle; presumably caused by chronic "friction" of iliotibial band rubbing over bony prominence of this area (see Fig. 55.7)

Mechanism of injury: Overuse; most cases caused by running

Predisposing factors: Varus alignment of the knee; running on sloped surfaces

Presentation: Lateral knee pain on activity, occasional popping

Examination: Tenderness over lateral femoral epicondyle, tight iliotibial band, and absence of intra-articular findings

Imaging: Not helpful

Differential diagnosis: Other causes of lateral knee pain, particularly popliteus tendinitis; lateral meniscus disorders, lateral patellofemoral joint sources such as VL tendinitis

Treatment: Iliotibial band stretching exercises, anti-inflammatory treatment, ultrasound to lateral femoral epicondyle, and corticosteroid injections; rarely, surgery to release area of tightness

ACKNOWLEDGMENT

The authors would like to acknowledge the contributions of **W. Michael Walsh, MD,** in the previous edition.

RECOMMENDED READINGS

Available online.

56 ANKLE AND LEG INJURIES

Christopher Kim • Annunziato Amendola • John E. Femino

GENERAL PRINCIPLES

- Leg and ankle injuries often occur concomitantly. Evaluation of one must include the other (Fig. 56.1).
- A neurovascular examination is essential in addition to making note of the amount of swelling.
- Injuries that require immediate treatment include open fractures, dislocations, neurovascularly compromised extremities, and acute compartment syndrome.
- Ankle sprains are the most common injury of the ankle.
- Chronic pain and disability may result from missed injuries, delayed treatment, or inadequate rehabilitation.

History

Acute Injuries

- Collect the detailed pain history, including onset, quality, severity, location, radiating and associated symptoms, and exacerbating and relieving factors.
- Mechanism of injury will give clues as to the type of injury
- Determine whether there is a history of prior injury or surgery. Prodromal symptoms may suggest stress fracture.
- In open fractures, determine the timing of injury and environment in which the injury occurred to help guide antibiotic use.

Chronic Injuries

- Obtain the detailed history of training activities, including frequency, duration, and intensity.
- Collect a detailed pain history.
- Type of shoe worn and use of orthotics should be considered.

Physical Examination

Inspection

- Evaluate the skin for lacerations and bleeding. Bleeding with fat globules suggests an open fracture.
- Evaluate for a deformity that may indicate a displaced fracture or dislocation.
- Note excessive swelling or skin tenting because these may lead to open wounds.

Palpation

- Palpation should be systematic, anatomically based, and end with the most painful area.
- Palpation of pulses may be limited because of the location of pain: the posterior tibial artery is palpated behind the medial malleolus, the anterior tibial artery is palpated beneath the extensor hallucis longus or over the first intercuneiform joint at the dorsalis pedis, and the peroneal artery pulse is found anteriorly over the syndesmosis (Fig. 56.2A and C).
- Neurologic examination should include the deep and superficial peroneal, saphenous, sural, and posterior tibial nerves.
- Palpation of bony prominences should include the tibial crest from the knee to the ankle (see Fig. 56.2B). Check the joints above and below the site of injury. Palpate the medial and lateral malleoli, beginning at the distal tips and moving proximally. Palpate the forefoot and midfoot.
- Palpation of leg compartments should reveal supple compartments; firm compartments may indicate compartment syndrome.
- Palpate the lateral ligaments. Tenderness of the syndesmosis is palpated anteriorly between the tibia and fibula just above the ankle joint line and extending proximally several centimeters. Palpate the medial ankle ligaments, including the superficial and deep deltoid ligaments. The anterior band of the deltoid between the medial malleolus and navicular is superficial and can be directly palpated (see Fig. 56.2D).
- Palpation of the tendons should include the Achilles, posterior tibial tendon, flexor hallucis longus (FHL), and the peroneals. Anterior tibial tendon and digital extensors can be individually palpated but are less frequently injured (see Fig. 56.2C).
- The ankle joint is directly palpated medial to the anterior tibialis over the anteromedial recess and lateral to the peroneus tertius over the anterolateral recess; joint effusion can be detected in these two areas.
- Palpation of the ankle posteriorly on either side of the Achilles tendon may reveal tenderness caused by a fracture or injury of the trigonal process of the talus, os trigonum, FHL tendonitis, or posterior ankle impingement.

Range of Motion

- Ankle range of motion is assessed for dorsiflexion and plantarflexion with the knee flexed and extended.
- Limitation of dorsiflexion with the knee extended may indicate contracture of the gastrocnemius.
- Subtalar joint motion can be isolated by stabilizing the ankle joint with one hand on the lateral side of the ankle and calcaneus. The subtalar joint is then inverted and everted, while the tibiotalar joint is fixed.

Muscle Testing

- Resisted ankle and toe dorsiflexion and plantarflexion should be tested. Tension in the tendons can be assessed at the same time.
- Weak plantarflexion and loss of resistance to passive ankle dorsiflexion are hallmarks of Achilles tendon rupture. However, patients may demonstrate minor strength by using toe flexor tendons, posterior tibial tendon, or an intact plantaris muscle.
- Resisted inversion with the foot plantarflexed and everted isolates the posterior tibialis muscle.
- Resisted eversion tests the peroneals, and detection of instability is enhanced with the ankle in dorsiflexion as well; peroneal tendons can be palpated with the opposite hand from behind the ankle.

Special Tests

Anterior drawer test: Best performed seated with the knee flexed to relax the gastrocnemius muscle; the ankle is plantarflexed, and the examiner stabilizes the tibia with one hand, while the other hand is placed along the lateral side of the foot with the fingers wrapped around the heel. The ankle is then shucked back and forth gently with emphasis on detecting an anterior translation (Fig. 56.3A). This motion should be combined with internal rotation of the talus because true lateral ankle instability is a rotatory phenomenon. The examination is repeated on the contralateral ankle for comparison.

Talar tilt test: With the ankle in less plantarflexion, a varus force is applied to the hindfoot. Internal rotation can enhance the test, which is supposed to detect insufficiency of the calcaneal fibular ligament (CFL) (Fig. 56.3B).

External rotation stress test: Can reveal syndesmotic injury; stabilize the tibia and externally rotate the foot and ankle. This is performed with the knee flexed to 90 degrees and the heel locked in neutral. Pain and apprehension may indicate

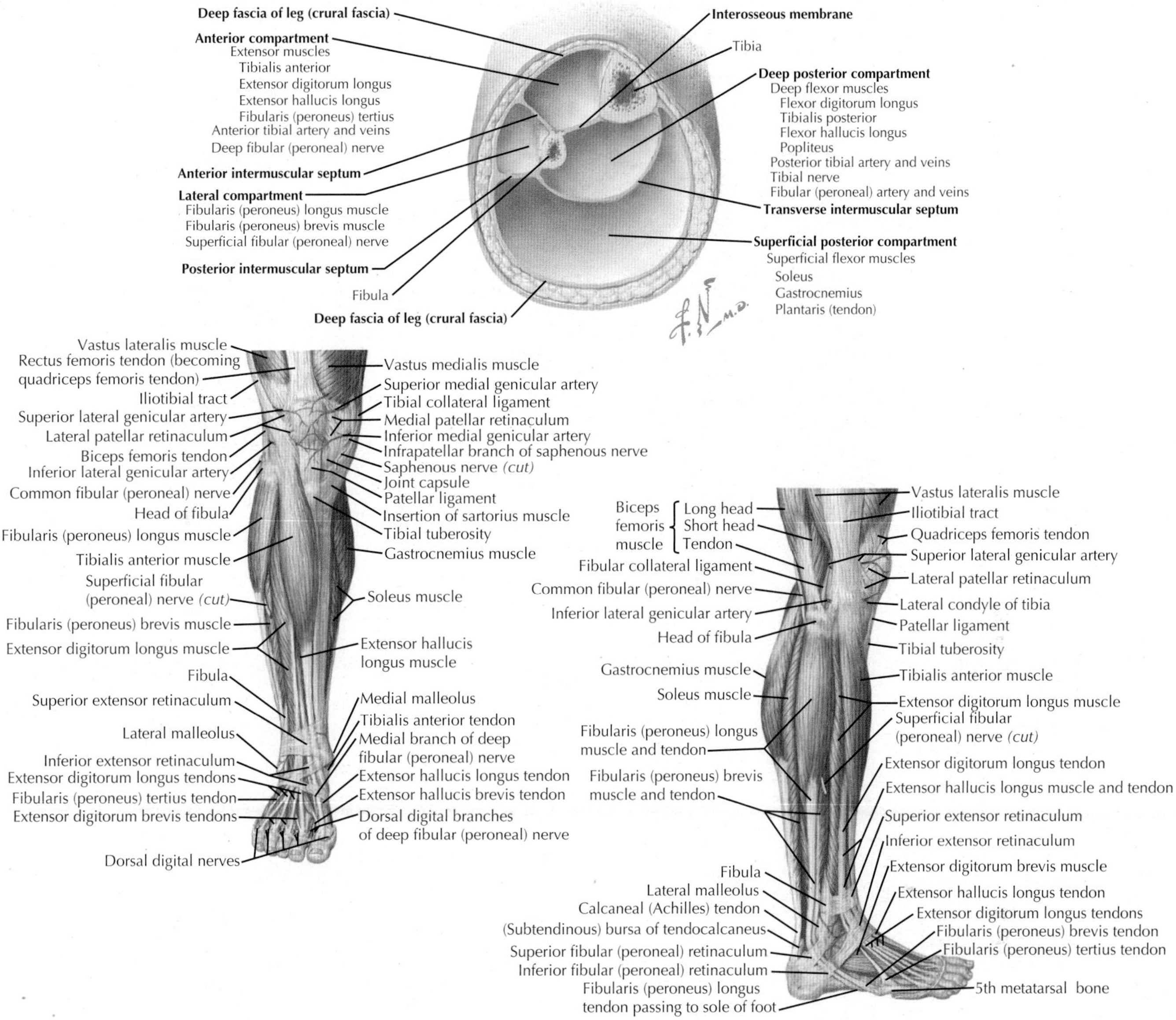
Deep fascia of leg (crural fascia)
Anterior compartment
Extensor muscles
Tibialis anterior
Extensor digitorum longus
Extensor hallucis longus
Fibularis (peroneus) tertius
Anterior tibial artery and veins
Deep fibular (peroneal) nerve
Anterior intermuscular septum
Lateral compartment
Fibularis (peroneus) longus muscle
Fibularis (peroneus) brevis muscle
Superficial fibular (peroneal) nerve
Posterior intermuscular septum
Fibula
Deep fascia of leg (crural fascia)
Interosseous membrane
Tibia
Deep posterior compartment
Deep flexor muscles
Flexor digitorum longus
Tibialis posterior
Flexor hallucis longus
Popliteus
Posterior tibial artery and veins
Tibial nerve
Fibular (peroneal) artery and veins
Transverse intermuscular septum
Superficial posterior compartment
Superficial flexor muscles
Soleus
Gastrocnemius
Plantaris (tendon)
Vastus lateralis muscle
Rectus femoris tendon (becoming quadriceps femoris tendon)
Iliotibial tract
Superior lateral genicular artery
Lateral patellar retinaculum
Biceps femoris tendon
Inferior lateral genicular artery
Common fibular (peroneal) nerve
Head of fibula
Fibularis (peroneus) longus muscle
Tibialis anterior muscle
Superficial fibular (peroneal) nerve (cut)
Fibularis (peroneus) brevis muscle
Extensor digitorum longus muscle
Fibula
Superior extensor retinaculum
Lateral malleolus
Inferior extensor retinaculum
Extensor digitorum longus tendons
Fibularis (peroneus) tertius tendon
Extensor digitorum brevis tendons
Dorsal digital nerves
Vastus medialis muscle
Superior medial genicular artery
Tibial collateral ligament
Medial patellar retinaculum
Inferior medial genicular artery
Infrapatellar branch of saphenous nerve
Saphenous nerve (cut)
Joint capsule
Patellar ligament
Insertion of sartorius muscle
Tibial tuberosity
Gastrocnemius muscle
Soleus muscle
Extensor hallucis longus muscle
Medial malleolus
Tibialis anterior tendon
Medial branch of deep fibular (peroneal) nerve
Extensor hallucis longus tendon
Extensor hallucis brevis tendon
Dorsal digital branches of deep fibular (peroneal) nerve
Biceps femoris muscle
Long head
Short head
Tendon
Fibular collateral ligament
Common fibular (peroneal) nerve
Inferior lateral genicular artery
Head of fibula
Gastrocnemius muscle
Soleus muscle
Fibularis (peroneus) longus muscle and tendon
Fibularis (peroneus) brevis muscle and tendon
Fibula
Lateral malleolus
Calcaneal (Achilles) tendon
(Subtendinous) bursa of tendocalcaneus
Superior fibular (peroneal) retinaculum
Inferior fibular (peroneal) retinaculum
Fibularis (peroneus) longus tendon passing to sole of foot
Vastus lateralis muscle
Iliotibial tract
Quadriceps femoris tendon
Superior lateral genicular artery
Lateral patellar retinaculum
Lateral condyle of tibia
Patellar ligament
Tibial tuberosity
Tibialis anterior muscle
Extensor digitorum longus muscle
Superficial fibular (peroneal) nerve (cut)
Extensor digitorum longus tendon
Extensor hallucis longus muscle and tendon
Superior extensor retinaculum
Inferior extensor retinaculum
Extensor digitorum brevis muscle
Extensor hallucis longus tendon
Extensor digitorum longus tendons
Fibularis (peroneus) brevis tendon
Fibularis (peroneus) tertius tendon
5th metatarsal bone

Figure 56.1 Compartments of the leg and ankle.

syndesmotic injury. If controlling tibial rotation is difficult, have the patient stand on the involved leg and rotate externally on the foot; this places a more realistic force across the syndesmosis.

Impingement testing: Performed in four locations with the joint in an "open" position and placing mild digital pressure at the point of impingement; the starting position is plantarflexion for anterior impingement and dorsiflexion for posterior impingement. With pressure held, the ankle is then passively moved into a "closed" position, which can then entrap the redundant tissue, reproducing the soft tissue impingement and pain. For bony impingement, the talar osteophyte can often be palpated while moving the ankle in dorsiflexion or plantarflexion with the examiner's finger over the anteromedial or lateral recess of the ankle. This same maneuver can be performed for the subtalar joint with the foot in an inverted, plantarflexed position and moved into a dorsiflexed and everted position.

Compartment pressure measurement: Most common measuring devices are solid-state battery powered units that use a side-slit catheter (see Fig. 56.3C). Compartment syndrome is a clinical diagnosis. Compartment pressure measurements should be used as adjuncts to a thorough clinical assessment. Measuring compartment pressures are particularly useful in obtunded or unconscious patients in whom an accurate clinical assessment is not possible. An absolute pressure >30 mmHg or a difference between the compartment pressure and a diastolic blood pressure <30 mmHg are very concerning. Hallmarks of compartment syndrome include pain out of proportion to the presenting injury, with particularly excruciating pain with passive stretching of the muscles in the affected compartment. Other features include firm compartments, pallor, paresthesia, paralysis, and loss of pulses. A diagnosis of compartment syndrome warrants emergent surgical release in the form of fasciotomies.

Radiologic Tests

Plain radiographs: Should include area of injury and the joint above and joint below; a minimum of two views should be performed for each area. Standard views for feet include anteroposterior (AP), lateral, and oblique. Standard views for the ankle include AP, lateral, and mortise (30-degree oblique) views. Radiographs are often performed while patient is bearing weight.

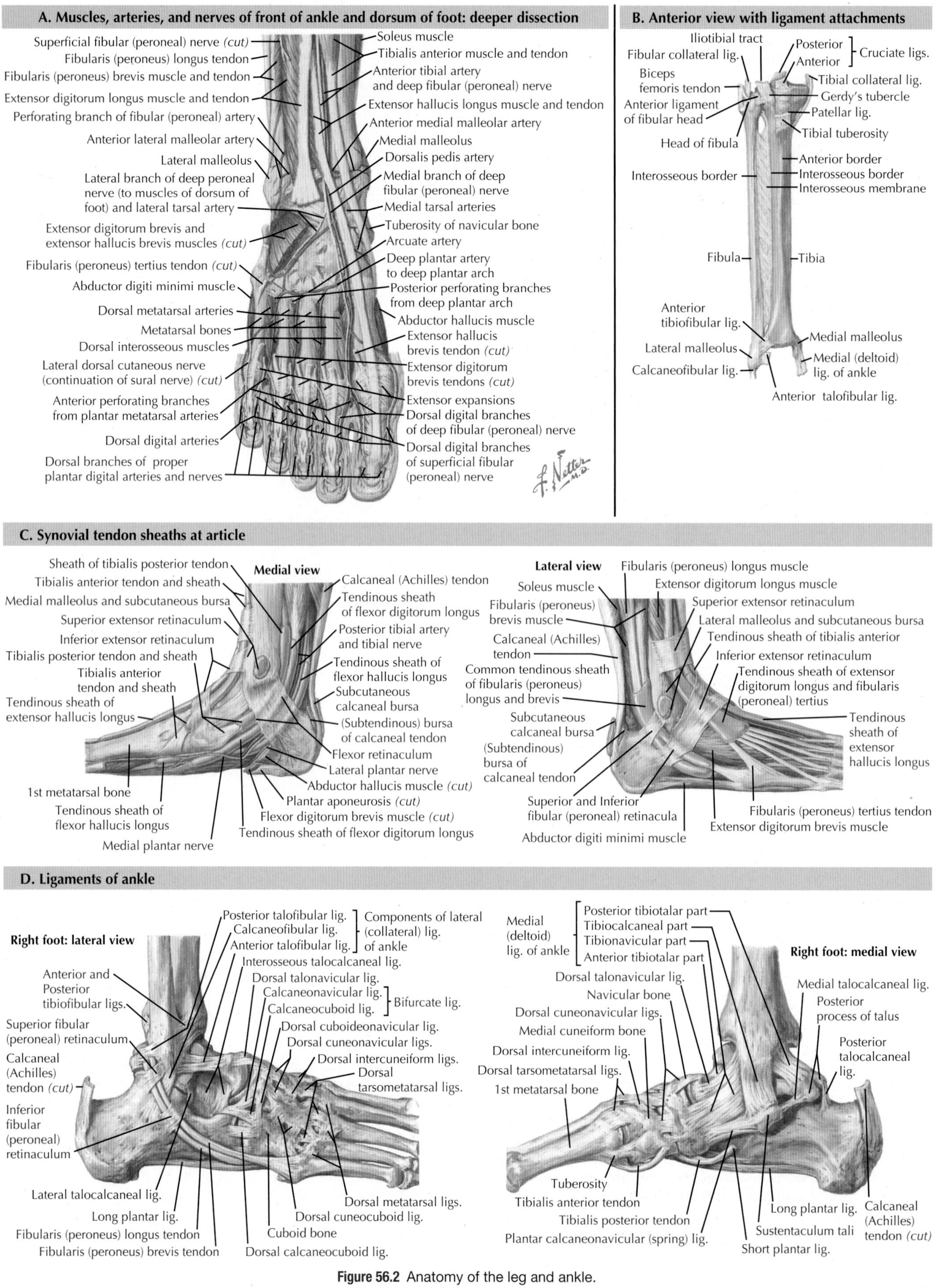
A. Muscles, arteries, and nerves of front of ankle and dorsum of foot: deeper dissection
Superficial fibular (peroneal) nerve (cut)
Fibularis (peroneus) longus tendon
Fibularis (peroneus) brevis muscle and tendon
Extensor digitorum longus muscle and tendon
Perforating branch of fibular (peroneal) artery
Anterior lateral malleolar artery
Lateral malleolus
Lateral branch of deep peroneal nerve (to muscles of dorsum of foot) and lateral tarsal artery
Extensor digitorum brevis and extensor hallucis brevis muscles (cut)
Fibularis (peroneus) tertius tendon (cut)
Abductor digiti minimi muscle
Dorsal metatarsal arteries
Metatarsal bones
Dorsal interosseous muscles
Lateral dorsal cutaneous nerve (continuation of sural nerve) (cut)
Anterior perforating branches from plantar metatarsal arteries
Dorsal digital arteries
Dorsal branches of proper plantar digital arteries and nerves
Soleus muscle
Tibialis anterior muscle and tendon
Anterior tibial artery and deep fibular (peroneal) nerve
Extensor hallucis longus muscle and tendon
Anterior medial malleolar artery
Medial malleolus
Dorsalis pedis artery
Medial branch of deep fibular (peroneal) nerve
Medial tarsal arteries
Tuberosity of navicular bone
Arcuate artery
Deep plantar artery to deep plantar arch
Posterior perforating branches from deep plantar arch
Abductor hallucis muscle
Extensor hallucis brevis tendon (cut)
Extensor digitorum brevis tendons (cut)
Extensor expansions
Dorsal digital branches of deep fibular (peroneal) nerve
Dorsal digital branches of superficial fibular (peroneal) nerve
F. Netter M.D.
B. Anterior view with ligament attachments
Iliotibial tract
Fibular collateral lig.
Biceps femoris tendon
Anterior ligament of fibular head
Head of fibula
Interosseous border
Fibula
Anterior tibiofibular lig.
Lateral malleolus
Calcaneofibular lig.
Posterior
Anterior
Cruciate ligs.
Tibial collateral lig.
Gerdy's tubercle
Patellar lig.
Tibial tuberosity
Anterior border
Interosseous border
Interosseous membrane
Tibia
Medial malleolus
Medial (deltoid) lig. of ankle
Anterior talofibular lig.
C. Synovial tendon sheaths at article
Medial view
Sheath of tibialis posterior tendon
Tibialis anterior tendon and sheath
Medial malleolus and subcutaneous bursa
Superior extensor retinaculum
Inferior extensor retinaculum
Tibialis posterior tendon and sheath
Tibialis anterior tendon and sheath
Tendinous sheath of extensor hallucis longus
1st metatarsal bone
Tendinous sheath of flexor hallucis longus
Medial plantar nerve
Calcaneal (Achilles) tendon
Tendinous sheath of flexor digitorum longus
Posterior tibial artery and tibial nerve
Tendinous sheath of flexor hallucis longus
Subcutaneous calcaneal bursa
(Subtendinous) bursa of calcaneal tendon
Flexor retinaculum
Lateral plantar nerve
Abductor hallucis muscle (cut)
Plantar aponeurosis (cut)
Flexor digitorum brevis muscle (cut)
Tendinous sheath of flexor digitorum longus
Lateral view
Soleus muscle
Fibularis (peroneus) brevis muscle
Calcaneal (Achilles) tendon
Common tendinous sheath of fibularis (peroneus) longus and brevis
Subcutaneous calcaneal bursa
(Subtendinous) bursa of calcaneal tendon
Superior and Inferior fibular (peroneal) retinacula
Abductor digiti minimi muscle
Fibularis (peroneus) longus muscle
Extensor digitorum longus muscle
Superior extensor retinaculum
Lateral malleolus and subcutaneous bursa
Tendinous sheath of tibialis anterior
Inferior extensor retinaculum
Tendinous sheath of extensor digitorum longus and fibularis (peroneal) tertius
Tendinous sheath of extensor hallucis longus
Fibularis (peroneus) tertius tendon
Extensor digitorum brevis muscle
D. Ligaments of ankle
Right foot: lateral view
Anterior and Posterior tibiofibular ligs.
Superior fibular (peroneal) retinaculum
Calcaneal (Achilles) tendon (cut)
Inferior fibular (peroneal) retinaculum
Lateral talocalcaneal lig.
Long plantar lig.
Fibularis (peroneus) longus tendon
Fibularis (peroneus) brevis tendon
Posterior talofibular lig.
Calcaneofibular lig.
Anterior talofibular lig.
Components of lateral (collateral) lig. of ankle
Interosseous talocalcaneal lig.
Dorsal talonavicular lig.
Calcaneonavicular lig.
Calcaneocuboid lig.
Bifurcate lig.
Dorsal cuboideonavicular lig.
Dorsal cuneonavicular ligs.
Dorsal intercuneiform ligs.
Dorsal tarsometatarsal ligs.
Dorsal metatarsal ligs.
Dorsal cuneocuboid lig.
Cuboid bone
Dorsal calcaneocuboid lig.
Medial (deltoid) lig. of ankle
Posterior tibiotalar part
Tibiocalcaneal part
Tibionavicular part
Anterior tibiotalar part
Dorsal talonavicular lig.
Navicular bone
Dorsal cuneonavicular ligs.
Medial cuneiform bone
Dorsal intercuneiform lig.
Dorsal tarsometatarsal ligs.
1st metatarsal bone
Tuberosity
Tibialis anterior tendon
Tibialis posterior tendon
Plantar calcaneonavicular (spring) lig.
Right foot: medial view
Medial talocalcaneal lig.
Posterior process of talus
Posterior talocalcaneal lig.
Long plantar lig.
Sustentaculum tali
Short plantar lig.
Calcaneal (Achilles) tendon (cut)

Figure 56.2 Anatomy of the leg and ankle.

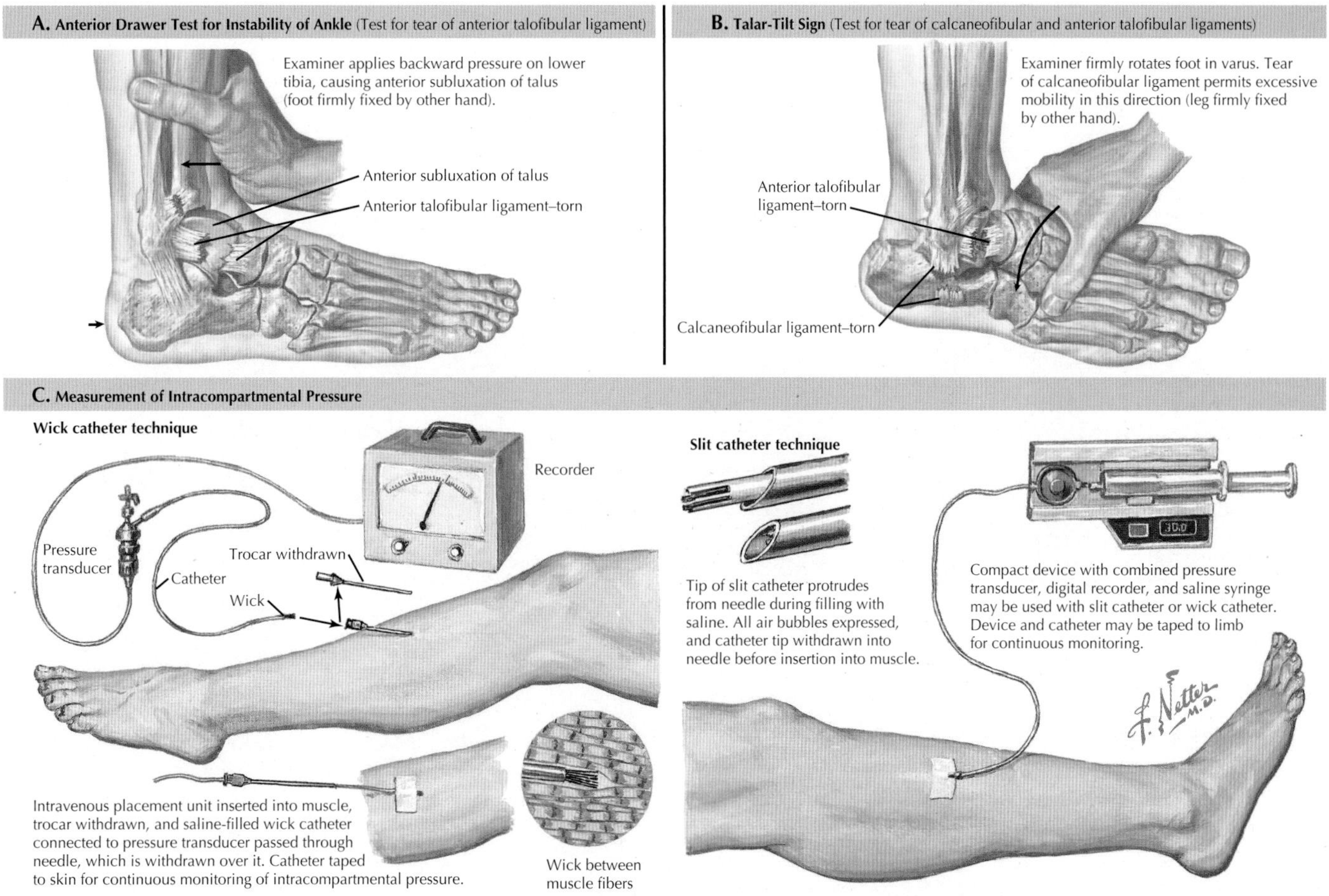
A. Anterior Drawer Test for Instability of Ankle (Test for tear of anterior talofibular ligament)
Examiner applies backward pressure on lower tibia, causing anterior subluxation of talus (foot firmly fixed by other hand).
Anterior subluxation of talus
Anterior talofibular ligament–torn
B. Talar-Tilt Sign (Test for tear of calcaneofibular and anterior talofibular ligaments)
Examiner firmly rotates foot in varus. Tear of calcaneofibular ligament permits excessive mobility in this direction (leg firmly fixed by other hand).
Anterior talofibular ligament–torn
Calcaneofibular ligament–torn
C. Measurement of Intracompartmental Pressure
Wick catheter technique
Recorder
Pressure transducer
Trocar withdrawn
Catheter
Wick
Intravenous placement unit inserted into muscle, trocar withdrawn, and saline-filled wick catheter connected to pressure transducer passed through needle, which is withdrawn over it. Catheter taped to skin for continuous monitoring of intracompartmental pressure.
Wick between muscle fibers
Slit catheter technique
Tip of slit catheter protrudes from needle during filling with saline. All air bubbles expressed, and catheter tip withdrawn into needle before insertion into muscle.
Compact device with combined pressure transducer, digital recorder, and saline syringe may be used with slit catheter or wick catheter. Device and catheter may be taped to limb for continuous monitoring.
F. Netter M.D.

Figure 56.3 Special tests.

Stress radiographs: Helpful to document instability about the ankle, which may often guide treatment decisions; best compared with a normal contralateral part

- Anterior drawer test will show anterior translation of the talus relative to the tibia.
- Talar tilt test will show varus tilting of the talus within the mortise.
- External rotation stress test will show syndesmotic or medial ankle widening.

Nuclear medicine scans: Helpful to pinpoint bone pathology that is not seen on radiographs; positive findings often nonspecific, and several experts will prefer magnetic resonance imaging (MRI) before this modality

Computed tomography (CT) scans: Often used in the foot and ankle to confirm and better delineate fractures; excellent in showing bony details in three dimensions

MRI: Excellent visualization of soft tissue structures and bone marrow, making it very good at detecting early stress fractures

COMMON INJURIES AND MEDICAL PROBLEMS

Acute Fractures

Tibia Fractures

Description: Tibia is often divided into thirds, and fractures are described as proximal, middle, or distal. Numerous fracture patterns are seen, including spiral, oblique, transverse, and comminuted fractures. Open fractures are common because there is little soft tissue surrounding the bone in this area (Fig. 56.4A).

Presentation: Patients present with pain and deformity and are unable to bear weight. Swelling is common, and it is important to check for open wounds that may suggest open fracture.

Treatment: Displaced fractures require provisional reduction and immobilization. Open fractures require immediate irrigation and debridement. Fractures associated with neurovascular compromise require immediate reduction, with urgent surgical treatment if pulses do not return with provisional reduction. Undisplaced or minimally displaced fractures may be treated with cast immobilization. Fractures that remain displaced or with inappropriate alignment require open reduction and internal fixation; should always monitor for compartment syndrome in tibia fractures

Fibular Shaft Fractures

Description: Often associated with tibia fractures; with weight bearing, the fibula will take up to 20% and the tibia up to 80% of the load; fibular shaft fractures may indicate syndesmotic injury

Presentation: Fractures often occur with twisting or a direct blow to the lower leg. Twisting injuries will produce spiral fractures, whereas direct blows will cause transverse or comminuted fractures.

Treatment: A majority of fibular shaft fractures are nonsurgically treated. If associated with other injuries, such as tibial shaft fractures, treatment of the other injury will often be sufficient; must be suspicious and check for associated injuries, such as syndesmotic or ankle injuries

High Fibula Fracture With Syndesmosis Injury

Description: Difficult injuries with often significant instability; usually involves injury to the medial ankle such as medial malleolus fracture or deltoid ligament rupture

Examination: Crucial to examine the ankle and syndesmosis in the presence of a high fibula fracture; common peroneal nerve

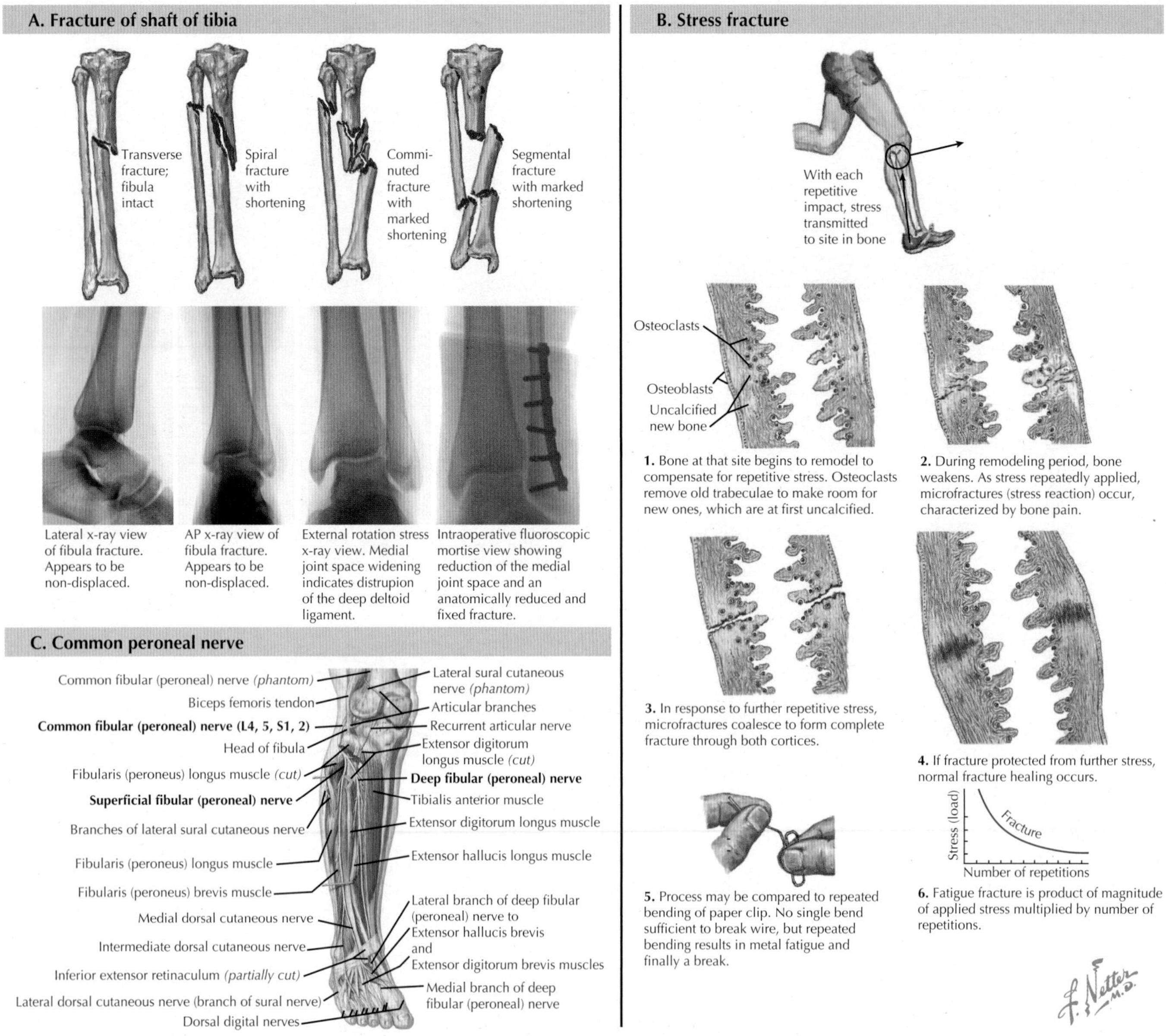
A. Fracture of shaft of tibia
Transverse fracture; fibula intact
Spiral fracture with shortening
Comminuted fracture with marked shortening
Segmental fracture with marked shortening
Lateral x-ray view of fibula fracture. Appears to be non-displaced.
AP x-ray view of fibula fracture. Appears to be non-displaced.
External rotation stress x-ray view. Medial joint space widening indicates distrupion of the deep deltoid ligament.
Intraoperative fluoroscopic mortise view showing reduction of the medial joint space and an anatomically reduced and fixed fracture.
B. Stress fracture
With each repetitive impact, stress transmitted to site in bone
Osteoclasts
Osteoblasts
Uncalcified new bone
1. Bone at that site begins to remodel to compensate for repetitive stress. Osteoclasts remove old trabeculae to make room for new ones, which are at first uncalcified.
2. During remodeling period, bone weakens. As stress repeatedly applied, microfractures (stress reaction) occur, characterized by bone pain.
3. In response to further repetitive stress, microfractures coalesce to form complete fracture through both cortices.
4. If fracture protected from further stress, normal fracture healing occurs.
5. Process may be compared to repeated bending of paper clip. No single bend sufficient to break wire, but repeated bending results in metal fatigue and finally a break.
Stress (load)
Fracture
Number of repetitions
6. Fatigue fracture is product of magnitude of applied stress multiplied by number of repetitions.
C. Common peroneal nerve
Common fibular (peroneal) nerve (phantom)
Biceps femoris tendon
Common fibular (peroneal) nerve (L4, 5, S1, 2)
Head of fibula
Fibularis (peroneus) longus muscle (cut)
Superficial fibular (peroneal) nerve
Branches of lateral sural cutaneous nerve
Fibularis (peroneus) longus muscle
Fibularis (peroneus) brevis muscle
Medial dorsal cutaneous nerve
Intermediate dorsal cutaneous nerve
Inferior extensor retinaculum (partially cut)
Lateral dorsal cutaneous nerve (branch of sural nerve)
Dorsal digital nerves
Lateral sural cutaneous nerve (phantom)
Articular branches
Recurrent articular nerve
Extensor digitorum longus muscle (cut)
Deep fibular (peroneal) nerve
Tibialis anterior muscle
Extensor digitorum longus muscle
Extensor hallucis longus muscle
Lateral branch of deep fibular (peroneal) nerve to Extensor hallucis brevis and Extensor digitorum brevis muscles
Medial branch of deep fibular (peroneal) nerve

Figure 56.4 Conditions of the leg.

traverses at level of proximal fibular neck and should be examined if injury is close to this region

Imaging: In the presence of a high fibula fracture, it is very important to also image the ankle to rule out associated injuries. Radiographs may demonstrate subtle widening of the mortise or a medial malleolus fracture. Stress views may be required to rule out syndesmotic injury.

Ankle Fractures

Description: Any fracture that directly enters the ankle or is associated with a ligamentous injury that compromises the ankle mortise

Treatment: Dislocated or subluxated ankles require immediate reduction and immobilization. Open fractures require immediate irrigation and debridement. Fractures or dislocations with neurovascular compromise require immediate reduction. Completely undisplaced fractures may be treated nonsurgically using a cast. Syndesmotic injury, disruption of the mortise, or displaced fractures require surgical fixation. Stress-view radiographs may be necessary to rule out mortise instability. Syndesmotic injuries usually require prolonged nonweight-bearing periods after surgery.

Chronic Exercise-Induced Leg Pain

Tibial Stress Fractures

Description: Commonly seen in athletes who perform repetitive running and jumping such as track athletes (see Fig. 56.4B)

Presentation: May present with low-level aching pain with early stress fractures or acute intense pain if fracture progresses; athletes often have period of prodromal symptoms

Examination: Tenderness and pain at location of stress fracture

Imaging: Begin with radiographs. If not visualized on radiograph and suspicion remains high, an MRI may show bony edema in early stress reactions or a fracture line in early stress fractures.

Treatment: Early stress reactions or fractures can be treated nonsurgically with rest and immobilization. Patients may return to activities as symptoms allow. Repeat imaging may be necessary to assess progress of healing. Stress fractures that have progressed to fully displaced fractures may require surgical fixation.

Patient factors should be optimized to promote early healing, such as adequate sugar control in diabetes or smoking cessation.

Medial Tibial Stress Syndrome

Description: Common cause of exercise-induced leg pain in athletes; seen in sports wherein repetitive running and jumping are required; considered a periostitis caused by traction of posterior leg muscles

Presentation: Pain along the posteromedial border of the mid-tibia, which worsens with activity; pain improves with rest but often does not completely resolve

Imaging: MRI is the best confirmatory test. Characteristic MRI finding is linear longitudinal edema of the periosteum; this can clearly differentiate medial tibial stress syndrome from a tibial stress fracture, which would show marrow edema and a transverse line of signal change within the bone.

Treatment: Initial treatment is rest and evaluation of training methods. If no response, surgery may be considered. Results have been mixed. Most common surgical procedure is fasciotomy adjacent to the area of pain, but this should be reserved for the most recalcitrant cases.

Chronic Exertional Compartment Syndrome (CECS)

Description: Activity-related increase in lower leg intracompartmental pressures leading to ischemic-like pain; symptoms slowly improve with rest but may remain quite bothersome to patients

Examination: Compartment pressure measurements before and after exercise can be used for diagnosis. A pre-exercise resting pressure >15 mmHg, a 1-minute postexercise pressure >30 mmHg, and a 5-minute postexercise pressure >20 mmHg have been suggested as diagnostic thresholds.

Treatment: Nonsurgical treatment comprises activity modifications. Fasciotomy is the surgical treatment of choice, which can be performed using open, mini-open, or endoscopic techniques. Surgical risks include damage to the peroneal nerves. Incomplete release is a common cause for persistent symptoms after surgery.

Peroneal Nerve Entrapment

Description: Common peroneal nerve is vulnerable at the lateral knee as it passes around the fibular neck and divides at the intramuscular septum between the anterior and lateral compartments (see Fig. 56.4C). Superficial peroneal nerve is most vulnerable at the fascial exit, but it may pass through a fibrous tunnel before exiting to the subcutaneous tissues. The nerve may become tethered or entrapped within this tunnel.

Presentation: Symptoms may be vague and poorly defined. Patients may complain of sensory changes, particularly at the dorsum of the foot. They may have weakness in the muscles of the anterior or lateral compartment.

Examination: May have tenderness at site of entrapment; symptoms may be reproduced with direct pressure over area of entrapment. Tinel sign may be positive, particularly after running, when symptoms are usually present. In severe cases of common peroneal nerve entrapment, transient foot drop and weakness of the anterior and lateral compartments may be presenting complaints. Nerve conduction and electrodiagnostic studies may help to delineate the location of entrapment.

Treatment: Nonsurgical treatment comprises rest and activity modifications. Physical therapy with desensitization therapy may help. Surgical treatment involves nerve release at the areas of entrapment or tethering.

Tendon Problems Around the Ankle

Achilles Tendon Rupture

Description: Frequently seen in athletes, particularly in males in the fourth decade; usually occurs in a zone approximately 6 cm above the calcaneal insertion, which is considered a hypovascular region of the tendon. Rupture of the tendon probably requires 50% of the tendon to be degenerative.

Presentation: Patients may admit to prodromal symptoms before the rupture; usually occurs during push-off during running or a hard lateral movement. Patients may hear a "pop," often described as a sensation of getting hit in the back, before realizing that they are unable to push off with the ankle and that the pain is localized to the heel.

Examination: Most reliable finding is loss of resistance to passive dorsiflexion or loss of active plantarflexion. There may be a palpable gap. Bruising is present. Thompson test is often positive.

Imaging: MRI is helpful in preoperative planning to determine the extent of tendon degeneration and the level of rupture.

Treatment: Both surgical and nonsurgical treatments can be considered. Nonsurgical treatment initially begins with immobilization in plantarflexion, with progressive dorsiflexion as healing progresses. Early functional rehabilitation has produced excellent results, with re-rupture rates similar to those with surgical treatment. Surgical treatment primarily consists of repairing the ruptured ends of the tendon using sutures. Re-rupture rates are low with surgical repair. Disadvantages of surgical management include wound healing problems, infection, and sural nerve injury. Minimally invasive percutaneous repair tries to avoid these complications and has been increasing in popularity. Early functional rehabilitation has also been achieved after surgical management.

Achilles Tendinopathy (Noninsertional)

Description: Tendinitis is a thickening and inflammation of the peritendinous tissue and is associated with acute pain; tendinosis is a degenerative condition that occurs within the tendon substance with mucoid degeneration, chondroid metaplasia, and fatty degeneration.

Examination: Collect the history of exercise and warm-up activity. Physical examination findings typically show thickening of the involved area with tenderness and varying degrees of local inflammation. Pain is enhanced with dorsiflexion and placing tension on the tendon (Fig. 56.5A). Biomechanical evaluation for hypermobile pes planus is important because corrective orthoses and shoe wear to control motion may be beneficial. MRI is the imaging modality of choice to assess inflammation or the extent of tendon degeneration.

Treatment: An improved stretching program, night splints, nonsteroidal anti-inflammatory drugs (NSAIDs), ice, rest, and even immobilization for a period of 2–4 weeks can be helpful. Surgical treatment involves debridement of inflammatory and degenerative tissue.

Posterior Tibial Tendonitis and Tears

Description: Uncommon in athletes under 30 years of age; unlike adult-acquired flat foot deformity, numerous cases of acute tendonitis do not involve a flat foot deformity. However, such injuries may indicate the earliest point in the development of this problem. A hypovascular zone of the tendon, behind and below the medial malleolus, is thought to be most susceptible to injury (see Fig. 56.5B).

Presentation: Focal pain with activity on the medial side of the ankle; may be particularly painful during push-off

Examination: Weakness, pain against resistance, and tenderness along the course of the tendon are strong diagnostic findings. Focal pain near insertion of the tendon, particularly with bony prominence, may indicate accessory navicular bone.

Imaging: Standing radiographs to determine alignment of foot and ankle; will also show accessory navicular. MRI will show status of the tendon and peritendinous tissue.

Treatment: Tendonitis can be treated with rest. An orthosis to unload the posterior tibial tendon may be helpful. When pain

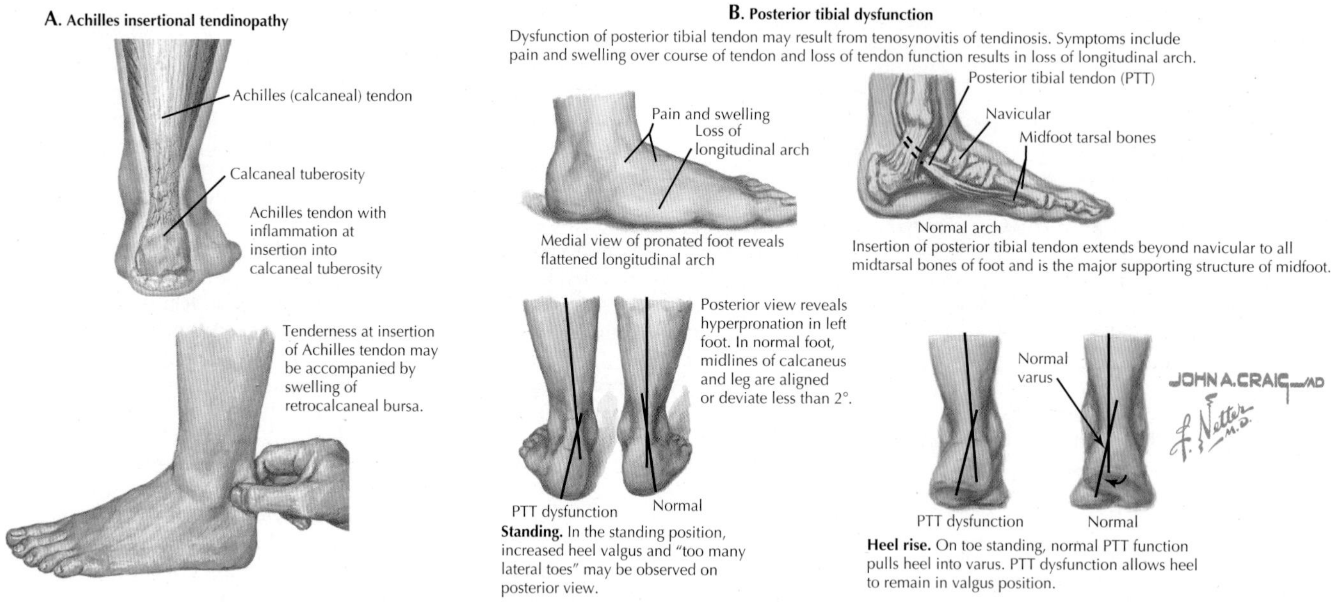
A. Achilles insertional tendinopathy
Achilles (calcaneal) tendon
Calcaneal tuberosity
Achilles tendon with inflammation at insertion into calcaneal tuberosity
Tenderness at insertion of Achilles tendon may be accompanied by swelling of retrocalcaneal bursa.
B. Posterior tibial dysfunction
Dysfunction of posterior tibial tendon may result from tenosynovitis of tendinosis. Symptoms include pain and swelling over course of tendon and loss of tendon function results in loss of longitudinal arch.
Pain and swelling
Loss of longitudinal arch
Medial view of pronated foot reveals flattened longitudinal arch
Posterior tibial tendon (PTT)
Navicular
Midfoot tarsal bones
Normal arch
Insertion of posterior tibial tendon extends beyond navicular to all midtarsal bones of foot and is the major supporting structure of midfoot.
Posterior view reveals hyperpronation in left foot. In normal foot, midlines of calcaneus and leg are aligned or deviate less than 2°.
PTT dysfunction
Normal
Standing. In the standing position, increased heel valgus and "too many lateral toes" may be observed on posterior view.
Normal varus
PTT dysfunction
Normal
Heel rise. On toe standing, normal PTT function pulls heel into varus. PTT dysfunction allows heel to remain in valgus position.
JOHN A.CRAIG_AD
F. Netter M.D.

Figure 56.5 Tendon problems around the ankle.

is too severe, cast immobilization for a period of 2–4 weeks may be necessary. Steroid injections may lead to tendon rupture and should be avoided. Physical therapy can be very helpful. Orthotics to support medial column can also help.

Flexor Hallucis Longus Tendonitis

Description: Seen in many athletes and classically in ballet dancers

Presentation: Symptoms may be vague and located medially or behind the ankle. Pain is usually activity related and may be severe enough to limit further participation in the competition.

Examination: Findings may include focal pain over the FHL, including behind the talus or medially between the Achilles and neurovascular bundle. Tenderness is increased with passive dorsiflexion of the hallux as the tendon is brought under tension. Motion of the hallux metatarsophalangeal joint may be decreased with ankle dorsiflexion compared with when the ankle is in plantarflexion.

Imaging: Radiographs may reveal a large trigonal process of the posterior talus or an os trigonum. MRI may show edema and fluid around the tendon behind the talus.

Treatment: Stretching, rest, night splints, and NSAIDs can lead to resolution of symptoms. Appropriate shoe wear is essential. A period of immobilization may be necessary to decrease any acute inflammation. Surgical release of the tendon sheath and tenolysis may be necessary if the patient fails nonoperative treatments. A symptomatic os trigonum should be considered for excision. Both open and posterior arthroscopic techniques have been described, and the choice of procedure depends on the experience of the surgeon and location of the pathology.

Peroneal Tendon Problems

Description: Include acute and chronic dislocations and tears; often occur with inversion injuries or other trauma such as calcaneal fractures

Presentation: Typically, a chronic problem that develops in the setting of other injuries may present as an acute injury. Patients will complain of pain to the lateral ankle as the tendon subluxates or dislocates. They are often able to voluntarily dislocate the tendon.

Examination: Cavovarus foot posture may be a risk factor for developing peroneal tendon pathology. Pain in the lateral retromalleolar region that is reproduced with palpation and resisted eversion is typical of peroneal tendon pathology. Testing for transient dislocation or subluxation is essential in evaluation of the integrity of the superficial peroneal retinaculum. This can be performed with the ankle starting in dorsiflexion and inversion and application of resistance as the patient tries to evert the foot. Often the dislocating tendon can be visualized and felt.

Imaging: MRI is the modality of choice for assessing pathology of peroneal tendons. Ultrasound is also helpful because it can be adjusted to the obliquity of the tendons. It is also dynamic and allows direct visualization of the dislocating tendon.

Treatment: Rest and brief immobilization may initially help to diminish pain. Orthoses with a lateral forefoot post can help offload the peroneals in a cavus foot. Gross instability or fixed dislocation warrants surgical consideration. Surgery for recalcitrant pain is performed to debride and repair longitudinal tears and, in certain cases, debulk the tendons if tendinosis has led to gross thickening.

Ankle Joint Problems

Osteochondral Lesions of the Talus

Description: Seen in several ankle injuries, but particularly inversion injuries; medial talar lesions typically have no history of trauma. Lateral talar lesions are typically associated with inversion injuries.

Presentation: Present with pain and swelling of the ankle joint; may have mechanical symptoms of clicking, catching, and locking

Imaging: Radiographs are helpful in diagnosing lesions. CT or MRI is preferred to better delineate the lesion and to assess for intra-articular loose bodies (Fig. 56.6). When combined with intra-articular contrast, can show the status of the cartilage; a segment is considered unstable if the dye tracks beneath the osteochondral fragment.

Treatment: Osteochondral lesions that are small, stable, and asymptomatic may be nonsurgically treated. Small lesions considered unstable can be excised; larger osteochondral lesions that are displaced may be fixed back into their native positions. Microfracturing can be performed in the presence of a healthy bone bed. Osteochondral autograft and allograft transplantation is also available, particularly in larger lesions or those that have failed previous surgical treatments. Autologous cartilage

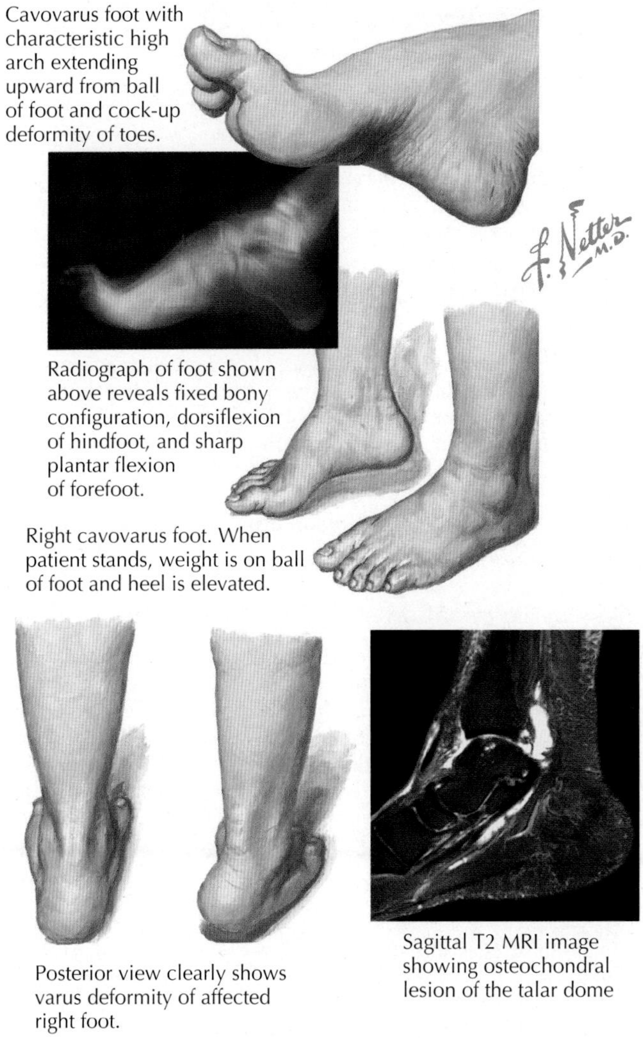
Cavovarus foot with characteristic high arch extending upward from ball of foot and cock-up deformity of toes.
Radiograph of foot shown above reveals fixed bony configuration, dorsiflexion of hindfoot, and sharp plantar flexion of forefoot.
Right cavovarus foot. When patient stands, weight is on ball of foot and heel is elevated.
Posterior view clearly shows varus deformity of affected right foot.
Sagittal T2 MRI image showing osteochondral lesion of the talar dome
F. Netter M.D.

Figure 56.6 Ankle joint problems.

implantation may also be an option. Surgery is performed using either arthroscopic or open techniques.

Chronic Lateral Ankle Instability

Description: The most common ligament to be injured is the anterior talofibular ligament (ATFL), and the second most common is the CFL. Chronic instability may result because of incomplete healing; often associated with other ankle pathology, such as talar osteochondral lesions or talar process fractures.

Presentation: Patients will complain of persistent instability with numerous inversion episodes. Instability may be exacerbated with small events such as stepping on a pebble or walking on uneven ground.

Examination: Always compare with the contralateral side. Stress examinations will reveal increased translation or subluxation of the talus.

Treatment: Nonsurgical treatment is the mainstay for acute ankle instability. Initial management focuses on controlling pain and swelling. Early functional rehabilitation has shown excellent results. Patients will work on strengthening, range of motion, balance, and proprioception training. Excellent results can be obtained with appropriate physical therapy. An orthosis may be necessary if subtle cavus foot is present and contributing to inversion events (see Fig. 56.6). Failure of nonsurgical treatments with ongoing symptomatic instability is an indication for lateral ligament reconstruction.

Soft Tissue Impingement

ANTEROMEDIAL AND ANTEROLATERAL IMPINGEMENT

Description: May occur after inversion injuries; anterior impingement caused by tearing of anterior capsule and synovial tissues; lateral impingement caused by torn ATFL or tearing of anterior inferior fascicles of syndesmosis; medial impingement less common and caused by tearing of anterior band of deltoid ligament; capsule and synovium may also cause impingement at this location

Examination: Physical examination can be very specific in reproducing the pain. Patients are often able to reproduce the pain and describe its exact location.

Imaging: MRI and arthrograms may show the lesion but are not very specific.

Treatment: Usually, arthroscopic debridement is adequate. Open debridement with arthrotomy is rare.

POSTERIOR ANKLE IMPINGEMENT

Description: Uncommon; caused by tearing of the posterior tibiofibular ligament, which forms a labrum-like structure at the posterior tibial plafond

Mechanism: Can be torn with ankle trauma; the unstable tissue can flip into the posterior ankle and become entrapped with plantarflexion.

Examination: Test for impingement with plantarflexion. Patient is often able to reproduce symptoms.

Imaging: MRI findings on the sagittal view can suggest the presence of an impingement lesion if the labral rim is seen to be detached in this view.

Treatment: Arthroscopic debridement is possible posteriorly with the patient in the prone position. Open debridement is also appropriate.

RECOMMENDED READINGS

Available online.

57 CARTILAGE PROBLEMS IN SPORTS

Courtney A. Quinn • Mark D. Miller

TYPES OF CARTILAGE

Hyaline Cartilage

- Functions to decrease joint friction and distribute load across the joint; also referred to as *articular cartilage*
- **Composition:** Water (65%–80%), collagen (10%–20%, predominantly type II), proteoglycans (10%–15%, aggrecan is most responsible for the hydrophilic property), and chondrocytes (5%) (Fig. 57.1)
- **Viability:** Articular cartilage is avascular, and chondrocytes are nourished via diffusion from synovial fluid
- **Structure:** Organized into three primary layers—superficial, middle, and deep; the tidemark separates these layers from the calcified cartilage and subchondral bone (see Fig. 57.1)
- **Location:** Articular surfaces, ribs, and nasal septum

Fibrocartilage

- Functions in direct tendon and ligament insertions and helps in the healing of articular cartilage lesions. Less durable than hyaline cartilage.
- **Composition:** Primarily type I collagen, extracellular matrix, chondrocytes, water
- **Location:** Tendon/ligament junction with bone, menisci, and annulus fibrosis of the intervertebral disc

Elastic Cartilage

- Strong but flexible cartilage that can withstand repeated bending
- **Composition:** Primarily type II collagen, elastin fiber network, extracellular matrix, chondrocytes, water
- **Locations:** Pinnae of ear, epiglottis

TYPES OF CARTILAGE ISSUES IN THE ATHLETE

Articular Cartilage Injuries

- Can be caused by either acute injury or a more chronic, avascular process
- **Deep lesions:** Cross the tidemark and penetrate the subchondral bone; vascularity from the subchondral bone promotes fibrocartilage healing (type I collagen) rather than the preferred articular cartilage
- **Superficial lesions:** Do not penetrate the subchondral bone and therefore have no intrinsic healing potential secondary to the avascular nature of articular cartilage
- Healing is enhanced by motion of the involved joint to encourage diffusion of nutrients and to trigger mechanoreceptors in the cartilage that promote matrix synthesis

Apophyseal Injuries

- An apophysis is a normal developmental outgrowth of cartilage adjacent to the physis that serves as the attachment site for major tendons and ligaments
- Is a separate secondary ossification center from the epiphysis and does not contribute to longitudinal growth of the bone
- Fuses with the bone later as skeletal maturity is reached
- **Traction apophysitis:** Repetitive microtrauma caused by the pull of attached tendons; results in partial avulsion and inflammation of the apophysis; common in active children and adolescents; excessive force may result in avulsion fracture of the apophysis
- **Osteochondrosis:** General term for disorders affecting one or more ossification centers in children; encompasses conditions such as traction apophysitis and avascular necrosis

HISTORY AND PHYSICAL EXAMINATION

History

- A detailed description of the onset of symptoms, mechanism of injury, duration and quality of symptoms, and any relieving or exacerbating factors should be obtained
- Symptoms may include pain with activity, swelling of the affected joint, and mechanical complaints, such as clicking and locking
- Overuse injuries typically have an insidious onset with no identifiable precipitating injury

Physical Examination

- Few, if any, physical examination tests are highly specific for the evaluation of articular cartilage injury
- A complete examination of the involved joint should be conducted, including range of motion, assessment of pain with resisted motion, focal tenderness, and presence of an effusion
- Apophyseal injuries can present with pain upon palpation of the affected apophysis and pain with resisted motion of the muscle or ligament that attaches at the apophysis

Imaging Studies

- Imaging studies are essential for the evaluation of cartilage injuries
- **Plain radiographs:** Useful in ruling out fractures and identifying various osteochondroses and osteochondral lesions such as osteochondritis dissecans (OCD); also beneficial in identifying intra-articular loose bodies, assessing limb alignment, and evaluating joint space
- **Computed tomography (CT):** Helpful in assessing cartilage lesions with associated osseous involvement
- **Magnetic resonance imaging (MRI):** Gold standard for the evaluation of articular cartilage; can identify subchondral edema; focal chondral defects may be underestimated (Table 57.1). Newer MRI techniques such as delayed gadolinium-enhanced MRI of cartilage can identify proteoglycans, and the measurement of T2 relaxation times are sensitive to collagen architecture

SPECIFIC INJURIES AND PROBLEMS

Hip

Focal Chondral Defect

Description: Localized, full-thickness loss of articular cartilage with exposed subchondral bone (Fig. 57.2)

Mechanism of injury: Typically, a direct blow to the greater trochanter; forces are transferred to the articular surfaces of the femoral head and acetabulum

Presentation: History of injury with failure of full recovery, catching or locking with vague hip and groin pain

Physical examination: Nonspecific; pain with range of motion, possible block to motion

Differential diagnosis: Avascular necrosis, femoroacetabular impingement (FAI), hip dysplasia, degenerative arthritis, labral pathology, and femoral neck stress fracture

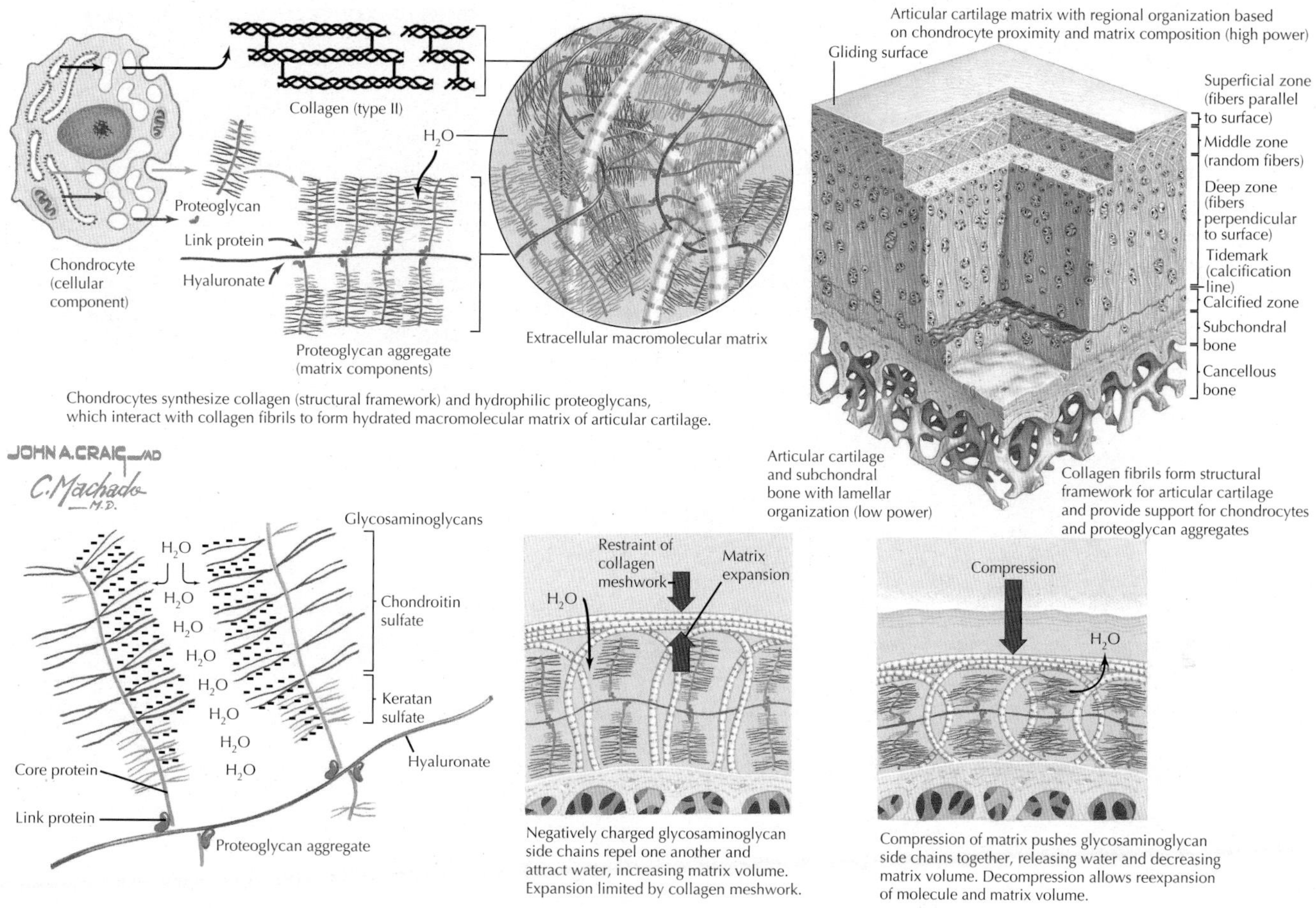
Collagen (type II)
H2O
Proteoglycan
Link protein
Hyaluronate
Chondrocyte (cellular component)
Proteoglycan aggregate (matrix components)
Extracellular macromolecular matrix
Chondrocytes synthesize collagen (structural framework) and hydrophilic proteoglycans, which interact with collagen fibrils to form hydrated macromolecular matrix of articular cartilage.
Articular cartilage matrix with regional organization based on chondrocyte proximity and matrix composition (high power)
Gliding surface
Superficial zone (fibers parallel to surface)
Middle zone (random fibers)
Deep zone (fibers perpendicular to surface)
Tidemark (calcification line)
Calcified zone
Subchondral bone
Cancellous bone
Articular cartilage and subchondral bone with lamellar organization (low power)
Collagen fibrils form structural framework for articular cartilage and provide support for chondrocytes and proteoglycan aggregates
JOHN A.CRAIG_MD
C.Machado M.D.
Glycosaminoglycans
Chondroitin sulfate
Keratan sulfate
Hyaluronate
Core protein
Link protein
Proteoglycan aggregate
Restraint of collagen meshwork
Matrix expansion
Negatively charged glycosaminoglycan side chains repel one another and attract water, increasing matrix volume. Expansion limited by collagen meshwork.
Compression
Compression of matrix pushes glycosaminoglycan side chains together, releasing water and decreasing matrix volume. Decompression allows reexpansion of molecule and matrix volume.

Figure 57.1 Composition and structure of articular cartilage.

Table 57.1 CARTILAGE SIGNAL INTENSITIES ON MRI

	T1-Weighted Images	T2-Weighted Images
Hyaline cartilage	Gray	Gray
Fibrocartilage	Dark	Dark

Diagnostics: Radiographs are helpful in evaluating joint space and ruling out other conditions. MRI may demonstrate localized defect or subchondral edema. MRI arthrography has higher detection rates for cartilage and labral pathologies

Treatment: Arthroscopic chondroplasty, drilling, or microfracture for localized lesions; excision of unstable or loose fragments to alleviate mechanical symptoms (see Fig. 57.2)

Prognosis and return to sport: Return to sport when symptoms allow after debridement or excision of fragments. Chondral reparative procedures such as microfracture require partial weight bearing for 6–8 weeks; early range of motion encouraged

Femoroacetabular Impingement

Description: Abnormal contact between the femoral head–neck junction and acetabulum; results in injury to the articular cartilage and labrum; may be a cause of chronic hip pain in athletes; three types defined based on the primary location of pathology (see Fig 57.2):

- **Cam type:** Femoral deformity; "pistol grip" deformity of the femoral head with decreased head–neck offset and asphericity, leading to abutment of this region with the normal acetabulum
- **Pincer type:** Acetabular deformity; increased acetabular retroversion leading to abutment of the normal femoral head–neck junction on the acetabular rim
- **Mixed type:** Combined deformity of femoral head and acetabulum; most common (up to 80%)

Mechanism of injury: Etiology unknown

Presentation: Anterior hip pain with difficulty squatting, cutting, and starting/stopping

Physical examination: Pain with flexion, internal rotation, and adduction indicate a positive impingement test; range of motion often limited.

Differential diagnosis: Traumatic chondral defect, hip dysplasia, hip osteoarthritis

Diagnostics: Radiographs demonstrate the "pistol grip" deformity of the femoral neck or signs of acetabular retroversion such as a crossover or posterior wall sign. MRI may help identify chondral injury and labral tears.

Treatment: Nonsurgical options include activity modification, anti-inflammatory medication, adductor strengthening, intra-articular steroid injections, and hip-motion exercises. Typical surgical options include arthroscopic osteoplasty for cam type lesions and acetabular rim trimming for pincer-type lesions. Chondral lesions are addressed as described previously with chondroplasty, drilling, or microfracture. Labral repair or debridement is also usually required.

Prognosis and return to sport: FAI may be a precursor to osteoarthritis. When chondral lesions are addressed, partial weight bearing for 6–8 weeks is necessary, with progressive activity to follow and return to sport around 3–6 months.

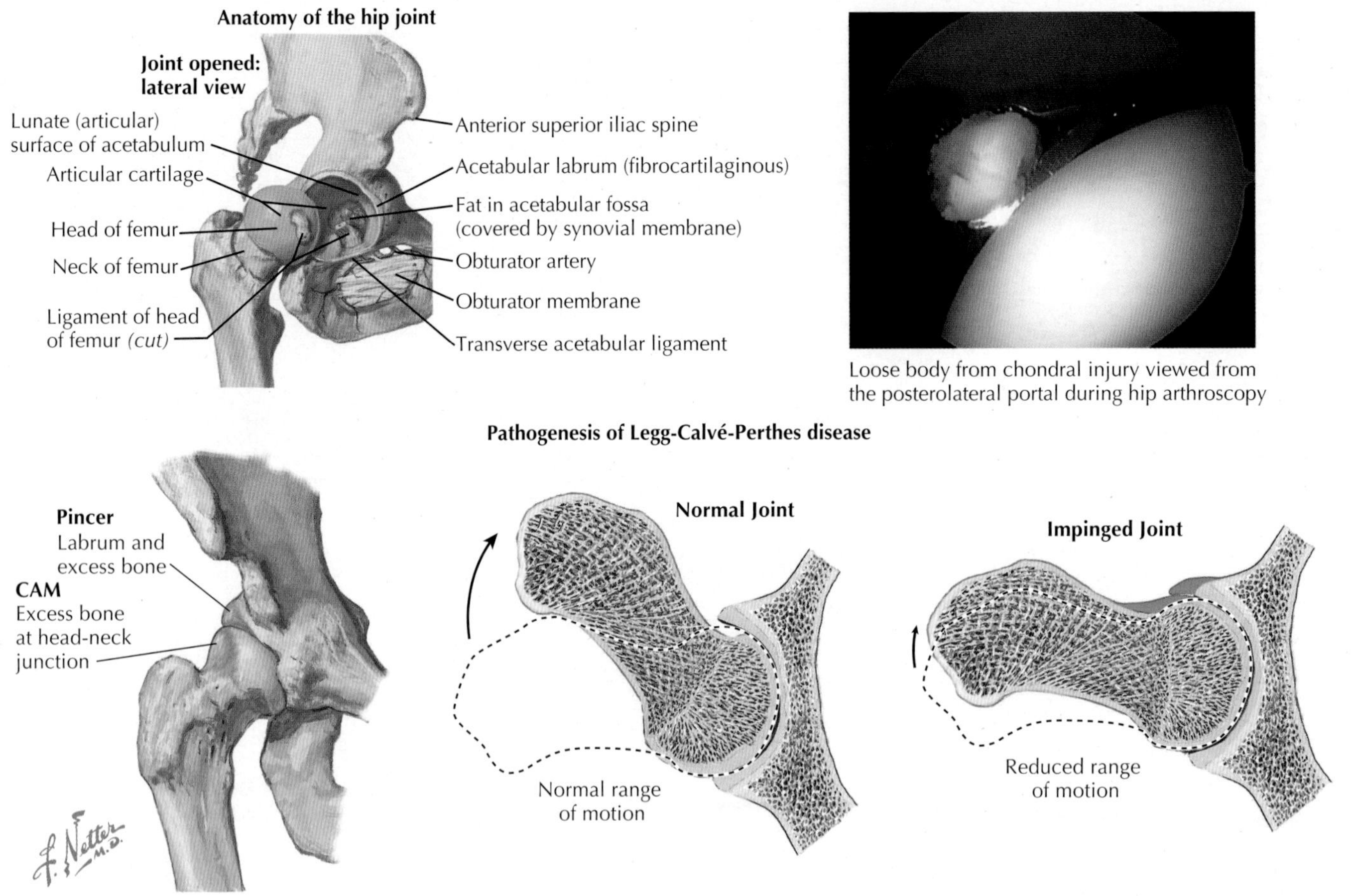
Anatomy of the hip joint
Joint opened: lateral view
Lunate (articular) surface of acetabulum
Articular cartilage
Head of femur
Neck of femur
Ligament of head of femur (cut)
Anterior superior iliac spine
Acetabular labrum (fibrocartilaginous)
Fat in acetabular fossa (covered by synovial membrane)
Obturator artery
Obturator membrane
Transverse acetabular ligament
Loose body from chondral injury viewed from the posterolateral portal during hip arthroscopy
Pathogenesis of Legg-Calvé-Perthes disease
Pincer
Labrum and excess bone
CAM
Excess bone at head-neck junction
Normal Joint
Normal range of motion
Impinged Joint
Reduced range of motion
F. Netter M.D.

Figure 57.2 Hip anatomy and femoroacetabular impingement. (Arthroscope image from Miller M, Cole B. *Textbook of Arthroscopy*. Philadelphia: Saunders, Elsevier; 2004.)

Table 57.2 TRACTION APOPHYSES OF THE HIP

Traction Apophysis	Muscle Attachments
Iliac crest	Internal and external obliques
Anterior superior iliac spine (ASIS)	Sartorius and tensor fascia lata
Anterior inferior iliac spine (AIIS)	Rectus femoris
Ischial tuberosity	Hamstrings
Greater trochanter	Abductors
Lesser trochanter	Iliopsoas

Apophyseal Injuries Around the Hip

Description: Several traction apophyses are present in the hip and pelvis of skeletally immature patients; ischial tuberosity is most commonly involved (Table 57.2).

Mechanism of injury: Traction apophysitis secondary to overuse in adolescent patients; common in running sports

Presentation: Activity-related pain, particularly when the musculotendinous unit attached to the apophysis is activated

Physical examination: Localized tenderness, discomfort with range of motion, and tension on the involved musculotendinous unit

Differential diagnosis: Apophyseal avulsion fracture, muscle strain, or rupture

Diagnostics: Radiographs may show irregularity of the involved apophysis and rule out avulsion fractures

Treatment: Activity modification, local modalities, and anti-inflammatory medications

Prognosis and return to sport: Return to sport as symptoms allow

Knee

Focal Chondral Defect

Description: Localized, partial- or full-thickness loss of articular cartilage

- If full thickness, can have exposed subchondral bone (Fig. 57.3A and B)
- Medial femoral condyle most commonly involved, followed by lateral femoral condyle, femoral trochlea, and patellar facets
- The proximal tibial articular surface is relatively protected by the overlying meniscus and thus less susceptible to injury

Mechanism of injury: Generally traumatic injury with shear or rotational forces

Presentation: History of injury, possible delayed effusion, pain with persistent weight bearing, and mechanical symptoms

Physical examination: Possible effusion and tenderness to palpation at the site of cartilage loss, occasional mechanical block to motion

Differential diagnosis: Meniscal tear, OCD, ligament injury, and degenerative arthritis

Diagnostics: Not visualized on radiographs unless there is bony involvement; MRI best delineates cartilage lesions, but may underestimate the involvement and size of focal lesions (see Fig. 57.3C)

Treatment: Nonsurgical treatment (anti-inflammatory medications, steroid and hyaluronic injections, and physical therapy)

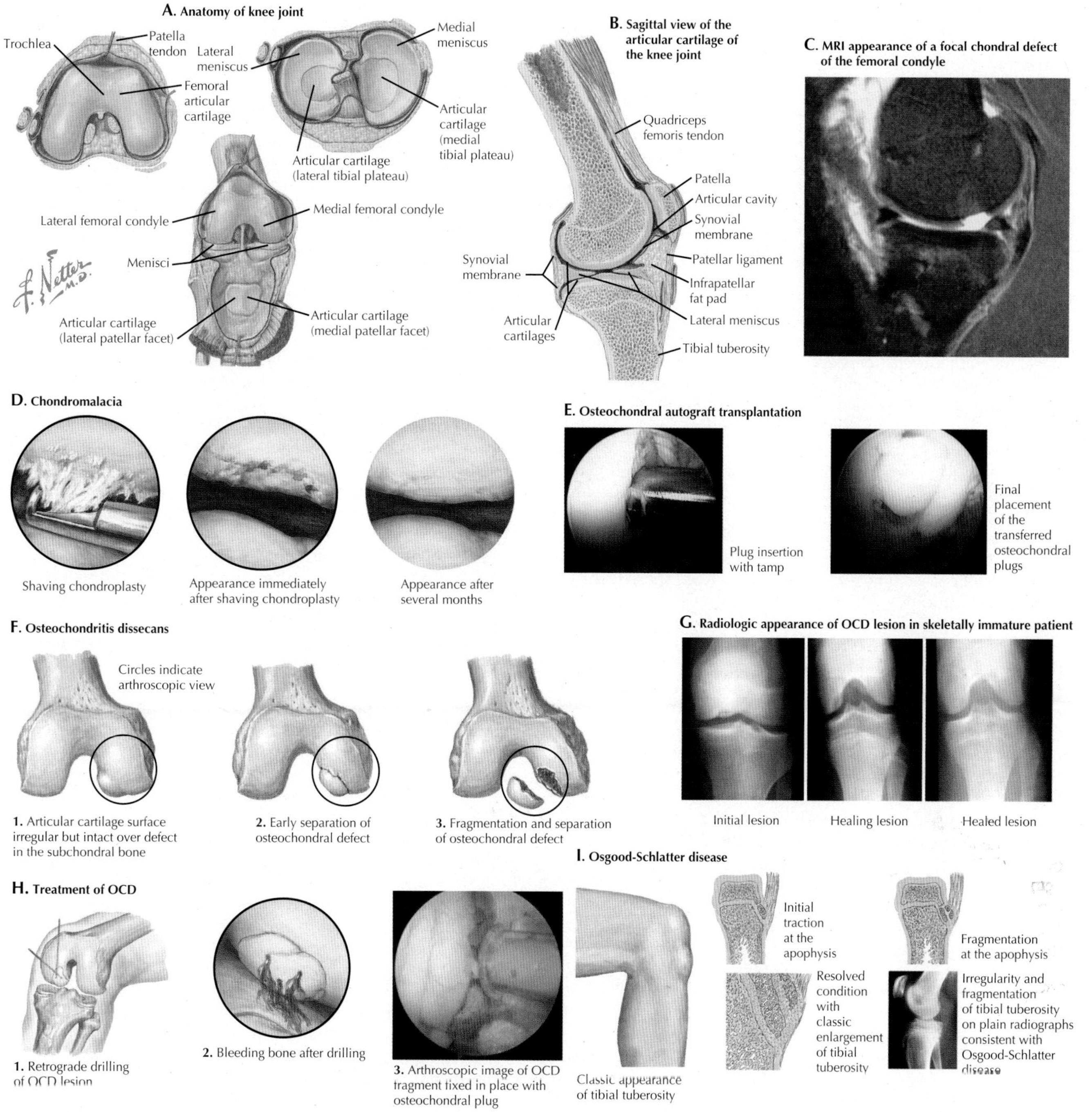
A. Anatomy of knee joint
Trochlea
Patella tendon
Lateral meniscus
Femoral articular cartilage
Medial meniscus
Articular cartilage (medial tibial plateau)
Articular cartilage (lateral tibial plateau)
Lateral femoral condyle
Medial femoral condyle
Menisci
Articular cartilage (lateral patellar facet)
Articular cartilage (medial patellar facet)
B. Sagittal view of the articular cartilage of the knee joint
Quadriceps femoris tendon
Patella
Articular cavity
Synovial membrane
Patellar ligament
Infrapatellar fat pad
Lateral meniscus
Tibial tuberosity
Synovial membrane
Articular cartilages
C. MRI appearance of a focal chondral defect of the femoral condyle
D. Chondromalacia
Shaving chondroplasty
Appearance immediately after shaving chondroplasty
Appearance after several months
E. Osteochondral autograft transplantation
Plug insertion with tamp
Final placement of the transferred osteochondral plugs
F. Osteochondritis dissecans
Circles indicate arthroscopic view
1. Articular cartilage surface irregular but intact over defect in the subchondral bone
2. Early separation of osteochondral defect
3. Fragmentation and separation of osteochondral defect
G. Radiologic appearance of OCD lesion in skeletally immature patient
Initial lesion
Healing lesion
Healed lesion
H. Treatment of OCD
1. Retrograde drilling of OCD lesion
2. Bleeding bone after drilling
3. Arthroscopic image of OCD fragment fixed in place with osteochondral plug
I. Osgood-Schlatter disease
Classic appearance of tibial tuberosity
Initial traction at the apophysis
Fragmentation at the apophysis
Resolved condition with classic enlargement of tibial tuberosity
Irregularity and fragmentation of tibial tuberosity on plain radiographs consistent with Osgood-Schlatter disease

Figure 57.3 Knee injuries and problems. (C and E, from Miller M, Cole B. *Textbook of Arthroscopy*. Philadelphia: Saunders, Elsevier; 2004.)

often provides limited benefits. A spectrum of arthroscopic options exists when nonsurgical measures fail:

- **Chondroplasty:** Loose chondral flaps debrided with careful preservation of surrounding normal articular cartilage (see Fig. 57.3D)
- **Microfracture:** Considered first line of treatment for small symptomatic lesions; multiple holes created to penetrate subchondral bone to promote bone marrow stimulation; bleeding into the defects promotes influx of pluripotent mesenchymal cells with resultant fibrocartilage formation, which is less desirable than hyaline cartilage.
- **Osteochondral autograft transfer (OAT):** Transfer plugs of normal osteochondral tissue from less essential weight-bearing regions of the knee into the defect. Bony healing occurs while articular gaps are filled with fibrous tissue; limited by donor site availability (see Fig. 57.3E).
- **Fresh osteochondral allograft (OCA) transplantation:** Defect filled with an osteochondral plug from a cadaver; main advantage is a single-stage procedure that allows replacement of a large defect with viable hyaline cartilage; primary concerns include host incorporation, potential disease transmission, immunologic reactions, and can be technically demanding.
- **Autologous chondrocyte implantation (ACI):** Two-stage procedure; first, chondrocytes are harvested and cultured from the patient from a nonweight-bearing zone of the

knee. After several weeks, the cultured cells, which contain pluripotent mesenchymal stem cells, are reimplanted under a patch or as a scaffold matrix. The chondrocytes proliferate and produce hyaline-like cartilage.

Prognosis and return to sport: No weight bearing for up to 8 weeks; early range of motion encouraged, and continuous passive motion may be beneficial; first line of therapy is microfracture, but certain studies have suggested young athletes experience the best results with restorative procedures (e.g., OAT and ACI); return to sport typically delayed by 3–6 months

Osteochondritis Dissecans

Description: Localized separation of subchondral bone and overlying articular cartilage (see Fig. 57.3F); typical location is lateral aspect of the medial femoral condyle. Usually occurs in skeletally immature patients aged 10–15 but can present later in life if asymptomatic and undiagnosed in early years.

Mechanism of injury: Can be caused by repetitive trauma, endocrine disorders, vascular insufficiency, and familial predisposition

Presentation: Often vague activity-related pain, possible effusion, and mechanical symptoms if the affected fragment becomes loose within the joint

Physical examination: Effusion and tenderness to palpation

Differential diagnosis: Meniscal tear, focal chondral defect, and intra-articular loose body of other etiology (e.g., subsequent to patellar dislocation)

Diagnostics: A tunnel (notch) view best demonstrates OCD lesions on radiographs (see Fig. 57.3G). MRI is better for delineating size and stability of the lesion. Synovial fluid behind the lesion indicates poor healing potential with nonsurgical management.

Treatment: Adolescents with open physes have a better prognosis, which may be observed with restricted weight bearing. Surgical treatment options recommended for unstable or loose fragments, failure of conservative management, and lesions in skeletally mature patients; consists of debridement, drilling, and internal fixation with addition of bone grafting in select cases (see Fig. 57.3H).

Prognosis and return to sport: Prognosis best in patients with open physes; return to sport when symptoms abate; with surgical fixation of lesions, return to sport often delayed 3–6 months to allow adequate healing of the lesion.

Osgood–Schlatter Disease and Sinding–Larsen–Johansson Syndrome

Description: Osteochondroses that occur at traction apophyses in knees of skeletally immature patients; Osgood–Schlatter affects the tibial tuberosity (patellar tendon insertion), and Sinding–Larsen–Johansson the inferior pole of the patella (patellar tendon origin); most common during periods of rapid growth (see Fig. 57.3I)

Mechanism of injury: Traction apophysitis secondary to mechanical stress from the extensor mechanism and chronic avulsion of the tibia

Presentation: Activity-related anterior knee pain, particularly with jumping and kneeling

Physical examination: Localized tenderness, prominent tibial tuberosity, and pain with resisted knee extension

Differential diagnosis: Patellar tendonitis, tibial tubercle physeal injury, and patellar sleeve fracture with acute injury

Diagnostics: Radiographs may show fragmentation or irregularity of the tibial tuberosity or inferior patellar pole and associated soft tissue swelling (see Fig. 57.3I)

Treatment: Activity modification, hamstring stretching, local modalities, bracing with compression sleeve or Cho-Pat strap, anti-inflammatory medications; rarely, ossicle excision for recalcitrant cases

Prognosis and return to sport: Self-limiting condition; return to sport as symptoms allow

Foot and Ankle

Osteochondral Lesions of the Talus (OLT)

Description: Focal osteochondral defect involving the dome of the talus (Fig. 57.4A); anterolateral lesions are typically traumatic, shallow, and more likely to be displaced. Posteromedial lesions are more common, usually deeper, atraumatic, and nondisplaced.

Mechanism of injury: Often occur in the setting of ankle fracture or inversion ankle sprain with recurrent lateral ankle instability

Presentation: Persistent pain after an ankle sprain or healed fracture, possible mechanical symptoms if fragment is unstable or loose within the joint

Physical examination: Localized ankle tenderness and swelling, may have an increased talar tilt and anterior drawer sign consistent with associated lateral ankle instability

Differential diagnosis: Recurrent lateral ankle instability, peroneal tendon pathology, lateral talar process fracture, or ankle arthritis

Diagnostics: Radiographs often normal, rule out fracture; MRI better to delineate size, depth, and displacement of the lesion

Treatment: Observation with immobilization in skeletally immature patients and stable lesions in adults; unstable, displaced, and loose fragments require surgical intervention. Options include arthroscopic excision of the fragment with microfracture, OAT, osteochondral allograft transplantation, and cartilage regeneration procedures (autologous chondrocyte implantation/matrix-induced autologous chondrocyte implantation [ACI/MACI], concentrated bone marrow aspirate, etc.). Occasionally, large fragments may be reduced and fixed, if recognized acutely.

Prognosis and return to sport: Acute injuries are treated conservatively, and avoid weight bearing for 6 weeks in all surgically treated ankles. Return to sport is often possible at 3–6 months

Sever Disease

Description: Osteochondrosis at the insertion of the Achilles tendon on the calcaneal tuberosity in skeletally immature patients; most common during periods of rapid growth

Mechanism of injury: Traction phenomenon on the calcaneal apophysis from the strong gastrocsoleus complex; overuse syndrome

Presentation: Skeletally immature patient with activity-related posterior heel pain; bilateral in up to 50% of cases

Physical examination: Localized tenderness of the posterior heel, pain with medial-lateral compression, tight heel cords, pain on stretching of triceps surae, and positive squeeze test

Differential diagnosis: Achilles tendonitis, retrocalcaneal bursitis, calcaneal stress fracture, plantar fasciitis, and calcaneal bone cyst

Diagnostics: Diagnosis is based on clinical symptoms, but radiographs may show irregularity, sclerosis, and fragmentation of the calcaneal apophysis

Treatment: Activity modification, anti-inflammatory medications, heel cord stretching, and heel cups or lifts

Prognosis and return to sport: Self-limiting condition; return to sport as symptoms allow

Freiberg Infarction

Description: Osteochondrosis of the second metatarsal head; most common in adolescent and young adult females

Mechanism of injury: May be secondary to acute trauma, repetitive microtrauma, or other conditions leading to osteonecrosis and collapse of the subchondral bone

Presentation: Acute pain (metatarsalgia), worse with weight-bearing activities, and second metatarsophalangeal (MTP) stiffness

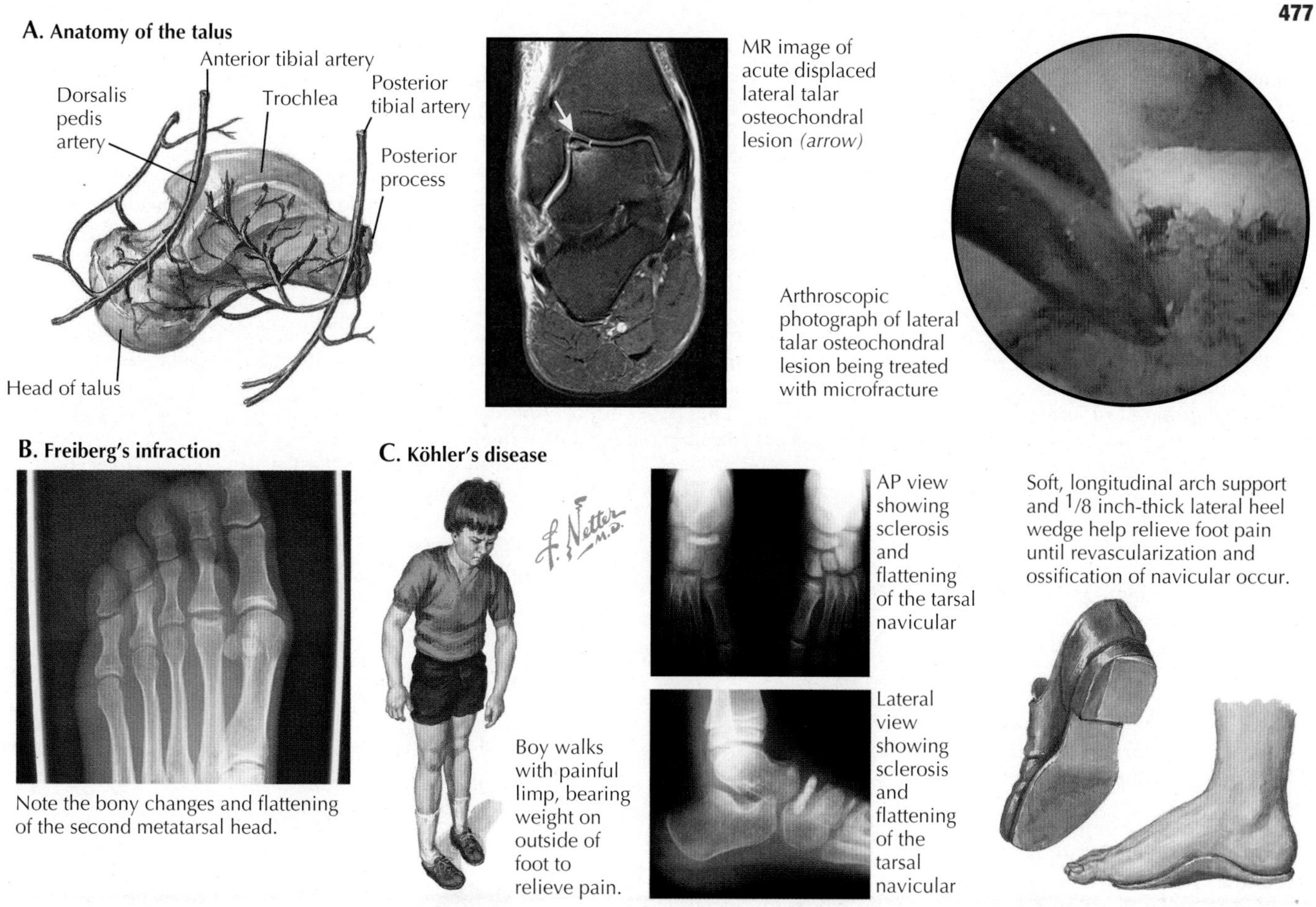
A. Anatomy of the talus
Anterior tibial artery
Dorsalis pedis artery
Trochlea
Posterior tibial artery
Posterior process
Head of talus
MR image of acute displaced lateral talar osteochondral lesion (arrow)
Arthroscopic photograph of lateral talar osteochondral lesion being treated with microfracture
B. Freiberg's infraction
Note the bony changes and flattening of the second metatarsal head.
C. Köhler's disease
Boy walks with painful limp, bearing weight on outside of foot to relieve pain.
AP view showing sclerosis and flattening of the tarsal navicular
Lateral view showing sclerosis and flattening of the tarsal navicular
Soft, longitudinal arch support and 1/8 inch-thick lateral heel wedge help relieve foot pain until revascularization and ossification of navicular occur.

Figure 57.4 Foot and ankle injuries and problems.

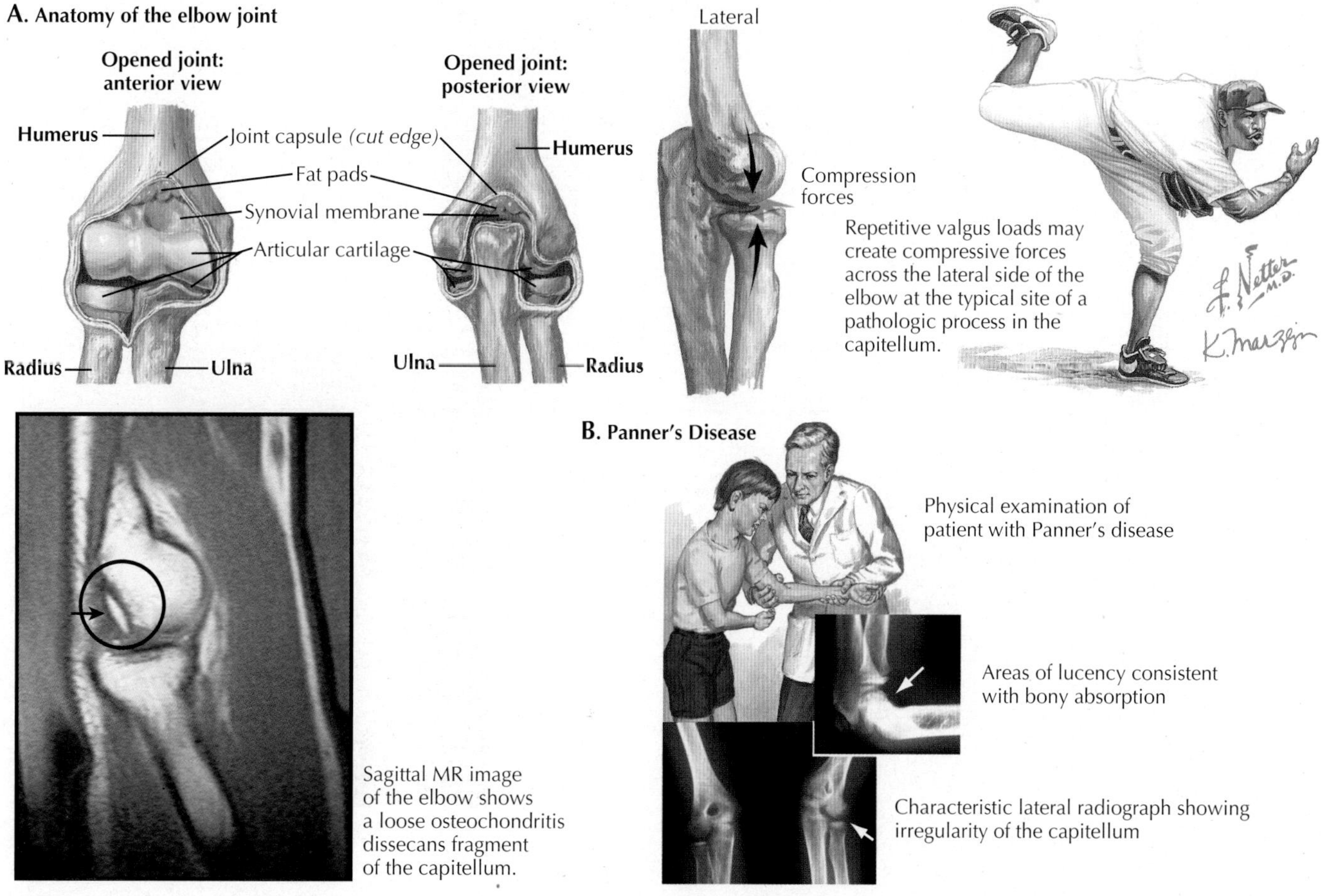
A. Anatomy of the elbow joint
Opened joint: anterior view
Opened joint: posterior view
Humerus
Joint capsule (cut edge)
Fat pads
Synovial membrane
Articular cartilage
Humerus
Radius
Ulna
Ulna
Radius
Lateral
Compression forces
Repetitive valgus loads may create compressive forces across the lateral side of the elbow at the typical site of a pathologic process in the capitellum.
Sagittal MR image of the elbow shows a loose osteochondritis dissecans fragment of the capitellum.
B. Panner's Disease
Physical examination of patient with Panner's disease
Areas of lucency consistent with bony absorption
Characteristic lateral radiograph showing irregularity of the capitellum

Figure 57.5 Elbow injuries and problems.

Physical examination: Localized tenderness of the second metatarsal head, swelling, and limited MTP range of motion
Differential diagnosis: Metatarsal fracture, stress fracture, and metatarsalgia of other etiology (e.g., transfer metatarsalgia secondary to conditions of the neighboring hallux)
Diagnostics: Early radiographs normal; radiographs later show collapse with flattening of the second metatarsal head, possible osteophytes, and articular cartilage destruction (see Fig. 57.4B)
Treatment: Protective footwear, orthotics such as metatarsal pads or bars, and anti-inflammatory medications often alleviate symptoms in mild cases. Advanced cases may require immobilization in a walking cast or surgical intervention. Surgical options can include synovectomy with core decompression of the metatarsal head, osteochondral plug transplantation, cheilectomy, osteotomy, or partial resection of the metatarsal head.
Prognosis and return to sport: Most patients show good prognosis with conservative management and may return to sport with resolution of symptoms

Köhler Disease

Description: Osteonecrosis of the tarsal navicular; usually presents in childhood
Mechanism of injury: Idiopathic
Presentation: Persistent midfoot pain in a young child (see Fig. 57.4C); more common in boys (approximately 80% of cases); may or may not recall an injury
Physical examination: Localized tenderness
Differential diagnosis: Accessory navicular and navicular stress fracture
Diagnostics: Radiographs show sclerosis and flattening of the navicular (see Fig. 57.4C).
Treatment: Immobilization and activity modification
Prognosis and return to sport: Self-limiting condition; navicular reconstitutes over time; return to activity when symptoms resolve, often 6–8 weeks

Elbow

Osteochondritis Dissecans

Description: Osteochondral fragmentation with localized separation of subchondral bone and overlying articular cartilage (Fig. 57.5A); typically involves the capitellum of dominant hand
Mechanism of injury: Repetitive trauma and compression across the lateral elbow may damage the blood supply to the capitellum; common in adolescent throwing athletes and gymnasts
Presentation: Lateral elbow pain; possible mechanical symptoms if the fragment is unstable or loose within the joint
Physical examination: Localized tenderness over radiocapitellar articulation, possible effusion, often lack full extension; posterolateral rotatory instability test should be performed to examine potential elbow instability
Differential diagnosis: Panner disease, lateral ligament injury or tendinosis, capitellum or radial head fracture, and loose body of other etiologies (e.g., after elbow dislocation)
Diagnostics: Radiographs may show sclerotic changes, loose bodies, and focal lesions in the anterolateral capitellum with rarefaction and irregularity of articular surface; MRI and CT useful for evaluation and classification of such lesions
Treatment: Conservative management in adolescents with stable lesions; large, unstable, or loose fragments typically require surgical intervention. Options include fragment removal with chondroplasty or microfracture versus fixation with drilling and possible bone grafting. Osteochondral autograft transplantation may reduce progression to osteoarthritis and lead to better long-term results.
Prognosis and return to sport: Return to sport varies based on treatment regimen. Conservative management allows return to sport when symptoms resolve. Surgical management warrants delayed return to sport, particularly if fragment reattachment is attempted. Early range of motion and strengthening are encouraged

Panner Disease

Description: Osteochondrosis of the capitellum in young children; an avascular segment develops and subsequently revascularizes over time
Mechanism of injury: Likely lateral compression overuse injury
Presentation: Activity-related lateral elbow pain; typically young patients with OCD lesions and generally not associated with trauma
Physical examination: Localized tenderness, may lack full extension (see Fig. 57.5B)
Differential diagnosis: Capitellum OCD, stress fracture, lateral ligament injury, or tendinosis
Diagnostics: Radiographs often normal, may show fissuring and fragmentation of the capitellum on initial radiographs (see Fig. 57.5B)
Treatment: Activity modification, local modalities, and anti-inflammatory medications
Prognosis and return to sport: Self-limiting condition; return to sport when symptoms resolve

Wrist

Kienböck Disease

Description: Avascular necrosis and collapse of the lunate
Mechanism of injury: Etiology still unknown; possible causes include disruption of vascular supply, abnormal lunate morphology, and negative ulnar variance
Presentation: Chronic wrist pain, stiffness, and weak grip

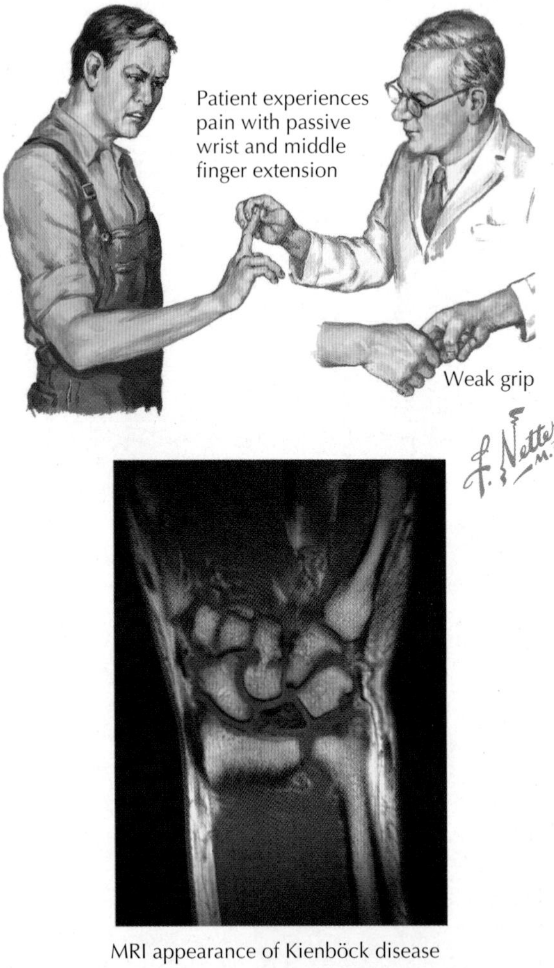
Patient experiences pain with passive wrist and middle finger extension
Weak grip
F. Netter M.D.
MRI appearance of Kienböck disease

Figure 57.6 Kienböck disease.

Physical examination: Tenderness and swelling localized over the lunate and the radiocarpal joint; pain and limited range of motion with passive flexion and extension of wrist (Fig. 57.6)

Differential diagnosis: Tendonitis, scapholunate dissociation, and ganglion cyst

Diagnostics: Radiographs may show sclerosis and collapse of the lunate in addition to ulnar negative variance. Advanced stages have associated degenerative changes. MRI may reveal diffuse signal changes over the lunate (see Fig. 57.6).

Treatment: Conservative measures as initial management, including immobilization and activity modification; if persistent or worsening symptoms, surgical options include radial shortening versus ulnar lengthening in early stages and intracarpal arthrodesis versus proximal row carpectomy in advanced cases

Prognosis and return to sport: Return to sport as symptoms allow

RECOMMENDED READINGS

Available online.

58 ACUTE FRACTURES AND DISLOCATIONS IN ATHLETES

James P. Stannard • Steven L. Martin • Dustin L. Richter

TRANSPORTATION OF AN ATHLETE WITH A FRACTURE OR DISLOCATION

- The need for and mode of transporting an injured athlete is determined after primary and secondary evaluations by the first responder. It must always be executed so that further injury is prevented.
- Planning the mode of transport and necessary equipment can help ensure that an appropriate technique is used (see Chapter 4: "Sideline Preparedness and Emergencies").
- An athlete with a suspected spinal injury should not be moved by anyone other than certified medical personnel with appropriate stabilization. An ambulance should be contacted immediately (see Chapter 46: "Neck Injuries"), if not already present.
- If a serious fracture, such as that of the tibia, femur, or pelvis, is suspected, the safest and most efficient mode of transportation for a short distance is by means of a stretcher that is taken onto a utility vehicle or preferably by an ambulance.
- Suspected extremity fractures must be immobilized before transport (Fig. 58.1).

Emergency Splint Equipment

- The ability to take care of an acute fracture in an athlete is directly related to one's level of preparedness and experience.
- Timely application of a splint to a fractured extremity minimizes the overall surrounding soft tissue injury and allows for safe transportation of the athlete for definitive care.
- Sports medicine providers (physician and trainers) should carry lightweight, easy-to-apply splint material in their sport medicine bag (see Chapter 4: "Sideline Preparedness and Emergencies").
- **Basic mobile splint kit for a medicine bag** (Table 58.1):
  - Arm sling/shoulder immobilizer (medium and large sizes)
  - Alumafoam padded splints (several lengths that can be cut to size)
  - Structural aluminum malleable (SAM) splint
  - Knee immobilizer (universal size)
  - Webril (cast padding) and Ace wraps (4 inch [10.16 cm] and 6 inch [15.24 cm])
  - Plaster or fiberglass splinting material for self-made splints (prepackaged splints are available)
- **Advanced facility kit** (available at all high-volume sports complexes or via emergency medical services [EMS]):
  - Extremity vacuum splints or air splints (total body kits)
  - Cervical collar
  - Spine board
  - Femoral (Hare) traction splint
  - Crutches

GENERAL PRINCIPLES

Overview

- Braces or orthoses stop or limit range of motion, facilitate movement, or guide a joint through an arc of motion.
- Splints are used to immobilize and position one or several joints (see Fig. 58.1).
- Splints and braces are prescribed after a fracture to protect a partially healed fracture or to prevent the pain and soft tissue damage that occur with motion.
- A cast is a stress-sharing device, allowing limited fracture motion and callus formation because of secondary bone healing. The joints above and below a fracture should be immobilized to prevent rotation and translation of the fracture fragments.

Splint Treatment

- Splints are beneficial because they provide some stabilization at the fracture site, but they may be removed for rehabilitation treatment.
- After a cast is initially removed, splints are frequently used during activity or at night to reduce pain and discomfort and allow additional fracture consolidation.
- Joint stiffness is common after cast removal and resolves after weeks to months of aggressive, but appropriate, rehabilitation.
- Immobilization of the joints above and below the fracture site often leads to stiffening and the need for a prolonged rehabilitation program.
- A cast brace can provide partial immobilization while allowing some range of motion and weight bearing on a limb.
- Once a fracture achieves an appropriate degree of stability as a result of callus formation, the cast can be replaced with a splint or brace, allowing motion of the joints proximal and distal to the fracture, without compromising the support at the fracture site.

Initial Evaluation

- Immediately after an athlete sustains a fracture or dislocation, the neurologic and vascular status must be evaluated and documented.
- Temporary immobilization measures should be employed as the patient is transported to the hospital (see Fig. 58.1).
- The mechanism of injury can provide clues regarding what type of injury has occurred.
- In all upper extremity fractures, assess the following:
  - Open or closed fracture
  - Pain, swelling, or paresthesias
  - Vascular status distal to the injury
  - Active and passive range of motion of wrist and/or digits
  - Radial, median, and/or ulnar nerve function and possible compression; axillary nerve function should also be documented with shoulder injuries
- In all lower extremity fractures, assess the following:
  - Open or closed fracture
  - Patient complaints of pain, swelling, or paresthesias
  - Vascular status distal to the injury
  - Active and passive range of motion of all metatarsophalangeal and interphalangeal joints
  - Nerve function and possible compression

UPPER EXTREMITY INJURIES

Humeral Shaft Fractures

Overview: Uncommon, accounting for approximately 1% of fractures in trauma registries (Fig. 58.2C).

Mechanism of injury: More frequently from a fall onto the involved extremity but can occur from a direct blow. On occasion, rotational injuries can also occur in some sports such as arm wrestling.

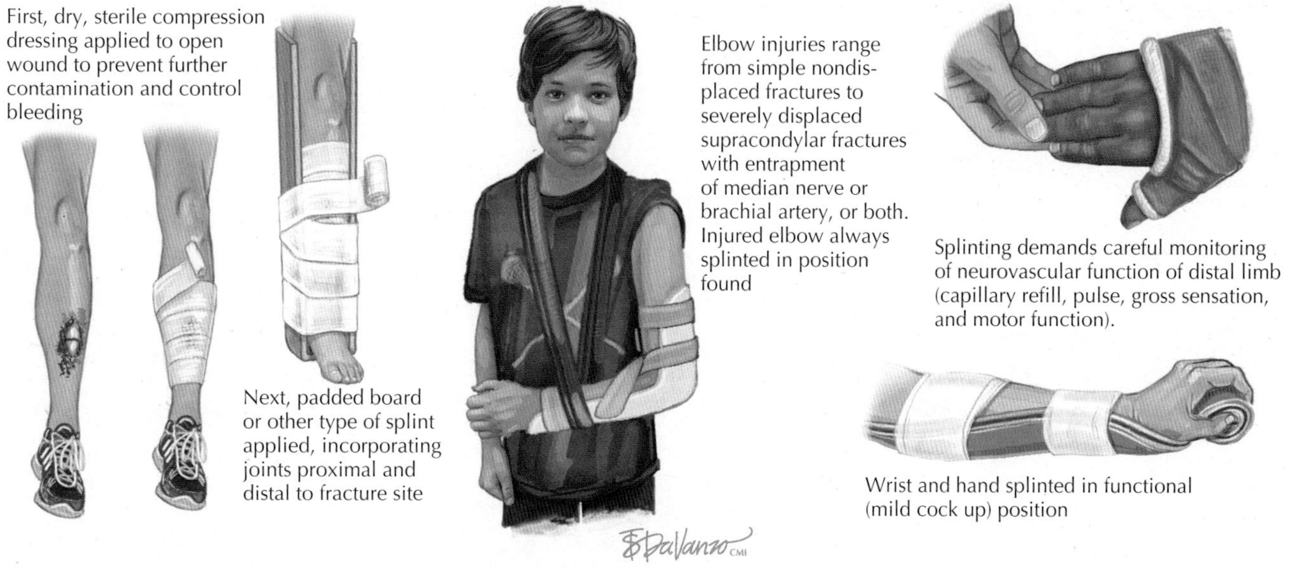
First, dry, sterile compression dressing applied to open wound to prevent further contamination and control bleeding
Next, padded board or other type of splint applied, incorporating joints proximal and distal to fracture site
Elbow injuries range from simple nondisplaced fractures to severely displaced supracondylar fractures with entrapment of median nerve or brachial artery, or both. Injured elbow always splinted in position found
Splinting demands careful monitoring of neurovascular function of distal limb (capillary refill, pulse, gross sensation, and motor function).
Wrist and hand splinted in functional (mild cock up) position

Figure 58.1 Prehospital care of fractures.

Table 58.1 SPLINTS USED PER INJURY LOCATION

Clavicle and Acromioclavicular (AC) Joint	Arm sling
Shoulder and Proximal Humerus	Arm sling and a 6-inch Ace wrap swathe
Distal Humerus and Elbow	Air or vacuum splint
Forearm and Wrist	Fiberglass/plaster splint, structural aluminum malleable (SAM) splint, prefabricated orthosis
Hand	Buddy taping, Alumafoam splint
Spine	Cervical collar and spine board
Hip and Femur	Femoral traction splint
Knee and Proximal Tibia	Knee immobilizer
Tibial Shaft, Ankle, and Foot	Air or vacuum splint

Presentation: Painful, unstable extremity with swelling and bruising.

Physical examination: Gentle palpation of the shaft of the humerus should be performed, noting any areas of malalignment and severe pain.

Associated injuries: Associated nerve injuries are relatively common and should be documented; radial nerve injuries are most common. Most common fracture type associated with a nerve injury is a transverse mid-diaphyseal fracture. Document a motor neurologic examination of the axillary, musculocutaneous, radial, median, and ulnar nerves. Skin should also be examined to rule out an open fracture. Shoulder and elbow joint should be examined and imaged.

Diagnostics: Anteroposterior (AP) and lateral radiographs of the entire humerus should be obtained. Additionally, radiographs of the shoulder and elbow should be taken.

Treatment: In most cases, nonoperative management of midshaft fractures is appropriate. Treat with functional bracing to allow active flexion and extension of the elbow during the healing process to prevent elbow stiffness; motion helps reduce the fracture and aids in the healing process. Isometric muscle exercises in the functional brace can aid in maintaining alignment and assist in fracture healing. Patients who have sustained significant nerve injuries that prevent active range of motion are not candidates for functional bracing. The humerus can heal with angulation of up to 30 degrees and shortening of 2 to 3 cm without functional problems in most patients. However, the functional needs of a high-performance athlete are different, and accepting that degree of malalignment is discouraged. If functional bracing is elected to treat an athlete, great care should be taken to follow the healing process and evaluate the alignment. If alignment is not maintained in the dominant arm of a skill athlete, consideration should be given to surgical stabilization of the fracture. Surgical treatment usually involves either plating or use of an intramedullary nail (see Fig. 58.2C). Shoulder pain is the most frequent complication after intramedullary nailing. It is important to warn an athlete of the risk of shoulder pain if intramedullary nailing is elected.

Prognosis and return to play: Prognosis for healing and good functional return after isolated humerus shaft fractures is good. Patients who have associated nerve injuries or shoulder dislocations have a less favorable prognosis, but still may be able to return to competition if the nerve injury resolves.

Distal Humerus Fractures

- Fractures that have minimal displacement and are in near anatomic alignment can be treated with casting or splinting if they are stable enough to allow early elbow motion.
- Elbow stiffness and permanent motion loss are significant risks after elbow trauma.
- Cast or splint treatment of these injuries should initially allow no motion at the elbow.
- Most distal humerus fractures require surgical stabilization, followed by early functional motion of the elbow.

Olecranon Fractures

- Minimally displaced fractures of the olecranon with <2 mm displacement and intact elbow extensor mechanism can be treated with cast or splint immobilization.
- Early elbow motion is necessary for good functional results.
- The cast should be adequately padded to avoid skin breakdown at the edges of the cast or splint.
- The cast should volarly extend to the proximal palmar crease and dorsally to the metacarpophalangeal joints to allow full motion at the interphalangeal and metacarpophalangeal joints.

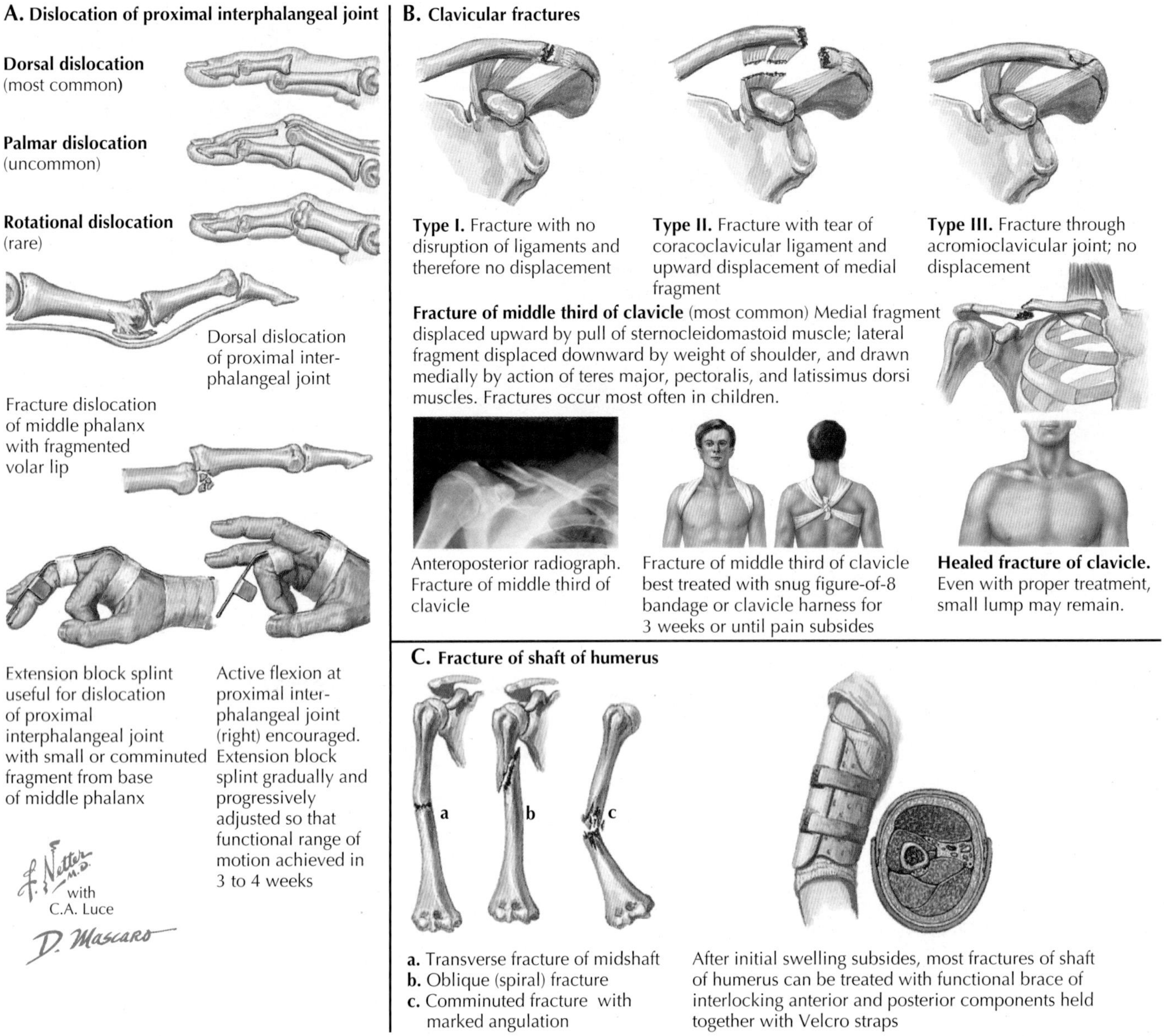
A. Dislocation of proximal interphalangeal joint
Dorsal dislocation (most common)
Palmar dislocation (uncommon)
Rotational dislocation (rare)
Dorsal dislocation of proximal interphalangeal joint
Fracture dislocation of middle phalanx with fragmented volar lip
Extension block splint useful for dislocation of proximal interphalangeal joint with small or comminuted fragment from base of middle phalanx
Active flexion at proximal interphalangeal joint (right) encouraged. Extension block splint gradually and progressively adjusted so that functional range of motion achieved in 3 to 4 weeks
F. Netter M.D.
with C.A. Luce
D. Mascaro
B. Clavicular fractures
Type I. Fracture with no disruption of ligaments and therefore no displacement
Type II. Fracture with tear of coracoclavicular ligament and upward displacement of medial fragment
Type III. Fracture through acromioclavicular joint; no displacement
Fracture of middle third of clavicle (most common) Medial fragment displaced upward by pull of sternocleidomastoid muscle; lateral fragment displaced downward by weight of shoulder, and drawn medially by action of teres major, pectoralis, and latissimus dorsi muscles. Fractures occur most often in children.
Anteroposterior radiograph. Fracture of middle third of clavicle
Fracture of middle third of clavicle best treated with snug figure-of-8 bandage or clavicle harness for 3 weeks or until pain subsides
Healed fracture of clavicle. Even with proper treatment, small lump may remain.
C. Fracture of shaft of humerus
a
b
c
a. Transverse fracture of midshaft
b. Oblique (spiral) fracture
c. Comminuted fracture with marked angulation
After initial swelling subsides, most fractures of shaft of humerus can be treated with functional brace of interlocking anterior and posterior components held together with Velcro straps

Figure 58.2 Upper extremity fractures and dislocations (proximal interphalangeal, clavicle, and humeral shaft).

- Once there is early evidence of healing, the elbow should be mobilized to prevent stiffness.
- An elbow-hinged brace can protect the fracture and maintain motion of the elbow. Often, some terminal extension is lost, but functional range of motion is maintained.
- Aggressive rehabilitation is critical, as the loss of some terminal extension may have implications on athletic performance even if it does not affect activities of daily living.
- Displaced fractures of the olecranon require open reduction and internal fixation (ORIF), followed by early elbow range of motion to minimize the development of elbow stiffness.

Radial Head Fractures

- Minimally displaced fractures can be treated in a sling with early elbow range of motion.
- For fractures requiring ORIF, short-term immobilization is needed, followed by early bracing mobilization.
- A hinged elbow brace is typically used to allow protection of the fixation during initiation of early range of motion.
- Most severe fractures have better outcomes with radial head replacement than with ORIF, even in young patients, although only about 50% of patients return to sport.

Distal Radius Fractures

- Minimally displaced fractures can be treated with a long-arm or Münster cast, followed by a short-arm cast.
- Rigid immobilization for 4–6 weeks, followed by a removable splint, is recommended.
- Displaced fractures require reduction before splinting and should be immobilized in a long-arm splint.
- The cast should be volarly trimmed to the proximal palmar crease and distally to the metacarpophalangeal prominences to allow free finger movement and full thumb opposition with the small finger.
- Distal radius fractures requiring ORIF require long-arm splints in the immediate postoperative period, followed by short-arm casting or removable gauntlet splint depending on the pattern of injury.

Scaphoid Fractures

- Most scaphoid fractures (including minimally displaced) are treated surgically with ORIF to allow expedited return to play in competitive athletes.
- Return-to-play decisions must be individualized and vary depending on fracture morphology, displacement, and type of sport for the returning athlete. Athletes that can wear a protective splint may be allowed to return almost immediately if the fracture has minimal displacement.
- As for unprotected play, one article notes that 24% returned within 4–6 weeks, 49% at 6–12 weeks, and 27% at greater than 12 weeks.
- Computed tomography (CT) scan may be used to follow healing and assist with return-to-play decisions.

Metacarpal and Phalangeal Fractures

- Dislocations of the proximal interphalangeal (PIP) joint should be immobilized using static dorsal extension splinting (see Fig. 58.2A).
- It is important to secure the proximal phalanx to the splint to ensure that the PIP joint does not extend when a patient flexes the metacarpal phalangeal (MCP) joint.
- Metacarpal neck and shaft fractures are best treated with a cast or splint.
- The splint is applied with the hand in "safe" position with the wrist in extension, the MCP joints flexed, and the proximal and distal interphalangeal joints in extension. Displaced fractures require reduction before splinting.
- Phalanx fractures that are minimally displaced can be treated with "buddy taping," wherein the fractured finger is taped to an adjacent finger. The adjacent finger functions as a splint but allows continued range of motion. Displaced fractures require reduction before splinting.

Clavicle Fractures

Description: The most common fracture, accounting for approximately 10% of all athlete fractures; 30% of all clavicle fractures occur during sports participation; 85% involve the middle third of the clavicle (see Fig. 58.2B)

Mechanism of injury: Most result from a fall onto the ipsilateral shoulder.

Initial on-field management: The fracture displacement and pain level are significant, and clinical diagnosis can be made on the field; the athlete should be assisted off the field with the arm held at his or her side. Initial management with a sling, with or without a swathe, is sufficient. A 6-inch (15.24-cm) Ace wrap can be used for a swathe and improves comfort by supporting the elbow and immobilizing the arm to the body.

Evaluation:

- **Inspection:** Look for obvious deformity and inspect for skin breakdown or tenting.
- **Palpation:** Check for neck, sternoclavicular joint, midclavicle, acromioclavicular joint, scapula, and proximal humerus tenderness.
- **Neurovascular examination:** Evaluate the upper extremity, including the axillary nerve (motor as sensation is not always reliable).

Radiographs: An AP and an AP with a cephalic tilt of 20 degrees are sufficient.

Treatment: Treatment for many closed clavicle fractures is nonoperative with application of an arm sling. Indications for operative treatment include skin compromise secondary to severe displacement, open fractures, shortening, and overlap greater than 2 cm in an active individual and a floating shoulder with neurovascular compromise. Displaced clavicle fractures are frequently managed with ORIF in athletes and active individuals. Operative management of displaced midshaft fractures offers improved return rates and times to sport compared with nonoperative management. The method of fracture stabilization is generally with a contoured plate, although intramedullary devices may also be used. Suture fixation and non-acromioclavicular (AC) joint spanning plates show promise with lateral clavicle fractures. Problems with conservative care include a higher incidence of nonunion and malunion.

Prognosis and return to sport: Several recent reports suggest a faster return to sport with surgical intervention than with conservative care. One report with intramedullary fixation reported a return to training in 6 days and a return to competition in 17 days with 12 high-performance athletes. Prognosis for athletes is very good after clavicle fractures.

Forearm Fractures

Description: Forearm injuries represent approximately 5% of all fractures and include isolated ulnar fractures and fractures of both the radius and ulna. Monteggia and Galeazzi fractures involve the proximal and distal radioulnar joints, respectively (Fig. 58.3A–C). Monteggia fractures involve fracture of the ulna with dislocation of the radial head. Galeazzi fractures involve fracture of the radius shaft (usually at the level of the junction of the middle and distal third) with injury to the distal radioulnar joint.

Mechanism of injury: Isolated ulnar fractures are seen in contact sports athletes resulting from a direct blow to the arm (see Fig. 58.3D). Moreover, fractures of both radius and ulna are seen in contact athletes, which may be open or closed.

Initial on-field management: The injured extremity should be stabilized with a splint, and the athlete must be taken off the field for further evaluation.

Evaluation:

- **Inspection:** Determine if the fracture is open or closed.
- **Palpation:** Assess both the elbow and wrist of the injured forearm to be sure there is no damage to either the proximal or distal radioulnar joint.
- **Neurovascular examination:** Check vascular status of the arm (pulses, capillary refill) distal to the site of the injury. Radial, ulnar, and median sensation should be assessed.

Radiographs: Include two views of the forearm and must always include adequate views of both the elbow and wrist.

Treatment: In skeletally mature athletes, surgical treatment is recommended to restore anatomic alignment in **displaced radial and ulnar shaft fractures.** The musculature of the proximal forearm makes maintenance of closed reduction difficult. For **nondisplaced fractures of the ulna,** management of injury is symptomatic and includes prohibition of sporting activities until clinical and radiographic evidence of fracture union is obtained; bracing or casting is used. Serial radiographs are recorded to ensure no further displacement and to monitor eventual healing. **Displaced fractures** may require surgical fixation. Isolated ulnar fractures are at risk for delayed or nonunion.

Return to sport: In general, a minimum of 4–6 weeks

Forearm Compartment Syndrome

Description: An increase in pressure in a muscle compartment leading to damage to the structures within the compartment, including muscles and nerves

Mechanism of injury: Typically the result of high-energy impact (either forceful or crushing) to the forearm and occurs more frequently in the volar compartment; in athletes with forearm injuries, a tense swelling and an out-of-proportion pain may suggest compartment syndrome. Excessive pain, particularly

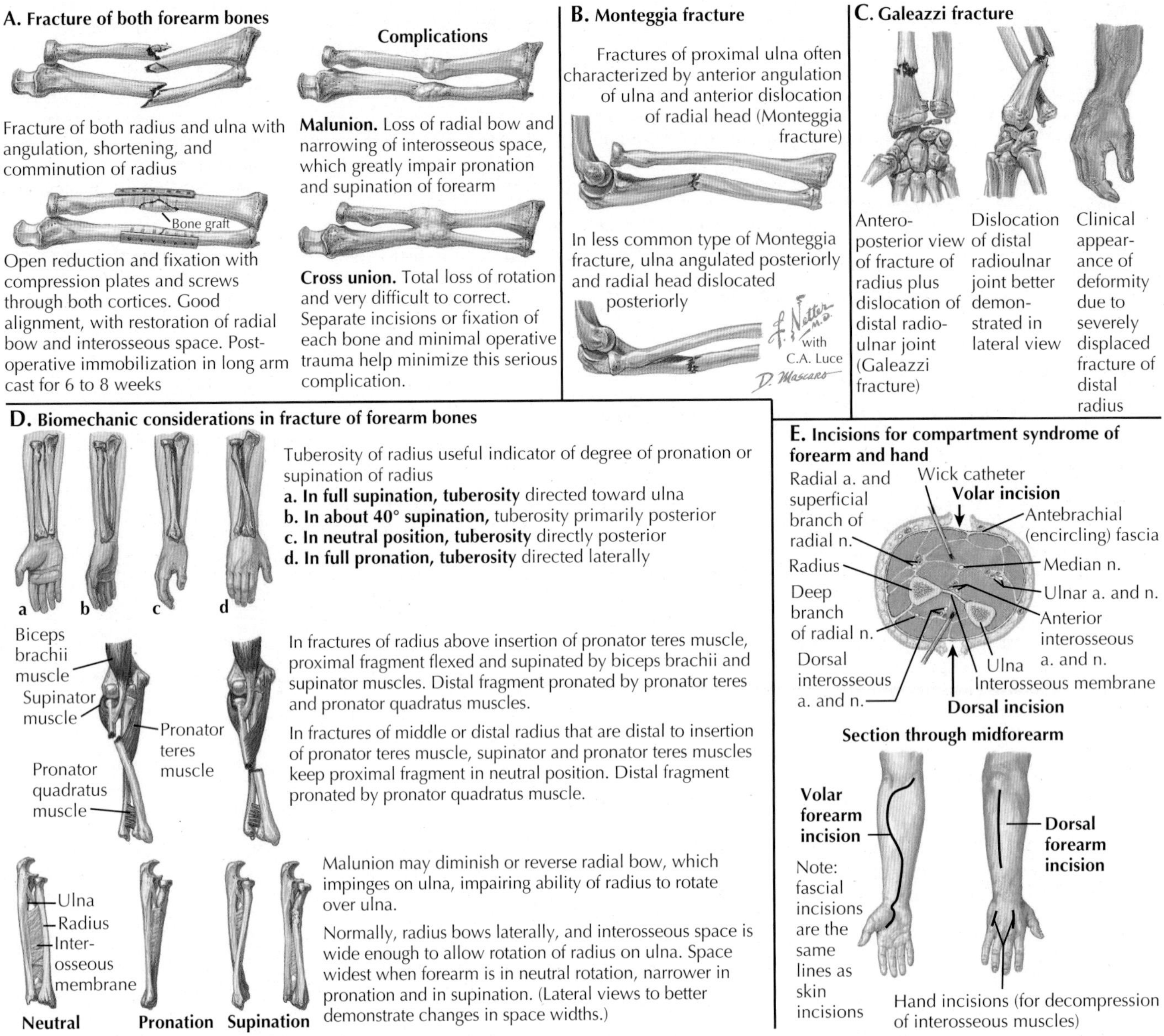
A. Fracture of both forearm bones
Fracture of both radius and ulna with angulation, shortening, and comminution of radius
Bone graft
Open reduction and fixation with compression plates and screws through both cortices. Good alignment, with restoration of radial bow and interosseous space. Post-operative immobilization in long arm cast for 6 to 8 weeks
Complications
Malunion. Loss of radial bow and narrowing of interosseous space, which greatly impair pronation and supination of forearm
Cross union. Total loss of rotation and very difficult to correct. Separate incisions or fixation of each bone and minimal operative trauma help minimize this serious complication.
B. Monteggia fracture
Fractures of proximal ulna often characterized by anterior angulation of ulna and anterior dislocation of radial head (Monteggia fracture)
In less common type of Monteggia fracture, ulna angulated posteriorly and radial head dislocated posteriorly
with C.A. Luce
C. Galeazzi fracture
Antero-posterior view of fracture of radius plus dislocation of distal radio-ulnar joint (Galeazzi fracture)
Dislocation of distal radioulnar joint better demon-strated in lateral view
Clinical appear-ance of deformity due to severely displaced fracture of distal radius
D. Biomechanic considerations in fracture of forearm bones
Tuberosity of radius useful indicator of degree of pronation or supination of radius
a. In full supination, tuberosity directed toward ulna
b. In about 40° supination, tuberosity primarily posterior
c. In neutral position, tuberosity directly posterior
d. In full pronation, tuberosity directed laterally
a
b
c
d
Biceps brachii muscle
Supinator muscle
Pronator teres muscle
Pronator quadratus muscle
In fractures of radius above insertion of pronator teres muscle, proximal fragment flexed and supinated by biceps brachii and supinator muscles. Distal fragment pronated by pronator teres and pronator quadratus muscles.
In fractures of middle or distal radius that are distal to insertion of pronator teres muscle, supinator and pronator teres muscles keep proximal fragment in neutral position. Distal fragment pronated by pronator quadratus muscle.
Ulna
Radius
Inter-osseous membrane
Neutral
Pronation
Supination
Malunion may diminish or reverse radial bow, which impinges on ulna, impairing ability of radius to rotate over ulna.
Normally, radius bows laterally, and interosseous space is wide enough to allow rotation of radius on ulna. Space widest when forearm is in neutral rotation, narrower in pronation and in supination. (Lateral views to better demonstrate changes in space widths.)
E. Incisions for compartment syndrome of forearm and hand
Radial a. and superficial branch of radial n.
Wick catheter
Volar incision
Antebrachial (encircling) fascia
Radius
Median n.
Deep branch of radial n.
Ulnar a. and n.
Anterior interosseous a. and n.
Dorsal interosseous a. and n.
Ulna
Interosseous membrane
Dorsal incision
Section through midforearm
Volar forearm incision
Dorsal forearm incision
Note: fascial incisions are the same lines as skin incisions
Hand incisions (for decompression of interosseous muscles)

Figure 58.3 Upper extremity fractures and dislocations (forearm and compartment syndrome).

with passive stretch of the digits, may be the first clue to an early compartment syndrome and cannot be ignored in athletes. A higher muscular volume may put the athlete at an increased risk of compartment syndrome.

Evaluation:

- **Inspection:** The forearm should be evaluated for swelling accompanied by severe pain.
- **Palpation:** Assess the compartment compressibility by gently pressing against the forearm compartments and comparing it to the contralateral side. Tense, noncompressible compartments or severe pain with passive motion of the fingers out of proportion to the injury should increase suspicion for compartment syndrome.
- **Neurovascular examination:** Check vascular status of the arm (pulses, capillary refill) distal to the site of the injury. Radial, ulnar, and median nerve sensation should be assessed.

Radiographs: Two views of the forearm should be obtained to ensure that there is no fracture.

Treatment: If compartment syndrome is diagnosed, emergent fasciotomies should be performed (see Fig. 58.3E).

LOWER EXTREMITY INJURIES

Tibial Plafond Fractures

- A long leg cast is only suitable for fractures with minimal displacement and no damage to the articular joint surface.
- Comminuted fractures usually have soft tissue damage that requires delayed surgery, which requires spanning external fixation before surgical fixation to allow soft tissue recovery and avoid complications.

Foot Fractures

- Fractures involving the forefoot, midfoot, or hindfoot can be immobilized using a short leg splint until swelling subsides.

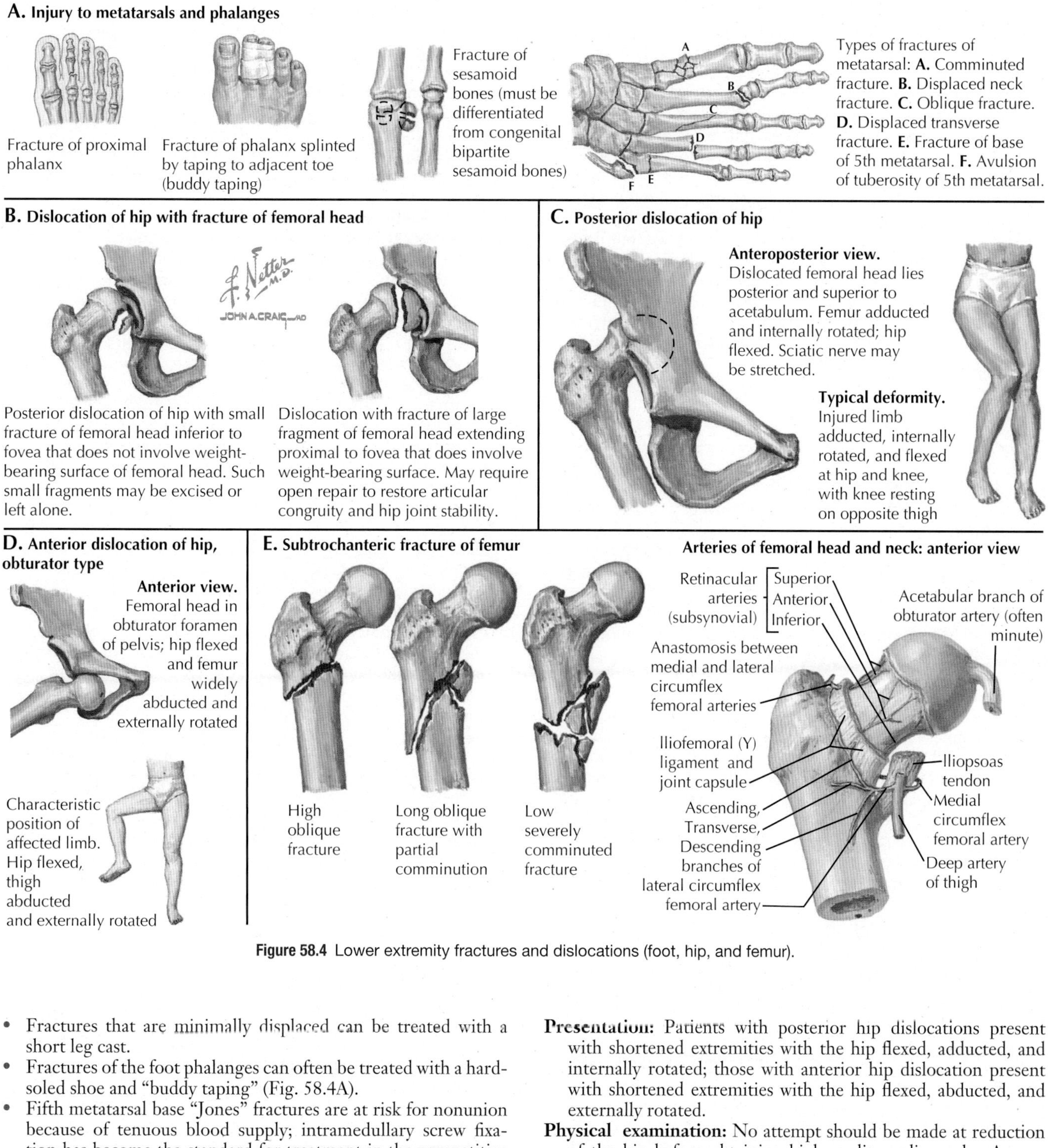
A. Injury to metatarsals and phalanges
Fracture of proximal phalanx
Fracture of phalanx splinted by taping to adjacent toe (buddy taping)
Fracture of sesamoid bones (must be differentiated from congenital bipartite sesamoid bones)
A
B
C
D
E
F
Types of fractures of metatarsal: A. Comminuted fracture. B. Displaced neck fracture. C. Oblique fracture. D. Displaced transverse fracture. E. Fracture of base of 5th metatarsal. F. Avulsion of tuberosity of 5th metatarsal.
B. Dislocation of hip with fracture of femoral head
Posterior dislocation of hip with small fracture of femoral head inferior to fovea that does not involve weight-bearing surface of femoral head. Such small fragments may be excised or left alone.
Dislocation with fracture of large fragment of femoral head extending proximal to fovea that does involve weight-bearing surface. May require open repair to restore articular congruity and hip joint stability.
C. Posterior dislocation of hip
Anteroposterior view.
Dislocated femoral head lies posterior and superior to acetabulum. Femur adducted and internally rotated; hip flexed. Sciatic nerve may be stretched.
Typical deformity.
Injured limb adducted, internally rotated, and flexed at hip and knee, with knee resting on opposite thigh
D. Anterior dislocation of hip, obturator type
Anterior view.
Femoral head in obturator foramen of pelvis; hip flexed and femur widely abducted and externally rotated
Characteristic position of affected limb. Hip flexed, thigh abducted and externally rotated
E. Subtrochanteric fracture of femur
High oblique fracture
Long oblique fracture with partial comminution
Low severely comminuted fracture
Arteries of femoral head and neck: anterior view
Retinacular arteries (subsynovial)
Superior
Anterior
Inferior
Acetabular branch of obturator artery (often minute)
Anastomosis between medial and lateral circumflex femoral arteries
Iliofemoral (Y) ligament and joint capsule
Iliopsoas tendon
Medial circumflex femoral artery
Ascending, Transverse, Descending branches of lateral circumflex femoral artery
Deep artery of thigh

Figure 58.4 Lower extremity fractures and dislocations (foot, hip, and femur).

- Fractures that are minimally displaced can be treated with a short leg cast.
- Fractures of the foot phalanges can often be treated with a hard-soled shoe and "buddy taping" (Fig. 58.4A).
- Fifth metatarsal base "Jones" fractures are at risk for nonunion because of tenuous blood supply; intramedullary screw fixation has become the standard for treatment in the competitive athlete.

Hip Fractures and Dislocations

Description: Intertrochanteric hip fractures and femoral neck fractures are rare in athletes; hip dislocation and femoral head fractures are more common injuries among athletes and younger individuals (see Fig. 58.4B–D). Fracture dislocation of the hip in a young, athletic patient should be viewed as a surgical emergency and a career-threatening injury. There is a correlation between the duration for which a hip remains dislocated and the development of osteonecrosis of the femoral head.

Presentation: Patients with posterior hip dislocations present with shortened extremities with the hip flexed, adducted, and internally rotated; those with anterior hip dislocation present with shortened extremities with the hip flexed, abducted, and externally rotated.

Physical examination: No attempt should be made at reduction of the hip before obtaining high-quality radiographs. A neurologic examination should be documented before attempting reduction.

Diagnostics: Radiographs are key and should be obtained before attempting reduction to prevent severe displacement of associated minimally displaced fractures. AP and lateral views of the hip joint, as well as Judet views (45-degree oblique views) of the acetabulum, must be recorded.

Treatment: After obtaining radiographs and ruling out an associated fracture, closed reduction of the hip can be attempted under conscious sedation. It is important to have complete relaxation of the hip muscles before attempting reduction. If the patient has an associated femoral neck fracture, he or she should be taken to the operating room expeditiously, although quality of reduction has been shown to be more critical than a short delay in fracture fixation. If there is an associated acetabulum fracture, it is reasonable to attempt a closed reduction if there are no large bone fragments in the joint that may block reduction. An attempt at a closed reduction should be made by an experienced physician. If that fails, the patient should be taken to the operating room for a reduction under general anesthesia. The most common method to achieve closed reduction of a posterior hip dislocation is the Bigelow maneuver.

Prognosis and return to sport: Long-term results after hip dislocations are poor, even if reduction is prompt and appropriate. Athletes who sustain a hip dislocation with or without fracture should be counseled that they may have sustained a career-ending injury. An initial period of protected weight bearing is advised. Close follow-up with magnetic resonance imaging (MRI) after dislocation may be used to evaluate for development of avascular necrosis (AVN), as well as soft tissue (labrum or capsule) injury and healing.

Femur Fractures

Description: Uncommon sports injury; requires high-energy trauma

Associated injuries: Carefully assess athletes for other injuries. Femur fractures can be associated with substantial blood loss. Common systemic injuries include head, chest, and abdominal injuries. The most important associated skeletal injury is a fracture of the femoral neck. It is critical to diagnose such injuries and avoid any additional displacement of the neck fracture; a displaced femoral neck fracture puts the blood supply to the femoral head at risk and may lead to AVN of the femoral head (see Fig. 58.4E).

Presentation: Severe pain and inability to bear any weight on the involved leg

Physical examination: Displaced femur fractures present with malalignment of the limb and severe pain. Document the neurologic and vascular status of the leg. Minimize movement of the injured extremity until radiographs can be obtained. Evaluate for skin lacerations, which can indicate an open fracture, and assess for compartment syndrome. Development of compartment syndrome represents a surgical emergency and should raise concern for vascular injury.

Diagnostics: Plain radiographs; AP and lateral views are generally adequate to characterize the injury. Imaging should include views of the femoral neck. Internal rotation radiograph of the femoral neck can be performed, or thin-cut CT or rapid limited-sequence MRI may be used to detect nondisplaced fractures. If the patient has an asymmetric pulse, emergent arteriogram or CT angiogram should be obtained.

Treatment: Initial treatment should concentrate on stabilization of the extremity (see Fig. 58.4E). Gentle longitudinal traction should be applied, and subsequently, a splint should be applied. A Hare traction splint or skeletal traction pin can help provide pain relief. Definitive treatment of femur fractures requires surgical stabilization. Intramedullary nails are the more commonly used implants.

Prognosis and return to sport: Long-term prognosis is good. Athletic activities should be deferred for 4–6 months. Abductor muscle weakness and dysfunction after antegrade intramedullary nailing is common. Knee pain is common after retrograde femoral nailing. Loss of muscular strength is common and may take ≥1 year to completely recover. Physical therapy should concentrate on rehabilitation of muscles around the hip, particularly the abductors.

Knee Dislocation

Description: Occurs when the tibia is no longer in contact with the femur; associated with ligament, nerve, and vascular injury (Fig. 58.5A); seen in contact sports such as football. Increasing incidence is being recognized with both high-energy mechanisms such as motor vehicle collisions and athletic injuries. Most dislocations spontaneously reduce and require careful evaluation to avoid missing the diagnosis.

Mechanism of injury: Result of a large force applied across the knee joint; knee joint is disrupted with dislocation of the tibiofemoral articulation with associated multiligament injury. Typical mechanism is hyperextension with the foot fixed in place.

Initial on-field management and evaluation:

- Gross deformity may be apparent, but it may look relatively normal if the dislocation has spontaneously reduced.
- **Palpation:** The knee joint, leg, and thigh should be palpated to assess for possible fracture or associated soft tissue injury.
- **Neurovascular examination:** The dorsalis pedis and posterior tibial pulse should be manually palpated and compared with the contralateral side. Careful sensory and motor examination should be performed and documented, with particular attention to peroneal nerve function. Ankle–brachial index (ABI) may also be documented and should be 0.9 or greater.
- **Ligament examination:** Careful knee ligament examination should be performed to assess any cruciate and collateral ligament injury.

Radiographs: Three views of the knee should be obtained to assess for fracture. The most common associated fracture is a tibial plateau fracture. Two views each of the femur and the tibia should also be obtained to check for associated injuries. MRI is recommended to confirm ligament injury and to assess the extent of the injury.

Treatment: Requires reduction of dislocation followed by assessment of vascular status (see Fig. 58.5A). Pulses of the involved extremity should be palpated and ABIs performed. Any discrepancy in pulse or ABIs should prompt immediate evaluation for vascular injury by means of diagnostic studies such CT or MR angiography. Neurologic evaluation should be performed to assess tibial and peroneal nerve function. If knee dislocation is suspected, the athlete should be immediately transferred to a medical facility for evaluation by an orthopedic and vascular surgeon. Vascular injury requires immediate intervention by the vascular surgery team. Multiple ligament injuries in knee dislocations will require surgical reconstruction. Rehabilitation after a knee dislocation is intensive and prolonged (see Fig. 58.5A).

Tibial Shaft Fractures

Description: Generally low- to medium-energy fractures in athletics; despite the lower energy mechanism, a tibial fracture can be a devastating and career-ending injury for an athlete. Early stabilization with a well-supervised rehabilitation program is critical for favorable outcomes (see Fig. 58.5B).

Mechanism of injury: Noncontact rotational injuries occurring in sports such as downhill skiing to direct blow-type injuries occurring in contact sports such as football or soccer

Initial management: Deformity, instability, and pain confirm the diagnosis. Immediate splinting before transportation is advisable; air or vacuum splints facilitate splinting and transportation. In general, splint the extremity as it lies. Gentle traction while the splint is applied limits the magnitude of deformity and limits ongoing soft tissue injury.

Evaluation:

- **Inspection:** Examine angulation and rotational malalignment, skin integrity, and the magnitude of initial soft tissue injury.
- **Palpation:** Check for other extremity injuries and compartment syndrome. Evaluate for pain with passive stretch of the great toe.
- **Neurovascular examination:** Document the neurovascular status on the field before transportation and before and after splint application.

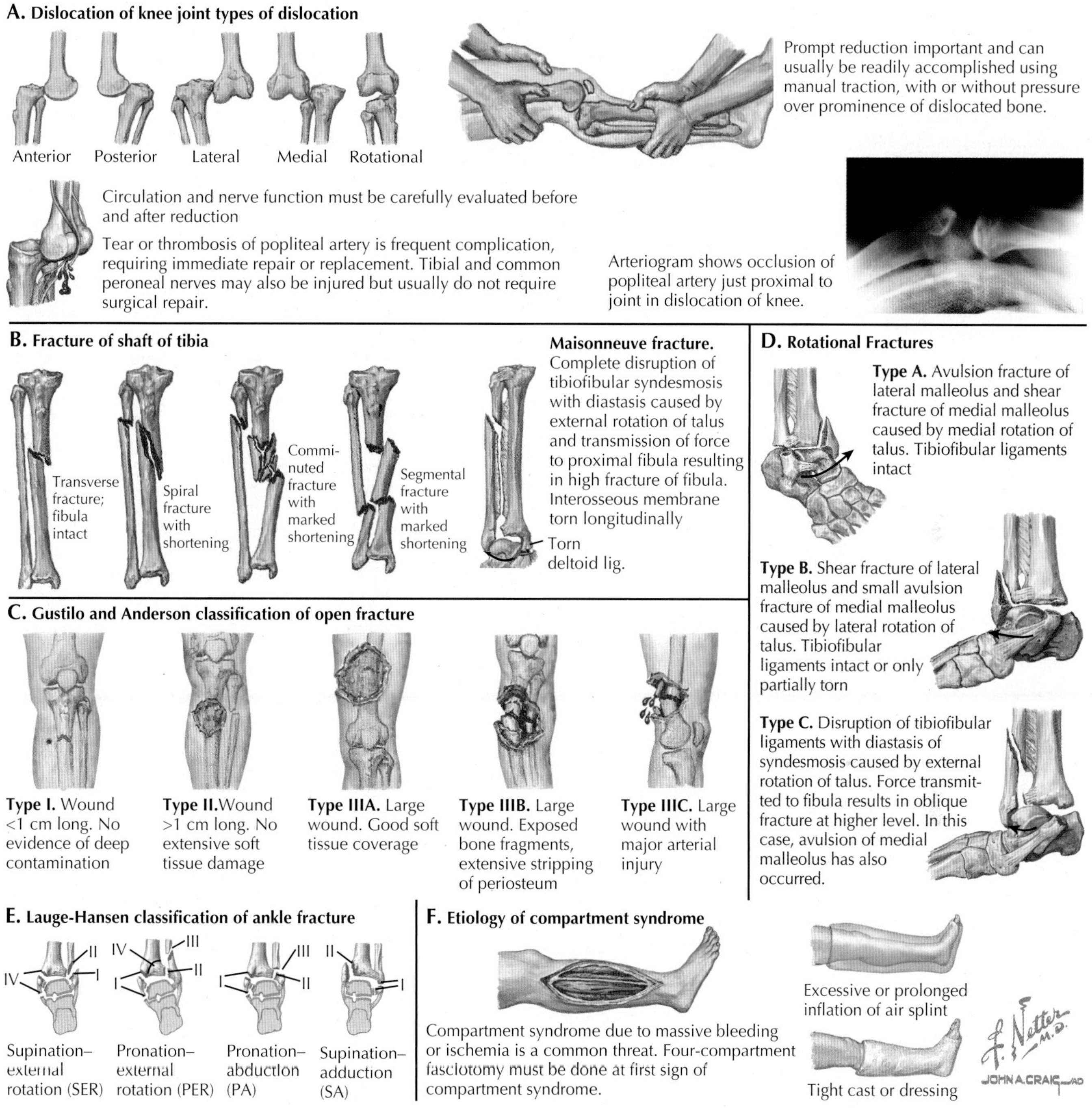

A. Dislocation of knee joint types of dislocation
Anterior
Posterior
Lateral
Medial
Rotational
Prompt reduction important and can usually be readily accomplished using manual traction, with or without pressure over prominence of dislocated bone.
Circulation and nerve function must be carefully evaluated before and after reduction
Tear or thrombosis of popliteal artery is frequent complication, requiring immediate repair or replacement. Tibial and common peroneal nerves may also be injured but usually do not require surgical repair.
Arteriogram shows occlusion of popliteal artery just proximal to joint in dislocation of knee.
B. Fracture of shaft of tibia
Transverse fracture; fibula intact
Spiral fracture with shortening
Comminuted fracture with marked shortening
Segmental fracture with marked shortening
Maisonneuve fracture. Complete disruption of tibiofibular syndesmosis with diastasis caused by external rotation of talus and transmission of force to proximal fibula resulting in high fracture of fibula. Interosseous membrane torn longitudinally
Torn deltoid lig.
C. Gustilo and Anderson classification of open fracture
Type I. Wound <1 cm long. No evidence of deep contamination
Type II. Wound >1 cm long. No extensive soft tissue damage
Type IIIA. Large wound. Good soft tissue coverage
Type IIIB. Large wound. Exposed bone fragments, extensive stripping of periosteum
Type IIIC. Large wound with major arterial injury
D. Rotational Fractures
Type A. Avulsion fracture of lateral malleolus and shear fracture of medial malleolus caused by medial rotation of talus. Tibiofibular ligaments intact
Type B. Shear fracture of lateral malleolus and small avulsion fracture of medial malleolus caused by lateral rotation of talus. Tibiofibular ligaments intact or only partially torn
Type C. Disruption of tibiofibular ligaments with diastasis of syndesmosis caused by external rotation of talus. Force transmitted to fibula results in oblique fracture at higher level. In this case, avulsion of medial malleolus has also occurred.
E. Lauge-Hansen classification of ankle fracture
Supination–external rotation (SER)
Pronation–external rotation (PER)
Pronation–abduction (PA)
Supination–adduction (SA)
F. Etiology of compartment syndrome
Compartment syndrome due to massive bleeding or ischemia is a common threat. Four-compartment fasciotomy must be done at first sign of compartment syndrome.
Excessive or prolonged inflation of air splint
Tight cast or dressing
F. Netter M.D.
JOHN A.CRAIG—AD

Figure 58.5 Lower extremity fractures and dislocations (knee, tibia, ankle, and compartment syndrome).

Radiographs: AP and lateral radiographs of the entire tibia are required. Radiographs of the joint above and below are mandatory with all long-bone injuries.

Classification:

- **Tscherne classification**
  - **Grade 0:** Minimal soft tissue damage
  - **Grade 1:** Abrasion/contusion of skin with moderate swelling
  - **Grade 2:** Deep abrasion/contusion with significant swelling and potential for compartment syndrome
  - **Grade 3:** Severe swelling, shearing injury, or compartment syndrome
- **Gustilo classification of open fractures:** An open wound over the fracture remarkably increases the likelihood of an infection; the more severe the open wound, the greater the likelihood of infection (see Fig. 58.5C).
  - **Type I:** Open wound <1 cm
  - **Type II:** Larger open wounds (1–10 cm) with slight contamination
  - **Type III:** Severe soft tissue damage
    - **A:** Can be closed primarily
    - **B:** Severe soft tissue wound with one or all the following: severe contamination, significant periosteal stripping, flap coverage, or wound vacuum-assisted closure (VAC) device required
    - **C:** Vascular repair or reconstruction required

Treatment: **Closed stable fractures** can be treated with casting and functional bracing. However, athletic individuals frequently benefit from surgical stabilization that allows early functional rehabilitation. Locked intramedullary nailing is the treatment of choice for most closed **unstable diaphyseal tibial fractures.** Open reduction with plate osteosynthesis is used in cases in which the fracture extends too close to the adjacent joint for adequate intramedullary nailing. **Open fractures** are treated with appropriate antibiotic coverage and aggressive soft tissue management with debridement and irrigation and early closure or coverage. The success of treatment is related more to the adequacy of the soft tissue management than it is with the fracture fixation method. External fixation is reserved for **high-energy, severe open grades** of tibial shaft fracture where the extent of the soft tissue zone of injury demarcation is poorly defined during initial debridement.

Ankle Fractures

Description: Ankle injuries are among the most common injuries treated by the sports medicine physician (see Fig. 58.5D).

Mechanism of injury: Most ankle injuries involve a planted fixed foot with a rotational force applied to the leg. The position of the foot and the magnitude and direction of the force determine the pattern of injury. How quickly the foot can disengage from the turf often determines whether an ankle sprain or an ankle fracture occurs.

On-field management: Unstable ankle injuries and those associated with obvious deformity should be splinted on the field before transportation. With a stable ankle injury, the athlete can be assisted to the sidelines where further treatment can be administered. Initial management includes neurovascular evaluation, splint application, extremity elevation, and ice therapy.

Evaluation:

- **Inspection:** Look for deformities, including foot alignment. Note areas of swelling, including the syndesmotic region and foot. Document any areas of skin contusion, abrasion, or disruption.
- **Palpation:** Start by checking for associated injury to the knee or proximal fibula. Palpate the medial side, lateral side, syndesmosis, hindfoot, and midfoot. Localize all areas of direct tenderness and try to differentiate ligamentous areas versus bone.
- **Stability:**
  - **Squeeze test:** Squeeze the midleg, compressing the tibia and fibula together, looking for syndesmotic pain.
  - **External rotation stress test:** In the absence of any obvious deformity, a lightly applied external rotation force to the foot can help identify a fracture. Stability and the absence of pain on external rotation rule out most unstable ankle fractures.
  - **Drawer test:** Stabilize the tibia with one hand and pull the foot forward. Look for excessive anterior translation of the talus out of the mortise and compare with the uninjured ankle.
- **Neurovascular examination:** Document the presence or absence of pedal pulses, capillary refill, and color of the toes. Check all sensory dermatomes of the foot and ankle.

Radiographs: Key examination findings that indicate a need for radiographs in the absence of deformity include pain at the malleoli, tenderness at the tip or posterior edge of the malleolus, severe swelling, and inability to bear weight. **Initial radiographs** should include an AP, a mortise (AP with the leg 15 degrees internally rotated), and a lateral radiograph. CT scans and MRIs are occasionally required for occult fractures and to rule out osteochondral lesions of the talus. Typically seen in patients with a large ankle joint effusion.

Classification:

- The **Weber/AO system** depends on the level of the fibular fracture.
  - Type A: Fibular fracture is below the level of the plafond.
  - Type B: Fibular fracture is at the level of the plafond.
  - Type C: Fibular fracture is above the level of the plafond and is generally associated with an injury to the syndesmotic ligament.
- **Lauge–Hansen classification** is based on the position of the foot and the direction of the deforming force (see Fig. 58.5E).
- **Anatomic classification** is based on the number of malleoli fractured and the level and pattern of fracture: isolated lateral malleolus, bimalleolar, and trimalleolar.
- **Syndesmotic ligament injury:** Examination findings suggestive of injury include tenderness over the anterior aspect of the syndesmosis and a positive squeeze or external rotation test. Radiographic findings include an increase in the medial clear space (distance between the lateral wall of the medial malleolus and medial wall of the talus) of >4 mm and the distal tibiofibular space (distance between the posterior border of the tibia and the inner border of the fibula) of >6 mm. However, injury may not be radiographically apparent; thus, routine external rotation stress radiographic testing is necessary to detect any instability.
- **Maisonneuve fracture:** Fracture of the proximal fibula associated with a rotational injury to the ankle; this is often overlooked. Patients often do not complain of pain in the region of the proximal fibula when more painful distal injuries are present; more likely when deltoid ligament is ruptured or the medial malleolus is fractured without a fracture of the lateral malleolus. Full-length AP and lateral radiographs of the tibia and fibula should be obtained in such cases.

Treatment:

- **Isolated lateral malleolus fracture:** Nonsurgical treatment of isolated distal fibular fractures without an injury to the medial side (supination-external rotation type II) is successful in most cases. The fracture can be treated with casting or an ankle orthosis with early weight bearing and early ankle range of motion.
- **Bimalleolar and trimalleolar fractures:** Displaced bimalleolar and trimalleolar fractures are best treated with ORIF to re-establish the integrity of the ankle mortise and joint congruity. Fixation of the posterior malleolus is indicated with an articular surface involvement of >25% and with persistent posterior talar subluxation.
- **Associated soft tissue ligamentous injuries**
  - **Deltoid ligament disruption:** Such injuries are nonsurgically treated if the medial clear space reduces anatomically with reduction and fixation of the lateral malleolus. Persistent medial widening demands inspection of the syndesmosis. After internal fixation of the lateral malleolus, external rotation stress radiographs should be re-recorded to confirm stability of the syndesmosis. If syndesmotic instability is present, indicative of a SER IV injury, this should be addressed as noted next.
  - **Syndesmosis:** Fixation of the syndesmosis is indicated when evidence of a diastasis is present. Fixation methods are evolving, but start with anatomic restoration of both fibular length and the tibiofibular relationship at the mortise. Suture repair devices such as the TightRope (Arthrex, Naples, FL), with or without repair of the syndesmotic ligaments, is the treatment of choice. Early data suggest that suture fixation devices might yield better functional results than screws, particularly in athletes.

Compartment Syndrome of Lower Limb

Description: Surgical emergency usually associated with fracture of the involved extremity. Acute compartment syndrome represents myoneural ischemia that is caused by elevated intracompartmental pressure. Exertional compartment syndrome is a related entity that involves athletes, but it does not represent an emergency.

Presentation: Can be initiated by several conditions, including fractures, crush injuries, severe contusions, or vascular injuries (see Fig. 58.5F); reported in almost every muscle compartment of the arms, legs, and trunk; most cases involve the legs. The earliest and most reliable symptom is pain that is out of proportion with the injury and pain with passive stretch. The classic five Ps (pain, pallor, pulselessness, paresthesia, and poikilothermia) are typically seen in acute ischemia and may only manifest in the late stages of compartment syndrome. Do not wait to see if the other symptoms occur before making the diagnosis and initiating treatment.

Physical examination: Primary diagnosis is based on physical examination, not compartment pressure measurements, in the mentally intact patient. Firm compartments and severe pain, particularly with passive stretch, are adequate to make the diagnosis. Possible loss of pulses distal to the compartment, pallor of the extremity, or nerve dysfunction in the form of either paresthesia or paralysis are late findings.

Diagnostics: Various commercial devices have been developed to measure compartment pressures in limbs; the pressure threshold that requires a fasciotomy is extremely controversial and should mainly be based on clinical examination. Compartment pressure measurement may be useful in the altered or sedated patient.

Treatment: Surgical emergency requires surgical release of the fascia over the entire length of the involved compartment; both skin and fascia should be left open after release. Negative pressure wound therapy to aid in the management of fasciotomy wounds can be very helpful.

Prognosis and return to sport: Prognosis is highly variable and largely depends on the timing of the diagnosis. This is a limb-threatening condition with a high likelihood that the athlete will not be able to function at the same level as before the injury. Prognosis is favorable in patients who undergo an early fasciotomy. As noted previously, a higher muscular volume within the compartment may put the athlete at an increased risk of compartment syndrome. Possibility of an evolving compartment syndrome must be considered and dealt with after injury before the athlete can fly home after a competition.

Open Fractures

Overview: Can be severe injuries that threaten the athlete's career, and possibly the athlete's leg; it is critical that every team physician understand certain key principles regarding the treatment of open fractures. The team physician should not hesitate to engage trauma surgeons, who have substantial experience with severe open fractures, to assist and provide the ideal treatment.

Presentation: Significant bleeding and an obviously open wound, or it may involve virtually no bleeding and only a small wound or abrasion (see Fig. 58.5C). Always assume a fracture is open until proven otherwise.

Physical examination: Remove all clothing and pads to allow careful evaluation of the skin; inspect for lacerations and abrasions. Open fractures should be classified according to the system developed by Gustilo and Anderson (see Fig. 58.5C).

Diagnostics: Orthogonal radiographs of the fracture are the primary diagnostic studies required. Compartment syndrome can occur in both open and closed fractures.

Treatment: Should be initiated on an urgent basis; although present data suggest that several open fractures do well as long as they are treated within the initial 24 hours; optimally, the patient should be taken to the operating room as soon as the appropriate team and equipment can be assembled. Appropriate antibiotics should be administered immediately and tetanus immunization status confirmed. Initial management of the wound, including thorough examination with gentle cleansing of any gross contamination, if possible, is key. Several open fractures that occur during athletic competitions are grossly contaminated with soil and grass; it is critical to perform an aggressive and thorough irrigation and debridement to avoid osteomyelitis. Several new treatment options have been developed that may be useful with the most severe open fractures.

- The use of negative pressure wound therapy has been reported to be associated with a decreased incidence of osteomyelitis after severe open fractures.

Prognosis and return to sport: Prognosis for a severe open fracture is driven by both the type of fracture and the open wound. It may be a career-ending injury, and the athlete and coach need to understand that. However, with aggressive treatment and incorporating contemporary treatment methods, complete recovery is possible, and the athlete can thus successfully resume his or her athletic career.

RETURN TO SPORTS AFTER EXTREMITY FRACTURE

General Principles

- Return to sport must be individualized based on the type of fracture, fixation method, healing, and type of sport activity and position played.
- Returning to a noncontact overhead sport such as tennis is much different than returning to a collision sport such as football.
- The individual and the team physician must weigh the benefits of an early return against the short- and long-term risks of reinjury.
- The overriding principle is the health and well-being/safety of the athlete.
- The sport-specific evaluation on the field or court is more important than any test in the office environment. Feedback from the athletes themselves is also crucial.

Upper Extremity

- In most cases, the time to return to sport with an upper extremity fracture is much less than that with a lower extremity fracture.
- A certain degree of cardiovascular fitness, speed, and agility can all be maintained from the beginning.
- In addition, the injury can be protected with taping, padding, splinting, and bracing.
- Return to sport is often a multiple of the time required for fracture union (0.5–1.0 times the fracture healing duration).
- The lower extremity rule would apply to an overhead athlete.

Lower Extremity

- Rehabilitation starts immediately, but because there is a period of limited weight bearing, return of full strength, speed, and agility takes longer.
- Generally, time taken to return to sport is a multiple of the time required for fracture union (1.5–2.0 times the fracture healing duration).
- Rehabilitation goes through three major phases: protected phase, partial protected phase, and unprotected phase.
- Fixation method and fracture healing determine how long each phase lasts and must be guided by experience, clinical examination, and radiographs.
- Biologically friendly anatomic reduction and biomechanical sound initial fixation allow faster progression to the unprotected phase of rehabilitation and shorten the return-to-play duration.

Hardware

- **Hardware left in situ:** Playing with hardware must be individualized, based on the type of sport (collision, contact, or noncontact), type of hardware, location of hardware, and stress concentration.
- **Type of hardware:**
  - **Plate:** Stress shielding occurs under a plate, and an area of stress concentration exists at the end of the plate. Risk of fracture at the end of the plate goes up in collision sports such as football. Protective padding to distribute loads over a broader surface area is advisable.
  - **Intramedullary nail:** Minimal stress shielding occurs with a load-sharing device such as an intramedullary nail, and stress concentration is better tolerated in the metaphyseal and epiphyseal regions at the ends of the nail. Minimal protection is required after fracture union.
- **Hardware removal:** Most hardware is left in place until the athlete finishes competitive sports. Symptomatic hardware, particularly intramedullary nail interlocking screws, can be removed in the off-season.
  - Refracture after plate removal occurs through screw hole sites. An extended period of protection may be required after removal, particularly with forearm fractures.
  - Refracture after screw removal for fifth metatarsal base fractures has been reported, and screws should be left in place until the athlete has finished competitive sports.
  - Intramedullary devices pose minimal risk and are left in place until competitive sports are finished.

RECOMMENDED READINGS

Available online.

STRESS FRACTURES 59

Christopher C. Kaeding • Kurt P. Spindler

GENERAL PRINCIPLES

Definition

Stress fractures are fatigue-failure injuries of the bone affecting physically active people, including military recruits, track and field athletes, and ballet dancers. With the increased role of exercise for elderly people and patients with chronic disease, stress fractures should not be overlooked in nontraditional populations.

Etiology

- Stress fractures are overuse injuries that present over a continuum of fatigue failure of the bone, from microfracture to complete structural failure. Excessive repetitive stress alters the balance of bone remodeling. Bone formation (osteoblastic activity) lags behind resorption (osteoclastic activity). Stress can be compressive, tensile, or rotational.
- Initially, increased osteoclastic activity at a site of stress leads to a more porous, weakened cortex. Above a certain threshold, additional stress cycles lead to the development of microscopic cracks, further decreasing bone strength. Continued repetitive stress leads to microfracture propagation and coalescence, resulting in a stress fracture. With further stress, frank fracture and displacement can occur (Fig. 59.1).

Epidemiology

- Individual sports place stress on specific anatomic sites, which are at increased risk of stress fracture. Site specificity is determined by the athletic population (Table 59.1).
- Certain sports are more commonly associated with stress fractures: **running (69%)**, fitness class (8%), racket sports (5%), basketball (4%), and other sports (14%).
- Female military recruits have 10 times the fracture risk of males; female athletes have 3.5 times the fracture risk of males.
  - Risk is activity dependent: higher risk for female runners and gymnasts.
  - Females' higher risk may be related to underlying menstrual irregularities and associated decreases in bone density (e.g., with female athlete triad) or anatomic and biomechanical factors specific to females.
- The most common bones injured, reported as a percentage of all stress fractures: tibia (49.1%), tarsals (25.3%), metatarsals (8.8%), femur (7.2%), fibula (6.6%), pelvis (1.6%), sesamoids (0.9%), and spine (0.6%); bilateral injuries in 16.6% of cases
- Age relationship: Femoral and tarsal fractures more common in older patients; tibial, fibular, and upper extremity fractures more common in younger patients

PROTECTIVE AND RISK FACTORS

See Table 59.2.

Bone Characteristics

- **Composition:** Mineral deposition around collagen matrix; the bone resists compression; the collagen matrix (connective tissue) resists tension
- **Bone remodels in response to stress** (Wolff law).
- Allows protective increases in cortical thickness, density, and diaphyseal diameter (Fig. 59.2)
- Remodeling is a function of number, frequency, and duration of loading cycles. It is influenced by strain volume, application rate, and duration per cycle.
- Osteoclasts activated by stress result in increased activity over 30–45 days, resulting in increased bone porosity.
- Osteoblasts migrate into porous areas and build matrix. This process begins approximately 30 days after stress and culminates with new bone formation over approximately 180 days.
- If a weakened bone is subject to additional stress, **osteoclastic activity can overwhelm osteoblastic activity, resulting in further weakened bone and microfractures.** Each load cycle may propagate microfractures until symptomatic stress fracture results. Increased microfractures have been demonstrated in areas of bone porosity.
- **Bone geometry** may determine the risk.
  - Larger and higher-density bones are more resistant to fatigue fractures
  - Long bones with increased diameter resist bending in response to load. During basic training, recruits with tibial stress fractures had significantly smaller tibial widths and cross-sectional areas than those without stress fracture.

Soft Tissues (Intrinsic Factors)

- Good muscle strength is protective. Muscle contractions attenuate ground reaction forces developed at impact during running and jumping.
- Bone strain increases as muscles fatigue.
- Contraction of strong opposing muscle groups on a single bone may produce tension across the bone and promote stress fracture.
- No relationship between stress fracture and muscle size or flexibility.
- General fitness is protective. Military recruits with higher activity levels before enlistment developed fewer stress fractures during basic training.

Endocrine

- Low testosterone or estrogen levels can increase the risk of stress fractures.
- Oligomenorrheic or amenorrheic female athletes are at a risk secondary to decreased estrogen levels and increased osteoclastic activity.
- High-intensity training may suppress menses.
- Delayed menarche, often observed in athletes, may result in decreased bone density but probably does not increase the risk of stress fractures.
- Cigarette smoking lowers estrogen levels in a dose-dependent manner, resulting in higher osteoclastic activity.

Nutritional

- Stress fractures are associated with a lower fat intake, a lower caloric intake, eating disorders, and weight <75% of the ideal body weight.

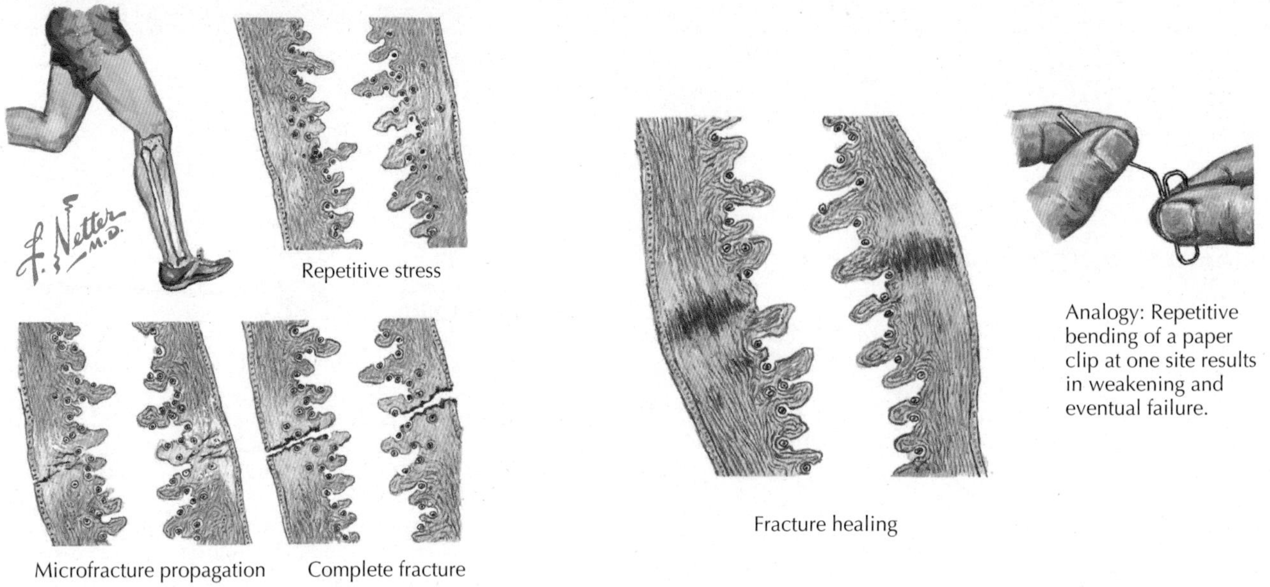
Repetitive stress
Analogy: Repetitive bending of a paper clip at one site results in weakening and eventual failure.
Fracture healing
Microfracture propagation
Complete fracture

Figure 59.1 Etiology of stress fracture. Site specificity of stress fractures in track and field athletes is determined by the anatomic stress demanded by the sport.

Table 59.1 STRESS FRACTURE SITES ASSOCIATED WITH SELECTED SPORTS

Track	Football	Basketball	Gymnastics	Softball (Fast-Pitch)	Dance	Running
Navicular	Tibia	First rib	Pars interarticularis	Rib	Metatarsals	Tibia
Tibia	Pars	Tibia	Radius	Ulna	Fibula	Fibula
Metatarsals	Fifth metatarsal	Fifth metatarsal	Midfoot	Humerus	Pars interarticularis	Metatarsals
Fibula		Tarsal	Navicular		Tibia	

Table 59.2 ETIOLOGIC FACTORS FOR STRESS FRACTURES

Intrinsic Factors	Extrinsic Factors
Alignment abnormalities	Overt
Femoral neck anteversion	Continued self-abuse
Pronation/supination	Inappropriate training
Tibial torsion	Inappropriate technique
Leg length discrepancy	Inappropriate equipment
Muscle imbalance	Harsh environment
Muscle weakness	Covert
Flexibility	Joint instability
Genetic predisposition	Extrinsic pressure
Aging/hormonal	Biomechanical fault

- Calcium intake correlates with bone density; low calcium intake does not correlate with stress fractures.

Training Intensity

- Training errors include rapidly escalating frequency, duration, and intensity of training; 60% of running injuries are associated with training errors.
- Stress fractures are increased during the initial 2 weeks after increased training intensity, with increases >30% in duration or intensity over a single season and in freshman runners adjusting to collegiate training demands.
- Multiple factors compound the risk

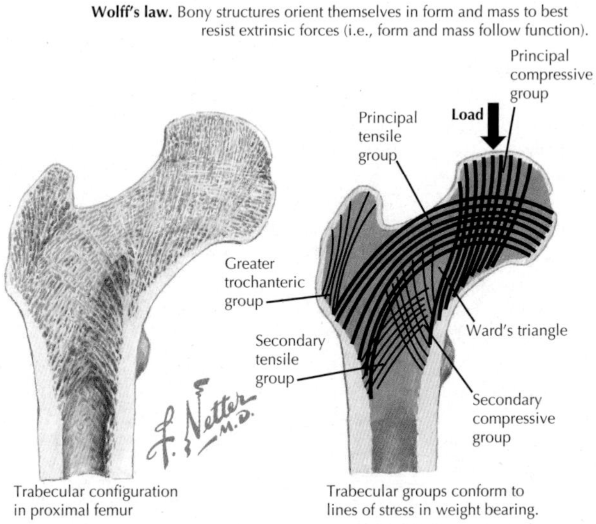
Wolff's law. Bony structures orient themselves in form and mass to best resist extrinsic forces (i.e., form and mass follow function).
Principal compressive group
Load
Principal tensile group
Greater trochanteric group
Secondary tensile group
Ward's triangle
Secondary compressive group
Trabecular configuration in proximal femur
Trabecular groups conform to lines of stress in weight bearing.

Figure 59.2 Bone architecture in relation to physical stress.

- Independent of risk associated with menstrual dysfunction, athletes training >5 hours/day have a sixfold increased risk of stress fractures.
- A dancer who is both amenorrheic for >6 months and training >5 hours/day is 93 times more likely to develop a stress fracture than an eumenorrheic counterpart who trains less.

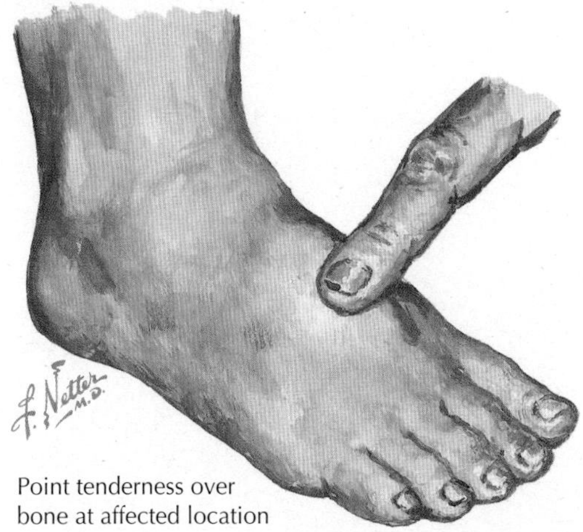
Point tenderness over
bone at affected location

Figure 59.3 Physical examination of stress fracture.

Extrinsic Factors

- **Surface**
  - **Hard running surfaces** increase impact forces.
  - Unidirectional running on **cambered track surfaces** may predispose to injury.
  - Large epidemiologic studies reveal no association between stress injury and running surface.
- **Environment** (e.g., hills or uneven terrain)
- **Technical faults in training or performance**—may predispose to stress injury

DIAGNOSIS

Time to Diagnosis

- It takes an average of 5–16 weeks to diagnose a stress fracture. Delayed diagnosis can be detrimental, particularly with high-risk stress fractures.

History

- Maintain a high index of suspicion.
- Certain affected anatomic areas are particularly challenging to diagnose.
- Recall of specific detailed historical facts may be challenging for athletes.
- Recent change in activity level over the past 2 months and preseason training
- Recent change in equipment or playing surface
- Activities added to already demanding physical performance
- **Insidious onset of pain,** usually initially after activity; with fracture progression, pain moves earlier into activity and may eventually occur with minimal activity (e.g., walking) or even at rest
- Vague pain in affected region, occasionally localized
- Pain relief with rest and/or reduced activity
- Prior stress fractures
- **Females:** Menstrual irregularities, recent weight changes, eating disorder history or behaviors, and nutrition
- **Older athletes,** particularly **females:** osteoporosis risk factors (e.g., smoking, family history, corticosteroid use, body weight, Caucasian race, menopause, and hormone replacement)

Physical Examination

- Point tenderness, edema, warmth, and palpable callus in certain cases (Fig. 59.3); in areas where bone not easily palpated, such as femoral neck, gentle range of motion (ROM) may elicit pain
- Tenderness with percussion or with sound waves (tuning fork or ultrasound)

Table 59.3 CLASSIFICATION OF STRESS FRACTURES

Grade	Pain	Imaging Findings (Radiograph, Bone Scan, CT, MRI)
I	(–)	Evidence of stress injury
II	(+)	No fracture line
III	(+)	Fracture line
IV	(+)	Displaced
V	(+)	Nonunion

- Specific tests:
  - **Stork test or one-legged standing hyperextension test:** Back extension with resultant hip flexion while standing on one leg increases pain in pars interarticularis stress fractures.
  - **Fulcrum test:** Performed by placing fist or arm of examiner under suspected fracture site and applying "bending" force to distal extremity while proximal extremity is kept relatively immobilized by anatomic restraints; positive test results in pain over the fracture site; commonly used to evaluate femoral shaft stress fractures, but may be used in other "long bone" areas
  - **Hop test:** Hopping on affected leg reproduces pain at the fracture site, usually with femoral shaft stress fractures.
  - **Tuning fork test:** Vibrating tuning fork over fracture site results in pain at the fracture site; high rate of false positives

Radiologic Studies

- **Plain radiographs** usually negative in the early phase, particularly during initial 2–3 weeks; two-thirds of initial radiographs are negative, but half ultimately prove positive; radiographs are specific but not sensitive.
- **Ultrasound:** Not reliable for diagnosis; several studies in progress.
- **Bone scan:** Approximately 100% sensitive but not specific; not helpful for guiding return to play; uptake on bone scan normalizes over 12–18 months, often lagging behind resolution of clinical symptoms; particularly useful in tarsal, femur, pelvis, and tibial plateau fractures; helps differentiate stress fractures from periostitis (shin splints). Stress fractures are **usually positive in all phases of triple-phase technetium bone scan** (angiogram, blood pool, delayed). Periostitis is often negative in the angiogram and blood-pool phase and positive in the delayed image phase.
- **Single-photon emission computed tomography (SPECT):** More specific than planar bone scan; particularly helpful in detecting stress fractures of the pars interarticularis, pelvis, and femoral neck
- **Computed tomography (CT):** Delineates bone well, useful when diagnosis is difficult (e.g., tarsal navicular stress fractures); helpful with spinal or linear stress fractures
- **Magnetic resonance imaging (MRI):** Superior sensitivity and specificity over bone scan and CT for soft tissue abnormalities and edema; may delineate early injury. Findings include periosteal or marrow edema. MRI may be highly useful with certain stress fractures (such as hip and pelvis).

CLASSIFICATION

- Reproducible classification system of stress fractures is important for accurate communication between clinicians and the study of stress fractures.
- Classification system should have implications for the treatment and prognosis of a stress fracture.
- Table 59.3 outlines a reproducible and generalizable classification system.

GENERAL TREATMENT

- Because they are overuse injuries, most stress fractures respond well to relative rest and gradual reintroduction of sport. High-risk stress fractures demand rapid diagnosis and specific intervention to avoid complications.
- Stress fractures frequently heal in 6–8 weeks (usually low-risk), but certain fractures (mostly high-risk) heal more slowly over ≥3–4 months.

Suggested Phases of Treatment

- **Phase I:** Pain control, usually 10–14 days
  - Controversial to use nonsteroidal anti-inflammatory drugs (NSAIDs) at analgesic doses. Use with caution because prolonged high doses of NSAIDs may inhibit bone healing.
  - Physiotherapy (may include bone stimulator)
  - Flexibility and strengthening
  - Complete or relative rest depending on fracture site and severity of symptoms
  - Bracing may speed return to play in specific cases (e.g., long-leg pneumatic splint with anterior buttress in tibial shaft fractures)
- **Phase II:** Reintroduction of activity; may last for several weeks depending on the location and type of stress fracture; initiation of phase II varies with patient symptoms and depends on size and type of stress fracture.
  - Continue phase I treatment
  - Maintain aerobic fitness through pool running and cycling; newer elliptical trainers may also be helpful.
  - Gradually add impact activity, altering surface or equipment if possible. Run short distances on grass or soft surfaces and gradually increase running time.
  - Resume sports-specific training in noncompetitive settings.
  - Work out on alternating days and maximize rest between bouts of exertion.
- **Phase III:** Preparation for return to competition
  - Increase sports-specific plyometric conditioning drills. Add running drills, cutting drills, and selected skill work.
  - Begin lower-level competitive challenges.

SPECIFIC STRESS FRACTURES

Upper Extremity

Although much less common than in the lower extremities, stress fractures of the upper extremities should be included in the differential diagnosis for athletes who perform repetitive throwing, swinging, or overhead activities. Gymnasts and cheerleaders who use the upper extremities for weight bearing and twisting are at a risk of stress fractures below the elbow. Young athletes and throwing athletes (e.g., goalkeepers or javelin throwers) develop stress fractures of the humerus and shoulder girdle. Swinging athletes (golf and rowing) are at risk of rib fractures.

Humerus

Description: **Proximal** and **medial epicondyle** fractures seen in younger throwing athletes and gymnasts. **Midshaft** fractures seen in adult throwing athletes and workers who perform heavy lifting

History: Pain with throwing or lifting heavy weights; may involve entire upper arm

Examination: Normal or pain on palpation or resisted motion

Treatment: Rest; immobilization, such as fracture brace; 6–8 weeks for healing; correction of biomechanical and technical faults

Ulna

Description: Reported in baseball and softball pitchers, rodeo riders, bowlers, golfers, and volleyball players

History: Pain over ulnar shaft during and after activity; fracture location varies by activity. Fractures develop proximally in volleyball players secondary to repetitive and explosive wrist flexion. Fractures occur distally in softball players (underhand activity). Midshaft stress fractures reported in tennis; pronation with backhand stroke at ball strike and follow-through are painful

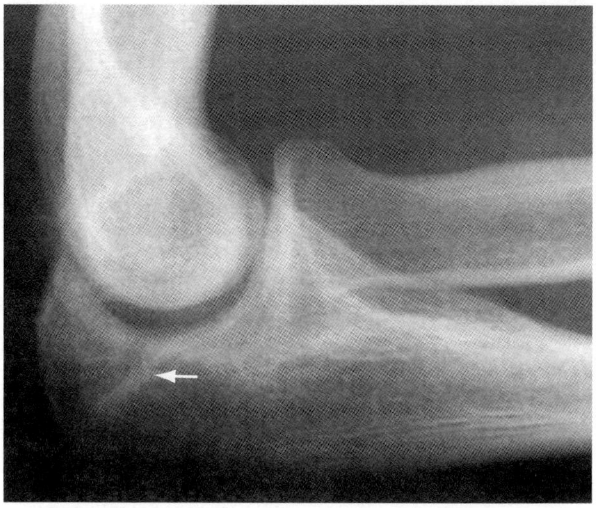

Figure 59.4 Lateral elbow, olecranon stress fracture *(arrow)*.

Examination: Pain, edema, and local heat over involved areas; painful pronation and supination

Radiographic studies: Radiographs typically helpful, show periosteal reaction; bone scan or MRI used to confirm. MRI may demonstrate edema in interosseous membrane.

Treatment and return to play: Rest from activity, resume gradual activity when pain free. Extension block splints used sometimes; correction of biomechanical or technical faults; in all reports, return to play was in 4–6 weeks

Olecranon

Description: Occurs in throwing athletes; caused by recurrent valgus extension overload; young gymnasts may injure olecranon physis.

History: Pain with elbow extension/throwing

Examination: Point tenderness and pain with triceps extension against resistance

Radiographic studies: Radiographs may be negative. Nonunion risk is higher if radiograph shows sclerosis around area of lucency. Fracture site is under tension. Radiographs demonstrate unique transverse radiolucency extending from posterior nonarticular to articular surface (Fig. 59.4)

Treatment: Short-term immobilization to reduce triceps pull; surgery may be required for nonunion.

Radius

Description: Uncommon; reported in military personnel, cheerleaders, gymnasts, tennis players, volleyball players, softball players, pool players, and cyclists

History: Pain in shaft of radius with aforementioned activities, particularly with wrist supination

Examination: Pain over involved area

Radiographic studies: Radiographs show periosteal thickening and occasionally bowing; bone scan or MRI confirms diagnosis

Treatment: Rest for 6 weeks; repetitive wrist weight bearers (e.g., gymnasts or cheerleaders) may require longer rest

Shoulder Girdle and Trunk

Clavicle

Description: Cases reported in javelin throwers and springboard divers; mechanism of injury hypothesized to be repetitive deltoid and pectoralis major contractions during javelin throw and repeated water entry (diving) with wrists extended and forearms pronated

History: Insidious onset of pain over clavicle

Examination: Pain reproduced with abduction of the shoulder above horizontal plane of shoulder

Radiographic studies: Radiographs show periosteal reaction. Bone scan or CT is used to confirm diagnosis.

Treatment: Rest from activity; return to play in 8 weeks

Scapula

Description: Stress fracture of coracoid process reported in female trapshooters secondary to repetitive impact of rifle butt; stress fractures at other scapular sites reported in gymnasts, joggers who carry dumbbells (superomedial scapula), and football players (associated with weightlifting; acromion)

History: Gradual-onset deep aching in shoulder

Examination: Pain with palpation of coracoid process and bicipital groove; painful resisted adduction and forward flexion of arm

Radiographic studies: Axillary view necessary for plain radiographic diagnosis; West Point axillary and modified oblique views helpful for acromial stress fractures; MRI or bone scan confirms diagnosis

Treatment: Rest from trapshooting for 6 weeks; at 6 weeks, patient is usually pain free with full ROM and can gradually resume shooting. Other fracture sites: Return to play in 8 weeks with rest; consider butt modification or padding when returning to play.

Ribs

Description: First-rib fracture most commonly seen in baseball pitchers and basketball players; reported in weightlifting, tennis, table tennis, rugby, judo, gymnastics, and ballet; other rib fractures seen in softball (pitchers), golf, tennis, and rowing; diagnosis often delayed because misdiagnosed as back strain; typically posterolateral, although anterolateral and rib neck stress fractures have been reported in rowers; possibly related to serratus anterior fatigue in golfers

History: Insidious onset, but occasionally presents acutely without preceding symptoms

Examination: Pain with arm motion over supraclavicular area (first rib) or over the affected area; pain with trunk rotation (lower ribs); serratus anterior weakness

Radiographic studies: Radiographs often negative; usually positive if fracture is over a broad, flat, and thick portion of the first rib. Other ribs are difficult to diagnose using radiographs; bone scan or MRI helpful to confirm diagnosis.

Treatment: Rest, avoidance of overhead and swinging activity, maintenance of aerobic fitness, general conditioning and strengthening of serratus anterior; gradual return to play when pain free

Spine

Spondylolysis: Pars Interarticularis Stress Fractures

Description: Most common in athletes undergoing repetitive hyperextension of spine (gymnasts, cheerleaders, divers, and weightlifters); L4 and L5 are most commonly affected vertebrae levels; common cause of pediatric low back pain. In orthopedic referral population, 47% of pediatric patients with low back pain had spondylolysis, compared with only 5% of adults.

History: Athletes usually involved in certain repetitive back **extension load** activities; insidious onset of low back pain; patient ultimately complains of significant back spasms (often misdiagnosed as lumbar strain); short periods of rest may temporarily relieve the pain, but return to activity results in immediate exacerbation of symptoms

Examination: May have clinical hyperlordosis; pain to palpation over affected vertebrae; pain and muscle guarding with one- and two-leg standing trunk extension test (one-leg usually worse), trunk rotation and extension, hip extension test (prone), trunk extension test (prone), and combined hip and trunk extension test (prone); neurologic examination usually normal; occasionally may have associated radiculopathy

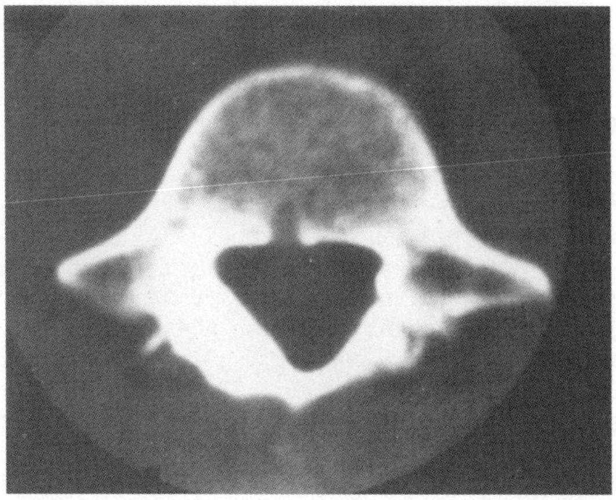

Figure 59.5 Axial CT image, pars interarticularis stress fracture with sclerosis.

Radiographic studies: Radiographs have low sensitivity. Anteroposterior (AP), lateral, bilateral, and oblique views; if positive, classic defect of "collar" on neck (pars interarticularis) of Scotty dog is seen on oblique views; falling out of favor because of low sensitivity and high radiation. SPECT scan has a greater sensitivity and is becoming the gold standard for diagnosis. Thin-cut CT scan (1.5- to 2-mm cuts) may help identify the extent and age of fracture, partial versus complete, and sclerosis (Fig. 59.5). Combination of SPECT and CT findings may help determine the likelihood of healing and may help design the treatment protocol.

Treatment: Somewhat controversial; initially, modify activity and avoid back hyperextension; some consider nonrigid bracing if pain persists. At 2–4 weeks, begin physical therapy; if pain present at 4 weeks, thoracolumbosacral orthosis (TLSO) or low-profile antilordotic Boston brace is an option to unload posterior elements and prevent hyperextension. Treat until patient is symptom free. Healing can take 3–6 months and may not correlate with symptoms. Consider CT scan to assess healing. Consider surgical spinal evaluation if persistent pain after rigid bracing, particularly if neurologic symptoms appear or progress.

Return to play: As early as 8 weeks if patient remains pain free at rest, in hyperextension, and while performing aggravating activities

Pelvis

Description: **Pubic ramus** usually involved; uncommon; seen almost exclusively in women, military recruits, and long-distance runners or joggers

History: Pain in the inguinal, perineal, or adductor region that is relieved by rest; seen in female British Army recruits forced to match official 30-inch stride length while marching; when stride length decreased to 27 inches, no further stress fractures were reported, suggesting increased stride length may promote biomechanical stress at the pubic ramus

Examination: Antalgic gait, full ROM, pain over pubic ramus, and positive "standing sign" (inability to stand unsupported on affected side)

Radiographic studies: Radiographs initially negative; late in course, may show abundant callus; bone scan or MRI needed for early diagnosis

Treatment: Brief nonweight-bearing and rest from running; healing variable, typically 3–5 months

Sacral Stress Fractures

Description: Fatigue fractures reported mainly in runners; high index of suspicion required; insufficiency fractures more common in osteoporotic bone (elderly)

History: Vague, poorly localized pain in the gluteal or groin area; rapid increase in mileage or training schedule often associated

Examination: Positive figure-4 (flexion, abduction, external rotation [FABER]) test and hopping test; normal ROM, but deep groin pain at extremes of motion

Radiographic studies: Radiographs usually negative; bone scan or MRI used for diagnosis

Treatment: Cessation of running, protected weight bearing, and relative rest lasting from 6 weeks to 8 months

Femoral Stress Fractures

Femur sites most commonly involved with stress fractures, from most to least common: shaft, lesser trochanter, intertrochanteric region, neck, and greater trochanter; missed diagnosis of a femoral neck fracture can lead to high morbidity

Femoral Neck

Description: Seen most frequently in runners, dancers, and military recruits; diagnosis is typically delayed 5–13 weeks. Severe complications arise with progression to complete fracture and displacement. Complications may include avascular necrosis, nonunion, varus deformity, and chronic pain. **Superior** neck fractures are under tension and are a high-risk area for progression to complete fracture. **Inferior** neck fractures are compression-sided and are often conservatively managed.

History: Earliest sign: 87% report inguinal or anterior groin pain; aching pain precipitated by weight-bearing activities: 40% reported symptoms after long run, between 6 and 8 weeks of training. Symptoms appear with increase in training schedule; diagnosis often delayed

Examination: Antalgic gait (22%); pain with palpation in groin, hip, or anterior thigh (70%); pain at extremes of hip ROM (79% of 39 patients in one study); subtle limitation of flexion and internal rotation

Radiographic studies: Radiographs have a high false-negative rate, particularly early; bone or SPECT scan for early diagnosis; false negatives reported for up to 12 days after fracture. MRI is becoming more popular and is a sensitive study for identifying early marrow edema, which typically resolves in 8–12 weeks.

Treatment (Blickenstaff criteria modified by Fullerton): Complications in up to 30% of patients; return to play may be delayed for up to 2 years

- **Compression-sided fractures** (Blickenstaff type I): inferior neck
  - Type Ia: Callus without fracture line and positive bone scan; managed conservatively with nonweight-bearing and/or bed rest; gradual activity progression when pain free; weekly radiographs until patient can walk without pain using a cane
  - Type Ib: Definite fracture line but no displacement; treat with nonweight-bearing, or surgery; serial radiographs
- **Tension-sided fractures** (Blickenstaff type II): superior neck (Fig. 59.6)
  - A positive bone scan without a visible fracture line on radiographs is treated with bed rest or nonweight-bearing and crutches; serial radiographs to look for developing fracture lines
  - If fracture lines present, higher risk of displacement, avascular necrosis, nonunion, and malunion; early diagnosis and surgical management usually required; if no displacement, some experts advocate bed rest as first-line treatment in lieu of immediate surger
- **Displaced** (Blickenstaff type III): surgical fixation recommended

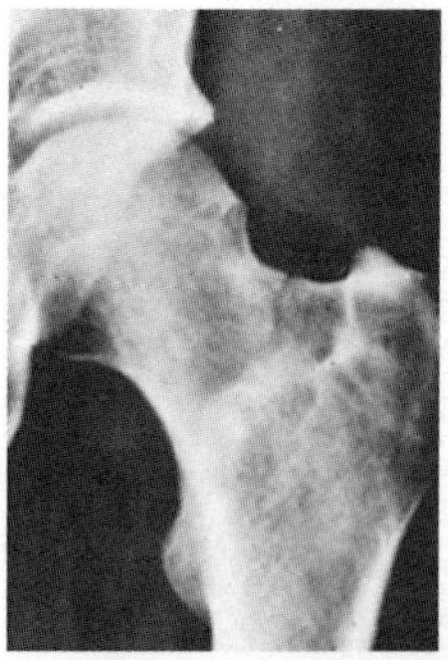

AP hip, superior femoral neck (tension-type fracture).

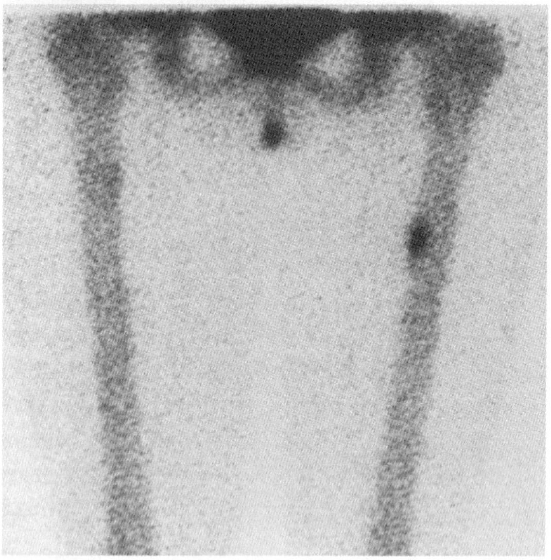

Bone scan, increased uptake femoral shaft.

Figure 59.6 Femoral stress fractures.

Femoral Shaft Stress Fractures

Description: Seen mostly in runners, particularly females; most common location is at the junction of proximal and middle thirds of the femoral shaft

History: Sudden increases in frequency, intensity, or duration; pain with running progresses to pain with activities of daily living

Examination: Antalgic gait (22%); normal ROM (94%); pain with palpation in groin, hip, or anterior thigh (70%); hopping on affected leg reproduces pain (hop test); positive in 70%; positive fulcrum or "hanging leg" test

Radiographic studies: Early radiographs negative; callus and lucent fracture line in 2–6 weeks; bone scan or SPECT scan for early diagnosis (see Fig. 59.6); MRI is much more sensitive; clearly identifies bone edema, which typically resolves in 8–12 weeks

Treatment: Conservative management of shaft stress fractures is successful; first-line interventions include protected weight bearing with crutches for 1–4 weeks (length of time depends on resolution of pain); activity modification; maintenance of aerobic fitness, skill, and strength; if pain free during day-to-day activities at 14 days, begin rehabilitation with low-impact, minimal weight-bearing exercise (cycling, swimming, pool running); time to full recovery varies, but reported as 5–10 weeks from diagnosis; resumption of athletic activity may take 8–16 weeks.

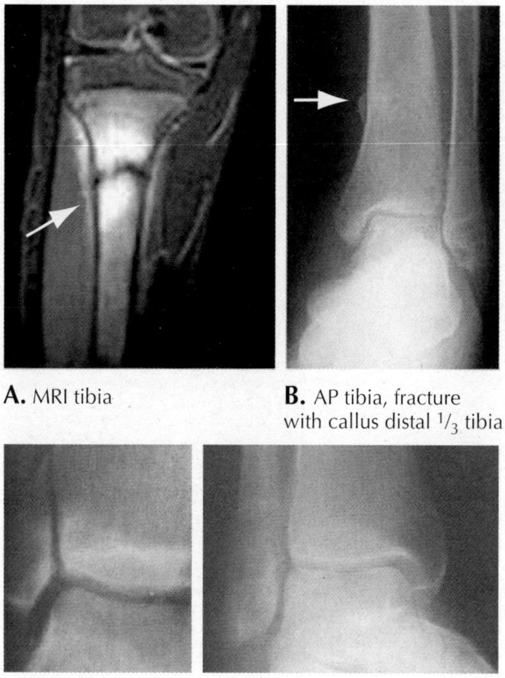

A. MRI tibia
B. AP tibia, fracture with callus distal $^1/_3$ tibia
C. Medial malleolus fracture
D. AP ankle, distal fibula stress fracture

Figure 59.7 Knee and lower leg stress fractures.

Knee and Lower Leg Stress Fractures

Patella

Description: Rare; reported in basketball, soccer, and high jump; may be longitudinal or transverse; reported after anterior cruciate ligament (ACL) and patellar tendon graft repair in patients with cerebral palsy and in young athletes

History: Anterior knee pain, worse with jumping, may have had prior bone tendon bone graft harvest for ACL reconstruction

Examination: Pain to palpation, pain with resisted knee extension

Radiographic studies: Radiographs may show definite fracture lines; must differentiate from bipartite patella; bone scan; MRI clarifies diagnosis and identifies bone edema

Treatment: **Transverse fractures** prone to displacement; nondisplaced fractures are treated with long leg or cylinder cast immobilization with the knee in full extension for 4–6 weeks, followed by quadriceps rehabilitation. Displaced fractures are treated with open reduction and internal fixation (ORIF). **Longitudinal fractures** occur in lateral patellar facet; if displaced, excise lateral fragment.

Proximal Tibia Fractures

Description: Infrequent; incidence unknown

History: Pain in anteromedial aspect of proximal tibia; weight-bearing precipitates pain

Examination: Localized tenderness and edema; need to differentiate from pes anserinus tendinitis, bursitis, and saphenous nerve entrapment

Radiographic studies: Acute stress fracture often has no radiographic findings. MRI is the most sensitive study (Fig. 59.7).

Treatment: Modification of offending activity usually by decreasing frequency and duration

Tibial Shaft Stress Fractures

Description: Need to differentiate between compression stress fracture and tension stress fracture ("dreaded black line")

- **Compression stress fractures:** MRI suggests continuum between medial tibial stress syndrome and stress fracture, with varying degrees of periosteal edema; common sites include proximal or distal third of tibia, posteromedial tibia (see Fig. 59.7); common in runners
- **Tension stress fractures:** Located in anterior or anterolateral cortex in central third of tibia; common in ballet dancers and jumpers

History: Initially, pain occurs after activity; later pain occurs with activity and activities of daily living

Examination: Localized pain, anterior or medial tibia; edema, palpable periosteal thickening, and pain with percussion; positive "tuning fork test" (beware of false negative; useful if pretest probability is high)

Radiographic studies: Radiographs may be positive if symptoms have persisted for 4–6 weeks; bone scan shows fusiform uptake, which differs from linear uptake of medial tibial stress syndrome. False-negative bone scans have been reported. MRI is more sensitive; used for grading and prognosis for return to play (grades 1 and 2 less symptomatic, return to sport 4–6 weeks; grades 3 and 4 often need more time for healing)

- Grade 1: mild periosteal edema (T2), normal marrow (T1, T2)
- Grade 2: moderate periosteal edema (T2), marrow edema (T2)
- Grade 3: severe periosteal edema (T2), marrow edema (T1, T2)
- Grade 4: severe periosteal edema (T2), marrow edema (T1, T2), distinct fracture line visible

Treatment: Control pain, stop running, and use crutches if necessary

- **Compression lesions** may take 2–12 weeks to heal. Return to play is faster with three-panel, long-leg stirrup brace. Correct amenorrhea in females. Calcium supplementation recommended; correct biomechanical faults (consider foot orthotics); in general, return to play guided by MRI grade:
  - Grade 1: return to play in 2–3 weeks, after rest
  - Grade 2: return to play in 4–6 weeks
  - Grade 3: return to play in 6–9 weeks (initially painful with ambulation)
  - Grade 4: return to play in 12 weeks, after casting for 6 weeks and 6 weeks of nonimpact rehabilitation (single case)
  - When pain free: cross-training, nonimpact, and reduced-impact aerobics training; progress to alternating-day graded return to running
- **Tension lesions** achieve faster return to play with intramedullary rod. Conservative treatment may heal in 6 months but has a high rate of recurrence; may progress to complete fracture if missed

Prevention is the best treatment: strength and flexibility of gastrocnemius and soleus; correction of poor running technique; correction of biomechanical issues (e.g., pronation or pes planus) at preparticipation evaluations, particularly with history of stress fracture

Medial Malleolar Stress Fractures

Description: Extend obliquely from plafond; inherently unstable and prone to nonunion; high index of suspicion key to early diagnosis

History: Insidious-onset medial ankle pain, increased with exercise and relieved by rest

Examination: Tender over medial malleolus, ankle effusion

Radiographic studies: Radiographs usually negative early; bone scan or MRI usually required for diagnosis

Treatment: MRI or bone scan positive, no fracture on radiographs: stirrup immobilization for 4–6 weeks. Radiographs or CT demonstrate the fracture; consider ORIF (see Fig. 59.7). Nonunion requires bone graft and screw fixation.

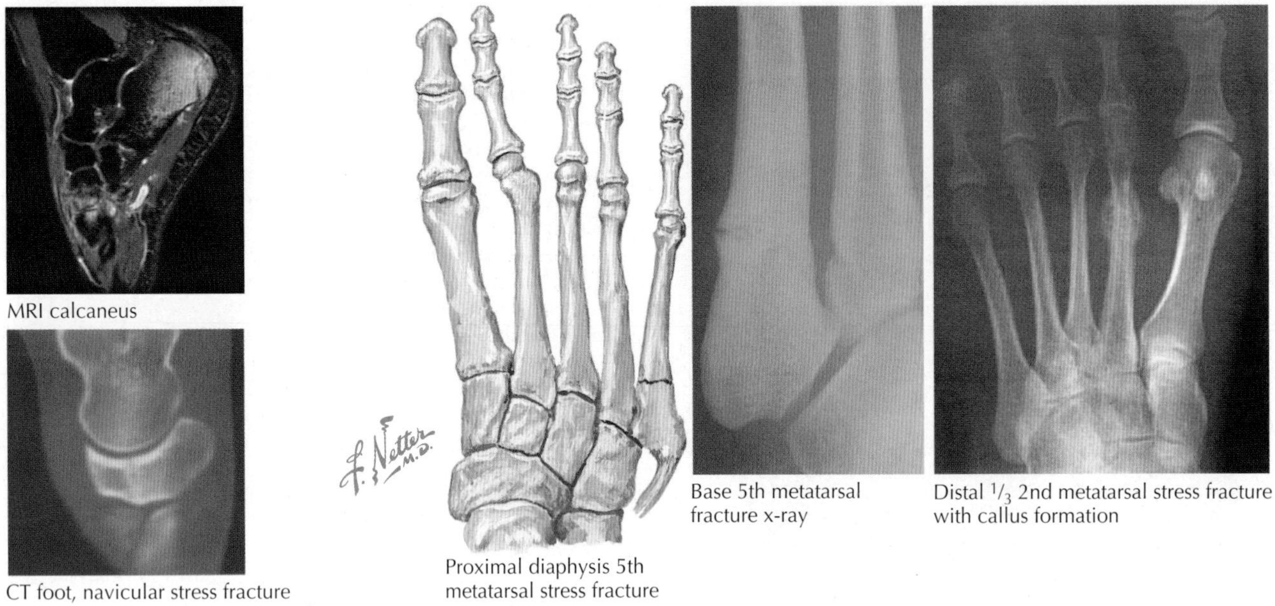
MRI calcaneus
CT foot, navicular stress fracture
Proximal diaphysis 5th metatarsal stress fracture
Base 5th metatarsal fracture x-ray
Distal 1/3 2nd metatarsal stress fracture with callus formation

Figure 59.8 Stress fractures in foot.

Fibular Stress Fractures

Description: Most common in distal third just proximal to distal tibiofibular syndesmosis
History: Limp, swelling
Examination: Point tenderness, localized edema; foot overpronation with hindfoot valgus common, as lateral malleolus is at risk
Radiographic studies: Radiographs not positive for 3–4 weeks (see Fig. 59.7); bone scan can assist with diagnosis.
Treatment: Conservative; for distal fractures, pneumatic ankle brace may be helpful.

Stress Fractures in Foot

Calcaneus

Description: Seen in military recruits and runners
History: Insidious onset of heel pain with running
Examination: Positive heel squeeze test; may have positive hop test; edema
Radiographic studies: Radiographs show endosteal callus perpendicular to the long axis of calcaneus; bone scan, MRI, or CT to confirm diagnosis (Fig. 59.8)
Treatment: Rapid healing with conservative treatment, including relative rest and activity modification; brief period of nonweight-bearing if ambulation painful; return to activity in 3–4 weeks

Tarsal Navicular Stress Fractures

Description: Previously thought uncommon, now recognized in jumping and running athletes, soccer, basketball, and track athletes; vague symptoms often lead to delayed diagnosis. Complications include nonunion and chronic pain. Most fractures in sagittal plane and middle third secondary to poor blood supply; diagnosis requires a high index of suspicion and early imaging (bone scan, MRI)
History: Insidious-onset forefoot/midfoot pain, particularly with running and jumping; pain occasionally mild and usually relieved with rest
Examination: Pain at the "N spot" (dorsal aspect of the navicular); pain may be diffuse rather than localized.
Radiographic studies: Radiographs usually negative; bone scan or MRI can confirm diagnosis. CT or MRI helps determine the fracture site and the extent of healing (see Fig. 59.8).
Treatment: If no bicortical fracture, then nonweight-bearing cast immobilization for 6–8 weeks; if pain free (best guide to healing), a 6-week graduated program of weight-bearing activity. Consider foot orthotics on return to play. ORIF with bone graft for displaced fractures, failure of nonsurgical treatment, delayed union, and nonunion.

Metatarsal (MT) Stress Fractures

PROXIMAL DIAPHYSIS OF FIFTH METATARSAL

Description: Distal to the tuberosity and prone to nonunion; seen in basketball and, less commonly, football
History: Insidious onset of lateral foot pain, worse during and after activity; pain steadily worsens; occasionally, there is acute fracture
Examination: Point tenderness distal to the tuberosity, usually in zone 3 (proximal diaphysis)
Radiographic studies: Radiographs usually show sclerotic changes around the fracture site. Bone scans are only occasionally necessary (see Fig. 59.8).
Treatment:

- Torg classification (proximal fifth MT fractures)
  - Acute: sharp fracture line with no sclerosis or cortical hypertrophy
  - Delayed union: history of previous injury, wide fracture gap, and intramedullary sclerosis
  - Nonunion: recurrent symptoms, wide fracture gap, and sclerosis
- In high-demand and recreational athletes, intramedullary screw has been demonstrated to permit faster return to play and decrease the nonunion rate. Usually weight-bearing activity in 7–14 days, with training progression to completely unrestricted activity over 6–9 weeks; a small risk of fracture nonunion and fatigue fracture of the screw.
  - In nonathletes, a short-leg, nonweight-bearing cast for 6–8 weeks may be considered.

OTHER METATARSALS

Description: First metatarsal MT: Ten percent of MT stress fractures; associated with overpronation
Second, third, and fourth MTs: Ninety percent of MT stress fractures; associated with running and training >20 miles/week; flatfeet (pes planus) increases impact stress to the MT. Most

fractures in runners are distal (see Fig. 59.8). In ballet dancers, fractures occur proximally and often involve medial second MT secondary to en pointe work.

History: Localized pain and edema; onset insidious, worse after increase in training

Examination: Pes planus or overpronation; point tenderness and localized edema over MT

Radiographs: Weight-bearing AP, lateral, and oblique radiographs; in dancers with second MT pain, consider internal and external oblique radiographs; usually positive; bone scan helpful if negative

Treatment: Rest and a stiff-soled shoe or low-tide cast boot; gradual reconditioning to repetitive stress (at 2–3 weeks), such as pool running performed first in chest-deep water and progressing to more shallow depths as symptoms allow; gradual progression to biking, then running. Consider foot orthotics. In distal first MT stress fractures, dorsal displacement may require casting with dorsal pressure to prevent lateral metatarsalgia. In dancers, proximal second MT stress fractures may progress to nonunion and must be aggressively managed with casting or ankle–foot orthosis for 8 weeks.

SESAMOIDS

Description: Difficult diagnosis; differentiate from sesamoiditis and bipartite and tripartite sesamoids; 30% of population have bipartite sesamoids

History: Pain over the plantar aspect of first metatarsophalangeal (MTP) joint; pain with "toe-off"

Examination: Pain on palpation, pain with resisted first toe plantarflexion, and pain over sesamoids with stretch into extreme of dorsiflexion

Radiographic studies: Diagnosis of sesamoid stress fracture by plain radiographs is challenging, and additional imaging (e.g., bone scan or MRI) is often required to differentiate stress fracture from bipartite sesamoid. MRI helps identify marrow edema.

Treatment: Conservative, initially nonweight-bearing cast for 6 weeks to prevent dorsiflexion of the first ray; gradual return to sports over several months; consider foot orthotics after casting; rarely surgical excision for delayed union or chronic pain

RECOMMENDED READINGS

Available online.

60 FOOT PROBLEMS

Kenneth J. Hunt • Thomas O. Clanton

GENERAL PRINCIPLES

Overview: Injuries and disorders of the foot can impose considerable dysfunction in an athlete. Although most foot problems will improve with appropriate care, a clear understanding of normal anatomy and physical examination findings is vital to recognize injuries and abnormal processes to prevent worsening and long-term damage.

Anatomy and Physiology of the Foot

Bones: Normal bony architecture includes 28 bones (7 tarsals, 5 metatarsals, 14 phalanges, and 2 hallux sesamoids) (Fig. 60.1A).

Accessory bones: Common accessory bones that can create symptoms in athletes are the accessory navicular (see Fig. 60.1B), os trigonum, os peroneum, and os vesiculanum.

Muscular anatomy: Most lower leg extrinsic muscles have tendinous attachments on the foot. Foot intrinsic muscles are important for normal function (see Fig. 60.1C).

Neurovascular structures: Three primary arteries/veins provide blood supply and five primary nerves provide innervation to the foot (see Fig. 60.1C).

Sport- and Athlete-Specific Issues

Overview: Most foot injuries in athletes are caused by acute or repetitive trauma. Several intrinsic and extrinsic factors can increase the risk of injury.

Intrinsic factors: Foot posture, hindfoot alignment, joint laxity and stiffness, nutrition, fitness level, training regimen, biochemical deficiencies, age, and body mass index

Extrinsic factors: Coaching, technique, environmental factors, footwear and equipment, and safety hazards

Running and jumping sports: Increased risk of bone stress injuries, tendinopathies, and fasciopathies

Impact/collision sports: Increased risk of acute fractures, tendon ruptures, ligament tears, and joint injuries

HISTORY

Overview: An athlete's recollection of injury onset, mechanism, and location is an important part of the diagnostic process.

Mechanism: Acute, chronic, or acute on chronic; position of the foot during injury; was a pop felt or heard?

Severity: Was the athlete able to ambulate on his or her own after the injury? Was there an obvious deformity, swelling, or discoloration?

Location: Ask the athlete to indicate "with one finger" the location of the injury, pain, or symptoms.

Previous injury: Has the athlete experienced a similar injury in the past? Tendinopathies can flare up or rupture, or bone stress injury can lead to fracture.

PHYSICAL EXAMINATION

Observation and Measurement

Standing Examination

Alignment of the lower extremities: View the patient from the front and back. Check for limb length inequality, pelvic tilt, genu varum, genu valgum, flexion, extension, and rotational abnormalities of both lower extremities.

Foot alignment and mechanics: Evaluate the medial longitudinal arch for pes planus, pes planovalgus, pes cavus, forefoot abduction, and forefoot varus (Fig. 60.2A). Check single- and double-leg heel rise to confirm that the heels invert and arches increase. Evaluate the forefoot for hallux valgus (or varus) and pronation; toe crossover, cock-up, hammering, or clawing of lesser toes (see Fig. 60.2B); and metatarsus adductus.

Gait Analysis

Inspect ambulation: Assess all phases of gait for asymmetric movement on either side of the body, degree of toeing in or out, inversion of the heel, and supination of the foot. Observe the medial longitudinal arch during the stance phase. Assess for antalgic, neuropathic (e.g., steppage), and myopathic (e.g., Trendelenburg) gait and symmetric strength during push-off.

Seated Examination

Visible abnormalities: Note varicosities, erythema, ecchymosis, edema, and muscle wasting.

Vascular: Palpate posterior tibial and dorsalis pedis pulses. Assess capillary refill time. Absence of hair distally may indicate peripheral vascular disease.

Skin: Note the location of callus formation, scars, wounds, blisters, ulcerations, and discoloration. Visualize toenails and nail beds.

Range of motion: Check active and passive ankle, subtalar, and transverse tarsal and first metatarsophalangeal joint (MTPJ) motion; compare them with the uninjured side. Notable crepitus during range-of-motion examination can indicate degenerative changes, fracture, or tissue thickening.

Strength testing: Test muscle groups against resistance—dorsiflexion, plantarflexion, inversion, and eversion; compare with the contralateral side.

Palpable Anatomic Structures

Bones: Fifth metatarsal base, peroneal tubercle, first tarsometatarsal joint, navicular tuberosity, head of talus, sustentaculum tali, lateral malleolus, medial malleolus, and metatarsal heads (see Fig. 60.1A)

Ligament attachments: Calcaneofibular ligament, anterior talofibular ligament, superficial deltoid ligament, spring ligament, and plantar fascia (see Fig. 60.1C)

Tendons: Posterior tibialis, flexor hallucis longus (FHL), anterior tibialis, peroneal brevis and longus, extensor hallucis longus, and Achilles (see Fig. 60.1C)

Bursae: Calcaneal, retrocalcaneal

Special Tests/Signs

Thompson test: Patient prone with affected leg extended; squeeze calf muscles to indirectly plantarflex the foot; failure of the foot to plantarflex (a positive test)

Abduction stress test: Manual abduction of the forefoot while stabilizing the hindfoot; assess for pain clinically and widening of Lisfranc joint on radiographs

Calcaneal compression text: Squeeze the posterior heel simultaneously from medial and lateral sides. Pain is a positive test and suggests stress fracture.

Too many toes sign: View the patient from behind; three or more toes visible lateral to the heel suggests forefoot abduction, often seen with posterior tibial tendon or spring ligament dysfunction (see Fig. 60.2A)

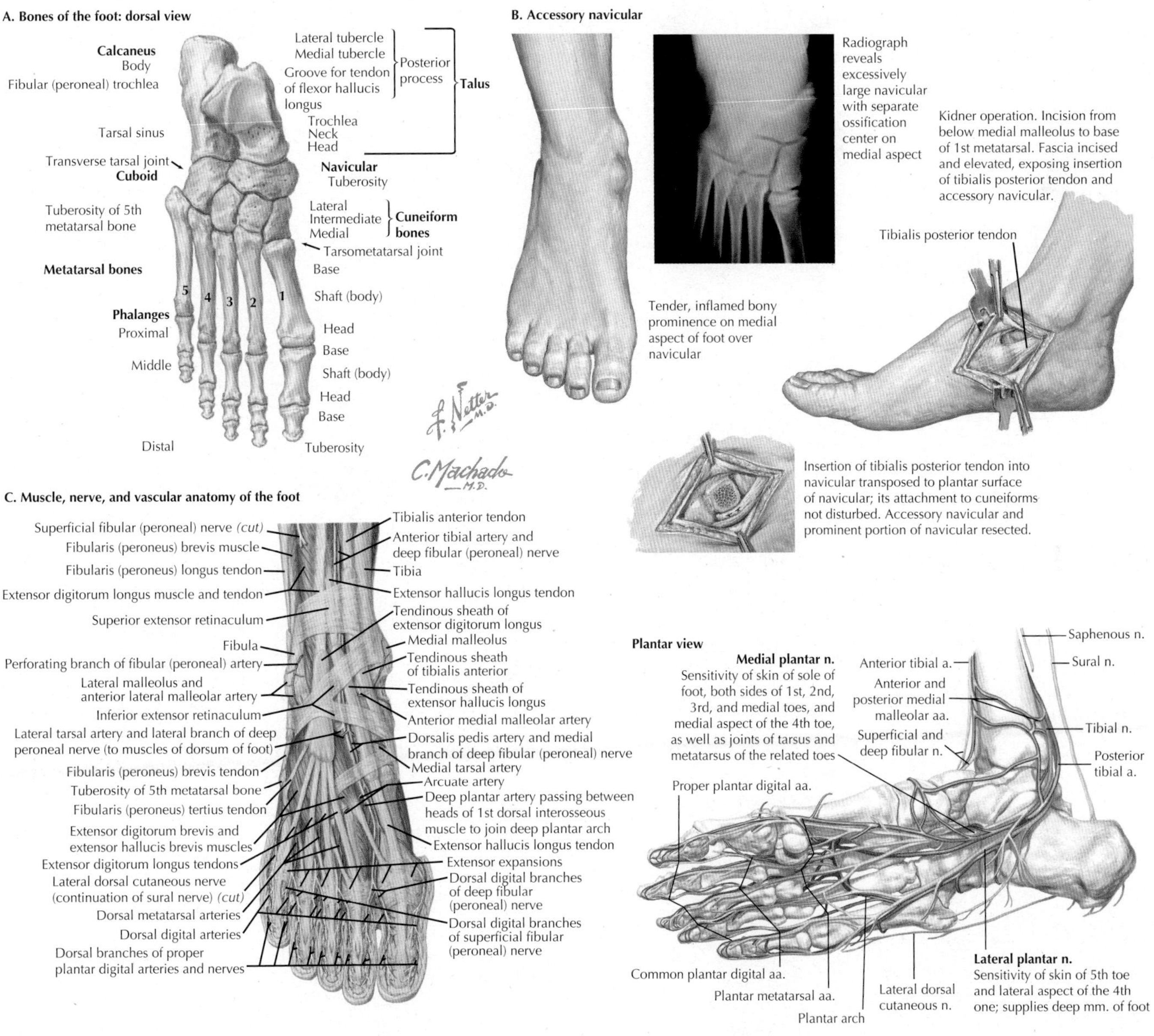
A. Bones of the foot: dorsal view
Calcaneus
Body
Fibular (peroneal) trochlea
Tarsal sinus
Transverse tarsal joint
Cuboid
Tuberosity of 5th metatarsal bone
Metatarsal bones
Phalanges
Proximal
Middle
Distal
Lateral tubercle
Medial tubercle
Groove for tendon of flexor hallucis longus
Posterior process
Talus
Trochlea
Neck
Head
Navicular
Tuberosity
Lateral
Intermediate
Medial
Cuneiform bones
Tarsometatarsal joint
Base
Shaft (body)
Head
Base
Shaft (body)
Head
Base
Tuberosity
5 4 3 2 1
B. Accessory navicular
Radiograph reveals excessively large navicular with separate ossification center on medial aspect
Kidner operation. Incision from below medial malleolus to base of 1st metatarsal. Fascia incised and elevated, exposing insertion of tibialis posterior tendon and accessory navicular.
Tibialis posterior tendon
Tender, inflamed bony prominence on medial aspect of foot over navicular
Insertion of tibialis posterior tendon into navicular transposed to plantar surface of navicular; its attachment to cuneiforms not disturbed. Accessory navicular and prominent portion of navicular resected.
F. Netter M.D.
C. Machado M.D.
C. Muscle, nerve, and vascular anatomy of the foot
Superficial fibular (peroneal) nerve (cut)
Fibularis (peroneus) brevis muscle
Fibularis (peroneus) longus tendon
Extensor digitorum longus muscle and tendon
Superior extensor retinaculum
Fibula
Perforating branch of fibular (peroneal) artery
Lateral malleolus and anterior lateral malleolar artery
Inferior extensor retinaculum
Lateral tarsal artery and lateral branch of deep peroneal nerve (to muscles of dorsum of foot)
Fibularis (peroneus) brevis tendon
Tuberosity of 5th metatarsal bone
Fibularis (peroneus) tertius tendon
Extensor digitorum brevis and extensor hallucis brevis muscles
Extensor digitorum longus tendons
Lateral dorsal cutaneous nerve (continuation of sural nerve) (cut)
Dorsal metatarsal arteries
Dorsal digital arteries
Dorsal branches of proper plantar digital arteries and nerves
Tibialis anterior tendon
Anterior tibial artery and deep fibular (peroneal) nerve
Tibia
Extensor hallucis longus tendon
Tendinous sheath of extensor digitorum longus
Medial malleolus
Tendinous sheath of tibialis anterior
Tendinous sheath of extensor hallucis longus
Anterior medial malleolar artery
Dorsalis pedis artery and medial branch of deep fibular (peroneal) nerve
Medial tarsal artery
Arcuate artery
Deep plantar artery passing between heads of 1st dorsal interosseous muscle to join deep plantar arch
Extensor hallucis longus tendon
Extensor expansions
Dorsal digital branches of deep fibular (peroneal) nerve
Dorsal digital branches of superficial fibular (peroneal) nerve
Plantar view
Medial plantar n.
Sensitivity of skin of sole of foot, both sides of 1st, 2nd, 3rd, and medial toes, and medial aspect of the 4th toe, as well as joints of tarsus and metatarsus of the related toes
Proper plantar digital aa.
Anterior tibial a.
Anterior and posterior medial malleolar aa.
Superficial and deep fibular n.
Saphenous n.
Sural n.
Tibial n.
Posterior tibial a.
Common plantar digital aa.
Plantar metatarsal aa.
Plantar arch
Lateral dorsal cutaneous n.
Lateral plantar n.
Sensitivity of skin of 5th toe and lateral aspect of the 4th one; supplies deep mm. of foot

Figure 60.1 Bones, muscles, and vessels of the foot.

Peek-a-boo heel sign: Viewed from the front, indicates hindfoot varus alignment (Fig. 60.3)

COMMON INJURIES AND DISORDERS OF THE FOOT

Skin and Nail Problems

For details, see Table 60.1, Fig. 60.4, and Chapter 40: "Skin Problems in the Athlete."

Tendinopathies (Table 60.2)

Etiology: Repetitive or abnormal stress on a tendon causes macrotears (acute trauma) or microtears (chronic overuse) with resulting inflammation (tendinitis) and ultimately tendon degeneration (tendinosis).

Common tendinopathies: Posterior tibial, Achilles, peroneal, anterior tibial, and FHL tendinopathy

Diagnostic considerations: Plain radiographs show alignment, mechanical risk factors, bony avulsions, and bony contributions (e.g., Haglunds and/or calcification at Achilles tendon insertion, os trigonum). Magnetic resonance imaging (MRI) and ultrasound best to assess tendon status and confirm partial or complete ruptures.

Treatment: Most tendinopathies will resolve with rest, protected weight bearing, ice, nonsteroidal anti-inflammatory drugs (NSAIDs), and addressing the risk factors. Acute tendon ruptures should typically be repaired in athletes (i.e., Achilles, posterior tibial, anterior tibial); peroneal tendon transfer can be considered in attritional peroneal ruptures and/or with advanced degenerative changes; surgery for tendinopathy only if conservative treatments fail.

Heel Pain in the Athlete

Plantar Fasciopathy

Etiology: Excessive tightness of gastrocsoleus complex pulling into Achilles tendon causes overload at plantar fascia origin on calcaneus during weight-bearing activities; results in microtears and inflammation (Fig. 60.5)

Symptoms/signs: Point tenderness/start-up pain, usually along medial tubercle of calcaneus; sometimes relieved with movement

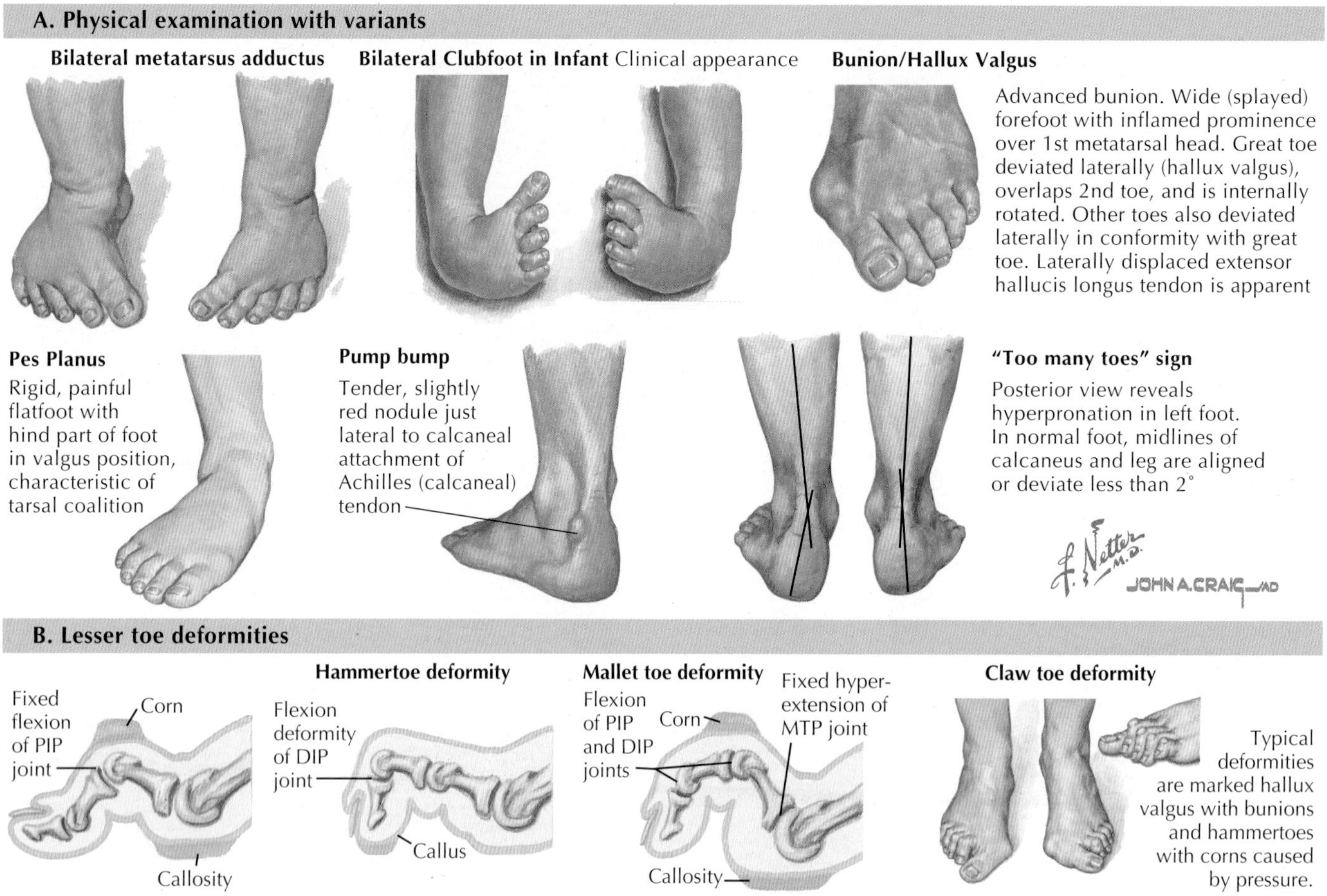
A. Physical examination with variants
Bilateral metatarsus adductus
Bilateral Clubfoot in Infant Clinical appearance
Bunion/Hallux Valgus
Advanced bunion. Wide (splayed) forefoot with inflamed prominence over 1st metatarsal head. Great toe deviated laterally (hallux valgus), overlaps 2nd toe, and is internally rotated. Other toes also deviated laterally in conformity with great toe. Laterally displaced extensor hallucis longus tendon is apparent
Pes Planus
Rigid, painful flatfoot with hind part of foot in valgus position, characteristic of tarsal coalition
Pump bump
Tender, slightly red nodule just lateral to calcaneal attachment of Achilles (calcaneal) tendon
"Too many toes" sign
Posterior view reveals hyperpronation in left foot. In normal foot, midlines of calcaneus and leg are aligned or deviate less than 2°
JOHN A.CRAIG MD
B. Lesser toe deformities
Fixed flexion of PIP joint
Corn
Callosity
Hammertoe deformity
Flexion deformity of DIP joint
Callus
Mallet toe deformity
Flexion of PIP and DIP joints
Corn
Callosity
Fixed hyper-extension of MTP joint
Claw toe deformity
Typical deformities are marked hallux valgus with bunions and hammertoes with corns caused by pressure.

Figure 60.2 Physical examination of the toe and deformities.

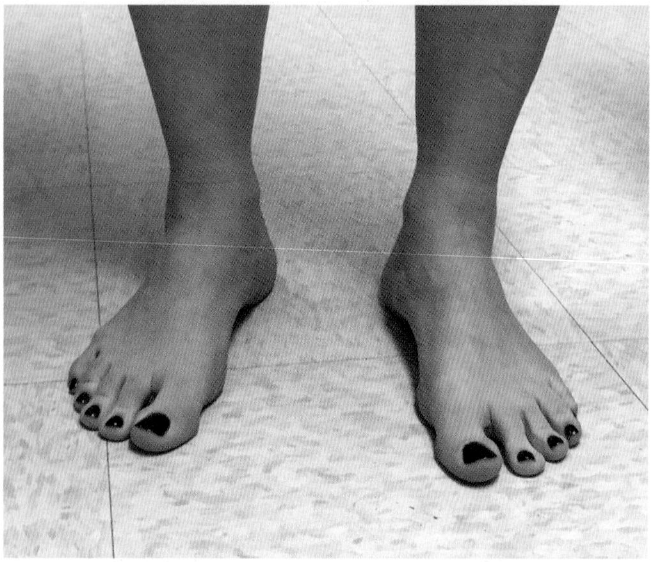

Figure 60.3 Peek-a-boo heel sign in hindfoot varus.

Imaging: Radiographs may show plantar calcaneal enthesophyte (usually not the cause of pain). MRI (see Fig. 60.5) or ultrasound can show thickening of plantar fascia/partial tear.

Differential diagnosis: Plantar fascial rupture; tarsal tunnel syndrome; calcaneal stress fracture; heel pad atrophy; and Baxter nerve entrapment

Treatment:
- Stretching, cushioned heel pad or orthoses, and supportive shoes (see Fig. 60.5)
- Decrease impact activities, ice/massage, and dorsiflexion night splint
- Refractory cases:
  - Corticosteroid injection: use with caution, risk of fat pad atrophy or plantar fascia rupture
  - Walking cast
  - Extracorporeal shock wave treatment
  - Percutaneous ultrasonic probe
  - Platelet-rich plasma injection
  - Endoscopic calcaneoplasty with partial fasciectomy

Sever Disease (Calcaneal Apophysitis)

Etiology: Heel pain in children between 9 and 14 years of age participating in running sports; often biomechanical abnormality contributing to poor shock absorption, such as equinus, hallux valgus, pes cavus, and pes planus; occasionally, acute trauma (e.g., violent heel strike)

Symptoms/signs: Posterior heel pain, worse during and after activity and improves with rest, tender to palpation at or just inferior to Achilles insertion. Positive "squeeze" test: compression of medial and lateral aspects of calcaneal apophysis produces pain. Positive "Severs test": heel pain aggravated by heel rise.

Imaging: Radiographs characterized by fragmentation, sclerosis, and increased density of apophysis that mimic the appearance of osteonecrosis; changes are best viewed on lateral radiographs

Table 60.1 SKIN AND NAIL PROBLEMS

Type	Cause	Signs and Symptoms	Treatment
Calluses and corns	Excessive localized friction or pressure from tight shoes or structural abnormalities of feet, such as hammertoes	Pain; thickening and hardening of skin (soft corns between toes because of moisture)	Appropriate shoe fitting, padding (e.g., doughnut pad), pumice stone, resection of bony prominences, metatarsal pad, Budin splint
Blisters	Friction, pressure Epidermal/dermal separation by serous fluid	Painful vesicles	Unruptured: sterile dressing, pressure relief Ruptured: sterile cleansing, dressing (consider antibiotics for diabetic patients or signs of infection in any patient)
Warts	Virus (papilloma)	Pain at site; skin thickening with central core; flat or raised	Trichloroacetic acid or salicylic acid, liquid nitrogen
Tinea pedis (athlete's foot)	Fungus	Dry or vesicular lesions; scaling, peeling, and cracking fissures in skin; deformed nails, hyphae, and buds on KOH wet mount	Dry: miconazole, clotrimazole, terbinafine, salicylic acid Vesicular: wet dressings with Burrow solution Erythema or other signs of infection: consider antibiotics
Paronychia	Soft tissue infection around the nail	Inflamed nail margin with or without drainage	Warm water soaks, antibiotics; partial nail resection; appropriate nail-cutting techniques
Subungual hematoma	Trauma	Dark blood under nail; pain/pressure at site	Drainage (insert no. 18 needle or drill sterilely through nail) Note: Ensure traumatic history to distinguish from subungual melanoma

Differential diagnosis: Achilles tendinitis/strain, heel pad pain, retrocalcaneal bursitis, calcaneal stress fracture, and plantar fasciitis

Treatment: Rest (crutches in severe cases), activity modification, ice, heel lifts or cups, stretching and strengthening, NSAIDs; if still resistant—dorsiflexion night splint and rarely, short leg cast for 2 weeks, orthoses

Forefoot Disorders

Turf Toe

Etiology: Hyperextension of MTPJ of great toe leads to a spectrum of injuries from plantar plate tear to dislocation (Fig. 60.6)

Mechanism of injury: Typically, an axial load on a foot fixed in equinus with MTPJ in hyperextension (e.g., football linemen during push-off)

Symptoms/signs: Pain, tenderness, and swelling at great toe MTPJ and plantarflexion weakness; positive great toe Lachman test; compare with the contralateral side

Imaging: Radiographs may show proximal migration of sesamoids with plantar plate rupture (see Fig. 60.6). Stress fluoroscopy to evaluate sesamoid tracking of the sesamoids; MRI (see Fig. 60.6) to determine injury severity and surgical planning.

Differential diagnosis: Phalangeal or metatarsal fracture, osteochondral injury, hallux rigidus, osteoarthritis, and gout

Treatment: Rest, ice/NSAIDs acutely, taping to limit MTPJ motion, walking boot until pain free, metatarsal pad to unload first metatarsal may be helpful; rigid shoe or insert to limit MTPJ hyperextension; surgery considered in complete rupture, unstable joint, sesamoid fracture, traumatic hallux valgus, or chondral injury with loose body

Hallux Valgus (Bunion)

Etiology: Associated with increased ligamentous laxity, inappropriate shoe fit, pes planus, heredity, posttraumatic, and/or inflammatory conditions; more common in females

Symptoms/signs: Pain usually secondary to pressure and friction on prominent medial eminence (i.e., bunion); soft tissues may become inflamed, thickened, and painful (Fig. 60.7), causing nerve irritation; secondary deformities (e.g., hammertoes, callosities, and metatarsalgia) may contribute to pain and discomfort.

Imaging: Standing radiographs to assess hallux valgus and intermetatarsal angles, MTPJ congruity and arthritis, distal metatarsal articular angle (DMAA), and sesamoid position (see Fig. 60.7)

Treatment: Conservative measures to provide pain relief: shoes with adequate forefoot width and arch support; pads to cushion bunion, toe separators, and orthoses to help redistribute weight; surgery for cases that fail conservative management and limit sports participation and should be avoided in sprinters, high jumpers, pole vaulters, and ballet dancers if possible because of the risk of decreased MTPJ range of motion; wait until end of athlete's career or until whenever possible

Hallux Rigidus

Etiology: Limitation of MTPJ motion, particularly dorsiflexion; mechanical block because of periarticular osteophytes; usually posttraumatic, but can result from chronic turf toe, repetitive microtrauma (runners), primary arthrosis

Symptoms/signs: Tender palpable MTPJ osteophyte(s); decreased and painful first MTPJ dorsiflexion; pain increased with running, incline training, and wearing shoes with elevated heels (Fig. 60.8)

Imaging: Weight-bearing anteroposterior (AP), lateral, and oblique views; may be normal initially; nonuniform narrowing of first MTPJ with widening and flattening of the metatarsal head, loose body, marginal osteophytes; dorsal exostosis of first metatarsal is the hallmark.

Treatment: Shoe modifications (stiff sole, rocker bottom, extradepth toe box), metatarsal bar, NSAIDs, orthoses with Morton extension, and intra-articular steroid injections; surgical options include cheilectomy or fusion to relieve impingement and decrease pain; proximal phalanx osteotomy may benefit a running athlete by improving dorsiflexion movement. Arthroplasty procedures are available but not optimal in athletes.

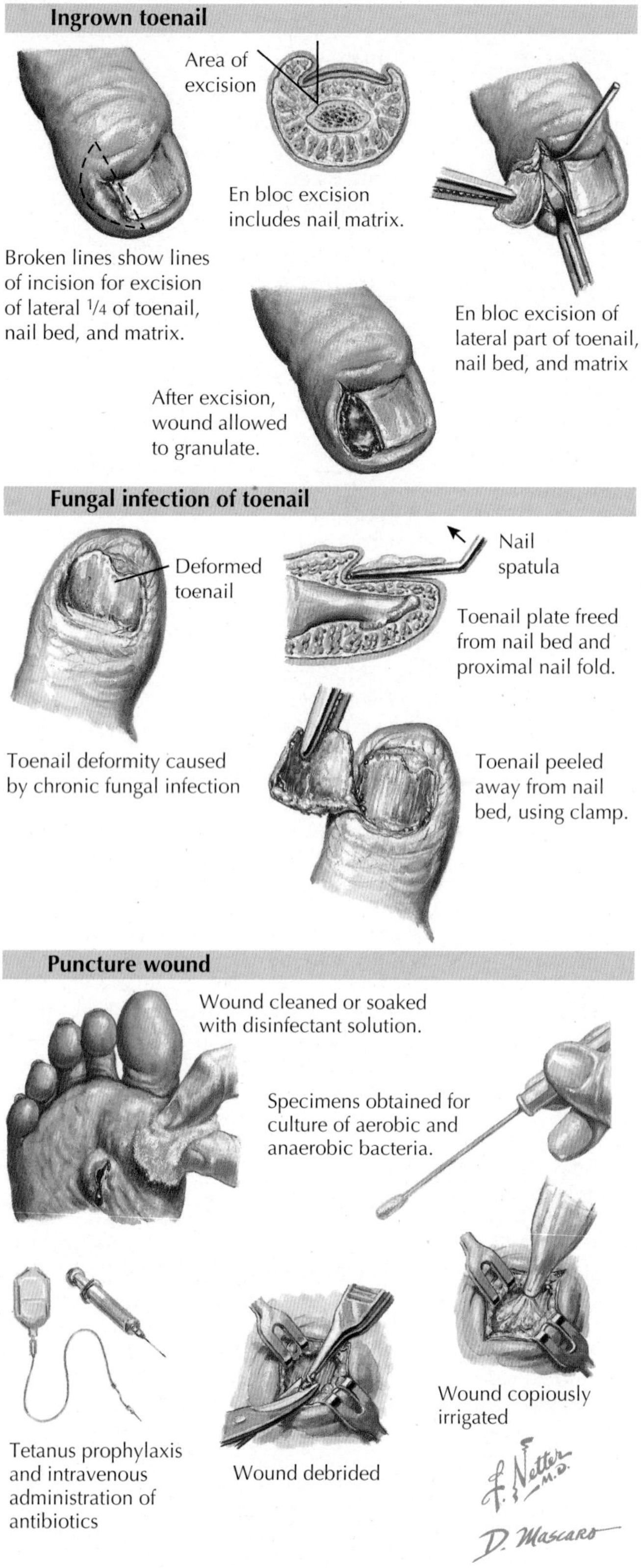
Ingrown toenail
Area of excision
En bloc excision includes nail matrix.
Broken lines show lines of incision for excision of lateral 1/4 of toenail, nail bed, and matrix.
En bloc excision of lateral part of toenail, nail bed, and matrix
After excision, wound allowed to granulate.
Fungal infection of toenail
Deformed toenail
Nail spatula
Toenail plate freed from nail bed and proximal nail fold.
Toenail deformity caused by chronic fungal infection
Toenail peeled away from nail bed, using clamp.
Puncture wound
Wound cleaned or soaked with disinfectant solution.
Specimens obtained for culture of aerobic and anaerobic bacteria.
Wound copiously irrigated
Tetanus prophylaxis and intravenous administration of antibiotics
Wound debrided

Figure 60.4 Nail problems in the foot.

Lesser MTPJ Instability

Etiology: Overload of metatarsal head leading to repetitive stress and attritional tear of MTPJ plantar plate

Symptoms/signs: Pain under metatarsal head (second most common), hammertoe deformity, swelling, and toe subluxation or dislocation

Imaging: Radiographs often show long second metatarsal and MTPJ subluxation or dislocation. MRI shows the grade of plantar plate injury.

Treatment: Rest, ice, splinting of toe, and stiff-soled shoes; surgery to repair plantar plate in recalcitrant cases

Bone Stress Injuries

Navicular Stress Fracture

Etiology: Common in running and jumping athletes; repetitive cyclic loading, explosive push-off; unique vascular anatomy results in relatively avascular central one-third; more common in cavus foot; frequently missed, delay in diagnosis by up to 4–7 months reported

Symptoms/signs: Ill-defined midfoot to anterior ankle soreness and cramping; insidious onset, progresses to frequent pain with activity; pain with percussion over navicular, N-spot tenderness to palpation, and symptom exacerbation with single-leg hop

Imaging: Foot radiographs often negative; bone scan highly sensitive, uptake seen in all three phases; MRI highly sensitive; computed tomography (CT): gold standard, defines location, completeness, direction, and displacement; fracture line usually proximal-dorsal to distal-plantar

Treatment: Nonweight-bearing short leg cast for 6–8 weeks; if remains tender to palpation, replace in cast; otherwise, progressive return to activity; persistent symptoms, delayed union, or displaced fractures require surgery (internal fixation with or without bone grafting); recovery can take up to 1 year.

Calcaneal Fractures

Etiology: Acute fractures are rare in athletes. Stress fractures more common, usually in endurance sports.

Symptoms/signs: Localized pain in heel, accentuated by weight bearing; mild swelling; pain with medial-lateral compression of calcaneus

Imaging: Stress fracture: May see line at posterior-superior aspect of the calcaneus perpendicular to the trabeculae; if negative, bone scan or MRI

Treatment: Modified rest with cessation of impact activities; cast or walking boot with crutches may be appropriate; gradual return to activity when clinical symptoms abate and serial radiographic assessment documents healing. Full healing can take 2–3 months. Consider shock-absorbing orthotic devices on returning to activity.

Traumatic: Closed or open treatment depending on severity of fracture

Jones Fracture

Etiology: Stress fracture of the fifth metatarsal at metaphyseal-diaphyseal junction in the region of or just distal to the fourth-to-fifth metatarsal articulation (Fig. 60.9); frequently seen in sprinters and jumpers; foot posture is a contributing factor; often have difficulty healing because of poor blood flow.

Imaging: Plain radiographs usually sufficient to show fracture; cortical thickening a sign of chronic stress; MRI can show bone stress injury or incomplete stress fracture.

Treatment: Cast for 4–6 weeks, followed by 4–6 weeks in walking boot; approximately 75% will heal with nonsurgical treatment, but 30%–50% will refracture. Surgical stabilization with intramedullary screw for acute fracture in athletes, nonunion, refracture, and cavovarus foot with lateral overload; plantar lateral plating an option; bone grafting considered when treating delayed union or nonunion.

Sesamoiditis

Etiology: Usually repetitive trauma in running/jumping sports; contributing factors include mechanical overload caused by pes cavus, ankle equinus, and poor footwear. Anatomic variations that can contribute to mechanical overload include absent crista, variations in sesamoid size, and significant metatarsal rotation.

Table 60.2 INFLAMMATORY CONDITIONS

Type	Signs and Symptoms	Treatment
Posterior tibial tendinitis	Medial arch pain, swelling, pain with resisted inversion, painful or inability to perform single heel rise, medial arch collapse, "too many toes sign": when viewed from behind, abducted forefoot allows more toes to be seen on the affected side	Initial: rest, ice, NSAIDs, orthoses with arch support, and medial heel wedge Rehabilitation[a]: plantarflexion and inversion strengthening exercises, heel cord flexibility Surgical: treatment ranges from osteotomy with tendon transfer to arthrodesis
Peroneal tendinitis	Lateral pain, particularly with active and resisted eversion; swelling; may complain of snapping sensation in cases of peroneal tendon subluxation; may be the result of underlying tendon tear	Initial: rest, ice, NSAIDs, orthoses, cast, or boot Rehabilitation[a]: eversion strengthening exercises; surgery may be required for recalcitrant cases, tears, or subluxation
Anterior tibial tendinitis	Pain in anterior medial foot, worse with active dorsiflexion; swelling and crepitation; seen in runners, hikers, and racquet sports	Initial: activity modification, ice, NSAIDs, and walking boot Rehabilitation[a]: dorsiflexion strengthening exercises
Achilles tendinitis	Decreased gastrocnemius flexibility; pain, tenderness, swelling, and crepitation; pain with active plantarflexion; radiographs to look for Haglund deformity or insertional calcifications	Rule out systemic conditions such as gout or spondyloarthropathy Initial: rest, ice, NSAIDs, and heel pads Rehabilitation[a]: heel cord stretching and strengthening exercises; possible surgical debridement in chronic cases
Retrocalcaneal bursitis	Posterior heel/ankle pain; tenderness and swelling in bursa located between the Achilles tendon and the calcaneus	Initial: rest, ice, NSAIDs, heel cup, and shoe modification Rehabilitation[a]: heel cord stretching, modalities, strengthening exercises
Sesamoiditis	Generic term; local tenderness (tibial side most common); pain worse with weight bearing; rule out avascular necrosis, sesamoid fracture. Bipartite sesamoid reported 10% tibial, rare fibular.	Reduce weight-bearing stress at site; orthoses with sesamoid relief or Morton extension; ice, NSAIDs, use of stiff-soled shoe or walking boot; if conservative treatment fails: bone scan, computed tomography, or MRI to rule out stress fracture
Metatarsophalangeal joint synovitis	Pain at metatarsophalangeal joint (second most common), positive Lachman test (increased anterior-posterior translation), and joint crepitus; distinguish from interdigital neuroma	Metatarsal pad, figure-of-eight taping, Budin splint, NSAIDs, steroid injection (with caution), and surgery for failed nonsurgical treatment

MRI, Magnetic resonance imaging; *NSAIDs,* nonsteroidal anti-inflammatory drugs.
[a]Rehabilitation includes maintenance of aerobic, well-leg, and upper-body fitness; physical therapy modalities, such as phonophoresis and iontophoresis, may also be useful.

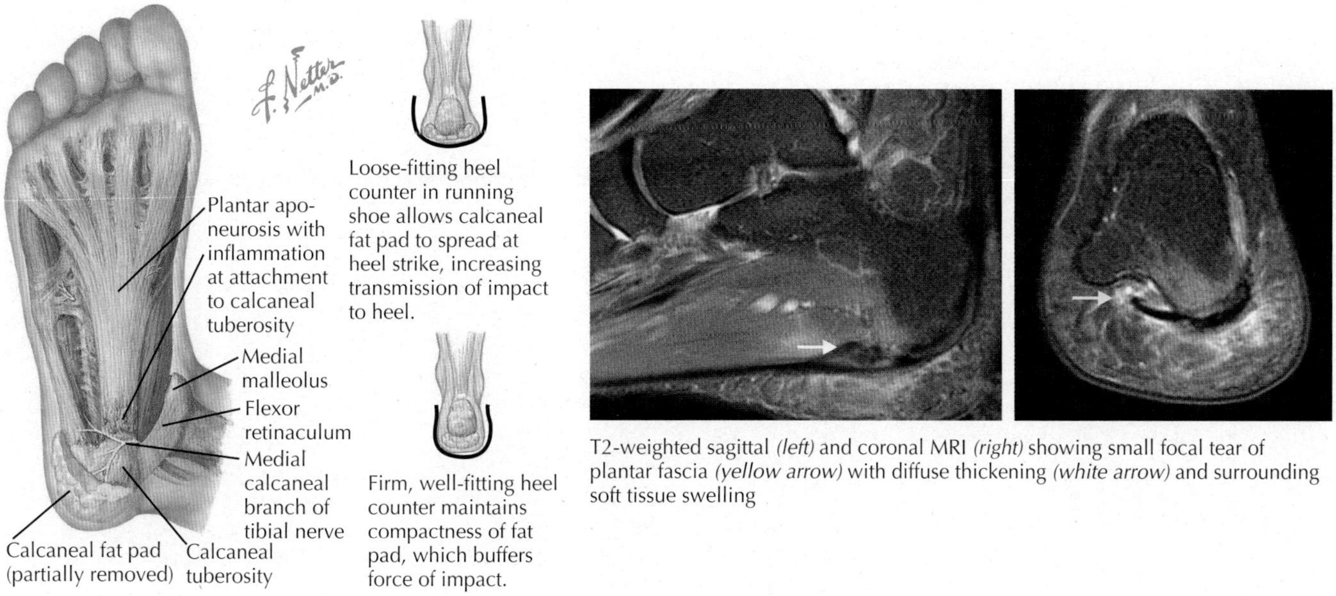

F. Netter M.D.
Plantar aponeurosis with inflammation at attachment to calcaneal tuberosity
Medial malleolus
Flexor retinaculum
Medial calcaneal branch of tibial nerve
Calcaneal fat pad (partially removed)
Calcaneal tuberosity
Loose-fitting heel counter in running shoe allows calcaneal fat pad to spread at heel strike, increasing transmission of impact to heel.
Firm, well-fitting heel counter maintains compactness of fat pad, which buffers force of impact.

T2-weighted sagittal *(left)* and coronal MRI *(right)* showing small focal tear of plantar fascia *(yellow arrow)* with diffuse thickening *(white arrow)* and surrounding soft tissue swelling

Figure 60.5 Plantar fasciitis.

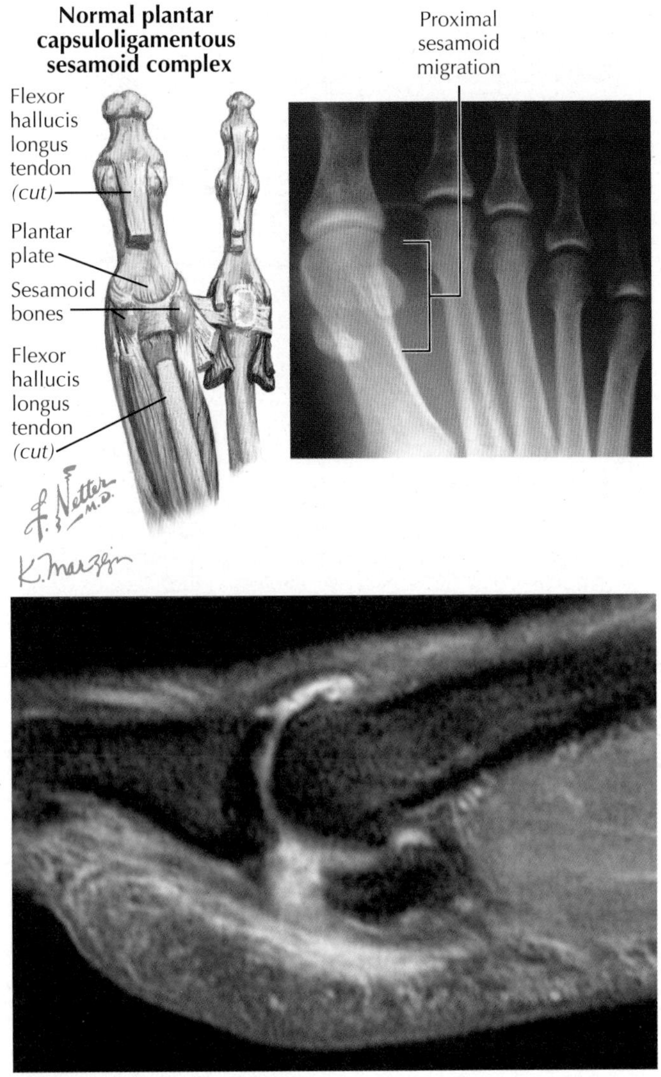
Normal plantar capsuloligamentous sesamoid complex
Flexor hallucis longus tendon (cut)
Plantar plate
Sesamoid bones
Flexor hallucis longus tendon (cut)
Proximal sesamoid migration

Plantar plate injury on MRI scan

Figure 60.6 Turf toe.

Symptoms/signs: Insidious, unilateral plantar forefoot pain with weight bearing, exacerbated by certain shoes or activities, focal to one or both sesamoids (tibial sesamoid most common); range of motion of the hallux MTPJ usually painless; direct tenderness and tenderness on resisted plantarflexion of the hallux indicate sesamoid pathology; attention to mechanical alignment of the foot is important.

Imaging: Plain radiographs (AP, lateral, and sesamoid views) show bony contour, bipartite sesamoid, fracture, and advanced avascular necrosis (AVN); MRI more sensitive for AVN, stress fracture, and injury acuity; bone scan and CT scan can also identify stress fracture and differentiate between bipartite and fracture.

Treatment: ***Sesamoiditis:*** Reduce weight-bearing stress at site; orthoses with sesamoid relief or Morton extension; ice, NSAIDs, use of stiff-soled shoe, carbon fiber insole, or walking boot; if conservative treatment fails, bone scan, CT, or MRI to rule out stress fracture.

Fracture: Immobilization, protected weight bearing (cast or boot), custom-molded orthosis to address mechanical contributors; if conservative treatment fails, surgical options include partial or complete sesamoidectomy. Beware of transfer sesamoiditis and alignment changes.

Acute Fractures

Talus Fractures

Etiology:

- **Acute trauma:** Rare in sports, often a surgical emergency; talar neck fractures are associated with severe foot dislocation
- **Stress fractures:** Also rare; symptoms/signs include diffuse midfoot pain, anterior ankle tenderness on palpation, and painful active and passive motion of subtalar joint
  - *Note:* Subtalar joint allows eversion/inversion.
- **Lateral process fractures:** "Snowboarder's fracture"; frequently misdiagnosed as a lateral ankle sprain; mechanism is acute dorsiflexion with inversion of foot and axial load.

Imaging: Radiographs usually provide definitive diagnosis. Subtle or stress fractures usually require bone scan or CT. Lateral process fractures are seen best on coronal CT images (Fig. 60.10).

Treatment:

- **Talus fractures:** Nondisplaced or stress fractures require rest, cessation of weight-bearing activity for 6 weeks followed by walking boot; displaced fractures usually require surgical open reduction and internal fixation (ORIF).

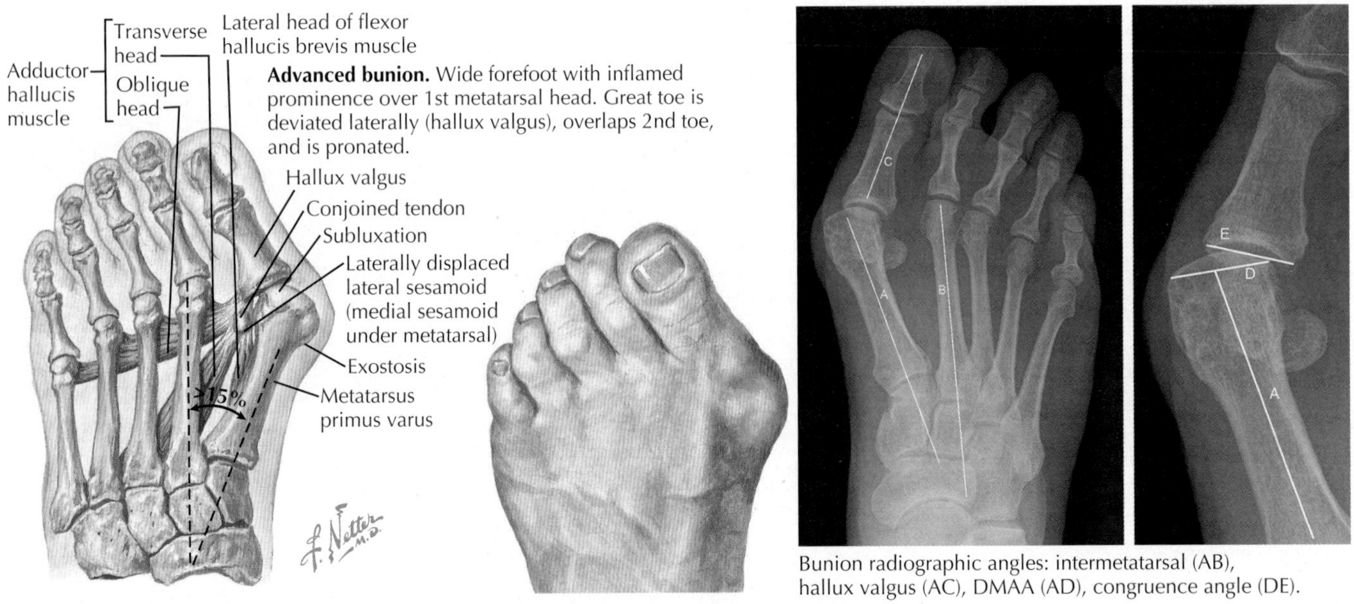
Adductor hallucis muscle
Transverse head
Oblique head
Lateral head of flexor hallucis brevis muscle
Advanced bunion. Wide forefoot with inflamed prominence over 1st metatarsal head. Great toe is deviated laterally (hallux valgus), overlaps 2nd toe, and is pronated.
Hallux valgus
Conjoined tendon
Subluxation
Laterally displaced lateral sesamoid (medial sesamoid under metatarsal)
Exostosis
Metatarsus primus varus
15%
C
A
B
E
D
A

Bunion radiographic angles: intermetatarsal (AB), hallux valgus (AC), DMAA (AD), congruence angle (DE).

Figure 60.7 Bunions and hallux valgus.

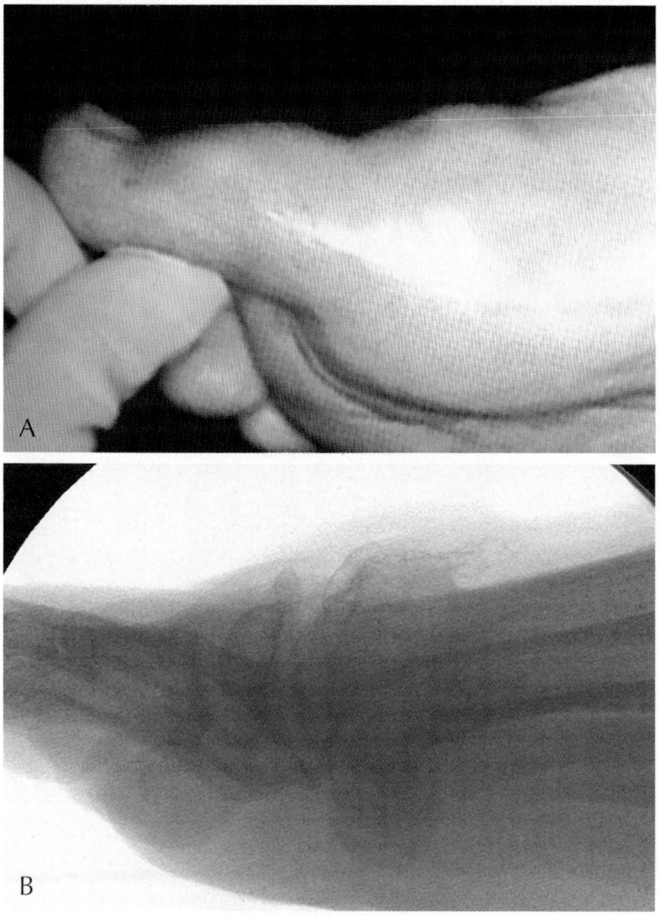
A
B

Figure 60.8 Hallux rigidus.

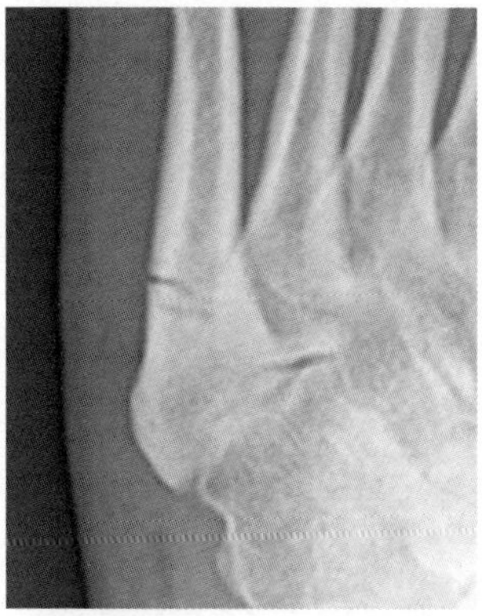

Figure 60.9 Jones fracture.

- **Lateral process fractures:** Treatment determined by fragment size, comminution, and displacement; nondisplaced—nonweight-bearing boot or cast for 6 weeks; displaced—ORIF or excision of fragment(s)

Midfoot/Forefoot Fractures

Lisfranc Injury

Etiology: Traumatic injury: (1) twisting of forefoot (e.g., equestrian foot caught in stirrup during fall); (2) axial load with foot in equinus (e.g., football and soccer); and (3) crush injury (Fig. 60.11). Lisfranc ligament runs from plantar-medial cuneiform to the base of the second metatarsal; no intermetatarsal ligament between the first and second metatarsals; important to identify the injury, particularly in subtle cases.

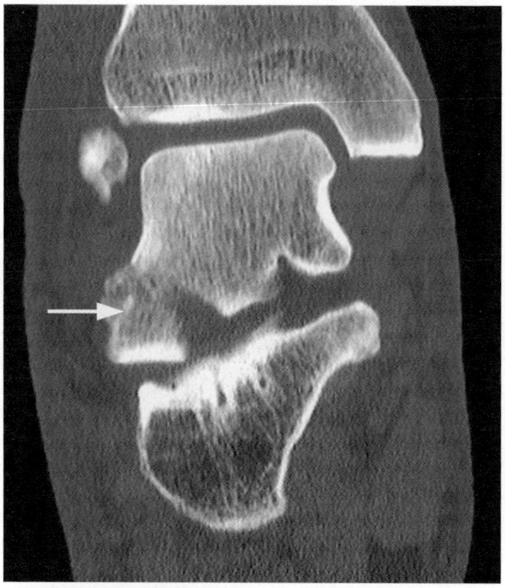

Figure 60.10 Coronal CT lateral process fracture.

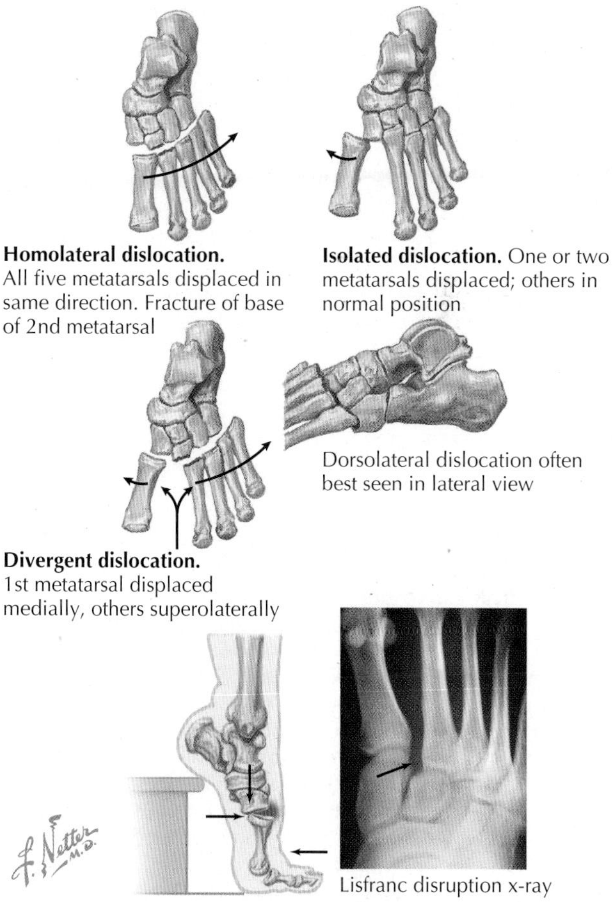
Homolateral dislocation. All five metatarsals displaced in same direction. Fracture of base of 2nd metatarsal
Isolated dislocation. One or two metatarsals displaced; others in normal position
Divergent dislocation. 1st metatarsal displaced medially, others superolaterally
Dorsolateral dislocation often best seen in lateral view
Lisfranc disruption x-ray

Figure 60.11 Lisfranc injuries.

Symptoms/signs: Pain and inability to bear weight or push off; swelling and gross deformity if severe; may have spontaneous reduction after injury

Imaging: Weight-bearing AP, lateral, and oblique radiographs; compare with contralateral side; medial border of second metatarsal should parallel medial border of the middle cuneiform on AP; medial border of fourth metatarsal should parallel medial

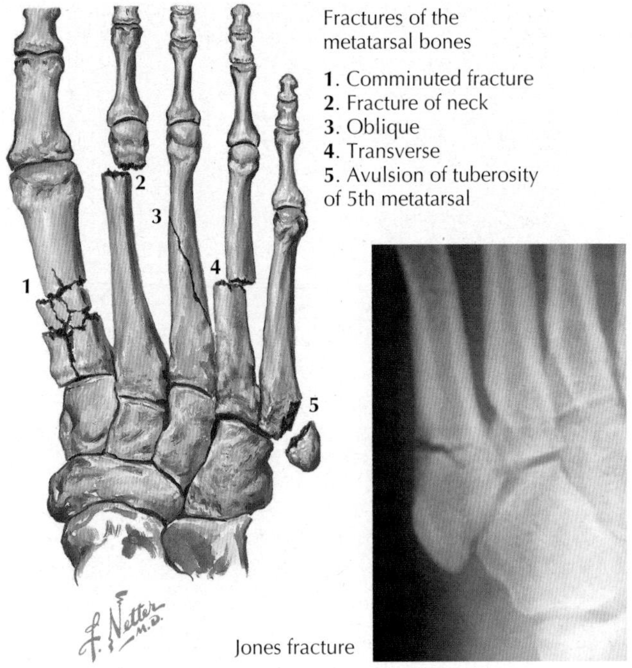
Fractures of the metatarsal bones
1. Comminuted fracture
2. Fracture of neck
3. Oblique
4. Transverse
5. Avulsion of tuberosity of 5th metatarsal
1
2
3
4
5
Jones fracture

Figure 60.12 Metatarsal fractures.

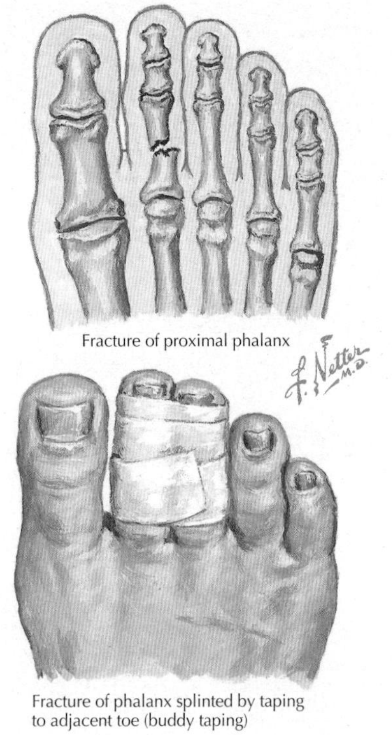
Fracture of proximal phalanx
Fracture of phalanx splinted by taping to adjacent toe (buddy taping)

Figure 60.13 Phalangeal fractures.

border of cuboid on oblique. Look for widening between first and second metatarsals and medial and middle cuneiform, small fracture fragment pathopneumonic; MRI if suspicion is high and radiographs are equivocal

Treatment: Sprains can be placed in a CAM boot. Nondisplaced with ligament disruption in nonweight-bearing cast; displaced injuries require ORIF using screws, plates, or flexible devices.

Metatarsal Fractures

Etiology: **Traumatic:** Direct blow to the foot or hard landing on forefoot

Stress: More common and the result of repetitive loading; associated with increased mechanical loading; seen in endurance running and jumping sports. Be aware of female triad (anorexia, amenorrhea, and osteoporosis).

Symptoms/signs: Localized pain with weight bearing, swelling, and tenderness

Imaging: Plain radiographs confirm most acute fractures (Fig. 60.12); may be negative for stress fractures; bone scan or MRI may be necessary to detect early stress lesions; CT more specific for stress fractures

Treatment:

- Acute fractures: ORIF if displaced or intra-articular
- **Second through fourth metatarsal stress fractures:** Nonsurgical treatment (first metatarsal stress fracture rarely seen); modified rest with cessation of weight-bearing activities and immobilization in cast or boot for 3 weeks may be used depending on the pain control needs; gradual return to activity when symptoms subside; base of the second metatarsal may show delayed or nonunion, thus requiring bone grafting and/or ORIF
- **Avulsion fracture of the base of the fifth metatarsal:** Common with ankle sprains; nonsurgical treatment successful in most cases; consider ORIF if displaced or nonunion

Phalangeal Fractures

Etiology: Trauma such as crush, direct blow, or jamming

Symptoms/signs: Pain, deformity, swelling, and ecchymosis

Imaging: Plain radiographs confirmatory

Treatment: Conservative unless open fracture or intraarticular fracture of great toe with displacement

- **Nondisplaced:** Buddy taping to adjacent toe and protection in stiff-soled shoe; symptoms dictate activity restrictions (Fig. 60.13)
- **Displaced:** Reduced by manipulation; subsequent buddy-taping/splinting
- **Complications:** Intra-articular fractures can result in joint stiffness and arthritis: consider ORIF.

Neurologic Injuries

Tarsal Tunnel Syndrome

Description: Entrapment of posterior tibial nerve at flexor retinaculum behind medial malleolus

Etiology: Trauma (subtalar dislocation or fractures); compression from space-occupying lesion (e.g., ganglion); systemic disorders (e.g., diabetes mellitus); biomechanical dysfunction (e.g., hindfoot valgus or tarsal coalition); idiopathic

Symptoms/signs: Aching pain at the medial foot, aggravated by prolonged weight bearing, radiating to plantar foot, plantar foot numbness/tingling; positive Tinel sign (tapping over tibial nerve causes radiating pain along nerve distribution); Valleix phenomenon (neural percussion causes radiation of pain proximally along course of nerve)

Diagnostics: Radiographs obtained to assess foot alignment, malunion, and exostosis; MRI visualizes soft tissue space-occupying lesions (Fig. 60.14); electromyography (EMG) and nerve conduction studies are abnormal in 80% of cases.

Differential diagnosis: Posterior tibial tendinitis, calcaneal stress fracture, gout, plantar fasciitis, and herniated lumbar disc

Treatment: Rest, NSAIDs, graduated return to activity; orthoses; local steroid injection; surgical decompression for intractable cases; best results with surgical decompression in cases caused by space-occupying lesions without nerve damage

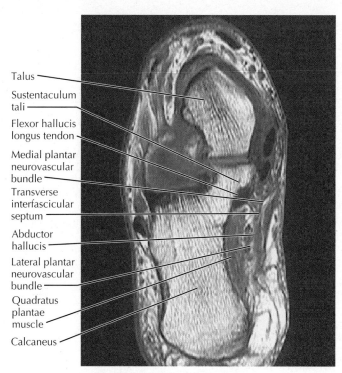

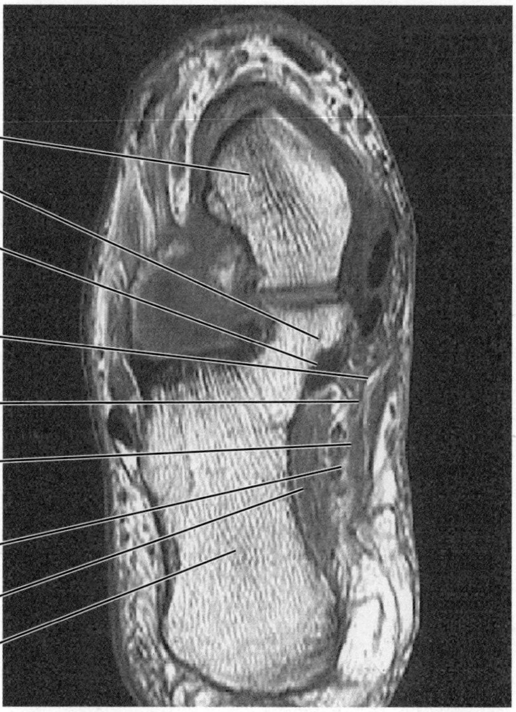
Talus
Sustentaculum tali
Flexor hallucis longus tendon
Medial plantar neurovascular bundle
Transverse interfascicular septum
Abductor hallucis
Lateral plantar neurovascular bundle
Quadratus plantae muscle
Calcaneus

Figure 60.14 Tarsal tunnel anatomy.

Interdigital (Morton) Neuroma

Description: Impingement of interdigital nerves as they bifurcate at metatarsal heads

Etiology: Trauma and/or repetitive stress leads to chronic irritation of nerves as they cross under transverse metatarsal ligament to toes; fusiform swelling and pathologic changes occur in nerves.

Symptoms/signs: Pain, burning neuralgia with radiation into involved toes; symptoms worse with activity and narrow shoes; sensation of "walking on marbles"; third interspace most common (Morton), followed by second interspace; tender to palpation between metatarsal heads, pain with squeeze of metatarsals; Mulder click: squeeze the forefoot from medial to lateral while palpating the web space; positive test is a click or gritty sensation

Differential diagnosis: Metatarsalgia, metatarsal stress fractures, MTPJ synovitis, and neuropathy

Radiographic assessment: Usually negative; evaluate for stress fracture, MTPJ synovitis, and compression from exostosis

Treatment: Initial: NSAIDs, metatarsal pads, wide toe-box shoes, lower heel, corticosteroid injection

Chronic: Surgical excision of nerve; patient may lose sensation between involved toes but no functional deficits; recurrence from stump neuroma may occur

Chronic Regional Pain Syndrome (CRPS)

Description: Pain syndrome accompanied by evidence of autonomic dysfunction

Etiology: **Type I:** unknown etiology, insidious onset; **type II** can occur after injury or trauma; likely results from dysfunction of autonomic nervous system

Symptoms/signs: Onset is heralded by severe, diffuse, unrelenting pain with exquisite tenderness to even light touch out of proportion to original injury; decreased range of motion and autonomic vasomotor signs, including warm or cool skin temperatures and decreased peripheral pulses. Skin may be moist/sweaty or dry/scaly with discoloration and swelling.

Imaging: Radiographs may reveal diffuse osteopenia of the involved foot. Bone scan may show delayed pattern of diffuse increased tracer throughout the foot, with juxta-articular accentuation of tracer uptake.

Differential diagnosis: Peripheral nerve injuries, polymyositis, lupus, Raynaud disease, gout, and thrombophlebitis

Treatment: Prompt diagnosis and therapy improve the chances of permanent relief. Refer to a pain management specialist. Sympathetic blockade relieves pain. Physical therapy includes vigorously active exercises, weight-bearing activities, and direct stimulation of skin. Adjuvant pharmacologic agents and psychological evaluation required in more difficult cases. Occasionally, chemical or surgical sympathectomy is required.

RECOMMENDED READINGS

Available online.

61 TAPING AND BRACING

Rebecca Ann Myers

GENERAL PRINCIPLES

- Taping and bracing are used as **adjuncts** to sports protective equipment, treatment, and rehabilitation of an injury.
- Should not take the place of appropriate diagnostic, treatment, and rehabilitation of an injury
- Role in prevention, treatment, rehabilitation, and return-to-play decisions

Functions of Taping and Bracing

Prevention: Aid in stabilization, support, and protection of uninjured or fully rehabilitated joints and soft tissues

Treatment: Minimize pain and swelling in the acute phase, aid in unloading painful structures, and provide support to unstable joints

Rehabilitation: Aid in early mobilization, muscle imbalances, neural control, proprioception, and protect healing injuries

Physician's Role in Taping and Bracing

- **Determine the appropriateness of taping/bracing.**
- **Facilitate the selection process.**
  - **Identify** available options.
  - **Communicate** with the treatment team: athlete, parent, certified athletic trainer, physical therapist, and coach
- **Evaluate effectiveness** of the selected support.

Implementation of Taping and Bracing

- **Athlete's acceptance:** Involve the athlete in the decision-making process; must be comfortable and functional; realize positive psychological effects of taping and bracing, which may improve athlete's confidence on returning to competition
- **Sporting equipment regulations:** Know the sport's regulations. Equipment modifications may be needed. Use materials that do not endanger other athletes. Exposed metal must be covered during contact sports. The environment will affect options.

Practical Considerations

Prescription: Braces may require physician prescription, which needs to include diagnosis code, type of brace, length of need, and, occasionally, statement of medical necessity.

Cost: Taping materials and braces can be costly. Athletic departments may or may not cover full expense. Insurance coverage varies, and durable medical equipment may not contribute toward the patient's deductible.

Marketing: Types of tape, taping techniques, and braces are full of unsubstantiated claims and disclaimers of liability. New products should be viewed with an open, but critical, mind.

PRINCIPLES OF TAPING

Preparation

Decide on an appropriate technique. Gather required tape supplies. Place the athlete's body part in position of function and/or protection. Use an appropriate table height to optimize the taper's body mechanics.

Types of Tape

- Nonstretch tape: good tensile strength with cloth backing that gives mechanical support to ligaments and joints; can also be used to reinforce stretch tape (e.g., standard trainer's athletic tape)
- Stretch tape: may be a one-way stretch (in length or width) or two-way stretch (in length and width); conforms to contours of the body and allows normal tissue expansion; typically requires scissors to tear and is more expensive (e.g., Kinesiotape, Elastikon, Lightplast, or Cover-Roll)
- Cohesive bandages: sticks to itself, waterproof, and reusable; may be used in place of stretch tape (e.g., Coban or Co-Flex)
- Hypoallergenic tape: alternative to standard zinc oxide non-stretch tape
- Size of body part determines the appropriate width.

Skin Care

Preventive measures:

- **Shave hair:** Increases adhesion of the tape and reduces irritation and build-up of residue
- **Apply taping base** (e.g., tincture of benzoin): Increases adhesion of the tape and provides a protective layer between the tape and skin
- **Apply tape underwrap** (e.g., thin polyester urethane foam): Decreases skin problems and increases athlete's comfort; may not be appropriate for all uses
- **Apply lubricant to possible areas of irritation** (e.g., lace and heel areas of the ankle)

Appropriate tape removal: Use scissors or cutters with a blunt tip. Teach the athlete the appropriate removal technique. Cleanse the skin to remove tape residue. Treat skin irritations and wounds promptly; these problems can prevent further taping.

Allergic reactions to tape materials: Recognize and treat problems. Consider alternative tape supplies. Investigate other forms of support and protection.

Application

- **Requires skill; proficiency results from practice**
- **Elements of appropriate taping technique:**
  - Tearing tape is a basic skill; tape must be torn often.
  - Every piece of tape should have a distinct purpose.
  - Place anchor strips proximal and distal to the injured area directly on the skin.
  - Bridge across injury; duplicate anatomy needing support
  - Weave strips to add strength, overlapping by at least one-half the width of the tape
  - Adapt two-dimensional tape to three-dimensional body part
  - Limit pressure around body prominences, particularly when vascular and neural structures are superficial.
  - Use stretch tape over muscle bellies to allow normal muscle expansion.
  - Inspect for and tape over any gaps in taping to prevent blisters and tape cuts.
- Avoid common problems that restrict circulation: applying too much tape; applying repeated circumferential strips without tearing between turns; forcing tape to go in desired direction; be careful if using tape with acute injuries because swelling causes tightness

PRINCIPLES OF BRACING

- Bracing material should be functional during sport and daily activities; comfortable, lightweight, and moldable braces enhance their functionality.
- Braces should fit appropriately and be adjusted as swelling improves and activity progresses.
- Braces may migrate during activity. Tape, straps, and undergarments may be used to decrease unwanted migration.
- Brace evaluation over time is necessary to ensure appropriate function and to assess need for part replacement.
- Over-the-counter braces are instantly available, less expensive, and efficient to use, but may not offer as much support as more specialized braces.
- Custom applications constructed from thermoplastic and other materials available for specific athlete needs (e.g., ankle–foot orthosis). Consultation with experienced orthotist, prosthetist, or occupational therapist recommended.

PROPHYLACTIC TAPING/BRACING

Knee

- Controversial whether knee braces prevent knee injuries.
- Hinged knee braces are commonly used by football linemen with the rationale that they will reduce the valgus force on the joint, preventing medial collateral ligament (MCL) sprains.
- Biomechanical studies show that braces can provide greater resistance to a valgus force, protecting the MCL and in certain cases, even the anterior cruciate ligament (ACL), but whether this translates to injury prevention is unclear.
- Braces have also been shown to impair performance and increase the incidence of injury in certain player groups. There are several variables in such studies (position, player size, and type of brace), and even when they are accounted for statistically, it is difficult to make clear conclusions.
- Prophylactic knee braces are used by 89% of Division I National Collegiate Athletic Association (NCAA) football teams compared with 28% of National Football League (NFL) teams.

Ankle

- Prophylactic ankle taping and braces are used in several sports. Many studies show a lower incidence of ankle injury with taping and bracing, especially in athletes with previous ankle injuries. Whether one method is superior to the other remains unclear; consider athlete preference and cost.
- Certified athletic trainers frequently use prophylactic taping (Fig. 61.1A).
- Lace-up ankle braces and hinged stirrup braces are often used (Fig. 61.1 B and C).

Wrist

- Wrist taping, wraps, or braces are commonly used in various sports (gymnastics, weightlifting, football linemen, and snowboarding).
- Wrist guards in snowboarding reduce the risk of wrist injury, particularly in children and beginner riders.

SELECTED TAPING/BRACING OF UPPER EXTREMITY INJURIES

Glenohumeral Instability

- Shoulder stabilization brace (Fig. 61.2) often used in sports
- Harness attaches upper arm to chest, preventing forceful abduction and external rotation of shoulder.

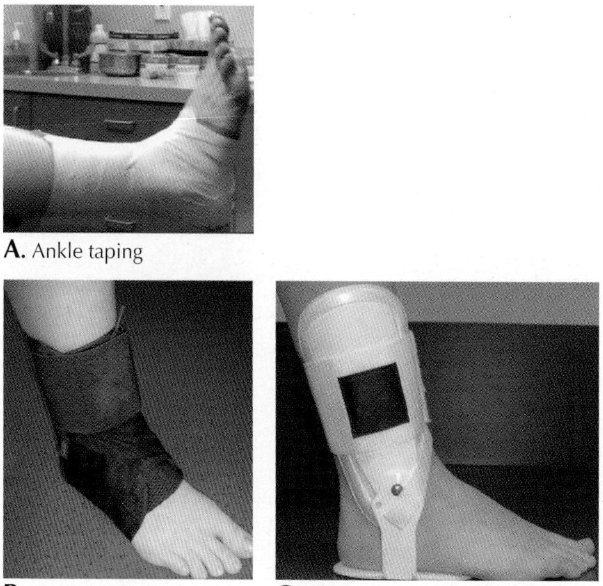

A. Ankle taping

B. Lace-up ankle brace C. Hinged stirrup ankle brace

Figure 61.1 Ankle taping and bracing.

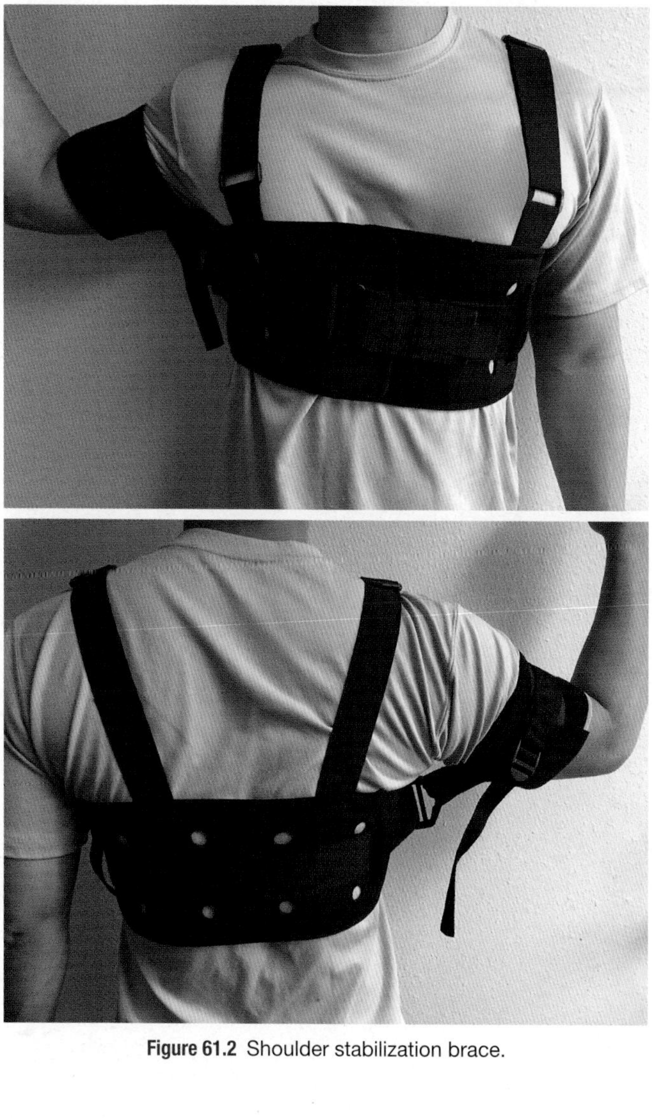

Figure 61.2 Shoulder stabilization brace.

- Because shoulder joint is multidirectional, taping typically does not give enough support.
- Time and effort are probably better spent on rehabilitation.

Elbow Hyperextension

- Taping technique (Fig. 61.3A): Use circumferential anchor strips around mid-upper arm and mid-forearm; criss-cross strips in "X" pattern over ventral elbow to limit elbow extension.
- Hinged elbow brace (see Fig. 61.3B): Brace with medial and lateral supports; ventral straps in "X" pattern limit elbow extension. Hinges may also be locked to restrict flexion and extension. Medial and lateral supports prevent varus and valgus motion, which can protect radial or ulnar collateral ligament sprains, respectively.

Lateral/Medial Epicondylosis

- Counterforce strap (Fig. 61.4) frequently used
- Velcro or elastic strap placed circumferentially around proximal forearm; designed to reduce contractile force on wrist extensor or flexor tendon attachment at the elbow.

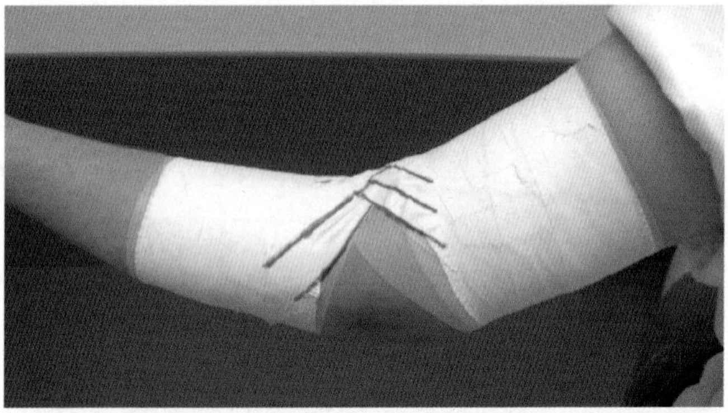

A. Elbow hyperextension taping

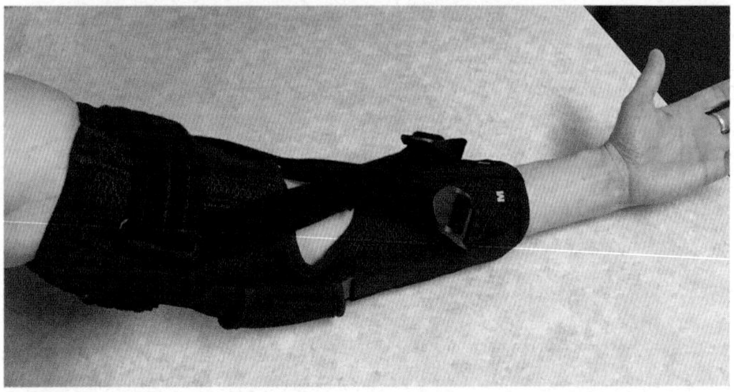

B. Hinged elbow hyperextension brace

Figure 61.3 Elbow hyperextension taping and bracing.

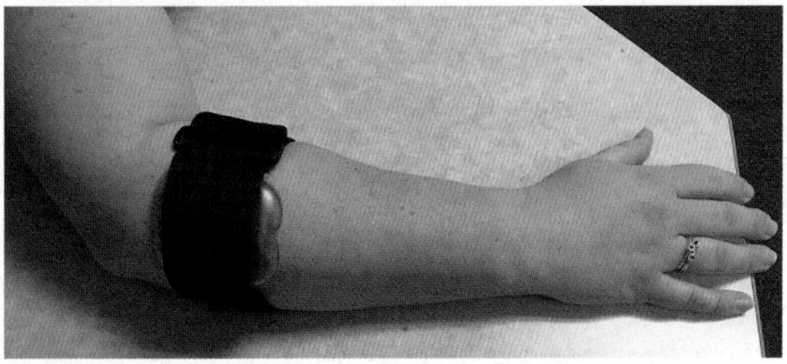

Figure 61.4 Counterforce strap for lateral epicondylosis.

Wrist Sprain

- Taping technique (Fig. 61.5A): Tape wrist circumferentially; may use a foam pad or "fan" of tape over the ventral or dorsal wrist to prevent flexion or extension
- Wrist brace (see Fig. 61.5B): Soft elastic support with or without plastic or metal ventral and/or dorsal support; braces that include the thumb (thumb spica splint extending across wrist to distal forearm, see Fig. 61.6C) are necessary to support radial-sided carpal bones such as the scaphoid.

Thumb Sprain

- Thumb spica taping (Fig. 61.6A): Pieces of tape encircle the thumb in a teardrop pattern, anchoring ends on wrist; traction may be placed on either end of the tape, offering support to any part of the first metacarpophalangeal joint.
- Thumb spica splint (see Fig. 61.6B and C): Neoprene wrap or brace with or without plastic or metal supports, which may extend to just below the radiocarpal joint or across the wrist to include the distal third of the forearm

Proximal/Distal Interphalangeal Sprain

- Buddy taping is used to tape the injured finger to the adjoining uninjured finger. The tape joins the fingers at the proximal and intermediate phalanges (Fig. 61.7).

SELECTED TAPING/BRACING OF LOWER EXTREMITY INJURIES

Hip Injury

- Multidirectional hip joint and adjacent buttock make bracing and taping of this area difficult. Elastic hip and groin spica wraps may be used in a figure-of-eight pattern around the waist and upper thigh.

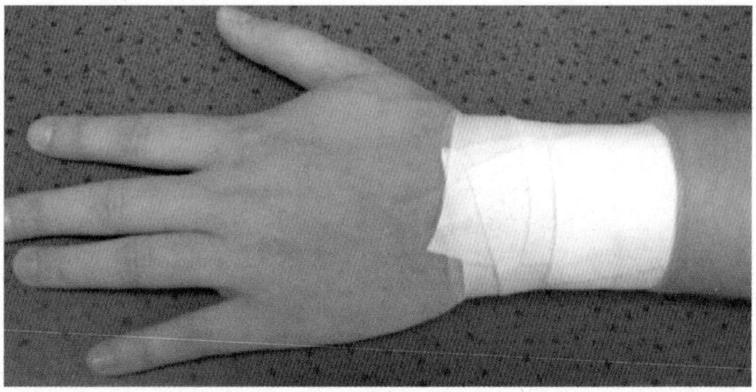

A. Wrist taping

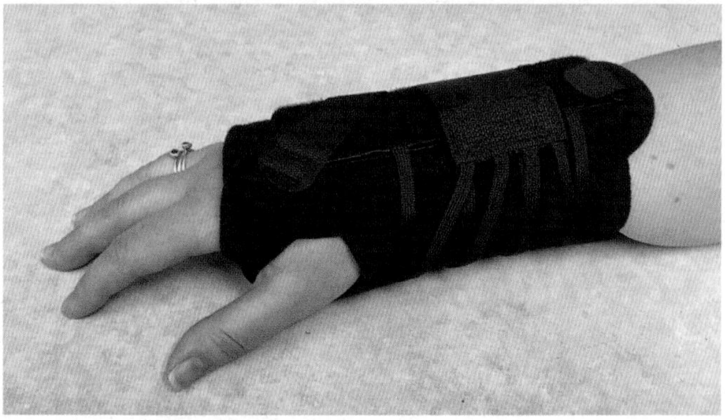

B. Wrist brace

Figure 61.5 Wrist taping and bracing.

ACL Injury

- Hinged knee brace (Fig. 61.8A): May be used for initial compression, support, and stability.
- Custom brace (see Fig. 61.8B): May be used when returning to sport. Functional bracing has been shown to prevent subsequent knee injuries in ACL-deficient and reconstructed knees while skiing. Evidence supporting prevention of injury in other sports is limited.

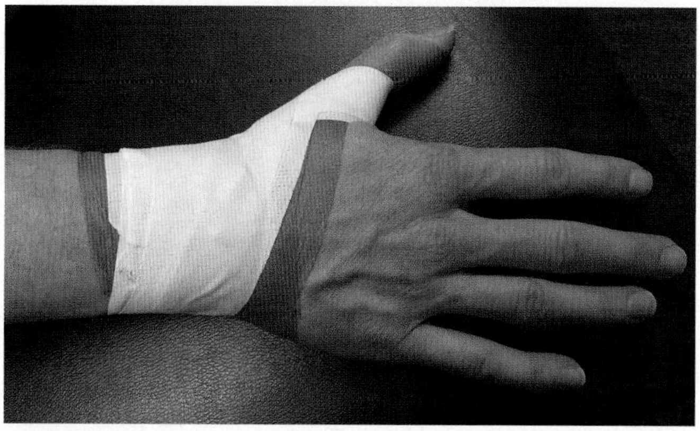

A. Thumb spica taping

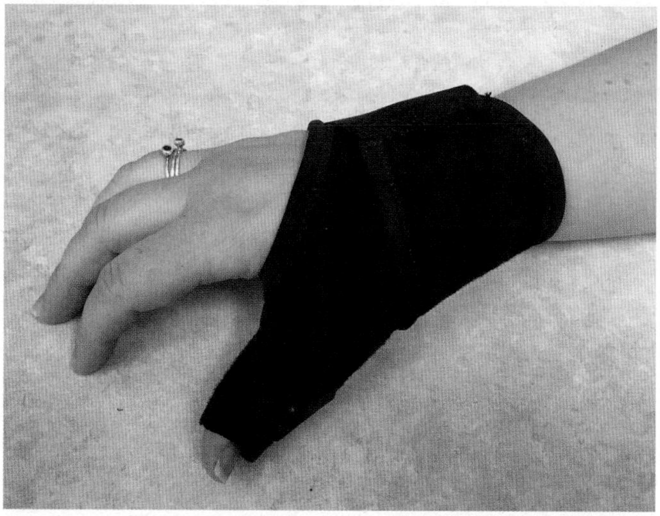

B. Thumb spica brace

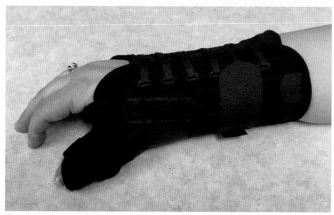

C. Thumb spica brace

Figure 61.6 Thumb spica taping and bracing.

Medial or Lateral Collateral Ligament (MCL/LCL) Injury

- Hinged knee brace (see Fig. 61.8A): Metal hinges provide medial and lateral support. Range of motion can be restricted using flexion and/or extension stops in order to decrease traction/stress on MCL or LCL.

Patellofemoral Pain/Injury

- Patellofemoral taping (Fig. 61.9): Used for patellar maltracking, fat pad impingement; Cover-Roll stretch tape is used over the anterior knee to protect the skin. Nonstretch tape is used to "pull" the patella into appropriate alignment. Patella may be pulled in any direction; important to assess mechanics with single- or double-leg squatting before and after taping.
- Medial/lateral patella-stabilizing brace (Fig. 61.10): Foam/plastic buttress provides medial or lateral patellar support; many are adjustable. Certain braces use a pulley system that offers more support as the knee moves into flexion; can be used for patellar maltracking, instability and subluxation, or dislocation.

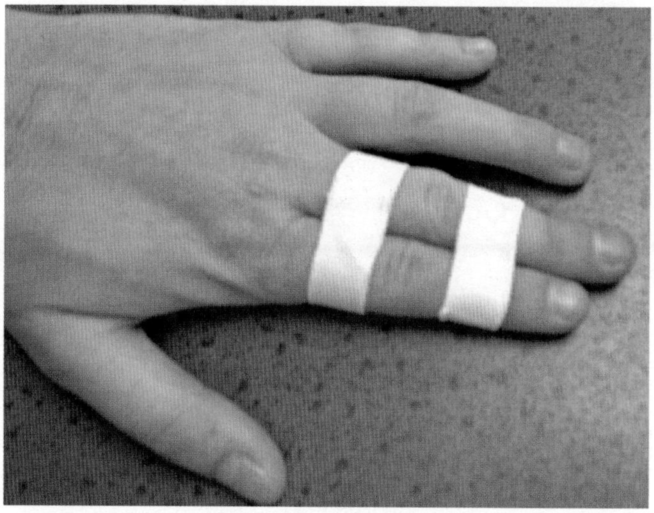

Figure 61.7 Buddy taping.

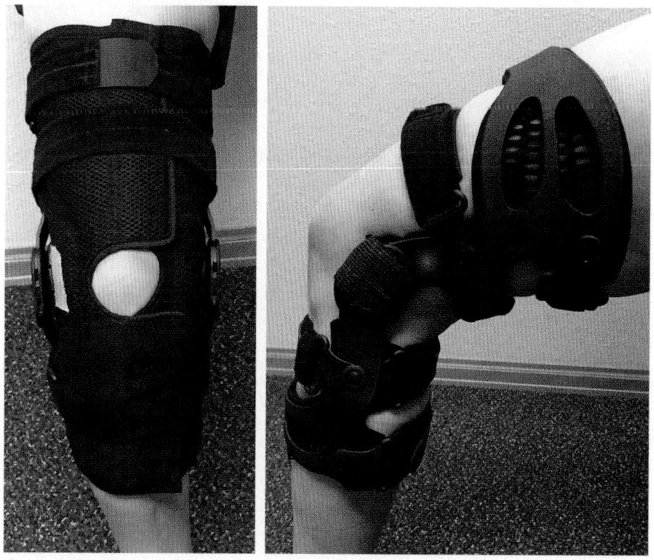

A. Hinged knee brace **B.** Custom ACL knee brace

Figure 61.8 ACL injury bracing.

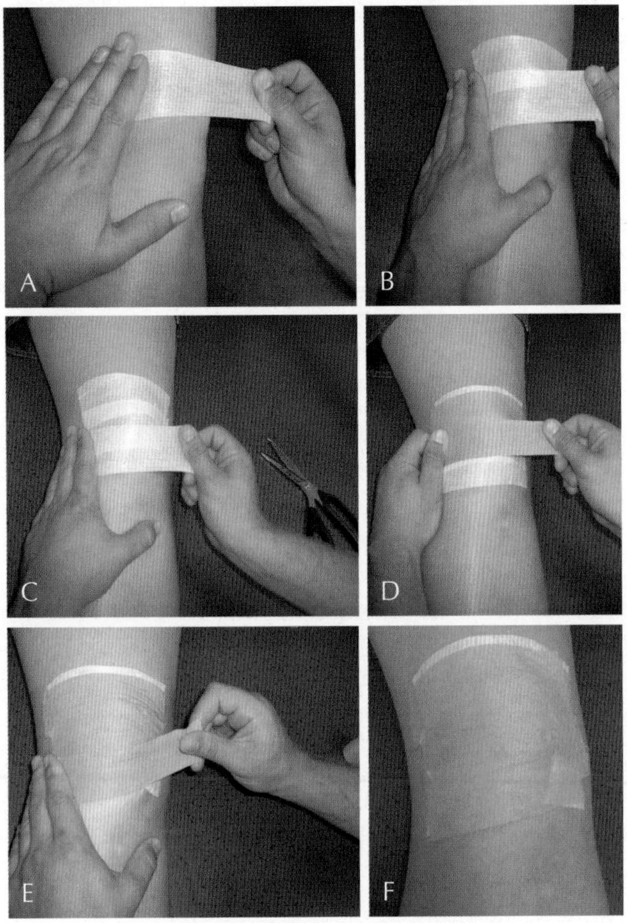
A
B
C
D
E
F
Figure 61.9 Patellofemoral taping.

Patellar Tendinopathy

- Patellar strap (Fig. 61.11): Circumferential elastic strap around the proximal leg beneath the patella; designed to reduce contractile force on the patellar tendon

Knee Osteoarthritis

- Braces may be used to "unload" the affected medial or lateral compartment. Certain braces use a pulley system that allows more "unloading" as the knee moves into flexion. These braces may also be used for condylar bone bruises and after meniscal or cartilage repair procedures.

Ankle Sprain

- Taping should not be performed on an acute sprain.
- Various taping techniques are used to support and provide protection to injured structures when an athlete returns to activity.
- Slip-on elastic support provides even compression to decrease edema in an acute sprain.
- Lace-up ankle brace uses medial and lateral stays and sometimes additional straps to restrict inversion/eversion (see Fig. 61.1B).
- Stirrup splints, based on semirigid orthosis, use Velcro straps to hold in place; designed for rehabilitative and functional uses. All are universally sized.
- Inflatable ankle air cast/brace uses adjustable air pressure linings to improve individual fit, decrease edema, and prevent excessive inversion/eversion (Fig. 61.12).
- Gel cast/brace uses gel-filled linings to improve individual fit; can be placed in freezer to be used as a form of cryotherapy.

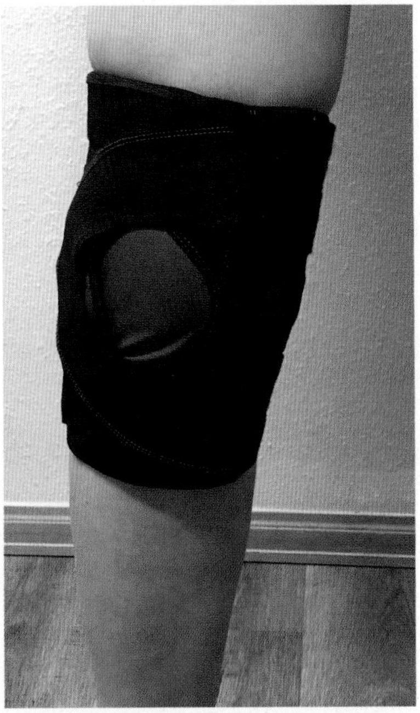
Figure 61.10 Patella-stabilizing brace.

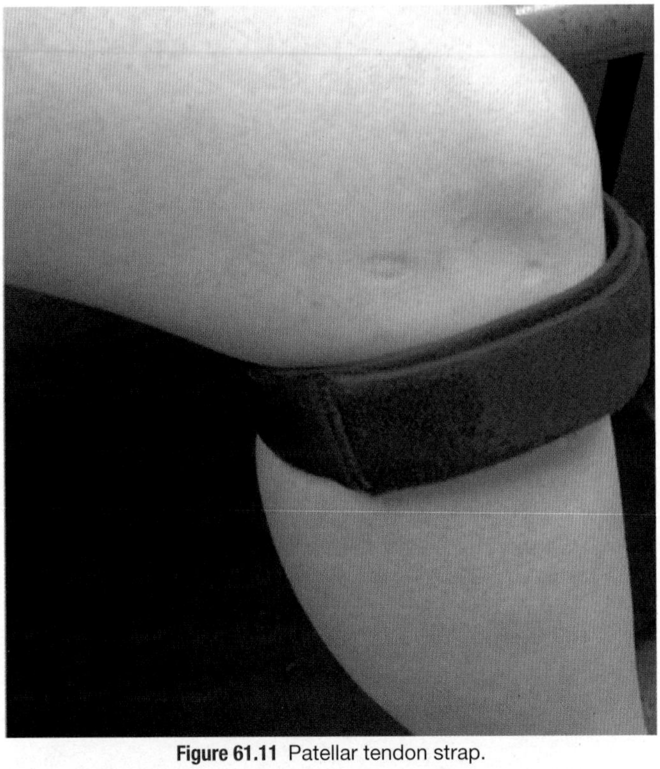
Figure 61.11 Patellar tendon strap.

Plantar Fasciitis

- Arch taping (Fig. 61.13): Supports longitudinal and transverse arch, which relieves strain on the plantar fascia
  - Patient lies prone with foot off the end of the examination table
  - A nonstretch, 0.5- to 0.75-inch athletic tape is used to support the longitudinal arch by taping from the plantar aspect of the first metatarsal head around the posterior heel to the plantar aspect of the fifth metatarsal head.

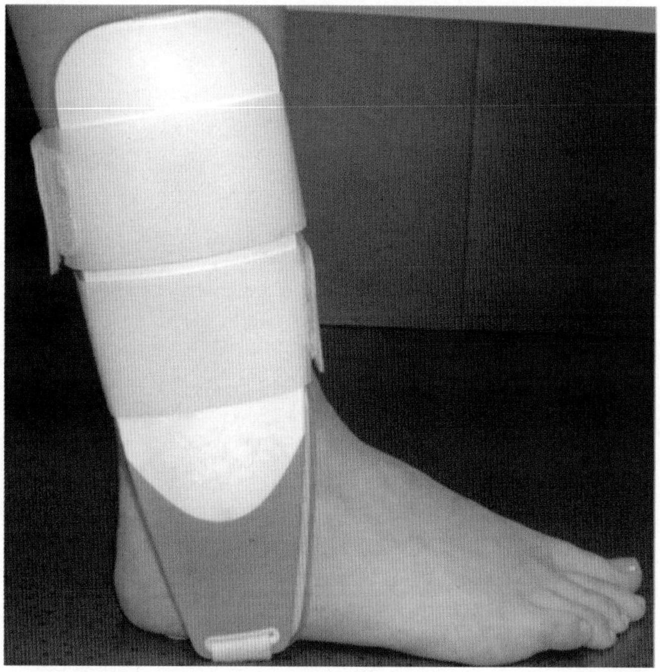

Figure 61.12 Ankle air cast.

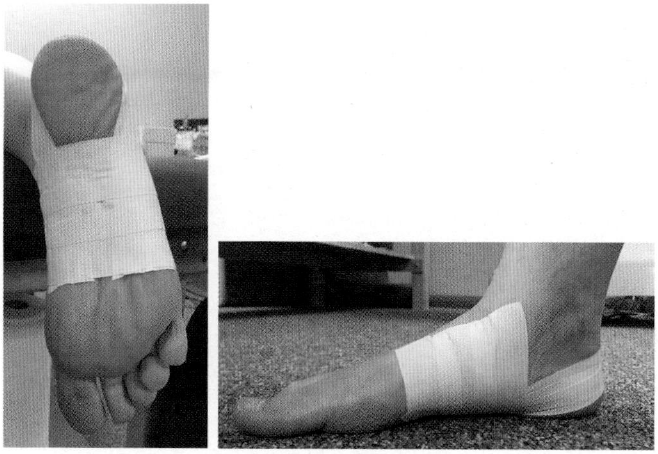

Figure 61.13 Arch taping.

- A nonstretch, 1- to 1.5-inch athletic tape is used to support the transverse arch by taping from the lateral to the medial arch.
- Distal and proximal ends of the strips supporting the longitudinal arch may be removed for comfort.

- Dorsal night splint (Fig. 61.14): Keeps the ankle at 90 degrees while sleeping, thus preventing ankle plantarflexion and offering gentle stretch of plantar fascia to reduce swelling at its medial calcaneal attachment.

Turf Toe

- Taping (Fig. 61.15): Anchor placed circumferentially around forefoot; pieces of tape placed in a teardrop pattern with ends attaching either to dorsal or plantar side of the foot depending on the need for dorsal or plantar first metatarsophalangeal joint support and whether dorsiflexion or plantarflexion of the toe is being restricted.

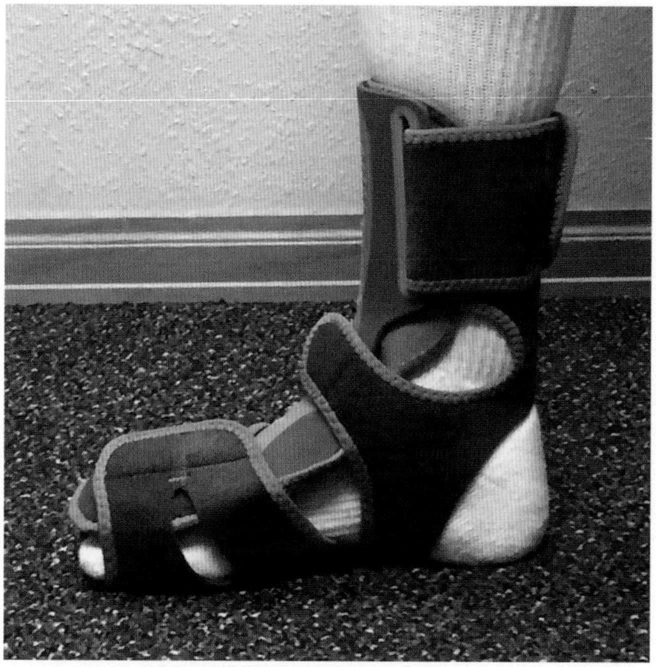

Figure 61.14 Dorsal night splint.

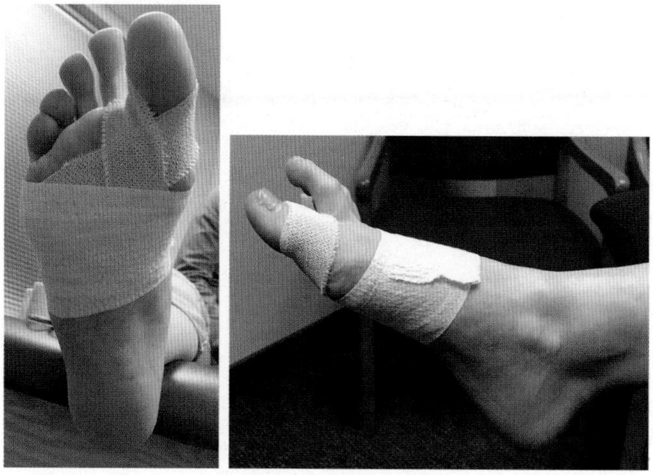

Figure 61.15 Turf toe taping.

Orthotics

- **Common indications:** Lower extremity kinetic chain conditions resulting from excessive pronation, cavus foot, or other foot dysfunctions or mechanical faults
- **Soft orthotics** provide inexpensive over-the-counter solution; easy break-in, have a limited lifespan
- **Rigid/hard orthotics** provide customized solution for certain athletes, particularly road runners not involved in agility activities; good motion control, minimal cushioning
- **Semirigid orthotics** provide support similar to rigid/hard orthotics for athletes involved in agility sports; good combination of support and cushioning; most popular for athletes
- **Sorbothane viscoelastic insoles** reduce impact-loading forces, particularly at the heel; provide minimal support
- **Steel or carbon (e.g., Dynaflex or Spring Plate) shoe inserts** provide support to metatarsal fractures, midfoot sprains, and limit dorsiflexion of first metatarsophalangeal joint; essentially convert normal athletic shoe to "stiff" shoe and may be used in weaning from cast or boot

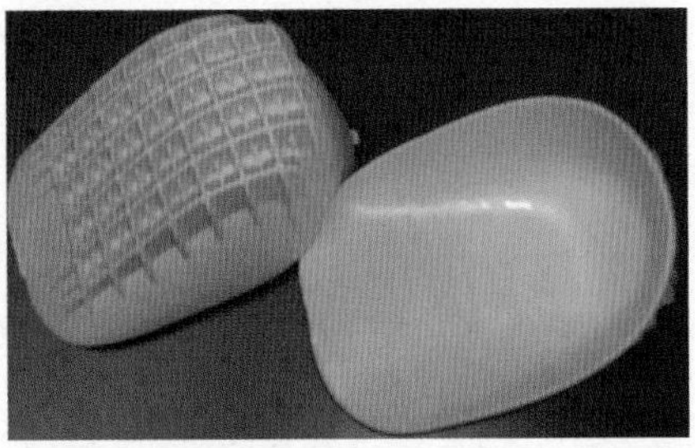

Figure 61.16 Tuli heel cups.

- **Heel cups** (e.g., Tuli) decrease impact and improve shock absorption capabilities of calcaneal fat pad (Fig. 61.16)
- **Longitudinal arch pads** or Barton wedges provide symptomatic relief from painful foot conditions; may be held in place with tape or glue, or may use a self-adhesive to affix to shoe or orthotic
- **Metatarsal arch pads** and bars provide symptomatic relief from painful foot conditions such as interdigital neuroma and metatarsalgia; may be held in place with tape, glue, or self-adhesive (Fig. 61.17); used to splay and elongate metatarsals and tarsals

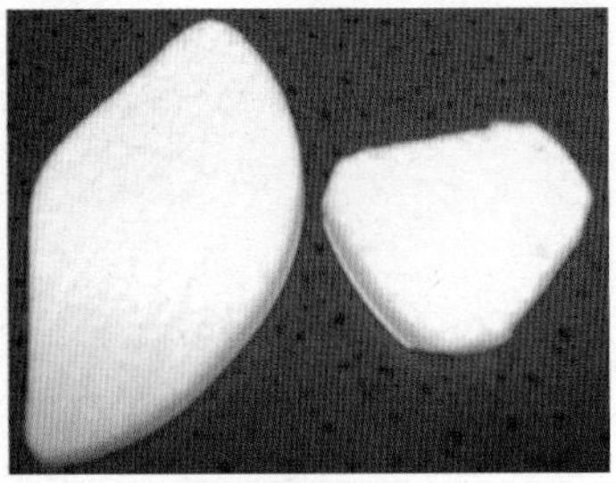

Figure 61.17 Metatarsal arch pads.

ACKNOWLEDGMENT

The author would like to acknowledge **Thomas A. Frette, MD,** for his contribution to the previous edition.

RECOMMENDED READINGS

Available online.

INJECTIONS IN THE ATHLETE 62

Andrew V. Pytiak • Andrew S. Maertens • Armando F. Vidal • Michelle Wolcott

GENERAL PRINCIPLES

- Knowledge of anatomy is essential in administering injections safely and effectively.
- Use of local anesthetic injections in athletes may reduce the number of games missed because of injury but carries a theoretical risk of worsening the injury.
- Corticosteroid injections are widely used in the treatment of athletic injuries because of their potent anti-inflammatory properties, but these are not without undesirable side effects.
- Corticosteroid injections may not offer a clear therapeutic advantage over anti-inflammatory medications alone.
- Both physicians and athletes should be aware of any restriction regarding the use of corticosteroids during a competition.
  - The World Anti-Doping Agency requires the completion of therapeutic use exemption before administration of corticosteroids.
  - The International Olympic Committee Medical Code requires that any team doctor wishing to administer corticosteroids to an athlete by local or intra-articular injection must give written notification to the relevant medical authority before the competition. A therapeutic use exemption is also required.
  - **National Collegiate Athletic Association (NCAA) statement on corticosteroid injections:** Corticosteroid injections should only be administered if a therapeutic effect is medically warranted and the student-athlete is not subject to any significant short- or long-term risks.
  - After careful consideration, the physician and athlete must determine that the benefits outweigh the risks before proceeding with an injection.

STERILE TECHNIQUE FOR INJECTIONS

- Mark the injection site by pressing the tip of a capped needle against the skin.
- Prep the injection site with Betadine or another appropriate antiseptic solution.
- Use prepacked sterile needles and syringes.
- Use single-dose vials of an injectable agent whenever possible.
- Change needles after drawing up the solution.
- Wear sterile gloves.

COMFORT MEASURES

- **Ethyl chloride** is a topical spray that rapidly cools the skin, providing topical anesthesia.
- Benefit of a **subcutaneous local anesthetic** may be limited by subcutaneous injection pain.
- **EMLA cream** must be applied at least 1 hour before injection but has been shown to be highly effective.

ACCURACY OF INJECTION

- Knowledge of surface landmarks and tactile feedback are essential for accurate needle placement.
- Clinician experience alone does not necessarily improve the accuracy of an injection.
- Joint aspiration in the presence of an effusion may assist in intra-articular needle placement but is not a guarantee.
- Injecting 1–2 mL of air with the injection may help verify intra-articular injection of the knee or shoulder. The presence of an audible "squishing" with range of motion indicates a successful intra-articular injection.
- Ultrasound guidance has been shown to improve the accuracy and clinical effects of certain injections in the hands of a skilled ultrasonographer.
- Image guidance has not shown a definitive advantage over traditional techniques for most injections, although it may be useful in certain situations, such as in obese patients or in patients who have failed to respond to previous injections.

COMMON AGENTS

Local Anesthetics

- **Lidocaine (Xylocaine)** is the most widely used anesthetic. Rapid onset of action with limited duration, approximately 30 minutes; maximum dose: 300 mg (30 mL of 1% lidocaine)
- **Bupivacaine (Marcaine)** has a slow onset of action with prolonged duration of effect, up to 8 hours; maximum dose: 175 mg (70 mL of 0.25% bupivacaine)
- A combination of lidocaine and bupivacaine allows the rapid onset of action with a prolonged duration of effect.

Corticosteroids

- Less soluble
  - Methylprednisolone acetate (Depo-Medrol)
  - Triamcinolone acetonide (Kenalog)
  - Triamcinolone hexacetonide (Aristospan)
- More soluble
  - Betamethasone sodium phosphate (Celestone)
  - Dexamethasone sodium phosphate (Decadron)
  - Prednisolone sodium phosphate (Hydeltrasol)
- Dosage
  - Dosage requirements vary and should be individualized on the basis of the condition being treated and the response of the patient (Table 62.1).
  - In chronic cases, injections may be repeated at intervals ranging from 1 week to ≥5 weeks depending on the degree of relief obtained from the initial injection.
  - No clear safety guidelines exist regarding the frequency and maximum number of injections. Judicious use of injections is recommended.

MECHANISM OF ACTION

Local Anesthetics

- Membrane-stabilizing agents cause a reversible conduction block along nerve fibers.
- Smaller nerve fibers are more sensitive, allowing inhibition of pain signals while sparing pressure and proprioceptive fibers.
- Maximum plasma concentrations of local anesthetic are achieved within 10–25 minutes.
- Avoid preparations containing epinephrine for intra-articular or soft tissue injections; epinephrine causes vasoconstriction, which prolongs the anesthetic effect when used in the skin.

Corticosteroids

- Interfere with inflammatory cell-to-cell adhesion and migration through the vascular endothelium.
- Inhibit the synthesis of cyclooxygenase-2 (COX-2) and various proinflammatory cytokines.

Table 62.1 SUGGESTED DOSES FOR CORTICOSTEROID PREPARATIONS

Corticosteroid Agent	Large Joint	Medium Joint	Small Joint	Soft Tissue
Methylprednisolone acetate (Depo-Medrol)	20–80 mg	10–40 mg	4–10 mg	4–30 mg
Betamethasone sodium phosphate (Celestone)	1.0 mg	0.5–1.0 mg	0.25–0.5 mg	0.5–1.0 mg

- Stimulate gluconeogenesis and catabolic activity in muscle, skin, lymphoid, adipose, and connective tissue
- Solubility determines duration of action and extent of systemic effects.
  - **Insoluble:** Average duration of action is longer for less soluble agents; primarily display local effects
  - **Soluble:** Diffuse more readily from the injected region and may exert greater systemic effects; may be more useful in extra-articular or soft tissue injections
- Average duration of action is 1–3 weeks and is longer for less soluble agents.

SIDE EFFECTS

Local Anesthetics

Anaphylaxis: Occurs from acute mast cell degranulation and is characterized by laryngeal edema, bronchospasm, and hypotension; the cause of local toxicity is allergic reaction to paraaminobenzoic acid (PABA). PABA is a metabolic product of the degradation of the ester class of local anesthetics, such as procaine (Novocain), and to a lesser extent, amide-class anesthetics such as lidocaine; it is also a metabolic by-product of methylparaben, a preservative in multidose vials of lidocaine.

Toxicity: Usually the result of inadvertent intravenous injection; primary target organ is central nervous system, resulting in altered speech, muscle twitching, and seizures. Cardiovascular toxicity (e.g., ventricular arrhythmias) may also occur. Aspirate before injection to avoid inadvertent intravenous injection. Compared with other local anesthetics, bupivacaine is markedly cardiotoxic.

Chondrotoxicity: Emerging evidence suggests that both lidocaine and bupivacaine may have negative effects on articular cartilage health and chondrocyte viability.

Corticosteroids

Postinjection flare: Most common side effect; related to steroid crystal synovitis; self-limiting; typically lasts for <12 hours; analgesic therapy and ice packs offer effective relief.

Facial flushing: Subjective sensation of warmth in the face and upper trunk

Poor diabetic control: May increase hepatic glucose production and antagonize insulin effects; close monitoring is suggested after a corticosteroid injection

Subcutaneous fat atrophy and skin depigmentation: May occur after a single injection; avoid repeated subcutaneous or superficial injections. Subcutaneous fat atrophy is particularly problematic in the plantar surface of the foot. Skin depigmentation occurs more commonly in dark-skinned individuals.

Tendon rupture: Dose-dependent decrease in tenocyte proliferation and reduced collagen production by tenocytes. Care should be taken to avoid direct intratendinous injection, which can result in this complication.

Steroid-induced arthropathy and cartilage damage: Destruction of articular cartilage and a decrease in cartilage matrix production has been shown in animal studies. Although not reported in humans, a theoretical risk remains.

Infection: Incidence of joint sepsis varies from 1 in 3000 to 1 in 50,000 for corticosteroid injections. Informed consent should be obtained before any invasive procedure. Use of good sterile technique minimizes this risk.

Anaphylaxis: May occur even after previous uneventful injections

Hypothalamic–pituitary–adrenal axis suppression: Suppression is mild and transient. Avoid simultaneously injecting multiple large joints. Prolonged suppression has been reported.

Drug interaction: Corticosteroids should be avoided in patients taking concurrent medications with significant liver enzyme CYP450 interaction, as this will affect corticosteroid clearance and may result in significant adrenal suppression.

Other

Syncope: Patients who feel lightheaded or overly apprehensive should lie down. Protect the airway in the event of loss of consciousness. Reassure the patient.

CONTRAINDICATIONS

Infection: Overlying cellulitis, bacteremia, or septic arthritis

Fracture or unstable joint: Risk of worsening injury

Tendinopathy: Risk of tendon rupture if injected directly into tendon (e.g., Achilles tendon)

History of medication allergy or anaphylaxis after injection: Previous uneventful injection does not eliminate possibility of future reactions

Coagulopathy or anticoagulation therapy: Risk of bleeding at the injection site

Poorly controlled diabetes: Corticosteroids may result in temporary exacerbation of diabetes. Blood glucose levels typically peak 48 hours postinjection.

Medication use: Corticosteroids should be avoided in patients taking certain medications including the antidepressant nefazodone, antifungals (itraconazole, ketoconazole), protease inhibitors (ritonavir, cobicistat), and some macrolide antibiotics (clarithromycin, telithromycin) to prevent significant adrenal suppression and potential adrenal crisis.

Prosthetic joint: Risk of infection

UPPER EXTREMITY INJECTIONS

Shoulder

Subacromial Space

Indications: Subacromial bursitis and rotator cuff tendinitis

Technique:

1. Allow the arm to hang at the patient's side to open up the subacromial space.
2. Palpate the lateral border of acromion.
3. The subacromial bursa is deep to the acromion and superficial to the rotator cuff (Fig. 62.1A).
4. Insert the needle angled slightly superiorly at the midpoint of the acromion and approximately 2–3 cm lateral to the lateral border of the acromion
5. Slowly withdraw the needle while injecting.

Considerations: Insertion of the needle too far medially may result in injection into the supraspinatus muscle belly. Up to 30% of subacromial injections may miss the subacromial space. Ultrasound guidance has been shown to improve the accuracy of subacromial injections.

Glenohumeral Joint

Indications: Labral tears, chondral defects, bone contusions, diagnostic injections

A. The subacromial bursa lies deep to the acromion and superficial to the rotator cuff. The glenohumeral joint is approached anteriorly through the interval between the supscapularis and supraspinatus tendons.

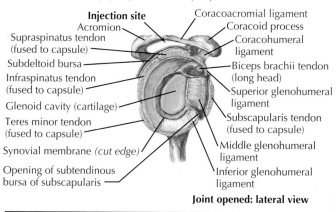

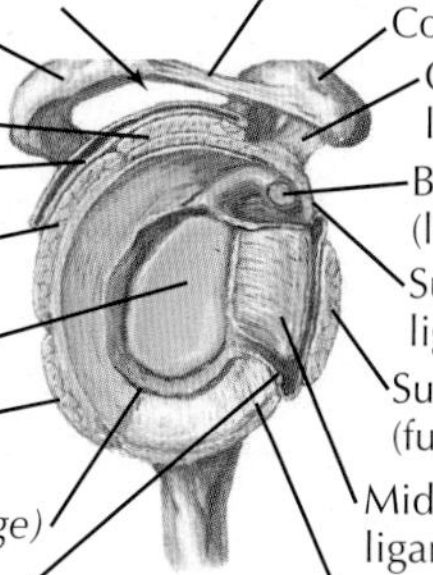
Injection site
Coracoacromial ligament
Acromion
Coracoid process
Supraspinatus tendon (fused to capsule)
Coracohumeral ligament
Subdeltoid bursa
Biceps brachii tendon (long head)
Infraspinatus tendon (fused to capsule)
Superior glenohumeral ligament
Glenoid cavity (cartilage)
Subscapularis tendon (fused to capsule)
Teres minor tendon (fused to capsule)
Middle glenohumeral ligament
Synovial membrane (cut edge)
Opening of subtendinous bursa of subscapularis
Inferior glenohumeral ligament
Joint opened: lateral view

B. The acromioclavicular joint is identified by palpating medially from the anterolateral border of the acromion.

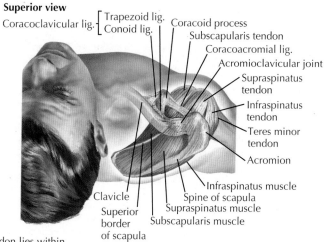

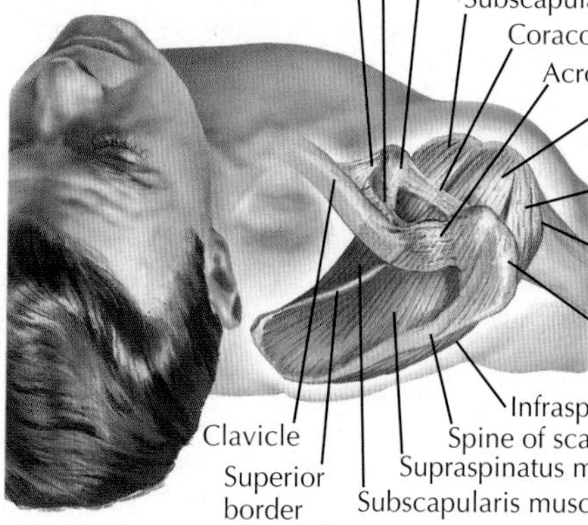
Superior view
Coracoclavicular lig.
Trapezoid lig.
Conoid lig.
Coracoid process
Subscapularis tendon
Coracoacromial lig.
Acromioclavicular joint
Supraspinatus tendon
Infraspinatus tendon
Teres minor tendon
Acromion
Infraspinatus muscle
Spine of scapula
Supraspinatus muscle
Subscapularis muscle
Clavicle
Superior border of scapula

C. During an AC joint injection, the needle is directed at a 30° angle from the vertical to follow the normal anatomic orientation of the AC joint.

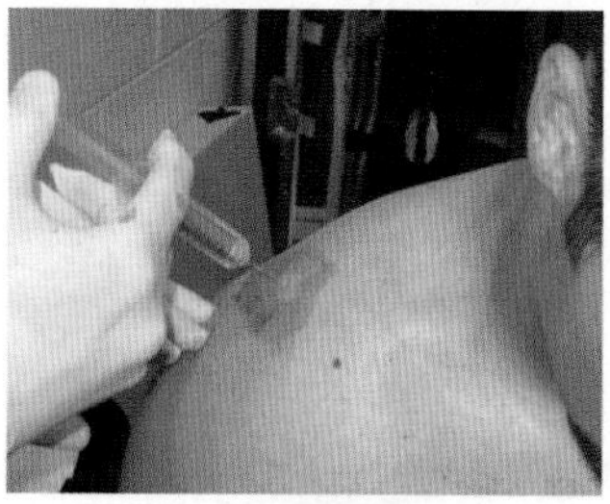

D. The long head of the biceps tendon lies within a sheath in the bicipital, or intertubercular, groove.

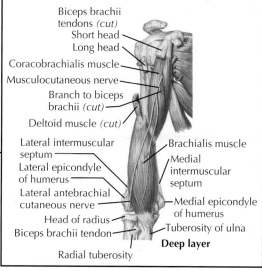

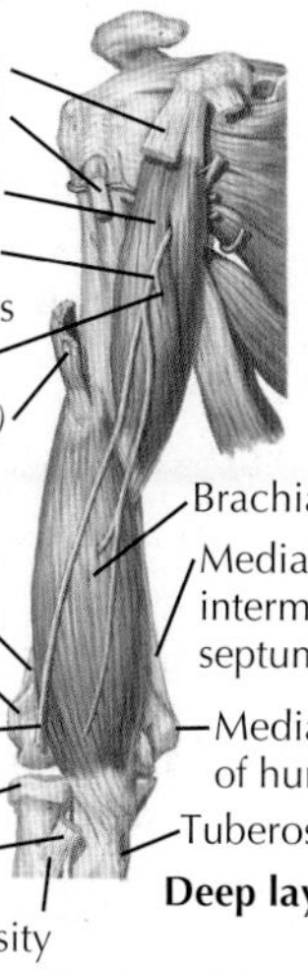
Biceps brachii tendons (cut)
Short head
Long head
Coracobrachialis muscle
Musculocutaneous nerve
Branch to biceps brachii (cut)
Deltoid muscle (cut)
Lateral intermuscular septum
Lateral epicondyle of humerus
Lateral antebrachial cutaneous nerve
Head of radius
Biceps brachii tendon
Radial tuberosity
Brachialis muscle
Medial intermuscular septum
Medial epicondyle of humerus
Tuberosity of ulna
Deep layer

E. Approach the elbow joint through the soft spot between the olecranon, lateral epicondyle, and radial head. The area of maximum fluctuance is identifed for needle placement into the olecranon bursa.

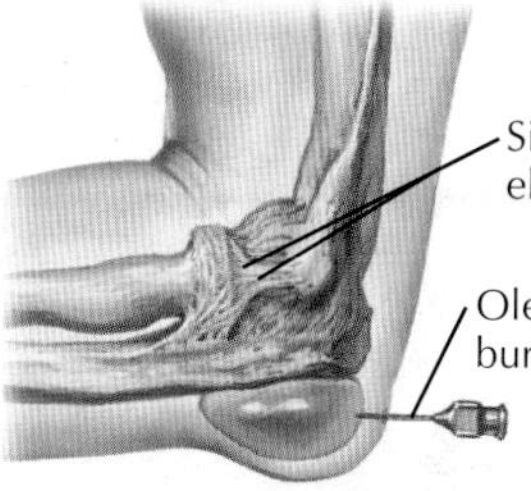
Sites for tennis elbow injection
Olecranon bursa aspiration

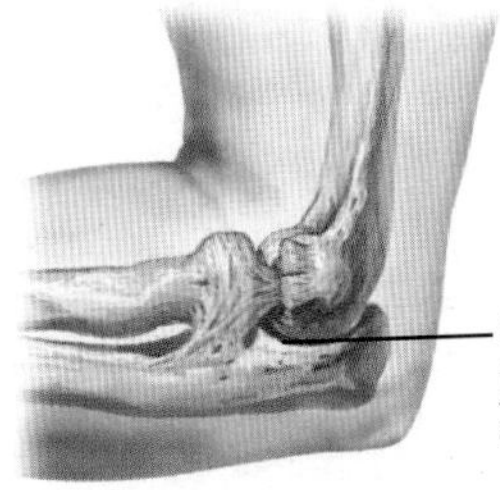
Elbow joint aspiration

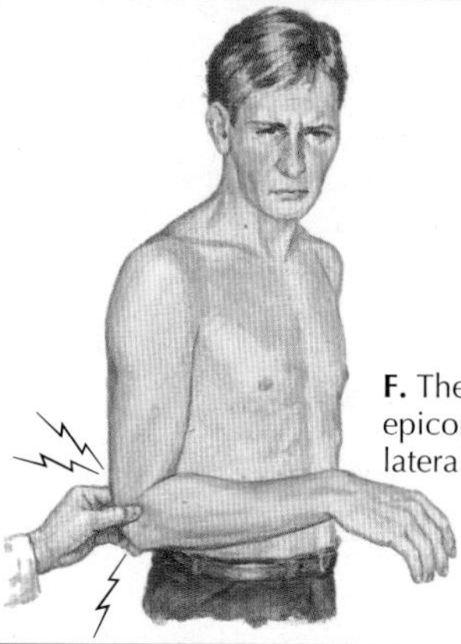

F. The point of maximum tenderness in lateral epicondylitis typically lies 1 cm distal to the lateral epicondyle.

Epicondylitis (tennis elbow)
Exquisite tenderness approximately 1 cm distal to the lateral epicondyle

G. The needle is inserted ulnar to the palmaris longus tendon to avoid direct injury to the median nerve.

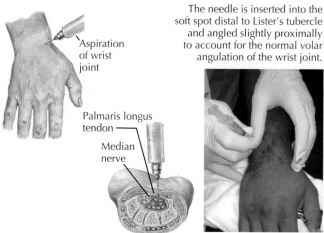

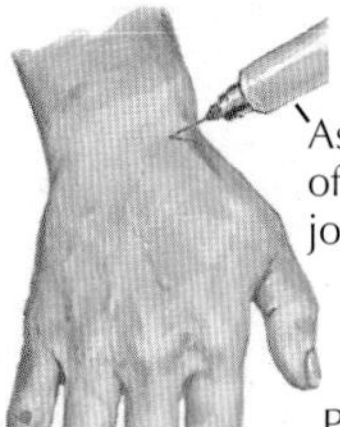
Aspiration of wrist joint

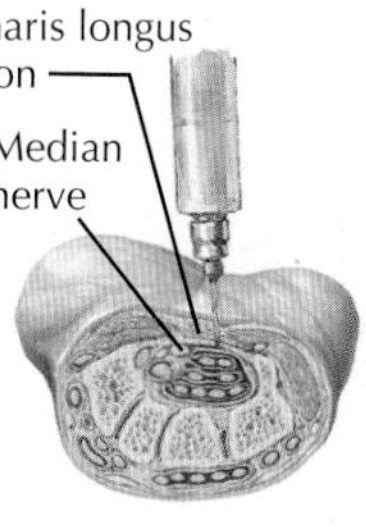
Palmaris longus tendon
Median nerve

The needle is inserted into the soft spot distal to Lister's tubercle and angled slightly proximally to account for the normal volar angulation of the wrist joint.

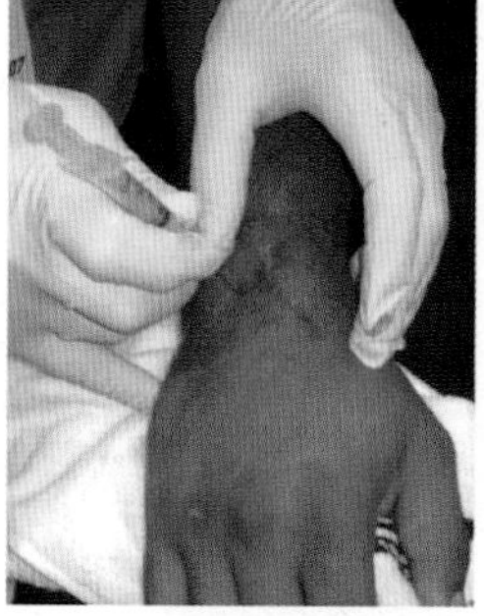

The injection is placed into the gap between the abductor pollicis longus and extensor pollicis brevis tendons at the base of the thumb metacarpal and directed proximally at a 30° angle. The superficial branch of the radial nerve lies in close proximity to the injection point.

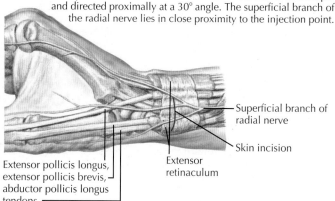

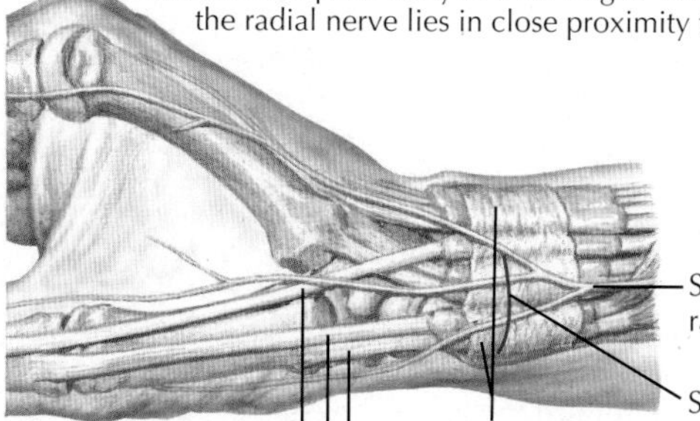
Superficial branch of radial nerve
Skin incision
Extensor retinaculum
Extensor pollicis longus, extensor pollicis brevis, abductor pollicis longus tendons

Figure 62.1 Upper extremity injections.

Technique (anterior):

1. Approach the glenohumeral joint through the rotator interval between the superior border of the subscapularis tendon and the anterior border of the supraspinatus tendon (see Fig. 62.1A).
2. Insert the needle at the midpoint between the anterolateral border of the acromion and coracoid, directing the needle slightly medially. Typically, a soft spot can be palpated in this region.

Technique (posterior):

1. Palpate the posterolateral corner of the acromion.
2. Palpate the soft spot of the glenohumeral joint approximately 1–2 cm medial and 2–3 cm inferior to the posterolateral corner of the acromion.
3. Palpate the coracoid anteriorly with the opposite hand.
4. Insert the needle into the soft spot, directing the needle toward the coracoid.

Considerations: Use caution to avoid direct injury to the articular cartilage of the humeral head and glenoid. Anterior injections may offer a higher rate of accuracy than posterior injections.

Acromioclavicular (AC) Joint

Indications: AC joint sprain, grades I and II AC joint separation, AC joint arthropathy, and distal clavicle osteolysis

Technique:

1. Identify the lateral border of the acromion anteriorly and palpate medially to identify the superior aspect of the AC joint (see Fig. 62.1B and C).
2. The AC joint articulation runs obliquely medially from superior to inferior.
3. Direct the needle medially at a 30-degree angle from the vertical (i.e., parallel to the joint line) (see Fig. 62.1B and C).
4. May inject lidocaine subcutaneously to locate the joint and switch syringe to inject steroid

Considerations: Use a smaller total volume for the AC joint, typically 1–2 mL.

Long Head of the Biceps

Indications: Biceps tendinopathy

Technique:

1. The biceps tendon lies within a sheath in the bicipital groove (see Fig. 62.1D).
2. Palpate the point of tenderness at the anterior aspect of the shoulder.
3. Insert the needle at the most superior point of tenderness, and direct the needle inferiorly, parallel with the tendon.

Considerations: Withdraw the needle slightly if resistance is encountered to prevent intratendinous injection. Ultrasound guidance may be useful to confirm needle placement in the tendon sheath.

Elbow

Elbow Joint

Indications: Chondral defects, bone contusions, posteromedial osteophytes, aspiration of effusion, and synovitis

Technique:

1. Position patient in slight elbow flexion with hand resting in lap.
2. Palpate the soft spot between the olecranon, lateral epicondyle, and radial head (see Fig. 62.1E).
3. Insert the needle into the center of the triangle formed by the aforementioned landmarks.
4. Direct the needle toward the medial epicondyle.

Considerations: The joint is relatively superficial—repeated injections may result in subcutaneous fat atrophy or skin depigmentation. Avoid overpenetration of the needle to prevent any direct injury to the articular cartilage of the elbow.

Olecranon Bursa

Indications: Olecranon bursitis

Technique:

1. Position the elbow in slight flexion with the hand resting in the lap.
2. Insert the needle into the area of maximum fluctuance (see Fig. 62.1E).

Considerations: Attempted aspiration before injection may be helpful in determining whether an infection is present. Avoid injection in the setting of infection.

Common Flexor and Extensor Origin

Indications: Medial epicondylitis, lateral epicondylitis

Technique:

1. Position elbow in slight flexion with hand resting in lap.
2. Supinate the forearm for common flexor origin injection. Pronate the forearm for common extensor origin injection.
3. Insert the needle at the point of maximum tenderness, typically 1 cm distal to the epicondyle (see Fig. 62.1F).

Considerations: Radial tunnel syndrome is a rare compression neuropathy that may be confused with lateral epicondylitis.

Wrist

Wrist Joint

Indications: Triangular fibrocartilage complex (TFCC) tear, scapholunate ligament sprain, bone contusion

Technique:

1. Position the wrist in slight flexion.
2. Palpate the Lister tubercle on the dorsal surface of the distal radius.
3. Identify the soft spot approximately 1 cm distal to Lister tubercle.
4. Direct the needle slightly proximally to account for the 11 degrees of volar angulation at the distal radius (see Fig. 62.1G).

Considerations: Scaphoid fracture must be ruled out definitively before proceeding with wrist joint injection.

Carpal Tunnel

Indications: Carpal tunnel syndrome

Technique:

1. Position wrist in 30 degrees of dorsiflexion.
2. The proximal border of the carpal tunnel lies at the distal wrist crease. The median nerve is ulnar to the flexor carpi radialis and deep to the palmaris longus (see Fig. 62.1G).
3. Palpate the palmaris longus tendon at the proximal wrist crease. Use the wrist midline if the palmaris longus tendon is absent.
4. Direct the needle distally toward the middle/ring finger at a 30- to 45-degree angle.
5. Insert the needle 1–2 cm until no resistance.

Considerations: Paresthesias indicate that the needle is in the median nerve—withdraw the needle and redirect more ulnarly. Direct injection into the median nerve can cause irreversible damage. Avoid injecting large volumes into the carpal tunnel because this may exacerbate compression of the median nerve.

First Dorsal Compartment

Indications: De Quervain tenosynovitis

Technique:

1. Position the thumb in abduction and extension to facilitate identification of the radial wrist tendons.
2. Palpate the abductor pollicis longus and extensor pollicis brevis tendons in the first dorsal compartment (see Fig. 62.1G).

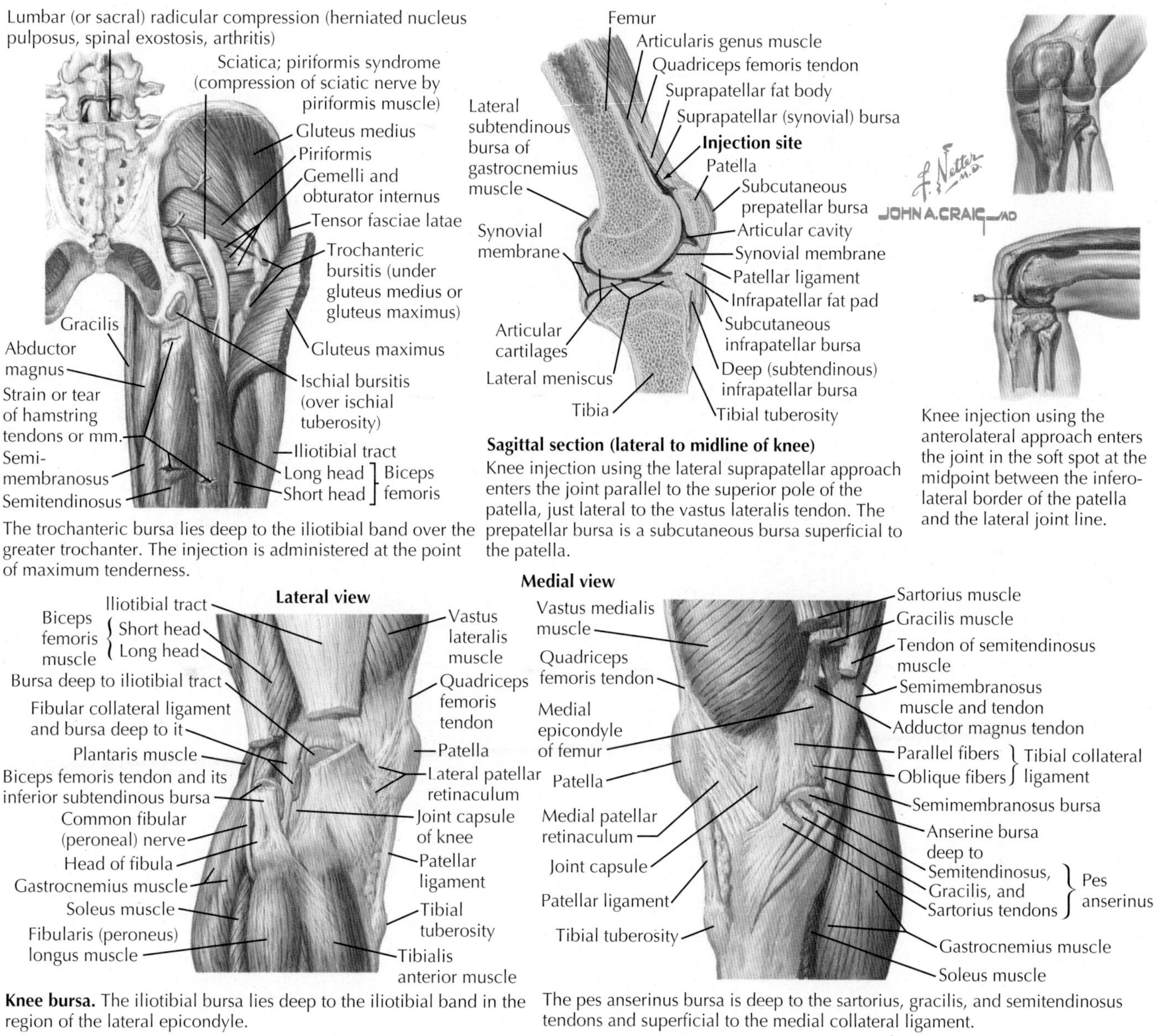
Lumbar (or sacral) radicular compression (herniated nucleus pulposus, spinal exostosis, arthritis)
Sciatica; piriformis syndrome (compression of sciatic nerve by piriformis muscle)
Gluteus medius
Piriformis
Gemelli and obturator internus
Tensor fasciae latae
Trochanteric bursitis (under gluteus medius or gluteus maximus)
Gracilis
Abductor magnus
Gluteus maximus
Strain or tear of hamstring tendons or mm.
Ischial bursitis (over ischial tuberosity)
Semi-membranosus
Semitendinosus
Iliotibial tract
Long head
Short head
Biceps femoris
Femur
Articularis genus muscle
Quadriceps femoris tendon
Suprapatellar fat body
Suprapatellar (synovial) bursa
Lateral subtendinous bursa of gastrocnemius muscle
Injection site
Patella
Subcutaneous prepatellar bursa
Synovial membrane
Articular cavity
Synovial membrane
Patellar ligament
Infrapatellar fat pad
Articular cartilages
Subcutaneous infrapatellar bursa
Lateral meniscus
Deep (subtendinous) infrapatellar bursa
Tibia
Tibial tuberosity
Sagittal section (lateral to midline of knee)
F. Netter M.D.
JOHN A.CRAIG_AD
Lateral view
Iliotibial tract
Biceps femoris muscle
Short head
Long head
Bursa deep to iliotibial tract
Fibular collateral ligament and bursa deep to it
Plantaris muscle
Biceps femoris tendon and its inferior subtendinous bursa
Common fibular (peroneal) nerve
Head of fibula
Gastrocnemius muscle
Soleus muscle
Fibularis (peroneus) longus muscle
Vastus lateralis muscle
Quadriceps femoris tendon
Patella
Lateral patellar retinaculum
Joint capsule of knee
Patellar ligament
Tibial tuberosity
Tibialis anterior muscle
Medial view
Vastus medialis muscle
Quadriceps femoris tendon
Medial epicondyle of femur
Patella
Medial patellar retinaculum
Joint capsule
Patellar ligament
Tibial tuberosity
Sartorius muscle
Gracilis muscle
Tendon of semitendinosus muscle
Semimembranosus muscle and tendon
Adductor magnus tendon
Parallel fibers
Oblique fibers
Tibial collateral ligament
Semimembranosus bursa
Anserine bursa deep to
Semitendinosus,
Gracilis, and
Sartorius tendons
Pes anserinus
Gastrocnemius muscle
Soleus muscle

The trochanteric bursa lies deep to the iliotibial band over the greater trochanter. The injection is administered at the point of maximum tenderness.

Knee injection using the lateral suprapatellar approach enters the joint parallel to the superior pole of the patella, just lateral to the vastus lateralis tendon. The prepatellar bursa is a subcutaneous bursa superficial to the patella.

Knee injection using the anterolateral approach enters the joint in the soft spot at the midpoint between the inferolateral border of the patella and the lateral joint line.

Knee bursa. The iliotibial bursa lies deep to the iliotibial band in the region of the lateral epicondyle.

The pes anserinus bursa is deep to the sartorius, gracilis, and semitendinosus tendons and superficial to the medial collateral ligament.

Figure 62.2 Knee injections.

3. Insert the needle in the gap between the two tendons at the base of the thumb metacarpal.
4. Direct the needle at a 30-degree angle proximally toward the radial styloid.

Considerations: Redirect the needle slightly if resistance is encountered to prevent intratendinous injection. Paresthesias may indicate that the needle is in the superficial branch of the radial nerve.

Flexor Tendon Sheath

Indications: Trigger finger
Technique:

1. Position patient with forearm supinated and fingers extended.
2. Palpate the nodule in the flexor tendon.
3. Insert the needle at the distal palmar crease.
4. Direct the needle distally at a 30-degree angle into the flexor tendon sheath.

Considerations: Withdraw the needle slightly if resistance is encountered to avoid intratendinous injection. Digital nerve anesthesia occurs with injection of local anesthetic.

LOWER EXTREMITY INJECTIONS

Hip

Trochanteric Bursa

Indications: Trochanteric bursitis, bone contusion
Technique:

1. Place patient in lateral decubitus position with hip and knee flexed.
2. Insert the needle perpendicular to the skin at the point of maximal tenderness over the greater trochanter.
3. Inject deep to the iliotibial band into the trochanteric bursa (Fig. 62.2).

Considerations: If the needle is advanced into the bone, withdraw slightly and inject. In larger patients, consider using a spinal needle.

Knee

Knee Joint

Indications: Bone contusion, meniscus tear, chondromalacia patellae, plica syndrome

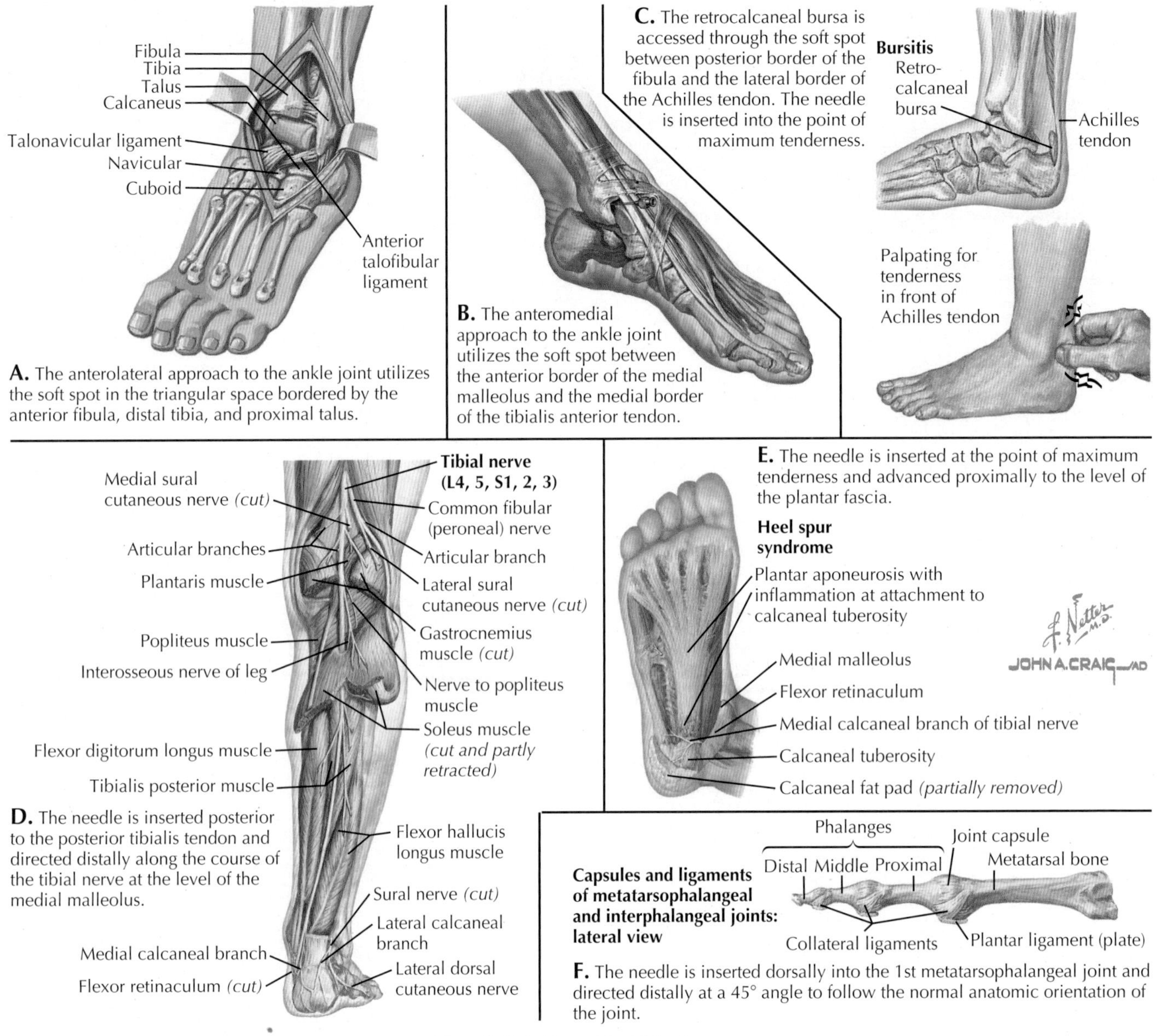
Fibula
Tibia
Talus
Calcaneus
Talonavicular ligament
Navicular
Cuboid
Anterior talofibular ligament
A. The anterolateral approach to the ankle joint utilizes the soft spot in the triangular space bordered by the anterior fibula, distal tibia, and proximal talus.
B. The anteromedial approach to the ankle joint utilizes the soft spot between the anterior border of the medial malleolus and the medial border of the tibialis anterior tendon.
C. The retrocalcaneal bursa is accessed through the soft spot between posterior border of the fibula and the lateral border of the Achilles tendon. The needle is inserted into the point of maximum tenderness.
Bursitis
Retro-calcaneal bursa
Achilles tendon
Palpating for tenderness in front of Achilles tendon
Tibial nerve (L4, 5, S1, 2, 3)
Medial sural cutaneous nerve (cut)
Common fibular (peroneal) nerve
Articular branches
Articular branch
Plantaris muscle
Lateral sural cutaneous nerve (cut)
Gastrocnemius muscle (cut)
Popliteus muscle
Interosseous nerve of leg
Nerve to popliteus muscle
Soleus muscle (cut and partly retracted)
Flexor digitorum longus muscle
Tibialis posterior muscle
Flexor hallucis longus muscle
Sural nerve (cut)
Lateral calcaneal branch
Medial calcaneal branch
Flexor retinaculum (cut)
Lateral dorsal cutaneous nerve
D. The needle is inserted posterior to the posterior tibialis tendon and directed distally along the course of the tibial nerve at the level of the medial malleolus.
E. The needle is inserted at the point of maximum tenderness and advanced proximally to the level of the plantar fascia.
Heel spur syndrome
Plantar aponeurosis with inflammation at attachment to calcaneal tuberosity
Medial malleolus
Flexor retinaculum
Medial calcaneal branch of tibial nerve
Calcaneal tuberosity
Calcaneal fat pad (partially removed)
JOHN A.CRAIG_AD
Capsules and ligaments of metatarsophalangeal and interphalangeal joints: lateral view
Phalanges
Distal Middle Proximal
Joint capsule
Metatarsal bone
Collateral ligaments
Plantar ligament (plate)
F. The needle is inserted dorsally into the 1st metatarsophalangeal joint and directed distally at a 45° angle to follow the normal anatomic orientation of the joint.

Figure 62.3 Ankle and foot injections.

Technique (lateral suprapatellar):
1. Position patient with the knee in full extension.
2. Palpate the superior border of the patella.
3. Push the patella laterally to tent the capsule.
4. Insert the needle inferior to the vastus lateralis tendon and parallel to the superior border of the patella (see Fig. 62.2).

Technique (anterolateral):
1. Position patient with the knee flexed to 90 degrees and the leg hanging off the examination table to distract the joint.
2. Palpate the lateral border of the patellar tendon.
3. Palpate the soft spot at the midpoint between the inferolateral border of the patella and the lateral joint line (see Fig. 62.2).
4. Direct the needle toward the notch approximately 0.5–1 cm lateral to the patellar tendon.

Considerations: The lateral suprapatellar approach may allow for more accurate intra-articular placement of the needle. With an anterolateral approach, use caution to avoid direct injury to the articular cartilage of the lateral condyle.

Prepatellar Bursa

Indications: Prepatellar bursitis
Technique:
1. Position patient with the knee extended.
2. Prepatellar bursa is superficial to the patella (see Fig. 62.2).
3. Insert the needle into area of maximum fluctuance.

Considerations: Attempted aspiration before injection may be helpful in determining whether an infection is present. Avoid injection in the setting of infection.

Pes Anserine Bursa

Indications: Pes anserine bursitis
Technique:
1. Position patient with the knee in 90 degrees of flexion.
2. The pes anserine is the insertion of the sartorius, gracilis, and semitendinosus tendons. The bursa is deep to the tendons and superficial to the medial collateral ligament (see Fig. 62.2).

3. Insert the needle perpendicular to the skin at the point of maximum tenderness deep to the pes anserine tendons.

Considerations: Advance needle until no resistance is met to avoid intratendinous injection. If the needle is advanced into the bone, withdraw 2–3 mm and inject.

Iliotibial Bursa

Indications: Iliotibial band syndrome

Technique:

1. Place patient in lateral decubitus position with hip and knee slightly flexed.
2. Palpate the lateral epicondyle of the femur. The bursa lies deep to the iliotibial band in the region of the lateral epicondyle (see Fig. 62.2).
3. Insert the needle perpendicular to the skin at the point of maximum tenderness and inject.

Considerations: Inflammation of the iliotibial band may occur more distally near its attachment at the Gerdy tubercle.

Ankle

Ankle Joint

Indications: Osteochondral defect, bone contusion, ankle sprain

Technique (lateral):

1. Position the ankle in slight plantarflexion.
2. Identify the soft spot in the triangular space bordered by the anterior fibula, distal tibia, and proximal talus (Fig. 62.3A).
3. Direct the needle slightly proximally and medially.

Technique (medial):

1. Position the ankle in slight plantarflexion.
2. Palpate the soft spot between the anterior border of the medial malleolus and the medial border of the tibialis anterior tendon (see Fig. 62.3B).
3. Direct the needle slightly proximally and laterally.

Considerations: Use caution to avoid direct injury to the articular cartilage of the tibial plafond or talar dome.

Retrocalcaneal Bursa

Indications: Retrocalcaneal bursitis

Technique:

1. Place the patient in the prone position with the foot in slight dorsiflexion.
2. Palpate the soft spot between the posterior border of the fibula and the lateral border of the Achilles tendon (see Fig. 62.3C).
3. Insert the needle at the point of maximum tenderness anterior to the Achilles tendon.

Considerations: Withdraw the needle and redirect if resistance is encountered to prevent intratendinous injection. Avoid overpenetration to prevent inadvertent injection into the medial neurovascular structures. Retrocalcaneal bursitis may be difficult to distinguish from Achilles tendinitis.

Tarsal Tunnel

Indications: Tarsal tunnel syndrome

Technique:

1. Palpate the posterior tibialis tendon.
2. Insert the needle posterior to the posterior tibialis tendon at the level of the medial malleolus (see Fig. 62.3D).
3. Direct the needle distally at a 30-degree angle from the skin surface, parallel to the posterior tibialis tendon.

Considerations: Aspirate before injecting to avoid inadvertent intravascular injection. Paresthesias indicate that the needle is in the tibial nerve. Withdraw the needle slightly and redirect if resistance is encountered to prevent intratendinous injection.

Foot

Plantar Fascia

Indications: Plantar fasciitis

Technique:

1. Place the patient in the prone position with the foot in slight dorsiflexion.
2. The area of inflammation typically occurs at the medial aspect of the plantar fascia near the medial process of the calcaneal tuberosity, just distal to the heel pad (see Fig. 62.3E).
3. Insert the needle at the point of maximum tenderness and advance proximally at a 45-degree angle to the level of the plantar fascia.

Considerations: Avoid injection into the heel pad to prevent subcutaneous fat pad atrophy. If the needle is advanced into the bone, withdraw slightly and inject.

First Metatarsophalangeal (MTP) Joint

Indications: Turf toe, chondral defects

Technique:

1. Position the great toe in slight plantarflexion. Passively flex and extend the great toe to aid in identifying the joint space.
2. Insert the needle on the dorsal surface of the MTP joint (see Fig. 62.3F).
3. Direct the needle distally at a 45-degree angle.

Considerations: Ultrasound can be particularly useful to visualize and avoid dorsal osteophytes. The joint is relatively superficial—repeated injections may result in subcutaneous fat atrophy or skin depigmentation. Avoid deep penetration with the needle to prevent direct injury to the articular cartilage.

RECOMMENDED READINGS

Available online.

63 DIAGNOSTIC IMAGING IN SPORTS MEDICINE

Corey K. Ho • Colin D. Strickland

GENERAL PRINCIPLES

- Imaging in sports medicine plays an increasingly important role in the diagnosis of injury and decision-making regarding return to play.
- Increasingly sophisticated imaging modalities allow for precise diagnosis of various patterns of injury but also present the care provider with a bewildering range of tests.
- The continued participation of older athletes in sporting activities makes the interpretation of imaging studies challenging as degenerative findings become intermingled with those of sports-related injuries.

INDICATIONS FOR IMAGING

- The approach to imaging in sports medicine mirrors the philosophy applied in clinical medicine as a whole. Imaging should primarily be pursued only when it is likely to alter the patient management and when benefits outweigh risks. The cost and availability of imaging studies are also important factors to consider (Box 63.1).
- It is important to consider risk of exposure to ionizing radiation, particularly in young or pregnant patients. In addition, discomfort, expense, and inconvenience of imaging to the patient are valid concerns.

IMAGING TECHNIQUES

- Musculoskeletal imaging techniques used in sports medicine provide excellent depiction of anatomic structures and often facilitate precise diagnostic accuracy. Imaging modalities differ in the technique of image generation and in terms of cost and radiation exposure.
- Radiography (plain radiographs) creates two-dimensional images of anatomy and typically serves as a first-line imaging study. Computed tomography (CT) also creates two-dimensional images, but in cross-section. Nuclear medicine examinations (including bone scintigraphy/bone scan) detect gamma rays emitted from a radiopharmaceutical administered intravenously to patients. Each of these modalities requires exposure to ionizing radiation.
- Magnetic resonance imaging (MRI) does not use ionizing radiation but is contraindicated for certain patients with metallic implanted medical devices. Ultrasound is generally safe, although tissue heating may be a concern.
- The use of the modern picture archiving and communication system (PACS) software allows diagnostic images to be stored and shared widely, which has greatly increased the portability of imaging information. As PACS software becomes available on a wide range of portable devices, it should be remembered that diagnostic radiology workstations are required to utilize special high-resolution graphics hardware and monitors.
- The judicious use of ionizing radiation is critical in protecting the safety of sporting patients, particularly the young who face greater theoretical lifetime risks from exposure to ionizing radiation. Some common examinations and typical dose levels are listed in Table 63.1.
- The diagnosis and management of injuries in sports medicine greatly rely on accurate history and physical examination findings in addition to an understanding of the mechanism of injury. Communicating this information at the time of an imaging request allows the radiologist to interpret studies in the appropriate clinical context and provide the most accurate and relevant report.
- A close working relationship among sports medicine providers, radiologic technologists, and diagnostic radiologists helps foster an efficient system and ensure that appropriate care is delivered to the patient.

RADIOGRAPHY

- Radiography (plain radiographs) uses ionizing radiation and provides an excellent depiction of bony anatomy with very high spatial resolution. PACS software allows radiographic images to be windowed and leveled, which reveals additional detail in the soft tissues.
- **Advantages:** The benefits of radiographic evaluation are the high spatial resolution and high sensitivity in detecting subtle fractures or dislocations. Osseous structures are well evaluated. Radiography is widely available, and a multitude of standardized views have been developed to evaluate each bone and joint.
- **Disadvantages:** Radiography generates images through the use of ionizing radiation, and thus, care must be exercised in its use, particularly in young athletes. However, the overall dose is small, particularly when imaging extremities (see Table 63.1). Dose is more substantial when imaging the hip, pelvis, or spine because these structures are deeper in the patient and require a greater radiographic exposure to penetrate surrounding soft tissues in order to provide images of diagnostic quality. Exposure of radiosensitive organs (such as lymphatic tissues and gonads) should be minimized.
- Although the spatial resolution is high, soft tissue contrast is limited, and radiographs are typically not diagnostic in assessment of soft tissue injuries. In some cases, however, the exclusion of a bony component to an injury is sufficient to direct appropriate management.
- **Common indications:** When an imaging study is required in the evaluation of an injured athlete, radiographs are almost always the starting point. Even if no fracture or dislocation is present, other features such as a joint effusion may direct the provider to suspect an occult intra-articular injury or other internal derangement.
- Fractures are well depicted by radiographs, and at least two orthogonal views are required to depict any displacement or angulation that may be present. When the patient requires additional imaging with another modality such as MRI, the radiographs still play an important role in depicting the bony anatomy and may improve the accuracy of MRI interpretation. Small avulsion fractures may not be evident on MRI.
- Certain diagnoses such as an anterior shoulder dislocation may be obvious by clinical examination, but radiographs confirm the diagnosis and are critical for demonstrating significant fractures that may accompany the dislocation (Fig. 63.1A).
- Scaphoid fractures may be radiographically occult, and repeat radiographs in 10–14 days may better show a nondisplaced fracture once bony resorption around the fracture and early new bone formation are evident (see Fig. 63.1B). This visible pattern of healing on radiographs can also be used to follow nondisplaced fractures in other locations over time as an alternative to more advanced imaging.
- Chronic injuries associated with sports may also be demonstrated by radiographs such as cortical thickening in a patient with a tibial stress fracture. It is important to recognize that certain features such as a thickened tibial cortex may persist beyond the period of

injury and subsequent healing; thus, correlation between imaging findings and the clinical picture remains critical, as always.

- As a subset of radiography, dual energy x-ray absorptiometry (DEXA) and trabecular bone score (TBS) can be used to assess the bone mineral density of a patient, which can influence the healing potential of the injured athlete, especially in regard to stress injury.

COMPUTED TOMOGRAPHY

- CT scans use a similar technique to radiography but generate cross-sectional images from which multiplane reformatted images can be created. Surface-rendered 3D images can also be created, which are often useful in surgical planning.
- **Advantages:** CT scans show anatomy and injury patterns in cross-section, which allows greater detail than is possible with planar imaging by radiographs alone. Complex fractures that involve an articular surface or have impacted fragments are often better depicted by CT because the cross-sectional capabilities facilitate a more complete characterization of the injury and guide appropriate management.

BOX 63.1 INDICATIONS FOR MEDICAL IMAGING IN SPORTS MEDICINE

- Imaging likely to change clinical management
- When diagnosis is established but extent of injury and associated injuries must be defined
- When conservative management has failed
- When atypical or systemic symptoms are present that cast doubt on a common diagnosis
- When additional information is needed for surgical planning
- Follow-up for healing or reinjury over time

Table 63.1 COMMON EXAMINATIONS AND TYPICAL DOSE LEVELS

Examination	Average Effective Dose (mSv)
Chest (Posteroanterior and Lateral)	0.05
Extremity Radiograph	0.005
Abdomen, Hip, or Pelvis Radiograph	0.7
Thoracic or Lumbar Spine Radiographs	1.25
CT Thoracic or Lumbar Spine	6
CT Abdomen/Pelvis	8–14
Bone Scan	6.3

- **Disadvantages:** The use of CT is limited by expense and more restricted availability compared with radiography. In addition, the dose of ionizing radiation to the patient may be significantly higher with CT, and thus, judicious use of the modality is important. Imaging of the hip, pelvis, and spine in particular results in exposure of a significant radiation dose and should only be performed when necessary. Metallic hardware produces artifact, obscuring adjacent anatomy.
- **Common indications:** CT plays a role in sports imaging in the characterization of complex fractures where radiographs alone are insufficient to fully depict the fracture features necessary to guide treatment. The depiction of calcific density by CT may also be useful in confirming certain diagnoses such as myositis ossificans or in the characterization of certain bone tumors and infections.
- A vast majority of fractures in the setting of sports medicine are adequately characterized by radiographs; however, complex fractures of joints such as the knee, ankle, and wrist may require CT (Fig. 63.2). In addition, CT is occasionally useful in the monitoring of fracture healing in the scaphoid and in regions of hardware fixation.
- Surgical planning may require CT to fully characterize a bony fragment, as in the case of a bony Bankart fracture of the glenoid suffered in the setting of an anterior shoulder dislocation. In such a patient with ongoing instability for whom a stabilizing procedure is being considered, a CT scan may depict the degree of glenoid insufficiency and whether the distracted fragment is of sufficient size that reduction by surgical means is possible (Fig. 63.3).
- In some cases, where patients have a contraindication to MRI or are unable to tolerate such an examination, CT arthrography can serve as an alternative method for evaluating soft tissues of a joint such as articular cartilage or the shoulder rotator cuff (Fig. 63.4). This technique requires the intra-articular injection of contrast using fluoroscopy or ultrasound guidance.

MAGNETIC RESONANCE IMAGING

- MRI generates images by exposing the patient to a powerful magnetic field and using radio waves to excite tissues. Extensive computer processing then generates cross-sectional images. The technique provides a high degree of soft tissue contrast and is thus unparalleled in its ability to depict ligament, tendon, and cartilage abnormalities. Numerous diagnoses can be made with MRI that previously required arthroscopic or open surgical inspection.
- **Advantages:** MRI images can be generated in any plane, and numerous sequences have been developed to characterize soft

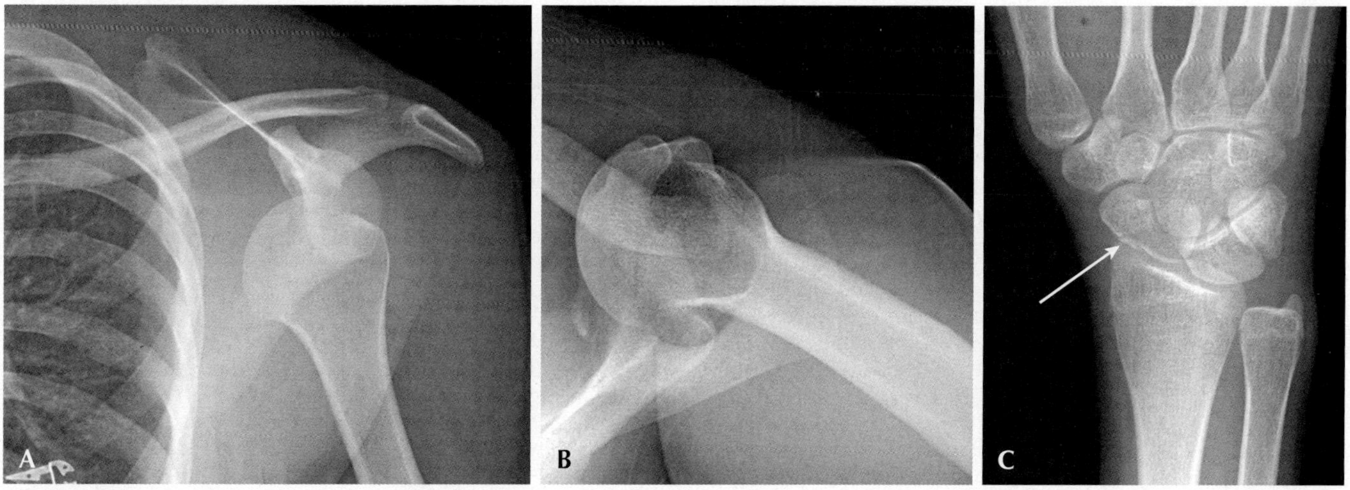
A
B
C

Figure 63.1 Anteroposterior **(A)** and axillary **(B)** radiographs of an anterior glenohumeral shoulder dislocation. Note the subtle fracture fragment on the axillary view arising from the anterior rim of the glenoid. An oblique radiograph of the wrist **(C)** shows a subtle nondisplaced scaphoid waist fracture *(arrow).*

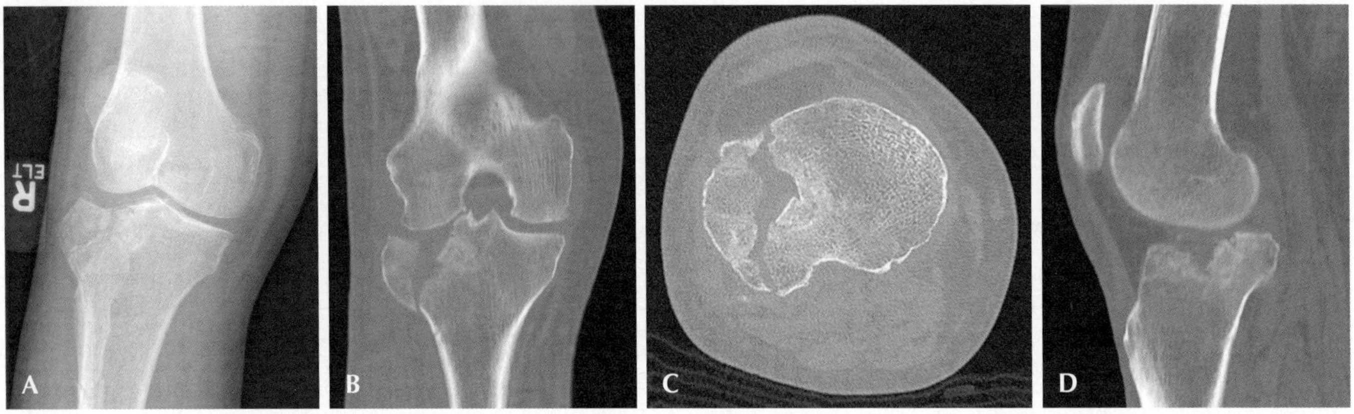
A
B
C
D

Figure 63.2 A knee radiograph **(A)** shows a lateral tibial plateau fracture. Computed tomography (CT) images in the coronal **(B)**, axial **(C)**, and sagittal **(D)** planes more completely characterize the injury, facilitating appropriate treatment.

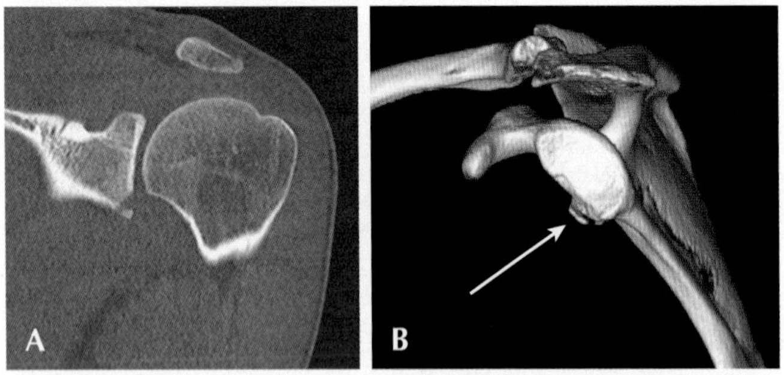
A
B

Figure 63.3 A coronal computed tomography (CT) image **(A)** and 3D surface-rendered reconstruction **(B)** of bone (with the humerus subtracted) shows the small glenoid rim fracture (bony Bankart lesion) related to a prior anterior shoulder dislocation *(arrow)*.

tissues. The technique does not use ionizing radiation, which is also an attractive feature, particularly when working with young athletes. Contrast agents exist and may be useful in evaluating infections and tumors and some inflammatory conditions.

- **Disadvantages:** Disadvantages of MRI include a more limited availability and high expense. Certain implanted medical devices (such as cochlear implants) are contraindicated in the magnetic environment, which can prevent the use of MRI in certain cases. Certain patients are unable to hold still for the required examination, which may be for >30 minutes. The MRI scanner itself has an enclosed patient compartment, and numerous patients find the scanning experience claustrophobic and uncomfortable.
- **Common indications:** The role of MRI in modern sports imaging is central. Injuries of soft tissues such as the cruciate ligaments, meniscus of the knee or labrum of the shoulder are well demonstrated by MRI. MRI arthrography involves intra-articular injection of contrast agents and is occasionally used to diagnose injuries of cartilage or labrum at the hip and shoulder. MRI arthrography can also play a role in evaluation of the post-operative meniscus.
- An acutely injured knee with suspected cruciate ligament and meniscus tearing is a common indication for MRI, and the examination can clearly depict internal derangements (Fig. 63.5), which is useful for planning conservative or surgical intervention. Commonly, a diagnosis or anterior cruciate ligament tear may be confirmed from physical examination findings, but an MRI may reveal associated meniscus or cartilage injuries that will alter planned surgical management.
- Large tendons such as the biceps tendon (Fig. 63.6) are also well depicted by MRI, and the degree of tendon retraction can be clearly seen. Soft tissue injuries such as muscle tears are also well demonstrated and easily differentiated from a fracture that might otherwise be clinically suspected.

ULTRASOUND

- Ultrasound is an increasingly used modality in sports medicine. The development of high-frequency linear transducers and greater portability of ultrasound units have led to widespread adoption of musculoskeletal ultrasound imaging.
- **Advantages:** Unlike the imaging modalities previously discussed, ultrasound images are generated in real time, allowing a provider to directly examine the site of injury and discuss findings with the patient while the study is performed. This unique aspect allows a dynamic assessment of painful maneuvers and comparison with the unaffected contralateral structure when necessary. Tendons and ligaments tend to be echogenic and bright on ultrasound images, whereas fluid is anechoic and dark. Muscle and fat are more intermediate in echogenicity and appear toward the center of the gray scale. However, the appearance of each of these structures is partially dependent on the scanning parameters and the probe used to acquire images.
- **Disadvantages:** Although ultrasound depicts superficial structures with high spatial resolution, deeper structures are not well demonstrated. The ultrasound beam cannot penetrate bone, and thus only the surface of bone can be seen. Given the small portion of the body shown on any ultrasound image, it is also critical to understand bony landmarks and to review radiographs and other imaging studies, if available, before an ultrasound examination. In addition, appropriate documentation of findings and labeling of images is necessary to maintain continuity of care.
- **Common indications:** Ultrasound is well suited for evaluation of superficial tendons and ligaments. Small portable ultrasound units have seen use in acute settings for evaluating sports injuries and may show the presence of an effusion or torn structure. An acutely ruptured patellar tendon or Achilles tendon (Fig. 63.7) is an example of an injury well demonstrated by ultrasound.
- Ultrasound is also uniquely suited to guide procedures such as a subacromial/subdeltoid bursa injection at the shoulder (Fig. 63.8). Depiction of muscle planes and tendons allows the operator to precisely guide a needle into a thin bursa or joint for a selective injection.

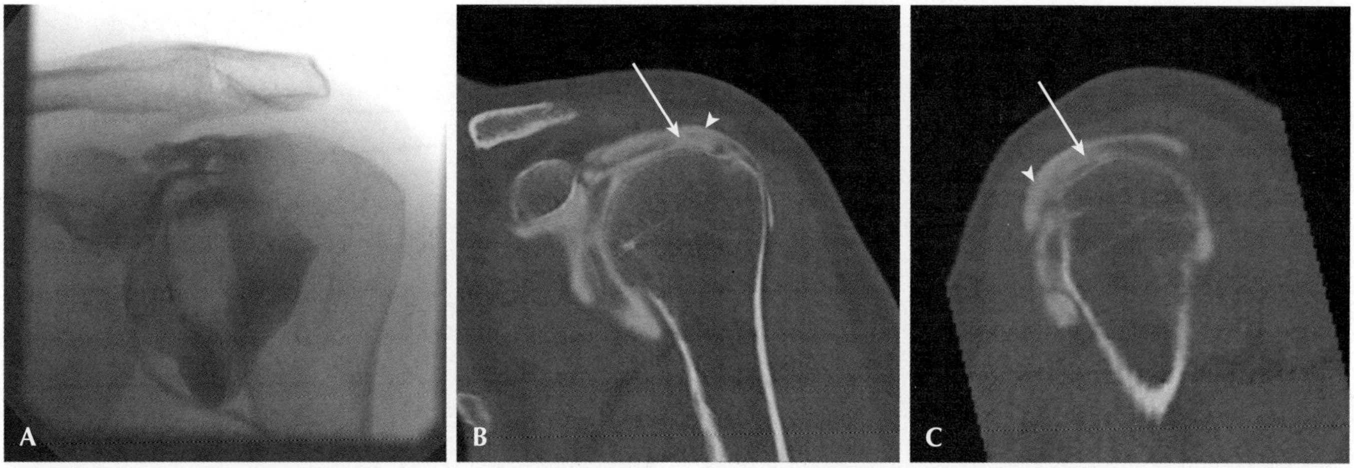
A
B
C

Figure 63.4 Images of a fluoroscopically guided shoulder arthrogram for purposes of CT arthrography **(A)**. Subsequent CT arthrography images show full-thickness supraspinatus tearing in the coronal oblique **(B)** and sagittal **(C)** planes, as depicted by the *arrow*. Contrast fills the cleft created by the supraspinatus tear extending into the subacromial/subdeltoid bursa *(arrowhead).*

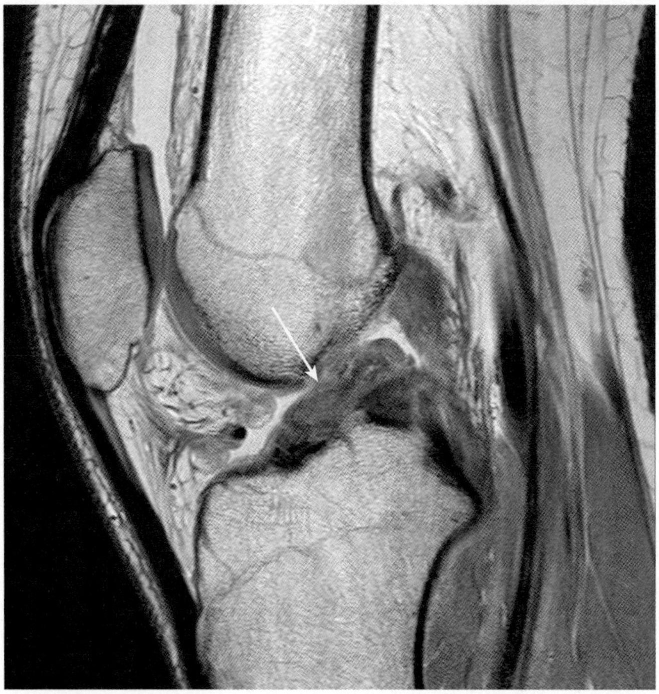

Figure 63.5 Sagittal proton density-weighted image of the knee showing a complete anterior cruciate ligament (ACL) rupture *(arrow)* with an associated effusion.

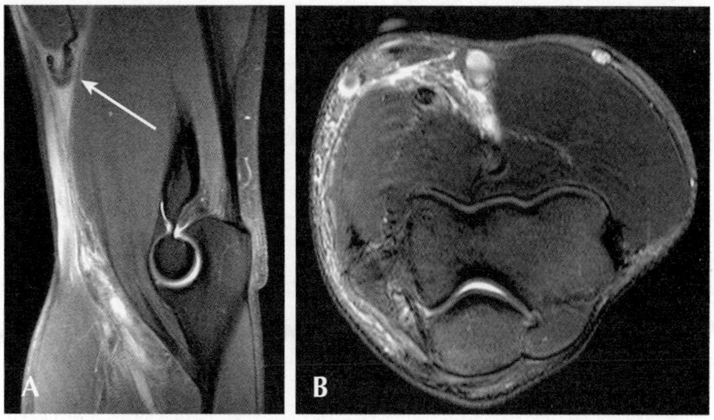
A
B

Figure 63.6 Sagittal **(A)** and axial **(B)** proton density fat-saturated images of the elbow show complete rupture of the biceps tendon with significant retraction *(arrow).* Note the fluid and swelling in the antecubital fossa.

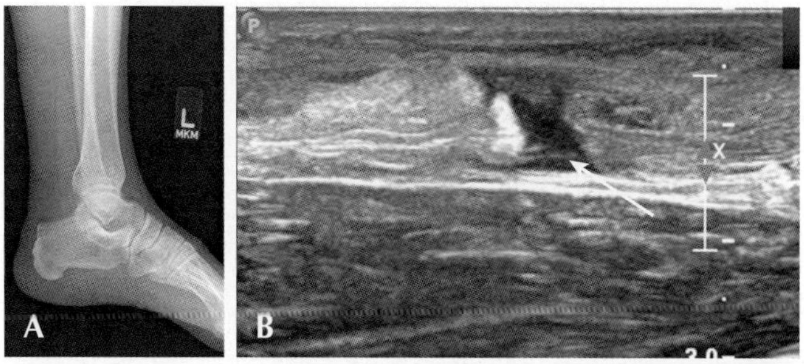
L
MKM
A
B

Figure 63.7 A lateral ankle radiograph **(A)** shows no fracture, but there is soft tissue swelling in the region of the Achilles tendon. A longitudinally oriented ultrasound image **(B)** in the same region shows a retracted, brightly echogenic Achilles tendon with dark anechoic fluid in the tendon gap *(arrow).*

NUCLEAR MEDICINE

- Nuclear medicine techniques are also used in sports medicine to depict stress fractures and localize infections. MRI has increasingly supplanted the use of nuclear medicine in sports medicine, but knowledge of the modality and potential uses remains important.
- The nuclear medicine technique used most commonly in the evaluation of sports injuries is the bone scan, which involves the intravenous administration of a radiopharmaceutical (typically technetium-99m tagged to hydroxymethylene diphosphonate or methylene diphosphonate), followed by imaging with a gamma camera. The radiopharmaceutical is taken up in bone and emits gamma rays as it decays, which are detected by the camera.
- Imaging the body part in question may begin in seconds, minutes, or hours after the administration of the radiopharmaceutical as a "3-phase" bone scan, which provides information about blood flow, inflammation, and bony abnormalities. A cross-sectional technique (single-photon emission computed tomography [SPECT]) can also be performed.

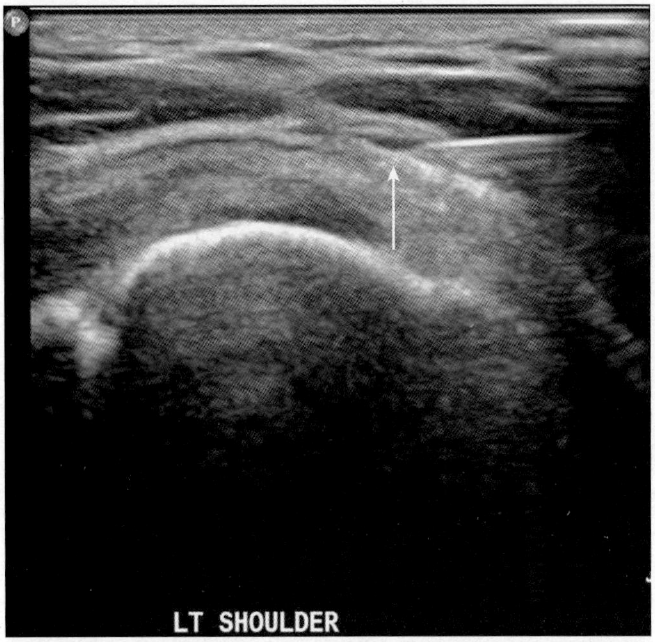
LT SHOULDER

Figure 63.8 An ultrasound-guided subacromial/subdeltoid bursal injection is demonstrated with placement of the needle tip (the bright linear structure at the upper right of the image) between the deltoid muscle and rotator cuff. This image is of the shoulder in the coronal plane, and the echogenic bright surface of the superior humeral head is visible at the bottom of the image. Anechoic fluid is visible in the bursa *(arrow)*.

- **Advantages:** Bone scan examinations are highly sensitive to any injury or abnormality of bone. However, they are relatively nonspecific, as an infection, tumor, or fracture all result in uptake of the radiopharmaceutical in regions of active bone turnover.
- **Disadvantages:** The lack of specificity limits the utility of bone scan techniques, and the dose to the patient can be substantial. For this reason, most diagnoses of stress fractures or suspected infections are currently made using MRI. In addition, the spatial resolution of a bone scan is low, providing less detail in regard to precise size and location of abnormalities.
- **Common indications:** Bone scans are highly sensitive in the detection of stress fractures (Fig. 63.9) and become positive soon after the onset of injury when no abnormality may be apparent on radiographs.

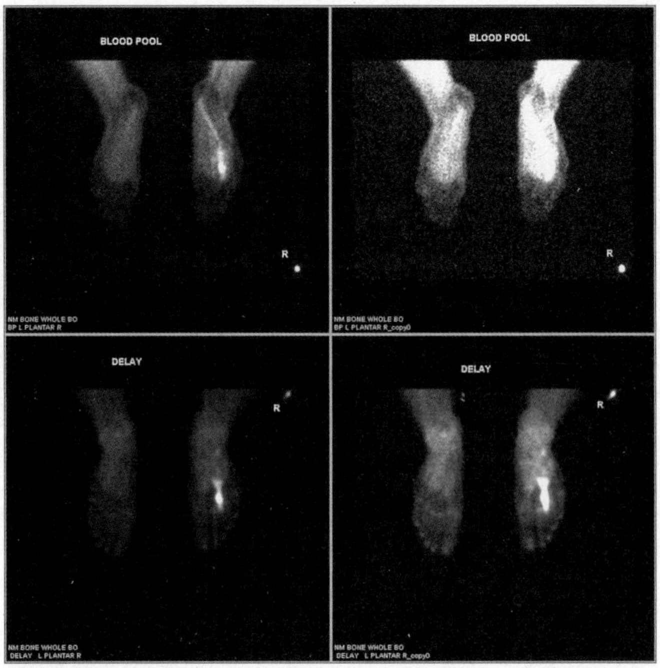
BLOOD POOL
BLOOD POOL
DELAY
DELAY
R

Figure 63.9 A bone scintigraphy scan shows increased activity on blood pool and delayed images in the region of the left third metatarsal, consistent with a stress fracture.

SUMMARY

- Imaging of an injured athlete typically begins with radiographs, although several diagnoses may be made without imaging of any kind.
- Imaging findings must be interpreted in the appropriate clinical setting because certain injuries may have persistent findings after symptoms or dysfunction have resolved.
- Each imaging modality has unique features that are well suited to answer certain clinical questions, and an understanding of their utility is crucial to the sports medicine provider.
- Open communication between radiologists and the sports medicine team is critical in determining accurate diagnosis and treatment.

RECOMMENDED READINGS

Available online.

SPORTS ULTRASOUND

64

Mederic M. Hall • Jeremiah W. Ray

SPORTS ULTRASOUND

- The use of ultrasound to evaluate and guide treatment for injuries and medical conditions associated with sport and exercise; this may involve both clinical and in-the-field applications.
- Evaluations are most often performed to answer a specific clinical question; need for further imaging and involvement of other medical imaging experts should be considered

GENERAL PRINCIPLES

Physics

- Electric **voltage from the base unit is converted to sound waves by the reverse piezoelectric effect.** Sound waves are reflected at tissue boundaries, producing echoes. Sound wave echoes returning to the transducer are converted to volts via the piezoelectric effect, and these volts are assigned a gray-scale color and location on the screen to produce an image.
- **A medium** is required for sound waves to pass through (acoustic coupling gel, water, etc.).
- Degree of reflection dependent upon **acoustic impedance**; similar acoustic impedance results in less reflection. Greater difference in acoustic impedance results in more reflection.
- The angle at which a sound wave strikes a tissue interface is referred to as the **angle of incidence. Perpendicular incidence** refers to a sound wave traveling perpendicular to the boundary between two media; this maximizes the amount of echoes reflected back to the transducer and optimizes the image. **Oblique incidence** occurs when the sound wave is not traveling perpendicular to the boundary between two media and some echoes are reflected away from the transducer; this can result in the artifact of **anisotropy** (discussed later).

Terminology

Short axis: Target structure (e.g., Achilles tendon) imaged in cross-section to the structure
Long axis: Target structure (e.g., Achilles tendon) imaged parallel to the structure lengthwise
Transverse: Anatomic region (e.g., knee) imaged in cross-section to the region
Longitudinal: Anatomic region (e.g., knee) imaged parallel to the region lengthwise
Anechoic: Black (i.e., no reflection)
Hypoechoic: Dark relative to the surrounding structures (i.e., less reflection)
Isoechoic: Same shade of gray as another structure
Hyperechoic: Bright relative to the surrounding structures (i.e., high reflection)

Transducers

- Higher frequency results in better resolution but lower penetration; recommended for imaging superficial structures
- Lower frequency results in lower resolution but improved penetration; recommended for imaging deep structures
- Linear array transducers: Flat transducer surface; sound waves exit perpendicular; minimizes anisotropy but produces a smaller field of view; recommended for superficial structures
- Curvilinear array transducers: Transducer surface curved with sound waves exiting in fan shape; increases the risk of anisotropy but produces a larger field of view; recommended for imaging deep structures and guiding procedures at steep angles

Artifacts

Anisotropy (Fig. 64.1)

- Sound waves reflected away from the transducer; result in an artifactual hypoechoic/anechoic appearance; risk of false-positive interpretation
- Results from oblique angle of incidence
- Tendons are most susceptible, followed by ligaments and then nerves
- Most common artifact in musculoskeletal imaging

Posterior Acoustic Shadowing

- Hypoechoic/anechoic region deep to the area of high reflectivity or high attenuation
- Commonly deep to a bone or calcium (may also be seen deep to scar tissue or normal fibrous septae)

Edge Shadowing

- Refraction artifact secondary to velocity change deep to a curved interface
- Helpful in identifying torn tendon edges
- Can obscure imaging deep to edges of both normal and abnormal structures

Acoustic Enhancement

- Also referred to as increased **through transmission**
- Hyperechoic region deep to an area of low attenuation
- Commonly deep to fluid collections

Reverberation

- Multiple internal reflections from highly reflective surface
- Commonly seen with metal from needles or orthopedic hardware

DIAGNOSTIC SPORTS ULTRASOUND

Musculoskeletal

- Provides detailed evaluation of musculoskeletal structures and offers several advantages compared with other imaging modalities, including high-resolution imaging (submillimeter), ability to image in real time and interact with a patient during the examination, contralateral comparison examination, minimal metal artifacts, portable, relatively inexpensive, and no radiation or known contraindications.
- Inherent limitations include limited field of view, limited penetration, incomplete evaluation of bones and joints, variability in equipment, and operator dependence.
- Diagnostic musculoskeletal ultrasound examinations are either a complete assessment of a joint or anatomic region (e.g., anterior knee) or a focused, limited assessment of a specific structure (e.g., Achilles tendon). Complete examinations should include all relevant structures within the anatomic region, including muscles, tendons, joints, other soft tissue structures, and any identifiable abnormality. Although most joint regions are divided into quadrants, a complete examination of the shoulder should include all relevant structures.

Tendon

NORMAL SONOGRAPHIC APPEARANCE

- High-frequency linear array transducer recommended
- Exceptions are in certain deep tendons in patients with large body habitus (iliopsoas, gluteals, etc.)
- Long axis (LAX): Fibrillar pattern of hyperechoic, tightly packed linear echoes
- Short axis (SAX): Stippled clusters of dots resembling a "broom end"

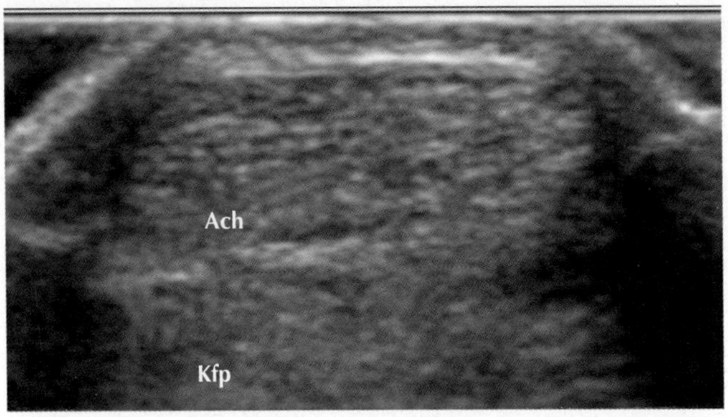
Ach
Kfp

A. Sound waves exiting transducer are perpendicular to the short axis of the Achilles tendon resulting in optimal image represented as hyperechoic uniform echotexture.

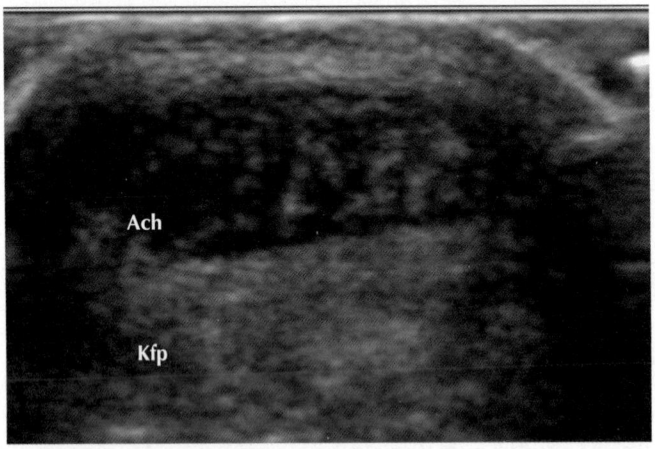
Ach
Kfp

B. Slight angulation of the transducer with oblique angle of incidence resulting in artifactual hypoechogenicity of the Achilles tendon.

Figure 64.1 Anisotropy. *Ach,* Achilles tendon; *Kfp,* Kaeger fat pad.

GENERAL PATHOLOGIC FEATURES

Pathologic findings are similar across tendons. Location of injury within specific tendons will vary and often are affected by zones of relative hypovascularity, biomechanical factors, and repetitive trauma.

Tendinosis: Features include thickening/swelling of the tendon, hypoechogenicity, and heterogeneity with loss of usual fibrillar echotexture. In chronic cases, the tendon may appear atrophic instead of thickened. Intratendinous calcifications may be identified; power or color Doppler imaging may demonstrate intra/peritendinous hyperemia, termed *neovascularity.*

Tendon tear: Classified as partial, full thickness, and complete:
- **Partial-thickness tear:** Well-defined focal defect in tendon confirmed in two planes; often seen as progression of tendinosis
- **Full-thickness tear:** Tear extends across full thickness of the tendon (deep to superficial) but may not involve full width of tendon
- **Complete tear:** Full thickness and full width of tendon; retraction of torn tendon fibers; this will appear as a gap within the tendon or complete nonvisualization of the tendon

Calcific tendinopathy: Calcium hydroxyapatite deposition within tendon; appearance is hyperechoic with variable amounts of posterior acoustic shadowing dependent upon type and phase of calcification; symptoms typically related to mass effect/impingement or inflammatory response in resorptive phase; may be asymptomatic

Tenosynovitis: Inflammation of tenosynovial lining of tendon sheath represented as complex fluid and hyperemic tissue adjacent to tendon within sheath; pain with transducer pressure helpful in distinguishing symptomatic tenosynovitis from other secondary causes of tendon sheath fluid (e.g., communicating joint fluid)

PEARLS AND PITFALLS
- Anisotropy can mimic tendinosis or tear and is common, particularly in the rotator cuff; confirmation in two planes and careful scanning technique are critical.
- Edge shadowing artifact can be useful in identifying torn tendon ends.
- Dynamic imaging is helpful in identifying complete tears.
- Clinical significance of neovascularity is controversial.

SPECIFIC PATHOLOGIES
- Rotator cuff tendinopathy and tears (Fig. 64.2)
- Proximal biceps tendinopathy (Fig. 64.3)
- Common extensor tendinopathy (Fig. 64.4)
- De Quervain tenosynovitis (Fig. 64.5)
- Gluteal tendinopathy (Fig. 64.6)
- Proximal hamstring tendinopathy (Fig. 64.7)
- Patellar tendinopathy (Fig. 64.8)
- Fibular (peroneal) tendinopathy (Fig. 64.9)
- Achilles tendinopathy and tears (Fig. 64.10)
- Plantar fasciopathy (Fig. 64.11)

Muscle

NORMAL SONOGRAPHIC APPEARANCE
- Hypoechoic muscle fibers/fascicles and hyperechoic septa of peri/epimysium form a pennate pattern on LAX and "starry night" pattern on SAX.

GENERAL PATHOLOGIC FEATURES
- **Strain:** Focal disruption of normal fiber pattern/structure; in an acute injury, there will be swelling of muscle with possible focal defect in higher-grade injuries. If fibers are torn, hemorrhage may be identified as hypo/anechoic compressible fluid collection at the site of injury; will begin to organize into mixed echogenic hematoma and eventually form hyperechoic scar tissue. Hyperemia on power and color Doppler imaging is common in acute injury.
  - Hamstring muscle tear (Fig. 64.12)
  - Medial gastrocnemius muscle tear (Fig. 64.13)
- **Contusion:** Typically involves deep muscle fibers adjacent to bone (e.g., vastus intermedius in the thigh); myositis ossificans will appear as a hyperechoic, linear calcific density within the zone of muscle injury; demonstrated earlier on ultrasound than radiograph
  - Quadriceps contusion and myositis ossificans (Fig. 64.14)

Ligament

NORMAL SONOGRAPHIC APPEARANCE
- Identify bony landmarks and align transducer with ligament; LAX most useful imaging plane
- Fibrillar echotexture pattern is less compact than tendon
- Typically hyperechoic, but depending upon surrounding tissue, may appear hypoechoic

GENERAL PATHOLOGIC FEATURES

Grade I: Swollen and hypoechoic without fiber disruption or laxity on dynamic stress imaging

Grade II: Partial tear/evidence of fiber disruption; may have some laxity on dynamic stress imaging, but end point appreciated

Grade III: Complete tear; dynamic stress imaging demonstrates laxity and absence of bridging fibers.
- High ankle sprain (Fig. 64.15)
- Ulnar collateral ligament of elbow sprain (Fig. 64.16)

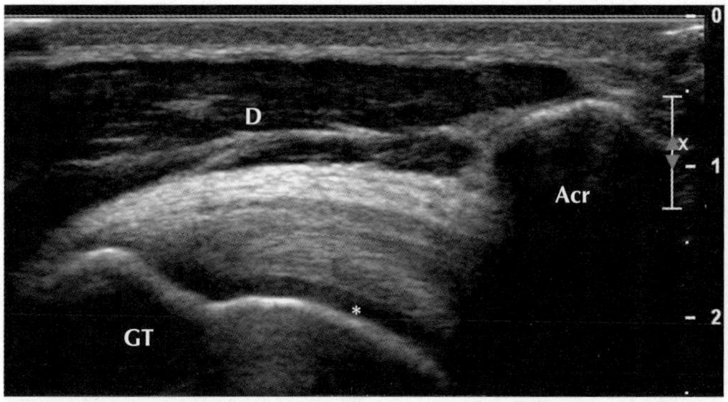
D
Acr
GT

A. Long axis view of normal supraspinatus tendon. Often referred to as "bird's beak" appearance. Note homogenous echotexture and smooth cortical margin.

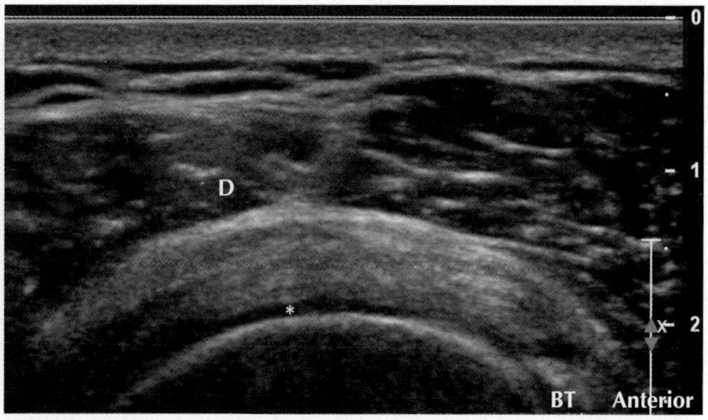
D
BT
Anterior

B. Short axis view of normal supraspinatus tendon. Note uniform thickness of tendon overlying anechoic rim of cartilage *(asterisks)*. Often referred to as "tire on a wheel." Identification of the long head of the biceps tendon (BT) is key to ensuring adequate evaluation of the leading anterior edge of the supraspinatus.

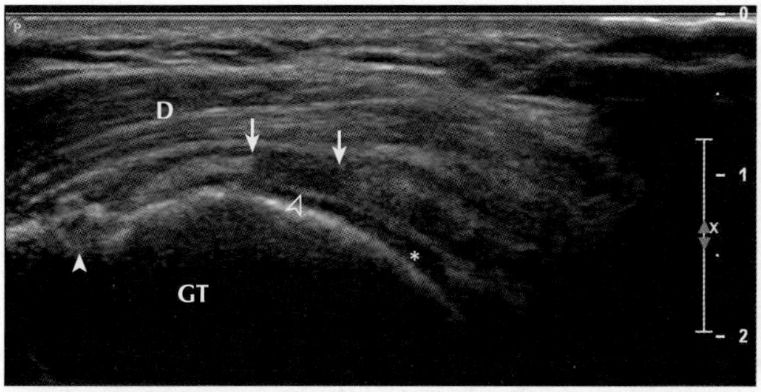
D
GT

C. Full thickness tear *(arrows)* of supraspinatus tendon in long axis. Cortical irregularities *(solid arrowhead)* at the greater tuberosity foot print and cartilage interface sign *(open arrowhead)*, both secondary signs of rotator cuff tear, are present.

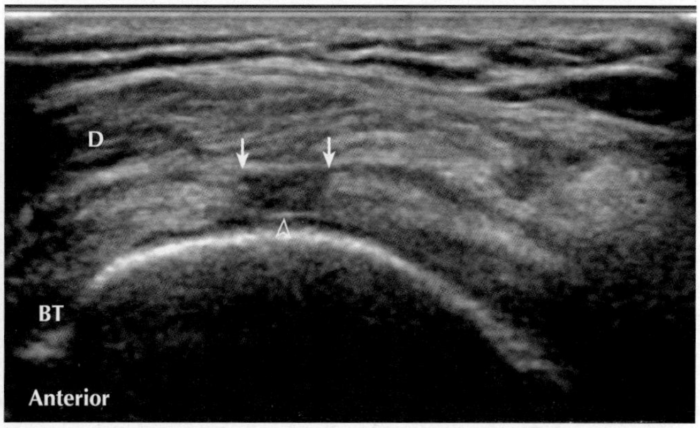
D
BT
Anterior

D. Corresponding short axis view of full thickness supraspinatus tear. Note volume loss at site of tear *(arrows)* and cartilage interface sign *(open arrowhead)*.

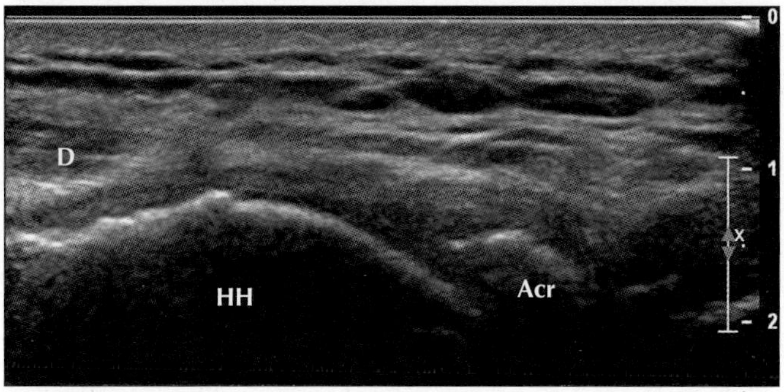
D
HH
Acr

E. Chronic complete supraspinatus tear in long axis. There is non-visualization of the rotator cuff with the humeral head (HH) high riding in relation to the acromion (Acr).

Figure 64.2 Rotator cuff tendinopathy and tears. *Asterisk* indicates articular cartilage. *Acr,* Acromion; *BT,* long head biceps tendon; *D,* deltoid; *GT,* greater tuberosity; *HH,* humeral head.

Nerve

NORMAL SONOGRAPHIC APPEARANCE

- Hypoechoic nerve fascicles and hyperechoic intra/extraneural epineurium form a "honeycomb" appearance on SAX; fascicular appearance on LAX (less tightly packed than ligament); typically adjacent to vessels, which may be easier to identify

GENERAL PATHOLOGIC FEATURES

- Swelling and hypoechogenicity, often accompanied by loss of normal fascicular pattern
- May demonstrate focal swelling proximal to entrapment site or focal narrowing ("notch sign") at the entrapment site
- Dynamic testing may demonstrate subluxation/dislocation or hypomobility and adhesion to surrounding structures.

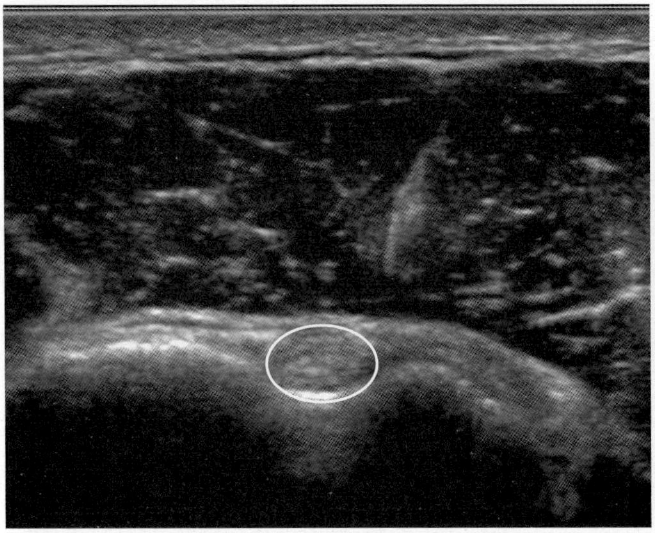

A. Short axis view of normal long head of the biceps tendon *(open oval)* at intertubercular groove.

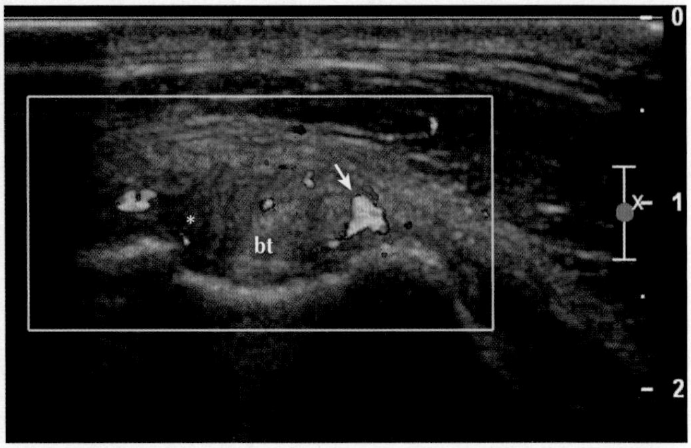
0
*
bt
1
2

B. Biceps tenosynovitis is identified as hyperemic tissue *(arrow)* and complex fluid *(asterisks)* within tendon sheath on color Doppler evaluation.

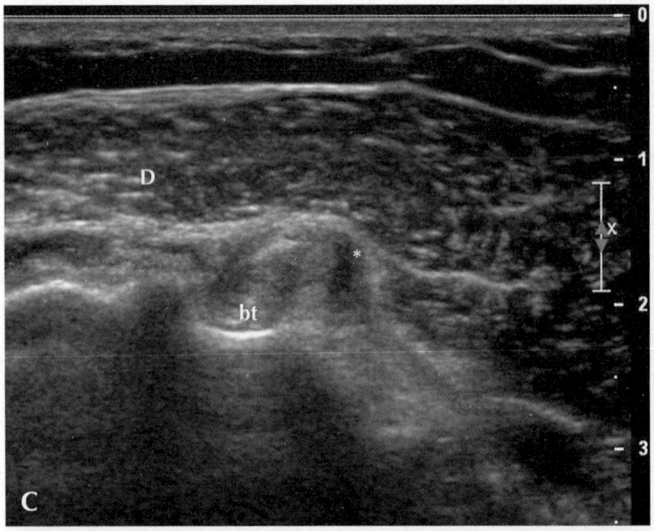
0
1
D
*
bt
2
3
C

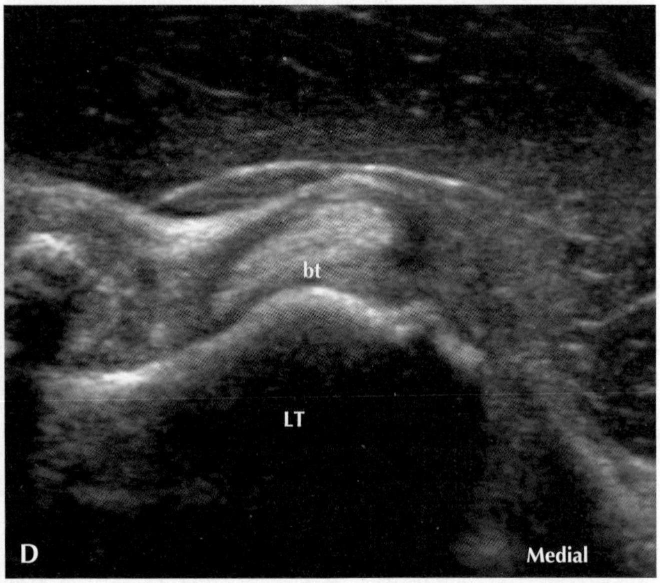
bt
LT
D
Medial

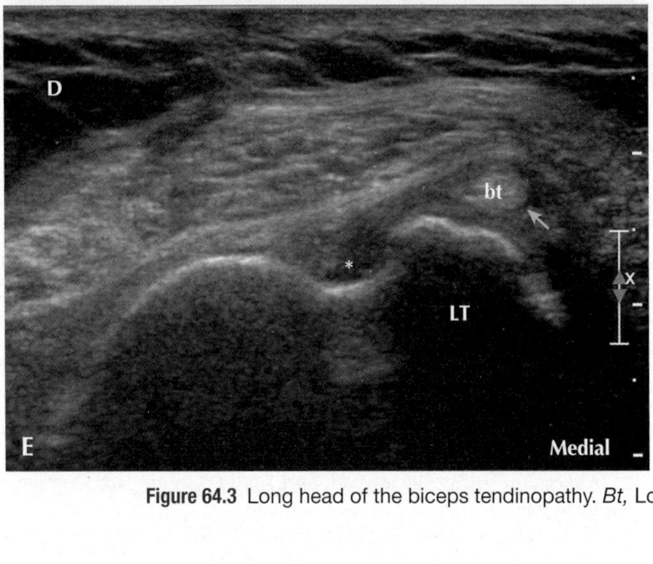
D
bt
*
LT
E
Medial

C–E. The biceps tendon (bt) is enlarged and heterogenous with hypoechoic fissurations representing tendinosis. Instability of the biceps tendon can be seen as subluxation onto the lesser tuberosity (LT) as seen in **D**, or frank dislocation medially as seen in **E** with empty groove *(asterisks)*.

Figure 64.3 Long head of the biceps tendinopathy. *Bt,* Long head biceps tendon; *D,* deltoid; *LT,* lesser tuberosity.

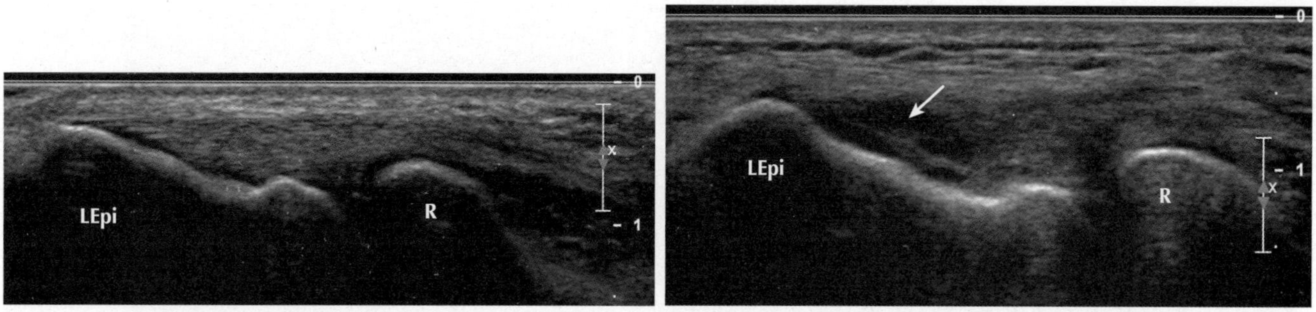
LEpi
R
LEpi
R

A. Long axis view of normal common extensor tendon.

B. Severe tendinosis of the common extensor tendon origin in long axis. Note the complete loss of fibrillar echotexture and hypoechogenicity *(arrow)*.

Figure 64.4 Common extensor tendinopathy. *LEpi,* Lateral epicondyle; *R,* radius.

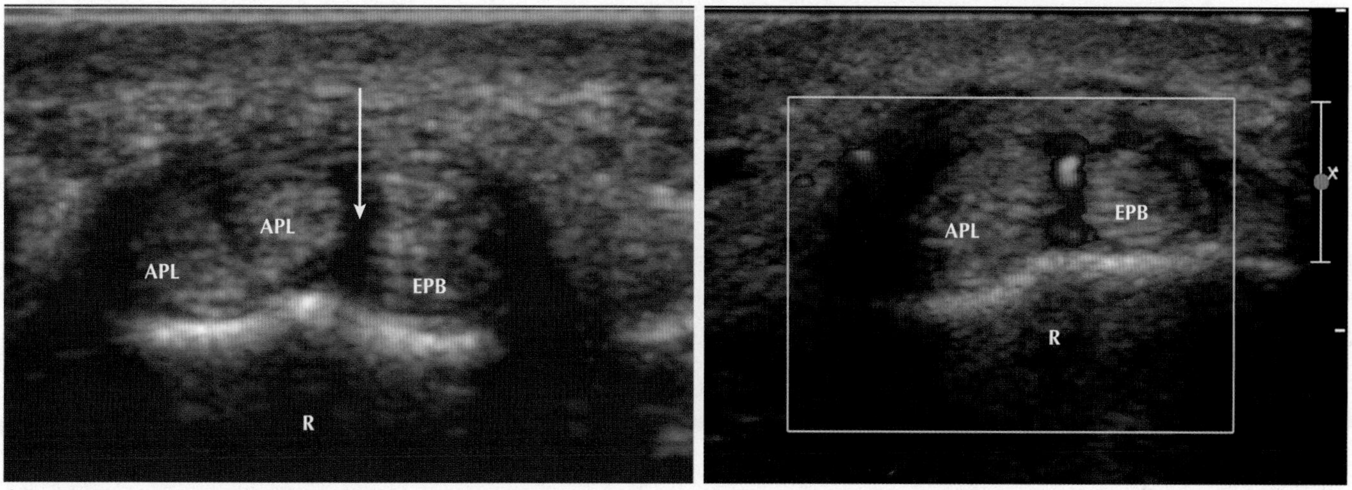
APL
APL
EPB
R
APL
EPB
R

A. Short axis view of normal first dorsal compartment tendons. Note the multiple slips of the abductor pollicis longus (APL) which is a normal variant as well as the hypoechoic vertical septum *(arrow),* which sub-compartmentalizes the sheath.

B. Power Doppler image of DeQuervain's tenosynovitis demonstrating hyperemia within the tendon sheath.

Figure 64.5 De Quervain tenosynovitis. *APL,* Abductor pollicis longus; *EPB,* extensor pollicis brevis; *R,* radius.

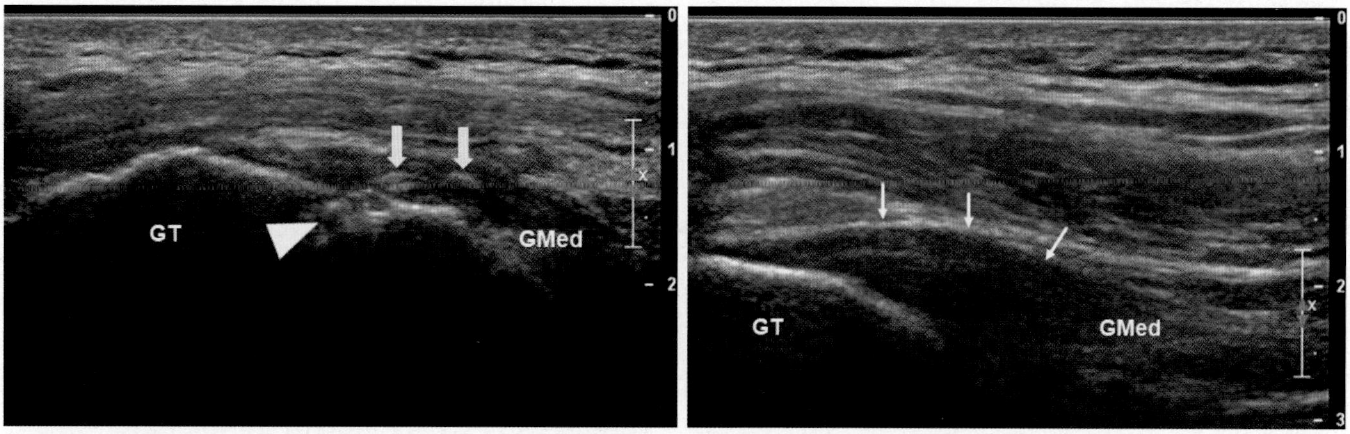
GT
GMed
GT
GMed

A. Long axis image of the anterior band of gluteus medius at the lateral facet of the greater trochanter. Hyperechoic linear calcifications are present *(arrows)* with associated bone irregularity *(arrowhead).*

B. Long axis view of the posterior band of gluteus medius tendon *(arrows)* at the superoposterior facet of the greater trochanter. Note hypoechoic thickening consistent with tendinosis.

Figure 64.6 Gluteus medius tendinopathy. *GMed,* Gluteus medius tendon; *GT,* greater trochanter.

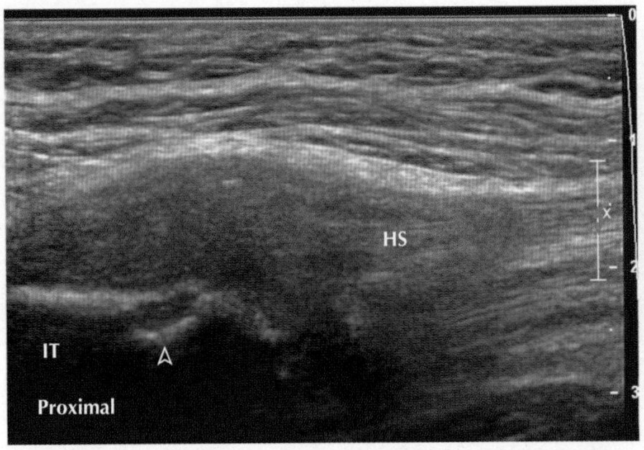
HS
IT
Proximal

A. Long axis view of proximal hamstring tendon demonstrating changes of tendinosis including thickening, hypoechogenicity, and cortical irregularities *(open arrowhead)* at the ischial tuberosity.

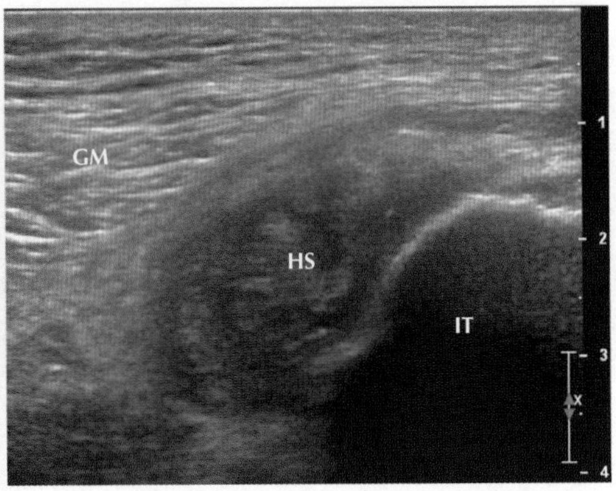
GM
HS
IT

B. Corresponding short axis image of tendinosis.

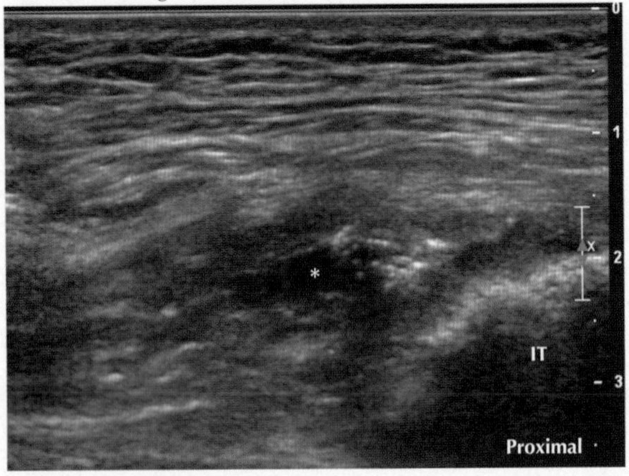
IT
Proximal

C. Severe tendinopathic changes are noted with focal partial thickness tear represented as anechoic region of fiber disruption *(asterisks)*.

Figure 64.7 Proximal hamstring tendinopathy. *GM,* Gluteus maximus; *HS,* proximal hamstring tendon; *IT,* ischial tuberosity.

SPECIFIC PATHOLOGIES
- Carpal tunnel syndrome (Fig. 64.17)
- Ulnar neuropathy and instability at the elbow (Fig. 64.18)

Bone

NORMAL SONOGRAPHIC APPEARANCE
- Evaluation limited to superficial portion because of inability of sound waves to pass through bone
- Surface of the bone should appear hyperechoic, smooth, and linear

GENERAL PATHOLOGIC FEATURES

Fracture: Disruption of smooth cortical surface; hypoechoic hematoma at the fracture site; hyperemia common; pain with transducer pressure
- Ultrasound appearance of fractures (Fig. 64.19)

Stress fracture/reaction: Periosteal thickening with (fracture) or without (reaction) cortical discontinuity

Joint and Cartilage

NORMAL SONOGRAPHIC APPEARANCE

Joint: Incomplete evaluation because of same limitations as bone; can identify hypo/anechoic joint effusions, certain synovial disorders, and loose bodies within the visualized portion of a joint

Hyaline cartilage: Hypo/anechoic and noncompressible (helpful distinction from fluid collection); uniform thickness

Fibrocartilage: Hyperechoic or mixed echogenicity with uniform echotexture ("salt and pepper" appearance)

GENERAL PATHOLOGIC FEATURES
- Joint effusion, nonspecific sign of intra-articular dysfunction
- Hyperemia within synovium consistent with synovitis
- Nonuniformity of hyaline cartilage can be seen with chondral injuries
- Focal hypoechoic defect in fibrocartilage with or without secondary signs of parameniscal cyst, joint effusion, etc.

SPECIFIC PATHOLOGIES
- Acromioclavicular (AC) joint disorders (Fig. 64.20)
- Knee joint effusion (Fig. 64.21)

Vessels

NORMAL SONOGRAPHIC APPEARANCE
- Hypo/anechoic tubular structures
- **Arteries:** Pulsatile, thicker walls, less compressible
- **Veins:** Thinner walled, easily compressible, nonpulsatile

GENERAL PATHOLOGIC FEATURES
- Typically limited to evaluation of acute thrombus and referred for formal vascular study as needed (see "Trauma and Other Acute Conditions")
- Focal enlargement concerning for aneurysm; noncompressibility concerning for thromboembolism

TRAUMA AND OTHER ACUTE CONDITIONS

- Sports ultrasound has become established as an on-site imaging tool for the point-of-care evaluation of many traumatic and acute conditions on the field and in the training room
- The fields of emergency medicine, critical care, and global health, among others, have defined best practices for many ultrasound techniques relevant to the sports medicine physician caring for the acutely injured athlete. These include ocular

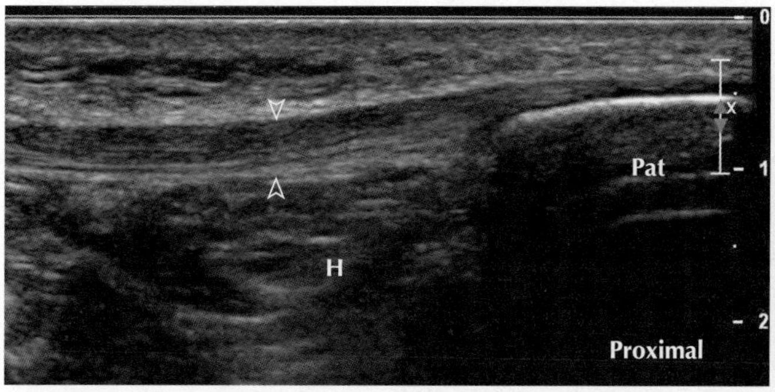
Pat
H
Proximal

A. Long axis view of normal patellar tendon *(open arrowheads).*

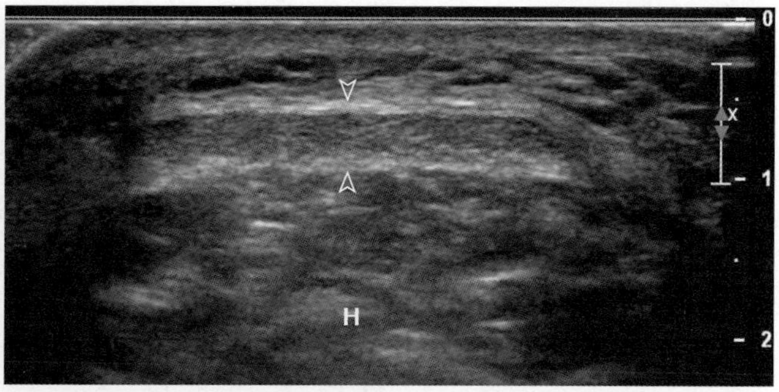
H

B. Short axis view of normal patellar tendon *(open arrowheads).*

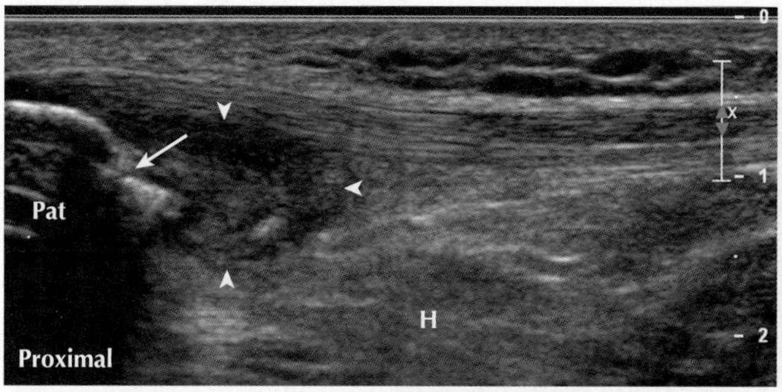
Pat
Proximal
H

C. Severe tendinosis of the proximal patellar tendon *(arrowheads)* demonstrated in long axis. Cortical irregularity is present at the patella *(arrow).* Note the superficial fibers are spared.

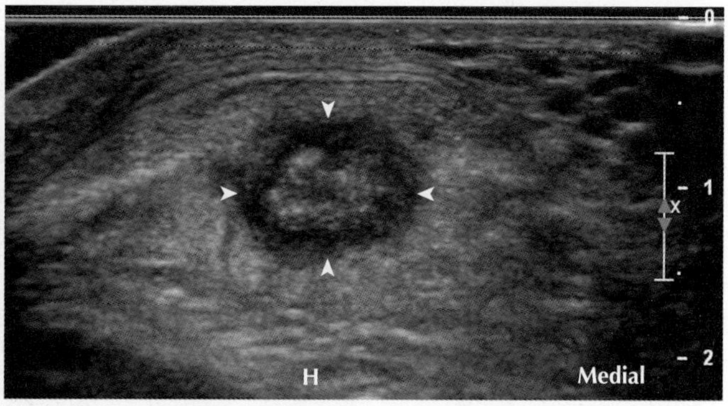
H
Medial

D. Corresponding short axis view of severe tendinosis *(arrowheads).* Note the nodular involvement of the deep central aspect of the tendon. This is the classic pattern of involvement in clinical "Jumper's Knee."

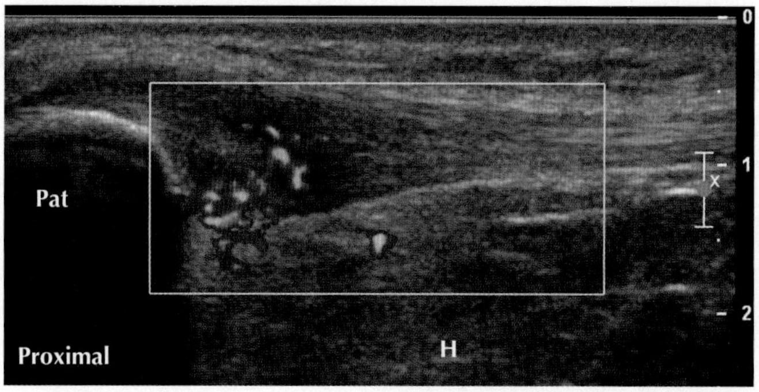
Pat
Proximal
H

E. Power Doppler image demonstrating neovessels invading the patellar tendon from the posterior Hoffa's fat pad.

Figure 64.8 Patellar tendinopathy. *H,* Hoffa fat pad; *Pat,* patella.

trauma; optic nerve sheath diameter (ONSD) assessment in increased intracranial pressures (ICP); the extended Focused Assessment with Sonography for Trauma (eFAST); the bedside lung ultrasound in emergency protocol (BLUE protocol) to evaluate high-altitude pulmonary edema (HAPE); volume/fluid assessment; skin and soft tissue evaluation; and deep venous thrombosis (DVT) evaluation.

Thoracoabdominal Evaluation

Extended Focused Assessment With Sonography for Trauma

- Goal is to identify pneumothorax, intraperitoneal free fluid (which in the setting of trauma is presumed to be because of a hemoperitoneum), or pericardial effusion in order to expedite the time to definitive care; low sensitivity but high specificity; negative study does not exclude the potential for serious injury. This ultrasound technique can also identify hemothorax and solid organ injury, including injury to retroperitoneal structures such as kidneys.
- Six standard views: anterior lung fields bilaterally; hepatorenal recess (Morison pouch), also called the *right upper quadrant (RUQ)* view; splenorenal recess, also called the *left upper quadrant (LUQ)* view; suprapubic view; and subxiphoid view, also called the *pericardial view.*

Pneumothorax

- Sensitivity and specificity significantly better than chest radiograph
- **Criteria for diagnosis:** (1) absence of lung sliding (identification = 100% negative predictive value), (2) disappearance of "B-lines" (visualization = 100% negative predictive value), and (3) M-mode transition from "sandy beach" in normal lung to "barcode" in pneumothorax (Fig. 64.22)

Pulmonary Edema

- Sensitivity 97%, specificity 98%
- Criteria for diagnosis: increased frequency of B-lines (>5) within intercostal space or increased pleural comet tail artifact. More sensitive with multiple intercostal spaces evaluated (>8).
- Particularly useful in differentiating HAPE from alternative etiologies of dyspnea such as reactive airway

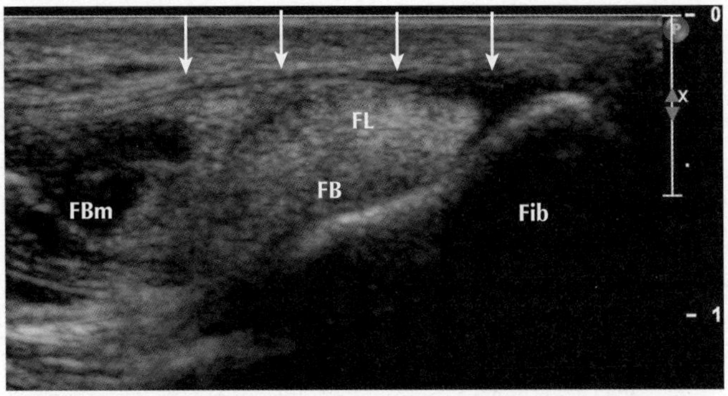
FL
FB
FBm
Fib
0
X
1

A. Short axis image of normal fibular tendons at the retro-malleolar groove. Arrows identify the superior fibular retinaculum.

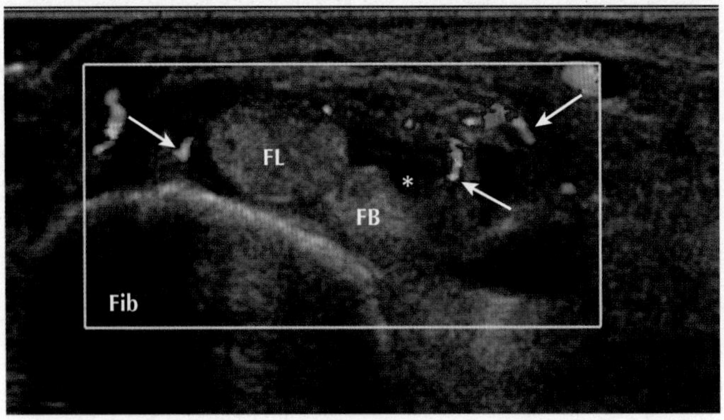
FL
*
FB
Fib

B. Fibular tenosynovitis is identified as hyperemic tissue *(arrows)* on color Doppler within the tendon sheath. Note small amount of anechoic free fluid adjacent to tendons *(asterisks)*.

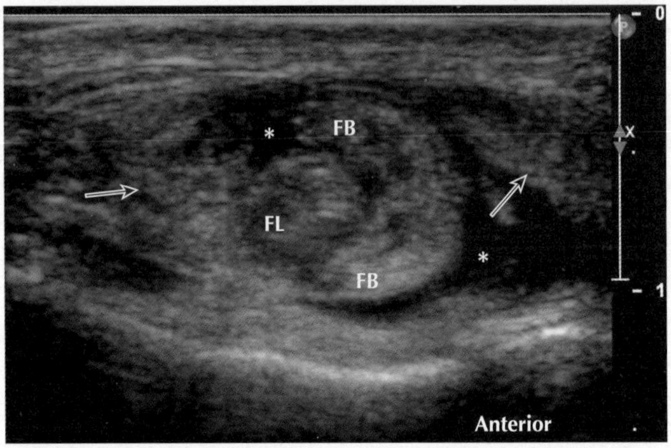
0
*
FB
X
FL
*
FB
1
Anterior

C. Short axis image of fibularis brevis longitudinal split tear in the infra-malleolar region. The fibularis brevis has taken a "boomerang" shape as the fibularis longus has invaginated into the tendon. Note the hypoechoic regions of tendinosis within the fibularis brevis. Free fluid *(asterisks)* and thickened tenosynovial tissue *(open arrows)* are seen within the tendon sheath.

Figure 64.9 Fibular (peroneal) tendinopathy. *FB,* Fibularis brevis; *FBm,* fibularis brevis muscle. *Fib,* fibula; *FL,* fibularis longus.

Ocular Trauma

- Evaluation of posterior chamber trauma for retinal detachment/tear and vitreous hemorrhage (Fig. 64.23)
- Anterior chamber difficult to assess but can detect lens dislocation
- Normal posterior chamber is anechoic. Any echogenic material is suggestive of injury and requires immediate referral

Optic Nerve Sheath Diameter

- Evaluation of optic nerve sheath; measurement taken 3 mm posterior to junction of globe and optic nerve. A value of >5–6 mm is suggestive of increased ICPs. However, it is more clinically useful to measure ONSD changes over time rather than an absolute value threshold of >5 mm because of variability of baseline ONSD.

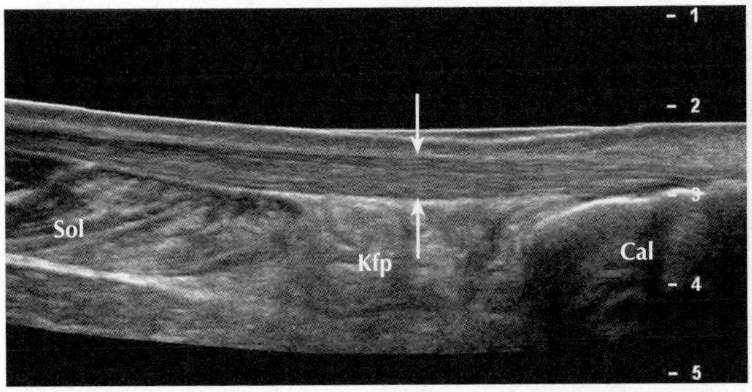
Sol
Kfp
Cal

A. Long axis extended field of view image of normal Achilles tendon *(arrows)*.

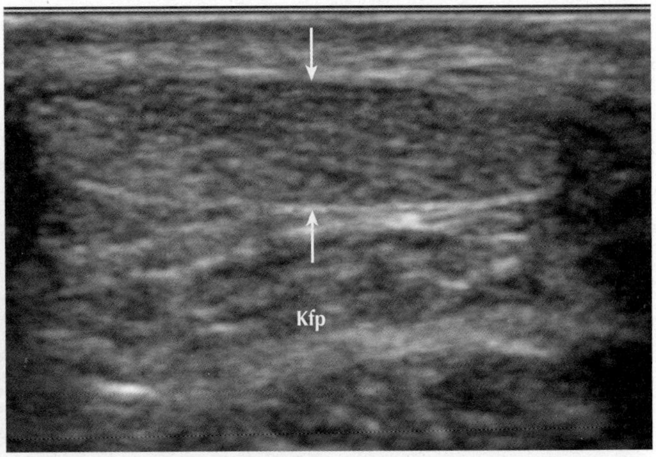
Kfp

B. Short axis image of normal Achilles tendon *(arrows)*.

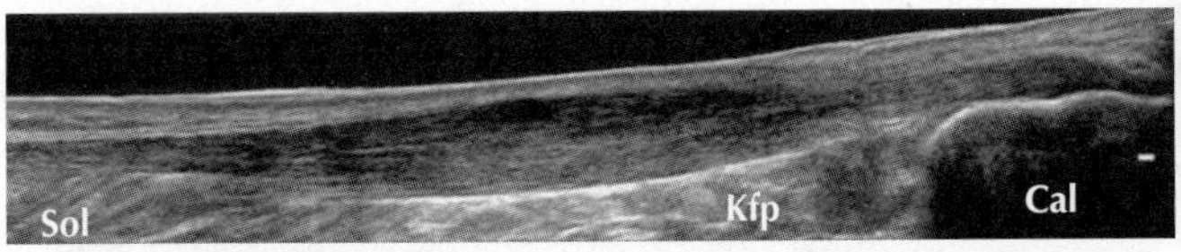
Sol
Kfp
Cal

C. Long axis extended field of view image demonstrating tendinosis of the midsubstance of the Achilles tendon.

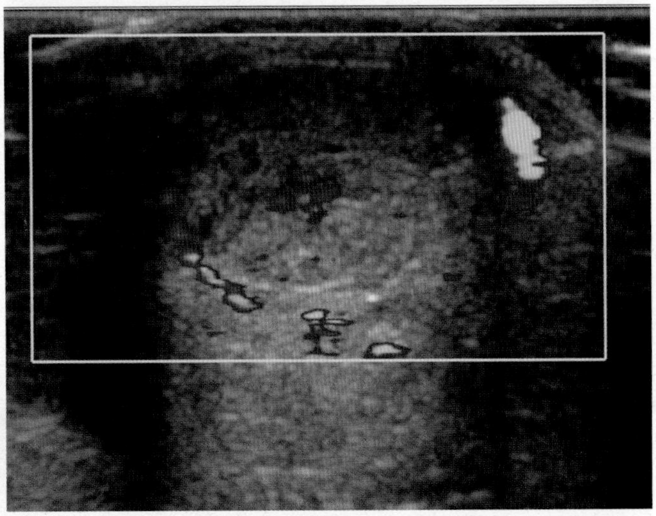

D. Power Doppler image of the Achilles tendon in short axis with intra- and peri-tendinous hyperemia referred to as *neovascularity*.

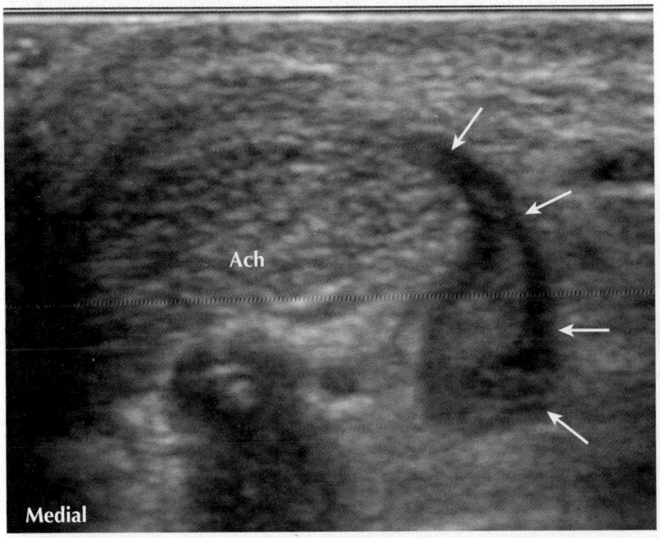
Ach
Medial

E. Complex fluid collection *(arrows)* along the lateral border of the Achilles tendon representing acute paratenonitis. Note the normal appearance of the Achilles tendon in short axis.

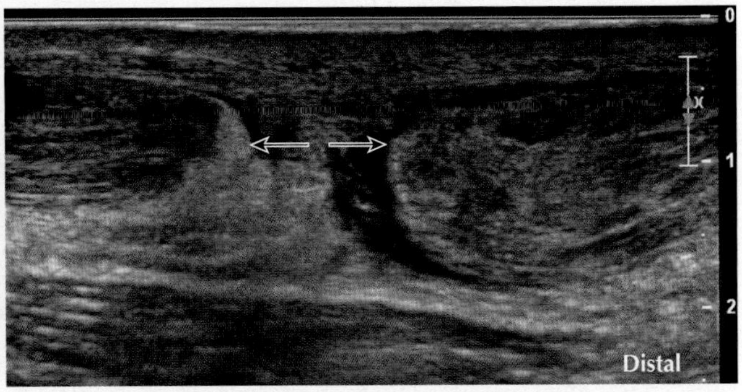
Distal

F. Acute rupture of the Achilles tendon in long axis. *Open arrows* identify the torn tendon edges.

Figure 64.10 Achilles tendinopathy. *Asterisk* indicates retrocalcaneal bursa. *Cal,* Calcaneus; *Kfp,* Kaeger fat pad; *Sol,* soleus.

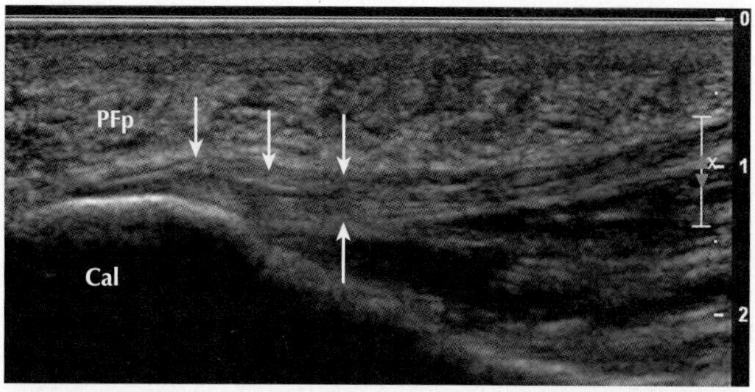
PFp
Cal
0
1
2

A. Long axis image of normal plantar fascia origin *(arrows)*.

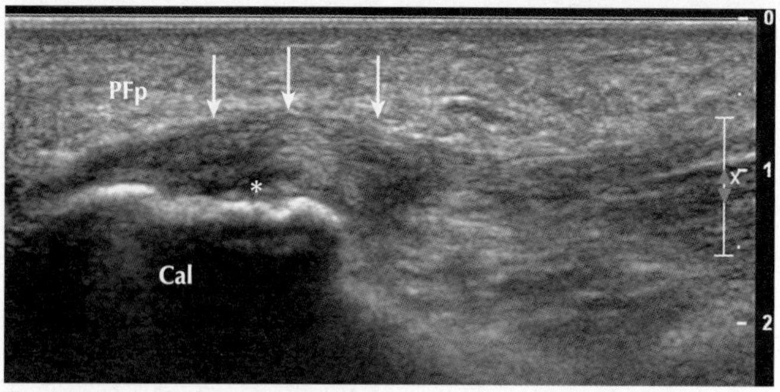
PFp
*
Cal
0
1
2

B. The plantar fascia origin *(arrows)* is thickened and hypoechoic consistent with degenerative fasciosis. A focal anechoic region devoid of fibers *(asterisks)* is consistent with a partial thickness tear.

Figure 64.11 Plantar fasciopathy. *Cal,* Calcaneus; *PFp,* plantar fat pad.

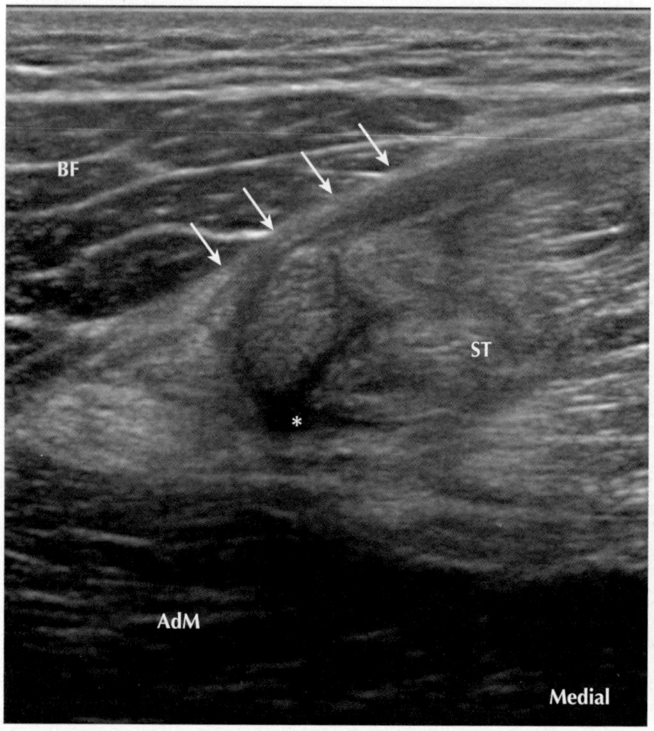
BF
ST
*
AdM
Medial

A. Short axis image of an acute partial muscle tear of the semitendinosus at the aponeurosis with the biceps femoris *(arrows)*. Note the anechoic free fluid *(asterisks)* at site of tear and disruption of normal echotexture at site of injury. The entire semitendinosus muscle is hyperechoic in relation to the surrounding biceps femoris and adductor magnus representing muscular edema.

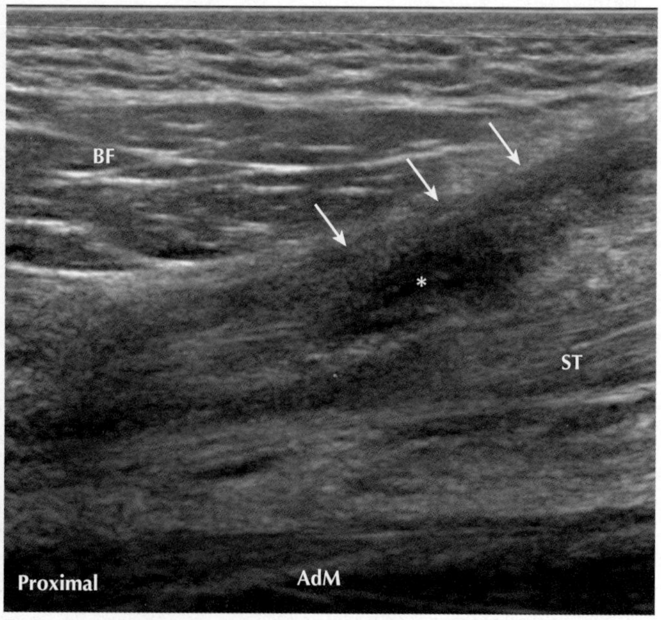
BF
*
ST
Proximal
AdM

B. Corresponding long axis view of the same injury.

Figure 64.12 Hamstring strain. *AdM,* Adductor magnus; *BF,* biceps femoris; *ST,* semitendinosus.

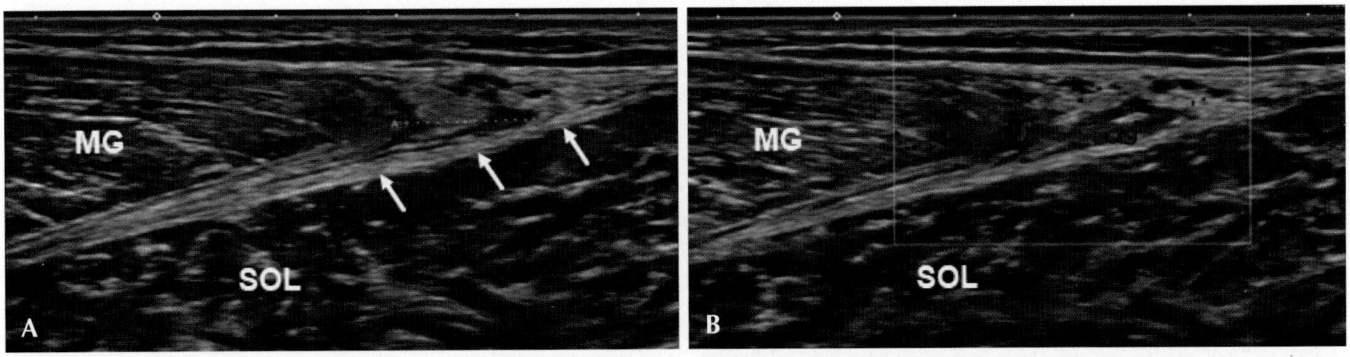
MG
SOL
A
MG
SOL
B

Long axis images of acute medial gastrocnemius tear at the distal myotendinous junction. Note disinsertion of the distal fibers from the aponeurosis (*arrows*) with retraction (calipers) (**A**). Minimal hematoma has formed as injury was < 2 hours old, but hyperechoic edema is appreciated within the torn fibers and hyperemia is already present on Doppler (**B**).

Figure 64.13 Medial gastrocnemius muscle tear. *MG,* Medial gastrocnemius; *SOL,* soleus.

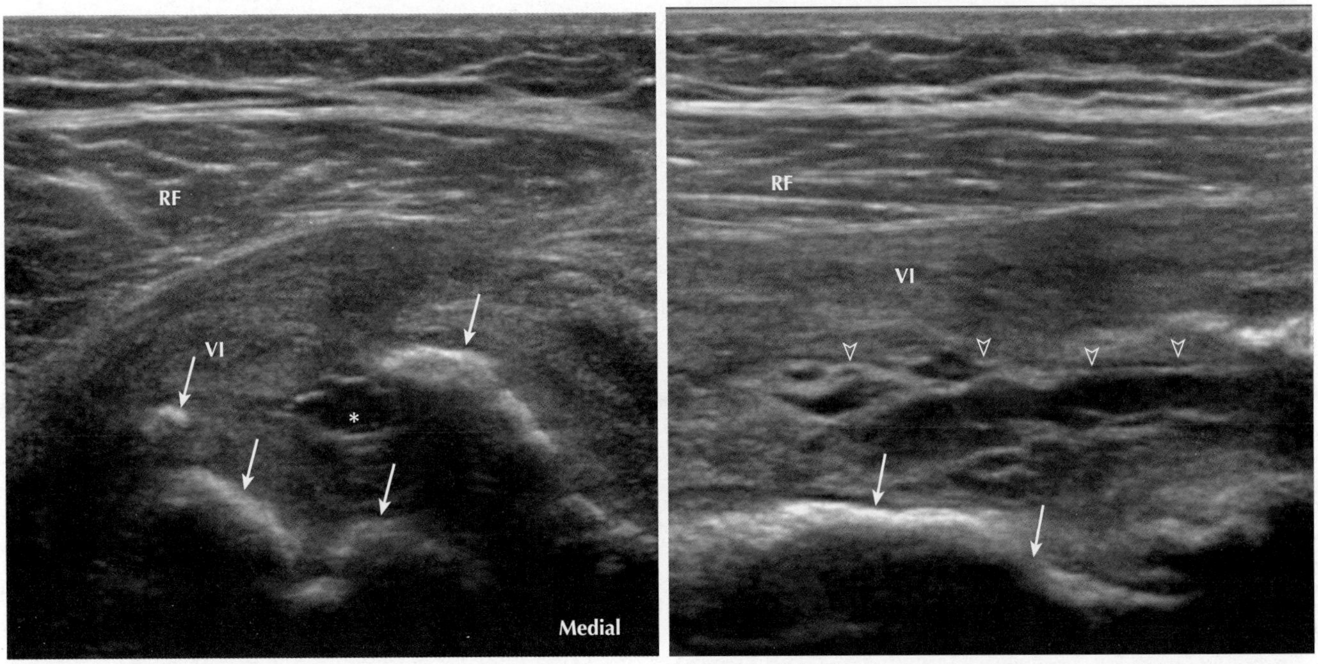
RF
VI
*
Medial
RF
VI

A. Short axis image of subacute quadriceps contusion with early myositis ossificans formation. The vastus intermedius is significantly swollen in comparison to overlying rectus femoris, which is normal in appearance. A central region of anechoic free fluid *(asterisks)* is noted with disruption of muscle fibers. Hyperechoic calcific tissue *(arrows)* representing myositis ossificans is seen throughout the vastus intermedius. Note posterior acoustic shadowing deep to the regions of calcification.

B. Corresponding long axis image of the same injury. The extent of the muscle fiber disruption is more apparent *(arrowheads)*. A large calcific lesion *(arrows)* shadows the underlying femur.

Figure 64.14 Quadriceps contusion. *RF,* Rectus femoris; *VI,* vastus intermedius.

Fluid/Volume Assessment

- Inferior vena cava (IVC) evaluation provides rapid global assessment of fluid status. Hypovolemia is confirmed if the IVC is less than 2 cm in anterior-posterior diameter and is seen to collapse >50% with respiratory variation.
- Use the curvilinear transducer over the hepatic window to follow the IVC to the right atrium and evaluate IVC collapsibility approximately 3–4 cm from the junction of the IVC and the right atrium.
- Ideal study would be to incorporate the Rapid Ultrasound in Shock and Hypotension (RUSH) examination to rapidly evaluate the collapsed athlete. The RUSH examination incorporates views from the eFAST with evaluation of the IVC and the aorta.

Skin and Soft Tissue

- High-frequency, linear-array transducer recommended for superficial evaluation
- Consider transducer cover when evaluating potentially infected tissues or over open lesions
- Differentiate abscess (hypoechoic or heterogenous mixed echogenic complex fluid collection) from cellulitis ("cobble-stone" perilobular edema without focal fluid collection)
- Useful in evaluation of foreign body (Fig. 64.24). Nonvegetative foreign bodies (i.e., glass, metal, rock/gravel) will appear as hyperechoic structures, commonly with surrounding cobblestoning and Doppler flow. Vegetative foreign bodies (sticks, grass, dirt) are commonly isoechoic and more difficult to

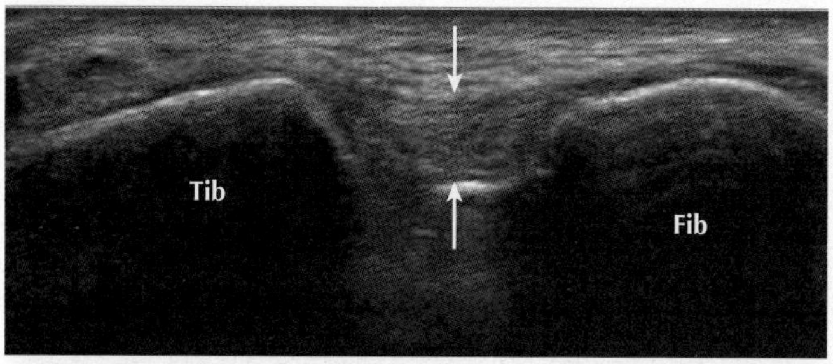
Tib
Fib

A. Normal image of the AITFL *(arrows)*

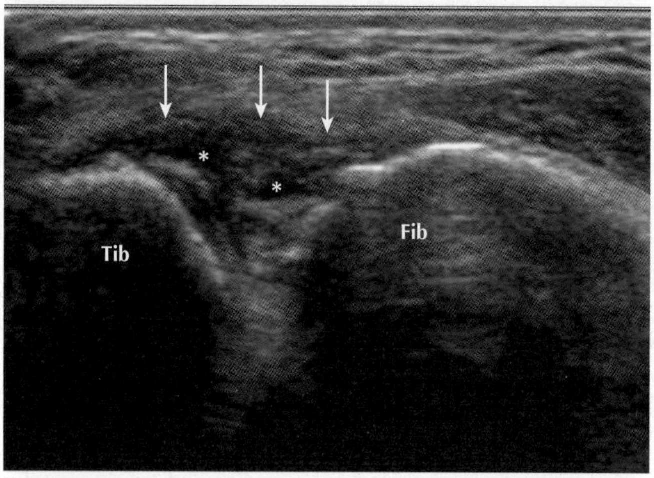
Tib
Fib

B. High-grade sprain of the AITFL *(arrows)* in collegiate football running back. Note disruption of the fibers, swelling, and anechoic regions of acute fluid *(asterisks)*. Dynamic stress imaging demonstrated laxity with external rotation stress.

Figure 64.15 Anterior inferior tibiofibular ligament (AITFL) tear. *Fib,* Fibula; *Tib,* tibia.

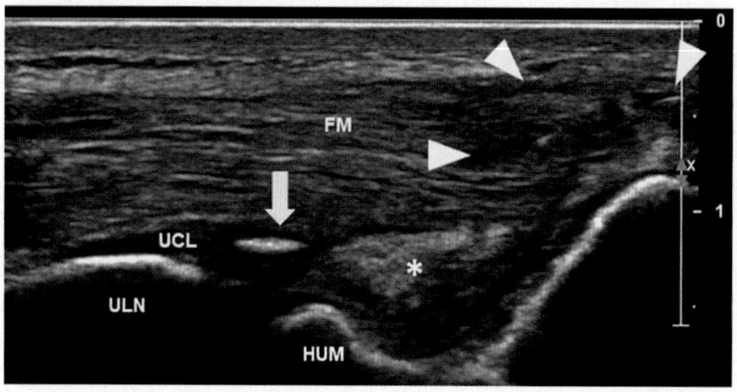
FM
UCL
ULN
HUM
0
1

Long axis image of an acute tear of the ulnar collateral ligament of the elbow. There is hyperechoic hematoma proximal (*asterisks*) and no visible ligament fibers. The distal attachment appears intact but is swollen and there is a hyperechoic linear density (*arrow*) overlying the joint space likely representing chronic calcific changes. Also note the associated muscle injury of the common flexor/pronator group (*arrowheads*).

Figure 64.16 Ulnar collateral ligament sprain. *FM,* Flexor muscle; *HUM,* humerus; *UCL,* ulnar collateral ligament; *ULN,* ulna.

visualize. Surrounding hypoechoic granulation tissue with Doppler flow aids in identification.

Vascular

- Significant heterogeneity in sensitivity and specificity based upon provider skill and experience.
- Evaluation of deep venous thrombosis is with high-frequency, linear-array transducer.
- A negative study reveals fully anechoic intraluminal appearance with complete collapsibility of the two venous walls with compression of the transducer.
- A positive study shows isoechoic or hyperechoic structures within the venous lumen and is not fully collapsible with compression.
- Three-point method is preferred with visualization and compression of the entire common femoral vein and visualization and compression of the popliteal vein.

INTERVENTIONAL SPORTS ULTRASOUND

Injections: General Considerations

Indications for Ultrasound Guidance

- No universally accepted indications
- Common indications may include the following:
  - Failed palpation-guided injection
  - Diagnostic aspiration without clinically present effusion
  - Diagnostic injections wherein accurate placement is required for diagnosis
  - Inability to identify surface/palpation landmarks because of body habitus, deformity, or deep location of target structure
  - Therapeutic injection where benefit requires accurate placement (i.e., no regional or systemic effects)
- Reduce risk of complication (proximity to neurovascular structures or organs at risk, anticoagulation, and bleeding diathesis)

Contraindications for Ultrasound Guidance

- General procedural contraindications apply. There are no known contraindications specific to ultrasound.

Technique

- Authors' preferred technique is presented, but alternative techniques may be preferred in certain clinical situations.
- Sterile technique is preferred, including sterile transducer cover, sterile acoustic coupling gel, and sterile gloves. However, this is an individual practice decision. The patient's skin should always be cleansed with an antiseptic cleanser before puncture.
- Needle size is determined by location of target, patient body habitus, and clinician preference. In general, smaller-gauge needles are more comfortable for patients and are readily identified with appropriate scanning technique. In cases of aspiration, a ≥20-gauge needle is typically required.
- Injectate volume will depend on clinical scenario and practitioner preference. One should always consider the goals of the injection and proceed accordingly (e.g., diagnostic vs. therapeutic injection). Certain injection sites, such as the AC joint, will accept a very limited volume, and overdistension can be uncomfortable and limit the diagnostic utility of injection.

Specific Injection Techniques

Subacromial–Subdeltoid Bursa Injection

Patient position: Supine, head of the bed elevated 30–45 degrees
Preferred transducer: High-frequency linear array
Technique: Transducer placed in the LAX of the supraspinatus tendon with the acromion in view to identify the subacromial bursa in the tissue plane between the rotator cuff and the deltoid. Needle is advanced in-plane with transducer from anterolateral to posteromedial.

Glenohumeral Joint Injection

Patient position: Side-lying
Preferred transducer: Curvilinear array transducer will allow better needle visualization secondary to steep angle required

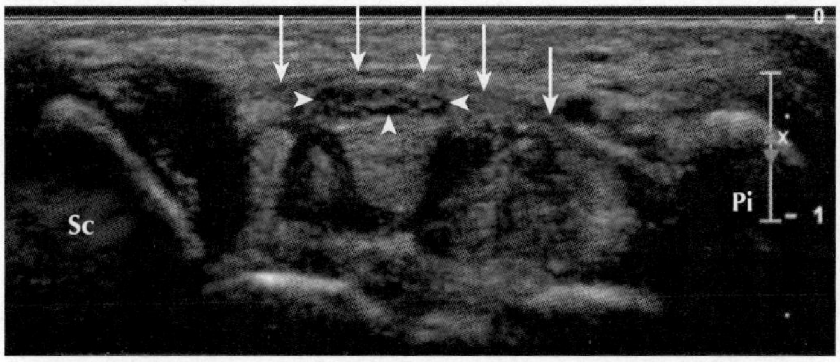
Sc
Pi

A. Short axis image of normal median nerve *(arrowheads)* under the transverse carpal ligament *(arrows)* at the carpal tunnel inlet.

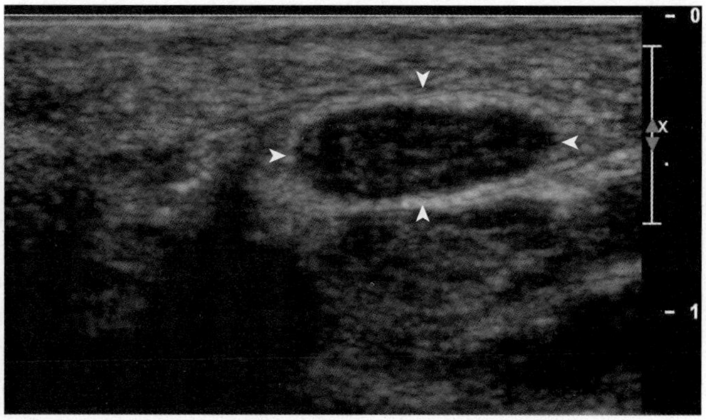

B. Short axis image of enlarged and hypoechoic median nerve *(arrowheads)* at carpal tunnel inlet in patient with carpal tunnel syndrome. Note fascicular loss.

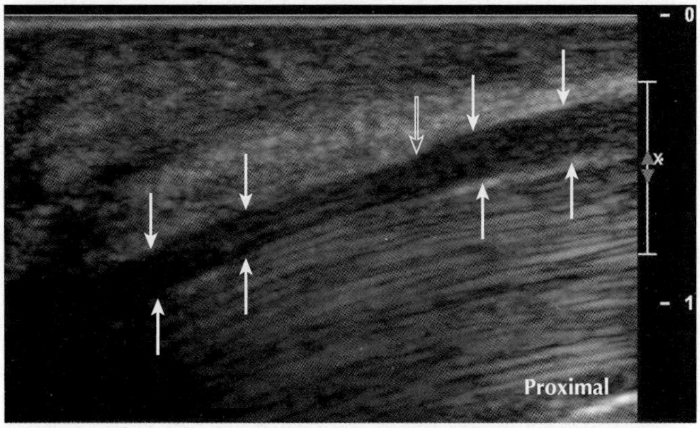
Proximal

C. Long axis image of median nerve *(arrows)* at carpal tunnel inlet demonstrating "notch sign" *(open arrow)* where the nerve is compressed at the transverse carpal ligament.

Figure 64.17 Carpal tunnel syndrome. *Pi,* Pisiform; *Sc,* scaphoid.

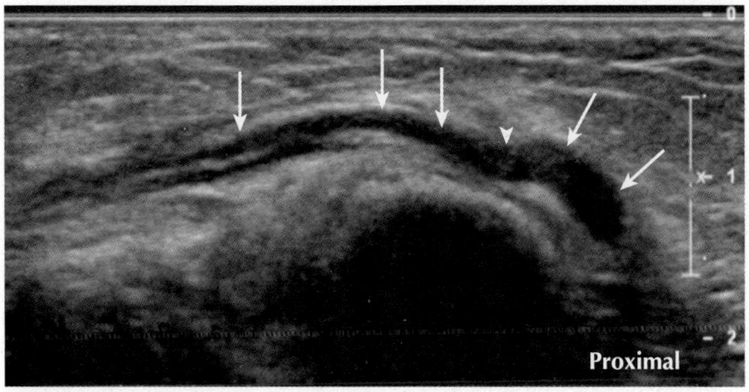
Proximal

Long axis image of the ulnar nerve *(arrows)* at the elbow status post ulnar transposition performed at time of ulnar collateral ligament reconstruction in a collegiate baseball pitcher. Patient presented with complaints of ulnar distribution paresthesia and grip weakness during his postoperative rehabilitation. Kinking of the nerve *(arrowhead)* was demonstrated distal to transposition site with proximal swelling consistent with ongoing compression.

Figure 64.18 Ulnar neuropathy at the elbow.

Technique: Transducer placed in the anatomic transverse oblique plane over the posterior glenohumeral joint in LAX of the infraspinatus tendon. Needle is advanced in-plane posterolateral to anteromedial as needle tip is guided between the humeral head and the glenoid labrum (Fig. 64.25).

Acromioclavicular Joint Injection

Patient position: Supine, head of the bed elevated 30–45 degrees
Preferred transducer: High-frequency linear array
Technique: Transducer is placed in an anatomic sagittal plane over the AC joint. It may be helpful to identify the clavicle and translate the transducer laterally until the joint space is identified. Needle is advanced in-plane anterior to posterior (Fig. 64.26).

Bicipital Tendon Sheath Injection

Patient position: Supine, head of the bed elevated 30–45 degrees, forearm in supination
Preferred transducer: High-frequency linear array
Technique: Transducer is placed in an anatomic transverse plane to visualize long head of the biceps tendon in SAX within bicipital groove. Ascending branch of the anterior humeral circumflex artery should be identified with Doppler and avoided. Needle is advanced in-plane from lateral to medial as the needle tip is guided into the tendon sheath and care is taken to avoid intratendinous injection.

Elbow Joint Injection

Patient position: Supine, elbow flexed 30–45 degrees with palm resting on lower abdomen
Preferred transducer: High-frequency linear array
Technique: Transducer is placed transverse to posterolateral aspect of radiocapitellar joint. Needle is advanced out-of-plane using a walk-down technique into the joint.

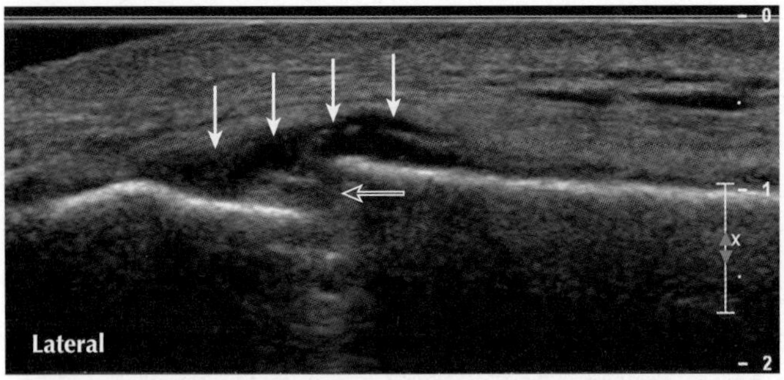
Lateral

A. Acute acromial fracture after mountain bike crash. Note the cortical step-off *(open arrow)* and the peri-fracture hematoma *(arrows)*.

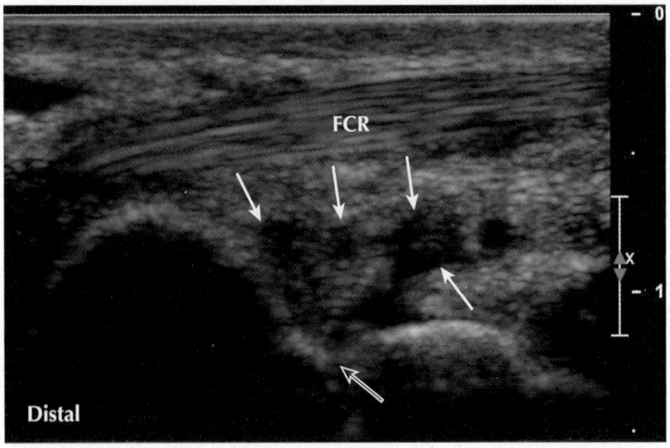
FCR
Distal

B. Radiographically occult acute scaphoid fracture *(open arrow)* demonstrated on volar wrist sonogram. Peri-fracture hematoma *(arrows)* is a helpful secondary sign of fracture.

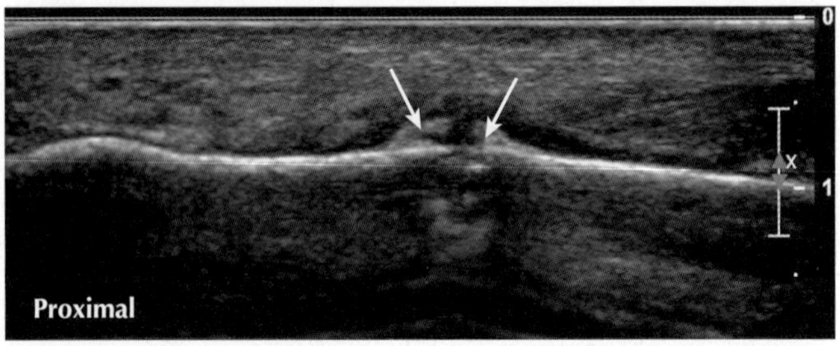
Proximal

C. Long axis image of subacute 5th metatarsal fracture with early callus formation *(arrows)* at fracture site.

Figure 64.19 Acute acromial fracture. *FCR,* Flexor carpi radialis.

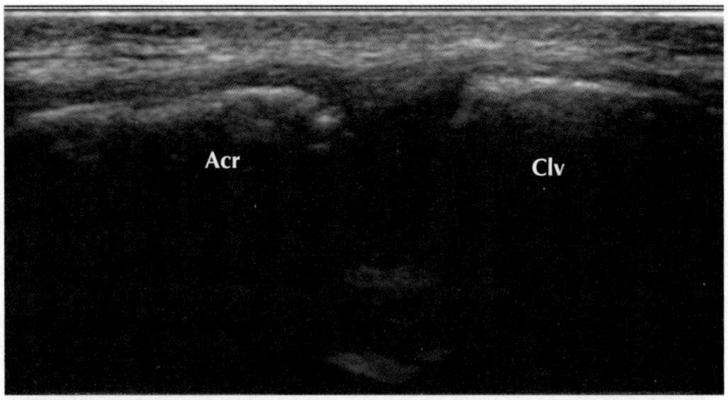
Acr
Clv

A. Normal image of acromioclavicular joint.

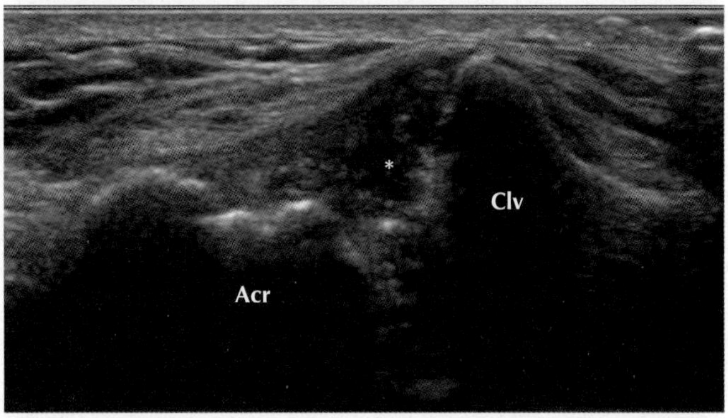
*
Clv
Acr

B. Osteoarthritis of the acromioclavicular joint with hypoechoic effusion *(asterisks)* and cortical irregularity.

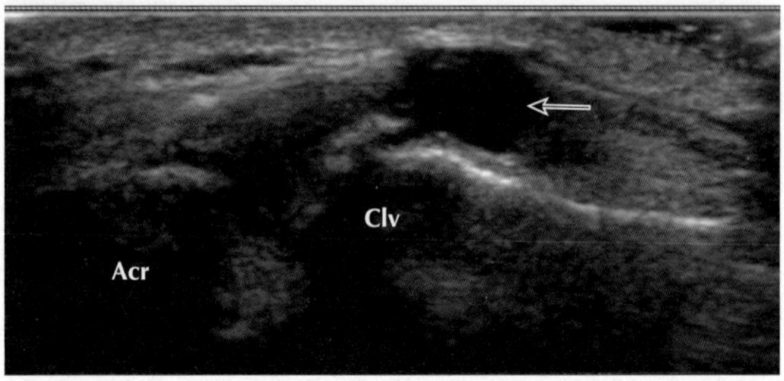
Clv
Acr

C. Distal clavicular osteolysis with associated ganglion cyst *(open arrow)* presenting in a competitive bodybuilder. Note the fragmentation at the distal clavicle.

Figure 64.20 Acromioclavicular joint disorders. *Acr,* Acromion; *Clv,* clavicle.

Carpal Tunnel Injection

Patient position: Seated or supine with forearm supinated (palm up)

Preferred transducer: High-frequency, linear-array transducer; a small-footprint transducer (i.e., "hockey stick") is preferred, if available.

Technique: Transducer is placed in an anatomic transverse plane over proximal carpal tunnel inlet, and the median nerve is identified in SAX. Needle is advanced in-plane from ulnar to medial superficial to the ulnar nerve and artery into the carpal tunnel adjacent to the median nerve. An "oblique stand-off" technique, where ample sterile acoustic coupling gel is used to identify the needle before skin puncture, should be considered. Depending on physician preference and skill level, hydrodissection of the median nerve may be performed as the injectate is placed both above and below the nerve, and any adhesions to the transverse carpal ligament are freed.

Wrist Joint Injection

Patient position: Seated, wrist flexed 20–40 degrees with forearm pronated and supported on a pillow

Preferred transducer: High-frequency, linear-array transducer; a small-footprint transducer (i.e., "hockey stick") is preferred, if available.

Technique: Transducer is placed in anatomic sagittal plane over the wrist (radiolunate). Needle is advanced in-plane from distal to proximal into radiocarpal joint. An "oblique stand-off" technique, where ample sterile acoustic coupling gel is used to identify needle before skin puncture, should be considered.

First Dorsal Compartment Tendon Sheath Injection

Patient position: Seated or supine with forearm in neutral position

Preferred transducer: High-frequency, linear-array transducer; a small-footprint transducer (i.e., "hockey stick") is preferred, if available

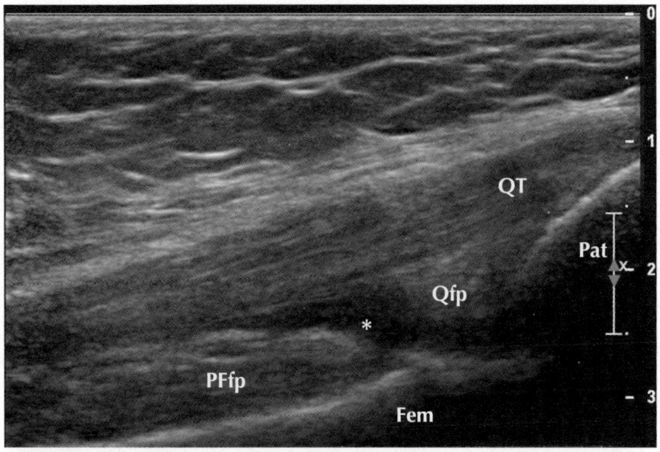
QT
Pat
Qfp
*
PFfp
Fem
0
1
2
3

A. Longitudinal image of the knee demonstrating small effusion in the suprapatellar recess *(asterisks)*. The locations of the pre-femoral and quadriceps fat pads are key to identifying the suprapatellar recess. The quadriceps tendon is seen in long axis inserting onto the patella.

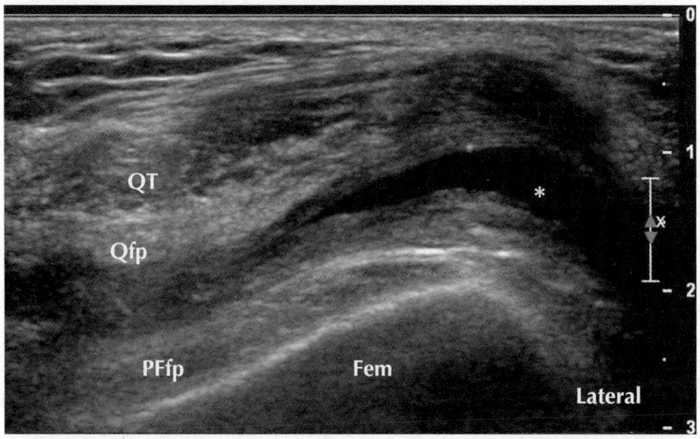
QT
Qfp
*
PFfp
Fem
Lateral
0
1
2
3

B. Corresponding transverse image of the knee demonstrating effusion within the superolateral recess *(asterisks)*.

Figure 64.21 Knee joint effusion. *Fem,* Femur; *Pat,* patella; *PFfp,* prefemoral fat pad; *Qfp,* quadriceps fat pad; *QT,* quadriceps tendon.

Technique: Transducer is placed in an anatomic transverse plane over distal radius and tendons of first dorsal compartment identified in SAX. Superficial radial nerve and radial artery should be identified during preprocedural planning. Needle is advanced in-plane from volar to dorsal as needle tip is guided into tendon sheath. Note should be made of any subcompartmentalization within the first dorsal compartment, and injectate spread around both tendons should be documented.

Hip Joint Injection

Patient position: Supine, hip in neutral rotation
Preferred transducer: Curvilinear array transducer
Technique: Transducer is placed in anatomic transverse oblique plane over anterior hip (axis of femoral neck), and the femoral head–neck junction is identified. Position of femoral neurovasculature should be noted medial to the target. Needle is advanced in-plane from inferolateral to superomedial as the needle tip is guided into the anterior joint recess near the femoral head–neck junction (Fig. 64.27).

Greater Trochanteric Bursa Injection

Patient position: Side-lying
Preferred transducer: High-frequency, linear-array transducer is typically preferred; however, body habitus may necessitate a lower-frequency, curvilinear-array transducer in certain patients.

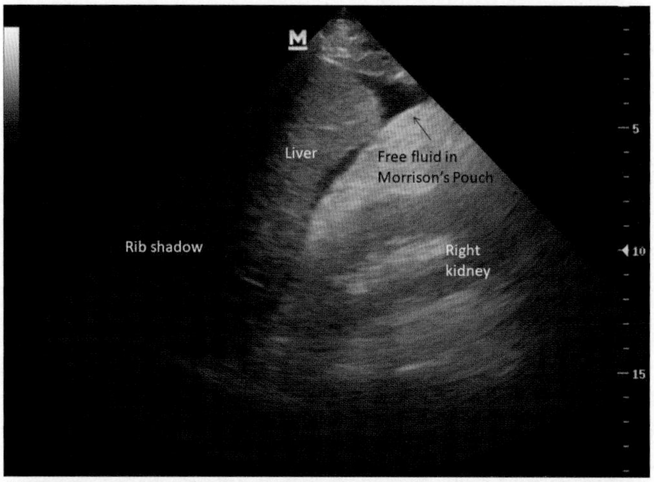
M
Liver
Free fluid in
Morrison's Pouch
Rib shadow
Right
kidney
5
10
15

A. Right upper quadrant view demonstrates anechoic intraperitoneal free fluid in Morrison's Pouch (*arrow*).

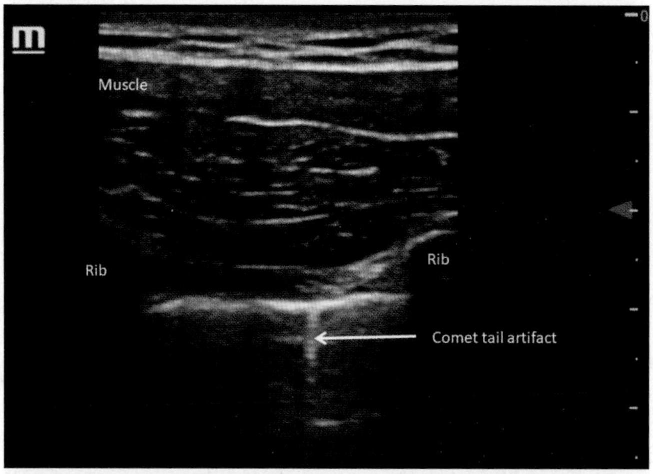
m
Muscle
Rib
Rib
Comet tail artifact
0

B. Normal pleural image with B line or "comet tail" artifact. The presence of B-lines excludes the possibility of pneumothorax.

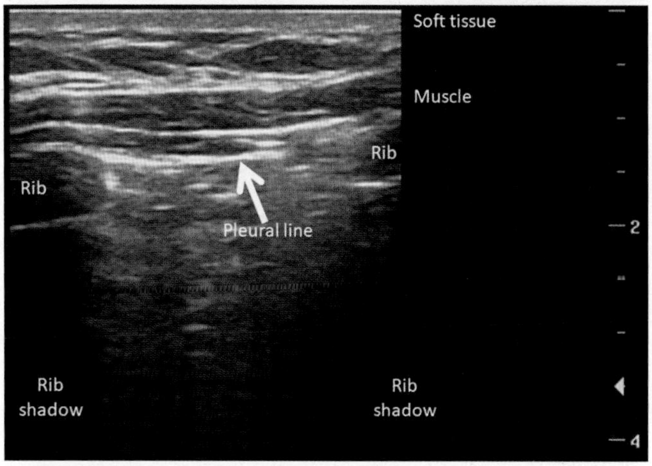
Soft tissue
Muscle
Rib
Rib
Pleural line
Rib
shadow
Rib
shadow
2
4

C. Positive eFAST for pneumothorax demonstrates a fixed pleural line without B lines.

Figure 64.22 eFAST.

Technique: Transducer is placed in an anatomic transverse plane over the greater trochanter, and the lateral and posterior facets of greater trochanter are identified. Gluteus medius tendon lies on the lateral facet, and gluteus maximus muscle overlies the posterior facet. Needle is advanced in-plane from posterior to anterior as the needle tip is guided into the subgluteus maximus

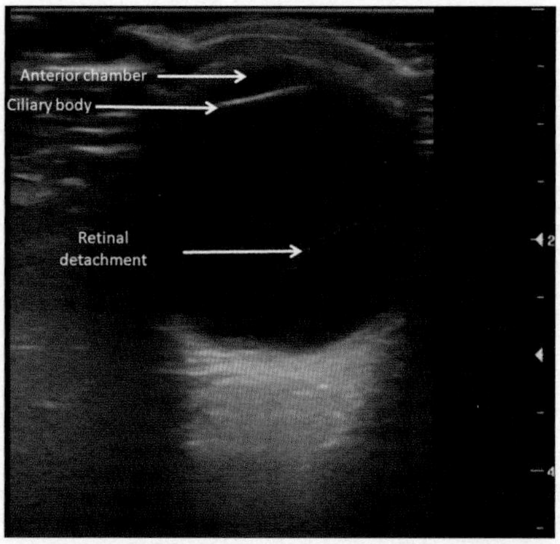
Anterior chamber
Ciliary body
Retinal
detachment

Figure 64.23 Retinal detachment appears as a linear hyperechoic structure within the anechoic vitreous body, fixed to the posterior globe.

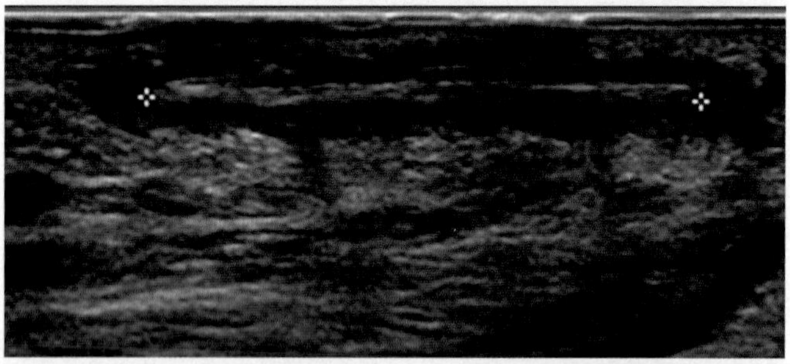

A. Linear hyperechoic wood splinter (calipers) is surrounded by hypoechoic granulation tissue.

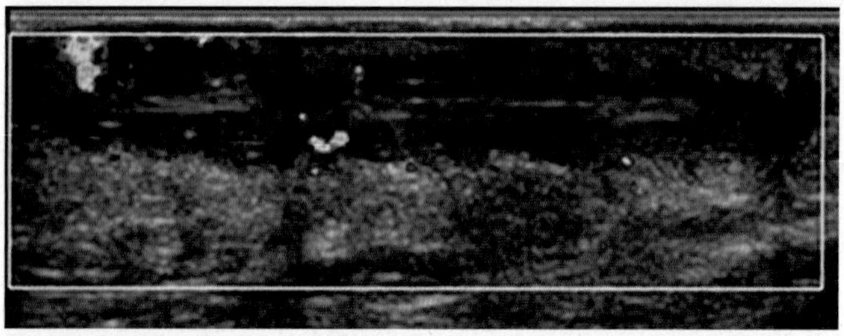

B. Color Doppler image of the same foreign body demonstrating surrounding hyperemia.

Figure 64.24 Long-axis image of a foreign body in the plantar foot.

bursa (the tissue plane between the gluteus maximus/iliotibial band superficially and the deep gluteus medius tendon).

Knee Joint Injection

Patient position: Supine, knee flexed 20 degrees and supported on pillow

Preferred transducer: High-frequency linear array

Technique: Transducer is placed in an anatomic transverse plane over the distal femur, and the suprapatellar recess is identified deep to quadriceps tendon (or quadriceps fat pad if transducer is closer to patella) and superficial to the prefemoral fat pad. Needle is advanced in-plane lateral to medial as the needle tip is guided into the joint recess (Fig. 64.28).

Iliotibial Band Bursa Injection

Patient position: Side-lying, knee flexed 20 degrees

Preferred transducer: High-frequency linear array

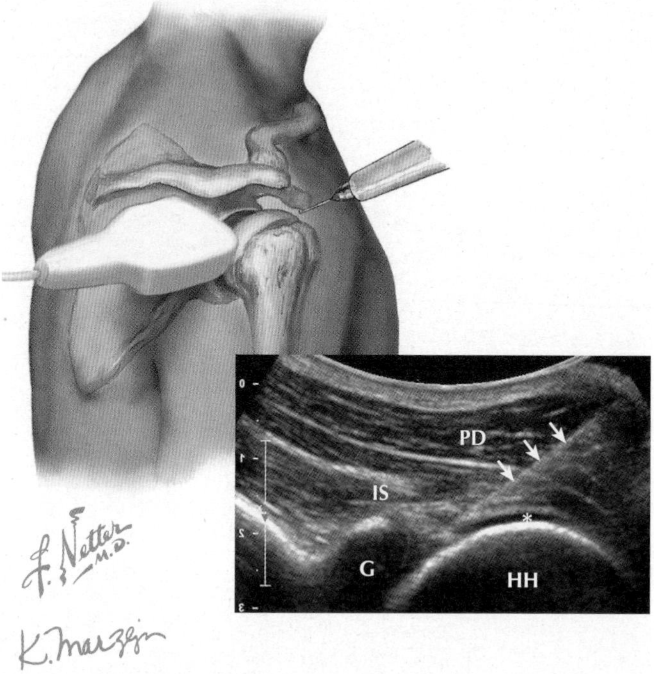
PD
IS
G
HH

Figure 64.25 Glenohumeral joint injection: posterior approach. *Arrows* indicate needle and *asterisks* indicate articular cartilage. *G,* Glenoid; *HH,* humeral head; *IS,* infraspinatus; *PD,* posterior deltoid.

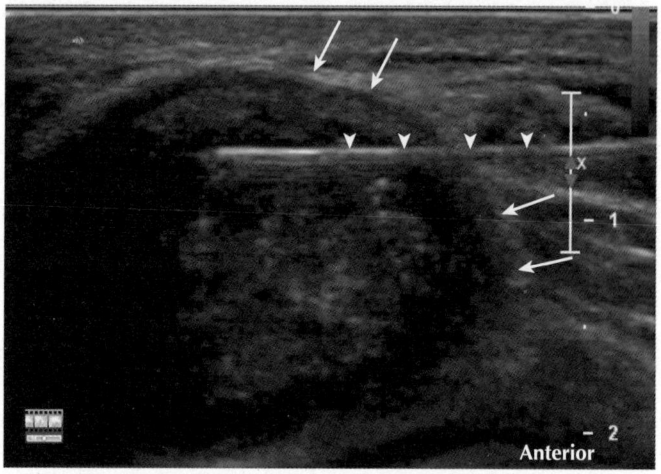
Anterior

Figure 64.26 Acromioclavicular joint injection: anterior approach. *Arrowheads* indicate needle; *arrows* indicate hip joint capsule.

Technique: Transducer is placed in an anatomic transverse plane over the lateral femoral condyle, and the iliotibial band is identified in SAX. Needle is advanced in-plane posterior to anterior as the needle tip is guided just deep to the iliotibial band into the region of the bursa. Common fibular nerve should be identified during preprocedural planning to ensure typical location posterior to the needle entry site.

Tibiotalar Joint Injection

Patient position: Side-lying, ankle in slight inversion supported by pillow

Preferred transducer: High-frequency linear array

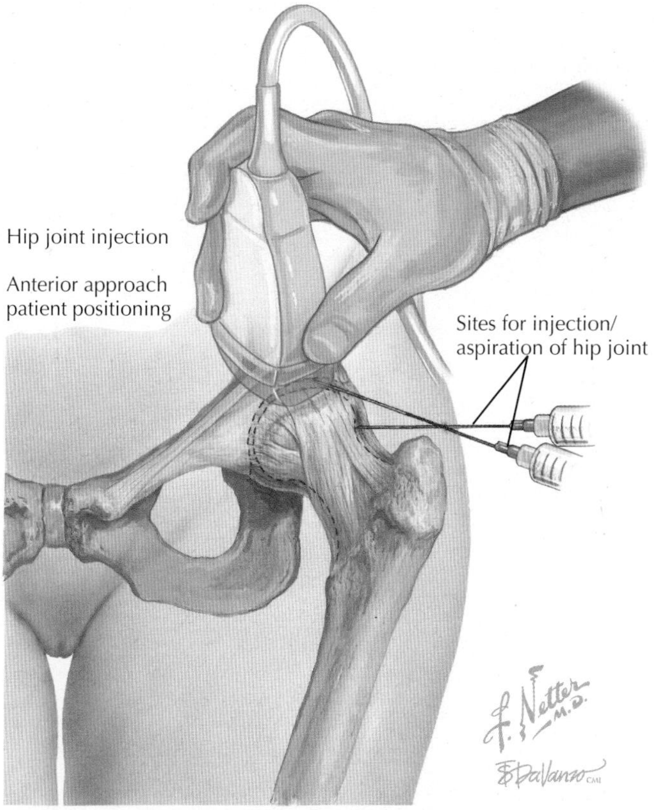
Hip joint injection
Anterior approach
patient positioning
Sites for injection/
aspiration of hip joint

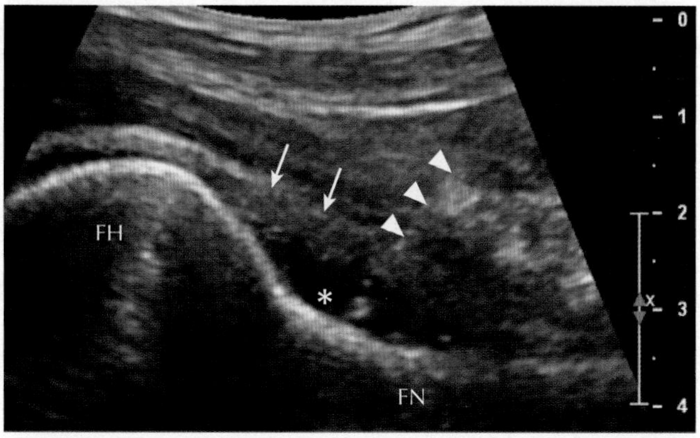
FH
FN
*

Figure 64.27 Hip joint injection: anterior approach. *Arrowheads* indicate needle, *arrows* indicate hip joint capsule, and *asterisks* indicate injectate within anterior hip recess. *FH,* Femoral head; *FN,* femoral neck.

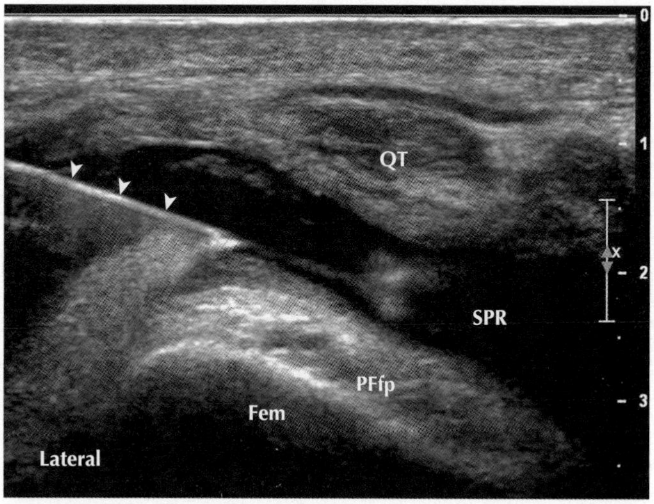
QT
SPR
PFfp
Fem
Lateral

Figure 64.28 Knee joint injection: superolateral approach. *Arrowheads* indicate needle. *Fem,* Femur; *PFfp,* prefemoral fat pad; *QT,* quadriceps tendon; *SPR,* suprapatellar recess.

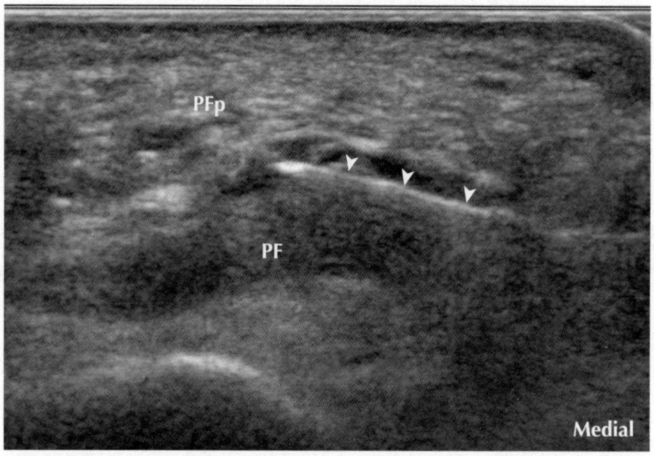
PFp
PF
Medial

Figure 64.29 Plantar fascia injection. *Arrowheads* indicate needle. *PF,* Plantar fascia; *PFp,* plantar fat pad.

Technique: Transducer is placed in an anatomic transverse oblique plane over the fibular tip, and the lateral gutter of the tibiotalar joint is identified deep to the anterior talofibular ligament (ATFL). Needle is advanced out-of-plane anterolateral to posteromedial into the lateral joint recess.

Fibular (Peroneal) Tendon Sheath Injection

Patient position: Side-lying, ankle in slight inversion supported by pillow

Preferred transducer: High-frequency, linear-array transducer; a small-footprint transducer (i.e., "hockey stick") is preferred, if available

Technique: Transducer is placed in an anatomic transverse plane just inferior to tip of the lateral malleolus, and the fibular tendons are identified in SAX. Needle is advanced in-plane anterior to posterior into the tendon sheath.

Plantar Fascia Injection

Patient position: Prone, foot hanging free off the end of examination table

Preferred transducer: High-frequency linear array

Technique: Transducer is placed in an anatomic transverse plane over the plantar heel, and the plantar fascia origin is identified in SAX at the calcaneus. Needle is advanced in-plane medial to lateral as the needle tip is guided to the superficial/plantar surface of the plantar fascia. Care should be taken to avoid injection into the plantar fat pad (Fig. 64.29).

Advanced Procedures: General Considerations

- Earlier advanced procedures such as calcific tendinopathy barbotage and percutaneous needle tenotomy have proven safe and effective means of treating certain tendinopathies in an outpatient clinical setting.
- Techniques and more specialized equipment continue to evolve with the general principle of taking proven surgical concepts

and making these less invasive via a percutaneous approach and live ultrasound guidance.
- Examples include tenotomy with or without debridement, tendon scraping, carpal tunnel release, trigger finger release, peripheral nerve hydroneurolysis, fascial release for chronic exertional compartment syndrome, and various regenerative medicine and orthobiologic techniques.
- Potential for decreased morbidity, improved patient outcomes, and overall cost savings, but definitive evidence for these claims is currently evolving

RECOMMENDED READINGS

Available online.

INJURY PREVENTION PROTOCOLS 65

Kevin E. Wilk • Adam N. Finck • Paul S. Fuller

INTRODUCTION

Sport-specific injury prevention training programs are used across the country as an aid to increase performance and decrease injury rates. Two common areas of injury include the athletic shoulder and knee. Among the athletic population, injuries to the throwing shoulder are becoming more apparent as a result of overuse and poor conditioning. Likewise, anterior cruciate ligament (ACL) knee injuries continue to rise each year among the athletic population. The focus of this chapter is aimed at specific prevention protocols for reducing the likelihood of injury in the athletic knee, specific to ACL pathology, and in the throwing shoulder of the youth and elite athlete.

ACL INJURY PREVENTION

Epidemiology and Injury Statistics

- Injury to the ACL can be functionally debilitating and often requires surgical intervention.
- ACL injuries are common in sports and strenuous work activities.
- Approximately 200,000 ACL injuries occur annually in the United States (Fu: *AJSM* 1999).
- Over a 20-year period, ACL surgery procedures have increased by 58%, with 148,714 ACL surgeries performed in 2013 (PearlDiver Technologies. PearlDiver supercomputer database. Available at: http://www.pearl-diverinc.com/).
- One in 3500 people will sustain an ACL injury (Baer, Harner: *Clin Sports Med* 2007).
- Sixty-two to sixty-six percent of ACL injuries are sports related, often in a noncontact manner (i.e., running, cutting, or landing from a jump).
- The incidence of ACL injury and reconstruction seems to be increasing because of an increasing number of youth engaging in high-level athletics and older individuals remaining active longer (Mall et al: *AJSM* 2014).
- Females are four to six times more likely to sustain an ACL injury compared with their male counterparts.
- There are 43,125 ACL injuries annually in high school–aged athletes (Joseph et al: *J Athl Train* 2013).
- High school–aged athletes, especially the female high school athlete, appear to be at the highest risk. The rank order for high school–aged athletes at highest risk are as follows (Yard et al: *J Athl Train* 2009):
  - Girls' soccer—11.7 per 100,000 athletic exposures (AEs)
  - Boys' football—11.4 per 100,000 AEs
  - Girls' basketball—11.2 per 100,000 AEs
  - Girls' gymnastics—9.9 per 100,000 AEs
  - Boys' lacrosse—7.4 per 100,000 AEs
- Ten times greater risk of developing osteoarthritis in an injured ACL knee (Fleming et al: *JOSPT* 2003).
- By 7–11 years after ACL injury, a cohort study reported a 50 times increased risk of radiographic changes on the lateral femoral condyle, 30 times increased risk on the retropatellar surface, and 19 times on the medical femoral condyle (Potter et al: *AJSM* 2012).
- Sixty-seven percent of ACL injuries occur in individuals between 15 and 29 years of age.
- At an increased risk of contralateral ACL injury after first-time ACL injury.
- Young, active athletes have high second-injury rates for the ACL, with the range of one-quarter to one-third. Most of these occur within 2 years after the first injury (Webster, Feller: *AJSM* 2016).

Risk Factors for ACL Injury

- Improper running, change of direction, or landing from a jump.
- Increased knee valgus with running, cutting, and jump landing.
- Poor body position awareness, proprioception, and dynamic stabilization.
- Decreased knee flexion angles with jump landing. This is often present in a quadriceps-dominant knee.
- Decreased hamstring-to-quadriceps strength ratios. Females rely more on their quadriceps to stabilize their knee joints and tend to have lower hamstring-to-quadriceps muscle strength ratios. Hamstring-to-quadriceps ratios less than 75% and bilateral hamstring difference of more than 15% have been correlated with a higher incidence of ACL injuries in female athletes (Knapik et al: *AJSM* 1991).
- Neuromuscular control deficits can create difficulty generating muscular force. This limits the ability to resist displacing loads through dynamic stabilization of the knee.
- Smaller intercondylar notch. A narrower intercondylar notch has been found to be associated with the risk of ACL rupture in a skeletally immature population.
- Lateral trunk displacement with jump landing.
- Poor hip/core strength and control.
- Excessive subtalar joint pronation.
- Ligamentous laxity. Athletes with greater generalized laxity demonstrate increased midfoot loading and valgus collapse. This valgus force can be most apparent during running, cutting, or landing from a jump.
- Hormonal changes.
- Higher-than-average body mass index (BMI) and fat mass indexes put youth athletes at a higher risk of ACL and knee injuries (Toomey et al: *JOSPT* 2017).
- In addition to anatomic and biomechanical risk factors, environmental risk factors of meteorologic conditions, surface conditions, footwear, and knee bracing may influence the risk of ACL injuries.

Review of Literature

- A 6-week prevention program focusing on plyometrics, neuromuscular and strength training, flexibility, and proper body mechanics reported that subjects of an untrained group had a 2.4 to 3.6 times higher ACL injury rate (Hewett, Lidenfeld, Noyes: *AJSM* 1999).
- In a study of trained soccer players between the ages of 14 and 18 performing preventive stretching, strengthening, plyometrics, and agility drills, there was an 88% reduction rate in ACL injuries over 1 year and a 74% reduction in ACL injuries over 2 years. Those in the untrained group were at a 10 times greater risk of ACL injury (Mandelbaum et al: *AJSM* 2005).
- In a study of the Norwegian team handball players analyzed over 3 years, significantly fewer noncontact injuries were reported in participants of the intervention group. Subjects performed proprioceptive, agility, plyometric, and balance drills three times a week for 5–7 weeks before the season and then once a week during the season (Myklebust et al: *Clin J Sports Med* 2003).
- In a program of 4700 ski instructors and patrollers that consisted of educational training on avoiding high-risk behaviors, recognizing potentially dangerous situations, and how to respond to situations, a reduced injury rate of 62% over the span of 3 years was described (Ettlinger, Johnson, Shealy: *AJSM* 1995).
- A study of 600 Italian semiprofessional and amateur soccer players participating in a proprioception and balance training

program reduced ACL injury rates by 87% over a duration of three seasons (Caraffa et al: *Knee Surg Sports Traumatol Arthrosc* 1996).

- An 8-week preseason program for German female team handball players reported significantly lower rates of ankle and knee injuries. Significant emphasis was made on educational training in regard to injury mechanisms. Subjects participated in balance board training drills that consisted of double- and single-leg stance, catch with a partner, and throws at a goal. Jump training exercises were also performed consisting of forward, backward, and lateral jumps; drop jumps onto a mat; and jump landing with eyes closed.
- A recent systematic review and meta-analysis found that exercise-based ACL prevention programs emphasizing neuromuscular training were most effective targeting younger athletes (13–19 years old), especially females. They emphasized that trained implementers should be used, while incorporating the lower body strength exercises, with a specific focus on landing stabilization, throughout their sport seasons (Petushek et al: *AJSM* 2019).
- ACL injury prevention programs have been shown to change the biomechanics of landing tasks, resulting in decreased risk factors for ACL injury. A systematic review and meta-analysis showed that after injury prevention programs, participants landed with increased hip and knee flexion (decreasing the quadriceps-dominant landing) and decreased peak knee abduction moment (Lopes et al: *AJSM* 2017).
- The current evidence supports several exercise-based knee/ACL prevention programs in athletes. Individual studies and systematic reviews have demonstrated significant reduction in overall knee injuries through injury prevention programs of FIFA 11, 11+, and HarmoKnee, among others. Furthermore, the Prevent Injury and Enhance Performance (PEP) and Sportsmetrics programs have overwhelming evidence supporting the reduction of ACL injuries (Arundale et al: *JOSPT* 2018).

Prevention Training

- ACL prevention training should focus on:
  - Dynamic stretching/flexibility
    - Aimed to promote muscle activation before athletic activity.
    - Target muscle groups should include those of the lower extremity that are used extensively during athletic activities: quadriceps, hamstrings, hip adductors, hip flexors, and calf muscles.
    - Example exercises include walking stretches for quadriceps/hamstrings/calf, standing side lunges for hip adductors, and standing dynamic stretches for hip flexors.
  - Hip/core strength and control:
    - Aimed to prevent valgus knee collapse.
    - Target muscle groups should be those that control hip abduction, hip external rotation, and hip extension.
    - Example exercises include: hip ER/IR with tubing, TheraBand lateral slides (Fig. 65.1), unilateral Romanian deadlifts (RDLs), side-lying manual resistance clams, and bridging.
    - Emphasize exercises/drills that improve core strength and trunk control.
    - Example exercises include bridging, dead bug drills, single-leg stance with side bends, planks, and balance drills on an unstable surface.
  - Neuromuscular control and proprioception
    - Athletes should be aware of where their knee is relative to their body in space and correct if the knee joint moves in a dangerous way that may cause injury.
    - Athletes must improve dynamic stabilization through balance, proprioception, neuromuscular control drills, and perturbation training.
    - Dynamic joint stability is dependent on neuromuscular response time.

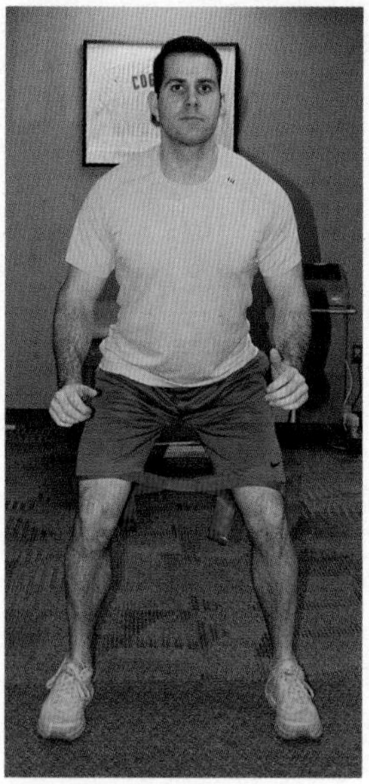

Figure 65.1 Lateral slides with resistance bands (TheraBand CLX; Performance Health, Akron, OH) around the distal femur to strengthen gluteus medius musculature of the hip.

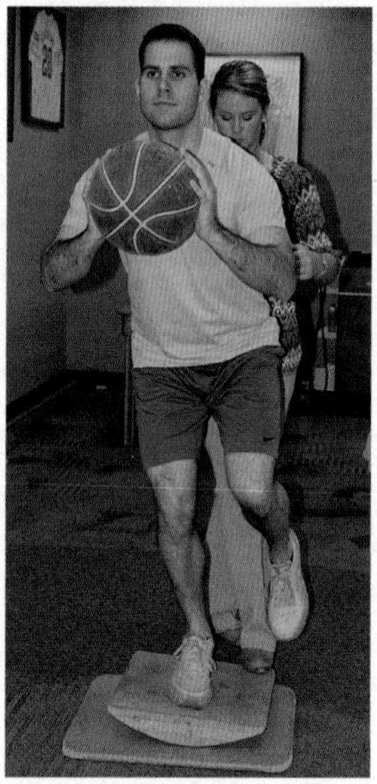

Figure 65.2 Manual perturbations with ball catches.

    - Example exercises include balance board drills with double- or single-limb stance. The difficulty of this activity can be progressed by having the athlete play catch with a partner. Difficulty can be further enhanced by having the athlete maintain balance while stabilizing against manual perturbations, while also playing catch with a partner (Fig. 65.2).
  - Trunk control and core strengthening
    - Important in preventing lateral displacement.
    - Females tend to land from jumping with greater lateral trunk motion than males.
    - Example exercises include prone or side planks, single-leg medicine ball trunk rotations on a foam disc (Fig. 65.3), and bridging.
  - Hamstring strengthening
    - Dependent on muscular coactivation to maintain appropriate knee joint dynamic stabilization.
    - The goal is to eliminate a quadriceps-dominant knee and establish an appropriate hamstring-to-quadriceps muscle strength ratio.

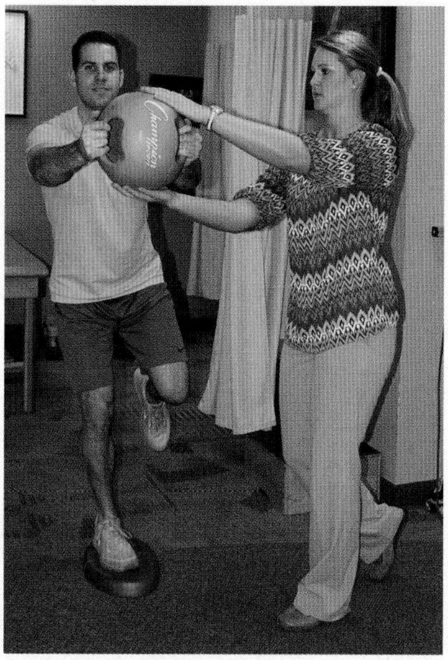
Champion

Figure 65.3 Single-leg cross pattern on a foam disc to alter the patient's center of gravity.

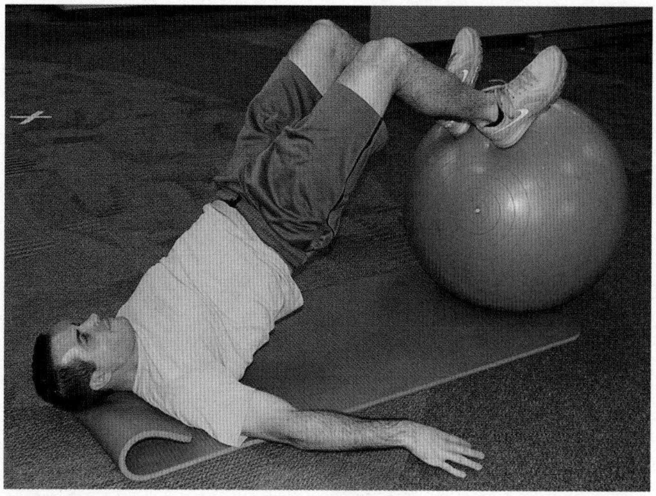

Figure 65.4 Stability ball hamstring curl to enhance recruitment of gluteus maximus and hamstring musculature.

    - Examples exercises include physioball bridging with concomitant hamstring curls (Fig. 65.4), prone machine hamstring curls, and eccentric Nordic hamstring drills.
  - Proper running, cutting, and landing mechanics
    - Fatigue is a risk factor for musculoskeletal injury; therefore, endurance training plays a key role in injury prevention.
    - Lower extremity muscle fatigue alters knee kinematics and kinetics during landing from a jump stop. This creates an increase in peak tibial anterior shear forces, increase in valgus knee moment, and decreased knee flexion.
    - Encourage a balanced positioning of the hip and knee in a flexed position.
    - Example exercises include agility ladders, line jumps, change-of-direction drills, deceleration drills, plyometric box jumps, bounding, single-leg hopping, and sport-specific drills with emphasis on appropriate body mechanics during landing and cutting.
- Exercise-based ACL injury prevention programs should be performed before athletic training sessions and games. Athletes should perform them multiple times per week, with each session lasting at least 20 minutes.
- Despite the overwhelming evidence documenting the efficacy and societal benefit of ACL prevention programs, ACL injury rates have not decreased. A primary reason is that the use of ACL prevention programs is very low nationally and very low in rural areas (Petushek et al: *AJSM* 2019).

PREVENTION OF THROWING INJURIES

Epidemiology and Injury Statistics

- Shoulder and elbow injuries are common in baseball and appear to be increasing year to year.
- In Major League Baseball (MLB) (Posner et al: *AJSM* 2012, Wilk et al: *AJSM* 2011, Conte et al: *AJSM* 2001):
  - Sixty-seven percent of all injuries to pitchers are to the upper extremity, with the shoulder being the most commonly injured joint.
  - Pitchers are 2.5 times more likely to sustain an upper extremity injury compared with position players.
  - Sixty-six to seventy percent of all injuries to pitchers are to the shoulder and elbow.
  - Seventy-two percent of all disabled list days are the result of shoulder and/or elbow injuries.
  - Sixty-one percent of all disabled list days are pitchers.
  - Elbow surgeries, specifically ulnar collateral ligament (UCL) surgeries, are increasing every year.
  - Elbow surgeries are presently the most common surgery performed to professional baseball pitchers.
  - Hodgins et al. reported a 193% increase in the number of UCL surgeries in the state of New York from 2002 to 2011, with the most common age group being 18–19 years old (Hodgins et al: *AJSM* 2016).
- In youth baseball:
  - Over 17 million kids play youth baseball in the United States.
  - Fifty percent of players (ages 9–14) complained of shoulder or elbow pain (Lyman et al: *AJSM* 2001).
  - Surgeries appear to be increasing in youth baseball players (Fleisig et al: *J Sports Health* 2012).

Risk Factors to Throwing Injuries

- Pitching at maximum effort can overload the stabilizing structures and lead to an accelerated rate of degradation to the soft tissue intrinsic stabilizers.
- Ball velocity has been shown to be the number-one risk factor for elbow injuries in professional baseball pitchers (peak velocity was first risk factor followed by mean velocity as the second risk factor) (Chalmer et al: *AJSM* 2016).
- Pitching too many innings throughout the season can also result in overutilization of static and dynamic stabilizing structures.
- Increased pitch counts during a single bout of throwing have been associated with shoulder and elbow injury in youth and high school pitchers (Bakshi et al: *AJSM* 2020).
- Pitching while fatigued can result in alteration of throwing mechanics directly affecting performance. Effects of fatigue can result in an increase of superior humeral head migration with arm elevation, diminished proprioception, and altered scapular position. Injury can often occur as a result of these alterations. Pitching with arm fatigue has been associated with shoulder and elbow pain or injury, regardless of pitch count in youth baseball players (Bakshi et al: *AJSM* 2020).
- Pitching year round. It is encouraged that no overhead throwing be performed for at least 4 months throughout the year. Furthermore, 2–3 months of rest from throwing is encouraged at the end of a baseball season.
- Usage of breaking ball pitches in the immature thrower alters throwing kinetics, especially in the presence of poor throwing mechanics.
- Improper throwing mechanics can lead to excessive strains in the upper extremity. Appropriate mechanics should be emphasized throughout the entirety of the throwing motion.

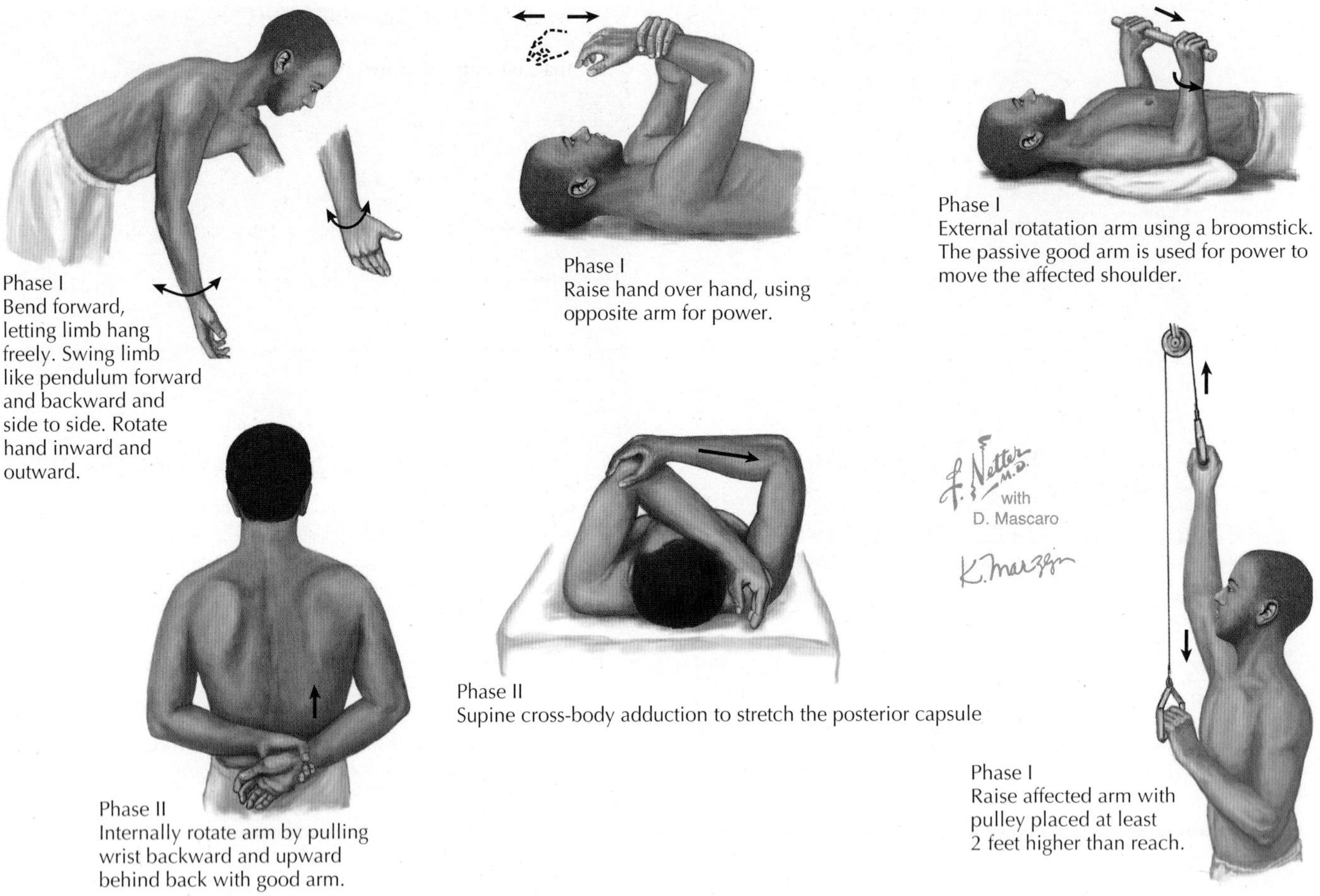
Phase I
Bend forward, letting limb hang freely. Swing limb like pendulum forward and backward and side to side. Rotate hand inward and outward.
Phase I
Raise hand over hand, using opposite arm for power.
Phase I
External rotatation arm using a broomstick. The passive good arm is used for power to move the affected shoulder.
Phase II
Internally rotate arm by pulling wrist backward and upward behind back with good arm.
Phase II
Supine cross-body adduction to stretch the posterior capsule
Phase I
Raise affected arm with pulley placed at least 2 feet higher than reach.
with
D. Mascaro

Figure 65.5 Basic, passive, and active assisted range-of-motion exercises.

- Participating as a pitcher and catcher throughout the season drastically increases throwing volumes. A Little League baseball rule since 2010 prohibits a pitcher from going to catcher, and vice versa, during the same game.
- Playing on multiple teams in various leagues increases the volume of throws on the upper extremity.
- Poor conditioning as a result of inadequate shoulder mobility and strength, neuromuscular control, dynamic stability, core and lower extremity strength, and posture.
- Weighted ball throwing programs. Using weighted baseballs to increase ball velocity has been shown to increase injuries in young baseball players (Reinold, Macrina, et al: *J Sports Health* 2018).

Review of Literature

- Prevention programs addressing posture, strength, endurance, power, mobility, and flexibility have been proficient at reducing injury rates while also enhancing performance.
- In adolescent baseball players (11–15 years of age), performance of the Thrower's Ten program over a span of 4 weeks demonstrated a 2% increase in throwing velocity (Escamilla: *J Strength Cond* 2010).
- A 2% increase in throwing velocity was also demonstrated in adolescent baseball players with performance of a 6-week plyometric training program (Escamilla: *J Strength Cond Res* 2012).
- Stretching and flexibility programs have demonstrated improvements in total rotation motion (TROM). TROM is a total motion concept that combines ER and IR. A TROM greater than 5 degrees, comparing dominant with nondominant shoulders, can place throwers at a 2.5 times greater risk of upper extremity injury (Wilk et al: *AJSM* 2011).
- In youth baseball players (9–11 years of age), a prevention program consisting of stretching, dynamic mobility, and balance training exercises during the warm-up before throwing reduced throwing injuries to the shoulder and elbow by 48.5% and improved ball velocity (Sakata et al: *AJSM* 2019).

Prevention Training

- Pitch counts
  - Pitch count charts can be used (game, season, and year) to maximize the longevity of the thrower.
  - The Little League Pitch Count Rule limits the number of throws a pitcher is allowed per game. Those aged 7–8 years are allowed 50 pitches, 9–10 years 75 pitches, 11–12 years 85 pitches, 13–16 years 95 pitches, and 17–18 years 105 pitches.
  - Studies using surveys of players and coaches have demonstrated poor knowledge of and compliance with pitching guidelines. Therefore, it is of the utmost importance to educate players, coaches, and parents about the recommended pitch counts and the injury implications associated with exceeding the pitching workload guidelines (Bakshi et al: *AJSM* 2020).
- Rest
  - Rest allows appropriate recovery to occur for the athlete.
  - The Little League Pitch Count Rule requires 4 days rest when a pitcher throws more than 66 pitches in a game, 3 days rest with 51–65 pitches, 2 days rest with 36–50 pitches, and one day rest with 21–35 pitches.
- Physical characteristics
  - Range of motion and flexibility exercises should target motions of shoulder flexion, shoulder ER, shoulder IR, and horizontal adduction (Fig. 65.5).

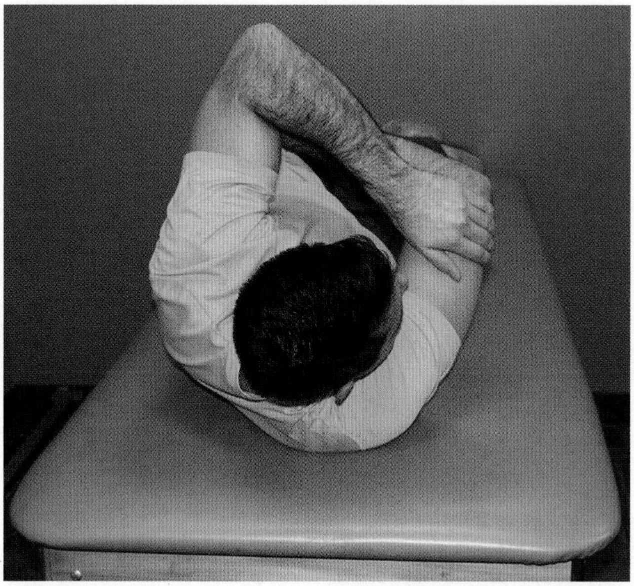

Figure 65.6 Modified cross-body stretch. The athlete passively and horizontally adducts the shoulder as the scapula is stabilized against the table, while IR is passively performed with counter-pressure of the opposite forearm.

- Emphasis to pectoralis minor stretching should be included as well. A wall corner stretch is an effective technique at maintaining and improving pectoralis minor flexibility.
- The modified sleeper stretch or cross-body stretch is effective at improving the flexibility of the posterior rotator cuff after episodes of throwing (Fig. 65.6).
- Stretching exercises should be held for a minimum of 30 seconds to promote plastic deformation and repeated three times.
- Throwers should emphasize proper shoulder and elbow range of motion.

- Neuromuscular control
  - Neuromuscular control is an efferent motor output in response to afferent sensory stimuli.
  - Neuromuscular control is fundamental in the generation of dynamic shoulder stability to minimize the potential for injury in the act of throwing a baseball.
  - The rotator cuff muscles aid in dynamic stability of the shoulder through continuous interplay of synergistic muscles, providing compression and congruency to the glenohumeral joint (Fig. 65.7).
  - Effective neuromuscular control drills for the shoulder include rhythmic stabilizations, closed kinetic chain exercises, and plyometric training.
  - Closed kinetic chain exercises stress the joint in a load-bearing position, resulting in joint approximation, stimulating receptors, and facilitating in the co-contraction of the

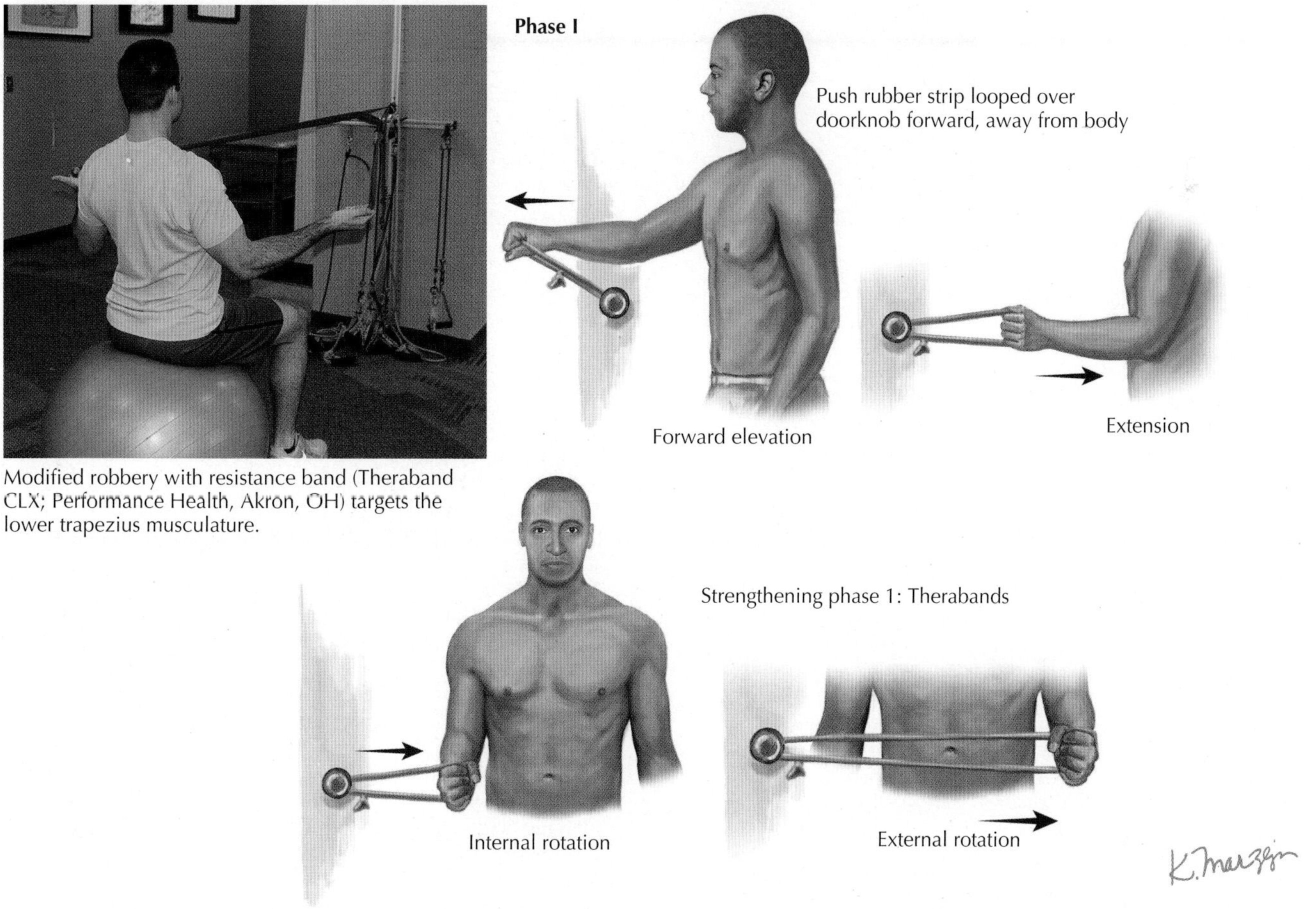
Phase I
Push rubber strip looped over doorknob forward, away from body
Forward elevation
Extension
Modified robbery with resistance band (Theraband CLX; Performance Health, Akron, OH) targets the lower trapezius musculature.
Strengthening phase 1: Therabands
Internal rotation
External rotation
K. Marzen

Figure 65.7 Shoulder and lower trapezius musculature strengthening.

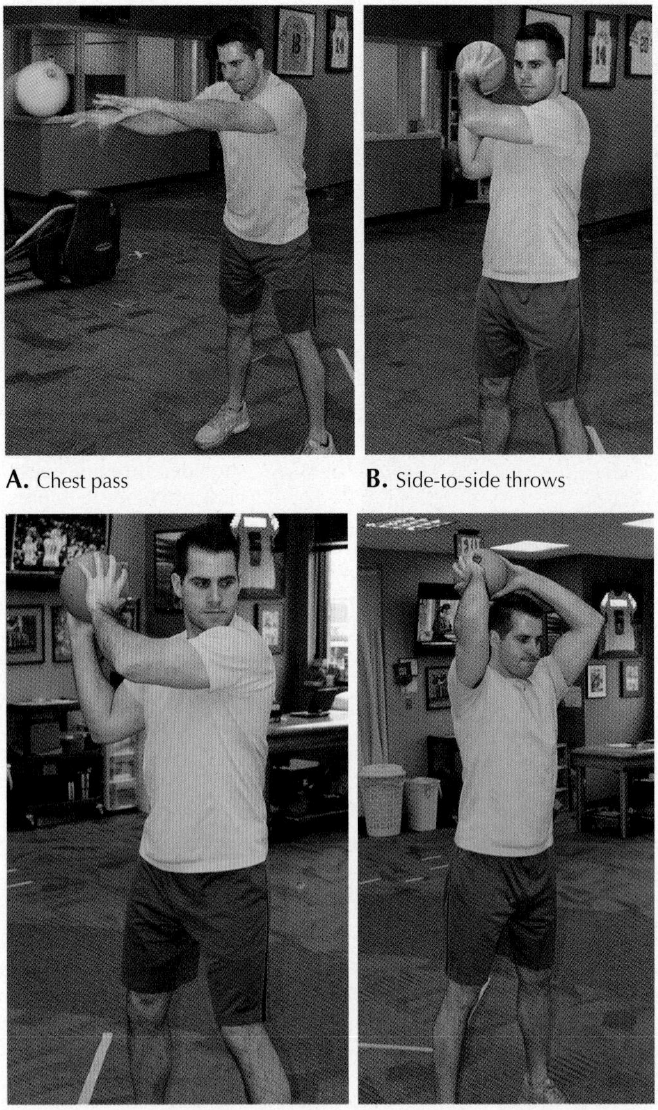

A. Chest pass **B.** Side-to-side throws

C. Side throws **D.** Overhead soccer throws

Figure 65.8 Two-handed plyometric drills.

shoulder force couples (Perry J 1988, Wuelker N: *J Biomech* 1995).
  - Plyometric exercises provide quick, powerful movements using the elastic and reactive properties of the muscle to generate maximum force production. These exercises increase the speed of the stretch reflex, desensitize the Golgi tendon organ, and increase neuromuscular coordination (Wilk KE: *JOSPT* 1993).
  - Plyometric training should begin with two-handed drills. Exercise examples include chest pass, side-to-side throws, side throws, and overhead soccer throws (Fig. 65.8).
  - Once the athlete is comfortable with two-handed drills they can progress to one-handed drills. Exercise examples include standing one-handed throws, wall dribbles, and plyometric step throws (Fig. 65.9).
- Total body conditioning
  - Proper training programs that apply periodization and proper training principles should be used.
  - The core and lower extremities are of utmost importance in the development and transfer of power in the act of throwing. Thus, the training program must have an emphasis on the hips, core, and legs.
  - Adolescent and preadolescent athletes often present with poor core, hip, and leg strength, as well as poor single-leg balance.
  - Poor strength, endurance, and/or neuromuscular control of the lower body can have a significant impact on the forces experienced by the upper extremity and influence pitching mechanics.
  - Proper exercises should focus on linking the shoulder and lower extremities because of the energy transfer that occurs with overhead throwing.
  - Exercises such as front step-downs (Fig. 65.10), TheraBand lateral slides, TheraBand or manual resistance hip ER, side-lying clams, and single leg RDLs are all excellent exercises to enhance lower body strength.
- Endurance
  - Motion analysis studies reported shoulder ER and ball velocity decreased once a thrower became fatigued (Murray et al: *AJSM* 2001).

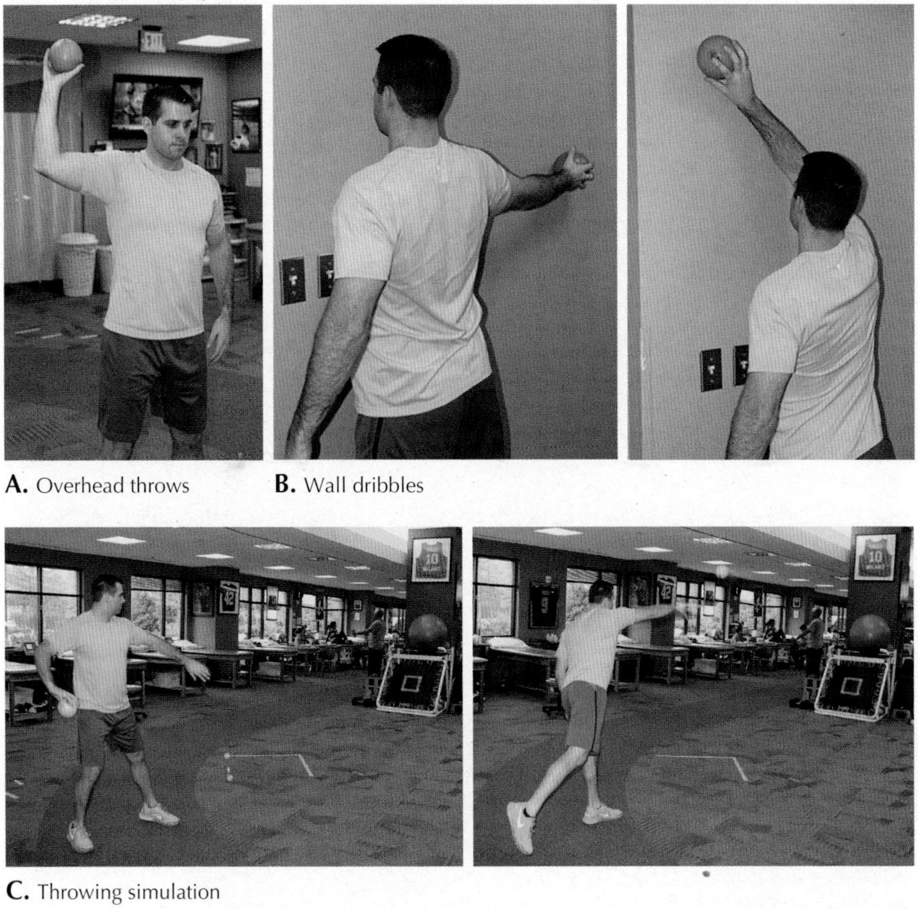
A. Overhead throws
B. Wall dribbles
C. Throwing simulation

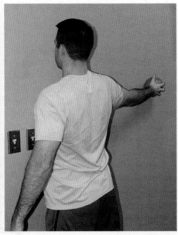

Figure 65.9 One-handed plyometric drills. **A,** Overhead throws. **B,** Wall dribbles. **C,** Throwing simulation.

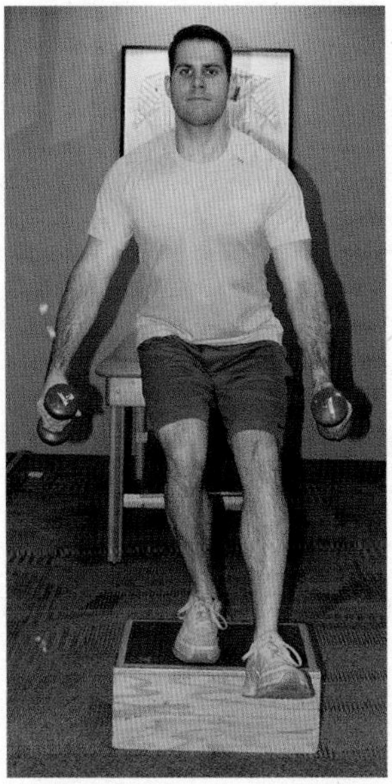

Figure 65.10 Front step-down. The athlete is instructed to maintain proper alignment of the lower extremity to prevent valgus knee collapse or pelvic drop during the lowering phase of the exercise.

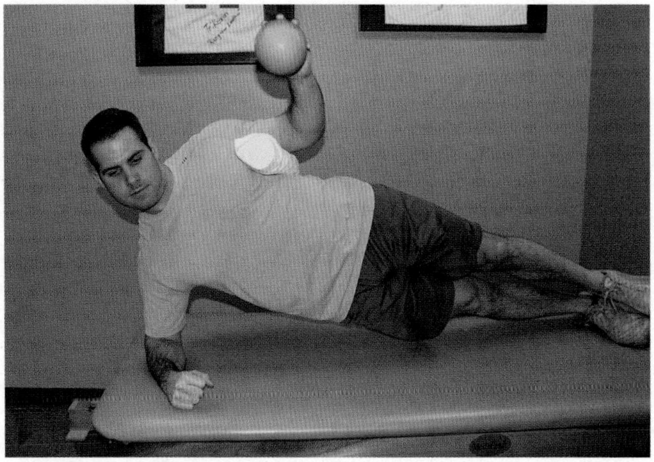

Figure 65.11 Side-lying ER ball flips with #2 plyoball for endurance training of shoulder external rotators.

- Muscle fatigue has also been shown to attribute to superior humeral head migration upon initiation of arm elevation, which can contribute to subacromial impingement (Chen et al: *J Shoulder Elbow Surg* 1999).
- Training activities that can help improve endurance of the shoulder joint complex include wall dribbles with a plyoball, ball flips (Fig. 65.11), upper body cycling, and the Advanced Thrower's Ten exercise program.
- Throwing mechanics
  - Learn good throwing mechanics as soon as possible. It is encouraged that athletes learn, in order, basic throwing, fastball pitching, and change-up pitching.

RECOMMENDED READINGS

Available online.

SECTION
VIII

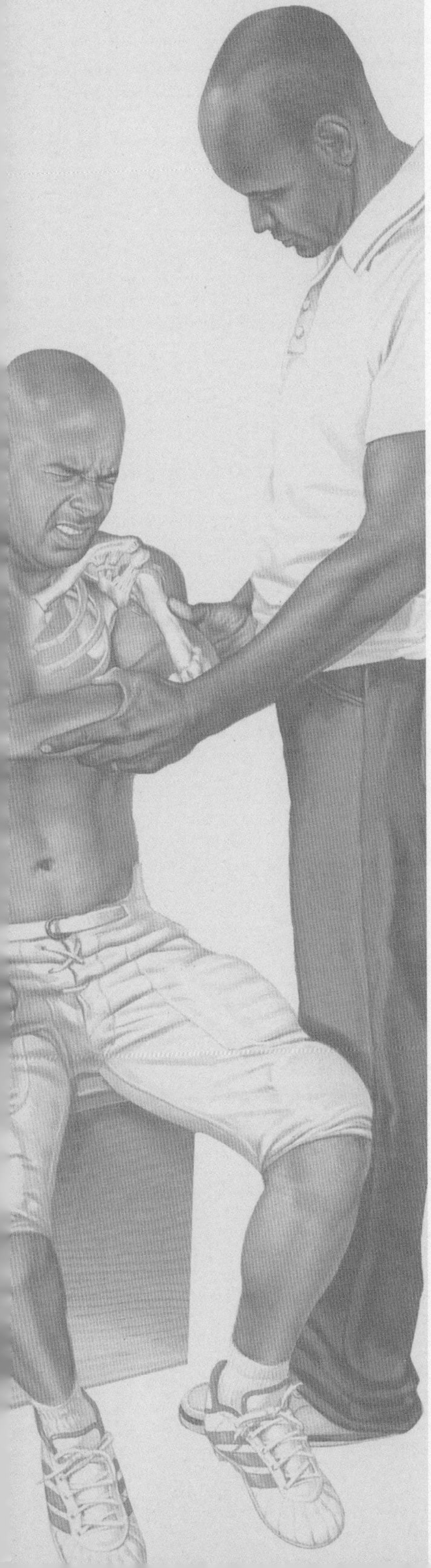

Specific Sports

FOOTBALL 66

Edward J. Smith • Margot Putukian • Eric C. McCarty, Jr. • Eric C. McCarty

INTRODUCTION

- Football developed in the United States, in what is commonly recognized as the first American football game between Rutgers and Princeton, on November 6, 1869.
- Since its inception, over 1.5 million athletes participate today and contribute to football being considered the most popular sport in the United States.
- There are well over 700 schools sponsoring varsity college football, which represent approximately 70,000 student-athletes involved in the sport.

GENERAL PRINCIPLES

History

- The flying wedge was a V-shaped formation used by Harvard in a game against Yale in 1892 and was thought to be associated with significant brutality and injuries. This technique was banned in 1894, just 2 years later.
- Years later, the National Collegiate Athletic Association (NCAA) was formed because of rising concerns of significant injuries associated with the sport.

Rules

- There are different objectives for each team depending on which portion of their team is on the field. Offensively, the objective is to move the ball down the field and score. Defensively, the objective is to prevent the offense from doing so.
- There are four "downs" per possession, each with the goal of moving the ball a minimum of 10 yards to acquire another set of "downs."
- Teams score by either moving the ball past the goal line (touchdown) or by kicking the ball through the goal post (field goal). The former is worth 6 points, and the latter is worth 3. After a touchdown, teams can opt for an additional point by kicking a point-after-touchdown (pat) or crossing the goal line again for a 2-point conversion.
- Different rules regarding the length of the game, overtime, and possession are determined by the level of play (high school, college, and professional).

Specific Training and Skills

- Football is a high-velocity collision sport with an increased risk of injury. Proper strength and conditioning are necessary to minimize injury.
- All players, regardless of position, should maintain a good level of flexibility in conjunction with overall body strength.
- Specific drills should be implemented based on the player's position, but endurance work should also be emphasized as the foundation.
- Explosive speed is needed and can be obtained by interval training, stair/stadium running, and hill training.
- Increases in lean body mass by means of supervised weight-training programs are recommended.

Nutrition

- The athlete should be counseled on the basic understanding of nutritional balance and their own specific needs based on their goals and the requirements of their position.
- A healthy, natural, well-balanced diet should be emphasized. (See Chapter 5: "Sports Nutrition.")
- The need for strength/weight gain often puts athletes at risk of potential abuse of performance-enhancing supplements. Therefore, the use of unsupervised nutraceuticals should be discouraged.
- **Fluids:** A study in high school football players in a 50-play simulation scrimmage found no difference in aerobic performance with a 7% glucose polymer beverage containing electrolytes compared with water, but the beverage had a positive effect on maintaining plasma volume during recovery.

PROTECTIVE EQUIPMENT

Football Helmet

- Purpose of the helmet is to prevent traumatic skull fractures.
- Must meet National Operating Committee on Standards for Athletic Equipment (NOCSAE) specifications.
- Construction
  - Outer shell is made of polymer plastic that is both lightweight and able to withstand high impact.
    - It is imperative to check for cracks in outer shell, as this can lead to loss of protection from the entire unit.
  - Inner shell is composed of padding, air/fluid-filled cells, or a combination of cells and pads.
    - Air cells can be inflated or deflated to provide a better fit.
    - Must check for leaks in the inner shell to prevent protective compromise.
- Helmet fitting
  - Helmet should be donned by grasping ear holes and pulling apart with thumbs. Helmet should have minimal sliding/turning during rotation of the athlete's head.
    - There should be no space between jaw pads and face or back of head.
    - There should be one to two fingerbreadths between bottom of forehead pad and athlete's eyebrows. Helmet should not cover eyes when downward pressure is applied to the top of the helmet.
    - Base of skull should be fully covered, but helmet should not impinge on cervical spine with full neck extension.
    - Helmet should have NOCSAE label on outer shell warning of potential head or spine injury with inappropriate helmet size.
  - Hair should be the same length at time of fitting as it will be throughout the season. Long hair should be wet when fitting to simulate sweaty conditions.
  - Chin strap (four-point more secure than two-point) helps prevent forward and backward rocking of the helmet. These should always be appropriately fitted and secured during competition.
  - A plethora of face masks are available and are generally position-dependent. Ball carriers require masks that provide protection but are open enough to allow clear vision. Lineman require masks that provide additional protection from eye and facial injuries.
  - Helmet visors, made of clear plexiglass, are also available for those seeking additional eye protection. Tinted visors, of the same material, can be worn by players needing special assistance for elimination of sun because of a medical condition. They require a physician's approval, and use is determined at the time of play by officiating staff.

- Mouth guards (required in high school and college) can be custom-made, formed by the mouth with heating, or obtained in standard sizes. They help dissipate blows to the chin, reducing intraoral and mandible injuries.

Shoulder Pads

- Two standard types of shoulder pads: cantilever and noncantilever (flat) pads.
  - Noncantilever pads are worn by those with positions that have a greater need for glenohumeral circumduction (quarterbacks, receivers, kickers).
  - Cantilever pads are worn by those in positions that require constant contact, thus needing additional protection (lineman and linebackers).
  - Modifications can be made to pads depending on position and preference (e.g., linebackers hit from a standing position so pads can be slightly tilted forward and larger anteriorly).
  - Appropriate fitting can be done by measuring from acromioclavicular (AC) joint to AC joint and comparing with manufacturer's size chart.
  - Neck opening should be large enough to prevent impingement when lifting arm overhead, but not so large that excessive sliding occurs.
  - Lateral aspect of pad should be just lateral to the shoulder, with epaulets large enough to cover the deltoid region.
  - Axilla straps should be adjusted snugly, but comfortably, to distribute impact across the entire chest area of pads.
  - When laced, anterior pads should meet but not overlap.
  - Bottom of chest plate and posterior plate should end just below the nipple line anteriorly and 1 cm below the scapula posteriorly, respectively.

Other Protective Equipment

- Standard equipment
  - Hip pads are used to protect iliac crest and tailbone from injury.
  - Thigh and knee pads are inserted into the pants. These should fit snug and not allow easy slippage. These pads have become smaller in size over the past decade and often do not cover much of the anterior knee or thigh.
- Special equipment
  - Neck rolls and collars are frequently used by players who have experienced "stingers" or those who seek prevention from this. The efficacy in these for prevention remains debatable. Neck rolls in high school are often ineffective because of inappropriate fit of shoulder pads.
  - Shoulder restraint harnesses restrict abduction and external rotation in chronic shoulder dislocations. The downside is that these devices may affect the capabilities of the athlete in several positions.
  - Padded gloves and upper extremity accessories are worn to prevent finger injuries, contusions, and myositis ossificans.
  - Flak jackets are commonly worn by quarterbacks to prevent rib injuries.
  - Mandatory knee bracing is not recommended for prophylactic prevention of knee injuries.

INJURY STATISTICS

- At the college level, in a report published by the Centers for Disease Control and Prevention (CDC) reviewing sport-related injuries from 2009 to 2014, football accounted for the largest annual estimated number of injuries per year, the highest competition injury rate (39.9 per 1000 athlete-exposures [AEs]), and the third highest overall injury rate (9.2 per 1000) (Table 66.1). Football also accounts for the largest proportion of injuries requiring >7 days before return to full participation (26.2%), surgery (40.2%), or emergency transport (31.9%).

Table 66.1 INJURY RATES (PER 1000 ATHLETIC EXPOSURES)

Sport	Practice	Game
Football	5.8	39.9
Wrestling	9.0	38.5
Men's Ice Hockey	3.2	26.3
Men's Soccer	5.2	17.9
Women's Soccer	5.3	17.2
Men's Basketball	5.8	15.0
Men's Lacrosse	4.9	13.7
Women's Gymnastics	2.9	13.2
Women's Ice Hockey	3.2	11.2
Women's Field Hockey	5.1	10.5
Women's Basketball	4.9	10.4
Men's Tennis	2.9	10.0
Women's Lacrosse	4.2	9.7
Women's Cross-Country	3.4	7.7
Women's Tennis	3.1	7.6
Men's Baseball	3.0	6.8
Men's Indoor Track	3.1	6.5
Women's Softball	3.5	5.9
Women's Volleyball	5.6	5.9
Men's Outdoor Track	2.3	5.4
Men's Cross-Country	3.2	5.2
Women's Outdoor Track	2.7	5.1
Women's Indoor Track	3.8	4.4
Men's Swimming and Diving	2.1	2.0
Women's Swimming and Diving	2.1	1.9

Modified from National Collegiate Athletics Association. *NCAA Handbook 2014-2015*. 25th ed. Indianapolis, IN: National Collegiate Athletics Association; 2014; Kerr ZY, Marshall SW, Dompier TP, et al. College sports-related injuries—United States, 2009-2010 through 2013-2014 academic years. *Morb Mortal Wkly Rep*. 2015;64(48):1330–1336.

- Between 1988–1989 and 2003–2004, preseason injury rates were higher than both in-season and postseason injury rates (7.05 vs. 2.02 and 7.05 vs. 1.70 per 1000 AEs, respectively). Preseason, therefore, is a critical time to emphasize appropriate warmups, fluid and nutrition replacement, technique, stretching, and recovery.
- Internal knee derangements, ankle sprains, and concussion account for most injuries in games (17.8%, 15.6%, and 6.8%, respectively).
- Internal knee derangements, ankle sprains, and upper leg muscular injuries account for most injuries in practice (12%, 11.8%, and 10.7%, respectively).
- Cervical spine injuries can have catastrophic potential, but the prevalence has decreased since the induction of rule modifications, improved athlete fitness, and substantial equipment upgrades.
- Direct player-to-player contact is the most common mechanism for injury in football. This holds true regardless of competitive environment (practice, scrimmage, or games).
- Player position plays a factor in the likelihood of injury. Running backs are the most injured position during games (19.6%), followed by quarterbacks (17.5%), linebackers (15.5%), wide receivers (14.4%), defensive backs (11.7%), defensive linemen (11.3%), then offensive linemen (9.9%).
- Fatalities have been reported in both high school and collegiate football players. From 1990 to 2010, 243 fatalities were reported to the National Center for Catastrophic Sports Injury Research. Of these 243, 164 were indirectly related and 79 were related. The most common causes of fatalities in the review were cardiac failure (41.2%), brain injury (25.5%), heat illness (15.6%), sickle cell trait (4.5%), asthma and commotio cordis

(2.9%), blood clot (2.1%), and cervical fracture (1.7%). Intra-abdominal injury, infection, and lighting completed the remaining causes, each accounting for 1.2%.

COMMON INJURIES AND MEDICAL PROBLEMS

This section will describe various common injuries encountered in the sport of football. The treatment and return to play for many of the musculoskeletal conditions may vary by the position that the athlete plays on the football field. A right thumb injury to an offensive lineman can likely be treated differently than the same injury in a quarterback's throwing hand, and the injury will affect the athlete with a much different level of significance. In this example, the lineman might be able to return to the same game in a cast, whereas the quarterback might take several weeks to return, as their ability to hold a football is severely affected. Thus, the treatment and return to play of many of the conditions need to be evaluated on an individual and position-specific basis.

Head Injuries

Concussion (See Chapter 45: "Head Injuries" for Full Details)

Description: A transient change in neurologic function secondary to an acute force being applied to the head and/or neck. In sports, a concussion is usually the most common form of a traumatic brain injury. Football has a high rate of head injuries as monitored at the collegiate level (Table 66.2).

History: In football, player-to-player contact is the primary mechanism of action. A forceful blow to the head by another person or solid object (turf, goalpost, benches) elicits axonal damage and neurotransmitter release, leading to direct brain injury and concussive symptoms. Other mechanisms for concussion would be a "whiplash" injury to the cervical spine.

Physical examination: Acutely, primary evaluation of the athlete should ensue, taking into careful consideration the ABCs of emergency management (Airway, Breathing, Circulation). Secondary assessment once the player is off the field would consist of neurocognitive testing with a Standardized Concussion Assessment Tool (SCAT5).

Diagnostic considerations: Usually not necessary for concussion. If concerns for neurologic deterioration exist, emergent Computed Tomography (CT) should be obtained to rule out cerebral hemorrhage.

Treatment: Rest until asymptomatic. Postconcussion complications are discussed in Chapter 45.

Return to play: If there are concerns for concussion, the athlete should be promptly removed from the field of play. General agreed-upon consensus is that no athlete should be allowed to resume play on the same day that a concussion has been suffered. Graded return to activity based on symptom severity has been used to assist athletes in obtaining level of function before injury. Special consideration should be measured with football players and specific positions. Graded return to play may be earlier for sport-specific drills in noncontact positions (quarterbacks, kickers, punters) than in contact positions (defensive linemen, offensive linemen, running backs).

Prevention: Efforts have been made throughout collegiate and professional levels to reduce the number of concussions obtained. In 1976, spearing became officially banned in football, with the goal of reducing brain trauma and catastrophic cervical injuries. Head-to-head injuries remained after the rule change, and in 2008 officials were able to label these as fouls. The NCAA (Safety in College Football Summit) and the NFL Foundations, USA Football (HeadsUpFootball) have made strides to decrease the amount of contact exposures, increase education about proper tackling mechanics, and have a formal concussion plan in place that brings the signs and symptoms of a concussion to the forefront.

Table 66.2 NCAA DATA ON CONCUSSION INJURIES: 2009–2010 THROUGH 2013–2014

Concussion[a]	Game	Practice	Overall
Sports With No Head Protection			
Field hockey	11.10	1.77	4.02
Women's lacrosse	13.08	3.30	5.21
Men's soccer	9.69	1.75	3.44
Women's soccer	19.38	2.14	6.31
Women's basketball	10.92	4.43	5.95
Men's basketball	5.6	3.42	3.89
Wrestling	55.46	5.68	10.92
Sports With Head Protection			
Men's ice hockey	24.89	2.51	7.91
Football	30.07	4.20	6.71
Women's ice hockey	20.10	3.00	7.50
Men's lacrosse	9.31	1.95	3.18
Women's softball	5.61	1.75	3.28
Baseball	1.20	0.72	0.90

[a]Concussion as a subset of all head injuries; rates are per 10,000 athlete-exposures.

From Zuckerman SL, Kerr ZY, Yengo-Kahn A, et al. Epidemiology of sports-related concussion in NCAA athletes from 2009-2010 to 2013-2014: Incidence, recurrence and mechanisms. *Am J Sports Med*. 2016;43(11):2654–2662.

Cervical Spine

Cervical Strain

Description: Musculotendinous injury to the cervical spine. Typically, the most common form of neck injury.

History: Athlete will present with paravertebral pain with or without spasm, depending on acuity, and decreased range of motion. Radicular and neurologic symptoms are usually absent.

Physical examination: Decreased range of motion on the contralateral side to the soft tissue injury (inability to side-bend head to the left or rotate the head to the left would indicate a cervical strain to the posterior right paravertebral muscles). Hypertonic paravertebral muscles would be palpable, with tenderness to palpation of the same soft tissue region.

Diagnostic considerations: Usually not indicated unless noticeable midline tenderness or bony prominence, feelings of instability from the athlete, or neurologic deficits associated. If necessary, plain radiographs should be used to rule out instability or fracture.

Treatment: Nonsteroidal anti-inflammatory drugs (NSAIDs), rest, and physical therapy using soft tissue treatment and stretching.

Return to play: Full, unrestricted range of motion without pain. Normal posture, physical examination, and absence of neurologic deficits should be obtained before returning to competition.

Prevention: Typically acute in nature. Maintain proper conditioning and posture. Thorough warm-up before intense practice or competition.

Brachial Plexus Injuries (Burners/Stingers)

Description: Typically occurs from acute traumatic distraction of the neck or shoulder, leading to stretching or pinching of the brachial plexus.

History: Can be seen from a player landing on the superior aspect of the shoulder or from a direct blow to the side of the helmet leading to excessive side-bending of the cervical spine. Athlete will present with electric shocklike radiating pain from neck to arm. May also experience numbness or paralysis in the affected extremity. Careful consideration should be taken for bilateral symptoms, as this could be suggestive of transient quadriparesis.

Physical examination: Athlete may hold arm adducted and flexed, close to body. May also notice athlete "shaking" arm in attempt to regain sensation or correct paresthesia. Full neurologic assessment for strength and sensation should take place to isolate nerve root affected.

Diagnostic considerations: Usually not necessary unless recurrent, physical examination yields bony tenderness, or symptoms are bilateral. Plain radiographs should be the test of choice if these symptoms are present.

Treatment: NSAIDs, rest, and physical therapy focusing on stretching hypertonic neck muscles and strengthening the same muscles that may have been weakened during the injury.

Return to play: Once full strength and resolution of neurologic symptoms have been obtained. Athlete should be reexamined 24 hours after injury because of phenomenon of delayed weakness.

Prevention: Protective equipment with a neck roll or soft collar. Shoulder pads must be well-fitting, as loose pads diminish the effect of the neck roll.

Cervical Fractures and Dislocations

Description: Fracture of either the spinous process or transverse process of the cervical vertebrae.

History: Less frequent since "spearing" has been removed. Can still inadvertently happen with secondary hyperflexion and compression of the cervical spine, as seen when one player encounters another by using the crown of the helmet.

Physical examination: Athlete will have pain in the neck, noticeably worse with cervical flexion. Assess for neurologic injury!

Diagnostic considerations: Imaging needed. Plain radiographs AFTER immobilization and transfer. Magnetic Resonance Imaging (MRI) if neurologic symptoms.

Treatment: Removal from play. Immobilization of the spine must be obtained. Pads and helmet should not be removed until spine is immobilized. Face mask should be cut if airway management is necessary. Be aware of emergency action plan and emergency personnel guidelines.

Return to play:

- Absolute contraindications for return to collision sports
  - Any C1–C2 injury with ligamentous instability or fusion
  - Unstable ligamentous injuries to C2–C7
  - Vertebral body fractures with displacement into the spinal canal
  - Healed fractures with residual instability
  - Disc herniation with neurologic findings or limited motion
  - Postoperative fusion of more than three levels
- Relative contraindications for return to collision sports
  - Full, pain-free range of motion without neurologic deficits with a healed vertebral body compression fracture or neural ring fracture
  - Postoperative fusion of two to three levels
- No contraindication for return to collision sports
  - Full, pain-free range of motion without neurologic deficits and a healed, stable compression fracture of spinous process
  - Postoperative fusion of one level after a discectomy of a vertebrae at or higher than C3

Shoulder

Clavicle Fractures

Description: Fracture to the clavicle from direct or indirect trauma. Roughly 90% occur in the middle third of the clavicle.

History: Most common from a direct blow to the clavicle. Also occurs while falling directly on to lateral aspect of shoulder with an adducted arm.

Physical examination: Bruising and tenderness to palpation over the clavicle. If severe enough, may notice tenting of the overlying skin.

Diagnostic considerations: Plain radiographs should be obtained.

Treatment: Majority can be treated nonsurgically with arm sling and immobilization. If fragments are overlapping >1.5 cm (Bayonet deformity), surgical fixation is recommended.

Return to play: Faster healing time and return to play with surgical fixation, usually 8–12 weeks. Athlete should have full range of motion, strength, and imaging evidence of healed fracture.

Prevention: Sudden injury without much anticipation. Ensuring athletes are wearing all proper protective equipment is first line.

Incomplete AC Joint Separation

Description: Referred to as grade I and II AC strains. Coracoclavicular ligaments may be intact or sprained without disruption. (See Chapter 49: "Shoulder Injuries.")

History: Most commonly results from fall onto the point of the shoulder (Fig. 66.1).

Physical examination: Athlete will have tenderness over AC joint. Will notice pain with cross-body test (resisted adduction of arm across the chest).

Diagnostic considerations: Plain radiographs with weight in arm to distinguish grade III from grade IV.

Treatment: Conservative therapy with rest, ice, compression, and elevation (RICE). Physical therapy also beneficial.

Return to play: After full strength and range of motion have been obtained. Pain tolerance is a key factor in regaining

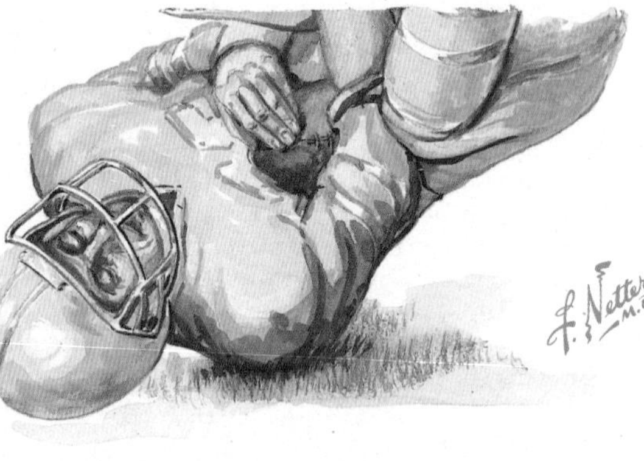

Injury to acromioclavicular joint with direct mechanism of fall on to top of shoulder causing sprain of acromioclavicular ligaments.

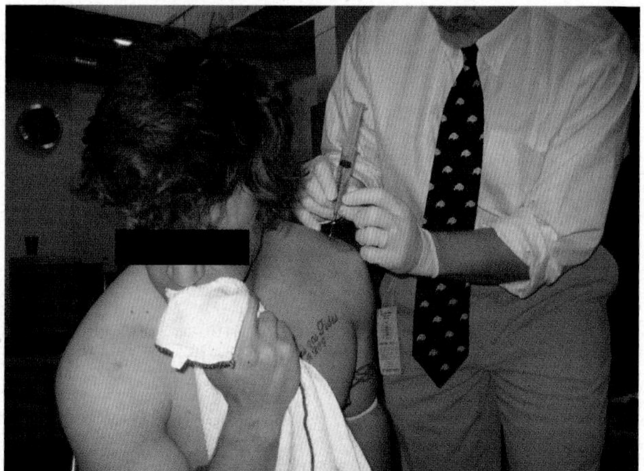

Anesthetic injection during game for grade I acromioclavicular joint sprain with proper sterile technique.

Figure 66.1 Acromioclavicular injury.

strength and motion and then returning to play. Pain tolerance is variable across all athletes. AC padding after restoration of strength. In resolving semiacute phase, local anesthetic injection can be used judiciously to allow in-game return or to enable play.

Prevention: Sudden and unexpected. Ensure athletes are wearing all properly fitted protective equipment.

Complete AC Joint Separation

Description: Referred to as grade III–grade VI AC sprains. Coracoclavicular ligaments are disrupted. (See Chapter 49: "Shoulder Injuries.")

History: Same mechanisms of action as incomplete AC joint separations.

Physical examination: Tenderness at AC joint. Palpable step-off between clavicle and acromion.

Diagnostic considerations: Plain radiographs.

Treatment: Grade III separations are controversial. Unless extensive muscle injury present or distal clavicle has penetrated the trapezius, conservative measures are appropriate. Grade IV–VI separations require surgical fixation.

Return to play: Once athlete has full restoration of strength and motion. Again, as in incomplete AC separations, pain tolerance will be a factor in return to play. AC padding should take place with return.

Prevention: Sudden and unexpected. Ensure athletes are wearing all properly fitted protective equipment.

Glenohumeral Instability

Description (common football injury usually seen as either anterior or posterior):

- Anterior: Most common secondary to abduction/external rotation force; can result from inappropriate tackling technique.
- Posterior: Traumatic posterior dislocation is uncommon. However, instability/labral tears are common in offensive linemen.

History:

- Anterior: Occurs secondary to a fall on an outstretched hand. Also can happen when an athlete lunges for a tackle with the arm abducted forcibly.
- Posterior: Athlete will have pain in posterior shoulder after arms have been extended forward and presented with a direct posterior force (offensive lineman when blocking or an athlete performing a heavy bench press), leading to posterior displacement of the shoulder.

Physical examination:

- Anterior: Athlete will have a prominence in the anterior of the shoulder. Arm will be visibly held in abduction and external rotation, with limited internal rotation. Be sure to assess neurovascular function.
- Posterior: Athlete will visibly hold arm in adducted, internally rotated position with lack of external rotation. Palpation of an anterior prominent coracoid. Posterior jerk test will reproduce symptoms.

Diagnostic considerations:

- Anterior: Plain radiographs to evaluate for reduction, Hill–Sachs, or Bankart lesions. MRI recommended to evaluate extent of cartilage injury.
- Posterior: Plain radiographs are needed to avoid a missed diagnosis.

Treatment:

- Anterior: On field, acute injury can be treated by experienced physician using gentle reduction. Early rehabilitation is important. Immobilization after acute injury is controversial. Bracing can control external rotation/abduction movement and allow earlier return to play (Fig. 66.2). Neither immobilization nor therapy has been shown to decrease the redislocation rate in young people. Arthroscopic stabilization has been shown to decrease the dislocation rate, but decision-making on surgery is case-dependent. Factors include timing, risk factors, and career goals.
- Posterior: Should consist of rehabilitation. There is no bracing that can control a posterior-directed force on the shoulder. If athlete remains symptomatic, then surgical stabilization is the treatment of choice. Usually a labral tear is associated, and players have been shown to have a successful return to football after surgery.

Return to play: Once athlete has regained full strength and range of motion with minimal apprehension, but little evidence exists for a formal recommendation as to return criteria. Athletes with previous instability episodes have a high rate of recurrence.

Prevention: Sudden and unexpected on first attempt. Educate on proper tackling technique. Surgical referral for episodes of repeat instability.

Rotator Cuff/Biceps Tendinopathy

Description: Overuse injuries involving rotator cuff tendonitis, biceps tendonitis/rupture, and shoulder impingement. Relatively uncommon pathology in younger populations but rotator cuff tendon involvement can occur in quarterbacks.

History: Athlete will have concerns for shoulder pain, usually with an insidious onset. Identifying positions played, and repetitive training, can lead to a specific diagnosis.

Physical examination: Evaluate for supraspinatus weakness by testing resisted abduction with arm in 30 degrees of forward flexion and 90 degrees of scapular plane abduction. Evaluate for bicep involvement with Speed and Yergason testing. Evaluate for impingement with Neer and Hawkins testing. (See Chapter 49: "Shoulder Injuries," for full description.)

Diagnostic considerations: MRI if tear suspected. Helpful to rule out large intra-articular tendon fragment if biceps rupture is suspected.

Treatment: Impingement with rotator cuff tendinopathy is usually responsive to physical therapy; surgical repair is generally indicated if full-thickness tear in the young population. Bicep tendonitis and proximal rupture are generally responsive to rest, followed by strengthening program; surgical tenodesis indicated in select high-demand positions, to include arthroscopic debridement of symptomatic intra-articular tendon fragment.

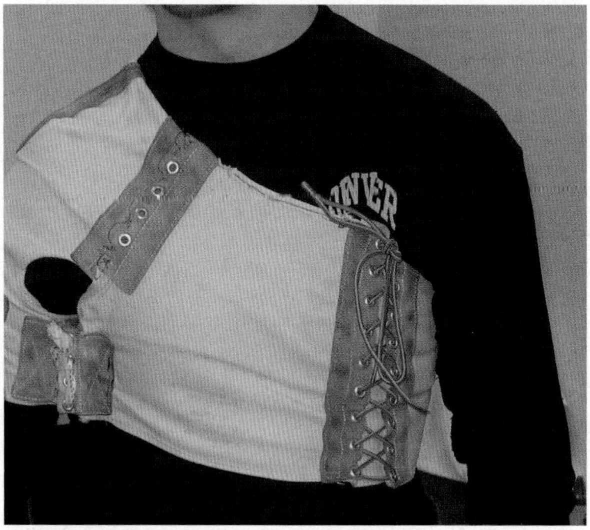

Example of shoulder harness to help assist player with anterior shoulder instability in preventing abduction and external rotation during competition.

Figure 66.2 Anterior shoulder instability.

Return to play: Early emphasis on strengthening and range of motion to prevent adhesive capsulitis. Return to play once range of motion and full strength have been achieved.
Prevention: Proper exercise mechanics, frequency, and duration to minimize overuse.

Shoulder Contusions

Description: Injury of the shoulder resulting from a direct blow to it. Common, particularly in linebackers.
History: Athlete will have weakness and tenderness in deltoid and rotator cuff region.
Physical examination: Physical examination like that of someone with a rotator cuff tear. May also notice bruising of the deltoid region.
Diagnostic considerations: Imaging usually unnecessary.
Treatment: Initial management with rest, ice, and anti-inflammatory agents. If a large hematoma is present, aspiration is indicated.
Return to play: Once full strength and range of motion have been obtained. If hematoma present, this should be resolved before return of contact.
Prevention: Sudden and unexpected. Ensure athletes are wearing all properly fitted protective equipment.

Elbow and Forearm

Valgus Injuries of the Elbow (Overuse)

Description: Occasional injury that happens in quarterbacks from repetitive throwing motion.
History: Athlete will present with pain on the medial aspect of the elbow and forearm. Typically, will have a history of repetitive throwing.
Physical examination: Noticeable tenderness to palpation distal and posterior to the medial condyle with valgus stress and occasional ulnar nerve irritation.
Diagnostic considerations: Because of concerns for laxity, MRI is gold standard for verification.
Treatment: Conservative treatment involves rest, ice, NSAIDs, physical therapy, and protective function. Surgery indicated if adequate therapy has failed and athlete desires to continue as a high-demand thrower.
Return to play: Activities that involve valgus stressing are restricted for a minimum of 6 weeks. Prolonged therapy and sport-specific training may be needed for 4–6 months before full return can be obtained.
Prevention: Proper throwing mechanics, frequency, and duration to minimize overuse.

Hyperextension/Dislocation Injuries of the Elbow

Description: Separation of the humerus and radial/ulna articulation resulting from a fall on an outstretched hand.
History: Typically results from a fall or from forced extension of the lower arm during a tackle.
Physical examination: Physical deformity will be visualized. Examine for open wounds and skin breakdown. Assess neurovascular status of median nerve and brachial/ulnar arteries.
Diagnostic considerations: Both hyperextension and dislocation injuries require radiographs to rule out fracture and assess neurovascular status of hand and forearm.
Treatment: Most common dislocation is a posterior dislocation. These can be reduced by experienced physician by using gentle traction with the athlete's elbow in a semiflexed position. Early protected range of motion recommended.
Return to play: Once strength and range of motion have been restored, return to sport with protective bracing (usually 3–6 weeks for dislocation and sooner with a hyperextension injury) (Fig. 66.3).
Prevention: Sudden and unexpected injury.

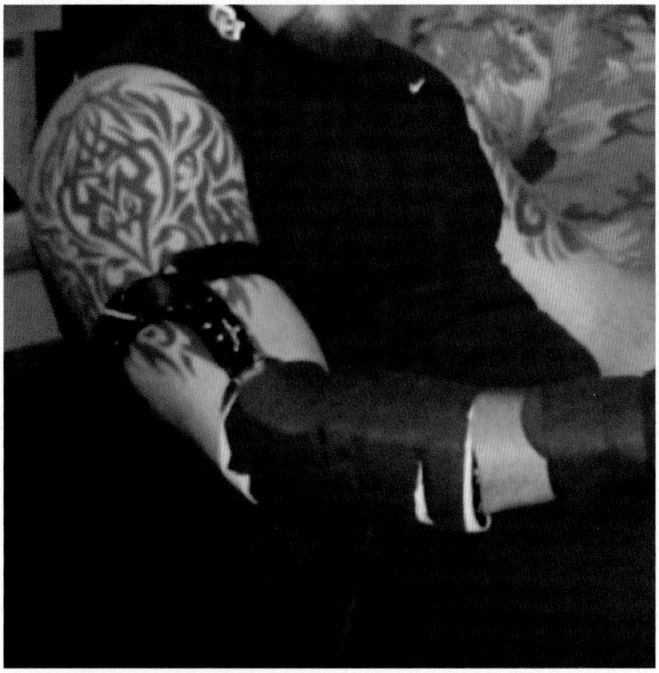

Hinged elbow brace utilized to protect player's elbow that has valgus laxity after elbow dislocation.

Figure 66.3 Valgus laxity.

Olecranon Bursitis

Description: Swelling of the superficial bursal sac over the olecranon process.
History: Common, traumatic bursitis, secondary to impact with tackling.
Physical examination: Careful examination of the skin to rule out an open communication with the bursa.
Diagnostic considerations: Plain radiographs should be considered to evaluate the presence of bony spurs.
Treatment: Initial aspiration if persistent or large effusion noted. If continual recurrence, consider a sclerosing agent or surgical excision of the bursa.
Return to play: Early return to sport with protective padding is reasonable.
Prevention: Traumatic, sudden, and unexpected injury in football.

Wrist and Hand

Scaphoid Fractures

Description: Common injury in athletes after falling on an outstretched hand. (See Chapter 51: "Hand and Wrist Injuries.")
History: Athlete will typically have pain in the anatomic snuff box.
Physical examination: Tenderness to palpation on the distal radius around the fracture.
Diagnostic considerations: Plain radiographs should be obtained.
Treatment: An acute nondisplaced fracture can be treated with a long arm cast for 4–6 weeks, followed by short arm thumb spica until healed. High-demand athletes are currently being treated by means of surgical fixation to facilitate earlier return to play.
Return to play: Position dependent. Linemen typically have faster return with appropriate outer cast padding. Displaced or symptomatic nonunion should have surgical fixation. After adequate healing and strengthening, return to sport with appropriate padding can be obtained.
Prevention: Traumatic, sudden, and unexpected injury in football.

Distal Radius and Ulna Fractures (See Chapter 51: "Hand and Wrist Injuries," for Full Details)

Treatment: Conservative vs. surgical treatment depends on fracture pattern and stability.

Return to play: Dependent on player position and fracture stability. May need 2–3 months before sufficient healing and stability before full return.

Prevention: Traumatic, sudden, and unexpected injury in football.

Carpal Fractures Other Than Scaphoid (See Chapter 51: "Hand and Wrist Injuries," for Full Details)

Description: Avulsion fractures are typically the most common in football.

Diagnostic considerations: Plain films are first line. MRI if plain films are inconclusive. Important to rule out carpal dislocations (lunate/perilunate) or ligamentous injuries (scapholunate).

Treatment: Avulsion fractures should be managed with immobilization.

Return to play: Position specific, but early return if tolerable.

Collateral Ligament Injuries

Description: Common injuries. Typically result from adduction (radial) or abduction (ulnar) forces applied to the metacarpophalangeal (MCP) joint.

History: Athlete will have pain at the distal aspect of the MCP joint, radial, or ulnar aspects.

Physical examination: Palpation of the ulnar/radial aspects of the MCP joint will yield pain. Stress testing of these joints will also yield reproducible tenderness.

Diagnostic considerations: Plain imaging recommended to rule out osseus pathology. Stress imaging also recommended to determine complete tears of the ulnar collateral ligament (UCL) injury.

Treatment: Radial ligament injuries, and incomplete ulnar ligament injuries, can be managed with protective splinting. Complete UCL tears are typically managed surgically because of the high prevalence of Stener lesions.

Return to play: Early return to play for radial ligament injuries and incomplete UCL injuries. For complete UCL tears, casting and early return to sport AFTER surgery are recommended.

Prevention: Traumatic, sudden, and unexpected injury in football.

Thumb Fractures/Dislocations (See Chapter 51: "Hand and Wrist Injuries," for Full Details)

Description: Because of perilous position of the thumb in football, this is a relatively common injury. MCP dislocations are most commonly dorsal, and it is important to differentiate simple (reducible) vs. complex (nonreducible). Bennett fracture is an unstable fracture of the intra-articular joint space.

Treatment: Complex MCP dislocations and Bennett fractures require surgical fixation.

Return to play: Early return to play for MCP dislocations with protective splinting for 4–6 weeks. Bennett fractures typically require 4–6 weeks of immobilization before gradual return to play.

Prevention: Traumatic, sudden, and unexpected injury in football.

Other Hand Fractures/Dislocations

Description: Most commonly occurs as a result of direct contact.

History: Will notably have pain and resistance to movement after direct contact with ground, helmet, or another player.

Physical examination: See Chapter 51, "Hand and Wrist Injuries," for full details

Diagnostic considerations: Plain radiographs recommended. For dislocations, radiographs should be obtained after the game to rule out bony injury.

Treatment: Fourth and fifth metacarpal fractures can be manually reduced to an acceptable level. Second and third metacarpals are less tolerant to manual reduction. Proximal phalanx fractures require surgical fixation to maintain appropriate length and rotation. Middle phalanx fractures are amendable to manual reduction. Distal tuft fractures should be treated as soft tissue injuries with examination of the nail bed and repair, or removal of the fracture site if incarcerated. Volar dislocations in the proximal interphalangeal (PIP) joint are rare and should be treated the same as a rupture of the central slip in the extensor tendon.

Return to play: Most hand fractures can be treated with protective splinting and early return to play. Dislocations are most commonly dorsal, can be manually reduced, and the continuous use of buddy taping for 3–6 weeks with early return to play is an appropriate approach.

Prevention: Traumatic, sudden, and unexpected injury in football.

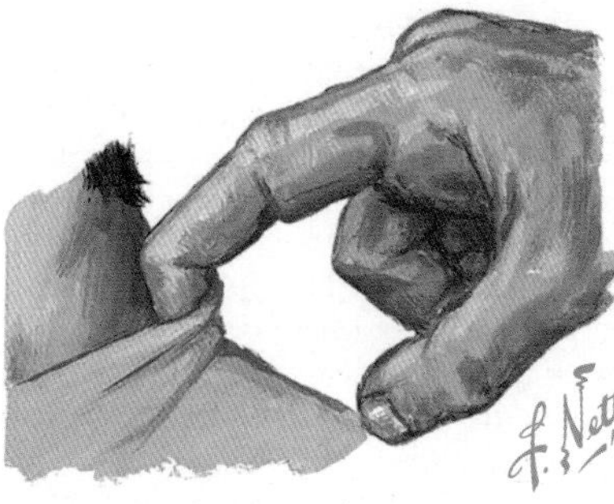
F. Netter M.D.

"Jersey Finger," example of injury to flexor tendon of hand while player trying to tackle opponent and finger getting stuck in jersey.

Figure 66.4 Jersey finger.

Flexor Tendon Injuries

Description: Flexor tendon injuries typically occur when a player attempts to grab another player's jersey or padding to make a tackle.

History: Athlete will have pain and an inability to flex the distal interphalangeal (DIP) joint of the involved finger (Fig. 66.4).

Physical examination: Important to assess and determine the level of retraction of the tendon. If tendon is retracted to the palm, blood supply is significantly compromised.

Diagnostic considerations: Radiographs should always be obtained to evaluate for bony avulsions.

Treatment: Fully retracted flexor tendons into the palm need urgent surgery, within 7 days. Less retracted tendons can be repaired later, but best results happen with earlier diagnosis and repair.

Return to play: Typical return after 4–6 weeks postoperatively. Athlete will need hand therapy during the recovery.

Prevention: Traumatic, sudden, and unexpected injury in football.

Extensor Tendon Injuries (Distal Phalanx)

Description: Extensor tendon avulsions of the distal phalanx typically occur by "jamming" finger.

History: Athlete would have experienced forced flexion of the distal phalanx (from a fall, tackle, or an attempt to catch a pass).

Physical examination: Will notice an inability of the athlete to extend the DIP.

Diagnostic consideration: Radiographs should always be obtained to evaluate for bony avulsions.

Treatment: Continuous splinting of DIP joint with a splint. Free range of motion should be maintained at the PIP joint.

Return to play: Early return to play recommended.

Prevention: Traumatic, sudden, and unexpected injury in football.

Extensor Tendon Avulsions (Central Slip)

Description: Avulsions of the central slip also occur with the same mechanism of action as distal injuries, a "jamming" injury. These are often misdiagnosed as a capsular sprain.

Diagnostic considerations: Radiographs important to rule out fracture.

Treatment: PIP joint should be held in continuous extension with the DIP joint free for a minimum of 6 weeks.

Return to play: Early return with proper splinting.

Prevention: Traumatic, sudden, and unexpected injury in football.

Chest and Abdomen

Rib Fractures

Description: Happens from direct trauma or impact to the rib cage.

History: Athletes will have chest wall pain, worse with breathing.

Physical examination: Tenderness to palpation of the chest wall or rib cage in the area of trauma.

Diagnostic considerations: Plain radiographs are needed to make the diagnosis.

Treatment: Removal from play. Conservative treatment for pain relief.

Return to play: Typically 6–8 weeks are needed in football. Protective "flak jacket" can be worn when symptoms are tolerable.

Prevention: Sudden and unexpected. Ensure athletes are wearing all properly fitted protective equipment.

Sternoclavicular Injuries

Description: Dislocations or injuries caused by an indirect blow to the shoulder or a direct blow to the upper chest.

History: Athlete will have pain with or without swelling to the sternoclavicular region.

Physical examination: Tenderness to palpation in the sternoclavicular area with exacerbation during range-of-motion testing of the arm.

Diagnostic considerations: CT scan is necessary to rule out posterior dislocation.

Treatment: Posterior dislocations require emergent surgical reduction to avoid injuries of the major vessels. Anterior dislocations are most common and are typically treated conservatively.

Return to play: Athletes with an anterior dislocation can return to play once strength and full range of motion have been restored.

Prevention: Sudden and unexpected. Ensure athletes are wearing all properly fitted protective equipment.

Pectoralis Major Ruptures

Description: Tears in the pectoralis muscle anywhere from the belly of the muscle to the musculotendinous attachment occurring from forceful extension/external rotation of the arm.

History: Will usually happen suddenly secondary to a forceful blow to the shoulder while arm is abducted.

Physical examination: Athlete will have pain and ecchymosis along the anteromedial aspect of the arm and an inability to flex the pectoralis muscle with arm adduction and internal rotation.

Diagnostic considerations: MRI typically needed to visualize extent of injury.

Treatment: Incomplete tears can be treated conservatively. Complete ruptures are treated surgically because of deficits in strength if treated conservatively.

Return to play: Athletes with incomplete tears can return to play once strength and range of motion have been achieved.

Prevention: Traumatic, sudden, and unexpected injury in football.

Abdominal Wall Injuries

Description: Two of the more common abdominal wall injuries in football are rectus abdominus strains and athletic pubalgia (sports hernia).

History: Rectus abdominal strains happen after a forceful, resisted contraction of the abdominal musculature. Athletic pubalgia happens secondary to explosive, twisting movements of the pelvis (repetitive sprinting in football).

Physical examination: Strains will have palpable tenderness around injury with flexion of the trunk. Athletic pubalgia can be difficult to diagnose, but ruling out a true "hernia" in the athlete is necessary for the physical examination.

Diagnostic considerations: Abdominal strains are a clinical diagnosis. Athletic pubalgia requires imaging. Radiographs should be obtained to rule out symphysis pubis changes. MRI is the gold standard for diagnosis.

Treatment: Rectus abdominus strains can be treated conservatively with ice and stretching. Athletic pubalgia often needs surgical intervention. Conservative management is usually prolonged and delays the athlete from returning to competition.

Return to play: Abdominal strains do well with trunk taping to limit flexion during play. Surgical treatment of athletic pubalgia can typically allow the athlete to return to play within 6–12 weeks.

Prevention: Proper running/exercise mechanics, frequency, and duration to minimize overuse.

Thoracolumbar Spine

Thoracic and Lumbar Strains

Description: Most common injury to spine in football. Often secondary to fatigue and poor conditioning; strains occur with bending or twisting of the torso during forceful activities.

History: Athlete will have pain with stiffness or tightness in the paraspinal musculature.

Physical examination: Visual decreased range of motion of the spine with tenderness to palpation of the paravertebral muscles. Check for radicular symptoms; strains often occur without these. Any radiation into the lower extremities should be suspicious for disc pathology.

Diagnostic considerations: Plain radiographs are helpful in ruling out osseous pathology, neural arch involvement, or Scheuermann kyphosis.

Treatment: Most uncomplicate strains resolve in 7–10 days with conservative management.

Return to play: Typically limited by pain. Progression to back rehab program when tolerated. Athlete can return when full strength and range of motion have been obtained.

Prevention: Flexibility and conditioning program during season, and off-season, is incredibly important.

Disc Herniation

Description: Herniation of the nucleus pulposus through the annular ligaments. Mechanism of injury mimics that of a lumbar strain.

History: Athlete typically has neuropathy findings of one or both legs with or without low back pain.

Physical examination: Complete neurologic assessment, including sensation, motor, and reflexes of the lower extremities. Can isolate level of herniation(s) based on area of deficits.

Diagnostic considerations: Plain radiographs and MRI helpful in documenting injury.

Treatment: Initial treatment is the same as for lumbar strains. Consider epidural injections or disc excision if no improvement with conservative care or if persisting or progressive neurologic deficits.

Return to play: Progressive long-term rehabilitation can lead to return.

Prevention: Proper exercise mechanics, frequency, and duration to minimize injury.

Spondylolysis/Spondylolisthesis

Description: Common in linemen secondary to repetitive loading of the posterior elements of the spine while in an extended position.

History: Athlete will have low back pain, much like that of a lumbar strain.

Physical examination: Palpable hamstring hypertonicity and reproducible pain with resisted back extension. Stork test will also yield pain for the athlete.

Diagnostic considerations: Anterior/Posterior (A/P)/lateral/oblique radiographs important to look for spondylolysis and spondylolisthesis. CT is often helpful in differentiating acute versus chronic injury of the neural arch.

Treatment: Restriction from play, abdominal and lumbar stretching, strengthening exercises, and occasional use of orthotics are the mainstays of treatment. Physical therapy can begin once resolution of hamstring spasm has been obtained. Skeletally immature patients with a high-grade spondylolisthesis (greater than 50%) are candidates for fusion.

Return to play: Clinical progress is more important than radiographic evidence of healing. Known presence of spondylolysis or spondylolisthesis in an asymptomatic player is not a contraindication for return.

Prevention: Sudden and unexpected injuries. If athlete is having signs of low back pain from overuse, early intervention with conservative treatment can be helpful in preventing the risk of fractures.

Thoracolumbar Fractures

Description: Infrequent injuries that can occur after direct impact to the spine or by way of violent muscle contractions.

History: Athlete will complain of severe back pain exacerbated by any movement.

Physical examination: If any concern for fracture present during initial evaluation, it is imperative to maintain spine precautions before moving the patient. Once this has been done, complete neurologic assessment should ensue.

Diagnostic considerations: Any suspected fracture should warrant further evaluation with AP/lateral/oblique radiographs of the concerning region. MRI should be obtained if any neurologic deficit accompanies the fracture. CT or MRI should be obtained if concern for injury of visceral structures.

Treatment: Isolated stable transverse fractures are amendable to a brief period of rest. Acute fracture with no history of prodromal symptoms can often heal if adequate immobilization and lumbar orthosis. Treatment should follow generally accepted guidelines for fracture management.

Return to play: Isolated transverse fractures usually do well with a return to play, after rest, within 3–6 weeks. Any patient requiring lumbar fusion should not be allowed to return to football.

Prevention: Sudden, unexpected, and traumatic injuries.

Hip and Pelvis

Hip Pointers

Description: A relatively common injury in football resulting in a contusion to the iliac crest or greater trochanter secondary to a direct impact. Rarely, hip pointers can lead to avulsion fractures.

History: Athlete will have a sharp pain around injury with possible bruising and loss of motion.

Physical examination: Tenderness to palpation in the area.

Diagnostic considerations: Often clinical diagnosis. Skeletally immature athletes should have radiographs obtained to rule out displaced apophysitis from avulsion injuries.

Treatment: Consists of rest, ice, stretching, and NSAIDs. Widely displaced avulsions or apophyseal fractures should be surgically repaired.

Return to play: Padding, heat, and stretching before play when symptoms are tolerable. Athlete can ice after activity to calm inflammatory response. Can consider injections with local anesthetic pregame/during game to mitigate symptoms from iliac crest contusions.

Prevention: Sudden and unexpected. Can reduce incidence by wearing all proper protective equipment and padding.

Groin Strain

Description: Common term for injury of the iliopsoas or adductor muscles in the leg. Happens secondary to forced abduction and external rotation of the leg.

History: Athlete will have pain in the anterior hip, exacerbated by abduction and adduction movements.

Physical examination: Tenderness and hypertonicity of the hip flexors. Pain with resisted adduction and passive abduction of the affected leg.

Diagnostic considerations: Radiographs should be considered to rule out an avulsion fracture.

Treatment: Initially use ice and rest, then follow with stretching and strengthening when symptoms allow. Most avulsion injuries are treated the same way unless there is significant displacement.

Return to play: Symptoms can be persistent depending on severity. Full strength should be obtained before allowing the athlete to return to competition.

Prevention: Effective, and proper, preseason conditioning program is the best means of prevention.

Osteitis Pubis

Description: Common in football players and weightlifters. Exact cause not clear but thought to be secondary to overuse of adductors and gracilis with gradual resorption of bone at the medial aspect of the pubis.

History: Athlete will generally present with insidious onset of groin pain, worsened by adduction of the leg.

Physical examination: Palpable tenderness along the inferior and medial aspects of the pubic bone. Forceful resisted adduction will reproduce the pain.

Diagnostic considerations: Diagnosis mostly clinical. Radiographs may show bone resorption at pubic symphysis with concomitant widening and sclerotic bone of the inferior ramus.

Treatment: Mainstay is relative rest and NSAIDs to assist with this overuse injury.

Return to play: Generally, takes 2–3 months to resolve. Can return when symptoms allow and full strength and range of motion have been obtained.

Prevention: Proper exercise mechanics, frequency, and duration to minimize overuse

Hip Subluxation/Dislocation

Description: Rare but potentially devastating injury because of the possibility of osteonecrosis of the hip. A posterior subluxation is the most common form.

History: Player experiences severe hip pain with any movement.

Physical examination: Examiner will notice a shortened and internally rotated leg on the side of the dislocation. Thorough neurovascular examination should be performed.

Diagnostic considerations: Radiographs should be obtained before attempts at reduction to rule out a femoral neck fracture.

Treatment: One attempt at closed reduction should be performed urgently, in an emergency room, after neurovascular examination and radiographs by an experienced physician.

Return to play: Orthopedic consultation should be highly favored in hip dislocations. Patient may need at least 2 weeks of nonweight-bearing before any progressive attempts at strengthening or therapy.

Prevention: Sudden, unexpected, and traumatic injury.

Thigh

Quadriceps Contusion

Description: Occurs after direct impact onto quadricep muscle belly, usually from a lower body tackle attempt.

History: Athlete will have pain with or without bruising around injury.

Physical examination: Tenderness in the quadricep muscle belly, decreased range of motion, and an occasional palpable mass.

Diagnostic considerations: Clinical diagnosis; radiographs are rarely needed.

Treatment: Immobilization of the leg in flexion overnight to minimize formation of hematoma. Avoid heat, ultrasound, and painful exercise. Ice can be used liberally to decrease swelling and pain.

Return to play: Once full strength, function, and range of motion have been achieved. Can use extra-protective thigh padding when returning to play.

Prevention: Ensure athletes are wearing all properly fitted protective equipment.

Hamstring Injuries

Description: Sudden injury in posterior thigh occurring secondary to rapid hamstring contraction. Associated with fatigue, poor conditioning, and inadequate stretching. Short head of the biceps is the most common site.

History: Athlete will have posterior leg pain and a hesitancy to fully straighten the leg.

Physical examination: Tenderness to palpation in the hamstring. May notice ecchymosis around the injured muscle.

Diagnostic considerations: Usually unnecessary. Imaging warranted if pain and bruising exist in the proximal origin of the hamstring tendon.

Treatment: Initially treat with RICE.

Return to play: Can progress to jogging and pain-free functional rehab when hamstrings are at 70% recovery. Baseline hamstring-to-quadricep ratio should be greater than 0.6. Full return to play can happen once isokinetic strength returns to at least 0.6.

Prevention: Effective off-season conditioning program is the mainstay of prevention. Nordic hamstring exercises can be greatly beneficial.

Knee and Leg

Medial Collateral Ligament

Description: Commonly caused by direct impact onto lateral aspect of knee.

History: Athlete presents with pain and a sensation of instability to the medial aspect of the knee.

Physical examination: Noticeable tenderness to palpation along the medial aspect along the course of the medial collateral ligament (MCL). Ligament laxity with applied valgus stress. Ligament laxity with knee in full extension is notable for a higher severity of injury (often cruciate and/or capsular disruption).

Diagnostic considerations: Radiographs can be useful if suspected epiphyseal fracture.

Treatment: Nonsurgical treatment with protected weight bearing, NSAIDs, and range-of-motion exercises. Progression to resisted exercises when symptoms allow.

Return to play: Early return with functional knee brace as symptoms allow. Grade III injuries often require 4–6 weeks until full return with knee bracing.

Prevention: Sudden and unexpected injury.

Anterior Cruciate Ligament

Description: Common injury in football resulting from either a noncontact twisting mechanism or a direct blow to the knee.

History: Athlete will commonly complain of instability in the knee and hearing/feeling a "pop" during the inciting injury.

Physical examination: Rapid effusion is a sign of an anterior cruciate ligament (ACL) disruption. Will notice a positive Lachman and pivot shift test.

Diagnostic considerations: Radiographs generally negative but may show a small proximal tibial plateau avulsion fracture (Segond fracture).

Treatment: Surgery is typically recommended for football because of the cruciate-dependent activity involved with the sport. It is rare, but very few football players have been able to play with ACL-deficient knees. After injury, most surgeons will delay surgery until knee range of motion is from full extension to more than 110 degrees of flexion to prevent arthrofibrosis. Preferred ACL graft choice for NCAA and professional football orthopedic team physicians is bone–patellar–bone autograft.

Return to play: Eight to twelve months with rehabilitation is needed before return.

Prevention: Sudden and unexpected injury.

Posterior Cruciate Ligament

Description: Mechanism of injury mostly occurs with a direct blow to the anterior tibia while the knee is hyperflexed and the foot is firmly planted.

History: Subtle signs occur, which makes diagnosis more difficult. Effusion may be present but is often not as prominent as other soft tissue injuries of the knee.

Physical examination: High degree of suspicion is needed, as this injury is often missed. Notice increased posterior tibial translation at 90 degrees of flexion. If posterior sag does not improve with internal rotation of tibia, suspect more severe injury.

Diagnostic considerations: MRI is gold standard.

Treatment: Treatment for isolated posterior cruciate ligament (PCL) injuries is controversial. Conservative treatment is the most common implemented approach with a focus on functional restoration.

Return to play: No clear clinical criteria for competition return. If surgery was performed, the athlete can expect 6–9 months of rehabilitation before return.

Prevention: Sudden and unexpected injury.

Meniscal Injuries

Description: Common injuries that occur by contact and noncontact mechanisms (twisting-type injury).

History: Athlete will present with joint line pain, swelling, and mechanical symptoms (catching, locking, and buckling). Unless a tear is in the periphery, an effusion is not noticed until 24 hours after injury.

Physical examination: Joint line tenderness, effusion, pain with flexion, lack of extension, and pain with circumduction maneuvers of the knee joint.

Diagnostic considerations: MRI is gold standard.

Treatment: Arthroscopic surgical repair of the torn portion is generally recommended over excision whenever feasible.

Return to play: After 6–8 weeks of rehabilitation status–postsurgical repair.

Prevention: Sudden and unexpected injury.

Patellar Dislocations

Description: Commonly noncontact, external rotation, leg injury leading to lateral displacement of patella.

History: Athlete presents with excruciating anterior knee pain with buckling and an inability to bear weight.

Physical examination: Will show a diffusely edematous knee with tenderness along the medial retinaculum, lateral trochlea, and patellar articular surfaces. Will also notice apprehension with attempts at patellar translation.

Diagnostic considerations: Radiographs are needed to rule out patellar and trochlea ridge fractures.
Treatment: RICE, with progression to range-of-motion exercises and strengthening after initial injury.
Return to play: Generally, requires 3–6 weeks.
Prevention: Unexpected injury. Repetitive dislocations often require surgery to reconstruct medial structures and alter mechanical alignment.

Patellar/Quadriceps Tendonitis

Description: Common overuse injury in football. Happens secondary to frequent stopping/starting and loading of extensor mechanism.
History: Athlete will present with anterior knee pain, above or below the joint line.
Physical examination: Tenderness to palpation superior to the patella if quadricep tendon involved or below the patella in the case of the patella tendon.
Diagnostic considerations: Diagnosis is often clinical. Ultrasound can be useful.
Treatment: Relative rest, NSAIDs, and subsequent progression to concentric and isometric strength training for symptomatic players. Athletes can progress to eccentric training when asymptomatic. Platelet-rich plasma has shown potential benefit in refractory cases.
Return to play: Once symptom free and full strength has been obtained.
Prevention: Optimal treatment is prevention. Focus on proper conditioning, including eccentric strength training and effective stretching.

Ankle and Foot

Ankle Sprains

Description: Most common ligamentous injury. Structures injured are dependent on force applied and direction of injury.
History: Pattern of injury is of extreme importance.

- Plantarflexion and inversion injuries typically involve the anterior talofibular ligament (ATFL), with progressive forces involving the calcaneofibular ligament (CFL) and posterior talofibular ligament (PTFL).
- Inversion injuries in a neutral position are suspicious for the CFL.
- Dorsiflexion injuries typically involve the tibiofibular ligament.
- Eversion and external rotation are concerning for deltoid ligament medially and the tibiofibular ligament laterally. These are often accompanied by a fibular fracture.

Physical examination: Athlete will have tenderness to palpation in the injured ligament. Stress testing is highly beneficial in isolating area of injury.

- Anterior drawer with 30 degrees of plantarflexion to assess ATFL; compare with contralateral side.
- Inversion test: Grasp heel and apply inversion stress; ability to palpate talar head indicates complete tears of both ATFL and CFL.
- Squeeze test: Squeeze tibia and fibula together near ankle joint; reproducible pain indicates probably syndesmosis/tibiofibular ligament injuries.
- Evaluate for other associated injuries, including peroneal tendon dislocation, fifth metatarsal fracture, posterior tibial rupture, and midfoot sprains.

Diagnostic considerations: Radiographs are necessary to rule out fracture. Stress radiographs are occasionally helpful in chronic instability. External stress radiographs with mortise view are helpful to evaluate syndesmosis. MRI is useful to evaluate talar dome osteochondral injuries when suspected.
Treatment: NSAIDs, early restoration of range of motion, and functional management depending on severity for acute injuries. Ankle braces useful to limit inversion/eversion stress on grade II and III sprains. Proprioceptive and peroneal strengthening immediately for grade I sprains, immediate to 7 days for grade II sprains, and 7 days to 30 days for grade III sprains. Unstable fracture patterns and syndesmotic injuries require surgical intervention.
Return to play: Dependent on athlete's ability to adequately perform position-specific drills with absent, or minimal, symptoms. Generally, 7 days or less for grade I sprains, 7–14 days for grade II, and 30 days for grade III.
Prevention: First-time occurrence is typically an unexpected injury. In repetitive injuries, ligament laxity can lead to chronic instability; these may require surgical intervention.

Fifth Metatarsal Base Fractures

Description: Three different types:

- Tuberosity fractures from traction/avulsion-type injuries involving the peroneus brevis tendon or other ligaments
- Metaphyseal fractures occurring from adduction and inversion forces
- Jones fracture (roughly 3 cm distal to the tuberosity) by way of repetitive insult or a single sharp-turning force

History: Athlete will have pain on the plantar aspect of the foot, worsened by weight bearing.
Physical examination: Tenderness to palpation over the fifth metatarsal base worsened with eversion forces.
Diagnostic considerations: Radiographs are necessary to determine the fracture site/type.
Treatment: Walking boot necessary for tuberosity and metaphyseal fractures. Jones fractures can be surgically fixated in high-demand athletes by means of an intramedullary screw; this has been shown to increase healing time. Surgical fixation also recommended for fractures with significant sclerosis or those that have delayed healing with conservative management.
Return to play: Once radiographic evidence of healing is noted and athlete can perform functional tests.
Prevention: Sudden and unexpected injury.

Turf Toe

Description: Hyperextension and, less commonly, hyperflexion injury to the first metatarsophalangeal joint (MTP). Associated with flexible footwear and, more commonly, artificial turf. Severity of injury can range from ligamentous sprains to MTP dislocation.
History: Athlete will generally report pain, tenderness, and swelling of the first MTP joint.
Physical examination: Reproducible pain of the first MTP with passive dorsiflexion. Will also notice decreased range of motion and decreased strength in flexion.
Diagnostic considerations: Plain radiographs needed to rule out bony injury. If plantar tenderness is present, obtain sesamoid views with radiography.
Treatment: Severity dependent.

- Capsular and ligamentous sprains can be treated conservatively with ice and continuous taping during competition.
- Partial or complete capsular tears should be treated with NSAIDs, protective footwear, and restriction of play until symptoms allow (typically 3–6 weeks).
- Chondral and dislocation injuries are treated with limited weight bearing and immobilization.

Return to play: Symptom dependent, but can often be prolonged. Will typically need a functional progression ranging from 7 days to 2 months.
Prevention: Typically, an unexpected injury. Can be mitigated with properly fitted athletic footwear.

Infections

- General recommendation is for athletes to avoid competition during acute infections with a fever >100°F (37.7°C). To prevent spread of waterborne illnesses, it is ideal for players to not share water bottles.
- Infections leading to **myocarditis** need to be taken seriously, as this has been a reported cause of sudden cardiac death in athletes.
- **Skin infections** such as herpes gladiatorum, Methicillin-resistant *Staphylococcus Aureus* (MRSA), and ringworm often spread from person-to-person contact. Risk of MRSA is of significant concern because of the number of athletes participating in football and the close environment in which these athletes exist. It is important to avoid sharing towels, razors, and toothbrushes to minimize transmission. Rigorous cleansing of shared athletic training facilities and ensuring appropriate hygiene are of extreme importance. Antiviral, antifungal, and antibacterial treatment is necessary with protective covering to prevent transmission.
- **Infectious mononucleosis** is concerning for splenic rupture because of the high-collision frequency in football. Athletes should be withheld from participation for the initial 3–4 weeks of symptoms. Further participation should be evaluated based on the athlete's clinical condition and the presence or absence of splenomegaly, which is present acutely in the majority of Epstein-Barr Virus (EBV) infections. Abdominal ultrasound can be useful for accurate assessment but is generally unnecessary. Position stand from the American Medical Society for Sports Medicine (AMSSM) regarding mononucleosis in the athlete was written and published in 2008. Recent systematic review involving 81 cases of splenic rupture secondary to mononucleosis between 1984 and 2014 revealed that 84% occurred within 4 weeks of symptom onset.
- **Human immunodeficiency virus (HIV)** is not an absolute contraindication for participation and does not exclude an athlete from play. A study in professional football players found that 3.7 bleeding injuries were found per game for each team involving 3.5 players. The study further noted that 88% of injuries were abrasions, with the remainder being lacerations. Risk of HIV transmission is estimated to be less than 1 per 85 million game contacts. Universal precautions should be used in general for all body fluid contact. It is imperative to consider off-field risk factors in the total care of the athlete.

RECOMMENDED READINGS

Available online.

SOCCER

67

Chitra Kodery • Margot Putukian

INTRODUCTION

- Soccer, or football, is the world's most popular sport. Although its origins trace back over 3000 years, the current organized form of soccer originated in 1863 in Britain.
- Federation Internationale de Football Association (FIFA) is the governing body for soccer in the world, and it includes 211 affiliated national associations. There are six different confederations within FIFA, and the United States is a member of the Football Confederation in North and Central America and the Caribbean (CONCACAF).
- The laws of the game are formed by the International Football Association Board (IFAB), which was formed in 1886 for this purpose. According to FIFA, there are 265 million registered soccer players in the world, including 26 million females and 22 million youth participants. Between 2000 and 2006 there was a 21% and 254% increase worldwide in the number of male and female participants, respectively, that registered.
- The popularity of soccer has steadily risen in the United States, with over 25 million Americans playing at all levels.
- Professional soccer in the United States includes Major League Soccer (MLS), United Soccer League (USL), and the National Women's Soccer League (NWSL). In 2021 the MLS will have 28 teams, USL has more than 100, and the NWSL has 9 teams. MLS has more diversity than any other professional male sport league in North America, with players from more than 70 countries.

GENERAL PRINCIPLES

Rules of the Game

- Objective of the game: To win the game by outscoring your opponent, which is achieved by hitting the ball into the opponent's goal
- Game lasts for 90 minutes; divided into two 45-minute halves
- Eleven players on the field—10 field players and one goalkeeper
- The ball cannot be played by the hands (except goalkeeper), but all other surfaces of the body can be used.
- Rules protect against rough play—there are direct and indirect fouls.
  - **Direct fouls** include kicking the opponent, tackling from behind, using hands, and pushing.
  - **Indirect fouls** include offside, obstruction, and certain unintentional fouls.
    - Offside rule: must have two players between an offensive player and the goal; this often includes the goalkeeper
- Required equipment: Ball, uniforms, and goalposts; most leagues require shin guards
- There are different methods of putting the ball back in play when it goes out of touch (out of bounds):
  - **Throw in:** when the ball goes out over the sideline
  - **Goal kick:** when the ball goes out over the endline, last touched by an offensive player; kicked in from the goal box by the defensive team
  - **Corner kick:** when the ball goes out over the endline, last touched by a defensive player; kicked in from the field corner by the offensive team

Sport-Specific Demands and Skills

Physical demands: Players engage in discontinuous, high-output activity that involves aerobic and anaerobic metabolism.

- At the elite level, players typically cover 8–10 km during a game, making soccer an endurance sport. Two-thirds of this distance is spent in low-intensity activity such as walking and jogging.
- The aerobic system is heavily involved, with heart rates around 85% of the maximum rate and oxygen demand about 70% of maximum oxygen uptake ($\dot{V}O_2$ max).

Strength demands: High demand on trunk and lower extremities. Most skills require balancing on one leg, which emphasizes lower extremity strength and proprioception.

Soccer-specific skills: Various surfaces of the lower extremity are used to strike or control the ball and tackle, thus putting various structures at risk.

- **Inside of foot pass/block tackle:** Foot and hip externally rotated, knee flexed, foot "locked" in dorsiflexion (Fig. 67.1). Results in significant valgus stress at the knee, which may be associated with traumatic injury such as a sprain of the medial collateral ligament (MCL).
- **Outside of foot pass/shot:** Internal rotation of the leg, foot in inversion, plantarflexion. Results in increased risk of forceful inversion plantarflexion injuries, mid/forefoot injuries, ligament sprains, and peroneal tendon problems (see Fig. 67.1). In younger athletes, this may lead to apophysitis or avulsion fractures.
- **Instep of foot:** Extreme plantarflexion in "locked" foot, hip flexors, quadriceps, rectus, and hamstrings (see Fig. 67.1); ball velocity at release is between 17 and 28 meters/second.
- In the approach and ball strike phase of an instep kick, a varus torque of >200 newton meters (Nm) and extension torque of >280 Nm is generated on the proximal tibia.
- A total of 2000 Nm is generated during a soccer kick. Only 15% is transferred to the ball; the remainder is absorbed by the eccentric contraction of the hamstrings.
- **Heading:** Purposeful, forceful striking of the ball with a player's head to control, clear, or redirect on goal; increases the risk of head and neck injuries because of player contact (head to head or other body part, or head to goal post or ground) that occurs while fighting for possession in the air (see Fig. 67.1)
- **Appropriate technique is important in all skills to avoid and decrease injuries.**

Factors Affecting Performance and Recovery

Fatigue

- **Fatigue** or decreased performance in soccer players is multifactorial—can be related to environmental or nutritional factors, including dehydration, glycogen depletion, aerobic fitness, and mental fatigue.

Dehydration

- Occurs when sweat losses exceed fluid intake, which is particularly a concern in warm weather
- A decrease in performance is noted when there is fluid loss of >2% of an athlete's body weight. At >3% loss, more serious consequences can arise such as exertional heat illness.

Heat Illness

- Risk factors for development of heat illness include preexisting medical disease, age, poor conditioning, inadequate

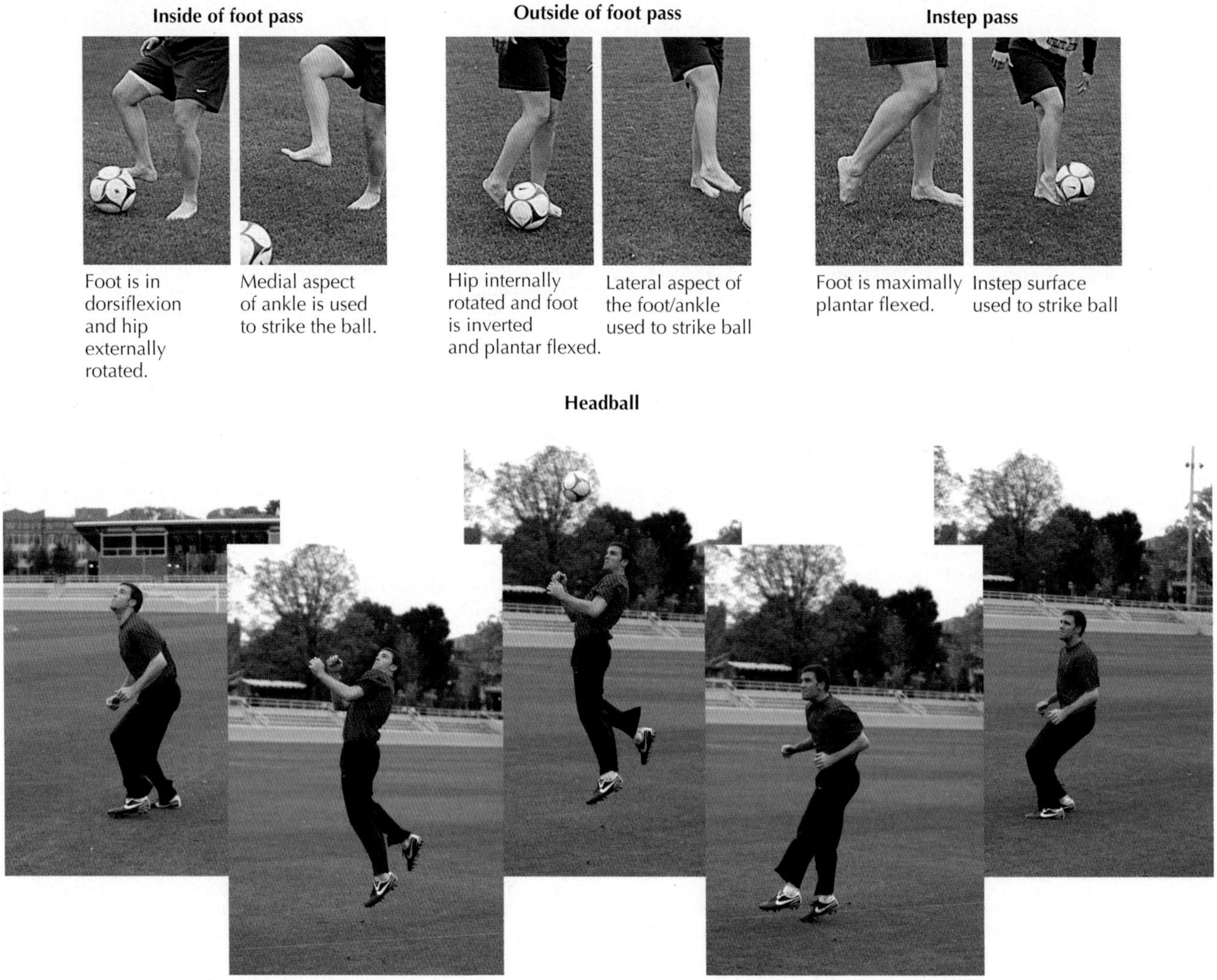
Inside of foot pass
Outside of foot pass
Instep pass
Foot is in dorsiflexion and hip externally rotated.
Medial aspect of ankle is used to strike the ball.
Hip internally rotated and foot is inverted and plantar flexed.
Lateral aspect of the foot/ankle used to strike ball
Foot is maximally plantar flexed.
Instep surface used to strike ball
Headball

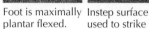

Jumping header. These photographs show the series of technique involved in the jumping header. The ball is struck when the player is at the maximal height of the jump, with the player's eyes open. Impact with the ball is made at the forehead/hairline with the head striking forward through the ball. The arms are held up for balance and to create space for the player and thus protect him from inadvertent contact with another player.

Figure 67.1 Soccer-specific demands and skills. (Photographs © 2008 Beverly Schaefer.)

acclimatization, dehydration, obesity, fatigue, prior heat injury, febrile illness, and medications.

- Modifications should be made to decrease the risk of heat injury: more water breaks, change game times, and shorten the length of play.
- Studies have investigated the effect of hyperhydration on improving thermoregulation.

Nutrition

CARBOHYDRATE INTAKE

- **Glycogen constitutes the major energy source for muscles.**
- Muscle glycogen is depleted within 90–180 minutes of exercise at 60%–80% $\dot{V}O_2$ max or 15–30 minutes of exercise at 90%–130% $\dot{V}O_2$ max. Glycogen stores take approximately 2–3 days to fully recover.
- Athletes need 10–12 g of carbohydrate per kg/day to maximize glycogen stores (see Chapter 5: "Sports Nutrition").
- Numerous studies have looked at the difference between a low- vs. high-carbohydrate diet and have consistently shown an increase in total distance covered in addition to an increase in high intensity and intermittent running with a high-carbohydrate diet.

Recovery

- Refers to physical and mental restoration to maximize performance and minimize potential for injury
- **Active recovery**
  - Active recovery, often referred to as *cool-down* or *warm-down*, after the conclusion of intense exercises is widely used despite the lack of clear evidence supporting its benefits.
  - Whereas numerous studies have found that active recovery enhances removal of blood lactate, other studies have reported decreased glycogen stores with this strategy.

Cold-Water Immersion

- Cold-water immersion (CWI) has gained tremendous popularity among athletes to minimize fatigue and enhance postexercise recovery.
- CWI protocols typically involve immersion into 48.2°F–50°F (9°C–10°C) water for 5–20 minutes immediately after exercise.
- Studies have suggested an effect on short- and long-term recovery by:
  - Ameliorating hyperthermia and rapidly reducing the body temperature, which, in turn, decreases central nervous

Table 67.1 SOCCER OVERALL INJURY RATES IN MALES AND FEMALES FROM THE NATIONAL HIGH SCHOOL SPORTS-RELATED INJURY SURVEILLANCE STUDY 2005–2006 TO 2013–2014

	Total	Competition	Practice
Number of injuries	6154	3949	2205
Number of athletic exposures (AEs)	2,985,991	894,441	2,091,550
Injury rate	2.06	4.42	1.05

Data from Khodaee M, Currie DW, Asif IM, et al. Nine-year study of US high school soccer injuries:
Data from a national sports injury surveillance programme. *Br J Sports Med.* 2017;51(3):185–193.

system (CNS) fatigue and possibly decreases cardiovascular strain
- Facilitating the removal of muscle metabolites, which may lead to delayed-onset muscle soreness
- Enhancing parasympathetic reactivation, which leads to a decrease in heart rate and is associated with improved long-term recovery

GENERAL INJURY PATTERNS

Overall Injury Incidence

- Overall injury incidence in soccer is favorable (much lower than in American football).
- Number of injuries increases as skill and age increase—low levels of injuries are seen in children aged <10 years, with the rate increasing 10-fold at the high school level.
- A 9-year surveillance study done in high school athletes from 2005 to 2014 done by Khodaee et al. found an overall injury rate of 2.06/1000 athletic exposures (AEs), with rates higher in competition than in practice and higher in girls over boys.
    - The most common injuries seen included ligament strains, concussions, and muscle strains, and the most common body sites injured included the head/face (20.8%), ankle (20.6%), and knee (16.5%) (Tables 67.1 and 67.2).
    - Player-to-player contact was the most common mechanism of injury, and injury patterns were found to be similar among the sexes.
- At the collegiate level, gender differences are less striking, with the exception of anterior cruciate ligament (ACL) injuries. Female soccer players are noted to have a higher incidence of ACL injuries compared with their male counterparts.
    - A 2005 study by Angel et al. reviewed ACL injuries in National Collegiate Athletic Association (NCAA) male and female basketball and soccer athletes from 1990 to 2002 and found that females sustained 67% of all noncontact ACL injures compared with 58% in males.
- **NCAA** data from 2009–2010 to 2014–2015 seasons showed an overall injury rate of 8.07/1000 AEs in men's soccer and 8.77/1000 AEs in women's soccer.
    - Lower limb injuries (foot/ankle, knee, hip/groin) were most common and accounted for 74.1% of men's injuries and 68.0% of women's injuries (Table 67.3).
    - Men were noted to have higher rates of hip/groin injuries in competition and practice compared with women, whereas women were noted to have higher rates of head/face and knee injuries in competition.
    - The largest proportions of injuries noted occurred from player-to-player contact in competition over practice.

Table 67.2 SOCCER INJURY SITES FROM THE NATIONAL HIGH SCHOOL SPORTS-RELATED INJURY SURVEILLANCE STUDY 2005–2006 TO 2013–2014

	Boys (%)	Girls (%)	Overall Number (%)
Head/face	568 (19.5)	710 (21.9)	706,572 (20.9)
Ankle	521 (17.9)	703 (21.7)	693,323 (20.6)
Knee	409 (14.1)	637 (19.7)	557,899 (16.5)
Thigh/upper leg	363 (12.5)	339 (10.5)	385,635 (11.4)
Lower leg	229 (7.9)	222 (6.9)	248,938 (7.4)
Foot	202 (6.9)	177 (5.5)	216,554 (6.4)
Hip	148 (5.1)	93 (2.9)	131,598 (3.9)
Hand/wrist	146 (5.0)	119 (3.7)	143,173 (4.2)
Trunk	140 (4.8)	97 (3.0)	124,861 (3.7)
Shoulder/clavicle	98 (3.4)	57 (1.8)	71,694 (2.1)

Data from Khodaee M, Currie DW, Asif IM, et al. Nine-year study of US high school soccer injuries:
Data from a national sports injury surveillance programme. *Br J Sports Med.* 2017;51(3):185–193.

Table 67.3 NCAA DATA OF INJURY PERCENTAGE BREAKDOWN FROM THE 2009–2010 TO 2014–2015 SEASON

Men's Soccer		Women's Soccer	
Ankle	18.3%	Knee	20.2%
Upper leg/thigh	17.2%	Ankle	18.1%
Head/face	12.5%	Head/face	17.9%
Knee	12.2%	Upper leg	11.6%
Hip/groin	10.6%	Lower leg	7.3%
Foot	8%	Foot	5.9%

Adapted from NCAA Data, 2009–2010 through 2014–2015; National Collegiate Athletic Association.

    - Nearly half (47.2% of men's injuries and 47.5% of women's injuries) were non-time-loss injuries in which no time off from sport was needed.
- Soccer players are three times more likely to be injured during a match compared with practice (Table 67.4).
- Studies have compared overall injury rates in indoor soccer compared with outdoor soccer and have found no significant differences.
- Data evaluating injury incidence, severity of injury, and mechanisms of injury on natural grass versus third-generation artificial turf by male and female players demonstrated no significant differences between these surfaces.

Injury Surveillance System

- The NCAA has used the Injury Surveillance System (ISS) to collect injury and exposure data from intercollegiate athletes since 1982. Injury is defined as time loss.
    - **Advantages:** Data are shared with NCAA sport and policy committees and individual institutions to make evidence-based decisions regarding health and safety issues.
    - **Disadvantages of ISS:** Injuries without time loss are missed, certain injuries may not be "time loss injury" (i.e., no time loss if in season but time loss if off season).
- Despite these limitations, ISS data provide a denominator (number of AEs) and are thus useful for comparing sports, genders, and injury types.

Table 67.4 INJURY DATA FROM NCAA INJURY SURVEILLANCE SYSTEM 2009–2010 THROUGH 2013–2014

Sport	Event	Avg. Annual Estimate of Injuries	Avg. Annual Estimates of No. of Athlete-Exposures	Estimated Injury Rate Per 1000 Athlete-Exposures
Men's Soccer	Competition	6458	360,880	8.0
	Practice	6977	1,323,974	
	Overall	13,435	1,684,854	
Women's Soccer	Competition	7434	432,347	8.4
	Practice	7679	1,367,650	
	Overall	15,113	1,799,997	

Adapted from Kerr ZY, Marshall SW, Dompier TP, et al. College sports-related injuries—United States, 2009-10 through 2013-14 academic years. *Morb Mortal Wkly Rep*. 2015;64(48):1330–1336.

SPECIFIC INJURY PATTERNS

Knee Injuries (See Table 67.3)

Overall Injury Patterns

- One needs only to watch soccer players pivot and cut back and forth, change direction while decelerating, take a cross with half-volley, or cross the ball from one side of the field to another to understand why they may be at an increased risk of knee pathology.
- Knee injuries account for 8%–18% of injuries in practices and games (NCAA, 1988–1989 through 2002–2003).

ACL Injuries

- May occur via contact or noncontact mechanisms.
- Eighty-five percent of ACL injuries in soccer players occur via noncontact mechanisms
- Female soccer athletes at the elite level represent a high-risk group for ACL injuries. Many studies have proposed anatomic differences in addition to possible differences in neuromuscular patterns, which may put female athletes at higher risk.
- Prevention is key, and many training protocols such as FIFA 11+ have been adapted to reduce the risk of injury.
  - FIFA 11+ consists of a 20-minute program that should be performed twice a week before each training session. It consists of 15 exercises that are divided into three components: 8 minutes of running exercises followed by 10 minutes of strength, plyometric, and balance exercises followed by an additional 2 minutes of running exercises.
  - Studies evaluating the efficacy of this program in varied settings (high school, collegiate, and professional levels) have showed lower extremity injury prevention by up to 30%–50%.
  - There has been extensive research specifically targeted to the use of neuromuscular training in women in reducing the number of ACL injuries.
    - Mandelbaum et al. (2005): Studied a neuromuscular and proprioception training program in 1041 females over the course of 2 years. Found a 74% decrease in ACL injuries in the first year and an 88% decrease in the second year compared with an age- and skill-matched control group (see Recommended Readings).

Meniscal Injuries

- May be isolated or in conjunction with ACL injuries.
- Coexistence of meniscal and ligamentous injuries to knee should not be underestimated in soccer players; isolated injury may not prohibit activity, whereas additional injuries make it difficult to return to high-level play.
- Meniscal deficiency is often a precursor to osteoarthritis, as the articular cartilage is subject to a higher biomechanical loading force in the elite athlete. Therefore, repair techniques of the meniscus are preferred over meniscectomy whenever possible.

Medial Collateral Ligament Injuries

- Inside of foot pass/block tackles and direct valgus trauma put soccer athletes at risk of an MCL injury.
- Soccer has the highest sport-specific injury rate of MCL tears among high school and collegiate athletes.
- Risk increases with poor technique, tentative athlete, and leg extended away from the body.

Osteochondral Injuries

- Injuries involving the bone and overlying articular cartilage
- Most commonly occurs in the knee at the medial femoral condyle and presents as pain and/or swelling with activity
- Diagnosis made with plain radiographs, although may need additional testing such as magnetic resonance imaging (MRI) (Fig. 67.2)
- Treatment depends on clinical presentation and diagnostic tests. If significant lesion and/or separation of fragment, arthroscopic treatment with microfracture procedure versus osteochondral autograft transfer system (OATS) procedure is often indicated.

Muscle Contusions

- Common injury in soccer and most common in pediatric age group
- Rate of injury increases with age; boys at a greater risk than girls
- Shin guards significantly decrease the risk of contusions (and fractures) to the lower leg.
- Treatment: rest, ice, compression, and elevation (RICE); avoidance of aggressive passive stretching in acutely injured muscle
- For large contusions of quadriceps, flex knee 120 degrees and use compressive wrapping in this position for 24 hours (stops bleeding, avoids more significant injury)
- Reinjury to the quadriceps is a major factor in developing **myositis ossificans**, also called *heterotopic (ectopic) ossification*.
  - Defined as new bone formation in a muscle after injury
  - Occurs in 9%–20% of all quadriceps contusions; average time of disability is 73 days

Muscle Strains

- Muscle strains often result from excessive stretch while muscle is activated.
- Tears tend to occur near the muscle–tendon junction.
- Risk factors for muscle strain include:
  - Eccentric contraction of a muscle
  - Increased type II muscle fibers
  - Biarthrodial (crosses two joints) muscles
  - Insufficient joint range of motion
  - Fatigue/overuse or inadequate recovery
    - Studies have shown that fatigued muscles are able to absorb less energy before reaching the degree of stretch that causes injury
  - Previous injury

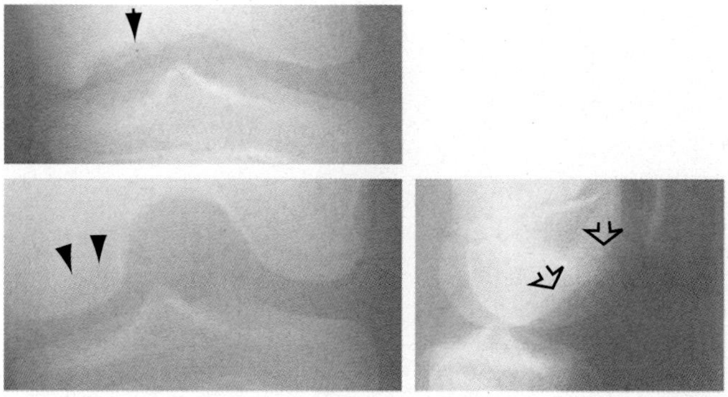

A. Radiographs of a 12-year-old soccer player with symptomatic medial femoral osteochondritis dissecans.

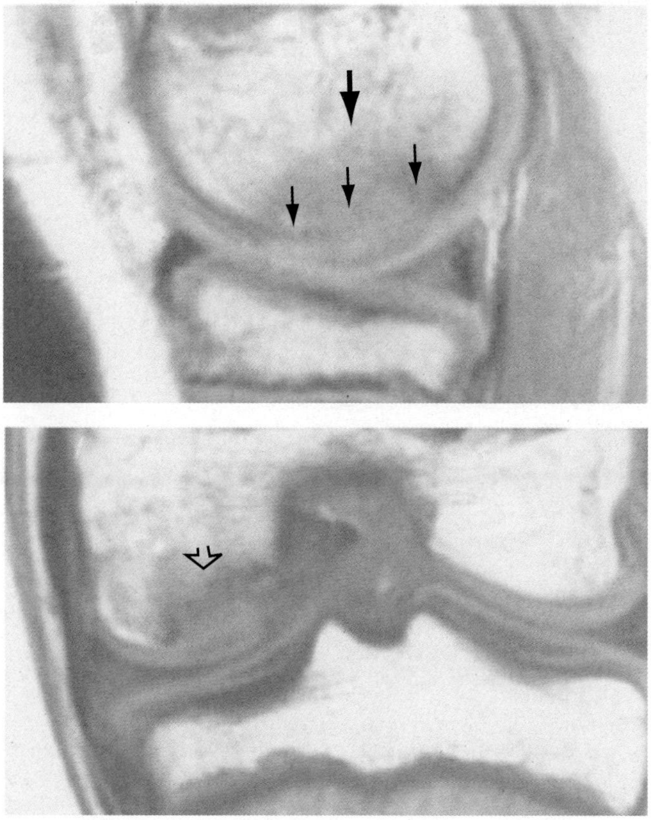

B. Magnetic resonance imaging shows loss of articular surface continuty *(small arrows)*. *Open and larger arrows* indicate the osteochondritis dissecans fragment subchondral junction.

Figure 67.2 Knee injuries. (From DeLee J, Drez D, Miller M. *DeLee and Drez's Orthopaedic Sports Medicine*. 2nd ed. Philadelphia: Saunders; 2002.)

- Rectus femoris crosses two joints, has a high content of type II fibers, and contracts eccentrically in decelerating the hip and knee
- Hamstring muscles contract eccentrically with running and deceleration and have a high content of type II fibers. **Hamstring injuries are one of the most common injuries in soccer and tend to recur.**

Prevention of Muscle Injury

- Emphasize beneficial effects of warm-up, temperature, and stretching on mechanical properties of muscle.
- Much research has gone into the prevention of muscle injury given its high incidence.
- Several factors protect muscle: strength, endurance, and flexibility.
- Arnason et al. showed that eccentric hamstring strengthening ("Russian hamstring curls or Nordic hamstrings") combined with warm stretching has been useful in preventing hamstring injuries.

Stress Fractures

- Represents overuse injury to the bone; generally caused by training regimen.
- Bone scans indicate that most overuse injuries and stress fractures occur in lower extremity: tibia (49.1%), tarsals (25.3%), femur (7.2%), metatarsals (8.8%), fibula (6.6%), pelvis (1.6%), sesamoids (0.9%), and spine (0.6%).
- Fifth metatarsal stress fractures, specifically Jones type (metaphyseal–diaphyseal junction), have unpredictable healing, and thus screw placement for internal fixation should be considered (Fig. 67.3).
- Training errors accounted for 22.4% of fractures.
- Other factors: playing surface, cleat and indoor shoe requirements, changes in training regimen/intensity, and (in female athletes) hormonal and/or nutritional influences.
- Address biomechanical issues (leg length discrepancies, femoral anteversion, foot pronation, and increased knee valgus) during preparticipation physical examination.
- Consider female athlete triad (disordered eating, menstrual dysfunction, and decreased bone mineral density [BMD]).
  - Although more common in sports emphasizing leanness (cross-country running and swimming) and sports with subjective scoring (gymnastics and skating), triad occurs in all sports.
  - Menstrual dysfunction and eating disorders are associated with low BMD at axial and at appendicular sites.
  - Optimize prevention and early treatment through education.

Groin Injuries

- Common injury in soccer, especially in males. Return to play can be difficult.
- Direct trauma can result in injury to external genitalia, muscles, vessels, or joints.
- Other injuries include osteitis pubis (symphysis pubis instability); adductor, rectus, or iliopsoas muscle strain; stress and avulsion fractures; hernia; and sportman's hernia/inguinal disruption (ID).
  - Osteitis pubis: low-grade inflammation at symphysis
  - Pain at adductor insertion and symphysis for >2 months; pain at morning or night, with cough/sneeze; positive bone scan and radiograph
    - Treated with either standard physical therapy (stretching, friction massage, and other modalities) or active training (strengthening, proprioceptive neuromuscular facilitation, and balance)
    - Seventy-nine percent of those treated with active training (vs. 14% treated with standard physical therapy) returned to play

Sportsman's Hernia (Inguinal Disruption)

- Defined as pain, either of insidious or acute onset, that occurs predominantly in the groin region near the pubic tubercle; diagnosis of exclusion after other pathology (i.e., hernia) ruled out
- Ninety percent male, 70% insidious onset, and 30% report injury
- Affects soccer, rugby, track, and hockey athletes; muscular imbalance common
- Diagnosis can be made if three out of five clinical signs are detected: tenderness over the pubic tubercle, palpable

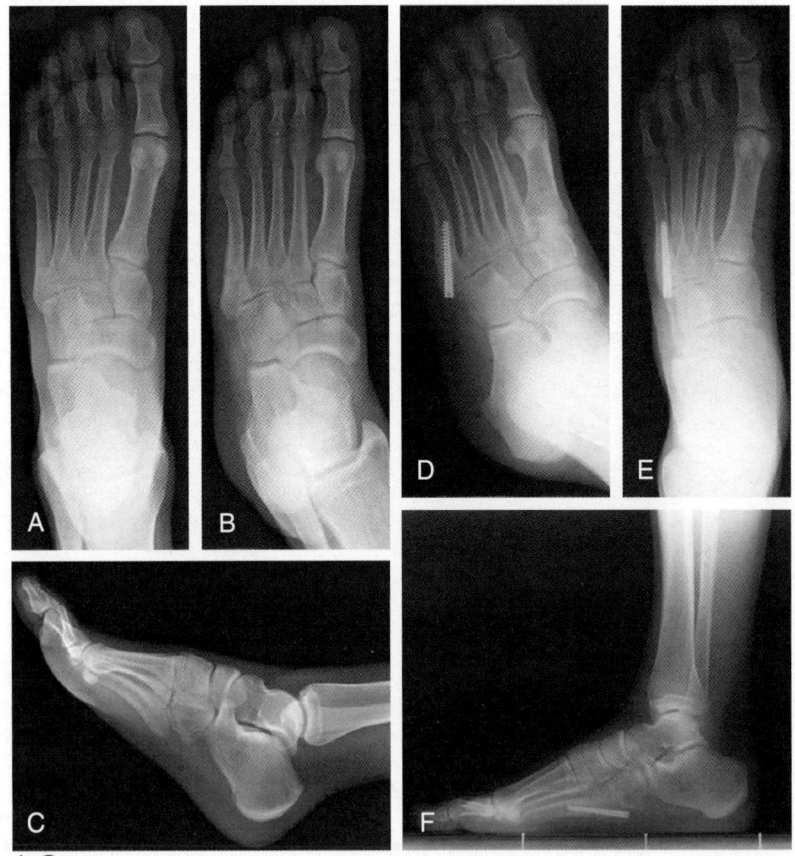
A
B
C
D
E
F

A-C. Type IA (DeLee) fifth metatarsal fracture in collegiate soccer player.
D-F. After fixation with variable pitch compression screw.

Figure 67.3 Stress fractures. (From Canale T, Beaty J. *Campbell's Operative Orthopaedics*. 11th ed. Philadelphia: Mosby; 2007.)

tenderness over the deep inguinal ring, pain or dilation over the external ring with no obvious hernia, pain at origin of the adductor longus tendon, and dull diffuse pain in the groin with possible radiation to the perineum (see Recommended Readings for British Hernia Society's 2014 Position Statement).

- Pain worse with activity, particularly sudden movement, twisting, striding, sprinting, long or dead ball kicks, sidestepping, coughing/sneezing, and sit-ups.
- Radiographs, bone scans, and MRI often used to exclude other diagnoses; newer use of ultrasound to diagnose sportsman's hernia
- Treatment: Initially conservative rehabilitation with strengthening, relative rest, and nonsteroidal anti-inflammatory drugs (NSAIDs); if no improvement and workup otherwise negative, surgical treatment indicated
- Surgery: In an 8-year study, 97% successful; return to play within 6 weeks

Ankle Injuries and Impingement Syndromes

- Ankle sprains are one of the most common injuries in soccer and thus are important to detect and treat appropriately
- Usual mechanism is inversion plantarflexion injury; other mechanisms in soccer include outside of foot pass/shot
- Because soccer players rely on mobility and "touch" on ball, challenge often lies in returning athletes to 100% functional activity
- If significant ankle laxity is detected during preparticipation examination, strengthening and proprioceptive programs should be initiated and also consider prophylactic taping or bracing.
- Athletes with ankle sprains who experience pain and disability after injury develop "ankle impingement" syndromes, which are a difficult problem in soccer players.
  - Consider impingement in patients with anterolateral pain but no instability or history of prior sprains
  - Soccer players complain of pain while trying to pivot or push off one foot or with instep shooting
  - Causes of impingement include hypertrophic scar formation, synovium, and fibrocartilage in anterolateral tibular–talar space from the anterior capsule into the lateral gutter
  - Occasionally described as "meniscoid" lesions in soccer players

Heading and Concussions

- Heading is a soccer-specific skill wherein the head is used to redirect the ball.
- In recent years, heading has become an area of controversy, given the potential adverse effects, including concussions, especially in youth players.
- As we have learned more about the repercussions of repetitive head trauma, concussion identification and prevention have become a key topic in all sports.
- Soccer is no exception, and joint ventures between MLS, USL, and NWSL have aimed to review these key issues and adapt best practices to the sport (see Recommended Readings).
- Sport-specific guidance for soccer and head injuries was published in 2020.

Epidemiology of Head Injuries

- Rate of concussion increases with age and level of competition.
- Increased rates of concussion reported during games compared with practices.
- Multiple studies have evaluated the mechanism of injury that causes concussion and have shown that very few occur with purposeful heading of the ball. Rather, the most common mechanism of concussion is from player-to-player contact and collision.
  - **Kontos et al:** Surveyed 101,699 youth soccer players aged 7–14 during the 2016 season. Total concussion incidence for the sample was 8.48/10,000 AEs. Games (rather than practices) and older age (11–14) had higher rates of concussion. Fewer than 1 in 5 concussions (47/253; 19%) occurred during attempted purposeful heading of the ball.
  - **Comstock et al. (2015):** Retrospective analysis of longitudinal surveillance data of high school soccer players from 2005–2006 to 2013–2014. Overall, there were 627 concussions per 1,393,753 AEs among girls and 442 concussions per 1,592,238 AEs among boys. Heading was the most common soccer activity that led to concussions, with collision with another player being the most common mechanism of injury in heading-related concussions (78.1% in boys and 61.9% in girls).
- The NCAA ISS data indicate that concussion rates are higher in competition when compared with practice in both women's and men's soccer. Summary data of injury mechanisms from the NCAA Injury Surveillance Program over multiple years shows that most concussions do not occur during successful, purposeful heading. The majority of concussions that do occur are from player-to-player contact.
  - A 2017 study by Chandran et al. looked at the sex differences between head injuries and concussions among NCAA soccer players between 2004 and 2009 and found a significantly higher rate of head injury in women during games compared with men.
- Among professional leagues, concussion was found to be the fifth most common injury in MLS. In a study by Ramkumar et al., of the 1784 eligible MLS and eligible English Premier League (EPL) players evaluated over a 10-year period, the incidence of concussion was 20.22 and 18.68 per 1000 AEs, respectively.

Assessment and Management of Head Injuries

- Assessment and treatment of head-injured athletes and return-to-play issues are no different in soccer players than in other athletes (see Chapter 45: "Head Injuries")
- Neuropsychological testing techniques attempt to quantify brain function by examining brain–behavior relationships (see Chapter 45: "Head Injuries"). These tests aim to compare data from baseline tests with postconcussion results and guide return-to-play decisions.
  - Milhalik et al. looked at the effects of sex, sport, and preexisting histories on baseline clinical concussion assessments in soccer and lacrosse athletes. They compared results of the 22-item symptom checklist, Standardized Assessment of Concussion (SAC), Balance Error Scoring System (BESS), Generalized Anxiety Disorder 7-item scale (GAD-7), and Patient Health Questionnaire (PHQ-9). Female athletes were noted to have a higher total symptom score and higher number of BESS total errors. Higher symptom and anxiety scores were also noted in those with history of migraines and previous concussion. These differences highlight the need for individualized concussion assessment and management.
- There have been discussions at numerous levels, including by the Concussion in Sport Group (CISG), FIFA, national governing bodies, and the NCAA, about possible rule modifications to allow sufficient time for medical staff to conduct an accurate evaluation when an injury is suspected. Unlike other sports, the lack of time outs and the current substitution rules may put undue pressure to assess quickly and return the player. IFAB has recently agreed to allow trials for a "concussion substitute" based on the concerns for head injury and concussion in soccer.

Prevention and Risk Reduction

- The Recognize to Recover (R2R) program has been established by the US Soccer Federation to improve the safety of soccer players of all ages and reduce injuries. It aims to strengthen the role of parents, players, coaches, and officials and educate them regarding injury prevention.
- Concussion awareness has led to adaptations in youth training.
- Recommendations from the R2R program include:
  - Children aged ≤10 years: no heading in games and practices
  - Children aged 11–13 years: heading training limited to maximum of 30 minutes/week and 15–20 headers per player per week
- There has been good adherence to these recommendations and appropriate introduction of heading to youth players across the country.
  - A study by Kaminski et al. (2020) surveyed 8104 players from teams across 55 state youth soccer associations to examine the frequency and characteristics of purposeful soccer heading in youth players (ages 7–14) in the United States and to better understand adherence to the 2015 US Soccer heading guidelines.
  - Seventy-two percent of respondents (4860) reported that they did not participate in soccer heading drills as part of their practice.
  - Of the percentage that did participate in heading drills in practice, the number of drills devoted to this skill was limited 1–2 each week.
- The United Soccer Coaches organization has created an online diploma program called "Get aHEAD Safely in Soccer" to educate coaches on how to teach safer heading techniques for players ages 11–13.
- Neck strength has been shown to reduce overall concussion risk by reducing the postimpact linear and rotational accelerations.
- The use of headgear in soccer to reduce the risk of concussion has been examined and is not currently supported.
  - McGuine et al. looked at 2766 participants (67% female) and randomized them to a headgear (HG) vs. no headgear (noHG) group. One hundred and thirty participants (5.3% female, 2.2% male) sustained a sport-related concussion (SRC). The incidence of SRC was not different between the HG and NoHG groups for males, and there was no difference in days lost because of SRC.
- Mouth guards: decrease the risk of dental injury; however, not effective in reducing the risk of concussion

IMPACT OF THE CORONAVIRUS PANDEMIC (COVID-19) ON SOCCER

- The global pandemic that began in 2019 affected all sports and sporting events around the world, bringing them to a halt.
- The highly infectious and deadly nature of this virus caught the world off-guard, and suddenly, new guidelines needed to be implemented to safely return to sport.
- In the United States, MLS and NWSL resumed their disrupted 2020 season by playing all of their games in a tightly controlled environment/bubble with strict COVID testing guidelines.
- Like many other sports organizations, US Soccer released guidelines called *Play On* for resuming safe play. These recommendations include five phases to help guide players, coaches, and parents on return to play if deemed safe by local and state COVID regulations.
- The long-term health implications for athletes after COVID-19 infection are still being investigated.

- A 2021 study by Martinez et al. looked at 789 professional athletes who tested positive for COVID-19. Testing with troponin, electrocardiogram (ECG), and echocardiogram was performed 19 days after a positive result. Abnormal screening was noted in 30 athletes (6 with troponin elevations, 10 with abnormal ECGs, and 20 with abnormalities on their echocardiogram). Five of these athletes underwent further cardiac imaging with cardiac MRI and were found to have inflammatory cardiac disease (myocarditis or pericarditis).
- No cardiac adverse events occurred, and thus far safe return to play has been achieved.

GUIDELINES FOR SUCCESSFUL PARTICIPATION IN SOCCER

- Preparticipation physical examination: focus on previous ankle or knee injuries, careful assessment for ligamentous laxity and history of concussion
- Prophylactic taping or bracing for ankle laxity
- Ensure adequate equipment, including shoes, clothes, and shin guards; consider mouth guards
- Optimize sport-specific cardiovascular training; endurance and intermittent sprints
- Appropriate 15- to 20-minute warm-up and flexibility programs (e.g., FIFA 11+) before practice and game with emphasis on adductors, hamstrings, gastrocsoleus complex, iliotibial band, neck, and upper extremities
- Proprioceptive training for injury prevention with stress on jumping skill and technique; particularly important for ACL injuries in women
- Ensure appropriate technique for all skills, particularly heading, blocking, and tackling
- Appropriate nutrition and hydration; education about performance enhancement
- Use smaller balls for younger participants
- Appropriate education of athletes, parents, and coaches about injury and prevention; explain the increased risks with foul play
- Appropriate supervision of practice sessions by certified athletic trainer and of games by trainer and physician

SUMMARY

- Soccer enjoys a relatively low injury profile, making it an ideal sport for youngsters and adults. There are significant physiologic demands, requiring both aerobic and anaerobic metabolism and adequate balance and proprioception.
- Soccer-specific nutrition is important and may improve performance.
- Lower extremity injuries predominate; ankle most common, knee most severe.
- ACL injuries in female players remain of paramount concern.
- Head injuries are of increasing concern, particularly in youth soccer; limiting/banning of heading in children aged <14 years may decrease concussion rates. Long-term effects of severe or cumulative concussions is less certain, and additional studies are warranted to determine the same.

RECOMMENDED READINGS

Available online.

RUGBY 68

Jon S. Patricios • William Dexter

INTRODUCTION

- Rugby union (rugby) is a continuous, multiple-sprint, unhelmeted (padded headgear is permitted) collision team sport (>200 tackles per game) played by men and women, boys and girls, in 120 countries across six continents.
- Rugby has unique metabolic demands, requiring fitness in multiple domains (aerobic, anaerobic, strength, power, endurance).
- The original 15-a-side game lasts for 80 minutes with a 10-minute half-time interval.
- The 15-a-side version is the traditional and most popular version, but 7-a-side ("Sevens," lasting 7 minutes per half) and 10-a-side versions are also played.
- Sevens has increased in popularity, has its own professional world circuit, and is a recognized Olympic sport.
- Apart from a lack of protective body equipment, the differentiating feature from American football is that rugby is continuous in nature with no "time outs"; this requires injured players to be assessed during play before a decision is made whether to replace them with one of eight reserves.
- The international federation, World Rugby (WR) (formerly the International Rugby Board), governs the sport.

EPIDEMIOLOGY

- Rugby has one of the higher overall rates of injury (around 70/1000 player hours) compared with soccer (28/1000 player hours) and ice hockey (53/1000 player hours).
- Risk of injury increases with age and rugby level; this has been attributed to greater size, speed, increased competitiveness, more aggression, and foul play.
- Risk of injury is higher in men than in women, with the distribution of injuries varying by sex; females are injured more in training than men and less in tournament play.
- Different facets of the game allow players of differing physiques and talents to contribute to different positions. All players may run or kick the ball, tackle, and be involved in rucks and mauls.
- The forwards are divided into tight forwards comprising two props, a hooker, and two locks; they are largely responsible for the set pieces of play such as scrums and lineouts, and three "loose forwards" who are also involved in set pieces but who have a mandate to roam more.
- Forwards tend to be heavier and place an emphasis on strength and power.
- The seven backs tend to be smaller in stature with speed, agility, and skill being the assets.
- These large discrepancies in size may result in physical challenges for smaller players.

GENERAL PRINCIPLES

Rules

- Field-based team sport lasting up to 80 minutes with 30 players involved in continuous play interrupted only by:
  - Set play: scrums and lineouts
  - Penalties
  - Injury
  - Half-time (10 minutes)

Terminology

Scrum: Formation used in the set play restarting play after a knock-on (spilling the ball forward) or forward pass; the forwards from each side bind together, and then the two packs (groups of forwards) come together to allow the scrum-half to deliver the ball to the scrum. A scrum can also be awarded or chosen in different circumstances by the referee (Fig. 68.1A and B).

Lineout: The set play restarting play after the ball has been carried or kicked to touch (out of bounds); both sets of forwards will line up opposite each other with one team throwing the ball between the two lines of forwards. The throw must be directly down the middle of the two lines (see Fig. 68.1C).

Ruck: Typically, after a runner has made contact with another player and the ball has been delivered to the ground, once any combination of at least three players have bound themselves over the ball, a ruck has been formed. The primary difference from the maul is that the ball is on the ground.

Tackle: Act of physically bringing opposing player who has the ball to the ground; the rugby tackle involves leading with shoulder and wrapping arms around and placing the head behind the ball carrier; legal tackles must not be around the neck or head, and tacklers are required to use both arms and not tip the tackled player head first into the ground (see Fig. 68.1D)

"Blood bin": A 15-minute period during which players who are bleeding or have open wounds may be removed from the field and temporarily replaced while their wounds are attended to and the bleeding stopped

Head Injury Assessment (HIA): A 12-minute period during which players suspected of having suffered a concussion may be removed from the field and evaluated; this applies only to professional rugby.

Injuries

- Injury patterns are influenced by position: forwards suffer more knee, shoulder, and ankle injuries, whereas backs have a greater incidence of thigh (particularly hamstring) injuries.

Injury Prevention

- Rugby is the first professional sport to produce tournament player welfare standards, a compulsory checklist for players before international competition. These include:
  - Confirmation before a tournament by the team doctor or Union chief medical officer that all players are medically, mentally, dentally, and physically fit to participate
  - Confirmation that each player has completed the WR cardiac screening questionnaire and examination (which includes a mandatory electrocardiogram [ECG])
  - Completion by all team and match-day medical staff of the following WR education modules: Concussion Management module, Keep Rugby Clean anti-doping module, and Keep Rugby Onside anti-corruption module. These can be accessed at https://www.world.rugby/the-game/training-education/elearning.
  - Completion of WR Level 2 Immediate Care in Rugby (ICIR) accreditation (or equivalent) by all team medical staff and match-day doctors
  - The host union must indicate to WR what medical staff will be in place on match day at each venue. The following medical staff must be in attendance: match doctor, surgery doctor, surgery nurse, advanced life support (ALS) paramedic, a staffed on-site ILS ambulance, and minimum of four basic life support (BLS) paramedics.
  - Completion of a concussion education session by all players and team management within a year of the tournament's

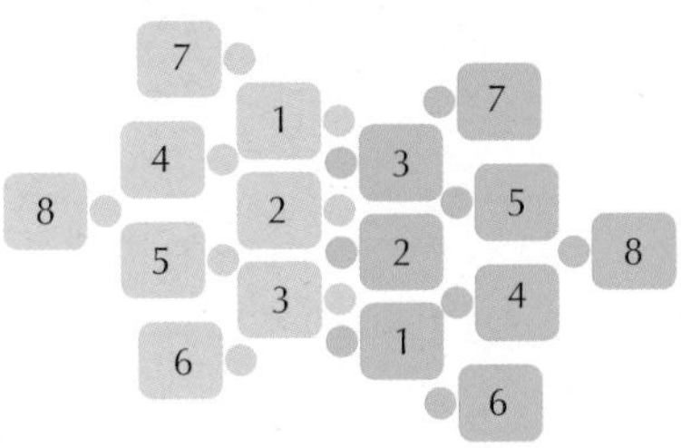

A. Positions adopted by opposing forwards in a scrum

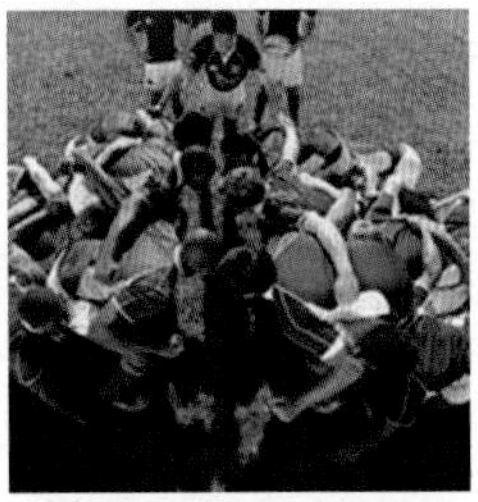

B. Setting a scrum

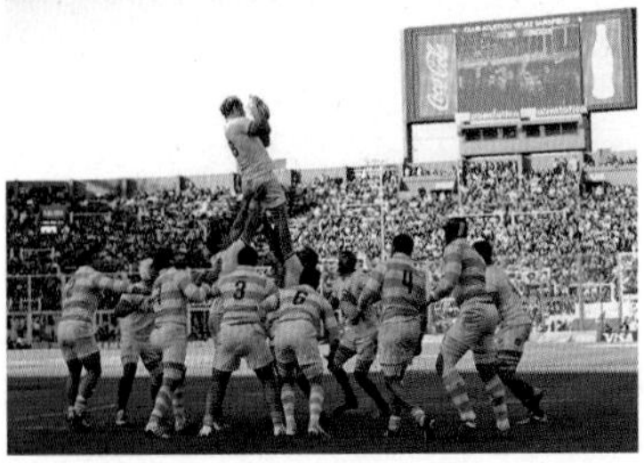

C. A lineout

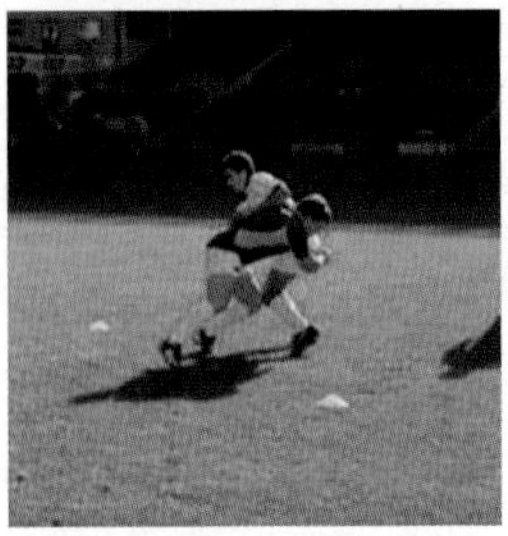

D. Correct tackle technique

Figure 68.1 Position terminology. (B and D, from South African Rugby Union; C, reused with permission from Gallo Images.)

commencement; this education session must cover the essential information outlined in the HIA protocol document.
- Completion of a baseline concussion assessment for each player; ideally with neurocognitive computer assessments, but at minimum with the Sport Concussion Assessment Tool (SCAT-5/6).
- Confirmation that a concussion risk stratification has been completed on all players to support concussion management on an individual basis.
- Acknowledgement that the tournament has an untoward incident review system for potential medical mismanagement and specifically for incidents where criteria, identified in the HIA, for permanent removal from play after a head injury are not enforced. All team staff acknowledge that they will participate if requested in any untoward incident review and that a charge of misconduct can be applied after an untoward incident review.
- Acknowledgement that the match-day doctor has the power to unilaterally remove an injured player from further game participation.
- Capturing all match injury data on an Injury Data Capture app required for the Injury Surveillance Monitoring System.

Neck Strengthening

- Research suggests that specific neck strengthening programs may help reduce the incidence of neck injuries.

Equipment

- Neither rugby headgear nor mouth guards have been shown to prevent concussion in rugby.
- Mouth guards have been unequivocally shown to reduce the incidence of dental and orofacial injuries. Customized mouthguards may be better tolerated and improve compliance.

TRAUMATIC INJURIES

Collisions are more likely to result in injury, whereas tackles are the game event responsible for the highest number of injuries and the greatest loss of time in rugby because they are by far the most common contact event.

Head Injuries

- Rugby has taken the lead in head injury management.
- WR has focused on head injuries as part of its Player Welfare initiative (http://playerwelfare.worldrugby.org/concussion)
- National programs such as BokSmart (www.boksmart.com) cover all areas of player wellness and injury intervention, but place an emphasis on head and neck injuries
- These interventions have significantly reduced the incidence of catastrophic injury in rugby over the last decade

Concussion

- Concussion is relatively common in rugby; the incidence has been reported as up to 1.2/1000 player hours in amateur rugby and 3.8/1000 player hours in professional rugby.
- Incidence appears to be increasing because of enhanced awareness and reporting.
- The most intense area of recent focus in WR has been head injuries, particularly concussion.
- An independent Concussion Advisory Group consisting of a neurosurgeon, sports physician, neuropathologist, and epidemiologist were consulted in devising all rugby concussion protocols.
- The tackle is the situation of greatest risk for head injuries. Player body position is a significant risk factor, with an injury risk that is 1.5 times greater when tacklers and ball carriers are upright, rather than bent at the waist. Based on this research, WR has made law changes and a launched global awareness program to change player behavior to lower the height of the tackle.
- Return-to-play (RTP) decisions after concussion should be individualized, considering player symptom score, general and neurologic examination, balance assessment, and verbal and possibly computerized cognitive scores.
- Recent rugby-specific research on the SCAT-5 has shown the expanded word recall list to have greater sensitivity for the verbal cognitive aspects of this tool.
- Minimum guidelines for RTP after concussion have been determined by WR (adults: a minimum 1-week complete rest followed by 5-day graduated return to play [GRTP]; 2 weeks minimum complete rest for <18 years followed by 5-day GRTP)
- Advanced Care Settings (ACS) are "gold standard" criteria determined by WR as being necessary for optimal concussion management, which include the following:
  - Medical doctors with training and experience in recognizing and managing concussion and suspected concussion
  - Access to brain imaging facilities and neuroradiologists
  - Access to a multidisciplinary team of specialists, including neurologists, neurosurgeons, neuropsychologists, neurocognitive testing, and balance and vestibular rehabilitation therapists
  - ACS must be in place for any deviation from the minimum criteria

HEAD INJURY ASSESSMENT

- HIA has been developed for elite-level adult players where experienced healthcare professionals support the teams (Fig. 68.2).
- Recognizing that concussion may have a variable natural history, with transient, fluctuating, delayed, and evolving signs or symptoms, WR promotes a three-stage approach to assessment, diagnosis, and monitoring of head injuries.
- HIA process reinforces review of injured players at specific points in time in order to increase the recognition of concussion:
  - Stage 1: pitch-side assessment using HIA Form 1 (12 minutes)
  - Stage 2: postgame, same-day assessment using HIA Form 2

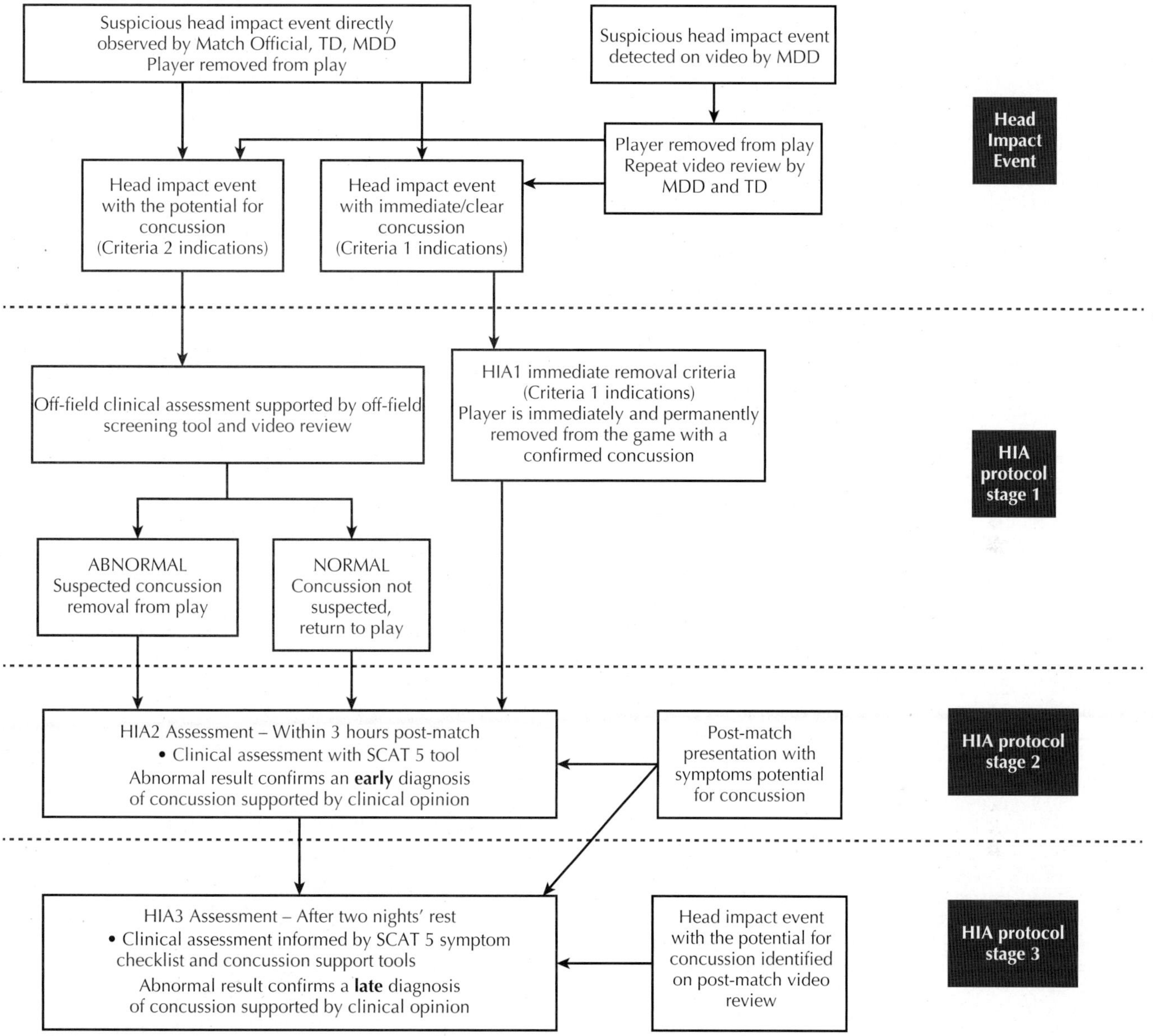
Suspicious head impact event directly observed by Match Official, TD, MDD Player removed from play
Suspicious head impact event detected on video by MDD
Player removed from play Repeat video review by MDD and TD
Head Impact Event
Head impact event with the potential for concussion (Criteria 2 indications)
Head impact event with immediate/clear concussion (Criteria 1 indications)
Off-field clinical assessment supported by off-field screening tool and video review
HIA1 immediate removal criteria (Criteria 1 indications) Player is immediately and permanently removed from the game with a confirmed concussion
HIA protocol stage 1
ABNORMAL Suspected concussion removal from play
NORMAL Concussion not suspected, return to play
HIA2 Assessment – Within 3 hours post-match
• Clinical assessment with SCAT 5 tool
Abnormal result confirms an early diagnosis of concussion supported by clinical opinion
Post-match presentation with symptoms potential for concussion
HIA protocol stage 2
HIA3 Assessment – After two nights' rest
• Clinical assessment informed by SCAT 5 symptom checklist and concussion support tools
Abnormal result confirms a late diagnosis of concussion supported by clinical opinion
Head impact event with the potential for concussion identified on post-match video review
HIA protocol stage 3

Figure 68.2 Summary of the HIA protocol for evaluating head impact events with the potential for concussion. (Reused with permission from World Rugby. https://playerwelfare.worldrugby.org.)

  - Stage 3: 36–48 hours postinjury assessment using HIA Form 3
  - Confirmed cases of concussion then must still undergo GRTP process
- WR recommends that players with head injury be regularly monitored for evolving signs and symptoms between these identified time frames.
- WR has introduced video analysis of suspected cases of concussion as an additional triage tool.

THE SIX "RS" OF RUGBY CONCUSSION MANAGEMENT

1. **Recognize:** Learn the signs and symptoms of a concussion so that you understand when an athlete might have a suspected concussion.
2. **Remove:** If athlete has a concussion or even a suspected concussion, he or she must be removed from play immediately.
3. **Refer:** Once removed from play, the player should be immediately referred to a qualified healthcare professional who is trained in evaluating and treating concussions.
4. **Rest:** Players should rest from exercise until symptom free and then start a GRTP program; WR recommends minimum rest periods for different ages (U/6 to U/18: 2 weeks minimum rest; adults: 1-week minimum rest).
5. **Recover:** Full recovery from concussion is required before RTP is authorized; this includes being symptom free. Rest and specific treatment options are critical for the health of an injured participant.
6. **Return:** For safe RTP, an athlete must be symptom free and should be cleared in writing by a qualified healthcare professional who is trained in evaluating and treating concussions. The athlete completes the GRTP protocol.

Spinal Cord Injury

- Result from a combination of distraction and compression forces in either flexion or extension depending on scenario.
- The tackle is now the area with the highest risk. The scrum was previously the greatest area of risk, but rule changes have reduced both the number of scrums and the risk.
- Intervention programs have been successful in reducing incidence of spinal cord injuries (SCIs); these include BokSmart

(South Africa), RugbySmart (New Zealand), and May Day Safety Procedure (Australia).
- Recommended organogram for management of SCIs in rugby is illustrated in Fig. 68.3.

Musculoskeletal Injuries

- Injury incidence is higher in professional rugby than in academy and school rugby.
- Match incidence is higher than training incidence (2/1000 player hours) and has been reported as 91/1000 player hours in professional rugby, 47/1000 player hours for academy rugby, and 35/1000 player hours for school rugby.
- Rugby 7s (Sevens World Series, Rio Olympics) injury incidence ranges from 88 to 109 injuries per 1000 match hours (women) to 108 to 124 (men), with the tackle accounting for 56% of injuries. Rugby 7s seemed to have similar time-loss injury rates as other contact collision Olympic sports. Considering injury severity, the burden of injury is two to three times higher in 7s than in Rugby World Cup (RWC) 15s.
- Longitudinal studies have shown a trend to increasing incidence injury but not severity
- Injuries differ by gender: females have up to five times the incidence of anterior cruciate ligament (ACL) injuries; male rugby players suffer more shoulder girdle injuries and fractures.
- Knee injuries account for the highest number of days absent because of injury and the longest time out followed by upper limb fractures and dislocations.
- Although medial collateral ligament injuries are more common, ACL injuries cause the greatest number of days missed.
- Shoulder injuries are associated with acute and repeated tackling, causing superior labrum anterior and posterior (SLAP) lesions, Bankart injuries, and rotator cuff tears. The acromioclavicular joint is the most common shoulder injury and one of the most common injuries seen in rugby.

WOUND MANAGEMENT

- WR emphasizes strong preventive measures against the spread of bloodborne diseases.
- Players with open or bleeding wounds must leave the field and have a 15-minute "blood bin" to control bleeding and to cover the wound.
- Players may not wear clothing contaminated by blood.

ILLNESS IN RUGBY

- Incidence of illness in rugby is higher than that of injury, particularly when frequent travel is involved.
- Most frequently affected are respiratory (31%), gastrointestinal (28%), and dermatologic systems and subcutaneous tissues (23%)
- The COVID-19 pandemic resulted in the cessation of rugby worldwide for varying periods of time. Extensive screening protocols were introduced and, in some areas of the world, so-called "biologically safe environments" (BSEs) were created to facilitate the resumption of professional rugby.
- Although the long layoff allowed for a rare uninterrupted period for the rehabilitation of injuries, it also necessitated the development of customized rugby-specific conditioning programs to maintain the key physical attributes associated with the game (e.g., strength, power, high-speed running ability, acceleration, deceleration, and change of direction), and game-specific contact skills (e.g., tackling) to mitigate injury risk on return.

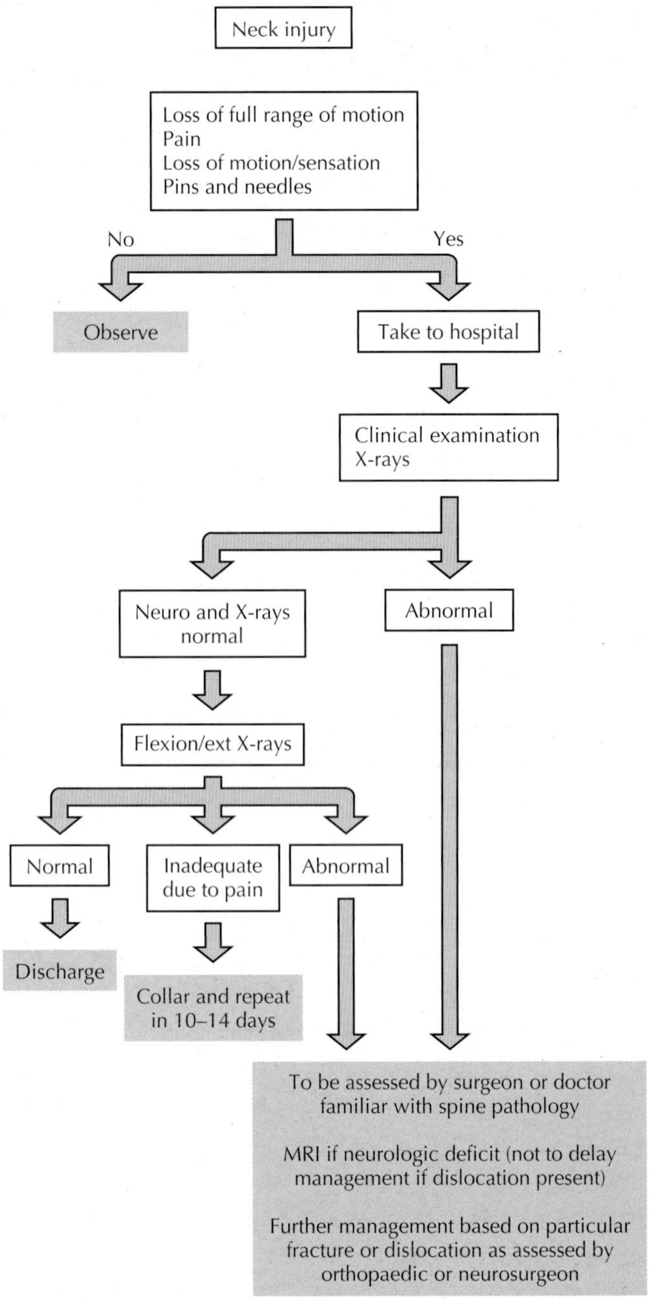

Neck injury
Loss of full range of motion
Pain
Loss of motion/sensation
Pins and needles
No
Yes
Observe
Take to hospital
Clinical examination
X-rays
Neuro and X-rays normal
Abnormal
Flexion/ext X-rays
Normal
Inadequate due to pain
Abnormal
Discharge
Collar and repeat in 10–14 days
To be assessed by surgeon or doctor familiar with spine pathology
MRI if neurologic deficit (not to delay management if dislocation present)
Further management based on particular fracture or dislocation as assessed by orthopaedic or neurosurgeon

Figure 68.3 An approach to managing neck injuries in community rugby. (From Dunn R. BokSmart: medical management of suspected serious acute spinal cord injuries in rugby players. *SAJSM*. 2009;21[3]:91–96.)

RECOMMENDED READINGS

Available online.

LACROSSE

69

Eugene S. Hong • Karen M. Sutton • Sarah M. Cheney

INTRODUCTION

- *US Lacrosse* is the governing body for all disciples of lacrosse in the United States, including men's and women's field lacrosse and indoor (box) lacrosse. *World Lacrosse* is the international federation responsible for providing governance and leadership for 66 member nations.
- Over the past 2 decades, lacrosse has been one of the fastest-growing team sports in the country at all levels.
- Lacrosse is known as a later-specialization sport, where many athletes compete in multiple sports throughout youth and into high school. Even as opportunities to play lacrosse exist year-round, lacrosse athletes are encouraged to play different sports in off-seasons to minimize burnout and prevent injuries.
- Approximately 830,000 athletes played lacrosse in 2018, a 20% increase since 2011 and a 227% increase since 2001.
- Despite a plateau in growth rate in recent years, over 50% of all lacrosse athletes are under the age of 16 years; hence, the continued growth of lacrosse is expected.

GENERAL PRINCIPLES

Men's Lacrosse

- **Men's lacrosse** is a moderate-risk sport where contact is allowed by the body and stick. The object of the game is to shoot the ball into the opponent's goal.
- In boys' lacrosse, stick checks are permitted at the U11 (age 9–10 years), U13 (age 11–12 years), and U15 (age 13–14 years) levels. Body checks are allowed at the U13 and older age groups.
- Each team has 10 players on the field at once, including one goalkeeper, three defenders, three midfielders, and three attackers.

Women's Lacrosse

- Women's lacrosse is a moderate-risk sport that allows for incidental contact to occur through controlled checking with the stick to another stick to dislodge a ball. Intentional body contact is prohibited.
- There is a theoretical 7-inch "bubble" around the head that cannot be invaded by the opponent's stick.
- The women's stick pocket is shallower than the men's stick pocket, allowing easier dislodging of the ball by an opponent and decrease in ball velocity as it is passed or shot on goal.
- Each team has 12 players on the field at once, including one goalkeeper, four defenders, three midfielders, and four attackers.
- Protective equipment required in the United States for women's field lacrosse players includes mouthguards and lacrosse eyewear. Women's lacrosse helmets are permissible, but not required.

Indoor or Box Lacrosse

- Indoor lacrosse, also known as *box lacrosse*, is a collision sport, mostly mirroring the rules of the men's game. The difference between the field and box games is that box is considered a rougher and more physical play of lacrosse. The game is more contact based and allows stick play not allowed in field lacrosse.
- The indoor game is played inside a multisport rink on artificial turf or a hard surface floor surrounded by boards (3′6″–4′ high).
- Each team has six players on the floor at once, including one goalkeeper and five runners.
- The goal is 4 feet tall, smaller than the 6-foot goal of the outdoor game.

Protective Equipment

- Men's lacrosse equipment protects against trauma caused by the stick, ball, and body contact.
- In men's lacrosse, field position players are required to wear a mouth guard; a lacrosse helmet with a full face mask and a four-point chin strap that meets the National Operating Committee on Standards for Athletic Equipment (NOCSAE) standard; mouthguards; gloves; and arm, elbow, and shoulder pads (Fig. 69.1).
  - In 2014, US Lacrosse mandated that young male players wear protective cups to prevent testicular trauma.
  - Beginning in 2021, all goalkeepers must wear goalie chest protectors that meet NOSCSAE certification standards to protect against commotio cordis (see later). In 2022, all boys' field players must wear shoulder pads that meet the NOCSAE specification to protect against commotio cordis.
  - Goalkeepers are required to wear arm pads, throat and chest protectors, and an athletic cup (Fig. 69.2). In the indoor game, the goalkeeper's additional padding and equipment resembles that used in ice hockey.
- In women's lacrosse, goalkeepers must wear a lacrosse helmet with a full face mask, throat protector that meets the NOCSAE standards, gloves, leg pads, and a chest protector. Starting in 2021, all goalies must wear chest protectors that meet NOSCSAE certification standards to protect against commotio cordis (see later). Field players are required to wear mouth guards and ASTM women's lacrosse eye protectors (Fig. 69.3). Field players have the option of wearing ASTM women's lacrosse headgear (Fig. 69.4).
- In 2014, the three rule-making bodies for lacrosse play in the United States—the National Collegiate Athletic Association (NCAA), US Lacrosse, and the National Federation of State High School Associations (NFSHA)—mandated the use of a lacrosse ball meeting the NOCSAE standard.

Rules Related to Safety and Injury Risk Reduction

- Youth lacrosse rules at ages 6U and below, provided by US Lacrosse, state that body-to-body contact is NOT permitted for boys. Intentional crosse-to-body or crosse-to-crosse contact is not permitted at 6U for girls' or boys' lacrosse. No player from either team may enter the crease at any time at 6U.
- Men's lacrosse has both technical and personal fouls, which may result in 1- to 3-minute penalties (removing the offending player from the game temporarily creating a "man down" situation), loss of possession, and even ejection.
- Women's lacrosse has minor and major fouls, which result in free position and possible loss of possession or removing the offending player.
  - For women's and girls' lacrosse, lacrosse penalizes dangerous play via time-loss cards. If a player receives two yellow cards, she is suspended from further participation in that game but does not have to sit out the next contest.
    - Dangerous contact is defined as any action that thrusts or shoves any player, with or without the ball, who is in a defenseless position.
- Men's lacrosse rules penalize dangerous play and provide points of emphasis annually that focus on minimizing the potential for injury. Examples of safety rules and points of emphasis provided by the NFHS for boys' lacrosse include:
  - Issuing penalties for excessive contact to the head/neck area and hits on defenseless players

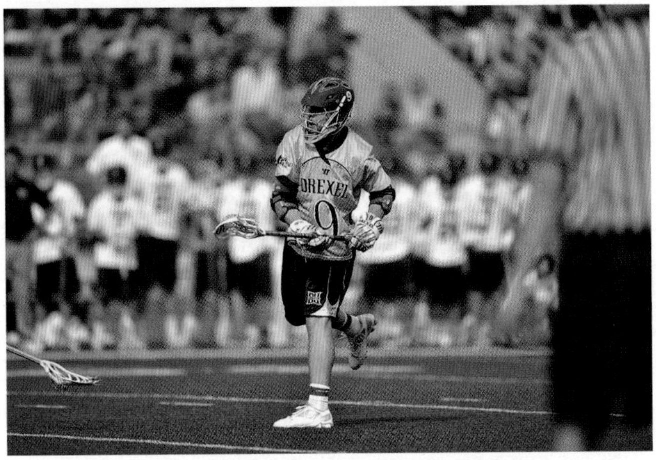

Figure 69.1 Men's lacrosse. (Courtesy of Sideline Photos, LLC.)

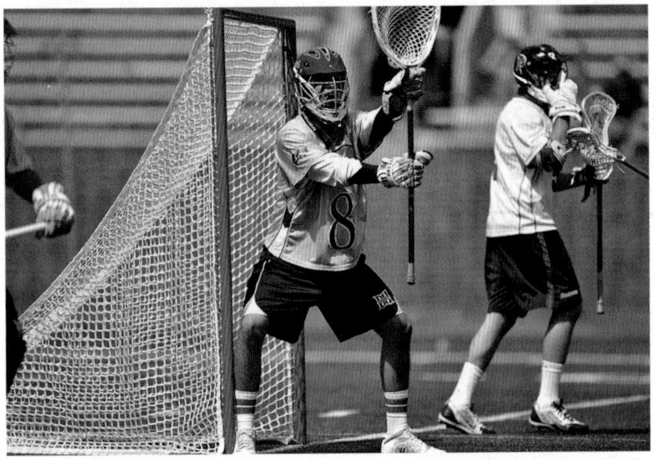

Figure 69.2 Men's goalkeeper. (Courtesy of Sideline Photos, LLC.)

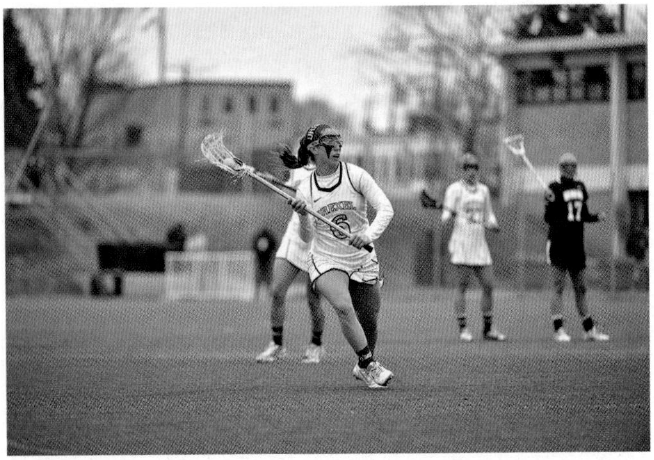

Figure 69.3 Women's lacrosse. (Courtesy of Sideline Photos, LLC.)

- Ensuring appropriate helmet fitting
- Using the final 3 minutes of halftime as a warm-up to help with injury prevention
- Using safety equipment use during pregame and practice
- Discouraging field players from defending the crease because they do not have the same degree of protective equipment as goalies to defend shots on goal

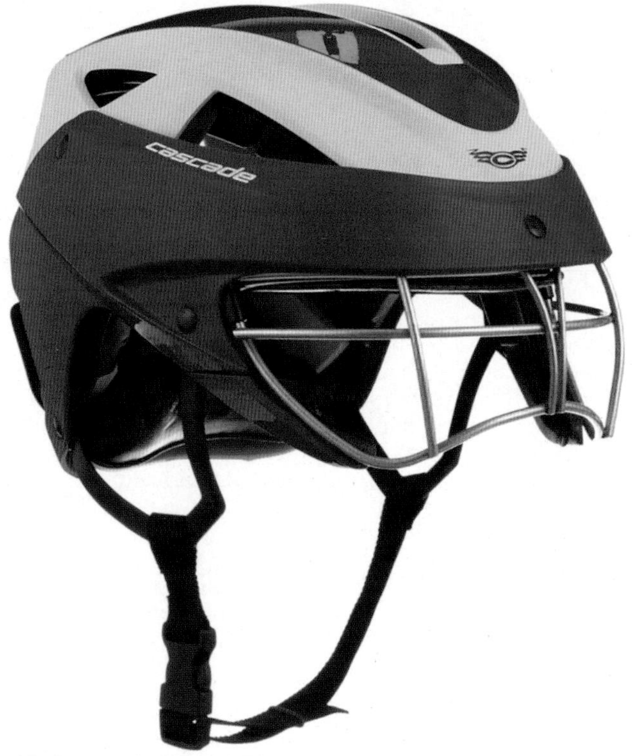
cascade

Figure 69.4 Women's lacrosse helmet. (From Cascade Lacrosse. https://cascadelacrosse.com/product/lx-headgear/.)

    - Prohibiting excessive body checks, issuing minimum penalties for checks involving the head/neck, and emphasis on prohibition of slashing
- NCAA rule changes, aimed at reducing head injuries, implemented in 2014 include increased and nonreleasable penalty time for offending players who target an opponent's head or neck by initiating contact with a stick or any part of the body

Injury Epidemiology

- Competition tends to result in higher injury rates than practice at all levels of play.
- The rate of time-loss injuries increases with age, from youth to high school to college to the international level.
- When directly compared, men/boys tend to have a higher injury rate than women/girls at all levels of play.
- Data collected from the 2018 Men's World Championship and 2019 Men's Indoor World Championship found an injury rate of 19.6 and 22.2 per 1000 athlete exposures (AEs), respectively.
- The NCAA Injury Surveillance System collects data on collegiate lacrosse injuries.
    - Over the 2009/2010–2014/2015 seasons, men's collegiate lacrosse had a total injury rate of 5.29 per 1000 AEs, with practice and game injury rates of 3.90 and 12.35 per 1000 AEs, respectively.
- Over the same time frame, women's collegiate lacrosse had a total injury rate of 4.93 per 1000 AEs. In 2009, women's lacrosse had 2.8 and 6.8 per 1000 AEs for practice and game injury rates, respectively.
- Data published in 2019 captured injury rates of high school lacrosse from the 2008/2009 to 2013/2014 seasons
    - Boys' high school lacrosse had 2.12 per 1000 AEs, and girls' high school lacrosse had 1.45 per 1000 AEs.
    - Common injuries among both boys and girls were strains/sprains (boys: 35.6%; girls: 43.9%) and concussions (boys: 21.9%; girls: 22.7%).

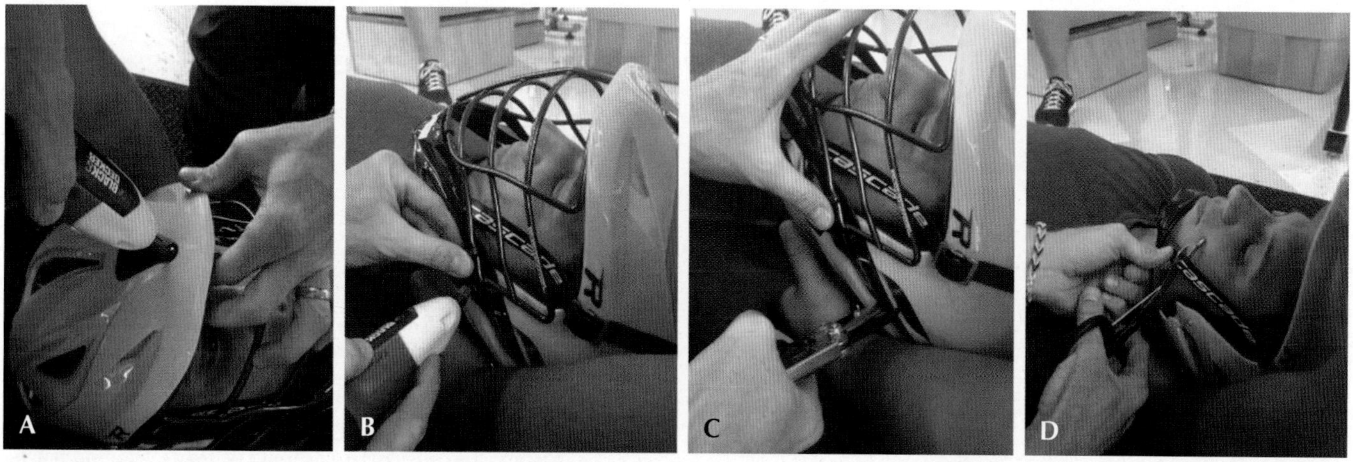
A
B
C
D

Figure 69.5 Steps of face mask removal with spine stabilization. This helmet has three screws that need to be removed, a top screw **(A)** and one on each side **(B)**. The side projections off the chin guard, along with the area where the chin guard interlocks with the shell, are unique to this model and require practice with face mask removal and helmet removal to ensure that optimal spinal motion restriction is maintained. Face mask and helmet removal may be facilitated by cutting through the side projections running from the chin guard back to the side of the helmet with pruning shears **(C)**. This will release the mask from the shell in most cases. The chin straps are cut if the helmet is being removed **(D)**. If the sizing/locking mechanism on the posterior (occiput region) of the helmet is accessible, releasing it may allow for easier helmet removal. (Reused with permission from US Lacrosse. Facemask and Helmet Removal: A Guide for the Medical Professional. https://www.nfhs.org/media/3609513/us-lacrosse-face-mask-and-helmet-removal-guidelines-for-an-injury-2019.pdf.)

- Data published in 2014 on youth lacrosse found injury rates of 8.7 injuries per 1000 AEs for boys and 3.4 per 1000 AEs for girls.
  - Most injuries were diagnosed as contusions (boys, 53.7%; girls, 47.2%)
  - Concussions occurred only in boys, and none were reported in girls
- In men's and women's lacrosse, the most common injury occurs at the lower extremity. This is likely because of the sharp cutting and dodging movements required to play the game.
- The most common injuries for men's and women's lacrosse are ligament sprains (particularly the ankle), muscle–tendon strains, knee internal derangement, and concussion.
- Men's and women's lacrosse differ in rules and equipment requirements in addition to some specific injury patterns.
  - Women sustain a higher percentage of head and facial injuries relative to male lacrosse players.
  - Because of its unique overhead contact nature, shoulder, trunk, and back injuries are also of concern in the men's game.
    - Noncontact injuries primarily occur at the lower extremity, whereas contact injuries primarily occur at the upper extremity, specifically the shoulder.
  - Although less common, upper extremity injuries such as hand or finger fractures are also present in both the men's and women's game.
- Lacrosse injuries treated in emergency settings are most commonly sprains/strains, contusions/abrasions, and fractures. Other serious injuries of concern include ocular/nasal injury and concussion.

SELECTED INJURIES AND MEDICAL PROBLEMS

Head and Neck

- Above-the-neck injuries account for one-fifth of all game-related injuries in women's lacrosse.
  - After implementing mandatory use of protective eyewear for women's lacrosse in 2004, rates of catastrophic eye injury dramatically decreased.
  - Although rare, females may have a higher incidence of facial fractures, possibly attributable to the lack of any required protective head equipment for field players.
- Sports-related concussions occur in lacrosse. In men's and women's lacrosse, the mechanism of concussive injury varies: in men, the primary cause is player-to-player contact, whereas in women, the primary cause is incidental contact with the stick or ball.
  - College concussion rates in competition: men 2.5/1000 AEs and women 1.2/1000 AEs
    - Concussion rates in men's lacrosse is below football but higher than men's ice hockey, wrestling, and soccer.
    - In women's lacrosse, rates are higher than women's field hockey, basketball, softball, and volleyball but remain lower than women's ice hockey and soccer.
  - In high school lacrosse:
    - Concussion rates for boys' lacrosse are 0.4/1000 AEs, making lacrosse the next highest concussion rate after football and hockey.
    - Concussion rates for girls' lacrosse may be comparable to girls' soccer (0.35/1000 AEs vs. 0.34/1000 AEs, respectively).
    - Forty percent of concussions resolve within 1–3 days.
    - Fifty-five percent return to play in 1–3 weeks.
- The potential for cervical spine injuries is concerning in all contact and collision sports.
  - The lacrosse helmet design is different from that used in football.
  - The decision to remove a player's helmet and shoulder pads may be made on a case-by-case basis (Fig. 69.5).
  - The face mask alone may be removed using appropriate tools.
  - Emergency preparedness by medical staff can include face mask removal, helmet and shoulder pad removal, and spine boarding. When appropriate, removal of face mask or helmet will ensure adequate ventilation and compression.

Eye

- In 2004, protective eyewear was mandated for women's lacrosse at the college level—high school and youth levels followed suit in subsequent years—to reduce the risk of catastrophic eye injury.
- There was an 84% reduction in serious eye injuries after the mandated protective eyewear rule change.

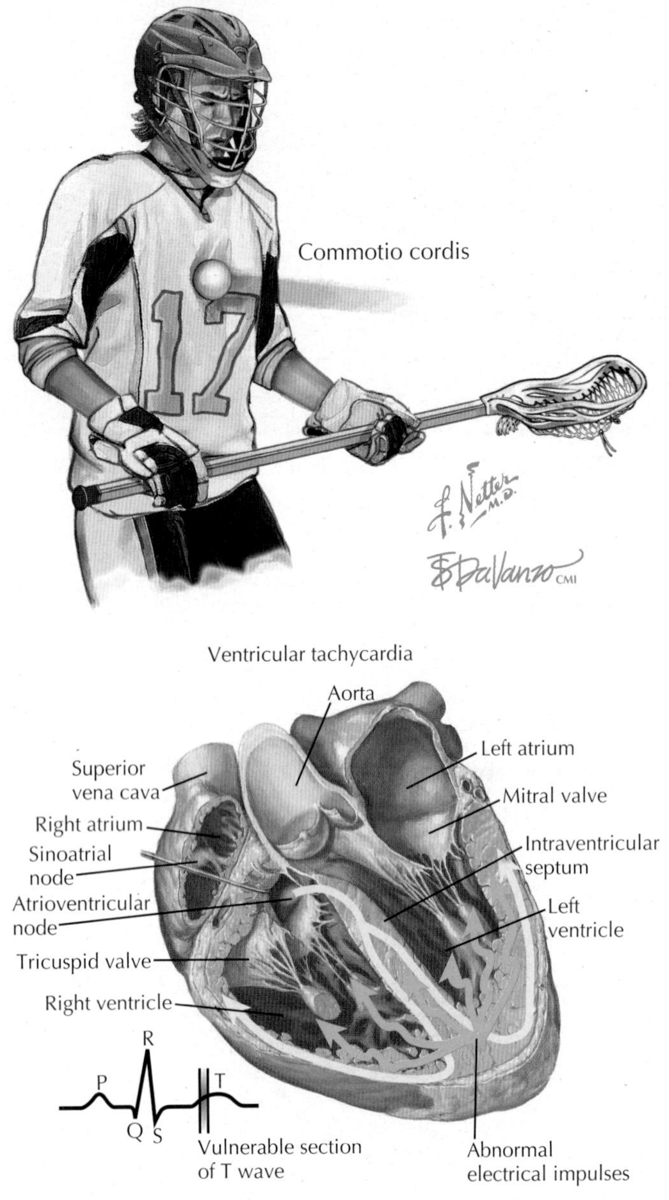
Commotio cordis
Ventricular tachycardia
Aorta
Left atrium
Superior vena cava
Mitral valve
Right atrium
Sinoatrial node
Intraventricular septum
Atrioventricular node
Left ventricle
Tricuspid valve
Right ventricle
R
P
T
Q
S
Vulnerable section of T wave
Abnormal electrical impulses

Figure 69.6 Mechanism of sudden cardiac death in commotio cordis.

Cardiac

- Commotio cordis is a cause of sudden cardiac arrest (SCA).
  - May occur in sports where a projectile is used.
  - Commotio cordis can occur when the ball impacts over the cardiac silhouette in a specific phase of the cardiac cycle (Fig. 69.6).
    - The impact causes an electrical disruption, resulting in an abnormal rhythm (most commonly ventricular fibrillation).
    - Animal studies demonstrate that an impact at a speed >40 miles/hour is more likely to induce an arrhythmia.
    - Harder lacrosse balls have a higher incidence of inducing arrhythmia based on animal studies.
  - If an athlete sustains a blow to the chest and collapses, the emergency action plan should be immediately initiated, emphasizing early access to defibrillation.
    - Significant consideration should be made when preparing emergency action plans to having an automatic external defibrillator (AED) present or location identified at the playing location.
    - In 2019, US Lacrosse launched a new initiative called "A Player's Pulse" to expand AED funding and awareness.
  - Commotio cordis may have a high mortality rate even with early cardiopulmonary resuscitation.
    - Mortality rate estimated at 16%.
  - According to an animal model, the survival rate is 90% if defibrillation is performed within 2 minutes; however, it drops to 40% if defibrillation occurs after 4 minutes.
  - Education is key to prevention; athletes should be discouraged from attempting to block shots with their chest.

Hand

- Fifty-nine percent of hand injuries in men's lacrosse are thumb injuries. Thumb injuries are higher in lacrosse than in other gloved, stick-handling sports.
- Lacrosse goalkeeper's thumb is described as a fracture of the distal or proximal phalanx of the thumb.
  - Typical mechanism is ball impact on the thumb tip as the goalie attempts to save a shot on goal. An axial load across the interphalangeal joint (IPJ) causes a fracture of the distal or proximal phalanx (Fig. 69.7).
  - Injury is managed according to standard fracture management protocols:
    - If >2 mm displacement or if >25% of joint surface involvement, open reduction with internal fixation is considered.

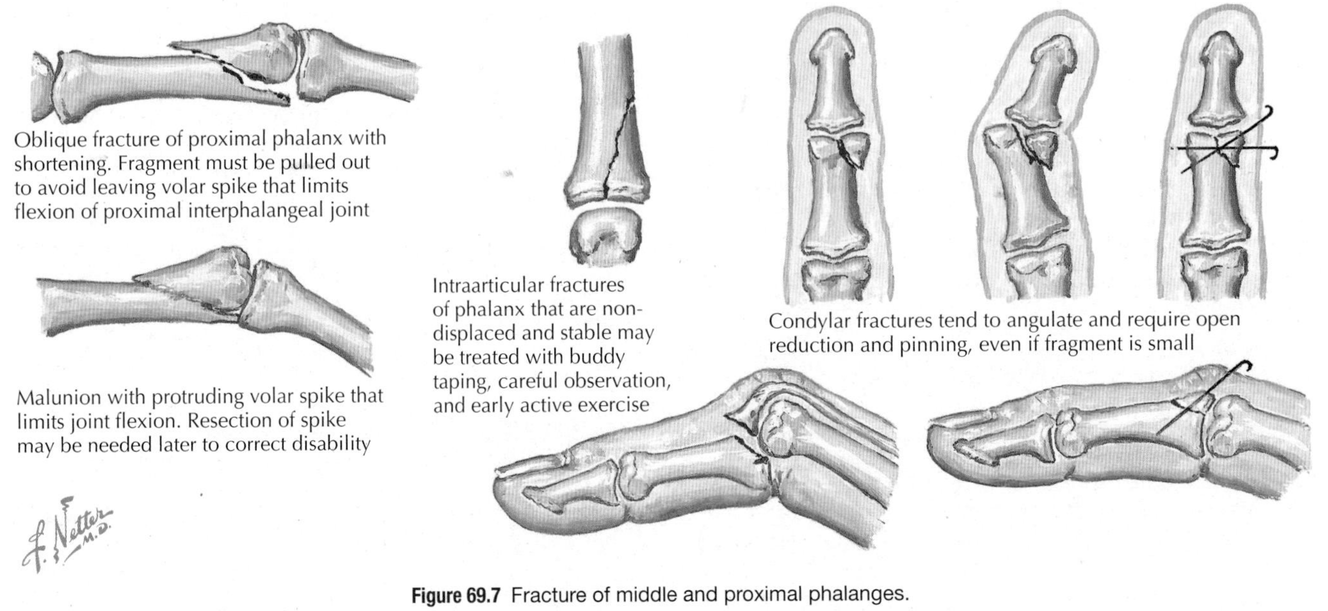
Oblique fracture of proximal phalanx with shortening. Fragment must be pulled out to avoid leaving volar spike that limits flexion of proximal interphalangeal joint
Malunion with protruding volar spike that limits joint flexion. Resection of spike may be needed later to correct disability
Intraarticular fractures of phalanx that are non-displaced and stable may be treated with buddy taping, careful observation, and early active exercise
Condylar fractures tend to angulate and require open reduction and pinning, even if fragment is small

Figure 69.7 Fracture of middle and proximal phalanges.

  - Nondisplaced fracture with minimal articular surface involvement can usually be treated with immobilization and protection.
- Injury risk may be reduced by using a molded, hard, protective splint or shell within the goalie's gloves.

Lower Extremity

- As with many explosive running and cutting-type sports, strained hamstrings, anterior cruciate ligament (ACL) tears, and ankle sprains are common lower limb injuries in lacrosse.
- The mechanism for a majority of lower extremity injuries in lacrosse, including ACL injury, is noncontact, most likely the result of cutting or pivoting.
- ACL injury rates for both men's and women's lacrosse place them in the middle third of 16 surveyed NCAA sports.
  - Although many studies find an increase in ACL injury in women's sports when compared with their men's counterpart, the ACL injury incidence is similar in lacrosse.
  - Men's lacrosse has an ACL injury rate of 0.12/1000 AEs (rank 10th), whereas women's lacrosse has 0.17/1000 AEs (rank 11th).
  - Decreased knee flexion angle during landing, consistent with sport-specific playing postures, may contribute to the higher incidence of ACL injury in female lacrosse players relative to field hockey.
  - See Chapter 55: "Knee Injuries."
- For ankle sprains, similar injury rates are noted in the NCAA.
  - Women's lacrosse ranks ninth and men's eighth, with injury rates of 0.70 and 0.66 per 1000 AEs, respectively.

BASICS OF THE GAME

Available online.

RECOMMENDED READINGS

Available online.

70 FIELD HOCKEY

Andrew Reisman • Chaney G. Stewman

GENERAL PRINCIPLES

History

- Oldest known stick and ball game in history, existing in the BC era.
- Became a popular British sport in 1861, entering as an outdoor Olympic sport for males in 1908 and for females in 1980.
- Primarily an outdoor sport, indoor field hockey (FH) is becoming more popular, with an Indoor Hockey World Cup in place since 2003. Although both bear many similarities, this chapter is specific to outdoor FH.

Equipment

Stick: Consists of a handle and J- or U-shaped curved head; flat only on the left-hand side; maximum length of 41 inches; made of composite materials.

Ball: Spherical, hard, and smooth (indentations permitted); circumference between 8-13/16 and 9-¼ inches; weight between 5-½ and 5-¾ ounces (slightly larger than a baseball).

Goal cage: Seven feet high, 12 feet wide, and 4 feet deep; consists of posts and surrounding nets; 18-inch high side- and backboards are positioned inside the bottom.

Outdoor field/pitch: Artificial turf or grass; measures 100 yards long by 60 yards wide; divided by a centerline and 25 yard lines on each side; "circles" are marked 16 yards from each goalpost. Penalty spots are marked 7 yards from the center of each goalline. Artificial turf is water- or sand-based for player safety (allowing slide with stop) and improved flow of game (providing a smooth, faster surface).

Goalkeeper: Footwear, kickers, leg guards, and headgear with fixed full-face protection and circumferential cover (international); throat, chest, and hand protectors (college); and wrap around the throat protector and attached mouth guard (high school [HS]) (Fig. 70.1). Although previously allowed, there can no longer be a field player with designated goalkeeping privileges.

Field players: Footwear, shin guards, mouth guards (international and college), and eye protectors (HS); flat, conforming face masks may be worn for defending penalty corners. National Collegiate Athletic Association (NCAA) players may wear soft-covered frame goggles with a plastic (not caged) frame. Soft headgear may be worn at all levels. Left-handed foam-padded gloves are encouraged but not mandatory.

Basic Rules of the Game

- Four 15-minute quarters with an interval of 2 minutes between quarters (collegiate and HS); two 35- (international) with a 5- (international) or 10-minute (collegiate and HS) half-time officiated by two umpires.
- Up to 11 players per team, including a goalkeeper, whose presence is only required in HS. A minimum number of seven players are required in HS. Tied games in the NCAA go into overtime with each team consisting of seven players including a goalkeeper.
- The ball can be touched only with the flat side of the stick and passed or dribbled down the field. The ball may be played above the shoulder as long as it is blocked to the ground and not hit in mid-air (Fig. 70.2). Players must not approach within 5 meters of an opponent receiving a falling raised ball until it has been received, controlled, and is on the ground.
- All players must have an equal chance to play the ball and may not shield the ball with their body or stick. Players cannot intentionally come into physical contact with an opponent's body or stick. Players may not intentionally raise the ball off of the ground in a manner deemed dangerous to surrounding players.
- No offside rule, and self-pass is allowed to restart play.
- Penalties/fouls occur only when a player or team has been disadvantaged by the opponent breaking the rules. Penalties include a free hit, penalty corner, and penalty stroke (Fig. 70.3).
- A goal is scored when the ball is played within the circle and crosses the goal-line.

Injury Epidemiology

- Injury patterns found in FH are similar to other field-based sports, except for a higher rate of hand/finger and head/face injuries compared with other stick-held sports.
  - The overall injury rate in 2004–2009 NCAA field hockey was 6.3 per 1000 athletic exposures (AEs) (injuries per 1000 AEs).
    - 18.7% of injuries are ball-contact injuries (NCAA 2009–2010 through 2014–2015)
    - Second highest women's sport for ball-contact injuries (first is softball): 7.71/10,000 AEs
- A majority of injuries occur during competition (two-thirds), and most occur within the circle (one-half).
  - Competition: 9.8 per 1000 AEs
  - Practice: 5.1 per 1000 AEs
- Major international FH tournaments injury data demonstrate differences between women's and men's competition.
  - Women's: 0.7 injuries per match
    - Head and face injuries are most common (40%–50%).
    - Most common mechanism of injury is an elevated ball (52%).
  - Men's: 1.2 injuries per match
    - Head/face and lower extremity injury rates are equal (22%–28%).
    - Most common mechanism of injury is an elevated ball (37%).
      - Stick contact and player collisions also significantly contribute (25% and 23%, respectively) to injury.
- NCAA injury data from 2004–2009 demonstrate:
  - Fifty-three percent involve lower limb.
  - Thirteen percent involve upper limb.
  - Thirteen percent involve torso and pelvis.
  - Nine percent involve head, face, and neck.
  - Six percent are concussions.
- NCAA 2009–2014 female sports-related concussion data indicated lower overall rates of concussion (4.2/10,000) compared with ice hockey, soccer, lacrosse, and basketball.
  - FH, however, had the highest overall rate of recurrent concussions in women's sports (13.3%).
- National Center for Catastrophic Sport Injury Research 1982–2013 data demonstrate:
  - One nonfatal catastrophic event at the college level
  - Three direct nonfatal catastrophic events at the HS level
    - One indirect fatality in 2007
  - No direct or indirect catastrophic injuries at either level since 2008
- Injuries by playing position:
  - Goalies have the highest injury rates of 0.58 injuries/athlete year.
  - Midfielders have 0.46 injuries/athlete year.
  - Forwards and defenders have equal rates at 0.36 injuries/athlete year.
  - Defenders have higher rates of lower limb injuries.
  - Forwards have higher rates of head and face injuries.

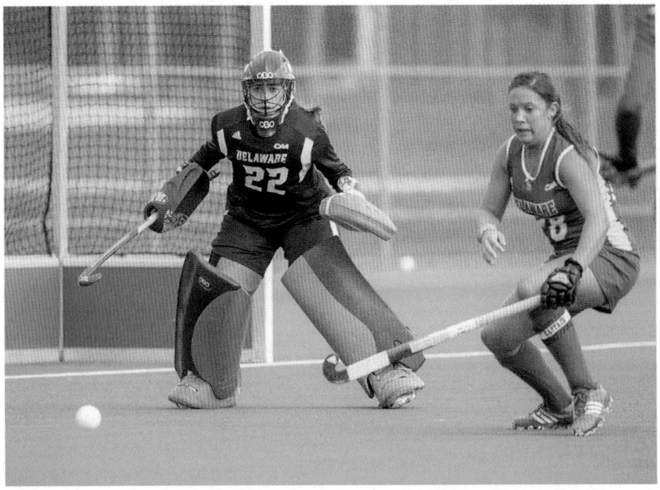

Figure 70.1 Players during competitions exemplifying protective gear worn by the goalkeeper and field player. (Courtesy of Mark Campbell, University of Delaware Athletics.)

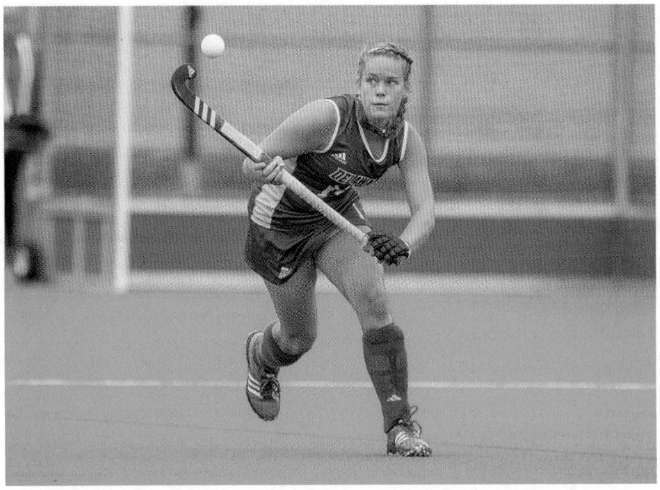

Figure 70.2 Permissible playing of a high ball being controlled to the ground. (Courtesy of Mark Campbell, University of Delaware Athletics.)

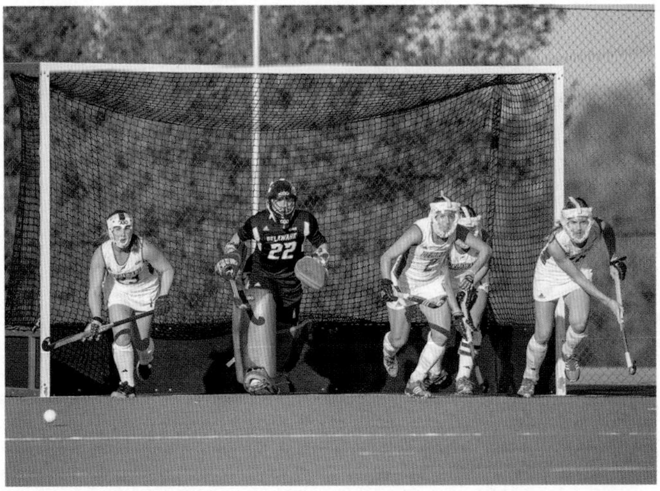

Figure 70.3 Defensive team flying out from the goal crease during penalty corners with protective equipment worn by the goalkeeper and field players. (Courtesy of Mark Campbell, University of Delaware Athletics.)

- Activity at time of injury:
  - General field play: 45.6%
  - Defending: 22.5%
  - Ball handling: 7%
  - Blocking a shot: 5.6%
  - Goaltending: 4.2%
- Time lost
  - A majority of injuries (32.2%) cause 3–6 days of time lost.
  - 13.1% of injuries result in ≥21 days of time lost.

SPORT-SPECIFIC INJURIES

Lower Extremity

- Over half of injuries involve the lower extremities (53.2%) and have multiple causes.
- Overall, upper thigh/leg strains and contusions and ankle sprains are the most common FH-related injury.
- Contusions and abrasions are frequent from contact with the ball, stick, and field.
  - Injury data comparing grass to artificial-turf injuries are limited but not significantly different.
- Exercise-related leg pain (ERLP), encompassing lower extremity overuse injuries, including medial tibial stress syndrome, chronic exertional compartment syndrome, stress fractures, and tendinopathies, is a common complaint.
  - A typical midfielder runs 5.6 miles (9 km) per game.
  - Rigorous conditioning for all players is necessary to keep up with the demands of this fast-paced sport.
- Incidence of noncontact first-time anterior cruciate ligament (ACL) injury at the college and HS levels is lower compared with women's soccer (according to a single state-wide epidemiologic study between 2008 and 2012).
  - College injury rate per 1000 person-days: 0.391 (soccer) and 0.038 (FH)
  - HS injury rate per 1000 person-days: 0.131 (soccer) and 0.048 (FH)

Torso/Pelvis

- Lower back pain is a common complaint among players. Although commonly experienced, it is rarely an acute injury.
  - The inherent trunk flexion and rotation required to play in a semicrouched, primarily right-handed position, hypothetically places players at an increased risk (Fig. 70.4).

Hand

- All types of hand injuries to metacarpals, fingers, and thumbs were almost two times higher in FH players compared with men's ice hockey and men's and women's lacrosse based on pooled NCAA data from 1986 to 2002.
- Phalangeal injuries are the most common injury overall to the hand; phalangeal fractures are the most common hand fracture.
  - Foam-padded gloves are frequently worn on the left hand, which is particularly exposed while block tackling (Fig. 70.5).
  - Right-hand gloves, although not commonly worn, are theorized to decrease the injury risk to these fingers, as they grasp the flat side of the stick close to the ground during play.
- Hand injuries represent 34% of pediatric American FH- and 32% of Australian FH-related injuries resulting in presentation to the emergency department.

Head/Face

- Lacerations and contusions are the most common injury to the head and face.

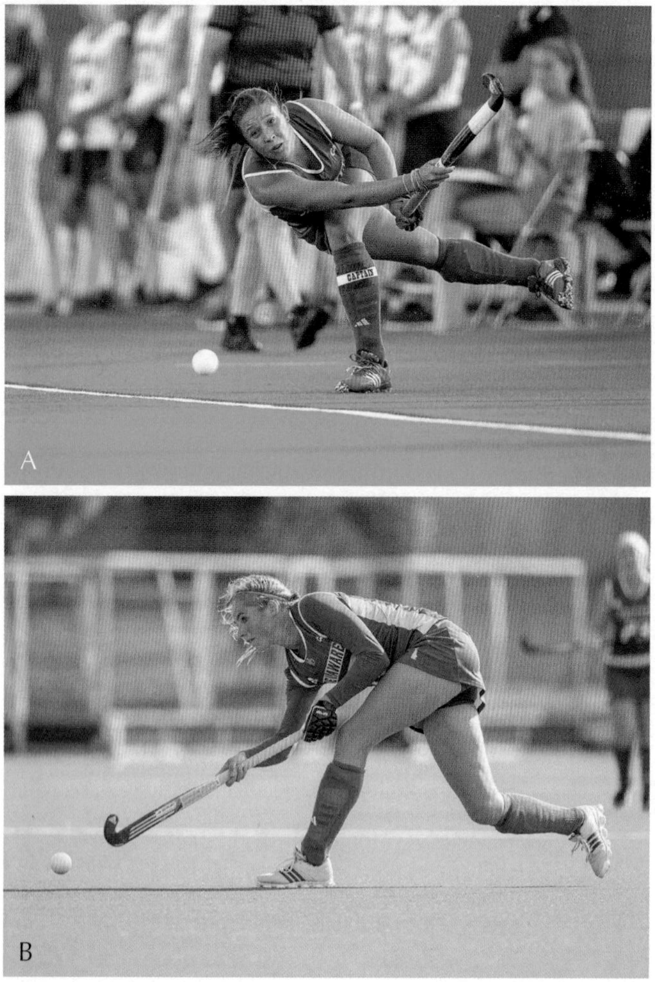
A
B

Figure 70.4 Common forward-flexed and axially rotated position noted during different aspects of the game. (Courtesy of Mark Campbell, University of Delaware Athletics.)

- Represent 21% of pediatric American FH-related injuries resulting in presentation to the emergency department
- Facial fractures occur relatively infrequently, representing 13% of head/face injuries in a two-season study of NCAA Division 1 players.
  - A majority (50%) involved the nose.
  - Sinus, zygomatic arch, and orbital fractures also occurred.
- Dental injuries denote a small proportion of injuries and are more common in elite players (men more than women) where mouth guard usage is not obligatory.
  - Represent 6% of head/face injuries in a two-season study of NCAA Division 1 players
  - Decreased rates from the 1980s to 2000s as mouth guard usage has increased from 31% to 85% among elite players
- Approximately two-thirds of injuries to the head and face occur during competition instead of practice, primarily because of contact with the ball (see Fig. 70.2 and Fig. 70.6).

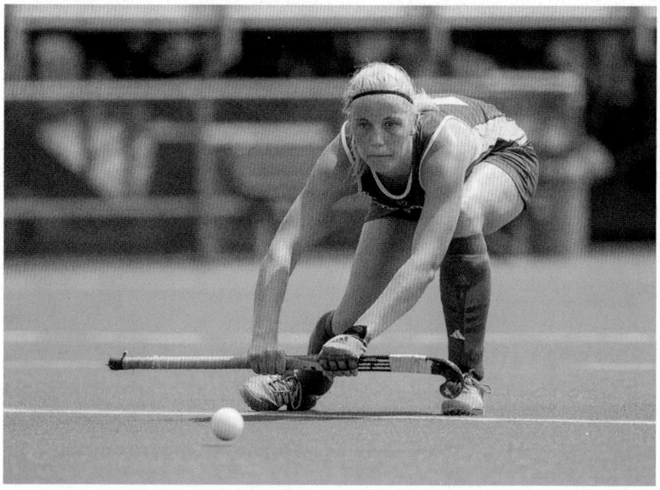

Figure 70.5 Ball stop by the offensive team at the top of the circle during a penalty corner. (Courtesy of Mark Campbell, University of Delaware Athletics.)

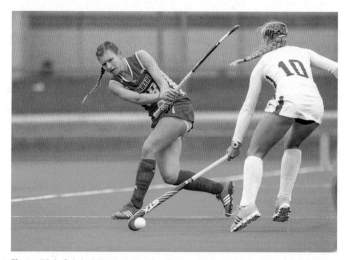
10

Figure 70.6 Stick follow-through after a pass can lead to risk of injury to the head and face area. (Courtesy of Mark Campbell, University of Delaware Athletics.)

Concussions

- NCAA 2009–2014 sports-related concussion data showed a low overall rate of concussions in FH (4.2/10,000). However, FH had the highest recurrent concussion rate in women's sports (13.3%).
  - Two-thirds occurred during competition.
  - Etiologies include player-to-player contact (53.3%), stick contact (20%), and ball contact (7.9%).
- Soft molded head gear is allowed for field players, but there is no evidence to show it reduces the concussion incidence.

RECOMMENDED READINGS

Available online.

ULTIMATE FRISBEE

71

Eric Traister

INTRODUCTION

- A group of students at Columbia High School in Maplewood, New Jersey, first played Ultimate Frisbee in 1968.
- Commonly referred to as "Ultimate."
- Distinct from disc golf.
- Played from the recreational to the international level.
- Most commonly played outdoors on grass or turf fields, but variations include indoor and beach Ultimate.
- In 2017, approximately 3.13 million participants in the United States, which includes all ages and genders.

EPIDEMIOLOGY

- Few studies in the literature regarding Ultimate.
- Noncontact sport with a high injury rate.
- One study reported out of 32 club college teams, Ultimate was second only to rugby for the number of injuries. Ultimate accounted for 31% of the injuries, whereas rugby accounted for 33.8% of the injuries.
- Another study noted that competitive collegiate club sports, which include Ultimate, have an injury rate equal to nonclub collegiate sports.
- 12.64 injuries per 1100 athlete exposures.
- Players are 43% more likely to be injured in a game than in practice.
- Multiple studies show that the most common injuries are sprains and strains.
- Lower extremity injuries account for up to 67% of injuries, with knee and ankle injuries being the most common.
- Men are more likely to be injured during a layout than women.
- Men are three times more likely to suffer a shoulder separation or dislocation.
- Women are seven times more likely to suffer an anterior cruciate ligament (ACL) injury than men.
- Overall women may be at more risk for injury than men.
- Concussions are likely prevalent, with one study showing 26% of competitive Ultimate athletes (male and female) sustaining one concussion and 43% sustaining multiple concussions during their playing career. More studies are needed to determine true incidence because of lack of standardized reporting.

GENERAL PRINCIPLES

Terminology

Backhand: Most common and basic throw. Throwing arm starts in an adducted position and brought across the body as the shoulder goes into external rotation. Power and distance are achieved through proper biomechanics transferring power through the hips and shoulder, ending with forcefully snapping the wrist upon release of the disc. Similar to backhand in tennis (Fig. 71.1A).

Forehand: Second most common throw. Also referred to as a "flick." Shoulder starts in external rotation, elbow flexed, and wrist supinated. Most of the power and distance are achieved with the wrist snapping upon release (see Fig. 71.1B).

Hammer: Overhead throw with shoulder adducted and elbow flexed. Disc is released at an oblique angle relative to the ground. Most of the power and distance are achieved with the wrist snapping upon release (see Fig. 71.1C).

Layout: Dive at the end of a run where a player leaves their feet, going horizontal to the ground in an attempt to catch or defend the disc. A significant number of injuries occur during a layout because of contact with another player and the ground (see Fig. 71.1D).

Mark: Person guarding the player with the disc. Players have 10 seconds to throw the disc (see Fig. 71.1B).

Pull: Starts every point. Defensive team throws the disc to the offensive team. Both teams start on their respective goal lines and cannot pass the goal line until the disc is released. Similar to a kickoff in football.

Organizations and Levels of Competitions

Nationally

- The governing body in the United States is a nonprofit organization called USA Ultimate.
- In 2014, USA Ultimate became a member of the US Olympic Committee (USOC) as a recognized sport organization.

College Division

- College Ultimate started in 1984 as a club sport.
- Over 18,000 student athletes from over 800+ colleges compete, which accounts for USA Ultimate's largest member segment. These student athletes make up multiple conferences within multiple regions nationwide.
- Student athletes have 5 years of eligibility.
- Men's and women's divisions.
- Regular season is from January to March (see "Specific Training, Physiology Issues, and Unique Environmental Issues" for competition format).
- Postseason is from April to May and includes conference championships, regional championships, and a national championship.
- Starting in 2010, a championship tournament was specifically created for Division III colleges.
- Starting in 2017, the college championships were live on ESPNU for the first time. Before that the college championships have been streamed on ESPN3 since 2015.

Club Division

- Open to any age group.
- Over 700 teams compete in four different tiers: pro, elite, select, and classic based on a point system. More points equal a higher tier.
- Each tier has a men's, women's, and mixed (co-ed) division.
- Regular season is from June to August where teams compete in tournaments to earn points, which determines postseason seeding.
- Postseason is from August to October and includes sectional and regional tournaments culminating in a 16-team national championship bracket.

Masters Divisions

- Started in 1991 as an age-restricted division of play at the club championships and evolved over time to include multiple age-restricted divisions.
- Masters division is 33+ for men's and 30+ for women's.
- Grand Masters division is 40+ for men's and 37+ for women's.
- Great Grand Masters division is 50+ for men's and 45+ for women's.
- Mixed (co-ed) mirrors the same age requirements for all three Masters divisions.
- Regional and national championships take place during the summer.

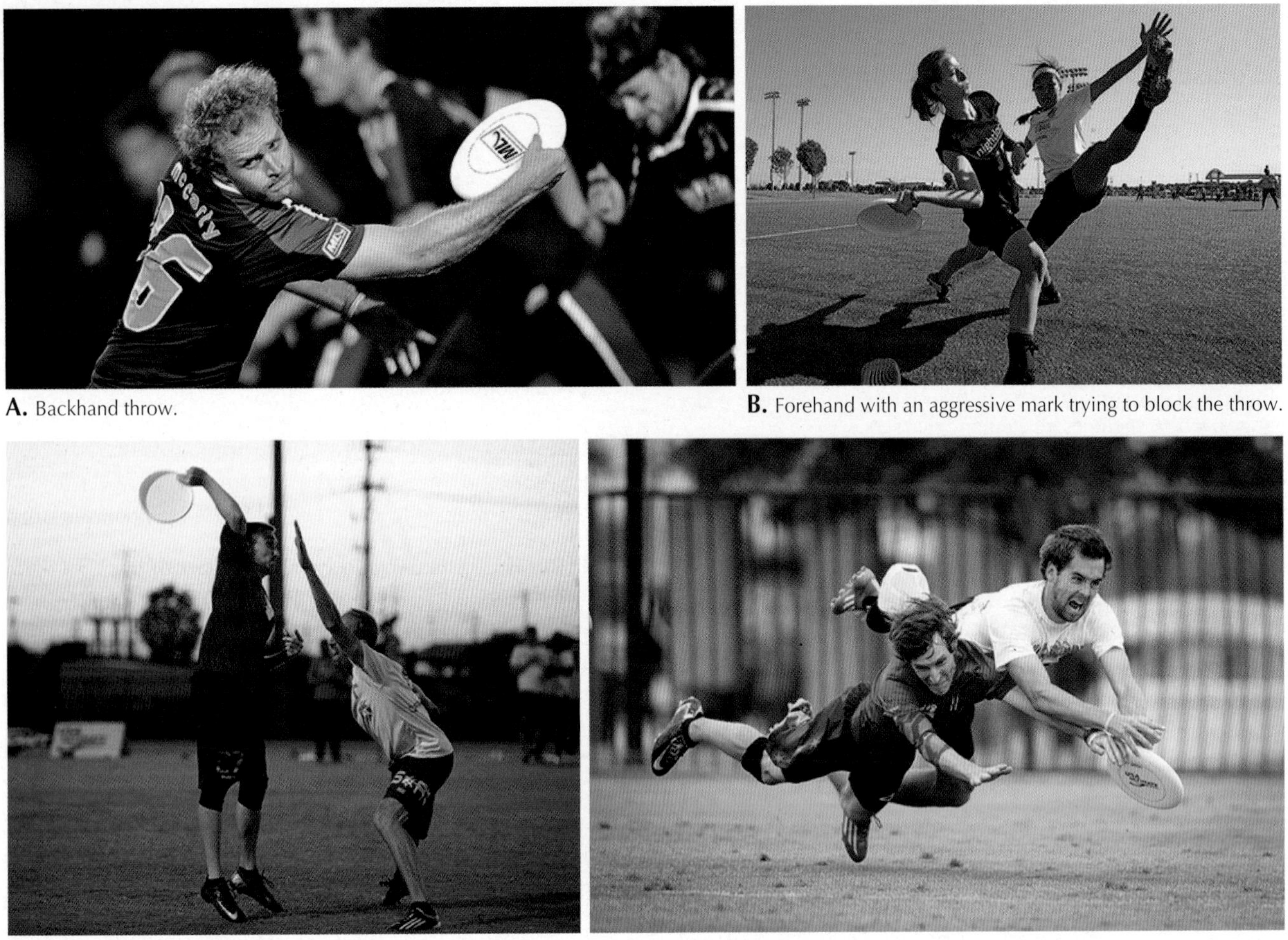

A. Backhand throw.

B. Forehand with an aggressive mark trying to block the throw.

C. Hammer throw.

D. Layout showing contact between players, disc and ground.

Figure 71.1 Ultimate Frisbee position terminology. (Photographs from Ultiphotos.com courtesy of photographers: **A,** Scobel Wiggins at Ultiphotos.com; **B,** Alex Fraser; **C,** Kevin Leclaire; and **D,** Paul Andris.)

Youth Division

- Started in 1988.
- Currently over 15,000 student athletes from over 400 club- and school-based teams.
- Divisions include boys, girls, and mixed.
- Includes championships at the high school, under 20, and under 17 level.
- There is also a developmental program for elementary and middle school players.

Professional

- A professional Ultimate league started in 2012 called the American Ultimate Disc League (AUDL). It is both the first and largest professional Ultimate league.
- AUDL functions independently of USA Ultimate.
- Consists of 22 franchises across four conferences in the United States.

International

- The world governing body of Ultimate is the World Flying Disc Federation (WFDF).
- Sixty-five countries on five continents represented in the WFDF.
- The International Olympic Committee fully recognized the WFDF in 2015.
- Multiple international tournaments that include under 20, under 23, club, and world game competitions and occur every 2–4 years.
- The 2018 World Championships had over 2500 participants with 128 teams representing 36 countries across three divisions: men's, women's, and mixed.

Equipment

- Only official equipment is a 175-g disc and cleats.
- The 175-g disc is standardized across all competitions except in youth competitions, where a lighter disc is used.

Rules

- Spirit of the game is the concept of putting sportsmanship and fair play at the forefront of Ultimate.
- Most games are self-officiated with players settling disputed calls among themselves.
- The highest levels of competition use observers to make rulings on out-of-bounds calls and goals. They also help settle calls between players if the players cannot reach an agreement.
- An Ultimate field is 40 yards wide, 70 yards goal line to goal line, and 25-yard-deep end zones. In general two Ultimate fields can fit on one soccer field.
- Teams play seven versus seven.
- Game is played to a specific number of points or time limit.
- Each point starts with the defense throwing (pulling) the disc to the offense.
- Play is continuous until one team completes a pass (scores) in the defense's end zone.

- Disc can be thrown in any direction at any time. Players have 10 seconds to throw the disc, which is counted by the mark. Running with the disc is not allowed.
- A pass is incomplete when it is dropped, blocked, or intercepted. After an incompletion, possession changes, where the defense becomes the offense and tries to score in the opposing team's end zone.
- Substitutions only occur after a goal or for injury.
- No intentional physical contact is allowed. Picks and screens are prohibited. Incidental contact is allowed.

Specific Training, Physiology Issues, and Unique Environmental Issues

- Most Ultimate competitions are in a tournament format played over 2 days. A total of six to nine games are played with each game lasting 1–2 hours.
- One study of a men's tournament showed average distance run in a single game is approximately 2.9 miles. Approximately 0.4 miles of that is high-intensity running and 0.1 miles is sprinting.
- Extrapolating over the course of a typical tournament, a player could run 17.5–26.3 miles with 2.4–3.6 miles classified as high intensity and 0.8–1.2 involving sprinting.
- Games are played outdoors and only cancelled for lightning. Players must be prepared to play in adverse conditions, including rain, snow, wind, and freezing temperatures.
- Ultimate requires a significant baseline aerobic capacity (similar to soccer) with the capability of making frequent sprints, jumps, and layouts.
- Aerobic training with running, biking, and swimming is common.
- Anaerobic training with high-intensity intervals, plyometrics, and running stairs and hills is common.
- Nutrition is geared for prolonged aerobic activity and quick recovery, as tournaments can consist of multiple games over several days.

INJURIES AND MEDICAL PROBLEMS

Skin Abrasions

- Common injury in Ultimate because of layouts. Worse abrasions occur on turf fields. Hips, lower abdomen, lateral leg, and forearms are the most common sites.

Head Injuries

- Concussions typically occur because of contact with another player or the ground during a layout.

Upper Extremity Injuries

- Shoulder injuries are common during layouts. These include acromioclavicular sprain/separation, glenohumeral subluxation/dislocation, and clavicle fractures.
- Repetitive overhead throws (hammer) can lead to rotator cuff tendinopathy, impingement, and subacromial bursitis.
- Elbow subluxations and dislocations are rare but usually occur during a layout.
- Wrist sprains and triangular fibrocartilage complex (TFCC) injuries are common because of forceful impact of the wrist on the ground during a layout.
- Finger and thumb sprains, contusions, fractures, and dislocations can occur during impact with disc, other players, or ground.

Pelvis and Hip Injuries

- Hip pointers are common because of a player laying out into another player's hip or direct impact with the ground during a layout.
- Constant running with repetitive acceleration, deceleration, sprinting, and change of direction lead to a high rate of hip flexor, quadricep, hamstring, adductor, and calf strains.

Lower Extremity Injuries

- Lateral sprained ankles are the most common injury seen overall.
- Traumatic knee injuries (ligament tears and meniscus injury) are common. Mostly occur during noncontact pivoting, landing from a jump, or change of direction. Also occurs during impact from a player laying out into another player.
- Patellar tendinopathy and patellofemoral syndrome are common because of the amount of running and jumping Ultimate players do.
- Overuse injuries such as medial tibial stress syndrome and stress fractures are common secondary to the high volume of running during typical competition.
- Achilles tendon injuries (tendinopathy and ruptures) are common, especially in the Masters divisions, where players will compete well into their 40s and 50s.

SUMMARY

Ultimate Frisbee is a sport that is played all over the world. It appeals to athletes of all ages and genders. There are youth, high school, college, club, masters, and professional leagues and competitions. It requires a significant baseline aerobic capacity with the ability to perform repetitive explosive movements such as sprinting, jumping, and laying out. Ultimate is classified as a noncontact sport but has a high injury rate. The high injury rate is at least partially the result of competitions comprising multiple games over a 2- to 4-day period. More studies are needed to determine actual injury epidemiology.

RECOMMENDED READINGS

Available online.

72 BASKETBALL

Justin J. Conway

INTRODUCTION

- Physical education teacher James Naismith invented basketball in 1891 as a noncontact sport wherein teams competed to throw a ball into opposing peach baskets.
- Since then, basketball has become increasingly physical, with regular contact between players yielding one of the highest overall injury rates among noncollision sports.

EPIDEMIOLOGY

- Most basketball injuries are sustained in the lower extremity, with contact mechanisms accounting for the majority of acute injuries (Table 72.1)
- Ankle sprain is the most common injury (Table 72.2)

GENERAL PRINCIPLES

Terminology and Rules

- Although the fundamental goal of putting the ball in the basket and scoring more points than the other team has remained unchanged since its inception, the rules of basketball have evolved over the past century. These changes have placed higher demands on individual participants (Table 72.3).
  - For example, initial rules written by James Naismith did not allow for dribbling.
  - Three-point line added by National Basketball Association (NBA) in 1979 and National Collegiate Athletic Association (NCAA) in 1987.
  - Dunking banned in NCAA 1967–1976 (the "Lew Alcindor rule").
- In standard play, five players per team are allowed on the court at one time with unlimited substitutions.
  - However, "3-on-3" competitions played on a half-court are a common variation sanctioned by many leagues and named an official Olympic sport in 2017.

Biomechanical Principles

- Basketball requires a high frequency of vertical movements, including single- and two-footed jumps and landings.
- Noncontact lower extremity injuries are more common in ball handlers compared with defenders.

Sport-Specific Training and Physiology

Sudden Cardiac Death (See Chapter 35: "Cardiac Disease in Athletes")

- Basketball athletes of all ages have a high risk of exertional-related sudden cardiac arrest and death (SCA/D) compared with other athletes.
- Black male NCAA Division 1 basketball players have highest risk of SCA/D among US high school and NCAA athletes (Table 72.4).
- The addition of 12-lead electrocardiogram (ECG) to preparticipation screening has been shown to increase the likelihood of recognizing potentially deadly cardiac disorders compared with history and physical alone.
- Regardless of preparticipation screening strategy or setting, a detailed and rehearsed emergency action plan should be in place, including easy access to an automated external defibrillator (AED).

Infectious Disease

- Basketball is a high-contact sport most commonly played indoors, thus creating a high-risk setting for the spread of communicable infectious disease.
- In response to the COVID-19 pandemic, the NBA and Women's National Basketball Association (WNBA) were able to successfully complete their 2020 seasons using a protected ("bubble") environment through a combination of strict quarantine rules and frequent testing.
- At the time of this writing (December 2020), collegiate, high school, and youth basketball leagues are grappling with whether they can safely compete, given high rates of COVID-19 infection throughout the United States.
- Changes in infection control practices are likely to persist beyond the COVID-19 pandemic.

COMMON INJURIES

Concussion (See Chapter 45: "Head Injuries")

- Basketball has second highest rate of concussion reported among female high school sports and sixth among males (Kerr et al. 2019).
- Adequate assessment for suspected concussion may require escorting the player to the locker room for off-court evaluation.
- Return-to-play protocol should include basketball-specific tasks and drills, including jumping, shooting, dribbling, and lateral movements, in addition to progressive increase in exertion and risk for contact.
- No difference in player performance postconcussion among NBA athletes (Patel et al. 2019).
  - Mean 7.7 days (median 5 days) missed postconcussion before return to play.

Ankle Sprain (See Chapter 56: "Ankle and Leg Injuries")

- A majority of ankle sprains in basketball occur when landing from a jump or planting on another player's foot.
- Most commonly inversion-type injury resulting in sprain of lateral ankle ligaments (anterior talofibular ligament [ATFL], calcaneofibular ligament [CFL], and posterior talofibular ligament [PTFL]) (Fig. 72.1).
- Risk factors include a history of ankle sprain, decreased ankle dorsiflexion strength, and decreased range of motion.
- Incidence of ankle sprains can be decreased by prophylactic ankle bracing or taping.
  - McGuine et al. (2011) found that using a lace-up ankle brace reduced the incidence of acute injuries by >50% in US high school athletes both with and without a history of prior ankle injury.
  - No clear evidence that ankle taping is superior to a functional lace-up brace for injury prevention during play.
- Neuromuscular training programs can effectively decrease the rate of ankle sprains in basketball players.
  - FIFA 11+ injury prevention programs have proven to reduce lower extremity injury rates in both female and male elite basketball players; efficacy in youth and high school athletes is unclear.

Achilles Tendon Rupture (See Chapter 56: "Ankle and Leg Injuries")

- Typically a noncontact injury that occurs when pushing off on a dorsiflexed foot from a stopped position.
- Increased risk with age.

Table 72.1 EPIDEMIOLOGY OF BASKETBALL INJURIES IN US SECONDARY SCHOOL AND NCAA ATHLETES

Level of Competition	Event Type	Time-Loss Injury Rate (Per 1000 AEs)	Total Injury Rate (Per 1000 AEs)
Female			
Secondary school	Practice	1.22	7.02
	Competition	3.13	11.84
	Overall	1.73	8.30
NCAA	Practice	2.39	5.34
	Competition	4.46	10.46
	Overall	2.87	6.54
Male			
Secondary school	Practice	1.25	6.57
	Competition	2.38	9.40
	Overall	1.53	7.28
NCAA	Practice	2.80	6.41
	Competition	4.56	13.61
	Overall	3.18	7.97

AE, Athlete exposure.
Data from Allen AN, et al. Epidemiology of secondary school boys' and girls' basketball injuries: National Athletic Treatment, Injury and Outcomes Network. *J Athl Train*. 2019;54(11):1179–1186; Zuckerman SL, et al. Injuries sustained in National Collegiate Athletic Association men's and women's basketball, 2009/2010-2014/2015. *Br J Sports Med*. 2018;52(4):261–268.

Table 72.2 COMMON INJURIES IN NCAA MEN'S AND WOMEN'S BASKETBALL 2009/2010–2014/2015

Injury	N (%)	Rate Per 1000 AEs	Most Common Injury Mechanisms (% Within Injury)
Men			
Ankle sprain	414 (17.9)	1.43	Player contact (54.6) Noncontact (27.8)
Hand/wrist sprain	119 (5.2)	0.41	Player contact (40.3) Surface contact (34.5)
Concussion	106 (4.6)	0.37	Player contact (79.3) Surface contact (18.9)
Hip/groin strain	83 (3.6)	0.29	Noncontact (61.5) Overuse (18.1)
Knee internal derangement	79 (3.4)	0.27	Player contact (44.3) Noncontact (34.2)
Women			
Ankle sprain	270 (16.6)	1.08	Player contact (49.6) Noncontact (27.0)
Concussion	136 (8.3)	0.55	Player contact (69.1) Surface contact (22.1)
Knee internal derangement	92 (5.6)	0.37	Noncontact (51.1) Player contact (32.6)
Thigh strain	75 (4.6)	0.30	Noncontact (61.3) Overuse (16.0)
Hip/groin strain	61 (3.7)	0.24	Noncontact (55.7) Overuse (21.3)

AE, Athlete exposure.
Data originate from the Datalys Center for Sports Injury Research and Prevention Injury Surveillance Program, 2009/2010–2014/2015; adapted from Zuckerman SL, et al. Injuries sustained in National Collegiate Athletic Association men's and women's basketball, 2009/2010-2014/2015. *Br J Sports Med*. 2018;52(4):261–268.

  - Career-ending injury in over 20% of NBA players (Lemme et al. 2019).
- Nonoperative and operative treatment are both shown to be effective in the general population, but surgical repair is standard of care in elite athletes.

Anterior Cruciate Ligament Injuries (See Chapter 55: "Knee Injuries")

- Anterior cruciate ligament (ACL) tears are more than three times more common in female than male basketball players at all levels of competition.
- Among US high school athletes, basketball has the second highest incidence of ACL tears in female athletes (after soccer) and the fourth highest in males (after football, lacrosse, and soccer).

Patellar Tendinopathy ("Jumper's Knee") (See Chapter 55: "Knee Injuries")

- Repetitive vertical jumping and squatting (defensive stance) required in basketball puts a high degree of stress on the patellofemoral joint and quad/patellar tendon.

Table 72.3 COMPARISON OF BASKETBALL RULES AND REGULATIONS IN COLLEGIATE AND PROFESSIONAL LEAGUES (2020 RULES)

Rule	NBA	WNBA	FIBA	NCAAM	NCAAW	US High School
Court length	94′ × 50′	94′ × 50′	91′0″ × 49′2″ (28 × 15 m)	94′ × 50′	94′ × 50′	84′ × 50′
Width of lane	19′	19′	16′1″ (4.9 m)	16′	16′	16′
Rim height (floor to rim)	10′	10′	10′ (3.05 m)	10′	10′	10′
Free throw line distance (from backboard)	15′	15′	15′1″ (4.6 m)	15′	15′	15′
Three-point FG distance (top)[a]	23′9″	22′1.75″	22′1.75″	22′1.75″	20′9″	19′9″
Game duration	48 min (4 × 12-min quarters)	40 min (4 × 10-min quarters)	40 min (4 × 10-min quarters)	40 min (2 × 20-min halves)	40 min (4 × 10-min quarters)	32 min (4 × 8-min quarters)
Shot clock	24 sec	24 sec	24 sec	35 sec	30 sec	none[b]
Back court violation	8 sec	8 sec	8 sec	10 sec	10 sec	10 sec
Player foul limit	6	5	5	5	5	5
Ball size (circumference)	29.5″	28.5″	29.5″	29.5″	28.5″	29.5″ boys 28.5″ girls
Size of basket (circumference)	30″	30″	30″	30″	30″	30″

[a]Measured from center of basket.
[b]Varies by state. Shot clock not currently mandated by US National Federation of High School Sports.

Table 72.4 RATE OF SUDDEN CARDIAC ARREST AND DEATH IN US HIGH SCHOOL AND COLLEGE ATHLETES

Athlete Population	Incidence Rate Per AE	Athlete Population	Incidence Rate Per AE
US High School		**NCAA**	
Overall	1:65,872	Overall	1:50,768
Female	1:203,786	Female	1:123,278
Male	1:43,932	Male	1:34,906
Male basketball	1:39,811	Male Caucasian	1:38,641
		Male African American	1:18,413
		Male Caucasian basketball	1:15,098
		Male African American basketball	1:4810
		Male Division 1 African American	1:2087

AE, Athlete exposure.
Data from Peterson DF, et al. Aetiology and incidence of sudden cardiac arrest and death in young competitive athletes in the USA: a 4-year prospective study. *Br J Sports Med*. 2020:bjsports-2020-102666.

- Biomechanical risk factors include tight quadriceps and hamstrings.
- Early single-sport specialization and a lack of rest periods throughout the year increase risk of overuse injury among youth athletes.
  - Osgood–Schlatter disease common in this population (Fig. 72.2).

Jones Fracture (See Chapter 60: "Foot Problems")

- Transverse fracture of the proximal fifth metatarsal at the metaphyseal-diaphyseal junction.
- High risk of nonunion, as injury is within the vascular watershed area (Fig. 72.3).
- Surgical fixation usually preferred over nonsurgical management, particularly in elite athletes participating in jumping sports:
  - Reduces the risk of nonunion and allows earlier return to weight-bearing.
  - Review of Jones fractures in NBA players over 19 seasons revealed that 85% of players returned to preinjury levels of competition in the season after injury (Begly et al. 2015).

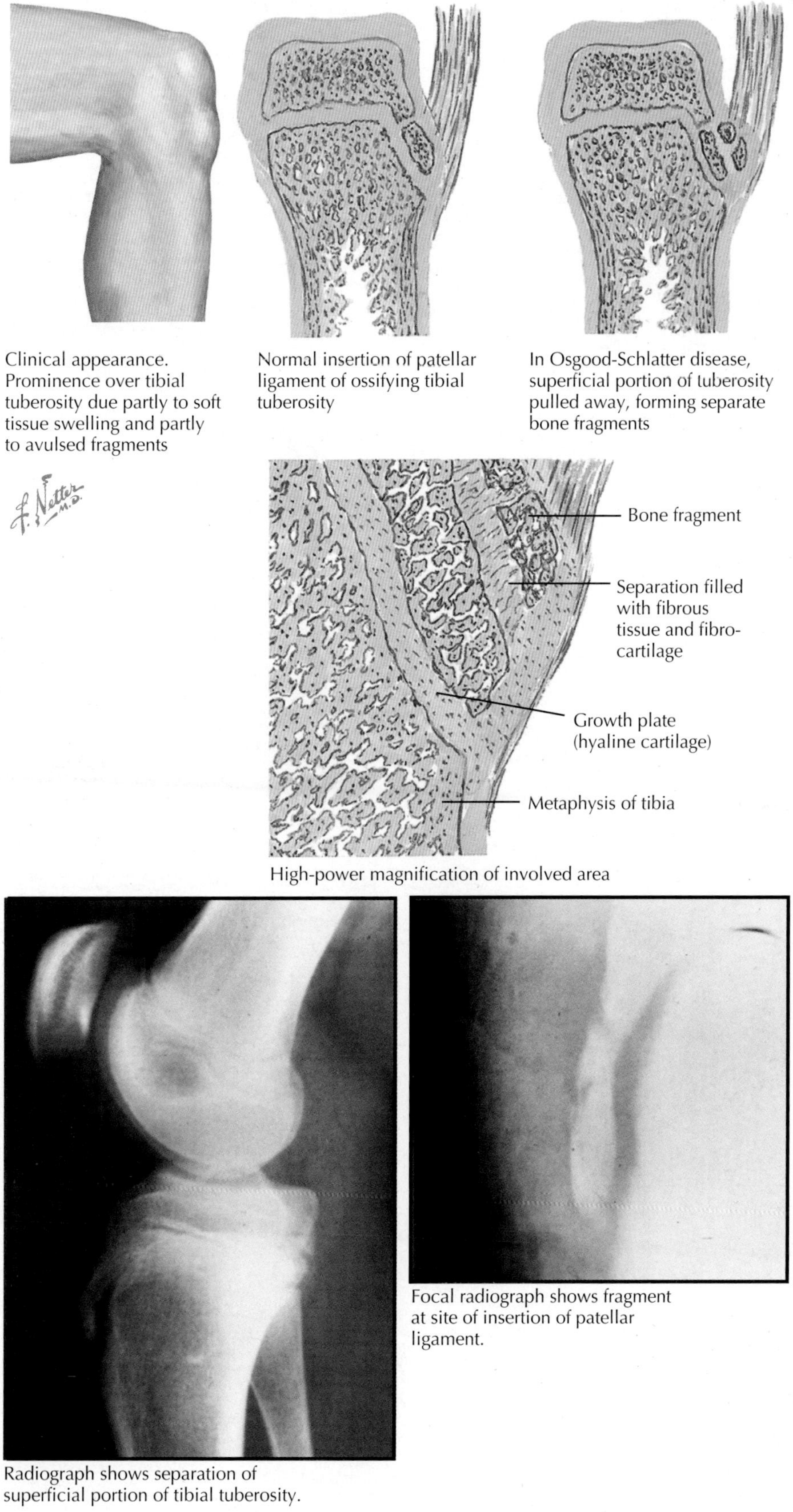
Clinical appearance. Prominence over tibial tuberosity due partly to soft tissue swelling and partly to avulsed fragments
Normal insertion of patellar ligament of ossifying tibial tuberosity
In Osgood-Schlatter disease, superficial portion of tuberosity pulled away, forming separate bone fragments
F. Netter M.D.
Bone fragment
Separation filled with fibrous tissue and fibro-cartilage
Growth plate (hyaline cartilage)
Metaphysis of tibia
High-power magnification of involved area
Focal radiograph shows fragment at site of insertion of patellar ligament.
Radiograph shows separation of superficial portion of tibial tuberosity.

Figure 72.1 Osgood–Schlatter lesion.

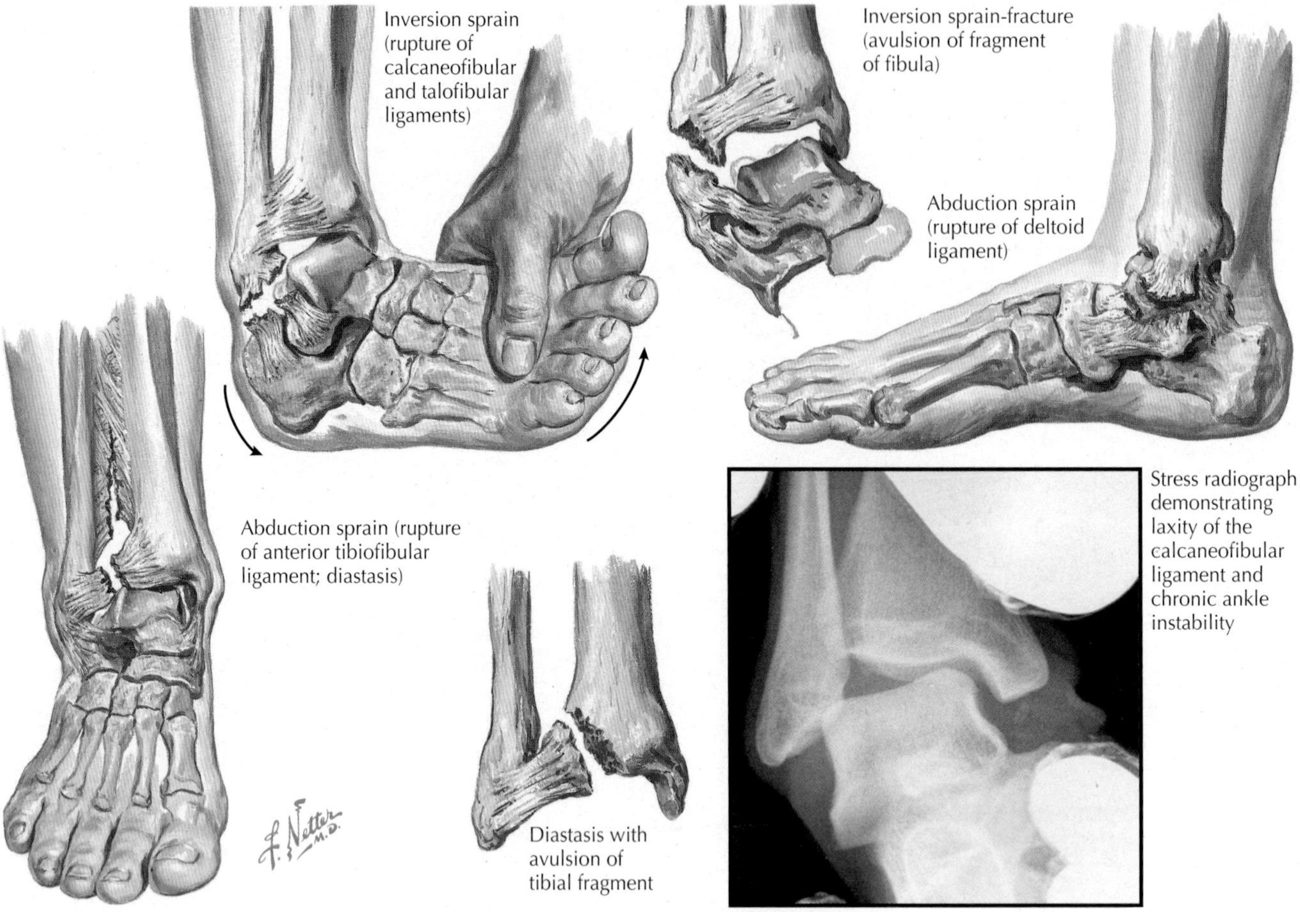
Inversion sprain (rupture of calcaneofibular and talofibular ligaments)
Inversion sprain-fracture (avulsion of fragment of fibula)
Abduction sprain (rupture of deltoid ligament)
Abduction sprain (rupture of anterior tibiofibular ligament; diastasis)
Diastasis with avulsion of tibial fragment
Stress radiograph demonstrating laxity of the calcaneofibular ligament and chronic ankle instability

Figure 72.2 Ankle sprains and associated fractures.

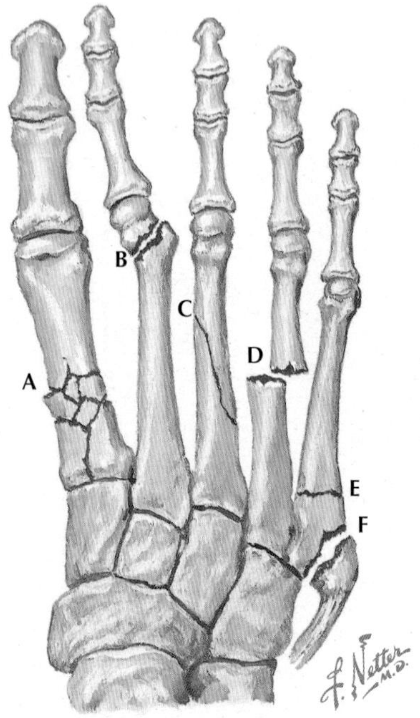
A
B
C
D
E
F

Types of fractures of metatarsal: A. comminuted fracture, B. displaced neck fracture, C. oblique fracture, D. displaced transverse fracture, E. fracture of base of 5th metatarsal, F. avulsion of tuberosity of 5th metatarsal

Figure 72.3 Metatarsal fractures.

RECOMMENDED READINGS

Available online.

VOLLEYBALL

73

Ryan J. Wagner • Kevin Eerkes

INTRODUCTION

- Volleyball is a popular sport played worldwide both recreationally and professionally.
- Volleyball is a truly American game with origins back to the 1890s.
- Made its debut at the Olympic Games in 1964.
- It requires quick and explosive movements.
- Volleyball is considered a noncontact sport.

EPIDEMIOLOGY

- Most injuries occur to blockers and hitters as opposed to passers and setters.
  - Certain positions are associated with specific injuries (Table 73.1).
- Most injuries are related to jumping and landing.
  - A player landing from a jump near the net may accidentally come down on an opponent's foot.
- Acute injuries
  - Ankle and finger sprains make up a majority of acute injuries.
  - Most acute injuries occur near the net.
  - Serious injuries requiring significant time away are rare.
- Overuse injuries
  - More common than acute injuries
  - Knee and shoulder injuries make up majority of overuse injuries
  - Patellar tendinitis is the most common
  - Occur more often in elite players because they spend more time doing drills than recreational players

GENERAL PRINCIPLES

Terminology

- Positions (see Table 73.1)
- Serve types
  - Float serve
    - The server immediately retracts the arm after hitting the ball.
    - This causes the ball to "float" through the air because it has no spin, making it hard to return, like a knuckleball.
  - Jump serve
    - The server gets a running start and then jumps high into the air, with the serve taking place at the top of the jump
    - Results in greater velocity and a sharp downward trajectory
- Dig
  - Pass of a ball that was spiked very hard
- Shank
  - When the ball goes in the wrong direction while attempting to pass

Equipment and Safety Issues

- Players often wear a long-sleeved jersey to allow for safer sliding on the court during dives and slides.
- Elbow and knee pads can be worn (Fig. 73.1).
- Padded pants can help prevent contusions to the greater trochanters, iliac crests, and anterior aspect of the knees.
- Sand socks can be worn during beach volleyball to protect the feet.
- Calling the balls (i.e., yelling "mine") helps reduce the chance of colliding with another player.

Rules

- Players are generally not allowed to cross the center line, as this can lead to injuries when a player comes down on an opponent's foot. The exception to the rule is doubles and beach volleyball.

COMMON INJURIES AND MEDICAL ISSUES

Foot and Ankle Injuries

Ankle Sprain

- Most common acute injury in volleyball, accounting for up to half of all acute injuries.
- Often occurs when a spiker or blocker lands from a jump around the net on another player's foot, causing an inversion injury.
- After first ankle sprain, player has increased incidence for recurrence.
- Ankle rehabilitation should focus on physical therapy emphasizing joint proprioception.
- Prevention
  - Wearing an ankle brace after an ankle sprain has been shown to reduce the incidence of recurrence in volleyball players.
  - Evidence suggests that preseason plyometric exercises, similar to those used to prevent anterior cruciate ligament (ACL) injuries, may help prevent ankle sprains.

Stress Fractures

- Most commonly involve metatarsal, navicular, and sesamoid bones.

Sand Toe

- Can occur during beach volleyball where shoes are not worn.
- Hyperplantarflexion injury to the first metatarsophalangeal joint.
- Increased pain with push-off, running, and jumping.
- Nonoperative treatment with toe strengthening, rest, ice, and anti-inflammatory medications. Need for surgical intervention is rare.

Wrist and Hand Injuries

Finger and Thumb Sprains, Fractures, and Dislocations

- Most common finger injuries are sprains and strains followed, in frequency, by fractures and contusions.
- Most acute finger injuries are the result of contact with the ball instead of contact with another player.
- When blocking, fingers are spread apart and vulnerable to injury from the ball or the opponent's hand (Fig. 73.2).
- If the fingers are below the ball while the player is attempting to block, they are prone to injury because of the downward trajectory of the ball onto the fingertips.
- Injuries may also occur when the fingers hit the net or another player during the follow-through phase of the swing.
- Injuries to thumb, index, and middle fingers are particularly bothersome for overhead setters because they use those three fingers to set.
- Prevention:
  - Appropriate blocking and hitting techniques may decrease the frequency of injury.
  - Keeping the fingers rigid during blocking can also help.

Table 73.1 INDOOR VOLLEYBALL

Position	Location on Court	Function	Injuries
Setter	Front court	Set ball to hitter	Wrist tendinitis Finger injuries
Hitter (spiker)	Front court	Spike ball into opposing court	Ankle sprains Shoulder instability/ impingement Spondylolysis Patellar tendinitis
Server (all players)	Back court	Serve ball	Shoulder instability/ impingement
Blocker	Front court	Block or alter ball hit by opponent	Finger injuries Ankle sprains Patellar tendinitis
Passer	Back court	Receive serve Pass ball to setter May need to dive for or "dig" ball	Contusions Injuries of upper extremities Patellofemoral syndrome Low back pain

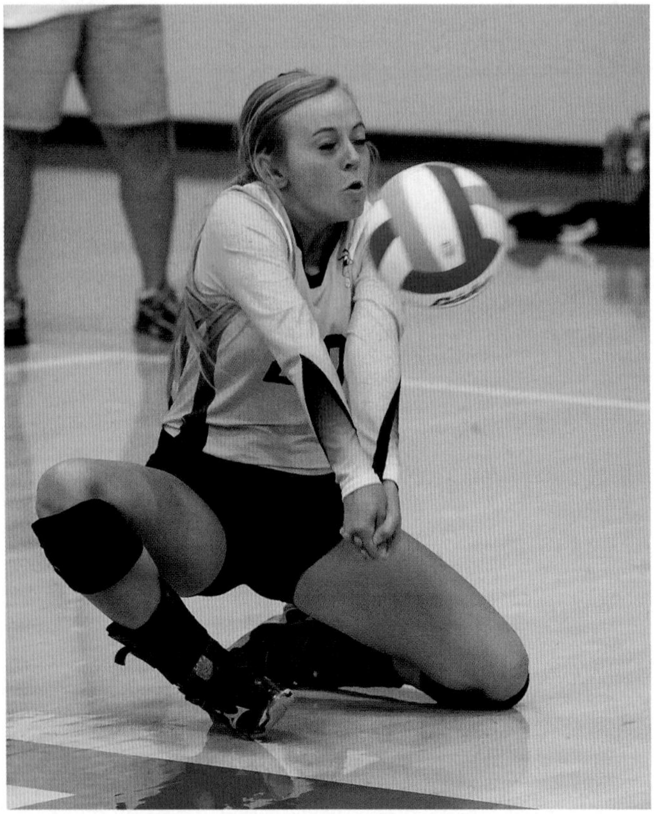

Figure 73.1 Prevention of injuries. Knee pads can offer protection when digging balls. (Copyright © P. Zivnuska 2016.)

Wrist Fractures

- From falling on outstretched hand when losing balance while coming down from a jump or tripping
- **Kienbock disease (idiopathic avascular necrosis of the lunate bone)**

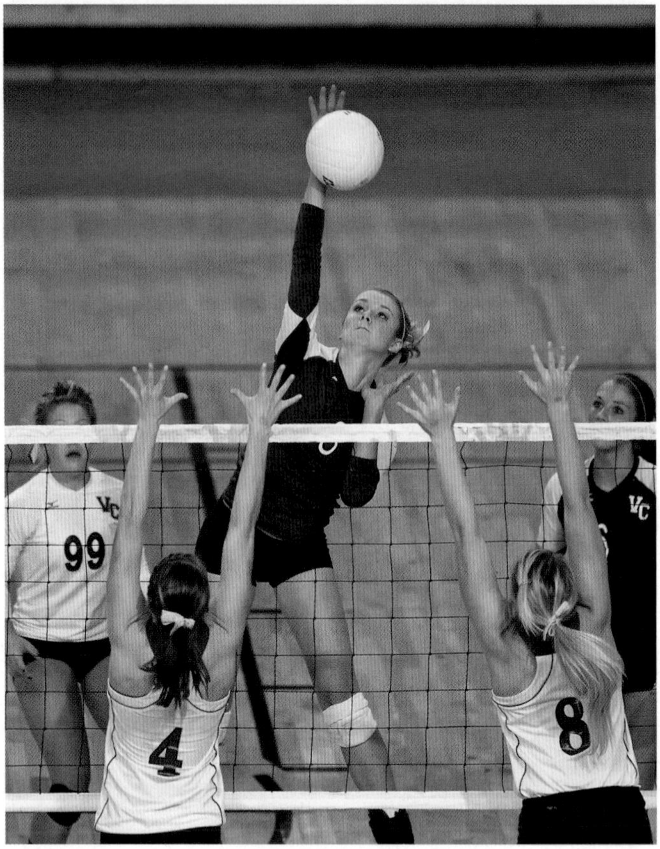

Blockers are prone to finger injuries from the ball.

Figure 73.2 Finger and thumb sprains. (Copyright © P. Zivnuska 2016.)

- In volleyball players, repetitive wrist trauma is a likely contributing factor

Wrist Tendinitis

- In overhead setters who frequently use wrists

de Quervain Tenosynovitis

- When passing, the ball is supposed to hit the fleshy part of the forearm. If the ball instead repeatedly impacts the radial aspects of the wrists, not only does the ball shank but tenosynovitis can develop as well.

Neuritis of the Superficial Branch of the Radial Nerve

- From repeated ball impact to dorsoradial aspect of distal forearm
- Decreased sensation and paresthesias over the dorsoradial hand
- Treatment involves improving technique so ball impacts more proximally on the forearms

Shoulder Injuries

Shoulder Instability

- During the early acceleration phase of hitting and serving, the arm is in extreme extension and external rotation (Fig. 73.3). During these maneuvers, the humeral head is levered anteriorly in the glenoid, which can lead to shoulder pain.
- Rotator cuff impingement and tendinitis may occur.
- Jump serving places higher loads on the shoulder than the traditional overhead serve or float serve.
- Treatment involves strengthening of the rotator cuff.

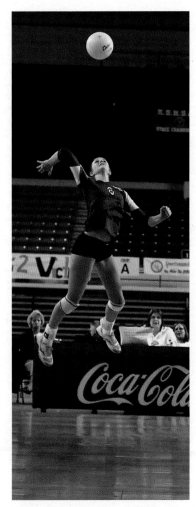
Coca-Cola

Extreme external rotation and extension during hitting can cause shoulder problems due to anterior instability and overuse of the rotator cuff.

Figure 73.3 Shoulder injuries. (Copyright © P. Zivnuska 2016.)

Internal Impingement

- When the humeral head translates anteriorly during hitting and serving, the articular side of the rotator cuff and labrum can become impinged at the posterosuperior aspect of the glenohumeral joint.
- Pain at the posterior shoulder.
- May lead to tearing of the rotator cuff and labrum.
- Treatment involves strengthening the rotator cuff and stretching the posterior capsule if tight.

Glenohumeral Internal Rotation Deficit (GIRD)

- Seen in hitters and servers.
- Have decreased internal rotation of the shoulder resulting from contracture of the posterior capsule; this results in obligatory posterosuperior shift in the humeral head during arm elevation.
- Associated with various shoulder problems such as internal impingement, external impingement, and tears of the labrum and rotator cuff.
- Treated with rest, stretches of the posterior capsule (sleeper stretches), and periscapular strengthening.

Suprascapular Neuropathy

Description: In most people, irritation of the suprascapular nerve (C5, C6) occurs at the suprascapular notch, but in volleyball

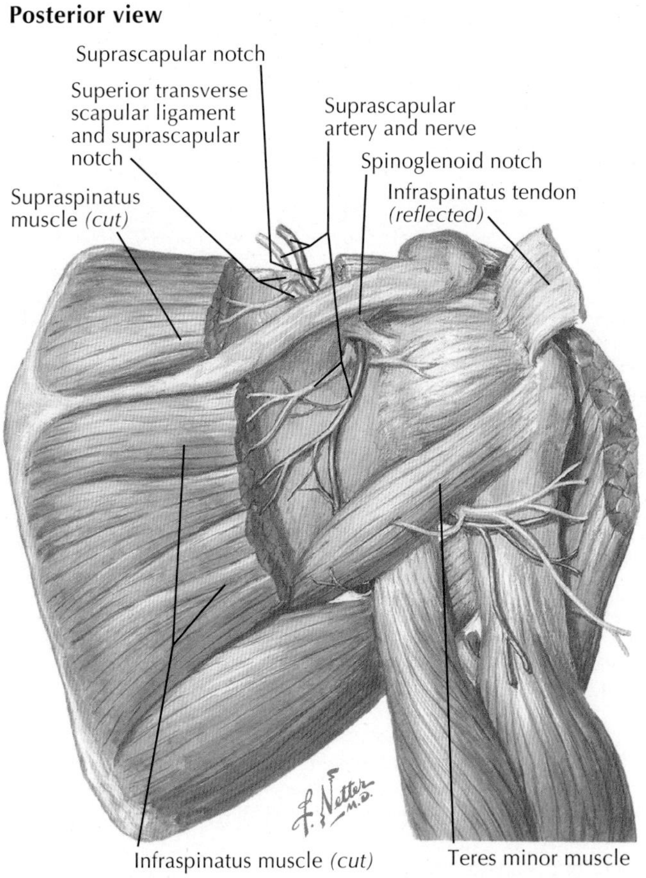
Posterior view
Suprascapular notch
Superior transverse scapular ligament and suprascapular notch
Suprascapular artery and nerve
Spinoglenoid notch
Infraspinatus tendon (reflected)
Supraspinatus muscle (cut)
Infraspinatus muscle (cut)
Teres minor muscle
F. Netter M.D.

Figure 73.4 Suprascapular nerve traversing the spinoglenoid notch, where it can be entrapped.

players, it occurs more distally at the spinoglenoid notch (Fig. 73.4). This leads to atrophy of the infraspinatus muscle and weakness of external rotation.

Mechanism of injury: Thought to occur from traction and/or compression of the nerve while serving and hitting because of the extreme position of the arm during the cocking phase or with the arm swing during the follow-through phase. Float serves require forceful eccentric contraction of the infraspinatus muscle to stop the arm, potentially creating a traction force on the nerve.

Incidence: Occurs in the dominant upper extremity in 12%–30% of high-level volleyball players.

History: Occasionally may cause posterior shoulder pain, but usually asymptomatic. Athletes are still able to play at a high level; proposed reasons for why it does not usually bother the athlete:

- Nerve lesion is usually incomplete, so certain functions of the muscle remain.
- Teres minor muscle, which is innervated by a branch of the axillary nerve, compensates.
- External rotation strength is much less important for performance in volleyball than is internal rotation.

Physical examination: Varying degrees of atrophy of the infraspinatus muscle along the posterior scapula (Fig. 73.5), weakness with external rotation, and some athletes may have point tenderness over the spinoglenoid notch. Supraspinatus muscle strength is normal.

Diagnostic considerations: Electromyography (EMG) and nerve conduction study (NCS) can usually confirm the diagnosis, but not necessary in most cases; if an athlete is not improving and is symptomatic, consider radiographs to check for a bony lesion

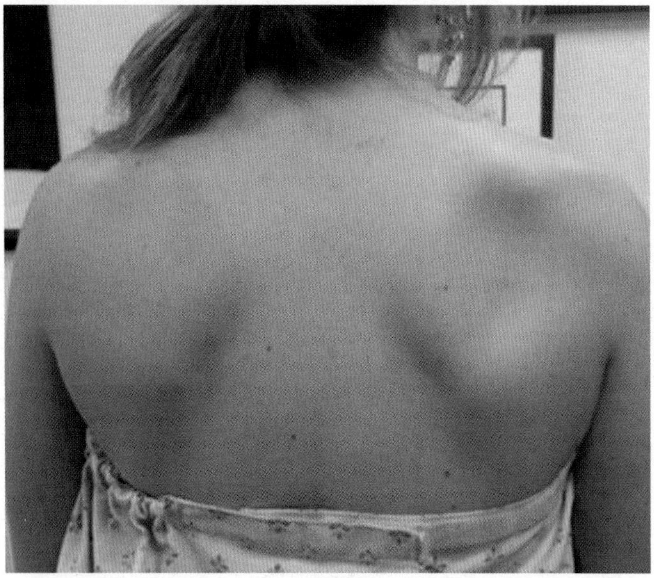

Figure 73.5 Atrophy of the infraspinatus muscle along the posterior scapula (Reused with permission from Plancher KD, Petterson SC. Posterior shoulder pain and arthroscopic decompression of the suprascapular nerve at the spinoglenoid notch. *Oper Tech Sports Med.* 2014;22[1]:73–87, Fig. 9, © K. Plancher.)

compressing the nerve (Bennett lesion) or magnetic resonance imaging (MRI) to check a space-occupying lesion (ganglion) compressing the nerve; differential diagnosis of infraspinatus atrophy:

- Infraspinatus tendon tear
- Brachial neuritis affecting the suprascapular nerve

Treatment (if symptomatic):

- **Nonsurgical treatment**
  - Restricting overhead hitting
  - Nonsteroidal anti-inflammatory medications
  - Physical therapy to strengthen the rotator cuff and periscapular muscles, improve posture, and stretch posterior capsule, if tight
  - Repeat EMG at 6 months, if performed initially, to assess recovery
  - If patient is not improving or has significant initial disability, consider obtaining an MRI
- **Surgical treatment**
  - Possible indications
    - Significant pain and decreased performance despite 6 months of nonsurgical treatment
    - Space-occupying lesion (cyst) compressing the nerve
  - Is rarely needed
  - Surgical procedure involves spinoglenoid ligament release with nerve decompression.

Prognosis/return to play: Most symptomatic cases respond to nonsurgical treatment, but may take up to a year for maximal recovery; an exception is a space-occupying lesion compressing the nerve, which often will not resolve without surgery. Although pain usually improves with nonsurgical or surgical treatment, muscle atrophy may not resolve. Most athletes are able to return to full function despite the persistent atrophy.

Lumbosacral Spine Injuries

Mechanical Low Back Pain

- Passers are susceptible because of repetitive lumbar flexion with arms held in front of the body (Fig. 73.6).
- Jumping positions are also susceptible because repeated landing places high forces on the spine.

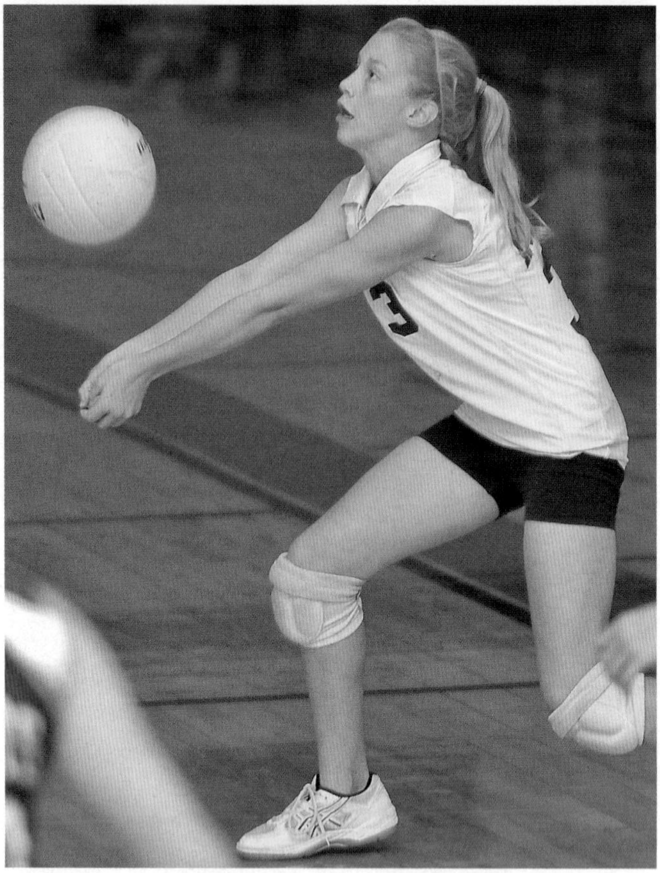

Repetitive flexion of the lumbosacral spine in under hand passing can lead to low back pain.

Figure 73.6 Lumbosacral spine injuries. (Copyright © P. Zivnuska 2016.)

Spondylolysis

- A stress fracture at the pars interarticularis of the vertebra, most commonly of the fifth lumbar vertebra.
- Occurs with repetitive hyperextension of the low back, most commonly associated with hitting (Fig. 73.7) but also with overhead setting and blocking.

Knee Injuries

Patellar Tendinitis (Jumper's Knee)

- Most common overuse injury of the knee in volleyball
  - Affects approximately 50% of elite players
- The result of repetitive eccentric quadriceps contraction with jumping (blockers or hitters)
- Usually an insidious onset with pain localized over the patellar tendon

Patellofemoral Syndrome

- Particularly common in volleyball positions that require jumping and squatting (hitting, blocking, and passing).

Anterior Cruciate Ligament Tear

- Occurs more frequently in female volleyball players than in male players.
- Reconstruction is usually required if return to a sport such as volleyball is desired.
- Preseason proprioceptive and plyometric training programs can significantly reduce the incidence of ACL tears in women.

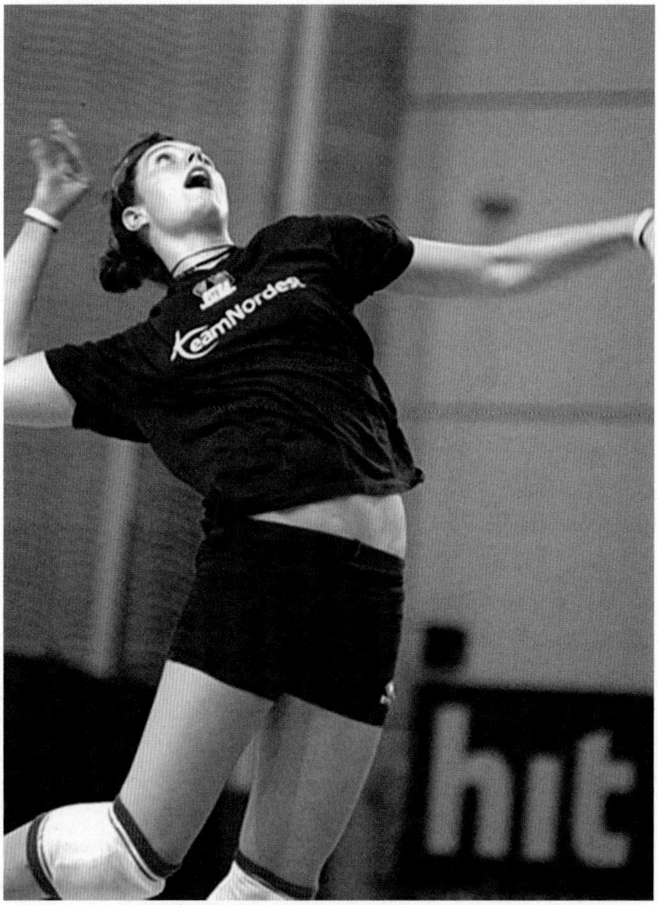
hit

Figure 73.7 Lumbar hyperextension with hitting.

Medial Collateral Ligament Tear

- From valgus force to the knee as a result of landing off balance

Meniscus Injuries

- Volleyball requires pivoting and rapid changes in direction, which can lead to meniscal tears

Leg Injuries

Tibial Stress Fracture

- May be found in positions requiring frequent jumping

Gastrocnemius Muscle Strain

- Associated with an eccentric load to the muscle–tendon unit

Achilles Tendon Problems

- **Acute Achilles rupture**
  - The result of rapid, forceful eccentric loading of the tendon when landing from a jump or from sudden acceleration
- **Achilles tendinitis**
  - The result of repetitive eccentric loads from jumping
- **Achilles tendinosis**
  - Degeneration and microtearing of the Achilles tendon at its insertion to the calcaneus

Concussion

- Can occur from impacting the head against the pole, the floor, or being hit by a player's arm

Heat Illness

- Can occur with beach volleyball during hot conditions

RECOMMENDED READINGS

Available online.

74 BASEBALL

William G. Raasch • Taurean G. Baynard

GENERAL OVERVIEW

- Baseball, the great American pastime, was first described by Abner Doubleday in 1839.
- Shoulder and elbow problems became a familiar part of the game in the 1880s with the advent of overhand pitching.
- Although ballplayers suffer the usual sports-related strains and sprains, it is in understanding common shoulder and elbow throwing injuries that the baseball team physician is defined.

THROWING BIOMECHANICS AND ASSOCIATED PATHOLOGY

- Throwing is all about the transfer of energy from the body to the ball. A smooth transition will maximize ball velocity while reducing the risk of injury.
- Injury anywhere along the kinetic chain (e.g., ankle sprain, hip labral tear) may result in decreased performance and injury down the chain.
- The mechanics of throwing can be separated into five phases (Fig. 74.1).
  - Because certain structures are susceptible to injury during each phase of throwing, determining the phase in which injury or pain occurs may help make a diagnosis.

Windup

- Varies from pitcher to pitcher.
- Description:
  - Begins from set position with ball in pitcher's glove.
  - Arms drop and body rotates 90 degrees (see Fig. 74.1).
  - Stride leg is elevated and flexed.
  - Provides rhythm and balance.
- Injury risk: minimal

Stride

- Description:
  - Begins when supporting leg flexes, lowering body.
  - Stride leg moves toward plate. Stride length averages 75% of body height, with an offset of 0.4 cm (i.e., lead foot lands almost directly in front of back foot).
  - Trunk remains back.
- Injury risk:
  - Stride too long: athlete will be unable to rotate hips, resulting in a loss of velocity. This is known as "arm throwing." Pitcher may compensate by overloading shoulder; may result in rotator cuff strain.
  - Stride off line to first base side (right-handed pitcher): torso will be ahead of shoulder, resulting in "opening" too soon and stressing the anterior capsule; may result in shoulder instability.
  - Stride off line to third base side (right-handed pitcher): "throwing across body" may result in labral shearing.
  - Altered stride may be a sign of hip contracture or hip labral pathology. Physical examination is required to assess overall range of motion and to rule out femoral acetabular impingement.

Cocking

- Places arm in maximum external rotation while abducted.
- Description:
  - Begins when stride foot makes contact with mound.
  - Hip rotation begins, followed by the trunk (speed of hip rotation correlates well with ball velocity).
  - Ends when shoulder reaches maximum external rotation.
  - External rotation in professional pitchers may approach 180 degrees.
- Injury risk:
  - When shoulder is in maximum external rotation and 90 degrees of abduction, internal impingement may occur: undersurface of superior rotator cuff impinges against posterior/superior labrum. This may result in undersurface tearing of rotator cuff and posterior/superior labrum fraying.
  - Anterior capsule stretching may occur over time and result in increased anterior/inferior laxity and possible glenohumeral instability (see Fig. 74.1).

Acceleration

- Generates ball velocity.
- Description:
  - Begins with initiation of shoulder internal rotation.
  - Ends with ball release.
- Injury risk:
  - Primary movers and stabilizers of shoulder are stressed by rapid acceleration that occurs (internal rotation velocity goes from 0 to 7000 degrees per second in less than one-tenth of a second).
  - Rotator cuff strain—primary stabilizer.
  - Latissimus dorsi, teres major strain—internal rotation and adduction.
  - Labral injury if humeral head does not remain centered during rapid acceleration. Risk is increased with cuff fatigue and subsequent loss of dynamic centering of the head.
  - Elbow is placed under significant valgus stress—ulnar collateral ligament (UCL) is under tension while the radiocapitellar articulation is under compression. Thus, UCL is at risk of tearing, and radiocapitellar articulation is at risk for osteochondral injury.
  - Valgus extension overload: as elbow extends under valgus load, posteromedial olecranon may impinge against olecranon fossa, resulting in posteromedial elbow pain. Over time, spurring and degenerative changes may occur at posteromedial ulnohumeral articulation (see Fig. 74.1).

Deceleration

- Dissipation of energy as ball is released.
- Shoulder undergoes a distraction force equal to body weight
- Description:
  - Begins at ball release.
  - Final elbow extension occurs.
  - Final shoulder internal rotation occurs.
  - Ends when internal rotation velocity reaches zero.
- Injury risk:
  - Superior labrum anterior to posterior (SLAP) lesion: traction injury to superior labrum at long head of the biceps tendon insertion.
  - Bennett lesion: traction osteophyte of posterior glenoid lip with thickening of posterior labrum and capsular attachment resulting from repetitive traction.

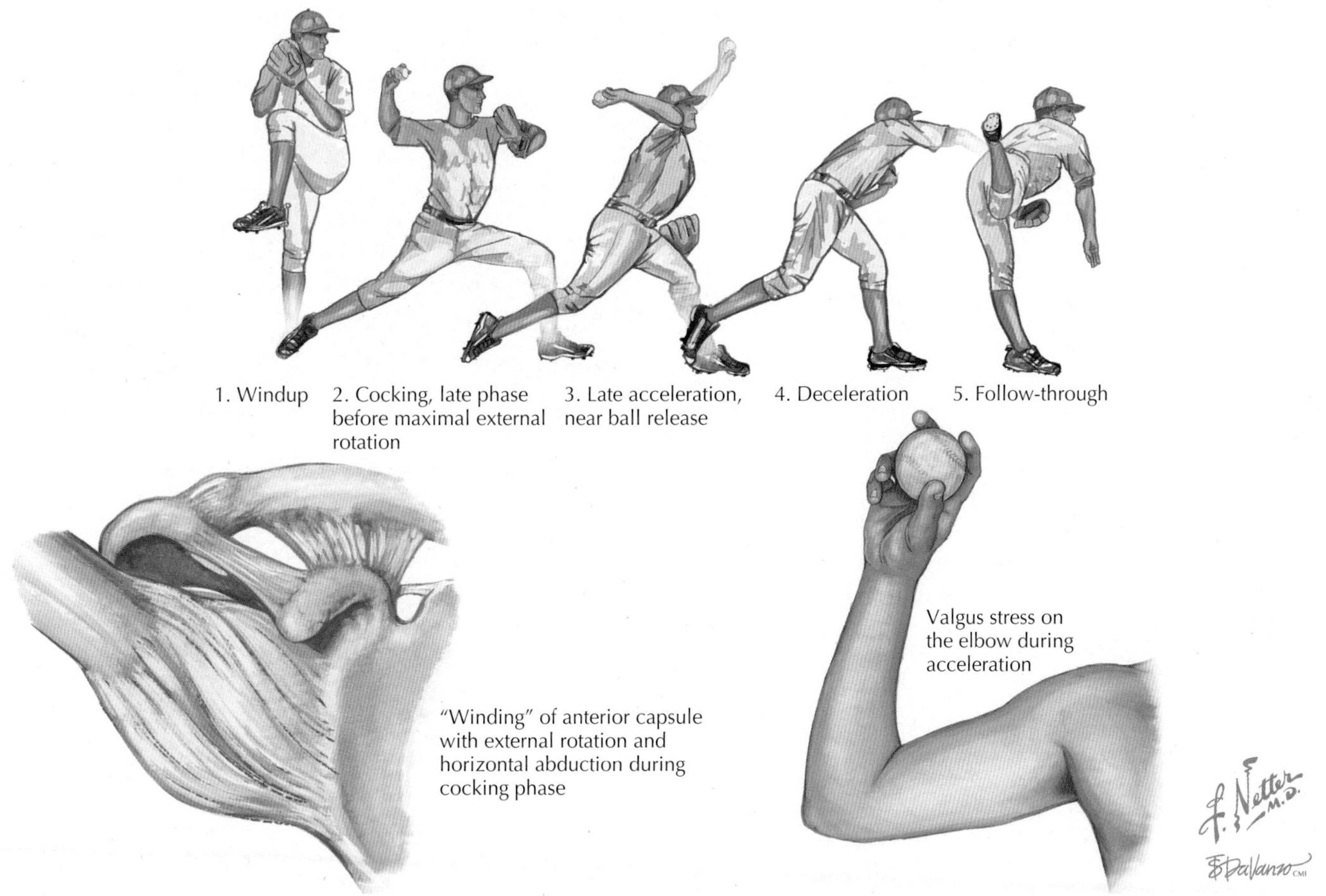
1. Windup
2. Cocking, late phase before maximal external rotation
3. Late acceleration, near ball release
4. Deceleration
5. Follow-through
"Winding" of anterior capsule with external rotation and horizontal abduction during cocking phase
Valgus stress on the elbow during acceleration

Figure 74.1 Phases of the overhead throw.

Follow-Through

- Allows for dissipation of energy
- Description:
  - Begins at end of shoulder internal rotation.
  - Ends when trailing leg touches the ground.
- Injury risk:
  - A proper follow-through reduces injury risk by gradual dissipation of the body's kinetic energy.

COMMON BASEBALL THROWING INJURIES

- Overhead throwing motion results in preponderance of upper extremity injuries because of the significant forces generated.
- Underhanded pitching motion (e.g., fast-pitch softball) is typically not associated with significant overuse injury because it creates less stress on the shoulder and elbow structures. However, variations in throwing mechanics used to create more ball movement subject the UCL to greater stress and increased injury risk.

Shoulder

Rotator Cuff Injury

Description: The rotator cuff is key to a healthy throwing shoulder, centering and controlling the humeral head as the arm accelerates. With weakness, the cuff may impinge against the acromial arch, the capsule may stretch, or the labrum may tear (Fig. 74.2). With subsequent labral and capsular injury, loss of proprioception may occur, resulting in diminished cuff function and creating a cycle of injury (Fig. 74.3). With extreme external

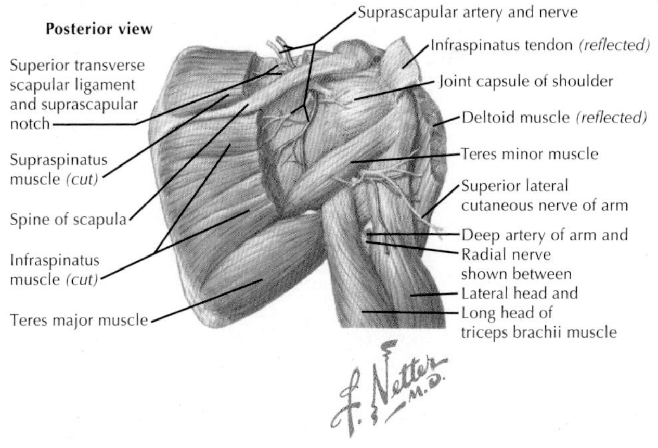
Posterior view
Suprascapular artery and nerve
Infraspinatus tendon (reflected)
Superior transverse scapular ligament and suprascapular notch
Joint capsule of shoulder
Deltoid muscle (reflected)
Supraspinatus muscle (cut)
Teres minor muscle
Superior lateral cutaneous nerve of arm
Spine of scapula
Deep artery of arm and
Radial nerve
shown between
Infraspinatus muscle (cut)
Lateral head and
Long head of
triceps brachii muscle
Teres major muscle

Figure 74.2 Rotator cuff anatomy.

rotation and abduction during cocking and early acceleration, undersurface tearing may occur. Rotator cuff injury should be at the top of the differential diagnosis for throwing discomfort.

Symptoms: Pain often referred to the lateral shoulder. Posterior/superior shoulder pain with arm in cocking position suggests internal impingement with possible undersurface cuff tear.

Diagnosis:

- Pain and/or weakness with resisted external rotation with elbow at side.
- Positive Jobe sign: pain from rotator cuff isometric contracture

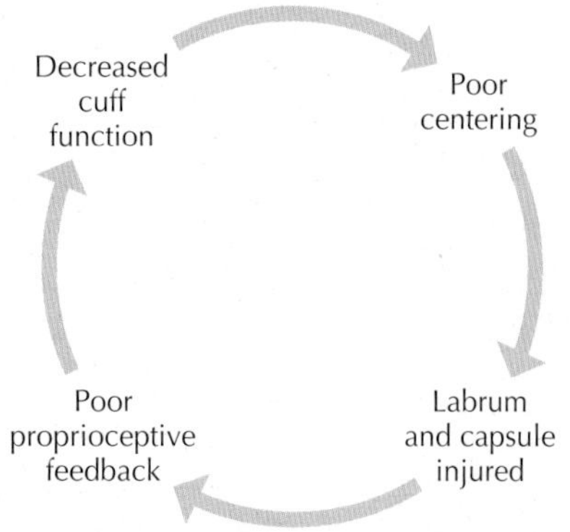
Decreased
cuff
function
Poor
centering
Labrum
and capsule
injured
Poor
proprioceptive
feedback

Figure 74.3 Cycle of injury. With decreased cuff function because of injury or fatigue, poor centering of the humeral head in the glenoid occurs, resulting in compression or tension to the labral and capsule and possible injury. With loss of labral and capsular proprioceptive feedback, the cuff's function is further diminished and the cycle continues. Note that the cycle may also begin with an acute injury to the labrum.

- Positive Hawkins sign: subacromial impingement of bursal side of cuff against acromial arch
- Pain with extreme abduction/external rotation: internal impingement of articular surface of the cuff against posterior/superior labrum
- Magnetic resonance imaging (MRI) to define extent of injury when nonsurgical management fails. History and physical examination directs initial treatment. MRI should be considered a presurgical study. When MRI is ordered, consider contrast to better define partial-thickness undersurface tears or associated labral pathology. The ABER view (shoulder abducted and externally rotated) is helpful to define posterior, superior labral, and undersurface cuff tears. MRI findings must correlate with physical examination and history, as there is a high incidence of degenerative labral and undersurface rotator cuff pathology present in asymptomatic throwing athletes.

Treatment:
- Relative rest: varies from complete shutdown of all throwing activity to shifting player's position (e.g., playing first base instead of pitching).
- Physical therapy
  - Rotator cuff strengthening
    - TheraBands with elbow at side
    - Advance to pulleys with arm in throwing position (e.g., shoulder abducted 90 degrees with arm internally rotating against resistance from 90 degrees of external rotation to neutral position).
    - High repetitions (30) with single set
    - Plyometrics before trial of throwing
  - Scapular stabilization: must rule out scapular dyskinesis
  - Posterior capsular stretch: must rule out tight posterior capsule
- Cortisone injection: subacromial for bursal-sided rotator cuff fraying and intra-articular for articular-sided undersurface partial tears
  - Only after failure to respond to physical therapy
  - Avoid activities using the shoulder for 5 days after injection
- Surgery if nonsurgical management fails
  - Arthroscopic debridement for partial-thickness tears
  - Arthroscopic or open repair for significant partial tears greater than 50%. Poor outcomes for return to pitching when rotator cuff requires repair.

Labral Injury

Description: Superior/posterior labrum can be injured by impingement during cocking phase or through distraction of biceps anchor during deceleration (i.e., tension from long head of biceps can pull labral attachment). The classic superior labral tear (type II SLAP) often seen in pitchers may be considered an adaptive change that allows for increased external rotation during cocking. With greater extension of tear posteriorly, limited surgical repair becomes a treatment option.

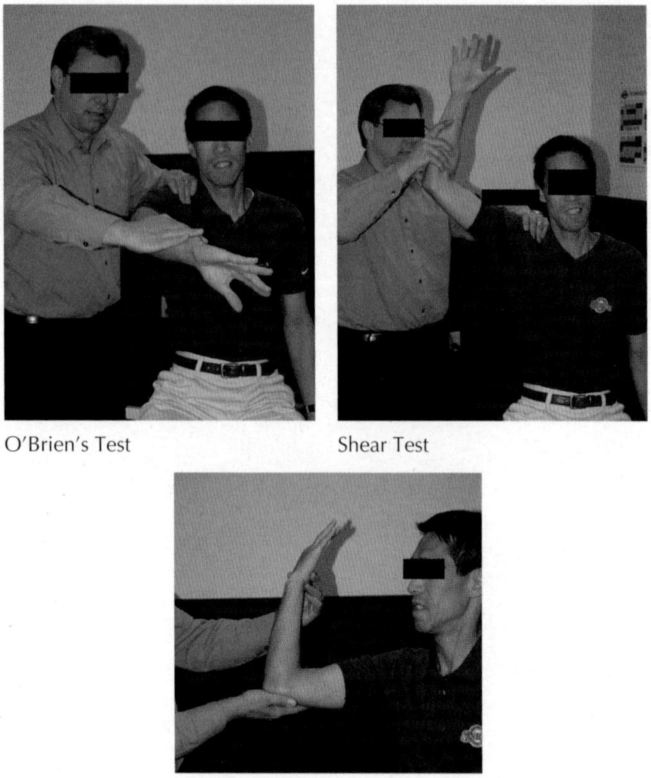
O'Brien's Test
Shear Test
Milking maneuver

Figure 74.4 Elbow examination tests.

Symptoms: Deep shoulder joint pain with throwing; typically not a problem with daily activities; pain is often positional and is not present at rest

Diagnosis: Positive provocative maneuvers with triggered pain located deep in shoulder joint (Fig. 74.4):
- O'Brien test: Pain while resisting downward force with arm extended in neutral position, horizontally adducted 30 degrees, and thumb pointing down.
- Shear: Pain with manipulation of shoulder in 90 degrees of abduction and maximal external rotation.
- Rotation/compression: McMurray of the shoulder—compress and rotate shoulder in an attempt to pinch labrum and trigger pain.

Treatment:
- Physical therapy
  - Correct anything that may increase the chance of labral pinching
  - Rotator cuff strengthening
  - Scapular stabilization
  - Posterior capsular stretch (with loss of internal rotation)
- Arthroscopic labral debridement or repair when nonsurgical management fails

Capsular Injury

CAPSULAR LAXITY

Description: Capsule may stretch anteriorly, resulting in anterior translation of the humeral head. Laxity itself is not the issue, but rather the inability to control the laxity that results in symptomatic instability. Although the rotator cuff is the primary stabilizer, the capsule will provide static stability at extremes of motion (e.g., cocking phase) and provides proprioceptive feedback.

Symptoms: Sensation of shoulder slipping, loss of velocity and control, tired arm (dead arm syndrome with subluxation)

Diagnosis: Made through history. Laxity is confirmed by physical examination: load and shift maneuver demonstrates laxity and apprehension with translation. Crepitation during load and shift maneuver may indicate labral injury.

Treatment: Control laxity by improving rotator cuff function with strengthening and proprioceptive training. Surgery with capsular placation for refractory cases with understanding that if shoulder is made too tight, return to throwing is at risk.

GLENOHUMERAL INTERNAL ROTATION DEFICIT (GIRD)

Description: During deceleration phase, posterior capsule is tensioned. With repetitive trauma to posterior capsule, thickening and contracture may occur. This is manifested by loss of internal rotation. With tight posterior capsule, humeral head translates anterior and superior, resulting in cuff impingement and possible superior labral injury. Check for loss of internal rotation whenever rotator cuff impingement symptoms are present. A traction osteophyte arising from posterior capsular attachment on the glenoid is known as a *Bennett lesion.*

Symptoms: Deep posterior shoulder pain; anterior lateral cuff pain secondary to impingement

Diagnosis: Examination reveals loss of internal rotation:

- Measurement is taken with arm abducted 90 degrees in scapular plane.
- Loss of ≥20 degrees (of total arc of motion, rather than isolated loss of internal rotation) is typically symptomatic. Must account for usual shift in rotation of throwing shoulder with entire range of motion shifted in external rotation.

Treatment: Physical therapy with stretching of posterior capsule includes adduction of arm across chest and internal rotation with arm abducted 90 degrees (sleeper stretch); surgical release in refractory cases—rarely required.

Scapular Dyskinesis

Description: Scapula is the anchor for arm during throwing motion. Incorrect scapular position or rhythm may lead to shoulder injury (e.g., cuff impingement, labral pinching).

Symptoms: Anterolateral cuff impingement pain, deep anterior shoulder discomfort, pain along scapular posterior/medial border.

Diagnosis: Physical examination reveals dyskinetic scapula.

- View patient from behind.
- Observe for differences in shoulder blade height and rotation.
- Observe for scapular winging when bringing arm down from forward elevated position.

Treatment: Physical therapy with scapular stabilization program.

Latissimus Dorsi/Teres Major Strain

Description: Strain at attachment site of proximal third of latissimus dorsi and teres major. May fail at bony insertion as the tendons become joined. Often misdiagnosed injury.

Symptoms: Pain localized to posterior inferior shoulder. May vary from complete avulsion to minor strain.

Treatment: Usually physical therapy; surgery is considered for complete avulsion of both the latissimus and teres major as anatomic variations with both tendons blending together before insertion may be present.

Elbow

- Valgus moment is produced with throwing; the UCL is stretched and the radial capitellar articulation compressed (Fig. 74.5).
- Valgus extension overload syndrome occurs from compression of the posteromedial ulnohumeral articulation that occurs with elbow extension under valgus stress (see Fig. 74.1).

Ulnar Collateral Ligament Sprain

Description: Valgus stress with throwing approaches ligament strength; may fail with single throw or attenuate over time; common flexors protect ligament.

Diagnosis:

- History of acute "pop" on medial side of elbow associated with acute complete rupture. Chronic medial-sided throwing pain with gradual ligament degeneration.
- Pain over UCL with palpation.
- Pain, increased laxity, and/or soft endpoint with valgus stress of the elbow in 20 to 30 degrees of flexion
- Pain with "milking maneuver" (valgus stress applied with elbow flexed 90 degrees and forearm in maximum pronation (see Fig. 74.5).
- Pain with moving valgus stress (same as milking maneuver but through a range of motion)
- With increased laxity, traction to ulnar nerve may occur, resulting in cubital tunnel syndrome—numbness in ulnar two digits of the hand.
- MRI with contrast to confirm the injury.

Treatment:

- Complete tear in a pitcher: UCL reconstruction ("Tommy John" procedure).
- UCL repair with internal brace when an avulsion is present.
- Partial tears:
  - Acute partial tear more likely to respond to nonsurgical management. Distal partial tears are less likely to respond to nonsurgical management compared with proximal tears.
  - Cessation of throwing for 6 weeks while emphasizing common flexor strengthening.
  - Plyometrics before throwing program.
    - Involves bouncing (and catching) weighted ball against angled trampoline with injured arm. This provides proprioceptive training while subjecting soft tissue to a ballistic load in preparation for throwing.
  - Progressive throwing program.

Common Flexor Strain

Description: Dynamic medial stabilizer for the elbow. Must differentiate from UCL sprain.

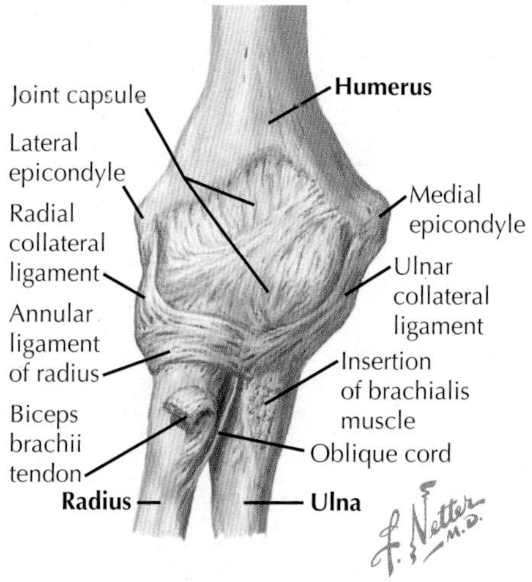
Right elbow: anterior view
Joint capsule
Humerus
Lateral epicondyle
Radial collateral ligament
Medial epicondyle
Ulnar collateral ligament
Annular ligament of radius
Insertion of brachialis muscle
Biceps brachii tendon
Oblique cord
Radius
Ulna
F. Netter M.D.

Figure 74.5 Anatomy of the elbow.

Diagnosis: Pain anterior and lateral to medial epicondyle, not over UCL; pain with resisted wrist flexion/pronation; negative milking maneuver.

Treatment: Activity restriction is important to prevent subsequent injury to UCL. Pain with throwing should not be allowed. Physical therapy with gentle common wrist flexor strengthening as symptoms allow. Transition to progressive throwing program after initial course of plyometric exercises. With significant common flexor tears and failed nonsurgical management, surgical repair may be considered.

Articular Surface Injury

Description: With elbow under valgus stress while in extension, the posteromedial aspect of the olecranon will grind against the medial olecranon fossa. This can lead to arthritis with spurring. Load can be increased with UCL laxity. With valgus stress, the radiocapitellar joint is under compression, which may lead to early articular wear.

Diagnosis:
- Posterior medial pain with throwing
- Discomfort and possible crepitation with valgus stress with extension
- MRI confirms extent of chondral injury and rules out UCL injury

Treatment:
- Rest, nonsteroidal anti-inflammatory drugs (NSAIDs), cortisone injection
- Treat any underlying UCL laxity
- Arthroscopic debridement

Olecranon Stress Fracture

Description: Repetitive loading of elbow with pitching may result in an olecranon stress fracture

Diagnosis:
- Discomfort along medial olecranon with throwing
  - Discomfort is poorly localized; negative milking maneuver
- UCL laxity may be a contributing factor
- MRI to confirm diagnosis

Treatment: Rest with no throwing, typically 4–6 weeks; consider intramedullary screw fixation for failed or recurrent stress fracture

Ulnar Nerve Neuropathy/Instability

Description: With valgus stress at elbow, the ulnar nerve can develop traction neuritis at the cubital tunnel. UCL laxity may contribute to the symptoms, and injury to UCL must be ruled out with ulnar nerve symptoms. Ulnar nerve subluxation may occur during pitching. The pitcher will experience a "zinger" down forearm with the subluxation.

Diagnosis:
- Dysesthesias in the ulnar two digits
- Tinel sign at the cubital tunnel
- Palpable subluxation of ulnar nerve perched on posterior aspect of the medial epicondyle with elbow in maximum flexion
- Nerve conduction velocities may be used to confirm diagnosis
- Must rule out UCL laxity as source of traction on nerve

Treatment:
- NSAIDs
- Night splinting
- Ulnar nerve transposition when nonsurgical management fails
- UCL reconstruction when laxity results in traction neuritis

Hand

Finger Flexor Pulley Injuries

Description: Traumatic rupture of middle finger A4 pulley because of repetitive extension force placed on finger during fastball pitch

Diagnosis:
- Tenderness to palpation over A4 pulley
- Pain with resisted finger flexion
- Dynamic ultrasound documents displacement with bowing of tendon
- MRI confirms pathology with volar subluxation of flexor tendon

Treatment:
- Two weeks rest with optional splinting
- Interval throwing program after rest
- Six to twelve weeks for full return to play

COMMON BASEBALL BATTING INJURIES

Batter's shoulder: Posterior subluxation of the lead shoulder while swinging the bat. Typically occurs when batter reaches out for a low-and-away pitch resulting in traction injury to posterior labral-capsular structure. Initially treated with rest followed by rotator cuff strengthening and proprioceptive training emphasizing dynamic control. MRI evaluation is considered with failure of initial management and before surgical repair of labrum if symptoms persist.

Anterior shoulder subluxation: With batting swing follow-through, the lead arm may end in an extremely abducted, externally rotated position. This especially occurs during a one-arm follow-through where the back hand releases the bat, placing all the decelerating force on a single shoulder. The bat weight combined with the significant bat speed generated during swing may result in injury to the anterior labrum and capsule. Initial treatment consists of rest, rotator cuff strengthening, and proprioceptive training. If nonsurgical treatment fails, MRI with subsequent arthroscopic labral repair may be indicated. Risk of reinjury may be reduced by keeping the back hand on the bat during follow-through.

Contusion/fracture: Baseballs weigh 5 ounces; Major League pitchers can throw the ball at up to 100 mph; when batter is hit by pitch or fouls off, a ball injury may occur. Hand, wrist, or forearm fractures may occur from direct impact by thrown ball. Foot fractures occur from indirect impact from ball fouled off bat.

Extensor carpi ulnaris subluxation: Typically occurs when wrist rolls over while swinging bat (i.e., ulnar deviation with forearm in pronation). Pain over extensor carpi ulnaris tendon at distal ulna. Subluxation may be reproduced with resisted forearm pronation while positioned in ulnar deviation. Acute injuries may respond to cast immobilization, but more often surgical repair/reconstruction of tendon sheath is necessary.

Hook of the hamate fracture: Hook of the hamate fractures occur when hook makes contact with nub of the bat during bat swing. May occur with single swing or as a result of repetitive trauma resulting in a stress fracture. Pain is located over hypothenar eminence. Hand radiographs, including carpal tunnel profile view, may provide diagnosis. Computed tomography (CT) will confirm diagnosis. MRI for stress fracture may be required. Excision is required with fracture.

Digital neuroma at ulnar base of thumb: Neuroma develops secondary to repetitive compression and impact from a bat handle. Dysesthesias over ulnar aspect of thumb with radiating discomfort. Tinel sign is often present on examination, and palpable nodular thickening of the nerve may be present. Initial treatment consists of rest, NSAIDs, and additional padding of batting glove. Cortisone injection may be used when padding is ineffective. Cryotherapy and surgical nerve transposition are options when previous treatments have failed.

Concussion/facial fractures: See Chapter 45: "Head Injuries" and Chapter 48: "Maxillofacial Injuries."

Table 74.1 LITTLE LEAGUE REST REQUIREMENTS

Age ≤16 Years	• If a player pitches ≥61 pitches/day, 3 calendar days of rest and a game must be observed. • If a player pitches 41–60 pitches/day, 2 calendar days of rest and a game must be observed. • If a player pitches 21–40 pitches/day, 1 calendar day of rest must be observed.
Age 17–18 Years	• If a player pitches ≥76 pitches/day, 3 calendar days of rest and a game must be observed. • If a player pitches 51–75 pitches/day, 2 calendar days of rest and a game must be observed. • If a player pitches 26–51 pitches/day, 1 calendar day of rest must be observed. • If a player pitches 1–25 pitches/day, no rest is required.

INJURIES UNIQUE TO YOUTH BASEBALL

Overview

- Skeletally immature athlete may incur injury to growth plates instead of the ligaments or capsule because the body will fail at the weakest site.
- Whenever evaluating a growth plate, comparison views are mandatory, using the nonthrowing extremity as a control.
- In an effort to reduce the risk of throwing injuries, Little League Baseball has instituted pitching limits based on pitch count, required rest, and age of the pitcher.

Little League Pitching Limits

- Age 17–18: 105 pitches/day
- Age 13–16: 95 pitches/day
- Age 11–12: 85 pitches/day
- Age 9–10: 75 pitches/day
- Age 7–8: 50 pitches/day
- **Exceptions:** Pitcher may continue to pitch until the current batter in which the limit is reached is put out or reaches base. A pitcher who delivers one or more pitches in a game cannot play the position of catcher for the remainder of that day.

Rest Requirements

See Table 74.1.

Common Injuries

Little Leaguer's Elbow (Medial Epicondyle Physical Injury)

- UCL is stronger than the epicondylar physis.
- May be acute or chronic injury. Acute injury represents avulsion fracture of growth plate with displacement. Chronic injury will show a widened physis on radiographs.
- Pain over medial epicondyle with pitching and palpation.
- Medial pain with valgus stress and milking maneuver.
- Medial laxity with valgus stress with avulsion fracture.
- For widened growth plate, treat with relative rest.
- For displaced fracture, treat with anatomic repair.

Little Leaguer's Shoulder (Proximal Humeral Physis Injury)

- Pain over proximal arm with throwing.
- Comparison radiographs required for diagnosis.
- Widening of proximal humeral growth plate on radiographs.
- Treat with relative rest (pitching with pain may lead to fracture).
- Four to eight weeks rest typically required for healing.

Table 74.2 TYPICAL PROGRESSIVE THROWING PROGRAM

Week 1	Warm-up throwing for 5 minutes 25 throws at 30 feet
Week 2	Warm-up throwing for 5 minutes 25 throws at 45 feet
Week 3	Warm-up throwing for 5 minutes 30–40 throws at 60 feet
Week 4	Warm-up throwing for 5 minutes 40–50 throws at 90 feet
Week 5	Warm-up throwing for 5 minutes 25 throws at 90 feet Rest 5 minutes 25 throws at 90 feet
Week 6	Warm-up throwing for 5 minutes 25 throws at 120 feet Rest 5 minutes 25 throws at 120 feet

Osteochondritis Dissecans of the Capitellum

- Osteonecrosis of the capitellum.
- Lateral elbow pain with throwing.
- Locking occurs with formation of loose bodies.
- Diagnosis with radiographs.
- MRI may be required for staging of lesion.
- Treat with rest with intact lesions.
- Excision or repair required with unstable lesions.

BASEBALL THROWING PROGRAMS (REHABILITATION AND CONDITIONING)

- After shoulder or elbow injury, a throwing program is initiated to regain strength, form, and control.
- Before initiation of throwing, the following should be accomplished:
  - No pain with palpation
  - No pain with resisted firing
  - No pain with passive stretch
  - No discomfort with plyometrics (e.g., bouncing a weighted ball against angled trampoline)
- The progressive throwing program
  - Soft toss
  - Progressive distance throwing
  - Long toss
  - Mound throwing
- Typical progressive throwing program (Table 74.2)

RECOMMENDED READINGS

Available online.

75 SOFTBALL

Aaron Lear • Andrew William Gottschalk

INTRODUCTION

First conceived as a way to play baseball indoors during months of harsh weather, softball has emerged over time as one of the most popular sports in the United States. Enjoyed by females and males of all ages and at all levels of competition, softball has proven itself distinct from its older cousin in terms of rules, biomechanical techniques, and injuries sustained during play.

INCIDENCE OF PLAY

- Softball is played in over 100 countries worldwide.
- Nine to twelve million Americans participated in softball annually between 2008 and 2018.
- Softball is one of the most popular sports in the United States partly because of its myriad variants, including:
  - Organized grade school and high school softball leagues
  - Organized college softball leagues
  - Female and male professional softball teams
  - Recreational female, male, and mixed-gender team leagues for all ages
  - Fast- and slow-pitch rule variations
- USA Softball (formerly the Amateur Softball Association of America) registers over 120,000 softball teams annually, comprising over 2 million players.
- As of 2017, 1678 universities fielded varsity softball teams.

GENERAL PRINCIPLES

Terminology and Rules

Overview

- The rules of softball are similar to those of baseball.
- Notable differences: softball uses:
  - A larger ball
  - A smaller playing field
  - Underhand pitching
  - Pitching area: pitchers stand in an 8-foot-diameter "pitcher's circle" that is flush with the field
- As with baseball, almost every softball league requires helmets for batters and base runners
- Mercy rules
  - National Collegiate Athletic Association (NCAA) softball: The game ends when one team wins by ≥8 runs after at least five completed innings.

Fast- Versus Slow-Pitch Softball

- The major variations are with respect to pitching.
- Rules common to fast- and slow-pitch softball.
- Field dimensions are the same with 60 feet between bases.
- Leading off a base is not permitted in softball. Base runners may leave the base after the ball has left the pitcher's hand in fast-pitch or once the ball crosses the plate in slow-pitch.
- Games are generally seven innings

FAST-PITCH SOFTBALL

- Primary variant used in competitive high school, college, and professional softball play.
  - Regulation NCAA softball dimensions are a 6½- to 7-ounce ball that is 11⅞–12¼ inches in circumference
- For the pitch the ball is launched underhand in a 360-degree windmill motion 40–46 feet away from home plate (vs. 60.5 feet in baseball). Distance depends on the league and player age. The pitched ball may have a trajectory that can have an upward, downward, or side-to-side motion. A strike is called if the ball passes over home plate in a zone between the batter's knees and chest.
- Bunting and base stealing are permitted offensive strategies in fast-pitch softball.
- "Slap-hitting" is a permitted offensive strategy, unique to fast-pitch softball, wherein the batter starts at the back of the batter's box and—once the pitch is thrown—advances toward the pitcher before aiming a bunt, or short "slap" swing, at the ball.
- "Drag-bunting" is a permitted offensive strategy, also unique to fast-pitch softball, wherein a left-handed hitting batter will essentially start running to first base as she or he is in the process of striking the ball.
- There are nine defensive players on the field at a time.

SLOW-PITCH SOFTBALL

- Main variant used in recreational softball league play in the United States (although certain recreational leagues do use fast-pitch)
- Whereas most slow-pitch softball leagues use a standard-dimension fast-pitch softball, certain leagues use larger balls up to 16 inches in circumference.
- For the pitch the ball is usually lobbed underhand in a "half-windmill" motion 50 feet from home base in an arc trajectory. The apex of the arc must be 6–12 feet high for the pitch to be legal.
- Unlike fast-pitch softball, bunting and base stealing are usually not permitted in slow-pitch softball leagues.
- There are 10 defensive players on the field at a time.
  - The tenth position is often a "short fielder," a fourth outfield player who stands in the outfield behind the shortstop or the second base position.
  - Alternatively, the defense will field both a right- and left-center fielder.
- Slow-pitch softball rules often allow for relatively heavier bats than those used in fast-pitch softball to help increase the power achieved when hitting a slower-moving ball.

History

Beginnings

- The sport that would come to be known as "softball" was first played in 1887 in Chicago, Illinois, as an indoor variant of baseball by using a larger ball and a smaller field.
- According to tradition, the first game was played using a wadded-up boxing glove and a broomstick handle and was invented by George Hancock.
- The term "softball" was first coined in 1926 and was in widespread use by 1930.
- In 1933 a slow-pitch softball tournament at the Chicago World's Fair ignited broader interest in the game; the Amateur Softball Association (ASA), the future parent of Team USA softball, was also created.
- In 1934 softball rules were standardized by the Joint Rules Committee on Softball.
- Fast-pitch softball was the dominant form until official ASA recognition of slow-pitch softball in 1953; thereafter, recreational slow-pitch league participation became dominant.

Softball at the Olympics

- The International Olympic Committee (IOC) included women's fast-pitch softball in the 1996 Summer Olympics in Atlanta, Georgia.

- The IOC removed softball and baseball from competition in 2012, but reinstated both sports for the 2020 Tokyo games.
- Since 2012, the World Cup of Softball held annually in the United States has been the premier international softball event.
- Professional women's leagues have existed in the United States since the mid-1990s. The National Pro Fastpitch league has been in existence since 2004.

BIOMECHANICAL PRINCIPLES

- The windmill pitching technique leads to injuries that are unique to softball play (see "Upper Extremity Injuries").
- The fast-pitch windmill motion can be broken down into six phases of delivery (Table 75.1 and Fig. 75.1) described as positions on a clock.
- Phases 1 and 2 produce the lowest kinetic and kinematic forces, whereas phases 4 and 5 produce the greatest force as the pitcher accelerates the arm and nears delivery of the ball. This differs from overhand pitching, which sees the greatest force during the deceleration phases.
- In fast-pitch softball pitchers, the measured distraction forces at the shoulder and elbow are similar to those measured for baseball. The windmill pitching motion has lower levels of torque at the shoulder and elbow compared with the overhead motion, which leads to less frequent pitching injuries compared with baseball.
- Ground reaction forces during pitching
  - Pitcher's leading lower extremity (the "stride leg") is subject to significant axial load forces. This may result in overuse or—less commonly—traumatic injuries, which most commonly involve the knee, especially the meniscus.

Table 75.1 DESCRIPTION OF WINDMILL PITCHING PHASES

Phase	Position	Motion
1	Windup	First ball motion forward to 6 o'clock, varied from subject to subject; arm extension ranged from 0 to 90 degrees
2	6 to 3 o'clock	Body weight placed on ipsilateral leg, trunk faced forward, arm internally rotated and elevated at 90 degrees
3	3 to 12 o'clock	Body weight transferred forward, body begins to rotate toward pitching arm, arm is elevated to 180 degrees, and the humerus is externally rotated
4	12 to 9 o'clock	Body remains rotated toward pitching arm, arm is adducted toward next position, body weight lands on contralateral foot
5	9 o'clock to release	Momentum is transferred to adducted arm, body rotated back to forward position, more power transferred to arm just before the ball is released
6	Follow-through	Arm contacts lateral hip and thigh, forward progression of humerus is halted, and ball release to completion of the pitch

Rojas IL, Provencher MT, Bhatia S, et al. Biceps activity during windmill softball pitching: injury implications and comparison with overhand throwing. *Am J Sports Med*. 2009;37:558–565.

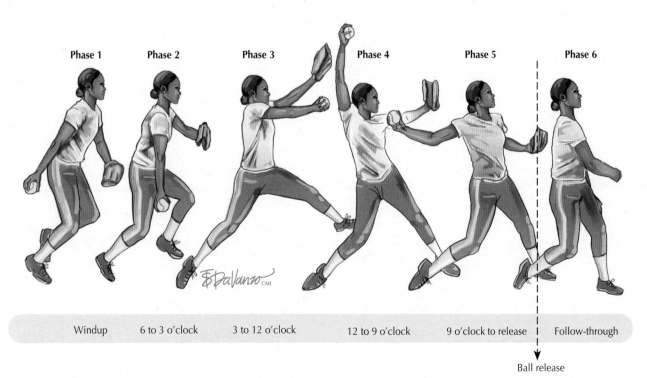
Phase 1
Phase 2
Phase 3
Phase 4
Phase 5
Phase 6
Windup
6 to 3 o'clock
3 to 12 o'clock
12 to 9 o'clock
9 o'clock to release
Follow-through
Ball release

Figure 75.1 Six phases of softball windmill pitch.

COMMON INJURIES AND MEDICAL PROBLEMS

Epidemiology

- Between 1994 and 2010, 2,107,823 patients aged 7–96 years were seen and treated for softball-related injuries in US emergency departments.
- On average, one person is seen every 4 minutes in an emergency department in the United States for a softball-related injury.
- High school fast-pitch players have injury rates reported between 1 and 5 per 1000 athlete exposures (AEs), whereas collegiate players are reported at 2–4 and professional players at 3.78 per 1000 AEs.

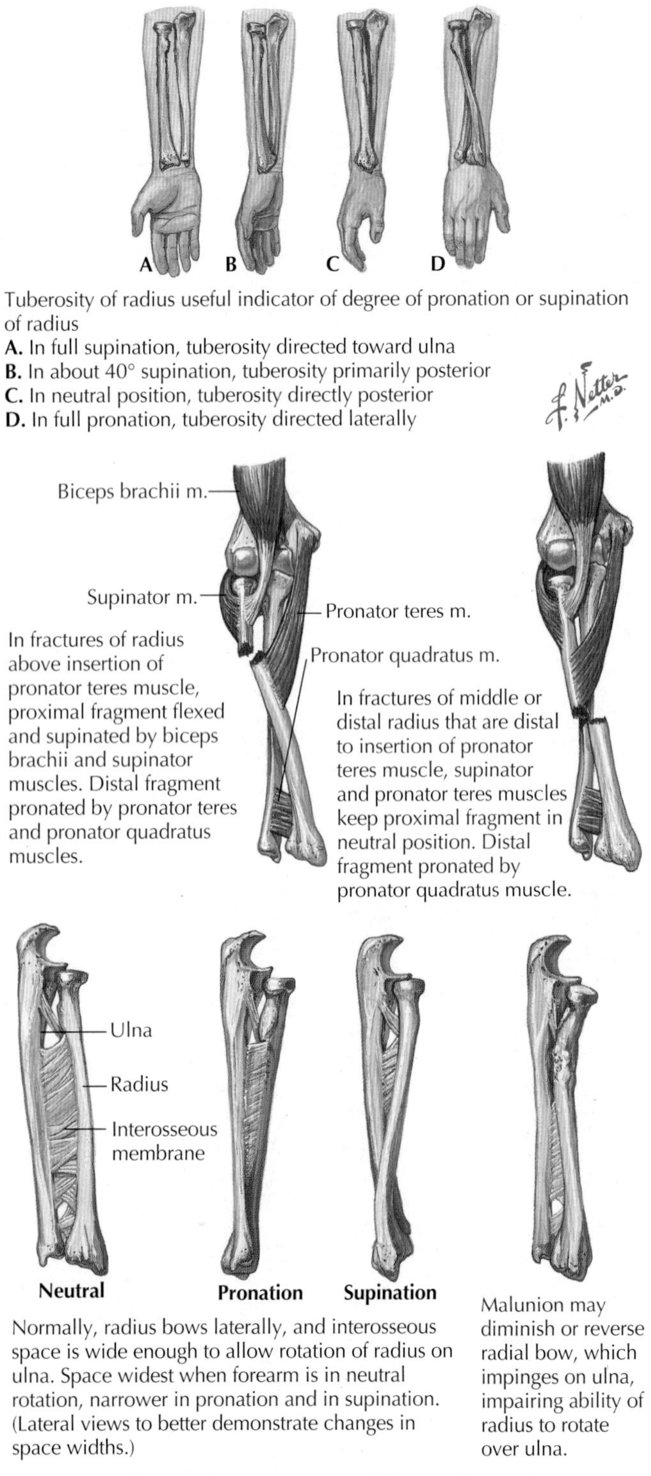
A
B
C
D
Tuberosity of radius useful indicator of degree of pronation or supination of radius
A. In full supination, tuberosity directed toward ulna
B. In about 40° supination, tuberosity primarily posterior
C. In neutral position, tuberosity directly posterior
D. In full pronation, tuberosity directed laterally
Biceps brachii m.
Supinator m.
Pronator teres m.
Pronator quadratus m.
In fractures of radius above insertion of pronator teres muscle, proximal fragment flexed and supinated by biceps brachii and supinator muscles. Distal fragment pronated by pronator teres and pronator quadratus muscles.
In fractures of middle or distal radius that are distal to insertion of pronator teres muscle, supinator and pronator teres muscles keep proximal fragment in neutral position. Distal fragment pronated by pronator quadratus muscle.
Ulna
Radius
Interosseous membrane
Neutral
Pronation
Supination
Normally, radius bows laterally, and interosseous space is wide enough to allow rotation of radius on ulna. Space widest when forearm is in neutral rotation, narrower in pronation and in supination. (Lateral views to better demonstrate changes in space widths.)
Malunion may diminish or reverse radial bow, which impinges on ulna, impairing ability of radius to rotate over ulna.

Figure 75.2 Biomechanics of forearm fracture.

- Injury rates in practice appear lower than during games; however, given the volume of practice compared with games, there are typically more practice injuries. Similarly, there may be more regular-season injuries, but rates of injury have been reported to be higher during the preseason.
- In professional female fast-pitch pitchers, it may be more common to report or have injury during practice than in games.
- Most common reported site of injury varies by level of play and position.
  - Noncontact and overuse injuries appear to be the most common cause of injury in high school and collegiate players, whereas acute injuries may be more common in professional female players.
  - Face and head injuries and hand/wrist injuries appear more frequent during games in comparison to practice.
  - Lower extremity injuries appear more common overall than upper extremity injuries.
- Recent reports suggest concussions account for around 11% of game injuries and 5% of practice injuries in high school and collegiate players.
- The risk of injury because of contact with a batted ball appears higher in college than in high school. This may be related to velocity of pitching and batted ball exit speeds, which are higher at more elite levels of play.
- Around three-fourths of softball injuries cause fewer than 10 days of time lost to injury.
- Injuries that result in longer time away from sport typically involve the knee/ankle or the hand/fingers. Player position/activity plays a role in injury rates (from highest to lowest incidence of injuries): base runners, batters, pitchers, catchers, infielders, and outfielders.
- Injury rates are greater for female softball athletes (9.56 per 1000 players) than for male softball athletes (7.93 per 1000 players).
- Catastrophic injury in softball is extremely rare. Between 1982 and 2018, the National Center for Catastrophic Injury Research reported rates of serious (nonpermanent disability) injury at 0.05 per 100,000 participants in high school and 0.58 per 100,000 in college, while reporting a single fatality in high school because of conditioning or indirect effects and only one serious (permanent disability) injury in college (0.01 per 100,000 in both cases).

Mechanisms of Injuries

- The mechanisms of softball injuries can be broken down into three categories: player-to-player contact, other contact, and noncontact.
- In games, "other contact" injuries are most frequent and include player contact with balls (particularly hit-by-pitch, or batted ball injuries), fences, equipment, bases, and sliding injuries.
- In practices, "noncontact" injuries are the most frequent and include overuse injuries, muscle strains, ligament sprains, and internal knee derangement.
  - Practices comprise more repetitive drills and stationary lower extremity plant-and-turn activities than typical game situations.

Upper Extremity Injuries

- Most commonly, overuse injuries of the shoulder and elbow.
- The shoulder injury rate for US high school softball was 1.14 injuries per 10,000 AEs.
- Approximately 1:20 US high school softball shoulder injuries required surgery (vs. approximately 1:10 for baseball).
- Upper extremity injuries occur in pitchers far more often than in nonpitcher positions.

- Little League of America has pitch count restrictions in youth baseball leagues. A similar rule was instituted for fast-pitch softball but then removed because of the belief among softball coaches that softball pitchers are not at risk of overuse injury to the same degree as baseball pitchers. Thus, it has been reported that youth fast pitchers can throw up to 1200 pitches in a three-day weekend tournament.

Forearm Stress Injury and Fracture

Description: The mid-diaphysis/third of the ulna is at risk of stress injury and fracture because of the repetitive forceful forearm pronation in softball windmill pitching (Fig. 75.2).

History: Nagging forearm/elbow pain with pitching (particularly throwing curveballs and fastballs) that becomes more intense and persistent. May eventually cause pain with activities of daily living.

Physical examination: Pain with active elbow range of motion and resisted pronation; tenderness along the anterior volar forearm/ulna.

Diagnostic considerations: Evidence of stress fracture may or may not be present on x-ray, and more advanced imaging is warranted if negative x-rays with high suspicion of injury. These include magnetic resonance imaging (MRI) or bone scan. If present, appropriate to screen for relative energy deficiency in sport syndrome.

Treatment: Initial treatment includes complete throwing rest (not just pitching), avoidance of upper body resistance/weight training, avoidance of batting, and appropriate caloric intake; consider bracing with wrist immobilization brace to prevent pronation. When the athlete is subjectively and objectively pain free, repeat imaging and progress to next phase. Once therapy program is ongoing and athlete remains pain free, throwing program can begin: short toss → long toss → easy pitching → harder pitching → pitches with pronation → competitive pitching. Return-to-throwing program should be specific to windmill pitching.

Return to play: Usually occurs after 6–8 weeks for osseous healing, then progress as tolerated; severe cases can take up to 10 months after presentation to return to competitive pitching

Tendonitis of the Long Head of the Biceps

- Softball pitchers activate their biceps brachii in eccentric loading to a much greater extent than do baseball pitchers; this leads to a greater relative incidence of biceps tendinitis in softball pitchers (Fig. 75.3; see Chapter 49: "Shoulder Injuries").

Ulnar Neuritis

- Repetitive stretching of the ulnar nerve at the medial elbow may occur in both softball and baseball pitchers.
- Softball pitchers may strike the medial elbow of the pitching arm against the lateral pelvis just before ball release, placing the ulnar nerve at a risk of injury (see Chapter 50: "Elbow Injuries").

Elbow Ulnar Collateral Ligament Sprain and Rupture

- Repetitive overhead throwing may lead to ulnar collateral ligament (UCL) inflammation, sprain, or rupture.
- Softball windmill pitchers are at a lesser risk than their baseball counterparts because the windmill technique avoids the more severe medial elbow stresses encountered with several baseball pitching techniques (Fig. 75.4; see Chapter 74: "Baseball").

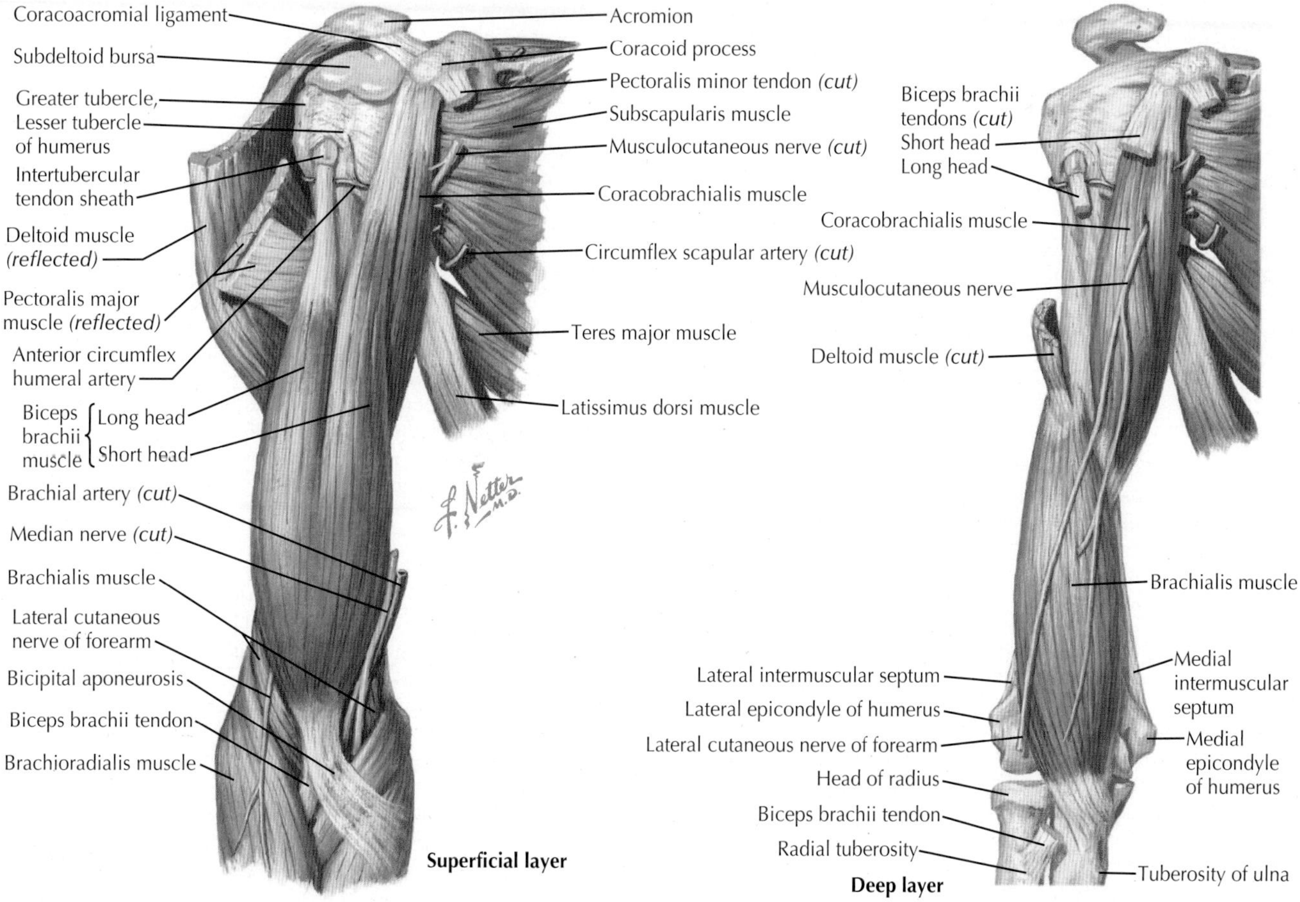
Coracoacromial ligament
Subdeltoid bursa
Greater tubercle,
Lesser tubercle
of humerus
Intertubercular
tendon sheath
Deltoid muscle
(reflected)
Pectoralis major
muscle (reflected)
Anterior circumflex
humeral artery
Biceps brachii muscle
Long head
Short head
Brachial artery (cut)
Median nerve (cut)
Brachialis muscle
Lateral cutaneous
nerve of forearm
Bicipital aponeurosis
Biceps brachii tendon
Brachioradialis muscle
Acromion
Coracoid process
Pectoralis minor tendon (cut)
Subscapularis muscle
Musculocutaneous nerve (cut)
Coracobrachialis muscle
Circumflex scapular artery (cut)
Teres major muscle
Latissimus dorsi muscle
Superficial layer
Biceps brachii
tendons (cut)
Short head
Long head
Coracobrachialis muscle
Musculocutaneous nerve
Deltoid muscle (cut)
Brachialis muscle
Lateral intermuscular septum
Lateral epicondyle of humerus
Lateral cutaneous nerve of forearm
Head of radius
Biceps brachii tendon
Radial tuberosity
Medial
intermuscular
septum
Medial
epicondyle
of humerus
Tuberosity of ulna
Deep layer
Figure 75.3 Muscles of the arm.

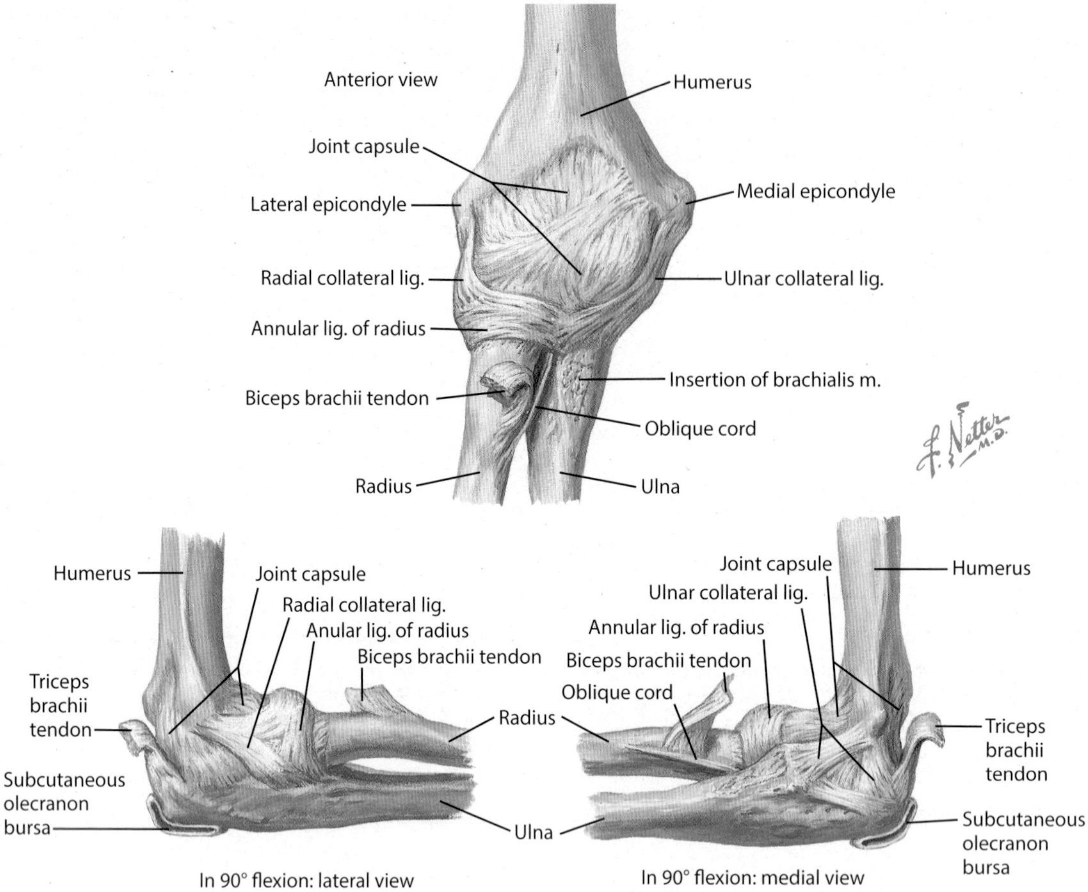
Anterior view
Humerus
Joint capsule
Lateral epicondyle
Medial epicondyle
Radial collateral lig.
Ulnar collateral lig.
Annular lig. of radius
Insertion of brachialis m.
Biceps brachii tendon
Oblique cord
Radius
Ulna
F. Netter M.D.
Humerus
Joint capsule
Radial collateral lig.
Anular lig. of radius
Biceps brachii tendon
Triceps brachii tendon
Radius
Subcutaneous olecranon bursa
Ulna
In 90° flexion: lateral view
Joint capsule
Ulnar collateral lig.
Annular lig. of radius
Biceps brachii tendon
Oblique cord
Humerus
Triceps brachii tendon
Subcutaneous olecranon bursa
In 90° flexion: medial view

Figure 75.4 Ligaments of the elbow.

Therefore, injury occurs in position players rather than pitchers in softball, unlike in baseball.

Thoracic Outlet Syndrome (TOS) (See Chapter 52: "Thorax and Abdominal Injuries")

- Seen in both softball and baseball players; in one report these two sports made up the greatest numbers of competitive athletes seeking treatment for the condition.

Lower Extremity Injuries

- In comparison with more softball-specific upper extremity injuries, lower extremity injuries are more frequent and are similar to the injuries seen in all sports (e.g., knee and ankle sprains; please see Chapter 55: "Knee Injuries" and Chapter 56: "Ankle and Leg Injuries" for information on knee and ankle sprains).
- Lower extremity injuries (42% of softball injuries) occur more frequently than upper extremity injuries (33%).
- Injuries in softball that keep a player out for >21 days are in the knee 31% of the time and the ankle 19% of the time.

Spondylolysis (See Chapter 53: "Thoracic and Lumbosacral Spine Injuries" and Chapter 59: "Stress Fractures")

- Related to extension in the lumbar spine associated with pitching motion.
- In one case series, in female athletes, softball was the third most common sport associated with spondylolysis.

Head Injuries

- Softball and baseball are the leading causes of sports-related facial trauma in the United States.
- Sixty-eight percent of craniomaxillofacial fractures in softball and baseball are caused by ball impact (see Chapter 48: "Maxillofacial Injuries").
- Concussion occurs in softball and occurs with player-to-player contact (e.g., collisions between same team fielders or when sliding into base between opponents); player-to-ground contact (e.g., diving for balls on defense or sliding into base); or ball-to-head injuries (e.g., batted balls when playing defense or as a batter by a pitched ball) (see Chapter 45: "Head Injuries").

Injury Prevention and Safe Play

- Appropriate maintenance of competition and practice ball fields helps prevent acute knee, ankle, and fall-related injuries.
- Appropriate coaching of proper sliding technique and use of breakaway bases are used for the prevention of ankle sprains.
- Consistent, appropriate use of protective gear (e.g., batting helmets) helps prevent and minimize dangers of projectile injuries. Use of face masks while batting and fielding can be worn to prevent facial injuries from pitched and batted balls. These are commonly worn in softball by infielders when playing their positions and by batters to prevent face contact by pitches.
- Overuse injuries are almost entirely preventable with good education.

- Proper coaching technique on pitching and pitching motions are thought to play a role in overuse injury prevention.
- Appropriate pitching volume and frequency are important, particularly at the youth level, to prevent overuse injury. There are no evidence-based pitch count recommendations for youth softball players. No clear limits on appropriate pitch count for youth players, but, at least in tournament settings, using a team of pitchers rather than a single pitcher for all games may limit injury risk.
- Attention to pitching fatigue and any pain developing in a pitcher is important, as there is good evidence noting the amount of both fatigue and pain that develop in pitchers over a tournament weekend.
- Encourage ongoing communication among the at-risk or injured athlete, the coaches, and the medical staff.

RECOMMENDED READINGS

Available online.

76 TENNIS

Marc R. Safran • Andrew Fithian

GENERAL

- 17 million people in the United States participate in tennis at least once a year (Fig. 76.1).
- 10 million people play tennis at least 10 times per year.
- 4.5 million youths play tennis annually.

EPIDEMIOLOGY OF TENNIS INJURIES

- Injuries to the lower extremity and spine account for 50%–75% of all tennis injuries.
- Elite players tend to have more injuries to the lower extremities and spine, whereas recreational players incur more injuries to the lower extremities.
- Most lower extremity injuries are acute sprains. Upper extremity injuries are more likely to be chronic overload injuries.

RULES OF TENNIS

- The court:
  - Tennis courts are 78 feet long and 27 feet wide for singles play, 36 feet wide for doubles play.
  - The court is divided by a net 3 feet tall at the center.
  - The lines around the end of the court are named *baselines* and *sidelines*.
  - Service lines are drawn 21 feet from and parallel to the net. On each side of the net, the area between the service line, the net, and the sidelines will be divided by a center service line.
  - Each baseline is divided in half by a center mark.
- Scoring
  - A standard game is scored with the server's score being called first:
    - No point – "love"
    - First point – 15
    - Second point – 30
    - Third point – 45
    - Fourth point – game
  - If each team or player has won three points, the score is "deuce." After deuce, the score for the next team or player to win a point is "advantage." If the player or team with advantage scores the next point, that player or team wins the game. If the opposing team scores before this, the score returns to deuce. Hence, a player or team must have a two-point margin to win.
  - An alternative method of scoring has the winner of the game winning four points. This type of game is called *no-ad scoring*. If both players gets three points each, then the person who wins the next, fourth, point wins the game, with no need to have a two-point margin.
  - There are different scoring methods in a set. The two main methods include "tie-break set" and "advantage set." Before a match, the method of scoring must be declared.
  - In an "advantage set," the first player to win six games wins the set (winner must have a two-game margin over the opponent).
  - In a "tie-break set," the first player to win six games wins the set, provided the winner has a two-game margin over the opponent. If each player wins six games, for a score of six-all, a tie-break game shall be played.
  - A player or team concedes a point if:
    - Two faults are incurred during the service of the ball.
    - The ball bounces twice consecutively before the return.
    - The ball is returned and hits the ground or an object outside the court of play.
    - The player hits the ball before it crosses the net.
    - In doubles, both players touch the ball when returning it.
    - The player, player's racquet, or clothing touch the net.
    - The player deliberately catches or carries the ball with the racquet or strikes the ball twice with the racquet.
- A match may be played to the best of three or five sets.
- The players or teams stand on opposite sides of the court. Players will change ends after the odd games of each set.
- The server is defined as the player or team that puts the ball into play, and the receiver is defined as the player or team who is ready to return the served ball. Players will switch roles after each game. In doubles play, each team will designate a player to serve a game first. They will then alternate games, serving the ball accordingly. Additionally, they will identify a player to return the first served ball. This, too, will be alternated in subsequent games.
- When serving a game, the server shall stand behind alternate halves of the court, starting with the right side every game. The server is allowed one fault each point. The second fault results in a loss of a point to the server. The ball should be served to the service court opposite to the server. The ball must be allowed to bounce once before the receiver striking the ball.

PHYSIOLOGY

- Tennis is a noncyclical anaerobic sport (10%–30%) with an aerobic recovery phase (70%–90%).
- Single rallies may only last 3–8 seconds, but complete matches may last 3 hours.
- Tennis requires physical elements of quickness, endurance, strength, flexibility, reaction time/speed, agility, and coordination.

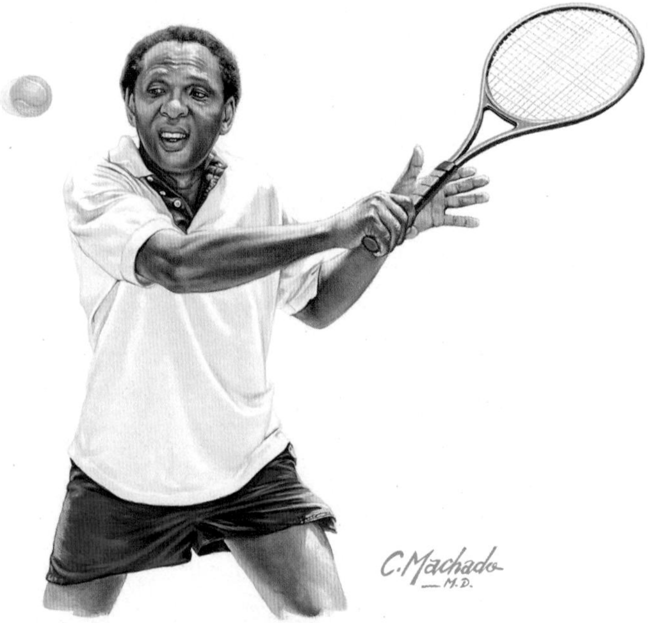
C. Machado M.D.

Figure 76.1 Tennis.

- Heart rate for singles tennis can average >160 beats per minute. Some skilled tennis players may average >80% of their maximal heart rate during a match.
- Depending upon conditioning, age, gender, intensity of play, hydration status, and environment, a player may lose 0.5–2.5 L of water per hour of play.
- Conditioning
  - Aerobic fitness
    - Aerobic intervals simulate intensity of play. Thirty-minute sessions, three times a week are required, at a minimum, for a conditioning effect.
  - Anaerobic fitness
    - High-intensity training performed at near-exhaustion levels with short work/recovery periods in a 1:2 ratio to mimic the tempo of match play (i.e., 15 seconds of work with 30 seconds of rest).
  - Progressive resistance strengthening of key muscle groups serves to prepare needed muscles for each tennis stroke and builds the body's tolerance for progressive tennis drills and match play. All muscles along the kinetic chain, including core muscle strength, are important for conditioning.
  - Functional mobility
    - Sufficient active range of motion of all joints in the kinetic chain is recommended to avoid injury at adjacent motion segments.

EQUIPMENT/FACILITIES

- **Racquets:**
  - **Composition:** Change in manufacturing materials has resulted in racquets that are larger, lighter, stiffer, and more powerful than racquets of the past. This predisposes some athletes to chronic overload injuries of the upper extremity.
    - **Stiffness:** Stiffness is the amount of bending a racquet does on ball impact. The more flexible a racquet is, the more time that is taken for the racquet to deform and return to its original shape. Flexible racquets decrease the shock of the impact and the vibrations felt by the player, which comes at a cost of power.
    - **Sweet spot:** Striking area of the racquet that provides the lowest transmission of vibrations to the upper extremity and allows for the ball to rebound with the highest velocity. The sweet spot will vary with each racquet and be dependent upon its size, stiffness, and shape.
    - **Weight:** Racquets currently on the market vary from 240 to 310 grams. Racquet weight and speed are factors that contribute to the velocity of the ball after impact.
    - **Balance:** Racquets with head weight equal to handle weight are considered balanced in regard to their geometric center and center of gravity. Alterations in this balance may allow for a racquet to be more maneuverable (handle heavy, head light).
    - **Grip size:** Scored 1–5 depending on circumference. The ideal circumference of the hand should equal the distance as measured from the tip of the ring finger to the proximal wrist crease. Materials may be added to alter the feel of the handle (less slippery) or to dampen vibrations felt after ball strike.
    - **String material:** Gut strings are more expensive and less durable than synthetic strings but provide better performance. String thickness is measured in gauges (16–18). A larger gauge string will be more durable but absorb less shock.
    - **String tension:** String tension is a very important part of the racquet. More loosely tensioned strings with longer ball dwell times will return more power at the cost of some control.
- **Tennis balls:**
  - **Nonpressurized:** Bounce created related to the thickness and suppleness of the rubber used to make the ball.
  - **Pressurized:** Bounce created is related to qualities of the rubber and the internal air pressure (which exceeds that of the external environment). Once the internal pressure is lost, the bounce will not be as high and the ball will feel "dead."
  - A nonpressurized ball must be hit harder than a pressurized ball, which places more load on the arm.
- **Tennis shoes:**
  - Important characteristics of a tennis shoe include cushioning, stability, stiffness, and design of the outsole.
  - Consideration to the amount of pronation/supination that a player endures during play will affect the decision to choose a shoe with material of higher density placed medially (to prevent excessive pronation) or for a shoe with a higher cut (to prevent excessive supination). A player should choose a shoe with an outsole that reflects the playing surface. Grass surfaces tend to have less friction and be more slippery, requiring a shoe with more grip. Carpet surfaces tend to have more grip; therefore, a shoe with less grip should be chosen to allow more twisting and turning.
- **Court surfaces:**
  - **Clay:** Red clay, green clay. Loose surface causes the ball to lose speed rapidly and bounce higher. Allows increased time for opponent to reach/return the ball. Considered a "slow" surface.
  - **Hard:** Concrete, coated asphalt, Rebound Ace. Balls bounce low, giving hard-hitting players an advantage. Considered a "fast" surface.
  - **Grass:** Grass grown on hard, packed soil. Balls tend to slide and bounce low, making returns difficult. Favors the serve-and-volley player. Considered the "fastest" surface.
  - **Indoor courts:** Allow for year-round play.
  - **Injury:** Data are equivocal on the overall rate of injury across different court surfaces. Injury rates in the lower extremity increase if the player changes surface to one with which they are unfamiliar.

TENNIS-SPECIFIC MECHANICS

Kinetic Chain

The kinetic chain is the transference of force efficiently from the ground to the racquet through the coordinated sequencing of the legs, hips, trunk, and upper extremity. Each segment adds additional energy to the previous one, resulting in maximal racquet acceleration. Fluid motion through the kinetic chain is essential to minimize the risk of injury.

Strokes

The Serve

- This stroke produces the highest ball speed and is most associated with injury.
- Particular serves, such as the kick, require hyperextension of the lumbar spine (increased lordosis) to be effective.
  - **Kick serve:** Produces top spin, which improves the ability to place the service in the service box. Similar to baseball's curveball, this serve places more stress on the upper extremity than other serve types and may place athletes (especially young players) at increased risk of injury
  - **Flat serve and slice:** These serves produce no topspin. These serves place less strain on the upper extremity, but shorter players may struggle to place them in the service box.
- **Four phases:**
  - **Wind-up:** Initiation of the serving stance to the toss of the ball by the contralateral extremity. The lower extremities prepare for the buildup of power that occurs in the cocking phase.

- **Cocking:** From the toss of the ball through the point where the dominant shoulder is in maximal external rotation. This phase is characterized by the buildup of power. Injuries are associated with the late-cocking phase.
  - **Subject to injury:**
    - Anterior shoulder capsule is tensioned to its physiologic limit, with the shoulder in maximum external rotation.
    - Glenoid labrum serves to prevent shoulder subluxation during external rotation.
    - Internal impingement may occur if the rotator cuff is pinched between the greater tuberosity of the humeral head and the posterior superior glenoid.
    - Muscles of the lower extremity during extension of hips and knees and ankle plantarflexion.
    - Intervertebral disc, pars interarticularis with hyperextension/rotation of the spine.
- **Acceleration:** From maximal external rotation through ball impact. High muscular activity is noted with peak activity immediately before ball impact. Internal rotation of the humerus is responsible for 40% of the racquet speed at impact. Fluid motion through the kinetic chain is crucial. Injury to one segment leads to a loss of power and places other segments at risk for injury.
  - **Subject to injury:**
    - Muscular overload of the abdominal muscles, rotator cuff, internal rotators, elbow extensors, and wrist flexors may occur
    - Labrum with extreme abduction and internal rotation of the humerus
    - Ulnar lateral collateral ligament and the flexor-pronator muscles of the elbow secondary to valgus stress
    - Extensor carpi ulnaris tendon at the wrist with hypersupination and ulnar deviation of the forearm and wrist
- **Follow-through:** Ball impact through completion of the stroke. Activation of shoulder musculature is required to decelerate the humerus to maintain glenohumeral stability.
  - **Subject to injury:**
    - The infraspinatus/posterior shoulder muscles and the biceps contract eccentrically to stabilize the shoulder, slow the internal rotation of the shoulder, and slow pronation of the forearm.
    - The posterior capsule is placed under tension.
    - Scapular motion combined with contraction of the infraspinatus muscle places the suprascapular nerve at risk for injury.

- **Biomechanics:**
  - Racquet speeds reach a peak velocity of 62–83 mi/hr.
  - Ball velocities reach 90–157 mi/hr.
  - These speeds are achieved in 0.2–0.3 seconds from the end of the cocking phase until ball contact.
  - Shoulder internally rotates at 1100–1700 degrees per second. Elite players achieve 1800–2400 degrees per second.
  - Elbow flexes to 120 degrees during late cocking and extends to 15–20 degrees of flexion at ball impact, resulting in an extension velocity of 1000–1400 degrees/second.
  - Forearm pronation has been recorded at 350–900 degrees per second before ball impact and has been documented to increase to 1300 degrees per second, 0.1 second after impact.
  - Wrist speeds exceed 1000 degrees/second, 0.1 second before ball impact; range of motion (ROM) of wrist during a serve is 90–100 degrees.

Backhand

- The backhand swing may be performed one-handed or two-handed. The one-handed backhand stroke allows the player to have a better reach and the ability to slice the ball. The two-handed backhand stroke requires less strength but requires more truncal rotation and places the nondominant arm at risk for wrist injury.
- The backhand has three phases: preparation, acceleration, and follow-through.
- There is an increased incidence of lateral elbow pain in novice players in the backhand stroke. This is attributed to the novice player's inefficient kinetic chain, placing more stress across the elbow joint, and from hitting the ball with the wrist in flexion (versus extension).
- In high-velocity games the time for a longer back swing is not always possible, and players compensate by "short-arming." Hence the player must accelerate the racquet faster, requiring more forceful muscular contractions. The player must consider and train appropriately for the increased muscular requirements of such movements.

Forehand

- Depending on surface/speed of play, players may hit the forehand shot with a continental, Eastern, semi-Western, or Western grip (Fig. 76.2). Each grip facilitates specific shots such as top spin and predisposes to different chronic overload injuries, especially at the wrist.
- The forehand shot has three phases: preparation, acceleration, and follow-through. Of note, during the acceleration phase the player may stand with an open or closed stance. Anterior hip pain may be seen in the players that use an open stance.

INJURIES

With injury to a player at any level, it is important to ascertain chronicity of symptoms, previous treatment, training schedule, neurologic symptoms, and mechanical symptoms.

Upper Extremity

Shoulder

- Thirty-five percent of junior tennis players complained of shoulder pain at some point in time.
- Over 50% of older players and elite athletes note shoulder pain at some point in their career.
- Quick acceleration/deceleration of the shoulder with focus on precision movement of the racquet places increased strain on the glenohumeral joint. **S**capular malposition, **I**nferomedial border prominence, **C**oracoid pain, and dys**K**inesis (SICK) scapula puts patients at risk of shoulder pathology through abnormal and unpredictable patterns of motion. Treatment is physical therapy to restore normal motor patterns.

Glenohumeral internal rotation deficit (GIRD): Posterior capsular tightness changes glenohumeral mechanics, putting athletes at risk of injuries at the shoulder and adjacent motion segments. Treatment is stretching of the posterior capsule.

King Kong arm: Drooping and hypertrophy of the musculature of the shoulder girdle of the dominant upper extremity from repetitive use.

Rotator cuff tendinopathy (Fig. 76.3): One of the more common causes of shoulder pain.

- Rotator cuff pain in the young player is more often the result of instability, whereas impingement and instability are factors in the older player.
  - Decreased strength of the scapular stabilizers and external rotators and decreased flexibility with internal rotation are associated with shoulder instability.
- Internal impingement of the rotator cuff between the acromion and humeral head is more likely to occur with overhead shots versus ground strokes.
- Players will present with subacromial pain and referred pain to the lateral arm. They may claim that their arm "feels dead" during play.
- Chronic symptoms may lead to tears of the rotator cuff.

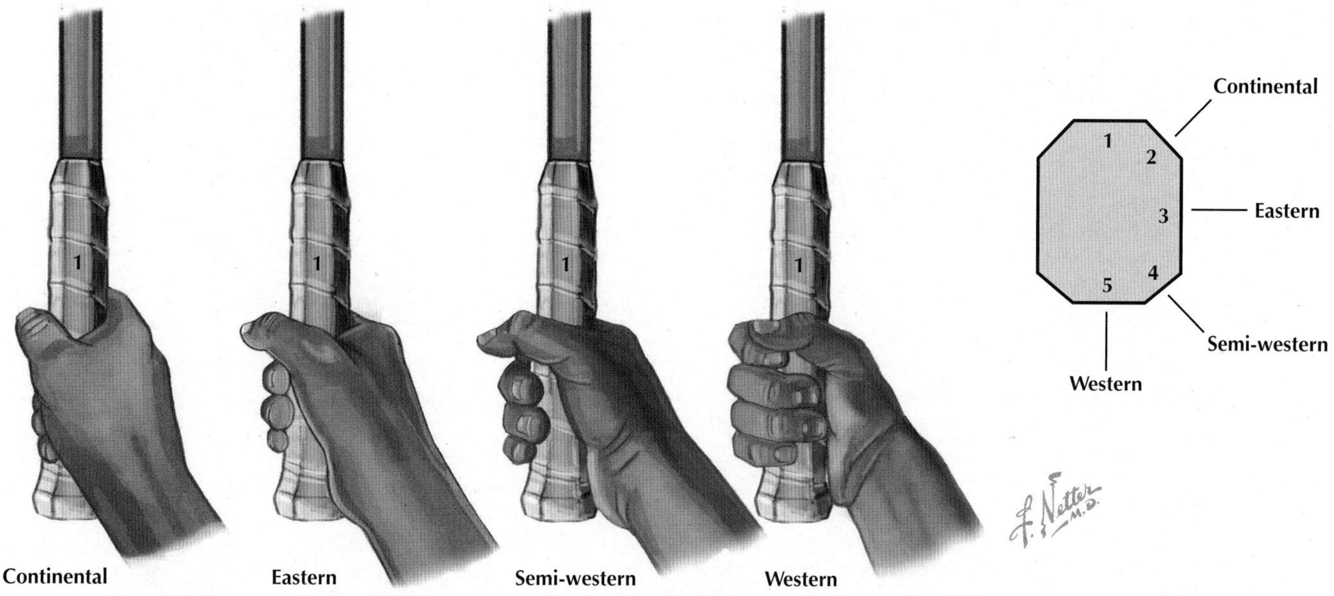
Continental
Eastern
Semi-western
Western
1
2
3
4
5
F. Netter M.D.

Figure 76.2 Tennis grip: continental, Eastern, semi-Western, and Western grips.

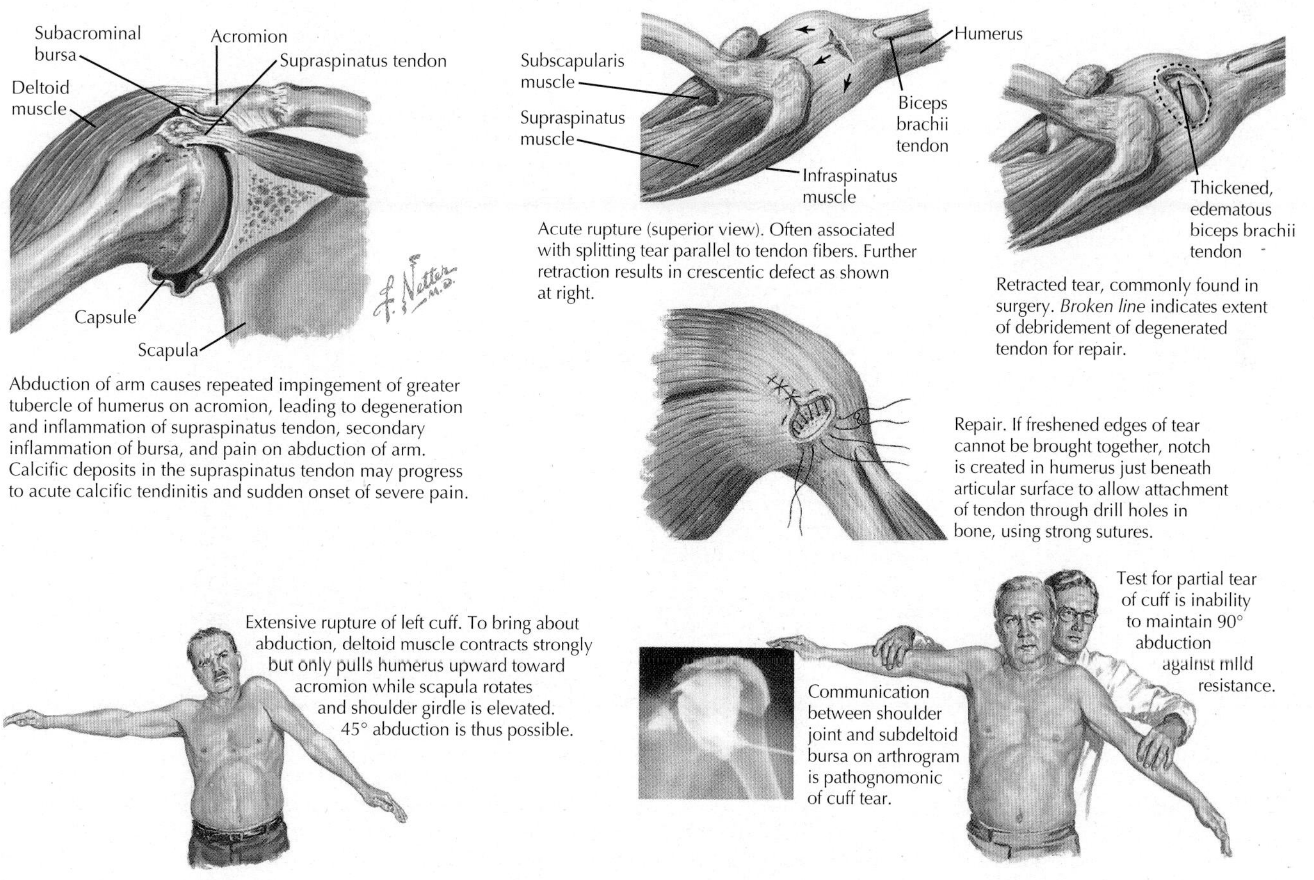
Subacrominal bursa
Acromion
Supraspinatus tendon
Deltoid muscle
Capsule
Scapula
F. Netter M.D.
Abduction of arm causes repeated impingement of greater tubercle of humerus on acromion, leading to degeneration and inflammation of supraspinatus tendon, secondary inflammation of bursa, and pain on abduction of arm. Calcific deposits in the supraspinatus tendon may progress to acute calcific tendinitis and sudden onset of severe pain.
Subscapularis muscle
Supraspinatus muscle
Humerus
Biceps brachii tendon
Infraspinatus muscle
Acute rupture (superior view). Often associated with splitting tear parallel to tendon fibers. Further retraction results in crescentic defect as shown at right.
Thickened, edematous biceps brachii tendon
Retracted tear, commonly found in surgery. Broken line indicates extent of debridement of degenerated tendon for repair.
Repair. If freshened edges of tear cannot be brought together, notch is created in humerus just beneath articular surface to allow attachment of tendon through drill holes in bone, using strong sutures.
Extensive rupture of left cuff. To bring about abduction, deltoid muscle contracts strongly but only pulls humerus upward toward acromion while scapula rotates and shoulder girdle is elevated. 45° abduction is thus possible.
Communication between shoulder joint and subdeltoid bursa on arthrogram is pathognomonic of cuff tear.
Test for partial tear of cuff is inability to maintain 90° abduction against mild resistance.

Figure 76.3 Rotator cuff injuries.

- Rehabilitation: Avoid activities that may further aggravate shoulder symptoms/pathology. Strengthen weak muscles, especially external rotators.
  - Additionally, strengthen:
    - Latissimus dorsi, serratus anterior for all strokes
    - Deltoids for overhead and backhand strokes
    - Rhomboids to counter drooping of the shoulder girdle

Infraspinatus atrophy: There is a high rate of incidental infraspinatus atrophy among top-level players. Incidence increases with career length and higher rank. Infraspinatus atrophy is typically asymptomatic.

Biceps tendinitis: An overuse injury leading to pain in the front of the shoulder with activities that flex the arm at the elbow and rotate the forearm such as hitting a high topspin forehand.

Activity modifications and antiinflammatories with eventual strengthening of the muscles of the shoulder, elbow, and scapula are recommended to prevent tendon rupture. Biceps tenotomy or tenodesis is contraindicated, as the tendon is an important stabilizer of the glenohumeral joint.

Superior labrum, anterior to posterior (SLAP) lesions: Tennis players are at risk for SLAP lesions during late cocking during serves. There is a high frequency of GIRD and SICK scapula in patients with symptomatic SLAP lesions, and early conservative therapy should address these pathologies if present. Failure of nonoperative management is an indication for arthroscopic labral repair.

Osteoarthritis (OA): There is a significantly higher rate of mild OA of the glenohumeral joint in the player's dominant shoulder. Instability resulting from high demands during play may be the underlying cause for the development of OA.

Elbow

- Biceps, triceps, wrist flexor, and wrist extensor strengthening with improved control over the elbow, helping to reduce injury risk
- Full pronation of the arm after impact will reduce excessive load and stress on the elbow

Lateral epicondylitis (Fig. 76.4): Fifty percent of players sustain injury to the origin of the extensor carpi radialis brevis (ECRB) tendon (and sometimes the extensor digitorum communis [EDC]) just distal to the lateral epicondyle leading to the formation of painful granulation tissue and adhesions.

- **Risk factors:** Age >30, improper grip size, tight strings, incorrect technique (wrist-flexed backhand), inadequate conditioning, practice >2 hr/day.
- **Improper technique:** Wrist flexed during backhand, premature truncal rotation, leading with the elbow during the backhand. Correction of technique in addition to rest, rehab, bracing, antiinflammatories is recommended.

Medial epicondylitis: Less common than lateral tennis elbow but more likely to occur in competitive and elite players. Usually the result of strain at the origin of the common flexor tendon at the medial epicondyle. Competitive players are prone to this injury from repeated wrist flexion from overhead serves or from pronation stress associated with placing top spin on the ball. Degenerative changes are seen in the tendons.

Valgus extension overload: Impaction of olecranon into the olecranon fossa of the humerus with repetitive, forceful extension of the elbow. Pain and tenderness occur about the elbow with repeated bony/soft tissue impingement. Activity modification to avoid leaning on the elbow and hitting the ball with the arm in full extension (e.g., Western forehand with fully extended arm) are recommended.

Ulnar collateral ligament (UCL) sprain: Over time, repetitive valgus stress to the elbow may stretch the UCL. This may lead to increased contact and cartilage wear of the radiocapitellar joint and to a stretch injury of the ulnar nerve. A ruptured UCL is rare but would require surgery. Avoid hitting the Western forehand with the arm fully extended.

Wrist/Hand

General: Injuries to the wrist and hand are common. In the absence of a clear injury mechanism, focal tenderness, dysesthesias, and numbness warrant further evaluation.

De Quervain stenosing tenosynovitis: Irritation to the abductor pollicis brevis and extensor pollicis brevis rubbing over the radial styloid with excessive ulnar deviation of the hand during grasping and swing of the racquet. Treatment may include periods of rest, injection to the tendon sheath, or release of the first dorsal compartment of the wrist.

Triangular fibrocartilage complex (TFCC) tears (Fig. 76.5): Painful or painless clicking noted on the ulnar side of the wrist from a tear in the TFCC. Increased association with

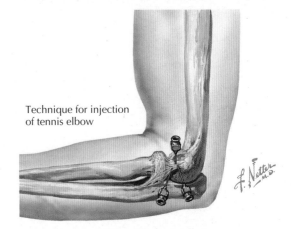

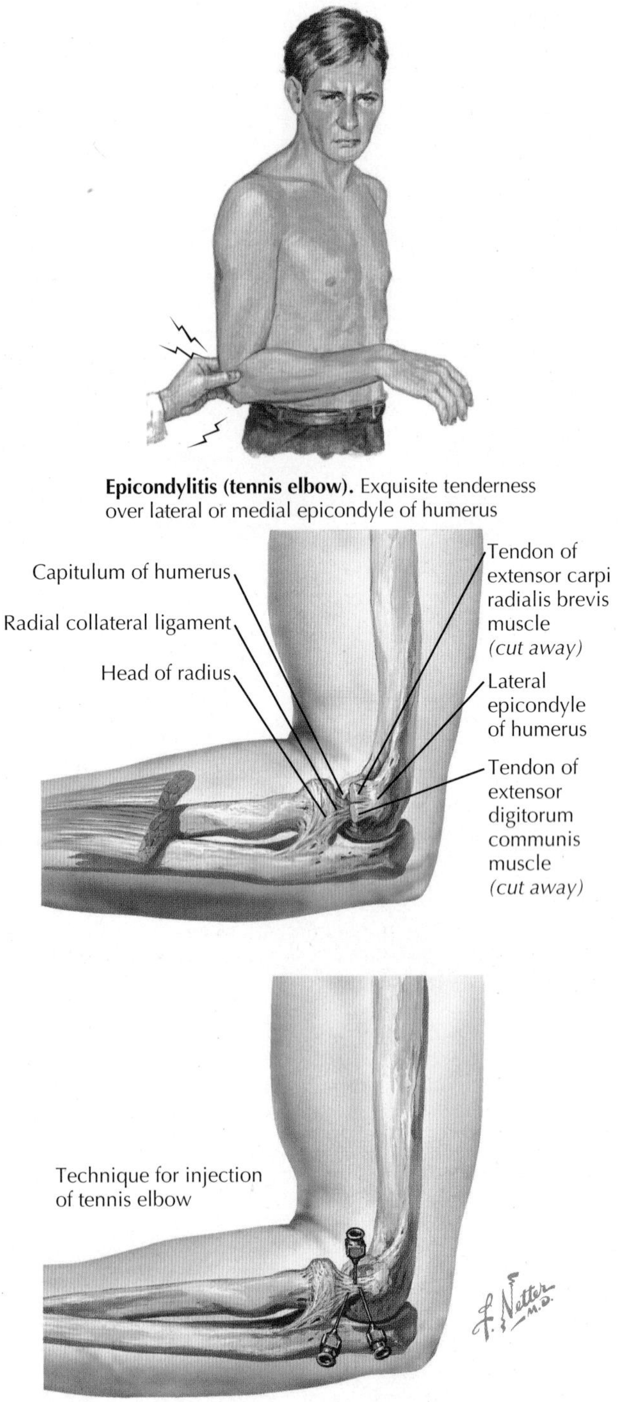
Epicondylitis (tennis elbow). Exquisite tenderness over lateral or medial epicondyle of humerus
Capitulum of humerus
Radial collateral ligament
Head of radius
Tendon of extensor carpi radialis brevis muscle (cut away)
Lateral epicondyle of humerus
Tendon of extensor digitorum communis muscle (cut away)
Technique for injection of tennis elbow

Figure 76.4 Lateral epicondylitis.

ulnar-positive variance (increased length of the ulna relative to the radius) and exacerbated by Eastern grip. Treatment with immobilization of the wrist for several weeks. If symptoms persist, surgery (arthroscopic vs. open) may be required. Prevention includes decreasing twisting motion at the wrist, functional bracing, and wrist strengthening exercises.

Lunate stress injury: Associated with negative ulnar variance and use of Western forehand grip.

Hamate fracture: The result of repetitive impaction of the butt end of the handle into the hook of the hamate.

Wrist ganglion cysts: May cause pain predominately in the dorsum of the wrist. They are treated by drainage, compression, antiinflammatories, splinting, and surgically. Recurrence rates are high.

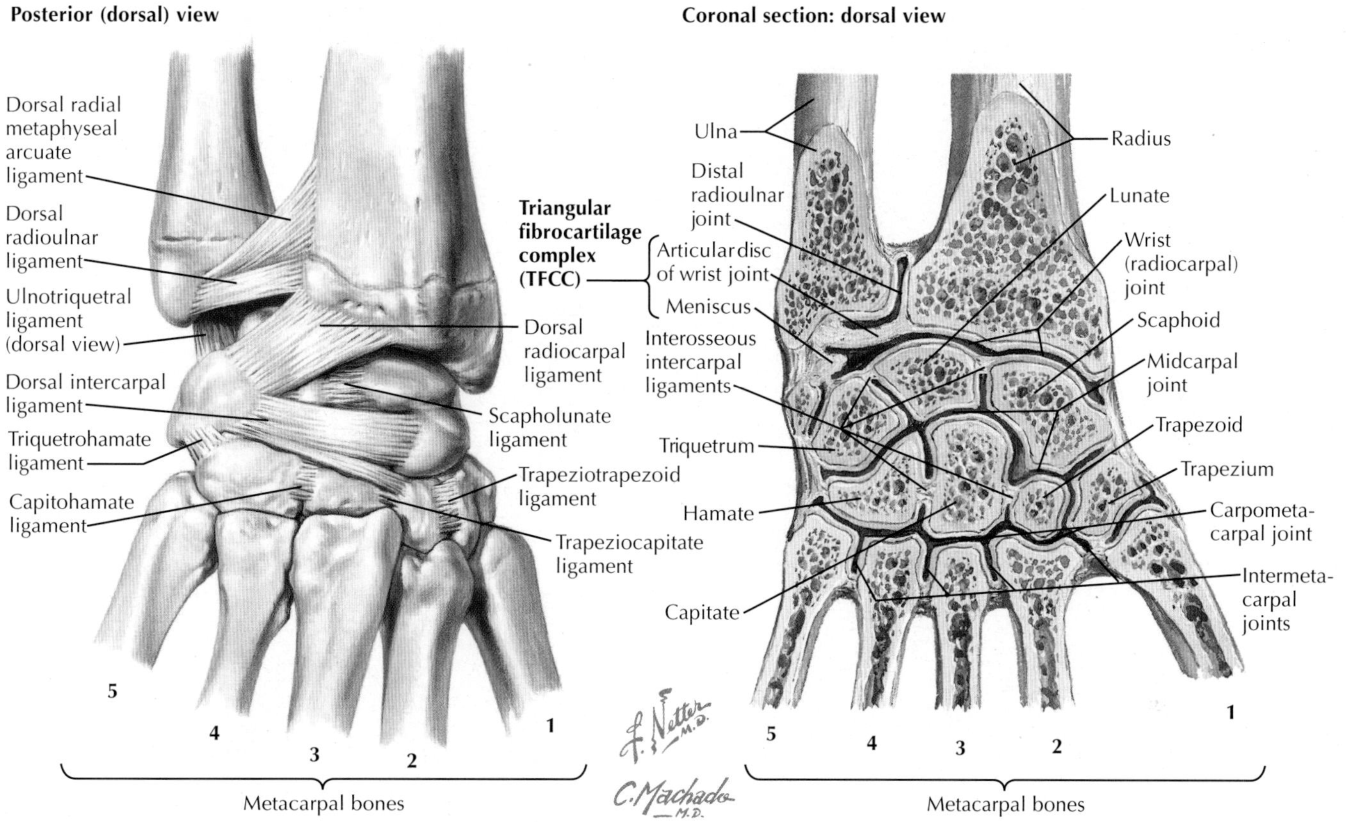
Posterior (dorsal) view
Dorsal radial metaphyseal arcuate ligament
Dorsal radioulnar ligament
Ulnotriquetral ligament (dorsal view)
Dorsal intercarpal ligament
Triquetrohamate ligament
Capitohamate ligament
Triangular fibrocartilage complex (TFCC)
Dorsal radiocarpal ligament
Scapholunate ligament
Trapeziotrapezoid ligament
Trapeziocapitate ligament
5
4
3
2
1
Metacarpal bones
Coronal section: dorsal view
Ulna
Distal radioulnar joint
Articular disc of wrist joint
Meniscus
Interosseous intercarpal ligaments
Triquetrum
Hamate
Capitate
Radius
Lunate
Wrist (radiocarpal) joint
Scaphoid
Midcarpal joint
Trapezoid
Trapezium
Carpometacarpal joint
Intermetacarpal joints
5
4
3
2
1
Metacarpal bones

Figure 76.5 Triangular fibrocartilage complex (TFCC) tears.

Wrist sprains: Acute overstretching or tearing of one or more ligaments of the wrist as the result of an unexpected twist, bend, or impact to the wrist. Pain, swelling, and bruising may follow with a decrease in the normal ROM. X-rays should be obtained to evaluate for a potential fracture. Treatment entails ice, rest, elevation, compressive bandage, antiinflammatories, and bracing. The player should not return to play until completely pain free.

Extensor carpi ulnaris subluxation: Tears or stretching of the extensor retinaculum allow for painful subluxation of the tendon in and out of its groove. The provocative maneuver is a forehand shot with the wrist in ulnar deviation and supination, as when imparting slice to the ball. Treatment entails immobilization of the wrist. If nonoperative treatment fails, surgery may be necessary to repair the retinaculum.

Vascular injuries: Injuries to palmar arteries should be considered with hand pain that increases with activity/play.

Neurologic injury: May include ulnar nerve (compression at the cubital tunnel or Guyon canal), median nerve (pronator teres syndrome, carpal tunnel syndrome), radial nerve entrapment (radial tunnel syndrome), axillary, or suprascapular nerve injury.

Lower Extremities

Ankle sprains: The most common acute injury in tennis and accounts for 20%–25% of all injuries. Inversion injuries predominate. Proper footwear, taping, and bracing may serve to prevent injury. Physical therapy for proprioception, strength, and balance is indicated for rehabilitation and secondary injury prevention.

Muscle strains: Partial muscle tears or pulls affecting the quadriceps, hamstrings, adductors, gastrocnemius, and soleus are common. Injury most commonly occurs at the muscle–tendon (myotendinous) junction. Muscles that span two joints are more susceptible to injury.

Femoroacetabular impingement (Fig. 76.6): Players will note a sharp pain when their affected hip is in a specific position. Clicking, popping, or catching may also be described. Physical examination findings such as a positive impingement sign (forward flexion, internal rotation, and adduction of the hip) are helpful. Surgical treatment via hip arthroscopy is advocated for athletes without acetabular dysplasia who fail conservative management.

Knee injuries: Common in tennis because of rapid and repeated pivoting and acceleration during play. Most common knee injuries include patellofemoral syndrome, patellar tendonitis, meniscal injuries, and bursitis. In a survey of the United States Tennis Association (USTA) national team, 19% of all injuries were knee related. Of these, 70% were traumatic and 30% were from overuse.

Tennis leg: Incomplete/complete rupture of the medial head of the gastrocnemius. Injury is acute with a forceful contraction of the gastrocnemius when the knee is extended and the foot is dorsiflexed. Physical examination findings of tenderness to palpation and/or ecchymosis over the site of rupture and loss of strength with plantarflexion are noted. Ultrasound and magnetic resonance imaging (MRI) may help establish the diagnosis.

Achilles tendon rupture: More commonly seen in the player over the age of 40 and is associated with movements that require a quick burst of speed.

Medial tibial stress syndrome (Fig. 76.7): Periostitis along the posterior medial border of the distal tibia from repetitive shock to the lower extremity. Muscles that normally absorb the shock in the leg fatigue, transferring the energy to the adjacent

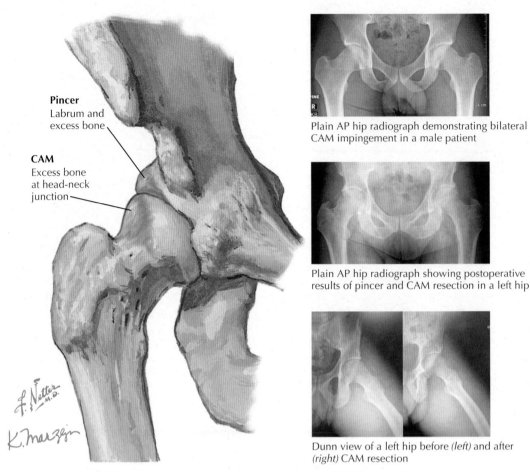

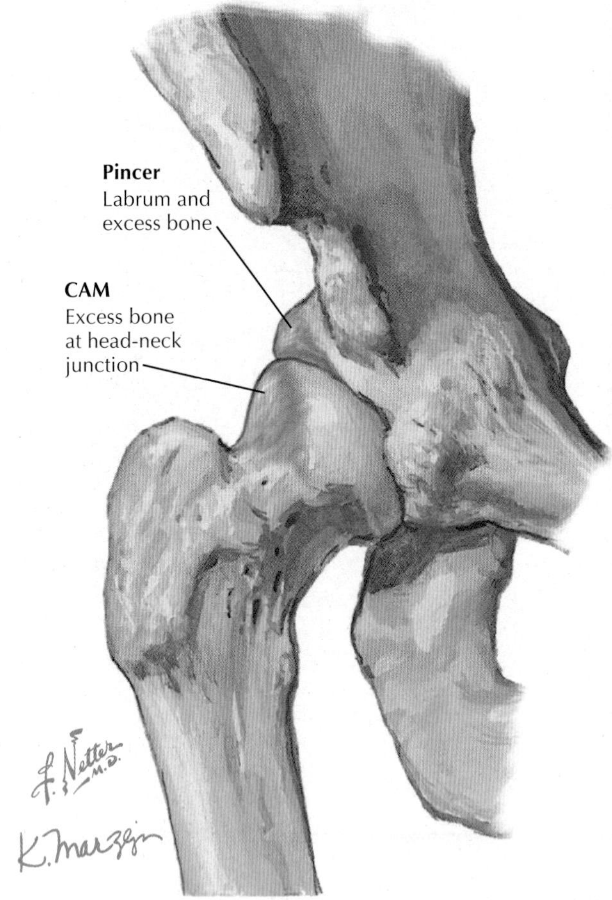
Pincer
Labrum and excess bone
CAM
Excess bone at head-neck junction

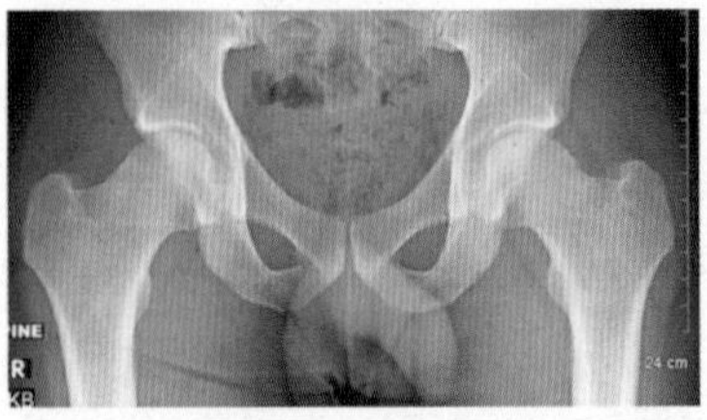

Plain AP hip radiograph demonstrating bilateral CAM impingement in a male patient

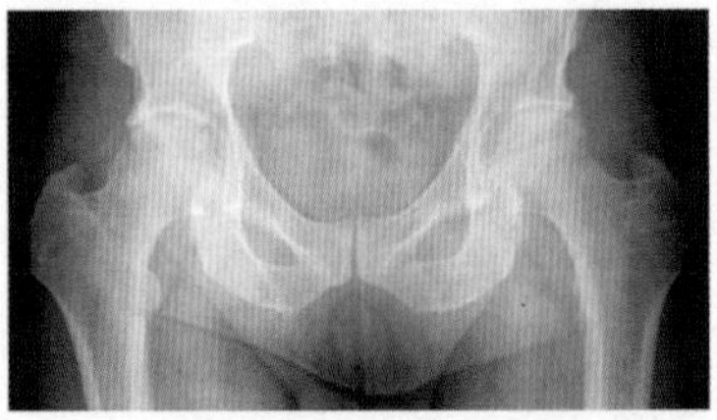

Plain AP hip radiograph showing postoperative results of pincer and CAM resection in a left hip

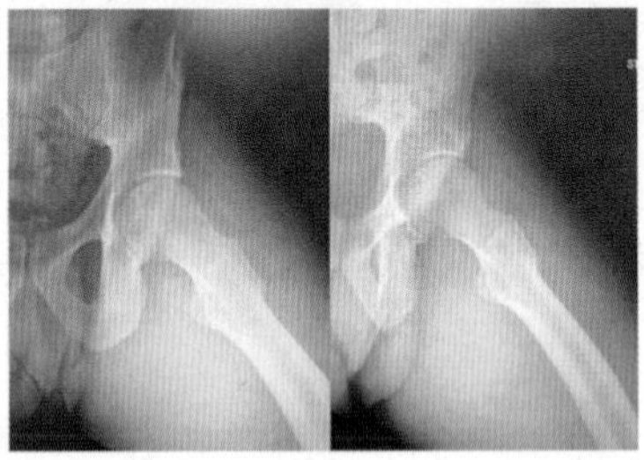

Dunn view of a left hip before *(left)* and after *(right)* CAM resection

Figure 76.6 Femoroacetabular impingement.

periosteum/bone. Rest, taping, and antiinflammatories may alleviate symptoms.

Plantar fasciitis: An overuse injury that occurs because of repetitive forefoot push-offs. Symptoms include sharp pain at posterior medial heel worse in the morning and with activity. Treatment includes activity modification, nonsteroidal antiinflammatories, and evaluation of heel and medial arch support. Changes in footwear or use of an insert may be required.

Posterior tibial tendon insufficiency and pes planovalgus: Pain is noted over the medial aspect of the ankle. Treatment is with the use of shoe inserts with a medial heel wedge, strengthening, and stretching.

Peroneal tendinitis: Frequently encountered in tennis players because of pivoting and rapid change in direction. Players should use tennis shoes appropriate for the surface of the court. Stabilize the ankle with braces, elastic bandaging, tape, or high-top athletic shoes. Exercises to strengthen peroneal muscles by eversion against resistance are indicated for treatment and secondary prevention.

Tennis toe: Repeated abutment of the great toe against the shoe may lead to a subungual hematoma. Players should wear appropriately sized shoes and keep their toenails cut short. Decompression may be indicated in severe acute cases of subungual hematoma.

The Trunk

Low back pain (LBP): Common in tennis players of all ages. Thirty-eight percent of professional, 47% of elite junior female, and 31% of elite junior male tennis players have missed a tournament secondary to LBP.

Lumbar strain: Symptoms often correlate to a change in intensity/duration of play. Repetitive truncal rotation and hyperextension place the erector spinae and multifidus muscles at risk for injury. When the player serves the ball, tossing the ball slightly ahead of the service line and using the lower extremities to launch into the service will decrease the amount of hyperextension of the lumbar spine.

Herniated disc: Repetitive hyperextension and rotational forces applied to the lumbar spine subject the annulus to microtrauma that could lead to a tear. Correction of form and biomechanics is important to prevent a recurrence in injury.

Rib stress fracture: Repetitive contraction of muscles that have origins or insertions onto the ribs places excessive stress on the ribs and may lead to a stress fracture. The fourth and sixth ribs are most frequently affected because of the action of the serratus anterior and external obliques. The player will have point tenderness over the site of the stress fracture. Rib fractures are commonly missed on plain x-ray; bone scans have a sensitivity that approaches 100%.

Spondylolysis (Fig. 76.8): Thought to occur in players secondary to repetitive hyperextension of the lumbar spine. Prevention is similar to that for lumbar strains.

Abdominal muscle strains: Partial muscle tear or pull of the abdominal musculature. Nondominant rectus abdominis is predominately affected. The internal and external oblique muscles are also prone to strains. Symptoms include sharp pain with contraction of the affected musculature.

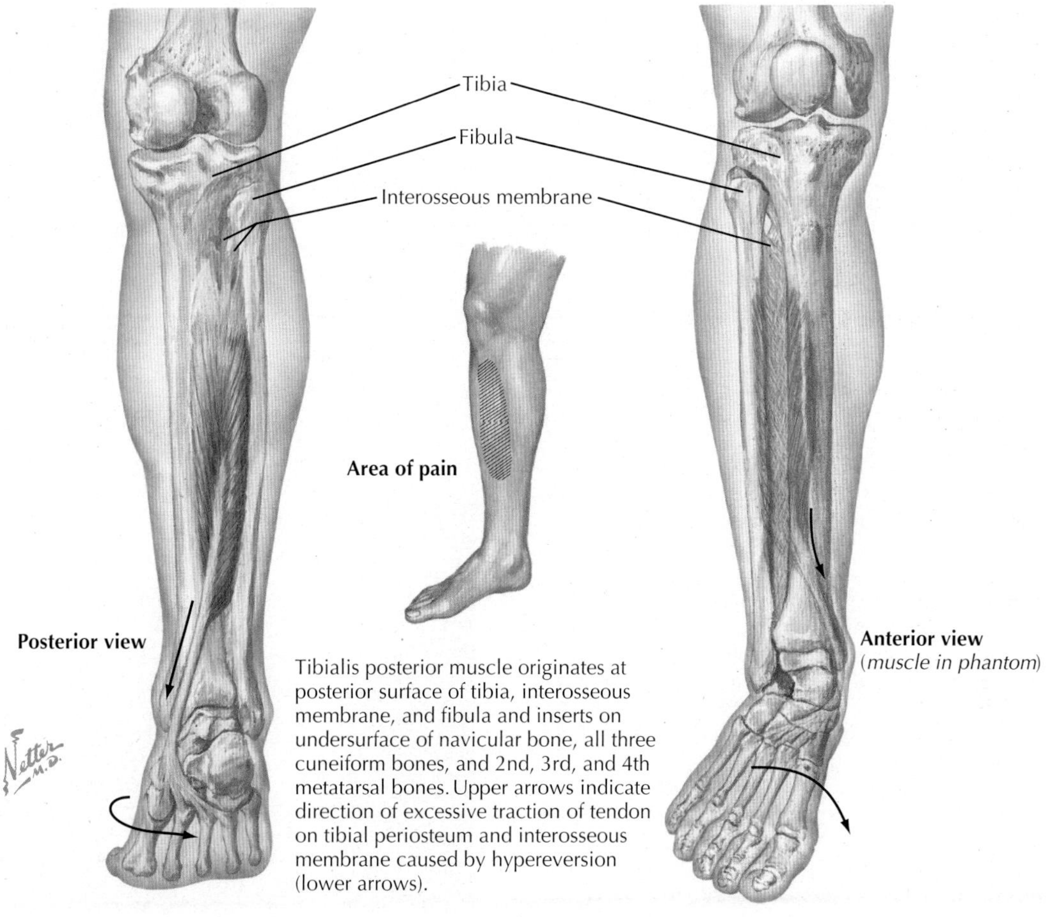
Tibia
Fibula
Interosseous membrane
Area of pain
Posterior view
Anterior view
(muscle in phantom)
Tibialis posterior muscle originates at posterior surface of tibia, interosseous membrane, and fibula and inserts on undersurface of navicular bone, all three cuneiform bones, and 2nd, 3rd, and 4th metatarsal bones. Upper arrows indicate direction of excessive traction of tendon on tibial periosteum and interosseous membrane caused by hypereversion (lower arrows).

Figure 76.7 Shin splints.

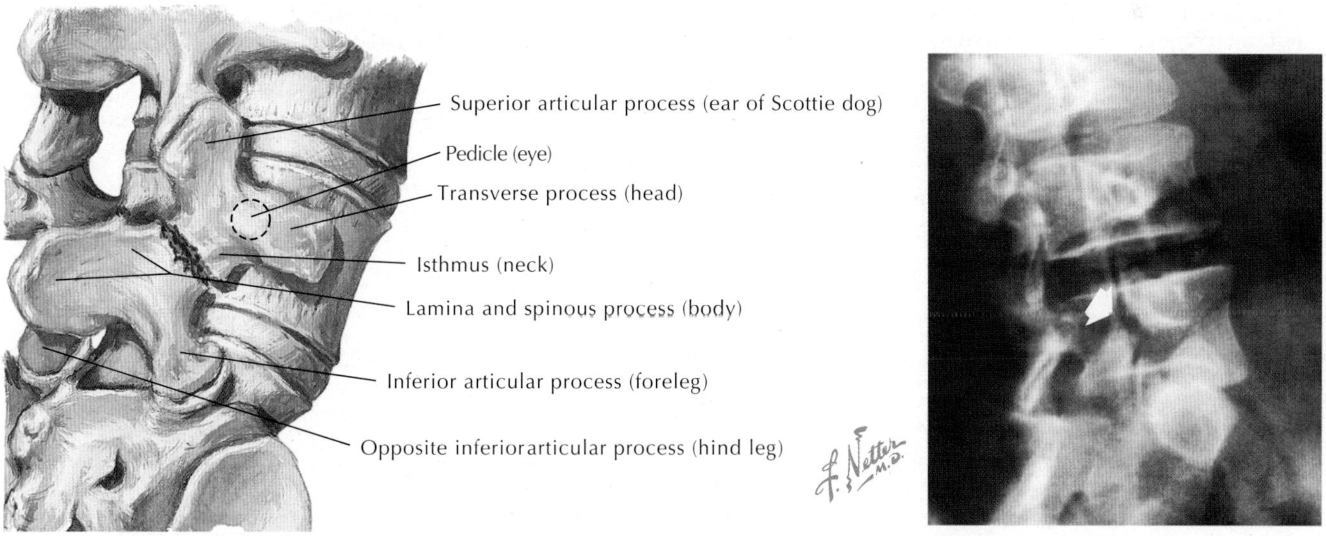
Superior articular process (ear of Scottie dog)
Pedicle (eye)
Transverse process (head)
Isthmus (neck)
Lamina and spinous process (body)
Inferior articular process (foreleg)
Opposite inferiorarticular process (hind leg)

Spondylolysis without spondylolisthesis. Posterolateral view demonstrates formation of radiographic Scottie dog. On lateral radiograph, dog appears to be wearing a collar

Figure 76.8 Spondylolysis.

Core muscle injury: Groin pain caused by shearing forces created across the pubic symphysis because of weak abdominal musculature, strong thigh adductors, and stiff hip joints. Players report unilateral, deep groin pain that is associated with activity and relieved with rest. Pain may radiate into the perineum, adductor region, rectus muscles, inguinal ligament, and testicular area. Patients will have local tenderness, and no palpable inguinal hernia will be identified. Conservative management begins with ice, rest, antiinflammatories, and physical therapy for core strengthening.

Injuries Common in the Adolescent Population

- Muscle and ligament strains and sprains from overuse predominate in the young player.
- Injuries to the lower extremity are twice as common as injuries to the spine and upper extremity.
- Injuries to the foot, leg, and wrist prevail in the female adolescent player, whereas injuries to the ankle, groin, hand, abdomen, and back prevail in the male adolescent player.

Physeal Injuries

Wrist epiphysitis (gymnast wrist): Repeated hyperextension and rotation of the wrist causing inflammation of the distal radius epiphysis. This is commonly seen in the dominant arm of adolescent players who put top spin on the ball. Premature closure of the growth plate is a potential complication. Players note a warm, swollen bump on distal radius that is tender to palpation. X-ray of the distal radius shows a widened physis. Players with wrist epiphysitis should avoid putting top spin on their strokes, and return to play should be delayed until symptom-free.

Proximal humerus epiphysiolysis (Little League shoulder): Chronic overuse injury may be associated with kick serves and top spin strokes. Rest and activity limitation are the mainstays of treatment. Upon return to play, the player should start with ground strokes only.

Medial epicondyle apophysitis (Little League elbow): Overuse injury resulting from the repetitive muscular contractions of the forearm and wrist flexors during forehands and serves. Players note a mildly swollen, tender prominence of the medial elbow. Players may sense a decrease in their ability to serve at full speed and to fully straighten the elbow. Activity limitations on the intensity of conditioning and play are necessary.

Osgood-Schlatter disease and Sinding-Larsen-Johansson disease (jumper's knee) (Fig. 76.9): Shoe wear modification for increased shock absorption and stability, stretching of the quadriceps and hamstring musculature to decrease tension on the patellar tendon, training on soft surfaces (clay or sandy surfaces), and use of a patellar tendon strap.

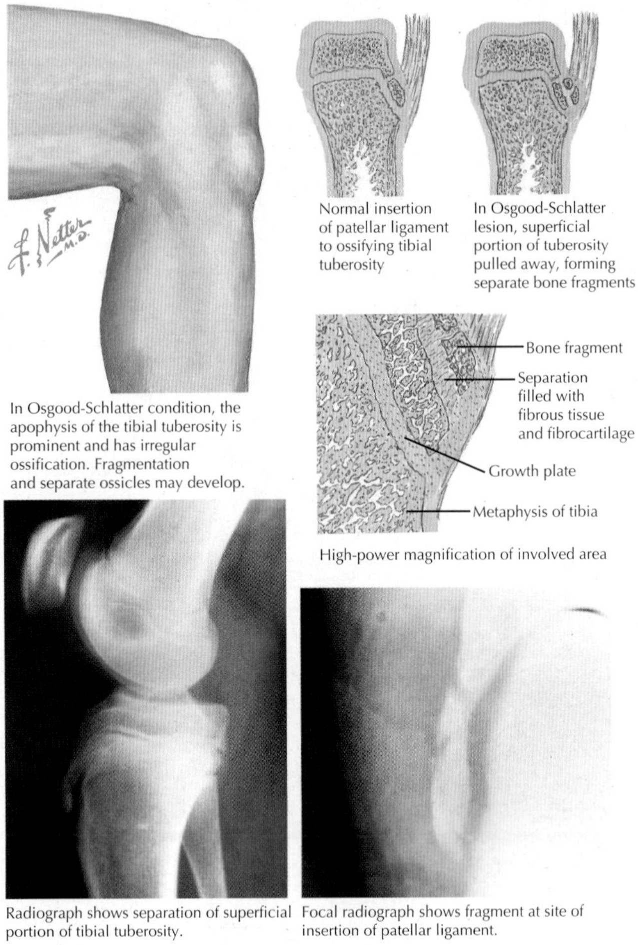
F. Netter M.D.
Normal insertion of patellar ligament to ossifying tibial tuberosity
In Osgood-Schlatter lesion, superficial portion of tuberosity pulled away, forming separate bone fragments
In Osgood-Schlatter condition, the apophysis of the tibial tuberosity is prominent and has irregular ossification. Fragmentation and separate ossicles may develop.
Bone fragment
Separation filled with fibrous tissue and fibrocartilage
Growth plate
Metaphysis of tibia
High-power magnification of involved area
Radiograph shows separation of superficial portion of tibial tuberosity.
Focal radiograph shows fragment at site of insertion of patellar ligament.

Figure 76.9 Osgood-Schlatter lesion.

Sever disease: Most common cause of heel pain in the adolescent player. Prevention and treatment entail proper stretching and use of a heel support that provides cushioning, shock absorption, and decreased tension on the Achilles tendon.

RECOMMENDED READINGS

Available online.

ALPINE SKIING

77

Matthew R. Gammons • Daniel C. Cole • John W. Karl

GENERAL PRINCIPLES

Background

- Alpine skiing is a popular sport worldwide, with approximately >200 million participants per year.
- High speeds, variable terrain, and weather conditions, combined with equipment, can create a significant opportunity for getting injured.
- Equipment changes have changed the nature of injuries, but with more recent studies showing some decline in injury rates.
- Lower extremity injuries are the most common, but upper extremity injuries are also frequent.
- Head injuries and chest wall/abdominal trauma are also of great concern because these injuries can be life threatening.
- Medical issues include cold exposure, sun exposure, altitude issues, and general travel-related problems.

Levels of Competition

- Alpine ski racing at its highest level is governed by Fédération Internationale de Ski (FIS).
- US Ski & Snowboard Association is the governing body in the United States.
- The US national team is divided into four groups: A–D. Athletes are ranked according to skill, with elite skiers in the A team, down to the development team (D team).
- Junior levels are divided by age groups (U21, U19, U16, U14, U12, U10, and U8).
- Often, there is overlap between collegiate levels, high school levels, and junior race clubs.
- Levels U12–U21 may compete locally, regionally, and nationally, with the best skiers competing internationally. U10 and younger usually compete locally and occasionally regionally.
- Recreational skiers can compete in the National Standard Race (NASTAR). The NASTAR is a program wherein recreational skiers of all ages and abilities can test their skills on courses set up at resorts across the country. Times and scores are compared under a universal handicapping system similar to that used in golf.

Events

Technical Events

- Slalom is the most technical of events and involves short arc turns around single turning poles, which are set 7–11 m apart, rather than gates.
- Giant slalom involves a course with technical turns marked by gates set 15–27 m apart.

Speed Events

- Downhill is the fastest event, with speeds reaching 90 mph and is the only event that allows on course training runs. All other events allow only course inspection.
- Super G combines downhill with giant slalom with gates that are farther apart, 25–45 m than those in the giant slalom, at speeds are slightly less than those in downhill.

Combined Events

- Classic combined races usually involve one downhill run and a slalom run; occasionally, they may combine a single slalom with a Super G race.

Event Coverage

- Planning and communication are key. Communicate with ski patrol and race staff before the event or training to learn established protocols and establish a chain of command in case an injury occurs.
- Ski areas may be located a significant distance away from medical or trauma facilities; this, along with winter weather, often mandates that stabilizing care and pain control be provided while transport is arranged.
- Medical personnel must be proficient in alpine skiing because courses are often steep and icy. Optimal course position will vary by event and location.
- Radios allow communication between the medical team and spotters on the course; these should be tested ahead of the training or race because most two-way radios are site-to-site and may have trouble transmitting in certain areas. Cell phone service is also inconsistent in several mountainous areas and should be investigated before the competition.
- Course should be clear of competitors before medical staff attends to injured athletes.
- Most injuries are best taken care of off the mountain; hence, if possible, the majority of care should be delayed until the athlete can be transported to lodge or medical facilities.

Epidemiology

- Rates of skiing injuries have declined over the last 50 years, from 4–5 per 1000 skier days to 2–3 per 1000 skier days.
- Injuries in elite skiers have not changed significantly in the last 10–15 years.
- Catastrophic injuries are rare: 0.01 per 1000 skier days, but have not decreased over the last several decades.
- Ratio of lower extremity to upper extremity injury is approximately 2:1.
- Location of most common lower extremity injury is to the knee.
- Rates and severity of injury are similar with snowboarding, although snowboarders have a higher rate of upper extremity injuries.

Equipment

- A common misconception is that modern equipment protects the knees when it is, in fact, designed to prevent ankle and tibia fractures. Although this appears to have been effective in reducing the number of injuries, it has caused a dramatic increase in knee injuries.
- Standard binding release is based on the skier characteristics such as skill level, boot size, height, and weight: most commonly adjusted based on the Deutches Institu für Normung (DIN) standard.
- Binding mechanism may not release at slow fall speeds because torque requirement is not met.
- Expert skiers and racers will often ski at DIN settings higher than recommended to prevent prerelease.
- Lower extremity injuries, excluding knee sprains, are often associated with inappropriate equipment adjustment.
- Modern skis, called *shaped skis*, have varying degrees of increased side cut when compared with traditional skis and have become the mainstay in all disciplines. Length varies by discipline. Although shaped skis are the most common type of ski used,

it is unclear if these skies have had any effects on injuries at the recreational level. FIS periodically modifies equipment requirements in an effort to make the sport safer, but this has not led to a significant decrease in injuries

Training and Physiology

- Skiing requires a good base of lower extremity and core strengthening and aerobic fitness to tolerate training loads.
- Large eccentric and isometric loads are placed on the lower extremity; hence, strength training should focus on these areas.
- Majority of any ski race occurs at the anaerobic threshold; hence, cardiovascular training regimens should focus on increasing this tolerance.
- The competitive season of elite skiers involves altitude and significant travel; therefore, training should be frequently adjusted to maximize performance while minimizing the risk of overtraining the athlete.

SPECIFIC INJURIES

Lower Extremity

Knee Ligament Injuries (See Also Chapter 55: "Knee Injuries")

- Not unique to skiing but the mechanism of injury differs because of the ski/binding/boot interface (Fig. 77.1)
- Injuries to the medial collateral ligament (MCL) are the most commonly reported, but anterior cruciate ligament (ACL)

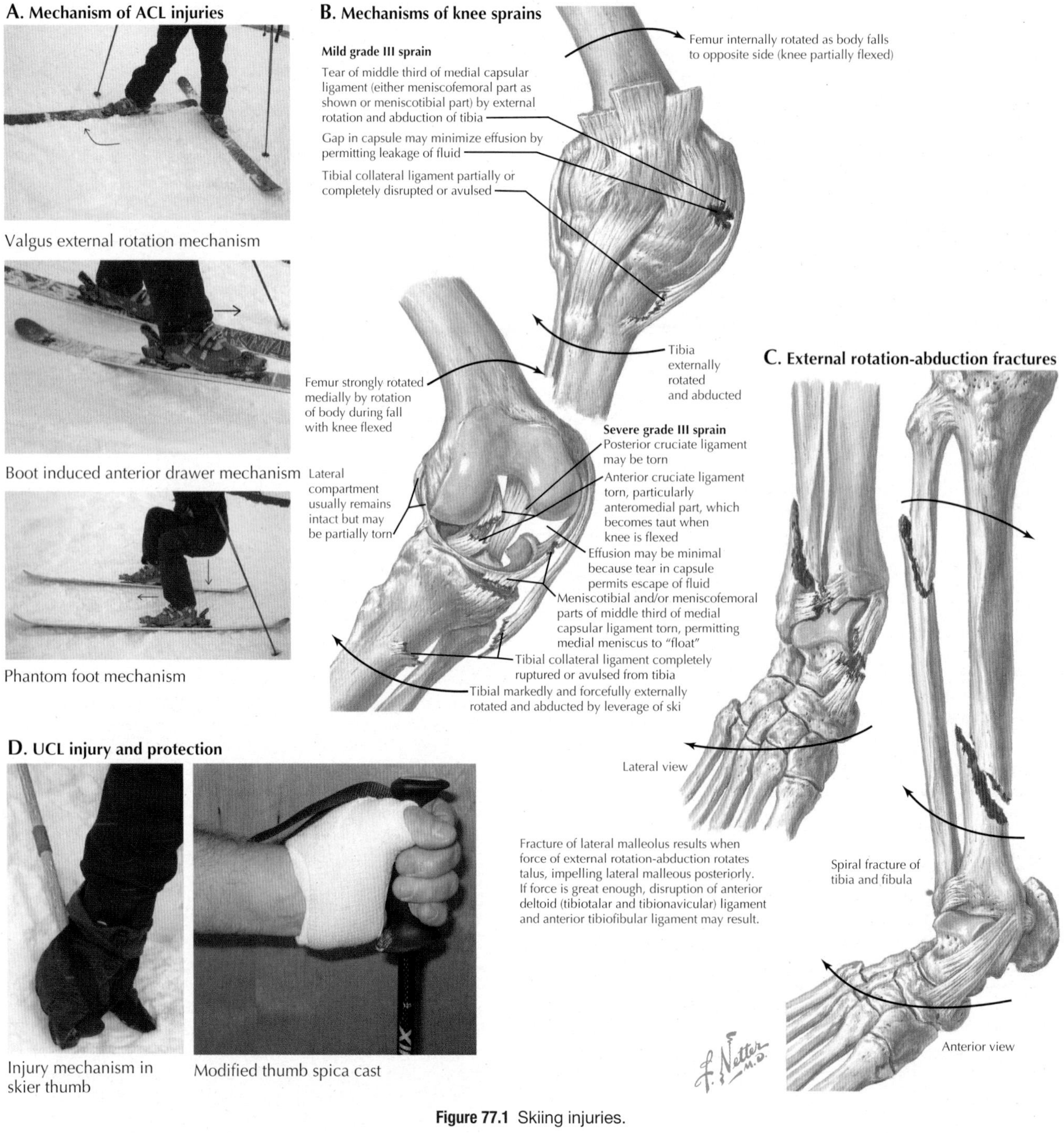
A. Mechanism of ACL injuries
Valgus external rotation mechanism
Boot induced anterior drawer mechanism
Phantom foot mechanism
B. Mechanisms of knee sprains
Mild grade III sprain
Tear of middle third of medial capsular ligament (either meniscofemoral part as shown or meniscotibial part) by external rotation and abduction of tibia
Gap in capsule may minimize effusion by permitting leakage of fluid
Tibial collateral ligament partially or completely disrupted or avulsed
Femur internally rotated as body falls to opposite side (knee partially flexed)
Tibia externally rotated and abducted
Femur strongly rotated medially by rotation of body during fall with knee flexed
Lateral compartment usually remains intact but may be partially torn
Severe grade III sprain
Posterior cruciate ligament may be torn
Anterior cruciate ligament torn, particularly anteromedial part, which becomes taut when knee is flexed
Effusion may be minimal because tear in capsule permits escape of fluid
Meniscotibial and/or meniscofemoral parts of middle third of medial capsular ligament torn, permitting medial meniscus to "float"
Tibial collateral ligament completely ruptured or avulsed from tibia
Tibial markedly and forcefully externally rotated and abducted by leverage of ski
C. External rotation-abduction fractures
Lateral view
Fracture of lateral malleolus results when force of external rotation-abduction rotates talus, impelling lateral malleous posteriorly. If force is great enough, disruption of anterior deltoid (tibiotalar and tibionavicular) ligament and anterior tibiofibular ligament may result.
Spiral fracture of tibia and fibula
Anterior view
D. UCL injury and protection
Injury mechanism in skier thumb
Modified thumb spica cast

Figure 77.1 Skiing injuries.

injuries have dramatically increased and now account for almost 20% of all skiing injuries.
- Injuries among elite skiers are reported at up to 16.5 per 100 skier seasons.
- Combination injuries (ACL/MCL) are common.
- Increased risk of ACL injury in elite female skiers compared with male, although the effect is not as dramatic as is seen in field sports.
- There appears to be no relationship between knee sprains and binding malfunction. ACL injuries in female recreational skiers have been reported to occur with slow speed falls and no binding release; this does not necessarily reflect binding malfunction, but indicates that torque release requirements, set to protect the leg and ankle, may not be met during this type of fall.
- Common mechanisms for knee ligament injuries (see Fig. 77.1)
  - **Valgus external rotation:** Occurs when ski edge catches, forcing the leg into abduction and external rotation; this is the most common mechanism for MCL injuries.
  - The boot-induced anterior drawer ACL injury occurs when the rear of the ski contacts the snow first after jump. The ski then levers the boot forward, creating the anterior drawer movement.
  - **The phantom foot:** Occurs when the skier's weight is posterior and the skier's hips drop below the level of the flexed knees; weight is on the downhill ski, and, as the skier attempts to recover, increased force to the downhill ski results in greater edge pressure. This causes an abrupt internal rotation force on the downhill knee. It was previously believed that this was the cause of most knee ligament injuries; however, more recent studies have challenged this theory.
  - Prevention is focused on education, avoidance of high-risk positions, and equipment adjustment. A small-scale study demonstrated a decrease in knee injuries with education on not trying to recover from a fall into the hill (phantom foot). It is unclear what effect these interventions may have on elite skiers.

Fractures

- Although lower extremity fractures have decreased, there are still two fractures commonly seen in skiers: spiral tibial shaft and tibial plateau.
- Spiral tibial shaft fractures are common in children and can also be seen in adults. They are caused by external rotation forces on the ski and have been associated with binding dysfunction (see Fig. 77.1).
- Incidence of tibial plateau fractures, most commonly of the lateral plateau, has increased along with knee ligament injuries.
- The increase of these fractures along with knee injuries likely represents a similar mechanism of injury—valgus/external rotation—as for knee ligament injuries.

Upper Extremity

- The shoulder, hand, and wrist constitute a majority of upper extremity injuries.
- The shoulder accounts for the largest overall number of upper extremity injuries in skiing. The most common shoulder injuries are listed in Table 77.1.
- Sprains of the ulnar collateral ligament (UCL) of the thumb are the most common single injury, at 8%.
- These injuries occur with a fall onto an outstretched hand with a pole in the palm (see Fig. 77.1).
  - This causes a radial stress on the ligament, sometimes resulting in a complete tear.
  - Treatment involves protection and sometimes surgical fixation.
  - There is no good evidence that risk of injury is reduced by breakaway straps or using a pole without straps.
  - A modified thumb spica splint, casted or removable, molded to a ski pole can allow continued skiing participation (see Fig. 77.1).

Table 77.1 COMMON SHOULDER INJURIES IN SKIING

Rotator cuff injuries	24%
Anterior dislocation/subluxation	22%
Acromioclavicular separations	20%
Clavicle fractures	11%

Data from Koehle MS, Lloyd-Smith R, Taunton JE. Alpine ski injuries and their prevention. *Sports Med*. 2002;32(12):785–793.

Trauma

Head Injuries (See Also Chapter 45: "Head Injuries")

- Account for a small portion of total injuries but for a majority of severe injuries.
- Concussions are relatively common, particularly in the adolescent age group.
- Helmets are mandatory in most competitions, but their role in prevention remains unclear. Several studies have shown a decrease in the risk of head injuries in helmet wearers. However, recent studies have not shown a decrease in severe traumatic brain injuries despite increased helmet use. Several confounding variables, including rates of helmet use, terrain, weather, conditions, and skill level, make it difficult to assess what overall protective effect helmets may have in skiing.

Spinal Injuries

- Severe spinal injuries are rare in alpine skiing: 0.001–0.004 per 1000 skier days.
- Spinal injury rates in snowboarding are higher than in skiing. The most common injury in both is a wedge compression fracture.
- Slope-side treatment of suspected spinal injuries can be difficult.
- Ski patrol members are usually the best personnel to accomplish boarding and spine stabilization on mountains.

Thoracoabdominal Trauma

- Minor chest wall, back, and abdominal trauma is relatively common in skiing and is generally not life threatening.
- However, because of the high speeds involved, physicians should always be aware of the possibility of severe trauma, particularly in cases of collisions.
- Severe injuries include aortic rupture and intra-abdominal organ trauma.

Medical Problems

- Medical problems inherent to skiing include cold-related injuries and altitude illness (see Chapter 22: "Exercise in the Cold and Cold Injuries").
- Elite athletes will often log several thousands of miles of travel during the year for both competitions and training camps. International travel is common, and general precautions should be taken to prevent travel-related illnesses such as traveler's diarrhea. Jet lag and fatigue can also be significant problems and are best managed on a case-by-case basis (see Chapter 24: "Travel Considerations for the Athlete and Sports Medical Team").
- Because of the cold weather climates, skiers often overlook the potential for sun-related skin problems.
- A combination of altitude and reflection off the snow can increase ultraviolet (UV) exposure to extreme levels.
- Education of both coaches and athletes on sun protection is important to help prevent acute sun exposure injuries and the potential for skin cancer.

RECOMMENDED READINGS

Available online.

78 CROSS-COUNTRY SKIING

David D. Cosca

GENERAL PRINCIPLES

- Cross-country or Nordic skiing is multifaceted and can be pursued either as a simple recreational outdoor activity or a vigorous competitive endurance sport.
- Cross-country skiing serves as an excellent means to develop and maintain cardiovascular fitness; most large muscle groups of the upper and lower body are used in a smooth, rhythmic, low-impact manner. A recent prospective study showed association with reduction in all-cause mortality.
- Injury rates are typically lower than those seen in alpine skiing and running.
- It is very popular in Scandinavian countries and is moderately popular in the northeastern and western mountain regions of the United States.

CROSS-COUNTRY SKIING VARIATIONS

Trail/Track Skiing

- Skiers use machine-groomed trails.
- Trails are compacted and rolled with heavy sleds pulled by snowcats or snowmobiles, leaving a set of parallel ski tracks and an 8-by-10-foot wide open lane for ski skating.
- Groomed trails are standard at cross-country ski resorts. Several communities set trails on snow-covered golf courses or bike trails for local citizen use, and some are lighted for night skiing.
- Trail skiing is suitable for a wide range of individuals, young and old, regardless of prior experience. Novices simply "ski-walk," employing a shuffling-like technique on the snow. More experienced skiers use tracks with a diagonal stride (classic) technique or groomed lanes with a ski-skate (freestyle) technique.
- Competitive ski racing and training require machine-groomed trails.

Backcountry Skiing/Ski Touring

- No groomed trail is required.
- Participants choose their own route (i.e., bushwhacking). Some enthusiasts pursue a midday trek in the woods and a picnic lunch, whereas others plan a multiday snow camping tour, and still others seek out backcountry slopes to climb and then descend using a telemark turn technique.
- A telemark turn is one wherein the skier thrusts the outside (or downhill) ski forward, assuming a lunge position with the front knee at approximately 90 degrees of flexion and the back knee in a kneeling position. The turn is carved while holding this position.
- Backcountry skiers typically choose skis with metal edges and relatively heavy, supportive boots.

Chair Lift–Facilitated Telemark Skiing

- Could be considered a variant of alpine skiing; participants opt for a chair lift at a ski area to repeatedly transport them to the top of a slope and then descend while making telemark turns (in contrast to the parallel turns of alpine skiers).
- Skiers use stiff plastic boots, wide metal-edged skis with a significant side cut, and strong three-pin or riveted toe cable bindings that still allow the heel to lift freely off of the ski. The three-pin and most other cable bindings are not designed to release during a fall, although newer binding designs do release.
- Skilled telemark skiers often reach speeds similar to alpine skiers and are subject to similar injuries.

COMPETITIVE CROSS-COUNTRY SKIING

Race Events

- There has been a recent trend toward using audience-friendly formats such as mass-start, sprint, relay, and pursuit (a race that involves switching skis and styles midway through the race).
- Venues for major ski races have been designed to allow better spectator viewing, with large sections of the course visible from the stands.
- World Cup and Olympic race events include (distance format for women and men, respectively) 1 km sprint, 2 × 1 km team sprint, 10 km/15 km individual start, 15 km/30 km pursuit, 30 km/50 km mass start, and 4 × 5 km/4 × 10 km relay.
- Citizen race distances vary from 5 to 55 km. Certain races are specifically designated as classical technique only, whereas most use a freestyle format.
- The largest event in the United States is the American Birkebeiner in Northern Wisconsin (52 km, with >7000 participants).

Equipment

Diagonal Stride (Classic)

Skis: Double camber, with central kick zone area for wax (waxless skis have a unidirectional texture, i.e., fish scale or micro-scale hair); when the skier's weight is evenly distributed between skis, the central kick zone should not contact the snow, thus allowing maximal glide. When the ski is aggressively weighted, the kick zone is engaged in the snow, thus allowing a push-off, or "kick." Skis are typically 20–25 cm longer than the skier's height, but the skier's weight should also be considered when choosing ski length and ski flex.

Boots: Lightweight, relatively low cut, flexible sole.

Bindings: Currently, there are two predominant systems: New Nordic Norm (NNN) and Salomon Nordic System (SNS). Both are lightweight and engage the ski boot at the toe alone, allowing the heel to lift freely off of the ski while striding. The two systems primarily differ by the ridges on the binding plate that fit into corresponding slots on the boot's sole.

Poles: Carbon fiber (preferred by elite skiers) or aluminum, with variable grip and strap systems. Pole length extends to a height between the skier's armpit and top of shoulder.

Ski Skating (Freestyle)

Skis: Typically 10–15 cm shorter than classic skis, with more torsional rigidity to accommodate the forces generated during skate push-off; ski design continues to evolve, particularly in relation to side cut and ski tip shape. Racing ski bases have specified "grinds" to enhance glide wax absorption and maximize glide when matched to specific snow conditions.

Boots: Skate boots are cut higher, with a stiffer upper boot that is hinged at the ankle, and provide more lateral support than classic boots. Skate boots also have a more rigid sole.

Bindings: Similar to classic bindings, but with a more rigid toe plate; the SNS Pilot system has a second attachment point to the boot under the toe that operates as a spring-loaded hinged plate and provides slightly more control over the ski.

Poles: Carbon fiber (best) or aluminum, with variable grip and strap systems, slightly longer than classic poles; typical height of a skate pole is skier's midchin.

Ski Base Preparation

Ski glide: Considerable effort is directed at maximizing ski glide during cross-country ski competitions. Most elite skiers carry several different pairs of skis with variable base compositions and stone ground patterns, or "grinds," each best suited to a particular snow condition. A "rill" pattern may also be pressed onto the ski base to facilitate channeling of melting snow and reduce friction on particularly warm and humid days.

Glide wax: Typically applied to the entire length of the base of skate skis and to the tips and tails of classic skis; layers of wax are melted in with an iron, scraped nearly clean between layers, and then the final layer is brushed and polished after it is ironed and scraped. High-performance ski waxes previously contained fluorocarbons, but these have been phased out because of environmental and health concerns.

Kick wax: Applied to the center section of classic skis to provide grip for forward propulsion; waxes are specifically formulated for different temperature ranges—harder for colder snow, softer for warmer snow—and can be rubbed on like a crayon, then melted with an iron. Certain conditions (icy or warm and wet) call for Klister wax—a sticky, gluelike paste squeezed from a tube.

Clothing

Fabric and fit: Cross-country skiing is a highly aerobic sport. Race participants typically wear light, form-fitting, synthetic clothing, although newer merino wool and silk alternatives are available.

Layers: Layered clothing is a key strategy to avoid either overheating or excessive cooling that might otherwise be caused by variations in exertion or variations in weather, particularly during training or casual skiing.

CROSS-COUNTRY SKI TECHNIQUES

- Ski racers use both classic and skating techniques in competitions (Fig. 78.1).
- Both require a dynamic body position, with forward lean and flexion at the waist.
- Both techniques rely on aggressive poling to generate forward propulsion, and therefore, both require good upper body and core strength.
- The technique of ski skating has evolved during the past 2 decades, with the result that skate skiing technique can be up to 25% faster than classic technique under certain conditions.

Classic Technique

Diagonal stride (classic): The skier keeps both skis in the groomed track, directed straight ahead, and obtains thrust by weighting one ski, engaging the kick zone for grip, and pushing off onto the other ski as it glides forward (see Fig. 78.1). The pole is planted on the opposite side of the kick ski, similar to the arm swing during running, and the body assumes a "diagonal" position relative to the snow.

Double pole: Both poles are simultaneously planted, while the skier vigorously flexes at the waist, leaving the elbows bent, and thrusts downward and backward onto the poles as the skis glide forward in the track (see Fig. 78.1). Double poling is often the predominant technique in a modern classic ski race.

Double pole with kick: Both poles are simultaneously planted as described earlier, but a single leg kick is made as the poles swing forward (see Fig. 78.1).

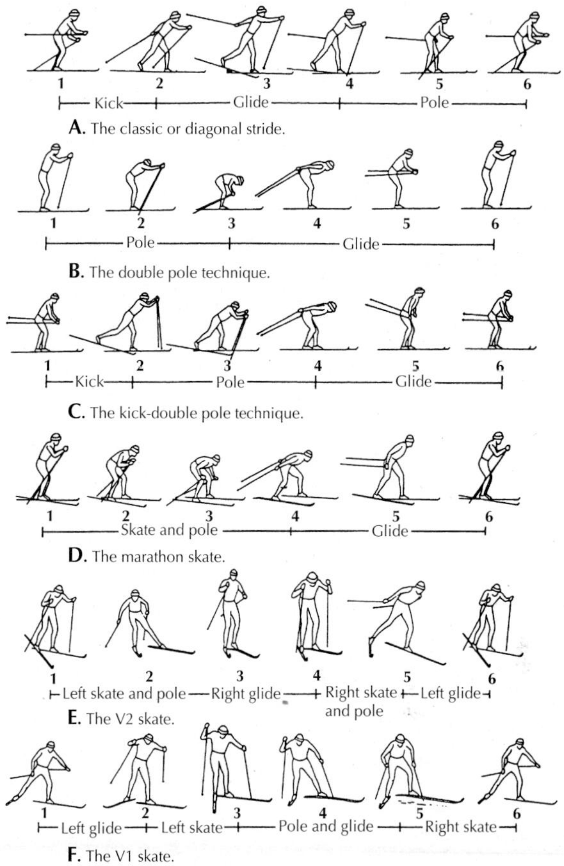

1 2 3 4 5 6
Kick
Glide
Pole
A. The classic or diagonal stride.
1 2 3 4 5 6
Pole
Glide
B. The double pole technique.
1 2 3 4 5 6
Kick
Pole
Glide
C. The kick-double pole technique.
1 2 3 4 5 6
Skate and pole
Glide
D. The marathon skate.
1 2 3 4 5 6
Left skate and pole
Right glide
Right skate and pole
Left glide
E. The V2 skate.
1 2 3 4 5 6
Left glide
Left skate
Pole and glide
Right skate
F. The V1 skate.

Figure 78.1 Cross-country skiing techniques. (From Elmquist LG, Johnson R, Kaplan MJ, et al. Alpine skiing. In: Fu FH, Stone DA, eds. *Sports injuries*. Baltimore: Lippincott, Williams, & Wilkins; 1994:481–500.)

Ski Skating Technique

Description: Skate skiing requires the skier to push one ski outward with the ski slightly angled, applying force to the inside edge much like an ice skater. Complete weight transfer onto the gliding ski is essential for fast and efficient skiing. Ski skating has different techniques for different terrain, much like changing gears on a bicycle.

V1 skate: The technique is asymmetric, with poling accompanying skating on one side but not the other. Double pole with arms in slightly offset position, simultaneously planted with every other step onto the glide ski, and the pole thrust timed with skating push-off (see Fig. 78.1); typically used for hill climbing, where poling contributes more than half of the propulsive force; requires good timing, cadence, and body position.

V2 skate: A symmetric technique with a double pole on every skating push-off, timed just before the step onto the gliding ski; used on flatland or gentle uphill (see Fig. 78.1); requires complete weight transfer, good balance, upper body strength, and aerobic fitness.

V2 alternate skate: An asymmetric technique with a double pole on every other skating push-off; timing similar to V2 skate, as opposed to V1 skate; used on flatland or downhill at relatively high speed.

Open field skate: Skate without poles; used on downhill at higher speeds.

TRAINING FOR CROSS-COUNTRY SKI RACING

Aerobic Capacity of Cross-Country Ski Racers

- Elite-level cross-country ski racers are among the most aerobically fit athletes in the world.
- Olympic gold medal–winning male ski racers have $\dot{V}O_2$ max levels that range from 85 to 92 mL/kg per minute.
- World-class female ski racers have mean $\dot{V}O_2$ max levels in the mid 70 mL/kg per minute range.
- Elite-level masters citizen ski racers in the United States in the 50- to 60-year-old age group have been shown to have $\dot{V}O_2$ max levels in the low-to-mid 60 mL/kg per minute range for men and low-to-mid 50 mL/kg per minute range for women (unpublished data from the University of California–Davis Sports Performance Lab).

Endurance Training

- Exercise training, in season and out, must be specifically targeted to maximize both aerobic fitness and skiing efficiency (technique) in order to improve race performance. Roller skiing is the most sport-specific off-season training activity, although cycling, ski bounding, and uphill ski walking are also good cross-training modalities.
- Most elite coaches recommend that 70%–90% of the total training volume be dedicated to a mix of long-distance, low- and medium-intensity training at levels below the respiratory compensation threshold (variably referred to as "maximal lactate steady state" or "anaerobic threshold"). The remaining training volume should consist of a progressive incorporation of fast distance training at intensities near race pace (slightly above threshold and with close attention to good technique) and short bouts of high-intensity training to improve $\dot{V}O_2$ max.
- Cardiopulmonary exercise testing on a treadmill using expiratory gas measurements can be used to measure aerobic fitness ($\dot{V}O_2$ max) and ventilatory thresholds and provide specific heart-rate training zones. Lactate threshold testing can be performed either on roller skis or on the snow and can also provide accurate heart-rate training zones.
- Ski racing does require anaerobic efforts during sustained hill climbs and end-of-race sprints, and therefore, skiers should include training to improve this capability.
- Upper body and core strength are key contributors to ski race performance; therefore, sufficient effort must be directed at improving these parameters during the off-season. Core strengthening may also reduce the incidence of back pain, which is a relatively common complaint among ski racers.

Blood Doping

- Three medal winners in the 2002 Winter Olympic cross-country skiing events tested positive for darbepoetin, and seven skiers were disqualified in the 2006 Olympics.
- Skiing is an endurance sport, much like cycling, where the benefits of an elevated erythrocyte mass brought on by use of erythropoietin (EPO) or autologous blood transfusion can result in a significant competitive advantage.
- Drug testing at the world-class level is aggressively maintained, with fewer disqualifying results in the past decade.

ENVIRONMENTAL CONCERNS

- Terrain for cross-country skiing ranges from well-groomed flatland skiing in open fields to backcountry alpine wilderness, where hills, obstacles, and uneven snow surfaces factor into play.
- Participants are subject to the effects of altitude, humidity, sun exposure, temperature, and wind chill, each of which can vary during any particular outing.
- In certain backcountry areas, avalanche is a concern.
- Skier awareness of snow conditions, weather, and potential hazards are foremost in the avoidance of environment-related health hazards.

Sun Injury

Description: Up to 85% of ultraviolet (UV) waves reflect off the snow surface, which magnifies the effect of sun on exposed areas of skin and unprotected eyes.

Cold Injury

Frostnip: Freezing of superficial layers of skin causing burning pain and erythema that is completely reversed with rewarming

Frostbite: Ranges from first-degree injury to epidermis only and no resultant tissue loss to deep, penetrating fourth-degree wounds involving subcutaneous tissues, muscle, and tendon

Corneal freezing: Affected by wind chill, ground speed, temperature, and humidity; use of goggles or sunglasses is recommended, although evidence for primary prevention is lacking

Hypothermia: Cooling of core temperature with resultant physiologic changes, ranging from shivering, tachypnea, and poor judgment to stupor, bradycardia, and death

Risk factors: Exposed or inadequately protected skin, wet or inappropriately fitting clothing, altitude, humidity, and wind chill constitute the inherent risk factors for cold injury in skiing. Cold injury is more common in recreational or inexperienced skiers. Prevention strategies include wearing appropriately sized clothing in removable layers; using a base-layer garment designed to "wick" moisture away from skin is recommended. Synthetic fabrics such as polypropylene or naturals such as wool or silk are suitable options for next-to-skin wear. Appropriate nutrition and avoidance of alcohol and dehydration are highly recommended (see Chapter 22: "Exercise in the Cold and Cold Injuries").

Altitude

Acute Mountain Illness

- Estimated to occur in approximately 20%–25% of individuals with recent ascent above 2500 meters (8000 feet) but is relatively infrequent in Nordic skiing, given that most ski areas are at lower elevations
- Acute mountain illness (AMS) may develop in skiers at the lower elevations encountered at ski areas or race events, particularly if the skiers live at low elevation and travel quickly to higher elevations.
- Symptoms in such athletes are usually mild and self-limited. Altitude illness is less common in elite athletes because of experience, acclimatization, and training.
- Backcountry skiers, particularly those who enjoy mountaineering, are at a higher risk of more severe AMS.
- Only a fraction of participants (0.01%–0.05%) develop high-altitude cerebral edema (HACE) or experience high-altitude pulmonary edema (HAPE). Severe symptoms are best treated with rapid descent (see Chapter 23: "Altitude Training and Competition," for details on diagnosis, treatment, and prevention of altitude illness).

EPIDEMIOLOGY OF INJURY AND ILLNESS

- Frequency difficult to measure; skiers may not report minor injuries or illness, and certain cross-country skiers seek out remote locations that may lead to a delay or even failure to present for medical care.

- A prospective case study reported an injury rate of 0.72 per 1000 skier days in cross-country skiers compared with an injury rate of 3.4–7.4 per 1000 skier days in alpine counterparts.
- A 2012 study in the Czech Republic reported an injury rate of 0.1 per 1000 skier days over 7 years. A 2014 study from Germany found an injury rate of 0.09 per 1000 skier days in competitive skiers and 0.51 per 1000 skier days for recreational skiers.
- Most traumatic injuries occur during descents.
- Injuries and illness occurring in competitive skiers are common, yet often minor in nature.
- Complaints addressed during or after competition include muscle fatigue and soreness, tendonitis, and minor ligament injuries.
- Medical complaints such as dehydration, cold injury, gastrointestinal problems, and bronchospasm are also common.
- Exercise-induced bronchospasm (EIB) is estimated to occur in >30% of participants; EIB is more common in cross-country skiing than any other winter sport.
- Cross-country skiing is a winter sport that is pursued when the risk of viral upper respiratory illness is at its highest. The intense nature of endurance training may also lead to a diminished immune response.
- A common cold may strike just before a highly anticipated race event, negating months of training and resulting in a disappointing race result.
- During race season, skiers should use all common sense strategies to minimize the risk of cold and flu: good hand washing, avoidance of close contact with infectious individuals, a flu shot, and optimization of immune function with adequate sleep and good nutrition.
- If ill, skiers should appropriately reduce their training intensity.

MUSCULOSKELETAL INJURY

- Lower extremity injuries are consistently reported as more common than upper extremity injuries (approximately 55% vs. 35%).
- Injury type and relative frequency as described in a published meta-analysis are sprains (40%), fractures (27%), contusions (16%), lacerations (9%), dislocations (6%), and others (1%).
- Injury frequency and type are significantly influenced by skier experience and terrain conditions.
- Competitive athletes tend toward overuse injuries, whereas less experienced skiers are at a higher risk of traumatic injuries.
- Impact injuries from falls are most common and are predisposed by icy surfaces and obstacles buried in snow.

OVERUSE INJURIES

Upper extremity: Common injuries to all skiing styles include de Quervain tendonitis; wrist extensor tenosynovitis; rotator cuff, bicipital, and triceps tendinopathy; and medial and lateral epicondylitis. The longer poles used in **skating** predispose skiers to **triceps tendinopathy.**

Lower extremity: Strains to the hip adductors, internal rotators, and flexors are common, with **adductor strain** being particularly predisposed by **skating** technique. Injuries common to running sports are similarly found in Nordic athletes and include patellofemoral pain, patellar tendinopathy, medial tibial stress syndrome, stress fracture, Achilles tendinopathy, plantar fasciitis and rupture, sesamoiditis, and hallux rigidus (skier's toe) (Fig. 78.2).

Trunk and spine: Low back pain is a common complaint in competitive skiers, likely related to the aggressive forward-flexed skiing posture. Studies report variable frequencies between classic and skating techniques, with strongly conflicting data. Inappropriate technique, inexperience, and training errors are thought to be contributing factors regardless of the skiing style.

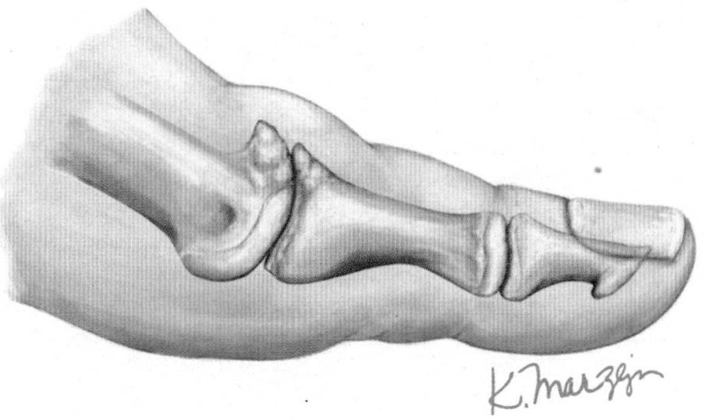

Figure 78.2 Skier's toe.

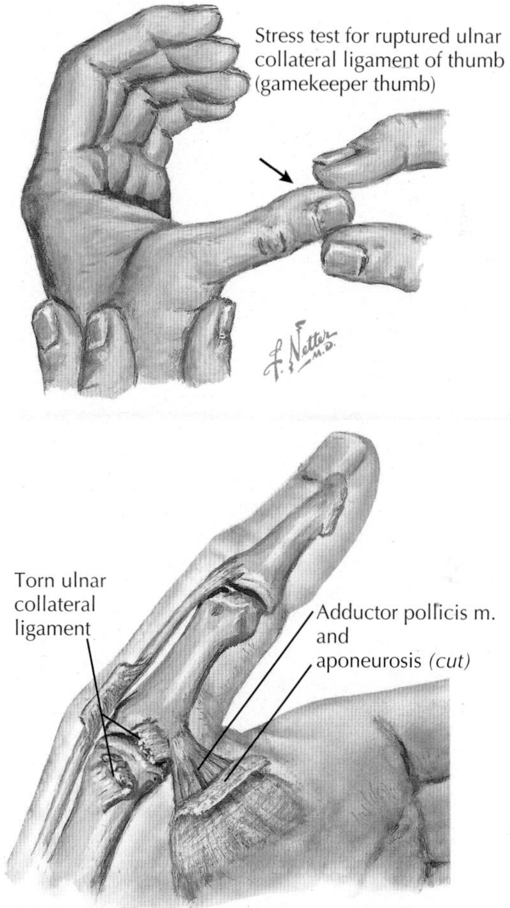
Stress test for ruptured ulnar collateral ligament of thumb (gamekeeper thumb)
Torn ulnar collateral ligament
Adductor pollicis m. and aponeurosis (cut)

Ruptured ulnar collateral ligament of metacarpophalangeal joint of thumb.

Figure 78.3 Skier's thumb.

TRAUMATIC INJURIES

Upper extremity: Mechanism for distal upper extremity injuries is most often a fall onto outstretched hand (FOOSH) or direct trauma and can result in ulnar collateral ligament sprain of the metacarpophalangeal (MCP) joint of the thumb **(skier's thumb),** or distal radius, carpal metacarpal, and phalanx fractures (Fig. 78.3). Proximal upper extremity injuries, often caused by direct shoulder trauma, include fracture of the clavicle, shoulder subluxation and dislocation, and acromioclavicular (AC) joint sprain or separation.

Lower extremity: Lower extremity traumatic injuries mimic those found in most high-velocity sports, and the risk is confounded by bulky equipment that may get caught in snow or obstacles, thereby acting as a lever and magnifying forces. Examples include femur fractures, knee sprains (medial collateral ligament [MCL] and anterior cruciate ligament [ACL]), meniscal tear, patellar dislocation, tibial and fibular fractures, ankle sprains, ankle fractures, calf strain, and plantar fascia rupture.

Trunk and head: Soft tissue trauma may cause contusions and lacerations. Direct blows to the head can result in mild traumatic brain injury (concussion). Current data suggest increasing use of helmets in snow sports, but current studies focus on alpine skiing and snowboarding. One report suggests a reduction in head injuries in helmeted alpine skiers when traveling at lower velocities, which might thus infer protection for Nordic skiers, particularly backcountry skiers and telemark skiers accessing ski lifts.

RECOMMENDED READINGS

Available online.

SNOWBOARDING 79

Rebecca Ann Myers • Thomas R. Sachtleben

GENERAL PRINCIPLES

Overview

- Snowboarding was developed in the 1970s, popularized in the 1980s, and became an Olympic sport in 1998 and a Paralympic sport in 2014.
- Recreational and competitive snowboarding has evolved over the past 2 decades because of increased popularity, equipment development, and new disciplines.
- Snowboarders ride on slopes, terrain parks, and half-pipes shared with skiers at winter resorts, as well as in the backcountry.

Equipment

- Standard equipment includes a snowboard, bindings, and snowboard boots (Fig. 79.1).
- Snowboard bindings and boots fix the feet to the board and transfer energy forces to the board.
- Snowboards are made of fiberglass with a wood or foam core and steel edges.
- Most riders wear soft boots, which are comfortable and allow increased foot and ankle movement.
- Hard boots are also available, which have a hard plastic shell similar to ski boots and are designed for increased control and precision of movements.
- Additional safety equipment includes helmets, wrist guards, goggles, and hip and knee pads.

Events

- Alpine-style races (parallel or giant slalom)
- Half-/super-pipe
- Snowboard cross—multiple riders race simultaneously through a course of ramps and jumps
- Big-air events—riders jump for maximum height with aerial maneuvers
- Slopestyle—snowboarders race through an obstacle course full of rails and tables

Biomechanical Principles

- Both feet are positioned nearly perpendicular to the long axis of the board and direction of movement (Fig. 79.2). This prevents the board from acting independently as a lever and applying torque on the knee, which occurs in skiing.
- Riders move with one shoulder and leg leading the way down the slope (see Fig. 79.2). This creates a partial blind side, increasing the risk of collision. Catching the toe or heel edge of the board on snow can cause falls forward onto the rider's hands and knees or backward onto the occiput, sacrum, and hands, respectively.

Injury Patterns

- Injury patterns vary based on skill level.
- Injury rate varies between 1 and 6 per 1000 snowboarder days.
- Upper extremity injuries are the most common injury in snowboarders regardless of skill level.
- Majority of beginner snowboarders' injuries are the result of falls forward or backward after one edge of the board suddenly gets caught on the snow surface, causing a loss of balance.
- Competitive riders have more lower extremity injuries, including knee injuries, because of falls from jumps/landings. As a result of increased velocity and aerials, competitive riders' injuries tend to be more severe.
- Wrist injuries are 10 times more common in snowboarders than in skiers.
- Flexible snowboard boots provide less support than ski boots, making snowboarders more susceptible to ankle injuries.
- Head and neck injury rates are higher in snowboarders than in skiers.
- Snowboarders are 2.5 times more likely to sustain a fracture than skiers, with the most common location being the wrist.

Risk Factors

- It is estimated that 40%–59% of all injuries occur in beginner snowboarders and that 13%–23% of injuries occur on the first day of snowboarding. Over half of injured beginners have never received formal instruction.
- Fast skill advancement and progression to aerials and jumping put numerous riders at risk of serious injury. During competitions, snowboard cross has the highest risk of severe injuries.
- Snowboarding often appeals to those seeking risky behavior. Recreational drug use, alcohol, sleep deprivation, using personal music players, and a rider's perception of these risk factors can contribute to injury.
- Additional risk factors include riding on hard, icy, or slushy terrain in addition to poor visibility/inclement weather.

INJURIES AND MEDICAL PROBLEMS

Upper Extremity Injuries

- Snowboarders reach out with their arms to aid in balance and to brace falls, causing upper extremity injuries. Backward falls cause twice as many fractures as forward falls.
- The shoulder is vulnerable, particularly in advanced riders (acromioclavicular joint separations, shoulder subluxations/dislocations, and clavicle fractures).
- Elbow fractures and dislocations occur frequently, particularly in children.
- Early detection of forearm intraosseous membrane injuries is essential, as delayed diagnoses lead to poor outcomes.

Wrist Injuries

- Wrist injuries occur frequently, particularly in children and beginners; one-fourth of all snowboarding injuries involve the wrist, and approximately 75% of these are fractures.
- Distal radius fractures are particularly common, with approximately two-thirds being intra-articular or comminuted fractures requiring surgical intervention.
- Wrists are often used for speed control in addition to pivoting and trick maneuvers. A majority of wrist fractures sustained by novice riders are a result of falls, whereas most wrist fractures seen in advanced riders are caused by jumping.

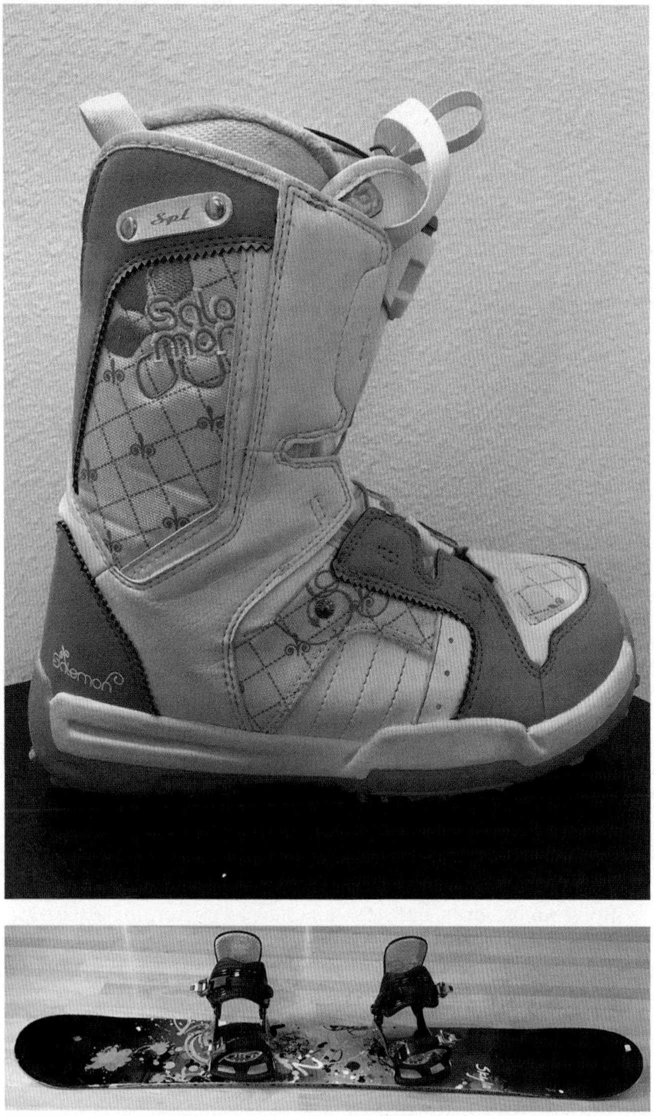
salomon
Spl

Figure 79.1 Snowboarding equipment.

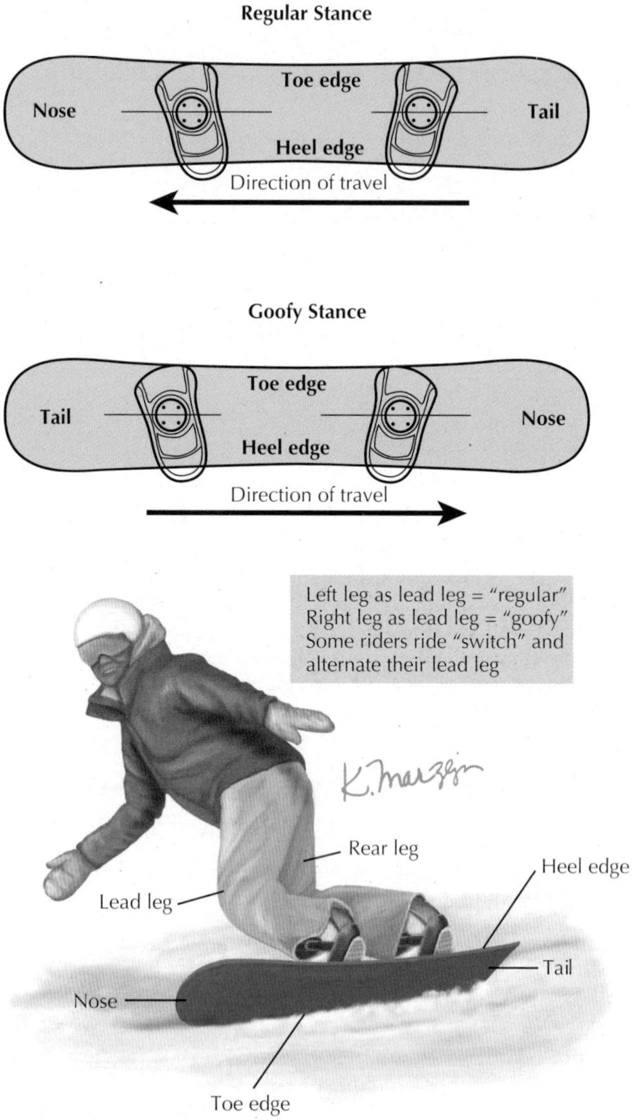
Regular Stance
Nose
Toe edge
Heel edge
Tail
Direction of travel
Goofy Stance
Tail
Toe edge
Heel edge
Nose
Direction of travel
Left leg as lead leg = "regular"
Right leg as lead leg = "goofy"
Some riders ride "switch" and alternate their lead leg
Rear leg
Heel edge
Lead leg
Tail
Nose
Toe edge

Figure 79.2 Snowboard stance.

Head Injuries

- Head injuries encountered in snowboarding include skull fractures, concussions, cerebral contusions, diffuse axonal injury, subdural (most common), epidural, and intracerebral hematomas.
- The incidence of traumatic brain injuries among adolescents is increasing.
- Traumatic brain injury is the leading cause of severe injury and death among snowboarders.
- Collisions with stationary objects (e.g., trees or lift poles) account for approximately half of head injuries.
- Acute subdural hematomas are more common in beginners, and fractures, epidural hematomas, and neurologic injuries are seen more often in intermediate and expert riders.

Spinal Injuries

- Spinal injuries constitute 2%–4% of all snowboarding injuries and are a major cause of permanent disability.
- Most spinal injuries involve compression, burst, or transverse process fractures.
- Half-pipe and "big-air" events are associated with an increased frequency of spinal injuries. Axial loads are transmitted to the spine when landing aerials and jumping in a flexed position. Spinal cord injuries usually occur at the thoracolumbar junction and involve an anterior fracture/dislocation.

Chest/Abdominal Injuries

- Snowboarders usually sustain injuries to the chest, including rib fractures and pneumothorax, as a result of collisions or falls while jumping.
- Blunt abdominal trauma, including liver lacerations, renal contusions, and splenic injuries, are also common in snowboarders, usually after falling from great heights while jumping.
- Contrast-enhanced computed tomography (CT) is best for rapid and accurate diagnosis of intra-abdominal injuries, and a follow-up CT is important when clinical examinations suggest possible delayed splenic rupture. These injuries can be life threatening, and plain radiographs detect an ominous sign such as pneumoperitoneum in only 30% of patients with visceral rupture. Ultrasound can be used when CT is not available or in patients who are hemodynamically unstable.
- Abdominal injuries may be initially overlooked because of concomitant distracting upper extremity injuries, head trauma, or when riders are under the influence of alcohol and/or drugs.

Lower Extremity Injuries

- Ankle injuries make up approximately 15%–20% of all snowboarding injuries, with half of these being fractures, primarily involving the lateral process of the talus (LPT).
  - Approximately one-third of ankle fractures in snowboarders involve the LPT.
  - This fracture is frequently seen in riders wearing soft boots that allow increased ankle flexibility.
- Snowboarders are also at a risk of malleolar bursitis and pseudotumor of the ankle.
- Malleolar bursitis develops as a result of repetitive friction from stiff snowboard boots, and pseudotumors occur as a result of compression of soft tissues between the lateral malleolus and snowboard boot.
- Approximately 75% of lower extremity injuries involve the lead foot.
- Anterior cruciate ligament (ACL) injuries are infrequent and are primarily seen in advanced snowboarders landing flat after a jump or riding in the terrain park. Novice riders are at a risk of ACL injury while getting on and off lifts because this action requires one leg free for self-propulsion.
- The incidence of hip dislocations in snowboarders is five times higher than in skiers.

Fracture of Lateral Process of Talus

Description: This injury is often referred to as "snowboarder's fracture" because it is relatively unique to snowboarding. This fracture occurs 15 times more frequently in snowboarders than in the general population. The LPT is a large, wedge-shaped prominence that articulates with the distal fibula and the posterior calcaneal facet (Fig. 79.3A). The lateral talocalcaneal ligament originates from the LPT, and it is important for hinge and rotatory movements.

Mechanism of injury: LPT fractures usually occur as a result of sudden dorsiflexion and hindfoot inversion with axial loading, although external rotation is thought to be a key component. Axial loading in this position, along with shearing forces transferred from the calcaneus, often occurs with landing after jumps.

Presentation: LPT fractures have a similar presentation as lateral ankle sprains. Persistent pain with weight bearing and severely limited range of motion should invoke a high index of suspicion for talar injury.

Examination: Swelling is anterolateral, with maximal tenderness inferior to the tip of the lateral malleolus. Significant pain is usually noted with attempts at weight bearing. The LPT stress test is performed by applying a dorsiflexed and everted stress to the foot while compressing the ankle in a cephalad direction and holding the lower leg in external rotation (see Fig. 79.3B). The LPT is compressed against the posterior calcaneal facet with this maneuver.

Differential diagnosis: Similar clinical presentations are seen with a lateral ligamentous sprain, subluxed peroneal tendon, lateral compartment syndrome, subtalar joint sprain, and Salter–Harris type 1 fracture of the lateral malleolus.

Diagnostics: The best radiographs for visualization of LPT fractures are the mortise view with 10–20 degrees of inversion or the Broden view. A posterior subtalar effusion should raise suspicion for a LPT fracture. However, the diagnosis of approximately 50% of LPT fractures is delayed because it is not visualized well on standard radiographs (see Fig. 79.3C). CT is often necessary to delineate fracture patterns (see Fig. 79.3D). Consider advanced imaging in snowboarders with positive Ottawa ankle rules with LPT fracture mechanism of injury. Concomitant injuries such as malleolar fractures, ligament sprains, and subtalar dislocations may also be present. LPT fractures are classified into three widely recognized patterns (see Fig. 79.3E): Type 1 fractures involve a small avulsion without extension to the talofibular articulation. Type 2 fractures involve a single large fragment extending from the talofibular joint to the subtalar joint. Type 3 fractures are comminuted.

Treatment: The management of LPT fractures is often challenging. Maintaining appropriate anatomic alignment is paramount to the management of LPT fractures. Type 1 fractures and nondisplaced type 2 fractures (<2 mm or extra-articular) are generally treated nonsurgically with 4–6 weeks of non–weight-bearing cast immobilization. After 2 additional weeks of a weight-bearing cast boot, patients should begin physical therapy to prevent stiff subtalar and tibiotalar joints. Surgical debridement of the LPT may be considered if symptoms persist >6 months. In type 2 fractures (particularly >2 mm or displaced), open reduction and internal fixation (ORIF) has been shown to reduce long-term morbidities (see Fig. 79.3F). Excision of small, displaced fragments is usually necessary with type 3 fractures, as patients treated with immobilization alone frequently have persistent symptoms. In displaced type 2 and all type 3 fractures, several authors recommend attempting closed reduction, with subsequent cast immobilization. If appropriate reduction is unsuccessful, secondary treatment with ORIF is generally required, followed by 4–6 weeks of non–weight bearing (see Fig. 79.3G). Delayed diagnosis of LPT fractures can lead to nonunion, avascular necrosis, and early degeneration of the subtalar joint. Surgical removal of multiple fragments and/or posttraumatic arthritis may result in instability and ultimately a subtalar arthrodesis. These potential complications can cause significant disability in a young, active population. Fortunately, early diagnosis and aggressive management typically result in good outcomes, with 80% of patients who sustained an LPT fracture returning to their previous sport level.

Other Risk and Prevention Measures

Environmental Risks

- Appropriate prevention and protection are necessary to prevent dehydration, hypothermia, and frostbite.
- Protection with sunscreen is particularly important because of high-altitude ultraviolet light exposure.
- Prevention of altitude illness and prompt recognition of symptoms is essential.

Backcountry

- Backcountry use by snowboarders continues to grow as riders seek more varied terrain and better snow conditions in unpatrolled areas.
- Avalanches claim the lives of numerous snowboarders each year, usually from suffocation and/or blunt trauma.
- Deep snow immersion can also cause asphyxiation as a result of a fall into a deep snowbank or tree well. Tree wells are deep depressions of loose snow that form around the base of a tree with low branches. Snowboarders who fall headfirst into a tree well or deep snowbank can be easily trapped and suffocate in as little as 15 minutes. These fatalities, also known as *nonavalanche-related snow-immersion deaths (NARSIDs)*, have become an increasingly recognized fatality pattern in snowboarders. Certain backcountry riders use strapless, releasable ("click-in") bindings or hand-accessible release cords to both bindings in an effort to get their board off quickly in emergent situations.
- Skill, knowledge, good judgment, and appropriate safety gear are crucial for the backcountry. Essential gear includes an avalanche transceiver, shovel, and probe in addition to appropriate avalanche training. Avalanche airbags (self-deployed bladders of air that can be used to keep avalanche victims closer to the surface) are gaining popularity, and certain riders use a device

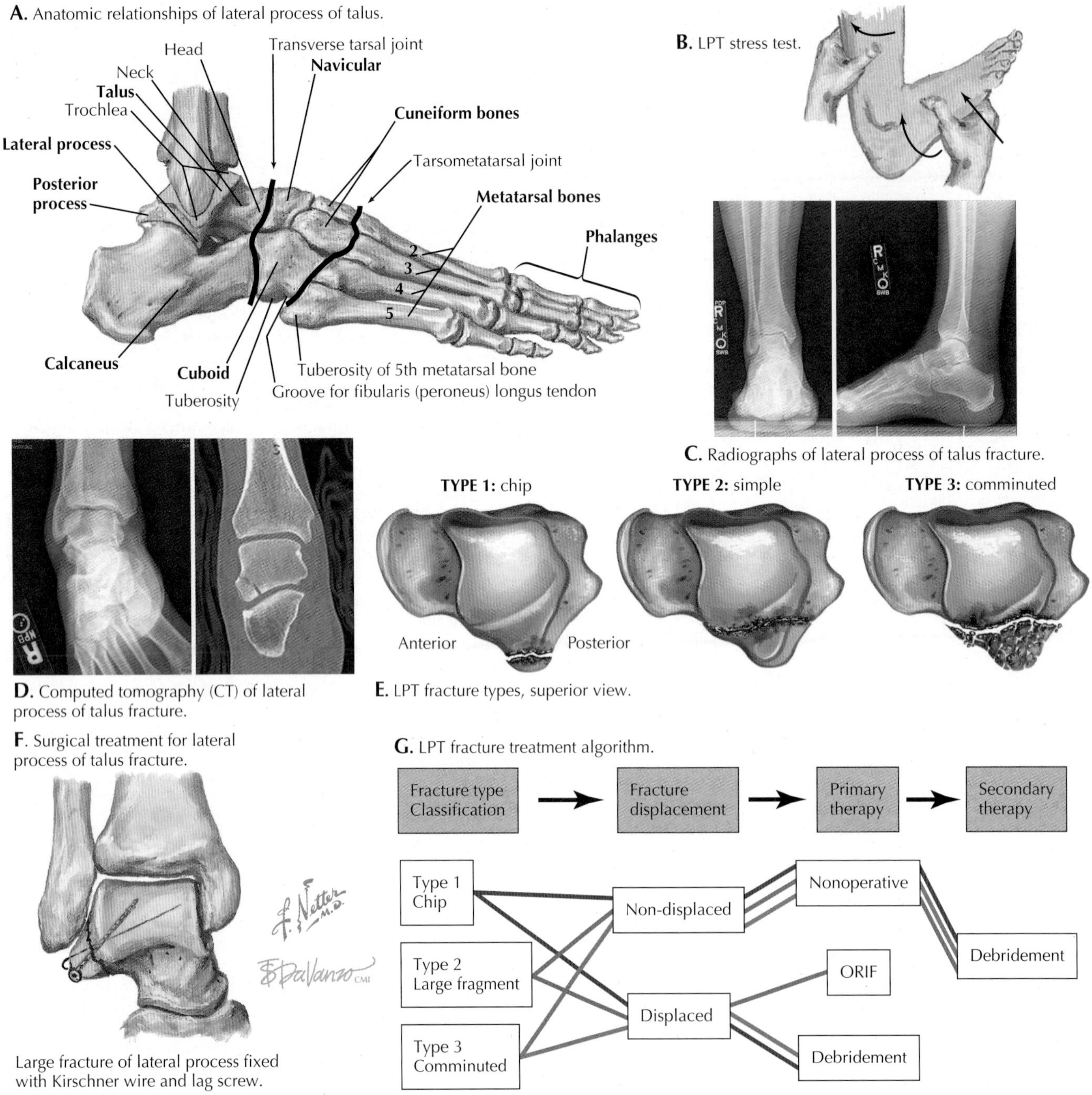
A. Anatomic relationships of lateral process of talus.
Head
Transverse tarsal joint
Navicular
Neck
Talus
Trochlea
Lateral process
Posterior process
Cuneiform bones
Tarsometatarsal joint
Metatarsal bones
Phalanges
2
3
4
5
Calcaneus
Cuboid
Tuberosity
Tuberosity of 5th metatarsal bone
Groove for fibularis (peroneus) longus tendon
B. LPT stress test.
C. Radiographs of lateral process of talus fracture.
D. Computed tomography (CT) of lateral process of talus fracture.
TYPE 1: chip
TYPE 2: simple
TYPE 3: comminuted
Anterior
Posterior
E. LPT fracture types, superior view.
F. Surgical treatment for lateral process of talus fracture.
Large fracture of lateral process fixed with Kirschner wire and lag screw.
G. LPT fracture treatment algorithm.
Fracture type Classification
Fracture displacement
Primary therapy
Secondary therapy
Type 1 Chip
Type 2 Large fragment
Type 3 Comminuted
Non-displaced
Displaced
Nonoperative
ORIF
Debridement
Debridement

Figure 79.3 Fracture of lateral process of talus. (Part G, modified from Valderrabano V, Perren T, Ryf C, et al. Snowboarder's talus fracture: Treatment outcome of 20 cases after 3.5 years. *Am J Sports Med*. 2005;33[6]:871–880.)

called an *AvaLung* that uses a shoulder sling, valve box, and tubing that allows fresh air intake and CO_2 displacement when buried. Backcountry riders should never ride alone.

Injury Prevention

- Effective education, including formal instruction and supervision, is important for young riders and beginners.
- Risk awareness in beginner and advanced snowboarders is paramount.
- Helmets are recommended. Wearing a helmet is associated with a reduced risk of head injury. Helmet use does not increase risk-taking behavior or cervical spine injury in riders. Helmets should fit appropriately.
- Wrist guards reduce the risk of wrist injury, particularly in children and beginner riders. Evidence is limited regarding what type of wrist guards is most effective.
- Further research is needed to evaluate the potential benefits of cardiovascular fitness, core strength, and neuromuscular training in injury prevention.

RECOMMENDED READINGS

Available online.

ICE HOCKEY 80

Robert Johnson

HOCKEY ORGANIZATION AND PARTICIPATION

- **USA Hockey,** located in Colorado Springs, Colorado, is the national governing body for ice hockey in the United States and the official representative of the US Olympic Committee and International Ice Hockey Federation. USA Hockey works in conjunction with the National Hockey League (NHL) and the National Collegiate Athletic Association (NCAA).
- During 1968–1969, 3800 teams were registered with USA Hockey. During 1993–1994, 21,150 teams with approximately 340,000 players were registered. Between 2005 and 2006, over 442,000 players and 58,000 coaches were registered. For 2014–2015, USA Hockey reported over 530,000 male registrants. USA Hockey had over 477,000 males participating in hockey in 2019–2020. Over 380,000 are age 18 or younger. According to the National Federation of High School Associations (NFSHA) statistics for 2018–2019, 1628 boys' teams representing 19 states and almost 36,000 players participated in interscholastic hockey.
- Women's hockey continues to grow in popularity. The number of female hockey players registered in 2014–2015 was almost 70,000. Of these, almost 52,000 were ≤18 years. In 2019–2020 USA Hockey registered over 84,000 females with over 65,000 age 18 or younger. NFHSA data show 642 girls' high school hockey teams representing 14 states with over 9600 participants. Between 1995 and 1996, 38 women's teams competed in an interscholastic competition held in Minnesota. During 2018–2019, 243 teams competed, representing over 2300 athletes. A first state high school tournament for girls was held in Minnesota in 1995. Despite the growth in women's hockey, in a few states, girls are still competing on boys' youth hockey teams.
- The NCAA has 41 women's teams competing in Division I and 67 in Division III. For men, the NCAA reports 61 teams competing in Division I and 84 in Division III. There are no Division II ice hockey teams.
- The Canadian Hockey Association, or Hockey Canada, represents the governing body for amateur hockey in Canada. They have over 621,000 registered players. Of these, approximately 522,000 are males.

Junior Hockey (Ages 16–21)

- Canada has two levels (Major Junior, Junior A)
- Unites States has three levels (Tiers I–III)

Professional Hockey

- Professional hockey in the United States and Canada is represented by the NHL and minor league affiliates.
- European professional leagues include teams from Russia, Norway, Sweden, Finland, Slovakia, Czech Republic, Switzerland, Germany, Austria, and Denmark.
- The National Women's Hockey League (NWHL) currently consists of six teams who play for the Isobel Cup as league champions. This has been contested since 2016, although women's professional hockey has been in existence since 1999.
- **Age range of organized competition: 5 to >50 years.**
- **Age group divisions** are determined by birth date as of August 31 of each year (Table 80.1).
- **Regarded by most as the fastest competitive team sport.**

GAME OF ICE HOCKEY

Structure

- **Professional, college, adult:** three 20-minute periods
- **High school:** three 17-minute periods
- **Youth:** three 12- to 15-minute periods

Team Composition

- Eighteen players and two goalkeepers (usual position distribution). Six players compete at one time: three forwards, two defensemen, and one goalie.
- **Goalkeeper (goalie):** The player who tends the goal to catch or deflect the puck and prevent the opponent from scoring
- **Forwards (left wing, center, and right wing):** Offensive-minded players who attack the opponent with an intent to score a goal; also assist defensemen in protecting their goal
- **Defensemen (left and right):** Primary responsibility is to protect their goal and the goalie to prevent the opponent from advancing to the net to score
- A **substitution** may occur during play ("on the fly") or during time stoppages for violations, goals, or penalties

Rink

- Should be 200 by 100 feet; smallest recommended dimensions are 185 by 85 feet.
- Should be surrounded by wooden or fiberglass boards 40–48 inches high with a yellow or light-colored kickplate at bottom; it is recommended that a safety glass or another protective screen encircle the rink.
- The goal should have dimensions of 4 feet high by 6 feet wide and should have metal goalposts and a crossbar and net surrounding the metal framework.

Special Equipment

- The **puck** is vulcanized rubber, 1 inch thick and 3 inches in diameter, weighing 5.5–6 ounces.
- **Hockey stick**
  - Forwards and defensemen: the blade is usually made of wood (the shaft may be made of other materials) with the shaft <63 inches, blade <12.5 inches long by 2–3 inches wide, and curve not exceeding 0.75 inches
  - Goalie: wood shaft <63 inches with the blade <15.5 inches long by 3.5 inches wide, and curve not exceeding 0.75 inches

Skills

- The skill in **skating** involves three factors: angle of propulsion (angle formed by the skate blade in the direction of the skate), angle of forward inclination (body lean), and length of the stride.
- **Shooting**
  - **Types of shots: standing wrist shot** (sweeping action with the stick terminating in wrist snap and follow-through), **skating wrist shot** (similar to a standing wrist shot except that a player has forward momentum while skating; most accurate), **standing slap shot** (the stick and blade are brought back a variable distance, followed by a vigorous forward motion and "slapping" at the puck like a golf swing; least accurate), and **skating slap shot** (greatest velocity)

Table 80.1 AGE GROUP DIVISIONS DETERMINED BY USA HOCKEY

Level	Boys (Years)	Girls (Years)
U8	≤8	≤8
U10	≤10	≤10
U12	≤12	≤12
U14	≤14	≤14
U16	≤16	≤16
U18	≤18	≤18
Senior	>19	>19

- **Maximal velocity** is the result of the strength of arm and shoulder muscles and full trunk rotation
- **Passing**
- **Stick handling:** Ability to advance the puck while maneuvering on ice
- **Checking:** Intentional contact with an opponent who is in possession of the puck, using the hip or shoulder; a player may check from the side, diagonally or frontally, approaching with no more than two skating strides. In 2011, USA Hockey changed the age at which checking could be introduced from PeeWee (U12) to Bantam (U14) based on injury data showing decreased injury and concussion rates at the U14 level.
- **Goal tending:** The goalkeeper (goalie) tends the goal and is protected by special equipment and pads to catch or deflect the puck from the goal.

Safety and Protection

Protective Equipment

- Goalie: helmet, mask, throat protector, chest protector, cup, thick-padded shin guards, blocker (worn on one hand), trapper (device to catch the puck, worn on the opposite hand), skates that are unique to protect the goal and goalie
- Forward and defense: helmet, shoulder pads, elbow pads, padded gloves, cup, breezers (padded hockey pants to protect the sacrum, coccyx, and pelvis), shin guards, and skates
- **Face masks**
  - Full face masks required at youth and high school levels in 1975; Eastern Collegiate Athletic Conference mandated use in 1977; NCAA required use in 1980; helmets required in NHL; visors (half-face shields) were required for all players new to the NHL as of the 2013–2014 season. For players entering the NHL before 2013–2014, face masks (visors) remain optional.
  - **Effects of full and half-face shields** (college level, Canada):
    - Full shield: 61.6% had at least one injury
    - Half shield: 63.2% had at least one injury
    - Risk of facial, dental injury: 2.3 times greater with half shield
    - Risk of concussion: Concussion rates are higher in those wearing the half shield compared with those wearing the full face mask

Rules to Protect Players

- Penalties: 2 minutes (minor), 5 minutes (major), 10 minutes (major), or a combination
  - Offending player must sit in a designated penalty box, and his or her team must play with one less player on ice ("shorthanded"). If two penalties are assessed against the team, it must play two players short. Team never has to play more than two players short.
  - For 10-minute penalties, offending team does not have to play shorthanded. They lose services of that player for that time interval.
  - Single or multiple game disqualifications may be assessed, depending on severity of infraction.
- Goaltender protection: no unnecessary body contact with goalie; the "crease" is the goalie-protected area in front of goal where opposing players cannot enter without a puck. If a goaltender loses his helmet, the play is immediately stopped.
- Common penalties enforced for protection of players:
  - **Cross-checking:** using shaft of stick with both hands to check opponent
  - **Hooking:** using blade of stick on opponent's body to block or impede opponent's progress
  - **Slashing:** striking or attempting to strike opponent by swinging stick
  - **Spearing:** poking or attempting to poke opponent with blade of stick
  - **Interference:** impeding progress of opponent not in control of the puck
  - **Charging:** using more than two skating strides to check the opponent
  - **Checking from behind**
- Officiating: Three to four officials enforce rules, assess penalties, and award goals

PHYSIOLOGY OF ICE HOCKEY

Skating Stride

- **Three phases:** Single leg support, single leg glide, and double leg support (preparation for propulsion)
- **Propulsion:** When extending knee joint in skating thrust, quadriceps develop largest contractile force. Hamstrings and gastrocnemius stabilize knee during weight shift and push-off.
- **Stride rate is related to skating velocity.** Stride length is unrelated except in young hockey players.
- Faster skaters show better timing in push-off mechanics, with resultant push-off in the direction perpendicular to the skating direction. Elite skaters sustain the gliding phase longer.
- In players aged 8–15 years, increases in velocity are accompanied by increases in stride length and no significant change in the stride rate.
- To accelerate quickly, players should attempt full extension of hip, knee, and ankle.
- With fatigue, decrease in skating velocity is caused by decreased stride rate (slower leg extension and longer glide phase) and excessive forward lean.
- Typical game skating behavior is a complex activity involving repeated accelerations, decelerations, turning, and stopping. Complicating skating behaviors are upper body activities of stick handling, shooting, passing, and checking.

Physical Characteristics of Hockey Players

- **Professional players** are taller and heavier on average than college and junior players.
- **Defensemen** are taller and heavier than forwards.
- **Body composition (% fat)**
  - Junior: 8.6%–13.6%
  - College: 8.6%–10.7%
  - Professional: 9.7%–14.2%
  - Forwards and defensemen have equal body compositions.
  - Goalies, on average, have higher body composition than forwards and defensemen.

Energy Expenditure

Physiology has been primarily studied in adult, elite hockey players, which underscores the uncertainty of applying this science to youth hockey.

Game

- Shifts
  - One shift averages 45–90 seconds, with an average of two to three play stoppages/shift, lasting an average of 27 seconds.

- Average playing time/shift is 40 seconds with recovery of 225 seconds between shifts.
- One shift plus recovery averages work capacity of 32 mL/kg/minute (66% of $\dot{V}O_2$ max).
- Average player plays 14–21 shifts each game, with an average playing time of 21–28 minutes/game (based on usual practice of alternating three "lines").
- Energy requirement estimated at two-thirds anaerobic metabolism and one-third aerobic metabolism. On-ice energy requirements of college players is estimated at 70%–80% $\dot{V}O_2$ max, and youth hockey players is estimated in excess of 80% $\dot{V}O_2$ max.
- On-ice heart rate averages 152 beats/minute.

Time–Motion Analysis

- Adult elite players average 6400–7200 meters/game (3.9–4.4 miles/game)
- Forwards demonstrate more anaerobic activity than other positions; aerobic system primarily used for recovery
- Defensemen have longer playing time (33%), more shifts (17%), and longer playing time/shift (21%) but less recovery time between shifts (35%); defensemen average approximately 62% of skating velocity of forwards
- Goalie's quick, explosive movements of short duration with rest periods of submaximal activity use primarily adenosine triphosphate–phosphocreatine (ATP-PC) energy system
- However, few physiologic studies of youth hockey (older age groups) had similar findings
- Adult recreational hockey players tend to stay on ice much longer per shift
- Time–motion analyses are based on use of alternating three lines. In adult recreational leagues, only two lines may be used. At collegiate and professional levels, four lines may be used.
- Heart rate telemetry estimates on-ice intensity averaging 70%–80% $\dot{V}O_2$ max during a 60-minute stop-time game. For 30 minutes of each game, players' $\dot{V}O_2$ max exceeds 90%. Adult recreational players average heart rate intensity in excess of 70%.

Muscle Glycogen Stores (Energy Source)

- Glycogen stores decline by an average of 60% for forwards and defensemen after one game.
- All muscle fibers (types I, IIa, and IIb) contribute glycogen; type I depletes (contributes) the most.
- Twofold increase in plasma free fatty acids suggests mild glycogen-sparing effects in the muscle.
- Consecutive-day games usually do not allow complete repletion of glycogen stores (based on diet as desired).

Lactate Accumulation

- Because anaerobic glycolysis is a major energy contributor, lactate accumulates over course of the game (8- to 10-fold increase). Because approximately 10 minutes are required to remove lactate from exercising muscle, there is inadequate time between shifts for full recovery. Result is mild metabolic acidosis.
- Lactate values usually higher in first and second periods; forwards and defensemen have similar levels
- Levels actually lower than predicted because each shift is interrupted by an average of two to three play stoppages, averaging 27 seconds; this usually allows approximately 60%–65% of PC to be resynthesized before the next shift.

Muscle Fiber Type

- Wide range of fiber composition
- No difference from general population; no position-to-position variation

Anaerobic Power and Endurance

- Forwards, defensemen, and goalies have similar results in peak power and endurance.
- Similar results occurred when younger, less experienced players were tested.

Aerobic Endurance

- Although hockey is largely anaerobic, improving aerobic capacity reduces fatigue and may enhance performance. Involvement of anaerobic system may depend on efficiency of the aerobic system.
- $\dot{V}O_2$ max ranges from 52 to 62 mL/kg/minute. Maximum aerobic capacities of youth hockey players are similar to those of adult players when adjusted for size and weight.
- NHL players have shown consistent increase in aerobic capacities over the past 15 years, presumably because of more effective off- and in-season conditioning strategies.

Muscle Strength and Endurance

- Professional players were stronger than amateurs based on each of the six tests used for comparison.
- Comparing defensemen and forwards at similar levels, data relative to body weight showed these to be equal.
- Compared with other sports, hockey players obtained high levels for total and relative leg force. Only elite canoeists and athletes from power events scored higher (Finnish study).

Flexibility

- Forwards and defensemen have similar flexibility.
- Goalies have significantly better flexibility (key element for that position).
- In general, flexibility of hockey players exceeds that of other elite athletes in wrist, hip, knee, and ankle.
- Other elite athletes exceed hockey players in flexibility on neck rotation, all shoulder and elbow actions, trunk extension-flexion, and lateral flexion.

Fatigue

- Hockey players at risk of fatigue; activities of ice skating require use of all major muscle groups. Hockey has heavy metabolic demands for energy *and* removal of waste products of energy metabolism.
- Studies of fatigue in hockey show failure of return of maximal muscle contractions to pre-exercise levels at 24 hours. Loss of ability to generate maximal force affects athlete's ability to perform peak-force activities to accelerate, stop, and turn.

Detraining

- On-ice practice and game play may not provide sufficient stimulus to maintain or improve fitness among hockey players.
- Studies suggest that additional aerobic activities may be necessary during competitive seasons.

Practical Application of Training Studies

- Programs that have **failed** to improve skating speed: leg squats using weights; pushing partner as technique of resistance skating; speed skating with instruction; skating with ankle weights
- Six-week preseason training program consisting of continuous running, stair running, flexibility, and strength training resulted in 11% increases in $\dot{V}O_2$ max. During subsequent season, gains in oxygen consumption were lost in the absence of any specific in-season aerobic training program.
- Hockey training stimulates improvement in cardiovascular conditioning similar to that of continuous training programs in untrained players. In fit elite players, there were no improvements in cardiovascular fitness over the course of the season.
- Hockey practice observations show 20 minutes of actual skating during 60-minute practice. Heart rate monitoring, however, provided sufficient stimulus for aerobic training effects.
- Anaerobic endurance improved over the course of the season by approximately 16% but not associated with increases in glycolytic enzymes.

- Muscular fatigue over 6-day routine of practices and games showed decrements in maximal voluntary muscle contractions, implying fatigue. Levels decreased through first 3 days, then reached plateau at a level lower than the baseline. After hockey practice, muscle output remains diminished over the practice–game cycle.

Nutrition of Hockey Players

- Dietary composition: protein, 14%–20.5%; carbohydrate, 38%–44%; and fat, 34%–43%
- Average daily intake is 2800–4900 calories

Environmental Factors

- Ice arenas usually have lower ambient temperatures than other athletic settings, which minimize the risk of heat-related injury.
- Hockey protective equipment reduces the ability to dissipate heat.
- Despite hydration between periods and shifts, hockey players lose 2–3 kg body weight through sweat each game.

Physiologic Studies and Their Implications for Shift Length

- Shorter shifts result in higher contribution of PC and oxidative phosphorylation to ATP (energy source) turnover, reducing contribution of anaerobic glycolysis, which reduces consumption of muscle glycogen.
- Shorter shifts result in less lactate accumulation in exercising muscles. Lactate accumulation causes muscles to be inefficient and fatigue more readily. If lactate levels are lower, lactate clears more quickly and muscles recover more quickly.

INJURIES IN ICE HOCKEY

Epidemiology

- **Incidence and rate:** In NHL, most recent data from the 2011–2012 season; injury incidence density 39.4 (per 1000 hours actual ice time) compared with 2007–2008, injury incidence density, 68 (Table 80.2)
  - NHL defensemen injured more often than forwards; goalies have greater time loss with injury than other positions.
- Collegiate injuries (Table 80.3)
  - Youth hockey injuries (Canada, 15-year study; Tables 80.4 and 80.5)
- Age group differences
  - Age 11–14 years: 1 injury/100 hours playing time
  - Age 15–18 years: 1 injury/16 hours playing time
  - Age 19–21 years: 1 injury/11 hours playing time
  - Professional: 1 injury/7 hours playing time
  - In Finland, youth hockey injuries occurred with an incidence similar to youth soccer and alpine skiing.
  - Under the age of 12 years, injury was infrequent. Beyond 12 years, injuries increased evenly over older age groups.
- Average injury risk of *all* sports is 1.37%. Hockey has an average incidence of 2.71% compared with an average risk of 3.95% in soccer.
- One study at the elite level showed 5% of all injuries were related to fighting.
- **Catastrophic injury rate:** 2.55 per 100,000 compared with football rate of 0.68 per 100,000; rules infractions related to 17% of all catastrophic injuries
- **Injuries per player per year:** youth hockey, 0.02; professional, 3.0
- **Descriptive injury data**
  - Twenty-four to forty-five percent of all injuries occur during practice (Table 80.6).
  - **Fifty-five to seventy-six percent of all injuries occur during games:** first period, 20.5%–31%; second period, 30%–38%; and third period, 28%–46.2%.

Table 80.2 NHL INCIDENCE RATE AT SITE OF INJURY AND MECHANISM

Injury Site	Incidence Rate
Head	17%
Thigh	14%
Knee	13%
Shoulder	12%
Ankle	6%
Foot	6%
Pelvis/low back	5%
Injury Mechanism	**Incidence Rate**
Checking	28.2%
Incidental contact	14.3%
Puck	13.5%

Table 80.3 COLLEGIATE INJURIES (BASED ON DATA FROM 2000–2001 TO 2006–2007 SEASONS)

	Men (Injury Rate Reported Per 1000 Athlete Exposures)	Women (Injury Rate Reported Per 1000 Athlete Exposures)[a]
Type	Game: 18.7 Practice: 2.23	Game: 12.1 Practice: 2.9
Position	Goalie: 2.7 Defense: 5.0 Forward: 5.1	Goalie: 14.0% Defense: 41.2% Forward: 44.7%
Period	First: 15.1 Second: 15.1 Third: 11.2	N/A
Location	Home: 11.9 Away: 15.6	N/A
Site	Knee/leg: 22% Head: 19% Shoulder: 15% Foot/ankle: 12% Hip/groin: 9% Back/spine: 9% Wrist/hand: 7% Other: 7%	**Game/practice**[b] Head/neck: 25.4/16.2 Upper extremity: 30.3/22.2 Trunk/back: 11.4/26.4 Lower extremity: 31.8/31.1 Other 1.1/4.2

[a]Checking is not permitted in women's hockey. Injuries are the result of "incidental" contact (collisions with other players, the boards, the ice, and the goal), the stick, and the puck. Fifty percent of injuries occur as a result of collisions.
[b]Concussion is the most common injury reported in both practices and games.
N/A, Statistics not available.

Table 80.4 YOUTH INJURIES

Years	Female (%)	Male (%)
Age 7–8	2.8	2.9
Age 9–10	9.3	8.6
Age 11–12	21.2	22.1
Age 13–14	34.7	35.6
Age 15–17	32	30.8

- In youth hockey, the rate of injury in games is four to six times the incidence in practices. The higher game rates occur at older, more competitive levels. Injury rates increased at ages when checking is introduced. House leagues had lower injury rates than the equivalent travel (more competitive) leagues.

Table 80.5 COLLEGIATE INJURIES BY INJURY SITE, MECHANISM, AND TYPE

Injury Site	Female (%)	Male (%)
Upper extremity	39.2	45.2
Head/neck	28.4	25.1
Lower extremity	23.2	21.4
Abdomen/thorax	25.3	17.8
Injury Mechanism	**Female (%)**	**Male (%)**
Collision	28.6	24.6
Checking	25.7 (illegal)	42.8
Falls	25.3	14.8
Other (puck, stick)	20.4	17.8
Injury Type	**Female (%)**	**Male (%)**
Soft tissue	39.8	32.6
Sprains/strains	21.1	17.6
Fractures	18.2	27.1

Table 80.6 PRACTICE VERSUS GAME (INJURIES/1000 PLAYERS): COLLEGE INJURY COMPARISON

Sport	Practice	Game	Total
Men's basketball	5.1	9.5	6.0
Men's gymnastics	4.7	14.8	8.9
Wrestling	6.8	28.1	8.9
Hockey	2.23	18.7	5.0

- **Injury incidence—time in period:** 0–7 minutes, 12.5%; 7–15 minutes, 40.6%; and 15–20 minutes, 46.9%
- **Acute versus overuse:** acute, traumatic, 80%; overuse, 13.5%–20%
- **Location on ice:** 40% in the defensive zone, 35% in the offensive zone, 25% in the neutral zone
- **Injury by position:**
  - Defensemen (107.8 per 1000 game hours): 55% minor, 30% moderate, 15% severe
  - Forwards (71.8 per 1000 game hours): 73% minor, 21% moderate, 6% severe
  - Goalies (39.2 per 1000 game hours): 83% minor, 17% moderate, 0% severe
- Male and female injury rates are similar in spite of "no-check" rules in women's hockey

- **Injury potential**
  - **Collisions** with players, boards, and goalposts
  - **Skating velocity** (examples): senior amateur players, 30 mph (48 km/hour); PeeWee (age 12–13 years), 20 mph (32 km/hour)
  - **Sliding velocity** (after a fall): 15 mph (24 km/hour)
  - **Hockey puck** (6 ounces [170 g] hard rubber) shooting velocity: professional, 120 mph (192 km/hour); senior recreational, 90 mph (144 km/hour); and PeeWee (ages 12–13 years), 50 mph (80 km/hour). Maximal impact force of the puck at its terminal velocity is 1250 pounds (567.5 kg). Hockey masks deform at puck speeds of 50 mph (80 km/hour).
  - **Hockey stick** velocity is measured at 100–200 km/hour during shooting.
  - **Hockey skates** often cause lacerations from sharp, steel blades.
  - **Nonimpact forces:** Vertical reaction force during skating stride is 1.5–2.5 times body weight compared with 3–4 times body weight in runners; posterior push force during skating measured at 150 pounds.

Table 80.7 MECHANISM OF INJURY IN ELITE ATHLETES

Mechanism	Beiner et al. 1973 (%)	Lorentzon 1988 (%)
Stick	25	11.8
Puck	17	14.5
Collision[a]	17	57.9
Skate	6	2.6
Other	36	13.2

[a]Thirty-three percent of injuries in adult hockey, with 14% of collisions unintentional.

Table 80.8 MECHANISM OF INJURY IN COLLEGE ATHLETES

Mechanism	%
Legal check	44.6
Accidental collision	28.6
Illegal stick check	12.2
Fighting	6.5
Illegal check	5.8
Noncontact	2.2

Table 80.9 MECHANISM OF INJURY IN YOUTH (SMALL STUDIES)

Mechanism	%
Collision[a]	50–86
Puck	14.3
Overuse	14.3
Stick	7.0
Skate	7.0

[a]Ten percent unintentional collision.

In one study, illegal checks and violations caused 66% of injuries, but penalties were assessed only 14% of the time.

- **Mechanism of injury** (Tables 80.7 to 80.9)
- **Anatomic sites** (Table 80.10)
- **Type** (Tables 80.11 and 80.12)
- **Severity**
  - **Minor (>7 days' absence):** 61%–73% (46% of all minor injuries caused by body checks)
  - **Moderate (8–30 days' absence):** 19%–22%
  - **Severe (>30 days' absence):** 8% (75% of all severe injuries caused by body checks)
- **Ice surface size and injury (Junior A)**
  - Injury rates: inversely proportional to ice surface size
  - Neurotrauma: no relationship to ice surface size
  - Aggressive penalties: no relationship to ice surface size
- **Incidence and severity of injuries are increasing.** Possible explanations: increased participation, increase in speed of game and size of players, longer seasons and more out-of-season participation at all levels, lack of appropriate training, and inconsistency in rule enforcement

Acute Traumatic Injuries

Acute traumatic injuries account for 80% of all hockey injuries.

Head

- Full spectrum of injury resulting from closed head trauma, including death
- NHL concussion rates: 5.8–6.1 per 100 games (forwards, 65%; defensemen, 32%; goalies, 3%) with mean time loss of 6 days

Table 80.10 ANATOMIC SITE OF INJURIES

Site	%
Professional[a]	
Head, scalp, and face	28.1–52.9
Eye	2.6
Shoulder	5.6–21.9
Hand	2.1–10.5
Thigh (groin)	15.3–35.7
Knee	11.6–17.0
Miscellaneous (back, foot/ankle, ribs)	3.6–23.3
College	
Knee	18.6
Face, eye, mouth, teeth	17.6
Shoulder, clavicle	14.9
Head, neck	10.6
Thigh, hamstring	9.0
Forearm, wrist, hand	6.9
Hip, groin, abdomen	6.4
Chest, back	4.8
Arm, elbow	3.7
Ankle	3.2
Youth[b,c]	
Head and neck	10–23
Upper body	23
Shoulder/arm	19–55
Trunk	13–17
Leg	17–19

[a]Range, four studies.
[b]Range, two studies.
[c]At Bantam level (ages 13–14 years), weight differences of 53 kg and height differences of 55 cm have been reported. Smaller players are more likely to be injured.

Table 80.11 TYPES OF INJURY

Type	%
Adult (Elite)[a]	
Contusion	25–47
Laceration	28–50
Fracture[b]	4–15
Dislocation	1–8
Muscle, ligament	3–12
Other	3–5
College	
Sprains, dislocations	22
Contusions	20
Lacerations	13
Strains	11
Fractures	10
Concussions	8
General trauma	6

[a]Range of three studies.
[b]Fractures are 12 times more common in leagues with checking.

- Study has shown no decrement in performance after return to play
- **Concussions account for 8%–28% of all hockey injuries,** with the highest incidence at the high school level. In males, data from the National High School Sports-Related Injury Surveillance System (NEISS) show the incidence of concussion in ice hockey ranks second behind football. Football has a game concussion rate of 22.9/10,000 athlete exposures (AEs) and a practice concussion rate of 3.6/10,000 AEs, accounting for 17% of all reported injuries. Hockey has a game concussion rate of 14.6/10,000 AEs and a practice rate of 1.1/10,000 AEs, representing 22% of all reported injuries. Lacrosse (10.4, 1.1), soccer (5.3, 0.4), and wrestling (4.8, 1.3) game and practice rates range third to fifth in terms of concussion. Similar data are unavailable for concussion rates in ice hockey for girls.
- Age-group concussion incidence (meta-analysis): 5–14 years, 0.0–0.8 per 100 player hours; high school, 0.0–2.7 per 1000 player hours; college, 0.2–4.2 per 1000 player hours; and elite adult, 0.0–6.6 per 1000 player hours.
- Frequency of closed head trauma has decreased because of mandatory use of helmets.
- Increased angular velocity of head and neck with helmet and face mask does not appear to increase head or neck injury risk.
- In an evaluation of sports-related head injuries reported from emergency departments (EDs) from 1993 to 1999 for the sports of ice hockey, soccer, and football, the overall head injury rate for ice hockey was 8.1–13.7 per 10,000 participants and 6.3–9.7 per 10,000 and 9.4–13.5 per 10,000 participants for soccer and football, respectively. The concussion rate was 2.0–3.5 per 10,000 for ice hockey, and 1.4–3.1 and 3.1–5.2 per 10,000 for soccer and football, respectively.
- Underreporting of concussions in youth hockey; study results of same populations differ depending on the sources reporting.
  - Official injury reports—0.25–0.61 concussions per 1000 player game hours
  - Volunteer observer reports—4.44–7.94 concussions per 1000 player game hours
  - Player surveys (elite level)—6.65–8.32 concussions per 1000 player game hours
  - Player surveys (nonelite level)—9.72–24.30 concussions per 1000 player game hours
  - Male high school hockey players have been observed to have more head impacts per game, but the head impact magnitude was greater in female high school hockey players
  - Although mouthguard use has not been shown to prevent concussion, a recent prospective cohort study shows mouthguard use was associated lower odds of concussion
- NCAA injury surveillance reports the following concussion rates: Division I men, 0.83/1000 AEs; Division III women, 0.78/1000 AEs; Division I women, 0.65/1000 AEs; Division III men, 0.64/1000 AEs.
- See Chapter 45: "Head Injuries," for information about diagnosis and treatment.

Neck

- **0.4%–9.2% of all hockey injuries**
- Based on NEISS data, ice hockey accounted for 1.5% of ED visits compared with basketball (46.6%) and football (32.6%), noting a decrease in ED visits over the last 10 years.
- If player has loss of consciousness, assume cervical spine injury.
- See Table 80.13 for ED data regarding neck injuries.
- **Since hockey helmets have been widely used, incidence of cervical spine trauma has increased; attributed to more aggressive play associated with better and more complete protective gear.**
- **Increased incidence of severe cervical spine injury since the early 1980s**; before 1973, no spinal cord injuries caused by hockey were reported. First published report in Canadian literature occurred in **1984. Between 1981 and 1985, 15 major cervical spine injuries reported each year were attributable to hockey.** From 2006 to 2011, 44 spinal injuries occurred (9.1% considered severe; 78.9%, cervical spine injuries).

Table 80.12 INJURY COMPARISON IN INTERNATIONAL WORLD HOCKEY CHAMPIONSHIPS (2007–2013)

	Men		Women	
Site	IR/1000 Player Games	IR/1000 Player Hours	IR/1000 Player Games	IR/1000 Player Hours
Face	3.5	12.7	0.2	0.5
Knee	2.0	7.5	1.3	4.6
Shoulder/clavicle	1.6	5.8	0.5	1.6
Head	1.6	5.7	1.1	3.8
Fingers/hand	0.8	3.1	0.3	1.0
Ankle/leg	0.7	2.5	0.8	2.7
Groin/hip/pelvis	0.6	2.3	0.3	1.2
Teeth	0.5	2.0	0.1	0.3
Thigh	0.6	2.2	0.2	0.8
Chest/throat	0.5	1.9	0.2	0.7
Foot/toes	0.4	1.6	0.1	0.4
Neck/back	0.4	1.6	0.6	2.0
Wrist	0.4	1.3	0.3	0.9
Arm/elbow	0.3	1.2	0.4	1.3
Abdomen/kidneys/genitalia	0.1	0.6	0.2	0.6
Eye	0.1	0.3	0.0	0.0
Total	**14.2**	**52.1**	**6.4**	**22.0**

IR, Injury rate.

Data from Tuominen M, Stuart MJ, Aubry M, et al. Injuries in women's international ice hockey: an 8-year study of the World Championship Tournaments and Olympic Winter Games. *Br J Sports Med*. 2015;49:1–7; Tuominen M, Stuart MJ, Aubry M, et al. Injuries in men's international ice hockey: a 7-year study of the International Ice Hockey Federation Adult World Championship Tournaments and Olympic Winter Games. *Br J Sports Med*. 2015;49(1):30–36.

Table 80.13 EMERGENCY DEPARTMENTS 1993–1999

Type of Injury	Ice Hockey	Soccer	Football
Sports-Related Neck Injuries			
Total neck injuries	5038	19,341	114,706
Fracture/dislocation	105	214	1588
Contusions/sprains/strains	4964	17,927	104,483
Lacerations	199	0	621
Rates of Injury			
Neck injuries	1.68–4.26	1.34–2.60	4.56–7.18
Fractures/dislocation	0.08–0.30	0.01–0.06	0.06–0.09
Strains/sprains/contusions	1.68–3.87	1.14–2.31	4.25–6.38

Data from Delaney JS, Al-Kashmiri A. Neck injuries presenting to emergency departments in the United States from 1990 to 1999 for ice hockey, soccer, and American football. *Br J Sports Med*. 2005;39(4):21–25.

- **Mechanism of serious injury:** Axial load of cervical spine with head in neutral alignment; in most situations, the player is pushed or checked from behind and slides headfirst into the boards.
- **Cervical spine injury data**
  - Ninety-six percent men, 4% women
  - Of 117 cases, 5 died; 48% had injuries to vertebrae C4–C5, C5, and C5–C6; with spinal cord affected in slightly over half of cases; 29 of 117 became permanently quadriplegic.
  - Causes: impact with boards, 65.0%; impact with player, 10.3%; impact with ice, 7.6%; impact with goalpost, 0.9%
  - Fifty percent of spinal cord injuries occur in the 16- to 20-year-old age group.
- **Factors affecting high incidence of spinal cord injuries:** player taller and heavier, skating faster; increased aggressive behavior at all levels (imitating style of professionals); rules not consistently enforced; insufficient emphasis on conditioning; and equipment problems (lack of shock absorption boards) (see Chapter 46: "Neck Injuries," for information about diagnosis and treatment).
- Cervical spine injury characteristics (1980–1996, Finland and Sweden): 16 cases with permanent disability; in 50% of cases, mechanism was checking from behind; 69% of vertebral injuries involved fractures and luxations between C5 and C7.
- Recent Canadian ice hockey data reflect a trend toward lower rates of catastrophic cervical spine injuries, perhaps reflecting more severe penalties for injurious behavior.

Eye and Face

- Significant injury reduction since mandatory face mask rule:
  - Unilateral injuries reduced from 478 to 42 in one season; blindness reduced from 37 to 12 in one season.
  - Hockey still accounts for 37% of eye injuries and 56% of blindness in sports.
  - **Face masks have been estimated to save in excess of $10 million/year in injury costs.**
- Injury types (before face mask rule): periorbital soft tissue trauma, 43%; hyphema, 19%; and iris damage, 13%; the stick responsible for more eye injuries than the puck

Throat

- Goalies particularly at risk of throat injuries (blunt trauma to larynx) from high-speed pucks
- Padded collars and other deflectors worn by both skaters and goalies to reduce injury risk

Shoulder

- **Acromioclavicular (AC) injuries**
  - Mechanism of injury: direct blows to shoulder and falls on outstretched hand
  - AC separation common
  - NCAA data show 29.1% of upper extremity injuries in men and 13.8% upper extremity injuries in women are to the AC joint

- In Norfray's 1977 study of 77 hockey players, 45% had asymptomatic radiographic abnormalities, including osteolysis of AC joint and callus from united and nonunited distal clavicle fractures
- In a study by Lorentzon and colleagues, only one of four players with AC separations missed >1 week of practice or games
- **Glenohumeral dislocation:** 8% incidence; greater morbidity than AC separations; high rate of recurrence

Elbow, Wrist, and Hand

- Twenty percent of moderate-to-severe injuries are a result of wrist and hand problems
- **"Skier's" or "goalkeeper's" thumb:**
  - Associated with fall on outstretched hand while hockey stick is still in possession
  - Treatment same as that outlined for other sports
  - It is possible to fashion splint of thermoplastic, plaster, or fiberglass to fit in a hockey glove; may be prohibited by rules or game officials
  - Nonsurgical as opposed to surgical therapy recommendations are changing for early versus late repair of grade III ulnar collateral ligament sprain; check with hand specialist
- Scaphoid fractures: uncommon
- **Metacarpal fracture:** usually related to stick trauma ("slashing")
- **Lacerations** of forearm, wrist, and hand may occur after fall if another player skates over fallen athlete. Skate blades can cut through thinner leather over palm of gloved hand. Wear and tear of leather of glove's palm makes it paper-thin—affords little protection.
- During fights and melees, gloves are often dropped, allowing other traumatic hand injuries plus risk of human bites. Usual human bite precautions are necessary.

Back

- Infrequent site of injury, 4.3%–7.0%.
- Spondylolysis can occur.
- Most back pain is probably of muscular origin and may be treated nonsurgically.
- Severe spinal injuries: T1–T11, 9.2%; T11–T12/L1–L2, 6.0%; L2–S5, 5.1%

Abdomen or Groin

- Common site of lower extremity injury because of forceful hip adductor contraction during skating stride; 10% of injuries in certain studies.
- Inguinal hernias, osteitis pubis, hip impingement, and pelvic or hip stress fractures have been reported in hockey players.
- Rectus abdominis muscle injuries can also be debilitating and chronic in hockey players. When nonsurgical treatment fails, surgical reinforcement has been necessary to permit athletes to return to skating.
- NHL experience (1991–1992 to 1996–1997)
  - Injuries per 1000 player hours: 1991–1992, 12.99; 1996–1997, 19.87
  - Preseason injury rate 5 times greater than the regular season and 20 times greater than the postseason play
  - 23.5% are recurrent injuries; >90% are noncontact injuries
  - Mean time loss: abdominal injury, 10.6 sessions; groin injury, 6.6 sessions
  - Groin injury accounts for 77% of injuries (68% were adductor strains)
  - Abdominal injury: 23%
  - Position: forwards, 60.6%; defensemen, 28.9%; goalies, 5.5% (4.9% not recorded)
- **Femoroacetabular impingement (FAI)** (includes cam and pincer deformities)
  - Identified with increasing frequency in ice hockey players, with a cam deformity occurring more commonly
  - A recent review showed ice hockey had the highest occurrence of hip impingement, with football and soccer lagging slightly behind. Goaltenders tend to have a higher incidence of FAI compared with position players.
  - Cross-sectional study of NHL players revealed cam morphology in 85%, acetabular retroversion (60%), and acetabular dysplasia (21%). Decreased hip external rotation and total arc of motion were predictive of pain and subsequent surgery.
  - Early sports specialization in ice hockey has been associated with increased occurrence of hip and groin pain in intercollegiate hockey players.
  - There are no data regarding the occurrence of FAI in women ice hockey players.
  - In general, women have a lower incidence of FAI when other similar sports are compared.
- **Sports hernia**
  - Common cause of groin pain that represents a hernia of the posterior wall of the inguinal canal with or without concomitant hip adductor muscle injury
  - Demand of certain sports such as ice hockey, soccer, and football seems to increase the rate of sports hernia diagnoses.
  - Male > female
  - Failing nonsurgical treatment with relative rest and physical therapy, surgical intervention may be necessary.

Thigh Contusions

- Hockey players are at a high risk because of high incidence of collisions with players, goals, and boards.
- In general, players are protected, but protective padding may slide to one side.
- Treatment of quadriceps contusions is no different from other collision sports.

Knee

- **Most common lower extremity injury**
- **Medial collateral ligament (MCL) sprain:** most common serious knee injury in most series; usually results from varus or valgus and rotational stresses
- Anterior cruciate ligament sprains: less frequent than MCL sprains
- Meniscal injuries usually occur in combination with ligamentous injuries
- Hockey poses a lower risk of injury to the knee than soccer

Ankle

- Sprains are less common than in other sports because of protection offered by skate boots.
- Lacerations just above boot often involve tendons.
- Ensure that players tuck tongue of skate boot under shin guards to minimize exposure of anterior ankle to laceration.

Foot

- Fractures of bones in the foot result from a direct blow, usually from the puck.
- Other foot injuries are uncommon.

Overuse Injuries

- Limited data, other than incidence, about types of overuse injuries.
- **Adductor tendinopathy and patellar tendinopathy are most common overuse injuries, specifically related to skating stride.**

Special Medical Situations

- **Commotio cordis:** Manifestation of concussive injury to heart resulting in ventricular dysrhythmia and cardiac asystole.
  - Despite protective equipment, rare case reports highlight a slight risk of such cardiac injury in hockey. Epidemiologic studies suggest that pediatric and adolescent athletes may be predisposed.
  - Seventy deaths (34 organized sports, 36 recreational activity) have been reported; 40 attributed to baseball and 7 to ice hockey; survival rate: 10%
- **Indoor air quality problems ("ice-hockey lung")**
  - Propane- or gasoline-propelled ice-resurfacing machines (known as *Zambonis*) have been implicated in causing illness when engines malfunction or ventilation within the arena is inadequate.
  - Players are at an increased risk of minimal exposures compared with spectators.
    - Nitrogen dioxide gas is heavier than air, found at higher concentrations at ice surface.
    - Thermic inversion occurs because of ice temperature.
    - Plexiglass shields along boards alter air circulation at the playing level.
    - During games and practices, players have minute ventilation up to 30 times higher than at rest.
- **Nitrogen dioxide–induced respiratory illness**
  - Nitrogen dioxide is a by-product of combustion
  - Recommended limit: <0.3 parts per million (ppm)
  - Common symptoms (acute onset after unknown indoor exposure after hockey practice or game): cough, hemoptysis, dyspnea, chest pain, headache, and weakness and pulmonary edema (rare)
  - Treatment: withdrawal from toxic environment, bronchodilators, and corticosteroids; untreated, most symptoms resolve within 2 weeks
  - Late complications of bronchiolitis obliterans may develop 2–6 weeks after initial symptoms
- **Carbon monoxide poisoning**
  - Source: inappropriate combustion of fuel of Zamboni; inadequate ventilation system for arena
  - Recommended limit: <20 ppm
  - Symptoms: acute respiratory (hemoptysis, dyspnea, chest pain, and coughing spells) and central nervous system (headache, dizziness, sleepiness, nausea, and vomiting)
  - Treatment: withdrawal from source of toxin; rarely requires emergency treatment
- **Safeguards**
  - Thirteen states have tested the indoor air quality of ice arenas.
  - Only three states have mandatory air quality testing in ice arenas (Massachusetts, Minnesota, and Rhode Island). Both Pennsylvania and Connecticut have nonbinding guidance for arena indoor air quality.
  - Adequate ventilation of indoor arenas should be ensured.
  - Regular inspection and maintenance of ice-resurfacing machines should be implemented, and indoor air quality should be regularly monitored.

Injury Prevention

- Continue to update protective equipment.
- Ensure use of mouth guards.
- Fabric designs with a high coefficient of friction are under evaluation to reduce the sliding speeds of fallen players.
- **Enforce rules.** One study suggests that 39% of all injuries were attributed to foul play.
- Effective training and conditioning may minimize the risk of injury. Adequate nutrition, training, and hydration may reduce third-period fatigue and reduce fatigue in situations when several games are played on consecutive days, as occurring in tournaments.
- Using fair-play rules for youth hockey tournaments has reduced injury rates.
- Advancing the age of checking from U12 to U14 has reduced injury risk in the U12 age group.
- Application of a "zero tolerance for head impact" rule did not reduce concussion rates in U12 and U14 male hockey players.

RECOMMENDED READINGS

Available online.

81 ICE SKATING (FIGURE SKATING AND SPEED SKATING)

Carole S. Vetter • Emily B. Porter

FIGURE SKATING

Introduction

- Figure skating is a sport that focuses on a unique combination of athleticism, strength, endurance, gracefulness, and artistry on ice.
- Today, over 203,000 members and 765 clubs are registered with US Figure Skating.

General Principles

History

- Began in the early 1800s; its name was derived from the complicated figures traced on the ice during its early years.
- Jumps and spins were introduced in the 1860s, with continuing development of more complex moves ever since.

Figure Skating Categories

- Singles skating: solo skater performing jumps, spins, and connecting steps
- Pairs skating: a male and female skater performing jumps, spins, and dance elements separately and in tandem along with overhead lifts, throws, and throw jumps
- Ice dance: a male and female skater performing intricate footwork and deep edges; partners have specific rules about lifts and the amount of time they can separately skate
- Synchronized skating: team comprising 8–24 skaters moving simultaneously as a group to form various moving patterns; team lifts and certain jumps are permitted

Discussion of Sports-Specific Skills and Other Considerations

- Majority of figure skaters are females who began skating when 5–8 years old. Competitive careers peak in teens or early 20s.

Biomechanical Principles

- At the senior level, men routinely perform at least one quadruple jump (4 revolutions), and several women have performed triple axels (3.5 revolutions).
- Jump landing impact forces can reach five to eight times the skater's body weight.
- Skaters can perform upwards of 50 jumps/session, with two to four sessions/day.

Equipment and Safety Issues

- Figure skates are traditionally composed of leather boots and steel blades. Certain newer skates use synthetic boot materials to decrease weight.
- Boots
  - For cosmetic reasons, traditionally have an elevated heel; however, this results in increased landing impact forces.
  - Becoming increasingly stiff to accommodate the stress placed on them during triple and quadruple jumps, which may contribute to weaker ankles and poorer proprioception.
  - Often custom-fit; may still fit suboptimally; boot shape makes the use of traditional orthotics difficult and may require special orthotics to be molded into the boot when needed.
- Figure skating blades have an inside and outside edge. They have a large front toe pick, which is used in jump landings and certain jump takeoffs.
- Boots are usually replaced every 6–12 months because of breakdown.
- Several lower extremity overuse injuries arise from interactions between the skater's body and the skate. Factors contributing to injury include:
  - Boot fit: Up to two-thirds of skaters may have boots that fit inappropriately
  - Tying technique
  - Boot condition
  - Blade mounting
  - Skating technique

Specific Training Issues

- Typical daily training comprises 2–4 hours of on-ice training and 1–3 hours of off-ice training, which includes strength and flexibility training, dance, conditioning, and choreography.
- Occurs ≥5 days/week throughout the year
- Can become all-encompassing to elite skaters and their families; not uncommon for young skaters to move to new cities or opt for home schooling in order to prioritize training.

Unique Environmental and Nutritional Issues

- Disordered eating is common in figure skaters. Weight and appearance may inappropriately be the primary focus of skaters and coaches over body composition and performance. Contributing factors include:
  - Major role that skater's appearance plays in judges' performance evaluation
  - Advantage of lighter body weight when jumping
- Delayed menarche may result from restrictive eating patterns. This is often perceived as an advantage by skaters because onset of puberty is accompanied by accumulation of additional body mass that must be lifted into the air with each jump in addition to wider hips that contribute to decreased rotational speed.
- Osteoporosis has not been frequently found among skaters.
- Screening for nutritional deficiencies (vitamin D, ferritin, etc.) should be considered in this population.
- Exercise-induced bronchospasm (EIB) and asthma may be triggered because of exposure to the cold, dry air found in ice rinks in addition to the chemicals used to maintain the ice surface or Zamboni fumes, which can contain air pollutants such as carbon monoxide and nitrogen dioxide.

Common Injuries and Medical Problems

- Factors contributing to injuries are the boot, training regimen, nutritional practices, environmental factors, and the culture of the sport that rewards high-risk moves and slender body type.

Foot and Ankle Injuries

- "Lace bite," or tendonitis of the tibialis anterior and toe extensors, can occur as a result of inappropriate placement of the tongue of the boot (Fig. 81.1). Impact from jump takeoffs and landings can also contribute.
- Ankle sprains are common; likely the result of weaker peroneal muscles from wearing stiff skating boots.
- "Pump bumps," or Haglund deformity, and Achilles tendonitis can occur with skate boots that inappropriately fit posteriorly (see Fig. 81.1).
- Bursitis (superficial calcaneal, retrocalcaneal, malleolar) can occur from friction from the boot.

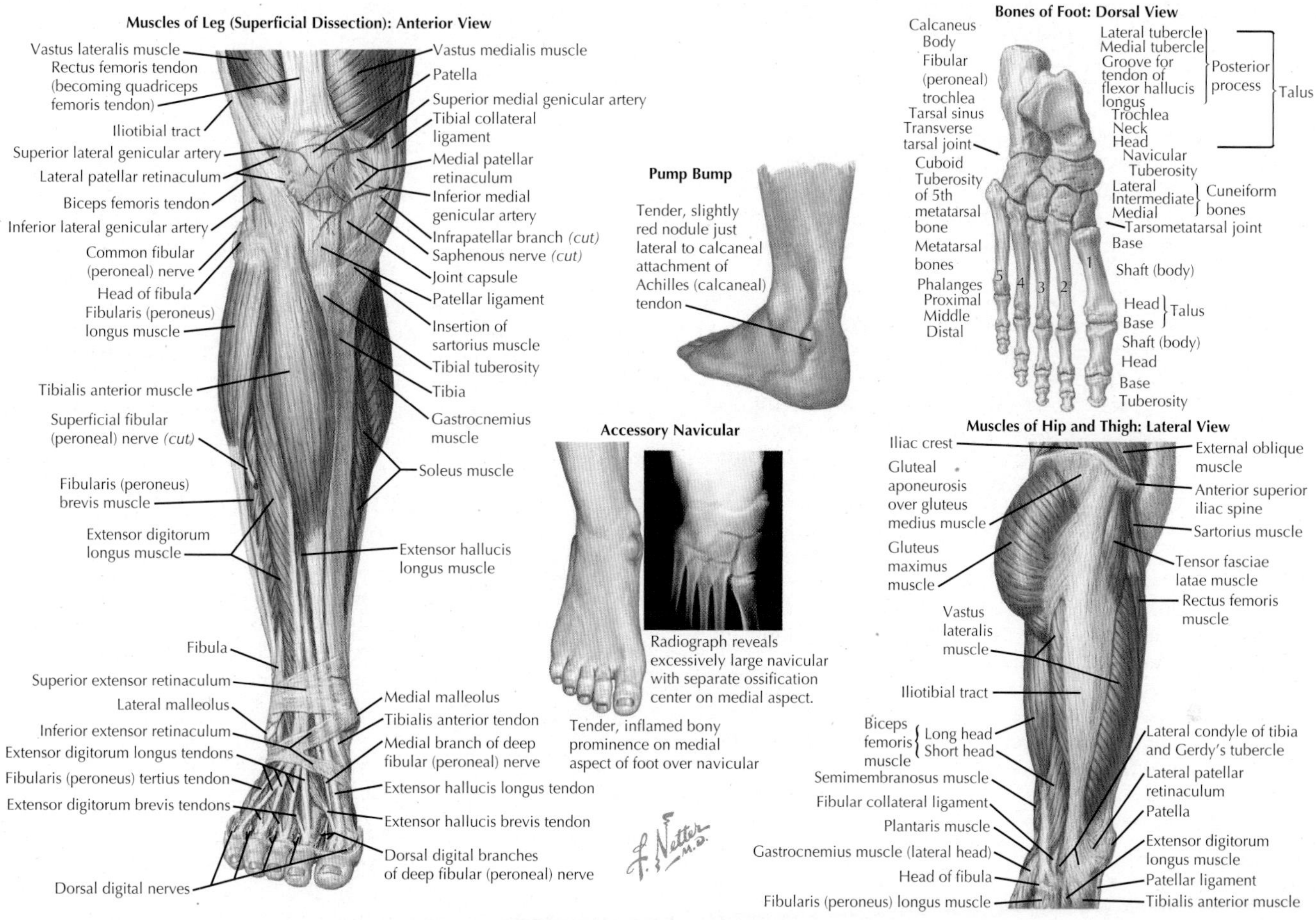
Muscles of Leg (Superficial Dissection): Anterior View
Vastus lateralis muscle
Rectus femoris tendon (becoming quadriceps femoris tendon)
Iliotibial tract
Superior lateral genicular artery
Lateral patellar retinaculum
Biceps femoris tendon
Inferior lateral genicular artery
Common fibular (peroneal) nerve
Head of fibula
Fibularis (peroneus) longus muscle
Tibialis anterior muscle
Superficial fibular (peroneal) nerve (cut)
Fibularis (peroneus) brevis muscle
Extensor digitorum longus muscle
Fibula
Superior extensor retinaculum
Lateral malleolus
Inferior extensor retinaculum
Extensor digitorum longus tendons
Fibularis (peroneus) tertius tendon
Extensor digitorum brevis tendons
Dorsal digital nerves
Vastus medialis muscle
Patella
Superior medial genicular artery
Tibial collateral ligament
Medial patellar retinaculum
Inferior medial genicular artery
Infrapatellar branch (cut)
Saphenous nerve (cut)
Joint capsule
Patellar ligament
Insertion of sartorius muscle
Tibial tuberosity
Tibia
Gastrocnemius muscle
Soleus muscle
Extensor hallucis longus muscle
Medial malleolus
Tibialis anterior tendon
Medial branch of deep fibular (peroneal) nerve
Extensor hallucis longus tendon
Extensor hallucis brevis tendon
Dorsal digital branches of deep fibular (peroneal) nerve
Pump Bump
Tender, slightly red nodule just lateral to calcaneal attachment of Achilles (calcaneal) tendon
Accessory Navicular
Radiograph reveals excessively large navicular with separate ossification center on medial aspect.
Tender, inflamed bony prominence on medial aspect of foot over navicular
Bones of Foot: Dorsal View
Calcaneus
Body
Fibular (peroneal) trochlea
Tarsal sinus
Transverse tarsal joint
Cuboid
Tuberosity of 5th metatarsal bone
Metatarsal bones
Phalanges
Proximal
Middle
Distal
Lateral tubercle
Medial tubercle
Groove for tendon of flexor hallucis longus
Posterior process
Talus
Trochlea
Neck
Head
Navicular
Tuberosity
Lateral
Intermediate
Medial
Cuneiform bones
Tarsometatarsal joint
Base
Shaft (body)
Head
Base
Talus
Shaft (body)
Head
Base
Tuberosity
5 4 3 2 1
Muscles of Hip and Thigh: Lateral View
Iliac crest
Gluteal aponeurosis over gluteus medius muscle
Gluteus maximus muscle
Vastus lateralis muscle
Iliotibial tract
Biceps femoris muscle
Long head
Short head
Semimembranosus muscle
Fibular collateral ligament
Plantaris muscle
Gastrocnemius muscle (lateral head)
Head of fibula
Fibularis (peroneus) longus muscle
External oblique muscle
Anterior superior iliac spine
Sartorius muscle
Tensor fasciae latae muscle
Rectus femoris muscle
Lateral condyle of tibia and Gerdy's tubercle
Lateral patellar retinaculum
Patella
Extensor digitorum longus muscle
Patellar ligament
Tibialis anterior muscle

Figure 81.1 Figure skating injuries.

- Calcaneal apophysitis can be seen in skeletally immature skaters.
- Other common foot issues include inflammation of an accessory tarsal navicular, prominence at the base of the fifth metatarsal, corns, and hammertoes (see Fig. 81.1). Most of these problems are treated with modification of the skate boot by locally "punching out" the leather by stretching or use of moleskin or foam/felt donuts to reduce friction or pressure.

Stress Fractures

- Lower extremity stress fractures were the most frequent overuse injury recorded in a 2003 study of elite junior women skaters.
- Common in the first and second metatarsals, particularly in the skater's takeoff leg for toe-pick jumps (see Fig. 81.1). Also common in the tibia, fibular, and navicular.

Knee Injuries

- Anterior knee pain (patellofemoral syndrome, Osgood-Schlatter syndrome, patellar tendinitis) is common, as in most jumping sports.
- Ligamentous and meniscal injuries are less common. This may be because of relative lack of fixation of the blade on the ice during landings, which decreases knee joint torque.

Hip Injuries

- Muscle strains of the hip flexor, adductor complex, and oblique abdominal muscles are commonly seen in skaters performing triple and quadruple jumps.
- Iliac crest apophysitis can be seen in skeletally immature skaters because of the repetitive stress from jump takeoffs or missed landings (see Fig. 81.1).
- Acetabular labral tears may occur, particularly in elite skaters. Contributing factors include repetitive forces from jump landings and hyperflexibility moves that are unique to figure skating.

Back Injuries

- Low back pain may be the result of acute trauma or overuse injury from repetitive falls or inappropriate equipment and is a common complaint of figure skaters.

Upper Extremity Injuries

- Wrist sprains and fractures may occur as a result of falling (more common at the recreational level).
- Rotator cuff injuries can occur in male pair skaters and synchronized skaters because of repetitive lifting or overhead use of arms.

Concussions

- Head trauma can occur during a fall or collision with another skater during practice or competition warm-ups.
- Figure skaters may have different recovery/return-to-play course because of impact forces, rotational forces, and multidirectional movements unique to the sport. Use a figure skating specific return-to-play progression (Table 81.1).

SPEED SKATING

Introduction

- Speed skating is the sport of competitive racing on specially designed skates, typically around an oval track.

Table 81.1 "RETURN-TO-SKATE" PROGRESSION FOR FIGURE SKATERS AFTER CONCUSSION

Phase 1	Rest from physical and mental activity until asymptomatic from concussion symptoms
Phase 2	Light aerobic exercise with light to moderate elevation of heart rate, off-ice stretching
Phase 3	Heavier aerobic exercise and sports-specific stretches with limited head and body movements off-ice; return to ice with managed sessions, forward skating only
Phase 4	Progressive managed time on the ice, forward and backward skating, changes of directions, choreography without spins and jumps; continue increased off-ice training
Phase 5	Full program run-throughs on the ice without spins or jumps, reintroduction of jumps outside of the program
Phase 6	Integration of jumps and spins into the program, with spins added last; full return to play

Epidemiology

- During the 2010 Winter Olympics, 27.8% of male short-track registered athletes sustained an injury, and <5% of all long-track athletes sustained an injury.
- Sixty-four to seventy-three percent of short-track speed skaters sustain at least one injury during a single competitive season.
- Upper respiratory tract infection is the most common illness, occurring more frequently around periods of competition and long-haul travel.

General Principles

History

- Early 13th century: Skating began as a mode of transportation across frozen lakes and rivers in Scandinavia using skates made of bone or wood.
- 1676: First known skating competition held in the Netherlands.
- Speed skating has been an Olympic event for men since the first Winter Olympics in 1924 and for women since 1960.

Review of Different Types of Speed Skating

LONG-TRACK SPEED SKATING

- A race against the clock.
- All events are run in a counterclockwise direction on a 400-meter oval track.
- Individual events:
  - Women 500, 1000, 1500, 3000, and 5000 meters
  - Men 500, 1000, 1500, 5000, and 10,000 meters
    - Pairs compete in separate lanes.
    - Contact is prohibited.
    - Each racer has only one opportunity to produce a winning time.
    - In order for the racers to skate the same distance, racers:
      - Must change lanes during each lap.
      - Begin from a staggered start.
      - Crossover occurs on the backstretch of the oval, with the racer in the outer lane having the right of way.
  - Mass start
    - Men's and women's event.
    - Up to 24 skaters line up in rows of 6.
    - No one can pass on the first lap of the 16-lap competition.
    - Skaters have four intermediate sprints (laps 4, 8, and 12) and the last lap (16), with points awarded for the top three finishers in each intermediate sprint and the top 6 for the final sprint.
    - Contact is allowed.
    - Race of strategy, drafting, and speed.
- Team event:
  - Team pursuit
    - Women race six laps, men race eight laps.
    - Team of three skaters.
    - Each round, two teams skate against each other starting on opposite sides of the track.
    - Head-to-head competition, single-elimination knock-out format.
    - Teams race without changing lanes. Last skater over the finish line gives the team their official finish time.
  - Team sprint
    - Women and men race three laps.
    - Team of three skaters.
    - First lap is skated with the skater assigned #1 leading the team.
    - Each lap the skater leading the team has to leave the outer part of the track and the next skater leads the team for the next lap.
    - Last assigned skater skates the last lap alone and finishes the race.
    - Team with the fastest time wins.

SHORT-TRACK SPEED SKATING

- An elimination race against other competitors.
- All events are run in a counterclockwise direction on a 111.12-meter oval track within an internationally sized 30-by-60-meter Olympic-sized ice hockey rink.
- Individual events:
  - Women and men race 500, 1000, and 15,000 meters.
  - Four to six racers compete per heat, with the first- and second-place finishers advancing to the next heat.
  - Skaters try to outskate and outwit the competition.
  - Lead skater has the right of way. Passing skaters must pass cleanly without body contact.
  - Skaters can skim their fingers along the surface of the ice inside the track but must skate around the outside of the blocks.
- Team event:
  - Relays
    - Women 3000 meters, men 5000 meters.
    - Four skaters skate per team competing against three other teams at the same time, with each team member skating at least once.
    - Skaters on the same team exchange by the incoming skater being pushed forward by the exiting skater.
    - Skaters can exchange anytime other than the final two laps.
    - One skater on each team races; others rest in the middle.

Discussion of Sports-Specific Skills and Other Considerations

- Average age of competitive long-track speed skaters is 20–24 years, short-track speed skaters is 19–22 years.
- An average of 8 hours of training per day, including on-ice and dry-land training.
- Competition season runs from September to April, and athletes travel an average of 2 weeks out of every month.
- Anthropometry studies show elite speed skaters have normal body height and mass; however, they have shorter legs and a longer trunk with better-developed thigh musculature compared with other elite athletes.

Biomechanical Principles

- Elite skaters generate the highest mechanical power output and the least loss of power to frictional forces.
- Speed skaters skate in a "crouched position" for aerodynamic and biomechanical advantage.
- Optimal trunk position is horizontal (trunk angle 15 degrees).

- Skaters generate power during push-off (skate in contact with ice) by nearly completely extending their knee (knee angle 171 degrees).
- Smaller knee angle at the onset of push-off results in better performance. Knee angle of elite skaters during the glide phase is typically 90–110 degrees.

Equipment and Safety Issues

LONG-TRACK SPEED SKATING

- Skaters wear skin-tight racing suits (skin suits) with hoods to decrease air resistance (Fig. 81.2). Racing suit must conform to the natural contour of the racer's body.
- Racers often wear glasses to protect their eyes from wind and ice chips and to reduce glare.
- The early 1990s brought a change in the skates for long-track racing from a "fixed blade" skate to a "klap blade."
  - Klap blades: only the toe of the blade is affixed to the boot (see Fig. 81.2).
  - At the end of each stride, the blade briefly disconnects from the heel of the boot.
  - When the ankle has fully extended and the heel is off the ice, the full length of the blade is still in contact with the ice.
  - At the moment the blade leaves the ice, the mounted spring mechanism snaps the blade back up to the boot, resulting in the clapping sound that gives the skate its name.
  - This mechanism keeps the blade on the ice longer, increasing the skater's pushing power and therefore speed.
- Pads to protect the athletes in case of falls surround the outer diameter of the track.
- For mass start and team events athletes must wear:
  - Cut-resistant racing suit or underwear
  - Knee and shin guards made of plastic or cut-resistant material
  - Cut-resistant gloves
  - Cut-resistant neck and ankle protection
  - A helmet that conforms to the shape of the head
  - The front and back of the skate blade must be rounded off with a radius of 10 mm

SHORT-TRACK SPEED SKATING

- Skaters wear similar skin suits as long-track skaters, but without a hood.
- Kneepads with or without a hard shell, shin protection, and cut-resistant neck guards fully covering the neck.
- Hard-plastic helmet that conforms to the head without protrusions (see Fig. 81.2).
- Cut-resistant gloves. Some have ceramic fingertips to allow the inside hand to skim on the ice and help maintain balance.
- Fixed-blade skate with boots that lace up higher on the ankle.
- Skates are constructed from customized foot molds to help stabilize the foot and ankle so that skaters can more tightly round corners.
- Skate blades are extremely sharp and are bent in at an arc that mirrors the direction of the turn to better grip the ice. Blades are placed left of center on the base of the skate to keep the boot from rubbing the ice when leaning into left turns at high speed. Blades must be fixed at a minimum of two points with no moveable parts. Blade ends must be rounded off in the front and the back with a minimum radius of 10 mm.

Specific Training and Physiologic Issues

- Skater's "crouched position" is a physiologic disadvantage to oxygenation of working muscles because of reduced blood flow.
- Deoxygenation of working muscles leads to faster fatigue compared with similar elite sports.
- Short-track skaters experience asymmetry of quadriceps muscle oxygenation, with the right leg having decreased blood flow. Skaters solely travel on their right leg during tight turns.

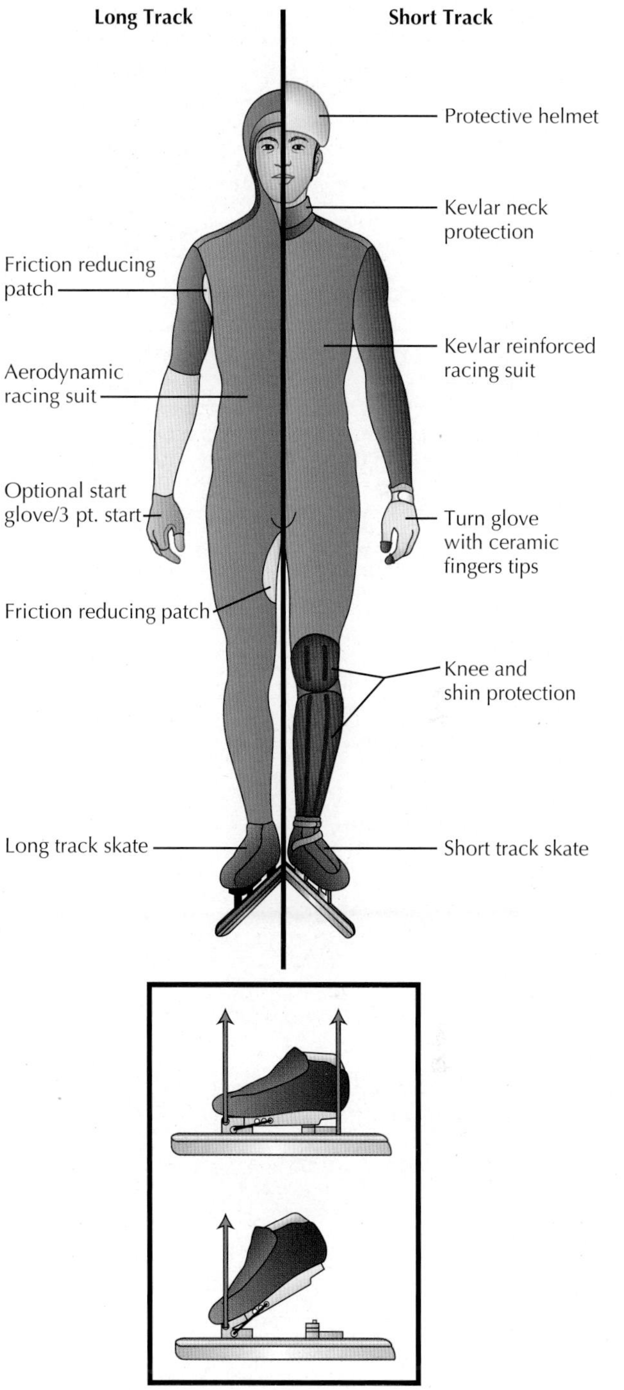
Long Track
Short Track
Protective helmet
Kevlar neck protection
Friction reducing patch
Kevlar reinforced racing suit
Aerodynamic racing suit
Optional start glove/3 pt. start
Turn glove with ceramic fingers tips
Friction reducing patch
Knee and shin protection
Long track skate
Short track skate

Figure 81.2 Speed skating equipment.

- Higher anaerobic demands for shorter race distances.
- Aerobic demands increase with increased race distances.
- Reduced blood flow to working muscles results in higher blood lactate concentrations.

Unique Environmental Issues

- Speed skaters are routinely exposed to cold, dry ice rinks during training and competition and to the chemicals used to maintain the ice surface and Zamboni fumes, including carbon monoxide and nitrogen dioxide.

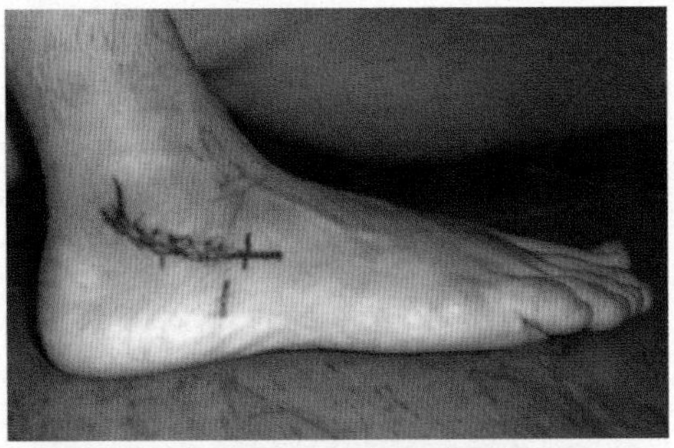

Lateral malleolus laceration from skate blade

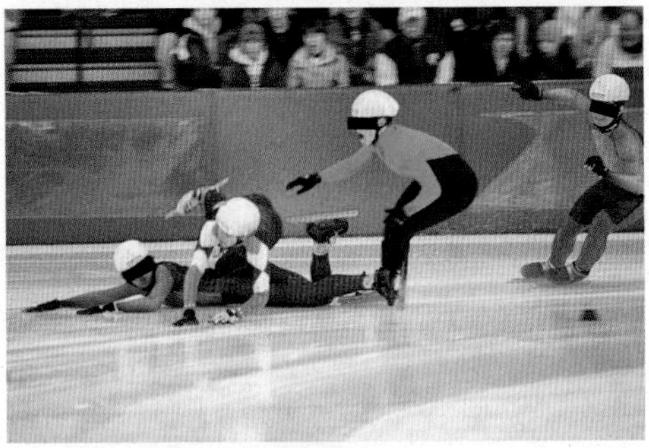

Short track skater collision

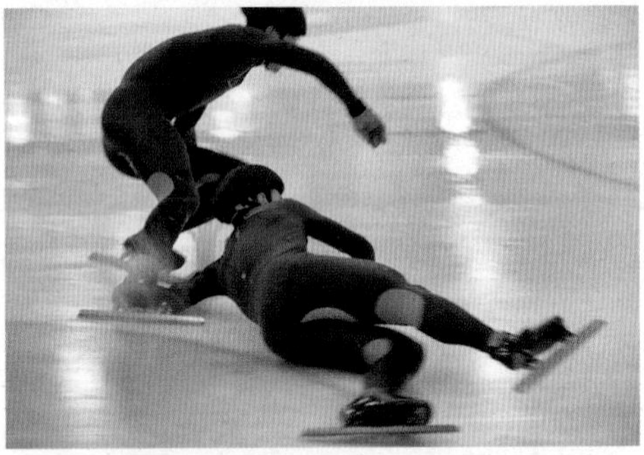

Skaters bracing for fall

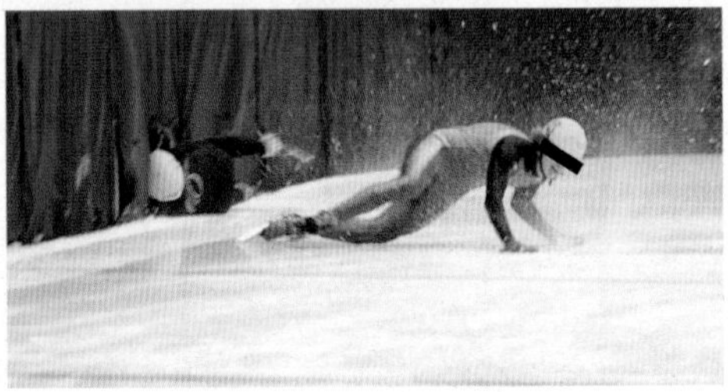

Skaters bracing for fall

Figure 81.3 Speed skating injuries.

Common Injuries and Medical Problems

Long-Track Speed Skating

- Numerous overuse injuries are secondary to the "crouching" and the constant repetitive motion of skating in the same direction.
- Mechanical low back pain and lumbar disc problems are common.
- Chronic hip flexor and iliotibial band (ITB) tightness, in addition to iliopsoas tightness, cause painful hip symptoms.
- ITB tightness and chronic knee flexion lead to the common problem of patellofemoral pain syndromes, patellar tendonitis, and ITB syndrome.
- Tightly laced skates often worn without socks, may also lead to certain common problems including callosities, corns, bunions, hammertoes, neuritis, and recurrent tinea pedis and can cause irritation to subcutaneous tendons, resulting in Achilles tendonitis/tenosynovitis and "lace bite," also known as *tibialis anterior*, *extensor hallucis longus*, and *extensor digitorum longus tendonitis*.
- The sprint start of a speed skating race involves an explosive sprint from a stationary position that can result in hip adductor and hip flexor strains.
- Most common injuries resulting from falls are lacerations, contusions, fractures, and joint sprains, particularly in the upper extremity because of skaters bracing for fall (Fig. 81.3).

Short-Track Speed Skating

- Similar to overuse injuries, including mechanical low back pain, lumbar disc problems, hip pain syndromes, and patellofemoral pain.
- Unique to the short-track skaters is peroneal tendonitis caused by repetitive, forceful dorsiflexion and eversion needed for the skate crossover on the short, tight curves.
- Traumatic injuries include shoulder dislocations, ankle and lower extremity fractures, concussions, cervical spine injuries, thoracic and rib contusions, and lacerations.

ACKNOWLEDGMENT

Dr. Porter would like to thank **Peter Zapalo,** director of Sports Science and Medicine for US Figure Skating, for his review and suggestions to the "Figure Skating" section of this chapter.

RECOMMENDED READINGS

Available online.

SWIMMING AND DIVING 82

Jennifer D. Stromberg • Nathaniel S. Jones

SWIMMING

Introduction

- Swimming is the most popular aquatic sports discipline and is an important part of triathlon and water polo.

Epidemiology

- At the international level, aquatic sports disciplines account for the second largest group of athletes at the Olympic Games and are governed by the Fédération Internationale de Natation (FINA).
- USA Swimming currently has over 400,000 registered athletes and 3100 clubs.
- US Masters Swimming consists of nearly 60,000 swimmers aged 18 years and older and provides support to more than 1500 clubs and workout groups.
- USA Artistic Swimming oversees competitive events for artistic (synchronized) swimmers who range in age from 12 to 20+ years.
- USA Triathlon (USAT) membership has more than tripled in the last 15 years, and there are more than 4300 sanctioned competitions each year.

General Principles

History

- Swimming has been a part of the Summer Olympic Games since its inception in 1896.
- Artistic swimming was first introduced to the Olympics in 1948, but solo and duet competitions did not become official events until 1984. Team artistic swimming was added in 1996.
- Swimming has been one of the most popular sports in the Paralympic games since their inception in 1960.
- Open-water swimming became a part of the Summer Olympic Games in 2008.
- The Ironman Triathlon began in 1978, and the number of participants continues to grow annually.

Types of Sports or Races

- Freestyle events do not require a particular stroke, but the front crawl is the most popular and commonly referred to as *freestyle.* Alternating arm strokes and an alternating or "flutter" kick propel the body forward in the prone position.
- Backstroke events are performed in the supine position with alternating arm strokes and "flutter" kick.
- Breaststroke events are performed by advancing the arms forward along the midline, then pulling to the sides without leaving the water while executing a "whip" kick by flexing the knees and hips and abducting the legs, and then "whipping" them back together.
- Butterfly events require the arms to be simultaneously advanced forward above the water and then pulled through underwater, while the legs kick up and down as a single unit similar to a tail in a "dolphin" kick.
- Relay competitions typically consist of four swimmers. In a medley relay, each swimmer performs one of the four different strokes.
- Artistic swimming events can consist of solos, duets, teams of 8, and combinations of up to 10 swimmers.

Discussion of Sports-Specific Skills and Other Considerations

- Successful swimmers are often lean and tall with long limbs, wide shoulders, and large palms with a large muscle mass in the middle and upper body.
- Elite swimmers tend to be more flexible than their nonelite counterparts.
- Artistic swimming requires exceptional breath control. Routines typically vary from 2 to 5 minutes in duration with 45%–50% of the time spent underwater.

Biomechanical Principles

- Achieving balance in the water is the base of swimming.
- Speed is gained by decreasing drag or resistance while moving through the water.
  - Form drag is body position–dependent water resistance. This type of drag is reduced by using a "streamlined" horizontal position with good body roll and remaining underwater when possible. Optimal hand positioning with slightly spread fingers and change in thumb position during the stroke are also of benefit.
  - Wave drag is caused by turbulence at the water surface. This type of drag is reduced by using deep pools with multiple lane lines, entering the water smoothly, and swimming in the wake of another swimmer ("drafting").
  - Frictional drag is caused by the contact of the body surface with the water and is reduced by shaving and using specially designed swimwear.
- Technique and efficiency play a greater role than power in performance.

Equipment

- Goggles protect the eyes from chlorine and aid in vision underwater.
- Caps decrease resistance and keep hair out of the face.
- Kickboards can be held in the arms while practicing kick techniques.
- Fins are used to increase kick propulsion in practice.
- Hand paddles add resistance to the pull during practice.
- Pull buoys are placed between the legs while practicing pull techniques.
- Wetsuits can be used for buoyancy and warmth, although studies suggest they do not raise core temperature significantly.

Safety Issues

- Neck injuries are uncommon, but they can be catastrophic. Preventive measures include a minimum pool depth of 5 feet for dives and flags placed 5 meters from the pool wall to help avoid collisions during backstroke. Backboards should be available and accessible on the pool deck.
- Sudden death in triathlon is most likely to occur during the swim, at rates more than double that reported in marathons. There is no clear association with skill level or medical problems. No athlete should swim without adequate supervision, which may include motorized and/or nonmotorized craft such as paddleboards or kayaks in larger bodies of water.
- Artistic swimmers practicing boosts and throws are at increased risk of traumatic injuries, including concussions.

Specific Training and Physiology Issues

- Although races typically range from 50 to 1500 meters, practices can range from 3000 to over 10,000 meters, which can predispose swimmers to overuse injuries.
- Several important physiologic changes occur with submersion in water.
  - Gravitational blood pooling in the venous system is decreased, shifting fluids to the central circulation and pulmonary vascular system.

    - Athletes with poor ventricular relaxation or increased pulmonary venous pressure may be at risk of swimming-induced pulmonary edema (SIPE) causing dyspnea and cough productive of pink, frothy, or bloody secretion (reported by 1.4% of triathletes).
    - Overhydration before competition should be avoided. Additional risk factors include older age, female sex, long course events, cold water, hypertension, valvular disease, fish oil supplement consumption, and wetsuit use.
  - The parasympathetic nervous system is activated via the diving reflex.
    - Heart rate is reduced, and vasoconstriction of muscle vasculature preserves blood flow to the brain and heart.
    - These adaptive changes allow for increased time underwater without additional breaths.
  - The sympathetic nervous system may be activated because of the cold shock phenomenon or event-related anxiety.
  - These changes can cause "autonomic conflict" and increase the risk of arrhythmia and sudden death, particularly in athletes with long QT syndrome and/or paroxysmal atrial flutter or fibrillation.
- Prolonged breath-holding in artistic swimmers can cause hypoxia and is often manifested by dizziness, disorientation, or even syncope.

Unique Environmental and Nutritional Issues

- Exercise-induced bronchospasm is prevalent in swimmers. Asthmatic children may be drawn to the sport by the warm, humidified air. There is concern exposure to airborne chlorine may lead to airway inflammation and bronchoconstriction in addition to rhinitis, but it is well-tolerated, with no evidence of adverse effects on asthma control in children and adolescents with stable asthma.
- Swimming with contact lenses has been associated with risk of microbial keratitis. This can be prevented by lens removal, use of goggles, or contact lens disinfection after swimming.
- Water immersion can expose athletes to a variety of dermatologic issues.
  - Infectious conditions include:
    - Swimmer's itch (schistosome dermatitis): pruritic, 3- to 5-mm erythematous papules in areas not covered by swimwear: lesions typically resolve spontaneously within 3–7 days
    - Swimming pool granuloma: verrucous nodules or plaques appear over bony prominences 6 weeks after inoculation with atypical mycobacteria; lesions may ulcerate and should be biopsied and treated with warm water soaks and antibiotics.
    - Diving suit dermatitis: diffuse erythematous papules in areas covered by swimsuits caused by *Pseudomonas*.
    - Seabather's eruption (sea lice): stinging sensation followed by pruritic vesiculopapular or urticarial rash on areas covered by a swimsuit within 24 hours of saltwater exposure; caused by larvae of thimble jellyfish trapped under swimwear; best treated with cold packs, antihistamines, and topical steroid; can cause febrile reaction.
    - Bikini bottom: firm, deep nodules along the inferior gluteal crease caused by *Streptococcus* or *Staphylococcus aureus* resulting from prolonged use of tight-fitting swimwear; best treated with systemic antibiotics and frequent warm soaks.
    - Swimmer's ear
    - Folliculitis
    - Molluscum contagiosum
  - Athlete's foot, warts, and pitted keratolysis may also result from skin contact with pool decks.
  - Contact dermatitis can occur from equipment or pool water. More severe forms include aquagenic urticaria, cold urticaria, and contact urticaria related to chlorine exposure.
  - Copper-chelating shampoos and hydrogen peroxide are used to treat the green hair caused by copper ions in pool water.
  - Prolonged water exposure commonly leads to dry, itchy skin, which is treated with application of petrolatum jelly and avoidance of long, hot showers.
  - Open-water swimmers may be at higher risk for skin cancer because of ultraviolet (UV) exposure. Sunscreen is recommended.
- Open-water swimmers are at increased risk of environmental injuries such as gastrointestinal infection, otitis, sunburn, jellyfish stings, dehydration, hypothermia, and hyperthermia.
  - "After-drop" refers to continued drop in core temperature, which can occur up to 1 hour after cold immersion as cooled peripheral blood returns to the core. Continued exercise, as in triathlon, can also shunt warmed core blood to the periphery.
  - Risk of hyperthermia occurs because of lost ability to regulate body temperature via sweating, radiant heat from the sun, and greater convection and conduction in warmer water. Wetsuits are typically illegal in competition at higher water temperatures to decrease this risk.

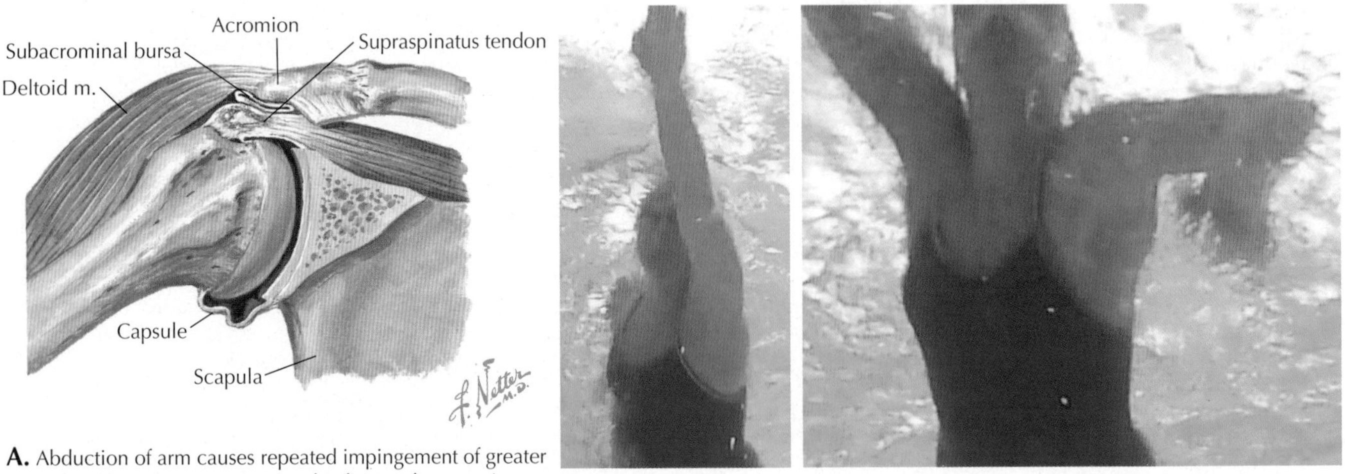
Acromion
Subacrominal bursa
Supraspinatus tendon
Deltoid m.
Capsule
Scapula

A. Abduction of arm causes repeated impingement of greater tubercle of humerus on acromion, leading to degeneration and inflammation of supraspinatus tendon, secondary inflammation of bursa, and pain on abduction of arm. Calcific deposits in the supraspinatus tendon may progress to acute calcific tendonitis and sudden onset of severe pain.

B. The catch occurs when the hand enters the water.

C. The hand reaches midpull when directly below the shoulder.

Figure 82.1 Swimmer's shoulder.

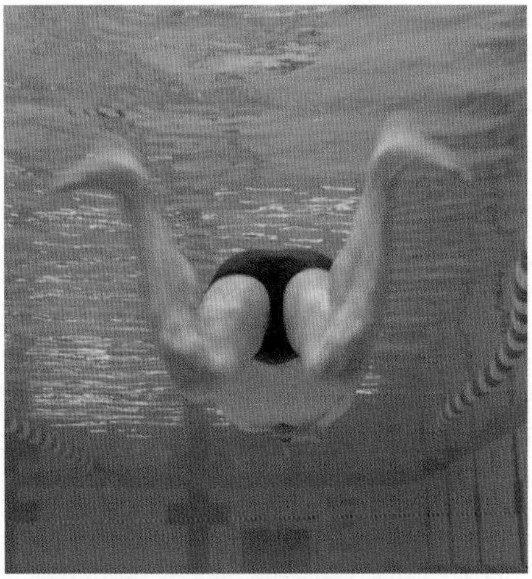

Correct alignment for breast stroke kick with hips held in closer adduction.

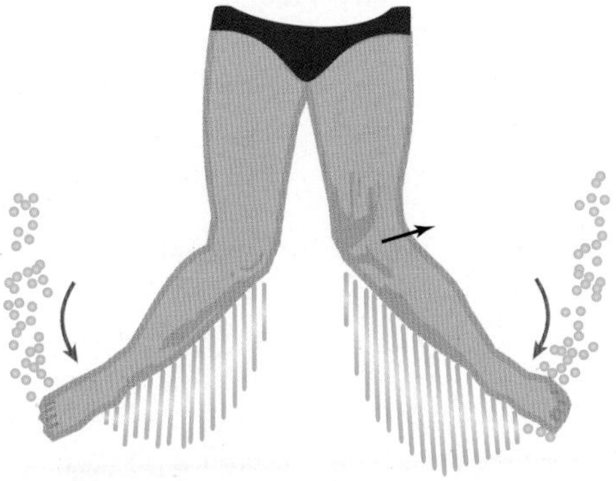

Lateral tracking of patella and/or medial knee stress with abnormal kick motion.

Figure 82.2 Knee pain associated with kick.

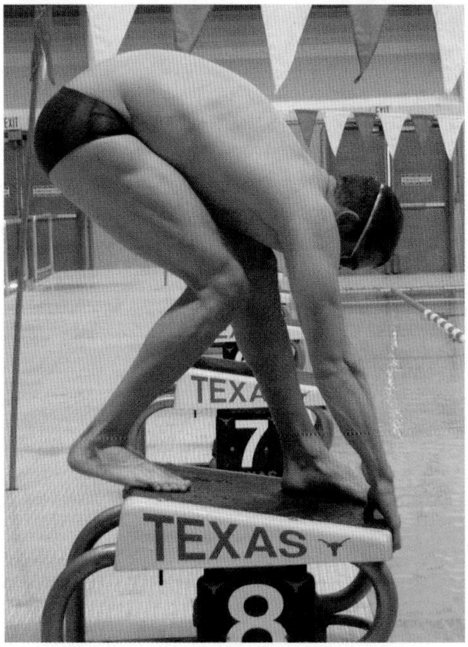
TEXAS
7
TEXAS
8

Extreme lumbar flexion seen in this swimmer on the block predisposes the athlete to lumbar injury when takeoff forces applied.

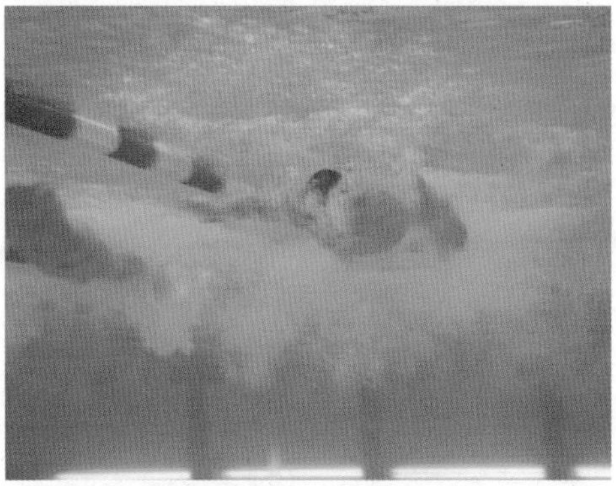

Center swimmer seen underwater with back flexed for butterfly stroke; swimmer on the left shows back extended with head and arms out of water for this stroke. Repetitive flexion and extension predisposed the athlete to lumbar back problems.

Figure 82.3 Low back pain.

- The necessity for revealing swimwear increases concern about body image and risk of relative energy deficiency, particularly in artistic swimmers.

Common Injuries and Medical Problems

Swimmer's Shoulder

Description: The most common musculoskeletal complaint in competitive swimming; typically results from some combination of intra-articular or subacromial impingement (Fig. 82.1A), scapular dyskinesis, overuse, and possible suprascapular nerve entrapment in the setting of joint laxity and rotator cuff muscle imbalance.

History: Pain is typically of gradual onset and often worse during the catch (see Fig. 82.1B) and early to mid-pull (see Fig. 82.1C) portions of the stroke. Poor body roll and unilateral breathing increase the propensity for impingement during freestyle.

Physical examination: Shoulder and/or core weakness, scapular dyskinesis, poor posture with tight pectoralis musculature, glenohumeral internal rotation deficiency (GIRD), positive impingement testing, dropped elbow during the recovery phase of the stroke, early exit during pull-through, scapular winging, excess body roll.

Treatment: Includes avoiding the use of hand paddles, correcting biomechanical deficits.

Return to play: Emphasize lower extremity training, avoid strokes that exacerbate pain, and focus on proper technique with good body roll (45 degrees along the long axis); bilateral breathing; and less internal rotation on hand entry for freestyle (fingers first, not thumb).

Prevention: Dry land training with stretching and strengthening program for rotator cuff, scapular stabilizers, and core; training distance should be increased by no more than 10% per week.

Breaststroker's Knee

Description: Medial and/or anterior knee pain; the second most common musculoskeletal complaint in competitive swimming

History: Results from repetitive valgus loading with breaststroke kick (Fig. 82.2) or the eggbeater kick used in artistic swimming and water polo

Physical examination: Medial collateral ligament (MCL) sprain, medial patellar facet tenderness, and/or inflamed medial synovial plica may be noted

Diagnostic considerations: More common in older, more competitive swimmers with more years of experience

Treatment: Cessation of breaststroke kick; lower extremity and core strengthening

Return to play: Gradual reintroduction of breaststroke kick with proper technique—hip abduction between 37 and 42 degrees, with good external rotation and dorsiflexion of the ankles

Prevention: Gradual increase in breaststroke distance; stroke diversity and stroke-specific warm-up; maintain quadriceps and hamstring flexibility

Spine Pain

Description: Occurs in approximately 20%–25% of swimmers in a single season; facet pain results from lumbar hyperextension required for streamlined position; pain may also result from repetitive flexion of the thoracic spine in butterfly stroke and with diving from the starting block (Fig. 82.3).

History: Pain is often accentuated by the use of the dolphin kick, in addition to fins, kickboards, and pull buoys, and increases with training intensity, duration, and distance. Flexion-based pain and facet joint injury can also result from spine rotation and flexion during flip turns.

Physical examination: Pain can be flexion-based or extension-based as detailed earlier

Differential: Spondylolysis/spondylolisthesis and discogenic pain

Return to play: Gradual reintroduction of butterfly, dolphin kick, and flip turns

Prevention: Gradual increases in butterfly and dolphin kick, stroke diversity, core strengthening and stabilization

Swimmer's Ear

See Chapter 48: "Maxillofacial Injuries."

Prevention: Dry canals with hair dryer, and maintain acidic environment with ear drops; use molded ear plugs in cold-water swimming.

Thoracic Outlet Syndrome

Description: Impingement of the brachial plexus and/or vascular supply to the upper extremity occurring in the interscalene triangle, the costoclavicular space, or the coracopectoral tunnel (Fig. 82.4)

History: Sensation of aching or coolness radiating down the arm associated with exertion and overhead activities

Physical examination: Findings include weakness or fatigue in the involved nerve root distribution, decrease in radial pulse in the affected arm noted while pulling down on the arm and having the patient inhale deeply and turn the head toward the affected side (Adson maneuver), and reproduction of symptoms by placing the arm in hyperabduction and external rotation (Wright test) or by manually compressing the clavicle.

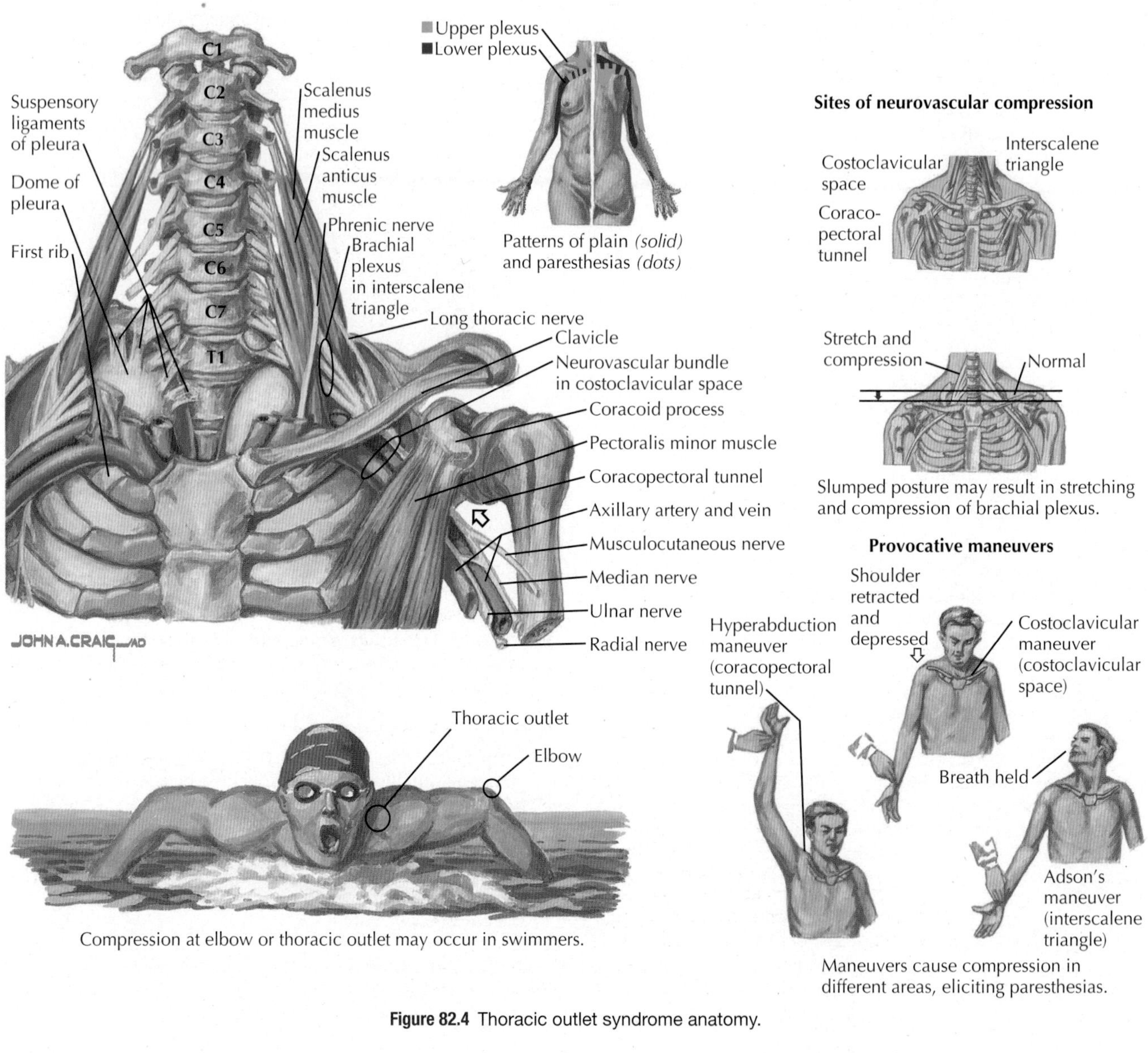
C1
C2
C3
C4
C5
C6
C7
T1
Suspensory ligaments of pleura
Dome of pleura
First rib
Scalenus medius muscle
Scalenus anticus muscle
Phrenic nerve
Brachial plexus in interscalene triangle
Long thoracic nerve
Clavicle
Neurovascular bundle in costoclavicular space
Coracoid process
Pectoralis minor muscle
Coracopectoral tunnel
Axillary artery and vein
Musculocutaneous nerve
Median nerve
Ulnar nerve
Radial nerve
JOHN A.CRAIG_AD
Upper plexus
Lower plexus
Patterns of plain (solid) and paresthesias (dots)
Sites of neurovascular compression
Costoclavicular space
Interscalene triangle
Coraco-pectoral tunnel
Stretch and compression
Normal
Slumped posture may result in stretching and compression of brachial plexus.
Provocative maneuvers
Shoulder retracted and depressed
Hyperabduction maneuver (coracopectoral tunnel)
Costoclavicular maneuver (costoclavicular space)
Breath held
Adson's maneuver (interscalene triangle)
Maneuvers cause compression in different areas, eliciting paresthesias.
Thoracic outlet
Elbow
Compression at elbow or thoracic outlet may occur in swimmers.

Figure 82.4 Thoracic outlet syndrome anatomy.

Diagnostic considerations: Imaging may include apical lordotic view of the chest to look for a cervical rib, plain films of cervical spine and shoulder, and/or arteriogram. Nerve conduction studies may be useful in brachial plexus involvement. Axillary vein thrombosis should be considered in patients with arm swelling and venous distension.

Treatment: Strengthen scapular elevators, stretch cervical girdle, address poor posture, and avoid provocative positions; surgical treatments include rib resection and scalene release.

Return to play: Stroke modification to minimize impingement

DIVING

Introduction

Diving is an aquatic sport that involves an aerial acrobatic maneuver after jumping or falling from a platform or springboard at measured height into water.

Epidemiology

- Approximately 12,000 athletes register with USA Diving each year.
- Typical age of Olympic-caliber divers: 12 years to mid-20s
- Most data on injury come from World Championships or Olympics
  - Injury rate 8.9% (female 5.9%, male 10.4%) with 8.3% in competition and 58.3% in training
  - Clinical incidence of injury in males is 1.94, and in females 2.49
  - Shoulder injuries are the most common injury in males, whereas trunk injuries are more common in females
  - Low back pain is the most commonly reported injury in elite competitive divers (38.4%–49%)
  - Most injuries are overuse injuries (male 24%, female 21.6%). Competitive divers train on average 40 hours per week, with springboard divers averaging 100–150 dives per day and platform divers averaging 100–150 dives per day.

General Principles

Terminology

- Save: in order to "save" a dive (avoid a nonvertical entry) a diver hyperflexes the shoulders and hyperextends the spine
- Swimout: occurs during entry into the water, where arms are forcibly pulled forward to the side in an attempt pull in the rest of the body with minimal splash
- Dive groups (designated by numbers 1–6) and dive body positions (designated by letters A–D) make up a dive (see Tables 82.1 and 82.2 and Box 82.1 for dive descriptions and examples)

History

- Early roots in mid-1800s in Europe with "fancy diving," where gymnasts performed acrobatics over water.
- Springboard diving became an Olympic sport in 1904, followed by platform diving at the 1908 London Olympics.

Biomechanical Principles

- Energy is transmitted along the kinetic chain from the hands, to the wrists, to the elbows, and to the shoulders.
- The upper extremity absorbs most of the water-entry axial loading.
  - Shoulder is stabilized by elevating the shoulder girdle with increased scapular abduction, so the glenoid fossa is behind the humeral head and is better able to absorb axial load impacts.
  - Inadequate scapular abduction increases the demands on the soft tissue, causing injury, ligament laxity, and, in turn, shoulder instability.
- Upon water impact, velocity is decreased by more than 50% within 1 second, with most injuries occurring during the first 600 ms and when the angle of water entry increases away from a vertical entry.

Competition Events

- Springboard: 1 meter and 3 meters
- Platform: 10 meters
- High dive: 27 meters for males and 20 meters for females

Equipment/Specific Training

- Pool with adequate depth; having a dark-colored bottom or a water surface agitator (bubbles) can help the diver visualize the surface.
- The water surface agitator can also reduce the axial load energy from water entry.

Table 82.1 DIVE GROUPS

Forward or front (Group 1)	A dive in which at takeoff the diver is facing the water with direction of rotation away from the board.
Backward or back (Group 2)	A dive where takeoff is from the end of the board with back toward water with direction of rotation away from the board.
Reverse (Group 3)	A diver has a takeoff facing the water, then using a forward approach rotates back toward the board.
Inward (Group 4)	The diver stands with back to the pool and rotates forward toward the board.
Twisting (Group 5)	A dive initiated by throwing one arm down and across the abdomen and one arm up and overhead and away from the body. Four types: forward, back, reverse, inward.
Armstand (Group 6)	A platform-only dive executed from an armstand position.

Table 82.2 DIVE BODY POSITIONS

Straight (Position A)	A dive position in which the body is straight at hips and knees with feet together pointing down. The arm position can vary.
Pike (Position B)	A dive position in which the legs are straight, body is bent at the waist, feet together and toes pointed. Position of the arms can vary.
Tuck (Position C)	A diver's body is bent at waist and knees bent with thighs drawn to chest and heels to buttocks.
Free (Position D)	Any combination of other positions and is restricted in its use in some twisting dives.

BOX 82.1 EXAMPLES OF DIVES

- A 5237D is a back dive with 1½ somersaults, 3½ twists, free position dive.
- A 301B would be reverse dive, with a half-somersault in the pike position.
- A 107B is a forward dive, with 3½ somersaults in the pike position.

- Dry-land equipment: trampolines with spotting rigs, landing pits, spotting harnesses, and poolside diving boards. Allow for a safe environment in which to learn new dives.

Nutrition

- Aesthetic-focused sport with emphasis placed on body type for performance and appearance can increase risk for disordered eating and diet restriction.
- Recommended daily energy/diet requirements are 3500 kcal for males and 2650 for females.
- Divers should consume 2–8 g/kg/day of carbohydrates and 1.2–1.7 g/kg/day of protein.

Common Injuries During Different Diving Components

TAKEOFF

- **Phases:** Approach (Fig. 82.5A), hurdle (i.e., jump onto end of board) (see Fig. 82.5B–D), and press (i.e., depression of board and upward acceleration of body) (see Fig. 82.5E). Timing is essential for maximal acceleration of body and efficient press.
- **Injuries during takeoff** (see Fig. 82.5F): Patellar tendonitis, quadriceps tendonitis, patellofemoral compression syndrome, Achilles and posterior tibialis tendonitis, and lumbar injuries resulting from compensatory hyperextension

FLIGHT OR MIDAIR MANEUVER

- Begins when a diver leaves the board or platform and ends with initial contact with water
- **Injuries during flight or midair maneuver:**
  - Spine and long head of biceps injuries because of torsional overload during twisting
  - Can strike the board midair, particularly the head, causing concussions and/or lacerations
  - Only two reported fatal head injuries, and both occurred from the 10-meter platform during a reverse 3½ somersault tuck dive attempt.

ENTRY

- Most injuries occur during water entry because of forces upon entry and during underwater maneuvers as diver attempts to have a splashless entry (Fig. 82.6).
- To protect the head and spine and dissipate energy, entry should be made with the arms extended and hands overlapping, maintaining a flexed wrist and extended elbows.
- **Injuries during entry:**
  - Can occur at any portion along the kinetic chain because of large forces, repetition, and overuse
  - Most injuries attributed to repetitive microtrauma: can include multidirectional shoulder instability, shoulder dislocations, shoulder impingement, elbow ulnar collateral ligament (UCL) strains/tears, ulnar neuritis from UCL laxity, scaphoid stress fracture, carpal instability, dorsal impaction syndrome, concussions, and lumbar spine injuries from attempting to save a dive

Common Injuries or Medical Problems

Lower Extremity Injuries

- Osteochondritis dissecans lesions can occur in the knees; consider keeping young athletes away from 10-meter platform during a growth spurt.
- Patellar tendonitis, quadriceps tendonitis, patellofemoral pain syndrome, Achilles and posterior tibialis tendonitis (most are secondary to overuse or incorrect technique with press on springboard)

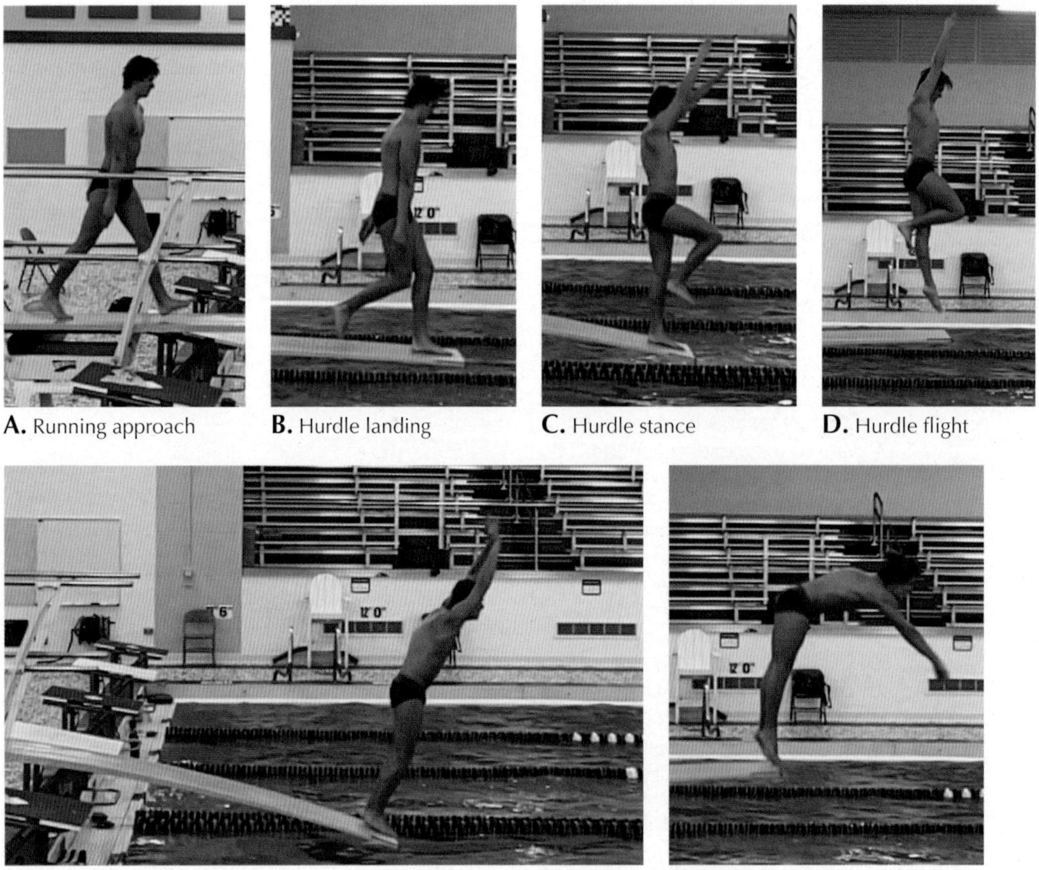

A. Running approach **B.** Hurdle landing **C.** Hurdle stance **D.** Hurdle flight **E.** Press (maximum depression) **F.** Takeoff

Figure 82.5 Phases of springboard dive approach.

- Ankle sprains and fifth metatarsal fractures with awkward landing on board
- Treatment: many of the standard treatments for knee and ankle injuries, such as braces or orthotics, are not viable options in diving. Therefore, taping of the knee and ankles can be attempted in addition to training modifications to avoid repetitive jumping stresses.

Shoulder Injuries

- Flexibility is important in diving but can also be a cause of problems, leading to glenohumeral joint instability and impingement.
- Multidirectional instability with associated microtrauma of repetitive diving can lead to shoulder instability.
- Mechanically at-risk position for shoulder: 180 degrees abduction, 180 degrees flexion, and maximum internal rotation, with no inferior support.
- When attempting to save a dive, there is usually hyperextension of the back and hyperflexion of the shoulder, increasing the risk of anterior glenohumeral subluxation.

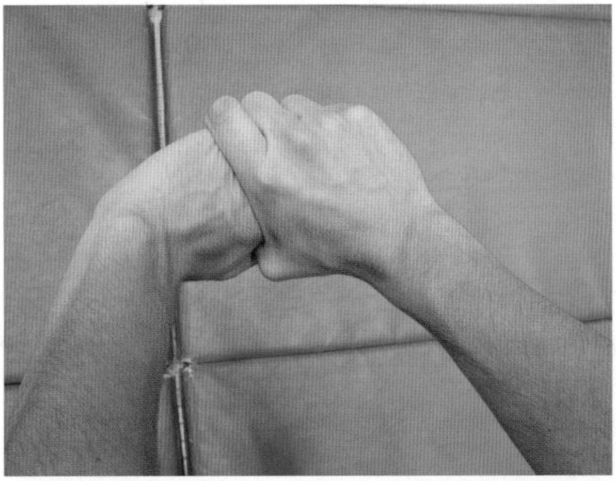

Flat-hand water entry postion on a dive (demonstrated on dry land)

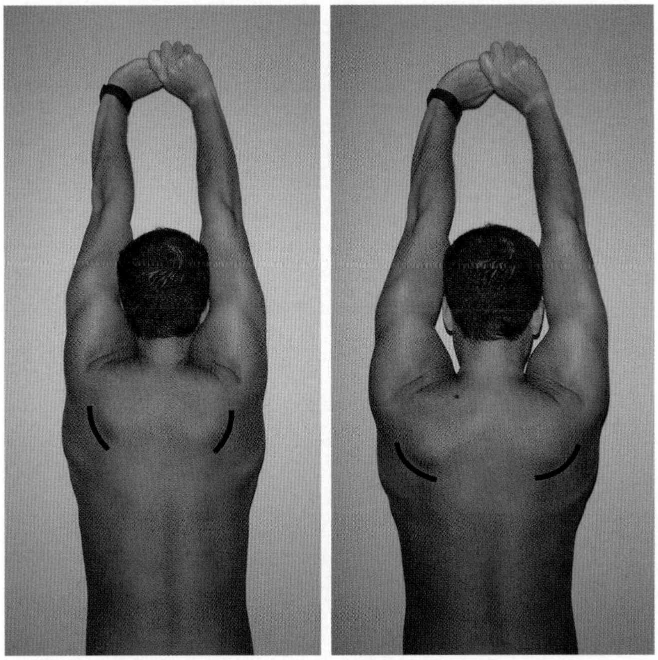

Flat-hand technique prior to entry At moment of water surface

Figure 82.6 Proper hand technique for entry.

Multidirectional Instability

History: Many times, divers have noted increasing soreness after diving early on; then, as instability increases, pain is noted with diving. Pain at rest points to advanced instability.

Elbow Injuries

- The elbow must be in extension upon water entry, taking on a large amount of stress.
- Instability is usually medial with concern for UCL injury and possible ulnar neuropathy.

Triceps Strain

Description: Seen in response to repetitive water entry forces; appropriate strength and range of motion are vital for the elbow to remain in extension upon contact with water. Often, injury occurs at the distal musculotendinous junction.

Return to play: When pain has improved and ability to lock in extension. Tendon rupture requires surgical intervention

Medial Collateral Ligament Injury

History: Pain at the medial elbow, affecting the UCL, particularly upon entry into water.

Return to play: Must be able to get elbow in full extension with appropriate strength to maintain extension during entry. Continued instability necessitates surgery.

Wrist Injuries

- Can be secondary to overuse versus trauma
- Can occur from hitting the board: fractures or UCL sprains of the thumb
- Overuse: carpal instability, ganglion cyst, and flexor carpi ulnaris tendonitis

Dorsal Impaction Syndrome

History: Pain at radiocarpal joint secondary to forced wrist dorsiflexion

Prevention: Taping of wrists can be helpful for prevention

Cervical Spine Injuries

- Most commonly seen in recreational diving where there is lack of experience, shallow water, inadequate supervision, and alcohol ingestion

Cervical Hyperflexion Injury

Description: Cervical hyperflexion injury secondary to poor technique

History: Pain, paresthesias, and radicular symptoms

Physical examination: Pain, restriction of cervical range of motion, specifically in extension; normal neck examination with neurologic findings in the upper extremity; consider a possible brachial plexus injury

Treatment: Rest, rehabilitation, and focus on proper technique with the neck in the neutral position, sitting protected in between the arms

Return to play: Pain-free, normal range of motion with normal strength

Lumbar Spine Injuries

- Flexion and extension with axial loading occur in most diving maneuvers along with shearing and torsional stresses at multiple spinal segments
- Anterior segments (vertebral body, vertebral endplate, and intervertebral disc) vulnerable to increases in loads, particularly during takeoff and entry
- Posterior segment (facet joints, pars interarticularis) is the more common cause of back pain because repetitive extension
- Low back pain is most frequently reported symptom in divers, with a rate of up to 38.4% in 13- to 17-year-olds. Lack

of flexibility at the shoulder joint translates into compensatory hyperextension of the lower back.
- Growing spine is highly vulnerable to trauma, particularly during the adolescent growth spurt. Most elite divers are in their teenage years.
- The reduction of speed upon water entry creates a tremendous amount of axial load.
- One study found 89% lifetime prevalence of back pain.
- Back pain is a common reason to retire from the sport.

Spondylolysis/Spondylolisthesis

Description: Considered to be more of a posterior element injury affecting the facet joints and pars interarticularis. Extension of the spine can occur throughout the diving process, but it most commonly takes place in takeoff for a back dive, a front spinning dive when the diver over-rotates, or most commonly, when trying to save a dive.

History: Diver presents with low back pain that worsens with activity, particularly extension. Many times, a decline in performance and technique because of pain is noted.

High Dive Injuries

Description: Divers enter water feet first from 27 meters (males) or 20 meters (females), with greater force and velocity, and are at higher risk of ligamentous knee injuries and lower extremity fractures, especially when dives go wrong.

Nonorthopedic Injuries

TYMPANIC MEMBRANE PERFORATIONS

Description: From landing directly on the ear

Treatment: Usually closes within 4 weeks; if not, consider surgery

Return to play: Use of ear plugs is recommended if continuing to dive

VESTIBULAR ABNORMALITIES

Description: Thought to be related to changes in linear acceleration and rotation in addition to water impact with rapid deceleration. In a forward somersault, there are 1260 degrees of rotation. Concussions can also occur. Therefore, anytime abnormal vestibular symptoms are reported, one should consider a concussion as the source. Visual orientation and cerebellar training come with time and experience and step-wise progression in dive complexity.

Treatment: Rest and vestibular rehabilitation; spotting techniques are helpful and can be taught with land-based techniques and spotting gear.

SCALP LACERATION

Description: More common with reverse and inward dives

CORNEAL EPITHELIAL INJURIES

Description: Occurs from repetitive trauma/impact to the water.

Treatment: Usually reversible with rest and improving timing of dive entry.

PULMONARY CONTUSION

Description: Rupture of pulmonary blood vessels and resultant hemoptysis secondary to landing flat, usually from a 10-meter platform dive.

Treatment/return to play: Resolution with rest; most return to play within 48 hours.

CONCUSSION

Description: Can occur from direct head impact with board/platform but also from water entry impact. Higher risk when learning new dives or when a dive does not go as planned.

Diagnostic consideration: High degree of suspicion anytime abnormal vestibular symptoms are reported.

ANXIETY AND PSYCHOLOGICAL STRESS

Description: Performance pressure and fear of hurting oneself because of the complexity of dives. Stress increases with age resulting from increasing dive complexity, sometimes leading to early retirement.

Treatment/return to play: Working with a sports psychologist to work on dive visualization can be very beneficial.

WATER POLO

Available online.

RECOMMENDED READINGS

Available online.

SCUBA DIVING 83

George A. Morris • Cynthia D. Dusel • Craig C. Young

GENERAL PRINCIPLES

Overview

- Diving includes multiple activities performed in an aquatic environment.
- Technology allows people to enjoy the underwater experience.
- An estimated 2.8–3 million US divers participate each year.
  - People dive for various reasons, including new experience, unique environment and surroundings, new challenges, jobs, military duties, sport, and environmental awareness.

Types of Diving

- Breath-hold diving (apnea, free, or skin diving)
  - Snorkel is the main piece of equipment used; may use fins for propulsion
  - Often performed in conjunction with spear fishing, shellfish gathering, snorkeling tours, and competitions
- Recreational scuba (self-contained underwater breathing apparatus)
  - Enjoyment of unique environments
  - Performed in several locations worldwide
- Commercial, technical, and advanced recreational diving
  - A wide range of gases used for respiration, depending on the characteristics of the event
  - Specialized training for wreck, cave, night, and exploratory diving
  - Various gases are used; decompression techniques may be required

Environments for Diving

- Multiple different underwater environments, each with different risks and techniques involved
- Ocean water is the most common location for recreational diving
- Freshwater lakes and rivers
- Ice diving
- Cave and wreck diving
- Pools for competition and training

Physiology of Diving

- Pressure at sea level on the surface is 1 atmosphere absolute (ATA).
  - Pressure in Denver, Colorado (elevation of 5280 feet) is 0.8 ATA, but at 6 feet under sea level, it will be 1.2 ATA.
  - Every 33 feet of seawater (FSW) below the surface increases the pressure by 1 ATA.
- Saltwater is approximately 775 times denser than air.
  - Increased density provides buoyancy to the diver.
  - Creates a sense of weightlessness, which can lead to disorientation or allow a freedom of movement for trained divers with neuromuscular disabilities.
- Increased viscosity of water increases resistance to movement.
  - Contributes to the need for increased physical fitness of the diver and importance of fitness for diving evaluation
- Increased heat capacity of water
  - Conductive heat loss in water is 25 times faster than that in air, which leads to an increased risk of cold illness and need for thermal protection while diving.
- Human body's response to the aquatic environment
  - Air spaces subjected to increased pressure and rapid pressure changes with depth changes.
  - Thermoregulation can be a challenge.
  - Shivering may hasten cooling in the water.
  - Diving reflex can occur as a response to facial immersion and leads to bradycardia, peripheral vasoconstriction, lower temperature, and shunting of blood to the core.

Physics of Diving

Boyle Law

- For a fixed amount of gas at a uniform temperature, volume (V) and pressure (P) are inversely related.

$$V_1 / P_1 = V_2 / P_2$$

- As diver descends and surrounding environmental pressure increases, the volume of air-filled flexible wall structures (e.g., lung or gastrointestinal tract) will decrease; the volume of these structures will subsequently increase on ascent.
- Liquid and liquid/solid organs (e.g., blood, bone, muscle, and organs) will equally transmit pressures in all directions according to the Pascal principle, which states that pressure is distributed equally over surfaces and transmitted equally through compartments containing gas or liquids.
- Air-filled rigid-walled structures (sinuses, middle ear, and face mask air space) will remain at surface pressure at a depth because of their inability to change volume.
- The pressure gradient is responsible for barotrauma injuries.
- The gradient can be resolved by equalizing spaces during depth changes.
- Gradient change is the greatest near the surface.

Dalton Law

- The total pressure exerted by a mixture of gases is equal to the sum of the pressures that would be exerted by each of the gases if it alone was present and occupied the total volume.
- Air pressure at sea level (1 ATA) is composed of nitrogen (0.79 ATA) and oxygen (0.21 ATA), with trace amounts of carbon dioxide (CO_2), water vapor, and other gases.
- At greater depths, the air will be breathed in at the ambient pressure.
  - 33 FSW has a pressure of 2 ATA, which will be composed of nitrogen (1.58 ATA) and oxygen (0.42 ATA).
- Increases the partial pressures of the inspired gases, and the body is sensitive to changes.

Oxygen (O_2)

- Our bodies tolerate a wide range of O_2 pressure (0.158–2 ATA) and extract enough to meet metabolic requirements without developing toxicity.
  - Below 0.158 ATA, the body will experience hypoxia, and the diver will develop air hunger, fatigue, confusion, loss of consciousness, and death of tissues.
- Brain cells are most sensitive and can die if deprived of O_2 for only 4 minutes.
- Oxygen toxicity can occur if the partial pressure is too high for too long.
  - Effects can include nausea, disorientation, visual changes, and seizures; life threatening underwater
  - Enriched air mixtures have varying concentrations of O_2 and different depth limits because of the increased partial pressures of O_2.

Henry Law

- The amount of gas that will dissolve in a liquid is directly related to the pressure (P) of the gas. Thus, $G_{(PD)}$::P, where $G_{(PD)}$ is the gas physically dissolved in a liquid phase and :: stands for *proportional*.
- With descent to greater depths and pressures, the number of molecules of each gas dissolved in body tissues increases.
- Factors that affect speed at which dissolution occurs include temperature, solubility coefficient, and cellular metabolism of the gas.
- Different tissues absorb and release gases at different rates.
- Tissue saturation eventually occurs if the diver stays at depth long enough.
- Upon ascent, partial pressure decreases and gas will leave the solution phase. If ascent is too rapid and/or decompression stops are not used, bubbles may form in the local tissue or the bloodstream.

Nitrogen

- Usually considered an inert gas because it does not unite chemically with other substances in the body.
- No effects at normal sea-level atmospheric pressures (0.79 ATA).
- Nitrogen can interact with cells at increased pressures and lead to nitrogen narcosis.
- Effects of nitrogen at depth are comparable to taking one alcoholic drink for every 50 FSW descended, and at 750 FSW, it has anesthesia-like effects. This effect is also called "rapture of the deep" and can cause confusion and strange behaviors.

Portions of the Dive

Surface: Surface swimming or wading before going underwater; uses energy and increases exposure to cold temperatures

Descent: Involves changes in pressures of 1 ATA per 33 FSW; need to have equilibration of pressure in closed air spaces

Bottom time: Traditionally, the amount of time spent at lowest depth; however, with the advent of dive computers, it has evolved to the amount of time spent underwater. Activity at depth can change respiratory needs and risks of complications. Good buoyancy management can decrease the O_2 consumption and conserve the air supply.

Ascent: Risk of injuries because of changes in pressure and release of absorbed gas back into local tissues and bloodstream.

Surface interval: Allows the body to resume its usual physiologic status and normalize tissue gas concentration before the next dive; complications or injuries encountered during the dive may not present until the diver is at the surface.

Incidence of Dive-Related Injuries

- Difficult to determine because exact number of divers and dives performed each year are unknown
- Decompression sickness (DCS)
  - Approximately 1.52 DCS events for males and 1.27 for females per 1000 dives
- The mortality rate for recreational divers is estimated to be 1 death per 200,000 dives
- Increased age, decreased physical conditioning, and history of chronic disease were risk factors
- Dehydration, exercise level during the dive, hypothermia, and hyperthermia may also play crucial roles

Safe Dive Profiles

- Follow standard recommendations on dive tables or dive computer algorithms for duration of dives at various depths, with decompression stops as needed.
  - US Navy Air Dive tables
    - Based on rectangular or square profiles that assume that the diver directly descends to the deepest depth and stays at that depth until returning to the surface.
    - Designed for safety to minimize risks of DCS, O_2 toxicity, and nitrogen narcosis.
- Dive computers are now very common and easy to use.
  - Allow flexibility in dive profiles
  - Potential for fewer calculation errors compared with tables
  - Provides planning information: dive profiles, safety stops, ascent rate alarms, decompression times, and dive intervals
- Recommended that most sport scuba divers perform only no-decompression dives to minimize risks
- No dive is 100% safe because of individual variation in conditions, health, physiology, and equipment.
  - Diving within skill limits, equipment, and certification makes diving safer.
  - Keep ascent rate below 30 feet/minute.
- Always dive with a buddy.

Importance of Basic Fitness for the Diver

- Metabolic equivalent (MET) level needed for typical diving activities
  - Average scuba and skin-diving activities use 7 METs.
  - Remaining stationary against a 1-knot current can take up to 13 METs, similar to the level required to run 7–7.5 mph.
  - Getting in and out of the water can require significant strength and coordination.

Guidelines for Diving

- Conditions that may disqualify the diver should generate discussion regarding risks versus benefits of recreational diving.
- Clearance for commercial, military, and technical divers is much more restrictive. Current US Occupational Safety and Health Administration (OSHA) and military guidelines should be reviewed.
- Divers Alert Network (DAN) is available for support if there are any questions about specific medical conditions and diving. A physician trained in dive medicine or appropriate specialist with knowledge of diving can be a local resource.

Medical Events During Diving

- Cardiovascular causes are implicated in approximately 40% of diving-related deaths.
- Important to evaluate underlying fitness for activities in a predive physical examination.
- Predive physical examination may only occur once in a person's lifetime; hence, it is important to educate the diver about ongoing monitoring of his or her health.

COMMON INJURIES AND MEDICAL PROBLEMS

Pressure-Related Diving Problems

Barotrauma

Ear squeeze: Most common pressure-related injury; occurs when the pressure inside the middle ear does not equilibrate with the ambient pressure and the tympanic membrane (TM) starts to displace inward, causing pain.

TM rupture: Pain of the ear squeeze is relieved, followed by a rush of cold water and dizziness; infection and chronic perforation can occur.

Inner ear barotraumas: Poor equalization can lead to rupture of the round or oval window. Perilymph may leak out. Tinnitus, dizziness, and hearing loss may occur. Chronic vestibular dysfunction or hearing loss may require surgical repair.

Return-to-dive recommendations after barotrauma: Divers with middle-ear symptoms may return to diving once TM is healed or protected, hearing has improved, and diver can equalize. Divers with chronic perforation or round or oval window rupture should not dive further because of risks of permanent impairment.

Sinus squeeze: Failure to equalize pressure in the sinuses can lead to pain and epistaxis.

Dental squeeze: May occur if there is a small amount of air trapped under a filling or presence of a dental abscess

Pneumothorax

Description: Can become a tension pneumothorax on ascent because of expansion of trapped air in pleural cavity (Fig. 83.1)

Return to dive: Consider no further diving if spontaneous; other causes, 3–6 months with documented healing, normal appearance on imaging, and normal function

Decompression Illness

Description: A major concern for divers because it is a potentially avoidable event with possible serious consequences. Decompression illness (DCI) encompasses events that include DCS and arterial gas embolus (AGE) in addition to other related events.

Etiology:

- Henry law is the primary factor playing a role in DCI.
  - On-gassing
    - Gas molecules dissolve into tissues as a diver descends.
    - Different tissues have different rates of gas permeability.
    - Fast—lung
    - Medium—blood and organs
    - Slow—joint capsules/ligaments
  - Off-gassing
    - Dissolved gas molecules diffuse back into the bloodstream and are transported to the lung for exchange/removal
    - Equilibration takes different amounts of time in different tissues
- Small venous bubbles are common during the ascent portion of a dive, and they are generally filtered or exchanged without problems in the lung.
  - Large bubbles can cause a problem if they enter the arterial side of the circulation, such as in a diver with a patent foramen ovale (PFO).
  - Local effects of nitrogen bubbles in the tissue can affect skin, peripheral nerves, joints, connective tissue, and muscles. This is the most common type of DCS.

DCS types: Can be divided into categories with overlap possible

- **Type 1 DCS, mild:** Characterized by one or more symptoms, including:
  - Arthralgia and myalgias that resolve within minutes
  - Pruritus and paresthesia
  - Rash, may be violaceous, mottled, and papular
  - Repeated or deep DCS exposure can lead to osteonecrosis
- **Type 2 DCS, serious:**
  - Pulmonary symptoms can include burning, substernal pleuritic pain; nonproductive cough; and severe respiratory distress.
  - Neurologic signs and symptoms can include focal spinal cord lesions with paresis, paresthesia, paralysis, loss of sphincter control, and impotence.
  - Symptoms do not always follow radicular or dermatomal patterns; may change over time.
  - Cerebral type 2 DCS may present with headaches, visual changes, dizziness/vertigo, nausea, vomiting, tinnitus, hearing loss, focal neurologic deficits, and changes in mentation.
  - Hypovolemic shock, circulatory collapse, and thrombus formation may occur.

Presentation: DCS injuries have been reported up to 36 hours after dive. AGE is a catastrophic event caused by rupture of alveoli with leakage of air into the pulmonary venous system, resulting in bubbles occluding the arterial circulation of the brain, heart, and other organs. Symptoms have an acute onset within 10–120 minutes of surfacing. Symptoms can begin with dizziness, anxiety, and headache and progress rapidly to loss of consciousness, seizures, shock, and death; often difficult to differentiate AGE from central nervous system (CNS) type 2 DCS. Treatment is similar: recompression and oxygenation. AGE can occur with any dive. DCS injuries often involve longer, deeper dives wherein tissue saturation occurs.

Prevention:

- Dive within tables/computer/conditions
- DCI has occurred in all types of dives, including free-diving
- Slow ascent with stops as required

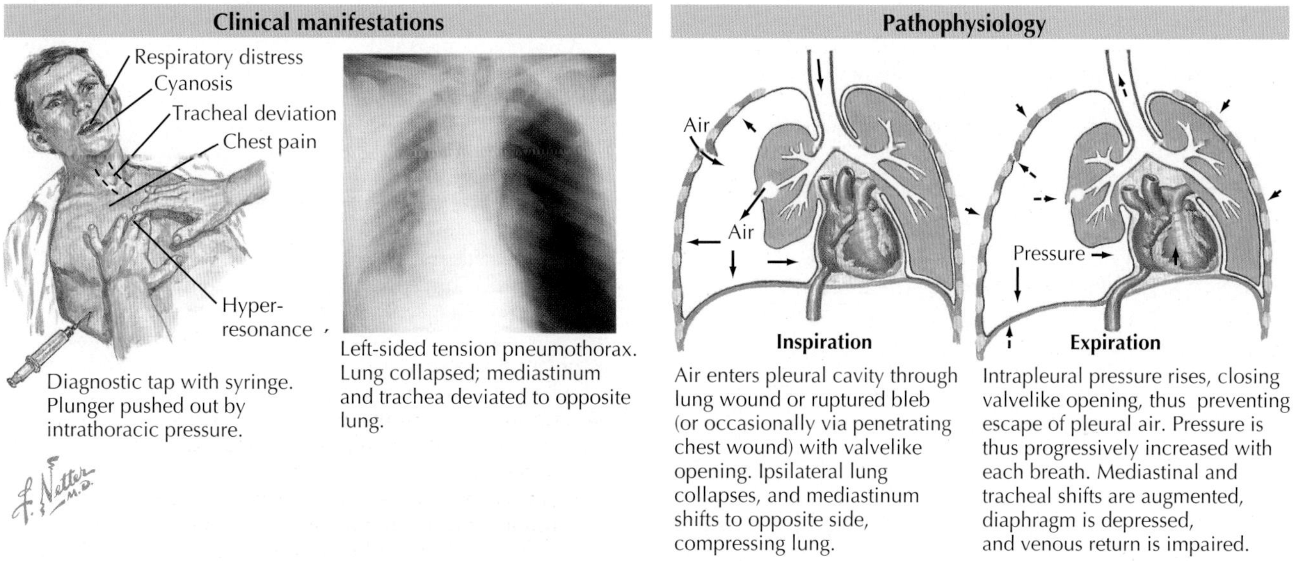

Clinical manifestations
Respiratory distress
Cyanosis
Tracheal deviation
Chest pain
Hyper-resonance
Diagnostic tap with syringe. Plunger pushed out by intrathoracic pressure.
Left-sided tension pneumothorax. Lung collapsed; mediastinum and trachea deviated to opposite lung.
Pathophysiology
Air
Air
Inspiration
Air enters pleural cavity through lung wound or ruptured bleb (or occasionally via penetrating chest wound) with valvelike opening. Ipsilateral lung collapses, and mediastinum shifts to opposite side, compressing lung.
Pressure
Expiration
Intrapleural pressure rises, closing valvelike opening, thus preventing escape of pleural air. Pressure is thus progressively increased with each breath. Mediastinal and tracheal shifts are augmented, diaphragm is depressed, and venous return is impaired.
F. Netter M.D.

Figure 83.1 Tension pneumothorax.

Risks of DCI:
- Dive profile that exceeds no-decompression limits for time and depth
- Rapid ascent, dehydration, and exertion at depth
- Age, fitness, obesity, lung disease, and cardiac defects
- Prior DCI

Treatment:
- Recompression via hyperbaric O_2 treatment (HBOT), which dissolves gases back into tissues and gradually returns the patient to atmospheric pressures.
- One hundred percent O_2 during transport can displace nitrogen from the tissues and decrease symptoms and complications.
- Correct hypovolemia with intravenous fluids.
- Aspirin may be considered for antiplatelet effects.
- Transportation and initial resuscitation should begin while HBOT facility is being arranged.
- Rapid symptom resolution with HBOT is a hallmark of DCI.

Return-to-dive recommendations after DCI: Should be evaluated for predisposing factors, including equipment, dive profile, and medical causes; medical causes should be evaluated and either corrected or decisions made regarding the advisability of further diving.
- **Type 1 DCS**—usually may dive in 2 days
  - Consider 2–4 weeks if symptoms are prolonged or if O_2 or recompression required
  - Joint involvement: 2–4 weeks
  - Paresthesia: 4 weeks
- **Type 2 DCS** with:
  - CNS involvement cleared with recompression: minimum of 4 weeks
  - Persistent or residual deficits: no further diving
- **AGE:** Minimum of 3 months if all symptoms cleared and no medical causes identified

Loss of Consciousness Underwater (LOCU)

Description: Life-threatening because of an individual's inability to protect the airway and return to the surface. Multiple causes:
- Seizures
- Hypoglycemia
- Syncope
- Cardiac event, ischemia, or arrhythmias
- Nitrogen narcosis
- Medication, alcohol, or drug use before diving
- Hypoxemia
  - Hyperventilation before breath-hold diving is common and results in decreased CO_2 levels; this leads to cerebral vasoconstriction and can reduce cerebral O_2 delivery; may lead to "shallow water blackout"
  - Carbon monoxide (CO) contamination can lead to hypoxemia despite adequate O_2.

Breathing/Air-Related Problems

- Air is the most common gas used and is composed of approximately 21% O_2 and 79% nitrogen.
- Oxygen toxicity can occur if pure O_2 is used or on prolonged deep dives with air.
- Nitrogen narcosis may occur on deep, prolonged dives.
- Nitrox is a gas with an increased percentage of O_2 (usually 32% or 36%) and may be used to prolong bottom time and decrease risks of nitrogen narcosis.
  - Different risks, including increased risk of O_2 toxicity; dive depth should be limited based on O_2 percentage.
  - Nitrox tanks should be specially labeled and not filled with air or vice versa.
- Heliox is a mix using helium as the inert gas, which can alleviate the risks of nitrogen.
  - It requires specialized support staff and equipment; hence, use is generally limited to commercial and technical divers.
  - Longer decompression time is required.
  - Increased risk of tremors, seizures, loss of consciousness, and even death, if diving on heliox below 660 FSW.
- Trimix is a blend with O_2, nitrogen, and helium, which also requires specialized equipment and training.
- Dirty air: If air compressor is incorrectly set up or malfunctioning, air may be contaminated with CO, which binds to hemoglobin molecules approximately 250 times stronger than O_2.
  - Symptoms may first start during bottom time with headache, confusion, and LOCU, and can lead to death.
- Bad tanks: Interior of tanks may expose the diver to contaminants via their air supply. Tanks can become rusted if the interior is exposed to moisture, leading to a decreased partial pressure of O_2 inside the tank. Tanks should be annually inspected and pressure-tested at least every 5 years. Tanks should be stored on their sides filled with approximately 500 pounds per square inch (PSI) of gas to prevent exposure to moist air.

Marine Animal Exposures

- Different types of marine creatures are encountered underwater. These need to be treated with respect and caution to minimize environmental degradation and risk to the diver.
- Underwater animals can move very quickly.
- Bites from animals such as eels, rays, sharks, groupers, and barracudas can occur.
  - Risks may be increased if spear fishing or in feeding zones.
  - Start with standard treatment for traumatic injuries. Remove diver from the exposure. Control bleeding and obtain treatment at nearest trauma center. Clean wound as able, and use broad-spectrum antibiotics that cover *Escherichia coli*, *Pseudomonas*, *Mycobacterium marinum*, *Staphylococcus aureus*, *Streptococcus*, *Clostridium*, and *Vibrio*.
- Jellyfish stings usually only cause discomfort, but certain types can be fatal. For most jellyfish:
  - Nematocysts on tentacles are responsible for envenomation.
  - Local inflammatory response with pain and erythema.
  - Neurologic and respiratory depression along with nausea, vomiting, and abdominal pain from certain species such as the Portuguese man-o-war.
  - Initial treatment is to remove diver from the exposure and gently remove tentacles to prevent further nematocyst firing.
  - Ice, flushing with saltwater or vinegar, meat tenderizer paste, or topical anesthetics are helpful. Rinsing with alcohol may worsen the symptoms.
  - Patients at risk of anaphylaxis should be monitored further.
- Box jellyfish, also called *sea wasp*
  - Multiple species; the most venomous are in the Indo-Pacific region with related species in the Gulf of Mexico.
  - Stings from multiple tentacles occur in linear whiplike arrangements on exposed skin.
  - Immediate and severe pain.
  - Hypotension, tachycardia, and respiratory distress may alternate with hypertension, bradycardia, and apnea.
  - Cardiogenic shock can progress quickly, and death can occur within 10 minutes.
  - Treatment must be initiated early. Remove the tentacles and get out of the water, administer vinegar to the stings, O_2, cardiopulmonary resuscitation (CPR), and treatment for anaphylaxis.
  - Parenteral pain medications and steroids may provide benefit along with intubation, sedation, administration of antivenom (if available), and intensive support in the hospital.

- Delayed problems can include paralysis, pulmonary edema, abdominal pain, irritability, and localized skin necrosis.
- Seabather's eruption is a reaction to thimble jellyfish larvae that can occur without the diver being aware of their presence because of their small size.
  - Larvae become trapped under wetsuit or bathing suit and discharge nematocysts into the skin when they are removed from seawater and exposed to air or freshwater.
  - Effects include erythema and pruritus.
  - Treatment can be initiated at the first sign of irritation and includes rinsing with saltwater, vinegar, 5% acetic acid solution, or using a meat tenderizer paste.
  - Topical corticosteroids generally help.
- Envenomation from fish, rays, and sea urchins
  - Shuffling feet and wearing thick protective footwear may minimize the risks.
  - Initial treatment: elevation and warm water or hot packs.
  - Barbs and spines can be considered for removal.
  - Antivenom for stone fish is available.

Dive Entry and Exit Injuries

- Low back pain from use of heavy and awkward equipment
- Exit and entering boat with equipment often requires maximum exertion from diver. Swells and waves increase risks.
- Shore dives have risks related to slipping on rocks or coral or being thrown into them by waves, stepping on objects, wave trauma, and rip tides.

Cardiovascular

Coronary artery disease (CAD): May allow if diver has adequate left ventricular ejection fraction (LVEF), no abnormalities with max stress testing to at least 13 METs, no recent ischemic events, and no history of exercise-associated events; should wait at least 6 months after percutaneous treatment or coronary artery bypass graft (CABG) and complete cardiac rehabilitation

Congestive heart failure (CHF): Advise against diving if New York Heart Association (NYHA) classification ≥II or if LVEF is <50% and requires medications. Fluid shifts may occur during diving with risk of immersion pulmonary edema.

Hypertension: May allow if well controlled, no trouble with exertion, and medications well tolerated with few side effects

Murmurs, structural, and valvular abnormalities:

- Atrial septal defect (ASD) and ventricular septal defect (VSD) should be a contraindication to diving if right-to-left shunting; may consider diving if there is a small membranous VSD without shunting.
- PFO is often undiagnosed and asymptomatic.
  - Can increase the risk of DCI because of right-to-left bubble shunting during Valsalva maneuvers or ascent
  - Discourage from diving if had DCI during a safe dive profile; commercial divers may be considered for repair
- **Aortic stenosis (AS):** Contraindicated if severe or if the diver has electrocardiogram (ECG) abnormalities, has poor blood pressure response to exercise, or is symptomatic
- **Mitral stenosis (MS):** Contraindicated if severe, symptomatic, or with an elevated pulmonary artery pressure
- **Mitral valve prolapse (MVP), mitral regurgitation (MR):** No contraindications unless associated with arrhythmias, dilated left ventricle, pulmonary hypertension, or syncope
- **Artificial prosthetic valve patients:** Generally disqualified because of anticoagulation
- **Transcatheter heart valve replacement:** Consult with cardiologist and consider maximum stress testing for exercise capacity and safety of required medications such as antiplatelets or anticoagulation, which place diver at risk of internal bleeding related to barotrauma
- **Hypertrophic obstructive cardiomyopathy (HOCM):** Disqualification
- **Marfan syndrome:** Disqualification
- **Congenital heart disease with cyanosis or decreased exercise tolerance:** Disqualification

Arrhythmias:

- **Long QT syndrome:** Contraindication to diving; patients with symptoms related to bradyarrhythmias or tachyarrhythmias should be disqualified from diving.
- **Atrial fibrillation:** If diver is asymptomatic, has adequate exercise capacity, rate well controlled, and no inducible cardiac ischemia and not on anticoagulation, may consider clearance.
- **Ventricular arrhythmias:** Should disqualify a diver, particularly if associated with structural abnormalities or reduced cardiac function. Pacemakers may be allowed for limited diving after an appropriate postoperative period, exercise testing, discussion with the cardiologist, and remaining below the depth limits to which the pacemaker has been tested. Diving with an implantable cardiac defibrillator (ICD) is not recommended.

Syncope: Contraindication to diving if triggers are unknown or if triggers may be encountered during dive-related activities.

Peripheral artery disease (PAD): Claudication can be worsened during a dive because of vasoconstriction from the dive reflex, cold temperature, and strenuous exercise, and symptoms may be mistaken for DCI.

Pulmonary

Asthma: Not an absolute contraindication; may be allowed to dive with mild, stable asthma if adequate lung function, no current wheezing or symptoms, and able to achieve appropriate levels on exercise testing. Cold triggers are potentially dangerous for divers. Risks associated with asthma and diving are related to air trapping and risks of alveolar rupture and AGE. Diving within 48 hours of rescue medicine use is not recommended.

Chronic obstructive pulmonary disease (COPD): In general, because of anatomic changes and alterations in function, COPD patients are unable to tolerate the exercise capacity needed to dive; generally contraindicated in patients with decreased exercise tolerance and significant airflow obstruction

Pneumothorax (PTX): Higher incidence of spontaneous PTX in tall, thin, young male smokers, and up to 40% experience recurrence; this is a contraindication to further diving. Traumatic PTX patients should not dive for a minimum of 3–6 months, with absolute contraindication to diving if pleurodesis is performed. If dive-related PTX, no diving for 3–6 months if cause can be determined and healing and normal lung function ensured.

Pulmonary embolism: No diving while on anticoagulants; no diving for 6–12 months until normal lung function and anatomy can be determined; underlying hypercoagulable state may represent a contraindication.

Immersion pulmonary edema (IPE): Edema and flooding of alveolar spaces resulting from pulmonary capillary failure from the pressure increase that occurs with water immersion, cold exposure, and exercise.

- Symptoms and signs: Dyspnea; cough productive of pink, frothy, or bloody secretion
- Risk factors: Older than 50 years, female sex, overhydration before exercise, tight wetsuits, cold water exposure, preexisting heart disease, nonsteroidal antiinflammatory drug (NSAID) use, and dive depth over 20 meters.

Central Nervous System

Seizure disorder: Risk of death is high if a seizure occurs underwater; seizure medications may have undesired side effects and increase the risk of nitrogen narcosis; may dive if stable and seizure free and off medications for 5 years. Febrile seizures as a child are not a contraindication.
Craniotomy: Generally, a contraindication to diving
Concussion: Avoid diving while symptomatic.
Cerebrovascular accident, transient ischemic attack (CVA/TIA): Need appropriate recovery and rehabilitation time; functional limits should be evaluated in light of specific needs of diving and whether equipment can be modified; if patient is cleared to dive, may need to consider having two dive buddies; presence of carotid stenosis >70% may disqualify diver.
Diving headache: Headache caused by diving to depth >10 m. Typically occurs during diving and intensifies upon surfacing. Usually accompanied by symptoms of CO_2 intoxication (e.g., mental confusion, lightheadedness, motor incoordination, dyspnea, facial flushing) and responds quickly to O_2 administration or spontaneously within 3 days. Must rule out other causes of headache, including barotrauma-related squeeze (e.g., sinus, ear, or dental) or overly tightened face mask strap.
Motor/nerve disorder (such as amyotrophic lateral sclerosis [ALS] or multiple sclerosis [MS]): May consider allowing if equipment needs can be met or modified; patients may have increased metabolic needs. Difficulty compensating for changes associated with diving, such as inability for the vascular system to adapt to the dive reflex; pulmonary, chest, or diaphragm muscle involvement may reduce respiratory capacity during the dive. Thermoregulation may be affected; extra dive buddy recommended

Gastrointestinal

Gastroesophageal reflux disease (GERD): Stomach squeeze after Nissen procedure may occur; reflux can increase because of frequent head-down position
Abdominal hernias: May have an increased risk of rupture or incarceration as the trapped air within the herniated segment expands upon ascent
Bariatric surgery: An uncomplicated surgery and successful postoperative course should not preclude diving; wait for 1 year after the procedure
Ostomies: Not a disqualification

Genitourinary

Menses: No increase in risk of shark attack during menstruation
Gas-filled penile implants: Contraindicated because of the risk of rupture
Pregnancy: Diving is contraindicated during all trimesters.

Ear, Nose, and Throat

Chronic sinus disease, allergies, or eustachian tube dysfunction: Can predispose the diver to problems
Sinus squeeze: Can cause headache, pressure, and bleeding
Otitis externa (OE): Common disorder in divers. Use of alcohol–vinegar drops in ears postdive will help with drying and prevention.
Exostoses (surfer's ear): Bony growths into external auditory canal. Common especially in professional divers. Prolonged exposure to cold water increases risk. Canal stenosis increases risk of cerumen impaction and OE. In severe cases with hearing impairment, consider surgical removal. Use of dive hood or beanie will decrease exposure and decrease risk of development or progression.
Middle ear squeeze: May cause pain and lead to TM perforation or round window or oval window rupture; equalization is best performed within the initial few feet of a dive and intermittently at the first sign of pressure.
TM perforation: No diving with an unprotected perforation because of middle ear exposure to water and contaminants.
Motion sickness: Primarily affects people in surface portions of dive; scopolamine is compatible with diving. However, several other antiemetics can increase risk of nitrogen narcosis.

Ophthalmology

Laser-assisted in situ keratomileusis (LASIK) procedure: Recommended to wait at least 2 weeks with final clearance per ophthalmologist.
Retinal tear and detachment: Diving should be avoided for at least 2 months.
Glaucoma: May be disqualifying if surgically treated.
Gas-filled prostheses: Contraindication to diving.
Corneal implants/rings or radial keratotomy (RK): Wait at least 3 months before returning to diving, with final clearance per ophthalmologist.

Psychiatry

Anxiety: Phobias and poorly controlled anxiety may lead to panic underwater and place the diver and buddy at risk. Medications often used to treat anxiety can affect diving performance and increase the risk of nitrogen narcosis.
Depression: If controlled, not a contraindication to diving; most antidepressants do not have significant adverse effects on diving.
Narcolepsy: Advisable to be episode free for 1 year.

Endocrinology

Diabetes mellitus (DM): Insulin use is not an absolute contraindication to recreational diving. Restrict diving if problems occur with unrecognized hypoglycemia or hypoglycemia requiring treatment by others within the past 12 months. Restrict diving if poorly controlled (e.g., hemoglobin A1c > 9%) or poor understanding of the disease and relationship to exercise; if allowed, the diver should monitor blood glucose levels before a dive.

- The dive should be canceled if ketones are present and delayed if blood glucose is not between 150 and 300 mg/dL (when checked 60 and 30 minutes and immediately before dive) and is not stable or slightly rising. Recheck postdive and monitor regularly for 12–15 hours.
  - Limit dive to 30 m depth with maximum dive time of 60 minutes.
  - Sugar and glucagon should be available.
  - Dive buddy should be aware of the disease and know emergency treatments.
  - Consider an extra dive buddy.

Thyroid disease: Thermoregulation may be an issue.

Musculoskeletal

- Should not dive with recent fractures or significant injuries because of an increased risk of DCI.
- Diving with an acute disc herniation or radicular symptoms is not advisable.
- Total joint replacement with solid components is not a contraindication to diving.

Hematologic

- **Sickle cell disease:** Contraindication

- **Sickle trait:** May be allowed to dive within certain depth and duration limits
- **Anemia:** Relative contraindication
- **Coagulopathy, therapeutic anticoagulation:** Contraindication

Rheumatology

- **Raynaud phenomenon:** May lead to pain and inability to use hands when diving, increased risk of injuries, or inability to perform safe diving
- **Lupus:** Depends on severity and extent of the disease

Medications and Diving

- Need to consider how pressure changes, O_2, nitrogen, potential for bleeding, and underlying disease may interact
- Medications generally considered safe for divers include:
  - Antidepressants, aspirin, cholesterol-lowering agents, nonsedating antihistamines, and NSAIDs
- Medications that are higher risk in divers and require risk–benefit discussions:
  - Anticoagulants, anxiolytics, and opioids
- Other medication considerations:
  - Decongestants: should be used with caution and consider not diving if symptoms are severe enough
  - Antihypertensives: angiotensin-converting enzyme (ACE) inhibitors and angiotensin receptor blockers (ARBs) are preferred.
  - Antibiotics appear safe, but ensure infection is controlled.
  - Phosphodiesterase type 5 (PDE5) inhibitors have not been associated with any adverse effects, although it may be prudent to avoid use within 2 hours of diving because of risks of hypotension.
  - Antioxidants have not shown any benefit in decreasing dive-related injuries.

Age-Related Concerns

- Professional Association of Dive Instructors (PADI) recommends that individuals must be at least 8 years old to participate in their Seal Team/Junior Divers program.
  - Divers aged 8 and over must have parental approval and can gain experience and become comfortable in the water.
  - Divers aged 10–11 years must dive with certified parent, guardian, or PADI professional, with dive depth limited to 40 feet.
  - Divers aged 12–14 years must dive with certified adult with dive depth limited to 60 feet.
  - A junior diver who has reached the age of 15 years may transition to a regular certification without any additional testing.
- No upper age limit to diving; base decisions on overall health and fitness.

Disabled Divers

- Fifteen percent of the US population is considered handicapped or disabled.
- Handicapped Scuba Association (HSA) International is a group of divers and trainers who have developed training programs and different levels of certifications to allow challenged/disabled individuals to enjoy opportunities to dive with safe and appropriate support.

Postdive Care

- New symptoms may present a long distance from water because of speed of travel and delay in symptom onset.
- DCI can present up to 36 hours after exiting the water.
- Safe interval before flying for no-decompression divers who have not experienced DCI symptoms and will be flying in airplanes pressurized between 2000 and 8000 feet.
  - A minimum 12-hour interval after a single dive
  - Eighteen hours minimum if multiple dives have been performed on the same day or during multiple days of diving
  - Longer intervals advisable for other situations; the longer the interval, the lower the chance of DCI

SUMMARY

- Dive training agency certification cards (C-cards) are required by dive shops in order to fill tanks.
- Do not dive when ill or with recent changes in health status.
  - Acute upper respiratory infection may lead to difficulty equalizing.
  - Bronchitis or pneumonia may lead to pulmonary air trapping because of bronchial edema and mucus.
  - Acute viral pneumonitis and postviral syndromes are often identified, and COVID-19 is the most recent example. Divers should not dive when symptomatic with fevers, cough, or shortness of breath. Chronic symptoms and respiratory compromise should be assessed with clinical examination and pulmonary function testing as indicated before return to diving.
  - Acute gastroenteritis may lead to dehydration, increasing the risk of DCS or aspiration by vomiting into the regulator.
- Diving is a very dynamic activity; diving conditions in the same area can be completely different on different days.
  - Unknown risks, dangers, or emergencies can be encountered underwater.
  - Dive buddy is depending on you; your fitness may affect your buddy's safety and your own.

RECOMMENDED READINGS

Available online.

84 SAILING

Joanne B. "Anne" Allen

INTRODUCTION

- Understanding the sport of sailing and the wide variations in sailboat classes, events, equipment, crew positions, and physical demands is essential to caring for a sailing team.
- The sport has evolved from early yacht racing in England in the 1600s, to Olympic-level racing and now, worldwide extreme endurance sailing.
- The recent advent of high-tech sailboats capable of increasing speeds and rapid maneuvers is now causing the sports medicine world to improve their efforts toward safety and injury prevention. As risk of acute injury increases, protective equipment (e.g., helmets) and quick access to emergency care are critical.
- The specific needs of a team competing in the Volvo Ocean Race, where sailors race offshore for weeks at a time but are able to communicate to a "home-base" hospital via satellite and require an on-board medic to be a member of the crew, will be different from the needs of an Olympic sailing team racing on small dinghies and keelboats in day races and from those sailing solo around the world in the Vendee race.
- All events require high-performance considerations in addition to emergency management preparations, particularly with the increase in popularity of extreme sailing. However, individual events and crew demands will differ significantly on a case-by-case basis.
- As the COVID-19 pandemic wreaked havoc on daily life throughout the world in 2020, focus on infectious disease prevention in sports became increasingly important. Adaptations have been necessary in order to continue competition and participation in the sport of sailing and will continue to evolve.

GENERAL PRINCIPLES

History

- Sailing has been a vital mode of transportation and trade since the dawn of history.
- Different types of sailboats have been developed through the centuries, ranging from the Polynesian outrigger proa and the Chinese lugsail, or "junk rig," to the Arabic triangular sail dhow.
- The first Dutch "yacht" arrived in England in 1660 as a gift to King Charles I.
- In 1661, two more yachts were built: *Catherine*, a second yacht to King Charles, and *Anne*, for the king's brother. A competition between the king and his brother ensued, and the vessels raced along the Thames in the first pleasure sailing race in history.

Competitive Sailing

- The first yacht club was founded in Ireland around 1720, and it was initially named the Water Club of Cork. It was later refounded as the Cork Yacht Club in 1828.
- The first club in England was founded in 1820 and was named the Royal Yacht Club. The first yacht club in the United States was founded in 1844: the New York Yacht Club.
- The golden age of yacht clubs and sailboat racing regattas started with the launching of the Royal Yacht Squadron's Cowes Week regatta, held annually since 1826 in Cowes, England.
- Competitive sailboat racing continued to grow in popularity with the America's Cup Race, which started in 1851 off the Isle of Wight, when the yacht *America* was victorious over the British competitors and claimed the "Hundred Guinea Cup," which is now the oldest continuously contested trophy in the world and known as the "America's Cup" (Fig. 84.1).
- As the sport of sailing grew, many other regattas and competitive events have developed, including offshore ocean racing, global solo-circumnavigation, and in-shore course racing.
- Well-known ocean racing events such as the Fastnet Race, Volvo Ocean Race, and Around Alone Race are aided by modern-day satellite navigation and other technologic advances.
- Sailing regattas have also been a part of the Olympic Games since 1900 and the Paralympic Games since 1992.
- Although professional sailors now dominate the sport in America's Cup, Grand Prix, and Volvo Ocean Race events, a vast number of amateur sailors continue to participate in and enjoy the sport through international- and national-class championships, college and high school events, regional race weeks, and local club regattas.

The Players

- The "players" in sailing are the sailors racing their boats in events governed by the international rules of the sport.
- Sailing is a sport played by all age groups, from junior sailors (8–16 years old) to masters and even great grandmasters (sailing into their 80s).
- Crews are often coed and open, but in some events and boat class there are sometimes men's and women's divisions.
- Weight may be a limiting factor (i.e., too heavy detracts performance in light air, but benefits in stronger winds), but there are no "weight classes," like there are in wrestling or rowing; combined crew weight is aimed to optimize the boat's performance.

The Playing Field

- The sailboat racing "playing field" is a body of water—whether a river, a lake, or the open ocean.
- A distance race is held in or on a "course" that can be influenced by an often constantly changing environment.
- Factors affecting the playing field include the wind strength, waves, current/tide, air and water temperature, visibility, and all types of weather systems, day or night.
- The "race course" itself varies depending on the type of event. It may be around a fixed buoy course of a half a mile or on a course of longer distances, perhaps from one seaport to another, or even from one part of the globe to another.

Rules

- The Racing Rules of Sailing (RRS) are governed by the International Sailing Federation, and there are slight variations to the basic RRS depending on the type of race or event. For example, match racing rules are slightly different from fleet racing rules because of the difference in format.
- Although a jury is often present to interpret the rules in case of protests, sailing is considered a Corinthian sport, in which participants are expected to abide by the rules and take their penalties when appropriate.
- Many sailboat races are similar to race car driving: the boat that completes the "course" quickest and crosses the finish line first, having followed the rules without infringement, wins.
- Some larger boat races have a "handicapping" system, requiring a rating system such as the Performance Handicap Racing Fleet

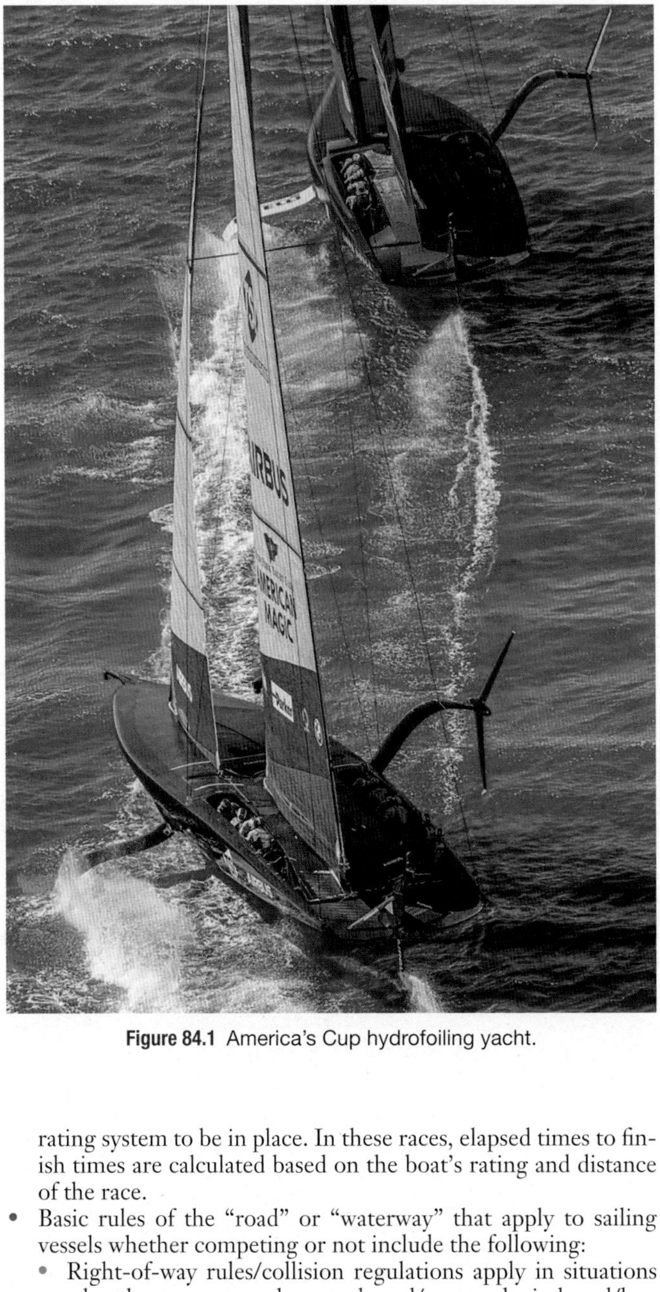

Figure 84.1 America's Cup hydrofoiling yacht.

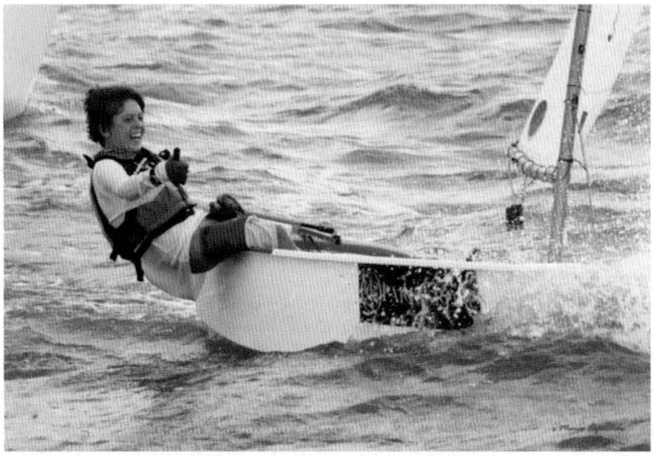

Figure 84.2 All smiles at the finish line!

rating system to be in place. In these races, elapsed times to finish times are calculated based on the boat's rating and distance of the race.

- Basic rules of the "road" or "waterway" that apply to sailing vessels whether competing or not include the following:
  - Right-of-way rules/collision regulations apply in situations when boats meet, such as starboard/port and windward/leeward convergences.
  - Knowledge of basic sailing techniques, including the points of sail, steering the boat through a tack or a jibe, and maneuvering the boat safely, is essential for anyone who is learning to race sailboats.

Sport Classes

Types of Races

- The most common types of races are fleet races, match races, team races, and distance races.
  - Fleet races involve multiple boats starting together and racing around a course (Fig. 84.2).
  - Match races are done in "flights," pitting two boats against each other in a round-robin format.
  - Team races involve teams of boats working together around the course to win a regatta.
  - Distance races are often from point to point and may even involve global circumnavigation.
- Events, known as *regattas*, vary in duration. Some are single-day events; others are weekend regattas, race weeks, or even part of a longer series that occurs over a few months.
  - America's Cup races are match races that involve both a series of races and an elimination ladder.
  - The Volvo Ocean Race is an around-the-world race with many individual legs and cumulative times.
  - Olympic and Paralympic races are a series of individual races with cumulative point totals.
- Races may involve many different types and sizes of boats competing against one another, with each having a "rating" or handicap assigned to level the playing field and even out the competition. Other races are "one-design," where all boats and equipment are almost identical.

Boat Classes and Crew

- There are many different types of boat classes—from the America's Cup class, which is currently a 75-foot hydrofoiling monohull sailboat with foil cant arms and an 87-foot mast crewed by 11 and reaching speeds of 50 knots, to the Volvo 70s, which require 13 crew members working together as a high-functioning team, to the Optimist dinghy class that junior sailors learn to race single-handed.
- The number of crew or team members varies according to the type of boat and the specific requirements of each individual class.
- The 2020 Olympic Games sailing program had 10 different disciplines. The boat class may change from one Games quadrennial to the next. For Tokyo 2020, the event program includes Laser (men's one-person dinghy), Laser Radial (women's one-person dinghy), Finn (heavyweight dinghy, men), 470 (men's and women's two-person dinghy), windsurfing RS:X (men's and women's board), 49er and 49erFx (men's and women's high performance), and NACRA 17 Foiling (multihull mixed class).
- Currently, Para World Sailing is applying to be reinstated in the Paralympic Games. The 2.4 mR class and the Sonar class are still sailed internationally by both able-bodied and disabled sailors. The RS Venture and Hansa 303, among other adapted boat classes, are still raced competitively worldwide in parasailing.
- Although the Laser is a single-person Olympic class boat, it is sailed very competitively all over the world by all age groups—from juniors to great grandmasters.
- Other boat classes that are very well known and participated in widely include J-24s, Etchells, Lightnings, Sunfish, 29er, Snipes, Melges 24s, Farr 40s, and TP-52s.

Equipment and Skills

- The basic equipment for sailing includes a boat that consists of a hull with a mast, sails, a keel or centerboard, a method to trim the sails to the wind, and a rudder attached to a steering mechanism or helm.
- Although some boats are very complicated with extremely advanced technology, hydrofoiling mechanisms, satellite navigational systems, and carbon fiber rigging, many competitive racing classes of sailboats control the equipment specifications, usually permitting only one common design.
- Many major one-design regattas require sail measurements and boat weigh-ins, and some also require crew to weigh in on a daily basis.
- Variations in sailing equipment exist depending on the type of boat sailed—whether it is a two-person dinghy that requires hiking straps, a multihull with trapeze capabilities, or a 10-person keelboat with large "coffee grinder" winch handles for trimming sails. Knowledge of the specific classes is essential for the proper care of the sailors.
- The skill sets required to competitively race sailboats at an advanced level are also variable but include helming (whether on a tiller or a wheel), trimming the sails (either on block systems or large winches), hoisting and dousing different types of sails, spinnaker pole/system management, rigging the boat and making fine-tune adjustments, hiking or trapeze work, maneuvering the boat with speed and agility, and navigation of the vessel. Navigation and tactical knowledge are also essential to the sport.

Protective Gear

- Sailor athletes often require protective equipment based on the environmental conditions in which they are sailing. For example, cold and wet weather requires proper foul weather gear, and offshore distance racing requires safety harnesses, lifejackets, helmets, etc.
- Extreme sailing, for example, through the intimidating Southern Ocean around Cape Horn in the Volvo Ocean Race, may require dry suits and head protection in addition to safety harnesses and other safety equipment because of high winds, volatile weather systems, and floating icebergs. On the other hand, a youth sailor racing a 420 dinghy in a summer regatta may only need a bathing suit, hiking shorts, sailing gloves, boat shoes, a hat, some sunscreen, and a lifejacket.
- There is constant debate over the "requirement" of wearing lifejackets/personal flotation devices (PFDs) in regattas.
  - Usually the decision to wear PFDs is primarily the responsibility of the sailor, although the race committee or regatta organizer may make it a mandatory requirement based on factors such as temperature, weather, and sea conditions.
  - Use of PFDs is encouraged because there are many documented instances of capsizes, even in favorable conditions, where a lifejacket saves a life (Fig. 84.3).
  - With the increasing awareness of concussion in sports, debate about the possibility of mandating helmet use for young sailors and in high-speed sailing has been escalating. Many athletes use water sport helmets, particularly in high-performance/high-speed racing.
  - Sun exposure is also a concern, and proper sunscreen in addition to ultraviolet A (UVA) and ultraviolet B (UVB) protective eyewear is recommended as ocular melanoma is on the rise in water activities.

Safety

- Safety is a major issue because the marine environment can be a hazardous playing ground (Fig. 84.4).
- Capsizes, collisions, and man overboard situations are the riskiest.

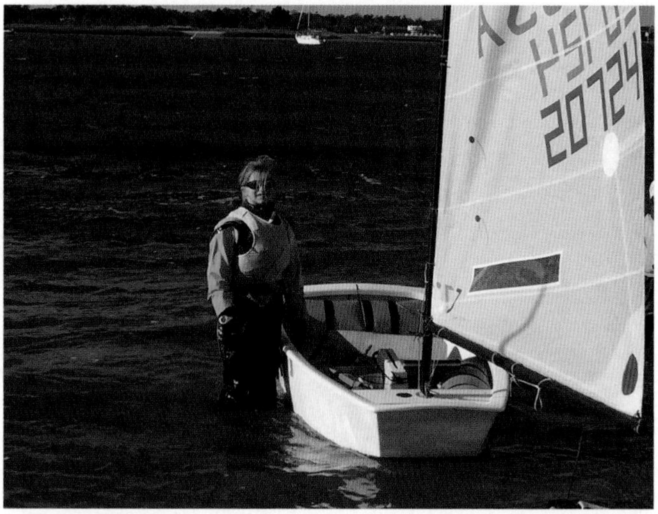

Figure 84.3 Lifejacket and foul weather gear in Opti sailor.

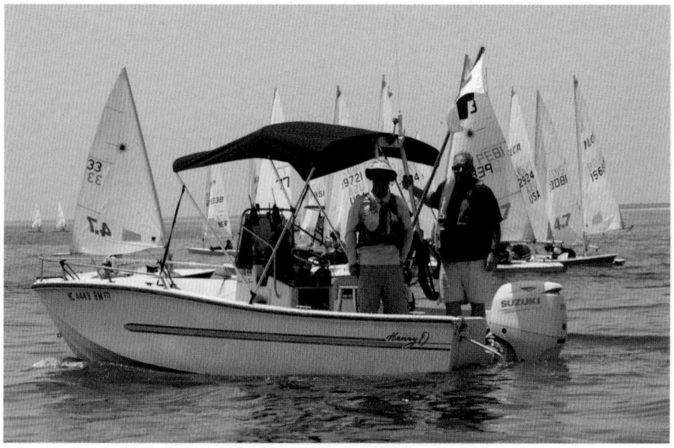

Figure 84.4 Medical safety team.

- An understanding of the properties of the body of water/geographic area where a competition occurs is essential.
- Along with emergency management plans, appropriate seamanship skills and water rescue skills are needed. Safety at Sea training assistance courses are readily available.
- The proper prevention of injury and illness is also a required element of safety in this sport.
- Understanding of right-of-way rules and avoiding collisions, knowledge of navigation signals, proper training, practice of man overboard rescue drills, and overall seamanship are important for safe participation in sailing.

SAILING-SPECIFIC MEDICINE

Epidemiology

- Efforts have been made to advance evidence-based knowledge of sailing and sports medicine over the last 20 years with an increase in research.
- Research by groups such as Olympic and America's Cup teams has produced many beneficial changes that have trickled down to high school and junior sailing.
- The overall injury rates have been estimated to be between 0.29 and 4.61/1000 days of athlete exposure. The incidence of injury in an America's Cup team was reported by Neville to be between 2.2 and 8.6 per 1000 hours in sailboat racing and training, with the most common injury being sprains and strains.

Nathanson reported fatality rates of 1.19 deaths per million sailing person-days, which is comparable to those in US football. The US Coast Guard (USCG) reported 23 deaths/year related to sailing.
- Because there are hundreds of boat classes, each with their own specific crew positions and demands, there are distinct injury profiles, optimal training regimens, and individualized physiologic stresses and demands that have been described.

Physical Demands

- Physical demands on sailors vary with boat class and crew position; injuries may differ on the basis of specific job stressors.
- Some injuries appear to be more related to overuse dynamics, causing sprains and strains usually in the upper extremities, yet others may be more acute because of accidents, with contusions and lacerations being the most common traumatic injuries. Falls on the deck or companionway and being hit by objects (including the boom) are common mechanisms of getting injured.
- Many actions in sailing are sudden and sporadic, which may place the sailor at high risk while performing explosive, powerful moves, particularly during a tacking or jibing maneuver. This is when concussions and man overboard issues that can lead to drowning can occur.
- Constant isometric contractions occur during hiking on a long upwind leg and result in significant strength and endurance requirements for sailors.
- Whether using the technique of straight-leg hiking or droop-seat hiking, sailors may be susceptible to back and knee problems (Figs. 84.5 and 84.6).
- Repetitive grinding on winches while trimming can result in shoulder and arm injuries.
- Inherent postures in many crew positions also play a role in musculoskeletal issues because some actions on a sailboat require twisting and hyperextension of joints and, in particular, may predispose a sailor to back injuries.
- Lifting sails and hoisting sails pose a particular risk, with difficulty in maintaining proper form on a moving vessel or using proper technique even on the docks.

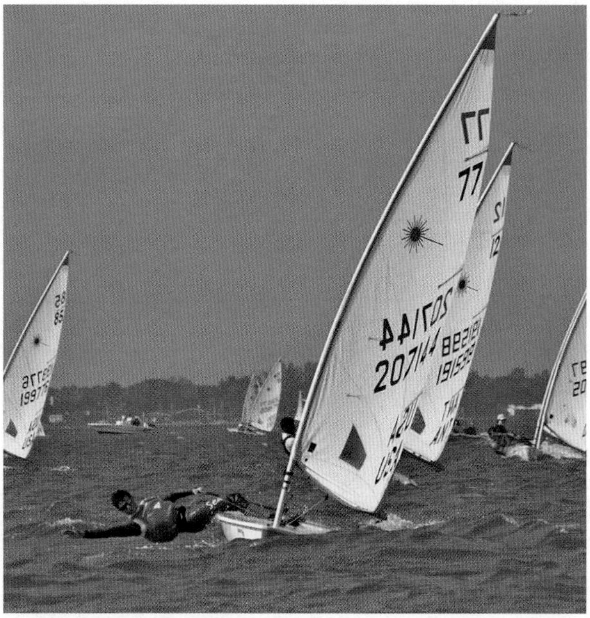

Physical demands of hiking out on a Laser.

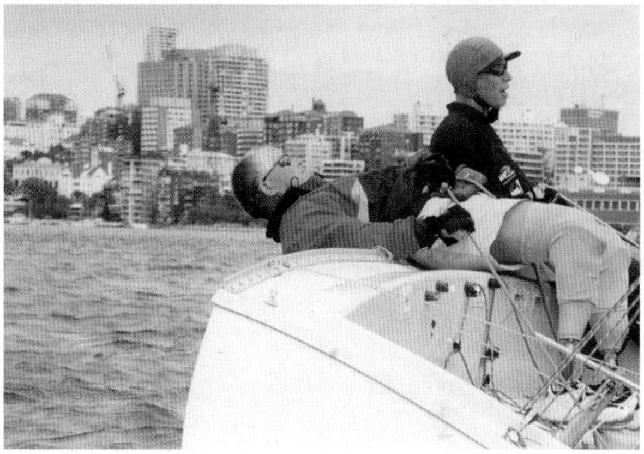

Paralympic amputee hiking on a Sonar in Sydney Games.

Figure 84.5 Biomechanics of hiking.

Injury Studies

See Table 84.1 and Fig. 84.7.

Environment and Illnesses

- Environmental issues concerning sailing include potential problems with polluted waters, such as those in Brazil at the Rio 2016 Olympic and Paralympic Games.
- Preventable illnesses have been prevalent among sailing teams working closely on a day-to-day basis, and proper hygiene always must be considered. The COVID-19 pandemic has been challenging for all athletes and sports, requiring adaptation to participation at all levels. As a sport, sailing has managed to maintain a high level of competition by adding precautions including mask wearing in crewed boats and maintaining physical distances among participants.
- Because elite sailors often travel internationally to training camps and events, consideration of water and food contamination and of jet lag is also essential.
- Environmental issues such as hypothermia, heat illness, dehydration, seasickness, poor nutrition, and sun-related problems are also prevalent within the sport of sailing. Nathanson reported that in the Newport to Bermuda race, cases of seasickness were more prevalent when the weather was stormier. In a recent Chicago to Mackinaw Island race, severe thunderstorms and wind gusts up to 60 mph caused a racing yacht to capsize, and two of the tethered crew could not free themselves and drowned.
- Other obvious risks at sea include water immersion, near-drowning, drowning, and contact with aquatic marine life such as jellyfish.
- A unique property of this sport is the field of play environment. Special consideration should be taken with regard to the amount of time spent on the water, and necessary preparations should be made regarding thermoregulation with cooling/heating units, hydration kits on and off the water, and sun protection (Fig. 84.8).
- Because most events require sailors to be on the water for extended periods without access to land-based facilities, it is necessary to also consider gastrointestinal issues, bladder problems in some disabled sailors, diabetic/blood sugar management, adequate nutrition, and the ability to readily manage minor emergencies on the water.
- Illness and environmental influences may affect healthcare within the sport of sailing. As such, appropriate preventive measures, including proper clothing, adequate nutrition, and safety regulations, are recommended.

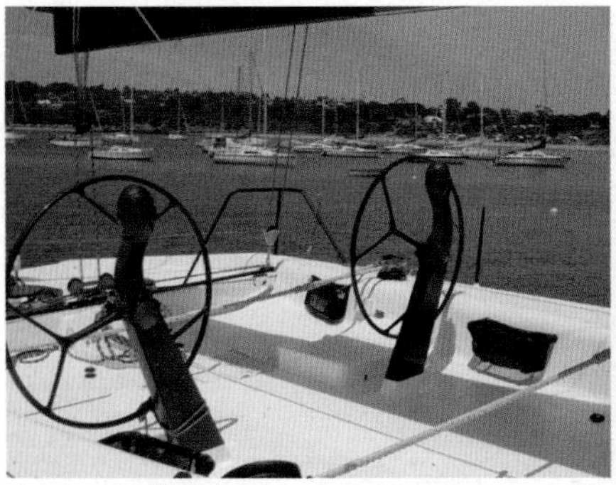

Helm on a Maxi-Yacht.

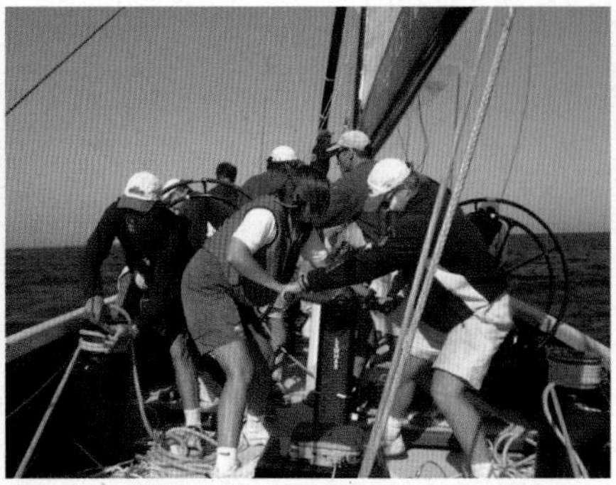

Grinding on pedestal winches aboard Stars and Stripes.

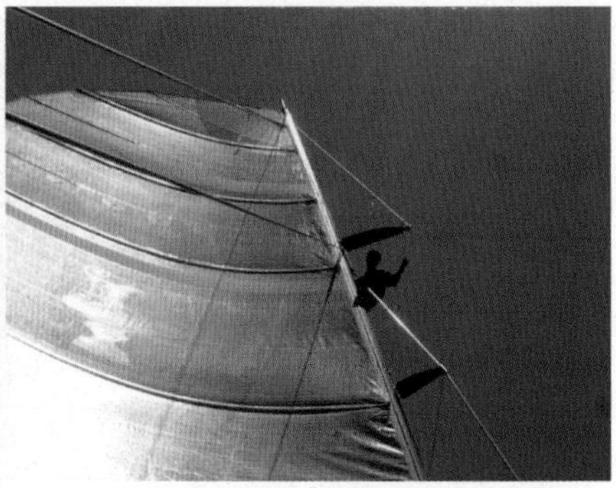

The Bowman lives dangerously up the rig.

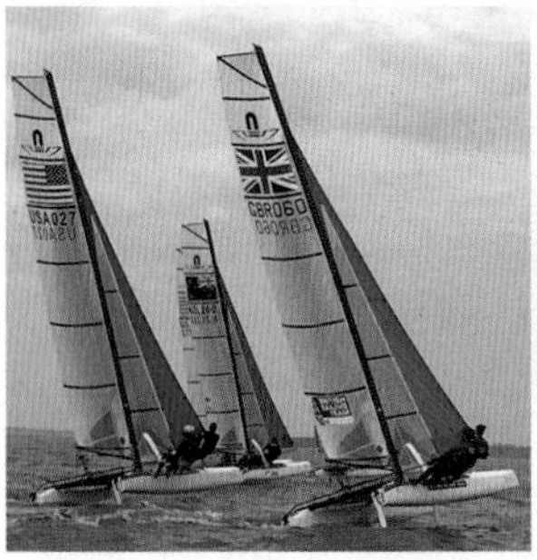

Trapeze work on the NACRA.

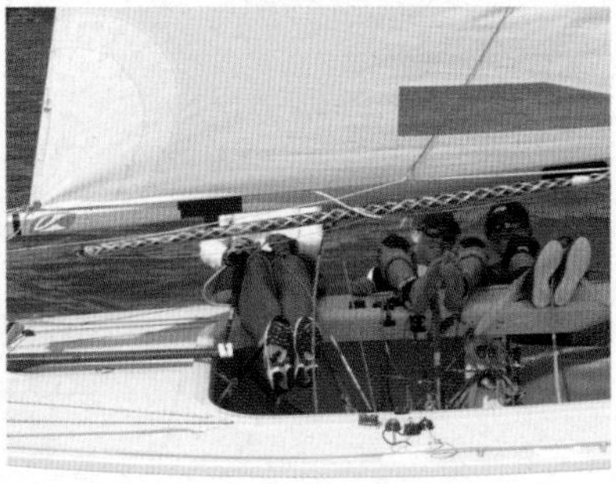

Hiking straps and foot position may affect knee injuries.

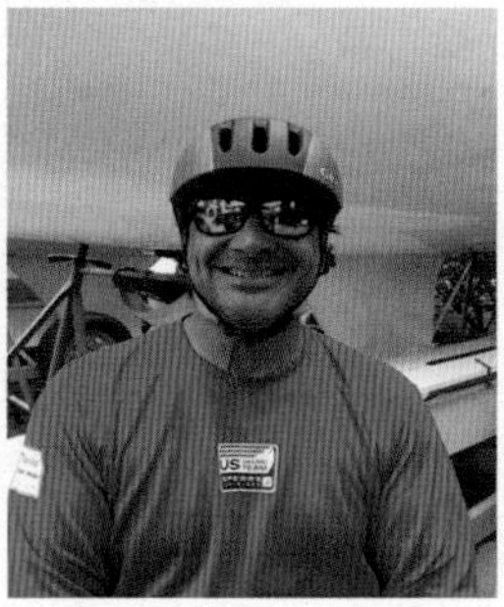

Protective helmet for Sonar Helmman.

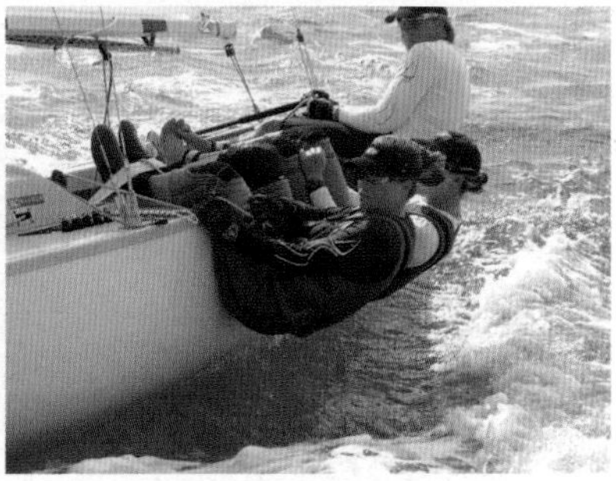

World Champion Yngling Team hiking out.

Figure 84.6 Crew positions and specific injury examples.

Table 84.1 COMMON AREAS OF INJURY/PAIN FOR SAILORS

Smaller boats	Lower back (52.9%)
Olympic classes	Other back areas (41.2%)
	Knees (25%–32%)
	Thigh/leg (26.5%)
	Neck (23.5%)
	Shoulder (23.5%)
	Forearm or elbow (20.6%)
Larger boats	Lumbar spine (16%)
America's Cup class	Shoulder (16%)
	Knee (10%)
	Cervical spine (8%)
	Hand (7%)
Offshore endurance races	Low back
(Volvo Ocean boats)	Shoulder
	Neck
	Skin lesions
Disabled sailors (Paralympic classes)	Upper extremity (60%)
	Spine (20%)
Boardsailing (Windsurfers)	Lower extremities (44.6%)
	Upper extremity (18.5%)
	Head and neck (17.8%)
	Trunk (16.0%)

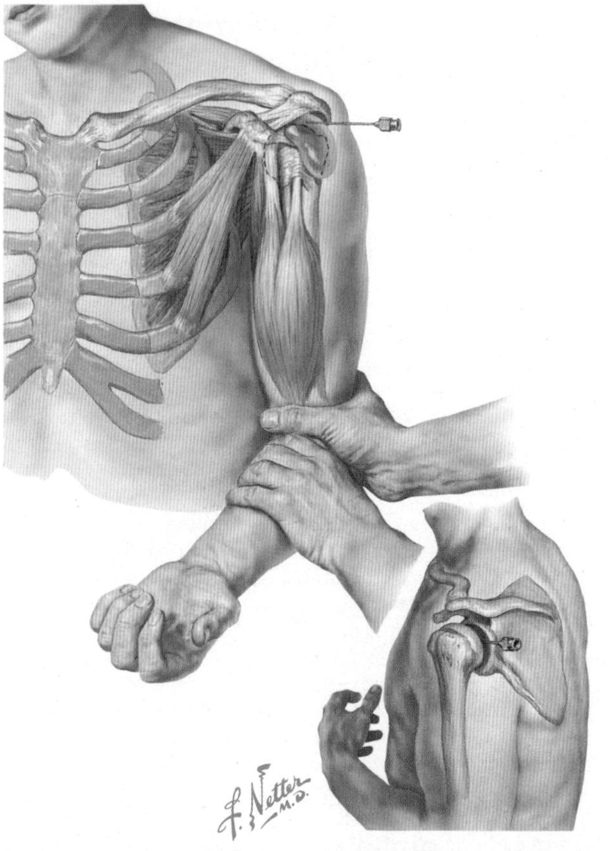
F. Netter M.D.

Figure 84.7 Injuries: Grinder's shoulder may require injections.

Physiology of Sailing

- Research addressing the biomechanics and physiology in the sport of sailing has been increasing as more scientists are analyzing the performance of the sailboat racer.
- In general, studies suggest that the most physiologically demanding positions are in the dinghy classes, which require more intense dynamic hiking maneuvers, and the big boat crew positions, which require the most agility or repetitive motion.
- One study of the 2002 Danish Olympic team showed that Laser sailors had the highest $\dot{V}O_2$ max at 58.3 ± 4.2 mL/kg/minute, whereas the Finn and Star sailors had the lowest, with an average value of 47.6 ± 3.5 mL/kg/minute. Helmsmen and crew on trapeze boats have had results of 55.3 ± 4.0 and 57.3 ± 3.7 mL/kg/minute, respectively.

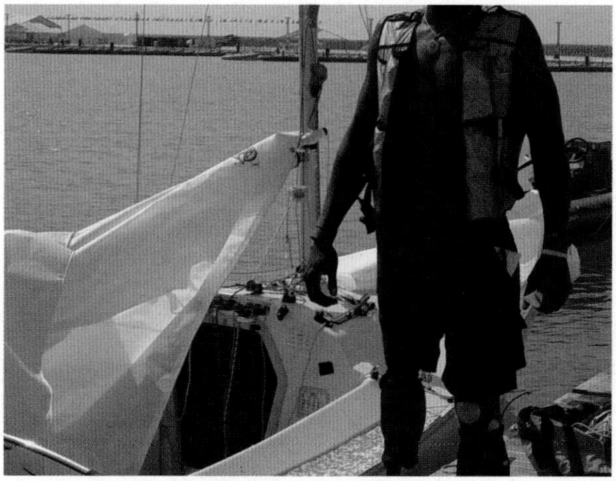

Figure 84.8 Cooling vest.

Biomechanics of Hiking

- The physical stress of hiking, which is using body weight to counterbalance the tilting forces of the boat, has been documented and is believed to be an important performance factor.
- Studies have recognized hiking as a dynamic activity, measuring physiologic responses and force demands within an active sailing environment, whether on a simulator or on the water.
- One study found that the elite status and national rankings of Laser sailors were strongly correlated to quadriceps maximal voluntary contraction, isometric endurance, and tolerance of muscular fatigue (see Fig. 84.5).
- Improper technique is commonly a factor in hiking-induced knee pain, resulting in unbalanced muscular forces around the knee joint.
- With fatigue, most sailors tend to isolate the vastus lateralis, leading to patellofemoral pain; turning out both feet with the legs extended increases the workload of the vastus medialis.
- Use of tight toe straps and plantarflexing the foot may help straighten the knees, centralize the force of gravity, and reduce the effort required by the quadriceps.
- The biomechanics of hiking in Paralympic sailing may change the dynamics because of the different force couples when using prosthetic legs, for example, and should be considered when working with athletes with disabilities (see Fig. 84.5).

Training for the Sport

- With physical fitness joining technical boat speed and tactical skill and mental performance as the main determinants of sailing performance, the issue of fitness training for sailors is accompanied by many opinion articles but very little scientific research.
- The existence of various boat classes, crew positions, racing conditions, and baseline fitness levels makes it unfeasible to provide a uniform recommendation for fitness requirements.
- Strength, power, muscle endurance, cardiovascular fitness, weight management, flexibility, and agility all play varying roles in sailors' training regimens.
- Agility exercises may improve hand–eye coordination and the efficiency of movement about a sailboat, especially in high-performance boats.
- Weightlifting routines should involve commonly used muscle groups, plus their antagonists, to maintain proper balance of strength and should include a core workout.
- Aerobic training and fitness has been directly correlated to sailors' reaction speed to wind shifts, in addition to enhanced

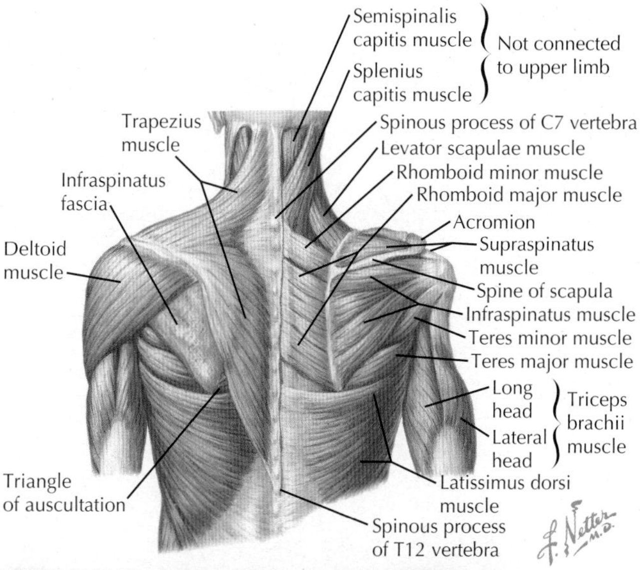
Semispinalis capitis muscle
Splenius capitis muscle
Not connected to upper limb
Trapezius muscle
Spinous process of C7 vertebra
Levator scapulae muscle
Infraspinatus fascia
Rhomboid minor muscle
Rhomboid major muscle
Acromion
Deltoid muscle
Supraspinatus muscle
Spine of scapula
Infraspinatus muscle
Teres minor muscle
Teres major muscle
Long head
Lateral head
Triceps brachii muscle
Triangle of auscultation
Latissimus dorsi muscle
Spinous process of T12 vertebra
F. Netter M.D.

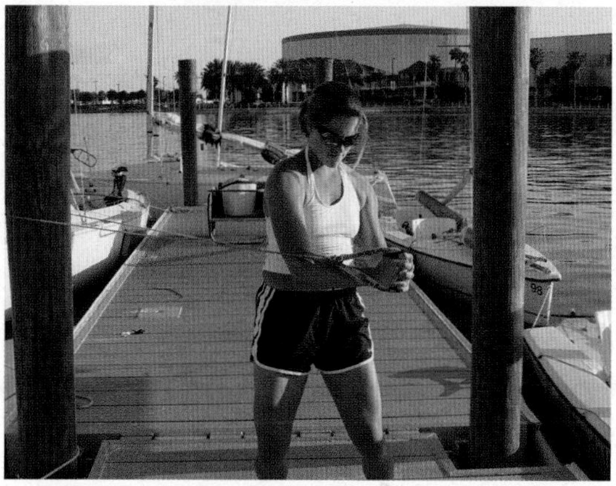

Trimmer demonstrates Thera-Band shoulder exercises on the docks.

Figure 84.9 Training for the sport.

endurance, decision-making, and concentration, particularly in the latter stages of longer races.
- Physical and mental recovery between races and regattas is critical and may improve with cardiovascular fitness.
- Position-specific fitness training:
  - Hiking training should include muscular strength and endurance of the core and lower extremities, maintaining balanced force and flexibility about each joint.
  - Sailors who hike rely on muscle groups in the thighs, abdominals, hips, and arms, whereas sailors on a trapeze may focus more on upper body strength/endurance, aerobic endurance, and agility.
  - Grinders (sailors who use their strength to power winches and mechanical systems that control the boat) and many other big boat sailors should address aerobic endurance in addition to muscular strength, power, and endurance, particularly in the upper body.
  - Board sailors require sustained isometric action of the pectoralis major, deltoid, and scapular stabilizers, and therefore training should involve the shoulder girdle (Fig. 84.9).
  - Sail trimmers (any boat size) should focus on training the arms, shoulders, and upper back (see Fig. 84.9).
- The proper timing of fitness training is important, whether that entails maintaining fitness in the off-season or reducing heavy training loads before regattas.

Nutrition and Weight

- Weight management issues for sailors commonly involve reaching a perceived ideal mass for racing a small boat or meeting the weight limits of a one-design class.
- Awareness of problems associated with relative energy deficiency in sport (RED-S) in sailors is also critical, because they are often required to "make weight," which can lead to eating disorders.
- Any weight loss should be gradual, focusing on reduced caloric intake while increasing aerobic exercise.
- Whether sailing in a 1-day regatta or a long-distance offshore race, adequate nutrition to sustain proper blood glucose levels throughout the event is important for maintaining concentration and coordination.
- America's Cup sailors have been found to average 56 kcal per kg of body weight in daily energy expenditure.
- Dehydration can hamper performance, including increasing cognitive impairment and increasing risk of injuries.
- General guidelines for hydration in sports apply to sailors.

Sports Psychology

- Mental skills training has been shown to be important, especially in high-level competition.
- Relaxation techniques, prerace routines, and mental rehearsal may be beneficial to sailors at any level.
- Sports psychology can facilitate effective goal setting; develop healthy relationships with coaches and teammates; prevent burnout; build resiliency; encourage teamwork, focus, and organization; and help athletes return to play after injury.
- Including sports psychology professionals as part of a performance enhancement team (PET) or integrated support team (IST) is essential to the health and wellness and sustained high levels of performance for sailors.

Injury Prevention

- Understanding and accounting for different skill sets and an attention to proper mechanics, technique, posture, and positioning will assist the clinician in injury prevention.
- Injury prevention is best addressed through appropriate fitness training and properly caring for prior injuries.
- Research supporting injury prevention programs in sailing is limited. It may be effective to include flexibility, hip flexor mobility, and core stability programs to reduce injury risk.
- Acute injuries are often related to accidents involving boat equipment and are difficult to prevent (e.g., lacerations from hitting sharp metal edges on the rig, abrasions from mishandling sheets, finger fractures from problems with winch overrides, contusions from free-flying winch handles, concussions from contact with an accidentally jibing boom, or slips and falls on a wet foredeck). Fisher reported that although head injuries only make up 10% of sailing-related injuries, many of these are severe, with >50% of them being fatal, usually caused by boom-related injuries. It is uncertain if helmet use would prevent these (see Fig. 84.6).
- Properly addressing ergonomic developments, particularly in big boat design, also holds potential for injury prevention.
- Certainly, although avoidance of accidents is preferable, overuse injuries may be more easily addressed.
- Returning to play is dependent on the nature of injury and the physical demands for which the athlete is returning to sail.

Crew Positions and Specific Injury Examples

Helm: Carpal tunnel syndrome (CTS) can be seen in both big boat sailing and dinghy sailing. Symptoms of CTS may be preventable by adjusting the grip width of the wheel at the helm of larger yachts; avoiding prolonged tight sustained grip positions on the tiller may decrease wrist and forearm stress in a dinghy (see Fig. 84.6). In distance racing, platforms for the helmsman have recently been used on large yachts in the Volvo Ocean Race to properly position the sailor's posture on long tacks, because standing in one place on a heeled boat for a prolonged period can lead to overuse problems for these drivers.

Grinders: Attention to grip size and angle of rotation on winch handles, and to height and angle of pedestal winches, may help prevent other overuse injuries such as lateral epicondylitis, often referred to as "grinder's elbow" (see Fig. 84.6). Lumbar spine injuries also frequently affect the grinder position, and the biomechanical forces required for this skill set should be considered. These athletes must be assessed on an individual basis because the height of the sailor, for instance, may directly affect both potential injury prevention and performance of peak power output on a pedestal winch if the height of the pedestal is not adjusted appropriately.

Mast: The mast man on larger yachts is also susceptible to injuries. Repetitive halyard hoisting at the mast with proper hand-over-hand technique, using the legs and trunk for strength and stability, may reduce overhead injuries to the shoulder.

Trimmer: "Trimmer's neck" has been described as neck pain related to the angle of cervical rotation and extension required to visualize the sail while constantly monitoring the tale-tells. Spinnaker trimmers may be especially susceptible to such problems because of the constant attention aloft that is required to fly this specialized sail.

Bow: One of the most frequently injured crew members on a sailboat is on the bow, primarily because of the multiple physical tasks required by this position (see Fig. 84.6). Safety is essential for the bow crew, who may be changing headsails in heavy weather and sea conditions or jibing the spinnaker pole when sailing downwind. Concussions have been reported in this position from contact with the spinnaker pole, and the bow crew must be clipped on with a safety harness in order to avoid falling overboard in heavy sea conditions.

Hiking crew: Hiking refers to using body weight as a lever for a righting moment. It is often required in heavy air conditions no matter what size boat is being sailed, but there is a difference in hiking out while sitting on a rail with a lifeline on a J-24 and hiking on a Laser. Dinghy sailing often requires a dynamic effort in heavy air conditions and will vary with the sailor and boat class. The hiking strap placement and foot position on the straps have been shown to be factors in forces generated at the knee and should be observed in any sailor with knee pain (see Fig. 84.6). The different hiking styles and torques placed on the knee when tacking the boat from a hiked-out position may affect development of meniscal injuries or patellofemoral injuries in these athletes. Hiking crew members are also susceptible to lumbar spine disc problems, and core stability is essential to preventing injury. In boats that use a trapeze, the harness fit may play a role in preventing low back pain, suggesting that custom-fit harnesses should be considered (see Fig. 84.6). Finally, hiking crew may also be susceptible to "rail rider's rump," or cutaneous rash, which can be worsened with unclean wetsuits or hiking shorts.

Shore crew: Unlike other sports, most sailors also have shore-based responsibilities for the boats on which they race, and proper caution when lifting boats onto trailers or moving large, heavy sails and equipment on and off larger vessels is essential to prevent lumbar strains and other injuries. Injuries occurring during fitness training can affect performance on the water and should be monitored adequately.

Boardsailing

- Because boardsailing is slightly different in its rules and techniques, the prevailing injuries may differ from other classes in the sport.

- The constant pumping action of the sail by the board sailor often causes increases in forearm compartment pressures, which can sometimes be relieved with daily massage and flushing.
- The newer segment of kite-boarding will have its own unique injuries, with problems including traumatic injuries from lofting and wind-shear dropping.

SUMMARY

- Although a team doctor's handbag for sailing will not differ from many other sports, his or her knowledge about the sport is critical for the successful caring for sailors.
- Injuries and illnesses will occur and will vary with the type of boat, the event, the crew position, and the environment.
- Finally, as with most teams, caring for the athlete on and off the field of play is essential to a healthy team.
- Prevention, whether through proper nutrition, adequate hydration, strength and endurance training, cardiovascular fitness, injury assessment, mental preparedness, environmentally appropriate clothing and equipment, or safety awareness, is the cornerstone to a healthy sailing team and the enhancement of the team's performance.

RECOMMENDED READINGS

Available online.

85 ROWING

Jane S. Thornton • Constance M. Lebrun

INTRODUCTION

- As a competitive sport, rowing dates back several hundred years and was an original sport in the modern Olympic Games.
- First intercollegiate sport in the United States; initial race held in 1852 (Harvard vs. Yale).
- With the adoption of Title IX regulations, the participation of women in collegiate rowing has surged, from roughly 1000 in 1981–1982 to approximately 7300 today, now surpassing males.

GENERAL PRINCIPLES

Physiology

Training

On-water: Usually high volume (one to three times daily, 1–2 hours in length), with higher-intensity pieces and intervals during the summer racing season.

Indoor: On rowing ergometer (dynamic and static options); simulates water training and monitors fitness.

Cross-training: Resistance training, running, cycling, and cross-country skiing; used to supplement water training or during winter. Injuries may result from inappropriate transition to cross-training from on-water practices (and vice versa) or via resistance training.

Racing

- Anaerobic portion 10%–30%; aerobic system supplies remainder.
- Ranks among the most strenuous of sports with high cardiovascular strain and lactate measurements of ≥15–20 mmol; $\dot{V}O_2$ max values can exceed 70 mL/kg/min in elite rowers.

Race Distances

2000 meters: Olympic distance and standard for collegiate and club spring/summer racing; boats line up side by side at starting gates in up to six lanes. Races typically last for ≥5.5–8 minutes, depending on event, weather, and rowers' ability. World record in Olympic men's eight event is under 5 minutes 20 seconds.

1000 meters: Paralympic distance and standard for adaptive (para-rowing) and Masters competitions.

Head racing: Predominantly in the fall season; distance usually is ≥3 miles against the clock from a moving start and involves steering on rivers that bend and turn.

Open water/coastal rowing: The "adventure" side of rowing—along a seacoast or inland on some lakes or rivers where water is rough. Boats are wider and sturdier: singles (solo) and doubles and coxed quadruple sculls (also used for recreational rowing touring). Requires knowledge of tides, currents, and maritime traffic. Races typically 4000 m for heats and 6000 m for finals, with buoyed turns. Beach sprints are shorter distances with a running start to the boats, sometimes relay format (Fig. 85.1).

Athlete Classification

- Rowers are classified by sex (male or female), age, weight, and ability (para-rowing).
- Age categories are Junior (age ≤18 years), Under 23 (<23 years), Senior (open), and Masters, ranging from "A" (age ≥27 years) to "M" (age ≥89 years).
- Weight categories are lightweight and heavyweight/open.
  - Both types of rowers have similar builds, although lightweights (because of the need to "make weight") typically have lower body fat, have more muscle mass, and may be slightly shorter.
  - Being tall and lean allows maximum stroke length while minimizing drag on the boat.
- Weight restrictions: Lightweight rowers typically weigh in 1–2 hours before racing at or below the maximal weight. Weight restrictions are as follows:
  - **Men:** 70-kg crew average, 72.5-kg individual maximum.
  - **Women:** 57-kg crew average, 59-kg individual maximum for an international competition. National rules vary.
- Coxswains: Steer the boat using a rope attached to the rudder; make technical and motivational calls and decisions about strategy; minimum weight is 55 kg (international regulations); if underweight, must carry weight for racing to a maximum of 15 kg. As of 2017, coxswains can be gender-neutral (i.e., women can cox men's crews, and vice versa).
- Para-rowing comprises three classifications based on the nature of the disability:
  - **PR1** (Para Rowing One, formerly known as AS or Arms and Shoulders): Rowers are effectively rowing with arms and shoulders alone.
  - **PR2** (Para Rowing Two, formerly known as TA or Trunk and Arms): Rowers whose movements include use of arms, shoulders, and trunk.
  - **PR3** (Para Rowing Three, formerly LTA or Legs, Trunk, and Arms): Rowers with essentially full range of movement with restricted ability in areas such as vision or digit loss on the hand.

Equipment and Safety Issues

Boat Types

Sweep: Rower uses one oar, placed on starboard or port (left and right, respectively, from rower's perspective); available boats: pair, four, and eight; the eight is the only boat to always use a coxswain (Fig. 85.2A).

Sculling: Rower uses two oars; available boats: single, double, and quadruple sculls (see Fig. 85.2B).

Rowing shell: Classically wooden, now constructed of synthetic materials such as carbon fiber; seats with wheels roll along fixed tracks. Athlete faces backward and pushes away from fixed shoes. The oar is held in an oarlock attached to a rigger that extends out from the shell. Equipment can be adjusted within a range (e.g., changing placement of feet or oar lengths to aid in loading), called "rigging" (see Fig. 85.2C).

Oars: Classically wooden, now primarily carbon fiber; consist of handle with varying grip sizes and material, collar and sleeve that fits into oarlock, and blade that enters water and provides resistance to move boat. Oar design has changed over time to generate more force per stroke, typically through shorter overall length and greater surface area, which may account for increase in injury rate.

Indoor rowing ergometer (colloquially "erg"): Used for fitness testing, training, and racing, primarily during winter, although erg testing is often used selectively throughout the year. Most common models consist of a sliding seat on rail, fixed footplate, and handle attached to a chain. The chain spins a flywheel that creates resistance, and a small monitor displays power output, split times, and stroke rate. In addition to stationary erg, dynamic erg systems are available where flywheel and footplate also move.

Phases of Rowing Stroke

Catch: Legs and back fully flexed, arms fully extended; rower's seat is at front of slides and the blade enters water in a "squared" position (blade perpendicular to water) (Fig. 85.3A).

Drive: Legs extend and back begins to extend slightly, while arms and shoulders remain relatively fixed; once back has extended to neutral position, arms begin to flex and continue acceleration of blade through water (see Fig. 85.3B).

Finish or release: Legs flat and fully extended, shoulders behind hips but back still slightly flexed, arms flexed; blade is removed from water by simultaneously putting weight on handle (tapping down) and feathering (turning the wrist so that the blade is parallel to water) (see Fig. 85.3C).

Recovery: Reverse of drive sequence; arms extend to move the oar handle forward, back becomes more flexed, and knees are flexed to bring rower into position for next catch.

APPROACH TO INJURY EVALUATION

- A vast majority of injuries to competitive rowers of all ages/abilities are overuse injuries.

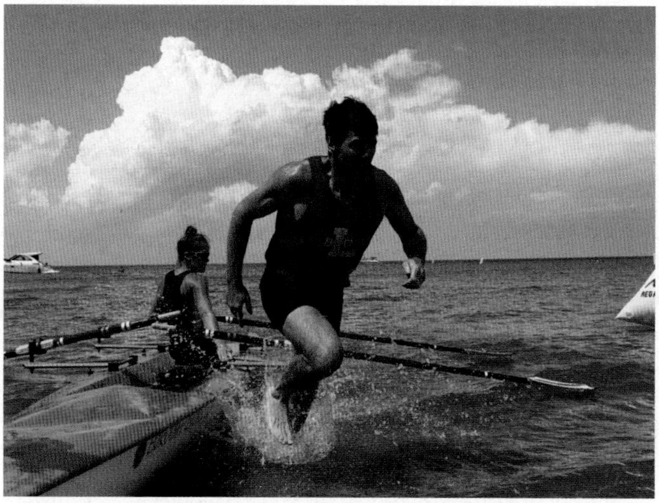

Figure 85.1 Coastal rowing: Beach sprint.

- Inappropriate stroke mechanics and asymmetries may predispose rower to injury.
- Other factors include poor weather conditions that affect stroke mechanics, fit of equipment and rigging, and transition from indoor to on-water training and vice versa.
- If possible, observe rowing technique on water or by using an ergometer. Watch for compensatory behavior related to poor mobility, muscle or strength deficiencies, abnormal asymmetrical movements, or undue force placed on the injury site.
- Most common injury sites: lumbar spine (2%–53%), chest wall (6%–22.6%), and forearm/wrist (2.3%–15.5%).
- Rib stress injury is typical and unique to rowing.

COMMON INJURIES AND MEDICAL PROBLEMS

Low Back

Description: Most frequently injured region, accounts for up to 53% of all reported rowing injuries.

Mechanism of injury: Large loads are placed on lower back; lower back muscles are relatively relaxed as rower approaches catch position. At catch, spinal extensors are quickly loaded with resulting compressive forces at the spine, building and reaching peak compressive forces mid-drive (estimated at >4 times rower's body mass). Sweep rowing introduces increased rotation through spine because rower reaches at catch to maximize stroke length. Fatigue of spinal extensor muscles, training intensity, and skill level may result in decreased ability of lumbar spine to resist forces during drive on passive spinal structures (e.g., ligaments and discs). Onset of low back pain is generally associated with prior history of injury and ergometer training sessions of >30 minutes.

Types of injury:

- **Muscle strain:** Most common injury; low back pain, involving erector spinae muscles, quadratus lumborum, and/or sacroiliac joints.
- **Sacroiliac joint pain:** Localized pain over buttock, lateral thigh, pelvis, and/or groin; contributing factors may include leg-length discrepancies, underlying hypermobility, or constant unforeseen balance changes.
- **Lumbar disc herniation:** Common; compressive loads applied to lumbar spine in flexion may contribute to disc bulge or herniation. This may be associated with or progress

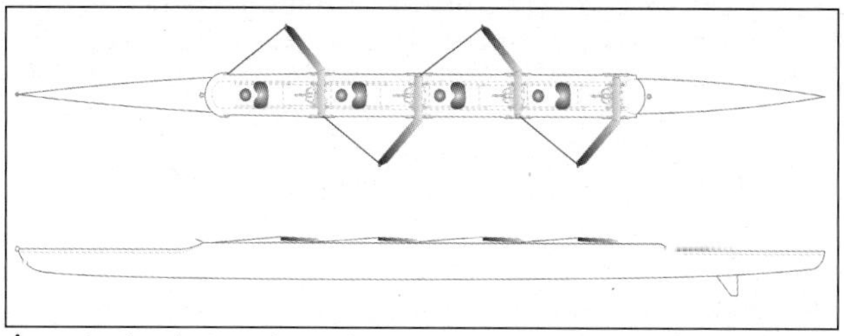

A. Example of sweep boat: the straight or coxless four.

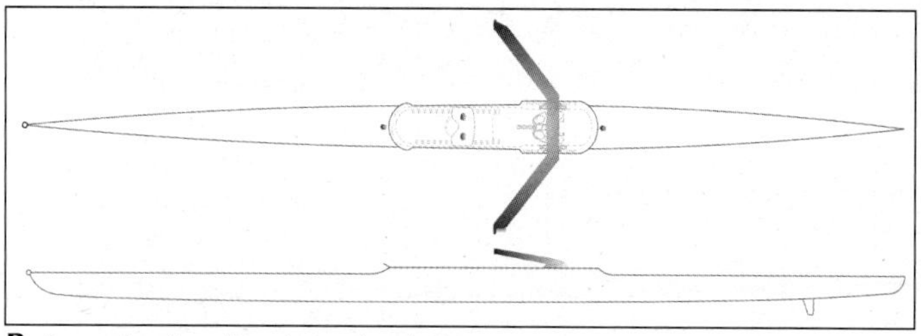

B. Example of sculling boat: the single.

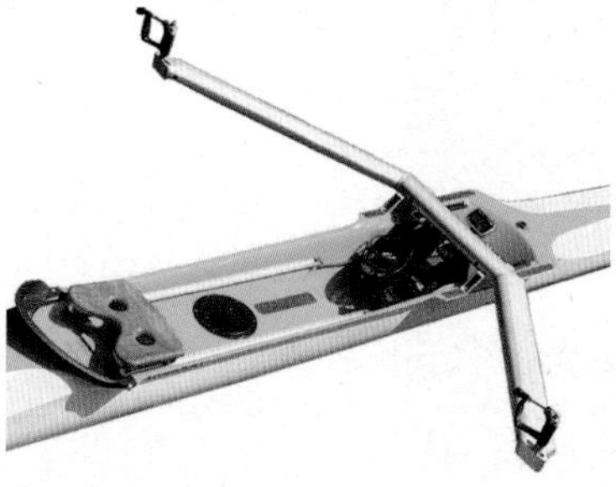

C. Inside of rowing shell.

Figure 85.2 Types of rowing boats. (Photographs © Dr. Volker Nolte.)

to spinal nerve impingement, causing radicular symptoms (pain or numbness radiating into legs) (Fig. 85.4A and B). However, initial symptoms may be limited to centralized back pain.

- **Spondylolysis:** Generally observed in young rowers, likely caused by repetitive axial loading of pars interarticularis; weight training rather than rowing induced all cases of spondylolysis seen in a group of rowers. If spondylolysis exists bilaterally at a particular level of the spine, spondylolisthesis can result (see Fig. 85.4C).

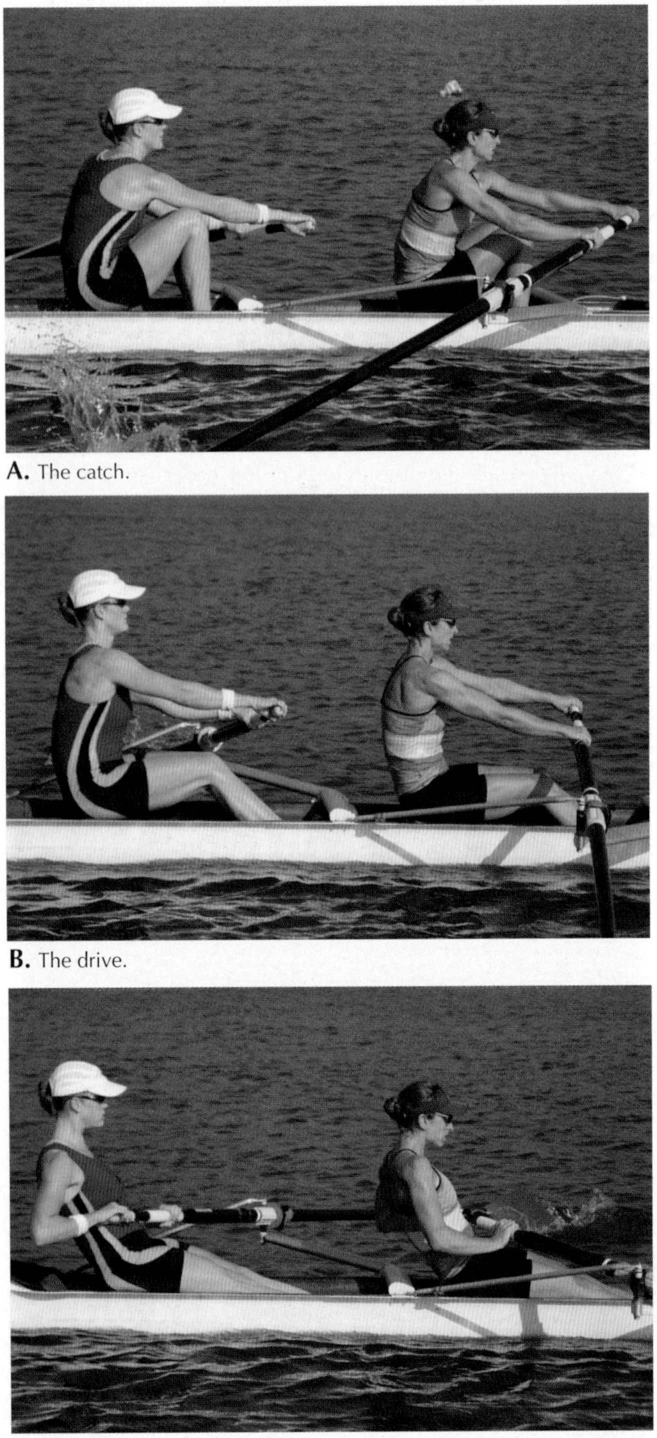

A. The catch.

B. The drive.

C. The release.

Figure 85.3 Phases of rowing stroke. (Photographs © Dr. Volker Nolte.)

History: Usually insidious onset during periods of high-volume or high-intensity training; pain may be localized to one region, and radicular symptoms may be present. If pain worsens with flexion and extending from the flexed position, suspect muscle origin and disc pathology; pain worsening with extension may indicate facet joint capsule strain, spondylolysis, or spondylolisthesis. In older rowers, pain may result from degenerative (bony/facet) changes.

Physical examination: Observe range of motion, reflexes, distal motor and sensory nerve function. Special addition: standing single-leg back extension for spondylolysis (worse back pain on side of standing leg indicates the side of spondylolysis); with spondylolisthesis, a "step" deformity may be visible or palpable; straight-leg raise, sitting root, and neural tension tests for discogenic and herniation problems.

Diagnostics: If indicated, begin with plain radiographs. Oblique views have been dropped because of high doses of radiation and minimal increase in sensitivity. The gold standard of a nuclear medicine single-photon emission computed tomography (SPECT) scan combined with limited-view computed tomography (CT) scan when SPECT scan is positive may also identify other causes of low back pain. Because the majority of these injuries occur in younger rowers, magnetic resonance imaging (MRI) is increasingly used in the diagnosis of this condition to avoid ionizing radiation. In young athletes with bilateral pars defects or spondylolisthesis, consider routine standing lateral radiographs every 6–12 months until skeletal maturity is reached to monitor for slip progression. If disc herniation suspected, proceed to MRI.

Treatment: Exercise therapy reduces pain and improves function in athletes with low back pain, which may incorporate dynamic "core stabilization" exercises. Activity and biomechanical modifications, manual therapy, and cortisone injections alone may be considered but require more evidence. Support gradual return to sport. Disc herniation infrequently requires surgical intervention, although outcomes are similar. Spondylolysis usually requires extended periods off from training (e.g., a full season). Spondylolisthesis infrequently requires surgical fixation (see Fig. 85.4D).

Technical changes: Analyze trunk movement, particularly lumbopelvic motion. Lumbar flexion and extension should be accompanied by hip range of motion; maintaining more neutral spine during stroke may help. Although equipment adjustments can lessen load per stroke, this may be unrealistic during racing season. Rigging changes may affect entire boat, affecting speed. However, lowering the load setting on the ergometer during indoor season is recommended and simple to perform. Address imbalances: low hamstring-to-quadriceps strength ratio, strength asymmetries between right and left erector spinae, and hip muscle imbalances in females. Emphasize appropriate breathing patterns: expiring through the drive phase may offset high levels of shear force and compression.

Chest Wall

Mechanism of injury: Broad differential as rowers use their upper bodies to apply force, provide stability, and breathe. Factors include weakness of surrounding musculature, specific rib architecture (angulation, diameter, etc.) and bone health, joint stiffness, and repetitive strain. Serratus anterior and external obliques historically implicated; more recently thought to be repetitive stress from external obliques and rectus abdominis (Fig. 85.5).

Types of injury:

- **Rib stress injury/fracture:** Increased incidence associated with introduction of more efficient blade design in 1992; occurs in 8.1%–16.4% of elite rowers, 2% of university rowers, and 1% of junior elite rowers; higher incidence in elite, heavyweight, and female rowers; most common in anterolateral/lateral aspects of ribs 5–9; equal incidence between

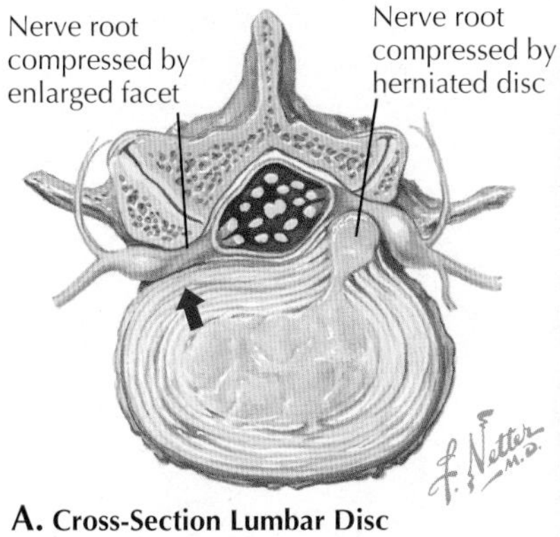
Nerve root compressed by enlarged facet
Nerve root compressed by herniated disc

A. **Cross-Section Lumbar Disc**
Pain sensation occurs in radicular pattern specific to distribution of a particular nerve root.

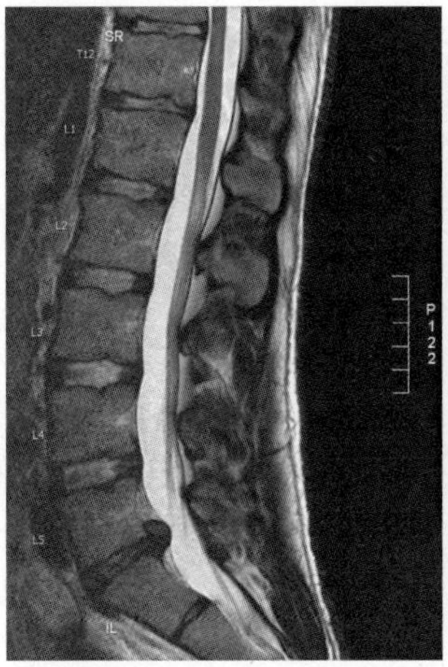

B. Disc herniation
(Courtesy of Grant James.)

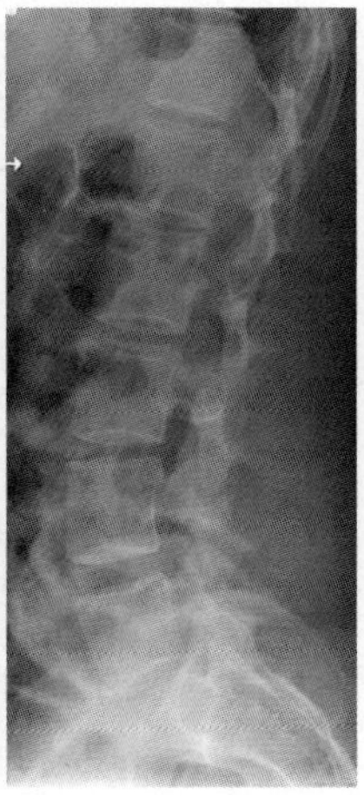

C. L4 bilateral spondylolysis (without spondylolisthesis)
(Courtesy of C. Lebrun.)

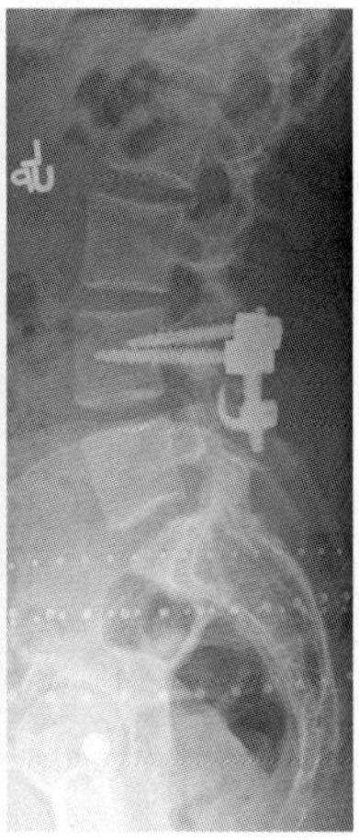

D. Spine fixation
(Courtesy of C. Lebrun.)

Figure 85.4 Low back injuries.

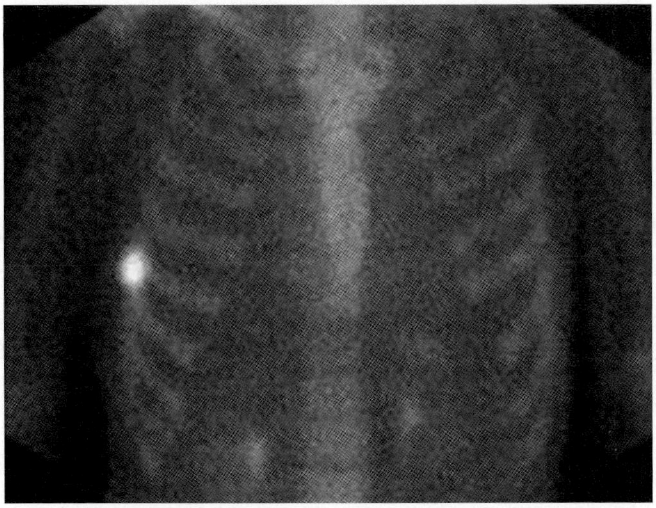

RSF bone scan (Courtesy of C. Lebrun.)

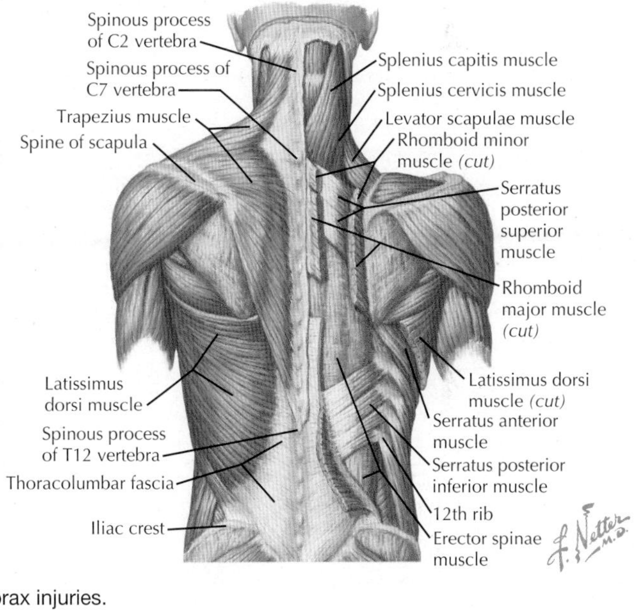
Spinous process of C2 vertebra
Spinous process of C7 vertebra
Trapezius muscle
Spine of scapula
Splenius capitis muscle
Splenius cervicis muscle
Levator scapulae muscle
Rhomboid minor muscle (cut)
Serratus posterior superior muscle
Rhomboid major muscle (cut)
Latissimus dorsi muscle
Spinous process of T12 vertebra
Thoracolumbar fascia
Iliac crest
Latissimus dorsi muscle (cut)
Serratus anterior muscle
Serratus posterior inferior muscle
12th rib
Erector spinae muscle

Figure 85.5 Thorax injuries.

sweepers and scullers, although location differs. Para-rowers (PR1 and PR2) may be at an increased risk because of compression of ribs from chest strapping that is used to secure athlete to boat.

- **Costochondritis:** Poorly understood condition, although most likely to occur during sweep rowing because of excessive rotation or altered thoracic spine and rib mobility.
- **Intercostal, rhomboid, and serratus anterior muscle strain:** Often confused with rib stress fracture at initial presentation; case study of complete avulsion injury of serratus anterior.

History: Usually insidious onset with generalized chest wall pain; worse with rowing, reaching, rolling over in bed. Over time, pain associated with stress fracture becomes more localized to a specific rib. Costochondritis will exhibit pain and tenderness on costochondral or costosternal joints without swelling. Muscle strain exhibits nonspecific tenderness on palpation.

Physical examination: Stress fracture: pain localized over rib; most commonly anterolateral ribs 5–9 but can be posterior; worse with rib compression. Athletes may have palpable rib callus. Costochondritis: adduction of arm on affected side and rotation of head toward affected side will reproduce pain.

Diagnostics: Important to exclude stress fracture; plain radiographs may detect callus formation (occurs late). Bone scan was the gold standard for timely diagnosis and management (see Fig. 85.5), recently, ultrasound and MRI have shown promise.

Treatment: For stress fractures: offload rib, initiate pain-free cross-training, analgesia for comfort (avoidance of nonsteroidal antiinflammatory drugs [NSAIDs]), taping for comfort and/or manual therapy, relative rest (3–6 weeks), with gradual return to sport; rowers should be evaluated for low calcium, vitamin D, disordered eating, relative energy deficiency in sport (RED-S), and hormonal disturbances such as oligomenorrhea/amenorrhea or low testosterone that can lead to decreased bone density and higher rate of fracture. Costochondritis: thought to be self-limiting; continue athletic participation as symptoms allow. Muscle strain: often rower is able to return to sport earlier, even with lingering pain (not indicated for stress fractures).

Technical changes: Address muscular or mobility imbalances in specific regions. Rowing on dynamic ergometers or with decreased load may reduce risk of overuse injury without compromising training efficiency and rowing performance. For para-rowers, adjustment of strapping may help, although this may be limited by rules and regulations.

Shoulder

Mechanism of injury: At catch, scapula is retracted and humerus is elevated to transfer forces from oar to legs and back. Most common pathology is a combination of anteriorly placed glenohumeral head, tight posterior capsule, tight latissimus dorsi, and weak rotator cuff muscles. Common technical error is to activate upper trapezius at catch instead of engaging mid-to-lower trapezius and latissimus dorsi, particularly in scullers; usually exaggerated in outside (farthest from blade) shoulder in sweep rowers.

Types of injury:
- **Rotator cuff tendinosis:** Overuse injury related to technical error and/or muscle strength imbalance.
- **Capsular instability:** May be exaggerated by reaching too far forward at catch or not extending fully at finish through the upper back.
- **Clavicular stress fracture:** Case report of lightweight rower with sudden resumption of training; uncommon but highlights the need to consider surrounding structures of shoulder girdle in differential diagnosis.

Physical examination: On physical examination, there will be localized tenderness over affected structures or muscle insertion (most commonly supraspinatus and/or biceps).

Diagnostics: Plain radiographs, diagnostic ultrasound, and/or MRI may be used to show affected structures and to help direct treatment.

Treatment: Rehabilitation should focus on stretching tight posterior capsule and correcting posture and muscle imbalance, with special attention to scapular stability. Surgical correction may be indicated in severe cases.

Technical changes: Limit overreaching at catch, and ensure linear motion of shoulder girdle through the entire drive.

Knee and Hip

Mechanism of injury: Inappropriate foot and knee alignment during each stroke cycle can lead to overuse injury and pain in knee and hip regions. Underdeveloped vastus medialis muscles in rowers may cause patellar tracking problems.

Types of injury:
- **Patellofemoral pain:** Two primary factors to consider: overcompression at catch, straining surrounding structures of flexed knee, and tendency of knees to slightly buckle or pop up at finish. If athletes cannot fully extend at finish, normal function of vastus medialis cannot occur; three remaining quadriceps muscles will cause lateral tracking of the patella. Certain females may be predisposed to patellofemoral pain because of wider pelvis (Fig. 85.6).
- **Iliotibial band (ITB) friction syndrome:** Compression at catch combined with varus knee alignment may cause friction and ensuing pain as iliotibial tract slides over lateral condylar prominence of the knee. Rowers who run for cross-training may encounter similar problems.
- **Labral tears:** May be caused by repetitive hip hyperflexion (± internal rotation) or underlying femoroacetabular impingement (FAI)—seen in young rowers—may be career-ending.

History: Patellofemoral: dull generalized pain in retropatellar area, worse on stairs or prolonged bent-knee position (positive "theater sign"); ITB: pain over lateral knee.

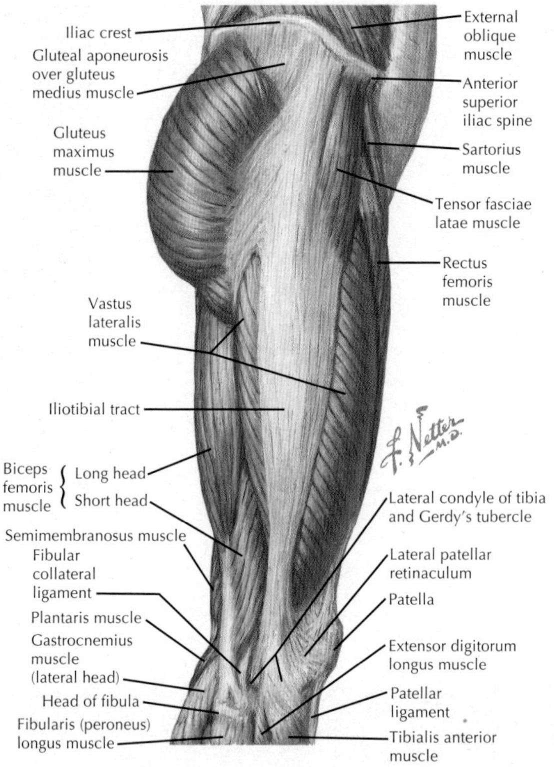

Iliac crest
Gluteal aponeurosis over gluteus medius muscle
Gluteus maximus muscle
Vastus lateralis muscle
Iliotibial tract
Biceps femoris muscle
Long head
Short head
Semimembranosus muscle
Fibular collateral ligament
Plantaris muscle
Gastrocnemius muscle (lateral head)
Head of fibula
Fibularis (peroneus) longus muscle
External oblique muscle
Anterior superior iliac spine
Sartorius muscle
Tensor fasciae latae muscle
Rectus femoris muscle
Lateral condyle of tibia and Gerdy's tubercle
Lateral patellar retinaculum
Patella
Extensor digitorum longus muscle
Patellar ligament
Tibialis anterior muscle
F. Netter M.D.

Figure 85.6 Knee and hip injuries.

Physical examination: Check for lateral tracking with bent knee, malalignment such as genu valgum or genu recurvatum, excessive pronation, or internal tibial and/or femoral torsion. ITB symptoms should prompt examination of possible leg-length discrepancy or pelvic malalignment.

Diagnostics: None indicated for patellofemoral pain, but large knee effusion or significant locking or catching may suggest meniscal or other knee pathologies. Plain radiographs, ultrasound, MRI may be required. MRI arthrograms will show hip labral tears best.

Treatment: Patellar taping to prevent maltracking useful in short term. Strengthening of vastus medialis and gluteus medius muscles; bracing not advised because of range-of-motion limitation; FAI and labral tears generally managed nonoperatively; however, symptoms may return if the aggravating activity is restarted. Surgical results for FAI (usually arthroscopic) vary from 70% to 96% success rate in higher-level athletes; positive (at least short-term) effect of intra-articular cortisone injection in elite rowers.

Technical changes: Modify shoe position (angle, distance between toes and heels, and height) or addition of heel wedges; wide foot placement may compound problems; modify position of tracks to ensure full knee extension at stroke finish.

Wrist and Forearm

Mechanism of injury: Relatively common, usually from excessive wrist motion during feathering/squaring actions, excessively tight grip of handle in rough water conditions or with inexperienced rowers; other factors: wrongly sized/slippery grips, poor rigging, and fatigue.

Types of injury:
- **Exertional compartment syndrome:** Often volar compartment, overuse injury that may occur because of repetitive and inappropriate initiation of pull-through with elbow instead of shoulder girdle at catch, or inability to relax forearm grip at release.

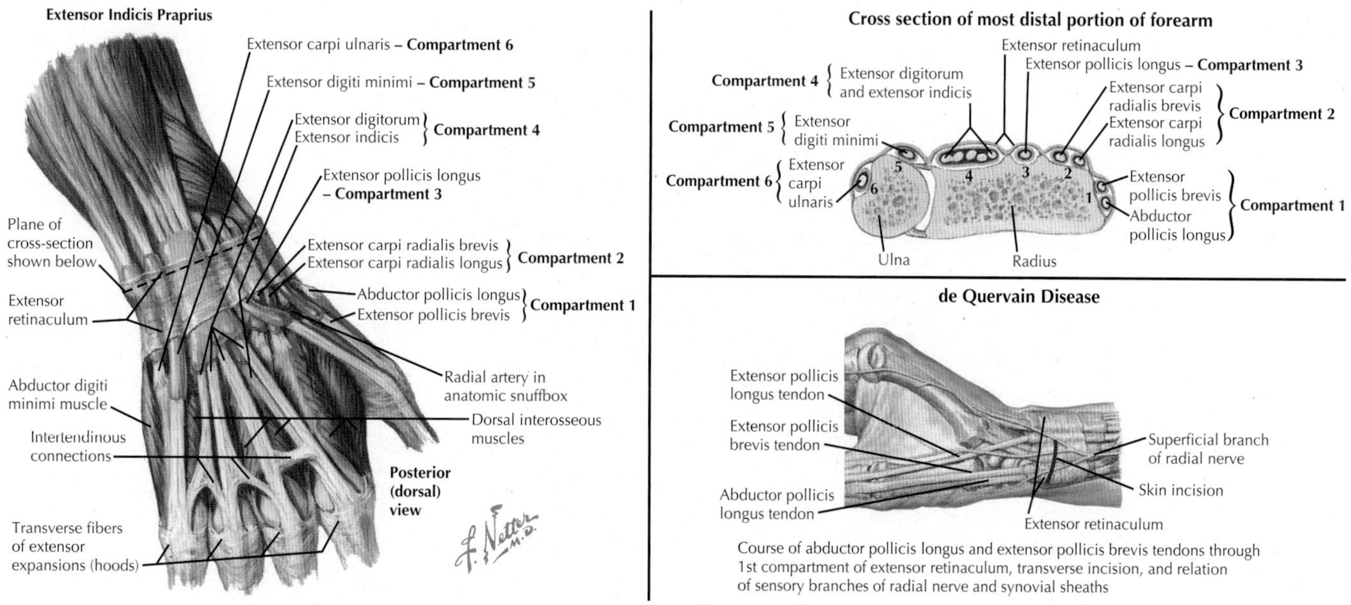
Extensor Indicis Praprius
Extensor carpi ulnaris – Compartment 6
Extensor digiti minimi – Compartment 5
Extensor digitorum
Extensor indicis
Compartment 4
Extensor pollicis longus – Compartment 3
Plane of cross-section shown below
Extensor carpi radialis brevis
Extensor carpi radialis longus
Compartment 2
Extensor retinaculum
Abductor pollicis longus
Extensor pollicis brevis
Compartment 1
Radial artery in anatomic snuffbox
Abductor digiti minimi muscle
Dorsal interosseous muscles
Intertendinous connections
Posterior (dorsal) view
Transverse fibers of extensor expansions (hoods)
Cross section of most distal portion of forearm
Extensor retinaculum
Extensor pollicis longus – Compartment 3
Compartment 4
Extensor digitorum and extensor indicis
Extensor carpi radialis brevis
Extensor carpi radialis longus
Compartment 2
Compartment 5
Extensor digiti minimi
Compartment 6
Extensor carpi ulnaris
Extensor pollicis brevis
Abductor pollicis longus
Compartment 1
Ulna
Radius
de Quervain Disease
Extensor pollicis longus tendon
Extensor pollicis brevis tendon
Superficial branch of radial nerve
Skin incision
Abductor pollicis longus tendon
Extensor retinaculum
Course of abductor pollicis longus and extensor pollicis brevis tendons through 1st compartment of extensor retinaculum, transverse incision, and relation of sensory branches of radial nerve and synovial sheaths

Figure 85.7 Wrist and forearm injuries.

- **Lateral epicondylitis:** May occur because of same factors; characterized by pain over lateral aspect of elbow and with resisted wrist extension.
- **De Quervain tenosynovitis and intersection syndrome:** Tenosynovitis of first and second dorsal compartments, respectively; intersection syndrome, often misdiagnosed as de Quervain, is also referred to as "oarsmen's wrist" (Fig. 85.7).
- **Tenosynovitis of wrist extensors or "sculler's thumb":** Swelling over dorsal aspect of forearm, caused by hypertrophy of abductor pollicis longus and extensor pollicis brevis muscle bellies; may be the result of inappropriate use of thumb to feather oar at finish or by allowing palm to slide down handle while keeping thumb rigid against handle end.
- **Carpal tunnel syndrome:** Pain over wrist and distal median nerve paresthesias; positive Tinel and Phalen signs; evidence of thenar eminence wasting in severe cases.

History: Pain in wrist or forearm region, particularly when rowing at high stroke rates or in cold or bad weather conditions; often, pain will lead to inability to appropriately feather or square and feeling of burning or swelling.

Physical examination and treatment: Pain and tenderness over affected muscles, with additional discomfort on resisted muscle testing; diagnosis of exertional compartment syndrome may require examination for pain and compartment tightness (and measurement of compartment pressures) before and immediately after exercise because there may be few physical findings at rest. If feathering action causes pain, advise athlete to row "on the square" or on ergometer. Lateral epicondylitis diagnosed by ultrasound (rather than MRI); management may include use of counter-force brace such as tennis elbow strap on the forearm for forceful activities, use of wrist splint at night to rest muscles and tendons, and specific physiotherapy and stretching. Corticosteroid injection only when conservative treatment fails; steroid injection (0.5–1 mL) into tendon sheath (for tenosynovitis) with return to rowing in 3 days; surgical intervention required only in more severe cases (i.e., fasciotomy for exertional compartment syndrome); early surgical intervention may provide benefit to elite rowers with intersection syndrome. Corticosteroid injections have been used into insertion of wrist extensors onto lateral epicondyle (for lateral epicondylitis), but repeated steroid injections into this area can cause atrophy of skin and subcutaneous fat. More recently, injection of orthobiologics such as platelet-rich plasma (PRP) have been used.

Technical changes: Encourage relaxed grip without excessive wrist motion. Ensure appropriate grip size/material. Advise the use of pogies (fleece or similar material coverings for hands and oar handle) in cold weather.

Sciatic Nerve Compression

Mechanism of injury: In general, rowers' seats are made of wood or carbon fiber specifically molded to accommodate ischial tuberosities; however, mold is usually generic and may not fit a particular rower's pelvic width, leading to constant compression of sciatic nerve. Different seat sizes are now available.

History: Numbness radiating down legs, only when rowing, without back pain or leg weakness.

Physical examination: As a standard, rule out radiculopathy, disc disease, and piriformis syndrome (compression of sciatic nerve by tight piriformis muscle) (Fig. 85.8).

Technical change: Change seats or use seat pads. Elevate or lower shoes in boat.

Hand Blisters and Skin Abrasions

Mechanism of injury: Most severe upon resumption of on-water training; blisters and abrasions can occur at any of the three points of contact: hands/oar, buttocks/seat, and feet/shoes; imperative to prevent secondary infection or scarring.

Types of injury:

- **Hand blisters:** Found on the anterior aspect of fingers and palm; caused by repetitive friction between skin and oar handle; usually only painful when rower resumes on-water training, but can be affected by heat, humidity, and change in grip size or material; may lead to infection (Fig. 85.9A).
- **Sculler's knuckles:** Superficial abrasions on dorsal aspect of right hand, caused by crossover of port and starboard handles mid-drive or mid-recovery; can cause significant bleeding and pain while rowing (see Fig. 85.9B).
- **Track bites:** Superficial abrasions on posterior aspect of lower legs, caused by tracks for sliding seat digging into calf muscles; can lead to scarring (see Fig. 85.9C).

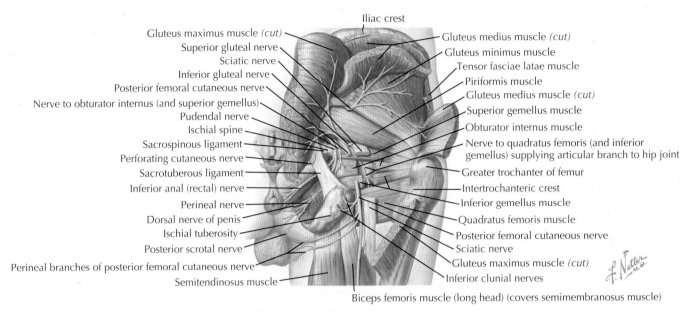

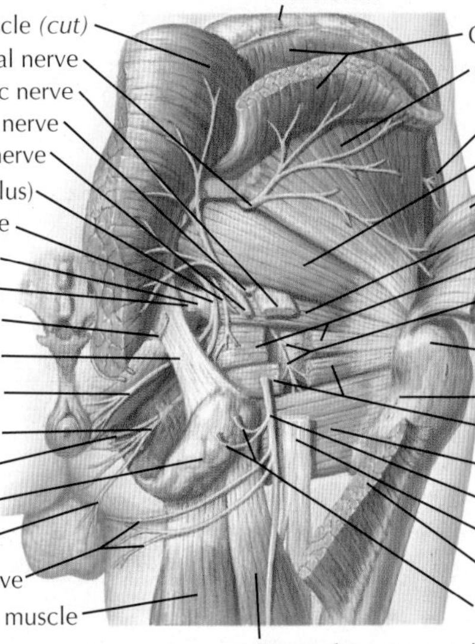
Iliac crest
Gluteus maximus muscle (cut)
Superior gluteal nerve
Sciatic nerve
Inferior gluteal nerve
Posterior femoral cutaneous nerve
Nerve to obturator internus (and superior gemellus)
Pudendal nerve
Ischial spine
Sacrospinous ligament
Perforating cutaneous nerve
Sacrotuberous ligament
Inferior anal (rectal) nerve
Perineal nerve
Dorsal nerve of penis
Ischial tuberosity
Posterior scrotal nerve
Perineal branches of posterior femoral cutaneous nerve
Semitendinosus muscle
Gluteus medius muscle (cut)
Gluteus minimus muscle
Tensor fasciae latae muscle
Piriformis muscle
Gluteus medius muscle (cut)
Superior gemellus muscle
Obturator internus muscle
Nerve to quadratus femoris (and inferior gemellus) supplying articular branch to hip joint
Greater trochanter of femur
Intertrochanteric crest
Inferior gemellus muscle
Quadratus femoris muscle
Posterior femoral cutaneous nerve
Sciatic nerve
Gluteus maximus muscle (cut)
Inferior clunial nerves
Biceps femoris muscle (long head) (covers semimembranosus muscle)

Figure 85.8 Sciatic nerve compression.

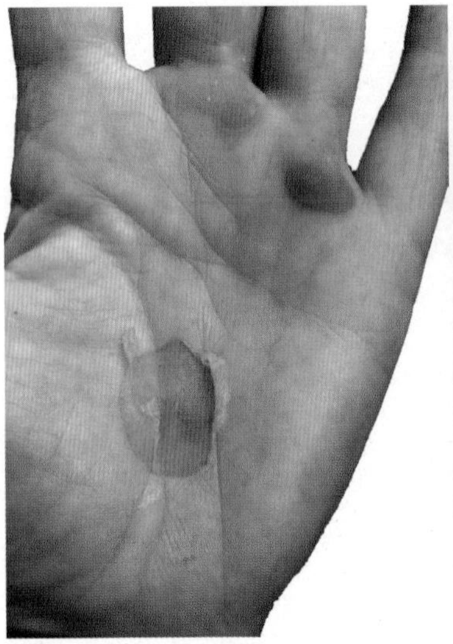

A. Blisters.

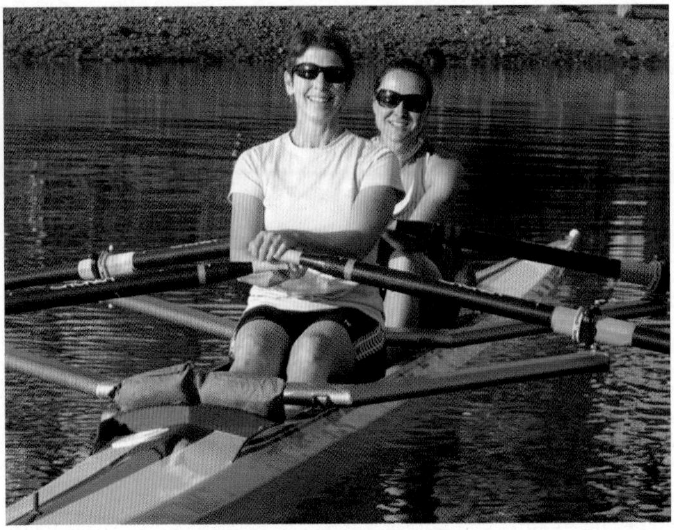

B. Crossover in sculling. (Courtesy of C. Lebrun.)

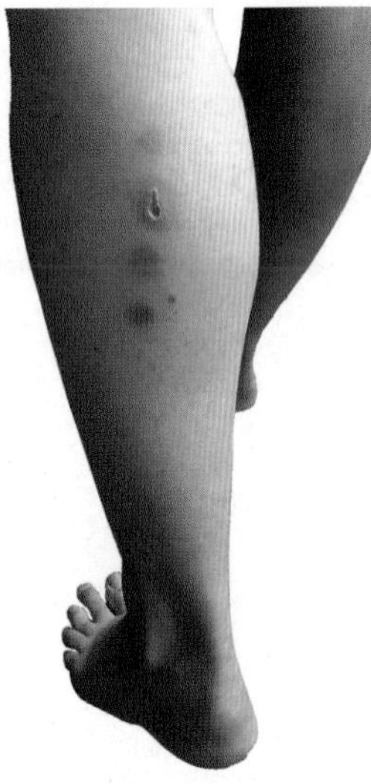

C. Track bites. (Courtesy of C. Lebrun.)

Figure 85.9 Hand blisters and skin abrasions.

- **Rower's rump:** Term coined for rowing-associated lichen simplex chronicus; uncommon, but several rowers have had superficial abrasions on buttocks, ranging from slight indentations to skin ulcerations, secondary to repetitive chafing caused by inappropriately fitted seats.

History: Recent resumption of on-water training, increase in training volume, or sudden shift in weather or equipment (sweep to sculling or grip change).

Physical examination and treatment: Monitor closely for signs of secondary infection (erythema, fever, and red streaking along lymphatic drainage route) and use of topical and/or oral antibiotics if appropriate.

Technical changes:

- **Hand blisters:** Change grip material and/or size of handles; several manufacturers offer a variety of grip material (wood, hard plastic, foam, etc.); in most cases, some blistering is unavoidable. Ensure scrubbing of oar handles after each use if shared among crew. Case study of spread of hand warts caused by oar sharing.
- **Track bites:** Use circumferential tape; consider moving tracks wider or toward bow of boat if possible.
- **Sculler's knuckles:** Oarlock height can be modified to increase gap between port and starboard oar handles. Circumferential tape may help for short term; extended use of gloves not advised because they may compromise proprioceptive feedback.
- **Rower's rump:** Regular application of corticosteroids in severe cases; in most cases, change seats or use seat pads.

Energy Availability, Body Composition Issues, and Disordered Eating

- Rowers, particularly lightweights and coxswains, may restrict calorie intake to the point of disordered eating; may be inadvertent.
- In females, resultant inadequate energy intake for energy needs can lead to menstrual dysfunction and altered bone mineral density (previously described as female athlete triad).

- Underlying cause is overall energy imbalance—termed RED-S: this condition can also affect males and their reproductive hormones.
- May result in lowered bone density and other musculoskeletal, cardiovascular, gastrointestinal, and electrolyte abnormalities, affecting performance in both female and male rowers.
- Prevent through education, awareness, nutritional counseling, gradual weight loss, and appropriate selection of athlete's natural weight.
- Need for healthcare professionals to be aware of energy imbalance/deficiency, disordered eating behaviors, menstrual dysfunction, and other hormonal abnormalities and potential for altered bone mineral density.
- Need for education of athletes, coaches, parents, etc., about health risks of these conditions.

ENVIRONMENTAL EXPOSURE AND SAFETY CONSIDERATIONS

Personnel: Coaches should always accompany or be in sight of rowing shells, with appropriate numbers of personal flotation devices (PFDs) and communication devices to call for outside help. Collisions may occur because of rowers facing backward and not checking course enough. Rowers should be advised never to attempt to swim away from swamped shell (even if shore is close by). If rescue is not imminent, rowers should attempt to get as much of their bodies on top of overturned shell to reduce heat loss.

Storms and wind conditions: High winds and choppy water can lead to swamping of boats because rowing shells sit very low in water. No boating should be attempted during thunderstorms.

Sun exposure: Athletes and coaches should wear water-/sweat-proof sunscreen, sunglasses, and hats during prolonged sun exposure.

Cold exposure: Rowers should dress in layers of synthetic clothing, avoid splashing with oars, and wear fleece pogies and hats.

Water conditions: Whitecaps signify high winds and should be avoided. For rowers who train on rivers, currents and eddies may be dangerous, particularly during flood conditions.

RECOMMENDED READINGS

Available online.

86 MARTIAL ARTS

Ian D. McKeag • Robert Virgil Masocol • Irfan Asif

INTRODUCTION

- Martial arts are bodies of codified practices or traditions of training for unarmed and armed combat, usually without the use of guns and other modern weapons.
- People study martial arts for various reasons, including improved fitness, self-realization (meditation), mental/character development, and self-defense.

EPIDEMIOLOGY

- There are over 140 martial arts styles practiced worldwide.
- Participants
  - Approximately 2–8 million participants in the United States
  - The male-to-female ratio is 5:1.
  - Judo, karate, and tae kwon do are now Olympic sports, which has increased the worldwide popularity of each sport.
- Injuries
  - Approximately 76,000 annual emergency department visits related to combat sports from individuals ages 5–24 years old between 2010 and 2016.
  - The actual incidence of injuries remains unknown because of a lack of reporting of injuries and lack of studies regarding the sport. However, it is thought to be low compared with other sports because most of the instructions and training are noncompetitive and noncontact.
- Fatalities
  - Catastrophic injuries and even deaths have occurred from participation in martial arts. Most catastrophic injuries involve massive direct trauma or fall with contact to the head or neck leading to an intracranial hemorrhage or a high cervical spine lesion.

FACTORS AFFECTING INCIDENCE AND PREVALENCE OF INJURY

Form of Participation in the Martial Arts

- Many participants train several times per week, year round, without a natural break in training for rehabilitation/recovery.
- Emphasis of training is often on personal development, both physical and mental, and not on competition.
- Muscle mass and strength are typically not as important as speed, strategy, technique, mental discipline, and flexibility.
- Individuals of different levels of training may "spar" (i.e., engage in practice competition with another individual to simulate competition or a bout) in practice, exploiting the mismatch in skill levels between participants.
- Incidence of injury is directly related to the amount of time spent in full-contact sparring, limited-contact sparring, or competition.
- A competition setting may also influence the injury rate and severity.
- Martial art style: tae kwon do has more severe injuries and greater incidence of multiple injuries than other disciplines. Three times injury rate and fourfold risk of multiple injuries compared with Shotokan karate
- Types of martial arts training include:
  - Kata—detailed choreographed patterns of movements/techniques used by practitioners to practice on their own
  - Basic hand strikes
  - Basic kicking
  - Strength training
  - Conditioning
  - Stretching
  - Flexibility
  - Breaking—using striking techniques to break boards or bricks
  - One-step sparring—noncontact sparring to practice techniques used during free sparring or competition
  - Grappling
  - Ground fighting
  - Joint locks—grappling technique involving manipulation of opponent's joint in such a way that the joint reaches a maximal degree of motion in order to induce submission or to injure opponent
  - Chokes—employed via various mechanisms using upper or lower extremities to temporarily disrupt vascular supply to brain or to compress trachea to prevent breathing
  - Free sparring—to engage in practice competition with another individual to simulate competition or bout
  - Point-scoring competition
  - Full-contact competition

Protective Equipment

Mouth guard: Risk of orofacial injury is 1.6–1.8 times greater when mouth guards are not worn. Use does not reduce the risk of concussion. Not widely used in martial arts.

Headgear: May reduce peak acceleration forces to the head; different brands have varying safety profiles (Fig. 86.1)

Hand and foot protection: Hand protection (as used in tae kwon do) and foot-padding gear have not been shown to reduce peak acceleration; combination of headgear and hand/foot protection superior to either used alone (see Fig. 86.1). Padding may lead to decreased inhibition and poorer control of striking, which may lead to greater number of blows with larger amount of force. Hand and foot padding are thought to decrease amount of superficial injuries, such as lacerations and abrasions, to both attacker and defender. Equipment varies with different martial arts.

Padded flooring: Padded flooring may reduce the intensity of a blow by absorbing some of the impact of falls and throws (see Fig. 86.1). The surface must be closely monitored for risk factors for fall, such as moisture (e.g., water, blood, or perspiration) or gaps between pads. Mat pads are common reservoirs for fungi and bacteria and therefore must be cared for in a similar manner to wrestling mats in order to prevent the spread of infections (e.g., community-acquired methicillin-resistant *Staphylococcus aureus*, herpes simplex virus, or tinea corporis).

Age

- Age is not a reliable predictor of the likelihood of injury, although one study reported decreased incidence of injury in adolescent karate practitioners during elite competitions.

Experience

- Experience and number of hours of participation appear to be associated with higher rates and severity of injury.
- A previous study reported a greater incidence of head injuries and fractures in professional Muay Thai kickboxers when comparing amateurs with beginners.
- Individuals with at least 3 years of experience were at twice the risk of injury than less experienced individuals.
- The number of tournaments and months of practice are directly and significantly associated with the likelihood of injury.

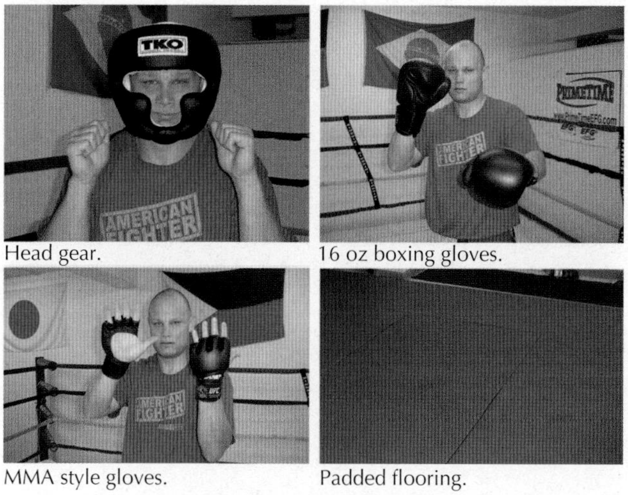
Head gear.
16 oz boxing gloves.
MMA style gloves.
Padded flooring.

Figure 86.1 Protective equipment.

Setting

- Tournament and competitive situations are associated with a lower absolute number of injuries but higher rate of severity. One study showed an injury rate six times higher during competition in tae kwan do compared with noncompetitive situations.
- Informal training sessions are associated with higher risk and severity of injuries compared with more formal supervised instructions.

Sex

- Males have higher rates and severity of injuries compared with females, probably related to increased aggressiveness, except in karate, where females have a higher injury rate than do males. However, with higher levels of competition, the discrepancy between the two sexes became insignificant.

Weight Class

- In competition, governing bodies of martial arts have established weight classes. Physicians must be aware of their athletes that are attempting to make different weight classes and provide appropriate counseling for weight maintenance.
- Muay Thai kickboxing participants who compete at a heavier weight are at a higher risk of injury.

Prevention

- American Academy of Orthopedic Surgeons (AAOS) tips for martial arts participants to safely train and compete:
  - Consult with a physician before beginning conditioning to establish readiness.
  - Train under the direction of an instructor who focuses on form and technique rather than competitive strategy.
  - Wear activity-appropriate protective gear (e.g., tae kwon do, a full-contact sport, requires head guard, body protector, forearm and shin guards, and groin guard).
  - Exercises that strengthen rotator cuff muscles and hip adductors/abductors are critical to martial arts for injury prevention, balance, and improved striking ability.
  - Maintain appropriate breathing techniques when practicing martial arts to avoid injury—breathing out during the contraction portion of any stretching movement, and breathing in during the extension portion of any stretching movement.

Coverage of Martial Arts Events

- General
  - Attending physician must be present when the rules of the competition are reviewed.
  - Important to identify yourself and briefly review certain medical considerations
- Prefight examinations
  - Perform in a quiet, well-lit environment.
  - Enquire about previous and/or recent concussions and "knockouts."
- Match stoppage
  - Typically by referee; however, the referee may consult with physician for medical guidance regarding whether match should continue
  - Interventions required for lacerations and bleeding
- Cervical spine injuries
  - Often teammates or coaches will want to attend to their fighter and may inappropriately move a fighter with an unstable cervical neck injury
  - Review rationale and need for appropriate cervical spine immobilization with all the participants and their teams
- Postfight examinations
  - After a loss or a knockout, the participant may be confused, belligerent, or emotional.
  - Important to maintain control of the situation to complete an appropriate examination.
- Medical kit suggestions: disposable gloves, gauze, silver nitrate, bandages, suture kits, sling, athletic tape, Coban, nonsteroidal antiinflammatory drugs (NSAIDs), cold/flu/allergy medication, antidiarrheal medication, shears, petroleum jelly, nasal plugs, otoscope/ophthalmoscope, tooth saver solution, syringes, needles, lidocaine with/without epinephrine, alcohol swabs, betadine, contact and eye wash solution, splinting material, oral airway, cervical collar, EpiPen, and albuterol

Martial Arts–Specific Injury Considerations

- It is critically important to understand unique aspects of each martial art discipline in order to best predict potential injuries.
- Certain martial arts disciplines focus more on contact and sparring, whereas others focus more on technique.
- When covering a competition or evaluating a martial artist, familiarize yourself with the techniques, emphasis, equipment, scoring, and target areas of each discipline in order to anticipate various possible injuries.

COMMON TECHNIQUES IN MARTIAL ARTS

Hand Strikes

Punching: Striking an opponent with closed fist (Fig. 86.2). Appropriate punching technique places wrist in slight volar flexion, with second and third metacarpals aligned with the forearm long bones. Contact is made with second and third metacarpal heads. A "boxer's fracture" of the fifth metacarpal typically results from poor punching technique, where contact occurs with the fifth metacarpal head instead of second and third metacarpal heads. Common injuries from poor punching technique include phalanx fractures, fourth or fifth metacarpal fractures, wrist sprains, extensor tendon injuries, and first metacarpal phalangeal ulnar collateral sprains.

Knife hand chop ("karate chop"): A strike with an open hand during which contact is made with the ulnar aspect of the fifth metacarpal head

Ridge hand (reverse knife hand chop): A strike during which the thumb is tucked into the palm and contact is made with the radial aspect of the second metacarpal head

Spear thrust: Open hand technique during which contact is made with the fingertips of the second, third, and fourth fingers, most commonly targeting the eyes and throat

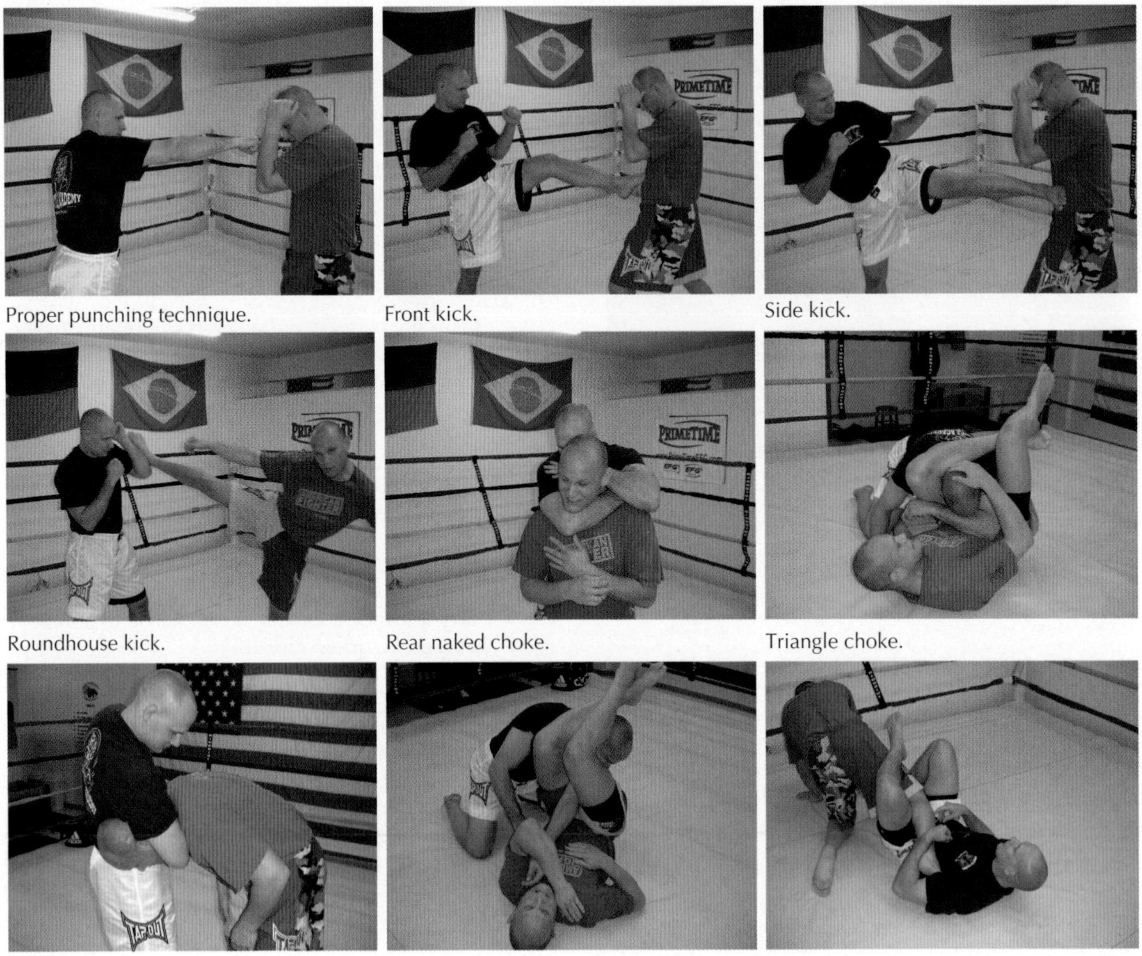

Proper punching technique. Front kick. Side kick.
Roundhouse kick. Rear naked choke. Triangle choke.
Guillotine choke. Arm bar. Leg lock.

Figure 86.2 Common techniques in martial arts.

Hammer fist: Closed-hand strike with the ulnar aspect of the fist

Spinning back fist: Attacker swivels 360 degrees and strikes opponent with dorsum of hand and second and third metacarpophalangeal (MCP) joints, employing great power and momentum.

Foot Strikes

Front snap kick: From a standing position, hip is flexed up to bring femur parallel to the floor (see Fig. 86.2). The leg is then extended, resulting in the ball of the foot making contact with defender's abdomen. If the target is the groin, the foot is plantarflexed and the point of contact is the dorsal aspect of the proximal first metatarsal. If the target is the face, the ankle is dorsiflexed and contact is made with the plantar aspect of the heel.

Side kick: Delivered sideways relative to the position of the person executing the kick; contact is made with the heel targeting the abdomen or face (see Fig. 86.2).

Back kick ("donkey kick," "mule kick," or "spinning back kick"): Kick is delivered backward, keeping kicking leg close to the standing leg and striking with the heel. Most often, it is delivered with a spinning motion generating great power.

Roundhouse kick: From a position with hip flexed up to 90 degrees, the attacker swings the lower leg up in a circular motion, striking with the dorsal aspect of the proximal first metatarsal (see Fig. 86.2).

Miscellaneous: Some martial arts disciplines encourage kicking with the shin instead of the ball of the foot or instep to reduce the likelihood of injury.

Chokeholds

Rear naked choke: Attacker approaches opponent from behind, wrapping arm around opponent's neck and then grasping the biceps of his or her other arm. Then, using free hand, the attacker forces the opponent's head into flexion, resulting in carotid artery compression, temporarily rendering opponent unconscious (see Fig. 86.2).

Triangle choke: Attacker is on his or her back (guard position) and wraps one leg around the neck and shoulder of the opponent with the knee next to the opponent's neck, the other leg crosses the ankle of the first leg, using the foot of the first leg to lock the second leg into position at the knee (see Fig. 86.2).

Guillotine choke: Applied from a standing position or the guard; the attacker faces the opponent and wraps an arm around opponent's neck so that the humerus is on the dorsal aspect of the neck and their forearm wraps around anteriorly to apply pressure to disrupt the vascular supply to the brain, temporarily rendering the opponent unconscious, or to compress the trachea in order to restrict breathing (see Fig. 86.2).

Joint Locks/Manipulation

Arm bar: A joint lock that hyperextends the elbow joint by placing the opponent's extended arm over a fulcrum such as an arm, leg, or hip (see Fig. 86.2). The opponent is controlled in this position, and if he or she does not tap out, continued force will result in dislocation of the elbow.

Leg lock: A joint lock that is directed at leg joints (i.e., knee or ankle). A kneebar is similar to armbar; it aims to forcefully hyperextend the opponent's knee (see Fig. 86.2).

Ankle lock: A submission applied to the opponent wherein the attacker uses the arm to secure opponent's ankle in his or her armpit. Once the ankle is secured, the attacker leverages his or her hip forward, which forcefully plantarflexes the ankle. The forearm serves as a fulcrum in leveraging and may cause severe pressure on the Achilles tendon.

Miscellaneous: Small joint manipulation is typically prohibited.

TYPES OF INJURIES

Contusions: Overall, the most common injury; orbital contusions can obstruct vision. Cold steel or ice can be employed between rounds to reduce edema.

Sprains/strains: Overall, second most common injury; commonly sprained joints include ankles and knees; hamstring and groin strains common from inappropriate stretching. Aikido has a higher incidence of sprains and strains than Shotokan karate.

Abrasions/lacerations: Laceration management: direct pressure, petroleum jelly, clotting agents such as silver nitrate or a vasoconstrictive agent; physician may only examine laceration during fight to determine whether the participant may continue and may not treat the laceration until after the round. Competition should be stopped if laceration bleeds to the extent that it will obstruct the vision of either competitor. Do not suture laceration until after the competition. Special attention may be warranted for suturing lip lacerations depending on lesion depth and whether the vermilion border is involved.

Epistaxis: Exceedingly rare to stop a competition for epistaxis. Direct pressure and petroleum jelly work well. Monitor for bleeding into either competitor's eyes such that it may obstruct vision. Careful examination to exclude septal hematoma or nasal fracture

Fractures: More common in experienced martial artists; finger and toe fractures common because of inappropriate kicking and striking techniques; rib fractures common from being kicked

Dislocations: Various digit dislocations can be immediately reduced with rapid return to competition. Postreduction radiography is recommended.

Mild traumatic brain injury (MTBI): Of severe injuries, concussion is the most common one. Increased rate of concussion in younger participants, in those who demonstrate poor blocking skills, and in association with receiving a kick to the head; decreased opportunities for head trauma in martial arts that emphasize grappling and joint locks over striking; individuals who regularly participate in full-contact sparring should consider baseline neurocognitive testing to aid future management of MTBI. Ringside physicians must always rule out more serious intracranial injuries. Proper return-to-play protocols should also be followed before return, to avoid prolonged or complicated recovery. Additional concussion guidelines are available through the Association of Ringside Physicians.

LOCATION OF INJURIES

Lower extremity: Common foot and ankle injuries are bruising, lacerations, ankle sprains, and digital fractures. Hamstring and adductor strains can occur secondary to overstretching or inappropriate stretching. A roundhouse kick is the most common type of kick to produce a lower extremity injury. In tae kwon do the foot instep is the most common location of lower extremity injury, with receiving or delivering a kick being the most common mechanisms of lower extremity injury.

Upper extremity:

- A unique injury with submission techniques is an arm bar. An arm bar hyperextends an already completely extended elbow, stretching the anterior capsule, and may result in complete rupture of the capsule and ligaments if continued force is applied and the participant does not tap out. If the elbow is rapidly extended, the capsule may tear and the elbow may dislocate. An arm bar may result in a humeral fracture, potentially causing damage to the radial nerve. Treatment of a simple arm bar with stretching of the capsule and anterior elbow pain consists of ice, NSAIDs, and a sling for comfort (be sure not to immobilize the joint to prevent stiffness). Complex arm bar injuries consisting of fractures and dislocations almost always require evaluation for cartilaginous, ligamentous, or nerve injury.
- Mixed martial arts (MMA) size gloves (4–6 ounces) are typically worn to prevent hand injuries to the individual wearing the gloves.
- Injuries that occur from striking or kicking rather than from being struck are typically caused by poor technique.

Head/neck: Increased frequency of head injuries in martial arts disciplines that emphasize striking and head contact; similarities in force, kinematics, and biomechanics that produce cervical neck injuries in motor vehicle accidents and common MMA maneuvers.

Dentofacial: Prevalence of dentofacial injuries (teeth, jaw, lips, zygomatic processes) was found to be ~30% throughout all combat sports via meta-analysis. Highest overall prevalence was seen in jiu-jitsu.

MARTIAL ARTS IN THE OLYMPIC GAMES

Judo ("Gentle Way")

- Country of origin and founder: Japan; Jigoro Kano
- Emphasis
  - Flexible or efficient use of balance, leverage, and movement in the performance of throws or techniques
  - Skill, timing, and techniques are emphasized over brute strength.
  - Soft method in which there is an indirect application of force applied to defeat an opponent
- Techniques
  - Throwing
    - Most throws are performed in a standing position.
    - Forceful throws are used in an attempt to render an opponent unconscious.
    - Increased points are given depending on the severity of the throw.
  - Strikes (kicks and punches) are practiced, but they are not permitted in competition.
  - Pinning
    - Attempt to hold an opponent to the mat
    - Pins of 25 seconds will win the match.
    - Pins of 10–25 seconds will score points.
    - Significant pressure is applied to the opponent with pain-generating techniques.
    - Certain body parts, particularly the ribs, are vulnerable for injury during these techniques.
  - Joint manipulation
    - Only elbow joint locks are permitted.
    - Leg locks, wrist locks, and spinal locks are not permitted.
  - Chokes (permitted depending on the age of the participants)
- Equipment: Judogi, "gi," traditional uniform, which is typically loose fitting and long sleeved, used in judo for practice and competition. Consists of two parts: a heavy fabric uwagi (jacket) and a lighter fabric zubon (pants).
- Medical coverage
  - Medical team not allowed on mat unless granted by referee; only one medical person on the mat
  - Bleeding: Same bleeding injury may be treated on two occasions. Third time of the same bleeding injury will be a medical disqualification

Tae Kwon Do ("The Way of the Feet and Fist")

- Country of origin and founder: Korea; unknown
- Emphasis
  - Kicking techniques are emphasized because the leg is the longest and strongest limb in the body and thus has the potential to deliver the most forceful blow, rendering one's opponent unable to retaliate.
  - Union of physical and mental strength in such techniques as breaking of boards
- Techniques
  - Hand techniques
    - Legal target areas: Front of the torso starting at the hipline and going up to the base of the throat from one side seam of the uniform to the other side seam
    - Legal hand techniques include typical punches and strikes.
    - Spinning back fists and finger strikes and other "blind techniques" are considered illegal.
  - Feet techniques
    - Legal target areas, front of torso as discussed earlier; the sides and back of the neck are legal, as are all areas of the head, including the face, mask, sides, and top.
    - Strikes only from below the ankle; no shin or knee striking.
    - Hand and standing-foot techniques to the legal torso area will score one point.
    - Standing kicks to head, face, and neck will score one point; jumping kick to body will score two points; jumping kick to head will score three points.
  - Breaking
    - Typically use hand or foot but may also use fingertip, toe, head, elbow, knuckle, or knee
    - It is postulated that the skeletal system, after being exposed to stress, will be stronger after it heals. Thus, many martial artists who practice breaking will continually stress their skeletal system and allow it to heal, allowing it to become stronger.
    - Many train to strengthen their fists by practicing bare knuckle push-ups, initially on a soft surface such as a carpet and then progressing to a harder surface such as concrete.
- Equipment
  - White American Tae Kwon Do (ATA) uniform
  - Headgear, mouthpiece, chest protector, and protective cup
  - Hand pads that cover the entire length of the fingers
  - Foot pads that cover the entire length of the toes
- Medical coverage
  - Medical director is appointed for international competitions
  - Team physician needs to get accreditation by attending the meeting before competition. Please see World Taekwondo Federation (WTF) medical code for further details.

Karate ("Empty Hand")

- Country of origin and founder: Ryukyu Kingdom of Japan; Tode Sakugawa or Gichin Funakoshi
- Emphasis
  - Striking art
  - Forms or techniques that demonstrate combat principles
  - Techniques must be performed with excellent control and good form
  - Injuring an opponent may result in point deduction
  - Light, but not full, contact is permitted and emphasized
- Techniques
  - Kicks: Kicks to head and neck score more points than kicks to body.
  - Punches: Punches to the back and back of the head score more points than punches to the head and trunk.
- Competition types
  - Kumite: Sparring against an opponent and based on points as described in the techniques section
  - Kata: Detailed choreographed patterns of movements practiced either solo or in a team

MARTIAL ART DISCIPLINES THAT FOCUS ON TECHNIQUE AND FORM

Aikido ("The Way of Harmonious Spirit")

- Country of origin and founder: Japan; Morihei Ueshiba
- Emphasis
  - Joining with an attacker and redirecting the attacker's energy
  - Moving together rather than clashing
- Techniques
  - Body throws and joint locks
  - Strong strikes or immobilizing grabs are employed but not emphasized

Jujitsu ("Art of Gentleness")

- Country of origin and founder: Japan; unknown
- Emphasis
  - The art of breaking balance
  - Yield force provided in an opponent's attack in order to apply a counter technique
- Techniques
  - Strikes, kicks, chokes, pins, and joint manipulation
  - Throws—perfect throws score more points than a throw that is strong but not perfect as deemed by the judges

Tai Chi Chuan ("Supreme Ultimate Boxing")

- Country of origin and founder: China; disputed—however, origins can be traced to the Chen and Yang families
- Emphasis
  - Receptive "ying"—slow, repetitive, meditative, slow impact
  - Active "yang"—active, fast, high impact
  - Health—relieve physical effects of stress on body and mind
  - Meditation—cultivate focus and calmness to maintain homeostasis and relieve stress
  - Martial art—change in response to outside forces
  - Do not resist a violent force; instead, meet force and redirect
- Techniques
  - Solo form: Slow sequence of movements that emphasize straight spine, abdominal breathing, and natural range of motion
  - Pushing hands for training in a practical form
  - Pushes and open hand strikes are more common than punches
  - Kicks are usually to leg and torso, never higher than hip
  - Fingers, fists, palms, forearms, elbows, knees, and feet are used to strike the eyes, throat, heart, and groin
  - Joint locks are also used

MARTIAL ARTS DISCIPLINES IN ADDITION TO JUDO, TAE KWON DO, AND KARATE THAT FOCUS ON SPARRING AND CONTACT

Brazilian Jiu Jitsu

- Country of origin and founder: Brazil; Carlos Gracie
- Emphasis
  - Ground fighting, grappling and leveraging opponents into a position of submission
- Techniques
  - Submission holds, including joint locks and choke holds
  - Guard position—advantageous grappling position where martial artist has his or her back to the ground and uses the legs to grip and control the opponent

- Side control—controlling an opponent on the ground from the side of the body
- Full mount—controlling an opponent from the top while sitting on their chest; most dominant position
- Competition types: Gi (with kimono) and No-Gi (inability to use clothing as leverage)

Kickboxing

- Founder: Unknown; the term was created by Japanese boxing promoter Osamu Noguchi as a variant of Muay Thai and karate
- Emphasis
  - Strikes with punches and kicks while standing up
  - Ground techniques and grappling are *not* permitted
- Techniques
  - Strikes above the hip with fists and feet
  - Using elbows and knees is forbidden; use of shins is seldom permitted
  - Spinning back-of-the-fist punches are permitted, as are traditional punches

Tang So Do ("Way of the Chinese Fist")

- Country of origin and founder: Korea; Hwang Kee
- Emphasis: Empty hand-and-foot fighting forms with emphasis on development of discipline, self-confidence, and self-defense
- Techniques
  - Emphasis placed on kicking techniques, particularly turning and spinning kicks to opponent's torso and head
  - Katas are used as training method for practitioners away from dojo
  - Techniques drawn from ancient Chinese and Japanese martial art traditions

Thai Boxing (Muay Thai) ("The Art of Eight Limbs")

- Country of origin and founder: Thailand; unknown—traced to Buddhist monks
- Emphasis: A distinguished art of fighting of attrition that employs strikes with fists, elbows, shins, and knees
- Techniques
  - Strikes: Fists, elbows, shins, feet, and knees are all permitted to strike an opponent.
  - Punching score lower than other striking techniques.
  - Emphasize entire body movements and hip rotation with strikes to increase strength.
  - Core body strength is essential.
  - Kicking techniques are encouraged to connect with the shin.
  - Grappling or clinching (Thai clinch): A clinch is not broken up as in traditional boxing because this can be an advantageous position from which knee strikes can be employed.

Krav Maga ("Contact Combat")

- Country of origin and founder: Israel; Imi Lichenfeld
- Emphasis
  - Counterattacking as soon as possible
  - Targeting attacks to the body's most vulnerable points
  - Maximum effectiveness and efficiency in order to neutralize opponent by any means
- Techniques
  - Kicks, punches, gouges, elbows, headbutts, and throws
  - Joint manipulation—less emphasized

Mixed Martial Arts

- Combat sport in which participants use a multidisciplinary approach to fighting that includes marital arts, boxing, wrestling, and other fighting disciplines in a supervised bout between two individuals (see Chapter 89: "Mixed Martial Arts").

SUMMARY

- Incidence of martial arts injuries varies with the quality of instruction, the level of experience, and the quantity and type of combative training practiced by the participant.
- Injury rates are much higher during competition compared with training.
- Injuries are very uncommon during practice sessions that primarily involve teaching and/or practicing techniques that do not involve full-speed contact.
- There are millions of martial artists practicing in the United States who do not compete or spar and therefore have a very low incidence of injury.
- Participation in martial arts training continues to grow, partly because of the emphasis on personal growth and improved self-confidence in addition to physical development and self-defense.
- Martial artists should be encouraged to use protective gear whenever possible because use decreases incidence of lacerations, contusions, and abrasions and may decrease peak acceleration forces to the head during kicks and strikes.
- Sports medicine providers should familiarize themselves with the rules and practices of different styles of martial arts and the terminology used to describe the types of training and the various kicks, strikes, and attacks used by martial artists.

RECOMMENDED READINGS

Available online.

87 BOXING

Yuka Kobayashi • Brian A. Jacobs

INTRODUCTION

- Boxing is one of the most ancient sports
- Marquis of Queensbury modified the rules in the early 1800s
- The 1904 St. Louis Olympic Games saw men's boxing introduced as a competition sport and women's boxing as an exhibition sport. Women's boxing became an official sport at the 2012 London Olympic Games.
- Boxing is a medically, ethically, and morally controversial sport because of the nature of the sport and risks of head injuries, especially in the pediatric and adolescent population. As such, the American Academy of Pediatrics and Canadian Paediatric Society oppose boxing as a sport for children and adolescents.

GENERAL PRINCIPLES

Equipment

- **Headgear (required):** Headgear should be properly fitted by trained coaches for sparring and competition. Fitted headgear reduces eye injuries, facial fractures, lacerations, cauliflower ear, and tympanic membrane perforations. There is no evidence to suggest protection from concussions.
- **Gloves (required):** Gloves, thumbless and those with thumbs attached, reduce both eye and hand injuries. Gloves with mobile thumbs are not authorized for use. Heavier gloves have decreased hand injuries and reduced impact forces. Two-toned gloves are easier to see for scorekeepers and officials. Gloves must remain clean, without scuffs and as close to "like new" condition as possible. In 2013, the Amateur International Boxing Association (AIBA) changed its rules and increased glove size to minimize injury.
- **Hand wrap (required):** Hands must be wrapped under supervision of certified official. Wrapping prevents hand injury by consolidating it as one unit and reduces force of blow delivered.
- **Mouth guard (required):** Custom-fitted mouth guards prevent dental and temporomandibular joint injuries. Mouthpieces also allow athlete to "set" their jaw, reducing likelihood of knockdowns by reducing intensity of the blow.
- **Cup protector (required for men)**
- **Groin protector (not required for women)**
- **Breast protectors (not required):** Must be well fitted, not extend beyond the clavicles or xyphoid, and not interfere with athlete's ability to move freely.

Specific Training and Physiology Issues

Amateur Boxing Weight Classifications

- Divided by age and weight classes (Table 87.1; Box 87.1)
- Experience and skills: details found at www.usaboxing.org

Weight Management

- Boxers try to compete in lowest weight class possible.
- Boxers do this to have an advantage over lighter opponents, and this practice is perceived as a psychological advantage of mental toughness.
- Data suggest heavier athletes are more successful within weight categories.
- A study of elite Olympic athletes found that the body mass of combat sport athletes was 4.3 ± 3.9% greater than their competitive division 7–21 days before competition, suggesting most athletes undergo significant decrease in body mass in a short amount of time.
- The most common methods of weight loss include cutting calories, plastic/rubber suits for sweating, and saunas. Less commonly, diuretics and laxatives are used.
- Rapid weight loss (>5% body mass loss) is known to have dangerous acute and long-term consequences.
  - Physiologic
    - Dehydration, increased heart rate, impaired thermoregulation, decreased plasma volume, muscle glycogen depletion
    - Over 5% of body weight loss in a short period (2 days) is associated with increased rates of injuries
  - Psychological
    - Decreased short-term memory, vigor, concentration, self-esteem
    - Confusion, rage, depression, fatigue, isolation
    - Long-term consequences of attention directed to body and body image have been proposed to have negative impacts, but longitudinal studies have not shown this to be true consistently
    - There is conflicting information on whether rapid weight loss negatively affects performance
      - Some studies report impairment of muscular endurance with moderate dehydration (3%–4% body weight) but not maximal muscular power
      - Other studies show no significant change in aerobic performance in rapid weight loss group versus control
- Despite known negative effects of rapid weight loss; unlike sports such as wrestling, there is no minimum body fat percentage allowed and weekly weight loss percentage allowed in boxing.
- National Collegiate Athletic Association (NCAA), International Olympic Committee (IOC), and American College of Sports Medicine (ACSM) have guidelines to safe weight loss

Physical Examinations

- In boxing, annual physical examination is required to be performed by a physician to certify that athlete is free of injury, disability, or infection that could jeopardize the boxer or their opponents.
- All athletes undergo pre- and postbout physicals for every bout.
- In tournament setting, athlete must have prebout physical and weight check each day they are competing.
- Ringside physician must clear each athlete and sign the Passbook before competition.
- At physical examination, pre- and postbout examinations and weigh-ins, boxer must present a USA Boxing Competition Record Book/Passbook with up-to-date information and sign-offs by either the secretary general or executive director of the boxer's national federation and is not allowed to compete without this document

Physician Clearance, Qualification, and Disqualification

Athletes are required to have clearance from their physician before competing. The American Board of Ringside Medicine and American College of Ringside Physicians both help determine ringside physician responsibilities for USA Boxing.

Disqualifying Conditions

- Acute and chronic infections (not limited to the list here)

Table 87.1 AMATEUR BOXING WEIGHT CLASSES

Male Olympic Boxers	48–52 kg, 52–57 kg, 57–63 kg, 63–69 kg, 69–75 kg, 75–81 kg, 81–91 kg, 91+ kg
Female Olympic Boxers	48–51 kg, 57–60 kg, 60–64 kg, 64–69 kg, 69–75 kg
Male Elite, Senior, and Youth Boxers	Up to 49 kg, 52 kg, 56 kg, 60 kg, 64 kg, 69 kg, 75 kg, 81 kg, 91 kg, 91+ kg
Female Elite and Youth Boxers	Up to 48 kg, 51 kg, 54 kg, 57 kg, 60 kg, 64 kg, 69 kg, 75 kg, 81 kg, 81+ kg
Boys and Girls Junior Boxers	Up to 46 kg, 48 kg, 50 kg, 52 kg, 54 kg, 57 kg, 60 kg, 63 kg, 66 kg, 70 kg, 75 kg, 80 kg, 80+ kg
Boys and Girls PeeWee, Bantam, and Intermediate Boxers (Prep)	Details can be found at www.usaboxing.org

BOX 87.1 AMATEUR BOXING AGE CLASSES[a]

- 8–14 years: Prep
  - 8–10 years: PeeWee
  - 11–12 years: Bantam
  - 13–14 years: Intermediate
- 15–16 years: Junior
- 17–18 years: Youth
- 19–40 years: Elite
- 40–45 years: Elite or Masters

[a]Age group class determined by actual birth date.

  - Illness causing fevers
  - Chest infection
  - Untreated tuberculosis
  - Gastrointestinal (GI) conditions with dehydration/malabsorption
  - Hepatitis
  - Open skin conditions (e.g., methicillin-resistant *Staphylococcus aureus* [MRSA], zoster, herpes)
  - Mononucleosis within the past 4 weeks
- Severe blood dyscrasias, conditions requiring anticoagulation, sickle cell disease
- Infection with hepatitis B virus (HBV), hepatitis C virus (HCV), or human immunodeficiency virus (HIV)
- Refractive or intraocular surgery, cataracts, retinal detachment
- Presence of myopia >–3.50 diopters, uncorrected vision worse than 20/200, or corrected vision worse than 20/60
- Significant cardiovascular or pulmonary abnormalities, including:
  - Severe chronic obstructive pulmonary disease (COPD), uncontrolled asthma with potential for hypoxemia, pulmonary hypertension
  - Severe aortic or pulmonic stenosis, myocarditis, pericarditis, recent embolic disease, high-grade atrioventricular (AV) block, complete left bundle branch block (LBBB), atrial or ventricular tachycardia, coarctation of aorta, corrected surgical conditions unless cleared by cardiovascular surgery
  - Uncontrolled resting blood pressure (BP) >160/100 (if >140/90, the boxer may compete if previous BP measures are normal, but physician follow-up is advised for persistent BP >135/85)
- Congenital/acquired musculoskeletal problems (e.g., spondylolysis, spinal fractures, atlantoaxial instability, and unstable joints)
- Unresolved concussion symptoms
- Significant intracranial mass lesions or bleeding, history of craniotomy, cerebral palsy, hypoxic brain injuries, neuropathies causing balance/coordination problems (benign smaller problems can be cleared by neurosurgery)
- Seizure within the past 3 years
- Hepatosplenomegaly, splenomegaly, ascites
- Pregnancy: Female boxers must present a Declaration of Non-Pregnancy. Ringside physician has the discretion to determine if acute conditions (such as abnormal menstrual bleeding or pelvic pain) is a disqualifying condition.
- Uncontrolled diabetes mellitus or thyroid disease
- Implantable devices interfering with physiologic process/enhancing performance
- Banned substances: In amateur and Olympic competitions, use of banned substances such as ergogenic aids and steroids are cause for disqualification. Refer to the appropriate authority (e.g., www.wada-ama.org) for comprehensive lists of banned substances, medications, and practices

Nondisqualifying Conditions

- Deafness—officials must be made aware of condition; official may tap boxer on shoulder to signal "break" or "stop"
- Dental braces/orthodontics if "Permission to Box with Braces or Orthodontic Appliances" form is attached to boxer's Passbook
- Single kidney
- Breast implants if "Permission to Box with Breast Implants" form is attached to boxer's Passbook
- Sex reassignment in accordance with IOC Consensus on Sex Reassignment and Hyperandrogenism

Ringside Personnel and Equipment

Coaches

- One coach and one assistant are allowed for each boxer in their corner
- Must remain seated during each round and not interact with fans or ringside officials
- Should have first aid supplies, clean white towels, sterile gauze pads, sterile cotton, cotton swabs, bags of ice
  - Banned substances include ammonia, ammonia inhalants, or smelling salts

Cutman

- Manages minor injuries that could otherwise disqualify a boxer during a bout
- Amateur boxing prohibits the use of medication to treat bleeding during a bout, but professional boxers are allowed any medication or topical treatment that the cutman or trainers have at their disposal

Official

- Serves to ensure safety of and hold best interests of boxers in the competition:
  - Ensures that rules of fair play are strictly observed
  - Responsible for maintaining control of athletes at all times
  - Responsible for preventing unnecessary punishment of a weaker opponent
  - Ensures that gloves, mouthpiece, and dress adhere to regulations

Physicians

- Serve as neutral advocate for boxers and provide care for boxers before, during, and after bouts
- Should pay close attention to bout because doing so will allow them to witness injury mechanisms and assess fatigue and other factors that contribute to injury

- Must be at least one physician at ringside at all times during competitions. Two physicians are preferable, as this allows one to care for an injured boxer after bout, while second physician attends to next bout.
- If ringside physician believes that a boxer is no longer capable of boxing, is in danger of further injury, or is outclassed, the physician may, at any time, signal the official to terminate the bout. However, only at the behest of the official can the physician enter the ring.

Competition

Surveying the Venue

- The ringside physician must be familiar with the venue; location of emergency medical services (EMS) providers and ambulances; the ring; and condition of turnbuckle padding, ropes, and mat
- The physician should meet with EMS and first aid personnel and be aware of location of first aid equipment, spine boards, oxygen, cervical collars, advanced cardiac life support equipment (including defibrillators, if available), and ensure adequate proximity to a communication device
- Ringside physicians are mandated to have an unobstructed view of the ring

Medical Supplies at Ringside

- Ringside physicians at amateur bouts are allowed the following:
  - Flashlight
  - Oral airway
  - Gloves
  - Stethoscope
  - Vaseline
  - Adrenaline chloride (1:1000) to control nosebleeds and cuts
  - Thrombin for dry cuts
  - Avitene (microfiber collagen hemostat) for active bleeding
  - Ice and ice bags
  - Clean sponges
  - Gauze pads
  - Enswell pressure plates to control hematomas
  - White towels
  - Scissors
  - Water in a clear plastic container
  - Adhesive athletic tape
- USA Boxing mandates that an oxygen tank, C-collar, and spine board be available ringside
- Physicians at professional matches may have additional supplies as they deem necessary

Evaluation During the Bout

- The physician can ask to evaluate an athlete or be called into the ring by the official
  - First identify yourself to the athlete
  - When there is concern for cervical spine injury or traumatic brain injury, stabilize C-spine immediately
  - Abide by basic life support/advanced cardiac life support (BLS/ACLS) principles
  - Practice universal precautions near blood or body fluids
  - If athletes do not require EMS transfer, have them return for re-evaluation during event. It is often helpful to talk to the coach to ensure this happens

Controlling Injury and Bleeding

- One minute is allotted to get bleeding under control
- Facial swelling is managed by pressure applied with an enswell, an iced metal spatula applied to hematoma that milks the blood to the surrounding tissues, or with a moldable ice bag
- Prevention of bleeding injuries can be attempted through the application of petroleum jelly
- Medications, only allowed in the professional world, to control bleeding include Avitene, Surgicel, Gelfoam, adrenaline hydrochloride, and thrombin; these are frequently mixed with petroleum jelly and applied with cotton swabs

Disqualification During the Competition

- The following injuries result in disqualification from the bout:
  - Excessive facial swelling that impairs vision
  - Presence of retinal detachment (permanent disqualifier)
  - Suspected or proven fractures or dislocations
  - Lacerations or wounds requiring dressings to control bleeding

Rounds and Standing Eight Count

- Amateur bouts are characterized by three rounds of 1–3 minutes separated by a 1-minute rest interval
- The official can institute a standing eight count whenever it is believed that a boxer has been stunned
- Should a boxer incur three standing eight counts in a given period or four in a given match, the bout is discontinued as referee stop contest–head (RSC-H)
- In the case of an unconscious boxer:
  - The official signals the physician to enter the ring
  - Only the official, ringside physician, and any assistants the physician deems necessary are allowed into the ring
- The official can stop a bout for other reasons/injuries that put a boxer at risk:
  - RSC: Boxer is outclassed by opponent and is thus at unreasonable risk
  - RSC-I: Boxer is unable to compete because of injury suffered during bout
    - Example: excessive swelling that impedes vision or bleeding that cannot be adequately controlled

Scoring

- In amateur boxing, points are awarded by three to five judges for number of blows to the upper body and head, regardless of force applied, technical and tactical superiority, and competitiveness
- Scores in professional boxing are also tabulated as noted, but greater weight is given to blows of greater force, knockdowns, and knockouts

Postbout Examination

- A medical survey is performed after every bout
  - All boxers should be assessed upon completion of a contest, with special attention focused toward neurologic and orthopedic status
  - All injuries suffered in bout should be recorded in Passbook
  - Any future medical suspension that results from bout should be noted in Passbook
- The coach is responsible for ensuring the boxer receives appropriate accommodations to return home safely.
- After bout, imperative that boxer's physician be contacted immediately if any of the following symptoms are present:
  - Headache or dizziness
  - Increasing drowsiness or change in mental status (i.e., irrational behavior, agitation, excessive restlessness, or persistent confusion)
  - Uncontrolled or persistent vomiting
  - Change in vision
  - Seizure
  - Inability to move a limb
  - Oozing of bloody or clear fluid from the nose or ears
  - Incontinence of bowel or bladder

Restriction From Boxing

- When the decision of a match is RSC because of mismatched skill of boxers, there is no need for a restriction to be placed on

Table 87.2 INJURY STUDIES IN BOXING

Amateur Boxing	A study of 1094 amateur boxers at the 1981 and 1982 USA/ABF championships observed: • 85 injuries of varying degrees of severity, 52 were considered notable • 48 matches were discontinued because of head blows, which occurred at a rate of 4.38% • All other injuries occurred at a rate of 4.75% • Soft tissue injuries of the hands accounted for the next largest category of injury in this study, comprising sprains of the first metacarpophalangeal (MCP) ligaments, subungual hematomas, contusions, and sprains of the carpus. Fractures of the hands and wrist accounted for three injuries; likewise, nasal fractures also accounted for three injuries A study looking at upper extremity (UE) injuries in boxers presenting to the emergency department between 2012 and 2016 showed: • Decrease in UE injuries from 865 to 656 per 100,000 person-years from 2012 to 2016. This correlates with rules changes made by AIBA in 2013. • Most common UE injuries (list correlates with the most common body parts involved): hand fractures, hand contusions, wrist sprains, shoulder dislocation, shoulder sprain
Olympic Boxers	A study conducted at the United States Olympic Training Center (USOTC) over a 15-year period from 1977 to 1992 showed the following injury trends: • Of 1776 reported injuries, only 6.1% met criteria for "serious injury," which was defined as a condition "which could not be remediated through the typical services of an athletic trainer at the USOTC" (concussions would fall within this definition) • Of all injuries, contusions, muscle strains, joint sprains, and tendonitis occurred with the greatest frequency, accounting for 71.9% of all injuries • Fractures were categorized as a group rather than by body region and accounted for 4.9% of all injuries. Lacerations accounted for another 4.1%, "neural disorders," including concussions for 1.4%, and all others for the remaining 17.7%. • The study also listed injuries by body region: UE injuries accounted for 24.8% of the total, head and facial injuries for 19.4%, lower extremity injuries for 15.0%, and spinal column injuries for 9.4% • Multiple examiners, with many specialties and many different levels of training, were involved in data collection
Professional Boxers	In a study of professional boxers conducted over a 16-year period (1985–2001) in Victoria, Australia: • Face and head trauma made up 89.8% of all injuries reported, with the eye, eyelid, and eyebrow injured most frequently • Concussions accounted for 15.9% of injuries • UE injuries accounted for 7.4% • 75% of all injuries were lacerations, abrasions, and hematomas • Other sites of injury mentioned include sprains of the ankle, muscular strains of the low back, perforations of the tympanic membrane, dental fractures, fractures of the ribs, and contusions to the lungs

Data based on studies from Estwanik JJ, Boitano M, Ari N. Amateur boxing injuries at the 1981 and 1982 USA/ABF National Championships. *Phys Sportsmed*. 12(10):123–128; Lemme NJ, Ready L, Faria M, et al. Epidemiology of boxing-related upper extremity injuries in the United States. *Phys Sportsmed*. 2018; 46(4):503–508; Zazryn TR, Finch CF, McCrory P. A 16 year study of injuries to professional boxers in the state of Victoria, Australia. *Br J Sports Med*. 2003;37(4):321–324; Timm KE, Wallach JM, Stone JA, Ryan EJ. Fifteen years of amateur boxing injuries/illnesses at the United States Olympic Training Center. *J Athl Train*. 1993;28(4):330–334.

that boxer. This means they will be allowed to box again as long as they did not sustain an injury that warrants restriction.

- It is the physician's discretion whether a restriction should be placed on a boxer for return to sport. For example, if a boxer sustains an injury such as a dislocated shoulder, the physician can place a 30-day restriction from competition. The minimum restriction time period is recorded in the Passbook.
- If a bout has ended by a knockout (RSC-H), the injured boxer receives a restrictions affidavit requiring signatures of the athlete, ringside physician, official, and coach. The athlete's Passbook is sequestered to USA Boxing Headquarters so that they may not compete during this restriction period.
- The USA Boxing Medical Rule Book is currently being updated based on the most recent information on treatment of mild traumatic brain injuries. There is no consensus on return to sport after RSC-H or technical knockout (TKO) in boxing that risks the well-being of the boxer. The most current guidelines are outlined in the USA Boxing Medical Handbook, with 30-, 60-, 90-, 180-, and 360-day suspensions placed depending on clinical picture. This rule does not align with the most recent guidelines on return to sport after a concussion.
- The Association of Ringside Physicians Concussion Management and Return to Play Guidelines for Combat Sport Athletes calls for all athletes with concussion to be suspended from sparring or competition until a physician familiar with concussion management clears the athlete.

COMMON INJURIES AND MEDICAL PROBLEMS

Comparing Injury Rates to Other Sports

Boxers suffer injuries at rates comparable to those found in other contact and noncontact sports (Tables 87.2, 87.3, 87.4, and 87.5)

Head and Brain Injury (See Chapter 45: "Head Injuries")

- Rate of head injuries suffered in boxers ranges from 27% to 94% of all injuries
- Most are minor, with contusions and lacerations being most common
- The Canadian Hospitals Injury Reporting and Prevention Program Database shows that between 1990 and 2007, prevalence of hospitalizations related to sports injuries were highest in boxing among all combat sports. Of those hospitalizations, facial fractures accounted for 58% and closed head injuries 25%. There was also a significant increase in overall number of injuries between 1999 and 2007 (16.4 per 100,000) compared with the decade previous (11.4 per 100,000).

Table 87.3 DEMOGRAPHIC CHARACTERISTICS OF INDIVIDUALS WITH BOXING INJURIES, US EMERGENCY DEPARTMENTS, 1990–2008

	Estimated No. of Cases (95% CI)	%[b]	Estimated Annual Average	Injury Rate Per 1000 Participants[a]
Age (Years)				
6–11	4724 (3363, 6085)	2.9	249	—
12–17	42,985 (34,493, 51,476)	26.0	2262	14.0
18–24	61,280 (48,518, 74,042)	37.0	3225	16.4
25–34	39,333 (31,219, 47,446)	23.8	2070	13.6
35–44	12,500 (9222, 15,778)	7.5	658	—
≥45	4780 (3032, 6529)	2.9	252	—
Gender				
Male	150,571 (123,260, 1,777,882)	90.9	7925	13.3
Female	15,025 (10,846, 19,204)	9.1	791	8.9
Total	165,602 (134,891, 196,313)		8716	12.7

[a]Injury rates were not calculated for categories with fewer than 20 unweighted cases. Injury rates were calculated from 2003 data only.
[b]Percentages may not total 100% because of rounding error.
From Potter MR, Snyder AJ, Smith GA. Boxing injuries presenting to U.S. emergency departments, 1990-2008. *Am J Prev Med*. 2011; 40(4):462–467.

Table 87.4 SELECTED DIAGNOSES AND INJURED BODY REGIONS FOR BOXING INJURIES: INJURIES RELATED TO PUNCHING BAGS COMPARED WITH INJURIES UNRELATED TO PUNCHING BAGS

	Injuries Related to Punching Bags			*Injuries Unrelated to Punching Bags*		
	Estimated No. of Cases (%)[a]	Average No./Year	Injury Rate[b]	Estimated No. of Cases (%)[a]	Average No./Year	Injury Rate[b]
Diagnosis						
STI	17,995 (29.6)	947	1.3	25,019 (23.9)	1317	1.8
Fracture	19,528 (32.1)	1028	1.4	25,941 (24.8)	1365	2.6
Laceration	2550 (4.2)	134	—	11,975 (11.5)	630	0.7
Strain/sprain	16,134 (26.5)	849	1.4	20,309 (19.4)	1069	1.0
Body Region Injured						
Head/neck	1491 (2.4)	78	—	35,800 (34.2)	1884	2.8
Wrist	13,543 (22.2)	713	1.0	8298 (7.9)	437	—
Hand	33,051 (54.3)	1740	2.5	21,647 (20.7)	1139	1.5
Finger	7340 (12.1)	386	—	9989 (9.5)	526	0.9
Shoulder	2204 (3.6)	116	—	10,204 (9.7)	537	1.0
Total[c]	60,881	3204	4.6	104,721	5512	8.1

[a]Percentage of injuries in each of the two categories of injury: those related and those unrelated to punching bags.
[b]Per 1000 participants per year. Injury rates were not calculated for categories with fewer than 20 unweighted cases. Injury rates were calculated from 2003 data only.
[c]Only commonly occurring diagnoses and injured body regions are included in the table. Therefore, numbers of injuries do not sum to the totals and percentages do not sum to 100%.
STI, Soft tissue injury.
Reprinted with permission from Potter MR, Snyder AJ, Smith GA. Boxing injuries presenting to U.S. emergency departments, 1990-2008. *Am J Prev Med*. 2011; 40(4):462–467.

Table 87.5 PERCENTAGE OF BOXING INJURIES ACCORDING TO BODY REGION INJURED, US EMERGENCY DEPARTMENTS, 1990–2008

Body Region	% of Injuries
Hand	33.0
Head and neck	22.5
Wrist	13.2
Finger	10.5
Shoulder	7.5
Trunk	6.3
Arm and elbow	3.6
Lower limb	3.3
Other	0.1

- Between 1950 and 2007, there were 339 mortalities in boxing
  - Sixty-four percent associated with knockout and 15% technical knockout
  - Sixty-one percent happened in the ring, 17% in locker room, and 22% outside the arena

Concussion

- Large organizations such as USA Boxing and Boxing Canada do not regularly report incidence or prevalence of concussions
- A large prospective cohort study found that more than 70% of amateur and professional boxing injuries were to the head, with concussions comprising of a third of those injuries
- Other reports show concussions range between 6.5% and 51.6% of all amateur boxing injuries
- Data are conflicting on whether there are acute cognitive changes after sparring or competition

- In 224 active professional boxers, increased exposure to repetitive head trauma (by bouts, years of boxing, or fight exposure score) was associated with decreased speed of processing using the CNS Vital Signs
- In a study of 38 amateur boxers, neuropsychological testing before and shortly after a boxing match resulted in impaired performance in planning, attention, and memory capacity when compared with controls
- There are studies that do not show this pattern of impairment acutely after boxing matches and instead show slight increase in scores, possibly because of learning effect

- Of note, there is a stigma surrounding reporting head injuries among the boxing community. A study of professional boxers found that there was a significant gap in athletes' perceived knowledge of concussion symptoms and long-term effects of multiple hits to the head
  - Forty percent of boxers reported returning to sparring or competition the same day of head injury
  - Twenty-one percent of athletes admitted to concealing symptoms from medical providers and their coaches

Second Impact Syndrome

- The injured boxer may appear initially stunned. Some have been witnessed to continue competing for a time
- Boxers usually remain conscious and may remain standing but then suddenly collapse and become comatose with rapidly dilating pupils, a fixed gaze, and imminent respiratory failure suggestive of diffuse and catastrophic cerebral edema over a 2- to 5-minute period

Intracerebral Hemorrhage

See Chapter 45: "Head Injuries"; Fig. 87.1.

Intracranial Epidural Hematoma

- Caused by accumulation of blood between skull and dura mater from ruptured middle meningeal artery because of overlying skull fracture. Injured boxer may suffer an immediate brief alteration or loss of consciousness, followed by a lucid phase (see Fig. 87.1). This is then followed by rapid deterioration in mental status with ipsilaterally dilated pupils (because of uncal herniation and oculomotor nerve compression), contralateral weakness, and progressive decline

Subdural Hematoma

- See Chapter 45: "Head Injuries"; Fig. 87.1.
- This is the most common cause of death associated with boxing

Intraparenchymal and Subarachnoid Hemorrhages

- Associated with extremely rapid deterioration without a lucid phase

Chronic Traumatic Encephalopathy

- An estimated 15%–40% of professional boxers demonstrate symptoms of chronic traumatic brain injury (CTBI)
- There is no predictable or sequential course to this disease process that presents with pyramidal, cerebellar, and extrapyramidal symptoms.
- There are countless anecdotal reports that boxing contributes significantly to late and debilitating CTBI. Long-term manifestations include altered affect and memory, Parkinson-type syndrome, slurred speech, loss of balance, loss of intellect, and Alzheimer syndrome.
- These reports are reinforced by retrospective studies conducted on retired boxers. However, the scientific literature lacks conclusive evidence regarding any association of these chronic brain injuries with boxing-related injuries.

EFFECTS OF REPETITIVE TRAUMA

- Most often observed in professional contact sport athletes, including boxers, with a history of repetitive head impacts
- Neurophysiologic changes in the brain consistent with chronic traumatic encephalopathy (CTE) have not been found in those without history of repetitive trauma. However, not everyone with a history of repetitive trauma develops CTE.
- Increased career length and mean number of boxing bouts may correlate with increased risk of CTBI.
- Comparing 1930 with 2002, the average professional boxing career has decreased from 19 to 5 years and career bouts from 336 to 13. However, the assumption that CTE is a manifestation of long careers and exposure to multiple hits needs to be further studied.

BIOLOGIC MARKERS FOR CHRONIC TRAUMATIC ENCEPHALOPATHY

- There is a unique pattern and accumulation of p-tau neurofibrillary tangles in CTE that is distinct from findings in Alzheimer disease and other neurodegenerative diseases.
- Apolipoprotein E-ε-4 assists with neural integrity and recovery after brain injury and has been linked to poor outcomes and activation of neurodegenerative mechanisms. This genotype has been linked to higher risk of developing CTE pathology.
- A study of 30 boxers showed greater cognitive impairments on the mean chronic brain injury scale for boxers with the apolipoprotein E-ε-4 allele compared with those without the allele

CAVUM SEPTUM PELLUCIDUM

- Changes on computed tomography (CT) and magnetic resonance imaging (MRI) have not been found to be useful for diagnosis of concussion. However, imaging changes for those with CTBI and CTE show there may be changes in the brain, specifically the cavum septum pellucidum (CSP), unique to those who experience repetitive head trauma.
- CSP is a normal variant of the cerebrospinal fluid (CSF) space between leaflets of the septum pellucidum.
- Studies show that the presence of CSP does not differ greatly between boxers and control groups, but the size of CSP is greater than controls. A study of 164 male boxers saw a high prevalence of CSP in both controls and boxers, with a higher trend towards enlarged CSP in the boxer group.
- Pathology study of 15 ex-boxers showed that 12 of the 13 cadavers with CSP was three times as wide as the control brains and 11 of 13 had gross fenestrations of the CSP.
- In boxers, this condition may be a marker of significant brain atrophy, presumably related to repetitive head trauma.

Neuroimaging

Positron emission tomography (PET) scans: Hypometabolism in frontal and parietal lobes has been observed in boxers with CTE, similar to patterns seen in Alzheimer disease

MRI: Useful in delineating contusions, subdural and white matter lesions, arachnoid cysts, and brainstem and cerebellar anatomy

CT: Useful in identifying acute bleeding injuries

Nasal Contusion, Fracture, and Septal Hematoma (See Chapter 48: "Maxillofacial Injuries")

- Assume fracture has occurred if there is crepitus and/or tenderness over bridge of the nose. Often associated with epistaxis, nasal airway swelling, and obstruction. Nasal asymmetry rarely obvious.
- Often, ringside physician will be asked to realign fracture at the event. Realignment is easier when done in a timely manner

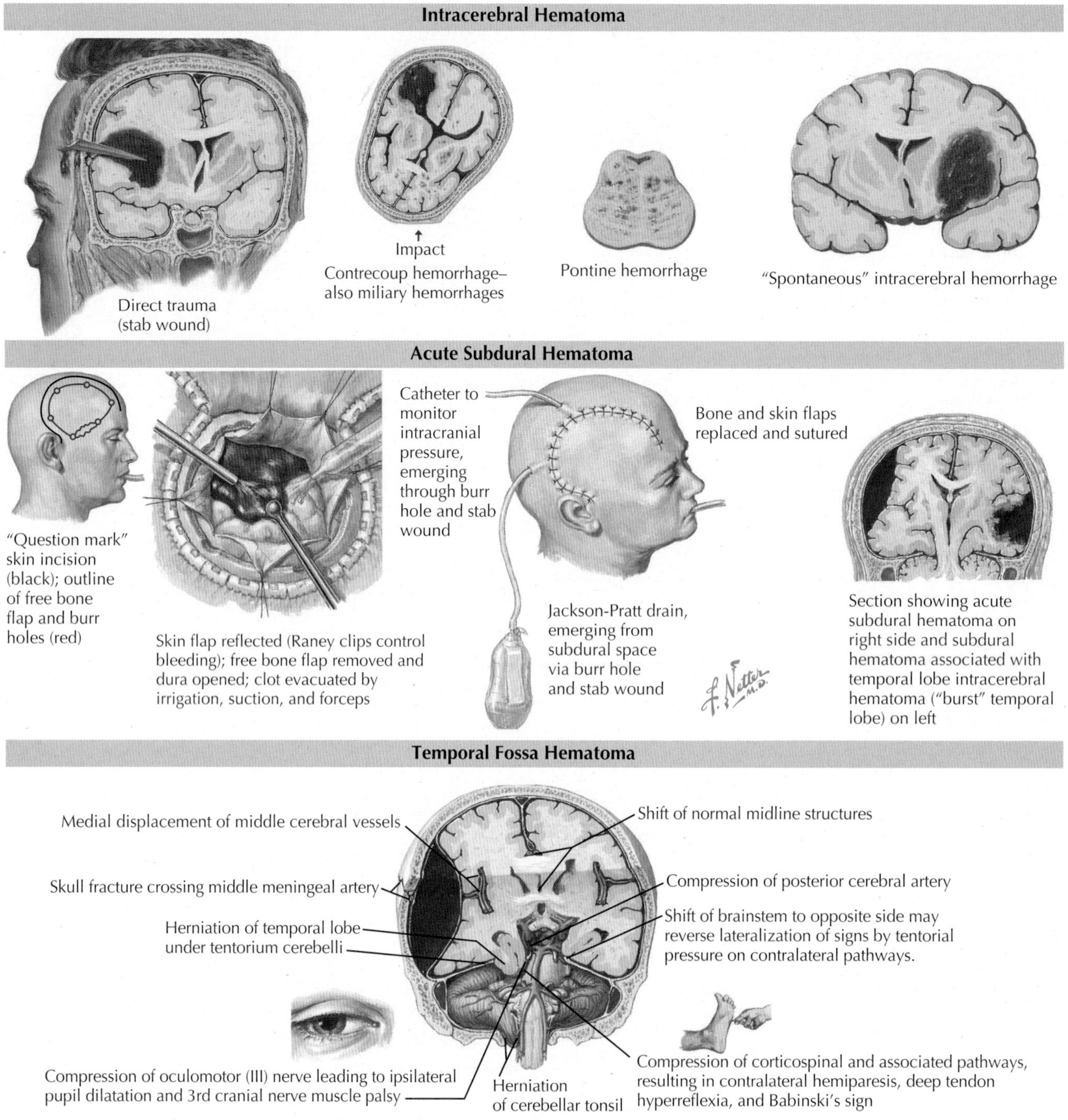
Intracerebral Hematoma
Direct trauma
(stab wound)
Impact
Contrecoup hemorrhage–
also miliary hemorrhages
Pontine hemorrhage
"Spontaneous" intracerebral hemorrhage
Acute Subdural Hematoma
"Question mark" skin incision (black); outline of free bone flap and burr holes (red)
Skin flap reflected (Raney clips control bleeding); free bone flap removed and dura opened; clot evacuated by irrigation, suction, and forceps
Catheter to monitor intracranial pressure, emerging through burr hole and stab wound
Bone and skin flaps replaced and sutured
Jackson-Pratt drain, emerging from subdural space via burr hole and stab wound
Section showing acute subdural hematoma on right side and subdural hematoma associated with temporal lobe intracerebral hematoma ("burst" temporal lobe) on left
Temporal Fossa Hematoma
Medial displacement of middle cerebral vessels
Skull fracture crossing middle meningeal artery
Herniation of temporal lobe under tentorium cerebelli
Shift of normal midline structures
Compression of posterior cerebral artery
Shift of brainstem to opposite side may reverse lateralization of signs by tentorial pressure on contralateral pathways.
Compression of oculomotor (III) nerve leading to ipsilateral pupil dilatation and 3rd cranial nerve muscle palsy
Herniation of cerebellar tonsil
Compression of corticospinal and associated pathways, resulting in contralateral hemiparesis, deep tendon hyperreflexia, and Babinski's sign

Figure 87.1 Acute traumatic brain injury.

unless there already is significant swelling. Realignment is followed by anterior packing and splinting.

- Crucial that septal hematoma be evaluated by an otolaryngologist specialist (ear/nose/throat [ENT]) within 24–48 hours to avoid saddle deformity. The ringside physician needs to communicate this clearly to athlete and their coach before departure from the competition.
- Simple nasal fractures take approximately 2 weeks to become stable, after which boxers can return to sport. However, close follow-up and clearance by the ENT should be obtained for septal hematomas.

Hand Injuries

Boxer's Knuckle

Examination: Marked swelling at metacarpophalangeal joint (MCPJ) and loss of range of motion (ROM), frequently with extensor lag; ulnar subluxation of extensor tendon (obvious when flexing MCPJ); tenderness at ruptured sagittal band (Fig. 87.2)

Imaging: X-ray may show subchondral cysts, which may indicate MCPJ osteochondral fracture

Treatment: Direct repair is performed through curvilinear incision, avoiding prominence of the knuckle. Repaired in 60–70 degrees

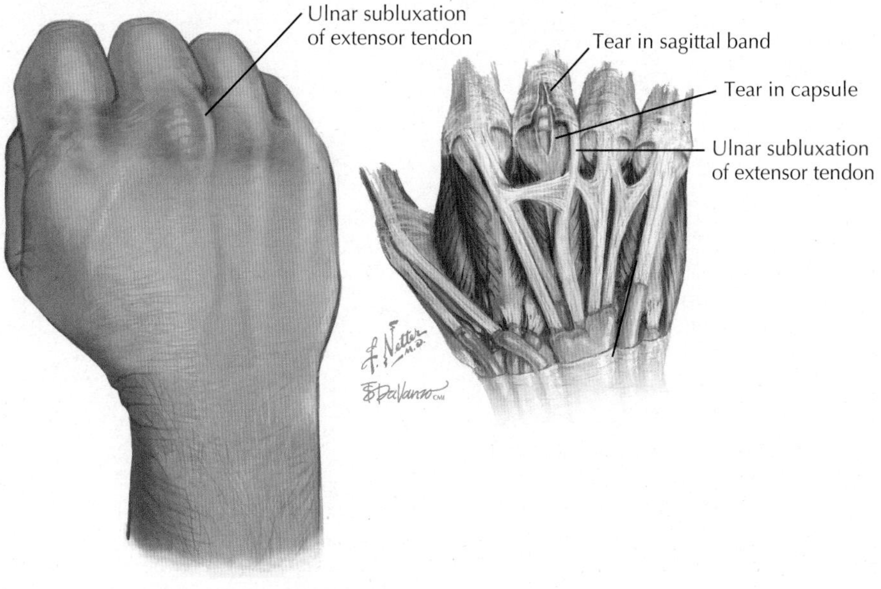
Ulnar subluxation of extensor tendon
Tear in sagittal band
Tear in capsule
Ulnar subluxation of extensor tendon

Figure 87.2 Boxer's knuckle.

of flexion; capsular tears, if present, are debrided but frequently are not repaired. Immobilized postoperation at 60–70 degrees for 6 weeks; occupational/hand therapy (OT) post-immobilization

Return to sport: Usually ready to return to punching at 8–12 weeks after immobilization when wounds are completely healed and pain-free and full ROM has been restored with normal strength

Traumatic Carpal Boss

Examination: Painful, bony prominence at carpometacarpal joint (CMCJ) either with or without a cyst, usually present in digits two and three

Imaging: X-ray shows hypertrophic bone adjacent to CMCJ and possibly widened CMCJ space. If the condition is chronic, obliteration of CMCJ should be noted

Treatment: Arthrodesis of affected joints, with removal of ganglion cysts (if present), and hypertrophic bone; K-wires for stability. The injured region is immobilized for 6–8 weeks, or until evidence of radiographic union. OT begins when cast and K-wires are removed.

Return to sport: Usually takes at least 6 months to achieve pain relief and regain satisfactory ROM and strength needed for competition.

RECOMMENDED READINGS

Available online.

88 WRESTLING

Robert Kiningham

INTRODUCTION

- Wrestling is widely considered to be the world's oldest sport, dating back to the ancient Greeks.
- It is a worldwide sport, with particular popularity in Eastern Europe, the Middle East, Asia, and North America.
- Men's wrestling was an original Olympic sport. Women's wrestling was added to the Olympics in 2004.

EPIDEMIOLOGY

- Ranks seventh among high school boys in participation, with almost 250,000 participants in 10,843 schools (2018–2019).
- Girls' participation in high school wrestling has increased 3.5 times since 2009–2010 and almost doubled since 2014–2015, with 21,124 participants from 2890 high schools in 43 states (2018–2019).
- A reported 249 National Collegiate Athletic Association (NCAA), 68 National Association of Intercollegiate Athletics (NAIA), and 62 junior college (JUCO) men's wrestling programs and 69 4-year college and 7 JUCO women's wrestling programs in the United States in 2020.
- High school boy injury rate of 2.38/1000 athletic exposures (AEs) per High School (HS) Reporting Information Online System (2005–2006 through 2013–2014 seasons)
- College male injury rate of 9.28 injuries/1000 AEs per NCAA Injury Surveillance System (2004–2005 through 2013–2014 seasons).
- Most common site of injury differs depending on level of competition.
  - Youth wrestling: Hand, wrist, and finger
  - High school: Head/face and shoulder
  - College wrestlers: Knee
- Most injuries occur during practices, but injury rate is much higher during competitions for both HS (1.91/1000 AE practice, 3.70/1000 AE competition) and college (7.02/1000 AE practice, 27.59/1000 AE competition).
- Injury rates appear to be rising for both HS and college wrestlers, primarily because of increased reporting of concussions.
- Concussion rate in HS boys wrestling (4.83/10,000 AE) is fourth highest among boy HS sports. Reports differ on the relative risk of concussion in men's collegiate wrestling, ranging from first to fourth highest concussion rate in collegiate sports.
- Approximately 7% of injuries are the result of illegal moves.
- Skin infections are the most common reason wrestlers seek medical attention and account for the most lost time from competitions and practices.

GENERAL PRINCIPLES

Wrestling Styles

- International wrestling: Freestyle and Greco-Roman
  - Greco-Roman: attacking opponent's legs is not permitted
  - Freestyle has both men's and women's divisions
- USA youth, HS, and college wrestling: folkstyle
- Greco-Roman and freestyle reward throws more than folkstyle, which leads to more high-velocity mat injuries, including head and neck injuries and concussions.
- Folkstyle allows wrestlers to be in a defensive down position for longer, which leads to more defensive injuries such as shoulder strains and subluxations.

Equipment and Safety Issues

- Most wrestling matches are contested in a singlet, which is a tight, one-piece uniform, whereas most wrestlers practice in shorts or sweatpants and a t-shirt.
  - Loose-fitting practice clothes can cause injuries (e.g., finger dislocations), so most wrestlers will tuck shirts into shorts and pant legs into socks.
- Wrestling shoes provide a light, but supportive, point of traction on a wrestling mat, which can be slippery when wet.
- Wrestling mats have greatly improved over the last 25 years and have become much more durable.
- Headgear is required in college and HS wrestling but is almost never worn in the international styles.
- Supportive braces will have to be approved by the referee and will likely be denied if there are any metallic pieces palpable because of the possibility of injury to the opponent.

Rules

- Governing bodies of wrestling in United States
  - High School
    - Most states adopt the National Federation of State High School State Associations (NFHS) rules. However, individual state HS athletic associations retain the power to determine their own state's rules. Physicians should check with their specific state's HS athletic association to see if their rules differ from NFHS rules.
  - College
    - NCAA Wrestling Rules Committee
    - The NAIA and National Junior College Athletic Association (NJCAA) both defer to the NCAA rules for wrestling.
    - Women's Collegiate Wrestling Association (WCWA) is the governing body for women's collegiate wrestling.
    - The NCAA designated women's wrestling as an Emerging Sport for Divisions I, II, and III in 2020.
  - International styles (Greco-Roman and freestyle)
    - USA Wrestling is the governing body for international style events
- Injury time during matches (Table 88.1)
  - Injury timeouts are stoppage of wrestling requested by a coach, wrestler, or referee.
  - Injury time is defined as the cumulative time spent being evaluated and recovering from an injury sustained during the match, including overtime.
- Recovery time
  - Time spent being evaluated and recovering from an injury that resulted from an illegal action by the opposing wrestler
- Bleeding time during matches
  - Time spent stopping bleeding and cleaning blood from mats, wrestlers, and equipment. Distinct from injury or recovery time.
  - NCAA does not limit bleeding time. Referee, in consultation with medical personnel, has authority to stop match and declare nonbleeding wrestler the winner by medical default if bleeding becomes excessive or causes an inordinate number of timeouts.
- Concussions
  - By NFHS, NCAA, and USA Wrestling rules, referee has the responsibility to stop the match if a concussion is suspected.

Table 88.1 INJURY ALLOWANCES PER WRESTLING MATCH[a]

	NFHS	NCAA	USA Wrestling
Injury Time-Outs	2	2	Unlimited
Cumulative Injury Time	90 sec	90 sec	Unlimited
Blood Time	5 min	Unlimited	Unlimited
Concussion Evaluation	Counts toward injury time	Unlimited	Unlimited
Recovery Time[b]	2 min	2 min	Unlimited

[a]Exceeding indicated values results in the wrestler losing the match by injury default.
[b]Time to recover from the opponent's illegal action. If the injured wrestler cannot resume wrestling within 2 minutes, he is declared the winner and the opponent is disqualified.
NCAA, National Collegiate Athletic Association. 2020–2021 NCAA Wrestling Rules and Interpretations; *NFHS,* National Federation of State High School Associations. NFHS 2020–2021 Wrestling Rule Book.

- NCAA makes distinction between injury time and time spent evaluating a concussion. Medical personnel have unlimited time to evaluate a wrestler suspected of sustaining a concussion. This time does not count against the wrestler's injury time or recovery time.
- Skin infections (see "Skin Infections" section)

Specific Training and Physiology Issues

Weight Classifications

Competitors are matched by weight classes in all styles:

- Men's freestyle: 6 weight classes (Olympics), 10 weight classes (World Championships)
- Women's freestyle: 6 weight classes (Olympics), 10 weight classes (World Championships)
- Men's Greco-Roman: 6 weight classes
- USA collegiate men folkstyle: 10 weight classes
- USA collegiate women folkstyle: 8 weight classes
- USA high school folkstyle: 14 weight classes

Weight Management

- Wrestlers have traditionally wrestled in the lowest weight class possible in the belief that this will give them a competitive advantage.
- Eighty-five percent of US HS wrestlers lose over 10% of body weight to achieve their competitive wrestling weight.
- In-season weight loss occurs through frequent weight cycles involving rapid weight loss and then weight gain after a competition.
- Surveys have found that HS and college wrestlers lose an average of 3.5–5.5 kg of weight in week preceding match.
- Most commonly used method of rapid weight loss is sweating combined with fluid and caloric restriction.
- Diuretics, laxatives, and vomiting are less frequently used, with 1%–5% of wrestlers using these methods.

Weight Loss and Health Concerns

- Rapid weight loss of greater than 5% of body mass in 1–2 days is cited as an acute health risk. During 1997–1998 season, three collegiate wrestlers died from complications of rapid weight loss. All three were attempting to lose greater than 5% of body mass through the traditional techniques of exercise and heat-induced sweating with fluid and caloric restriction.
- Long-term consequences of frequent weight cycling are unknown. Impaired growth, eating disorders, and obesity have been proposed, but not consistently found in longitudinal studies.

Weight Loss and Performance

- Impact on performance dependent on level of dehydration, glycogen stores, time for replenishment (i.e., time between the weigh-in and competition), and number of same-day matches.

BOX 88.1 NCAA AND NFHS WEIGHT MANAGEMENT PROGRAMS[a]

- Preseason establishment of minimum weight based on lean weight assessment
  - NFHS: 7% body fat (boys), 12% body fat (girls)
  - NCAA: 5% body fat (men)
- Urine specific gravity (Usg) at initial weight certification
  - NFHS: Usg <1.025
  - NCAA: Usg <1.020
- No more than 1.5% body mass loss per week
- Weigh-ins must occur within 1 hour of the start of dual meets (2 hours for tournaments)
- The use of laxatives, diuretics, emetics, excessive food and fluid restriction, self-induced vomiting, impermeable (plastic, rubber) suits, hot rooms, hot boxes, steam rooms, and saunas is prohibited.
- NFHS: The weight management program should include "a nutritional component developed at the local level."

[a]The NFHS is an advisory organization. Each state athletic association determines its own specific rules that may or may not incorporate the NFHS recommendations.
NCAA, National Collegiate Athletic Association. NCAA Wrestling 2020–2021 Rules and Interpretations; *NFHS*, National Federation of State High School Associations. NFHS 2020–2021 Wrestling Rule Book.

- Dehydration of 2%–3% has little effect on muscle strength and anaerobic power.
- Glycogen-depleted wrestlers reach a performance-limiting level of glycogen within 7 minutes of wrestling. Replenishment of glycogen stores takes 24–48 hours. Therefore, glycogen depletion can have a profound impact on performance during a multiple-match day (e.g., a tournament).
- Weight loss of 3%–6% body fat over 3–4 days even without dehydration significantly reduces average work performance for tasks as short as 6 minutes.

Weight Management Guidelines and Rules

- 1964: NFHS Athletic Associations urged states to pass regulations that included "weight control plans" that would decrease potentially dangerous rapid weight loss methods (Box 88.1).
- 1976: American College of Sports Medicine Position Stand on Weight Loss in Wrestlers called for weight certification based on a preseason measurement of body composition.
- 1991: Wisconsin becomes the first HS athletic association to implement a mandatory preseason body composition as the basis for weight certification. Minimum weight was based on 7% body fat. A nutrition education program for wrestlers and coaches was included. Subsequent studies found significant decreases in rapid weight loss and weight cycling in Wisconsin HS wrestlers. Michigan instituted a similar rule in 1997.
- 1997–1998: Deaths of three collegiate wrestlers while attempting rapid weight loss.
- 1998: NCAA implements five rule changes for 1998–1999 season, including minimum weight based on 5% body fat and moving weigh-ins to, at most, 1 hour before competition (see Box 88.1). NJCAA and NAIA both mandate that their member institutions adhere to the NCAA Weight Management Program for wrestlers.
- NFHS calls for each individual state HS athletic association to develop a program to "discourage excessive weight reduction and/or wide variations in weight." This recommendation became a national mandated rule for the 2006–2007 season. However, the NFHS is an advisory organization. Each state athletic association sets its own rules and regulations.
- Exception to minimum body fat certification for athletes who have <5% body fat (NCAA) or 7% body fat for boys and 12% body fat for girls (NFHS) at preseason body composition

assessment is that these wrestlers are allowed to wrestle at their preseason weight with a physician's statement that this weight is their "normal" healthy weight.

- Very unusual for postpubescent wrestlers to be <7% body fat in HS or <5% body fat in college. Studies of wrestlers at NCAA championships found no wrestlers with a percentage of body fat of <5%, and fewer than 5% of wrestlers with <7%.
- USA Wrestling, which governs international-style wrestling tournaments for all age groups, prohibits several rapid dehydration techniques, such as saunas, "hot boxes," and vapor-impermeable suits at their non–Senior-level competitions. However, there are no other weight loss rules, and there is no minimal weight certification.

Impact of Weight Management Rules in Wrestling

- Average weight gain the day after weigh-ins at NCAA championships decreased from 3.7 kg before implementation of weight management rules to 1.7 kg after implementation.
- Surveys in Wisconsin and Michigan done before and after implementation of their weight monitoring programs found significant decreases in average weekly weight loss, frequency of weight loss cycles, and use of potentially harmful weight loss methods.
- Studies have found that US HS wrestlers will use rapid weight loss methods at international-style tournaments where there are no weight loss rules. Indicates that despite educational efforts, HS wrestlers will revert to previous weight loss patterns if rules are not in place.

SKIN INFECTIONS

General Considerations

- Wrestlers at increased risk because of two factors
  - Repetitive skin trauma causes breakdown in natural skin barriers to infection
  - Close and prolonged exposure to potential skin infectious agents
- Locations: Most commonly infected areas are head, neck, and face, which are the areas of maximum skin-to-skin contact. This indicates that primary transmission is through skin-to-skin contact and not from mats and other environmental sources.
- Infectious agents
  - Viral (herpes simplex), bacterial, and fungal
  - In college wrestlers, herpes simplex virus (HSV) is the skin infection responsible for the most lost practice or game time, followed by bacterial and fungal skin infections.
- Wrestlers with skin infections should be withheld from contact with other wrestlers until it is determined they are no longer infectious. NCAA and NFHS both have specific criteria for return to competition after wrestler has been diagnosed with infectious skin conditions (Table 88.2 and later in the text).
- Designated on-site physician or certified athletic trainer for competition may exclude any wrestler deemed infectious even with documented appropriate treatment from the wrestler's personal or team physician (NCAA and NFHS).

Table 88.2 SKIN INFECTIONS: RETURN TO WRESTLING

Infection	NFHS	NCAA
HG primary	No competition for 10 days (uncomplicated) or 14 days (systemic symptoms)	No new lesions for 72 hr
HG primary and secondary	No systemic symptoms All lesions scabbed over; no new lesions for 48 hr Minimum 120 hr oral antiviral	No systemic symptoms All lesions scabbed over Minimum 120 hr oral antiviral
Molluscum contagiosum	24 hr after curettage	Lesions curetted or removed and covered
Bacterial	All lesions dry No new lesions for 48 hr. Oral antibiotic for minimum 3 days **MRSA: minimum 10 days oral antibiotic**	All lesions dry No new lesions for 48 hr Oral antibiotic for minimum 3 day
TG	Oral or topical antifungal for minimum of 72 hr (14 days for tinea capitis)	Oral or topical antifungal for minimum 72 hr (14 days **oral** therapy for tinea capitis) Participation allowed if active lesions are adequately covered

HG, Herpes gladiatorum; *NCAA*, National Collegiate Athletic Association. NCAA Wrestling 2020–2021 Rules and Interpretations; *NFHS*, National Federation of State High School Associations. NFHS 2020–2021 Wrestling Rule Book; *TG*, tinea gladiatorum.

Herpes Gladiatorum

Description: Cutaneous infection in athletes caused by herpes simplex virus-1 (HSV-1)

History:

- **Primary infection:** Often associated with mild systemic symptoms (fever, fatigue, myalgia) that occur 1–2 days before appearance of vesicles. Vesicles usually resolve within 10–14 days. After primary infection, virus lives dormant in trigeminal ganglion for facial lesions or in dorsal root ganglion for other areas.
- **Secondary infection:** Burning or itching usually occurs at outbreak site for 2–3 days before vesicle appearance. Reactivation can be induced by stress, trauma, temperature extremes, and/or immunosuppression.

Physical examination:

- **Primary infection:** Multiple clusters of vesicles that can be spread out over several dermatomes
  - Facial lesions often associated with cervical adenopathy
- **Secondary infection:** Vesicles localized to a specific dermatome
  - Herpetic lesions in wrestlers often are not vesicular because the lesions get deformed and abraded by local trauma induced by wrestling

Diagnostic considerations:

- High index of suspicion because lesions in wrestlers are often not vesicular.
- Tzanck staining from freshly unroofed vesicle is relatively insensitive.
- Viral cultures taken from the base of an unroofed lesion are most sensitive when done within 24–48 hours of their appearance. Can take up to 5 days to grow and become "positive."
- Polymerase chain reaction (PCR) testing is the most sensitive and specific laboratory test and can detect asymptomatic viral shedding. However, detection of HSV particles on PCR testing does not necessarily indicate infectivity.

Treatment:

- Oral antiviral treatment should be started as soon as infection (or reactivation) is suspected. Valacyclovir 500 mg twice a day for 7 days has been shown to reduce clinical clearance to 3 days (compared with 5.5 days) and PCR clearance to 6.4 days (compared with 8.1 days).

- Topical antiviral treatments have not been shown to reduce viral shedding or transmission, and their use in wrestlers is not recommended.
- Athletes with suspected HSV ocular involvement should be immediately referred to an ophthalmologist for evaluation because of the risk of dendritic keratitis and corneal scarring.

Return to play (see Table 88.2):
- Primary outbreak
  - NFHS: No competition for a minimum of 10 days if uncomplicated, 14 days if general body signs and symptoms (fever, adenopathy) are present. All lesions must be scabbed over with no oozing. No new lesions for at least 48 hours.
  - NCAA: Appropriate dosage of systemic antiviral therapy for at least 120 hours before and at the time of competition. No new blisters for 72 hours before competition, and no general body signs or symptoms. All lesions must have a firm adherent crust with no evidence of secondary bacterial infection.
- Recurrent outbreak
  - NFHS: Minimum of 120 hours or 5 full days of oral antiviral treatment. No new lesions for at least 48 hours. All lesions scabbed over.
  - NCAA: Minimum of 120 hours of oral antiviral treatment. All lesions must be scabbed over.
  - Covering an infectious herpetic lesion does not make the athlete eligible to participate (NCAA and NFHS).

Prevention:
- Herpes gladiatorum (HG) spreads very rapidly between wrestlers
  - Estimated that a wrestler exposed to another wrestler with active HG has a 32.7% chance of contracting HG.
  - Time from exposure to outbreak ranges from 4 to 11 days (average 6.8 days).
- Viral shedding occurs before the appearance of vesicles. Therefore, it is important to educate wrestlers, parents, and coaches about the signs/symptoms of primary and recurrent HG infections so that infected wrestlers can be excluded as soon as possible to minimize transmission to other wrestlers.
- Valacyclovir 500–1000 mg a day during the wrestling season has been shown to be highly effective in reducing recurrent outbreaks in wrestlers with a history of HG infection.
- Consider course of valacyclovir for a wrestler exposed to another wrestler with active HG.

Common Warts and Molluscum Contagiosum

Description: Viral skin infections that can be transmitted by skin-to-skin contact.

Physical examination: Molluscum appears as a round papule with a central keratotic plug, giving it an umbilical appearance.

Diagnostic considerations: Diagnosis is usually based on characteristic appearance. Lesions can be biopsied or excised and sent to pathology for confirmation of diagnosis.

Treatment:
- **Molluscum:** Curettage, cryotherapy with liquid nitrogen, or chemical destruction. Lesions usually spontaneously resolve within 6 months without treatment.
- **Common warts:** Cryotherapy, salicylic acid, hyfrecation.

Return to play (see Table 88.2):
- NFHS: Participation allowed 24 hours after curettage.
- NCAA: Lesions must be curetted or removed before the event and covered.

Prevention: Good skin care. Both molluscum and common warts tend to grow in areas of cracked or otherwise damaged skin.

Bacterial Skin Infections

Description: Classified by the depth of the infection and presence of systemic symptoms (e.g., fever, myalgia, fatigue).
- Impetigo
  - Superficial infection characterized by honey-colored crusting. Can have associated bullae.
  - Nonbullous impetigo: *Staphylococcus aureus*, *Streptococcus pyogenes*
  - Bullous impetigo: Always caused by *S. aureus*
- Folliculitis
  - Infection of a hair follicle that remains superficial and localized to the epidermis.
  - Most commonly caused by *S. aureus*
  - "Hot tub" folliculitis: *Pseudomonas aeruginosa*
- Furuncle
  - Infection that has spread from hair follicle deeper into dermis and subcutaneous tissue, forming a perifollicular abscess.
  - Almost always caused by *S. aureus*.
- Carbuncle
  - Group of interconnected furuncles.
  - Often associated with systemic symptoms (e.g., fever, myalgia, fatigue).
- Cellulitis
  - Diffuse infection of the connective tissue with inflammation of the dermal and subcutaneous skin layers.
  - Triad of erythema, edema, and warmth, with absence of a discrete focus of infection.
  - *S. aureus* or *S. pyogenes*
- Erysipelas
  - Superficial infection of the dermis that produces intracutaneous edema causing palpable skin margins.
  - Usually *S. pyogenes*
- Methicillin-resistant *S. aureus* (MRSA) infections
  - Infection by *S. aureus* species with *mecA* gene that confers resistance to most beta-lactam antibiotics
  - Typical presentation: pustular lesion with central necrosis
  - Can also present as cellulitis, folliculitis, furuncle, or carbuncle

History:
- Presence of fever, lethargy, and/or hypotension indicates deeper infection. Hospitalization should be strongly considered.
- MRSA: Athletes will often complain of pain out of proportion to size and appearance of the lesion. Complaint of a "spider bite" associated with 65% chance of MRSA.

Physical examination: See descriptions earlier.

Diagnostic considerations: Fluctuant lesions should be incised and drained, with purulent material sent for culture.

Treatment:
- Definitive treatment of fluctuant lesions, even MRSA lesions, is incision and drainage (I&D). Use of antibiotics after I&D does not improve cure rate, but may decrease formation of subsequent lesions.
- Nonfluctuant lesions should be treated empirically with a first-generation cephalosporin or amoxicillin-clavulanate unless MRSA is *strongly* suspected. Overuse of antibiotics leads to the creation of resistant organisms.
- If MRSA is strongly suspected, clindamycin, doxycycline, or trimethoprim/sulfamethoxazole should be prescribed. There is MRSA resistance to these antibiotics as well. Check with local public health or infectious disease experts for the MRSA resistance pattern in your area.

Return to play (see Table 88.2):
- Athletes with bacterial skin infections should be checked daily for their response to treatment.
- Wrestlers with bacterial skin infections should be prohibited from all contact wrestling activities until determined to be noninfectious.
- NFHS: No drainage from lesions or new lesions for preceding 48 hours. Oral antibiotics for 3 days minimum. If MRSA diagnosed or suspected, 10 days of oral antibiotics minimum before return to competition.

- NCAA: All lesions must be dry. No new lesions for 48 hours. Minimum of 72 hours of oral antibiotics.
- Covering an infectious lesion does not make the athlete eligible to participate (NCAA and NFHS).

Prevention:
- Most bacterial infections in wrestlers are thought to be transmitted by person-to-person contact, so the most important preventive measure is to identify infections early and immediately exclude athletes with infectious lesions from wrestling.
- MRSA has been transmitted by equipment and towels in other sports. Mats should be cleaned daily. Discourage towel and equipment sharing. All wrestlers should shower with soap after every practice and competition.
- Protocols for MRSA eradication in carriers have been published. However, effectiveness in wrestlers has not been studied. Prophylactic use of antibiotics has been shown to promote antibiotic resistance. A local infectious disease specialist should be consulted before instituting an eradication program in identified or suspected MRSA carriers.

Tinea Gladiatorum

Description: Cutaneous fungal skin infections (tinea corpora) in athletes. Survey reported that 60% of college wrestlers and 52% of HS wrestlers developed a fungal skin infection during the season.

History: Dermatophytes infect the outer epidermal layer. Arthrospores with extended survival time are shed in dead skin scales.

Physical examination:
- Classically described as erythematous, annular plaque with peripheral surface scale and central clearing.
- Tinea gladiatorum (TG) in wrestlers can have an atypical appearance with more irregular borders and less central clearing.
- Also check scalp for tinea capitis. Scalp can be an asymptomatic reservoir of fungus.

Diagnostic considerations:
- Diagnosis is usually made clinically based on appearance.
- KOH prep from a scraping of lesion's outer border can be done to confirm diagnosis, but not very sensitive.
- Fungal cultures are more sensitive and specific than KOH prep examination, but can take 1–2 weeks to grow.

Treatment:
- Topical antifungal creams are first line of treatment for TG.
  - Allylamines are fungicidal, and thereby more effective than the fungistatic imidazoles.
  - Treatment should be for a minimum of 14 days or a week after the lesion has faded (whatever is longer) to prevent recurrence.
- Oral antifungal agents can be used if there are an extensive number of tinea lesions or if there is a failure to clear with topical antifungals.
- Tinea capitis: Two weeks of an oral antifungal (e.g., terbinafine 250 mg a day for 2 weeks).

Return to play (see Table 88.2):
- Wrestlers should be withheld from physical contact activities until lesions have faded.
- NFHS: Oral or topical treatment for a minimum of 72 hours for TG, 14 days for tinea capitis.
- NCAA: Minimum of 72 hours of topical therapy for TG, 2 weeks of oral antifungal treatment for tinea capitis. ***NCAA allows participation if active lesions are in a location that can be adequately covered with a wrap that cannot be dislodged during match.***

Prevention:
- TG primarily transmitted by skin-to-skin contact, so the keystone of a prevention program is to identify and exclude wrestlers with active lesions.
- Prophylaxis with oral antifungal agents (itraconazole and fluconazole) has been found to effectively decrease TG outbreaks in wrestlers.
- Risk–benefit ratio of prevention of an essentially benign condition (HG) with a potentially liver-toxic agent (oral antifungals) must be considered.

Auricular Hematoma

Description:
- Blunt trauma to ear can cause accumulation of blood in subperichondrial space between the perichondrium and auricular cartilage, resulting in a hematoma.
- The perichondrium carries the auricular cartilage's blood supply. Formation of a hematoma separates the perichondrium from the cartilage, thereby interrupting the blood supply (Fig. 88.1).
- If persistent, an auricular hematoma can result in cartilage death. Over time, new abnormal cartilage with fibrosis will form, resulting in the characteristic deformity known as *cauliflower ear.*

Treatment:
- Goals of treatment: remove the blood and prevent re-accumulation.
- For acute hematomas, blood can be removed by aspiration with an 18-gauge needle. Hematomas may have to be evacuated through an incision.
- Removal of the blood leaves a potential space into which blood will rapidly re-accumulate with even minimal trauma. Therefore, treatment should include a technique to prevent blood re-accumulation. Most effective technique uses absorbable mattress sutures to close the space. Outcomes have been excellent, and wrestlers may immediately return to wrestling.

Prevention: NFHS and NCAA mandate wearing of headgear to prevent direct auricular trauma, but this rule is generally only enforced during official matches. International-style wrestling (freestyle and Greco-Roman) does not require headgear.

HEAD AND FACE INJURIES

Brow Lacerations

Description: Eyebrow lacerations make up the largest proportion of lacerations and are typically caused by two wrestlers striking heads. A knee or elbow to the brow is also a common cause of lacerations.

Physical examination: Assess for concussion, facial fractures. Assess depth of wound, presence of arterial bleeding, and neurologic function.

Treatment:
- During match
  - Control bleeding and protect wound by placing gauze over wound and tightly wrap head with elastic tape under athletic tape.
  - Ferric subsulfate (Monsel) solution and/or skin glue can control bleeding. However, these substances can complicate subsequent repair and healing. Ferric subsulfate solution creates necrotic subcutaneous tissue that potentially increases the risk of infection if sutured over.
- After match
  - Suturing the wound will allow the wrestler to continue wrestling and minimize subsequent bleeding.
  - Vertical mattress sutures are especially useful to withstand large amounts of tension placed on a wound during wrestling.

Epistaxis

Description: Usually unilateral and anterior involving Kiesselbach plexus.

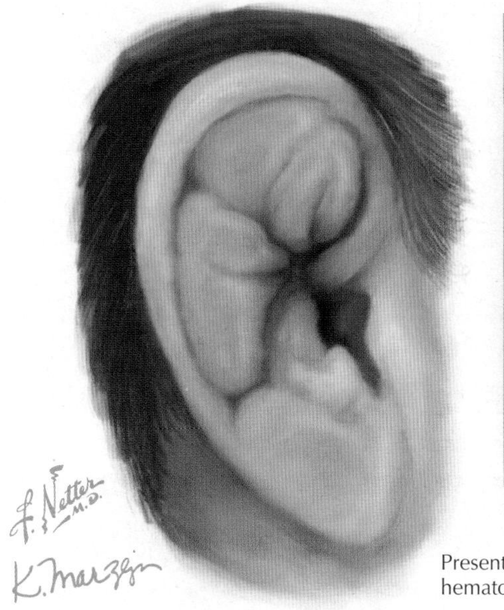
F. Netter M.D.
K. Marzen

Presentation of auricular hematoma (cauliflower ear).

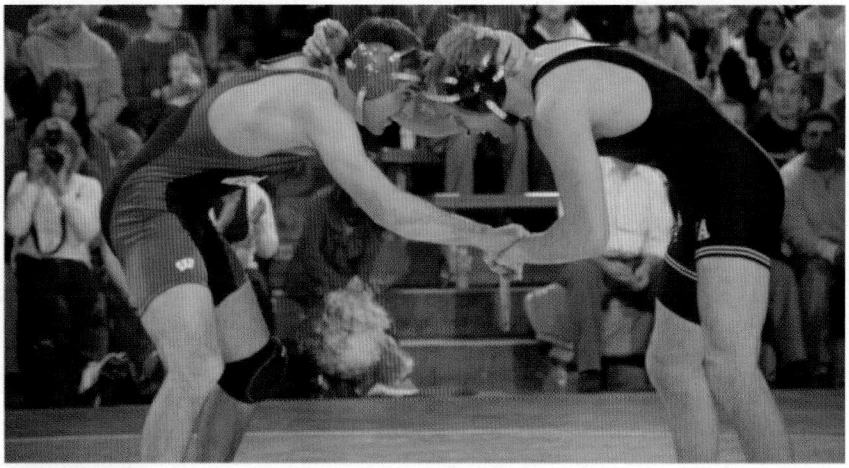

Protective headgear is worn to prevent auricular hematomas.

Figure 88.1 Auricular hematoma.

Physical examination: Make sure a septal hematoma is not present.

Treatment:
- During match, bleeding can usually be controlled with insertion of folded cotton roll to apply compression to the bleeding septum.
- NFHS allows 5 minutes cumulative blood time per wrestler, per match, beyond which the wrestler is disqualified.
- No blood time limit in NCAA wrestling.
- After the match, persistent bleeding can be stopped by vasoconstriction with 0.05% oxymetazoline nasal spray applied directly to the bleeding or used to soak a cotton roll that is placed in the nose for 4–5 minutes.
- Directly visualized bleeding vessels can also be stopped by gentle cautery with silver nitrate.
- Septal hematoma needs immediate drainage to prevent cartilage death. Refer to otolaryngology if not experienced in management.

Prevention: Petroleum jelly can be spread on septum to reduce dryness.

LOWER LIMB INJURIES

Prepatellar Bursitis

Description: The prepatellar bursa lies directly anterior to the patella and can be easily injured with direct trauma, most commonly from repeated striking of the knee on the mat. The bursa can fill with fluid and/or blood.

Physical examination:
- Swollen and tender area just anterior to the patella.
- May be associated with erythema and warmth of the skin.
- Typically, the knee is tender but not painful. Range of motion is normal, with pain only in full flexion because of stretching of the bursa.
- Must distinguish infectious bursitis from traumatic bursitis. Infections occur through a breakdown in overlying skin.
- Traumatic bursitis should not be aspirated because of the risk of introducing infection. Consider aspiration if infection suspected. Bursal fluid should be sent for Gram stain and culture.

Treatment:
- Treatment focuses on reducing bursal irritation through suspension of activity and wearing a knee pad.
- Typical wrestling neoprene knee pads will likely not provide enough padding once a traumatic bursitis has developed, so a large, volleyball-style knee pad is usually required.
- Off the mat, an elastic bandage, simple neoprene, or elastic knee sleeve will maintain compression and reduce the swelling and pain of bursitis.
- A week or two of immobilization and avoidance of direct trauma has been recommended to shorten the healing course, but many wrestlers will choose to practice and compete.
- Once bursal swelling has resolved, the wrestler should continue to wear a knee pad to prevent recurrence.
- Surgical bursectomy can be considered for wrestlers who develop chronic bursitis.

Return to play: Wrestlers may compete with a knee pad if bursal swelling is not excessive and there are no signs/symptoms of infection.

Prevention: Floors around wrestling areas need to be covered with mats to prevent knee trauma.

Medial Collateral Ligament Sprain

Description: Medial collateral ligament (MCL) of the knee is the major stabilizer against valgus force and is frequently placed under great stress in the sport of wrestling.

Physical examination: See Chapter 55: "Knee Injuries."

Treatment: Protocols for MCL injuries that emphasize early controlled motion and protected weight bearing have been found to be successful in returning athletes to full function. A hinged brace can be used to protect against valgus stress and external rotation.

Return to play: Return to wrestling is based on a functional assessment of the athlete more than a specific time frame. When a hinged knee brace has been used after a sprain, it may be used in wrestling competition if properly padded and must be approved by the referee before a match.

UPPER LIMB INJURIES

Shoulder Subluxation/Dislocation

Description: Shoulder injuries are common in wrestling because of extreme anterior flexion, abduction, and external rotation that occur frequently and increase the risk of subluxation or dislocation.

History: Wrestler with glenohumeral dislocation will present in acute pain with the arm typically held in a fixed position in slight internal rotation and abduction

Physical examination (see Chapter 49: "Shoulder Injuries"): Important to assess neurovascular status:

- **Axillary nerve:** sensation over lateral aspect of shoulder
- **Brachial plexus:** hand strength and sensation

Treatment:

- Ease of reduction is related to amount surrounding shoulder musculature spasm, which is often directly related to the amount of time since the injury. Therefore, prompt reduction has the advantage of avoiding muscular spasm and decreasing neurovascular compromise.
- Choice of reduction technique should be based on the familiarity and comfort level of the physician. Some of the older techniques, such as the Kocher and Hippocrates methods, have been associated with more postreduction complications and should be avoided.
- Immobilization in a sling for 3 weeks recommended by some orthopedic surgeons after a first dislocation.
- Physical therapy for rotator cuff strengthening and neuromuscular training.
- Surgery after an acute dislocation has been shown to reduce the risk of recurrence. Referral to orthopedic surgeon to discuss the potential risks and benefits of surgery should be considered.

Return to play: Full rotator cuff strength, absence of apprehension sign

Prevention:

- Shoulder flexibility: Shoulder joint stiffness may increase the risk of injury in wrestlers.
- Rotator cuff strengthening and neuromuscular control.

Cervical Strain/Sprain

Description: Cervical injuries can occur when wrestler tries to resist a force placed on his or her neck by the opponent or while being returned to the mat during a throw by the opponent.

History:

- The wrestler may recall the exact instant that pain began or may simply notice pain after a match.
- Wrestlers who compete in several matches in one day in a tournament may complain of neck pain by the end of the day because of overuse and fatigue.
- Numbness, tingling, paresthesia, and radicular pain should be investigated because these findings indicate irritation or injury of nerve roots.

Physical examination:

- Assess for spinous process tenderness.
- Assess active range of motion. Do not attempt to forcibly move the neck if pain or muscle spasm occurs.
- Assess upper extremity motion and strength
- Imaging studies indicated only after significant trauma, spinous process tenderness, or neurologic findings.

Treatment:

- Cervical immobilization with hard cervical collar indicated when there is concern for cervical spine injury associated with nerve injury.
- Spinal immobilization in absence of lower extremity neurologic signs is generally not recommended.
- Once significant cervical spine and nerve injury are ruled out by examination and/or imaging, treatment consists of pain control with analgesics, stretching, and mobilization techniques.

Return to play: Return is allowed when there is painless neck range of motion and full strength on resisted neck muscle testing.

Prevention: Neck strengthening and adherence (and enforcement) of rules regarding safe return to the mat of a controlled wrestler.

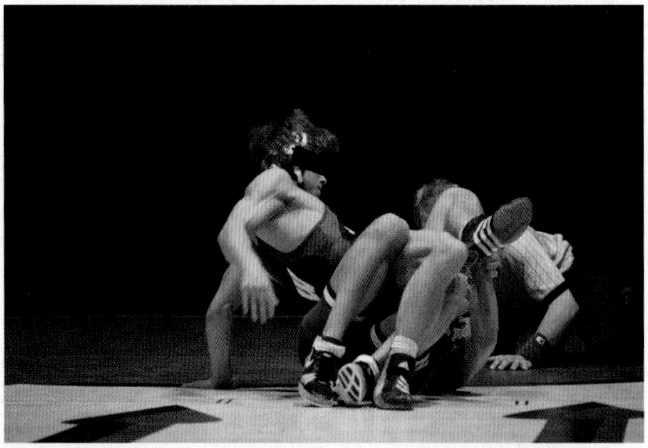

Elbow injuries often occur while attempting to break a fall.

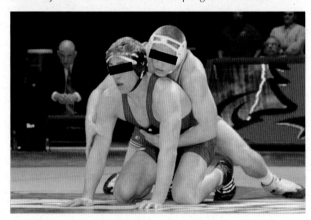

The "referee" position, also known as the *parterres* or *on-the-ground position.*

Figure 88.2 Elbow dislocation.

Elbow Dislocation

Description:

- Most elbow injuries in wrestling occur when wrestlers are lifted off their feet then attempt to catch themselves with an outstretched arm as they are returned to the mat.
- Approximately 80% of elbow dislocations are posterior and are associated with significant disruptions of the supporting ligaments.
- Commonly associated with fractures (Fig. 88.2).

Physical examination:

- The elbow appears swollen with a disruption of the normal bony landmarks.
- Examine the hand for vascular or neural compromise by testing the pulses of the radial and ulnar arteries; capillary refill in the fingers; and sensation and motor functions of the radial, ulnar, and median nerves.

Treatment: Imaging of the elbow with radiographs should be performed as soon as possible because of the high association with fractures. Relocation may be attempted before x-rays if there is a sign of neurovascular compromise.

Return to play: Painless range of motion of elbow; full strength of elbow flexion/extension and forearm pronation/supination.

Finger Dislocation

Description:

- The proximal interphalangeal joint is the most common dislocated finger joint.
- Medial-to-lateral plane dislocation: One or both of the collateral ligaments of the finger are damaged.

- Volar-to-dorsal plane dislocation: Volar capsular ligament is injured.

Physical examination: Neurovascular examination; assess for phalange shaft fracture

Treatment: Reduction can be attempted before x-rays if no bony tenderness or notable deformity of the phalanges. Buddy tape or splint after reduction.

Return to play: May return with buddy taping if no significant fracture or neurovascular injury.

ACKNOWLEDGMENT

The author would like to acknowledge the work of **Aaron Monseau, MD,** on the previous edition's chapter.

RECOMMENDED READINGS

Available online

89 MIXED MARTIAL ARTS

Bryant Walrod

GENERAL PRINCIPLES

Overview

- The popularity of mixed martial arts (MMA) has grown tremendously in the last 20 years.
- Despite this incredible growth, consensus with respect to management of common injuries and proper ringside management of these athletes is lacking.
- Coverage of MMA events can be overwhelming without any basic understanding of either the sport or the ringside considerations for the evaluation and management of competitors.
- Other considerations for ringside physicians covering MMA athletes include weight loss/hydration concerns before the competition and postinjury follow-up/return to training after competition.
- Ringside physicians need more input with respect to allowing a fight to continue and time off after knockout (KO)/technical knockout (TKO) and concussion.

Pertinent History

- Founded in 1993, the Ultimate Fighting Championship (UFC) is the largest organization in MMA. The other major US organizations promoting MMA on a large scale are Bellator MMA; the all-female organization, Invicta FC; and the tournament-style Professional Fighters League (PFL). There are numerous smaller international organizations such as One Fighting Championship and Rizin.
- MMA is defined as a combative sport between two individuals occurring in a ring or cage that uses fighting techniques from a variety of martial arts, including jujitsu, wrestling, boxing, kickboxing, and other martial arts, and follows the Unified Rules of MMA, which were developed to give some standardization to competitions and to attempt to make the sport safer.
  - These rules mandate that there are two contestants in each match who are paired by promoters and approved by the state commissions.
  - Bouts will typically be three or five rounds, with championship bouts most often being scheduled for five rounds.
  - Each round is 5 minutes in duration.
  - No contest should exceed five rounds or 25 minutes in duration.
  - No contestant shall exceed completing more than five rounds and/or 25 minutes of fighting in a 24-hour period.
  - These rules are continually reviewed and updated for optimal fighter safety.

Terminology

- Bouts can be declared by KO, TKO, submission, referee stoppage, doctor stoppage, corner stoppage, disqualification, or a judge's decision.

  KO: A competitor is knocked down and deemed unconscious or disoriented.

  TKO: The referee stops the bout when one competitor is unable to intelligibly defend himself or herself. These include strikes, laceration, corner stoppage, and did not answer bell.

  TKO because of medical stoppage: Laceration, doctor stoppage, or loss of control of bodily function

  Submission: One of the fighters signals to the referee, via either a tap or a verbal cue, that he or she no longer wants to continue.

  Referee stoppage: Referee calls an end to competition for any reason other than a TKO.

  Doctor stoppage: Ringside physician determines that it is unsafe for one of the combatants to continue because of injury.

  Corner stoppage: Combatant's corner "throws in the towel" to signify that they no longer want their competitor to continue fighting.

  Disqualification: Combatant is disqualified because of rules violation.

  Decision: Decision is based upon ringside judges' scorecards after the bout is successfully completed.

Weight Classes

- MMA competitors are divided into 15 weight classes:
  - **Bolded weight classes are the most typical and the classes used in the UFC**
  - Parentheses: uncommon in MMA
    - (Atomweight—up to and including 105 lb)
    - **Straw weight—over 105 to 115 lb**
    - **Flyweight—up to 125 lb**
    - **Bantamweight—over 125 to 135 lb**
    - **Featherweight—over 135 to 145 lb**
    - **Lightweight—over 145 to 155 lb**
    - (Super Lightweight—over 155 to 165 lb)
    - **Welterweight—over 155 to 170 lb**
    - (Super Welterweight—over 170 to 175 lb)
    - **Middleweight—over 170 to 185 lb**
    - (Super Middleweight—over 185 to 195 lb)
    - **Light Heavyweight—over 185 to 205 lb**
    - (Cruiserweight—205 to 225 lb)
    - **Heavyweight—over 205 to 265 lb**
    - (Super Heavyweight—over 265 lb)

Equipment and Safety Issues

- Competitors wear 4- to 8-oz open-finger gloves, supplied by the promotor and approved by the commission. These allow for greater punch velocity and lesser impact dissipation than 16-oz gloves (Fig. 89.1). The gloves have many functions, including protecting the hands of the striker and decreasing the risk of lacerations to the opponent's face.
- Competitors are also instructed to wear protective cup and mouth guard.
- No bracing is allowed, but soft neoprene sleeves can be used to cover knee and/or ankle joint.
- Hair is secured so that it does not interfere with the vision and safety of either competitor.
- Breast protectors, jewelry, shoes, and a "gi" are not permitted.
- No body grease is allowed to be applied to the body. Petroleum jelly may be applied solely to the facial area at cage side in the presence of an inspector, referee, or other commission designee.

Rules and Regulations

- Considerable state-to-state variation in rules and ringside physician's responsibilities; it is critical to be familiar with the state's rules in which the competition is held. Clarification on specific state rules, as well as the Unified Rules of MMA, is provided by the Association of Boxing Commission and Combative Sports (ABCCS) (www.abcboxing.com).

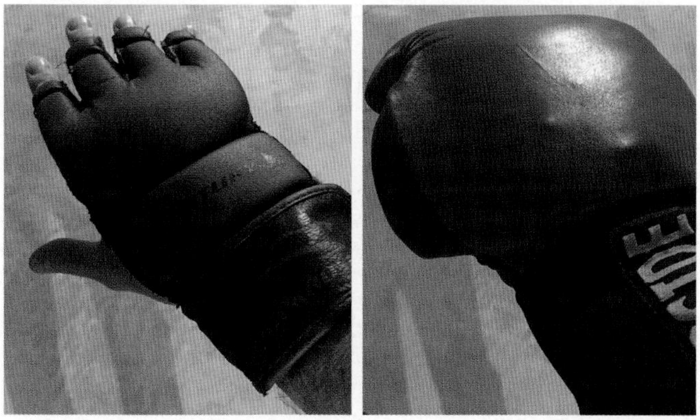
OUTSIDE

Figure 89.1 The glove on the left is a traditional 4–6 ounce MMA open finger glove; the glove on the right is a typical 10–16 ounce boxing glove.

BOX 89.1 LONGITUDINAL COHORT STUDY OF 257 FIGHTERS

- Sixty-two percent reported at least one concussion during their career
- Fifty-seven percent suffered a KO/TKO
- Twelve percent had five or more KO/TKOs
- Fifty-seven percent reported that they "usually" or "always" trusted ringside medical providers
- Forty percent returned to training or competition on the same day that they sustained a head injury
- Twenty-one percent reported that they had returned to training/competition earlier than was recommended by their medical provider
- Twenty-one percent of fighters hid symptoms from their medical providers

KO, Knockout; *TKO*, technical knockout.

- ABCCS has general forms that can be used for physicians to clear an MMA combatant before competition. These include forms for general physical examination, ophthalmologic examination, neurologic evaluation, electrocardiogram (ECG) interpretation, magnetic resonance imaging (MRI) interpretation, and computed tomography (CT) scan interpretation.

Ringside Physician Function Categories

- **Primary**
  - Health promotion
  - Risk factor reduction
  - Preparticipation physical examination (PPPE)
- **Secondary**
  - Early detection and treatment of problems
    - Ringside management
- **Tertiary (largest need for physician input)**
  - Reducing complications associated with previous problems
    - Injury follow-up
    - Concussion follow-up
    - Return to training and/or sparring
    - Return to competition
    - Hydration and weight loss concerns

Prefight Coverage and Examination

- Prefight physical examinations are usually completed the day before competition at the time of weigh-ins. However, sometimes logistics of coverage mandate that the examination be completed the day of competition.
- When preparing to cover an MMA competition, it is important to review the contents of the medical bag. See "Medical Bag Contents" section.

Unique Environmental and Nutritional Issues

- Dehydration is an important consideration during the prefight physical examination.
  - Although renditions of the unified rules of MMA mentioned weight loss and dehydration, the updated 2019 guidelines make no specific mention of hydration status at weigh-ins or at the time of the competition. No specific weight loss strategies are banned.
- Same-day weigh-ins are difficult in MMA because of the potential financial losses from pay-per-view audience reduction if an individual does not make weight and is thus removed from the fight card the day of the fight.
- The typical period between weigh-in and competition is much longer in MMA (24 hours) when compared with boxing, wrestling (7 hours), and Brazilian jujitsu (8 hours).
- When comparing MMA with other combative sports, MMA had the highest percentage of weight loss in the 24 hours before the competition, the highest weight gain between weigh-in and competition, and the highest weight regain 7 days after competition. Multiple studies have revealed that MMA fighters lost about 10% of their body weight before a competition.
- There is often no physician input with respect to weight loss strategies: MMA fighters are more often to consult their teammates, coaches, or even their opponent before consulting their physicians. One study specifically asked about physician input with respect to weight loss before a fight, and none of the self-reported professional MMA athletes asked for physician advice, but rather they relied on teammates and social media (Box 89.1).
- MMA fighters also very commonly report concerning methods of weight loss, with 75% admitting to using a sauna and 63% trained in heated rooms or with rubber plastic suits.
- Water loading is when athletes consume large volumes of fluid (7–10 L) for several days before beginning severe fluid restriction. The goal is to manipulate renal hormones and urine output and increase the amount of fluid lost relative to fluid restriction after excessive fluid intake. Sixty-seven percent of MMA fighters admit to water loading before a fight.
- In 2016 the UFC changed their weigh-in protocol
  - Moved the weigh-in to 10 AM on the day before the fight, extending the duration of time for rapid weight gain from 24 to 36 hours.
  - They will also have a 4-hour window in which to weigh in.
  - Ringside physicians will also have the ability to use urine specific gravity (USG) tests to determine a fighter's hydration status and will have the ability to pull the competitor out of the fight for safety reasons
- One championship instituted stricter measurements in 2015 after a Chinese fighter died from weight cutting.
  - Intravenous fluid hydration was banned
  - Fighters were subjected to multiple days of weigh-ins and USG tests to ascertain hydration levels and the fighter's "walking weight"
  - Athletes cannot drop a weight class less than 8 weeks out from an event
  - Final weigh-ins are 3 hours before a fight
- **For a study examining weight loss in MMA fighters, see Box 89.2**
- **For a hydration study in MMA fighters, see Box 89.3**
- **For a study examining rapid weight loss and weight gain on fight outcome, see Box 89.4**

BOX 89.2 EXTREME WEIGHT LOSS AND GAIN IN MMA FIGHTERS

- 8.0 ± 1.8% body mass loss in the rapid weight loss (RWL) period
- 11.7 ± 4.7% body mass gain in the rapid weight gain (RWG) period
  - One athlete lost 10.8% and gained 20.6%
- Urine osmolality: significantly increased from baseline to weigh-in and significant decrease from weigh-in to competition
- All admitted to using a sauna suit and water loading

Data from Barley OR, Chapman, DW, Abbiss, CR. Weight loss strategies in combat sports and concerning habits in mixed martial arts. *Int J Sport Physiol Perform*. 2018;13(7):933–939.

BOX 89.3 HYDRATION STUDY IN MMA FIGHTERS[a]

- Body mass increased 4.4% in the 22-hour period before the competition.
- Similar to a body mass increase in college wrestlers before new rule implementation (4.9%).
- After the rule change, college wrestlers now have 1.2% weight gain.
- Thirty-nine percent significantly dehydrated 2 hours before event (USG > 1.021)
- Eleven percent seriously dehydrated (USG > 1.030)
- Twenty-three percent well hydrated (USG < 1.010)
- It is yet to be determined if these findings will influence rule changes with respect to hydration and weight loss.

[a]Fighters were weighed at the official weigh-in (24 hours before the bout) and then reweighed about 22 hours later (2 hours before the bout). Fighters provided a urine sample at each of these times and had a skin fold analysis to determine body density during the official weigh-in.
USG, Urine specific gravity.
Data from Jetton AM, Lawrence MM, Meucci M, et al. Dehydration and acute weight gain in mixed martial arts fighters before competition. *J Strength Cond Res*. 2013;27(5):1322–1326.

BOX 89.4 RAPID WEIGHT LOSS AND WEIGHT GAIN ON FIGHT OUTCOME

- Body mass (BM) data from 75 MMA fighters (73 men, 2 women)
- All weights except heavyweight, amateur, and professional
- Self-reported precut body mass 7 days before competition
- Weighed 24 hours before and immediately after fight
- Fight outcome analyzed
- Cutting greater amounts of BM significantly correlates with losing fight
  - Loss: cut 10.6%
  - Win: cut 8.6%

Data from Brechney, GC, Chia, E. Moreland, AT. Weight cutting implications for competition outcomes in mixed martial arts cage fighting. *J Strength Cond Res*. 2019.

Day-of-Fight Considerations, Match Coverage, and Injury Patterns

- Important considerations for an emergency action plan:
  - The physician needs to ensure that they have a reserved seat ringside with an unobstructed view and easy access to the ring if they are called to enter.
  - Medical team: If a single person is covering, competition may need to be temporarily suspended if the need arises to attend to an injured fighter. This delay may not be acceptable to ringside fans or the television audience.
  - Emergency medical services (EMS) must be present. It is imperative for the physician to introduce themselves to the EMS team and cover specific responsibilities.
  - If the physician provides laceration repair or intravenous fluid replacement therapy, it is important to arrange for appropriate follow-up after the competition.
  - If there is a large card, consider contacting the closest level one trauma center to inform them of the local MMA competition that will be occurring.
- It is important to meet with the referee before the competition to review responsibilities and to provide an opportunity to ask any questions (i.e., appropriate equipment, roles of individuals at ringside [cutmen, cornermen])
- During the competition, the physician may be asked to enter the ring, but one may not do so unless summoned by the referee.
  - If the physician is asked to enter the ring during the competition, the physician may examine the fighter but not treat him or her (e.g., the physician can wipe away blood to examine a cut, but one may not actively treat the laceration).
  - The physician can only determine if the fighter is able to continue or should be disqualified for medical reasons.
- It is important to take control of the situation.
  - Often, the competitor's cornermen will attempt to enter the ring to assist their down fighter. This action must be prohibited because moving an injured fighter carries significant risk if not paying attention to cervical spine precautions.
- The establishment of a unified team approach, where each individual clearly knows his or her responsibilities, is paramount to the maintenance of fighter safety.

Groin Fouls (Time Considerations)

- Fighters injured severely enough by a groin foul to require medical consultation may be given up to 5 minutes, at the referee's discretion, for evaluation by the ringside physician before a decision to continue is rendered. If the competitor is able to continue, the contestant may have up to 5 minutes to recover.

Accidental Fouls

- If a fighter is fouled by a blow that the referee deems illegal, the referee should stop the action and call for time. The referee may have the ringside doctor examine the fighter to determine their ability to continue on in the contest. The ringside doctor has up to 5 minutes to make their determination. If the ringside doctor determines that the fighter can continue in the contest, the referee shall restart the fight as soon as practical. However, unlike the low blow foul rule, the fighter does not have up to 5 minutes of time to use at their discretion.

Loss of Bodily Function

- If a fighter, during the course of a round, visibly loses control of bodily function (e.g., vomitus, urine, feces), the fight shall be stopped by the referee and the fighter shall lose the contest by a TKO because of medical stoppage.
  - In the event a loss of bodily function occurs in the rest period between rounds, the ringside physician shall be called in to evaluate if the combatant can continue. If the combatant is not cleared by the ringside physician to continue, that combatant shall lose by a TKO because of medical stoppage.
  - If fecal matter becomes apparent at any time, the contest shall be halted by the referee, and the offending combatant shall lose by a TKO because of medical stoppage.

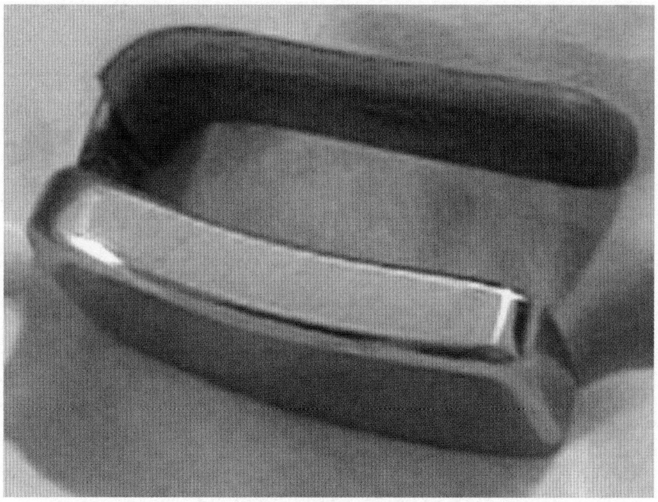

Figure 89.2 Enswell.

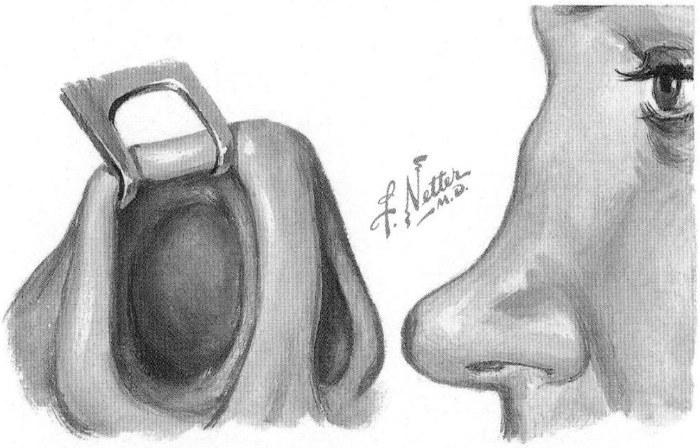
Examination for septal hematoma.
Cartilaginous deformity secondary to untreated septal hematoma.

Figure 89.3 Nasal fracture.

Laceration Management

- The ringside physician should be able to provide care for contusions and basic lacerations.
- Some teams and/or promoters will provide a "cutman" for the competitors.
  - The experience of cutmen varies greatly.
  - Cutmen do not replace a physician's medical expertise with respect to deciding whether a fighter is qualified to continue or whether a fighter should be disqualified because of a laceration.
- If the physician is asked to tend to a laceration, the physician may only treat the laceration in between rounds.
  - Applying pressure with sterile gauze or a large cotton swab is the best first-line treatment.
  - Also consider petroleum jelly.
  - The only substances that are permitted for administration are a solution of adrenaline 1:1000, Avitene, or thrombin.
  - An enswell is another helpful instrument to have in the medical bag (Fig. 89.2); it is a frozen piece of steel that can help reduce facial swelling and contusions.
  - Typically, lacerations involving the medial aspect of the eye and those that cross the vermillion border of the lip should be referred for subspecialty care.
- The presence of periorbital lacerations or contusions that obstruct vision form potential grounds to disqualify a fighter.
- Epistaxis is also common.
  - Application of direct pressure is typically effective; also consider petroleum jelly.
- Observe for presence of septal hematoma or nasal fracture (Fig. 89.3)

COMMON INJURIES AND MEDICAL PROBLEMS

- For summaries from studies of common MMA injuries and medical problems, see Boxes 89.5 to 89.13 and Table 89.1.
- Ringside physicians must be proficient in basic life support, cervical spine evaluation, and assisting with cervical spine immobilization and transport.
- Knowledge of basic fracture/dislocation and splint care is critical.
  - Finger and elbow dislocations (see Figs. 50.7, 51.4, 51.5, 51.10) from striking and arm bars are common.
  - An attempt to reduce the joint should be performed ringside, with subsequent postreduction radiographic films being obtained.

BOX 89.5 VIDEO ANALYSIS OF 642 MMA MATCHES

- Seventy-two percent ended secondary to injury.
- Twenty-eight percent of competitors suffered closed head trauma.
- Severity of injuries and concussion rate were difficult to ascertain secondary to video analysis.

Data from Buse GJ. No holds barred sport fighting: a 10 year review of mixed martial arts competition. *Br J Sports Med.* 2006;40(2):169–172.

BOX 89.6 RETROSPECTIVE REVIEW OF RINGSIDE PHYSICIAN REPORTS FROM 171 MATCHES

- Overall injury rate: 28.6/100 participants
- Facial lacerations: 47.9%
- Hand injuries: 13.5%
- Nose injuries: 10.9%
- Eye injuries: 8.3%
- Risk of injury increased with:
  - Age
  - Losing a match
  - Losing a match by KO or TKO
  - Match going into rounds 4 or 5
- Outcome of match:
  - TKO: 39.8%
  - Tap out: 30.4%
  - Decision: 18.1%
  - KO: 6.4%
  - Choke: 2.3%
  - Disqualification: 1.8%
  - Draw: 1.2%

KO, Knockout; *TKO,* technical knockout.
Data from Bledsoe GH. Mixed martial arts. *Combat Sports Medicine*. 2008;323–330.

BOX 89.7 RETROSPECTIVE REVIEW OF 635 MMA MATCHES

- Injury of 23.6/100 fight participants
- Lacerations and upper extremity injuries were the most common.
- Age, weight, and fight experience had no impact on injury rate.
- The losing fighter was 2.53 times more likely to be injured.

Data from Ngai KM, Levy F, Hsu EB. Injury trends in sanctioned mixed martial arts competition: a 5-year review from 2002 to 2007. *Br J Sports Med.* 2008;42(8):686–689.

BOX 89.8 RETROSPECTIVE REVIEW OF INJURY TRENDS WHILE TRAINING FOR MMA EVENTS

- Males were more likely to be injured.
- Seventy-eight percent occurred in training; 22% occurred in competition
- The most common areas to be injured were:
  - Head and neck: 38%
  - Lower and upper extremities: 30% and 22%, respectively
- The most common injuries were:
  - Contusions: 29%
  - Miscellaneous strains: 16%
  - Concussions: 1.8%
- MMA styles associated with the highest injury rates in descending order:
  - Jujitsu, freestyle wrestling, wrestling, and then kickboxing
- A lower belt rank correlated with an increased risk of injury.
- Professional fighters were three times more likely to get injured than amateur fighters.

Data from Rainey CE. Determining the prevalence and assessing the severity of injuries in mixed martial arts athletes. *N Am J Sports Phys Ther*. 2009;4(4):190–199.

BOX 89.9 DATA FROM 711 MMA BOUTS (2178 ROUNDS OF EXPOSURE)

The most common injuries were:
- Lacerations and abrasions: 38%
- Altered mental state: 21.5%
- Fractures: 16.5%.

Injuries were more common in:
- Professionals vs. amateurs
- Later rounds of the fight
- Bouts ending in KO/TKO

Injuries were less likely in bouts that ended in submission, decision, or disqualification compared with a KO/TKO.

The rate of injury in bouts ending in strikes was 9.1%, whereas the rate of injury in bouts ending by decision, choke, or lock was 4.0%.

A diagnosis of altered mental status was made in:
- 0.2% of bouts ended by submission, decision, or disqualification
- 4.2% of bouts decided by KO/TKO

A diagnosis of altered mental status was made in:
- 3.5% of bouts ended by strikes
- 0.2% of bouts ended by submission, choke, or lock

KO, Knockout; *TKO*, technical knockout.
Data from McClain R. Injury profile of mixed martial arts competitors. *Clin J Sport Med*. 2014;24(6):497–501.

  - Fractures of the metacarpals, carpals, metatarsals, and tarsals also occur commonly.
- The ringside physician should also maintain a high index of suspicion for orbital floor fractures (see Chapter 47: "Eye Injuries," "Orbital Fractures" section and Fig. 47.3)
- Head trauma
  - For summaries from studies of MMA head trauma, see Boxes 89.10 to 89.13.

Concussion Management

It is imperative to understand concussion management (see Chapter 45: "Head Injuries"); the official statement with respect to concussions from the unified rules of MMA is:

Before allowing a fight to continue, the Referee should consult with the Ringside Physician in all cases involving concussive head fouls. The Referee, in conjunction with the Ringside Physician, will determine the length of time needed to evaluate the affected athlete and his or her suitability to continue.

BOX 89.10 DATA FROM THE NEVADA ATHLETIC COMMISSION OBTAINED FROM UFC FIGHTS

- Sixty percent reported no injury
- Forty percent complained of injury
- Overall injury rate: 39.7/100
- The face, as well as the lower and upper extremities, was the most common location of injury.
- The types of injuries recorded were:
  - Facial laceration/soft tissue: 19.2%
  - Facial fractures: 4.6%
  - Eye injury: 2%
  - Knee, shoulder, and hand injury: 1%
- Ten percent of fighters were sent to the ED or were instructed to obtain x-rays.
  - Eleven percent had CT scans
  - Fifty-two percent were negative
  - Thirty-eight percent revealed a new fracture (facial bones)
  - One percent had soft tissue injury
  - No CT scan revealed any intracranial soft tissue or vascular abnormalities
- An increased injury rate was observed for losses via tap out by arm bar, TKO, or a decision.
- A loss via KO/TKO increased the risk of having a facial fracture 20-fold.

CT, Computed tomography; *ED*, emergency department; *KO*, knockout; *TKO*, technical knockout.
Data from Otten MH. Ultimate Fighting Championship injuries: a two-year retrospective fight injury study. *Osteopath Family Physician*. 2015;7:13–18.

Mandatory Time Off: Variable

- **There is significant variability from state to state with respect to return to practice/competition after a KO, TKO, or concussion.**
- The Association of Ringside Physicians (ARP) consensus statement says: "Currently, there are no general requirements for combat sports athletes to be evaluated by a licensed healthcare provider specifically trained in the evaluation and management of concussion as a part of medical clearance to RTS following a concussion or TKO/KO."
- The ARP recommends baseline neuropsychological (NP) evaluation and to consider baseline balance/vestibular testing. Repeat testing is recommended annually.
  - Currently, no known combat sports organization baseline offers formal NP or computerized NP testing.
- **ARP consensus statement recommendations**
  - If a fighter is exhibiting signs of a concussion during a bout, the fight should be stopped. These signs include but are not limited to headache, confusion, blurred/double vision, nausea/vomiting, and balance/gait issues.
  - If a combat sports athlete sustains a TKO secondary to blows to the head, the recommendation is suspension from competition and sparring for a minimum of 30 days.
  - If a combat sports athlete sustains a KO without loss of consciousness (LOC) secondary to blows to the head, the recommendation is suspension from competition and sparring for a minimum of 60 days.
  - If a combat sports athlete sustains a KO with LOC secondary to blows to the head, the recommendation is suspension from competition and sparring for a minimum of 90 days.
  - All combat sports athletes, including the winners, should be evaluated for signs and symptoms of concussion postbout.

BOX 89.11 VIDEO RECORDS OF 844 UFC MATCHES FOR THE IDENTIFICATION OF THE PRINCIPAL MECHANISMS AND SITUATIONAL FACTORS ASSOCIATED WITH KOs AND TKOs SECONDARY TO REPETITIVE STRIKES[a]

With respect to matches:
- 55% ended before their scheduled time
- 12.8% ended in KO
- 21.2% ended in TKO
- 90% ending in TKO were the result of repetitive strikes

They also found:
- Incidence of KO: 6.4/100 athlete exposures (AEs)
- Incidence of TKO: 9.5/100 AEs

Increased risk of KO was associated with:
- Previous KO/TKO: odds risk (OR) 1.30
- Age >35 years: OR 1.94

Decreased risk of KO was associated with:
- Middleweight class: OR 0.44
- Undercard match: OR 0.51
- Each additional minute of the round: OR 0.69
- Additional rounds: OR 0.36

Increased risk of TKO was associated with:
- Heavyweight class: OR 2.12
- Age >35 years: OR 1.96

Decreased risk of KO was associated with:
- Each minute of competition: OR 0.76
- Each additional round: OR 0.64

In KOs:
- The fist was the striking implement in 84% of the KOs.
- The head was the body part struck in all KOs.
- The most common region of head to be struck:
  - Mandible: 54%
  - Maxillary/temporal regions: 20% each
- 63% of those who lost by KO sustained a secondary head impact with the fighting surface (floor, cage, or post).
- The average time between KO strike and match stoppage was 3.5 ± 2.8 seconds; during that time, the competitors sustained an average of 2.6 ± 3.0 (range 0–20) additional strikes to the head.
- In the 30 seconds preceding the KO strike, the losing competitor sustained an average of 6.2 ± 7.3 strikes (range 0–35), with 82% of these strikes being to the head.

With respect to TKOs:
- The losing competitor sustained an average of 18.5 ± 8.8 strikes (range, 5–46) in the 30 seconds preceding TKO, with 92% of these strikes being to the head.

[a]It is critical that the ringside physician be aware of these findings and the significant head trauma that occurs in the moments preceding a KO/TKO. This should influence postfight evaluations and return to competition considerations.

KO, Knockout; *TKO,* technical knockout.

Data from Hutchenson MG. Head trauma in mixed martial arts. *Am J Sport Med*. 2014;42(6):1–7.

Evaluation should be performed immediately postbout ringside but also later repeated in a quieter, controlled environment (e.g., dressing room).

- Combat sports athletes may participate in noncontact training and conditioning 1 week after sustaining a concussion or loss via TKO/KO secondary to head strikes, provided his or her symptoms are improving and do not increase in severity with activity.
- A gradual activity progression of increased intensity is recommended, starting with light aerobic activity, progressing to more rigorous/combat sports–specific activity, and finally sparring when symptoms have completely resolved.
- Under no circumstances should a combat sports athlete compete or engage in sparring activity or competition if he or she is experiencing signs and symptoms of concussion.

BOX 89.12 RETROSPECTIVE REVIEW OF 1903 UFC MMA FIGHTS

Weight

- Males
  - Decreased risk of KO/TKO in Flyweight (−62%)
  - Increased risk of KO/TKO
    - Heavyweight (+206%)
    - Light Heavyweight (+100%)
    - Middleweight (+80%)
- Females
  - Bantamweight (+221%) increased risk of KO/TKO

Sex

- Seventy-five percent of male fights ended with strikes to the head
- Fifty-nine percent of female fights ended with strikes to the head

KO, Knockout; *TKO,* technical knockout.

Data from Follmer B, Dellangrana RA, Xehr EP. Head trauma exposure in mixed martial arts varies according to sex and weight class. *Sports Health.* 2019;11(3):290–285.

BOX 89.13 MUSCULOSKELETAL AND HEAD INJURIES IN THE UFC

- Two hundred and ninety-one injuries in 285 fights in 9 weight divisions
- Overall injury rate 51/100 AEs. More common in males (54/100) than females (30/100)
  - Head injury: 34/100 AEs
  - Lower limb: 9/100 AEs
  - Upper limb: 8/100 AEs
- KOs/TKOs were significantly more common in matches involving males (36%) than females (14%)
- Head injuries were significantly more common in matches that ended in KO/TKOs (38%) than decision (23%) or submission (6%)
- As weight division increased, KO injury rates increase, whereas submission and decision injury rates decrease

AE, Athletic exposure; *KO,* knockout; *TKO,* technical knockout.

Data from Fares MY. Musculoskeletal and head injuries in the UFC. *Phys Sportsmed*. 2019;47(2):205–211.

- In addition to the earlier mentioned periods of suspension, we recommended that a combat sports athlete's suspension continue until a specialist physician trained in concussion management clears the fighter. Specialist physicians trained in concussion management include neurologists, neurosurgeons, and primary care sports medicine physicians
- A physician may issue a medical suspension any time he or she believes it to be in the best interest for the safety of a boxer (i.e., high blood pressure at the prefight physical examination).
- In any and all cases, the decision by the physician to issue or extend a suspension is final.
- Returning to practice and competition can be logistically difficult for a fighter.
- Covering ringside physicians can provide recommendations with respect to return to practice; however, this can be difficult to enforce, and follow-up is difficult if the competitors are from different cities and states.
- MMA fighters do not typically have a "team physician" who can administer a baseline or a postfight Sport Concussion Assessment Tool 5 (SCAT 5), follow daily symptom scores, or oversee return-to-play considerations.
- The gym owner and promoter are not qualified to make these recommendations, and often, the fighter will return with no real guidance, which can put him or her at risk of injury.

Table 89.1 REASONS FOR ENDING A BOUT BY GENDER AND LEVEL

	KO/TKO	Submission	Decision	Referee Stoppage
Overall Bouts	29%	55.3%	14.9%	0.7%
Men	28.6%	56.6%	14.0%	0.8%
Women	35.2%	38.9%	25.9%	0.4%
Amateur	29.5%	58.1%	12.1%	11.9%
Professional	27.7%	45.2%	25.2%	1.0%

KO, Knockout; *TKO,* technical knockout.
Data from McClain R. Injury profile of mixed martial arts competitors. *Clin J Sport Med*. 2014;24(6):497–501.

BOX 89.14 PROPOSED RETURN TO FIGHTING PROTOCOL

Phase 1: Gradual return to fitness
- Step 1: Light aerobic exercise
- Step 2: Moderate aerobic exercise
- Step 3: Sport-specific activity

Phase 2: Gradual return to sparring
- Bag/mitt work with movement
- In the ring shadow boxing/drills with gloves and headgear
- One-sided sparring
- Sparring with short duration, long breaks
- Sparring with longer duration, short breaks
- Sparring with normal parameters/sport specific

Phase 3: Full return to all contact training activities

Data from Nalepa B, Alexander A, Schodrof S, et al. Fighting to keep a sport safe: toward a structured and sport-specific return to play protocol. *Phys Sportsmed*. 2017;45(2):145–150.

BOX 89.15 RETROSPECTIVE SELF-REPORTED SURVEY ABOUT MMA TRAINING REGIMENS AND MEDICAL RELATED ISSUES FROM 119 INDIVIDUALS CURRENTLY TRAINING IN MMA

- Fifteen percent reported a KO
- Twenty-eight percent reported a TKO
- Thirteen percent of those reporting concussion-like symptoms during training sought medical attention.
- Sixty percent with postconcussive symptoms returned to training in 2 days or fewer.
- This is an area of MMA ringside medicine that certainly must be addressed for the improvement of fighter safety.
- There must be improved regulations, especially with respect to concussion management, affecting return-to-play considerations after MMA competition to ensure that fighter safety is paramount.

KO, Knockout; *TKO,* technical knockout.
Data from Heath CJ, Callahan JL. Self-reported concussion symptoms and training routines in mixed-martial-arts athletes. *Int J Res Sports Med*. 2013;21(3):195–203.

- In 2016 a Return to Fighting Protocol was proposed for MMA fighters with specific guidance as to return to sparring; see Box 89.14 for more details.
- For a retrospective self-reported survey about MMA training regimens and medical-related issues from 119 individuals currently training in MMA, see Box 89.15.

SCORING

Available online.

PROHIBITED ACTIONS

Available online.

STATE OF OHIO PREFIGHT PHYSICAL EXAMINATION REQUIREMENTS

Available online.

MEDICAL BAG CONTENTS

Available online.

CERTIFICATION

Available online.

RECOMMENDED READINGS

Available online.

GYMNASTICS 90

Amy Jo F. Overlin

INTRODUCTION

- Disciplines: acrobatic, artistic, gymnastics for all, parkour, rhythmic, tumbling, and trampoline (Tables 90.1 to 90.5)
  - Olympic disciplines: artistic, rhythmic, trampoline
- Over 169,000 competitive gymnasts register yearly with USA Gymnastics, and up to 5 million recreational gymnasts in the United States.
  - USA Gymnastics current national governing board and oversees the majority of competitions within the United States.
    - New nationwide governing boards for competitive gymnastics are being founded and may change the landscape of gymnastics within the United States
- More than 70% are female artistic gymnasts

EPIDEMIOLOGY

- Injury rates: vary greatly depending on the level of the gymnast and hours spent training
  - 0.687–2.859 injuries per 1000 hours of training
  - 6.07–9.22 injuries per 1000 athletic exposures in collegiate athletes
  - 42.6–106.2 injuries/1000 registered gymnasts in Olympic-level gymnasts (artistic, rhythmic, trampoline)
- Higher incidence during dismounts and floor exercise in women and during vaulting in men
- Contributing factors:
  - Poor landing technique, including landing short
  - Landing with overly upright posture, decreased knee flexion, and relative joint stiffness
- Sprains most common, followed by strains
- The ankle/foot is the most commonly injured body part, except in nonelite male gymnasts and acrobatics (where it is the hand/wrist)
- Competition injury incidence approximately two times the practice incidence
- High incidence of growth plate injuries because of an immature skeletal system
- Injury risk factors:
  - Larger size
  - Rapid growth
  - Training for >15–20 hours/week
  - Life stress
- Gymnasts are both lower and upper extremity weight-bearing athletes; therefore, injuries incurred during gymnastics participation are comprehensive (Table 90.6).

COMMON INJURIES AND MEDICAL PROBLEMS

Mild Traumatic Brain Injury (MTBI)

Mechanism of injury: Hitting the head on the mat/floor or apparatus during a fall or dismount.

Incidence: One study on club female gymnasts found a 30% lifelong occurrence. An additional study on elite-level male gymnasts had an incidence rate of 5.7/1000 registered gymnasts.

Return to play: Several activities are aerial in nature; hence, the graduated return protocol will have to be modified to meet the demands of the gymnast while maintaining their safety until the athlete has been fully cleared.

Cervical Spine Fracture, Subluxation, and Dislocation

Mechanism of injury: Complex aerial and acrobatic nature of gymnastics places athletes at a risk of catastrophic neck injuries. Cervical spine fractures, subluxations, and dislocations can occur through various mechanisms:
- Landing head first in loose foam pit, on trampoline, or on mat
- Failure to complete rotation or over-rotating on aerial or salto maneuver
- Landing on upper back with neck in hyperflexed position
- Landing on chin or chest with neck in hyperextended position

Specific consideration to standard evaluation and treatment:
- Pediatric cervical spine collar availability
- Loose foam pit injuries:
  - Foam blocks that fill the pit are easily disturbed, and the athlete is typically buried in the blocks.
  - Avoid jumping into pit to help an injured athlete because the disruption of foam blocks could worsen the injury and make it more difficult to remove the athlete.
  - Considering the difficulty of removing a gymnast with a cervical spine injury from a loose foam pit, physicians, trainers, coaches, and local paramedics should practice emergency removal as part of an emergency action plan.
  - Gently placing a mat into the pit and then using this as a means to reach the athlete is one method to minimize disturbing the foam blocks.

Shoulder Injuries (See Also Chapter 49: "Shoulder Injuries")

Anterior Dislocation, Labral Tears, and Multidirectional Instability

- Important to differentiate between instability related to anatomical abnormality vs. generalized ligamentous laxity and multidirectional instability (MDI)
- Surgical fixation, when appropriate, should take into account the gymnast's need for stability vs. the range of motion required in competitive gymnastics

Rotator Cuff Syndrome, Impingement, and Tears

- More common in male gymnasts
- Rings, high bar, and parallel bars all put substantially increased stress on the shoulder

Elbow Injuries

Dislocation

- Upper extremity weight-bearing activities can be gradually introduced, once a gymnast has full range of motion (ROM) and strength in the upper extremity and is pain-free.

Ulnar Collateral Ligament Sprain

Mechanism of injury: Valgus stress to the medial aspect of the elbow causes traction injury to the ulnar collateral ligament (UCL); may occur acutely because of a fall on an outstretched hand or chronically because of repetitive upper extremity weight bearing.

Table 90.1 ACROBATIC GYMNASTICS (MEN AND WOMEN)

Events	Levels	
	Junior Olympic	Elite
Women's pairs Men's pairs Mixed pairs Women's group Men's group	Levels 1–10 Competitive levels: 2–10	Future Stars Junior Senior

See https://usagym.org/.

Table 90.2 ARTISTIC GYMNASTICS

Events	Women's Programs		
	Xcel Program: Competitive Recreation Tract	Junior Olympic	Elite
Vault Uneven bars Beam Floor exercise	5 Levels: Bronze–Diamond All levels competitive	Levels 1–10 Competitive levels: 2–10	Talent Opportunity Program (TOPS 7–10 years old) HOPES (10–12 years old pre-elite) Junior Pre-Elite Junior and Senior International
Events	**Men's Programs**		
	Xcel Program	**Junior Olympic**	**Elite**
Floor exercise Pommel horse Still rings Vault Parallel bars High bar	3 Levels: Bronze–Gold All levels competitive	Levels I–X Competitive levels: IV–X	Future Stars Program Junior National Team Senior Elite Team

Table 90.3 RHYTHMIC GYMNASTICS (WOMEN ONLY)

Events	Programs		
	Xcel Program	Junior Olympic	Elite
Rope Hoop Ball Clubs Ribbon	Levels A–D Competitive levels: A–D Individual and group competitions	Levels 1–8 Competitive levels: 3–8 Individual and group competitions	Future Stars Program Junior Senior Individual and group competitions

History: Valgus mechanism; may be acute or chronic

Physical examination: Findings typical of UCL injuries; evaluate for an increased carrying angle and elbow hyperextension bilaterally, which may be a risk factor for this type of injury

Imaging: Radiographs for evaluation of medial epicondylar avulsion fracture or chronic changes of the apophysis. A magnetic resonance imaging (MRI) arthrogram may be needed to determine the degree of ligamentous tear.

Treatment: Typically, nonoperative; surgery is reserved for complete rupture of UCL and chronic instability.

Table 90.4 TUMBLING AND TRAMPOLINE (MEN AND WOMEN)

Events	Levels	
	Junior Olympic	Elite
Double minitrampoline Synchronized trampoline Trampoline Tumbling	Levels 1–10 Competitive levels: 1–10 First competitive level: 1 (except synchronized trampoline: level 10)	Junior Senior

Table 90.5 GYMNASTICS FOR ALL (MEN AND WOMEN) AND PARKOUR

Programs			
Noncompetitive	Competitive	HUGS (Special Needs Program)	Parkour
Exhibitions and Shows	Power Team: Levels 1–10 Acrobatics and Tumbling USA Gym for Life	Has both recreational and competitive options	Newest discipline Only international-level competitions

Capitellar Osteochondritis Dissecans (OCD)

Mechanism of injury: Repetitive weight bearing causes valgus stress with medial elbow tension and lateral radiocapitellar joint compression.

History: Gradual onset, elbow pain with weight-bearing activities; pain relieved by rest; decreased elbow extension; in more advanced cases, mechanical symptoms of catching and locking.

Physical examination: Tenderness to palpation over radiocapitellar joint; effusion may be present; ROM, particularly extension, may be decreased.

Imaging: Radiographs: If positive will show a radiolucency or fragmentation within the capitellum, with irregular ossification and crater next to articular surface; MRI arthrogram helps determine integrity of articular cartilage or if radiographs are negative and there is a high clinical suspicion.

Classification and treatment of OCD lesions (Fig. 90.1):

- **Type I:** No displacement of lesion or fracture of the articular cartilage
  - Treatment: Nonoperative; no upper extremity weight bearing or strengthening activities until radiographs show evidence of healing and pain resolves completely; consider splint or brace if pain not relieved by discontinuing upper extremity weight-bearing activities or to improve compliance
- **Type II:** Evidence of fracture of articular cartilage or partial displacement of lesion
  - Treatment: Controversial; ranges from conservative to surgical
- **Type III:** Complete detachment of lesion with resulting loose body
  - Treatment: Typically, surgical
    - Osteochondral autologous transplant surgery (OATS) is showing promising outcomes in gymnasts, including improved return to sport with type III lesions

Complications: Loss of ROM, degenerative changes, chronic pain; can be career ending; imperative to identify these early in order to minimize complications; 40% of lesions in female gymnasts noted to be bilateral, highly consider bilateral evaluation given the incidence. Considering severity of outcomes in gymnasts with

Table 90.6 DIFFERENTIAL DIAGNOSIS OF GYMNASTICS INJURIES

Lower Extremity Injuries	
Foot	Base of the fifth metatarsal avulsion fracture
	Base of the fifth metatarsal apophysitis (Iselin's disease)
	Calcaneal apophysitis
	Calcaneal fat pad contusion
	Calcaneal stress fracture
	Lisfranc injury
	Stress fractures: navicular and metatarsals
	Toe fractures
	Turf toe
Ankle	Anterior and posterior ankle impingement
	Distal fibular Salter–Harris I fracture
	Ankle sprains: high, lateral, and medial
	Os trigonum fracture
	OCD of the talar dome
	Osteochondritis dissecans-talus
	Posterior tibialis tenosynovitis
Knee	ACL tear
	MCL/LCL sprain/tear
	Meniscal injuries
	Osgood-Schlatter syndrome
	Osteochondritis dissecans of the MFC
	Patellofemoral syndrome
	Patellar subluxation/dislocation
	Sinding–Larsen–Johansson syndrome
Hip	Acetabular labral tear
	Apophysitis
	Femoral acetabular impingement
	Femoral stress fracture
	Hip instability/hypermobility
Upper Extremity Injuries	
Hand/Wrist	Fractures related to grip lock
	Ganglion cysts
	Gymnast wrist
	Rips
	Scaphoid fractures/stress fractures carpals
	Scaphoid impaction syndrome
	Scapholunate dissociation
	TFCC tears
	Ulnar impaction syndrome
Elbow	Elbow dislocations
	Medial epicondyle apophysitis
	Medial epicondyle avulsion fractures
	Osteochondritis dissecans of the capitellum
	Ulnar collateral ligament injuries
Shoulder	Proximal humeral epiphysitis (Little Leaguer's shoulder)
	Impingement syndrome
	Labral tears
	Multidirectional instability
	Rotator cuff strain/tears
	Shoulder dislocations/subluxations
Other	
Head	Concussions
Cervical Spine	Cervical fractures
	Cervical strain
Lumbar Spine	Discogenic back pain
	Facet syndrome
	Lumbar strain
	Mechanical lower back pain
	Sacroiliitis
	Scheuermann disease
	Spondylolisthesis
	Spondylolysis

ACL, Anterior cruciate ligament; *LCL*, lateral collateral ligament; *MCL*, medial collateral ligament; *MFC*, medial femoral condyle; *OCD*, osteochondritis dissecans; *TFCC*, triangular fibrocartilage complex.

high-grade lesions, maintain a high index of suspicion for this entity in a gymnast who presents with chronic elbow pain even with normal x-rays.

Grip Lock

Mechanism of injury: When gymnast performs circling elements on uneven bars or horizontal bar, overlapping of leather grip against itself causes grip to lock or catch in place. The hand remains stationary as body continues to swing, causing forearm to "wrap around the bar" and fracture.

Evaluation and treatment: Appropriate for type of fracture(s)

Prevention: Regular replacement of grips as leather stretches out over time; routine checks to ensure that grips are not long enough to overlap around bar. Avoid sharing of grips between gymnasts. Use caution if gymnast has been training on larger-diameter bar and then switches to smaller-diameter bar.

Wrist and Hand Injuries

Distal Radial Physeal Stress Injury (Gymnast Wrist)

Definition: Stress injury to distal radial physis

Mechanism of injury: Repetitive overuse of wrist as a weight-bearing joint; forces between two to six times the athlete's body weight can load wrist joint during gymnastic maneuvers

History and physical examination: Tenderness over distal radial physis, pain reproduced with wrist hyperextension and axial loading, wrist extension may be decreased

Imaging: Radiographic and MRI findings suggest chronic stress injury to physis (Table 90.7). Recommend radiographs of contralateral wrist to compare physes for subtle differences. Initial radiographs may be negative. Consider MRI for a more detailed evaluation of physis.

Treatment:

- Decrease or eliminate upper extremity weight-bearing activities until pain resolves; may take up to 12 weeks.
- Use a short arm cast or bracing, particularly if the athlete experiences pain outside of gymnastics or x-rays are positive. Helps to reduce "cheating" during non–weight-bearing period.
- Physical therapy (PT) addressing flexibility and strength deficits; include upper extremity kinetic chain evaluation and therapeutic exercises to correct additional deficits.
- Reintroduce weight-bearing activities gradually once pain subsides.
- Coach should review and correct poor technique.
- Specialized wrist splints (e.g., Ezy Pro brace, Lion-Paws, or Teurlings wrist brace) may be recommended on returning to gymnastics.
- In a cadaveric study the Ezy Pro wrist brace decreased wrist hyperextension and ulnocarpal joint forces during axial loading of a pronated and extended wrist.

Complications:

- Chronic wrist pain
- Abnormal closure of physis resulting in positive ulnar variance
- Triangular fibrocartilaginous complex tears
- Degenerative changes and/or stress fractures in triquetrum, lunate, and ulna
- Alterations in radioulnar articulation
- Extensor tendon ruptures

Scaphoid Stress Fractures

Mechanism of injury: Repetitive upper extremity weight bearing causing hyperextension and abduction of wrist, causing increased forces across the radioscaphoid articulation

History and physical examination: Chronic radial-sided wrist pain, worse with upper extremity weight-bearing activities; tenderness to palpation over the dorsum of scaphoid or anatomic snuff box

Imaging: Radiograph may show sclerosis of scaphoid waist, a fracture, or can be negative. MRI shows edema of the scaphoid consistent with a stress reaction with or without a definitive fracture line.

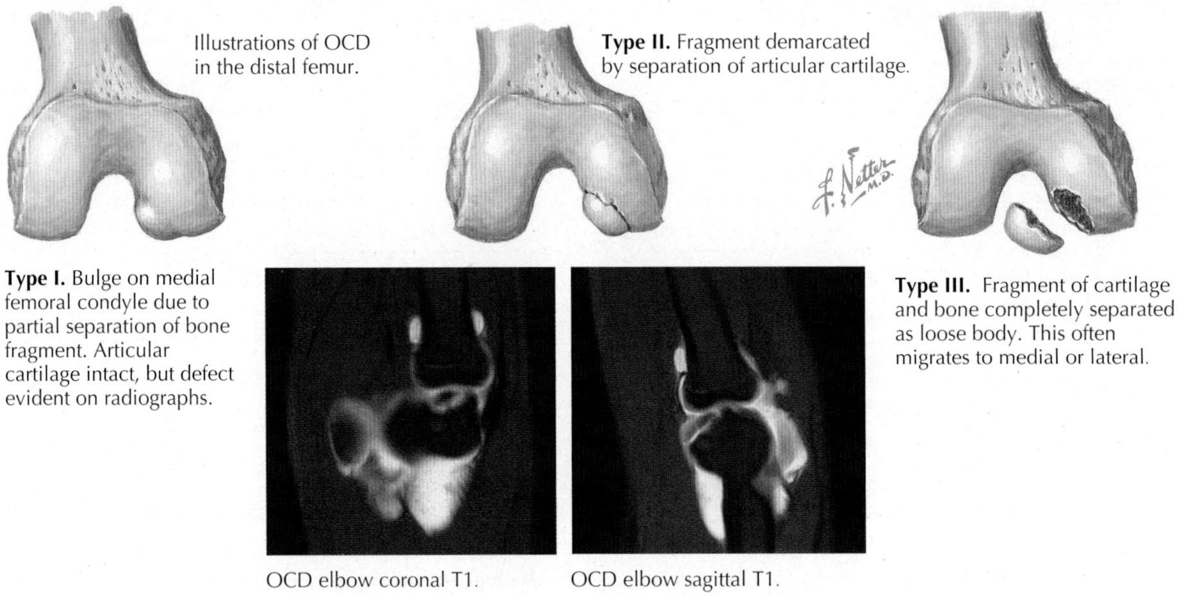
Illustrations of OCD in the distal femur.
Type II. Fragment demarcated by separation of articular cartilage.
Type I. Bulge on medial femoral condyle due to partial separation of bone fragment. Articular cartilage intact, but defect evident on radiographs.
Type III. Fragment of cartilage and bone completely separated as loose body. This often migrates to medial or lateral.
OCD elbow coronal T1.
OCD elbow sagittal T1.

Figure 90.1 Capitellar osteochondritis dissecans.

Table 90.7 RADIOGRAPHIC FINDINGS CONSISTENT WITH DISTAL RADIAL PHYSEAL STRESS INJURY

Radiograph	Magnetic Resonance Image
Growth plate widening	Growth plate widening
Haziness within physis	Lack of physeal homogeneity
Cystic changes on metaphysis	Physeal cartilage extension
Breaking of epiphysis	Metaphyseal "bone bruise"
	Linear striations

Treatment: Thumb spica cast 8–12 weeks; after immobilization PT, then gradual return to upper extremity weight bearing. Specialized wrist splints: see "Gymnast Wrist" earlier. Consider initial surgical fixation if athlete has a recurrent stress injury, has clinical high risk of recurrence, or has failed nonoperative treatment.

Calluses, Blisters, and "Rips"

Mechanism of injury: Several events in gymnastics require hanging, swinging, and support movements on hands while gripping apparatus. Friction between hands and apparatus causes soft tissue injuries to hands. Even with use of leather grips and chalk to decrease friction, skin develops calluses in response to repetitive forces. Calluses can tear ("rips") or blister.

Treatment: Most important principle: avoid infection. Trim torn skin from "rip" and clean with antibacterial soap and water. Protective padding and wrapping should be applied to prevent irritation and infection until the athlete can tolerate friction in area. Consider using DuoDerm Extra Thin CGF Spot Dressing:

- Apply to area of rip
- Athlete may swing bars with dressing in place, held on with athletic tape under grips.
- Change dressing after each bars practice or every 7 days if bars are not being practiced
- Drawback: expensive

Prevention: Calluses should be shaved down on a regular basis to decrease the frequency of "rips." Young gymnasts should avoid overtraining on swinging events, allowing time for calluses to appropriately develop.

Complications: Infection and injuries related to decreased ability to grip bar ("peeling off") secondary to pain

Lumbar Spine

- 5.2%–20% of injuries, lower back pain reported in 25%–85% of gymnasts.
- Weak core and muscle imbalances despite overall general body strength.
- Maintain a high index of suspicion for significant pathology. Gymnasts often present with chronic back pain despite training load modifications.

Spondylolysis and Spondylolisthesis

Epidemiology: Female gymnasts have a 10%–16% incidence of pars defects on radiographs. Rhythmic gymnasts considered highest risk because of skills requiring repetitive extreme lumbar hyperextension.

History and physical examination: Pain walking or sitting for long periods, worse with hyperextension maneuvers, tenderness to palpation over lumbar spine posterior elements, positive stork test, relative loss of hamstring flexibility

Differential diagnosis: Facet syndrome, sacroiliitis, mechanical lower back pain

Treatment: No gymnastics until pain-free; bracing is controversial; aggressive core strengthening program with focus on imbalances and flexibility; important to diagnose early in order to decrease risk of a nonunion.

Degenerative Disc Disease

Epidemiology: Repetitive hyperflexion, increased incidence because of larger focus on "hollow body" position loading the anterior vertebral bodies. A chronic pars defect, either congenital or acquired, increases the risk of degenerative disc disease (DDD) at the disc levels above and below the affected pars.

Hip Injuries

Pelvic Apophyseal Injuries

Definitions:

- **Apophysis:** Growth plate that adds contour and shape to bone without contributing to bone length (for pelvic apophyses, see Table 90.8)
- **Apophysitis:** Spectrum of injury from irritation of apophysis to stress injury

Mechanism of injury:

- **Acute:** Sudden, powerful contraction of involved muscle, avulses apophysis

Table 90.8 PELVIC APOPHYSES

Apophysis	Attachment(s)	Age of Appearance (yr)	Age of Fusion (yr)
Anterior superior iliac spine (ASIS)	Sartorius	13–15	21–25
Anterior inferior iliac spine (AIIS)	Rectus femoris	13–15	16–18
Ischial tuberosity	Hamstring	15–17	19–25
Lesser trochanter	Iliopsoas	8–12	16–18
Greater trochanter	Gluteus medius	2–5	16–18
Iliac crest	Internal and external obliques Transverse abdominis Tensor fascia lata Gluteus medius	13–15	15–17

- **Chronic:** Repetitive tensile forces from eccentric muscle contractions placing traction on involved apophysis

History:
- **Acute:** Sensation of popping with resultant pain in hip; pain may be severe
- **Chronic:** Insidious onset of pain and weakness of affected muscle group; possible recent growth spurt

Physical examination: Apophyseal tenderness; decreased ROM and strength, particularly with acute avulsions; antalgic gait

Imaging:
- **Acute:** Radiographs reveal avulsion
- **Chronic:** Radiographs normal or findings of chronic stress injury
- Bilateral radiographs may reveal subtle differences. MRI may help confirm the diagnosis.

Treatment: Protected or non–weight-bearing, especially in acute avulsions, but also beneficial in chronic injuries. PT to address kinetic chain issues; pain should resolve before beginning PT. Surgical treatment reserved for significant fragment displacement or chronic pain and disability despite adequate nonoperative treatment.

Femoral Acetabular Impingement (FAI)

Mechanism of injury: Congenital bony malformation of hip that with repetitive use causes breakdown of normal labrum and articular cartilage, leading to pain, dysfunction, and early osteoarthritic changes. Hypermobility syndromes with repetitive trauma to labrum and articular cartilage secondary to extraphysiologic ROM causes eventual hip degeneration. Because of the large ROMs required, this can be particularly debilitating to gymnasts.

Acetabular Labral Tears

Mechanism of injury: Repetitive extreme ROMs, including extreme hip flexion, abduction, and extension, increases the repetitive forces placed on the labrum, increasing the risk of tears, can also occur with an acute fall.

Hip Instability

Mechanism of injury: May be secondary to acetabular dysplasia or chronic laxity of the soft tissues of the hip; can be beneficial in attaining large ROM required for gymnastics but over time can cause overuse syndromes related to chronic instability in addition to labral tears and articular cartilage degeneration

Physical examination: Evaluate for hypermobility syndromes

Complications: Increases the risk of labral tear and/or FAI

Treatment: Physical therapy focused on stabilizing hypermobile joint; may require period of rest from exacerbating activities

Knee Injuries

Anterior Cruciate Ligament (ACL) Tear

Mechanism of injury: Landing without fully completing twisting elements, resulting in valgus, varus, or hyperextension of the knee; pure hyperextension mechanism

- Traction apophysitis of the knee
- Tibial tubercle apophysitis (Osgood-Schlatter disease)
- Inferior pole of the patella apophysitis (Sinding-Larsen-Johansson syndrome)

History: Pain with running, jumping, tumbling, and vaulting

Education: Inform gymnast and parents that the condition is limited and will resolve once apophysis fuses; symptom-guided modifications of training

Further workup warranted: Athlete has an acute injury with a pop (evaluate for an acute avulsion of the apophysis), new soft tissue swelling, pain remains unchanged despite training modifications, unable to train secondary to pain

Ankle Injuries

Inversion Sprains

Mechanism of injury: Inversion or inversion plantarflexion; landing with ankle/foot rolled under from jumps, saltos, and twists; stepping off landing mats; foot lands in the seams between mats

Treatment: Standard ankle sprain treatment with emphasis on high-level proprioception and evaluation and correction of entire kinetic chain; ankle taping/bracing may be used until the injured ankle is completely rehabilitated or with chronic instability

Complications: Missed diagnoses, including talar dome OCD, os trigonum fractures, chronic lateral ankle instability, or distal fibular physeal fracture; consider MRI in recalcitrant cases; recurrent ankle sprains most often secondary to inadequate PT

Distal Fibula Physeal Fracture

Mechanism of injury: Same as inversion ankle sprains, often misdiagnosed as a lateral ankle sprain

Imaging: Recommend bilateral radiographs for comparison; may be negative in Salter–Harris type I fractures; diagnosis based on physical examination

Treatment: Nondisplaced, low-grade Salter–Harris fractures are treated with short leg walking cast or walking boot for 3–4 weeks. Once immobilization is completed, treatment is identical to an inversion ankle sprain.

Anterior Ankle Impingement Syndrome

Mechanism of injury: Abutment of dorsal portion of talus and/or navicular against anterior lip of tibia; results from gymnasts landing "short" (i.e., athlete underrotates backward saltos and lands with ankles hyperdorsiflexed) increasing forces across anterior ankle structures; over time, bone responds by forming exostoses that produce anterior ankle pain with dorsiflexion. Cartilage overgrowths (synovial chondromatoses), chronic synovitis, and articular damage also can occur.

History and physical examination: History of repetitive short landings with chronic anterior ankle pain, decreased dorsiflexion, tenderness over anterior tibiotalar joint, and pain to forced dorsiflexion of ankle

Imaging: Lateral ankle radiographs confirm exostoses, can be negative if impingement consists only of soft tissue (Fig. 90.2).

Treatment: Land on soft surfaces; avoid short landings; improve ankle flexibility. Use ankle taping that includes prevention of full dorsiflexion. This includes using a cut-up tennis ball placed on the anterior ankle to prevent full dorsiflexion with landings (Fig. 90.3). In general, conservative treatment provides limited improvement. Consider steroid injection to reduce associated synovitis. Consider surgical intervention for complete resolution of symptoms.

Posterior Ankle Impingement

Mechanism of injury: Recurrent inversion ankle sprains; repetitively performing skills on ¾ pointe; posterior impingement may be caused by a combination of:

- Hypertrophy or tear of posterior inferior tibiofibular ligament or transverse tibiofibular ligament
- Pathology of os trigonum–talar process, subtalar joint disease, and fractures
- Flexor hallucis longus tenosynovitis

History and physical examination: Pain occurs with skills that require ¾ pointe or requires rebounding off ¾ pointe. Tenderness to palpation over posterior talus, posterior tibiofibular ligament, or os trigonum; swelling may be noted; pain reproduced by forced plantarflexion.

Imaging: Radiographs may show presence and/or fracture of os trigonum. Lateral ankle radiograph in full plantarflexion may be helpful to assess any overlapping posterior bony elements. **MRI:** consider to evaluate for stress injury, posterior chondral injury, tenosynovitis (see Fig. 90.2).

Treatment: PT, including entire kinetic chain, flexibility, and proprioception; taping of ankle to minimize full plantarflexion; corticosteroid injection around posterior talus; if a nonunion of an os trigonum is the source of pain, consider arthroscopy for removal.

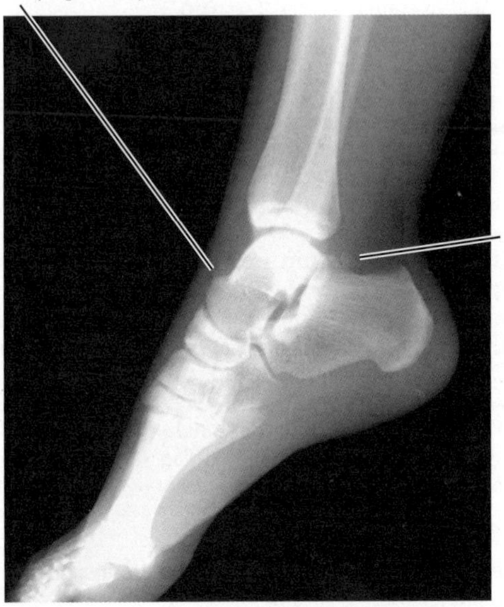
Bony exostoses consistent with chronic anterior ankle impingement syndrome
A non-union os trigonum noted, which can be consistent with chronic posterior ankle impingement

Figure 90.2 Ankle impingement.

Foot Injuries

Calcaneal Apophysitis (Sever Disease)

Treatment: Modification of training, including reducing high impact, perform landings on soft surfaces; use tumble track for tumbling and leaps; see the "Injury Prevention" section. Evaluate landing technique to ensure that the gymnast does not land back on heels; gastrocnemius–soleus complex stretching; tape on heel cups for practice or use Cheetah brace; work out in tennis shoes if symptoms are particularly bothersome.

Prognosis: Persistent pain is uncommon, but symptoms could mask an underlying calcaneal stress fracture, reported cases of subsequent avulsion fractures.

Further workup warranted: See section earlier on knee apophysitis, as same indications apply

Calcaneal Contusion

Mechanism of injury: Landing over-rotated on dismounts, tumbling, and vaults with body weight back on heels; hitting heels on various apparatuses; accidentally landing on a nonpadded gym floor

History and physical examination: Mechanism noted earlier; pain with ambulation, calcaneus tender to palpation and/or compression, and localized swelling and ecchymosis

Imaging: Radiographs if calcaneal fracture or stress fractures are suspected; MRI may be useful to diagnose calcaneal contusion or stress fracture not seen on radiographs

Treatment: Ice massage; padding during weight bearing; crutches (if very symptomatic); heel cups for practice, and/or knee pads (such as those used in volleyball) or Asher Athletic bar heel pads used to protect the heel on uneven, horizontal, or parallel bars; or use basket weave taping of the heel. Correction of poor landing technique and landing on soft surfaces are important to prevent reinjury.

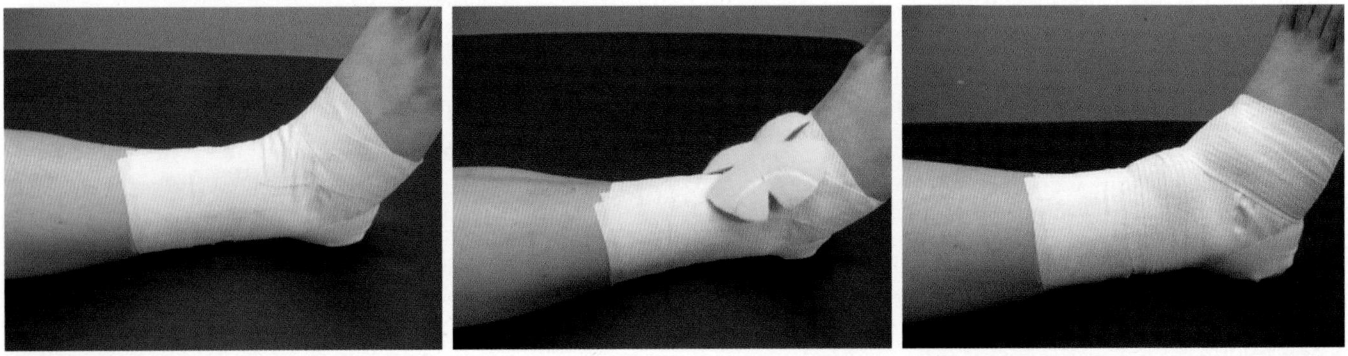

Traditional ankle taping. Cut tennis ball placed along anterior ankle joint. Tennis ball secured with Elastikon.

Figure 90.3 Ankle taping for anterior impingement syndrome. (Photo courtesy of Anna Thatcher, PT, ATC.)

RELATIVE ENERGY DEFICIENCY IN SPORTS

- Epidemiology: The prevalence of relative energy deficiency in sports (RED-S) in gymnasts is unknown. Studies have shown female gymnasts are at an increased risk of disordered eating and tend to have an increased drive for thinness and high rates of body dissatisfaction.
- High training demands with little nutritional education can increase the risk of nonpurposeful caloric deficits.
- Gymnasts have higher bone mineral density secondary to impact loading forces of the sport compared with other athletes and nonathletic controls. This may offer a certain level of bone protection for gymnasts even in the setting of RED-S.

GROWTH AND MATURATION

- Female gymnasts are short before beginning gymnastics.
- Studies suggest attenuated growth during training.
- Catch-up growth during reduced training or retirement
- Studies unclear if "catch-up" is complete
- Cause and effect of gymnastics training resulting in stunted growth has not been demonstrated
- Gymnasts tend to undergo menarche later than general female population
- Bone age lags 1–2 years behind general population, increasing the window for physeal and apophyseal injuries

Pelvic Floor Dysfunction

- High-impact sports, including gymnastics, increase risk of urinary incontinence in nulliparous women
    - Caused by recurrent increased intra-abdominal pressure without control of pelvic floor muscles
    - Stress-induced urinary incontinence most common type
    - May use coping strategies such as frequent bladder emptying during practices or competition events or using a thin menstrual pad
- Recommend pelvic floor muscle training for gymnasts for treatment and prevention

Vitamin D Status

- Studies in artistic gymnasts show an increased risk of vitamin D deficiency.
- Stress fractures in general are common in gymnastics. Besides overtraining or complications of RED-S, vitamin D deficiencies could be contributing.
- Consider checking vitamin D status in gymnasts presenting with stress fractures and treat appropriately.

INJURY PREVENTION

- Ankle strengthening, proprioception, and gastrocsoleus stretching
- Core programs to focus on relative muscle weaknesses or imbalances, including technique during gymnastics conditioning
- Correct hand placement on round-offs and offloading the elbow joint
    - T hand position versus parallel position
- Wrist and forearm stretching and strengthening
- Using sting mats, resi-pits, and alternative landing surfaces to help prevent overuse syndromes
- Use "no crack" training areas
- Teach correct landing biomechanics because of a higher risk of injury during dismounts
- Track gymnast height, may modify training during peak growth velocity with an aim to reduce incidence of injuries during adolescent growth spurt

GENERAL RETURN-TO-PLAY (RTP) GUIDANCE

Guided by the type of tissue injured, body part, and type of injury (acute vs. overuse):

- Tissue affected by compressive forces (joint surfaces, bones), use equipment that reduces impact forces; trampoline, tumble track, alternative landing mats, modify training numbers.
- Tissue that provides power, force, stability (muscle, tendon, ligament): introduce static skills on a stable surface moving towards dynamic skills on a compliant surface.
- Isolated injuries of the upper or lower extremity may allow modified training of skills or continued conditioning that do not require the involved body part, for instance, continuing to train uneven bars while recovering from an ankle injury. Be sure to avoid overtraining the opposite body part during recovery.
- Overuse injuries: key modification is altering volume of training.
- Higher-level gymnasts may have a longer RTP progression because of the complexity and difficulty of the skills they perform
- Sweeney et al. published a more in-depth guideline on RTP progressions for both men's and women's artistic gymnastics. See Recommended Readings for citation.

RECOMMENDED READINGS

Available online

91 CHEERLEADING

Casey G. Batten • Joshua C. Scott • Susan M. Joy

INTRODUCTION

- November 2, 1898, is considered cheerleading's official start date when the University of Minnesota organized a "yell leader" group of six male students for football games.
- By 1923, the University of Minnesota allowed women to participate in cheerleading, but female participation did not start to grow significantly until World War II. Popularity among women continued to grow in the latter half of the 20th century, and by the 1970s it was a female-dominated sport.
- Cheerleading involves a combination of dance, gymnastics, and overall athleticism and has evolved largely in the 1980s and 1990s to what we see today.
- Teams are found at the recreational, club, and varsity levels.
- All-Star teams are focused primarily on competition against other cheer teams rather than cheering for another sports team.
- Organized cheer may be found in three scenarios:
  - Competition
    - Routines are performed and judged based on difficulty and execution of maneuvers.
    - Events typically last 1–2 days.
    - Generally held on spring floors or gymnasium hardwood floors.
  - Performance
    - Participate in pep rallies or engage in sideline cheering and other events, rather than competition.
    - Occur on wide variety of surfaces (e.g., grass or turf, gymnasium hardwood, or cafeteria and multipurpose room flooring that ranges from linoleum to tile and carpet).
  - Practice
    - Regular practices occur at the high school and college levels, similar to that held for other sports teams.
- Growth of cheerleading
  - In 1995, there were 30,954 cheerleaders on competition squads registered in the National Federation of High Schools database.
  - By 2017, there were 3.82 million cheerleaders over the age of 6 in the United States and 7.5 million participants worldwide.

Glossary of Terms

Base: A person in direct contact with the performing surface and supporting another person's weight.
Basket toss: A stunt where bases interlock their hands and launch a flyer who performs a jump and returns to the cradle.
Cradle: A dismount from a partner stunt, pyramid, or toss, in which the catch is completed below shoulder height by a base or bases with a top person in a face-up open-pike position.
Dismount: Finishing the stunt by releasing top person down to performing surface or cradle.
Dive roll: Forward roll where feet leave the ground before hands reach the ground.
Drop: Landing on performance surface from an airborne position.
Elevator/sponge toss: Stunt in which top person loads into elevator/sponge-loading position and is tossed into air.
Extension: Extended stunt in which flyer has both feet in the hands of a base.
Flip: When a person is airborne while his or her feet pass over the head.
Flyer/top: A person who is not in contact with the performing surface and is being stabilized by another person or who has been tossed into the air.
Helicopter: Stunt in which top person is tossed into air in a horizontal position and rotates parallel to the ground in the same motion as a helicopter blade.
Inverted: Refers to a body position where the shoulders are below the waist.
Middle: A person who is being supported by a base while also supporting a top person.
Post: A person on the performing surface who may assist a top person during a stunt or transition.
Prep: A stunt in which one or more bases hold a standing top person at approximately shoulder height.
Prep level: When a top person's base of support is at approximately shoulder height.
Pyramid: Skill in which a top person is being supported by a middle and base layer person.
Quick toss/partner toss: Toss technique where top person begins toss with at least one foot on the ground.
Release stunt: A transition from one stunt to another (including loading positions) in which a top person becomes free from all bases, posts, and spotters.
Rewind: Skill in which top person starts with both feet on the ground, is tossed into air, and performs a backward or side rotation into a stunt or loading position. Flips are limited to one rotation, and twists are not permitted.
Spotter: A person who is responsible for assisting or catching top person in a partner stunt or pyramid. This person cannot be in a position of providing primary support for top person but must be in a position to protect the top person coming off of a stunt or pyramid.
Stunt/partner stunt: One or more persons supporting one or more top persons off of the ground.
Toss: Release stunt in which the base(s) begin underneath a top person's foot/feet and execute a throwing motion from below shoulder level to increase the height of the top person, and the top person becomes free from all bases, spotters, posts, or bracers.
Tumbling: Gymnastic skills that begin and end on the performing surface.

Governing Bodies

- **American Association of Cheerleading Coaches and Administrators (AACCA):** Founded in 1987 with a focus on promoting safety and safety education in cheerleading. Merged with USA Cheer in March 2018, and now safety rules and recommendations can be found at usacheer.org/safety.
- **US All-Star Federation:** Founded in 2003 to promote All-Star–style cheer as a competitive sport; governing body for cheer teams and competitions that are not associated with schools.
- **USA Cheer:** Founded in 2007 as the governing body for sport cheering in the United States.
- **National Federation of High School Sports (NFHS):** Provides rules for high school cheerleading as it does for other sports.
- **International Cheer Union (ICU):** Established in April 2004 and recognized as the world governing body of cheerleading, with over 7.5 million athletes in 70 countries.

Safety Rules

- Rules vary based on league and location, especially for recreational cheer teams.
- Rules for youth recreational (rec) sideline, junior high/middle school, high school, college, and All-Star/club cheer may be found at the website https://www.usacheer.org/safety/rules/cheerleading-rules.
- Youth recreational sideline cheer general rules for all levels:
  - Follow all direct governing association rules regarding age levels, concussion management, heat illness, etc.
  - All skills legal for sideline cheering can be performed on artificial/live grass, rubberized track, indoor basketball court, or a matted surface. No skills are allowed on asphalt, concrete, or any other similar surface.
  - Uniforms must be appropriate for youth rec cheerleading. When standing at attention, apparel must cover the midriff.
  - Fingernails, including artificial nails, must be kept short, near the ends of the fingers.
  - Hair must be worn in a manner that is appropriate for the activity involved. Hair devices and accessories must be secure. In general, hair should be pulled back away from the face and secured.
  - Supports, braces, soft casts, etc., that are unaltered from the manufacturer's original design/production do not require any additional padding. Supports/braces that have been altered from the manufacturer's original design/production must be padded with a closed-cell, slow-recovery foam padding no less than ½-inch thick if the participant is involved in partner stunts, pyramids, or tosses. A participant wearing a plaster cast or a walking boot must not be involved in partner stunts, pyramids, tosses, jumps, or tumbling.
  - Jewelry of any kind is prohibited except for the following: A religious medal without a chain is allowed but must be taped and worn under the uniform. A medical-alert medal must be taped and may be visible.
  - Use of mini-tramps, springboards, spring-assisted floors, or any height-increasing apparatus is not permitted for use at any time other than practices under the direct supervision of someone trained in their use.
  - Participants must not chew gum or have candy in their mouths during practice or performance.
  - Cheerleaders must remain outside of the playing area during a 30-second or less time-out during a basketball game.
  - The only props allowed to be used are megaphones, poms, signs, and flags. The only props allowed to be used while in stunts or pyramids are poms or signs in use by the top person only. A top can hand a sign to a base or spotter with the intent of immediately releasing it to the ground as long as the top is not extended.
  - Participants must not stunt or tumble when the ball is in play, including during free throws in basketball.
  - Participants are not allowed to be in the area directly beneath and behind the basketball goal, called the "free throw lane extended."
  - For youth recreational sideline cheer, allowable skills are dependent on level/age (Table 91.1).
  - In 2006–2007, a major rule change banning basket tosses on hard surfaces dramatically decreased catastrophic injury rates in cheerleading. In particular, there was an almost fourfold reduction in catastrophic injuries from basket tosses in high school and collegiate cheerleading.

EPIDEMIOLOGY

- Overall injury rate in cheerleading is 0.71 injuries per 1000 athlete exposures (AEs), which ranks 18 of the 22 high school sports evaluated.
- Injury rates are higher in competition than in other settings (Fig. 91.1)
  - 0.85 per 1000 AEs in competition
  - 0.76 per 1000 AEs in practice
  - 0.49 per 1000 AEs in performance
- Most recent data from 2018 to 2019 show high school cheerleading injury rates decreased to 0.67 per 1000 AEs (Fig. 91.2).

COMMON INJURIES AND MEDICAL PROBLEMS

- 96.8% of all injuries are in females, but the overall injury rate is higher in boys.
- Falls are the most common mechanism of injury (29.4%).
- Concussions and injuries to head are most common, followed by injuries to the ankle, knee, and hand/wrist.
- Parts of the body most commonly injured:
  - Head (30.8%)
  - Ankle (16.9)
  - Knee (10.8%)
  - Hand/wrist (7.7%)

Catastrophic Injuries in Cheerleading

- Given rule changes, restrictions, and coaches training, catastrophic injuries in cheerleading have dropped significantly. From 2014 to 2018–2019 there were two reported catastrophic injuries, similar to other female sports such as track and field, softball and gymnastics, and lower than football, baseball, wrestling, and female soccer.
- From July 2002 through June 2017 basket toss stunts accounted for the highest proportion of catastrophic injuries (n = 19, 35%).
- After the 2006–2007 rule change banning basket tosses performed on hard surfaces, there was a reduction of basket toss–related catastrophic injuries from 1.55 to 0.40 per 1,000,000 cheerleaders.
- Floor surface types may play a role in the potential for head injury, as different materials have different "critical heights," defined as the height above which life-threatening head injuries are more expected to occur if one is dropped. The most ideal surface is a spring floor, followed by a landing mat over a foam floor.
- An emergency action plan (EAP) should be written, available, and rehearsed for venues hosting cheerleading competitions, performances, or practices.
- Sample cheerleading EAPs may be found on the USA Cheer website at www.usacheer.org/safety/resources/cheerleading-emergency-action-plan.

Cheerleading and Concussion

- From 2009–2010 to 2013–2014, concussions accounted for 31.1% of all cheerleading injuries.
- High school Reporting Information Online (RIO) study: High school cheer female concussion rate 0.28 per 1000 AEs. Less than other female sports such as soccer (0.56), lacrosse (0.39), and basketball (0.33).
- Concussions account for about 6% of stunt-related injuries, but actual rates may be as high as 35%.
- Sixty-nine percent of concussions sustained during stunts, pyramids 15.7%, tumbling 15.7%.
- Most common mechanism of concussion is contact with another person (58.9%), followed by contact with playing surface (37.9%).
- Most concussions occur in practice versus competition and performances.
- A cheer-specific return-to-play sequence after concussion has been proposed.
  - Sequence follows the same principles of return to play in other sports.

Table 91.1 YOUTH REC SIDELINES RULES GRID FROM USA CHEER[a]

Category	Level 1 (10 and Under[b])	Level 2 (14 and Under[b])	Level 3 (18 and Under[b])
Jumps	All jumps and jump combinations allowed.	All jumps and connections to tumbling allowed.	All jumps and connections to tumbling allowed.
Tumbling	Forward and backward rolls. Forward and backward walkovers. Roundoffs. Cartwheels (series cartwheels allowed).	Nontwisting standing handsprings and standing back tucks allowed. No series or connected airborne tumbling and no twisting airborne skills.	Series tumbling allowed. No twisting airborne skills.
Stunts	No inversions (the head can never be below the hips). No release stunt transitions other than a reload from a cradle position.	No inversions (the head can never be below the hips). No release stunt transitions other than a reload from a cradle position.	No inversions (the head can never be below the hips). No release stunt transitions other than a reload from a cradle position.
	A spotter is required for all stunts.	A spotter is required for all stunts.	A spotter is required for all prep-level and above stunts.
	No spinning/twisting.	Half-twist loading allowed. Full twist to a loading position allowed.	Full twist from a loading position to double base prep and double base extension allowed.
	Allow all skills prep level and below. A standing stunt at prep level must be double based and standing on both feet.	Double base extensions allowed. Liberties and liberty hitches at prep level allowed.	Extended liberty/hitch allowed. Single base extensions allowed.
Dismounts	No spinning/twisting No released dismounts (bump down, regrab hands, use a post and pop down, etc.)	Nontwisting cradles and pop downs allowed.	Full-twisting cradles and nontwisting pop downs allowed.
Pyramids	Follow stunt rules.	Follow stunt rules.	Follow stunt rules. If two connected stunts are extended, the connection must be hand to hand/arm. Twisting while connected is not allowed.
Baskets	Not allowed.	Not allowed.	Pencil/timer and toe touch only. No twists.

[a]Skills not specifically allowed in the rules grid are prohibited. Skills from any lower level are allowed at the higher level.
[b]USA Cheer recognizes that there are different age brackets for each organization based on what works best for their teams. The age recommendations provided for Levels 1, 2, and 3 are recommendations and can be modified to best fit an organization. All athletes on a team are subject to the rules for that level, regardless of age. For example, a 10-year-old on a "14 and under" team may perform back handsprings. Regardless of the upper age in the group, coaches should always be mindful of the ability, maturity, and preparedness level of each individual and what skills they are performing.
Reused from USA Cheer. https://www.usacheer.org/youth-rec-cheer. Accessed June 1, 2021.

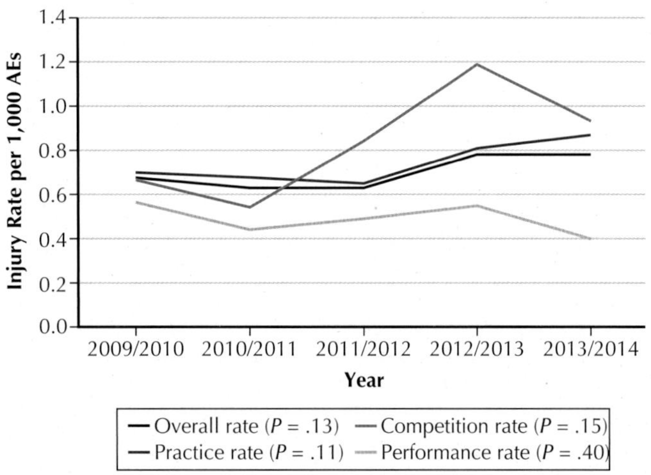

Injury Rate per 1,000 AEs
1.4
1.2
1.0
0.8
0.6
0.4
0.2
0.0
2009/2010
2010/2011
2011/2012
2012/2013
2013/2014
Year
Overall rate (P = .13)
Competition rate (P = .15)
Practice rate (P = .11)
Performance rate (P = .40)

Figure 91.1 Cheerleading injury rates over time by exposure type, National High School Sports-Related Injury Surveillance Study, United States, 2009/2010 through 2013/2014. Cheerleading Injuries in United States High Schools. (Reused with permission from Currie DW, Fields SK, Patterson MJ, et al. Cheerleading injuries in United States high schools. *Pediatrics*. 2016;137[1]:1–9, Figure 2.)

  - With progression, it is important to monitor for vestibular/ocular-based symptoms, especially with inversions.
- Cheer-specific concussion recommendations, including a sample stepwise return-to-cheer plan, are available on the USA Cheer website at www.usacheer.org/safety/resources/concussion-management-return-to-play.
- See Table 91.2 for concussion return-to-play progression.

Other Medical Concerns

- Body image dissatisfaction and female athlete triad:
  - Body dissatisfaction has been reported by 73% of Caucasian and 50% of African American female high school cheerleaders.
  - A study of collegiate cheerleaders has demonstrated that flyers not only had the lowest average body mass index (BMI) (20.8 kg/m^2) on a cheer squad but also had the highest risk of developing eating disorders compared with bases or back spots.
    - For each BMI unit increase, cheerleaders had an odds increase of 0.368 in their risk of developing eating disorders.
- Some cheer teams have coaching-imposed weight restrictions, often based on aesthetic beliefs or focused on flyers or top persons.

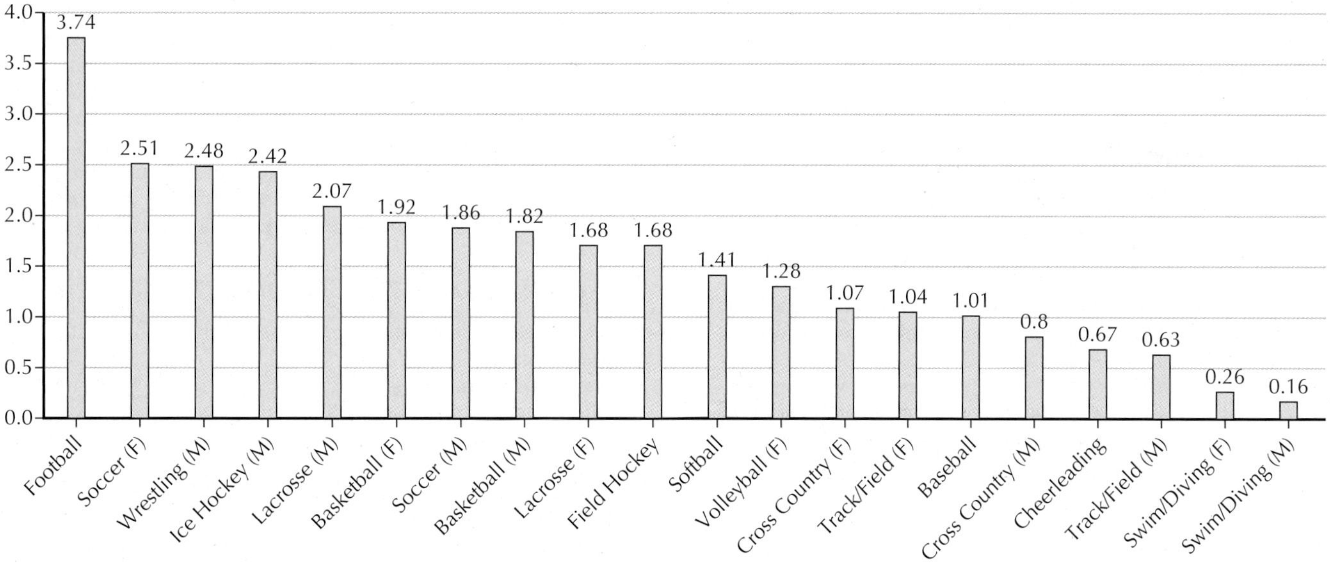
4.0
3.5
3.0
2.5
2.0
1.5
1.0
0.5
0.0
3.74
2.51
2.48
2.42
2.07
1.92
1.86
1.82
1.68
1.68
1.41
1.28
1.07
1.04
1.01
0.8
0.67
0.63
0.26
0.16
Football
Soccer (F)
Wrestling (M)
Ice Hockey (M)
Lacrosse (M)
Basketball (F)
Soccer (M)
Basketball (M)
Lacrosse (F)
Field Hockey
Softball
Volleyball (F)
Cross Country (F)
Track/Field (F)
Baseball
Cross Country (M)
Cheerleading
Track/Field (M)
Swim/Diving (F)
Swim/Diving (M)

Figure 91.2 2018–2019 high school sports injury rates per 1000 athletic exposures. (Reused from Comstock RD, Collins CL, McIlvain NM. National High School Sports-Related Injury Surveillance Study. https://coloradosph.cuanschutz.edu/research-and-practice/centers-programs/piper.)

Table 91.2 RETURN-TO-PLAY PROTOCOL[a]

Phase	Activity Level	Functional Exercise/Cheer Activities
Phase 1	Light aerobic exercise (Target HR: 30%–40% of maximum exertion)	• Slow walking on a treadmill or stationary bike (15 minutes) • Walk through cheers
Phase 2	Moderate aerobic exercise (Target HR: 40%–60% of maximum exertion)	• Stationary bike, elliptical, or jogging on a treadmill (15 minutes) • Cheer activity limited to sideline cheers/chants at a low volume • Include arm motions while allowing some positional changes and some head movement • Light upper-body weight training (50% or less of max)
Phase 3	Heavy aerobic exercise (Target HR: 60%–80% of maximum exertion)	• Stationary bike, elliptical, or jogging on a treadmill (20–30 minutes) • 15-yard sprints (as in tumbling passes) • Cheer activity limited to sideline cheers/chants including arm motions, but may now introduce quick head movement • Mark through dance activity • Begin light lower body weight training activities (50% of max) • May participate in crunches, push-ups, squats, etc. • Balance/proprioception exercises
Phase 4	Sport performance and training (Target HR: 80% of maximum exertion)	• Full weight lifting, agility, and conditioning activities • Light tumbling (hand-supported activities): cartwheels, roundoff walk overs, hand springs • Cradle catch (no basket tosses or flipping) • Simple dismounts for base and flyer • Stunting limited to double-legged, chest-level stunts with added spotter • Minimum 2-minute break between tumbling passes for a maximum of 30 minutes total participation • Moderate dance activity (at three-quarters effort) • Sideline cheers
Phase 5	Full practice, sport performance and training (Target HR: maximum exertion)	• Full weight lifting, agility, and conditioning activities • Limit stunting to double-legged, extension-level activities with simple dismounts and added spotter • Limit gymnastics to basic and moderate tumbling passes: maximum of two rotations with no twisting per any single pass (i.e., roundoff back tuck) • Minimum of 2-minute break between tumbling passes for a maximum of 60 minutes total participation • Full dance participation • Sideline cheers
Phase 6	Full sport/physical activity participation (Pending medical clearance)	• Return to full participation/activity, including advanced stunts, gymnastics, and dances • May practice, compete, and participate in sideline game activities

[a]For use by medical providers in conjunction with cheerleading coaches and advisors. The athlete should return to nonsports activities, such as school, with a greenlight from the healthcare provider to begin the return-to-play process outlined.
HR, Heart rate.
Reused from US Cheer, usacheer.org/safety, last updated February 27, 2020. https://www.usacheer.org/concussion. Accessed June 1, 2021.

- These restrictions, often out of concern for bases and spotters, are not supported by data.
- These practices should be discouraged because they may have detrimental effects on the athletes' body image.

STRENGTH AND CONDITIONING

- Few cheerleading-specific studies have been done; however, other sports such as gymnastics and dance may offer a guide to the development of a cheerleading strength and conditioning program, given the commonality of many of the movements.
- Given the frequency of strains and sprains in cheerleading, the following are recommended to help promote prevention of injury and reinjury:
  - Ankle sprains:
    - Balance and coordination training, in addition to strengthening and stretching.
    - Consideration of bracing or taping, in addition to orthotics and appropriate footwear.
  - Back strains and sprains:
    - Especially of concern for bases and spotters.
    - Training on proper lifting techniques.
    - Total body weight training to improve the strength of core musculature, in addition to that of the upper and lower extremities.
- A small randomized controlled trial in dancers demonstrated that a conditioning program that included aerobic endurance, strengthening, motor control, and proprioceptive training significantly reduced lower back injuries compared with a group randomized to the usual training and educational health promotion programs. These exercises may be especially helpful for spotters and bases who need to lift their teammates up in the air.
- Jump training in prepubertal, high-level female gymnasts has been suggested to improve flight time, which may also be beneficial in cheer.
- Arthrometer-measured shoulder laxity in a group of collegiate cheerleaders decreased after a strength training program, suggesting that this may be beneficial for shoulder stability.

CHALLENGES AND FUTURE DIRECTIONS

- As a relatively new sport, specific research on cheerleading has been limited.
- Data are difficult to collect, especially at the collegiate level, where cheer is often formally classified as an activity rather than a sport.
- Information is scarce for athletes before reaching high school, at which point they may be captured by the NFHS or the National High School Sports-Related Injury Surveillance Study.
- Cheerleading should be included in ongoing efforts of quantifying sports participation and related injuries, given its unique catastrophic injury profile and mix of other athletic disciplines.

RECOMMENDED READINGS

Available online.

DANCE

Craig C. Young • Selina Shah • Laura Gottschlich

INTRODUCTION

- Dance is an activity that can be found in most cultures dating back to ancient times.
- Dance is unique in its fusion of art and athletic activity.
- Dance can increase cardiorespiratory fitness, muscular strength and endurance, flexibility, and bone mineral density.
- Classical ballet provides a foundation for other dance forms.
- Other popular forms of dance include contemporary (modern), jazz, street, tap, Irish, folk dance, and ballroom. Although there is some crossover, each of these forms has unique features and injury profiles.

EPIDEMIOLOGY

A 2011 study of American adolescents found that 20.9% participated in dance, making it the third most common physical activity in girls.

Ballet

Demographics

- Professional female ballet dancers often start classes between ages 4 and 9, with males starting between ages 12 and 16.
- Preprofessional ballet training begins at about age 11 but can start as early as age 8.
  - There is an increase in the duration and intensity of training.
  - Training is conducted 5–6 days per week, ranging from 6 to 45 hours per week.
- The average age for professional ballet dancers is 26 to 27 years.
- The average female body mass index (BMI) is 18–19; that for males is 21–22.

Injuries

FREQUENCY

- Injury rate: 75%–95% of ballet dancers suffer at least one injury per year, with an average of 3.0 to 3.2 injuries per dancer per year
- 1.09 to 3.52 injuries per 1000 dance exposures
- 0.6 to 4.4 injuries per 1000 hours of training

TYPE

- 53.6%–85% of injuries are from overuse and 12%–45% from acute trauma
- Most injuries are of muscle strains, followed by ligament sprains and chronic inflammatory processes

SEVERITY

- The average time lost to injuries is 32.5 days in females and 21.6 days in males.

ANATOMIC LOCATION OF INJURY

- Most common: foot and ankle, low back, hip, and knee

RISK FACTORS

- Intrinsic risk factors for dance-related injuries include anatomic structure, inadequate strength and flexibility, improper technique, nutrition, previous injury, fatigue, inadequate turnout, higher rate of growth, and disordered eating behaviors.
- Extrinsic risk factors include choreography, cold environment, dance floor properties (e.g., surface, resilience).
- Students in summer intensive programs are at high risk of injury because of the sudden increase in hours of activity.

Modern

Demographics

- Professional female dancers start taking dance class at 6.5 years of age, whereas male dancers start at 15.6 years of age.
- Most professional female modern dancers began their dance careers by studying ballet, whereas men began by studying modern dance.
- The average age for female professional modern dancers is about 30 years; that for males is 31 years.
- The average BMI for females is 20.6; that for males is 23.6.
- Professional modern dancers study various forms of dance, including ballet, pointe, jazz, tap, hip hop, African, and ballroom, outside the time they spend in rehearsal for their companies.
- They spend an average of 8 hours taking various types of dance classes and about 17 hours in rehearsals for their companies.
- Most dancers also spend about 2–3 hours per week doing some form of exercise outside of dance such as yoga, Pilates, Gyrotonics, weightlifting, running, biking, and walking.

Injuries

FREQUENCY

- Up to 82% suffer injuries per year
- The annual incidence of injury is 1.2 in males and 1.7 in females
- Injury rate: 0.6/1000 hours of dancing
- The majority of injuries occur in class, followed by rehearsal and performance

TYPE

- Most injuries result from overuse or gradual onset (57%) rather than as a consequence of an acute or traumatic event (43%).
- The most common injury types are muscle strains, followed by ligament sprains, and then other chronic inflammatory processes.

SEVERITY

- Dancers can return to partial dancing after an average of 2–3 weeks post injury.
- Returning to full dancing can take an average of up to 2 months.
- Modern dancers admit to returning to dance with pain.
- Males miss fewer classes and rehearsals as a result of injury than females.

ANATOMIC LOCATION

- The most common sites of injury in descending order are ankle, low back, knee, and foot.

RISK FACTORS

- Intrinsic risk factors: self-pressure, ignoring pain, and fatigue
- Extrinsic risk factors:
  - The demands of the role and from the choreographer
  - Floor characteristics: surface, resilience, raked or not (floor angled down to audience for better viewing)

Irish

Demographics

- The age of professional dancers ranges between 17 and 34 years.
- The mean age of dancers first turning professional is 18.5 years.
- The age of competition-age dancers generally ranges from 4 to 21 years.

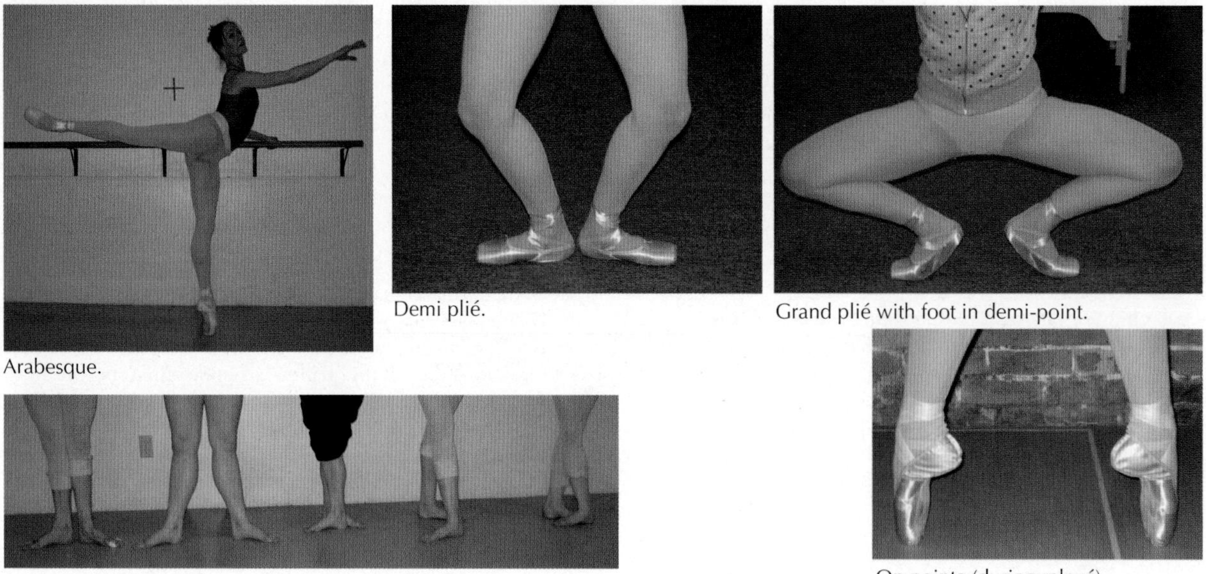

Arabesque.

Demi plié.

Grand plié with foot in demi-point.

Basic foot positions—first to fifth from left to right.

On pointe (during relevé).

Figure 92.1 Common terms in dance. (Photographs courtesy of Craig C. Young, MD, and Selina Shah, MD.)

Injuries

FREQUENCY

- Up to 60% of professional Irish dancers have suffered injuries.
- Up to 80% of competitive-level Irish dancers have suffered injuries.
- The lifetime risk of injury can be as high as 90%.
- 79.6% of injuries are categorized as overuse or chronic.
- 20.4% of injuries are categorized as traumatic or acute.

TYPE

- In descending order of frequency: tendon injury, apophysitis, patella pain or instability, stress injury, strain, and sprain

LOCATION

- Ninety-five percent of injuries involved the lower extremities. Frequency in descending order: foot, ankle, knee, and hip

RISK FACTORS

- Intrinsic: fatigue or overwork, ignoring early warning signs, improper or lack of warm-up and/or cool-down
- Extrinsic: accident, unsuitable floor, repetitive movement, unsuitable foot wear

GENERAL PRINCIPLES

Terminology

Arabesque: A pose in which the dancer stands on one leg and raises the other straight behind (at various angles); usually one arm is stretched out in front (Fig. 92.1)

Class: Lesson

- Barre—the first part of ballet class conducted using the railing for balance and technique training
- Center—the portion of class in which dancers perform dance movements in the "center of the room" without using the barre for assistance
  - Across the floor: A series of choreographed steps performed diagonally across the room in small groups, with choreography done on the right side in one direction and on the left side in the other

Demi-pointe: The foot is maximally plantarflexed with toes maximally extended—weight on metatarsal heads (see Fig. 92.1)

Foot positions: (see Fig. 92.1)

- First position—feet turned out with heels touching
- Second position—feet turned out with heels apart
- Third position—feet turned out, overlapping with right heel in hollow of left foot
- Fourth position—feet turned out, apart but with overlapping heels
- Fifth position—feet turned out, touching with right heel in front of left toe

Jeté: A jump where the legs are in a split position in the air

Plié: Bending of the knees and ankles with the legs turned out

- Grand plié—a large or deep plié where the knees are maximally flexed and the feet are in demi-pointe (see Fig. 92.1)
- Demi-plié—a "small" plié where the knees are only partially flexed and the feet are flat on the floor (see Fig. 92.1)

Pointe: Dancing while supporting the body on the tips of the toes (see Fig. 92.1)

Relevé: To rise up to the tiptoes or full pointe

Passé: Standing on one leg with the gesture leg externally rotated, abducted, and with the leg flexed so that the foot is plantarflexed and tips of the toes are touching the knee or higher, depending on style. The standing leg is flat or in relevé position. This position is used in pirouette turns (Fig. 92.2).

Turnout: A stance in which legs are rotated outward. Turnout is the sum of the external rotations of the hip, knee, tibia, ankle, and foot.

TYPES OF DANCE

Ballet

Background

- Classical ballet originated in the 1400s in Italy and blossomed in the 1600s in France.
- Traditionally, professional ballet companies perform story ballets. Some of the most famous ones are *The Nutcracker* (usually performed during Christmas), *Swan Lake*, and *Giselle*. They also will perform mixed programs consisting of a variety of choreographed dances.
- Ballet is a choreographed series of specific motions, with specific placement of all body parts from the head to the toes.

Technique

- Many positions require extreme external rotation of the hips (see Fig. 92.1).
- Flexibility is required to achieve 180-degree splits of the legs.

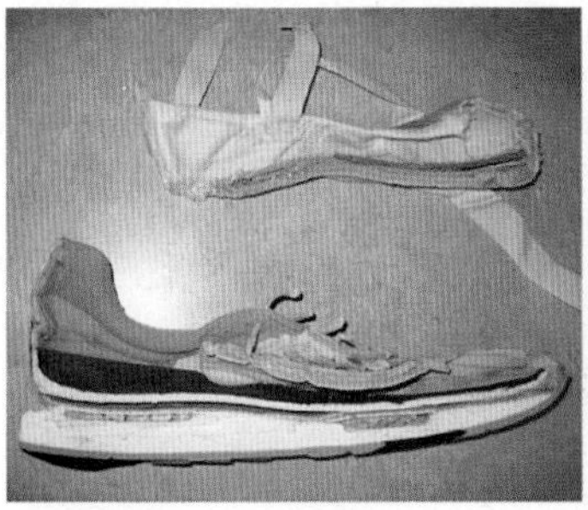

Ballet shoes: Pointe shoe cutaway-note lack of padding when compared to running shoe.

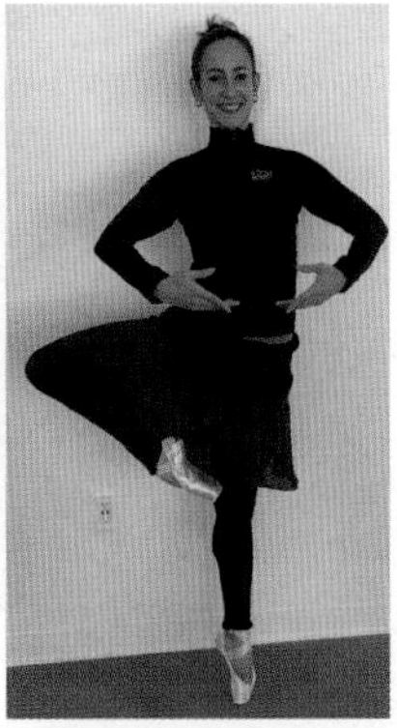

Ballet: Relevé passe.

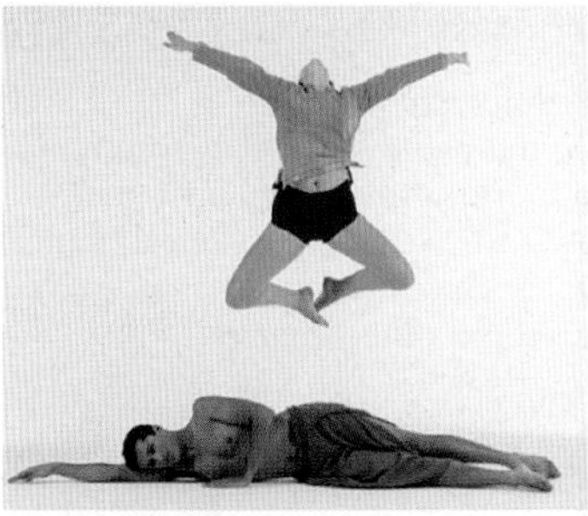

Modern dancers.

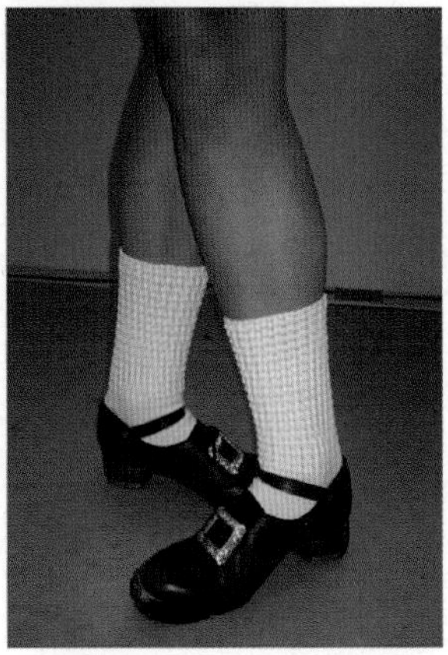

Irish dance hard shoes.

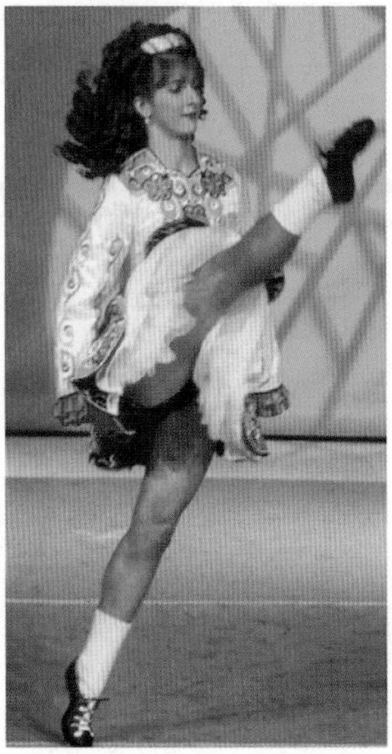

Typical Irish dance position (arms tightly adducted to side and elbows locked in extension. Neutral posture is held from the waist up during all dancing and hands are closed into fists).

Figure 92.2 Types of dance and equipment. (Ballet photographs courtesy of Craig C. Young, MD; modern dance photograph courtesy of Blue 13 Dance Company, Ryuichi Oshimoto; Irish dance photographs courtesy of Laura Gottschlich, DO.)

- Strength is required to hold the legs in extreme positions of hip flexion and in extension with extended knees and plantarflexed ankles and toes.
- Dancing on pointe consists of dancing while supporting the body on the tips of the toes. This is almost always done by women, but there is one professional male company, as well as a few other choreographed dances, where males perform pointe work.
  - Most young female dancers aspire to go on pointe.
  - Adequate skill, technique (including balance and core stability), strength, balance, alignment, maturity to apply teacher corrections, and at least 90 degrees of ankle plantarflexion to achieve full pointe are the basic requirements. More sophisticated tests that examine the dancer's ability to maintain proper alignment and balance while performing ballet jumps and combinations may also be useful (see Fig. 92.2, relevé passé).
  - Though age is not a requirement, most dancers are about 11 or 12 years old before they achieve all of the necessary criteria for pointe.

Equipment

- Both men and women wear ballet slippers for the majority of classwork. These are made of soft, supple material and a flexible, thin leather sole. They must fit snugly and are secured with elastic band(s).
- Pointe shoes are handmade from lacquered satin and burlap, with a stiff leather sole, which results in a hard but pliable shank and a rigid, unpadded toe box (see Fig. 92.2).

Jazz

- Jazz dance originated from the African-American dances of late 1800s and has led to the advent of tap dancing and some forms of ballroom (e.g., the swing and Lindy).
- Traditional jazz shoes—soft leather with a small heel
- Jazz sneakers—soft leather/canvas with a padded sole to increase shock absorption from jump landings
- Some positions require less external hip rotation than ballet.
- Jazz dancing is very free-form and includes kicks, falls, jumps, and slides; in general consists of quicker, sharper movements than ballet.

Modern (Contemporary)

- Originated at the turn of the 20th century in defiance of the rigidity of classical ballet.
- Unlike ballet, modern dance uses gravity and emphasizes freedom of movement, sometimes taken to bizarre extremes.
- Most professionals dance barefoot, although a few wear some type of jazz shoe, ballet shoe, foot thong, socks, or simply use duct tape (see Fig. 92.2).

Ballroom

- Ballroom dancing is a set of partner-based dances that were initially developed as social dances.
- Traditionally, the purpose of the dance was to show off the woman, who performs all the fancy moves, while the male acts as support and as the leader.
- Women wear high heels.

Types of Ballroom

- Smooth (waltz, foxtrot, tango)
  - These dances, especially waltz, involve lots of extension and flexion from the knees to create the rise and fall of the dancers.
- Latin (cha-cha, rumba, samba, jive, paso doble)
  - These dances emphasize hip motions.
- Rhythm (East Coast swing, mambo)
- Dance sport—competitive athletic-style dancing based on all of the earlier styles that typically involves more lifts, throws, and slides than traditional ballroom dances.
- Other ballroom dances include the polka, two-step, Lindy, and West Coast swing.

Folk

- A highly variable type of dance—depends on individual style
- Irish is the most common subtype of traditional folk dance.

Irish

- The earliest recording in literature of Irish dancing was in 1300.
- Became mainstream in 1994 with the production of *Riverdance*.
- Originated in Ireland, migrated first to England, and then to Australia, Canada, and the United States.
  - Schools are now established in 30 countries across five continents.
- Combines artistic elements of ballet with the rhythm of jazz and tap. Has had an important influence on American dancing—including square dance, clogging, jazz, and tap.
- Has a competitive and a professional element.
  - Professional/paid dancers are ineligible for competition.
- Shoes consist of a soft leather, lace-up slipper (soft ghille or reel shoes) and a leather shoe with fiberglass tips and heels (hard or jig shoes) (see Fig. 92.2).
  - The extremely snug fit gives a tight toe appearance in plantarflexion.
  - Recent adjustments of neoprene padding have slightly improved shock absorption.

Irish Competition

- Competitions exist at local *(Feis)*, regional *(Oireachtas)*, National, and World *(Rince Na Cruinne)* levels.
- Competition may be solo or in groups of up to 16 dancers.
- Dancers compete in multiple dances in both hard (Treble Jig, Hornpipe, Set Dances) and soft shoes (Reel, Slip Jig, Jig, Figures).
- Dancers are judged on timing to music, posture, position of feet and legs during execution of the dance, and style.

Biomechanical Principles

- There are some similarities between ballet and tap dancing.
- Most elements of Irish dancing are performed in the sagittal plane.
- Hamstring flexibility must be enough to afford approximately 0 to 135 degrees hip flexion.
- Dancing is performed in external rotation from the hip to approximately 70–80 degrees.
- The front foot is routinely crossed in front of the back foot, covering the back toe during most dance moves and in tight plantarflexion (see Fig. 92.2).
- The front knee is routinely covering the back knee during most dance moves.
- Most dancing is performed with arms tightly adducted to the side and elbows locked in extension. A neutral posture is held from the waist up during all dancing, and hands are closed into fists (see Fig. 92.2).
- Most dance moves are performed with rigid landing in point/demi-point positions and the knees tightly extended.
  - This is different from ballet where jump landings utilize a demi-plié so that shock is also absorbed through the knees.
- Repetitive pounding of the balls of the foot occurs for minutes at a time during rhythm moves with the hard shoes and during landing from jumps.
- Recent studies show many moves in Irish dance produce force of 2–4 times a dancer's body weight.
- Turning of the head for the purposes of spotting for jumps and spins is not allowed, unlike most other forms of dance.
- In the late 1980s, dancers began to dance on pointe in their hard shoes, often jumping, spinning, and running on the fiberglass tips.
- In 2002, the governing body of Irish dancing, *An Coimisiun*, banned toe or "block" movements for all children under the age of 12, citing concern over stress on immature bones with pointe movements.

Street Dance

- Street dance styles have evolved outside of formal dance programs. Many of the current styles evolved from the African American and Puerto Rican communities in the 1970s.
- Examples of street dance include hip hop, breaking, locking, popping, krumping, and Gangsta Walk.
- These styles are highly variable, improvisational, and tend to incorporate nontraditional dance moves, which may place these dancers at risk for unusual injuries.

Aerobic

- Differs from other form of dance because its purpose is primarily for exercise.
- Emphasizes quick motions to raise heart rate and tone muscles, rather than artistic form and performance.
- Exercisers wear shock-absorbing athletic shoes.

COMMON INJURIES AND MEDICAL PROBLEMS

Eating and Nutritional Disorders

- Very common, especially in adolescent dancers.
- Professional female dancers often believe that they weigh more than an "ideal" dancer should, even though audience members believe that most appear to be at the weight of an "ideal" dancer.
- Problems may start in preadolescent dancers.
- Increases risk of stress fractures and other injuries.

Menstrual Disorders

- Dancers are at increased risk for primary and secondary amenorrhea.
- Increases risk of stress fractures.

Smoking

- Higher prevalence in dancers compared with other athletic populations.
- Especially at risk—female dancers who are having difficulty maintaining weight.

Burnout

- Beware—especially in adolescent folk dancers who present with recurrent atypical injuries.

Osteopenia

- Amenorrheic female dancers at risk.
- Eumenorrheic female dancers and male dancers tend to have higher bone densities than nonathletes.

Musculoskeletal Injuries

Shoulder

- Rotator cuff problems, particularly in male dancers

Spine

- Neck and back strains (especially of the trapezius, rhomboid, and latissimus)
- Prevalence of "incorrect" lifting techniques—choreographers and artistic directors often value appearance over optimal lifting technique
- Other back problems—spondylolysis, spondylolisthesis, scoliosis, and facet syndrome
- Core stability tests (for at least 30 seconds)
  - Pike position—push up with forearms supporting (elbows bent 90 degrees) and on toes with ankles in neutral
  - Side lift—hold trunk linear facing side support on forearms

Hip and Groin

- Piriformis syndrome
  - Pain deep in gluteal or groin region

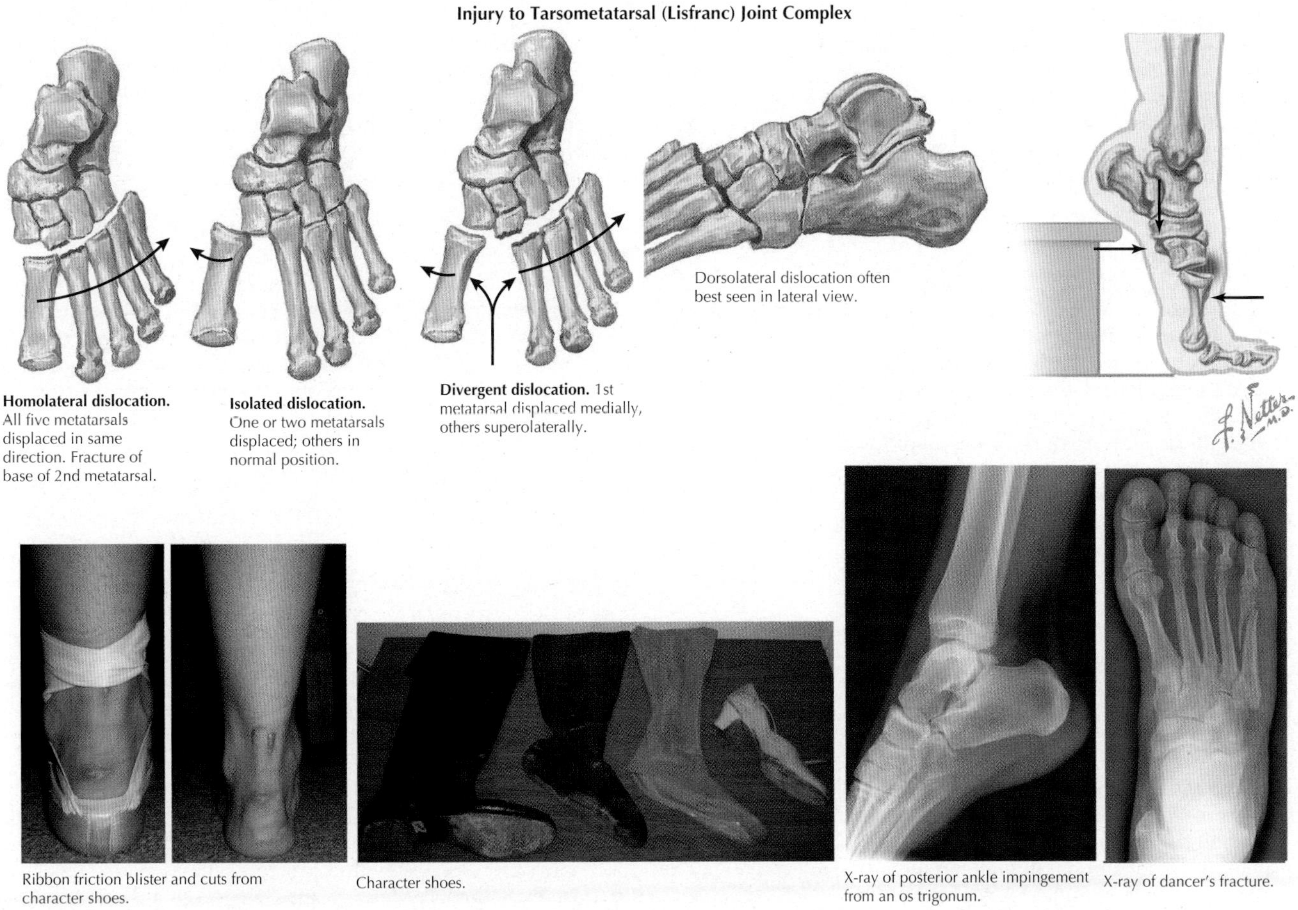
Injury to Tarsometatarsal (Lisfranc) Joint Complex
Homolateral dislocation. All five metatarsals displaced in same direction. Fracture of base of 2nd metatarsal.
Isolated dislocation. One or two metatarsals displaced; others in normal position.
Divergent dislocation. 1st metatarsal displaced medially, others superolaterally.
Dorsolateral dislocation often best seen in lateral view.
Ribbon friction blister and cuts from character shoes.
Character shoes.
X-ray of posterior ankle impingement from an os trigonum.
X-ray of dancer's fracture.

Figure 92.3 Musculoskeletal injuries in dance. (Photographs courtesy of Craig C. Young, MD.)

  - Pain worsens with stair climbing, standing up, or prolonged sitting
  - Pain with extreme passive hip internal rotation (flexed approximately 90 degrees) or resisted hip external rotation
- Snapping hip syndrome
  - External snapping hip—in most nondancers, snapping hip syndrome is of this type, which is caused by the iliotibial band (ITB) snapping over the greater trochanter.
    - Dancers with external snapping hip syndrome complain of snapping when landing jumps.
- Internal snapping hip syndrome is common in dancers and is caused by the iliopsoas.
  - Usually in the non–weight-bearing gesture leg (e.g., when bringing the hip from an externally rotated, abducted, flexed position to a neutral extended position)
  - Can be reproduced by bringing hip from flexed, externally rotated position to an extension with internal rotation
  - Sometimes reproduced with a resisted straight-knee sit-up
- Both can be clinically diagnosed and, if required, confirmed with ultrasound
- Hip labral tears and femoral acetabular impingement
  - Sharp, painful catch in groin
  - The majority can be confirmed with high quality 3 Tesla magnetic resonance imaging (MRI); however, to identify subtle tears or for better characterization of tears, an MR arthrogram may be needed.
- Sartorius tendonitis
  - From overuse of external rotator and flexor of the hip
  - Pain with external rotation, full flexion, abduction of hip
- Rectus femoris tendinitis
  - From repetitive forward extension of leg (e.g., battement or développé devant)
  - Groin pain, especially with knee extended

Knee

- Patellofemoral pain syndrome
- Patellar tendonitis

Leg

- Tibial stress fracture
  - Avoid rodding—this may cause loss of motion at knee; drilling out the fracture is a better option.
- Medial tibial stress syndrome

Ankle

- Achilles tendonitis
  - Ribbon friction—beware of where ribbons from slippers cross the Achilles tendon (Fig. 92.3).
  - Character shoes—often do not have Achilles tendon notch and may not have optimal sizing because the wardrobe department may have limited costumes (see Fig. 92.3).
  - Certain movements like the "rock" step in Irish dance puts up to 2700 N of force, or 14 times a dancer's body weight, on the Achilles tendon and the connecting muscles (see Fig. 92.2).
- Ankle sprains
- Ankle impingement
  - Anterior: especially aggravated by pliés; often associated with osteophyte at margin of anterior tibia and dorsum of talus
  - Posterior: especially aggravated by pointe and demi-pointe; often associated with os trigonum or prominent posterior process of talus

- Evaluation: lateral foot X-ray in maximal dorsiflexion (for anterior impingement) or maximal plantarflexion (for posterior impingement) (see Fig. 92.3)
- Treatment: although surgery in dancers is often career-ending, surgery for ankle impingement may be career-saving
- Peroneal tendonitis; subluxation, dislocation, and dysfunction
- Tarsal tunnel syndrome

Foot

- Cuboid subluxation
  - Plantar subluxation of the cuboid
  - Risk factors include the tendency to be in valgus position of forefoot at metatarsal joints
  - Can occur secondary to lateral ankle sprain
  - Symptoms: lateral foot pain, weakness with push-off, and inability to jump because of sharp pain
  - Diagnosis: pressing dorsally on cuboid from plantar surface reproduces pain and possibly produces visible depression. Radiographic studies are usually negative.
- Cuboid compression fracture; "nutcracker fracture"
  - Caused by axial loading
  - Often need computed tomography (CT) to diagnose
- Subtalar coalition
  - A bony connection that is between the calcaneus and either the navicular or the talus
  - Limits foot motion
  - May cause mechanical pain
  - Usually affects young dancers
- Navicular stress fractures
- Lisfranc joint injuries
  - Lisfranc joint: articulation of second metatarsal with first and second cuneiforms (see Fig. 92.3)
  - The Lisfranc joint has limited mobility
  - Pointe dancers at highest risk
  - Lack of dorsal support and immobility of second metatarsal causes dorsal displacement of second metatarsal with axial load in plantarflexion
  - Sprain: disruption at Lisfranc joint
  - Fracture/dislocation: diastasis between first and second metatarsal seen in standing anterior-posterior radiograph of foot. Line from medial edge of fourth metatarsal to cuboid is disrupted, as seen on standing medial oblique view of foot.
- Spiral fracture of shaft of fifth metatarsal (dancer's fracture) (see Fig. 92.3)
  - Etiology: inversion injury while on pointe
  - Treatment: cast shoe
- Metatarsal shaft stress fractures
  - Usually in second to fourth metatarsals
  - Especially in the longest toe
- Flexor hallucis longus tendonitis (dancer's tendonitis)
  - Usually occurs in demi-pointe
  - Pain posteromedial ankle: tenderness with active or passive motion
  - May have painful crepitus with active motion
  - Pain with resisted flexion of great toe
  - May present with a palpable nodule behind medial malleolus and triggering of the great toe with plantarflexion
- Morton neuroma and corns
  - Use of silicone spacers; check shoe size, especially pointe shoes; remember that each pair is handmade, thus variable in size.
- Bunion (hallux valgus), hallux rigidus, and hammertoes
  - Bunions are particularly a problem if the great toe is longer than the second toe.
  - Avoid bunion surgery—minimal loss of motion may result in the ending of a dance career.
  - Hammertoe usually occurs in second toe, particularly if it is the longest toe.
  - Shoe padding can be used to help spread the load on the toes.
  - Silicone pad (great toe) or sleeve (toes).
  - Orthotic with rigid extension in nondance shoes (rarely fits into dance footwear except some character shoes).
- Paronychia and subungual hematoma
  - The range of appropriate nail length is small; too short—paronychia/ingrown nails; too long—subungual hematoma/nail trauma.
  - File nails daily to maintain optimal length.
- Sesamoiditis and sesamoid fracture
  - Especially common in folk dancers; 27.7% of stress fractures of the foot in Irish dancers are in the sesamoid.
  - Most likely linked to repetitive pounding in demi-pointe and pointe with jumps, landing, rhythm sequences, increased loading with forced turnout, and weak control of external rotation at the hip.
- Plantar fasciitis and turf toe
  - Especially common in Irish dancers
- "Stone bruise"—metatarsal head contusion
- Calluses and corns

GENERAL TIPS FOR TREATING DANCERS

- Most dancers will consult with someone within 1 week of injury.
- Less than half of dancers will consult a physician because:
  - They think that physicians are not helpful or do not understand dancers.
  - They are worried that they will be told to stop dancing for too long.
  - They do not have health insurance.
  - Many dancers consult other individuals such as fellow dancers, choreographer, company director, instructor physical therapists, chiropractors, massage therapists, and acupuncturists.
- Respect dancers as artists, but also encourage them to think of themselves as athletes who need proper conditioning, nutrition, and rest.
- Most dancers actually adhere to the advice given to them.
  - Their main reasons for not adhering to the advice given to them include the lengthy amount of time recommended to refrain from dance, fear of being held out of class or rehearsal if the staff knew about the injury, not agreeing with the advice, and fear of losing their role in the performance to an understudy or rival.
- Evaluate the dancer's schedule. Many hours are spent in solo class, team class, private lessons, and cross-training.
- Most dance classes have multiple parts (barre vs. center class, warm-ups vs. full class, strength training, etc.), and it is often not necessary to have a dancer stop dance class completely. Even the observation of class or a walkthrough of rehearsal is often beneficial and may lead to increased compliance with the treatment plan.
- Evaluate the dance floor for overuse injuries.
  - Sprung floors have the best impact absorption.
    - This is particularly important because dance shoes have little or no cushioning.
  - Dancers may use different floors in the class area than in performance areas.
  - Dancers in smaller programs and folk dancers are much less likely to have the luxury of dancing on sprung floors.
    - Fifty percent of Irish dance schools are not in traditional studios.
- Evaluate footwear worn when dancer is not dancing.
  - Alteration of this footwear may allow the dancer to continue dance activities by allowing for more effective relative rest when not dancing.
- If you do not understand the names of the motions, have the dancers describe or demonstrate them.

  - The knowledge of aggravating motions is critical in designing rehabilitation and return-to-activity plans.
- In general, avoid surgery in dancers because even the minimal loss of range of motion may result in the end of a dance career.
  - Exceptions are "excisional operations" (e.g., excision of os trigonum, osteophyte shaving for ankle impingement syndrome).
  - Dancers also recover well from meniscus and hip labral surgery.

RECOMMENDED READINGS

Available online.

93 TRACK AND FIELD

Tauqeer Qazi

INTRODUCTION

Overview

- Track and field often attracts multisport athletes.
- The sport involves year-round competition and training.
- Differing athletic events subject athletes to differing demands. For example:
  - The shot put demands explosive power.
  - Endurance events demand high levels of aerobic conditioning and stamina.
  - Sprint distances (100 m, 200 m, and 400 m) demand explosive conditioning for power, flexibility, and anaerobic conditioning.
  - Middle distance races (800 m or 1500 m) demand a combination of anaerobic and aerobic conditioning to sustain power and stamina.
  - Distance events (3000 m, 5000 m, 10,000 m, and marathon) demand stamina, high levels of aerobic conditioning, and sustained power.
  - The 100 m and 400 m hurdles, in addition to relays (4 × 100 m, 4 × 200 m, 4 × 400 m, 4 × 800 m, 4 × 1500 m, distance medley, and sprint medley), demand mental concentration, power, and stamina.
  - Field events, such as long jump, high jump, triple jump, shot put, javelin, discus, hammer, heptathlon, decathlon, and pole vault, in addition to the track event 3000 m steeplechase, demand combinations of technique, stamina, power, and speed.

EPIDEMIOLOGY

- It is difficult to look at injury statistics given the lack of a common denominator (player hours or athlete exposures) and variability in methodology of studies.
- There are no National Collegiate Athletic Association (NCAA) data collected for track and field.
- For large track and field events, injury incidence is the greatest for minor orthopedic injuries (5.7 per 1000 athletes), followed by minor medical injuries (3.4 per 1000 athletes). Medical coverage should be planned to accommodate seven major orthopedic injuries and two major medical injuries per 10,000 athletes.
- Male athletes and masters athletes are at greater risk of injury than other categories of athletes.
- Of all participants in the 1985 Junior Track Olympics, 35% reported the need for performance-related medical treatment.
- In general, **most injuries are overuse injuries that occur during training. However, the risk of injury during competition is four times higher than that in training.**
  - Acute injuries are often muscle strains or avulsions or are related to stress fractures; other acute injuries are uncommon.
  - Majority of injuries involve lower extremities.
  - There is some risk for head and neck injury during the high jump and pole vault; there is a risk of blunt trauma with javelin, hammer, and discus.
  - Of particular concern are acute medical problems such as cardiovascular collapse secondary to underlying cardiac disease, dehydration, or other abnormalities related to environmental conditions.

Site of Injury

- The most common injury sites are the lower leg (28%), thigh (22%), and knee (16%).
- The most common injuries are hamstring muscle strains and stress reactions.
- **The knee is the most commonly injured joint in runners** (48% of all joint injuries).
- Overuse injuries are more common in distance runners, whereas acute injuries are more common in sprinters, hurdlers, jumpers, and multievent athletes. Recurrent injuries are common.

Specific Diagnoses

- Anterior knee pain accounts for 24% of running injuries in men and 30% of running injuries in women.
- Medial tibial stress syndrome accounts for 7.2% of injuries in men and 11.4% in women.
- Iliotibial band syndrome accounts for 7.2% of injuries in men and 7.9% in women.
- Patellar tendinosis accounts for 5.1% of injuries in men and 3.1% in women.
- Metatarsal stress syndrome accounts for 3.1% of injuries in men and 3.8% in women.
- Achilles tendinosis accounts for 4.7% of injuries in men and 2.7% in women.

MUSCULOSKELETAL ISSUES

Basic Running Mechanics

- It is important to understand the normal biomechanics of running to recognize abnormal biomechanics and how they can affect incidence of injury.
- **Foot strike:** At lower speeds, occurs with the heel, but at higher speeds, occurs with the forefoot
- Ground strike occurs 800 to 2000 times per mile for the average runner (5000 foot strikes per hour of running).
- **Reaction forces at foot strike are usually 1.5 to 5 times the body weight.** Joint shear forces during running increase to almost 50 times that of walking. These reaction forces are augmented considerably by different surface types.
- At the point of initial rearfoot contact, the foot is in supination. This is associated with the "closed-pack" position, a rigid positioning of the tarsal bones increasing stability.
- The foot then pronates with the tarsal joints, assuming an "open-packed" position, which is more accommodating and less rigid, allowing partial absorption of reaction forces. There is internal rotation of the tibia on the talus.
- As runners progress to the push-off, the subtalar joint supinates with external rotation of the tibia. The foot remains in supination during the airborne phase and forward swing of the leg.
- Major muscle groups all show increased electromyographic activity during running, and all lower extremity joints show increased motion during running.
- In the stance phase of running, the ankle contributes 60% of the power generation, whereas the knee and hip generate 40% and 20%, respectively.
- **The knee is the principal shock absorber during running, absorbing twice as much energy as the ankle and hip.**
- **Abnormal biomechanics can lead to overload of other structures.** Commonly, gluteus maximus weakness can lead to poor control of the lower limb and reaction forces being transmitted throughout the kinetic chain. As another example, an abnormal amount of rearfoot varus or pronation can abnormally

load structures higher in the kinetic chain, leading to increased valgus stress at the knee. This is an important etiologic factor in patellofemoral dysfunction (see the "Patellofemoral Dysfunction" section later in the chapter).

- **Orthotics** may help prevent injury if significant biomechanical abnormalities are present. Screen with gait assessment during the preparticipation examination.

Physiologic Issues

- **Demands depend on type of activity**
  - **Sprinters:** Energy requirements provided primarily by anaerobic energy pathways. Glucose is the major fuel source.
  - **Long distance events:** Energy requirements provided primarily by aerobic energy pathways, with fat and glucose derived from glycogen stores
  - **Middle distance and combination events:** Combination of both aerobic and anaerobic pathways
- Specificity of training, including periodization, to demands based on type(s) of energy pathways used.

Strengthening and Conditioning

- **Sport specificity in training is key in track and field. This differs for each event.** Most training continues year round. There is a need to emphasize variability in training and avoid overtraining.
- **Endurance and sprint athletes:** The selective strengthening of certain muscle fiber types (fast-twitch vs. slow-twitch) demonstrates specificity (i.e., endurance-type training leads to changes in slow-twitch fiber morphology and enzyme metabolism specific for endurance-type activities). Similarly, explosive strengthening programs specifically train fast-twitch muscle fibers and the metabolic functions used to sustain these activities. It is more beneficial to train with sport specificity in mind when designing strength and conditioning programs.
- **Use of the entire range of motion (ROM) for strengthening is important.** Strength gains observed are specific to the range and speed at which strengthening exercises are performed.
- **Field events:** The successful transfer of ground reaction force through the foot, ankle, knee, hip, trunk, shoulder, elbow, wrist, hand, and finally, to the implement is critical to success in throwing events. Maintain quadriceps–hamstring balance. Again, sport specificity is helpful. A shoulder scapular stabilization and rotator cuff strengthening program will be helpful for the shot put, javelin, hammer, and discus and the reproduction of shoulder movement with manual resistance. Proprioceptive work is helpful in hurdles, discus, javelin, triple jump, and long jump.
- **Develop smaller supporting muscles:** Strengthening prevents development of medial tibial stress syndrome, plantar fasciitis, patellofemoral dysfunction, and other overuse injuries.

Flexibility

- Despite a lack of reliable data about the effects of increased flexibility in preventing injury, most agree that the introduction and usage of a flexibility program helps avoid acute muscle strains. If the muscle length at which maximal stretch felt is greater, it takes larger acute overload to "stretch" the muscle past this length, leading to injury. Flexibility remains an essential tool in the treatment of muscle strains and joint protection.
- A flexibility program should be worked into strengthening programs such that strength is improved throughout the ROM without loss of motion.
- Ballistic stretching should be avoided.
- Stretching should be performed after warming up, rather than while "cold" at the start of practice.
- Stretch larger muscle groups first, followed by smaller groups.
- Hamstring flexibility is important in mechanical low back injuries. If hamstring flexibility is limited, a posterior pelvic tilt is created and the trunk flexion becomes limited, increasing stress in the lower back.

COMMON MEDICAL PROBLEMS

Preparticipation Physical Examination

- Stresses the importance of cardiac, musculoskeletal, and neurologic systems.
- Detailed family history is conducted, emphasizing any history of heart murmur, arrhythmia, sudden cardiac death, Marfan syndrome, hypertrophic cardiomyopathy, or premature atherosclerotic disease.
- Screen for possible anatomic abnormalities that may predispose to injury; consider use of orthotics and a flexibility/strengthening program in the presence of muscle imbalances, especially of the hip abductors and gluteal musculature, assessed both statically and dynamically.
- Assess for nutritional or training errors, including any "self-restricted" food types. Inquire about lactose intolerance. Screen for relative energy deficit syndrome (RED-S) (see Chapter 27: "Eating Disorders in Athletes").
- Rule out significant medical or orthopedic problems that would preclude activity or require restrictions.
- In female athletes, pay special attention to menstrual dysfunction, hypocalcemic diets, a history of disordered eating, and/or a history of stress reactions or fractures (see the "Female Athlete Triad" section later in the chapter).

Nutrition Issues

- It is important to consider nutrition and mental health when an athlete presents with symptoms of fatigue, burnout, or recurrent minor injuries (see Chapter 5: "Sports Nutrition" and Chapter 25: "The Role of Sport Psychology and Sports Psychiatry").
- Zinc, calcium, and iron are commonly deficient in athletes.
- Ideal nutritional intake: 6–13 g carbohydrates per kg body weight, 1.2–1.7 g protein per kg body weight, with the remainder of calories from fat. This translates into a diet of 60%–70% carbohydrates, 10%–15% protein, and 25%–30% fat. No performance benefit has been shown with diets consisting of 15% fat versus diets consisting of 20%–25% fat.
- If an athlete eats an adequate caloric intake from a variety of wholesome foods, nutritional needs are often met. Proper food selection, not supplementation, is the ideal form of nutrition.

Iron Deficiency

- Common in young athletes. Iron loss can be the result of hemolysis with hemoglobinuria, gastrointestinal (GI) losses, and excessive sweating. Female athletes are at increased risk of anemia because of the additional loss that occurs with menses. Athletes are not immune from other medical problems, and thus a complete workup of an iron-deficient athlete is important.
- Iron deficiency or decreased iron stores can occur without anemia in as many as 24%–47% of female athletes and 0%–17% of male athletes.
- The dietary recommended intake varies based on sex and age. Females aged 19–50 years require 18 mg of iron per day, and males aged 19–50 years require 8 mg per day.
- Pseudoanemia: an increase in plasma volume of 6%–25% with training results in hemoglobin and hematocrit appearing falsely low. Typically self-limited.
- Screening for iron deficiency is recommended in elite athletes and high-risk populations, such as vegan/vegetarian athletes, those with a history of iron deficiency, or athletes exhibiting an unexplained decrease in performance.

- Screening hemoglobin with a follow-up examination of ferritin is reasonable for assessing iron deficiency. Ferritin is a storage form of iron but can be transiently elevated in acute inflammation or after vigorous activity. Ferritin levels decrease, however, with longer-term aerobic training. Iron and total iron binding capacity can differentiate pseudoanemia from true anemia.
- Although anemia has been shown to affect athletic performance, the effect of iron deficiency alone is unclear.
  - Supplementation of 65 to 200 mg elemental iron per day is recommended if truly iron deficient. Increase intake of iron-rich foods and ensure adequate vitamin C intake.

Calories

- Although obtaining an adequate total caloric intake is obviously essential, this basic ingredient of good nutrition is often neglected.
- In an attempt to eat "healthy," many athletes restrict fat intake. This strategy results in the risk of fat-soluble vitamins (vitamins A, D, E, and K) being deficient. Diets with less than 15% fat have shown no gains in athletic performance or health.
- Some athletes experiment by restricting calories as a means of reducing body weight, thus improving aesthetics and performance. This can increase the risk for developing a frank eating disorder, along with its concomitant medical problems.
- Other deficiencies found in athletes include zinc, magnesium, folate, and vitamins B_6, C, and B_{12}. Athletes should consider a nutritional consultation to formally review food intake if concerned about vitamin and/or caloric deficiencies.

Protein Intake

- Often an issue in vegan/vegetarian athletes and those that restrict food intake
- Consult a nutritionist to ensure adequate intake.
- If vegetarian, protein complementarity with legumes and grains can ensure adequate protein intake, but it is still important to assess iron intake. Minimizing this potential deficit may minimize potential fatigue and diet-related conditions.
- Voluntary protein intake, along with fat and total energy intake, has been shown to be lower in athletes with menstrual irregularities than in normally menstruating athletes.

Calcium

- Dietary reference intakes (DRIs) vary based on age. The most recent guidelines suggest 1300 mg daily for ages 14–18 years, and 1000 mg daily for ages 19–50 (Fig. 93.1).
- Female athletes often consume less than the DRI for calcium.
- Calcium and estrogen are necessary in women for normal bone deposition. If depleted, this can lead to lower bone density. Peak bone density is reached in women in late teens to early 20s; thus, adequate intake in childhood and adolescence is critical.

Vitamin D

- Vitamin D is essential for bone health and the incorporation of calcium. Primary sources are sunlight and vitamin D-enriched foods such as milk.
- Vitamin D levels have been increasingly associated with generalized musculoskeletal pains.
- The DRI is 25 micrograms daily, and vitamin D-25-OH levels can be monitored.
- Athletes who practice and compete in indoor sports and those living in northern latitudes may be at risk. **Consider supplementation if levels are low.**

Nutritional Supplements and Ergogenic Aids

- Athletes are at risk for use and abuse of supplements and ergogenic aids.

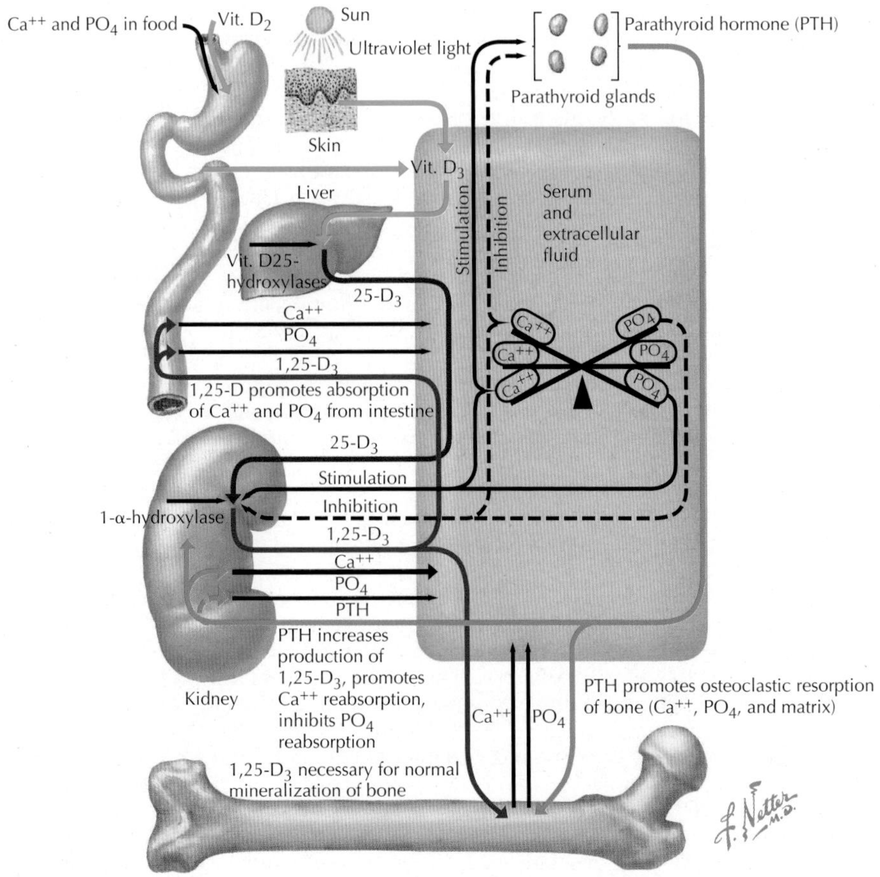

Ca++ and PO4 in food
Vit. D2
Sun
Ultraviolet light
Parathyroid hormone (PTH)
Parathyroid glands
Skin
Vit. D3
Liver
Stimulation
Inhibition
Serum and extracellular fluid
Vit. D25-hydroxylases
25-D3
Ca++
PO4
1,25-D3
1,25-D promotes absorption of Ca++ and PO4 from intestine
25-D3
Stimulation
Inhibition
1-α-hydroxylase
1,25-D3
Ca++
PO4
PTH
PTH increases production of 1,25-D3, promotes Ca++ reabsorption, inhibits PO4 reabsorption
Kidney
Ca++
PO4
PTH promotes osteoclastic resorption of bone (Ca++, PO4, and matrix)
1,25-D3 necessary for normal mineralization of bone
F. Netter M.D.

Figure 93.1 Normal calcium and phosphate metabolism.

- Some of these are restricted under US Olympic Committee and NCAA drug testing. Examples include ingesting excess amino acids, medium-chain fatty acids, vitamins, minerals, herb extracts, special proteins, and enzyme complexes.
- Often marketed to individual sports.
- There are reports suggesting that up to 62% of track athletes use supplements, including multivitamins.
- Specific questions related to pharmacokinetics, interaction with normal foodstuffs and prescribed medications, and side effect profile should be asked of the pharmacist.

SUPPLEMENTS

- The positive effects of supplementation are unproven if the athlete is not actually deficient in a vitamin.
- In the setting of dehydration, amino acid supplementation may be detrimental if kidney function is marginal.
- Protein and vitamin supplementation in great excess can be dangerous.
- Excesses of most vitamins are eliminated from the body.
- Fat-soluble vitamins are stored within the body, and thus toxicity is possible.
- Most methods of supplementation are expensive.

ERGOGENIC AIDS

- Erythropoietin, human growth hormone, and anabolic steroids.
- Erythropoietin is detected by a urine test; new tests being developed to detect biosimilar formulations.
- There is a blood assay to detect the use of human growth hormone.
- Anabolic steroids are detectable with urine drug testing.
- All are associated with significant side effects. Erythropoietin is associated with hyperviscosity syndrome and even death. Hyperviscosity syndrome is made worse with dehydration. Human growth hormone is associated with side effects that include acromegaly-like features and worsening of existing cardiovascular disease. Anabolic steroid side effects are well known.
- For up-to-date information, contact the US Anti-Doping Agency Drug Reference Line (800-233-0393).

Fluid Considerations

- During prolonged exercise, 2–4 pounds of body weight are lost per hour; equivalent to 1–2 L per hour.
- The rate of dehydration can be estimated by changes in nude body weight; each pound of weight lost equals 450–650 mL (16–24 ounces) of dehydration.
- Dehydration can incur physiologic changes: for every liter of water (2.2 pounds) lost while exercising in the heat, there is an increase in core body temperature of 0.3°C, increase in heart rate of 8 beats per minute, and decrease in cardiac output of 1 L per minute.
- Proper rehydration is essential before, during, after, and between events.
- Pre-exercise hydration should consist of 500–600 mL of water or sports drink 2–3 hours before exercise and 200–300 mL 20 minutes before exercise.
- To maintain hydration, ingestion of 200–300 mL every 10–20 minutes is required to prevent greater than 2% body weight reduction.
- Postexercise hydration should aim to restore fluid loss accumulated during the event.
- Thirst is a delayed sensation and therefore is not a good indicator of hydration status.
- Water temperature does not affect body heat storage, and thus water should be consumed at a comfortable temperature (50°F–59°F [10°C–15°C]) to promote hydration.
- Carbohydrates should be replaced if the exercise session lasts longer than 45 minutes or is high intensity.
- For an athlete who weighs 68 kg (150 pounds), the carbohydrate requirement is 30–60 g per hour. Carbohydrate and fluid needs can be met by drinking 625–1250 mL per hour of beverages with 4%–8% carbohydrate content.
- For a glycogen-depleted athlete, a postrace carbohydrate intake of 1.5 g per kg body weight during the first 30 minutes postrace and again every 2 hours for 4–6 hours will effectively replenish glycogen stores.
- Some studies document a decrease in gastric emptying once the glucose concentration is above 6%. Water is still an excellent source for short-distance events (<1 hour).

Nutritional Recommendations Are Different for Females and Males

- Societal influences have made constant dieting acceptable for girls and women, and athletes are even more likely to attempt to change body appearance if they think it will improve performance.
- Females are at increased risk of nutritional deficiency and eating disorders.

Relative Energy Deficiency in Sport (RED-S)

RED-S relates the impact of energy deficiency on physiological function including, but not limited to, menstrual function, bone health, metabolic rate, immunity, protein synthesis, and cardiovascular health. (See Chapter 12: "The Female Athlete" and Chapter 27: "Eating Disorders in Athletes.")

Female Athlete Triad

- Three interrelated conditions: low energy availability (with or without an eating disorder), menstrual dysfunction, and altered bone mineral density (BMD), each on a continuum from healthy to disease state (see Chapter 12: "The Female Athlete" and Chapter 27: "Eating Disorders in Athletes") (Fig. 93.2).
- Present in every sport, but most commonly seen in sports that select for a lean body weight (swimming, cross-country skiing, cross-country running) or in sports scored subjectively (gymnastics, figure skating, diving)

Low Energy Availability/Disordered Eating

- When energy availability falls below a threshold because of an imbalance in energy expenditure, cellular maintenance, growth, and reproduction are disrupted.
- Origins are multifactorial: genetics, perfectionism, personality traits, identity, self-esteem, family dynamics, coping skills, control issues, alterations of body image, and/or need for control. Patients often have a history of sexual or physical abuse. Societal pressures increase risk.
- Inadequate caloric intake can also result from lack of knowledge of proper nutrition.
- Prevalence estimates of disordered eating among high school and college athletes range from 15%–62% compared with 13%–20% in the general adolescent female population.
- Characteristics associated with successful athletes that lead to overlapping and increased risk for developing eating disorders include perfectionism, goal setting, and overachieving.
- Subtle messages by coach, parents, or teammates (often unintentional) can add to pressures that lead an athlete to experiment with pathogenic weight control behaviors:
  - Misconception that lower body weight improves performance
  - Educating coaches in how to recognize and prevent eating disorders is essential
- Difficult to identify; a team approach is often necessary for proper treatment
- The treatment team usually includes a physician, psychiatrist, and nutritionist. Additional support system includes coaches, sport psychologists, athletic trainers, and families. Psychological counseling is a cornerstone.
- Treatment usually not very successful, emphasizing the need for prevention through education and early identification.

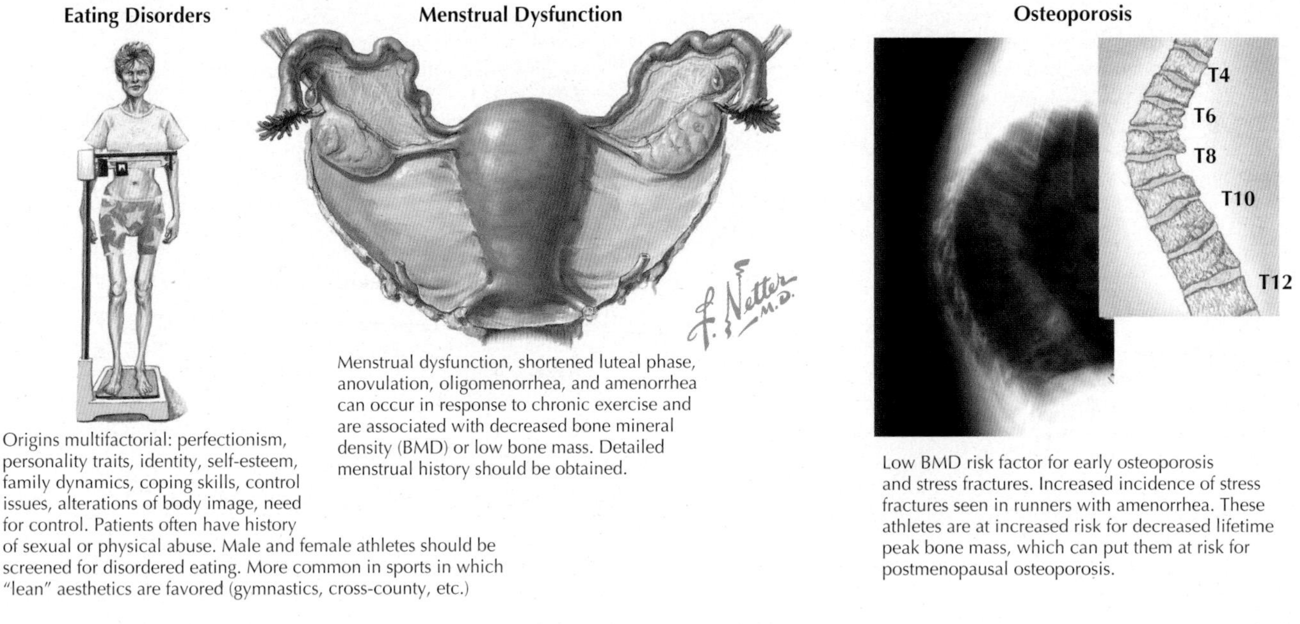
Eating Disorders
Menstrual Dysfunction
Osteoporosis
T4
T6
T8
T10
T12
Menstrual dysfunction, shortened luteal phase, anovulation, oligomenorrhea, and amenorrhea can occur in response to chronic exercise and are associated with decreased bone mineral density (BMD) or low bone mass. Detailed menstrual history should be obtained.
Origins multifactorial: perfectionism, personality traits, identity, self-esteem, family dynamics, coping skills, control issues, alterations of body image, need for control. Patients often have history of sexual or physical abuse. Male and female athletes should be screened for disordered eating. More common in sports in which "lean" aesthetics are favored (gymnastics, cross-county, etc.)
Low BMD risk factor for early osteoporosis and stress fractures. Increased incidence of stress fractures seen in runners with amenorrhea. These athletes are at increased risk for decreased lifetime peak bone mass, which can put them at risk for postmenopausal osteoporosis.

Figure 93.2 Female athlete triad.

- Screen for concomitant depression. Preliminary studies suggest a favorable response to antidepressants such as fluoxetine.

Menstrual Dysfunction

- Common in athletes, especially endurance athletes
- Menstrual dysfunction may include a shortened luteal phase, anovulation, oligomenorrhea, or amenorrhea.
- Strenuous training alone does not cause menstrual dysfunction; requires concurrent dietary restriction.
- Exercise-associated menstrual dysfunction remains a diagnosis of exclusion.
- The physician must rule out other conditions such as pregnancy, thyroid disorders, adrenal disorders, prolactin-secreting tumors, and/or ovarian disorders.
- Important to initiate workup and treatment because of the long-range consequences of menstrual dysfunction. Treatment must be individualized.
- "Progesterone challenge" helpful in functionally differentiating an estrogen-deficient state from an estrogen- and progesterone-deficient state.
- Referral to a sports dietitian and consideration of trial of increase in energy intake depending on other risk factors for bone health. Consider dual energy x-ray absorptiometry (DEXA) scan if concern for possible low bone density and screening for eating disorders. Close follow-up to include energy serial assessments important.
- The oral contraceptive pill (OCP) has a good side effect profile, is well tolerated, and has convenient packaging for females that are interested in contraception. Can complicate determination of energy availability status because masks menstrual dysfunction. Estrogen patch may provide improved bone health results compared with OCP if bone health concerns exist. If positive progesterone challenge, can use monthly progesterone alone.
- Other considerations: decrease training intensity; increase body weight if underweight; assess nutritional intake; maintain high index of suspicion for eating disorders.

Osteoporosis and Stress Fractures

- The bone is constantly remodeling; the process is a balance between osteoblast and osteoclast activity.
- Amenorrheic runners have lower estrogen levels and lower BMD than runners with normal menstrual cycles.
- An alteration in homeostasis because of low energy availability and low estrogen levels, which increases osteoclast activity, leads to decreased BMD.
- Stress fractures are caused by increased stress on normal bones (stress fractures) or normal stress on abnormal bones (insufficiency fractures) (Fig. 93.3).
- Low BMD is a risk factor of early osteoporosis and stress fractures. An increased incidence of stress fractures is seen in runners with amenorrhea. These athletes are at increased risk of decreased lifetime peak bone mass, which can put them at risk of postmenopausal osteoporosis.

Recognition and Treatment

- **Detection and education are critical.**
- A preparticipation physical examination offers a good opportunity to address these issues with female athletes and provides an opportunity to educate young athletes about the importance of maintaining normal menstrual function, risks of eating disorders, and the relationship of both to incidence of stress fractures and early low bone mass.
- Ask athletes who present with stress fractures about current and past menstrual history.
- Supplemental history for female athletes is a helpful screening tool during preparticipation physical examination.

Male Athlete Triad

- Parallels female athlete triad: inadequate nutrition, hypogonadotropic hypogonadism, and low BMD. There is a lack in the quality and quantity of studies in males.
- Similar to female athlete triad, each condition falls on a continuum of healthy to disease state.
- More prevalent in sports that emphasize leanness (running, cycling, wrestling, judo, horse racing).
- Subset of male endurance athletes has been shown to have lower testosterone levels and sperm counts.
- Screening for hypogonadism in male athletes has been proposed; however, no current evidence-based guidelines incorporate risk stratification or screening for male athletes.

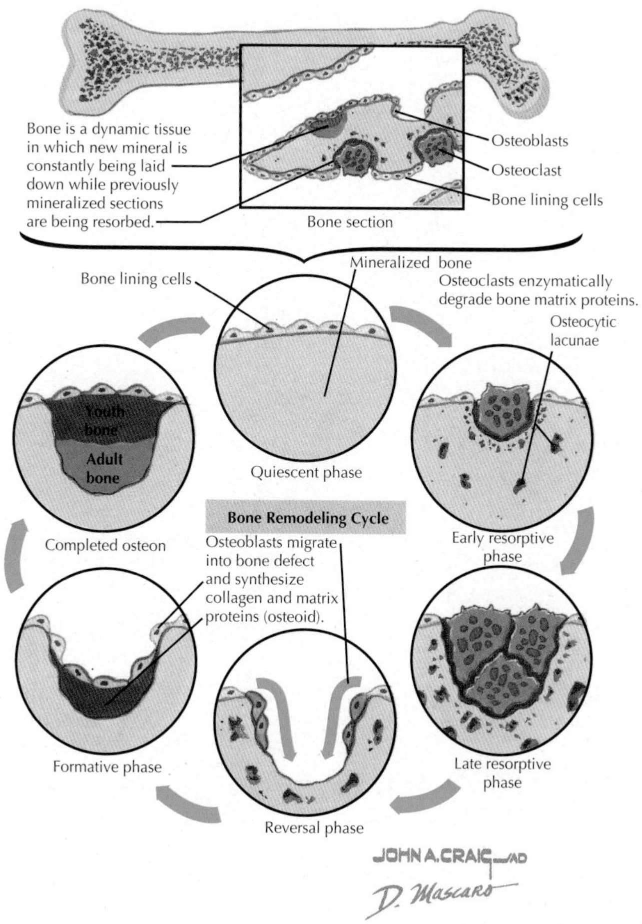

Bone is a dynamic tissue in which new mineral is constantly being laid down while previously mineralized sections are being resorbed.
Osteoblasts
Osteoclast
Bone lining cells
Bone section
Bone lining cells
Mineralized bone
Osteoclasts enzymatically degrade bone matrix proteins.
Osteocytic lacunae
Youth bone
Adult bone
Quiescent phase
Bone Remodeling Cycle
Completed osteon
Osteoblasts migrate into bone defect and synthesize collagen and matrix proteins (osteoid).
Early resorptive phase
Formative phase
Late resorptive phase
Reversal phase
JOHN A.CRAIG_AD
D. Mascaro

Figure 93.3 Bone remodeling.

- Proposed screening for athletes with recurrent stress fractures, especially in the presence of low body mass index (BMI), includes scanning bone densitometry (DEXA), 25-hydroxyvitamin D, and free and total testosterone levels.

Overtraining

Description: A spectrum of adaptations that includes functional overreaching, nonfunctional overreaching, and overtraining syndrome, where the balance of energy expenditure and recovery is disrupted (see Chapter 28: "Overtraining").
- **Functional overreaching (FOR):** Intensified training accompanied by a temporary decline in performance. With appropriate rest periods, the process leads to overall enhanced performance.
- **Nonfunctional overreaching (NFOR):** A *short-term* (several days to several weeks) decrease in performance related to stress from both training and nontraining sources that may lead to maladaptation.
- **Overtraining syndrome (OTS):** A *long-term* (several weeks to several months) decrease in performance related to stress from both training and nontraining sources that may lead to maladaptation.

Symptoms: Nonspecific, insidious symptoms include fatigue, mood disturbance, sleep difficulty, and performance decline.

Diagnostics: Generally a diagnosis of exclusion; presence of normal laboratory testing results. Important to assess for anemia, hypothyroidism, infection, collagen vascular disease, glucose abnormalities, and/or hormone deficiencies.

Treatment: Decrease in training, increase in carbohydrate intake, and a gradual return to activity. Sports psychologist referral should be made.

Associated conditions: Overtraining contributes to burnout, overuse injuries, stress fractures, menstrual dysfunction, iron deficiency, and long-lasting decrements in performance.

Syncope

Description: Common medical problem with multiple causes

Evaluation: Need to be rigorous in excluding the possibility of a serious medical problem, especially if syncope occurs in the midst of full exertion. Ask about history of associated chest pain, palpitation, shortness of breath, and dizziness.

Differential diagnosis:
- Dehydration
- Cardiac sources: long QT interval, arrhythmias, hypertrophic cardiomyopathy, anomalous coronary arteries, aortic stenosis or other valvular abnormalities, neurocardiogenic syncope
- Neurologic sources: seizures, arteriovenous malformations, aneurysm
- Hematologic (anemia) or electrolyte abnormalities (red flag for eating disorders)

Diagnostics: History is essential because syncope during exertion is much more concerning than syncope occurring after full exertion or standing still (common in neurocardiogenic syncope). Requires further workup and testing as indicated by history, family history, and physical examination. Often difficult to differentiate pathologic cardiac condition from "athlete's heart," which is a physiologic response to training. Both share common symptoms such as hypertrophy, prolonged electrocardiographic intervals, functional (nonpathologic) flow heart murmurs. Echocardiography, maximal exercise testing, and tilt-table testing are often useful adjuncts to the history and physical examination.

Return to play: Guidelines are unclear, but serious, life-threatening abnormalities must be ruled out first.

Gastrointestinal Problems

Alterations in GI function: 25%–50% of runners experience abdominal cramps, diarrhea, nausea, and abdominal pain. Blood flow to the gut typically decreases 50% during exercise.

Diarrhea: Typically self-limited and physiologic, tending not to cause dehydration or electrolyte imbalances. Antidiarrheal medications should be avoided whenever possible.

Celiac sprue (gluten-sensitive enteropathy): Can lead to decreased bone mass secondary to poor absorption of calcium. Athletes will typically complain of bloating and/or diarrhea and may have a family history. Consider this condition in athletes with these chronic symptoms. The athlete may also have electrolyte abnormalities and vitamin deficiencies. A diagnosis is made with serologic testing for immunoglobulin A and immunoglobulin G antitissue transglutaminase. If the test is positive, then a small intestinal biopsy is performed to establish a definitive diagnosis.

GI bleeding: Severe GI bleeding after endurance running has been reported, with rare occurrences of death secondary to acute hemorrhage, although these are reported as isolated cases. Reports of bright red blood per rectum must be rigorously worked up, and ulcerative colitis and Crohn disease must be ruled out. Occult forms of GI bleeding are common. Studies have reported anywhere from 8% to 22% rates of clinically detectable bleeding in marathoners after a race. If more sensitive assays are used, an increase in fecal heme concentrations is seen in 83% of marathoners. Thus, runners have an increase in stool heme after a race, and in approximately 20% it is detectable clinically. Bleeding is typically self-limited and resolves in roughly 72 hours. Bleeding can be associated with excessive iron loss and resultant iron deficiency, but must be differentiated from runner's pseudoanemia. Pathophysiology is unclear, but the physician must consider nonsteroidal antiinflammatory drug (NSAID) use, bowel ischemia, the traumatic shearing effect from running, and underlying GI abnormalities. A postexercise biopsy of the colon should be performed to reveal congestion and vascular lesions. The biopsy should be evaluated with appropriate imaging techniques. After GI pathology has been ruled out, treatment issues surround the presence/absence of iron deficiency and consideration of antimotility agents for diarrhea. Antidiarrheals inhibit heat dissipation and should be used with caution.

Reflux/delayed gastric emptying: A common complaint in endurance athletes and may result in nausea or vomiting. Exercise increases acid secretion and may lead to heartburn-type symptoms in some athletes. Symptoms can be exacerbated by precompetition nervousness. Thorough workup indicated to rule out GI pathology. Treatment centers on alteration in eating patterns, trials with magnesium or aluminum hydroxide and simethicone (Maalox), or H_2-blocker trial (1 hour before events).

Exercise-Induced Asthma

Description: Common in athletes, especially when exercising in cold. **Should be discussed during preparticipation physicals, including severity and current medications.**

Symptoms: Variable and occurring with exercise: wheezing, tightness, chest pain, shortness of breath. Symptoms can sometimes be vague: poor exercise tolerance, cough, or tightness after exercise. Symptoms aggravated by allergens, upper respiratory infections, and environmental conditions (humidity, cold air).

Diagnostics: Provocative testing helps make a diagnosis and assess response to bronchodilators: spirometry before exercise challenge, adequate exercise challenge (use whatever athlete describes as "typical" precipitant), postexercise spirometry. Look for a decrease in forced expiratory volume in the first second (FEV_1) and a decrease in FEV_1 as a fraction of total forced vital capacity.

Treatment: Beta-adrenergic receptor agonists, such as albuterol, are often helpful as pre-exercise medication to prevent exercise-induced asthma. Other medications include sodium cromolyn (Intal) or nedocromil sodium (Tilade) as premedication. Inhaled corticosteroids or the three to four times daily use of medications tends to be helpful for acute flaring of symptoms, baseline asthma (not only exercise-induced asthma), or allergen-induced asthma. Avoid known precipitants. Proper cardiovascular warmup can lessen symptoms and allow athlete to "run through" asthma: 15–20 minutes at approximately 70% $\dot{V}O_2$ max, using a series of 40- to 50-yard sprints. Minimize symptoms: use a scarf or other methods to warm inspired air; breathe through nose.

Drug testing concerns: The drugs permitted for the treatment of asthma change frequently. Athletes should be made aware of the acceptability of their current medications. All medication questions should be addressed to the US Anti-Doping Agency Drug Reference Line (800-233-0393).

Renal Issues

Pseudonephritis: Proteinuria, hematuria, and presence of cellular elements in the urine after exercise. Exercise is associated with decreased renal blood flow, and when coupled with dehydration, results in a decreased glomerular filtration rate as exercise continues. Proteinuria, hematuria, and pyuria, as well as cellular elements seen after intense exercise, are self-limited. Workup

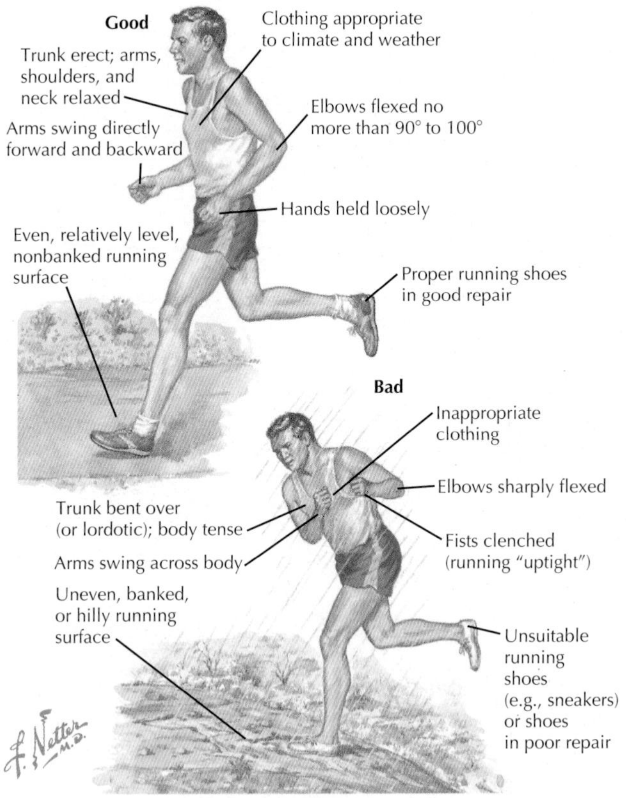
Good
Clothing appropriate to climate and weather
Trunk erect; arms, shoulders, and neck relaxed
Elbows flexed no more than 90° to 100°
Arms swing directly forward and backward
Hands held loosely
Even, relatively level, nonbanked running surface
Proper running shoes in good repair
Bad
Inappropriate clothing
Elbows sharply flexed
Trunk bent over (or lordotic); body tense
Fists clenched (running "uptight")
Arms swing across body
Uneven, banked, or hilly running surface
Unsuitable running shoes (e.g., sneakers) or shoes in poor repair

Figure 93.4 Good and bad running practice.

indicated if abnormalities persist after discontinuing exercise or if other symptoms or risk factors exist.

Gross hematuria: Reported in runners and often occurs without warning and without symptoms as painless clots of blood or grossly bloody urine. Possibly the result of a traction effect on bladder. Cystoscopy can sometimes detect the source of bleeding but is often negative. Further workup indicated if abnormalities persist despite stopping exercise or if other symptoms or risk factors are present.

COMMON MECHANISMS OF INJURY

Precipitating Factors

- **Training errors account for approximately 80% of injuries** (Fig. 93.4). Changing to a harder running surface, an abrupt increase in training mileage (10%), an abrupt increase in training intensity, hill running, consistent running on crowned roads, previous injury, inadequate rest/nutrition.
- **Uncorrected anatomic problems** include hip, pelvis, back, knee, foot, ankle, and leg length discrepancy.

Overuse

- Most common mechanism in track and field injuries
- Classified according to timing of pain in relation to onset of activity
  - Type 1: Pain after activity
  - Type 2: Pain during activity, not restricting activity
  - Type 3: Pain during activity, restricting activity, which restricts performance
  - Type 4: Chronic, unremitting pain

SPECIFIC MUSCULOSKELETAL INJURIES

Knee

The knee accounts for 30%–50% of all track and field injuries.

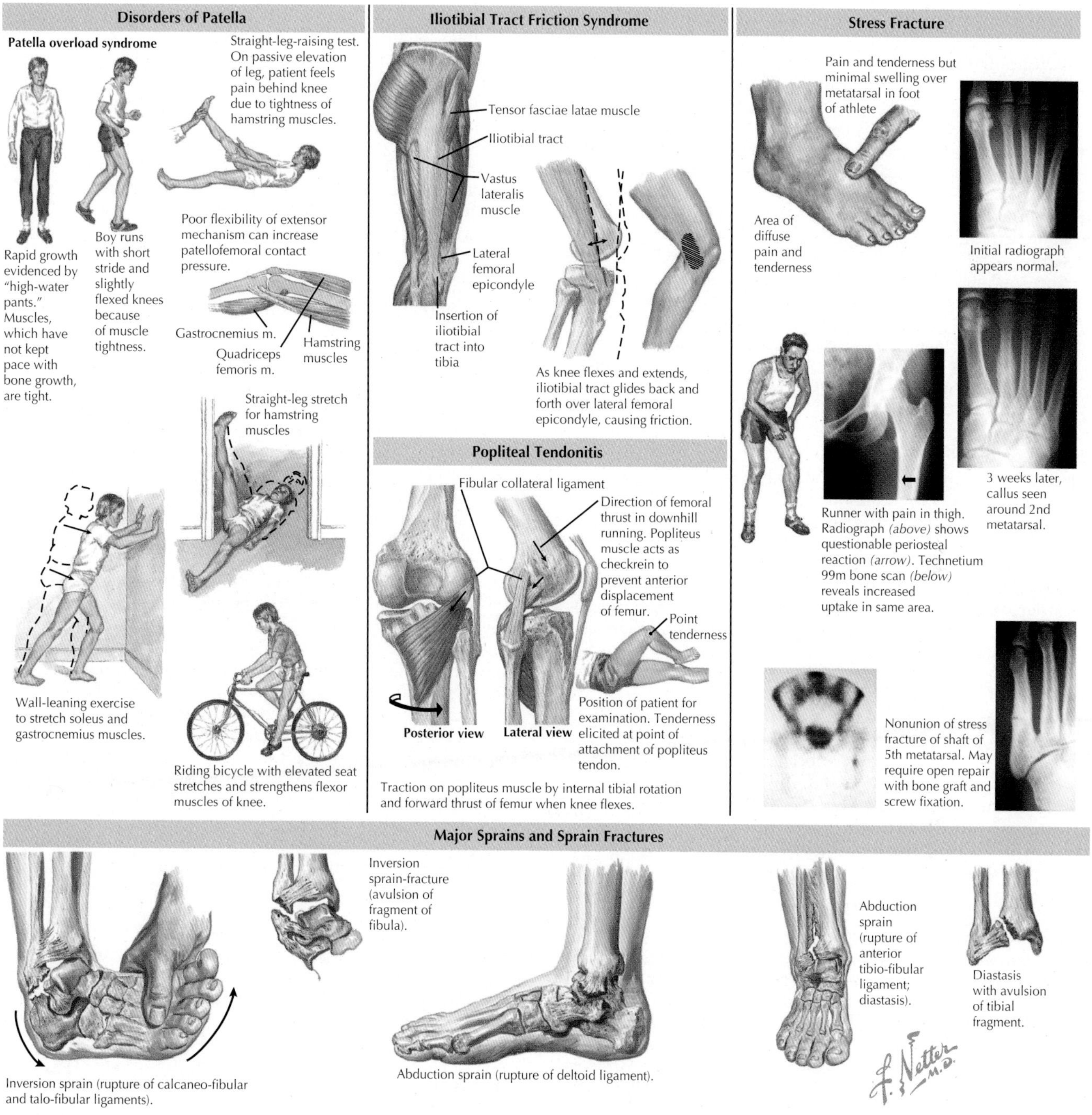
Disorders of Patella
Patella overload syndrome
Straight-leg-raising test. On passive elevation of leg, patient feels pain behind knee due to tightness of hamstring muscles.
Rapid growth evidenced by "high-water pants." Muscles, which have not kept pace with bone growth, are tight.
Boy runs with short stride and slightly flexed knees because of muscle tightness.
Poor flexibility of extensor mechanism can increase patellofemoral contact pressure.
Gastrocnemius m.
Quadriceps femoris m.
Hamstring muscles
Straight-leg stretch for hamstring muscles
Wall-leaning exercise to stretch soleus and gastrocnemius muscles.
Riding bicycle with elevated seat stretches and strengthens flexor muscles of knee.
Iliotibial Tract Friction Syndrome
Tensor fasciae latae muscle
Iliotibial tract
Vastus lateralis muscle
Lateral femoral epicondyle
Insertion of iliotibial tract into tibia
As knee flexes and extends, iliotibial tract glides back and forth over lateral femoral epicondyle, causing friction.
Popliteal Tendonitis
Fibular collateral ligament
Direction of femoral thrust in downhill running. Popliteus muscle acts as checkrein to prevent anterior displacement of femur.
Point tenderness
Posterior view
Lateral view
Position of patient for examination. Tenderness elicited at point of attachment of popliteus tendon.
Traction on popliteus muscle by internal tibial rotation and forward thrust of femur when knee flexes.
Stress Fracture
Pain and tenderness but minimal swelling over metatarsal in foot of athlete
Area of diffuse pain and tenderness
Initial radiograph appears normal.
3 weeks later, callus seen around 2nd metatarsal.
Runner with pain in thigh. Radiograph (above) shows questionable periosteal reaction (arrow). Technetium 99m bone scan (below) reveals increased uptake in same area.
Nonunion of stress fracture of shaft of 5th metatarsal. May require open repair with bone graft and screw fixation.
Major Sprains and Sprain Fractures
Inversion sprain-fracture (avulsion of fragment of fibula).
Abduction sprain (rupture of anterior tibio-fibular ligament; diastasis).
Diastasis with avulsion of tibial fragment.
Inversion sprain (rupture of calcaneo-fibular and talo-fibular ligaments).
Abduction sprain (rupture of deltoid ligament).
F. Netter M.D.

Figure 93.5 Lower extremity injuries.

Iliotibial Band Syndrome

Description: Common in runners. Iliotibial band inserts into Gerdy tubercle along the lateral tibia (Fig. 93.5). Often seen in conjunction with greater trochanteric bursitis.

Presentation: Lateral knee pain, often in midrange of knee flexion from 20 to 70 degrees, when the iliotibial band rubs across lateral femoral condyle.

Evaluation: Contributing anatomic factors (should be corrected if possible): leg length discrepancy, abnormal foot biomechanics (especially hyperpronation), tibia vara, scoliosis. Tightness of the musculature and/or muscle strength imbalances often seen; important to treat with corrective rehabilitation

Diagnostics: Ober test is useful for identifying tight iliotibial bands. Can reproduce the pain by resisting knee extension and looking for painful arc. This is sometimes difficult to differentiate from trochlear articular surface or an osteochondral defect.

Treatment: Stretching, ice, oral NSAIDs, phonophoresis, iontophoresis. Avoid running on beveled surfaces. Consider the use of corticosteroid and anesthetic agents if other measures fail.

Patellofemoral Dysfunction

Description: Generally thought to be caused by abnormal tracking of the patella with resultant patellofemoral irritation and pain (see Fig. 93.5). The proposed mechanism of patellofemoral dysfunction suggests that it results from activity that pushes the tissues of the knee beyond a "zone of homeostasis" rather than biomechanical alignment problems. Understanding the static and dynamic orientations of the patella is important in understanding the nature of a tracking dysfunction and in guiding rehabilitative treatment.

Contributing factors: Increased Q angle, deficient vastus medialis obliquus (VMO) or tight vastus lateralis musculature, patella alta, pronation (increases the functional Q angle), genu valgum, and recurvatum

Presentation: Anterior knee pain, which is often made worse by climbing or usually descending stairs, or prolonged sitting ("theater sign")

Treatment: Mainstay remains the strengthening of the VMO along with improved flexibility of lateral structures. There are various patellar taping methods to allow the patella to track more normally and facilitate pain-free strengthening of the VMO. Unclear how functionally effective taping is. Correction of leg length discrepancy or excessive pronation or other abnormal foot biomechanics, if present. Closed-chain kinetic exercises can be used in combination with physical therapy modalities, including ice, to decrease inflammation. Biofeedback is often helpful.

Patellar Tendinosis

Description: Common, especially in activities requiring jumping

Symptoms: Pain along the infrapatellar tendon, inferior pole of patella, or insertion of the patellar tendon into tibial tubercle; pain during knee extension, especially terminal extension

Treatment: Ice, stretching, NSAIDs, modalities (phonophoresis, iontophoresis), and decreased activity. Can use alternative cardiovascular equipment (bicycle, aqua arc, swimming, aquajogging). Avoid activities that aggravate pain, such as jumping and plyometrics.

Infrapatellar Fat Pad Impingement

Presentation: Anterior knee pain, similar in presentation to patellofemoral syndrome, except typically worse with standing and rapid knee extension. Often associated with an acute hyperextension injury.

Examination: Reveals tenderness at or below the inferior pole of the patella, often worse with passive, ballistic hyperextension

Treatment: Patellar taping, often by compressing the fat pad even further

Hamstring, Adductor, and Quadriceps Strains

Description: Common, especially in sprinters

Prevention: Eccentric hamstring exercise programs have been shown to reduce the risk of hamstring injury; specific exercises include Nordic hamstring exercises and yo-yo curls. Risk factors retrospectively associated with adductor strain include relative adductor weakness and decreased hip abduction ROM.

Presentation: A sudden pain in belly of affected muscle. Athletes often describe "pulling" or "tearing" sensations. Athletes often run through initial discomfort only to experience increasing pain and disability later.

Examination: Variable amounts of swelling and ecchymosis, depending on extent of muscle damage and exact location of injury. The size of the hematoma and cross-sectional damage can be assessed with magnetic resonance imaging (MRI), though it does not correspond well with future risk of injury. Diagnostic ultrasound, although operator dependent, can be useful in grading the extent of injury.

Most common hamstring injury: Short head of biceps femoris. Most often occurs at the proximal musculotendinous junction. As the athlete's velocity increases, the hamstrings take an increasingly active role in force production, leaving them prone to injury. Injuries typically occur during the eccentric phase of high-velocity movements. Although the data are speculative, incidence of hamstring strains appears to increase with inadequate flexibility, quadriceps–hamstring muscle imbalances, inadequate warm-up, prior injury, poor proprioception, and fatigue.

Treatment: All of these are extremely difficult to treat. Initial management: compressive wrap, ice, stretching. **Subsequent management:** use of NSAIDs, possibly ultrasound if scarring occurs. **Rehabilitation** should emphasize eccentric activity, reproduction of sport-specific demands, and maintenance of adequate ROM.

Prognosis and return to play: Gradually, as long as athlete has full ROM, full strength, and normal functional testing. Recurrence is common and often frustrating for the athlete. Progression back to full activity must be slow. Use of sport-specific progression helpful.

Lower Leg, Foot, and Ankle

Medial Tibial Stress Syndrome

Description: Pain over the medial third of the posteromedial tibia; association with excessive pronation.

Presentation: The area of tenderness is often located in the soleus muscle, which is involved in the inversion of subtalar joint and plantarflexion of ankle joint.

Diagnostics: X-ray findings have poor sensitivity (10%) in the early stages of stress reactions. Findings are typically very subtle and include the thickening of the medial tibial cortex common on plain radiographs; myositis and tendinosis are evident on bone scan (differentiated by increased blood pool phase). Order further imaging if clinical suspicion is high. Scintigraphy helps identify stress fractures. Plain radiographs may show evidence of stress fracture after 14 days, whereas bone scan is very sensitive but lacks specificity (statistics depend on site of fracture). Computed tomography (CT) scans with thin cuts over the suspected area are an option. However, false negatives are common, and stress reactions are not well visualized. Furthermore, radiation exposure is involved. MRI has several advantages: no radiation exposure, multiplanar imaging, high sensitivity, precise location of abnormalities, and the ability to detect early pathology. There are some reports of false-positive MRI results in asymptomatic patients. Fat-suppressed or short tau inversion recovery (STIR) images can be ordered. May also have the radiologists use MRI-visible markers to localize the painful area. Cost of bone scan and MRI varies based on institution.

Associated injuries: Progression from medial tibial stress syndrome to stress fracture is a major concern; treatment is aimed at preventing this.

Treatment: Ice; assessment of biomechanical abnormalities, focusing specifically on the need for orthotics; eccentric strengthening of antagonistic muscle groups and flexibility exercises, relative rest with alternative methods of training is useful (cycle, swim, aqua-jogging, Zuni unloader). Pain serves as a useful guide in injury management. Day-to-day, week-to-week adjustments in training regimen are often necessary. Athletes may continue pain-free activities (swimming, cycling, hand-cycle, pool running, ellipticals). Return to play is dictated by patient's ability to be pain-free during activities. Avoid NSAIDs, as they are felt to inhibit osteoblast activity.

Fractures and Stress Fractures

Description: Typically associated with mileage of more than 20 miles per week, changes in training volume and intensity, or underlying bone abnormalities (see Fig. 93.5).

Treatment: Depends on site, extent, and circumstances. Discontinue the offending activity, unload the affected extremity (walker-boot, crutches, even a wheelchair if bilateral involvement is present). Analgesia: NSAIDs have been shown to inhibit osteoblast activity in vivo in a rat model. Therefore, a non-NSAID may be a wiser choice. The same study demonstrated that low-intensity pulsed ultrasound facilitated the healing of stress fractures. Human studies on the efficacy of bone stimulators, via pulsed ultrasound or electrical field stimulation,

Table 93.1 FOOT FRACTURES

Fracture Type	Mechanism	Location	Chronicity	Prognosis
Avulsion	Hindfoot inversion	Tuberosity	Acute	Excellent
True Jones	Forefoot adduction	Metaphyseal-diaphyseal junction	Acute	Good
Diaphyseal stress	Cyclical loading	Proximal diaphyses		
Torg type I		Narrow fracture line, no medial sclerosis	Acute or chronic	Fair-good
Torg type II		Wide fracture line, some medial sclerosis	Delayed union	Variable
Torg type III		Complete medullary sclerosis	Nonunion	Variable

Adapted from Quill GE. Fractures of the proximal fifth metatarsal. *Orthop Clin North Am*. 1995;26(2):353–361.

are less conclusive. Low-intensity pulsed ultrasound did not affect the healing of stress fractures in a study of 26 midshipmen. Electrical field stimulation hastened healing in a small subset of acute, severe stress fractures but had no overall impact on healing for the whole study population. Consider use of a sports psychologist and nutritionist for support. Locate and correct any biomechanical abnormalities with orthotics, shoe-type changes, assess shoe age, and consider physical therapy for stretching and strengthening. Bisphosphonates should be used with extreme caution, given the negative impact on reproductive health; the agent has very little role in women of reproductive age. The navicular, tibia, and metatarsals are the most common sites of injury in track athletes. Distance runners are prone to tibial and fibular stress fractures. Studies suggest females are more susceptible than males. Likely multifactorial: the female athlete triad, baseline fitness level differences, training errors, and body geometry differences have all been cited as possible causes.

TUBEROSITY AVULSION FRACTURES

Description: **Most common fracture of the proximal fifth metatarsal** (Table 93.1). Often occurs where the plantar aponeurosis or peroneus brevis attaches. Fracture displacement rare.

Evaluation: Look for an associated lateral malleolus fracture. Can be differentiated from unfused tuberosity apophysis by the smoothness and orientation of the fracture line (fracture often perpendicular to shaft of bone). Differentiated from os peroneum by smoothness of edges and frequent presence of bilaterality.

Treatment: **Primarily symptomatic.** Can immobilize using a cast or molded hard-sole shoe for 1–2 weeks, followed by protected weight bearing to tolerance and close follow-up.

JONES FRACTURE

Description: **Acute forefoot injury of the proximal fifth metatarsal without prodrome. However, likely an acute-on-chronic phenomenon in an area of consistent microtrauma.** Occurs at the junction of metaphysis and diaphysis; no intermetatarsal extension

Treatment: Varies. Conservative management with casting for 6–8 weeks. If no improvement is observed, surgical consultation should be ordered.

PROXIMAL FIFTH METATARSAL DIAPHYSEAL STRESS FRACTURE

Description: A fracture resulting from repetitive cyclic forces applied to the foot

Presentation: Can have prodromal symptoms or acute or chronic presentation

Classification: Torg classification helps differentiate stress fractures by their potential to heal (see Table 93.1).

- Acute, early diaphyseal stress fracture (periosteal reaction)
- Delayed union (lucent fracture line and medullary sclerosis)
- Nonunion

Treatment: Depends on patient needs and expectations.

- Type I: treat as an acute nondisplaced Jones fracture
- Type II: treat operatively with bone graft or medullary screw fixation
- Type III: treat operatively; some prefer closed cannulated medullary screw fixation, others open methods

OTHER STRESS FRACTURES

Description: Runners account for 69% of all stress fractures because of increased stresses on normal bone, in addition to normal to increased stresses on weakened bone. Injury can occur throughout the lower extremity: tibia (34%), fibula (24%), metatarsals (18%), femur (14%), and pelvis (6%).

Evaluation and treatment: Pay particular attention to the location of femoral neck fractures. Fractures occurring on the superior/tension side of the femoral neck require prompt surgical evaluation. Fractures on the inferior/compression side of the femoral neck can be managed more conservatively.

Associated injuries: Associated with gait abnormalities, leg length discrepancy, poor surface, incompletely rehabilitated prior injuries, reduced bone mineral density, training errors, and abrupt changes in the volume or intensity of training.

Exertional Compartment Syndrome

Description: Reversible ischemia caused by a noncompliant osseofascial compartment that does not appropriately respond to the expansion of muscle tissue during exercise.

Presentation: A tight cramping ache over the involved compartment, with onset at a reproducible point during exercise, and resolution with rest. Presentation in the anterior compartment is most common (45%), followed by the deep posterior (40%), lateral (10%), and superficial posterior compartments (5%). Can present with associated weakness and paresthesias.

Diagnostics: Compartment pressures can be measured by a variety of methods, including a needle manometer, wick catheter, slit catheter, continuous infusion, and solid-state transducer intracompartmental catheter. Criteria for diagnosis include a pre-exercise pressure 15 mmHg or greater, 1-minute postexercise pressure 30 mmHg or greater, and 5-minute postexercise pressure 20 mmHg or greater. The more criteria met, the greater the confidence in the diagnosis. Testing may require sport-specific exercise to reproduce symptoms. Less invasive alternatives currently being explored include ultrasound, triple-phase bone scan, MRI, and near-infrared spectroscopy.

Treatment: Treatment can be surgical or conservative. Conservative measures include relative rest (limiting exercise to produce minimal symptoms), antiinflammatories, manual therapy, stretching, and strengthening. If symptoms persist beyond 6–12 weeks despite conservative treatment, or if diagnostic testing demonstrates severely elevated pressures, surgical release is recommended. Surgical remediation involves fasciotomy, with or without fasciectomy, by various techniques. Return-to-play period is approximately 3 months.

Peroneal, Anterior Tibialis, and Posterior Tibialis Strains

Description: Feature as common overuse injuries, in addition to acute overload injuries and strains. **Usually caused by training errors,** increase in training, change in shoes, poor flexibility.

Diagnostics: Can see avulsions or partial tears, especially of the peroneal tendons. Peroneal tendons run in the common tendon sheath until just posterior to the lateral malleolus, then bifurcate and run in their own tendon sheaths. MRI helps evaluate significant tendon injuries. Tendinosis is rarely detected by MRI. Musculoskeletal ultrasound can help diagnose these types of soft tissue injuries.

Treatment: Ice, stretching, addressing training errors or foot and ankle biomechanics.

Plantar Fasciitis

Description: Microtears caused by traction of the plantar fascia and associated structures at the calcaneal insertion.

Presentation: Heel or arch pain, often worst with first steps after getting out of bed.

Examination: Seen in both pes planus and pes cavus, although the latter is more common. A tight gastrocnemius–soleus complex and plantar flexors, as well as excessive pronation, increase the risk of developing plantar fasciitis. Pain to palpation along the plantar fascia, often at insertion into calcaneus. Pain with resisted toe flexion and passive toe extension.

Imaging: Radiographs may demonstrate heel spur, but this often presents bilaterally despite unilateral symptoms.

Treatment: NSAIDs, ice massage, arch stretches, heel cushioning, counterforce taping, phonophoresis, or iontophoresis. Corticosteroid injections can be useful if other modalities are not helpful but may increase risk of rupture. Surgery can be used to release the plantar fascia in severe, refractory cases. **Night splints** are useful to keep the plantar fascia at length by placing the foot at 90 degrees of dorsiflexion. Stretching of the gastrocnemius–soleus complex and hamstrings is also important, as is intrinsic strengthening of foot musculature. **Arch supports or orthotics can be used if other rearfoot abnormalities are present.**

Heel Pain: Fat Pad Contusion, Heel Spurs

Description: Common in hurdlers, jumpers, and endurance runners

Presentation: Pain along fat pad or at insertion of the plantar fascia into the calcaneus. Patients often have history of increased training or increased shoe wear and tear without replacement.

Evaluation: Consider calcaneal stress fracture in the differential. Presence of an exaggerated heel strike in gait is common.

Treatment: Ice massage, NSAIDs, shoe modification: soft cushioning, replacement of worn shoes (recommend changing shoes every 6 months or 300–500 miles).

Achilles Tendinopathy

Description: Common in events involving jumping, landing, and sprinting. Tendonitis represents an inflammatory process, whereas tendinosis refers to chronic intratendinous degenerative changes without acute inflammation. Pathology reveals no inflammatory cells involved.

Evaluation: Pain often presents approximately 2 cm proximal to the insertion of the Achilles tendon into the calcaneus or distal tendon. Palpation of nodularity may signify mucinous degeneration of the tendon and/or a partial tear. Can palpate crepitus along tendon sheath with a passive or active motion ("squeaking tendon"). Pain along the tendon is accompanied by resisted plantarflexion and passive dorsiflexion. A positive **Thompson test** signifies a complete tear. The patient is placed prone and the gastrocnemius is squeezed, which creates an automatic plantarflexion of the foot. A positive test occurs if no plantarflexion occurs. Test with the knee in full extension and in 90 degrees of flexion to confirm the diagnosis.

Treatment: Ice, relative rest, NSAIDs, bilateral heel lifts to put tendon at rest, eccentric rehabilitation program that emphasizes stretching, return to functional activities, slow progression. Modify activities to pain tolerance. Assess for training errors or anatomic precipitants. Treatment of Achilles rupture should be individualized. For a competitive athlete, surgical treatment may be the better option for an earlier functional recovery. Surgical debridement is sometimes considered for recalcitrant tendinosis.

Hip and Spine

- Hip and spine injuries **account for close to 20% of all injuries** in track and field athletes.

Muscular Imbalance

Description: Common cause of muscular strains and overuse injuries. Unclear cause but can been seen in association with an old injury or as a response to overload, muscular weakness, leg length discrepancy, or other asymmetric anatomic abnormalities. One theory is the "lower crossed syndrome," where tight hip flexors and erector spinae are associated with weak gluteals and abdominals. This can lead to an anterior pelvic tilt and dysfunctional lower extremity biomechanics.

Treatment: The most difficult aspect of treatment is the recognition of muscular imbalances. Treatment rests on the flexibility of tight structures, in addition to the strengthening of weak structures. The correction of anatomic or gait abnormalities is essential.

ENVIRONMENTAL ISSUES

Heat Injuries

General considerations: When an athlete exercises in the heat, as body temperature increases, physiologic mechanisms act to dissipate excess heat into the environment. These thermoregulatory adjustments impart physiologic strain and may lead to dehydration, which in itself can also lead to further thermal and cardiovascular strain.

Heatstroke: Body temperature above 104°F (40°C), altered mental status, absent sweating, seizures, and coma. Can be fatal and accounts for hundreds of deaths in the United States annually. Treat as medical emergency; assess renal, neurologic, hepatic systems, and hospitalize.

Heat exhaustion: Where body temperature does not exceed 104°F (40°C) and no mental status changes are observed. Symptoms include profound weakness, dizziness, syncope, muscle cramps, and nausea. Risks are similar to heatstroke if unrecognized. Treatment often similar: assessment by physician, rest in cool environment out of the sun, oral administration of fluids. Activity should be restricted for remainder of day, and athlete should be re-evaluated on the following day.

Heat cramps: Cramps often in abdomen and lower extremities; often related to fluid or electrolyte deficiency. Treat with fluid and electrolyte replacement.

Heat syncope: A decrease in vasomotor tone and venous pooling (especially immediately after stopping exercise), which leads to syncope; dehydration and increased body temperature contribute to development.

Heat tetany: Spasm, often in wrist, observed with heat; exacerbated by hyperventilation.

Heat edema: A swelling of the hands and feet in response to heat; often worst in initial phases of accommodation to new environment. Self-limited; often resolves with cold compresses and elevation. Diuretics not indicated and may exacerbate dehydration.

Risk factors: Very young or very old age; preexisting dehydration; obesity; a history of previous heat-related illnesses, heart disease, sickle cell disease/trait, alcohol use, or drugs (tricyclic antidepressants, amphetamines, LSD, PCP, cocaine, anticholinergics [previously discussed], antihistamines, diuretics, beta-blockers); increased humidity, temperature, no clouds or wind; poor physical conditioning; acute febrile illness.

Treatment: Generally focuses on rapid cooling using cold water immersion and timely transport to a medical facility. If rectal temperature is above 104°F (40°C), cooling should occur immediately with the goal of reaching a temperature of 102°F (38.8°C) within 30–60 minutes. Airway protection must be ensured. Electrolyte abnormalities common.

Prevention:

- Heat acclimatization: athletes planning to compete in heat should train for a minimum of 2 weeks for 60 minutes per day in a similar environment to the competition venue to allow for optimal physiologic adaptations.
- Hydration: before training or competing in the heat, athletes should consume 6 mL/kg fluid every 2–3 hours. Sodium supplementation may be required during training. Postexercise hydration should aim to replenish 100%–150% of body mass losses.
- Cooling strategies: combination of internal (ingestion of cold fluids) and external (iced garments, cold towels, water immersion, fans).

Cold Weather Injuries

- Heat production in the body is maintained by:

Basal heat production: Produced by metabolic processes; ineffective in maintaining body temperature when exposure to cold environment occurs.

Muscular thermoregulatory heat: Produced by shivering. Blood flow is preferentially shunted to vital organs. Can increase heat production threefold to fivefold but requires energy; also increases cooling of the distal extremities and skin.

Mild-to-moderate exercise-induced heat: Produced by low-intensity exercise; can increase heat production fivefold. Uses low-energy requirements and can thus be sustained for a long period.

High-intensity exercise-induced heat: Can increase heat production 10-fold but cannot be maintained for long periods because of higher energy requirements.

Specific Cold Weather Injuries

Frostnip: Reversible without permanent tissue damage; blanching of skin; slow, painless crystal formation on ears, face, toes, and fingertips; common in windy conditions.

Chilblains: Repeated exposure to cold water or wet cooling; a red, hot, tender, swollen extremity with numbness or tingling. Irreversible damage can occur to capillaries, muscles, and nerves innervating the extremity; may progress to gangrene.

Frostbite: The freezing of soft tissue; commonly involves the nose, fingertips, ears, and toes. Symptoms include local pain, numbness, redness, and superficial blistering. Deeper blistering and the involvement of deep soft tissue and bone occur with increased severity of exposure. Common in winter months and/or with windy and wet conditions. Frostbite may be permanent if not treated quickly.

Hypothermia: Occurs when the core body temperature drops below 95°F (35°C); significant cause of mortality.

Treatment of cold injuries:

- **The best treatment is prevention.**
- After a warm environment is secured, patient should be rewarmed slowly to minimize the risk of tissue damage.
- Removal of all wet clothing; proper measurement of core body temperature using oral, rectal, or auricular thermometer.
- Use of warm whirlpool, analgesics, skin protection.
- Other preventive measures: layered clothing; covering for head; protection of hands and toes; avoidance of wetness; proper nutrition and hydration; adequate warmup before activity; breathing through nose to warm inspired air; avoidance of alcohol, nicotine, and other drugs. Never train alone.

Table 93.2 COLOR-CODED FLAG SYSTEM

Color	Risk	Comments	Restrictions
Black	Extreme risk	WBGT >82°F (27.7°C)	Cancel race
Red	High risk	WBGT 73–82°F (22.7–27.7°C)	Be aware; high-risk athletes should not run
Yellow	Moderate risk	WBGT 65–73°F (18.3–22.7°C)	Heat-sensitive athletes should slow pace
Green	Low risk	WBGT 50–65°F (10–18.3°C)	No restrictions
White	Risk for hypothermia	WBGT <50°F (10°C)	Hypothermia possible, especially if wet or windy

WBGT, Wet bulb globe temperature.

Table 93.3 CORRECTED ESTIMATION OF THE RISK OF EXERTIONAL HEAT ILLNESS BASED ON THE WET BULB GLOBE TEMPERATURE (WBGT) TAKING INTO ACCOUNT THAT WBGT UNDERESTIMATES HEAT STRESS UNDER HIGH HUMIDITY

Estimated Risk	WBGT (°C)	Relative Humidity (%)
Moderate	24	50
Moderate	20	75
Moderate	18	100
High	28	50
High	26	75
High	24	100
Excessive	33	50
Excessive	29	75
Excessive	28	100

From Racinais S, Alonso JM, Coutts AJ, et al. Consensus recommendations on training and competing in the heat. *Br J Sports Med.* 2015;49(18):1164–1173.

Guidelines About Environmental Issues

- American College of Sports Medicine Guidelines remain standard.
- Use of wet bulb globe temperature (WBGT) ideal but has limitations
- WBGT = (0.7 Twb) + (0.2 Tg) + (0.1 Tdb), where Twb = wet bulb thermometer temperature, Tg = black globe thermometer temperature, and Tdb = dry bulb thermometer temperature
- Use color-coded flag system (Table 93.2).
- Use correction system to account for humidity (Table 93.3).

UPPER EXTREMITY INJURIES (SHOULDER IMPINGEMENT, ACROMIOCLAVICULAR INJURIES, FRACTURES, MEDIAL EPICONDYLITIS)

Available online.

KNEE INJURIES (GREATER TROCHANTERIC BURSITIS, LEG LENGTH DISCREPANCY, MENISCAL LESIONS)

Available online.

LOWER LEG, FOOT, AND ANKLE INJURIES (ANKLE SPRAINS, CHONDRAL AND OSTEOCHONDRAL LESIONS)

Available online.

HIP AND SPINE INJURIES (SPONDYLOLYSIS AND SPONDYLOLISTHESIS, HERNIATED NUCLEUS PULPOSUS, PARASPINAL MUSCULAR STRAINS)

Available online.

SAFETY AND EQUIPMENT ISSUES

Available online.

ACKNOWLEDGMENTS

The author would like to acknowledge the work of the previous edition authors, **Scott R. Laker, MD; Margot Putukian, MD; Deborah Saint-Phard, MD; and Adele J. Meron, MD.**

RECOMMENDED READINGS

Available online.

ROAD BIKING

94

Marc R. Silberman

GENERAL PRINCIPLES

Races

Road Racing

Stage races: Multiday races over consecutive days with daily stage winners and an overall winner based on cumulative time; mass start races where the athletes ride in a peloton.

Grand tours: Tour de France, Giro d'Italia, and Vuelta a España; usually include a prologue, flat stages for "sprinters," hilly stages for "climbers," and time trials.

Road races: Mass-start point-to-point races between 100 km and 298 km in length (Milan–San Remo, the longest professional 1-day race in modern times).

Circuit races: Multilap races of 100 km to 140 km on 5-km to 30-km courses. The World Championship and Olympic road races are circuit races. A kermesse is a common cycling race type in Belgium for amateurs, lasting 120–80 minutes.

Criterium: Multilap races of 40–80 km or miles, on 1-km to 1-mile courses containing tight cornered roads. A common cycling race for amateurs in the United States, lasting 60–90 minutes. Crashes are common.

Time trials (TTs): Individual races "against the clock"; riders start at 1- to 2-minute intervals on TT bikes. Drafting is prohibited. Distances range from 20 km to 50 km. **Triathlons** have TTs in lengths from 20 km (sprint distance) to 180 km (full distance).

Track Racing

Description: Held on a **velodrome** track (with banking, length 250–333 m); riders use **track bikes** (with no brakes and fixed gears).

Races: Match sprint, kilometer, pursuit, team pursuit, points race, miss and out, keirin, Madison.

Gravel Riding ("Gravel Grinding")

- Cycling, often long-distance events and/or racing over unpaved roads on a gravel bike (road bike designed for unpaved roads).
- Dropbar bike riding over any unpaved surface would constitute gravel riding.
- Roads range from well-maintained dirt roads, dry or muddy, to gravel, rocks, ruts, washboards, blown-out jeep tracks, potholes, and sand.
- Wider tire width commonly used: 33–38 mm.

Touring

- Self-contained noncompetitive cycling for pleasure, ranging from a day to multiday trips.
- Fully loaded or self-supported touring involves cyclists carrying everything they need—clothing, food, cooking equipment, and tents in panniers.
- **Cyclosportive (randonnee cyclosportive),** or cyclosportif, is a long-distance, annual, organized, mass-participation cycling event.
- The Italian term **Gran Fondo** is used to name these events in the United States.
- The true Italian Gran Fondos are long-distance bicycle races, whereas in the United States, they refer to something in between a race and a tour: a mass-participation ride of varying distance on open roads, with some racing for time.
- Both a cultural and a sporting event.

Riders

Sprinters: Possess high numbers of fast-twitch muscle fibers for explosive acceleration; can reach speeds of 66.1 ± 3.4 kph (57.1–70.6 kph), with peak power outputs at the end of a Tour de France Stage of 989–1443 W and average power of 865–1140 W for a duration of 9–17 seconds. Sprinters take calculated risks in maneuvering through the pack, waiting until the last possible moment to move out of another rider's slipstream and into the wind. A low shoulder, head-down position can lower the coefficient of drag area by about 10%, resulting in a more than 3-meter advantage over a 14-second sprint duration. The average professional male road sprint speed is 63.9 kph (53.7–69.1 kph) sustained between 9 and 17 seconds, and the average women's professional sprint speed is 53.8 kph (41.6–64 kph) for 10–30 seconds.

Climbers: Lightweight, possessing high levels of aerobic power, a high power-to-weight ratio, a VO_2 max of 75–85 mL/kg/min, and power output measurements of 7.4 W/kg over 5 minutes, 6.5 W/kg over 20 minutes, 6.1 W/kg over 30 minutes, and 5.7 W/kg over 1 hour.

Lead-out riders: Break the wind for their sprinters until the very last possible moment by sustaining high speed for a kilometer; generally lack the finishing top end speed of sprinters.

Time trialists: Ride at a steady state for long periods; physically larger cyclists who can push a big gear and produce greater absolute power outputs.

Team leaders: Riders for stage race overall classification; must be able to climb and TT.

Domestiques: Sacrifice themselves for the sprinters and leaders by chasing down breakaways, carrying water, blocking the wind, or even giving a wheel or bike up to their leader.

Organizations

USA Cycling (USAC): National governing body for bicycle racing in the United States.

Union Cycliste Internationale (UCI): World governing body for cycling. Issues licenses, enforces disciplinary rules, manages the classification of races and points ranking systems, and oversees the World Championships.

International Olympic Committee (IOC): Organization that oversees the Olympics.

United States Anti-Doping Agency (USADA): A nongovernmental agency responsible for implementation of the World Anti-Doping Code in the United States. The World Anti-Doping Code, which lists drugs and methods that are prohibited in sports, was developed by the World Anti-Doping Agency (WADA).

WADA: Independent foundation created through a collective initiative led by the IOC. In November 1999, the WADA was created to promote and coordinate the fight against doping in sports. In 2004, the **World Anti-Doping Code** was implemented by sports organizations before the Athens Olympics, standardizing regulations governing antidoping.

Court of Arbitration for Sport (CAS): International institution independent of any sports organization to facilitate the settlement of sports-related disputes through arbitration or mediation.

Epidemiology and Injury Statistics

- Traumatic injuries occur in 38%–48.5% of professionals.
- Overuse injuries occur in 51.5%–62% of professionals.
- Two-thirds of traumatic injuries involve the upper extremity.
- Two-thirds of overuse injuries involve the lower extremity.
- Touring cyclists on a 500-mile, 8-day ride sustained 57.2% of bicycle contact injuries (32.8% buttock, 9.1% groin, 10% palmar, 5.3% foot) and 42.8% of overuse injuries.
- A 4-year study of 51 top-level professionals found that 43 athletes sustained 103 injuries (50 traumatic and 53 overuse). Eight (16%) remained free of injury, 22 (43%) sustained both traumatic and overuse injuries, 13 (25.5%) sustained only traumatic injuries, and 10 (19.6%) sustained only overuse injuries. Twenty-nine (56.9%) sustained more than one injury. A survey of 81 cyclists in a well-established masters cycling club found:
  - Eighty-one percent had a racing license; average number of racing years was 9.5, with an average annual mileage of 6000 miles.
  - Seventy-nine percent were seen in an emergency room, 33% had been admitted to hospital, with 15% to the intensive care unit.
  - Fifty-four percent had sustained fractures: clavicle, 22 cyclists; upper extremity, 20 cyclists; ribs, 20 cyclists; lower extremity, 11 cyclists; vertebral, 11 cyclists; pelvis, 6 cyclists; skull, 6 cyclists.
  - Forty-five percent reported a head injury; 34% reported a concussion, with 9% reporting more than one.
  - Seventy-five percent reported breaking one or more helmets from a crash.
  - Ninety percent reported having road rash.
  - Thirty-seven percent of crashes involved motor vehicles, 9% were the result of road surface hazards, 12% were the result of skill errors, and 10% were the result of mechanical problems.
  - Seventeen percent occurred in a paceline, 12% in racing, often criteriums.

Equipment and Safety Issues

- Bicycles should be inspected regularly. Tire pressure (pounds per square inch [PSI]) should be set at the proper amount; lower PSI in wet road conditions.
- Protective gear:
  - **Helmets** manufactured after 1999 must meet the Consumer Product Safety Commission (CPSC) standard by law to be sold in the United States. There is no federal law in the United States requiring bicycle helmet use. Presently, 22 states, including the District of Columbia, have mandatory helmet laws. Helmets are designed for one crash only. No helmet design has been proven to prevent concussions. Helmets are designed to prevent skull fractures. Cyclists should write their name, contact information, and medical information in the helmet for emergencies.
  - Protective gear: helmet, gloves, tight-fitting cycling jersey and shorts, chamois padding in shorts, sunglasses, reflective gear, arm warmers and leg warmers, vest, tights, booties, and daytime running lights on the front and back of bicycle. Covering of skin is more important than type of material for prevention of road rash.

Biomechanical Principles

Bicycle Anatomy

ROAD BICYCLE

- **Key frame measurements** are seat tube length, seat tube angle, and top tube length.
- **Key component measurements**

Table 94.1 CRANK ARM

Height (in)	Crank Length (mm)	Inseam (in)	Crank Length (mm)
<60	160	<29	165
60–64	165–167.5	29–32	170
65–72	170	32–34	172.5
72–74	172.5	>34	175
74–76	175		
>76	180		

Modified from Burke ER. *High-Tech Cycling*. 2nd ed. Champaign, IL: Human Kinetics; 2003.

  - **Crank length:** Based on height of rider or inseam length (Table 94.1). Too long may predispose rider to fatigue and knee ailments. "Spinning" (pedaling with a higher cadence) is easier with a shorter crank.
  - **Crankset:**
    - Triple (three chainrings): Large chainring commonly has 52 teeth, medium has 39 teeth, and small has 30 teeth.
    - Standard (two chainrings): Large chainring commonly has 53 teeth and small 39 teeth.
    - Compact (two chainrings): Large chainring commonly has 50 teeth and small 34 or 36 teeth.
  - **Stem length and angle: Reach is determined by stem along with length of top tube.**
  - **Handlebar width** should be close to the width of the shoulders.
  - **Handlebar tilt:** Bars can slip and rotate into downward tilt, which can cause excessive reach, leading to hand, neck, and back symptoms.
  - **Gearing:** The number of gears on a bike is equal to the number of sprockets on the rear wheel multiplied by the number of chainrings. A double chainring on the front with an 11-speed cassette has 22 speeds. A high or big gear is achieved by riding the larger chainring on the front and a smaller cog on the rear, such as 53 × 11. The smallest chainring combined with the largest cog produces a small gear, used for climbing and spinning. Professionals are efficient in choosing the right gear to maintain a high cadence of 90 rpm or greater while maintaining a high speed for an extended period.
- **Key bicycle measurements**
  - Saddle height: center of the bottom bracket to the height of saddle where rider sits
  - Difference between saddle height and handlebar height
  - Saddle tilt
  - Saddle fore-aft
  - Plumb line from nose of the saddle, measure the distance to the bottom bracket
  - Distance from nose of saddle to handlebars

TRACK BICYCLE

- No brakes
- Fixed gear
- Major trauma risk with crashes

TIME TRIAL BICYCLE

- Steeper seat tube angle (78–84 degrees), aero bars, aero deep dish wheels and/or rear disc
- Designed to go fast and straight
- Goal is the reduction of frontal surface area, a flat back, narrow arm position, and elbow flexion of 90–110 degrees with the ear directly over elbow. The "Praying Mantis" and "Superman" positions are aero setups, and both are banned by the UCI.
- The narrow positioning of the arms does not restrict oxygen consumption and lung function.

Table 94.2 OVERUSE INJURIES: CONTRIBUTING BICYCLE POSTURE AND BICYCLE ADJUSTMENTS

Ailment	Contributing Position	Bicycle Adjustment
Posterior neck pain, may extend to head	Too great of a reach, handlebars too low, too stretched out	Ride more upright to shorten reach Raise stem height Shorten stem length Ride with hands on hoods or tops of bars
Scapular pain	Too great of a reach, handlebars too low, too stretched out	Ride more upright shorten reach Raise stem height Shorten stem length Ride with hands on hoods or tops of bars
Hand neuropathy (cyclist's palsy)	Too much pressure on bars, handlebars too low, saddle too far forward, excessive downward saddle tilt	Increase padding on bars and gloves Avoid prolonged pressure, change hand position often Raise stem height Move saddle back if too far forward If saddle is tilted down, position it level
Low back pain	Too stretched out	Ride more upright to shorten reach Raise stem height Shorten stem length
Tibialis anterior tendinopathy	Saddle height too high	Lower saddle height
Achilles tendinopathy	Saddle height too high (excessive stretch) Saddle height too low (with concomitant dropping of heel to generate more power)	Lower saddle height Raise saddle height
Morton neuroma/foot pain/ numbness	Cleat position Irregular sole Shoes too tight	Usually, move cleat back, but may be forward Check sole for inner wear or cleat bolts pressing inward Wider shoes, loosen Velcro straps/shoe buckle
Perineal numbness	Saddle too high Tilt angle excessively up or down	Lower saddle height Adjust angle closer to level with the ground

From Baker A. Medical problems in road cycling. In Gregor RJ, Conconi F, eds. *Road Cycling*. Oxford: Blackwell Sciences; 2000:18–45; and Silberman M, Webner D, Collina S, et al. Road bicycle fit: practical management. *Clin J Sport Med*. 2005;15(4):271–276.

Bike Fit

- A proper fit is essential for rider comfort, safety, injury prevention, and peak performance.
- The goal is the optimization of power and aerobic efficiency while avoiding injury (Table 94.2).
- Fit can be tested using static (at rest) or dynamic (while riding) measurements. Dynamic fit testing may involve video analysis; heart rate, wattage, pedal torque readings; wind tunnel testing.
- Changes should be made gradually.
- There are **three contact areas** where a rider interfaces with the bicycle: shoe–cleat–pedal, pelvis–saddle, and hands–handlebar (Fig. 94.1).

SHOE–CLEAT–PEDAL INTERFACE

- The first metatarsal head lies directly over the pedal axle (see Fig. 94.1).
- Leg length discrepancy: shims can be inserted beneath the cleat of the shorter leg, or the cleat may be moved forward (and the foot back) on the shorter leg when differences are small. One-third to half of the difference should be corrected with shim.
- Heel lifts and orthotics are not sufficient for cycling because the driving force is primarily through the first and second metatarsal heads. Varus forefoot wedges may be used.

PELVIS–SADDLE INTERFACE

- **Saddle height**
  - Traditional existing formulas are designed to fit a rider to produce the most power at the least aerobic cost.
  - Greg LeMond and Cyrille Guimard formula: rider's inseam length in centimeters (standing wearing thin socks floor to crotch) × 0.883 = saddle height (see Fig. 94.1).
  - Knee angle method: The knee should be flexed 25–30 degrees from full extension, with the pedal in the 6-o'clock position (also known as *dead bottom center* [DBC]) (see Fig. 94.1).
- **Saddle fore-aft**

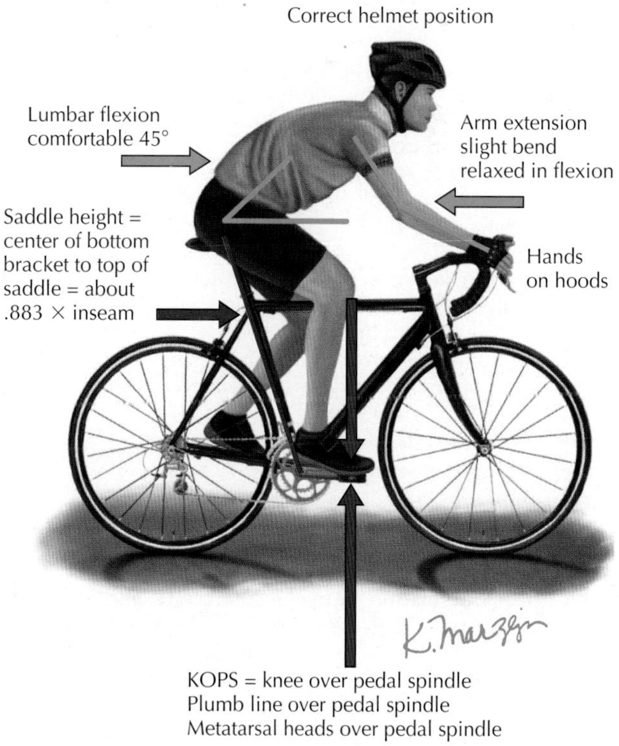
Correct helmet position
Lumbar flexion comfortable 45°
Arm extension slight bend relaxed in flexion
Saddle height = center of bottom bracket to top of saddle = about .883 × inseam
Hands on hoods
K. Marzen
KOPS = knee over pedal spindle
Plumb line over pedal spindle
Metatarsal heads over pedal spindle

Figure 94.1 Road bike fit.

- With the pedal positioned at 3 o'clock (knee over pedal spindle [KNOPS]), a plumb line dropped from the inferior pole of the patella should hang directly over the pedal axle (see Fig. 94.1).
- Time trialists and triathletes prefer a more forward position so that the plumb line falls in front of the axle.

- Moving the saddle forward lowers the saddle height, whereas moving it backward raises the saddle.
- To compete in a TT with aerobars mounted on their usual road bike, a rider may move the saddle slightly forward and higher.
- **Saddle tilt**
  - Saddle tilt should be close to level.
  - About 60% of body weight should be centered on the narrow saddle.
  - Time trialists riding on aerobars may prefer a slight downward tilt of the saddle or a saddle with a split nose to relieve pressure on the perineum.

HANDS–HANDLEBAR INTERFACE

- **Stem and handlebar height**
  - Stem height is a subjective measurement; is important in terms of aerodynamics, power production, comfort, and injury prevention (see Fig. 94.1).
  - With the hands positioned on the brake hoods and the arms slightly flexed, the torso should flex to about 45 degrees in relation to a nonsloping top tube. The majority of time cycling will be spent on the hoods.
  - When the hands are in the drops, the torso should flex to about 60 degrees.
  - The vertical distance, or drop, between the top of the saddle to the bars should be about 5–8 cm, approaching level as a rider ages.
  - A recreational rider may prefer to sit more upright with a shorter reach and higher-raised handlebars for comfort.
  - An average-sized male cyclist may decrease his frontal area by 30 degrees, moving from the upright touring position to a racing position.
  - If forward-flexed excessively, the maximal sustainable power may be reduced because of diminished blood flow and/or changes in muscle lengths.
  - **Handlebar tilt** is a personal preference, but most cyclists prefer the lower curve and brake hoods to be slightly elevated. Bar shape and size also play an integral role in comfort.
- **Stem length or extension**
  - A rider's reach is determined by the top tube length, stem length, and stem angle or rise (see Fig. 94.1).
  - Too short a top tube or stem length, and the rider will be bunched up. Too long, and the rider will be stretched out.
  - A good starting point is when the rider looks down with the arms slightly bent and the hands in the drops, the front hub should be obscured by the handlebars.
  - If the frame was properly fitted, the top tube length will allow an optimum position to be achieved with the use of a 100-mm to 120-mm stem.

TRAINING AND PHYSIOLOGY

Performance Testing

Conconi test: One of the first tests to determine lactate threshold (LT) without directly measuring lactate; the **pace at which the linear correlation between heart rate and velocity is lost is called the *deflection velocity* or *deflection point*,** and is said to occur at the LT; a ramp protocol of increasing watts is performed in the laboratory with measurement of heart rate (HR); numerous authors have found the Conconi test invalid.

Lactate threshold (LT) or anaerobic threshold (AT): There is no consensus definition. The original *incorrect* hypothesis: the point of exertion where the body goes **anaerobic or into "oxygen debt"** and rapidly produces **lactic acid,** causing **fatigue and leg burn.** The onset of blood lactate accumulation **(OBLA)** was originally referred to as the effort level that corresponded to the point at which lactate began to rise exponentially—a blood lactate level of 4 mmol. Most commonly, **LT** refers to the effort (watts) that an athlete can maintain without a rise in lactate. The USOC Sport Science and Technology Division identifies the LT as **the point at which a minimum increase of 1.0 mmol/L above baseline values is followed by another increase greater than 1.0 mmol/L.** Maximum lactate steady state **(MLSS):** the effort level at which there is an equilibrium between lactate production and clearance, such that prolonged exercise does not result in rising serum lactate. Critical lactate measurements are power output at 2 mmol and 4 mmol. Lactate is a useable fuel, and training helps the body become more efficient at shuttling lactate for utilization to other parts of the body.

$\dot{V}O_2$ max test: Traditionally a graded exercise test (GXT) with a ramp protocol lasting 8–12 minutes consisting of increasing load by 25 watts at 1-minute increments until athlete fails to maintain set cadence. There is no standard protocol. Measures oxygen consumption ($\dot{V}O_2$), $\dot{V}CO_2$, respiratory exchange ratio (RER), and HR at increasing workloads. Self-paced laboratory 5-km TT versus a GXT has been found to produce greater $\dot{V}O_2$ max and HR. Current research is also directed toward using a supramaximal verification protocol performed after a GXT to confirm attainment of $\dot{V}O_2$ max.

Maximum aerobic power (MAP) test with lactate: Incremental ramp protocol with increasing load of 25–40 watts (W) at 3- to 4-minute intervals until failure to maintain set cadence. Alternatively, a submaximal test can be performed with termination of the ramp at the end of the step that produces a blood lactate concentration of greater than 4 mmol, and then after a 15-minute period of active rest of cycling at less than 100 W and able to drink ad libitum, a maximal test can be performed starting at 150 W with increases of 30 W per minute until unable to maintain set cadence. Measures $\dot{V}O_2$, HR, W, and lactate. MAP is defined as the highest power output maintained during the test. Peak power output (PPO) is the highest 30-second power output from the maximal aerobic test. Higher power outputs are achieved during shorter ramp protocols of 1-minute stages of 25-watt increments versus 4-minute stages of 35-watt increments. PPOs of professional cyclists have been recorded to be as high as 525–585 W. When expressed in watts/kilogram body weight, the PPO of a Tour de France champion has been measured to be 7.5 W/kg. The workload at 4 mmol/L has been correlated to cycling performance, with values as high as 6.4 W/kg at 4 mmol/L measured in Tour de France champions. $\dot{V}O_2$ max values of greater than 70 mL/kg/min are found in elite and professional cyclists, with top Tour de France cyclists ranging from 76 to 82 mL/kg/min. Professional cyclists appear to have a decrease in the magnitude of the $\dot{V}O_2$ slow component compared with amateur elites (oxygen uptake slowly rises during prolonged exercise at submaximal intensity, attributed to recruitment of type II fibers because of fatigue of type I fibers).

Cycling economy (CE): Power output generated in watts at a cost of 1 L of oxygen per minute of exercise (Coyle). For a constant load test of 20 minutes at 80% of $\dot{V}O_2$ max, the economy of world-class cyclists averages 85 W/L/min.

Gross mechanical efficiency (GE): Ratio of work accomplished to energy expended; GE = 60 × W ÷ 20,934 × $\dot{V}O_2$ (Jeukendrup). For world-class cyclists, the GE is 25%. Both CE and GE are positively related to the percentage distribution of type 1 fibers in the knee extensors. Once a high level of fitness has been obtained, such as in the elite athlete, CE and GE performed at submaximal intensities of 70%–90% of maximum HR are more important determinants of cycling performance than $\dot{V}O_2$ max (Lucia).

Wingate anaerobic test (WANT): Developed in Israel during the 1970s and measures **peak anaerobic power** (highest mechanical power generated during any 3- to 5-second interval of the test), **anaerobic fatigue** (the percentage decline in power compared with PPO), and **total anaerobic capacity**

(total amount of work accomplished over 30 seconds); the athlete pedals on a mechanically braked ergometer for 30 seconds all out against a fixed resistance.

Training Periods of Professional Road Cyclists

- "Rest" (November to December)
  - Weekly average 200 km/week, gentle, easy
  - Ninety percent of the time spent in Zone 1, less than 70% of maximum heart rate (HRmax)
  - Ten percent of the time spent in Zone 2, 70%–90% HRmax
  - Zero percent of the time spent in Zone 3, greater than 90% HRmax
- Precompetition (December to mid-February)
  - Weekly average 700 km/week; building base mileage, long steady rides, no intervals before 1000 miles
  - Eighty percent of the time spent in Zone 1, less than 70% of HRmax
  - Fifteen percent of the time spent in Zone 2, 70% to 90% HRmax
  - Five percent of the time spent in Zone 3, greater than 90% HRmax
- Competition (mid-February to October)
  - Weekly average 800 km/week
  - Seventy-five percent of the time spent in Zone 1, less than 70% of HRmax
  - Fifteen percent of the time spent in Zone 2, 70% to 90% HRmax
  - Ten percent of the time spent in Zone 3, greater than 90% HRmax
- Most riders plan for two peaks during the season.
- Training prescription is traditionally not as precise as in other endurance sports; most build long steady low-intensity mileage in winter months; attend one or two 8-day training camps with higher intensity and mileage in the late winter; "race into shape" with early season races. Traditional programs are followed to prepare riders for grand tours, with generally 30 days of racing before Tour de France.
- With power measurements on the road, cyclists can follow stricter training programs.

Training Measurements

Perceived level of exertion: Simply monitoring how one feels. Borg 10- or 20-point scale.

Time: Measure ride duration only, not intensity. Hours per ride for recreational rider: 1–1.5 hours. Amateur: 2–3 hours per ride, 8–12 hours per week. Professional: 15–30 hours per week.

Speed: Training based on average speed. Generally a poor indicator of training intensity because of the effects of altitude, wind, terrain, road surface, and drafting. Using average speed as indicator of intensity will lead to overtraining.

Distance: Training based on weekly or daily mileage. Does not measure intensity.

HR: Closely correlates with exercise intensity, power output, or rate of oxygen consumption in the laboratory, correlation not as close out on the roads. Influenced by altitude, heat, hydration, illness, sleep, overreaching, and overtraining. HR responds relatively slowly to changes in exercise intensity and cannot be used to regulate the intensity of shorter efforts **(HR lag).** HR is not a direct determinant of performance but is a reflection of the strain imposed on the cardiovascular system for the level of exertion.

Power output: Provides a direct and immediate answer to exercise intensity. Measured on the road with bike-mounted power meter systems. Power at LT, or 4 mmol of lactate, is one of the most important physiologic determinants of cycling performance. Functional threshold power equals average power during a 40-km (50- to 70-minute) TT. Correlates very highly, slightly greater than, power at LT (defined as 1 mmol/L increase in blood lactate over exercise baseline). Estimates athlete's threshold power by measuring power athlete can routinely produce in training during long interval repeats of 2 × 20 minutes. Mean power for five mass start stages: 220 ± 22 W (range 190 W to 310 W), average HR: 142 ± 5 beats per minute (bpm). Mean power for uphill 13-km TT: 392 ± 60 W (5.5 ± 0.4 W/kg), average HR: 169 ± 3 bpm. Indirect measurement for 3-week stage races: 246 ± 44 W for high mountain stages, 234 ± 43 W for semimountainous stages, 192 ± 45 W for flat stages (Table 94.3).

Technique

Pedaling

- The driving force of forward motion is the downward push on the pedals.
- The muscles involved in the power phase drive the crank downward in an effort to rotate the crank, whereas the muscles active in the recovery phase are firing primarily to reduce resistance versus the contralateral propulsive limb.
- Most athletes who are clipped into pedal systems believe they are supposed to pull up on the pedals; **pulling up on the pedals is inefficient and may lead to overuse injury.**
- In elite cyclists, even on the upstroke, the vector of forces is downward in the opposite direction of the pedal motion (the leg in the recovery phase is not lifted as fast as the crank is rotating). The elite cyclist exhibits reduced negative force and time during the upstroke.
- **Maximal torque during the downstroke is what differentiates elite athletes from the recreational rider.**

Cadence (Revolutions Per Minute)

- To date, no optimal cadence has been determined. Experienced cyclists will spontaneously pick the cadence that appears to work best for them. The freely chosen cadence of elite cyclists is 90 rpm for group stages and TTs, 70–100 rpm for mountain ascents.
- Although low cadences (50–60 rpm) have been found to be more economical and efficient (lower $\dot{V}O_2$), most cyclists prefer to pedal at high cadences. Improved blood flow and reduced muscular stress are possible advantages at higher cadences.
- Blood flow oxygenation to the vastus lateralis is significantly reduced during the first third of the crank cycle, with a compensatory transient increase in blood supply during the relaxation phase of the upstroke.
- For a given power output, at faster cadences, the force on the pedals and of muscle contractions is reduced.
- Faster cadences may be beneficial because less intramuscular pressure causes less blood vessel constriction.

COMMON INJURIES AND MEDICAL PROBLEMS

General Overview

- Injuries can be classified into bicycle contact, traumatic, and overuse categories.
- There are few scientific studies regarding injuries.
- Two-thirds of traumatic injuries occur in the upper extremity, with the most common site being the shoulder.
- Two-thirds of overuse injuries occur in the lower extremity, with the most common site being the knee.
- Cycling is a nonimpact activity, *except when crashing*; overuse injury in cycling rarely prevents an athlete from continuing to ride. Stress fractures do not occur in cycling.
- The primary muscle action is quadriceps concentric activity; acute muscle tears rarely occur.
- Overtraining or staleness is common.

Table 94.3 POWER-BASED TRAINING LEVELS

Level	Name	% of Threshold Power	% of Threshold HR	Perceived Exertion
1	Active recovery	<56	<69	<2
2	Endurance	56–75	69–83	2–3
3	Tempo	76–90	84–94	3–4
4	LT	91–105	95–105[a]	4–5
5	$\dot{V}O_2$ max	106–120	>106[b]	6–7
6	Anaerobic capacity	>120	N/A	>7
7	Neuromuscular power	N/A	N/A	Maximal

Sample Workouts for the Athlete Who Time Trials at an Average Power of 300 W and HR 160

Level	Avg. Wattage	Avg. HR	Workout
1	<166	<111	1-hour ride
2	166–225	111–134	3-hour ride
3	226–270	135–152	Warm up 30 min at L1–2, then 1.5 hour at L3, 30-min cool-down
4	271–315	153–170[a]	Warm up 30 min as if for race, perform 2 × 20 minutes at level 4 with 5 minutes at level 1 between efforts, warm-down
5	316–360	>171[b]	Warm up as earlier, then 6 × 5 min at L5, with 5 min at L1 between efforts, warm-down
6	>360	N/A	Warm up as earlier, then 10 × 1 min at L6 with 3 min at L1 between, warm-down
7	N/A	N/A	Warm up thoroughly, then do 6–10 all-out 10-s sprints with complete recovery between efforts

Level	Description of Level
1	Easy spinning, light pedal pressure, minimal sensation of leg effort, active recovery after hard training or races
2	"All day" pace or classic long slow-distance training, sensation of leg effort low but may rise when climbing, frequent days in a row possible, but complete recovery may take more than 24 hours for very long rides
3	"Spirited group ride" or brisk paceline, requires concentration to maintain alone, consecutive days still possible if duration is not excessive and carbohydrate intake is adequate
4	Just below to just above TT effort, mentally very taxing, usually done in multiple repeats of 10–30 min duration, consecutive days possible if completely recovered from prior training
5	Intensity of long 3- to 8-min intervals designed to increase $\dot{V}O_2$ max, completion of 30–40 min total training difficult, consecutive days not necessary
6	Short 30-s to 3-min intervals designed to increase anaerobic capacity, HR not useful because of nonsteady-state nature of effort, consecutive days not necessary
7	Very short, high-intensity efforts (jumps, standing starts, sprints) stressing musculoskeletal system versus metabolic systems, power useful as guide to compare versus prior efforts

[a]May not be achieved during initial phases of effort.
[b]May not be achieved because of slowness of the heart rate response and/or ceiling imposed by maximum heart rate.
Data from Coggan AR. *Training and Racing With a Power Meter*. Boulder, CO: Velopress; 2006.

Contact Area Injuries

There are three areas at which a rider makes contact with the bicycle, and each of these areas lends itself to specific injuries.

Shoe–Pedal Interface

- Burning feet, numbness, or pain is common. Riders may unclip their cleats to shake their feet to relieve symptoms.
- Plantar radiculopathy, or a **Morton neuroma,** may result from the impingement of interdigital nerves, classically between the third and fourth metatarsal heads, from tight, rigid cycling shoes and pressure on the pedals.
- Bike fit remedies: adjust cleat, usually by moving farther back; wearing a shoe with a wider toe box; loosening straps on cleats; inspecting the shoe for compression points; using a wider platform pedal or a small metatarsal pad
- Treatment: Massage, manual therapy, nonsteroidal antiinflammatory drugs (NSAIDs), shoe inserts, injection therapies such as cortisone, nerve block, prolotherapy, platelet-rich plasma (PRP), or sclerotherapy injections; surgical excision considered as last resort if a mass is present.

Pelvis–Saddle Interface

PERINEAL VASCULOPATHY/NEUROPATHY

- The most common urogenital problem encountered is genital or perineal numbness; reported in as high as 91% in a study of 17 cycling policemen. Symptoms transient for most individuals, but the long-term risks are unknown.
- Ischemic neuropathy may result from the compression of the neurovascular bundle in the perineum or in Alcock canal.
- Compression, friction, and/or stretching hypothesized.
- "Cyclist's syndrome": pudendal nerve entrapment; results in pain, burning, numbness, and sometimes sexual dysfunction, impotence, and urinary incontinence.
- A 2018 cross-sectional study of female cyclists found that women cyclists were no more likely to report sexual dysfunction or urinary symptoms compared with runners and swimmers.
- Bicycle factors: excessive saddle tilt upward, saddle height too high, handlebars too low or too far forward; too much or too little saddle padding, narrow saddle, prolonged seated riding in one position; riding on rollers is worse than a stationary bicycle, which is worse than riding on the road.

- Effectiveness of ergonomic wide saddles—with a split nose, chopped nose, and central cutout designed to decrease compression—has not been scientifically proven.
- Treatment: Relative rest, physical therapy, adjustment of bike fit or riding technique, change of saddle type, nerve blocks, cortisone injection, Botox injection, surgical decompression for severe recalcitrant cases.

ERECTILE DYSFUNCTION

- There is anecdotal evidence of cycling-related erectile dysfunction (ED).
- A 2020 meta-analysis with systemic evaluation of 843 studies, with 6 meeting inclusion criteria, found limited evidence for any positive correlation between cycling and ED when adjusting for age and comorbidity.
- Reported to affect 13%–24% of male riders. True incidence unknown.
- Vascular and neurologic mechanisms are implicated.
- Compression of the perineal region during cycling may cause decreased penile perfusion.
- Prolonged hypoxemia has been associated with penile fibrosis, which is known to cause ED.
- Blunt trauma to the corpora cavernosa has been considered to be a risk factor for the subsequent development of ED.
- Penile blood flow decreases significantly while cycling in a seated position; as much as an 82% drop in transcutaneous penile oxygen pressure has been recorded.
- The elimination of the nose of the saddle results in a reduction in perineal pressure.
- An important factor in safeguarding penile perfusion is a saddle wide enough to support the ischial tuberosities without compression of the perineal region—*not* saddle padding.
- Scientific studies have been limited; most conducted in laboratory settings on stationary bicycles, without attention to technique and factors involved in road cycling.
- Recumbent cycling causes no compression of perineum.
- Perfusion is increased with standing; frequent position changes are beneficial.
- The TT position in the aerobars increases compression of the perineum; may be reduced with adjustment of saddle tilt and use of a split-nose saddle.
- Millions of cyclists are asymptomatic. Some appear at more risk than others. Obesity is a significant risk factor. Bike fit and technique play a role in prevention.

SADDLE SORES

- Moisture, friction, and pressure lead to skin ailments in the genital region.
- **Chafing** is its most common mild form. Relieved with 1–2 days off the bike.
- **Ulceration** or more severe friction injury may require local wound care.
- **Furuncles and folliculitis** (saddle sores). Very painful and may limit riding for long periods.
- **Perineal nodular induration (third testicle)** is the most severe form. Also called *ischiatic hygroma*, *accessory testicles*, and *biker's nodule*.
- Friction and pressure from the saddle induce collagen degeneration, myxoid changes, and pseudocyst formation.
- Histologically: presentation of a nodule with a dense fibrous capsule surrounding a central pseudocyst.
- Clinically: elastic 2- to 3-cm perineal nodules fixed to the underlying soft tissue.
- Time off from riding and cortisone injections are nonsurgical options. Surgical excision is definitive.
- Bike fit remedies: change or cut a hole in the saddle; check saddle height and tilt, raise handlebar height or shorten reach.
- Medical treatment: prevention; wear a dry, clean chamois; emollients; avoid shaving the area; warm soaks; topical cortisone, antifungal, antibacterials; oral antibiotics; surgical incision and drainage; excision.

PROSTATE DISORDERS

- No conclusive evidence linking bicycling to prostatitis or prolong increase in prostate specific antigen (PSA).
- A systemic review and meta-analysis in 2015 suggests that there is no effect of cycling on PSA; however, there are only a few, small studies, and none are randomized and controlled.
- Hormonal effects from strenuous exercise and local mechanical stress may increase PSA.
- Avoiding cycling before PSA sampling may be advised but is without any scientific basis.

FEMALE ISSUES

Description: The anatomic course of the pudendal artery and nerve is the same as in males; sexual and genitourinary complaints are similar.

Saddle discomfort: Women may find the saddle uncomfortable and experience sexual and urinary dysfunction. Study of 282 females found that 33% had perineal trauma, 19% associated with hematuria or dysuria, and 34% with numbness. Bike fit: women's specific frame with shorter top tube for decreased reach, women's saddles, shorts with padded chamois, saddle tilt down slightly.

Vulvar swelling: Mostly unilateral and caused by prolonged riding; no long-term sequelae.

Urethritis: May be caused from pressure, friction, or infection. Rule out genitourinary infection with a pelvic examination for vaginitis (yeast because of moisture) and urinalysis and culture. Hematuria and dysuria may be caused by local trauma alone. Treatment: improved bike fit and routine management.

Hands–Handlebar Interface

- **"Cyclist's palsy":** Prolonged compression of ulnar nerve in Guyon canal. Median nerve may also be compressed. Complaints of numbness, pain, and weakness; resolves with rest. Damage is rarely permanent.
- The distal motor latencies of the deep branch of the ulnar nerve to the first dorsal interosseous were significantly prolonged in a study of 28 riders in a 420-mile tour.
- Twenty-three out of 25 cyclists participating in a 600-km ride experienced compressive palmar symptoms, the majority in the ulnar distribution.
- Thirty-two of 89 touring cyclists on an 80-day tour of 4500 miles experienced hand numbness, 10 in the median nerve, with 1 unable to adduct his thumb, 1 unable to adduct his little finger, and 1 unable to abduct his little finger.
- Mononeuropathy of the deep palmar branch of the ulnar nerve in Guyon canal may cause clawing. In a type 1 lesion (mixed sensory and motor), compression is proximal (outside of Guyon canal) and clawing is not usual. In isolated lesions of the deep terminal motor branch with the distal sensory branches intact, the athlete is unaware of compression until severe motor lesion develops.
- Cycling factors: infrequent change of hand position, downhill cycling, stationary riding, prolonged saddle time, rough terrain, handlebars too low or forward, poor padding in gloves or bars.
- Bike fit remedies: frequent change of hand position, reduction of training volume, change ride terrain, increase padding, shorten reach or raise bars, introduction of aerobars. Gel padding may worsen problem.
- Medical treatment: rest, massage, injection therapies, night splint, hand therapy; surgery in severe cases.

Acute Traumatic Crash Injuries

Skin Abrasion ("Road Rash")

- Most common traumatic injury.
- Treatment: Rapid cleansing with scrubbing to prevent infection and staining ("tattooing"). Soap and water is best. Peroxide can inhibit healing. Use local anesthetic.
- The wound should not be left open to the air to heal because large scabs may form.
- Traditional method: Cover wound with a nonadherent dressing with antibiotic ointment or silver sulfadiazine, pad with gauze, wrap with stretch gauze, and cover with tube stretch gauze. Daily dressing changes with cleansing of exudates until pink healthy tissue emerges.
- Alternative: Semipermeable films, hydrocolloid dressings, or bioclusive bandages may be used and left in place for extended period until healing.

Handlebar Trauma

- More common in children with straight handlebars.
- Caused by a direct blow of the bars turning sideways into the abdomen.
- Injuries: **splenic, liver, pancreatic, renal, bowel,** and **urethral.**
- Presentation is often delayed.
- Most cases of organ contusion are handled with observation and serial computed tomography (CT); occasionally surgery.
- **Handlebar hernia** is a rare traumatic hernia involving disruption of the abdominal wall muscles with bowel loop herniation and potential volvulus. Treatment is primary repair.
- **Lacerations** result from the sharp metallic ends of the handlebar cutting through soft rubber handles or bars with no end plug.

Concussion

- From direct blow, fall over front of handlebars; most get up and ride concussed.
- May be overlooked because of concomitant injuries.
- If helmet has any surface scratch, look for interior damage.
- Discard helmet after one blow.
- Sample return-to-competition protocol:
  1. Complete physical and cognitive rest until symptom free; traditionally recommended but now questioned, may start with stage 2 at a level that does not worsen symptoms
  2. Stationary cycling on a trainer for 30–45 minutes at HR <70% of max
  3. Nongroup road riding of low intensity and duration once symptom free
  4. Nongroup road riding with bigger gears, hills, and/or intervals
  5. Group riding

Upper Extremity Injuries

CLAVICLE FRACTURES

- The most common cycling fracture, followed by the wrist, ribs, and elbow.
- Caused by a direct blow to the shoulder.
- Of clavicle fractures, 72%–80% occur in the middle third of the clavicle, 25%–30% in distal clavicle, and about 2% at the proximal clavicle.
- May be associated with **rib/scapula fractures and concussion.** Also rarely associated with **pulmonary contusion, pneumothorax, hemothorax,** and **neurovascular injury.**
- Historically, clavicle fractures have been considered to be best treated nonoperatively with a simple sling. A prospective randomized trial found that a simple sling caused less discomfort and fewer complications than a figure-eight brace.
- Slings are commonly used for 1–2 weeks until pain free, with early range of motion as pain allows.
- Most cyclists with nondisplaced fractures treated nonoperatively can ride on a trainer within 3 days to 1 week, outdoors within 2 weeks, and resume racing in 4–6 weeks.
- Professional and elite cyclists with displaced midshaft fractures treated with plate fixation have returned to cycling on the trainer on the second day after surgery, resumed training programs within 1 week, and returned to competition after 3 weeks.
- Current management of medial clavicle fractures remains nonoperative because significant displacement is rare as a result of ligament stability. If displacement is present or suspect sternoclavicular injury, image with CT.
- The ideal treatment of distal clavicle fractures remains controversial because of the existence of multiple subtypes of associated ligamentous injury; most cases treated nonoperatively.
- Treatment of middle third fractures is nonoperative, except when severe displacement, communition, or shortening is present.
  - Initial shortening of 20 mm or more significantly associated with nonunion and an unsatisfactory result.
  - Displacement of more than one bone width on an x-ray is a risk factor for nonunion.
- Late repair of painful nonunion displaced midshaft fractures has results similar to immediate fixation.
- Open reduction and internal fixation: Optimal method to treat displaced midshaft clavicle fractures is unknown. The two most commonly performed procedures are plate fixation and intramedullary nailing. Four different types of plates: reconstruction plates, locking reconstruction plates, dynamic compression plates (DCPs), and precontoured locking compression plates (LCPs). Purpose of surgery is to reduce rates of nonunion, enhance functional outcome, and return to cycling sooner. Risks include infection, migration of nail, implant irritation and pain requiring removal, implant failure requiring revision, fracture, and nonunion.
- Asymptomatic nonunion is not associated with significant disability.

OTHER UPPER EXTREMITY INJURIES

Acromioclavicular separation: Direct blow from fall on adducted arm. Requires brief use of sling for comfort. Stationary trainer workouts can begin within days, road riding in 2–3 weeks. Treatment is same as for noncyclists; grade I and II always nonsurgical. Even grade III, grossly visible in thin cyclists, is rarely surgical. For grades IV, V, and VI, internal fixation with a hook plate, sometimes temporary, may be considered.

Shoulder dislocation: Usually involves transient dislocation and relocation with bone bruising, **tear of ligaments and/or labrum, Bankart or Hill-Sachs lesions.** Cyclists can generally return quickly; instability in everyday activity is a considering factor for operative repair later.

Radial head fractures: Type I presents with hemarthrosis, decreased extension, and fat pad sign on x-ray. A short-term sling is employed with rapid commencement of range-of-motion exercises to achieve full extension. Aspiration of hemarthrosis with infiltration of anesthesia may check for mechanical block and aid in range of motion and pain relief. With nondisplaced fractures, the athlete can return to riding within 1–2 weeks.

Distal radius, scaphoid, or hook of hamate fracture: Falling on an outstretched hand. Magnetic resonance imaging (MRI) should be conducted if there is any suspicion of scaphoid fracture. In nonsurgical cases, a rapid return to training within 1–2 weeks is possible with casting.

Lower Extremity Injuries

Hip pointer and/or greater trochanteric bursitis: Common from a direct blow to the lateral aspect of pelvis/femur; large **hematoma** may result; have a high clinical suspicion for pelvic

Table 94.4 BICYCLE ADJUSTMENT BASED ON THE LOCATION OF KNEE PAIN

Location of Knee Pain	Bicycle Adjustment to Consider
Anterior	Raise saddle if saddle too low Move saddle back if saddle too far forward Spin higher cadence if cyclist "mashes" or cycles with low cadence Shorten cranks if cranks too long
Medial	Adjust cleat to point toes inward/neutral if toes pointing outward Consider floating pedals if pedals have no float Limit float to 5 degrees if excessive float is present in pedals Move cleats closer to cranks if feet too far apart
Lateral	Adjust cleat to point toes outward/neutral if toes pointing inward Consider floating pedals if pedals have no float Limit float to 5 degrees if excessive float is present in pedals Move cleats wider apart or shim pedal on crank 2 mm if feet too close
Posterior	Lower saddle if saddle too high Move saddle forward if saddle too far back Limit float to 5 degrees if excessive float is present in pedals

fracture—most are stable and treated with crutches and time; MRI and/or CT when in doubt; most are able to ride on a trainer before walking normally. Aspirations of greater than 60 cc of blood are common with hematomas.

Knee contusion: If there is a clinical suspicion for a patella fracture, take sunrise or merchant x-ray. Musculoskeletal (MSK) ultrasound is reliable in diagnosing cortical fracture. **Prepatellar bursitis** is common and can be treated with aspiration. Caution for infection. Wrapping the patella should not be done when cycling because restriction of patella movement may lead to patella–femoral pain.

Fractures of the femur and hip are less common; usually seen in high-speed collisions, simple falls at slow speed, and in those with osteoporosis. Occult pelvis fractures are common in masters athletes; have a high index of suspicion in any masters athlete who crashes with an antalgic gait and obtain MRI, as fracture is often missed on x-ray. Common if motor vehicles are involved in the incident.

Overuse

Knee Injuries

- The knee is the most common site of overuse injury in the cyclist.
- Simple bicycle adjustments may be made based on the location of knee pain (Table 94.4).

ANTERIOR KNEE PAIN

- Patella tendon strain, partial tears, tendinopathy ("tendonitis"):
  - Anterior knee pain in the tendon
  - May become chronic (tendinosis). MSK ultrasound is excellent for imaging the patella tendon.
  - Causes: Pushing big gears; cranks too long; steep, long hills; excessive head wind; rapidly increasing mileage or intensity; saddle too low or forward; acute forceful motion
  - Medical treatment: Physical therapy, eccentric one-legged squats, manual therapy, massage, assisted stretching, strapping; prolotherapy, PRP, tenotomy, or sclerosis of neovessels for tendinosis/partial tears; use of surgery is rare
  - Cycling treatment: Decrease mileage and intensity, avoid hills, and spin 80–90 rpm. Check saddle height and fore–aft position.
- **Patella femoral pain syndrome:** Presents as pain in the patella–femoral groove or patella facets. Similar to "tendonitis" in etiology and cycling treatment. Limit the use of cortisone injections.
- **Prepatellar bursitis:** Swelling overlying the patella. Caused by direct trauma or repetitive overuse. Treatment as noted earlier; occasional aspiration, injection, and/or culture.
- **Pes anserine bursitis/enthesopathy:** Swelling and/or pain at the pes anserine insertion. Use cortisone, prolotherapy, or PRP for recalcitrant cases; otherwise, treat as noted earlier.

LATERAL KNEE PAIN

- **Iliotibial band (ITB) syndrome:** Lateral knee pain with or without snapping; one of the most common complaints. Ultrasound may show anechoic fluid echotexture beneath ITB along femoral condyle or thickening of ITB when compared with contralateral side. Causes: High mileage and intensity, big gears, hills, prolonged steady-state riding, windy conditions, toes pointing inward, or a narrow bottom bracket.
- Cycling treatment: Adjust cleats; check bike fit; change pedaling technique.
- Medical treatment: Massage and assisted stretching form an effective first-line treatment. Physical therapy, foam rolling. Osteopathic manipulation of sacrum and pelvis. Leg length evaluation and correction. Orthotics. Use of cortisone, prolotherapy, and/or PRP a last resort.

MEDIAL KNEE PAIN

- **Medial collateral ligament (MCL) bursitis:** Often overlooked; responds well to relative rest, bike fit adjustment, massage therapy, and injection therapies.
- **Medial meniscus tear:** Not known to be primarily caused by pedal systems; if tear is present, take caution when unclipping. Often seen on MRI, but not often the cause of the cyclist's pain.
- **Medial plica** syndrome may cause anteromedial knee pain, in addition to snapping or clicking.
- Repeated irritation from cycling may lead to fibrosis with decreased elasticity and condylar cartilage damage.
- Presence of a plica alone on the MRI is not diagnostic.
- Symptoms similar to meniscal tear.
- If treatment with therapy, rest, and/or cortisone fails, arthroscopic resection of plica can be used, as it has a quick recovery.

POSTERIOR KNEE PAIN

- Not as common; hamstring tendinopathy, baker's cyst, or ganglion cyst.
- Contributing factors: saddle too high or far back, pedals with excessive float, improper technique of pulling up on the pedals, tight hamstrings.
- Treatment: Proper bike fit, relative rest, physical therapy, massage, injection therapies, and/or aspirations.

Hip Injuries

FLOW LIMITATIONS IN ILIAC ARTERIES

- Prevalence as high as 20% in top cyclists; underreported and unrecognized problem; have a high clinical suspicion.
- Presents as a sensation of dead leg, powerlessness, pain in thigh; disappears upon rest. Worsens with increased hip flexion while riding, time trialing, or climbing (steady-state riding).
- Physical examination is usually normal, may hear bruit in the inguinal region at rest or postexercise.
- Flow limitation may be caused by kinking (functional iliac artery obstruction) or endofibrosis (external iliac artery endofibrosis [EIAE]).

- Mechanical, anatomic, and hereditary factors
  - Anatomically, the external iliac artery (EIA) may be anchored to the psoas muscle and lengthened with multiple collateral vessels.
  - Mechanically, the middle part of the EIA kinks during flexion–extension of the hip, with stress lesions in the vessel wall from shearing forces created by constant cycling.
  - Hereditary and metabolic factors are implicated because 75% of surgical cases also presented with increases in homocystinemia and homocystinuria after a load test with methionine.
  - Histopathology: A nonatheromatous vascular lesion with intimal subendothelial fibrosis, leading to wall thickening and reduction of lumen caliber. May be caused by mechanical loading in susceptible individuals.
  - Functional kinking may lead to intravascular damage and poor perfusion.
  - Chevalier treated 334 lesions of endofibrosis surgically from 1991 to 2003. The first method of surgery, deemed conservative, involved endofibrosectomy with the shortening of excessive length and closing with a venous or arterial closing angioplasty. The second method involves saphenous bypass surgery. Mean return to competition time frame is 3 months.
  - Schep studied 80 suspected cases (92 symptomatic legs) and demonstrated a flow limitation in 58 legs (63%). In 40 of the legs (69%), the primary cause was kinking of the EIA because of a psoas muscle side branch or fibrous fixation of the iliac bifurcation. Twenty-three legs (40%) underwent surgical release, with 87% able to return to a high level of competition.
  - Testing
    - The provocative cycling test ankle–brachial index (ABI) is the most important clinical test and has a specificity and sensitivity in detecting moderate lesions of 90% and 87%, respectively. Twenty-watt per minute ramp protocol, ABI measured immediately postexercise while supine with 90-degree hip and knee flexion. The readings of the ankle pressures must be corrected for the height difference of the ankle from the arm (1 cm = 0.76 mmHg). Positive test: ABI less than 0.54, ankle difference greater than 23, ankle pressure less than 107; suspicious if ABI is 0.54–0.70.
      - Echo Doppler at rest and immediately after provocative exercise cycling test.
      - Magnetic resonance angiography immediately post provocative cycling.
      - Arteriography is the gold standard.
- Treatment: Surgical, one or more of the following: (1) release of artery (mobilization) for treatment of primary kinking when there is no structural narrowing or lengthening; (2) treatment of excessive length with shortening; (3) treatment of endofibrosis with endofibrosectomy with venous or arterial closing angioplasty, polyester patch angioplasty, or saphenous bypass surgery; and (4) inguinal ligament release. Angioplasty and stenting are NOT recommended.
- Medical treatment: Vitamin B_1, B_6, and folates when minor hyperhomocysteinemia is detected. Less hip flexion on bike. Retirement (unknown natural history, both untreated and treated).

GREATER TROCHANTERIC BURSITIS/GLUTEUS MEDIUS TENDINOPATHY, "PROXIMAL ITBS"

- **Proximal lateral thigh pain with or without snapping.**
- **Distal hip external rotator tendon involvement not uncommon.**
- Treatment: Relative rest, easy riding, physical therapy, stretching, massage, osteopathic manipulation, injection therapies.
- Iliopsoas bursitis rare compared with running; treatment as noted earlier for greater trochanteric bursitis.

LABRAL TEARS AND OSTEOARTHRITIS

- High incidence of asymptomatic labral pathology found on MRI. May not be underlying cause of the athlete's pain. May be found incidentally after a crash. If associated osteoarthritis is present, then pain is more likely from arthritis. First-line treatment involves physical therapy and/or injection therapies. Risks and benefits of surgery for labral tears should be discussed.
- Femoroacetabular impingement may also occur (see Chapter 54: "Pelvis, Hip, and Thigh Injuries").

Ankle Strains

- **Including Achilles, tibialis anterior, posterior tibialis.**
- Rare; usually the result of a cyclist running, an improper bike fit, or poor pedaling technique (excessive pushing down of heel in downstroke, or pulling with foot in upstroke), leg length inequality.
- Treatment: Physical therapy, massage, relative rest, cycling technique modification, bike fit adjustment, injection therapies.

Spine Injuries

- **Cervical strain with or without radiculopathy**
  - More common in older athletes with underlying spondylosis or disc disease.
  - Worsens with long rides, rough terrain, and handlebars too far forward or too low with hyperextension of the neck.
  - Cycling treatment: assume more upright cycling posture. Medical treatment: same as for noncyclists.
- **Thoracic strain,** may be associated with **scapula dysfunction and muscle spasm at the levator scapula,** worse with aerobars.
  - Treatment: Trigger point injections, manipulation, massage, physical therapy, bike fit adjustment, and strengthening exercises.
  - **Coronary artery disease** may present as scapula or upper back pain.
- **Lumbar spine and low back pain**
  - May be caused by strain, spasm, spondylosis, or disc disease.
  - Imaging should be performed more quickly for patients with risk factors of other medical conditions and always with trauma.
  - Cycling treatment: bike fit adjustment, avoiding hills and big gears, and shorten rides.
  - Medical treatment: same as for noncyclists.

Ischial Tuberosity Pain

- Discomfort in the "sits bones" where the rider makes contact with the saddle.
- Area can be tight and sore with or without bursitis.
- Risks: pushing big gears and time trialing, especially early in the season and/or on colder rides.
- Treatment: Relative rest, massage, extra padding with new chamois, a new saddle. Injection therapy, cortisone, prolotherapy, or PRP for severe cases.

MEDICAL CONDITIONS

Osteoporosis

- Masters cyclists with a long history of training exclusively in cycling had low bone mass density (BMD) compared with age-matched peers.
- Cyclists were seven times more likely to have osteopenia of the spine than runners, controlling for age, body weight, and bone-loading history.

- Several factors may play a role:
  - Bicycling is a nonimpact sport; cyclists avoid weight bearing when they are not training.
  - Calcium lost in sweat may play a role. Most cyclists live on a low-fat, high-carbohydrate diet with little extra calcium in the foods they eat.
  - Overtraining can lead to a sex hormone imbalance, increasing bone turnover and decreasing resorption.
- Performance-enhancing substances can accelerate bone loss.
- Unlike in running, where stress fractures are common, cyclists with osteoporosis are at risk of major fractures from crashes.

Asthma

- Forty to eighty percent of Tour de France riders reported to "have a diagnosis" or use inhalers during the race.
- The diagnosis of asthma requires supporting medical history with recurrent symptoms of bronchial obstruction (chest tightness, wheeze, or cough provoked by hyperventilation, exercise, or other stimuli), physical examination, and laboratory or field testing, especially if initially recommended treatment fails or if indicated by governing agencies.
- WADA recommends all athletes considering taking asthma medications seek a clear diagnosis from a specialist and undergo testing.
- Since 2010, salbutamol (not to exceed 1000 ng/mL in the urine) and salmeterol by inhalation were removed from the Prohibited List and no longer require a Therapeutic Use Exemption (TUE). Inhaled formoterol to a maximum dose of 54 mcg/24 hours is no longer prohibited. All other beta$_2$-agonists are prohibited and require a TUE.
- A positive response to any one of the following provocation tests is required to confirm airway hyperresponsiveness:
  - Exercise challenge tests (field or laboratory) ≥10% fall of FEV_1
  - The Eucapnic Voluntary Hyperpnea (EVH) test ≥10% fall of FEV_1
  - Methacholine challenge ≥20% fall of FEV; PC_2O <4 mg/mL if steroid naïve. If taking inhaled glucocorticosteroids longer than 1 month, then PD_2O should be ≤1600 mcg or PC_2O ≤16.0 mg/mL
  - Mannitol inhalation ≥15% fall in FEV_1 after challenge
  - Histamine challenge ≥20% fall of FEV_1 at a histamine concentration of 8 mg/mL or less during a graded test of 2 minutes
- A 12% or higher increase in FEV_1 after the use of an inhaled beta$_2$-agonist is considered the standard diagnostic test for reversibility of bronchospasm. Medication inquiries should be directed to the athlete's national antidoping organization. USADA's Drug Reference Toll-Free Line (866-601-2632) provides phone assistance Monday through Friday 8 AM to 5 PM MST. The Global Drug Reference Online (Global DRO, www.globaldro.org) provides support regarding the prohibited status of medications, but not supplements, based on the current WADA Prohibited List.

Exercise-Induced Laryngeal Obstruction (EILO) or Vocal Cord Dysfunction (VCD)

- EILO refers to symptomatic laryngeal obstruction during exercise because of narrowing or obstruction at the level of the vocal cords (glottis) and/or above the vocal cords (supraglottis).
- Exercise-induced inspiratory symptoms (EIISs) of EILO typically produce coarse or high-pitch stridor, peak during exercise, and stop 1–5 minutes after exercise. Exercise-induced bronchospasm (EIB) symptoms typically present with expiratory symptoms, peaking 3–15 minutes after exercise.
- EIB is overdiagnosed in athletes with upper airway obstruction.
- Flow volume loops are a useful tool in discriminating between EILO and asthma. With EILO, spirometry demonstrates decrease of forced vital capacity (FVC) in tandem with FEV_1, and flow volume loops demonstrate inspiratory loop flattening.
- Continuous laryngoscopy during exercise (CLE) test is a method that allows for continuous visualization during exercise on a cycling trainer using a laryngoscope.
- Speech therapy for respiratory retraining therapy is the first-line treatment in managing EILO.

Overtraining Syndrome

- Accumulation of training and/or nontraining stressors resulting in long-term performance decrement, with or without related physiologic and psychological signs and symptoms; restoration of performance capacity may take weeks to months; exclude organic disease.
- Disparity of load and load tolerance.
- Cyclists are prone to overtraining because long hours may be spent cycling without an MSK injury.
- Staleness and lack of improvement more common than frank overtraining syndrome.
- Pathophysiology: Damage in muscle fibers and mitochondria, impaired recruitment of muscle fibers, impaired hypothalamic–pituitary axis, and reduced sympathetic nervous system activity.
- Risks: High training load, nontraining stressors, sticking to a training program when sick or injured, making up lost time (to illness, injury, or missed training), increase in training because of poor performance, monotonous training, and **not enough rest.**
- Early signs: Performance decrement, progressive weight loss, poor sleep, increased resting HR, increased fluid intake in the evening.
- Symptoms: Loss of vigor, fatigue, depression, agitation, insomnia, irritability, restlessness, loss of motivation, poor concentration, heavy legs.
- Prevention: Individualize training, build base mileage before speed work, periodization, avoid monotony, rest, carbohydrate-rich diet, avoid overcompensating.
- Laboratory tests: **No single identifiable parameter;** exclude organic disease; complete blood count to rule out anemia, infection, cancer; complete metabolic profile to rule out renal or hepatic disease, electrolyte disturbance as clue to eating disorder; thyroid-stimulating hormones, Epstein-Barr virus titer, Lyme disease if in endemic region, vitamin D, magnesium levels. Also consider mycoplasma, cytomegalovirus, parvovirus B19, hepatitis, and chronic sinus or tooth infections. Consider hormonal workup. Glutamine/glutamate decreased. Salivary immunoglobulin A decreased. Consider electrocardiogram (ECG), echocardiogram (echo), $\dot{V}O_2$ max, stress test, pulmonary function test.
- Two best markers of overtraining: (1) decreased performance on standard exercise tests with HR, lactate, and $\dot{V}O_2$ max and (2) self-analysis of well-being by the athlete such as with Profile of Mood State (POMS).
- Best log book markers: mood, muscle soreness, stress, quality of sleep, and performance decrement.
- Overtraining should be discussed not only under the clinical aspect, but more under the aspect of training content.
- Late diagnosis may result in loss of months of racing.
- Cycling treatment: easy riding or complete time off the bike until fresh, return slowly with no hills or hard efforts for 1 month for severe cases. Three days off and 7 days easy spinning on a small gear is sufficient for mild cases of overreaching.

Gastrointestinal Distress

- Not as common as with running.
- Blood flow may be reduced to the gastrointestinal (GI) system by 40%–50% during exercise with shift toward working muscles, skin, and vital organs.

- In triathlon, majority of issues in the run section are related to the lower GI tract with diarrhea, and in the bike section are related to the upper GI tract with reflux and vomiting. Swallowing water and air during swimming contributes to this. Increased pressure on abdomen from cycling position may also contribute. Dehydration and nutrition contribute.

Nutrition

- A cyclist with average efficiency and aerodynamics requires about 21 kcal per minute to ride at 40 kph.
- Carbohydrate stores in the body (2000–3000 kcal) can fuel about 90 minutes of riding at 40 kph.
- During the Tour de France, cyclist energy expenditure may be as high as 9000 kcal per day.
- The training diet for a cyclist:
  - Sixty to seventy percent carbohydrates = 3.1 g per pound of body weight daily
  - Fifteen to twenty percent protein = 0.5–0.9 g per pound of body weight daily
  - Twenty to thirty percent fat = *not* less than 20 g per day
- Pre-exercise:
  - Intake of 150–300 g of carbohydrate 3 hours before exercise will increase muscle glycogen and performance.
- During exercise:
  - Sixty to seventy g carbohydrate per hour of training.
  - Use of carbohydrate levels off at 1 g per minute.
  - Glucose, maltodextrins, sucrose, maltose, and soluble starches oxidized at high rates versus fructose and galactose.
  - Three hundred to four hundred calories per hour of training.
  - Four hundred to six hundred mL of fluid per hour.
  - Drinking ad libitum (according to the dictates of thirst) has been shown to have no detrimental effect on performance.
  - Sodium intake of 0.15–0.45 g per L of fluid.
- Postexercise:
  - Maximum rate of muscle glycogen resynthesis is reached at intake of 1.2–1.4 g per minute (75–90 g of carbohydrate per hour).
  - Carbohydrate intake of 1.2 g per kg body weight per hour for 4 hours post exercise, preferably within 90 minutes.
  - Carbohydrate intake of more than 1.4 g per minute provides no additional benefits in glycogen storage and can increase GI distress.
  - Total carbohydrate intake of 8–10 g per kg of body weight within 24 hours.

RECOMMENDED READINGS

Available online.

MOUNTAIN BIKING 95

Michael K. Neilson • Christopher C. Bell • Christopher C. Madden

GENERAL PRINCIPLES

Definitions

- The term "mountain biking" broadly refers to riding bikes with specific design characteristics in various off-road settings.
- Mountain bikes generally differ from road bikes in several ways: a smaller frame, stronger wheels, larger range of gears, a wider flat or upright handlebar, hydraulic brakes, suspension, and wider, knobby tires.
- There are many riding and bike types, with some overlap between bikes and riding styles.
- The five main mountain biking categories are cross-country (XC), trail/all-mountain (AM), downhill (DH), Enduro (essentially hybrid between DH and AM), and freeride (FR), which includes trials and urban riding (TR) (Fig. 95.1).

Demographics

- Participation is open to all age groups, with the average age dependent on the type of biking; 22–36 years is the gross average, with most competitors aged between 19 and 44 years. There are more males than females, but female participation is increasing; the sport is especially popular among young males.
- Mountain bikes are the largest category of bikes sold in US bike shops.
- Racing/competition is now common in XC, Enduro, DH, FR, and other styles.
- The sport attracts risk-tolerant personalities.
- The number of noncompetitive mountain bikers is increasing; less is known about their injury epidemiology. The National Interscholastic Cycling Association (NICA), founded in 2012 in the United States and currently with individual leagues in 30 states, has led to an impressive upsurge in participation in mountain biking, primarily XC racing, in thousands of children and adolescents since its inception, both on junior developmental teams ("Devo," grades 7–8) and high schoolers. There were 22,752 participants nationwide in 2019 alone. The NICA has developed a surveillance system for coaches, riders, and parents to report and collect injury data for high school student-athletes to improve our knowledge of injury epidemiology, especially in young riders.

Research

- Injuries are reported inconsistently in the literature, ranging from specific injuries to general types of injury (e.g., laceration, fracture) to injured body areas (e.g., joint, upper or lower extremity, head).
- Early data are from competitive XC; more data are now available from all areas: XC, DH, Enduro, and FR. Although recreational data are still sparse, more large organizations and events (i.e., Enduro World Series, Olympic Games data) have begun surveillance and reporting injuries.
- Available studies are primarily descriptive and focus mainly on epidemiology or injuries themselves (generally defined by body or joint area); there are fewer details available regarding mechanisms of injury.
- Most injury studies have a preponderance of male participants (75%–80%). Many studies depend on victim recall.

Competition

- XC still popular, but a shift to Enduro, DH, and other events is being seen.
  - The origin of NICA has led to the addition of a number of high school races (XC) in participating leagues
- Categories are established based on age, gender, and rider skill.
- Rider skill categories were changed in 2009 (applicable to riders 15 years of age and above): Pro, Category 1 (previously Expert), Category 2 (previously Sport), and Category 3 (previously Beginner); previous riders classified as "Semi-Pro" must choose between the new Pro or Category 1 tiers. Some races still use classification categories of novice/beginner, sport, expert, and elite/pro.
- Age categories: Youth (<10 years old), Junior (10–18 years old), Under 23 (19–22 years old), Senior (23–29 years old), and Master (>30 years old)

Protective Equipment

Protective torso armor and extremity padding: Primarily for FR and DH; use of lighter, flexible pads increasing in XC

Helmet designs: Full face (mainly DH, FR) and standard (mainly XC, Trail/AM); helmets should be Snell-, Consumer Product Safety Commission (CPSC)-, or American National Standards Institute (ANSI)-approved and tested. Recommend replacement after any significant crash.

Shorts: Multiple types of synthetic moisture-wicking chamois; some have built-in hip padding; loose-fitting shorts with inner chamois are becoming more popular

Gloves: Varying thickness, with shell protection (dorsal fingers and hand) and padding

Eyewear: Ultraviolet protection, shatterproof, changeable light-reducing and colored lenses for varying conditions; clear lenses for night/low light riding; goggles in DH and extreme cold

Mountain Bike Fit

- May start with a professional fit (see Chapter 94: "Road Biking").
- **Mountain bike fit not as straightforward as road fit;** use the initial road fit to help achieve a mountain bike fit window (an ideal, individualized fit that may deviate slightly from a virtual perfect fit).
- Correct fit important for prevention and treatment of acute and chronic injuries

Mountain Bike Fit

Available online.

PHYSIOLOGY AND TRAINING

Physiology

- High-intensity sport—generally higher (especially XC) than road stage races
- XC circuits span 1–2 hours (depending on age/racing category), performed at a heart rate (HR) of approximately 90% (±3%) of HRmax, corresponding to a $\dot{V}O_2$ max of approximately 84%; more than 80% of race time is spent above the lactate threshold (LT).
- Intensity is related to a fast start, several climbs, rolling resistance, and isometric and eccentric arm and leg muscle contractions that are required for shock absorption, bike handling, and stability over rough terrains (increases HR response to submaximal cycling).

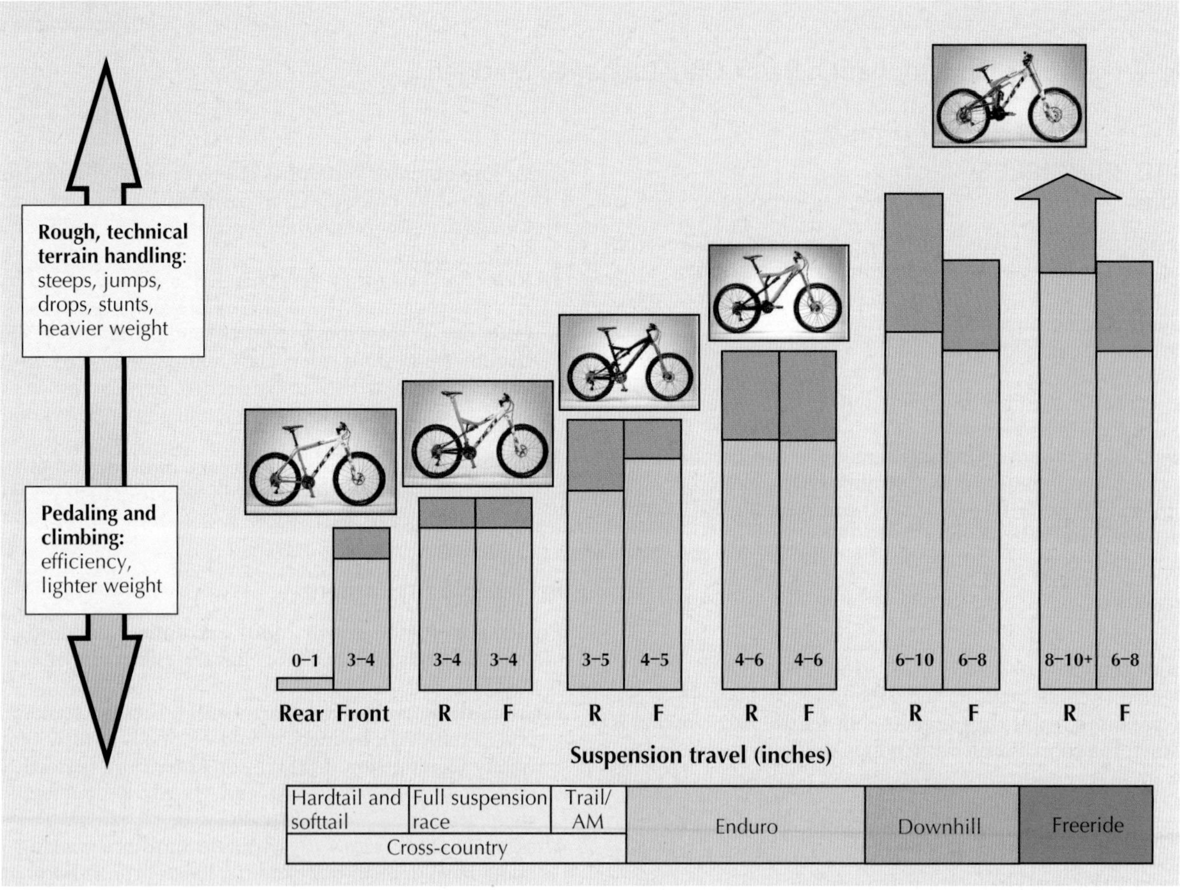
Rough, technical terrain handling: steeps, jumps, drops, stunts, heavier weight
Pedaling and climbing: efficiency, lighter weight
0–1
3–4
Rear
Front
3–4
3–4
R
F
3–5
4–5
R
F
4–6
4–6
R
F
6–10
6–8
R
F
8–10+
6–8
R
F
Suspension travel (inches)
Hardtail and softtail
Full suspension race
Trail/ AM
Cross-country
Enduro
Downhill
Freeride

Figure 95.1 Mountain bike styles and characteristics. (Photographs from Yeti Cycles with permission. Data from Lopes B, McCormack L. *Mastering Mountain Bike Skills: Techniques to Excel in All Riding Styles.* Champaign, IL: Human Kinetics; 2005.)

- Start has fundamental importance to the entire race. XC races are generally on single track (narrow trail where only one biker could fit); however, typically start on a wider course (either paved or dirt road) and race to the single-track portion to achieve a good position; fast starts and early steep climbs lead to high intensity and HRmax early in the race.
- Anaerobic energy systems taxed, especially during steep climbs (require high power output: up to 250–500 watts); anaerobic power and ability to sustain high work rates for prolonged periods are prerequisites for competing in high-level off-road cycling events.
- Various factors may affect off-road XC performance, especially in elite cyclists: $\dot{V}O_2$ max, peak power output (PPO), power output (PO), and $\dot{V}O_2$ at the ventilatory threshold (VT) and at the respiratory compression threshold (RCT); studies are conflicting regarding which is most important:
  - PO and $\dot{V}O_2$ at the RCT normalized to body mass are predictors of off-road performance times.
  - $\dot{V}O_2$ max, PPO, and LT normalized to body mass correlate with XC performance in some studies.
  - PO at the VT may correlate with time trial performance.
- Body mass is a factor: power-to-weight characteristics are important for success in off-road events; high power-to-weight ratio is good for strong hill climbing ability; higher mass may assist with rapid descents.
- Factors other than aerobic power and capacity may affect off-road cycling performance: cycling experience and economy (specificity of principle); technical ability; and nutrition before, during, and after competition.

Training

- Need to develop good aerobic endurance, anaerobic capacity, overall muscle strength, good coordination, balance, and bike-handling skills.
- Significant upper body and core muscular strength is necessary for repeated isometric and/or eccentric muscle contractions required to absorb shocks and constantly adjust to changing terrain; accomplished using weight training and riding off-road.
- Many competitive XC riders train for 10–14 hours weekly; some XC racers train systematically in a similar fashion to road racers. Others train with much less structure.
- Athletes ride at varying aerobic and anaerobic intensities (zones); it is helpful to use an HR monitor.
- Mountain bikers train both on- and off-road.
  - Use different types of training in a similar manner to other endurance events (listed in order of decreasing intensity): race pace, intervals and hills, speed and tempo, endurance, strength, and recovery.
  - Training cycle (depends on peaking goals): base (4 months), intensity (4 months), peak (4–6 weeks), racing (8–12 weeks), or recovery (4–6 weeks).
  - Off-road terrain incorporates various training types and is less flexible than road riding under controlled intensity.
  - Long off-road rides over rough, technical terrain, especially if at altitude, require longer recovery compared with equidistant road rides.
  - Use periodization and monitor overtraining, especially if training at high altitude and/or frequently on rough terrain.

- More injuries reported during training than during competitions, where there is less access to medical personnel and treatment.

INJURY OVERVIEW

Epidemiology

- Injury types and numbers likely grossly underreported secondary to varying and limited study design, difference in injury definitions, understudy of a large population of recreational and noncompetitive aggressive riders in all styles.
- Peak incidence: June to August
- Mixed competition and noncompetition data indicate that 50%–90% of riders have been injured in the previous year; one study showed 20% had a significant injury requiring medical attention and were prevented from cycling for at least 1 day; competitive cyclists were injured more than recreational cyclists in earlier studies, but unclear if this still reflects the current trend.
- Reported injury rates (multiyear data) is as low as 0.45%–0.6% per year in XC, DH, and DS competitions; 0.30% injury rate for recreational cyclists, but some reports are higher; definition of injury rate may vary (e.g., number of injured cyclists per number of starts per 100; number of injured cyclists per 100 hours of race time).
- Injury rates are greater for DH versus XC relative to time spent on bike (0.37 injuries per 100 hours on bike for XC vs. 4.34 injuries per 100 hours on bike for DH).
- There is a possible association between increased hours on bike and injury severity, but some data indicate the presence of fewer injuries in competitive cyclists who spent 1 hour per week more on the bike during the competition season and 3.5 hours per week more on bike during the off-season compared with those who experienced major injuries.
- A large study with 2029 competitive Enduro riders showed an injury rate of 8.9% in 10 events; almost a third of the injuries occurred in inexperienced riders (those who only raced one previous Enduro World Series event).
- Cannot extrapolate injury data from road bikers because road bike crashes are often specific to riding on pavement; many more collisions with motor vehicles, which is rare in off-road cycling (a few case reports of serious injury resulting from mountain bike–motor vehicle collisions do exist)
- Experienced cyclists injure bones and joints more frequently than beginners.
- Injuries tend to occur when riding downhill or losing control. Professional DH racers are more likely to sustain injuries than amateurs.
- Young males are the most frequently injured population because of the popularity of the sport in this group and the likelihood to engage in aggressive and technically demanding riding styles.
- In high school riders, most common injured areas include head/brain, wrist/hand, shoulder, and knee (in order).
- Injury risk in competing females appears higher than in males, but injury severity is higher in males than in females.
    - Risk factors in females: loss of bike control, poor upper extremity strength, fewer riding years
- The number of injuries occurring during racing and training are about equal, but traumatic injuries are more common in races, whereas overuse injuries are more common in training.

Mechanisms of Injury and Risk Factors

- Most commonly reported: **excessive speed, unfamiliar terrain, loss of control** (encompasses multiple factors), **inattentiveness, riding beyond ability,** and **riding DH, slippery terrain** (approximately 90% may be viewed as errors in judgment) (Table 95.1)

Table 95.1 SPECIFIC REPORTED CAUSES AND RISK FACTORS

Rider-related	Errors in judgment and riding technique Excessive speed Inattentiveness Riding beyond ability and loss of control Incorrect braking Improper training and overtraining Female or young male Intoxication No helmet; especially children
Bike/equipment-related	Mechanical failures (more common in DH): flat tires, brakes, chains, forks, handlebars, pedals, suspension parts, seatposts, frames Improper fit
Terrain-related	Surface: mud, gravel, loose dirt, wet Unfamiliarity Downhill Obstacles and jumps
Environment-related	Competition Heat Cold Sun Lightning Orienteering mishaps Animals and reptiles (attacks and collisions)

- **Most crashes occur while riding DH.**
- Injuries from loss of control, loss of traction, and mechanical failure result in similar injury patterns.
- Special attention is applied to the cyclist–bike–terrain interface and how it relates to injuries.

Falls

- Forward fall over handlebar ("endo")
    - **Most common direction of fall and mechanism of acute traumatic injury**
    - **Common causes:** rapid deceleration during downhill descent (most common cause of severe injury), hitting an object, improper jump landing, improper braking
    - **Reported injuries:** soft tissue injuries and trauma to head, torso, shoulder, upper extremity; head, neck, and face injury
- Side falls
    - **Common causes:** sliding out around corners (sideslip), misjudged handling resulting in tipping over, dabbing of hand after losing balance in technical terrain
    - **Reported injuries:** mainly soft tissue injuries; leg injuries, especially to knee and ankle; some upper extremity (reaching out or a fall on elbow or lateral shoulder)
- Rear falls
    - **Common causes:** forceful wheelie, preloading (compressing suspension) to adjust for change in terrain, jumping too early
    - **Reported injuries:** soft tissue, upper extremity (especially hand and wrist), head, spine and torso, tailbone

Collisions

- Other cyclists (common in XC/AM)
- Stationary object (trees or rocks)
- Bike parts; especially bar, stem, and pedals; frame, brakes, and seat less common
- Animals (prairie dogs and other)

- Injuries from collision and noncollision similar in severity and anatomic location
- One reported fatality in 2015 from blunt force trauma to the chest in an Enduro event

Evaluation

History

- Acute traumatic injury typically requires no specific history other than fall mechanism, whereas specific historical features are more useful when evaluating overuse injury.
- Review athlete **training history** to detect common errors (e.g., volume, intensity, hill work, periodization).
- **Bike fit** history (professional vs. self)
- Experience, type of bike and riding, type of terrain and challenges
- Helmet and other protective equipment use

Examination

- Use stationary trainer in the office for overuse and fit issues (dynamic evaluation); consider use of digital video.
- Evaluate on and off the bike. Identify anatomic variations or malalignments (e.g., excessive knee valgus, LLD) and errors in bike fit; adjust rider; evaluate shoes and orthotics if used.
- Helpful tools: bike trainer, plumb line, long carpenter's level, laser level, goniometer, suspension pump, zip ties (for sag settings), Allen wrenches and screwdrivers (for quick office adjustments)

General Treatment

- General treatment approaches for traumatic and overuse injuries in off-road cyclists are similar to approaches used with other athletes (e.g., physical therapy, cryotherapy, antiinflammatory medication).
- Specific cycling injury diagnosis and treatment is a highly individualized area; affected by multiple variables, including training, experience, riding style/type, and bike fit.
- **Treatment options**
  - Relative rest and activity modification: temporarily decrease mileage, intensity, hill work; spin using low-resistance and high-cadence pedaling; correct training errors.
  - Bike fit: consider placing rider back to neutral position, especially if bike was never fit; adjust from there
  - Medication: nonsteroidal antiinflammatory drugs (NSAIDs) for analgesia and inflammation, bacitracin ointment for soft tissue trauma
  - Heat and ice: ice appropriate overuse injuries after rides and intermittently throughout day; keep the affected joint warm during ride (e.g., knee warmers)
  - Physical therapy (see specific injuries)
    - Lower extremity (especially hamstring, iliotibial band) flexibility
    - Back and neck flexibility
    - Strengthening: lower extremity (eccentric programs for Achilles, patellar, and hamstring tendinopathy), dynamic core stabilization
    - Plyometrics, proprioceptive, and other cycling-specific coordination training
    - Deep tissue massage and release techniques
    - Neural stretching maneuvers
  - Bracing, strapping, or taping where appropriate
    - Knee: soft patellofemoral brace, infrapatellar strap, McConnell taping
    - Hand and wrist: use an off-the-shelf wrist or thumb spica splint (can bend steel stay to handlebar, most cycling gloves fit over), custom-molded orthosis (e.g., Orthoplast)
  - Corticosteroid injection
    - Upper extremity: carpal tunnel syndrome, de Quervain tenosynovitis, intersection syndrome
    - Lower extremity: pes anserine bursitis, trochanteric bursitis, iliotibial band syndrome, Morton neuroma

SPECIFIC INJURIES

- Injuries are divided into **overuse, acute traumatic,** and **environmental.**

Overuse Injuries

Epidemiology

- Retrospective questionnaire surveys indicate 45%–90% of mountain bikers have had an overuse injury in their career.
- Body regions most commonly involved (in order): **knee** and **low back,** hand, wrist, neck, and buttocks/saddle region
- Likely grossly underreported: poorly studied
- Many studies only capture injuries resulting in lost time on bike; this would exclude many overuse injuries
- **Bike fit is closely linked;** interaction between cyclist, bike, and terrain. See Table 95.2 for bike fit problems for common chronic injuries.
- Anatomic variations and fit errors (even by a few millimeters) are magnified by many hours of training and cumulative repetition, especially in the lower extremity
- Upper extremity injuries related to weight distribution over the front of the bike and are affected by bars, bar ends, grips, and stem height relative to saddle; also related to shifter type and front suspension (travel, preload, rebound)
- Causes and risk factors: **excessive training/racing, improper training progression** (e.g., sudden increases in mileage or riding intensity, climbing too many hills during the early season, inadequate recovery), **improper fit,** too many different types of riding, too much rough terrain, anatomic variations and faults, incorrect saddle position (dynamic), insufficient stretching, incorrect gear ratio (pushing large gears too much, especially during the early season), not enough warm-up, wrong shoes, inadequate preseason conditioning, cold weather
- **Treatment and prevention focus on training and fit.**

Knee

May be the most common joint affected by overuse; affects 30%–40% of mountain bikers

ANTERIOR KNEE CONDITIONS (PATELLOFEMORAL PAIN, PATELLAR TENDINOPATHY, QUADRICEPS TENDINOPATHY)

Causes: Saddle set too low and/or forward, aggressive sprinting, pushing big gears and aggressive climbing during the early season, pes planus and overpronation, excessive genu valgum, LLD, crank arm too long

Treatment: Pedal spacers, medial wedge, or a cycling orthotic for excessive knee valgus, raise seat, move cleats rearward, move seat back, set a higher cadence (90–100 rpm), easier gears, avoid hills, shorten crank arm, correct LLD (shim), correct training errors

PES ANSERINE BURSITIS

Causes: Saddle set too high, pedals with too much float, stance too wide on pedals, LLD, overpronation, tight hamstrings, cleats inappropriately neutral or internally rotated, external tibial torsion

Treatment: Lower saddle, correct LLD (short leg) and overpronation with an orthotic, shim, wedge, or by adjusting cleat position (move anterior); adjust cleats to match foot alignment (e.g., toes point out slightly)

Table 95.2 COMMON MODIFIABLE BIKE FIT PROBLEMS BASED ON COMMON CHRONIC INJURIES IN MOUNTAIN BIKERS

Injury/Interface	Saddle/Buttocks	Handlebar/Hand	Foot/Shoe/Pedal
Neck pain	Improper saddle tilt, too high	Long stem, low handlebar	NA
Ulnar/median neuropathy	Forward tilt, too aft	Low or narrow handlebar, thin grip	NA
Chronic LBP	Improper saddle height, fore/aft, tilt	Low handlebar	NA
Genitourinary complaints	Improper saddle height, fore/aft, tilt	Long stem, low handlebar	NA
Patellofemoral pain syndrome	Seat too low, fore	NA	Hyperpronation, improper cleat positioning, cleat valgus tilt
ITBFS at the knee	Seat too high, aft	Low handlebar	Hyperpronation, improper cleat positioning, and tilt, excessive float
Quadriceps/infrapatellar tendinopathy	Seat too low, fore	NA	Hyperpronation, improper cleat positioning and tilt, excessive float
Achilles tendinopathy	Too low	NA	Hyperpronation, posterior positioning, excessive float
Metatarsalgia	NA	NA	Cleat position too forward; shoe too narrow

ITBFS, Iliotibial band friction syndrome; *LBP*, low back pain; *NA*, not applicable.
From Ansari M, Nourian R, Khodaee M. Mountain biking injuries. *Curr Sports Med Rep*. 2017;16(6):404–412.

ILIOTIBIAL BAND FRICTION SYNDROME

Causes: Stance too narrow on pedals, cleats inappropriately neutral or internally rotated, saddle set too high, pedals with too little or too much float, genu varum

Treatment: Add a threaded spacer or washer between the crank arm and pedal (correct varus), adjust cleats to reflect foot alignment (toe out), lower the saddle, use pedals with appropriate float, introduce cycling orthotics to control excessive lower leg rotation

PLICA SYNDROMES (ESPECIALLY MEDIAL)

Causes: Saddle set too low, genu valgum, overpronation, internal tibial torsion, excessive pedal float

Treatment: Raise saddle, introduce cycling orthotics, adjust cleats to reflect foot alignment (toe in), decrease pedal float

HAMSTRING, POPLITEUS TENDONITIS, AND POSTERIOR CAPSULE STRAIN

Causes: Saddle set too high and/or posterior, riding a fixed-gear bike (hamstrings used to decelerate), genu varum, pedals with too much float, LLD

Treatment: Lower and/or slide the saddle forward, slide forward on seat during steep climbs in granny gear (increases quad workload), pedals with minimal float, use of a threaded spacer or washer between crank arm and pedal, correct LLD, eccentric strengthening program

Hip

GLUTEUS MEDIUS PAIN SYNDROME, TROCHANTERIC BURSITIS, ILIOPSOAS TENDONITIS, AND HIP EXTERNAL ROTATOR TENDONITIS

Causes: Weak and/or inhibited hip abductors and external rotators, genu valgus, overpronation, pedals with too much float, LLD, saddle set too high

Treatment: Strengthen hip abductors and external rotators, decrease pedal float, introduce a cycling orthotic, medial wedge or shim, lower the saddle, consider trochanteric bursa corticosteroid injection if there is evidence for bursal fluid on ultrasound (avoid multiple injections because of concerns for gluteus medius tendon rupture)

Leg and Ankle

ACHILLES TENDINOPATHY AND RETROCALCANEAL PAIN

Causes: Improper pedal form (drop heel, toe pedaling, or combination of both called *ankling*—excessive dorsiflexion and plantarflexion during pedaling), cleat too far forward, overpronation, tight Achilles, shoe rubbing (with Haglund deformity), saddle set too high or too low

Treatment: Correct pedal form, move cleat rearward, stretch Achilles, raise or lower saddle depending on problem

TIBIALIS ANTERIOR PAIN

Causes: Saddle set too high, ankling

Treatment: Lower saddle, anterior ankle stretching, tibialis anterior eccentric strengthening, establish proper pedal stroke

POSTERIOR TIBIALIS TENDINOPATHY

Causes: Overpronation, ankling

Treatment: Cycling orthotic or medial wedge, posterior tibialis eccentric strengthening, establish proper pedal stroke

Foot

HOT FOOT (FOREFOOT/TOE NUMBNESS AND PAIN, METATARSALGIA, PARESTHESIAS, AND MORTON NEUROMA)

Causes: Improper cleat position, irregular sole (cleat bolt causing localized plantar pressure), tight or narrow shoes, small pedal platform, toe clips, improper rotational cleat adjustment

Treatment: Move cleats back (lower saddle same amount) and adjust rotation to individual mechanics, loosen toe clips or convert to clipless pedal, install thinner insoles and/or add metatarsal or neuroma pad, larger pedaling platform, wider shoe or shoe with anatomic footbed, occasional corticosteroid injection

PLANTAR FASCIITIS

Causes: Tight plantar fascia, overpronation, excessive pedal float, saddle set too low

Treatment: Stretch plantar fascia, introduce night splint or sock, cycling orthotic or anatomic footbed, decrease pedal float, raise saddle, neutral position or dorsiflexion night splint or sock

Hand and Wrist

Wrist pain in 19%, hand numbness in 19%, and finger tingling in 35% of all mountain bikers.

ULNAR (CYCLIST'S PALSY) AND MEDIAN NEUROPATHY (CARPAL TUNNEL SYNDROME)

Description: Incidence of compression of nerves at Guyon canal and carpal tunnel syndrome is probably similar in road and mountain cyclists; presents with motor or sensory symptoms or both; ulnar nerve presents with the most sensory symptoms; experienced and inexperienced cyclists equally affected

Causes: Improper grips (size, shape, firmness), infrequent change in hand position, bumpy terrain, improper suspension settings and tire pressure relative to terrain, lack of suspension, "death grip," lack of glove padding

Treatment: Proper grip size and comfort fit, frequent changes in hand position (bar ends can be helpful), proper weight distribution on bars and seat (affected by fit and riding style), experimentation with bar angles, padded gloves, instructing the athlete to loosely grip bars, decrease suspension preload and tire pressure, consider front suspension if rigid, stretching while on the bike.

DE QUERVAIN TENOSYNOVITIS, EXTENSOR CARPI ULNARIS TENDINOPATHY, AND INTERSECTION SYNDROME

Causes: Occurs especially with grip shift, sometimes with integrated shifters

Treatment: Wrist and/or spica splint (dynamic) to minimize provocative motion, change shifters to trigger, consider a local steroid injection

Muscle Cramps

Description: Especially affects quads, hamstrings, and calves, some upper extremity (especially triceps)

Treatment: Hydrate with appropriate electrolyte drinks (especially when hot), decrease riding intensity slightly, soften suspension, ensure appropriate training volume, stretching

Low Back Pain

Description: 37% of cyclists are affected; one of the most common overuse complaints, **may be as common as knee pain**

Causes: Most frequently by improper fit, riding position, or inappropriate progression of training volume and intensity. Specific causes are overreaching (stem too long or seat too posterior), too much drop, rough terrain, incorrect suspension preload and tire pressure settings relative to terrain, and training errors (especially too many hills and long rides early in season).

Treatment: Proper fit, raise handlebars (especially during early season), shorten stem, correct LLD, core strengthening (also addressing abdominals and iliopsoas), adjust suspension setting to terrain, lower tire pressure slightly and consider changing to wider tires, hamstring flexibility, proper riding form, avoid excessive bumpy terrain and intense hill climbs early in season, change positions on the saddle during a ride and stand intermittently, sometimes may need to increase reach if pain is related to crowded position (lengthen stem). Disc injuries and radiculopathy frequently worsen with hills and rough terrain. Certain styles of yoga may be helpful.

Neck Pain

Description: Prevalence of 16%–43%, similar rider–bike causes and treatments to low back pain

Causes: Weakness and fatigue of cervical stabilizers lead to recruitment of accessory neck extenders, such as levator scapula and trapezius. Microtrauma and fatigue of these muscles may lead to myofascial pain and trigger points.

Treatment: Ride with elbows appropriately flexed, change neck positions frequently, avoid tensing. Hydration packs worn by most mountain cyclists can augment neck pain. Make sure pack straps are adjusted appropriately. Consider decreasing weight of or eliminating the pack by using water bottles and/or an under-the-seat storage pack. Postural corrective exercises, strengthening of cervical spine stabilizers, dry needling, and osteopathic manipulation can be helpful.

Scapulothoracic Pain

Causes: Common in mountain cyclists, similar causes to neck pain. Scheuermann kyphosis (classic or atypical) can worsen with mountain cycling, especially over more aggressive terrain. Hydration packs especially contribute to levator scapula, trapezius, and rhomboid myofascial pain and trigger points.

Treatment: Stretching, needling or acupuncture, fascial release, establishing proper rider form, stretching on the bike (especially during long rides)

Genitourinary

PUDENDAL NEUROPATHY

Description: Numbness in saddle region reported in 19% of cyclists. Males affected more than females; females report sensory symptoms.

Causes: Compression of the pudendal nerve (and possibly the artery), especially after repeated long hill climbs and many hours on the bike.

Presentation: Perineal, penile shaft, and scrotal numbness; impotence/erectile dysfunction and priapism (rare). In females, vulvar discomfort is common and more prevalent with increasing age.

Treatment: Ensure proper bike fit (especially seat height, fore-aft position, and tilt), proper weight distribution between bars and seat, make sure saddle not tilting up, lower seat, consider change to a softer seat with a central cutout, use quality cycling shorts with adequate padding, increase handlebar height (which distributes weight more posteriorly over ischial tuberosities), recommend standing during long climbs

SKIN PROBLEMS RELATED TO SADDLE

Description: Chafing, callus (ischial tuberosities), maceration and ulceration, and painful nodules. Painful nodules (saddle sores) likely inflammatory (repetitive friction of hair follicle with resultant inflammation and scarring), but can be infectious; considerations: folliculitis, furuncles, carbuncles, pseudocysts, hidradenitis suppurativa

Treatment: Mostly aimed at prevention. Proper seat height and fore-aft, level seat position; individualize saddle fit (consider softer saddle with center cutout and/or broader rear); proper reach and bar height; proper hygiene (skin and shorts, shower immediately after ride, and wash cycling shorts between every ride); intermittent standing; avoid wearing low-quality underwear; use well-padded cycling shorts; lubricants or chamois creams are frequently used (petroleum-based probably better than water-based); antibiotic ointments or gels (bacitracin, clindamycin) can be used for infection and for prevention if recurrent folliculitis or hidradenitis suppurativa; occasional corticosteroid injection of recalcitrant painful nodule; sometimes requires surgical resection

URETHRITIS

Description: Traumatic irritation of urethra from rough terrain and/or improper rider position and fit

Symptoms: Variable; urethral paresthesia, dysuria, hematuria, sometimes pyuria

Treatment: Similar to pudendal neuropathy

PROSTATE CONCERNS

Description: In healthy men, the measurement of total prostate specific antigen (PSA), free PSA, and complexed PSA is not disturbed by long-distance mountain biking or endurance exercise.

Treatment: Based on the present data, there is no evidence for a recommendation to limit bicycle riding or physical activity before any measurement of PSA.

SCROTAL ULTRASOUND

Description: One study compared mountain bikers with healthy males and found 94% of mountain bikers had abnormal findings compared with 16% of the control group. Another study compared mountain bikers with road cyclists and found that 94% of the mountain bikers had abnormalities versus 48% of the road cyclists. Most common abnormalities include scrotoliths, spermatoceles, and epididymal calcifications. The clinical significance of increased prevalence of these benign conditions is unclear.

Overtraining

Description: Aggressive terrain, often with repeated hill climbing, may contribute to overtraining in mountain bikers who are not careful to incorporate adequate recovery between rides. May especially be a factor during the early season, after a "melt out" in colder regions, when mountain bikers tend to get spring fever and increase their training volumes rapidly because of a desire for trail time. Altitude training may increase need for recovery.

Treatment: See Chapter 23: "Altitude Training and Competition" and Chapter 28: "Overtraining." Mountain cyclists often complain of "heavy" legs on the bike, especially during hill climbs (a loss of power is also noted) and with stairs.

Acute Traumatic Injuries

Epidemiology

- Most injuries are minor (e.g., skin and soft tissue wounds); second most common are orthopedic injuries such as fractures, sprains, and dislocations; most commonly affecting the upper extremity in XC and DH studies (Table 95.3).
- Reported more than overuse injuries in literature.
- Injury severity measures vary: level of treatment required, lost riding time, different injury registries.

Table 95.3 BICYCLING-RELATED INJURIES

Injury	%
Orthopedic	46.5
Fractures and dislocations	68
Lower extremity	29
Upper extremity	25
Soft tissue	29
Other (including nerves and tendons)	3
Head	12.2
Fatality	Rare, most commonly because of intracranial hemorrhage
Other	
Spine	12
Chest	10.3
Facial	10.2
Abdominal	5.4
Genitourinary	2.2
Neck	1

Most riding likely FR (north shore–style riding); from 1992 to 2002, 399 patients sustained 1092 injuries while mountain biking; 1037 total patients identified with bicycling-related injuries and 67% of patients required surgery.

Data from Kim PT, Jangra D, Ritchie AH, et al. Mountain biking injuries requiring trauma center admission: a 10-year regional trauma system experience. *J Trauma*. 2006;60(2):312–318.

- General trend of frequency for body area (not specific to riding style): upper extremity (fingers and wrist are most common) injuries are more common than lower extremity (knee and ankle are most common), which are more common than head and trunk injuries.
- **Extremity injuries** are more common than any other body area.
- General trend of injury type (listed first to last in order of greatest incidence):
  - Skin lacerations
  - Wounds and contusions
  - Joint injuries (ligament sprains and dislocations)
  - Fractures
  - Muscle injuries
  - Neck/spinal and brain injuries (concussions are most common)
  - Facial and dental injuries
  - Abdominal injuries
  - Genitourinary injuries
- Ligament injury trend by location (listed first to last in order of greatest incidence):
  - Acromioclavicular (AC) joint
  - Knee
  - Ankle
  - Fingers
- Off-road cyclists sustain more fractures, dislocations, and concussions than road cyclists.
- Causes and risk factors (see the "Mechanisms of Injury and Risk Factors" section): Often multifactorial with some connection to uneven terrain (e.g., rocks, roots), bike fit (related to bike control), falls/unscheduled dismounts, collisions, problems releasing from pedals (inexperience and release adjustments for some pedals are similar to ski bindings; avoid pulling up and off pedal), contact with rough terrain.

Skin and Soft Tissue

PREVALENCE/CAUSES

- **Contusions, lacerations, and abrasions are the most frequently reported injuries** (up to 65%–75% of reported injuries): contact with rocky, varied terrain, sometimes pedals and chainrings

INJURIES

- **Road or "rock" rash:** abrasions affecting small to large surface areas, usually the lower extremities (with some incidences of upper extremity and torso injury), caused by contact with rocks and other rough terrain. Lateral lower leg most common.
  - **Treatment:** appropriately irrigate and cleanse, cover with a hydrocolloid, protective dressing (e.g., Duoderm) and antibacterial ointment (bacitracin), oral antibiotics should be administered if infection is present.
- Other soft tissue injuries include blisters, chafing, Morel-Lavallée lesions, prepatellar bursa laceration, olecranon bursa laceration, scalp laceration, ragged lower leg lacerations (problems releasing from clipless pedals, injury on chainrings, grease in wound, skin loss, debridement, and delayed primary closure concerns)
- Considerations: protective pads to protect against lacerations and abrasions, especially in downhill or rocky terrain.

Upper Extremity

PREVALENCE/CAUSES

- Upper extremities (57%) injured more frequently than lower (21%) (not the case in FR), most commonly caused by fall over handlebars (70%) and DH riding (60%).

INJURIES

- **Shoulder: most frequently injured joint in mountain biking**

- Dislocation and rotator cuff injuries (arm raised during forward fall, anterior or posterior depends on arm position relative to body with fall)
- **Clavicle fracture** and acromioclavicular separation: falls on lateral shoulder are common; sometimes, force is transmitted through the arm axially; shoulder dislocation and clavicle fractures cause the greatest burden of time lost and days needed for recovery.
- **AC separation is the most common joint injury.**
- **Prevention:** learning how to fall and roll is key, especially over the bars: cyclist should snap the bike under the body like a center snaps a football, tuck and roll (can turn endo into two-footed landing or tuck and roll); fall to side: avoid locking elbow while reaching, absorb impact with whole body.

- **Finger** dislocations and fractures, metacarpal fractures
  - Caused mainly by falls or catching a finger on an object (e.g., sapling) while riding
  - Buddy taping, clamshell type, or custom-molded Orthoplast brace for protection (mold using handlebars)
- **Wrist injuries:** falls resulting in wrist hyperextension, bracing, and collisions
  - Sprains: distal radioulnar joint and intercarpal ligaments, also triangular fibrocartilage complex tears and extensor carpi ulnaris subluxation
  - Fractures make up 50% of hand and wrist injuries: radius most common, also ulna, scaphoid, hook of hamate
  - Prefabricated wrist splints and custom orthoses (Orthoplast) that limit provocative repetitive motion may allow an earlier return to riding
- **Elbow:** Falls resulting in direct impact or axial load
  - **Radial head fracture (most common elbow fracture), radial neck fracture**
  - Subluxation/dislocation
  - Olecranon fracture
  - Medial epicondyle fracture

Lower Extremity

PREVALENCE/CAUSES

- Lower extremity injury common with side falls and contact with terrain and bike.
- The knee is more frequently injured with falls in DH and FR, less than in XC

INJURIES

- Hip and pelvis: side fall with lateral impact
  - Trochanteric bursitis (traumatic)
  - Intra-articular injuries: labral tears, bone bruise, hip fractures
  - Pelvic fractures
- Knee
  - Ligament injury common (especially FR and DH); injury to collaterals (especially medial) probably more than to the anterior cruciate
  - Meniscal injuries occur, other intra-articular injures less common
- Ankle and foot: forward momentum can be augmented by bike rider plus bike weight, combined plantarflexion and inversion on contact foot/ankle
  - **Inversion sprains most common,** syndesmosis and medial sprains sometimes occur
  - Other intra-articular injuries (e.g., talar dome lesions)
  - Can sustain midfoot sprains, but are less common, probably the result of relative protection from torsional rigidity of cycling shoes
  - **Prevention:** Use of stable, torsionally rigid shoes with a strong heel counter, practice dismounts to enhance proprioception and reaction time, bracing, strengthening

Spine

PREVALENCE

- Cervical spine injury caused by fall over bars and landing on head
- Spinal cord injuries reported in FR (24% of total spine injuries)

INJURIES

- **Cervical** most common site of injury, followed by thoracic, then lumbar
- Cervical and lumbar fractures reported
- The cervical spine is the least protected and most mobile region of vertebral column.
  - Some paraplegics, quadriplegics, central cord syndromes, some nerve root injuries
  - About half of reported FR spine injuries required surgery.
    - Vertebrae C2–C3 subluxation with cord compression (halo traction treatment, result: incomplete C3 tetraplegia)
    - Vertebrae C6–C7 bifacetal dislocation with cord transaction and cord edema to C2 (halo traction treatment, result: C3 complete tetraplegia necessitating tracheostomy and ventilatory support)
    - Vertebra C4 burst fracture body, C3 lamina fracture, nondisplaced C1 arch fracture (C4 vertebrectomy with grafting and plating, result: C4 complete motor and incomplete sensory tetraplegia)
    - T5–T6 vertebral body fracture and lumbar fractures reported
  - All of the listed injuries involved falls on head; mechanism: flexion–compression and axial compression; helmet showed significant damage in all three cases.
  - Assume cervical spine injury if altered mental status and damaged helmet; have a low threshold to obtain computed tomography (CT) and/or magnetic resonance imaging (MRI) scans if plain radiographs are negative and suspicion high.

Brain

PREVALENCE

- Concussion incidence is common; a fall over the bars is the most common mechanism of injury.
- Intracranial hemorrhage rare, but occurs with helmet use, and is the most common cause of death; may be more common in FR than DH because of higher velocities and forces compared with XC
- Bleeding or contusion to the cerebral cortex more common than to the cerebellum, followed by the brainstem
- Most mountain bikers wear helmets (80%–90%), but they are less commonly used in children and during recreational riding. In one study of professional riders, 29.2% admitted to riding in the last year with a broken helmet; however, research is unclear if this confers a greater risk of injury.

INJURIES

- Concussion
  - Younger age has been identified as a risk factor for a diagnosed concussion when looking at a broad range of ages (17–69 years). Risk is not as clear when looking at younger interval populations.
  - Rate of concussion in professional riders low and relatively mild: 1 concussion for every 263 rider races.
  - One study with a 1-year duration suggests that more than 50% of riders who experienced concussion symptoms during that time continued to ride, demonstrating that rider education and concussion protocols can likely be improved (such as early recognition and removal from training and races).

Abdomen and Chest

PREVALENCE

- Uncommon in mountain biking; blunt trauma from bike bars and bar ends (exposed bar ends are uncommon now)
- Solid organ injuries more common than hollow viscus or abdominal wall injuries
- Small bowel most frequent viscus site of injury; then the mesentery, colon, and omentum

INJURIES

- Chest wall injuries most common: rib fracture, intercostal injury, sternum fracture
- **Spleen most frequent solid organ injured** (49%), then liver (15%); injury to adrenals and pancreas has been reported.
- Spleen injuries required surgery in 25% of cases; 17% of liver injuries and most bowel injuries also required surgery.
- Liver–subcapsular hematomas (straight bar ends)
- Pancreatic transaction
- Small bowel evisceration
- Renal laceration and hemorrhage
- Hemothorax, hemopneumothorax, pneumothorax
- Blunt cardiac injury and cardiac contusion

Other Body Areas

- Genitourinary
  - Straddling most common mechanism of injury
  - Cavernosal artery laceration
  - Perineal and vulva laceration, contusion, hematoma
  - Scrotal and testicular injuries more common than penile shaft
  - Ureter injuries
- Eye
  - Foreign objects: insects, gravel, tree branches, sleet
  - Shatterproof lenses and goggles (DH) help prevent eye injuries; should be breathable to avoid fogging
- Facial and dental
  - Usually caused by fall over handlebars
  - Facial and dental fractures, lacerations, and abrasions
  - Most common facial fracture: maxilla (FR)
- Fatal
  - Brain injury, ruptured diaphragm, transected coronary vessel, pulmonary contusion, and others are generally not reported.

Fractures

- **The second most common injury behind skin and soft tissue injuries**
- Upper extremity incidence greater than lower extremity overall
- Women affected more than men (bone mineral density issues have been suggested as a cause but has not been proven). Bone mineral density for male mountain cyclists higher than comparable road cyclists.
- **Clavicle is the most common fracture,** fingers may be second, radial head, distal radius (also common), olecranon, medial epicondyle, scaphoid, metacarpals, phalanges, and other forearm fractures.
- Other reported fractures:
  - Pelvis (few details available), proximal femur, open and closed tibia and patellar
  - Tarsometatarsal fracture–dislocation
  - Trunk: ribs and scapula
  - Cervical > thoracic, and lumbar spine
  - Various others less common

Muscle Strains

- Back, thigh, and calf common

BOX 95.1 BASIC MOUNTAIN BIKING SKILLS

- Mounting and dismounting in various situations
- Braking
- Cornering
- Wheelies and hops
- Drops (slow and fast)
- Jumping
- Line selection and flow
- Pedaling efficiency
- Climbing
- Switchbacks

ENVIRONMENTAL

- Not often reported in literature in association with mountain biking; however, should remain a concern, especially as long endurance rides gain popularity
- Injuries involved with mountain biking include altitude sickness (acute mountain sickness, high-altitude pulmonary edema [HAPE], high-altitude cerebral edema [HACE]), heat- and cold-related illness/injuries, dehydration, wildlife, collisions with terrain

Environmental Injuries

Available online.

INJURY PREVENTION

- Appropriate bike fit (helps prevent overuse injury more than acute traumatic injury)
- Mountain biking skills development (more effective in preventing acute traumatic injuries than overuse): workshops or clinics, skills manuals, home skills drills, and riding time and practice can assist in developing mountain biking–specific skills that will improve riding and reduce injuries (Box 95.1).
- **Riders, sponsoring organizations, manufacturers:** improvements in rider training, race course design, and safety equipment
- Rider-related: technical skill and neuromuscular coordination drills; strength and endurance training, especially the upper body and core; awareness of limitations (riding near "the edge"), especially when riding with more experienced cyclists or on unfamiliar terrain; avoid intoxicants.
- Bike/equipment-related: use of padded and rigid protection (e.g., bulky chest and shoulder protectors, shin guards), full-face helmets for DH and FR, appropriate shoes (clipless, stiff sole, flat bottom in DH and FR), padded shorts, padded gloves, regular bike inspection and maintenance, appropriate tire setup (tubeless conversion, appropriated width, tread, and compound for setting), ensuring wheel build strength matches riding type (rim strength, number and size of spokes, type of hubs), grips (cover ends, no-slip lock, curved bar ends [if used])
- Terrain-related: responsible race organizers; avoid exciting "spectator spots," adjust course and number of laps to skill and competition level; note risky surfaces (gravel, mud, wet)

TYPES OF MOUNTAIN BIKING

Available online.

BICYCLING MODERNIZATION AND SPECIALIZATION

Available online.

RECOMMENDED READINGS

Available online.

96 INLINE SKATING, SKATEBOARDING, AND BICYCLE MOTOCROSS

Erica L. Kroncke • Craig C. Young

INTRODUCTION

- Inline skating, skateboarding, and bicycle motocross (BMX) are relatively new sports that are often included in the category of adventure and extreme sports (AES). These sports have had increased participation and popularity in the last couple of decades, in part because of AES events (such as X-games); inclusion of some AES in the Olympic Games; and social media, Internet sites, sponsorships, television channels, and AES businesses.
  - Present unique challenges compared with traditional, team, or school- and club-based sports, including in terms of medical care.
  - Increased injury rates in new and inexperienced individuals and experienced athletes trying to push the boundaries of what is possible on their equipment.
  - Most injury data are from emergency department (ED) or hospital admission data, which do not account for injuries evaluated at urgent care or private physician offices.

INLINE SKATING

History

- Inline skates date back to 1849; Louis Legrange crafted skates with wooden wheels to simulate ice skates for an opera
- In the 1970s, inline skating was primarily limited to hockey players looking for ways to practice during summers.
- In 2019, there were an estimated 4.4–4.8 million inline skaters in the United States according to the Sports & Fitness Industry Association (SFIA) and National Sporting Goods Association (NSGA), with the largest participation in the youngest age groups (6- to 17-year-olds).

Equipment

Boots: Higher, firmer boots provide more ankle support and control; used by beginners and trick skaters. Lower boots allow more ankle flexion; used by speed skaters.

Frame: Shorter frames are more maneuverable; longer frames are faster and more stable. Most recreational skaters use four-wheeled frames. Speed skaters use five-wheeled frames. Artistic skaters use two- or three-wheeled frames.

Wheels: Wheel design: in a row for inline (rollerblades) compared with in side-by-side pairs for roller skates ("quads"). Wheel sizes vary by skating style. Harder wheels are faster and more durable, but soft wheels may have better grip.

Brakes: Some inline skates have a rubber brake built into the heel, creating friction against the pavement. Standard rear brake pressure does not allow efficient stopping. Older styles require the skater to lift the toe, causing loss of contact between the front wheels and the ground, reducing stability. Expert skaters, trick skaters, figure skaters, and speed skaters often use skates without brakes. Other braking techniques include spin stops, dragging the skate, or skating into grass.

Competitive and Noncompetitive Disciplines

- Speed skating (sprint and long-distance events); roller speed skating was part of the 2018 Summer Youth Olympic Games
- Team sports (inline and roller hockey, roller soccer, roller derby)
- Aggressive inline focuses on tricks. "Big air competitions" rate competitors on jump height, trick execution, and artistic performance. In half-pipe ("vert") competitions, tricks are performed at or above the pipe (ramp) rim
- Street: tricks, grinds, and jumps on railings, curbs, stairs, and obstacles found in typical urban settings
- Recreational (solo or group) skating
- Others: Freestyle and freestyle slalom skating; off-road skating; free skating (urban skating or "riking"); inline alpine; inline downhill; artistic/figure skating; skate cross (multiple skaters racing an obstacle course)
- Governing body: International Federation of World Skate (inline and skateboard)

Injury Patterns

Risk Factors

- Male
- Age: 10- to 14-year-olds account for a majority of injuries (according to Consumer Product Safety Commission [CPSC])
  - Inexperienced skaters are at increased risk of injury. Experienced skaters are also at increased injury risk related to performing tricks and dose-response skating (higher number of injuries the more hours per week spent skating, specifically >10 hours/week).
- Skitching: hanging on to a moving vehicle, can lead to speeds of >70 mph. Deaths from inline skating usually involve motor vehicle collisions (MVCs).

Injuries

- Primarily from falls and collisions.
- There was a significant downward trend in ED-treated inline skating injuries from 2005 to 2014 (CPSC). Medically attended injuries (which include ED, doctor's offices, clinics, and school nurses) in 2014 were estimated at 29,857, and 2018–2019 national estimates of ED-treated injuries are <5000/year.
- Severity: In a previous study, injury severity score (ISS) was 10.6 for inline skating compared with 10.5 for skateboarding and 12.7 for cycling.
- Wheeled sports (roller skating, skateboarding, and scooter) had highest rate of traumatic brain injury (TBI) on computed tomography (CT) (12%) and clinically important TBI compared with all other sports; wheeled sports also had a TBI hospitalization rate 10 times that of team sports. Approximately half of inline fatalities in the Centers for Disease Control and Prevention (CDC) database are from head injuries.
- Abdominal injuries are uncommon but may be significant. Five percent of clinically important intra-abdominal injuries (CIIAI) presenting to the ED were related to rollerblades, bicycles, or skateboards.

Location

- Upper extremity (UE, especially wrist and forearm) are the most frequent sites of injury, particularly more severe injuries (fractures and dislocations). Compared with other sports, skating sports have one of the highest frequencies of elbow dislocations.
- Knee and ankle are most common lower extremity injury sites

Prevention

Protective Equipment

- American Academy of Pediatrics (AAP) and American Academy of Orthopaedic Surgeons (AAOS) recommend personal protective equipment (PPE), which includes helmets, wrist guards,

and elbow and knee pads. American Dental Association (ADA) recommends mouth guards.
- Estimated that wrist guards and elbow pads can decrease UE inline skating injuries by 90%.
- Failure to wear wrist guards may increase the relative risk of injury by 10.4; nonuse of elbow pads may increase the relative risk of injury by 9.5.
- Cadaveric studies using high-speed impact loading suggest that wrist guards may reduce injuries.
- PPE has the potential to transmit forces to areas away from the impact site, placing other body areas at risk of injury (wrist guards may place skaters at risk of "splint-top" fractures). Helmets have been shown to reduce the risk of injury in bicyclists; this may be even more important for skaters who may reach speeds >40 mph.
- Fatally injured skaters universally seem to be nonhelmet wearers.
  - The CPSC contains information on helmet type, certification, and when to replace helmets.

Use of Protective Equipment

- Actual use: unknown. Helmets and wrist guards are the most commonly worn PPE; helmets are required in some competitions.
- Adolescent skaters are much less likely to use PPE.
- Most influential factors for adolescent PPE use: parents (40%), requirement of skating location (33%), friends and coaches (14%–15%)
- Common reasons for lack of PPE: lack of perceived need (47.3%), discomfort, and appearance. Formal school-based instructional programs may have a small but significant positive effect in attitude toward and use of PPE

OTHER

- Safe age for inline skating: unknown. AAOS does not recommend skating (inline or skateboarding) before age 5 and close supervision of 6- to 10-year-olds.
- Skate parks: advantages are smoother surface separate from traffic; however, some have concern for increased injuries.
- Beginners should consider lessons; learning how to fall can decrease injury.
- Small-scale study showed increased balance and strength in preteens in a 4-week instructional inline skating program.

SKATEBOARDING

History

- Modern-day skateboard is thought to be adapted from the scooterboard (wooden crate connected to a board and roller skates or wheels) or soapbox.
- Skateboarding experienced intermittent periods of popularity since the 1960s.
- There were an estimated 5.5–6.6 million skateboarders in 2019 (NSGA, SFIA; largest group of participants ages 7–17 years).

Equipment

- Skateboard parts:
  - Deck: made of aluminum, bamboo, carbon fiber, fiberglass, Kevlar, plastic, or wood. Longer, inflexible decks are safer for beginners; shorter, more flexible decks lead to increased maneuverability. Wider decks are used for vert (vertical) skating. Longboard ("sidewalk surfer") is a variant with a longer deck, larger wheels, and a more stable truck.
  - Wheels: Usually polyurethane or plastic; wide wheels ("stokers," 6–10 cm) provide more stability; narrower wheels ("slicks," 3–4 cm) increase maneuverability
  - Truck: Made up of axles, frames, and hardware; connects the wheels and deck
- Modern skateboards usually have nose and tail kicks (upward curves) with a concavity between them, allowing foot cupping for more control.
- Stance
  - Regular (left foot forward) most common
  - Goofy (right foot forward)

Competitive and Noncompetitive Disciplines

- Vert uses 8- to 10-foot-high ramps (usually half-pipes); involves "big air" flare
- Slalom skating (weaving between cones)
- Freestyle emphasizes technical flat-ground skating
- Street skating: boarding on sidewalks, streets, and parking lots; may include tricks
- Pool (drained swimming pool) or (skate) park skating named by location
- Other: downhill, off-road or dirt-boarding, cruising (usually longboards)
- Skateboarding made its Olympic debut at the Tokyo 2020 Olympic Games

Injury Patterns

Risk Factors

Male.

Age: 15- to 19-year-olds are the most often injured (CPSC). Despite number of injuries trending down for 5- to 14-year-olds and rising for ≥15-year-olds according to ED and hospital admission data, 10- to 19-year-olds are more likely to sustain a skateboarding injury when compared with older skaters.

Experience: Inexperienced riders still suffer injury; however, newer data suggest increased injuries in experienced skaters pushing the boundaries of their skills

Injuries

- Increases during periods of popularity: cyclical over the last 2 decades (27); increased from 2000 to 2008, then decreased from 2008 to 2017. There were an estimated 299,286 medically attended skateboard injuries in 2014 (CPSC).
- Majority of injuries are left sided because of regular stance.
- UE injuries are the most common
- Skateboard elbow: olecranon process fracture caused by fall directly on elbow
- Older age groups were more likely to sustain a head injury; younger skaters were more likely to sustain a UE fracture
- Skateboarding has higher risk of head or neck injury (HNI) compared with other AES. Approximately 11% of injuries in a subset of AES, including skateboarding, were HNI.
- Ankle sprains are common
- Majority of skateboarding deaths involve MVC

Prevention

- PPE use decreases the risk of injury
  - Injury less likely to require hospital admission if wearing PPE. One study showed that helmet use would have prevented all head injury admissions over a 30-month period.
- Recommended PPE
  - PPE recommendations, "safe age," helmet information (see "Inline Skating" section), and formal instruction.
  - Although multiple organizations recommend PPE (CPSA, AAP, AAOS), there is concern that helmet use may increase tactically risky behavior, and wrist protectors may transfer force to the forearm ("splint top fractures").
- Use of PPE: unknown. Earlier studies suggested 13%–33% of skateboarders of all ages wear PPE. Use of PPE less common as age increases.

- Certain skate parks and competitions require PPE
  - Requirement of skating location, parents, and peers are the most common reasons adolescent skateboarders wear PPE; discomfort, lack of perceived need, and appearance were the most commonly cited reasons by adolescents for nonuse of PPE.

BICYCLE MOTOCROSS

History

- Started in California in the 1960s. For riders who wanted to participate in motocross but did not have the means, BMX was an option. Riders dressed in motocross gear and raced on homemade tracks.
- Scot Breithaupt, considered the founder of BMX, organized the first race in 1971; manufacturers began constructing bikes with 20-inch wheels specifically for this growing sport.
- Union Cycliste Internationale (UCI, or International Cycling Association): governing body for cycling and classifies cycling disciplines (which includes BMX).
- US sanctioning bodies of BMX racing:
  - National Bicycle League (NBL), certified under the UCI
  - American Bicycle Association (ABA)
- International BMX Federation founded in 1981
- BMX was introduced in the 2008 Olympic Games in Beijing; BMX Freestyle was scheduled to make its Olympic debut at the 2020 Olympic Games
- BMX is among the top 10 most popular AES. The Outdoor Foundation considers biking (including BMX) a "gateway activity" to other outdoor activities; it is among the most popular outdoor activities. In 2019, there were an estimated 3.65 million BMX bikers in the United States, with the largest age group comprising 6- to 12-year-olds.

Competitive and Noncompetitive Disciplines

BMX Racing

- Track: Closed loop 300–400 meters in length and 5–10 meters wide with jumps and obstacles. Head-to-head competition of up to eight riders per heat; top four qualify for next round.
- Competition classes are based on age, gender, bike style, and level.
- May reach speeds >30 mph.
- Majority of racers are men.

Freestyle BMX

- Evolved from BMX racing when riders focused on aerial maneuvers and began to merge skateboard riding with stunts and tricks.
- Events are timed and judged based on difficulty, originality, creativity, style, flow, maneuvers, and height.
- Disciplines:
  - Street: street riding allows for creativity because almost anything can be an obstacle
  - Park (skate park)
  - Vert: Analogous to skateboarding discipline, riders perform tricks on a vert ramp (half-pipe)
  - Dirt: involves lines of jumps built from compact dirt; airborne riders often perform tricks before landing
  - Flat (flatland): riding terrain is smooth and flat

Equipment

- BMX bikes usually have 20-inch wheels
- Certain bikes are free-wheeling (wheels operate independent of pedals)
- Racing bikes tend to be lighter than freestyle and street bikes and have only a rear brake
- Freestyle and street bikes
  - Most freestyle bikes have front and rear brakes; handlebar is designed to completely spin around without twisting the front brake cable; has axle pegs for tricks
- Pedals
  - Platform (flat) pedals without a cage are most often used; offer grip when using short metal studs and do less damage if the rider is in an accident
  - Toe clips generally not used

Injuries

Risk Factors

- Male
- Stunts/tricks
- Poor technique
- Inexperience

Injuries

- Most injuries are acute. The 10- to 14-year-olds are the group most often injured on bicycles based on ED data (CPSC), which includes but is not specific to BMX.
- Among BMX injuries seen at EDs, mild injuries were most common, although 7% of injuries in one study were head injuries.
- Extremity injuries are most common; facial injuries are also common (21%–22%).
- Abdominal, scrotal/genitourinary, perineal, and spinal injuries are reported.
- Racing injuries at the 1989 European BMX Championships: 61 injuries/976 participants; injury breakdown: 42% abrasions, 29% contusions, 8% sprains, 4% fractures (majority UE), 2% concussion, and 2% other; injury rate: 1190 injuries per 1000 competition hours; higher injury rate in females.
- 6.2% of athletes were injured at the 2007 World Championships.
- BMX was among the sports with the highest injury risk at the 2012 London Summer Olympic Games; however, there was a similar injury incidence in new Olympic sports (includes roller speed skating and BMX freestyle) compared with other sports at 2018 Youth Olympic Summer Games

Personal Protective Equipment

- Helmets (see CPSC)
  - Full face or open face (latter must be used with mouth guards)
- Long-sleeved shirts and pants, gloves and elbow pads required at UCI-sanctioned races
- Knee pads
- Closed-toe shoes
- Chest protectors
- Shin guards

ACKNOWLEDGMENTS

The authors would like to acknowledge **Thomas Schroeder, CPSC, NSGA, SFIA, Worldskate, UCI, and Diane Giebink-Skoglind.**

RECOMMENDED READINGS

Available online.

MASS PARTICIPATION ENDURANCE EVENTS 97

William O. Roberts

GENERAL PRINCIPLES

- This chapter develops an algorithm for managing mass participation endurance events.
- The medical director is the safety and health advocate for athletes who participate in the race.
- The safety of athletes is the primary purpose of race medical operations.
- A central medical command structure can improve the efficiency of the medical team, integrate community resources into the medical plan, and reduce response times for emergencies during the event.

Events

- Road running
- Cycling
- Cross-country skiing
- Triathlon
- Wheelchair
- Swimming

Approach as a "Planned Disaster"

- Participant and volunteer safety is the primary goal of the race and race medical committees.
- Mass participation events should be approached as a "planned disaster" (potential mass casualty incident), which may adversely affect the community medical delivery system.
- Mass gatherings always have the potential for medical illness or injury.
- Potential casualties can occur in two groups of people: participants (a literature review allows estimation of injury type and incidence; individual race experience allows for more accurate estimates) and spectators (often not considered a part of race medical management).
- Endurance events share common injury and illness risks that must be addressed by medical management teams, but each event will also have a unique injury and illness profile.
- A comprehensive medical plan using a central command structure will decrease the community medical burden and reduce the potential for emergency room overload.
- A central command structure can respond to unexpected race-related or race course incidents by drawing on community emergency medical, public safety, and law enforcement assets.

Incidence and Risk

- Estimating medical encounters is best done with race data.
  - Anticipated number of starters multiplied by encounter incidence; a race with several years of start history will have an average "no show" rate for race registrants.
  - Project needs: staff, supplies, equipment
- Risk ranges (defined as a medical encounter during or immediately after the event)
  - Running (56 km): 13% risk of injury over 4 years
  - Running (42 km): 0.5%–20% risk of injury
    - Twin Cities Marathon (Minnesota): 0.5%–3% risk of injury (average 1.89% for entrants from 1983 to 1994)
    - Boston Marathon: 1.6%–10% risk of injury (data from recent races only, as the start time was moved from noon to 10 AM)
  - Running (≤21 km): 1%–5% for the 11.5-km Falmouth Road Race (Massachusetts), less than 1% severe injury incidence rate; 0.54% for 21-km Two Oceans Marathon (South Africa), with 0.05% serious injury rate
  - Women over age 50 had more medical encounters at Two Oceans Marathon
  - Triathlon (225 km): 15%–35% injury rate, 13%–21% injury rate among Kona Ironman participants from 1995 to 2014
  - Cross-country skiing (55 km): 5%
  - Triathlon (51 km): 2%–5%
  - Cycling (variable): 5%
- Variables and unknowns: race-day weather, event distance, event type, participant health and fitness, and participant acclimatization to race-day environment
  - Heat and humidity influence on marathon outcomes:
    - Medical encounters and race dropouts increase
    - Race times slower (increase)
    - Exertional heat stroke and exercise-associated hyponatremia (EAH) increase
  - Heat limits
    - Twin Cities Marathon data imply cancelling at wet bulb globe temperature (WBGT) near 70°F (21.1°C) may be better for nonelite runner safety and community emergency system response, especially for unacclimatized participants (early October race, 45 degrees N latitude).
    - The cancellation level is likely specific to each event, but the number of medical encounters and nonfinishers seems to accelerate with WBGTs above 60°F (15.5°C).
    - Elite runners seem to tolerate hotter and more humid conditions (elites are still at greater risk and will be slower); races may elect to run the elite race while cancelling the nonelite race (best done in advance of the event).
    - A WBGT measurement on site is best for event decision-making, but if not available, WBGT can be accessed for a given locale at https://www.weather.gov/tsa/wbgt. WBGT may become a part of local weather reporting and forecasting in the near future.

Anticipating Casualty Types

- Exercise-associated collapse (EAC) or exercise-associated postural hypotension (EAPH) is most common cause of collapse after an endurance running event. Body temperatures may be hyperthermic, normothermic, or hypothermic.
- Low-frequency but potentially fatal medical emergencies can occur, including cardiac arrest, exertional heat stroke, EAH, asthma, insulin shock, anaphylaxis (exercise associated or "bee" sting), and high-velocity or impact trauma.
- Macrotrauma: musculoskeletal (fracture, dislocation, sprains and strains, contusions), vascular (closed, open), head and neck (concussion, intracerebral bleed, fracture–dislocation), and visceral organs (contusions, laceration, rupture)
- Microtrauma: tendinitis, stress fracture, fasciitis
- Dermatologic trauma: blisters, abrasions, lacerations
- Drowning, near-drowning, and swimming-induced pulmonary edema can occur in water-based events.

Race Medical Operations Purpose

Prerace: Develop strategies to improve competitor safety and reduce race-related injuries and illnesses.

Race day: **Primary:** stop progression of injury or illness; evaluate casualties (triage, treat, transfer); reduce community medical burden. **Secondary:** prevent overloading of local emergency medical services and emergency departments.

Role in Race Operations

- Event and runner safety
- Medical decision-making
- Medical spokesperson
- Executive committee administrative functions
- Coordinate event transfer to "unified central command" if emergency situation develops

PREVENTION STRATEGIES

Primary

Definition: Prevent or reduce medical encounters, reduce severity of casualties

Passive: Participant cooperation or decision-making is not required. Examples: start times, course modifications, traffic control

Active: Participant cooperation or self-initiated behavior change is required. Examples: education, safety advisories.

Enforced active: Require helmets or wetsuits to participate in the event

Secondary

Definition: Early detection of injury or illness; intervention protocols to stop progression

Examples: Impaired runner policy; advanced cardiac life support (ACLS), advanced trauma life support (ATLS), or EAC protocol; on-course ambulance; finish line triage

Tertiary

Definition: Treatment and rehabilitation of illness or injury

Examples: Emergency department transfer, hospital admission, rehabilitation center

PREPARATION

Race Scheduling

- Location (latitude, longitude, and altitude)
- Season of year (temperature and relative humidity [median, mean, and range])
- Safest start and finish times (if average high temperature is >60°F [15.5°C], schedule race start for sunrise)
- Maximum time limit for competitors to remain on course

Competitor Safety

- Consider the safety of the athlete first and foremost in all race-related decisions.
- Use the safest start and finish times for both elite and nonelite competitors.
- Determine hazardous conditions and develop a written race administration plan to simplify decisions on race day.
  - Ensure volunteer and competitor safety.
  - Define heat, cold, traction, wind, wind chill, lightning, and torrential rain race limits.
  - Develop alternatives: alter course, postpone start, cancel event
  - Publish protocol in advance.
  - Announce event risks at start.
- Local incidents, such as residential or commercial building fires, gas line explosions, train derailments, etc., may require cancellation of the race if the local public safety personnel are called upon to respond, leaving the race "unattended"
- Natural disasters and terrorist activities can also shut down a race (COVID-19 pandemic, bomb detonation—Boston, Hurricane Sandy—New York)
- Pandemics—COVID-19 pandemic—affected most 2020 events.
- Impaired competitor policy:
  - Define an approach regarding an athlete who appears ill or injured during the competition, especially related to fluid balance abnormalities and heat or cold stress.
  - No disqualification for medical evaluation. Most event rules allow medical assessment of athletes who appear ill without automatic disqualification and allow athletes deemed fit to continue participation if they leave and enter the course in the same spot and receive no intravenous (IV) fluid. This is especially important for citizen-class (nonelite) runners.
  - Criteria to continue participating in the event: oriented to person, place, and time; straight line progress toward the finish; good competitive posture; clinically fit appearance
  - Publish policy in advance.
- Emergency department (ED) notification: notify local EDs of date, time, and duration of event; also estimate numbers and types of possible race casualties.
- Preparticipation screening
  - Decide whether event should require pre-event medical screening: Will it improve safety of participants? Will it be cost-effective? Will it protect event and volunteer staff from liability or disease transmission?
  - Generally not recommended beyond usual health screening or interventions by the participant's personal physician based on risk factors and symptoms.
  - COVID-19 or similar infectious disease agents may affect participant safety, and how to effectively assess participants before the event remains to be determined
- Data from South African distance running races suggest that an online, automated, and individually targeted medical screening and educational intervention program for runners reduces the incidence of medical complications, specifically serious life-threatening cardiovascular complications, during a race. This intervention program also included a prerace acute illness checklist with an educational handout for symptomatic runners.
- Competitor education: safety measures, risks of participation, fitness level recommended for participation, hydration and overhydration (drink to thirst, knowledge of sweat rate, ingestion of adequate fluid to nearly replace sweat losses without excessive intake), volunteer identification (standard colors, visibility), and nutrition recommendations.
  - Medical information should be registered with smart phone or computer apps designed for race medical care or placed on the back of race bibs and should include training weight, prerace weight, allergies, medications, chronic medical problems, and emergency contact phone number.
  - Medical alert tags should be worn during the race.
- Child and adolescent participation in endurance events: there are no data to support restricting participation of individuals under the age of 18 years for medical reasons, and children as young as 7 years have completed marathons without reported adverse effects. A motivated child (not parent), who is growing physically, physiologically, psychologically, and socially during training, should be allowed to participate if the race or event does not ban participation for administrative reasons.

Course

- Course survey: review the course for hills, turns, immovable objects, traffic control, altitude changes, and open water that may affect participant safety and alter environment factors
- Start: downhill starts increase risk for wheelchair, bike, inline skate, and Nordic ski competitors; wave starts should be employed to relieve congestion and risks associated with falls in mass starts
- Aid stations
  - Major: full medical care; equipped and staffed for most anticipated problems
  - Minor: comfort care, fluids, first aid, shelter
  - Location: start; every 15–20 minutes along course; finish line
  - Rolling aid: vehicle (bus or van) equipped and staffed to deliver medical care for expected injuries along the course; requires an open lane on the race course for the vehicle(s)
  - First-response teams: motorcycles, bikes, golf carts, or gators; 2- to 3-person cardiopulmonary resuscitation (CPR) and automatic external defibrillator (AED) trained teams; automatic defibrillator and first aid supplies
- Finish area (Fig. 97.1)
  - Triage: chute, postchute, and finish area triage (sweep teams in family meeting, clothing pick up, and "party" areas)
  - Field hospital: major aid station (see Fig. 97.1). Subdivisions may include triage, intensive medical, intensive trauma, minor medical, minor trauma, skin, and medical records.
  - Ambulance support for ED transfer (see Fig. 97.1)
  - Shelter for healthy finishers
  - Dry clothes shuttle; consider clothes dryer for wet or cold conditions
  - Fan out finish line area to spread out participants in hot races
  - Elevated spotters to identify downed participants in crowded areas (see Fig. 97.1)

Transportation

- Healthy competitors who abandon the race
  - Prevent new or exacerbation of previous injury by transporting to shelter or reducing repetitive stress: hypothermia, hyponatremia, stress fracture, muscle–tendon strain
  - Examples: vans, buses, golf carts, gators, snowmobiles, snowcats, public transportation, sled, toboggan, boat
- Ill or injured competitors
  - Prevent progression of illness or injury (both overuse and acute injuries) without increasing individual morbidity or mortality.
  - Access care for more severe acute illness or injury. Minor injury can use transportation for healthy athletes who abandoned race. Casualties requiring medical care need transport by ambulance to nearest ED or event medical station.
  - Examples of medically equipped vehicles for ill competitors who abandon the race: advanced life support (ALS) or basic life support (BLS) ambulance, life flight helicopter.
- Finish area
  - Access medical care in finish area.
    - Examples: wheelchair, litter, stretcher, manned carriers (Fig. 97.2)
    - Access tertiary care by ambulance: ALS, BLS

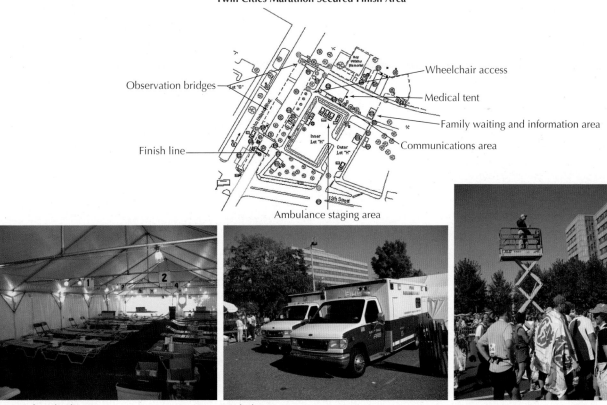

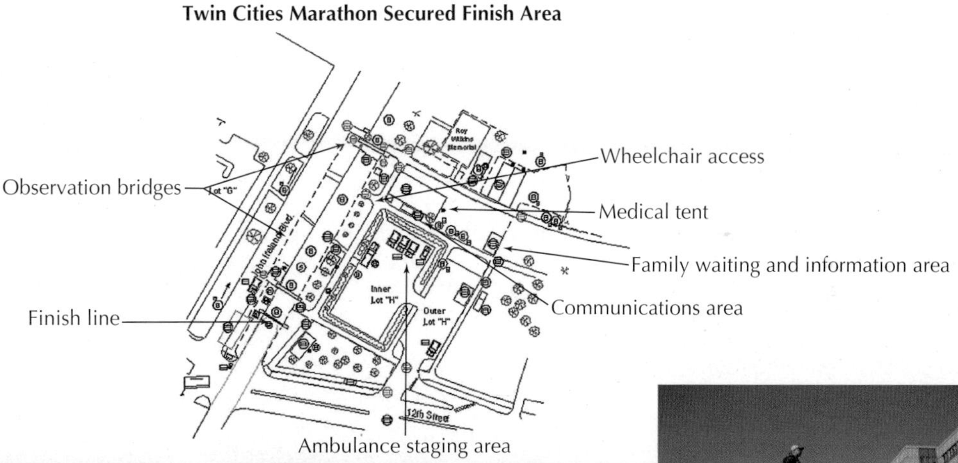
Twin Cities Marathon Secured Finish Area
Wheelchair access
Observation bridges
Medical tent
Family waiting and information area
Communications area
Finish line
Inner Lot "H"
Outer Lot "H"
12th Street
Ambulance staging area

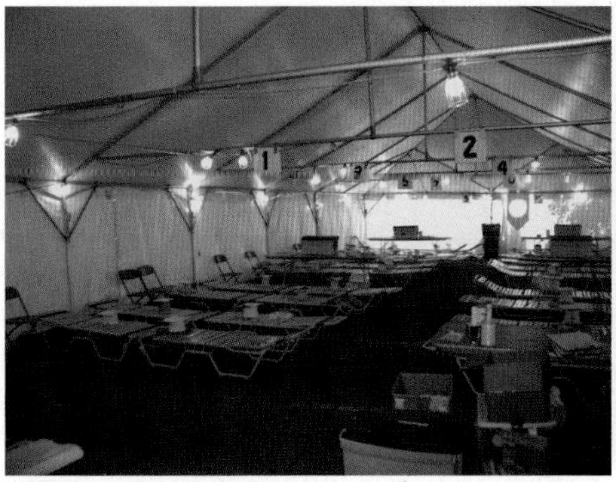
Interior of medical tent.

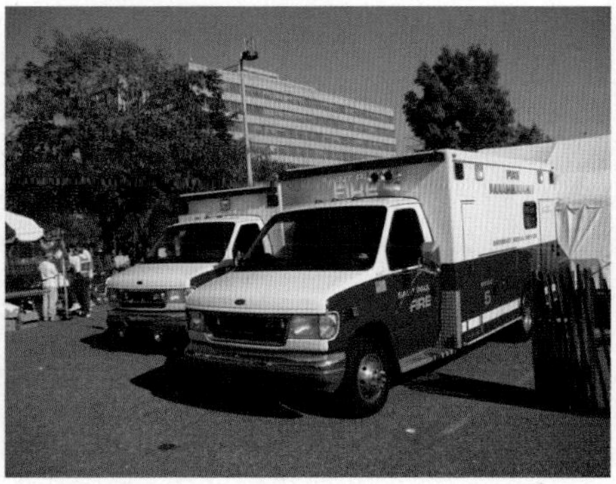
Ambulance support.

Elevated spotter to identify downed participants.

Figure 97.1 Finish area of mass participation events.

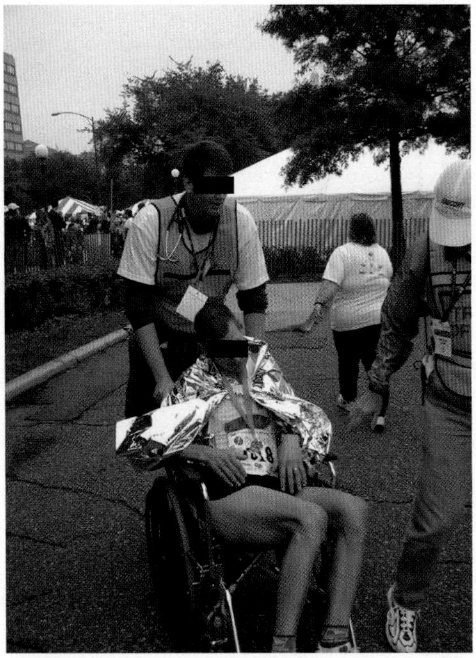

Figure 97.2 Finish area should be equipped with wheelchairs, litters, stretchers, and manned carriers.

Communications

- Type: phone (cellular/digital, hard wire), ham radio systems, two-way radio systems. Three-tiered system provides overlap and backup if a single system fails. It is common in disaster scenarios for cellular service to be shut down or be overwhelmed by user demand.
- Location: start; course (aid stations, pickup vans, course spotters, ambulance, race volunteers with cell phones forming a "line of sight" spotter network to blanket the course); finish area (field hospital [central dispatch for course], triage teams).
- 911 access: given to any volunteer to summon an ambulance, but must know exact location.
- Give runner number to ensure that the dispatched ambulance responds to the correct person. Notify race incident command central dispatch of pickup and disposition.
- Consider smart phone apps that can be used to access race communications and record participant medical encounters along the course and in the finish area.

Fluids and Fuel

Type: Water, carbohydrate–electrolyte solutions, high-carbohydrate foods or gels

Location: Start, aid stations, finish area (postchute area, medical area)

Amount: 6–12 ounces available for each competitor every 15–20 minutes. Double for start, finish, and transition areas. Total volume and course distribution can be estimated from similar events or past race needs. Competitors should know their individual needs based on sweat rate, and most are safest if drinking to thirst. A validated fluid calculator app described at https://sportssciencesynergy.com/road-race-water-planner/ and is available for purchase at https://apps.apple.com/us/app/rrwp/id1249618165.

Publish in advance: Fluid and food types, locations; risks and symptoms of underhydration and overhydration; calculation of personal sweat rate (measure nude weight, run at race pace for an hour in expected race conditions, strip down, towel off, and reweigh nude; difference in weight is the maximum fluid volume to be replaced every hour).

Equipment

- Shelter (tents, vehicles such as school buses, buildings) with heaters for cool weather and air conditioning for hot weather (if possible)
- Security fencing
- Cots (chaise lounges work well for leg elevation), chairs, tables
- Heating and cooling equipment (microwave to warm blankets; tubs for immersion cooling; coolers for ice)
- Generator
- Defibrillator (manual or automatic)
- Back boards
- Lights
- Portable sink
- Toilet
- Point-of-care laboratory measuring devices for serum sodium, blood urea nitrogen (BUN), potassium, hematocrit, glucose, oxygen saturation (if available)

Supplies

- Medical
- Trauma
- IV fluids (normal saline [NS] or 5% dextrose in NS)
- Medications (albuterol, epinephrine 1:1000, dextrose 50% in water, oxygen, midazolam, cardiac arrest drug kit, 3% NaCl solution, others)

Staffing

- Personnel located at start, throughout course, and at finish
    - Physicians; physician assistants, advanced nurse practitioners
    - Acute care nurses (intensive care unit, coronary care unit, ED)
    - Paramedics
    - Emergency medical technicians (EMTs)
    - Physical therapists
    - Athletic trainers
    - First aid personnel
    - Nonmedical assistants
- Sources for volunteers: hospitals, clinics, the American Red Cross, National Ski Patrol, National Mountain Bike Patrol, National Guard, Armed Forces Reserves, medical personnel training centers

Medical and Race Records

- Document care
- Calculate incidence and document types of medical encounters
- Project future needs
- Research injury/illness patterns
- Design a system to easily document care for common problems (eFig. 97.1).

MEDICAL PROTOCOLS

- **First aid:** Do no harm; stay within training level.
- **Basic problems:** EAC/EAPH, low-frequency life-threatening medical emergencies (cardiac arrest, exertional heat stroke, EAH, anaphylaxis, insulin-related hypoglycemia), trauma, repetitive use musculoskeletal (MSK) injury, and skin injury
- **Initial assessment of collapsed athlete (ABCDE):** **A**irway (cervical spine control), **b**reathing, **c**irculation (hemorrhage control), **d**isability (neurologic status), **e**xposure and examination

- **Initial disposition:** Race medical facility, transport to emergency facility. Decide if on-course problems are triaged in a race medical facility or moved directly to nearest ED. This will depend on both the medical capabilities and the accessibility of the race facility(ies) and the local ED(s).
- **Treatment and transfer protocols**
  - Decide on level of care (first aid vs. medical treatment) in the finish area and course aid stations.
  - Determine in advance medical problems warranting automatic transfers to an ED (cardiac arrest, respiratory arrest, shock, symptomatic hyponatremia, severe trauma) and problems better served in race medical facilities.
  - Keep treatment protocols simple.
  - Consider initiating treatment for exertional heat stroke and EAH in the race medical facility to avoid life-threatening treatment delays.
  - Integrate race-day evaluation and transfer protocols into emergency medical services (EMS) protocol.
- Medical precautions
  - Exposure to body fluids (blood, stool, emesis, respiratory droplets; *not* sweat) can transmit disease.
  - Modified universal precautions are most frequently used: hand washing, gloves, no food or eating in treatment areas; however, during the pandemic of COVID-19, more extensive personal protective gear may be required.
  - Risks: hepatitis B, C, D, others; AIDS/HIV, COVID-19
  - Disposal of contaminated waste: Red Bag materials, sharps containers
- Adverse event protocol
  - If a participant has a medical event with an adverse outcome resulting in death or catastrophic injury, a predetermined protocol should be in place to communicate with the family, public, and media.
    - Medical event is first reported to the medical director and head of event administration.
    - Medical event should not be discussed with or by volunteers outside immediate need for medical care.
    - Medical director or a designated alternative should present the incident to media.
  - Event administration and medical director should keep detailed records.

EXERCISE-ASSOCIATED COLLAPSE CLASSIFICATION AND TREATMENT SYSTEM

- **Based on symptoms and signs of collapsed finishers**
  - Simple treatment protocols should be in place.
  - Weather influences injury patterns, and warmer weather increases the number of medical encounters and participant abandons (start race, but do not finish).
  - Clinical classification system: varied presentation of symptoms within each temperature class; symptoms do not reflect body temperature; similar treatment for all classes; rapid recovery for most victims
- **Definition of EAC:** Requiring assistance during or after endurance activity; not orthopedic or dermatologic
- **Etiology:** Undetermined, but most cases are related to exercise-related postural hypotension because of sudden loss of muscle-pump blood flow from legs (secondary heart function of legs during exercise). Significant dehydration may be present in more severe cases but is not common.
- **Diagnosis:** Presence of signs or symptoms. Major criteria: body temperature, mental status, ambulation status
- **Clinical picture** (derived from clinical presentations of Twin Cities Marathon casualties)
  - Symptoms: exhaustion, fatigue, hot, cold, nausea, stomach cramps, lightheadedness, headache, leg cramps, and palpitations
  - Signs: abnormal body temperature, altered mental status, central nervous system changes, inability to walk unassisted, leg muscle spasms, tachycardia, vomiting, diarrhea, and unconsciousness
- **Classification scheme**
  - Types: **hyperthermic** (body temperature ≥103°F [39.5°C]), **normothermic** (temperature between 97°F [36°C] and 103°F [39.4°C]); **hypothermic** (temperature ≤97°F [36°C])
  - Severity ratings: **mild** (presence of any symptom or sign, able to walk with or without assistance, alert, systolic blood pressure greater than 100 mmHg, heart rate less than 100 beats per minute, weight loss <5%); **moderate** (no oral intake, extra fluid loss, unable to walk, severe muscle spasm, weight loss 5%–10%, temperature ≥105°F [40.5°C] or ≤95°F [36°C]); and **severe** (central nervous system changes, no oral intake, extra fluid loss, unable to walk, severe muscle spasm, weight loss >10%, temperature ≥106°F [41°C] or ≤90°F [32°C]). Runners classified as severe should be evaluated for exertional heat stroke, EAH, and hypothermia.

Management Protocol

Diagnosis and Documentation

- Initiate medical record; record presenting symptoms and medical history.
- Record vital signs.
  - Temperature: rectal measurement required for accurate core body temperature estimate; tympanic membrane, temporal artery, oral, and axillary measurements (shell temperatures) are not accurate for core estimates in athletes and should not be used.
  - Blood pressure (BP), pulse, respiration
  - Orthostatic BP and pulse changes
- Record mental status and orientation, walking status, and other physical examination findings.
- Record treatment and log times.

Fluid Replacement and Redistribution

- Supine position (nonambulatory): elevate legs and buttocks; restore pooled blood to circulation; if ambulatory and able, assist walking (Fig. 97.3)
- Oral fluids (preferred method): all mild cases; all moderate cases, if tolerated
- IV fluids: all severe cases not due to exercise associated hyponatremia; moderate cases if no response to oral fluids or unable

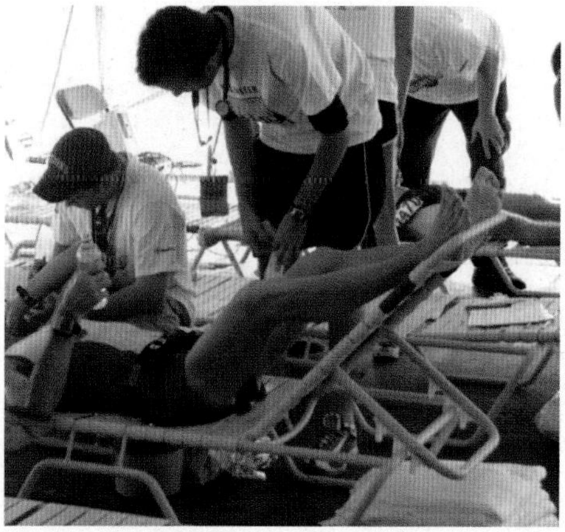

Figure 97.3 Fluid replacement and redistribution after exercise-associated collapse. Supine position (nonambulatory)—elevate legs and buttocks; restore pooled blood to circulation.

to tolerate oral fluids; IV access for EAH and casualties with undetermined fluid status

- **Recommended fluids**
  - **Oral:** start with hypertonic fluids like bouillon broth and then move to simple glucose–electrolyte drinks, fruit juices, or water
  - **IV:** 5% dextrose in NS for first liter if Na is normal or high, or if clinically dehydrated, then NS unless blood glucose is low (remember that lactated Ringer's solution contains potassium; avoid until potassium status known; do not use in hypothermic patient because a cold liver does not metabolize lactate)
- **IV access uses** (invasive procedure that should be used for set criteria)
  - Medication access
  - Measure serum electrolytes, BUN, glucose, and hematocrit.
  - Fluid replacement in participants with normal or high Na (most finishers are minimally to moderately dehydrated and improve rapidly with IV fluids when oral fluids fail)
  - Hypertonic (3%) NaCl solution for symptomatic hyponatremia (present in marathons usually because of inappropriate antidiuretic hormone (ADH) levels in the face of excess fluid intake, resulting in fluid overload; in hot condition Ironman triathlons or ultramarathons (long duration), may be related to sweat Na loss and dehydration (rare); initial treatment for symptomatic cases is the same as fluid overload).
  - Do not give IV fluids to any athlete who appears overhydrated or has increasing confusion, severe progressive headache, or vomiting without first checking Na levels.
- **Selection criteria for rapid IV fluid replacement** (based on data from the Twin Cities Marathon)
  - Administration should be considered after leg elevation for at least 10 minutes with no improvement (may take 20–30 minutes to resolve).
  - Systolic BP less than 100 mmHg (orthostatic BP drop after leg elevation)
  - Persistent heart rate greater than 100 beats per minute
  - Temperature above 104°F (40°C) or below 95°F (35°C), if not responding to initial therapy
  - Severe muscle spasms
  - Anorexia, nausea, diarrhea
  - Hypoglycemia (<60 mg/dL)
  - High sodium and/or hematocrit and BUN
  - Confusion with normal or high sodium levels
  - Not doing well and hyponatremia ruled out
- Other options: no IV starts for fluid replacement and send all who do not recover with simple first aid to ED (may potentially overwhelm EMS transport and ED centers)

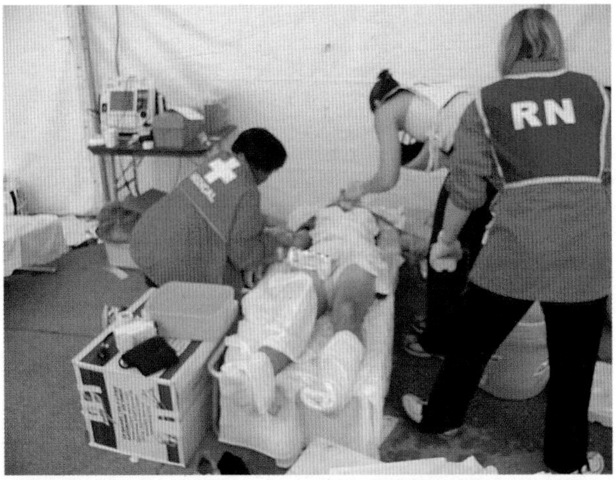
RN

Hyperthermic EAC. Rapidly rotate ice water soaked towels to the arms, legs, trunk and head to give adequate cooling rate.

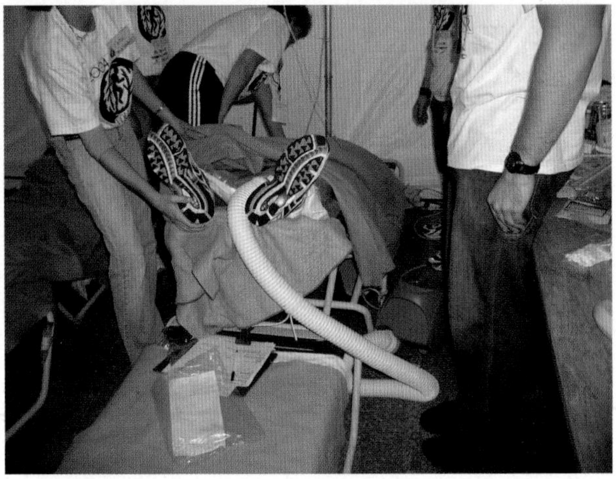

Hypothermic EAC. Use BairHugger™ or warm heater air to blow into blankets.

Figure 97.4 Temperature correction.

Temperature Correction

HYPERTHERMIC EAC

- Move to cool or shaded area, remove excess clothing.
- Active cooling (rectal temperature >105°F [40.5°C]) by any means possible: ice water tub immersion for fastest cooling rates; rapidly rotating ice water–soaked towels to the arms, legs, trunk, and head combined with ice packs in neck, axilla, and groin will give adequate cooling rate (Fig. 97.4)
- Control continued muscle contractions: shivering, muscle cramping, seizure (considerations include cardiac arrest, heat stroke, and hyponatremia). The following medications may be considered: midazolam (1 to 2 mg, slow IV push), repeat as needed (must be prepared to intubate and enforce no driving for 24 hours). Dantrolene may be considered in casualties who are resistant to cooling (ED administration) and is not generally recommended or practical for field use.
- Cool aggressively until athlete "wakes up," then monitor temperature every 10 minutes to assess efficacy of treatment and to reduce overcooling. End active cooling at 100°F–102°F (37.7°C–38.8°C). (Overcooling to 95°–97°F [35°–36.1°C] rectal temperature range probably not harmful.)
- Precool IV fluids.

HYPOTHERMIC EAC

- Move to warm area, remove wet clothing (use a clothes dryer in cold conditions).
- Dry skin and insulate with prewarmed blankets (use a clothes dryer or microwave).
- Use BairHugger or warm heater air to blow into blankets (see Fig. 97.4).
- Have patient breathe warmed, humidified air (Bennett or Bird respirator).
- Place warm packs (hot water bottles, warmed IV bags) in neck, axilla, and groin.
- Prewarm IV fluids.
- Consider IV dextrose 50% in water.
- Monitor temperature at regular intervals.
- Walk to generate intrinsic heat (if body temperature >95°F [35°C]).

NORMOTHERMIC EAC

- Maintain temperature; monitor temperature if not improving (postrace hypothermia, delayed hyperthermia [unlikely]).
- Check serum sodium if not improving.

LEG CRAMPS

- Neuromuscular inhibition techniques, salty fluid and glucose replacement, assisted walking.
- Avoid massage until patient is well hydrated.
- Can be a sign of hyponatremia or exertional heat stroke.
- Consider midazolam 1 to 2 mg IV push (be prepared to intubate and enforce no driving for 24 hours).

Fuel Supply

- Oral glucose solutions
- IV glucose solutions: dextrose 5% in stock IV NS solutions (no dextrose in water)
- IV dextrose 50% (indications for use): low blood glucose (measure with home glucose meter at toe and/or ear lobe), insulin reaction

Transfer or Discharge

- Transfer to an emergency facility if patient does not respond to usual treatment or if severe cases do not respond rapidly. Remember automatic transfer rules.
- Discharge clinically stable and normothermic patients with good cognitive function from race medical facility.
- Instruct in fluid and food replacement.
- Reevaluate if change in status.
- Recommend follow-up examination for severe cases (eFig. 97.2)

LOW-FREQUENCY MEDICAL EMERGENCIES

Cardiac Arrest

- Equipment and supplies: automatic or manual defibrillators, intubation equipment and induction medications, ACLS drug kits (aspirin 81-mg tablets, nitroglycerin spray or 0.4-mg tablets, dextrose 50% [dextrose 25% if treating pediatrics], naloxone 1 mg/mL (6), epinephrine 1:10,000 (3), atropine sulfate 1 mg (3), amiodarone 150-mg vial (4), solumedrol 125-mg vial, Benadryl 50-mg vial (2), adenosine 6 mg (4), Lopressor 10 mg (2), Cardizem 20-mg vial (2), Pronestyl [procainamide] 100 mg/mL vial (1), epinephrine 1:1000 (3) [check for updated ACLS recommendations]), oxygen and delivery system, and IV kits
- Assume that brief seizure-like activity is the result of cardiac arrest and apply AED; if pulse and breathing present, check rectal temperature; if normal, assume hyponatremia and check serum sodium
- ACLS standard protocol: ABCs (airway, breathing, circulation), defibrillation and CPR, cardiac monitor, IV access, intubation, medications
- In prolonged resuscitation of marathon or longer-distance runners, consider placement of pressure transducers in lower leg compartments to detect elevated compartment pressures.
- Sudden cardiac arrest (SCA) and sudden cardiac death (SCD) in marathon road racing:
  - Twin Cities Marathon and Marine Corps Marathon combined database 1982–2014: 2.45 SCA per 100,000 finishers and 1.14 SCD per 100,000 finishers
    - US marathons from 2000 to 2010: 1.01 SCA per 100,000 finishers and 0.63 SCD per 100,000 finishers
    - Successful resuscitation for race-related SCA: Twin Cities Marathon, 5 of 7; Twin Cities 10 Mile, 3 of 3; London Marathon, 6 of 11 (through 2006); Marine Corps Marathon, 6 of 11. (In major US metropolitan areas, nonrunners with out-of-hospital SCA have a 1 in 20 survival rate.)
- Road racing by trained individuals is safer than a sedentary lifestyle.
- Preventable
  - Can cardiac screening reduce deaths? Unknown; cost is a problem.
  - Close attention to symptoms and risk factors with appropriate diagnostics as needed based on specific case findings.
- Emerging data from South Africa suggest that integrating cardiac risk questions into the registration process with suggestions to be evaluated may reduce race-related SCA cases.

Cardiac Chest Pain (Acute Coronary Syndrome)

- Activate emergency response system
- Give 325 mg aspirin (chew)
- Start high-flow oxygen if available
- Attach AED if available
- Start IV line if available
- Transport to nearest cardiac center

Exercise-Associated Hyponatremia

Etiology: Water excess and serum sodium dilution because of overhydration combined with inhibition of renal water clearance (inappropriate ADH) is the most common cause; in very long events such as the Ironman distance triathlons, athletes with high sweat sodium concentrations may develop sodium depletion hyponatremia with or without dehydration (rare).

Incidence: Low in events less than 4 hours duration; more common in ultramarathon distances and long-distance triathlons (lasting more than 8 hours); five deaths in marathons since 1998, and reports are increasing in slower participants (3 symptomatic runners in 210,000 finishers at Twin Cities Marathon, but 12%–13% of Boston and London Marathon cohorts tested before and after the race [asymptomatic]).

Significance: Potential for fatal outcome is characterized by rapid deterioration, progression to seizure, respiratory distress, and coma because of worsening cerebral and noncardiac pulmonary edema; reason for transfer to ED. May present at home, in hotel, or in transit (subway, train, airplane, automobile) several hours postrace.

History: High fluid (sports drink or water) intake of 1–2 glasses at every aid station or lack of weight loss during event in dilutional hyponatremia; severe pounding headache that progressively worsens over time; feeling of "impending doom" or feeling scared; puffiness in extremities; muscle cramping; sleepiness; nausea and vomiting; confusion; slow times; small body habitus; inconsistent reports of nonsteroidal antiinflammatory drug (NSAID) use

Physical findings: Ashen skin (including lips), tight rings, watches, or shoes; vomiting; normal pulse, BP, and respiration (early); intact mental status (early); confusion, check for muscle spasms, tetany, clonus, seizure

Lab tests (if available): Sodium (<135 mmol/L); low hematocrit and BUN from fluid overload. Average sodium in fatal cases is between 121 and 122 mmol/L. It is desirable to have point-of-care sodium, BUN, and hematocrit measurements available in the medical area.

Treatment on site: If minimal symptoms, may treat on site with observation until urination or administration of hypertonic fluid (four bouillon cubes dissolved in 4 ounces water) and observation until urinating freely. If symptomatic and deteriorating mental or respiratory status, start high-flow oxygen supplementation and give 100 mL 3% NaCl IV push (can infuse two additional boluses or more if not responding) and continue hypertonic saline at 50 to 70 mL per hour during transfer to ED. The initial treatment for either water dilution or hyponatremia is hypertonic saline. Patients with sodium levels of <135, clinical signs of dehydration, and normal to high BUN/hematocrit levels may be treated on site with IV NS. Have midazolam and/or magnesium sulfate ready if clonus or seizure develops.

Disposition: Transfer runner with this clinical constellation to an emergency facility if no point-of-care laboratory tests are available. Start IV line for medication access but do not assume dehydration and do not administer hypotonic or isotonic fluids. Alert ED of transfer and expected treatment and complications (especially computed tomography [CT] or magnetic resonance imaging [MRI] delays). For athletes with improving clinical status and laboratory values who begin to urinate freely, on-site observation with discharge in the company of responsible family or friends is permissible.

Other

Anaphylaxis: Types (atopic, exercise-induced) and treatment (epinephrine, antihistamine)
Asthma: Inhalers (albuterol metered-dose inhaler with extender), oxygen high flow, nebulizer (albuterol), subcutaneous terbutaline or epinephrine
Insulin shock: Dextrose 50% in water, glucagon

TRAUMA

- **High-velocity activity collisions and falls:** biking, skiing, wheelchair racing
- **Vehicle on course** (pedestrian or bicycle–vehicle collision)
- **ATLS protocol**
  - Equipment: back boards, neck collars (semirigid), splints, cricothyroidotomy kit (with appropriate training), oxygen, IV fluids
  - Primary survey: airway and cervical spine control; breathing and ventilation; circulation and bleeding control; disability or neurologic status; exposure and examination
  - Initial resuscitation: high-flow oxygen, shock management (fluid therapy, position, shock trousers), cardiac monitor
  - Secondary survey: look for other problems
  - Definitive field care: temperature maintenance, pain control, splint
  - Transport to emergency medical facility (in all cases of major trauma)

POSTRACE REVIEW

- **What went right** (and can it be improved)?
- **What went wrong** (and why)?
- **Proposed changes** to improve safety and care of athletes

BUDGET FOR MEDICAL OPERATION COSTS

- Race or event should develop budgets that include medical equipment and supplies.
- Equipment and supplies can be purchased, donated, rented, or borrowed; cost of high-tech equipment makes it difficult to purchase or borrow.
- Volunteer time is usually donated, but the race should provide a T-shirt, poster, pin, or similar reward for volunteer personnel.
- Ambulance service should be enlisted to help with transport of athletes off course and from finish area to local hospitals (often the high-cost budget item for many events).

RECOMMENDED READINGS

Available online.

ULTRAENDURANCE AND ADVENTURE RACING AND EVENTS

98

Kathryn Alfonso • Chad Asplund

INTRODUCTION

- Ultraendurance and adventure races are prolonged events, usually longer than 6 hours (and some may be as long as 10 days) that usually take place in remote, austere, harsh, or extreme environments.
- These events include challenging terrain, extreme elevation changes, inclement weather, and on-course obstacles.
- Adventure races require participants to perform multiple disciplines that may include trail running, hiking, mountaineering, mountain biking, boating/rafting, climbing, caving, and/or orienteering.

EPIDEMIOLOGY/PARTICIPATION

- More than 100,000 ultramarathoners compete in more than 1000 races held annually worldwide.
- Adventure racing participation has increased by 211% in the last 5 years (1.3–2.2 million participants in 2013).
- Over the past few decades, there has been continual increase in the number of masters athletes (>40 years of age) and women participating in ultraendurance events.

GENERAL PRINCIPLES

Terminology/Event Types

- Adventure races
  - Sprint (2- to 6-hour races): 4–8 miles on foot, 15–25 miles biking, and 2–4 miles paddling
  - Endurance (12-hour races): 6–12 miles paddling, 8–14 miles trekking, and 25–50 miles biking
  - 24-hour races: 10–25 miles paddling, 10–25 miles trekking, and 50 miles biking
  - Expedition: 400+ miles of varied disciplines
- Ultraendurance races
  - Any running race longer than the standard marathon distance
  - Most common distances are 50 km, 100 km, 50 miles, and 100 miles.
  - 100 km is recognized as an official world record distance by the International Association of Athletics Federations (IAAF).
  - Other distances include double marathons, 24-hour races, and multiday races of 1000 miles or longer.
  - Many events involve challenges such as trails, variable terrain, altitude, weather, and variable aid and support

Equipment

- **Discipline-specific** (e.g., shoes, clothing, pack and tools, lights, bike, kayak, paddle, rope harnesses, compass)
- Participants must carry/provide their own food, water, protective clothing/footwear.
- Hydration system
- Water purification devices (e.g., iodine tablets, filter system, ultraviolet pen)
- Compass (global positioning system [GPS] is usually prohibited), maps, and race directions
- First aid kit and personal medications
- Boxed food, water, clothing, other apparel for resupply points
- Additional information can be found at http://www.usaranationals.com/gearlist.aspx.

Specific Training

- Need to think about physical, mental, and skills training
- Master the logistics of fluids, nutrition, use of equipment, and rest.
- Frequency, intensity, and duration of training should be balanced for fatigue management and avoidance of overtraining.
- Plan multidiscipline, multihour sessions so that athletes know how their bodies will react and feel after extended exertions in different disciplines (Table 98.1).

Nutritional Issues

General Guideline

- Aim for a healthy weight; avoid rapid weight loss.
- Choose foods sensibly and consume them during training to ensure body tolerance on race day.
- 60/20/20 split common (aim for 60% of calories from carbohydrates, 20% from protein, and 20% from fat)
- The International Society for Sports Nutrition (ISSN) recommends consumption of carbohydrate (~5–8 g/kg.day-1) and protein (~1.6–2.5 g/kg.day-1) to mitigate effects of chronic glycogen depletion during training for single-stage events.

Pre-event

- Carbohydrate loading: load muscles and liver with glycogen (stored carbohydrates) during the week before an event
- Consume a normal intake of carbohydrates (5–7 grams per kilogram of body weight) during the first 3 days of the taper week.
- Increase this amount to 10 grams of carbohydrate per kilogram of body weight for the next 3 days.
- Eat the last big, high-carbohydrate meal 2 nights before the race.
- Do not overeat night before race! Avoid items high in fiber or in fat, which may be hard to digest and may lead to gastrointestinal (GI) distress during the event.

During Event

- General carbohydrate needs vary but often range between 30 and 60 grams per hour or approximately one-quarter to one-third of body weight in pounds per hour.
- Some athletes also use small amounts of protein during events, up to 5–10 grams per hour.
- Athletes may need up to 300–400 calories per hour (with consideration of an additional 100 calories/hour per 1000 ft of elevation gain). This calorie intake may be difficult to achieve depending on GI tolerance with demands of exercise.
- Athletes must realize that the rate of loss will exceed rate of assimilation by approximately threefold during endurance events.
- Many athletes use sports bars, drinks, and gels to replace calories on event day. Make sure to test tolerance in advance to minimize GI distress during the event.
- Use of caffeine may be recommended towards the latter stage of the event when sleep deprivation may compromise the athlete's safety.

Post-event

- Important to replace calories, especially glucose, within the first few hours after training sessions lasting >90–120 minutes to ensure liver and body stores are replenished adequately before future training sessions.

Table 98.1 GUIDELINES FOR ADVENTURE RACES

Race Distance	Total Training Hr/Wk	Bicycling	Running	Paddling
Sprint	5–10	2–3	2–3	1–2
Endurance	10–20	4–5	4–5	2–4
Expedition	20+	5–7	5–7	4–6

- The American College of Sports Medicine recommends consuming 1.5 g/kg carbohydrates within the first 30 minutes after prolonged exercise, then every 2 hours for up to 4–6 hours.
- Protein should also be included as a refueling tool after prolonged exercise, with current recommendations of approximately 20 g or 0.25 g/kg/meal.

Train Low, Race High

- Some athletes train with low carbohydrate reserves/supplies to train the body to increase oxidative enzymes and use fat stores and to spare glycogen use for longer periods (fat adaption).
- These athletes then race while ingesting carbohydrates so that their bodies will burn the ingested carbohydrates but will be able to rely on fat stores for energy when the carbohydrate supply decreases.

Fluids

- Drink to thirst.
- Train with the fluids you will use during the event.
- Aim for no more than 2% weight loss during training/event; avoid weight gain, as too much fluid may lead to hyponatremia.
- If mixing calories in fluids, make sure to avoid >6% sugar solutions, because they can interfere with fluid absorption and cause GI distress.
- Using different types of sugars (e.g., glucose, fructose, maltodextrin) may be helpful.
- Maltodextrin is a complex carbohydrate that may be mixed at high percentages (e.g., up to 18%) without exceeding system osmolality, and it may cause less GI distress than other sugar types.

Electrolytes

- Mainly used by athletes for the prevention of exercise-associated muscle cramping.
- Larger athletes, faster athletes, and those who have high volumes or high concentrations of sodium in their sweat (white salt deposits on chin straps, headband, clothes, skin, etc.) may need to ingest additional sodium beyond what can be found in sports drinks, but the best method to ingest is in fluid or food form.
- Some athletes use salt tablets but can easily ingest too much; GI upset and cramping are common.
- Need to remember that muscle cramping is also frequently a result of exercise-associated muscle fatigue, excitability, dehydration, and heat illness.

Practical Issues

- Must experiment with a variety of different foods/nutritional items during training; essential to have a basic hydration and nutrition plan before entering competition.
- The amount of calories tolerated per hour is inversely related to the intensity of effort (harder the effort, fewer calories tolerated).
- Should assume that calorie and fluid deficits are inevitable even in ideal circumstances; must plan to minimize this as much as possible.
- In multiday events, the goal is to return to a state of euhydration before resuming competition the next day.
- Urine should be "clear and copious" before resuming competition.

Environmental Challenges

- Remember that the variables listed here are often a greater threat in ultraendurance athletes because of sustained exposure.

Heat

- The most serious temperature-related illnesses are heat stroke and hyperthermia.
- Heat acclimatization is an important adaptation but is unrealistic for many athletes who may live in variable climates; takes approximately 10–14 days training in heat to acclimate, loss of acclimatization is rapid once heat exposure is removed.
- See Chapter 21: "Exercise in the Heat and Heat Illness" for further details.

Cold

- Hypothermia and frostbite are the most serious cold-related illnesses.
- Need to factor in wind chill (especially when on a bike) and body heat loss in water, which is constantly displaced from body in swimmer (wetsuit helps).
- See Chapter 22: "Exercise in the Cold and Cold Injuries" for further details.

Altitude

- Altitude illness may occur above 2500 m; see Chapter 16: "The Wilderness Athlete and Adventurer."
- Acute mountain sickness (AMS), high-altitude pulmonary edema (HAPE), and high-altitude cerebral edema (HACE) may all occur.

Lightning

- Fifty-four running-related lightning deaths per year
- Strike types:
  - Direct strikes: lightning directly strikes the athlete
  - Ground strike: travels through ground and may be conducted through an object (body) nearby
  - Side flash: lightning strikes a taller object and part of the current jumps to the victim
- If feasible, suspend event start if thunder or lightning is in the area ("if you can hear it, clear it").
- Athletes should seek shelter if thunder heard or lightning seen while on course.
- Avoid ridgelines or summits, in addition to tall objects such as ski lifts, cell phone towers, or isolated trees.
- If lightning strike is imminent, assume lightning position:
  - Sitting or crouching with knees and feet close together to create only one point of contact with the ground; get as low as possible.

COMMON INJURIES AND MEDICAL PROBLEMS

Soft Tissue/Dermatologic Issues

The most commonly encountered complaint in ultramarathon running and one of the top reasons that adventure athletes seek medical care

Blisters

Description: Most common soft tissue injury in ultraendurance or adventure athletes (Fig. 98.1). Caused by repetitive friction between the skin and another surface.

History: Compose 20%–40% of injuries occurring during same-day ultramarathons; 35%–75% of injuries occurring during

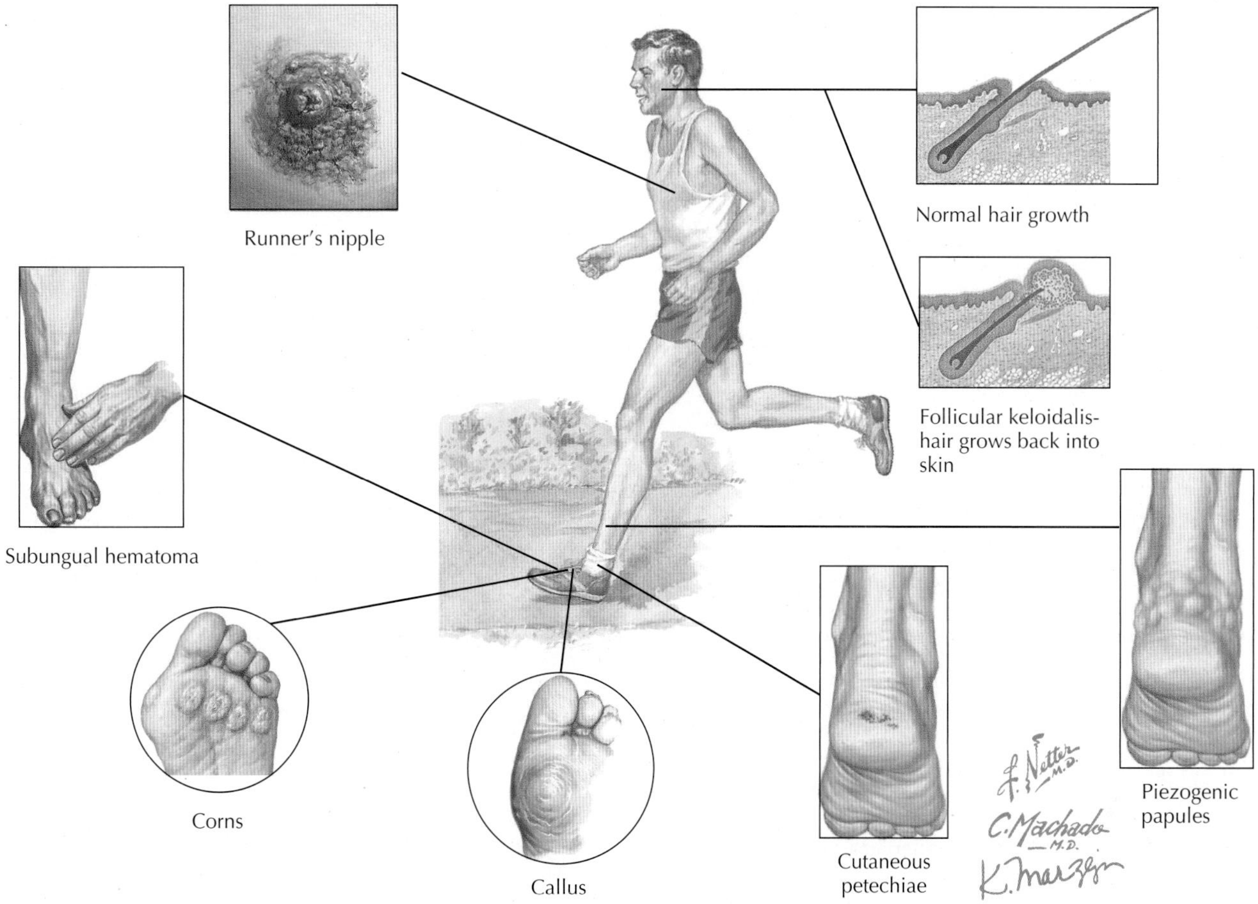

Runner's nipple
Normal hair growth
Follicular keloidalis-hair grows back into skin
Subungual hematoma
Corns
Callus
Cutaneous petechiae
Piezogenic papules

Figure 98.1 Common problems caused by friction and pressure.

multiday ultramarathons; most likely to occur during the middle of multistage races, as this is the time frame when accumulated friction and skin wetness reach critical levels to create the blister. Foot care accounts for up to 76% of all medical visits in multistage ultramarathons.

Physical examination: Common locations: distal aspects of toes, balls of the feet, and posterior heel. Areas of redness and chafing are precursors of blister formation and invite prevention.

Risk factors: Heat, moisture, ill-fitting shoes, anatomic abnormalities (e.g., calcaneal exostosis, accessory navicular, bunion), and increased running distance

Treatment: Painful nonbloody blisters can be drained in a sterile environment, taking care to preserve the overlying skin. A blister with murky or hazy fluid may be infected and should be opened (deroofed) and irrigated with the appropriate cleanser (e.g., saline with iodine, Hibiclens, etc.); the cavity should be then treated with bacitracin or another non-Neosporin antibiotic ointment before covering.

Prevention:

- Decreasing shear frictional forces on the skin
- Concept of a prevention layer at high-friction spot—may use tape, second skin, Tegaderm, Compeed products
- Moisture-wicking synthetic socks; ensure feet are dry
- Lubricants, although theoretically helpful, may paradoxically increase the rate of friction for long-duration events by trapping moisture and grit
- *Educating participants and encouraging them to carry their own blister care kit will greatly minimize the burden of the medical staff*

Subungual Hematoma

- Accumulation of blood underneath the nail bed
- Caused by repetitive contact between the longest toe and the toebox of the shoe, especially during predominantly downhill courses
- Occurs in 3%–10% of participants in ultraendurance events
- If painful, may be drained by piercing the nail with a clean wide-bore hypodermic needle or heated paper clip under sterile conditions
- Monitor closely for infection
- May be prevented by trimming toenails short before event

Chafing

- Superficial inflammatory dermatitis because of skin rubbing on skin or clothing
- Affects 9% of runners
- Mainly involving thighs, groin, back, axilla, and nipple areas
- Can be prevented by lubrication (e.g., Aquaphor), chamois cream, or taping
- May be treated with topical corticosteroid cream to reduce inflammation
- May be prevented by wearing dry, breathable, well-fitting clothing

Abrasions

- Damage to superficial layers of the skin usually caused by a fall
- May cause pain secondary to exposed nerve endings.
- Clean with soap and water.
- A semipermeable and/or hydrocolloid dressing such as Tegaderm, Duoderm, Bioclusive, or second skin may be used.

Respiratory Issues

- Respiratory illnesses, including upper respiratory infection (URI), bronchitis, and reactive airway disease, are common reasons for athlete withdrawal from adventure races.
- Heavy exercise, especially with inadequate recovery, may induce immune suppression and increase susceptibility to URIs and other respiratory infections. J-shaped curve: average risk of infection with moderate physical activity, increased risk of infection as intensity of exercise increases (Fig. 98.2).
- Endurance athletes are known to have a higher incidence of asthma and allergies than the general community.

Upper/Lower Respiratory Infection

- Majority are caused by viral pathogens and lead to inflammation of the respiratory tract.
- Hold febrile athletes out of competition because of risk of myocarditis.

Reactive Airway Disease, Asthma, and Exercise-Induced Bronchospasm

- Exercise-induced bronchospasm (EIB) is more common among ultramarathon runners than other athletes, although the exact reason is unclear.
- Predisposing factors include dust, allergens, cold weather, prolonged event duration, and high altitude.
- Runners with lower respiratory symptoms (shortness of breath and wheezing) should be evaluated for HAPE when participating at high altitude and/or for exercise-associated hyponatremia (EAH).
- Concurrent URI may exacerbate or cause EIB and may increase the risk for HAPE.
- Spacer-delivered beta$_2$-agonists provide effective and portable treatment for asthma and may reduce pulmonary arterial pressure with HAPE.
- Athletes who can identify exercise/event triggers should consider pretreatment with beta$_2$-agonists.

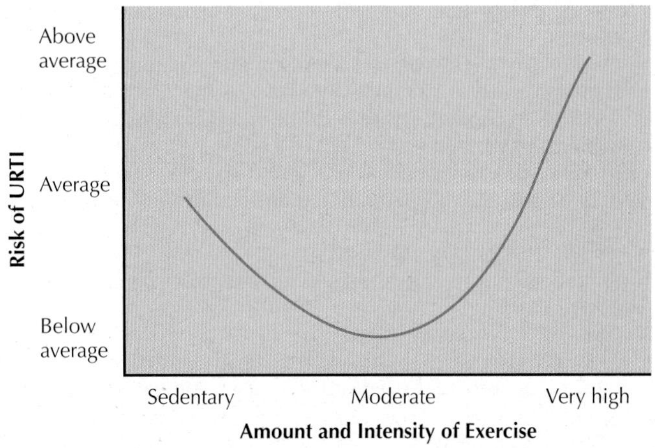
Above average
Average
Below average
Risk of URTI
Sedentary
Moderate
Very high
Amount and Intensity of Exercise

Figure 98.2 J-shaped model of relationship between varying amounts of exercise and risk of URTI. This model suggests that moderate exercise may lower risk of respiratory infection, whereas excessive amounts may increase the risk. *URTI,* Upper respiratory tract infection. (From Nieman DC. Exercise, infection, and immunity. *Int J Sports Med.* 1994;15[suppl 3]: S131–S141.)

- Long-acting beta$_2$-agonists may be more appropriate for pretreatment events lasting >5–6 hours.
- Asthma may actually improve at high altitude secondary to a reduction in pollen and pollutants at higher altitude.
- *Any runner requiring supplemental oxygen to maintain oxygen saturation should not be allowed to participate in/continue event.*

Gastrointestinal Issues

- GI distress, including nausea, vomiting, diarrhea, and gastroesophageal reflux disease (GERD), is prevalent among ultramarathon competitors.
- Vomiting is another common issue causing withdrawal from races and affecting race performance.
- Adherence to a diet low in fat and fiber before and during competition will reduce incidence of GI distress.

Upper Gastrointestinal Tract

- Nausea and vomiting may be the result of exercise-induced gastroparesis, catecholamine secretion, altitude exposure, pre-exercise consumption of fatty- or protein-rich foods, overdrinking, or drinking hyperosmolar fluids, resulting in unabsorbed fluid in the upper GI tract.
- Incidence of nausea is directly related to activity intensity.
- *Nausea may be an early sign of EAH, altitude illness, dehydration, or heat illness and should be further evaluated before returning the runner to competition.*
- Use of nonsteroidal antiinflammatory drugs (NSAIDs) during the race increases risk of upper GI distress.
- Infective causes of nausea and vomiting are more likely to occur in multiday races and can spread quickly from person to person through unwashed hands, close contact with infected individuals, consumption of spoiled food, contaminated water, or unclean eating utensils.
- Proper hydration with appropriate fluids and electrolytes is essential.
- Oral ondansetron (dissolvable tabs) can effectively reduce nausea and vomiting.
- Some athletes may benefit from pre-event proton pump inhibitors.

Lower Gastrointestinal Tract

- Dehydration and increased intake of simple sugars have been implicated in lower GI distress.
- Other risk factors include the female sex, younger age, history of abdominal surgery, history of irritable bowel syndrome, lactose intolerance, and dehydration.
- Transient lower GI bleeding is common in endurance athletes but is usually self-limited.

Cardiac Issues

Athlete's Heart—Normal Adaptations

- Demands of endurance sport training lead to physiologic changes to cardiac structure in endurance athletes.
- Right ventricular (RV) and left ventricular (LV) hypertrophy are common.
- Left atrial enlargement may also occur.

Proposed Mechanism of Cardiac Maladaptation

- Studies show that cardiac function (LV ejection fraction) is reduced and troponin release increases after prolonged endurance activity, which may be indicative of myocardial damage. These changes typically resolve within 72 hours.
- Prolonged exercise stress results in RV strain, right atrial and right ventricular dilation, and diastolic dysfunction.
- Persistent, intense efforts without adequate rest to facilitate heart recovery, in addition to long-term participation, may lead to the development of scarring or fibrosis within the cardiac muscle.

- Exercise-induced arterial hypertension (EIAH) has been associated with LV hypertrophy. Therapeutic intervention may be necessary to reduce cardiac muscle stiffening, which is thought to be likely cause of exercise-induced cardiac fatigue.
- Patchy areas of fibrosis may increase risk for arrhythmias (atrial and ventricular) in addition to sudden cardiac death (SCD).

Cardiac Biomarkers

- Troponin I is elevated after prolonged endurance racing.
- Algorithms have been proposed using high-sensitivity cardiac assays for evaluation of runners with cardiac symptoms during and after events.
- These algorithms are a proposed design to differentiate between exercise-induced troponin elevations and acute coronary syndrome after exercise. More research is needed in this area.
- Coronary calcium score is higher in endurance athletes compared with age-matched norms.

Arrythmias

- Bradyarrhythmias are very common and are typically benign in ultraendurance athletes if asymptomatic; sinus bradycardia, junctional bradycardia, first-degree atrioventricular (AV) block, and Mobitz type 1 block are common.
- Premature ventricular or atrial beats are common and typically benign.
- Tachyarrhythmias, including atrial fibrillation (AF), may occur and may be more problematic in endurance athletes.
- Studies show veteran endurance athletes are at a fivefold greater risk for AF.
- Majority of arrhythmias in endurance athletes originate in the RV (possible exercise-induced arrhythmogenic right ventricular cardiomyopathy [ARVC]).

Sudden Cardiac Death in Ultraendurance Athletes

- Myocardial scarring may trigger lethal arrhythmias
- Myocardial infarction more common in older athletes
- Autopsy data not always conclusive

Cardiac Risk Stratification of Veteran Ultraendurance Racers

- No proven method to evaluate for myocardial fibrosis/scarring
- Reasonable approach includes electrocardiogram (ECG), sometimes a graded exercise test
- A coronary calcium score may be helpful for athletes >50 years of age
  - A coronary artery calcium (CAC) score <100 is generally regarded as low risk.
  - Athletes with CAC >100 should be further risk stratified with an exercise test or catheterization as indicated.

Orthopedic Issues

- Although medical conditions result in the most withdrawals from competition in ultraendurance running events, orthopedic conditions, especially trauma, are a common reason for withdrawal from adventure races and ultraendurance mountain bike races.
- Major trauma in ultraendurance running races is rare but can result from falls, animal attacks, and lightning strikes.
- Traumatic musculoskeletal injuries tend to occur during the later stages of multiday races, likely because of fatigue.
- In adventure races, injuries are most likely to occur during the orienteering and/or mountain biking portions.

Acute Traumatic Musculoskeletal Injuries

UPPER EXTREMITY

- The arm/shoulder is the second most injured area, with strains/sprains occurring in kayaking/paddling events and traumatic injuries occurring secondary to falls.
- **Shoulder dislocation:**
  - Ninety-five percent are anterior dislocations secondary to external rotation and abduction at the shoulder
  - Common in kayakers
- **Clavicle fracture:**
  - Most common cause is a fall onto the shoulder, such as an "endo" injury on the mountain bike leg
- **Other fractures:**
  - Scaphoid, distal radius, and radial head most commonly fractured
  - Mechanism is typically via a fall onto outstretched hand (FOOSH).

LOWER EXTREMITY

- **Ankle**
  - Most common joint injured in the lower extremity (LE)
  - Ankle sprain
    - Most common acute injury in adventure racing
    - Typically caused by inversion injury as a result of uneven terrain
- **Knee**
  - Patellar dislocation
    - Caused by the powerful contraction of the quadriceps, combined with flexion and external rotation of the tibia on the femur (very steep downhill trail running), or by direct contact because of a fall onto the patella while knee is flexed
  - Anterior cruciate ligament disruption
    - Typically caused by noncontact, deceleration, pivot-type injuries

Overuse Musculoskeletal Injuries

UPPER EXTREMITY

- Shoulder overuse injuries are common in kayak/paddling disciplines
  - Rotator cuff tendinopathy most common overuse shoulder injury
    - Experienced paddlers: excess volume of paddling
    - Inexperienced paddlers: too much, too soon, or improper technique

LOWER EXTREMITY

- **Ankle/knee**
  - Achilles tendinopathy
    - Most common LE overuse injury in adventure racers
    - Occurs in 11.5% of ultramarathoners yearly
    - Midsubstance most common
    - Made worse by uphill running
  - Ultramarathoner's ankle
    - Peritendinitis of the extensor tendons at the extensor retinaculum as they cross over the anterior ankle
  - Patellofemoral pain syndrome (PFPS)
    - Most common cause of anterior knee pain in active adults
    - Typically occurs in events with running such as ultraendurance racing, common in cycling
  - Iliotibial band (ITB) syndrome
    - Common in events that require extensive running
    - Overuse injury that may present with pain at the lateral femoral epicondyle of knee
- **Other**
  - Stress fractures
    - Metatarsals most common location
    - Also seen in tarsals, tibia, femoral neck
  - Medial tibial stress syndrome (MTSS)
    - Repetitive stress-induced tenderness along the posteromedial aspect of the tibia after running
    - Poorly understood, but thought to be caused by chronic traction of the periosteum and fascia at the medial tibial border

Exercise-Associated Muscle Cramps

- Very common in ultramarathons
- Painful, involuntary muscle spasms during or immediately after exercise
- Occur primarily in gastrocnemius and soleus muscles, hamstring, or quadriceps muscle groups
- Most common mechanism is neuromuscular fatigue and increased activity of neuromuscular units
- Dehydration and sodium loss, particularly in salty sweaters, may also contribute

Renal/Electrolyte Issues

Exercise-Associated Hyponatremia

- Defined as a serum sodium level less than 135 mmol/L during or after endurance or ultraendurance events.
- May occur during or after prolonged activity (>4 hours) and can be detected up to 24 hours after exercise.
- Often asymptomatic and found in up to 50% of ultramarathon (161 km) participants
- Risk factors for EAH include event duration 4 hours or longer, female sex, low body weight, low body mass index (BMI), weight gain during exercise, slow running pace, extreme heat or cold, low competition experience, and intake of NSAIDs.
- See Chapter 97: "Mass Participation Endurance Events" for further details.

Dehydration

- Common during ultraendurance events
- Body weight losses of up to 8% or greater can occur.
- Oral hydration is the preferred route of fluid administration.
- IV fluids should only be administered in cases of significant hypovolemia and inability to tolerate oral fluid intake.
- In athletes who present with both dehydration and EAH, treatment should focus on EAH because isotonic IV fluids can worsen cerebral edema and lead to death.

Rhabdomyolysis

- Ultraendurance events can lead to exertional rhabdomyolysis and acute kidney injury.
- Heat stress, dehydration, and NSAID use increase risk.
- Serum creatine kinase (CK) concentrations over 20,000 IU/L are common in athletes without evidence for rhabdomyolysis and renal injury.
- CK readings over 160,000 have been reported without clinical consequences.
- If an athlete presents with dark urine, a urine dipstick with 1+ or greater protein, 3+ or greater blood, and a specific gravity greater than 1.025, further renal evaluation is warranted if there is suspicion for rhabdomyolysis.
- If aggressive fluid resuscitation is to be undertaken, it is important to measure the serum sodium to assess for EAH.

Vision/Eye Issues

Description: Transient vision problems have been reported among ultraendurance athletes

History and physical examination: "Hellgate eyes" is caused by corneal edema and drying. Symptoms typically begin during the nighttime hours with runners noticing halos around bright objects. Progresses to blurred vision and a slight gritty sensation in the eyes; the cornea may appear hazy in more severe cases.

Prevention: Protective eye wear, frequent blinking

Treatment: Stop activity and close eyes; this will resolve most symptoms within several hours. 5% hypertonic saline drops or ointment may also be helpful.

Psychological Challenges

Mental Health

- Athletes have higher rates of depression than the general population and often do not seek treatment.
- The Ultrarunners Longitudinal Tracking Study (ULTRA), published in 2014 by Hoffman, found that runners had relatively significant rates of depression, anxiety, and substance use.
- Risk factors to consider in elite athletes are injury longer than 6 weeks, age-related loss of performance, pregnancy, retirement, overtraining, perfectionist personality traits, recreational substance use, and anabolic steroid use.

Sleep Deprivation

- Fatigue, sleep deprivation, and a negative energy intake–expenditure balance can cause negative emotions during and after competition in ultraendurance athletes.
- Sleep deprivation can lead to involuntary microsleeps while exercising, hallucinations (3D), and eventually psychosis.
- A "sleep strategy" for multiday events is important for a successful competition.

EVENT COVERAGE ISSUES

Description: Event coverage for ultraendurance events, especially those held in remote areas, can be quite challenging.

Communications: Satellite phones or radios often necessary without cell phone coverage.

Allocation of resources: Events can be spread over a large geographic area with varied terrain and conditions. Discuss with race directors ahead of time where injuries and illnesses can be anticipated to occur on the course. Personnel and first responders should be positioned in those locations. Examples would include at the bottom of a steep technical mountain bike descent or at the end of a long trail section without water resources in anticipation of dehydration issues.

Search and rescue: Locating and extracting injured or ill competitors can be challenging. Have an emergency plan in place. It is helpful to have a search and rescue team available.

ACKNOWLEDGMENT

The authors would like to acknowledge **George Wortley, MD,** for work on the previous edition's chapter.

RECOMMENDED READINGS

Available online.

ROCK CLIMBING

99

Charles S. Peterson • Aaron D. Campbell • Anthony S. Ceraulo

INTRODUCTION

- Rock climbing popularity and access have opened the sport up to climbers of all ages.
  - Beginning with Tokyo 2020, sport climbing included in Summer Olympic Games
  - International Federation of Sports Climbing (IFSC) organizes senior and junior World Championships, World Cup, and international events
- Climbing requires strength, endurance, flexibility, agility, and courage
- Equipment advances have made climbing safer
- Overuse and climbing-specific injuries pose challenges to climbers and providers
  - Increase in adolescent overuse injury patterns

EPIDEMIOLOGY

- A 2015 systematic review in *British Journal of Sports Medicine* evaluated risk factors for injury:
  - Age, years of climbing experience, highest climbing grade achieved, high climbing intensity score, lead climbing, previous injury
  - No conclusive data regarding injury prevention
- Type of climb
  - Competition climbing: route climbing, speed climbing, bouldering
  - Indoor climbing is safer and more controlled, but adds risk for overuse, particularly to fingers.
  - Risk of death and serious injury greater in mountaineering (Table 99.1)
  - 3.1 injuries per 1000 climber hours in sport competitions (Table 99.2)
- Equipment
  - Regular inspection and replacement of damaged or expired equipment
    - Follow manufacturer's recommendation for soft and metal gear replacement
  - Proper use of protection
- Skill level
  - Elite climbers on more difficult climbs carry higher risk of overuse and exposed falls.
  - Most injuries occur at or below the climber's usual level.
  - Greater risk in male climbers who climb harder routes, have been climbing more than 10 years, and lead climb more than top rope climb.
- Environmental
  - Falling rocks
  - Isolation, weather, heat, cold (see Chapter 21: "Exercise in the Heat and Heat Illness" and Chapter 22: "Exercise in the Cold and Cold Injuries")
  - Altitude (see Chapter 23: "Altitude Training and Competition")
  - Plants and animals/insects

GENERAL PRINCIPLES

Terminology

Belayer: Controls the rope for a climber, uses a belay device
Rappel: To descend on the rope, regulating the rate with an ATC, figure 8, or other device
Pro: Protection, specialized equipment attaching rope to mountain or surface
Top rope: Rope placed through chains or metal loops at the top of a climb, alleviating the need to place protection
Lead climber: Assumes highest risk by "clipping-in" rope to protection on the way up. Subsequent climbers ascend using the top rope.
Problem: A term used in bouldering (see later) to describe a challenging route or segment that is worked on to mastery, often at lower heights and without a rope

Types of Climbing (Fig. 99.1)

Free Climbing (Traditional Rock Climbing, "Trad")

- Climbing without pulling or hanging on gear, rope, or stepping on anchors
  - True rock climbing, rope simply used as protection for falls
- Pro (protection) used for safety
  - Passive: nut/stopper/chock, hex, tricam (Fig. 99.2)
  - Active: "cam," spring-loaded camming device (see Fig. 99.2)
- Climbers ascend a single or multiple pitches, or 20- to 50-meter climbing sections
  - Gear and ropes "cleaned," or removed and carried to next pitch
  - Climbers belay up and either rappel down each pitch or walk off the top (hike down another route)

Sport Climbing

OUTDOOR (SEE FIG. 99.1)

- Established routes, often with ratings and maps
- Fixed protection—inspect for safety (should not be loose or spin)
  - Bolts: anchored often at 2- to 4-meter intervals, lead climbers clip in as they pass, ideally placed strategically to prevent ground falls
  - Chains: chains or welded loops anchored to the rock at the top

INDOOR

- "Rock gyms"
- Molded holds and bolts attached to climbing walls, ropes provided and maintained by gym
- Risk of overuse injury, as climbers can do multiple routes
- Skills augmented in a safe environment

Mountaineering/Alpinism

- Often requires travel to austere environments in remote areas (see Chapter 24: "Travel Considerations for the Athlete and Sports Medical Team")
- Variable techniques, from hiking to rock and ice climbing, often over multiple days
- Single push expeditions becoming more common and popular
- Injury risk:
  - Serious injury or death from falls, usually related to fatigue and human error
  - Minor injuries magnified by remoteness
- Environmental risks

Bouldering

- Indoor or outdoor (see Fig. 99.1)
- Problems, usually 3–4 meters high, contain traverses and overhangs, repeated to completion
- Spotting (partner standing below to protect from serious injury from falls) and mats prevent many lower extremity injuries

- Finger overuse injuries common
- Indoor and outdoor bouldering carry similar injury risk

Rappelling

- Descent from cliffs using rappel devices (Fig. 99.3)
- Rate of descent controlled via friction between rope and device by holding rope behind back
  - Use of gloves prevents friction burns.
- A prusik cord or a second rope can be attached with a belayer at the top or bottom for redundant safety measures.

Table 99.1 ACCIDENTS AND INJURIES IN NORTH AMERICAN MOUNTAINEERING AND ROCK CLIMBING

Year	Accidents Reported	Injured	Fatalities
2005	111 USA	85 USA	34 USA
	19 Canada	14 Canada	7 Canada
1951–2005	6111 USA	5158 USA	1373 USA
	958 Canada	715 Canada	292 Canada

Modified from Williamson JE. *Accidents in North American Mountaineering*. Golden: American Alpine Club, Inc.; 2006:97–98.

Table 99.2 2005 WORLD CHAMPIONSHIPS IN ROCK CLIMBING INJURY RISK

Year	2005
Climbers	443
Countries	55
Climbing days	520
Acute medical issues	18
Serious medical issues	4 (zero deaths)
Injury rate per 1000 climbing hours	3.1

Modified from Schoffl VR, Kuepper T. Injuries at the 2005 World Championships in rock climbing. *Wilderness Environ Med*. 2006;1(3):187–190, used with permission.

Canyoneering

- Descent into canyons or slots
  - Limited access and stretches without escape routes
- Combination of hiking, rappelling, climbing, swimming, camping, exploring, and courage
- "Pots" and "keepers," deep rock pockets, pose great danger to inexperienced explorers
- Pack rafting—canyoneering down to a river (such as the Colorado River in the Grand Canyon), floating down in a personal raft, then hiking or climbing out
- Flash floods pose great danger

Caving

- Cave explorers refer to less experienced counterparts as "spelunkers"
- Requires horizontal and vertical movement through caves with extensive use of ropes for pitches, crawling, and squeezing through narrow openings
- Experienced guides and terrain study
- Possible digging and diving (scuba diving for intense cavers, see Chapter 83: "Scuba Diving").
- Excellent light sources, specialized equipment, redundant safety measures essential

Solo Climbing

- No ropes or gear
- Highest risk of injury or death
- Unencumbered speed without ropes and gear, "street cred"
  - Excellent example in 2018 film, *Free Solo*

Ice Climbing

- Specialized equipment, including crampons and axes (see Fig. 99.1)
- Anchors screw into ice, or climber can thread a cord through holes cut into ice (V-thread)
- Unfavorable weather, melting/falling ice hazards

Difficulty Rating Systems

Yosemite Decimal System (YDS)

- Most common in United States, developed by Sierra Club in 1930s

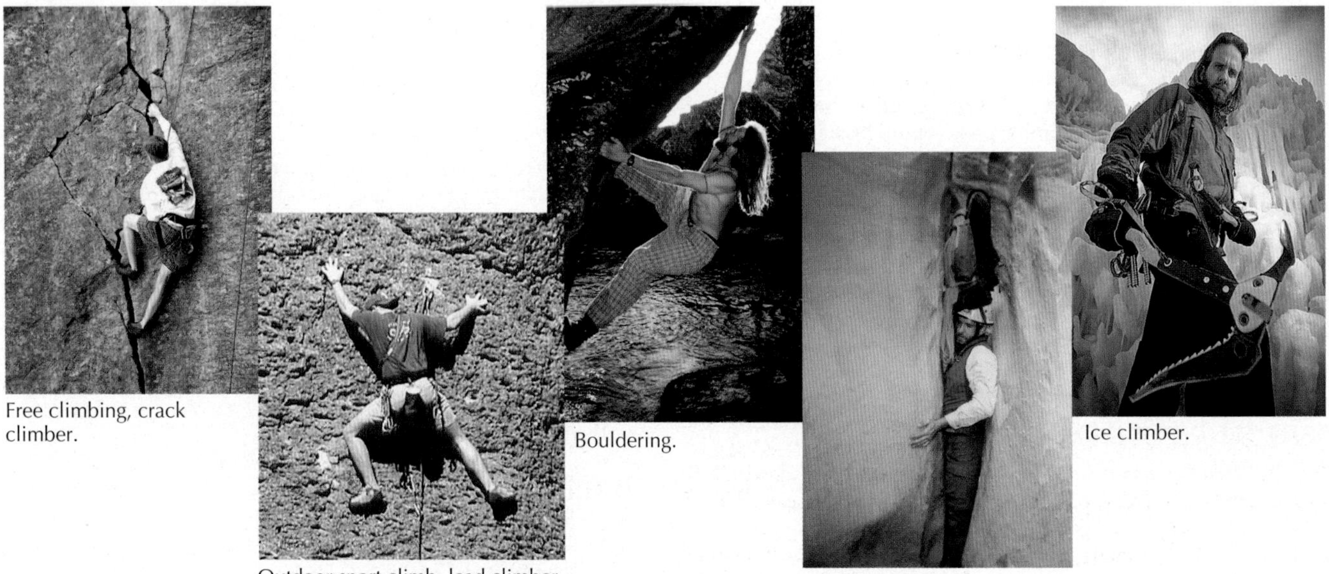

Free climbing, crack climber.

Outdoor sport climb, lead climber.

Bouldering.

Canyoneering.

Ice climber.

Figure 99.1 Types of climbing. (Figs. courtesy of Matt Turley.)

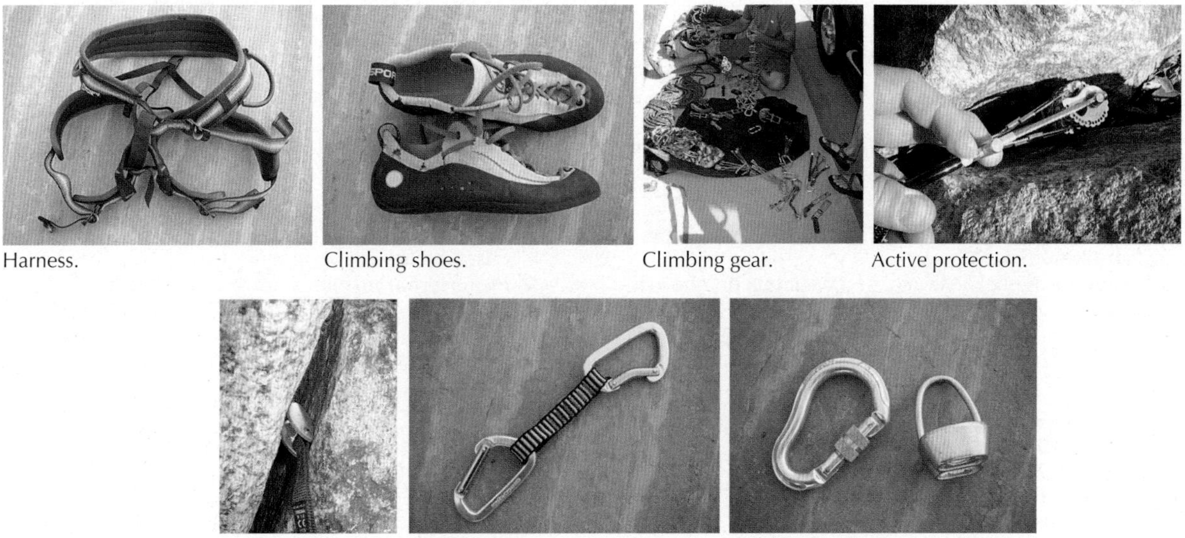

Harness. Climbing shoes. Climbing gear. Active protection.

Passive protection. Quick draw. Carabiner and ATC.

Figure 99.2 Climbing equipment.

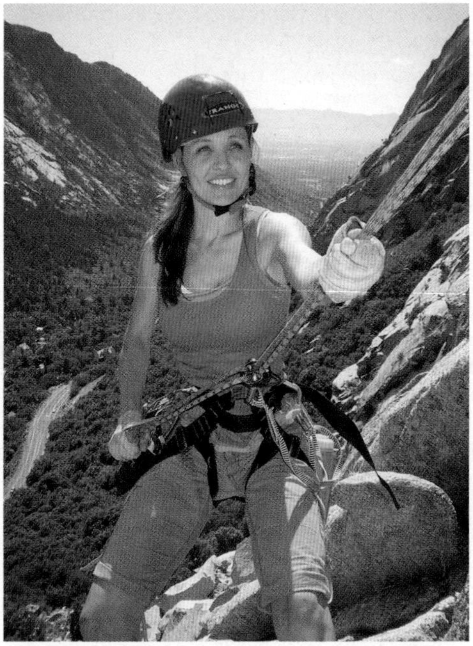

Figure 99.3 Rappelling from multiple pitch climb.

- **Classes**—rated by difficulty:
  - Class 1: Walking sufficient
  - Class 2: Hiking with scrambling; occasional use of hands required
  - Class 3: Scrambling with some exposure and use of handholds; rope not required
  - Class 4: Simple climbing with natural protection and exposure; ropes often used
  - Class 5: Technical free climbing with ropes; belaying and protection used
    - Rated from 5.0 through 5.15d, with letters (a–d) added at 5.10
  - Class 6: Aid climbing (rarely used; separate scale A0–A5 available)
- **Grades**—traditionally rated by time perceived to ascend (some longer climbs can be done faster or in single push attempts)
  - Grade I: 1–2 hours
  - Grade II: Less than half a day
  - Grade III: Half a day
  - Grade IV: Full day
  - Grade V: Two-day climb
  - Grade VI: Multiday climb
  - Grade VII: One week or longer
- **Protection**—rates spacing and quality of bolts/protection
  - Follows movie rating system: G, PG, PG-13, R, and X
  - Significant variation; climbers advised to avoid anything beyond PG-13

Bouldering Rating Systems

- Hueco Scale most commonly used rating system in North America, spans from V0 to V17

Other

- Ice climbing uses Water Ice (WI) Scale, 1–11+; Alpine Ice (AI) scale for glacial ice.
- International rating systems vary by country.

Equipment and Safety (Adhere to Manufacturer's Specifications)

- Rope
  - Dynamic (high stretch) ropes lessen impact of falls by 5%–7%.
    - Used in vertical rock/ice climbing
  - Static (low stretch) ropes better for rappelling; stronger and less supple
    - Used for rappelling, glacier travel, and rescue
  - Dry ropes specially treated to repel moisture, maintaining strength
  - Typical rope length 50 m, 55 m, 60 m, and 70 m
  - Diameter ranges from 7.5 mm to 11 mm
  - Standard rope has a length of 60 m and a diameter of 9–10 mm, but is determined by climber preference and style
  - Ropes rated by diameter and number of falls
    - Union Internationale des Associations d'Alpinisme (UIAA), governing body over climbing rope safety standards
- Harness (see Fig. 99.2)
  - Proper fit and sizing are essential for manufactured harnesses.
  - Should be inspected for damage and be retired according to manufacturer, regardless of damage
  - Climbers should also inspect each other's harnesses to ensure proper fit and safety.

- Shoes (see Fig. 99.2)
  - Tight-fitting, but should be bearable; smaller than a normal shoe
  - Creates a "hoof effect" of the foot to provide strength, grip, and protection
  - Slipper-like shoes for indoor climbing and bouldering, stiffer shoes or boots for outdoor climbing
- Belay device (see Fig. 99.2)
  - Controls rate of descent on the rope
  - ATC: "air traffic control"
  - Grigri: autolocking belay device, heavy, and technique critical for proper use
  - Figure-8: somewhat antiquated in modern climbing, twists the rope core
- Surface
  - Indoor, outdoor
  - Type of rock, condition
- Protection (see Fig. 99.2)
  - Active: cams with spring loading
  - Passive: chocks, nuts, stoppers, hexes, tapers, tricam
- Carabiner (see Fig. 99.2)
  - D, oval, or pear-shaped with hinged closure of the ring
  - Attaches the climber to a harness, bolt, or rope
  - Locking carabiners are stronger and safer for specific uses such as anchors and harnesses.
- Quick draw (see Fig. 99.2)
  - Two carabiners attached by sewn webbing, used to attach a rope to bolts or trad gear while climbing
- Chalk
  - Held in a pouch behind the back; used to improve hand friction and reduce moisture
- Webbing, cord, slings
  - Used to carry gear, attach protection, or create a top rope with a carabiner by tying onto a rock, tree, or other solid structure
- Helmet
  - An essential piece of equipment that is often overlooked
  - Should also be worn by the belayer to protect them from falling rocks, ice, and debris

Biomechanics, Training, and Physiology

- Training variables more important than anthropometric determinants
- Leanness, strength, flexibility, low body fat are characteristics of more successful climbers
- Energy expenditure:
  - Outdoor climbing expends greater energy than indoor.
  - Metabolic equivalent of task (MET) values less than those of running at same heart rate (HR).
  - $\dot{V}O_2$ max reaches a plateau during climbing.
  - Handgrip fatigue lasts 20 minutes.

CLIMBING INJURIES BY ANATOMIC REGION

Upper Extremity

More commonly overuse injuries

Shoulder (See Chapter 49: "Shoulder Injuries")

- Rotator cuff tendonitis, tear, or impingement
- Rupture long head biceps
- Superior labrum, anterior to posterior (SLAP) lesions
- Acromioclavicular (AC) sprain
- Dislocation
- Muscular strain: usually of the rhomboid, latissimus dorsi, or lower trapezius
- Rhabdomyolysis of shoulder/upper extremity from acute overtraining
- Paget–Schroetter syndrome, upper extremity deep venous thrombosis (UEDVT)
  - Nonspecific shoulder pain, pressure, and swelling; color change to arm after intense training

Elbow (See Chapter 50: "Elbow Injuries")

- Anterior
  - Climber's elbow: brachialis strain (see "Climbing-Specific Injuries" section)
  - Distal biceps strain or tear
  - Posterior interosseous nerve compression
- Medial
  - Forearm flexor strain, overuse leads to medial epicondylitis
  - Pronator teres strain or tear
  - Ulnar nerve compression
- Lateral
  - Extensor strain: lateral epicondylitis
  - Radiocapitellar compression
  - Superficial branch of radial nerve compression
- Posterior
  - Triceps tendonitis
  - Osteoarthritis
  - Stress fracture, osteochondritis dissecans (OCD)

Wrist (See Chapter 51: "Hand and Wrist Injuries")

- Tendonitis/tenosynovitis
  - Flexor carpi ulnaris most common
- Sprains
- Carpal tunnel syndrome, tendon hypertrophy, edema
- Triangular fibrocartilage complex (TFCC) injury
- Retinacular injury

Hand

- Climber's finger: flexor pulley injury (see "Climbing-Specific Injuries" section)
- "Sausage fingers"
  - Joint effusion with synovial irritation, cartilage damage
- Flexor digitorum superficialis (FDS) and flexor digitorum profundus (FDP) tendonitis, strain, tear, laceration (Fig. 99.4)
  - Tenoperiostitis, tears at insertion
  - Force loads on FDS and FDP at a mechanical disadvantage with certain grips
- Extensor hood syndrome (EHS)
  - Induced by use of a crimp hold
  - Degenerative spurring to the joints results in irritation to tendon sheaths
  - Often associated with chronic flexor mechanism injuries
  - Clinically see 3- to 5-degree extension deficits, in addition to morning stiffness
- Collateral ligament injury: pocket hold
- Flexion contracture
- Osteoarthritis (OA)
  - A 2018 prospective longitudinal study over 11 years in *Orthopaedic Journal of Sports Medicine* revealed 25% of former adolescent climbers performing at high level in youth showed mild form of OA to fingers.
  - Finger training (campus board training) can lead to early hand OA.
  - High UIAA climbing level correlates with risk for early-onset OA of the hand and fingers.
- Stress fracture
- Epiphyseal fracture
- Nodule/trigger finger (see Fig. 99.4)
- Dupuytren contracture
- Ganglion cyst (see Fig. 99.4)
- Mallet finger
- Lumbrical tear/lumbrical shift (see Fig. 99.4)
- Amputation

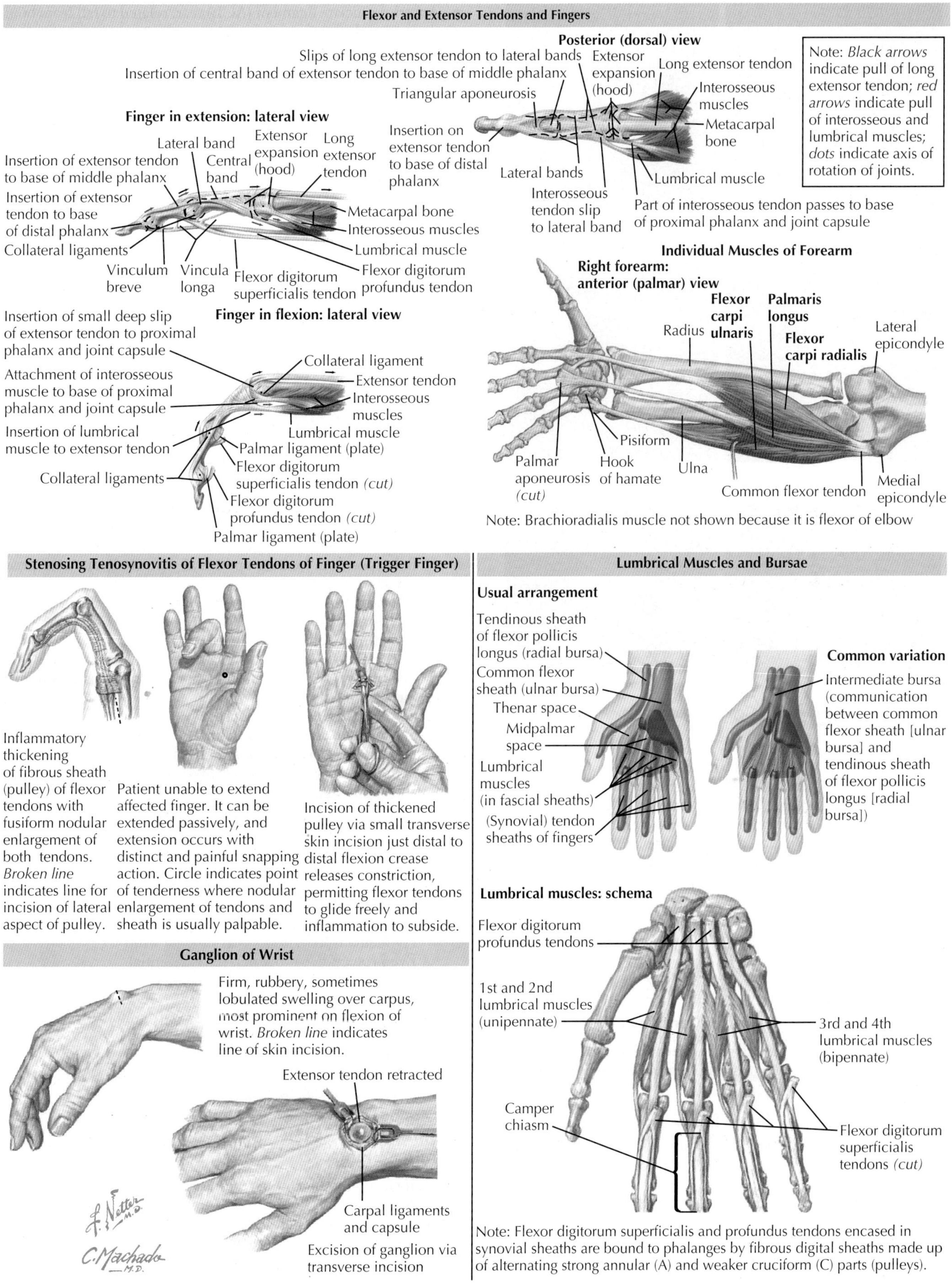
Flexor and Extensor Tendons and Fingers
Posterior (dorsal) view
Slips of long extensor tendon to lateral bands
Insertion of central band of extensor tendon to base of middle phalanx
Extensor expansion (hood)
Long extensor tendon
Triangular aponeurosis
Interosseous muscles
Metacarpal bone
Insertion on extensor tendon to base of distal phalanx
Lateral bands
Interosseous tendon slip to lateral band
Lumbrical muscle
Part of interosseous tendon passes to base of proximal phalanx and joint capsule
Note: Black arrows indicate pull of long extensor tendon; red arrows indicate pull of interosseous and lumbrical muscles; dots indicate axis of rotation of joints.
Finger in extension: lateral view
Lateral band
Extensor expansion (hood)
Long extensor tendon
Insertion of extensor tendon to base of middle phalanx
Central band
Insertion of extensor tendon to base of distal phalanx
Collateral ligaments
Metacarpal bone
Interosseous muscles
Lumbrical muscle
Flexor digitorum profundus tendon
Vinculum breve
Vincula longa
Flexor digitorum superficialis tendon
Finger in flexion: lateral view
Insertion of small deep slip of extensor tendon to proximal phalanx and joint capsule
Collateral ligament
Extensor tendon
Attachment of interosseous muscle to base of proximal phalanx and joint capsule
Interosseous muscles
Lumbrical muscle
Insertion of lumbrical muscle to extensor tendon
Palmar ligament (plate)
Flexor digitorum superficialis tendon (cut)
Collateral ligaments
Flexor digitorum profundus tendon (cut)
Palmar ligament (plate)
Individual Muscles of Forearm
Right forearm: anterior (palmar) view
Flexor carpi ulnaris
Palmaris longus
Radius
Flexor carpi radialis
Lateral epicondyle
Pisiform
Palmar aponeurosis (cut)
Hook of hamate
Ulna
Common flexor tendon
Medial epicondyle
Note: Brachioradialis muscle not shown because it is flexor of elbow
Stenosing Tenosynovitis of Flexor Tendons of Finger (Trigger Finger)
Inflammatory thickening of fibrous sheath (pulley) of flexor tendons with fusiform nodular enlargement of both tendons. Broken line indicates line for incision of lateral aspect of pulley.
Patient unable to extend affected finger. It can be extended passively, and extension occurs with distinct and painful snapping action. Circle indicates point of tenderness where nodular enlargement of tendons and sheath is usually palpable.
Incision of thickened pulley via small transverse skin incision just distal to distal flexion crease releases constriction, permitting flexor tendons to glide freely and inflammation to subside.
Ganglion of Wrist
Firm, rubbery, sometimes lobulated swelling over carpus, most prominent on flexion of wrist. Broken line indicates line of skin incision.
Extensor tendon retracted
Carpal ligaments and capsule
Excision of ganglion via transverse incision
F. Netter M.D.
C. Machado M.D.
Lumbrical Muscles and Bursae
Usual arrangement
Tendinous sheath of flexor pollicis longus (radial bursa)
Common flexor sheath (ulnar bursa)
Thenar space
Midpalmar space
Lumbrical muscles (in fascial sheaths)
(Synovial) tendon sheaths of fingers
Common variation
Intermediate bursa (communication between common flexor sheath [ulnar bursa] and tendinous sheath of flexor pollicis longus [radial bursa])
Lumbrical muscles: schema
Flexor digitorum profundus tendons
1st and 2nd lumbrical muscles (unipennate)
3rd and 4th lumbrical muscles (bipennate)
Camper chiasm
Flexor digitorum superficialis tendons (cut)
Note: Flexor digitorum superficialis and profundus tendons encased in synovial sheaths are bound to phalanges by fibrous digital sheaths made up of alternating strong annular (A) and weaker cruciform (C) parts (pulleys).

Figure 99.4 Upper extremity climbing injuries.

injury. At 90 degrees, the pulley sustains more tension than the tendon. Grading of the injury is very important (Table 99.3).

Presentation: The climber often presents with a history of feeling a "pop" related to the injury with associated swelling and pain. May present with a long-standing injury and/or chronic pain.

Physical examination: Bowstringing of the affected digit with acute pain and swelling. Most commonly affects the fourth digit of the nondominant hand (see Fig. 99.6).

Diagnostics: Magnetic resonance imaging (MRI), ultrasound. Dynamic ultrasound is 98% sensitive, 100% specific; user dependent (see Fig. 99.6).

Treatment:

Nonsurgical treatment (Table 99.4)

- Grade 1: pulley strain
  - No immobilization
  - Physical therapy for 2–4 weeks
  - Return to light climbing at 4 weeks
  - Full climbing at 6 weeks
  - Taping for 3 months
- Grade 2: complete rupture of the A4 pulley or a A2 or A3 partial rupture
  - Ten days immobilization
  - Physical therapy for 2–4 weeks
  - Return to light climbing at 4 weeks
  - Full climbing at 6–8 weeks
  - Taping for 3 months
- Grade 3: complete A2 or A3 rupture
  - Ten to fourteen days immobilization
  - Physical therapy for 4 weeks
  - Use of a thermoplast or soft-cast ring
  - Return to light climbing at 6–8 weeks
  - Full climbing at 3 months
  - Taping for 6 months

Table 99.3 GRADING OF FLEXOR PULLEY INJURIES

Grade	Flexor Pulley Injury Pattern
Grade 1	Pulley strain
Grade 2	Complete rupture of A4 pulley or partial rupture of A2 or A3
Grade 3	Complete rupture of A2 or A3 pulley
Grade 4	Multiple pulley ruptures or single pulley rupture with lumbrical or collateral ligament injury

From Schoffl V, Hochholzer T, Winkelmann HP, Strecker W. Pulley injuries in rock climbers. *Wilderness Environ Med*. 2003;14(2):94–100.

Surgical treatment (see Table 99.4 and Fig. 99.6)

- Grade 4: multiple pulley ruptures or a A2 or A3 pulley rupture with lumbrical or ligament injury
- Surgical repair:
  - Widstrom technique: loop and a half
  - Weilby repair can be used as an alternative
- Fourteen days immobilization
- Physical therapy for 4 weeks
- Thermoplast or soft-cast ring should be used
- Return to light climbing at 4 months
- Full climbing at 6 months
- Taping should accompany climbing for at least a year

Prognosis: Most climbers do well with conservative care. Ten percent experience persistent pain. Consider surgical treatment in climbers with residual pain or inability to return to prior climbing level.

Climber's Elbow

Description: Brachialis tendonitis or a tear at the muscle–tendon junction; caused by flexion and pronation of the elbow typical of climbing with traverses; insufficient firing of the biceps brachii in the flexed and pronated positions contribute to overuse of the brachialis (Fig. 99.7).

Presentation: Pain with climbing; typically presents after a prolonged, hard climb or a lengthier period of intense climbing with insufficient rest between climbs

Physical examination: Presence of pain to the anterior elbow that is worsened with elbow flexion and pronation. A partial tear or rupture will typically have swelling and/or ecchymosis.

Diagnosis: Physical examination and history often sufficient to reveal climber's elbow. MRI or dynamic ultrasound can aid in identifying the presence of tendonitis or a tendon tear (see Fig. 99.7).

Treatment: Most athletes with climber's elbow can be treated conservatively. Rest is the mainstay of treatment; typically 2–4 weeks of rest is sufficient for a strain. Modified climbing may be attempted if milder injury is present, but the athlete must be pain-free and climbing with diminished frequency/intensity and at two to three levels below normal. Physical therapy is highly beneficial but requires an experienced physiotherapist. Modality care; administration of oral anti-inflammatories for inflammation and pain. Strengthening of opposing muscle groups. Complete ruptures should be treated with surgical repair within a week or two of injury for best results. Patients who fail conservative treatment

Table 99.4 TREATMENT OF PULLEY INJURIES

	Grade 1	Grade 2	Grade 3	Grade 4
Injury	Pulley strain	Complete rupture of A4 or partial rupture of A2 or A3	Complete rupture of or A3	Multiple ruptures, such as A2/A3, A2/A3/A4, or single rupture (A2 or A3) combined with lumbrical muscle or ligament damage
Therapy	Conservative	Conservative	Conservative	Surgical repair
Immobilization	None	10 days	10–14 days	Postoperative 14 days
Functional therapy	2–4 weeks	2–4 weeks	4 weeks	4 weeks
Pulley protection	Tape	Tape	Thermoplastic or soft-cast ring	Thermoplastic or soft-cast ring
Easy sport-specific activities	After 4 weeks	After 4 weeks	After 6–8 weeks	4 months
Full sport-specific activities	6 weeks	6–8 weeks	3 months	6 months
Taping through climbing	3 months	3 months	6 months	>12 months

From Schoffl V, Hochholzer T, Winkelmann HP, Strecker W. Pulley injuries in rock climbers. *Wilderness Environ Med*. 2003;14(2):94–100.

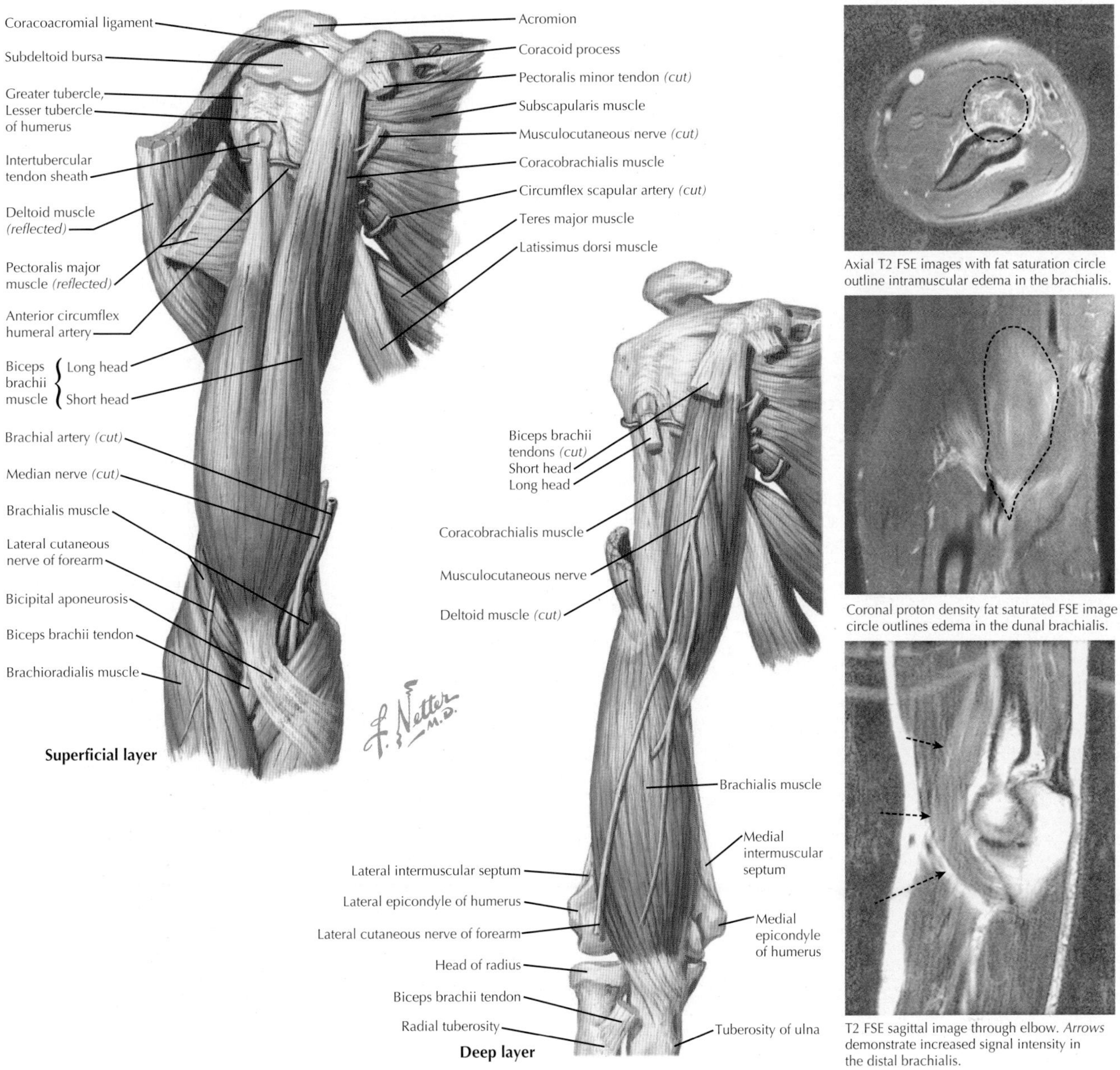
Coracoacromial ligament
Subdeltoid bursa
Greater tubercle,
Lesser tubercle
of humerus
Intertubercular
tendon sheath
Deltoid muscle
(reflected)
Pectoralis major
muscle (reflected)
Anterior circumflex
humeral artery
Biceps brachii muscle
Long head
Short head
Brachial artery (cut)
Median nerve (cut)
Brachialis muscle
Lateral cutaneous
nerve of forearm
Bicipital aponeurosis
Biceps brachii tendon
Brachioradialis muscle
Superficial layer
Acromion
Coracoid process
Pectoralis minor tendon (cut)
Subscapularis muscle
Musculocutaneous nerve (cut)
Coracobrachialis muscle
Circumflex scapular artery (cut)
Teres major muscle
Latissimus dorsi muscle
Biceps brachii
tendons (cut)
Short head
Long head
Coracobrachialis muscle
Musculocutaneous nerve
Deltoid muscle (cut)
Brachialis muscle
Medial
intermuscular
septum
Lateral intermuscular septum
Lateral epicondyle of humerus
Lateral cutaneous nerve of forearm
Medial
epicondyle
of humerus
Head of radius
Biceps brachii tendon
Radial tuberosity
Tuberosity of ulna
Deep layer
Axial T2 FSE images with fat saturation circle
outline intramuscular edema in the brachialis.
Coronal proton density fat saturated FSE image
circle outlines edema in the dunal brachialis.
T2 FSE sagittal image through elbow. Arrows
demonstrate increased signal intensity in
the distal brachialis.

Figure 99.7 Climber's elbow.

should also have surgical consultation. Surgery requires months for recovery.

Prognosis: With adequate rest period, physical therapy, and strengthening of opposing muscle groups, many climbers return to full activity pain-free, whether conservative or surgical treatment was used. Length of restricted activity depends on the severity of the injury and resolution of symptoms.

INJURY PREVENTION, DIAGNOSIS, AND TREATMENT

Medical Care of Climbers

- Physician inexperience or misconception
  - "What did you expect when you climb?"
  - Leads to delayed diagnosis and treatment
  - Many elite climbers find that health professionals do not understand climbing stresses and are not helpful in diagnosis or treatment
- Compliance is a significant issue with climbing overuse injuries.
- Climbers seek "street cred" from their peers by taking challenges and risk.
- Platelet-rich plasma (PRP), amnion allograft, stem cell injections, extracorporeal shockwave therapy (ESWT) as investigational treatments

Prevention

- Tendon strengthening, stretching, inclusion of opposing muscle groups
- Low-weight, high-repetition endurance training
- Heat before, ice after
- Taping: pulley protection, buddy taping when necessary
  - "H-tape" produces added protection
  - Division of tape into two strips with a bridge in the middle, placing the bridge at the volar proximal interphalangeal (PIP) joint, and then the strips are placed circumferentially on either side of the dorsal PIP
- Adequate rest period between climbs

Rest Guidelines

- Twenty-four hours should be taken for recovery after training.
- Forty-eight hours should be taken for recovery after climbing or hard training.
- Significant injuries require several months of rest.
- Splinting, ring to support pulley, taping
- Older climbers require more rest (double age = double rest).

Rehabilitation

- Can be for 2–3 months
  - Stretches
  - Range-of-motion exercises
  - Low weights
  - Gradually increased repetitions
- Strengthen muscle antagonists
- Change climbing technique (e.g., rely more on open than cling grip), slowly return to activity, start at lower level
- Formal physical therapy with an experienced therapist familiar with climbing injuries
- Rock climbing can aid the therapy of other injuries
  - Improves functional ankle instability with near-static movements, but care must be taken to not reinjure self with belaying to the ground

Repair

- Indication is based on injury grade and injury type
- Failure of conservative therapy
- Reconstruction of the fibro-osseous flexor sheath of fingers or repair of a brachialis tear; can fail with insufficient compliance/rehabilitation

Advice and Counseling for Climbers

- Adequate instruction
- Climb with trusted companions
- Climb to your ability, know your limitations
- Impeccable equipment use and safety
  - Protect equipment from moisture, sun, heat, dirt, water, oil, abrasion
  - Use appropriate protection, knots, equipment
  - Date ropes and harnesses, check damage after each use, replace according to manufacturer specifications
- Plan and leave an itinerary
- Carry a cell phone, map, global positioning system (GPS), satellite phone or SOS device
- First aid kit
- Food, water, sunscreen, eye protection, helmet

SUMMARY

- Climbing is a popular sport worldwide among all ages and genders.
- Climbing requires specific training, conditioning, and specialized equipment.
- The majority of climbing-specific injuries are overuse-related to the fingers.
- Providers should familiarize themselves with unique climbing injuries and be responsive to climbers' desires to return to their sport.

RECOMMENDED READINGS

Available online.

RODEO AND EQUESTRIAN SPORTS

100

Dawn Mattern • Kelly Ryan • Adrian McGoldrick

RODEO

Introduction

- Rodeo is a competitive sport with participants of all ages and at all competition levels.
- Athletes may compete in a single event or multiple events and may attend anywhere from one to four or five events in a single weekend.
- Most events are derived from skills needed to work cattle.

Epidemiology

- The composite injury rate for professionals is 16.6/1000 competitor exposures and for high school competitors is 8.2/1000 competitor exposures.
- The incidence of catastrophic injury is around 20/100,000, with a fatality rate of 7.29/100,000.
- The highest injury rates are found in roughstock events, with bull riding injury rates twofold greater than those in any other major rodeo event.
- When compared with the injury rates of all other contact sports, bull riding ranks as the most dangerous.

Events

Roughstock

Description: An 8-second duration is required for a qualified ride; one arm holds on to the animal, while the other is free and is not allowed to contact the animal. The score is based on the performance of the athlete and animal.

Bull riding: The rider hangs onto a rope tied to a bull (Fig. 100.1A).

Saddle bronc: The rider seated in a saddle, holding onto a rope attached to a halter.

Bareback riding: The rider holds on to a rigging attached to a horse's back (see Fig. 100.1B and C).

Steer riding: The rider hangs onto a rope tied to the steer (usually an event for younger athletes before starting bull riding).

Timed Events

Quickest time wins.

Steer wrestling: While atop a galloping horse, the athlete slides his or her arms onto the neck of a steer and throws it to the ground.

Calf roping: While riding a horse, the athlete ropes a calf, dismounts, and ties three of the four legs together.

Team roping: The header ropes the head of a steer, while the heeler ropes the heels.

Barrel racing: The rider races around three barrels in a cloverleaf pattern.

Steer roping: Similar to calf roping, except with a steer.

Goat tying: A youth event similar to calf roping.

Breakaway roping: Similar to calf roping, but the calf is not thrown and tied.

Pole bending: Riding a horse through six poles in a pre-established pattern.

Cutting: The rider separates a single animal from a herd.

Coverage

- Some rodeos are well covered by medical staff and services, but many are not covered at all, or maybe only by an ambulance crew.
- May be difficult to arrange follow-up care, as many rodeo athletes travel to multiple sites. Acute injuries commonly become chronic because of lack of or inadequate treatment in addition to pressure of competing.
- Rodeo athletes pay entrance fees to each rodeo; a withdrawal because of injury results in the loss of money. Competition is the best way to acquire skill and leads to greater exposure to risk.
- An athlete may request a medical release if unable to perform, but medical personnel cannot prevent an athlete from participating.

Common Injuries and Medical Problems

- Thoracic compression is the most common cause of catastrophic injury.
  - Unknown to what degree a rodeo protective vest reduces injury
- Roughstock athletes most common injuries: Contusion, concussion, sprains
- Timed athletes: Sprains, strains, contusions
- **Concussion**
  - Many know signs and symptoms of concussion, but may not report to medical staff
  - "Rodeo SCAT" modifies Maddock's questions to the sport of rodeo. (What rodeo are you at? What was your score/time? Where did you compete last? Who is traveling with you?)
  - Bareback riders experience 46× *g* of head acceleration, and bull riders experience 26× *g* (football players experience 21–23× *g* consistently and may sustain hits of 98–102× *g*).
  - In bull riding, helmet use does appear to reduce incidence of both catastrophic injury and fatality, currently required for those 18 years of age and younger, optional for those older than 18.
- Thumb amputations—combination of crush and avulsion mechanisms occurs in roping athletes, with high incidence of infection and failed replantation
- Pectoralis major/latissimus dorsi tendon ruptures—occurs in steer wrestling and is managed by surgical fixation
- Femoral acetabular impingement—exacerbated in the roughstock riding position
- Chronic neuropraxias
- Methicillin-resistant *Staphylococcus aureus* (MRSA)—livestock are frequently colonized; infections can be transmitted in both directions

HORSERACING

Introduction

- Horseracing is an immensely popular global sport with television audiences of over 100 million for major events (Melbourne Cup, Kentucky Derby), and annual attendance figures in Great Britain alone are over 5 million.
- It is a very exciting and physically demanding sport with high injury rates.
- Career-ending injuries and fatalities are not uncommon.

Epidemiology

- Horses weigh 1000–1200 lb (450–550 kg) and travel at speeds of 20–40 mph (32–64 km/hr)

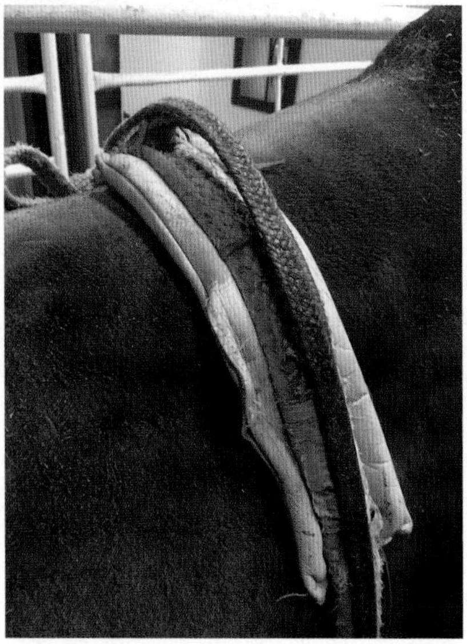

A. Bull rope.

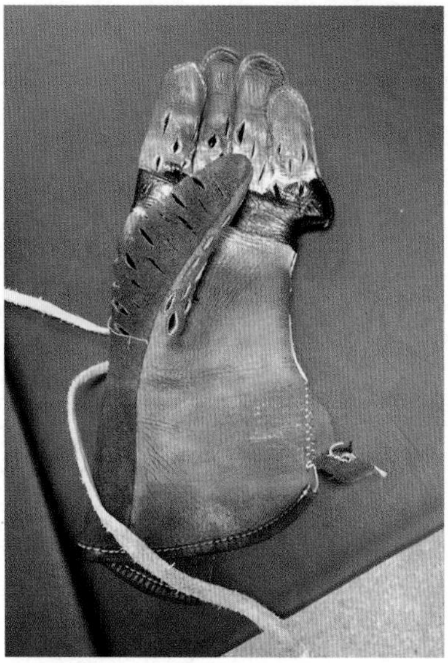

B. Bareback rider's glove.

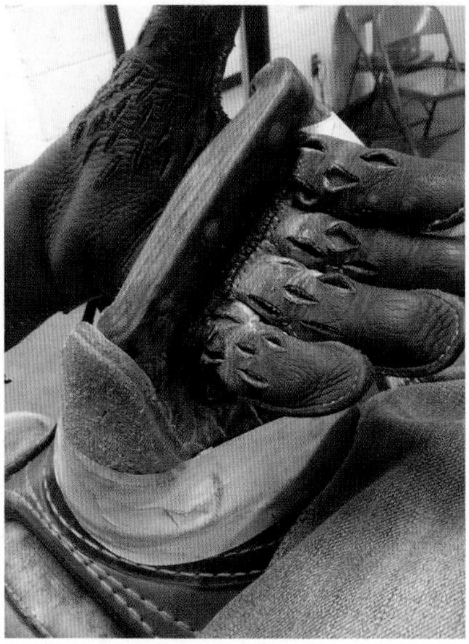

C. Glove in rigging.

Figure 100.1 Roughstock events.

- In flat racing, jockeys are seated approximately 6 ft (183 cm) above ground level and their head is approximately 8.5 ft (260 cm) above the ground (higher when jumping)
- Concussion rates in horseracing are the highest in the recorded literature
- Majority of professional jockey fatalities result from head injury
- Flat jockeys fall every 250 rides, with 35% of these resulting in injury
- Jump jockeys fall every 20 rides, with 20% of these resulting in injury
- Amateur jump jockeys sustain more falls than professional jockeys
- Concussion incidence is 0.2 concussions per 1000 rides and 28.6 concussions per 1000 falls
- Fatality rates are on the order 460–900/100 million rides. Comparable fatality rates/100 million participant days in other sports are >780 mountaineering, >640 air sports, 146 motor sports, 67.5 water sports, 15.7 rugby union, and 3.8 football (soccer).
- Jockey falls can be caused by horse stumbling, horse injury, jockey error, involvement of accidents, bad behavior of the horse, and other unspecified causes.
- In addition to the trauma caused by falls, the horse can inflict injuries by biting, pulling, kicking, standing, or rolling on the jockey, in addition to hitting the rider in the face with a sudden movement of the head.
- Injuries can also occur during the horse handling and other nonriding activities centered around horses, such as grooming, saddling, shoeing, loading/unloading, and stable work.

General Principles

- Horseracing is broadly divided into flat racing and jump racing (sometimes referred to as *National Hunt racing*).
- Trotting is not included in this review but is very popular with fewer injuries.
- Jockeys can generally start race riding at the age of 16 and are usually referred to as "apprentice jockeys" at the beginning of their careers (usually the first 5 years).
- Jump jockeys retire around the age of 40, but flat jockeys can continue past 50 years of age.
- Male and female jockeys compete on equal terms. The male:female jockey ratio tends to be closer to 50:50 in amateur racing and higher in professional racing.
- Flat racing generally takes place over a 12-month season, whereas jump racing tends to be limited to winter months when the ground is softer.
- Flat jockeys in Great Britain ride in an average of 600 races/year.
- Jump jockeys in Great Britain ride in an average of 300 races/year.
- Flat racing takes place over 0.625–2.75 miles (1–4.4 km).
- Jump racing takes place over 2–4.5 miles (3.2–7.2 km).
- The minimum riding weight varies considerably from country to country—Great Britain flat = 112 lb (51 kg) and Great Britain jump = 140 lb (63.5 kg). This weight must be achieved by the jockey wearing normal riding clothes and riding boots and carrying a saddle.
- Jump racing requires horses to jump over either hurdles (3.5 feet high; 101 cm) or steeplechase fences (4.5 feet high; 137 cm).

Safety Equipment

Helmets

- Helmets are designed to attenuate energy on impact by deformation of the helmet and in particular the inner lining, which is usually constructed from expanded polystyrene (EPS) foam.
- The prevention of skull fractures and catastrophic brain injury is the primary aim.
- To date, no helmet has been proven to prevent concussion, but research is ongoing to develop a tangential impact test with a view to reducing concussions.
- When designing a helmet, the criteria used are:
  - Shock absorption
  - Penetration of the shell
  - Lateral deformation
  - Load distribution
  - Area of protection
  - Retention system strength and effectiveness
  - Field of vision
  - Weight

- Current helmet standards:
  - Helmet standards vary from country to country, and riders wishing to compete outside the United States must ensure that their safety vests meet the required standard for participation.
  - Helmets in the United States are required to meet ASTM or SNELL standards. In some situations, other standards may also be acceptable (e.g., the interim European Standard VG1 01.040; Australian Standard AS/NZ; or specifications such as PAS015:2011, United States: ASTM F1163-13/ASTM F1163-04a, VG1 01.040/AS/NZ 3838:2006, and SNELL E2016).
  - Helmets should be replaced after they sustain an impact.

Safety Vests

- Safety vests are designed to reduce chest wall injuries (i.e., rib fractures) and are not capable of preventing spinal injuries.
- Lightweight vests (Level 1) are licensed for use during race riding only, with several European countries (Ireland, UK, France, and Germany) requiring Level 2 vests.
- Heavier vests (Levels 2 and 3) are required while riding out/barrier trials/breeze ups, etc.
- Current safety vest standards:
  - As with helmets, safety vest standards vary enormously from country to country, and riders wishing to compete outside the United States must ensure that their safety vests meet the required standard for participation. In the United States, safety vests are required to meet an ASTM or SNELL standard. In some situations, other standards may also be acceptable (e.g., the European Standard EN13158 or the Australian Standard ARB 1.1998).
  - United States: ASTM F2681-08/ASTM F1937-04/EN13158:2000 or 2009/BETA 2009 or BETA 2000 Body Protector Standard/Australian Racing Board (ARB) Standard 1.1998.

Goggles

- There are currently no equestrian goggle standards, but high-impact plastic or polycarbonate lenses are recommended to reduce the risk of shattering and resultant eye injury.

Racecourse Medical Coverage

- Medical coverage at racetracks varies across the globe. It is important to ensure that they have appropriate training and qualifications for prehospital care and that they have access to the necessary emergency equipment and supplies.
- In almost all countries a minimum of two ambulances follow the riders. In many countries it is standard to have two doctors on track also. However, in some countries such as New Zealand and Japan, only paramedics work on the track.
- Diagnostic equipment on the track varies from the very basic to full x-ray scanning facilities in Japan.
- Work with vets to create weather protocols such as heat, rain, snow, and lightning. There are two different types of athletes, horses and jockeys, and weather can affect them differently.

Racecourse Safety Arrangements

- Major changes have taken place over the last 15 years with the replacement of cement/steel running rails and railings with flexible plastic to reduce the risk of injury. Gates also continue to be improved to decrease noise, increase visibility, and avoid startling the horse.
- Provision of access to the racing surface has improved with the creation of ambulance roads or the deployment of four-wheel-drive vehicles in situations where access is difficult.
- In jump racing, rules are in place to bypass fences if a rider or horse is injured and cannot be moved before the horses complete the circuit and return to the site of the accident.

Insurance

- Race riding is a high-risk sport, and insurance can be difficult to arrange. In countries where there is an active jockeys association, insurance is usually available for death and disability, career-ending injuries, and private medical care.
- All medical staff must have suitable medical malpractice insurance if they wish to provide medical support on a racecourse.

Race Track Surfaces

- Most racing in Europe takes place on turf during the summer. During the winter months, some racecourses provide an "all-weather" racing surface that is constructed from a mixture of artificial frost-resistant materials.
- In the United States and Australia, racing also takes place on dirt or cinder tracks.
- The injury rates on turf tracks are similar to those found on all-weather tracks.

Common Injuries and Medical Problems

Concussions

- Concussions: 8% in professional racing Fig. 100.1 (18% in amateur racing)
- Concussion protocol should be established for racetracks and based off recommendations by current consensus statement on concussion in sport
- Active rehabilitation with sport-specific exercises, including cardiac, ocular, vestibular, and/or physical rehabilitation. These treatments should be used without putting the rider at risk for another head injury (back on horse too soon; Fig. 100.2).

Disordered Eating, Bone Health, and Energy Deficiency

- Nutritionist or nutrition programs should be used if possible
- Increased odds of osteoporosis: odds ratio (OR) = 6.5
- Consider vitamin D or other vitamin and mineral deficiencies
- Potential for jockeys to be affected by relative energy deficiency in sport (RED-S)

Mental Health

- Jockeys are affected by mental health disorders such as psychological distress (35.7%), depression (57.1%), generalized anxiety disorder (21.4%), and social phobia (38.1%). Professional jockeys have a greater prevalence of these disorders compared with amateur jockeys and other elite athletes.

Orthopedic/Trauma

- Soft tissue injuries: 75%–80% (muscle contusion, ligament sprains, ligament strains)
- Fractures: 10%–18% (less common but result in greater severity)
- Fractured vertebrae (cervical, thoracic, lumbar)
- Clavicle fractures, dislocated shoulders, acromioclavicular/sternoclavicular (AC/SC) injuries
- Pelvic fractures, femur fractures
- Distal radius fracture, scaphoid
- Dislocations: 1%–4%
- Intraabdominal bleeding (splenic and renal laceration/rupture, lung contusions)
- Increased odds of osteoarthritis: OR = 7.5

Career-Ending Injuries

- In Great Britain, from 1991 to 2005 there were approximately 1,113,500 rides, 32,445 falls, and 555 injuries. Of these injuries 45 (8.1%) were career ending (including 4 fatalities).
- Career-ending injury location distribution: 24.3% torso-pelvis, 22.1% upper limb, 20% head, 17.7% lower limb, 13.3% neck and spinal cord.

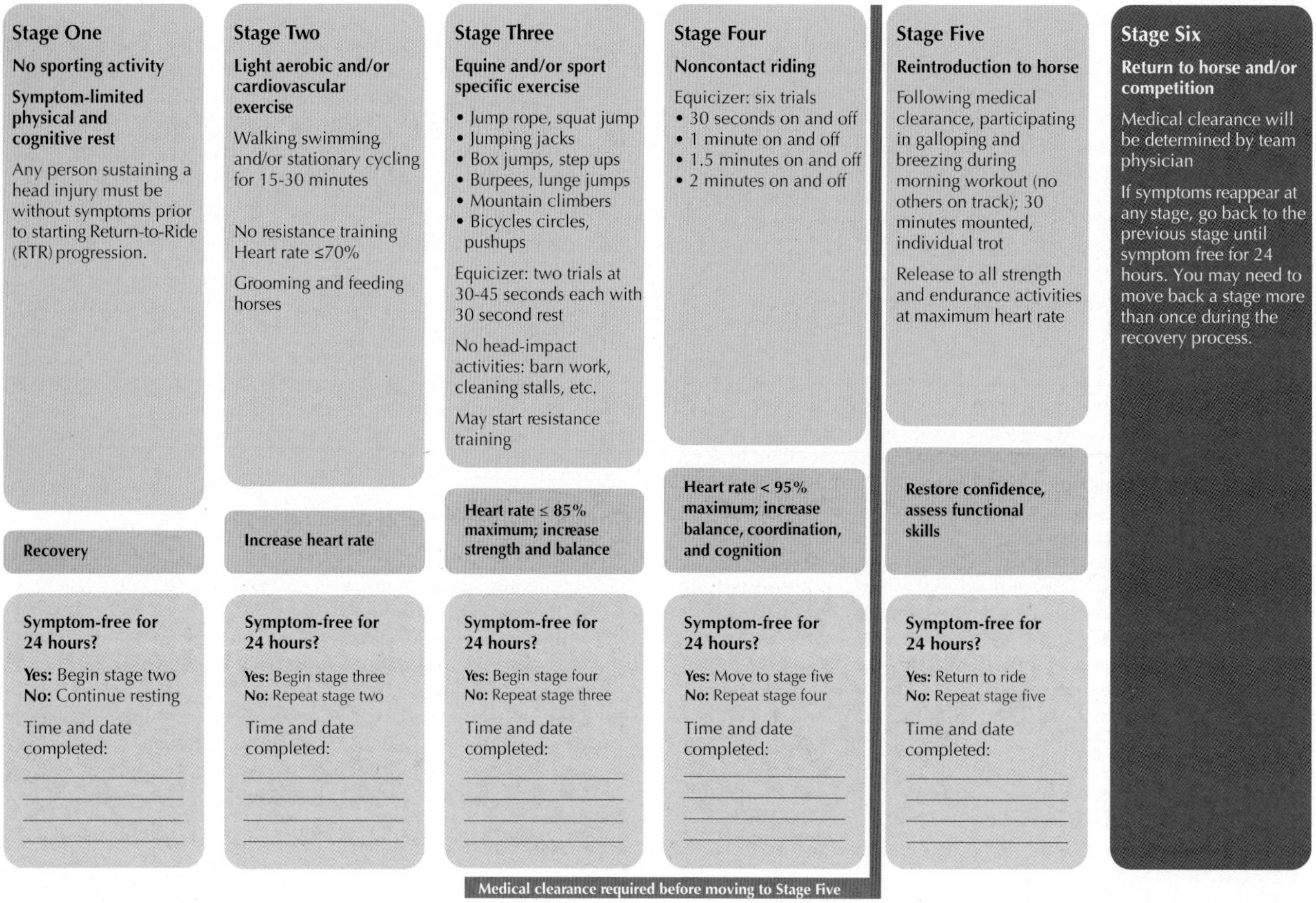

Stage One
No sporting activity
Symptom-limited physical and cognitive rest
Any person sustaining a head injury must be without symptoms prior to starting Return-to-Ride (RTR) progression.
Recovery
Symptom-free for 24 hours?
Yes: Begin stage two
No: Continue resting
Time and date completed:
Stage Two
Light aerobic and/or cardiovascular exercise
Walking swimming, and/or stationary cycling for 15-30 minutes
No resistance training
Heart rate ≤70%
Grooming and feeding horses
Increase heart rate
Symptom-free for 24 hours?
Yes: Begin stage three
No: Repeat stage two
Time and date completed:
Stage Three
Equine and/or sport specific exercise
• Jump rope, squat jump
• Jumping jacks
• Box jumps, step ups
• Burpees, lunge jumps
• Mountain climbers
• Bicycles circles, pushups
Equicizer: two trials at 30-45 seconds each with 30 second rest
No head-impact activities: barn work, cleaning stalls, etc.
May start resistance training
Heart rate ≤ 85% maximum; increase strength and balance
Symptom-free for 24 hours?
Yes: Begin stage four
No: Repeat stage three
Time and date completed:
Stage Four
Noncontact riding
Equicizer: six trials
• 30 seconds on and off
• 1 minute on and off
• 1.5 minutes on and off
• 2 minutes on and off
Heart rate < 95% maximum; increase balance, coordination, and cognition
Symptom-free for 24 hours?
Yes: Move to stage five
No: Repeat stage four
Time and date completed:
Stage Five
Reintroduction to horse
Following medical clearance, participating in galloping and breezing during morning workout (no others on track); 30 minutes mounted, individual trot
Release to all strength and endurance activities at maximum heart rate
Restore confidence, assess functional skills
Symptom-free for 24 hours?
Yes: Return to ride
No: Repeat stage five
Time and date completed:
Stage Six
Return to horse and/or competition
Medical clearance will be determined by team physician
If symptoms reappear at any stage, go back to the previous stage until symptom free for 24 hours. You may need to move back a stage more than once during the recovery process.
Medical clearance required before moving to Stage Five

Figure 100.2 Return-to-ride communication tool. (Reused with permission from Long L, Mattacola C, Ryan K. MedStar Health, Sports Medicine Research Institute.)

SUMMARY

- Horse racing is a very high-risk activity, and jockeys should wear the highest standard of protective equipment when riding (helmets and safety vests).
- Injuries are common, and medical staff providing coverage at racing events must be prepared to deal with fractures, dislocations, concussion, head injuries, and acute spinal trauma.
- All medical staff must be suitably trained in prehospital care and have the appropriate equipment on-site to manage the anticipated trauma. This should include a rapid method of transportation for critically injured jockeys (e.g., a fully equipped paramedic ambulance/air ambulance).
- Emergency action protocols are essential for critical intervention for severe trauma and should include a well-developed communication plan to notify, direct, and communicate with local emergency medical services (EMS) to transport riders in an expedited manner.

RECOMMENDED READINGS

Available online.

THE EXTREME ATHLETE 101

Lior Laver • Kai Fehske • Omer Mei-Dan

INTRODUCTION

- The definition of *extreme sports* (ES) includes any sport featuring high speed, height, real or perceived danger, a high level of physical exertion, highly specialized gear or spectacular stunts, and involving elements of increased risk for major injuries or fatalities. ES activities tend to be individual and can be pursued both competitively and noncompetitively.
- Often taking place in remote locations and in variable environmental conditions (weather, terrain), there could be little or no access to formal medical care, and even if medical care is available, it usually faces challenges related to longer response and transport times, access to few resources, limed provider experience because of low patient volume, and more extreme geographical and environmental challenges.
- Popular ES include mountaineering; hang-gliding and paragliding; free diving; surfing (including wave, wind, and kite surfing); personal watercraft; whitewater canoeing, kayaking, and rafting; BASE jumping and skydiving; extreme hiking; skateboarding; mountain biking; inline skating; ultraendurance races; alpine skiing and snowboarding; parkour; and all-terrain vehicle (ATV) and motocross sports.
- In the past 2 decades there has been a major increase in both the popularity and participation in ES, with dedicated TV channels, Internet sites, high rating competitions, and high-profile sponsors drawing more participants.
- The popularity of ES has been highlighted in recent years by the success of the X-games, an Olympic and Olympic like competition showcasing the talents in ES.
- Social media has had a major impact on ES because it enables extreme athletes to exhibit their talents to a wide audience on a regular basis. Maintaining their popularity on social media can often push extreme athletes to attempt new high-risk maneuvers.
- The risk and severity of injury in some ES are high, and participation in ES is associated with risk of injury or even death, and therefore the extreme athlete—amateur or professional—and the medical personnel treating these athletes must consider the risk of injury and measures for injury prevention.
- Medical personnel treating the ES athlete need to be aware of the numerous differences between the common traditional sports and this newly developing area. These relate to the temperament of the athletes themselves, the particular epidemiology of injury, the initial management after injury, treatment decisions, rehabilitation, and protective and injury prevention measures.

EPIDEMIOLOGY OF INJURIES IN EXTREME SPORTS

- Injury mechanisms in ES are less studied, particularly the injury pattern in many sports.
- The highest injury rates in ES are justifiably found in two groups: new and inexperienced athletes who have just started engaging in ES and experienced extremists who wish to push beyond their limits.
- Reported injury rates in ES may be expected to increase during competition rather than training—a trend well recognized in common team sports as athletes are trying to push their limits even further for prizes, audience, or fame.
- In some ES disciplines, the injury and fatality rates are hard to establish because of a lack of formal recorded events, hours of participation, or number of participants.
- In many situations, the extreme athlete competes against oneself or the forces of nature and the sport is practiced in relative isolation.
- Unlike expected terrain and environmental conditions, which are similar in most traditional sports (i.e., soccer is played on a real or synthetic grass field), comparison of injury rates across ES is difficult, given the large variance in terrain and environmental conditions—often changing variably during a single competition or event.

SPECIFIC EXTREME SPORTS AND THEIR ASSOCIATED INJURIES

Skydiving

- Skydiving is a sport of parachuting from a flying aircraft.
- It can be practiced both competitively and recreationally, with over 5.5 million jumps performed annually by over a million jumpers worldwide (including tandem jumps, which are commercially "one-off" jumps of an inexperienced person connected to an instructor).
- Focusing on skydiving, injury rates are relatively high.
- The majority of jumps are performed by a significantly smaller number of sports skydivers, whereas a larger number of participants perform fewer jumps.
- Recent fatality estimations are about 1 per 16,300 jumpers and approximately 1 fatality per 88,000 jumps, which increases to 1 per 4000 skydivers, excluding tandem jumps data.
- About 60% of fatalities are categorized as expert jumpers, whereas students account for about 20% of fatalities.
- Most fatalities (~70%) occur with the skydivers having at least one good parachute above them (i.e., not because of the parachute failing to open), and the majority have been caused by human error.
- Fatalities are mostly related to low or no pull of the parachute (~30%), malfunctions of the parachute system (~15%), reserve canopy problems (~15%), midair collisions (~20%), and landing errors (~20%).
- Fatalities are more common in experienced jumpers in their fourth to fifth decade of life and with on average 11 years in the sport.
- More than half of the fatalities occur in jumpers with the highest parachute license (USPA D-License).
- Injury rates in skydiving are around 170 per 100,000 jumps, whereas only about 30% of these require a visit to an emergency department and as little as 10% necessitate hospital admission.
- About two-thirds of injuries in skydiving are minor, with around a third of these commonly being abrasions and contusions, whereas lacerations constitute between 20% and 25% of all minor injuries.
- About 50% of injuries requiring emergency department follow-up treatment involve extremity trauma, with dominance of lower extremity injuries in as much as 80% of cases.
- Fracture rates in skydiving are estimated at 0.5 fractures per 100,000 jumps (mostly limbs but also spinal).
- The incidence of nonfatal events is estimated to be around 1 incident in every 2000 jumps and 1 per 3200 jumps in licensed jumpers.
- About 90% of the nonfatal injuries occur around the landing, with about 50% of injuries involving the lower extremities (Fig. 101.1), about 20% involving the upper extremities (Fig. 101.2), about 20% involving the back and spine, and <10% involving the head.

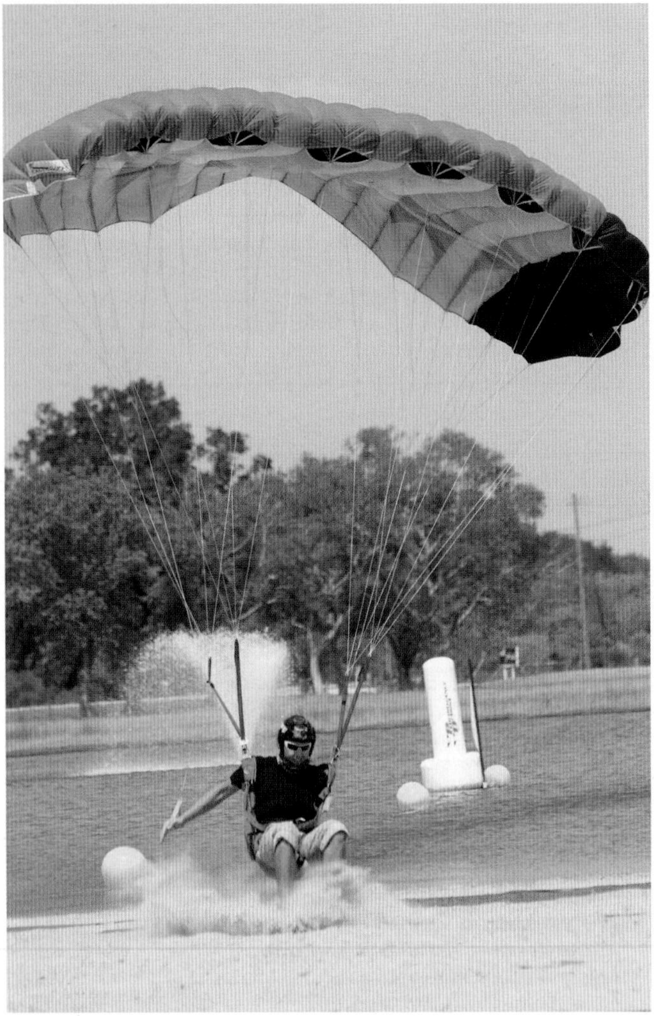

Figure 101.1 A hard-stop landing in skydiving (or in paragliding), which can lead to a knee ligament injury. (Courtesy of Ori Kuper. www.HOUvideographers.com and Omer Mei-Dan.)

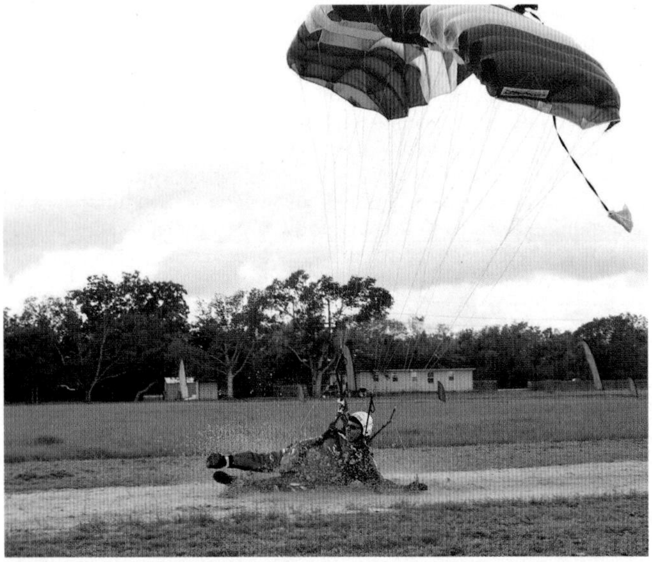

Figure 101.2 An off-balanced landing in skydiving (or in paragliding) can result in a forearm fracture or even a pelvic injury. (Courtesy of Omer Mei-Dan.)

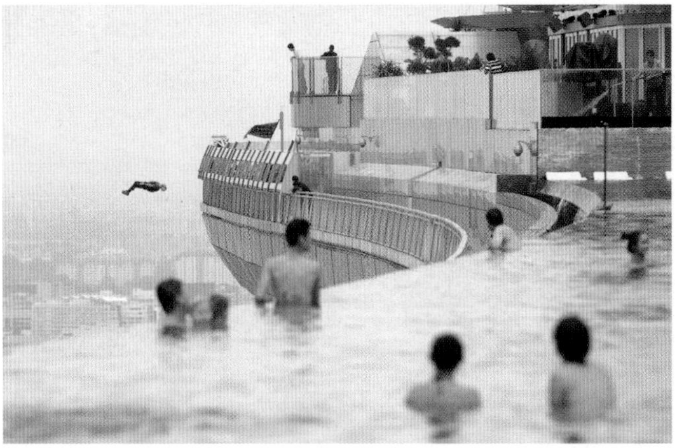

Figure 101.3 BASE jumping off a tall building. (Courtesy of Omer Mei-Dan.)

- Injury severity is normally equally distributed between minor and moderate, with around 40% of each, with severe injuries accounting for a little over 10%.
- Most serious injuries are experienced by licensed skydivers, whereas students in training have a six times higher injury rate.
- Women seem to be overrepresented with injuries, with a higher proportion of landing injuries than men.
- Although many parameters and participants have changed over the last 20 years, injury rates remain similar. Modern equipment has decreased overall morbidity and mortality, but it has also led to faster landings with increased limb injuries.

BASE Jumping

- BASE jumping (BASE = **B**uilding; **A**ntenna; **S**pan—a bridge, arch, or dome—and **E**arth—a cliff or other natural formation) is a sport that developed from skydiving and uses specially adapted parachutes to jump from fixed objects (see Fig. 101.3). A popular form of BASE jumping is wingsuit BASE jumping, using a special wingsuit that allows pilots to fly far away from the objects they jumped from and drastically increase their freefall time before deploying the parachute.
- Estimated to involve only about 2500–3000 active members worldwide, it is considered among the most dangerous adventure sports in the world and significantly more dangerous than skydiving, as BASE jumps are performed from much lower altitudes (often less than 500 feet above ground level, with a single parachute system [no reserve chute]).
- It seems the sport attracts predominantly male participants.
- Lower falling speeds with far less aerodynamic control and a high risk of losing flying stability leave little room for error. If the parachute is deployed while the jumper is unstable, there is a high risk of entanglement or malfunction. In such cases, the single canopy used may also be facing the wrong direction, which although not problematic in skydiving, in BASE jumping can cause head-on collision with the object one jumped from.
- Off-heading opening resulting in object strike is the leading cause of serious injury and fatality in BASE jumping.
- Taking place in close proximity to a cliff, a tower, or a building, which is used as a jumping platform, increases the risk of collision with the object in BASE jumping (Fig. 101.3).
- BASE jumping is associated with a fivefold to eightfold risk for fatality or injury when compared with regular skydiving.
- The fatality rate associated with BASE jumping was found to be 0.04%, although lacking information on demographic characteristics or jumpers' experience level.

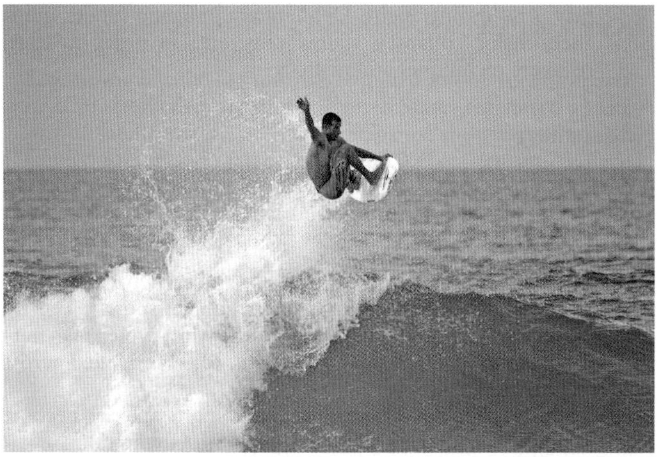

Figure 101.4 An aerial maneuver in surfing. (Courtesy of Shiran Valk and Omer Mei-Dan.)

- Several studies show estimated injury rates are around 0.4%.
- The majority of accidents (>50%) involve the lower limbs, about 30% involve the back\spine, <20% the upper limb, and about 3% are head injuries.
- Injury severity could vary according to the topographic conditions and altitudes involved, with higher altitudes (1000 m and above) offering relatively safe jumping conditions, allowing greater speed generation before parachute deployment and controlled landing, whereas lower-altitude jumping sites could result in more severe injuries.
- The rate of injuries requiring hospitalization in BASE jumping is estimated at around 300 per 100,000 jumps and is 16 times higher compared with the estimated rate of such injuries in freefall skydiving.
- Recently, a growing pattern of wingsuit-related fatalities has been shown in BASE jumping. It seems that most wingsuit-related fatalities are attributed to cliff or ground impact, being mostly the result of flying path miscalculations.

Surfing

- The sport of wave surfing is ever growing, with a huge market involved, commercialization of surfing apparel and the surfing lifestyle, fashion trends, and media coverage (Fig. 101.4).
- In 2009, it was estimated that there were more than 2.4 million surfers in the United States.
- There are four main board categories: longboards, shortboards, Stand Up Paddle board (SUP), and tow-in boards.
- Surfing is considered relatively safe compared with more traditional sports, with estimations ranging between 2 and 3.5 "moderate to severe" injuries (resulting in lost days of surfing or requiring medical care) per 1000 surfing days and around 0.25 injuries/surfer/year.
- The most common traumatic injuries requiring medical attention or resulting in inability to surf are lacerations (around 40%) and soft tissue injuries (around 35%).
- The majority of acute injuries are caused by striking a surfboard (a sharp fin, the tail, or the nose of the surfboard) or another surfer, with the rest from the sea floor.
- Lacerations, sprains, and contusions the most commonly encountered, but fractures and dislocations are also prevalent, with an estimated incidence of 10% for each.
- Injury rates in competitive surfing (professional and amateur) are higher, estimated at almost 6 per 1000 athlete exposures, or 13 per 1000 hours of competitive surfing, with >6 significant injuries per 1000 hours of competitive surfing—rates favorably comparing to those found in American collegiate football (33 per 1000 hours), soccer (18 per 1000 hours), and basketball (9 per 1000 hours).
- The relative injury risk is estimated to be 2.4 times greater when surfing in waves overhead or bigger and 2.6 times greater when surfing over a rock or reef bottom.
- More than one-third of acute injuries involve the lower extremities, and similar rates are found with relation to the head and neck.
- A considerable proportion of head injuries is found in surfing, in contrast to the fact that very few surfers use protective headgear.
- Fatality rates are not well documented in surfing; however, they have been reported in low numbers in ocean-related, mainly big-waves surfing drownings and shark attacks while surfing.
- As 50% of a surfer's time is spent paddling and 45% is spent remaining still, whereas only 3%–5% is spent actually riding waves, most overuse injuries derive from paddling.
- Overuse injuries in surfing are mostly found in the shoulder (~20%), back (~20%), neck (~10%), and knee (~10%).
- Injury prevention in surfing is practiced by following basic safety recommendations such as maintaining adequate swimming skills (the ability to swim 1 km in less than 20 minutes and being comfortable swimming alone in the ocean), familiarizing oneself with the surfing environment and conditions (entry and exit points, currents, and underwater hazards), avoiding surfing to exhaustion, and safely practicing breath-holding training.
- Using adequate equipment is also essential such as temperature-appropriate wetsuits protecting against hypothermia; protected, rounded, and shock-absorbing surfboard noses and fins trailing edges; and a board leash to keep the surfer's board close at hand. The board also can be used as a flotation device should a surfer become exhausted or injured.

Paragliding

- Paragliding is a recreational and competitive flying sport.
- It is defined as a sport using a single-seater, nonmotorized, foot-launched flexible aircraft, steered aerodynamically and able to start from ground level without requiring a free-fall phase.
- The paraglider, an advanced form of the parachute, consists of an upper and lower sail, with "ribs" dividing it into numerous separate compartments that are stabilized by air pressure.
- Accurate maneuvers are enabled using two steering lines attached to the rear corners of the parachute.
- Despite not having an engine, paraglider flights performed by an experienced pilot can last many hours and cover large distances (up to many hundreds of kilometers) because of the paraglider pilot's ability to gain altitude using air thermals, often climbing a few kilometers over the surrounding countryside/geographic surface.
- Paragliding accidents present a completely new injury pattern, not comparable to injuries associated with other air sports or even traffic accidents.
- Most accidents are caused by pilot errors, unpredictable meteorological changes, or wrong appreciation of environmental conditions.
- Accidents may occur in difficult terrain, making rescue operations often beyond the capacities of ground rescue services, necessitating helicopter rescue operations.
- The spine is considered the "Achilles heel" of the sport, sustaining the majority of impact during accidents and consequent injuries.
- **Spinal injuries** are relatively common, with an incidence ranging from 25% and up to around 50%.
- The thoracolumbar transitional region is most commonly involved (T12–L1).
- Spinopelvic dissociations can occur in a higher odds ratio than in the general trauma population, and even pelvic injuries can occur in up to 19%.

102 ESPORTS

Ahmed Emara • Michael Dakkak • David Graygo •
Jason Cruickshank • Jonathan Schaffer • Dominic King

HISTORY

- Electronic sports (esports), or competitive sports competition focused around video games, is a rapidly growing industry
- Esports athletes train 10–12 hours a day, crafting their skills in various console and computer-based video games, including *League of Legends*, *Counterstrike: Global Offensive*, *Rocket League*, *Overwatch*, and *Fortnite*.
- Top-performing esports athletes possess a specific skill set of enhanced neurocognitive processing speed, reaction time, and impulse control, making them "synaptic specialists."
- Secondary education institutions, colleges, and universities have begun to incorporate esports into their traditional varsity sports programs, with competitive scholarships being offered at 22 US colleges.
- In this regard, esports share descriptions and goals similar to that of traditional competitive sports; however, given their relatively new inclusion, there are few comprehensive recommendations for providing healthcare for esports athletes.

POTENTIAL HAZARDS AND INJURIES

- Similar to workplace hazards, esports hazards can be classified into musculoskeletal, sedentary status, psychosocial, and infectious risks

Musculoskeletal Hazards

Prolonged Aberrant Posturing

- Persistent cervical spine flexion: leads to a 10-pound increase in cervical muscle torque per inch of anterior cervical displacement. Persistent stress at cervicothoracic junction (Nintendo/gamer's neck) occurs with subsequent paraspinal muscle spasm. Cervical degenerative changes may occur, most commonly at the cervicothoracic junction. Cervical radiculopathy can be seen secondary to degenerative changes.
- Wrist (carpal tunnel) compression associated with median neuropathy.
- Elbow compression is associated with ulnar neuropathy secondary to compression between the two heads of the flexor carpi ulnaris, within the arcade of Struthers, between the Osborne ligament and medial collateral ligament, and at the medial epicondyle (Fig. 102.1).
- Pisiform (Guyon canal) compression secondary to mouse movement pivoting around the medial wrist is associated with distal ulnar neuropathy.

Repetitive Movement-Induced Microtrauma (200–500 Actions Per Minute)

- Rapid, repetitive, short-range mouse, keyboard, or controller motions are associated with de Quervain tenosynovitis (i.e., tenosynovitis of first and second dorsal compartments), carpal, and ulnar tunnel syndromes (see Fig. 102.1).
- Repetitive long-range, sweeping mouse movements and resisted wrist extension or flexion are associated with lateral and medial epicondylitis, respectively, which if long-standing can lead to degenerative epicondyle tendinosis.
- Intersection syndrome: tenosynovitis occurring at site where the extensor pollicis longus (EPL) tendon crosses over the extensor carpi radialis tendon (ECR) (Fig. 102.2)

Sedentary Status

- Although esports is a predominantly sedentary activity, esports participants often engage in high-exercise levels for in-game conditioning and lifestyle betterment.

Energy Intake/Expenditure

- The average collegiate esports participants invest >10 hours/day gaming.
- Esports players report increased appetite, despite an average of 61.8 calories/hour being expended during gaming.

Venous Thromboembolic Effects

- Dubbed *ethrombosis* and is promoted by prolonged immobilization and dehydration.
- Prolonged screen time associated with 2.8-fold increase in venous thromboembolism (VTE) risk.

Central Neurologic and Psychological Hazards

- A constellation of addictive tendencies, compromised sleep, and social anxiety are occasionally associated with gaming and have been designated as "gaming disorder."
- Prolonged screen time, along with microintensive rapid-paced games, cause eye fatigue (computer vision syndrome), the most common central neurologic complaint (up to 56% of gamers).
- Gamers may be at greater risk for "screen insomnia." Bedtime device use is associated with more than twofold increase in risk of poor sleep quantity and daytime sleepiness.
- Addictive behavior can be demonstrated through prioritizing videogaming over other interests, combined with gaming escalation despite negative consequences.

Infectious Hazards

- Infectious hazards are an emerging concern, especially with shared hardware or closed gaming spaces.
- Keyboard devices are often contaminated with skin commensals and potential pathogens, including methicillin-resistant *Staphylococcus aureus*, *Clostridium difficile*, vancomycin-resistant enterococci, and *Escherichia coli*.
- Despite being online, esports typically occur in local arenas to mitigate network latency and may be a source of infection transmission. Such concern has led to the cancellation or switching to a fully online format in 2019–2020 for fears over COVID transmission.
- Conventions typically involve large in-person gatherings that impede social distancing (6 feet) and are associated with frequent international travel.

PREVENTION AND HEALTH PROMOTION

Ergonomics

- Monitor distance should be approximately one arm's length away with the top of the monitor aligned at eye level and tilted 10–15 degrees.
- Mouse and keyboard variations to maintain neutral wrist alignment
- Chair settings and joint alignment
  - Trunk–hip angle: 90–110 degrees
  - Knee angle: 90–100 degrees

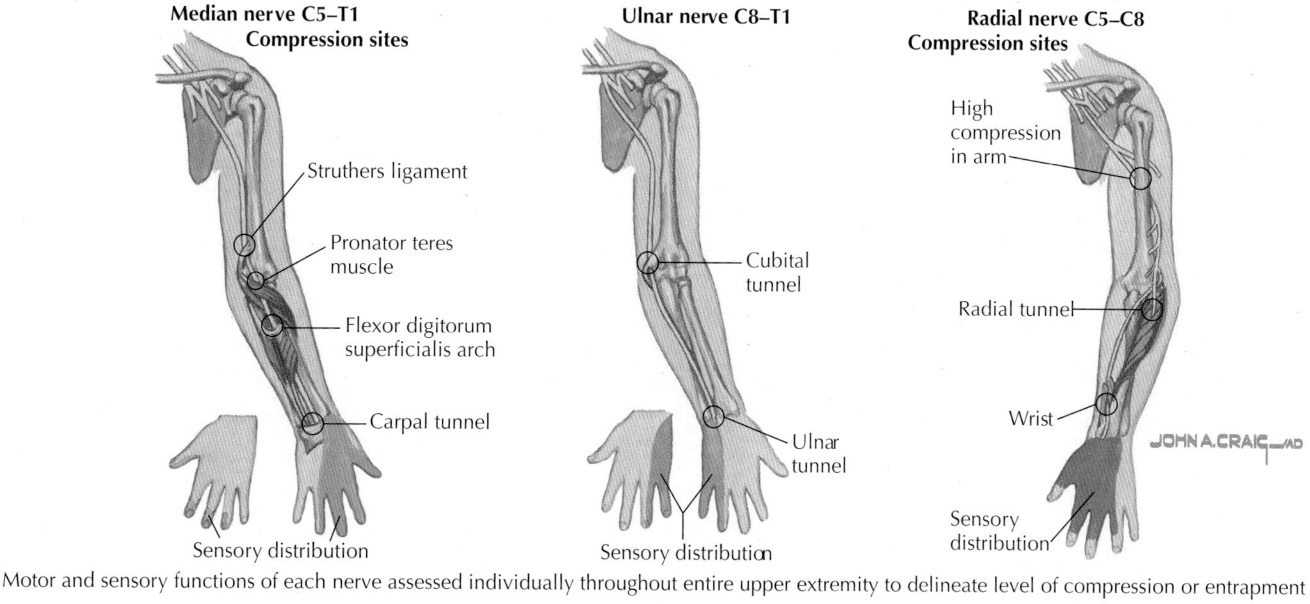
Median nerve C5–T1
Compression sites
Struthers ligament
Pronator teres muscle
Flexor digitorum superficialis arch
Carpal tunnel
Sensory distribution
Ulnar nerve C8–T1
Cubital tunnel
Ulnar tunnel
Sensory distribution
Radial nerve C5–C8
Compression sites
High compression in arm
Radial tunnel
Wrist
JOHN A.CRAIG_MD
Sensory distribution
Motor and sensory functions of each nerve assessed individually throughout entire upper extremity to delineate level of compression or entrapment

Figure 102.1 Common sites of upper extremity nerve entrapment.

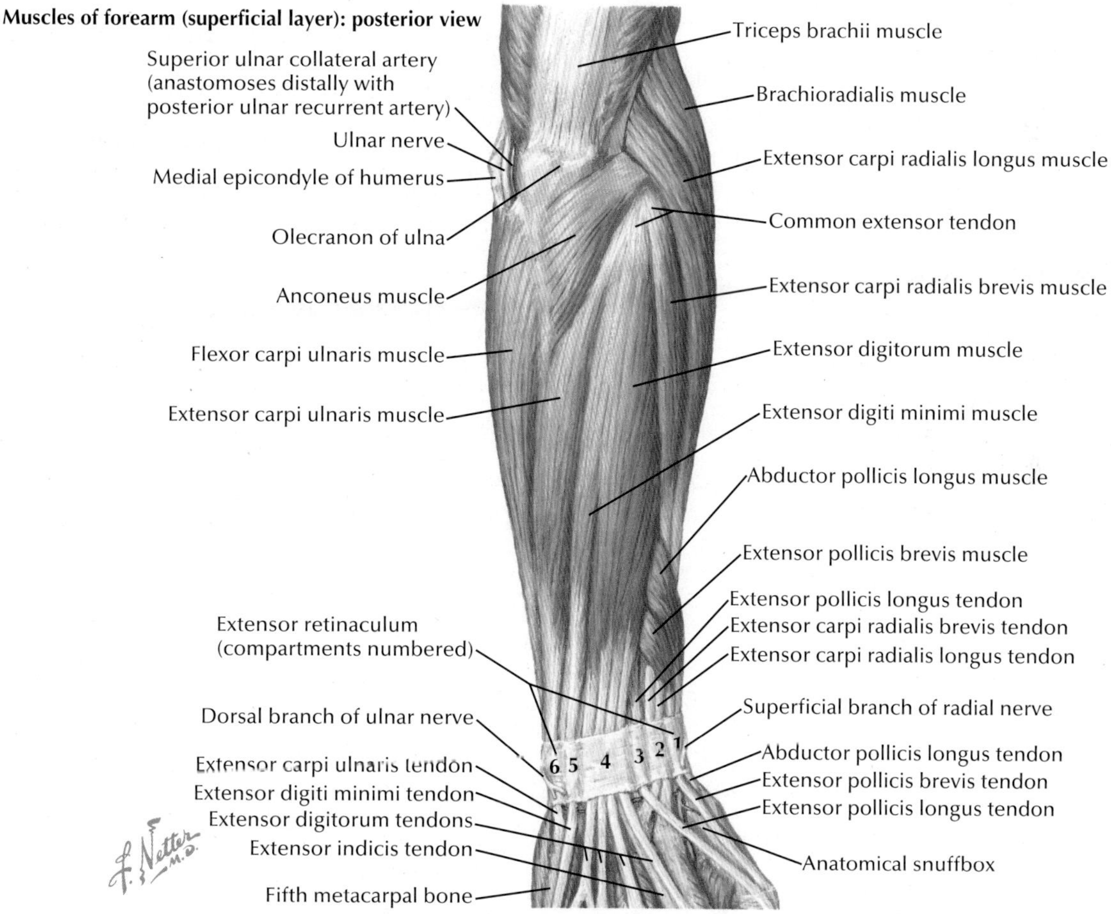
Muscles of forearm (superficial layer): posterior view
Triceps brachii muscle
Superior ulnar collateral artery (anastomoses distally with posterior ulnar recurrent artery)
Brachioradialis muscle
Ulnar nerve
Medial epicondyle of humerus
Extensor carpi radialis longus muscle
Common extensor tendon
Olecranon of ulna
Anconeus muscle
Extensor carpi radialis brevis muscle
Flexor carpi ulnaris muscle
Extensor digitorum muscle
Extensor carpi ulnaris muscle
Extensor digiti minimi muscle
Abductor pollicis longus muscle
Extensor pollicis brevis muscle
Extensor pollicis longus tendon
Extensor retinaculum (compartments numbered)
Extensor carpi radialis brevis tendon
Extensor carpi radialis longus tendon
Superficial branch of radial nerve
Dorsal branch of ulnar nerve
6 5 4 3 2 1
Abductor pollicis longus tendon
Extensor carpi ulnaris tendon
Extensor pollicis brevis tendon
Extensor digiti minimi tendon
Extensor pollicis longus tendon
Extensor digitorum tendons
Extensor indicis tendon
Anatomical snuffbox
Fifth metacarpal bone
F. Netter M.D.

Figure 102.2 Muscles of forearm (superficial layer): Posterior view.

- Ankle angle: 90–110 degrees
- Thighs parallel to the floor with feet resting flat and making use of an adjustable footrest as needed.
- Adjustable arm rests in width for various body types, height to be level with work surface but should also avoid placing the shoulders in a shrugged position, distance as not to limit the chair from the work surface.
  - Adjustable lumbar support with heights and depth.
- Establishing a gaming station with neutral spine positioning where head, chest, and hips stack on each other, with the chair

or couch adjusted so that knees are positioned horizontally relative to floor and upper extremities are in line with the torso.
- Maintain appropriate alignment while not sacrificing speed of action.
- Reinforcement with core and postural strength training.

Decrease Repetitive Strain

- Regular rest breaks approximately every 45 minutes as able and changes of posture during breaks in play.
- Use of padded wrist supports for better alignment.
- Limit use of the ulnar aspect of the wrist as a pivot for mouse flicking movements.
- Intermittent full range-of-motion exercises of the wrist should be a routine practice to mitigate the risk of developing carpal and ulnar tunnel syndromes and unload tissue stress.

Decrease Sedentary Status

- Esports athletes should be counseled to take short 5- to 10-minute breaks from gaming, ideally every hour, or 20 minutes every 3 hours, to decrease the axial stress placed on the back.
- Stretches throughout gameplay include 3–5 minutes of warm-up before starting with 2-hour intervals, including flexion and extension in the coronal and sagittal planes of the spine. These exercises should also include the cervical spine and major upper extremity joints (i.e., wrist and elbows) to reduce associated risk of musculoskeletal pain.
- Flexibility exercises should also be incorporated into daily workout sessions and include exercises targeting movement throughout the body.
- The seated athlete will have shortening of certain muscles while lengthening other muscles based on their postural position. These positions held for a prolonged period can potentially shorten tissues over time, creating dysfunction and eventually causing pain in different areas.

Core Muscle Training

- Train the deep core muscles to hold the body upright in a stable and balanced postural position to minimize the risk of musculoskeletal and spinal disc chronic injuries from prolonged sitting.

Upper Extremity Training

- Train the upper extremity complex used in the athlete's movement mechanics during competition.
- Evaluate from their fingers to their shoulders.
- Exercises can include stretching and strengthening for hand, wrist, forearm, and elbow to maintain appropriate alignment while not sacrificing speed of action.
- Eccentric load activities for the elbow can help prevent chronic injuries such as lateral epicondylitis.

Cardiovascular Training

- Thirty minutes of cardiovascular activity or high-intensity interval training each day.
- Individuals should perform at least 150–300 minutes of moderate-intensity exercise or 75–150 minutes weekly.
- Resistance training should occur at least two or more days a week.

Infectious Surfaces

- Regular sanitization of all surfaces and devices is essential, especially in the setting of shared consoles within a single team.

Additional Considerations

- Sports medicine physicians should be aware of the interdisciplinary and holistic approach to managing esports patients and referring to specialists when appropriate.
- Collaboration with the primary physician; referrals to ophthalmology/optometry for eye fatigue; and referral to psychiatry for potential psychiatric complaints ranging from depression, addictive tendencies, and social anxiety should also be considered.
- Appropriate nutrition education and recommendations should also be consistently imparted.

RECOMMENDED READINGS

Available online.

INDEX

Page numbers followed by "*f*" indicate figures, "*t*" indicate tables, "*b*" indicate boxes, and "*e*" indicate online content.